Become PRACTICE-READY using your PEARSON RESOURCES

Simplify your study time by using the resources included with this textbook at **http://nursing.pearsonhighered.com**.

Enhance your SUCCESS with the additional resources below.
For more information and purchasing options visit **www.mypearsonstore.com**.

For Your Success

MyNursingLab®

MyNursingLab provides a guided learning path that is proven to help students synthesize vast amounts of information, guiding them from memorization to true understanding through application.

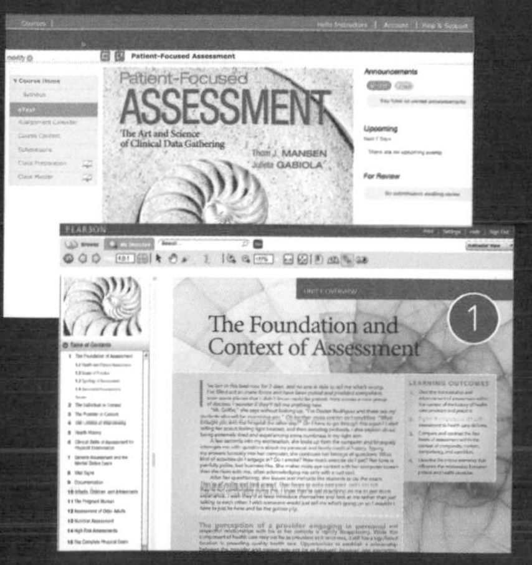

For Your Clinical Success

MyNursingApp™

www.mynursingapp.com

Clinical references across the nursing curriculum!

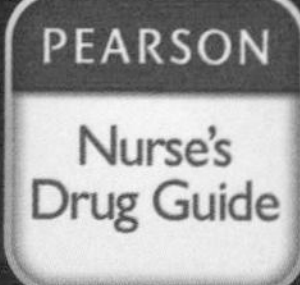

Clinical Handbook for Kozier & Erb's Fundamentals of Nursing, 9th edition

Clinical Handbook for Medical-Surgical Nursing, 5th edition

Clinical Handbook for Maternal-Newborn Nursing & Women's Health Across the Lifespan, 9th edition

Clinical Pocket Guide for Patient-Focused Assessment

Pearson Handbook of Laboratory and Diagnostic Tests

For Your NCLEX-RN® Success

MARY ANN HOGAN

COMPREHENSIVE REVIEW FOR NCLEX-RN®

PEARSON REVIEWS & RATIONALES

SECOND EDITION

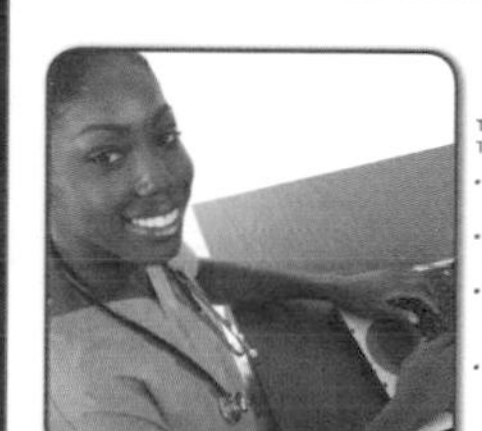

THE ONLY REVIEW BOOK THAT OFFERS:

- Unique organization by 2010 NCLEX-RN® Test Plan
- Over 1600 NCLEX®-style questions, comprehensive rationales & strategies
- Online MyNursingReview with additional 4,000 practice questions & eText
- Nursing Notes guide to the 2010 NCLEX-RN® Test Plan

Aligned to the 2013 NCLEX-RN® Test Plan

ALWAYS LEARNING

PEARSON

Patient-Focused ASSESSMENT

The Art and Science of Clinical Data Gathering

Thom J. **MANSEN,** PhD, RN
Associate Professor
University of Utah
Salt Lake City, Utah

Julieta **GABIOLA,** MD, FACP
Clinical Associate Professor of Medicine
Stanford University
Stanford, California

PEARSON

Boston Columbus Indianapolis New York San Francisco Upper Saddle River
Amsterdam Cape Town Dubai London Madrid Milan Munich Paris Montréal Toronto
Delhi Mexico City São Paulo Sydney Hong Kong Seoul Singapore Taipei Tokyo

Publisher: *Julie Levin Alexander*
Publisher's Assistant: *Regina Bruno*
Executive Acquisitions Editor: *Pamela Fuller*
Development Editor: *Jill Rembetski, iD8/TripleSSS Media Development, LLC*
Editorial Assistant: *Erin Sullivan*
Project Manager: *Cathy O'Connell*
Program Manager: *Erin Rafferty*
Production Editor: *GEX Publishing Services*
Manufacturing Buyer: *Maura Zaldivar-Garcia*
Art Director/Cover and Interior Design: *Mary Siener*
Director of Marketing: *David Gesell*
Senior Marketing Manager: *Phoenix Harvey*
Marketing Manager: *Deborah Doyle*
Marketing Specialist: *Michael Sirinides*
Assistant Editor for Media: *Sarah South*
Media Project Managers: *Karen Bretz and Tanika Henderson*
Composition: *GEX Publishing Services*
Printer/Binder: *Courier/Kendallville*
Cover Printer: *Phoenix Color/Hagerstown*
Cover Image: *David Muir/Getty Images*

Credits and acknowledgments borrowed from other sources and reproduced, with permission, in this textbook appear on appropriate page within text.

Notice: Care has been taken to confirm the accuracy of information presented in this book. The authors, editors, and the publisher, however, cannot accept any responsibility for errors or omissions or for consequences from application of the information in this book and make no warranty, express or implied, with respect to its contents.

The authors and publisher have exerted every effort to ensure that drug selections and dosages set forth in this text are in accord with current recommendations and practice at time of publication. However, in view of ongoing research, changes in government regulations, and the constant flow of information relating to drug therapy and drug reactions, the reader is urged to check the package inserts of all drugs for any change in indications of dosage and for added warnings and precautions. This is particularly important when the recommended agent is a new and/or infrequently employed drug.

Library of Congress Cataloging-in-Publication Data
Mansen, Thom J., author.
Patient-focused health assessment : the art and science of data gathering / Thom J. Mansen, Julieta Gabiola.
p. ; cm.
Includes bibliographical references.
ISBN 9780132239387e -- ISBN 0-13-223938-8
I. Gabiola, Julieta, author. II. Title.
[DNLM: 1. Diagnosis, Differential. 2. Data Collection--methods. 3. Diagnostic Techniques and Procedures. 4. Patient-Centered Care. WB 141.5]
RC71.3
616.07'5--dc23
2013043422

10 9 8 7 6 5 4 3 2 1

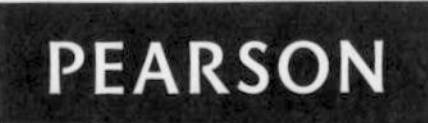

ISBN-10: 0-13-223938-8
ISBN-13: 978-0-13-223938-7

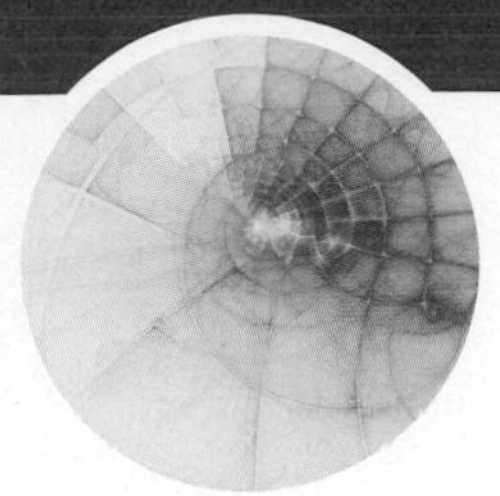

About the Authors

Thom J. Mansen

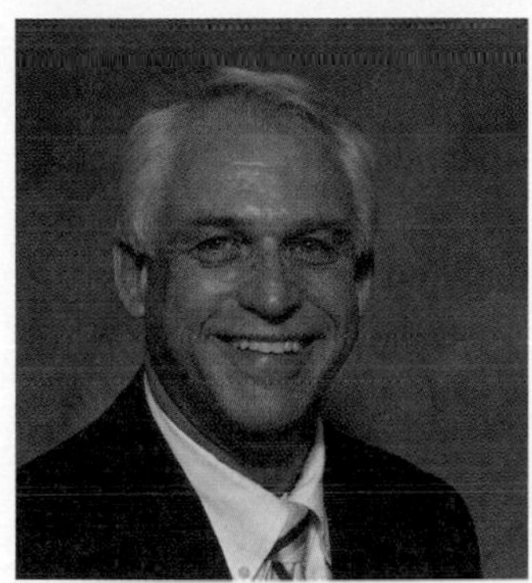

Thom J. Mansen graduated from the University of Michigan with a Bachelor of Science in Nursing degree. He went on to earn his MS degree from the University of Utah in cardiovascular nursing as a clinical specialist and worked as a clinical specialist in the MICU at University of Utah Hospital. He earned his PhD in nursing from the University of Texas at Austin with an emphasis in nursing education administration. Dr. Mansen has been a nursing educator for 35 years, having taught at Westminster College in Salt Lake City, Hope College/Calvin College in Holland/Grand Rapids, Michigan, and the College of Nursing, University of Utah. His primary classroom teaching responsibilities have been physical assessment, leadership/management (undergraduate/graduate), pathophysiology, medical-surgical nursing; and also clinical supervision of medical–surgical nursing students. He was also Program Director (Acting) and Baccalaureate Curriculum Coordinator.

Dr. Mansen has been actively involved in developing computer and video methods and techniques for teaching and assessing student's physical assessment skills. He developed the Head to Toe video disk with Dr. Sandra Haak, and later worked for Elsevier/Mosby in developing their Health Assessment Online. He also authored chapters for three editions of McCance & Huether's *Pathophysiology* textbook and *Understanding Pathophysiology*. Dr. Mansen has made international presentations at the first, second, and third Hacettepe University School of Nursing's International Nursing Management Conferences in Turkey. In 1996 he was awarded a Cockcroft Nursing Leadership Development Fellowship from the University of South Carolina, Charleston.

Dr. Mansen has also been active in community and nursing organizations. He was elected to the Gamma Rho (University of Utah) Chapter of Sigma Theta Tau and served as its president from 1989 to 1991. He is also active in the American/Utah Nurses Association and served as president of UNA from 1998 to 2001. He is active in musical activities; he plays piano and organ and has sung with the Oratorio Society of Utah and Utah Opera productions.

Julieta Gabiola

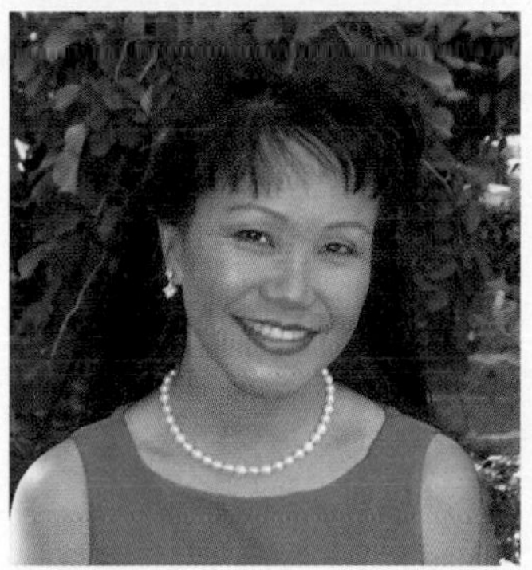

Julieta M. Gabiola is a Clinical Associate Professor of Medicine and teaches the Practice of Medicine (POM) at Stanford University. She is also involved in the Educators for CARE (**C**ompassion, **A**dvocacy, **R**esponsibility, and **E**mpathy) program at Stanford, which seeks to instill compassion, professionalism, values appropriate in becoming a good doctor.

Dr. Gabiola was raised in the Philippines, and long before she began teaching at Stanford, she obtained her bachelors in nursing at the Far Eastern University, Manila Philippines. She had diverse training in the medical field as a nurse, working in trauma at Temple University Hospital and Medical ICU and Operating Room at Rush Presbyterian St. Luke's and Cook County Hospital in Chicago.

While working fulltime as a nurse, she embarked in a rigorous preparatory training for medical school. She obtained her medical degree from Rush University Medical School and proceeded with her internship and residency in internal medicine at Stanford University. After her training, she worked for five years in the emergency department at Kaiser Permanente in Santa Clara, CA, followed by a fulfilling 15 year private practice in internal medicine in Salt Lake City. Dr. Gabiola's passion for lifelong learning prompted her return to Stanford University, where she currently teaches the practice of medicine course, taking medical students back to the very basic foundation of history taking, physical examination, and clinical reasoning. She extends her passion for teaching and humanitarian pursuits to the community by conducting health fairs in the Bay Area and medical missions and research in prevention of chronic diseases in the Philippines.

Her boundless energy, passion for learning, and diversity of experience—in patient care, classroom and bedside teaching, and in both the fields of nursing and medicine—have helped to shape this textbook. Dr. Gabiola believes that patient care is a collaborative effort, and she hopes this book will be a useful resource for all members of the healthcare team. She believes that nurses, doctors, pharmacists, nutritionists, discharge planners, social workers, and others play an integral role in patient care and should be given similar tools to evaluate the needs of patients.

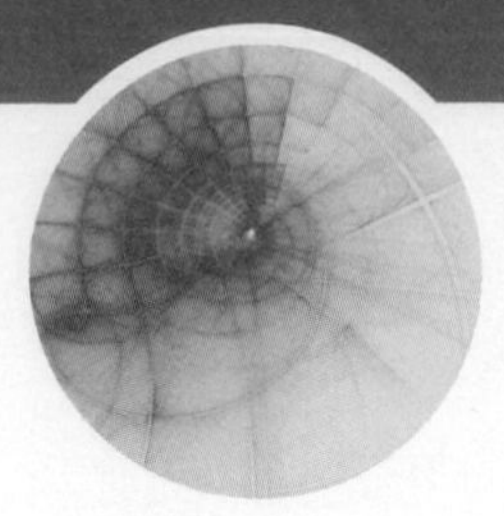

Thank You

We extend a sincere thank you to our contributors, who have given their time, expertise, and efforts to help create and make this textbook a reality. Most have been colleagues of mine (TJM) throughout my teaching career and I also appreciate their friendship and encouragement.

Linda Bergstrom, RN, CNM, PhD, FACNM
Associate Professor (Clinical)
College of Nursing
University of Utah, Salt Lake City, UT
Chapters 11, 30

Connie Madden, MS RN
Assistant Professor
University of Utah College of Nursing, Salt Lake City, UT
Chapter 12

Nanci McLeskey, MCG, MDiv, RN-BC, FNGNA
Clinical Instructor, Gerontology
University of Utah College of Nursing
Salt Lake City, UT
Chapter 12

Mary Molewyk Doornbos PhD, RN
Professor of Nursing
Calvin College
Department of Nursing, Grand Rapids, MI
Chapter 7

Marianne F. Moore PhD(c), CNM
Staff Midwife
Bay Area Birth Center, Houston, TX
Chapters 11, 30

Rachael J. Pohle-Krauza, PhD, RDN, LD
Associate Professor of Nutrition
Department of Human Ecology,
Youngstown State University, Youngstown, OH
Chapter 13

Katherine A. Sward, PhD, RN
Assistant Professor, College of Nursing and
Department of Biomedical Informatics
University of Utah, Salt Lake City, UT
Chapter 9
EMR Documentation sections in Chapters 16–30

Reviewers

We would like to thank the following individuals who graciously and generously gave of their time and expertise to provide excellent critiques and comments of our work. Their collective knowledge and experience helped to improve our efforts and the text wouldn't be what it is without their valuable input.

Jennifer Bailey DeJong, PhD, FNP-BC, CNE, CLE
Associate Professor
Concordia College, Moorhead, MN

Joan Carlson, RN, MSN, CNE
Professor
Harper College, Palatine, IL

Linda Cook, PhD, RN, CCRN, CCNS, ANCP-BC
Professor
Prince George's Community College, Kettering, MD

Tammi L. Damas, PhD, MBA, WHNP-BC, RN
Associate Professor
Howard University, Washington, DC

Ann Denney, MSN, RN
Associate Professor
Thomas More College, Crestview Hills, KY

Karlynne Galczyk, PhD (candidate), MSN, MPH, RN
Lecturer
Widener School of Nursing, Chester, PA

Sue K. Goebel, MS, RN, WHNP, SANE
Associate Professor
Colorado Mesa University
Grand Junction, CO

Jennifer Gwin, DNP, APRN, FNP-BC
Adjunct Professor
Maryville University, St Louis, MO

Karen L. Hessler, PhD, FNP-C
Assistant Professor
University of Northern Colorado, Greeley, CO

Rosemary Macy, PhD, RN, CNE
Associate Professor
Boise State University, Boise, ID

Lizy Mathew, EdD, RN, CCRN
Associate Professor
The William Paterson University of NJ
Wayne, NJ

Claudia Mitchell, PhD, MSN, RN
Executive Director
University of Cincinnati, Cincinnati, OH

Laurie J. Palmer, MS, RN, AOCN
Professor
Monroe Community College
Rochester, NY

Colleen M. Quinn, RN, MSN, EdD
Professor
Broward College, Fort Lauderdale, FL

Mary Rudnicki, MS RN
Instructor/ Student Success and Enrichment Coordinator
Northern Illinois University
DeKalb, IL

Sonya Saffell, CNP
Assistant Professor
Ohio University, Athens, OH

Colleen Sanders, RN, MS, FNP-BC
Instructor
Georgetown University,
Washington, DC

Kristi Schroeder, RN, MSN
Nursing Faculty/Program Coordinator
Southeastern Community College
Whiteville, NC

Ruth E. Schumacher, MSN, RN, CPN
Teaching Associate
University of Illinois, Chicago, IL

Christy Seckman, DNP, RN
Associate Professor
Barnes-Jewish College
St Louis, MO

Mary Shortreed, MSN, RN, CNE
Instructor
Youngstown State University
Youngstown, OH

Jennifer Sipe, MSN, RN, CRNP, ANP-BC
Assistant Professor
La Salle University, Philadelphia, PA

Valerie Steiner, RNC, MA, MSN, CNE
Director (Retired)
Midland College, Midland, TX

Marianne F. Swihart, RN, BSN, MEd, MSN, CRNI, PCCN, CWON
Associate Professor
Pasco Hernando Community College
New Port Richey, FL

Bonnie Thompson, MSN, RN
Full time Faculty, BSN program
Youngstown State University
Youngstown, OH

Marjorie Vogt, PhD, DNP, CNP, CNE, FAANP
Professor, Director, DNP Program
Otterbein University, Westerville, OH

Sandra K. Voll, MS, CNM, WHNP, FNP, RNC
Assistant Professor
Moravian College, Bethlehem, PA

B.J. Whiffen, DNP, RN, ACNP-BC, FNP-BC
Associate Professor, RN-MSN Cohort Coordinator
Southeast Missouri Hospital College of Nursing & Health Sciences,
Cape Girardeau, MO

Elizabeth Zion Stratton, RN, MS
Assistant Professor
Monroe Community College
Rochester, NY

Additional Thanks

Thanks is also extended to the Intermountain Simulation Lab of the College of Nursing, University of Utah for allowing us to use their facilities for our photo shoots, and to all those friends, students, family, and others who provided their services as models for the photo shoot. We would also like to thank London Roberts (student) who also provided her expertise as a photographer and worked with me (TJM) in photographing our students during the performance of their physical assessments and in other settings. Also thanks to the students who allowed themselves to be photographed. Thanks to Randy Carter, DO, for his expertise in eye conditions and disorders and providing valuable input and service in obtaining our eye photos. Thanks to Patrick Watson for his work taking the photos during our photo shoot.

Thanks to Dr. Nadim Mahmud, now a resident in internal medicine at Brigham, who was instrumental in helping create all the vignettes.

Thanks to the Educators for CARE at Stanford who gave us their critical comments and continued inspiration to many aspects of the book. Also thanks to Dr. Kathleen Kenny, Internal Medicine at Stanford, who helped review the clinical chapters, Dr. May Han, Neurology at Stanford, who reviewed Chapter 26, Dr. Mary Bronk, who reviewed the abdomen and breast chapters, and to Dr. Joslyn Woodard and Dr. Jay Nathan (now neurosurgical residents), who helped instill their medical students' perspectives while at Stanford. Finally, thanks to Dr. Abraham Verghese whom I (JG) consulted initially about the book.

Special thanks and gratitude to our developmental editor Jill Rembetski for assuming the position and responsibility as our third developmental editor. Jill worked around the clock, seeing this project to completion. Her dedication, efforts, patience, persistence and input were all graciously and thoughtfully provided. It was a great pleasure to work with her. Also thanks to Susan Geraghty and Karen Hoxeng, our previous developmental editors, for getting the project started. Great thanks goes to Pam Fuller, our acquisitions editor, who believed in the vision and overall concept of this text and took on the task of keeping us going in the right direction; we thank her for her patience and understanding when we weren't able to meet all of our deadlines.

I (TJM) also want to extend gratitude to June Thompson, who worked with me on other assessment projects and was instrumental in getting me in contact with Pam Fuller at Pearson. June has been a real inspiration and mentor, and I probably wouldn't be doing all of this if she hadn't initiated it.

Also thanks goes to my co-author, Julieta, who willingly jumped into the project mid-stream and persevered throughout all the changes and having to meet all of our deadlines "yesterday." Her ideas, insight, and suggestions were invaluable and made a significant addition to our team.

This book is dedicated to my wife, Cheryl, and son Cameron, who had to put up with my extended work hours. Their support and love has been immeasurable. My thanks and love to them.

—Thom Mansen

To my two children Sean and Micaela Finnegan who helped shape me to be one of the best single mothers after we lost their dad (Kevin Finnegan) to pancreatic cancer at such a young age of 47.

I would also like to dedicate this book to all the passionate educators, colleagues, students, and the members of health care teams. I am forever inspired by your dedication to teaching, learning, and excellence in patient care.

—Julieta Gabiola

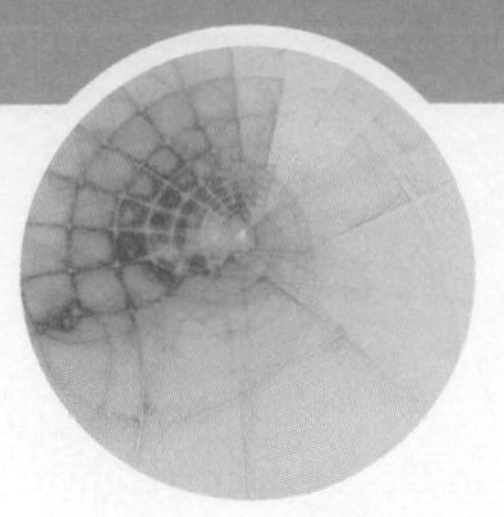

Preface

Patient-Focused Assessment: The Art and Science of Clinical Data Gathering is a text written for students new to health assessment and physical examination in undergraduate nursing programs, graduate nursing programs, as well as medical, physician assistant, physical therapy, and pharmacy programs. It is also an excellent reference for practicing health care providers who wish to develop their patient assessment skills. Patient assessment is critical for all providers of patient care, and the foundation for providing care, so the intent of this text is to focus on the patient.

Although the focus of health care may be shifting from identification and treatment to the prevention of specific diseases and conditions, the focus of the assessment does not change. The information required remains the same; what is done with this information may, however, differ within various health care disciplines, such as nursing, medicine, pharmacy, or physical therapy, depending on the discipline and how the data is used within that context. While disciplines may adhere to different methods of thinking and reasoning (e.g., the nursing process, diagnostic reasoning/formulation), the foundation for any and all of these methods is data from assessment. Categorization of data may also vary among and within the disciplines, but this does not change how or what data is obtained. What can be done with the data is determined by each discipline's scope of practice.

To assist students in all health care disciplines and at all levels, the assessment chapters in Unit IV provide a conceptual framework for assessment that is based on the fundamental physical examination skills used by nurses (Giddens, 2007; Secrest, Norwood, & DuMont, 2005) and the Stanford 25 used by physicians (Knox, 2010). This unit begins with Chapter 15, which presents a comprehensive head-to-toe approach to physical examination. The intention of this chapter is to present patient assessment of all body systems in a systematic manner as a means for helping the student understand how each system is assessed in an integrated approach. Chapters 16–30 next focus on specific areas of the body where the assessment techniques are organized by four levels of assessment that are based on the 1) provider's competency (skill level), 2) content (provider's discipline-specific knowledge), 3) complexity of the assessment techniques and procedures, and 4) patient's condition.

- The Level I assessment is designed for the beginning student provider who has minimal competency and knowledge base. This is the basic exam that may be performed at the bedside in a clinical setting or in an outpatient setting. The assessment techniques are relatively easy to perform. The Level I assessment requires a basic understanding of the skills and knowledge required in history taking, physical assessment, synthesis, diagnosis, and work up of common outpatient conditions.
- The Level II assessment is appropriate for an intermediate student or more experienced provider who has increased experience, skill, and knowledge. The techniques are more involved at this level, and the patient is in a more serious condition with health problems that concern multiple body systems.
- In the Level III assessment, the patient has the more complex conditions and care requirements that are commonly seen in an emergency department where immediacy of history gathering, physical assessment, synthesis, diagnosis, and actions take place almost simultaneously, requiring an advanced and more experienced provider with the knowledge and skills to perform more complex techniques.
- Finally, the Level IV assessment is directed at the provider who is proficient in performance of skills that are complicated or may require more complex thinking skills for interpretation.

Because the levels of these exams are not mutually exclusive, the student or provider must still determine the kind and amount of assessment data needed in relation to the patient's condition and care requirements. The four levels are also considered sequential and additive in their contexts, increasing in their scope and demands as well as the time required. Each level should be performed in a head-to-toe manner.

The most recent *Institute of Medicine* Report made recommendations that support the theme of this text. The IOM report emphasizes the need for nurses to assume more responsibility in providing health care, which implies the need for well-prepared nurses to take on the responsibility for health and physical assessment. To that end, this book was written to meet the needs of undergraduate nursing programs in the preparation of these nurses.

The IOM Report also emphasizes interdisciplinary education, which focuses on our similarities rather than our differences. In this spirit, our text was written to be discipline neutral and uses the term *providers*, which refers to any provider conducting a health assessment.

The primary focus of the text is the adult patient; however, the assessment needs for pediatric, geriatric, and pregnant patients are incorporated into each appropriate chapter. Unit II also includes individual chapters on each of these special populations to review their unique assessment related considerations.

Organization of this Textbook

This text is organized into four units. Unit I is a broad overview of assessment and the individuals involved. Chapter 1 focuses on the function and use of assessment within the context of providing health care. Chapter 2 focuses on the individual as a patient and/or provider, the uniqueness of each, and recognizing the unique characteristics associated with culture, beliefs, practices, experiences, etc., that each one brings to the relationship that develops during the history and physical examination, and delivery of care. Chapter 3 covers critical-thinking and decision-making skills, which are necessary skills for providers in delivering care. Chapter 4 focuses on the interviewing skills and communication techniques that are necessary to obtain patient-focused data.

Unit II focuses on the elements of the exam and comprehensive approaches and concepts needed in the process of data gathering. Chapter 5 provides a survey of the components of the health history and specific data that should be obtained. Chapter 6 introduces the four assessment techniques and their use during the physical examination. Chapter 7 presents the elements of the mental status exam as well as the general appearance exam. Knowledge of these two exams provides the foundation for overall assessment purposes, whether there will or won't be a structured history and physical. Chapter 8 covers assessment of vital signs and pain. Chapter 9 teaches how data obtained during the history and physical is documented in a meaningful and purposeful manner.

Unit III describes assessment of different groups or situations. Chapters 10, 11, and 12 provide details related to the assessment of pediatric patients (infants, children, and adolescents), pregnant women, and geriatric patients (older adults). Chapter 13 covers assessment of the patient's nutritional status. Chapter 14 covers assessment of high-risk situations and/or high-risk individuals. These situations or individuals demonstrate high-risk behaviors such as alcohol/drug abuse, unsafe sexual activity, abusive situations (child, intimate partner, elder), and suicide.

Unit IV, Chapters 15–30, details assessment of each body system. Chapter 15 provides a structured approach to integrating the assessment of each individual system into an organized, comprehensive physical examination presented in a head-to-toe approach. It is our philosophy that understanding and recognizing how one goes about assessing a patient in a systematic manner will better help the student to comprehend how each system is assessed in an integrated approach. The process is much like putting a jigsaw puzzle together. One has to look at the picture of the puzzle to help put all the pieces together; trying to put the puzzle together without knowing what it is supposed to look like is not conducive to success or satisfaction. Chapters 16–30 are each devoted to an individual system or physical location of the system. Each chapter begins with a brief review of the structure and function of a specific body system that includes a special focus on the developmental variations that occur throughout a person's lifespan or during pregnancy. This is followed by a discussion of the key objectives related to that body system as identified by *Healthy People 2020*. Students will next encounter patients who present with health care needs in a series of clinical context scenarios with critical thinking questions at end of each scenario before they begin the subjective and objective assessment of patients with manifestations of disorders related to that body system.

Within Chapters 16–30, the history (subjective data) and physical (objective data) are presented in two columns. For the subjective data, the first column identifies the appropriate questions (inquiries) to ask, and the second column provides the rationale (clinical reasoning/logic) for the questions.

The objective assessment sections in these chapters each begin with a table that identifies the specific skills related to the four different assessment techniques (inspection, palpation, percussion, auscultation) used in the assessment of that body system. These skills are then further subdivided into assessment levels, providing students with a framework to identify what assessment skills are appropriate and what data is needed for patients who have varying needs, conditions, and acuities. For the objective data, or physical assessment, the first column identifies and describes the specific techniques that are used with the expected findings related to each procedure. The second column presents the unexpected findings that may be associated with specific pathologies. When relevant and appropriate, photos, figures, and tables are included to illustrate concepts or findings.

Although the organization of this text differs from other texts on assessment, the content remains the same. The intent of the organizing framework is to provide a format for helping students identify specific skills that they need to focus on for learning physical assessment of patients in various clinical experiences. The format is also meant to be helpful in developing teaching methods (e.g. organizing content for lectures, application exercises, etc.).

It may also be noted that there is no use of the terms "normal" or "abnormal" throughout the system chapters. While we may think that we know what normal is when we see it, there really is no specific criterion to define or delineate normal. *Normal* implies that some type of measurement exists that can be used to establish what normal is. In reality, normal is relative and not absolute. For this reason, we have chosen to use the terms *expected* and *unexpected*.

Chapter Features

Vignettes

Each chapter begins with a vignette that presents a provider's and/or patient's thoughts and reactions to a situation within a context unique to each chapter.

> I review the patient's record before entering his room. Apparently 3-year-old Jack has had a 6-month history of runny nose, congestion, and fevers. A list of diagnoses swirl through my mind, and I already feel overwhelmed. Purulent discharge from the right nostril...MRI confirms acute sinusitis. The most recent note seems to be particularly useful: "Symptoms persist despite antibiotics… follow-up imaging strongly suggests chronic sinusitis." I smirk with a sudden omniscient confidence, and enter his room. Jack is occupied with the buttons on the examination chair, so I ask his foster mother for an update. She says the antibiotics still aren't working, and wants another opinion. I distract Jack with a stuffed monkey before tilting his head back and quickly slipping my otoscope into his right nostril. Just as I suspected—copious pus on an erythematous background. "It looks like it could be chronic sinusitis," I say flatly. "Let me bring in the attending physician for a quick look."
>
> Upon seeing Jack, the first thing Dr. Cox has him do is blow his nose, hard. Greenish pus coats the tissue. "Now lean your head back for me," he says sweetly. Craning his neck just slightly, Dr. Cox eases his otoscope into Jack's nostril and does a slow visual sweep. "Take a look at this," he motions to me. Lining up my eye with his scope, I see, to my utter amazement, what looks like the ashen stub of a cigarette butt. "Do you have something up your nose?" Dr. Cox asks, peering sternly over his

Symptom Analysis (COLDERRA)

In each system assessment chapter, each symptom is presented with a consistent approach (COLDERRA) to symptom analysis (Characteristics, Onset, Location, Duration, Exacerbation, Relief, Radiation, and Associated signs/symptoms). Each component of COLDERRA presents related questions with appropriate rationale (clinical reasoning/logic). The consistent use of COLDERRA symptom analysis framework helps students to recognize the essential information needed for symptom analysis.

Provider Inquiries	Clinical Reasoning/Logic
Characteristics: Is the blood red or brown? Does the blood include clots? Have you experienced oozing or spurting?	Anterior nosebleeds are common and arise from the watershed area known as Keisselbach's plexus. Posterior nosebleed arises commonly from the sphenopalatine artery or carotid artery.
Onset: When did this nosebleed start? When did you first start having nosebleeds? Frequency of nosebleeds? Anything noted that brings on nosebleed (trauma, picking nose, dry air, forceful blowing, allergies, coughing)? Any foreign object placed in nose (primarily related to children)?	Nasal inflammation from rhinosinusitis related to bacterial, viral or allergic origin causes dilation of blood vessels, which may rupture and cause epistaxis. Dry climate dries out nasal membranes, causing them to become irritated. Household heaters during the winter are a frequent cause of nasal dryness.

Physical Assessment

A table describing the specific levels of assessment appears in each system assessment chapter. These provide a framework that helps students and faculty identify what assessment skills are appropriate and what data is needed for patients with varying needs, conditions, and acuities.

Nose, Mouth, Sinuses, and Throat				
	Level I	**Level II**	**Level III**	**Level IV**
Inspection	Nose/sinuses Position, shape, symmetry, patency, discharge	Nose/sinuses Mucosa/turbinates, septum	Nose/sinuses Nasal, oral trauma	Nose/sinuses Sinuses: Transillumination
	Mouth–external Lips: color, shape, moisture symmetry, lesions			
	Mouth–internal Buccal mucosa: color, condition, state of hydration, surface characteristics	Mouth–internal Buccal mucosa: Hard palate	Mouth–internal Dental trauma	
	Teeth/gums: presence (number, missing), alignment, color, condition, surface characteristics,			Occlusion Malocclusion

Clinical Context Exemplars

Multiple Clinical Context Exemplars in Chapters 16–30 stimulate students' critical thinking by exposing them to realistic situations that they may experience in their clinical education. Each one provides a short case study and a series of critical-thinking questions.

Clinical Context Exemplars

Situation A

A 30-year-old woman with history of migraine headaches comes in with unrelenting, pulsating daily headaches associated with nausea, vomiting, and photophobia. She has been taking Excedrin, Maxalt, Vicodin, and tramadol with no relief.

1. What other history might you ask for?

Situation B

A 14-year-old young woman was brought in by her parents to the emergency department with cold symptoms, fever, and headaches of 12-hour duration. Many of her classmates have the similar symptoms. At the ED, the patient is noted to have fever and a stiff neck, is toxic appearing, and has no focal neurologic findings. An antibiotic was started, CT was done, and lumbar puncture (LP) was performed. The patient became obtunded and died within 10 hours of admission.

1. As you reflect on how you took care of the patient, is there anything that you could have done differently to change the course?
2. What would you predict to be the lumbar puncture results?

Situation C

A 60-year-old man presents with a sudden episode of severe headache, the worst headache in his life.

1. Is there any significance to the age of this patient? Why or why not?
2. How would you differentiate primary headaches from secondary headaches? What questions would you want to ask to help determine which type of headache this might be?
3. What pain characteristics would help you differentiate between the three major primary headache types?

Situation D

A 40-year-old woman noted painful swallowing, ear pain, and 8-pound weight loss in one week, which she attributed to not eating much due to pain when swallowing and stress. She tells you that she just returned from scuba diving to relieve stress and attributes her ear pain to scuba diving.

1. What else will you ask about her history, and what will the focused exam look like?

Think Links

Think Links in each chapter point out unique attributes of chapter topics/systems that help explain and/or clarify concepts associated with each topic/system.

THINK LINK: Meningitis

Patients with meningitis may present with fever, headache, nuchal rigidity [resistance to neck flexion], and altered mental status. However, these symptoms are only present in about 44% of adults with bacterial meningitis and even fewer children. No single sign is pathognomonic, and symptoms may vary and may be nonspecific depending on the host response and age of the patient. Symptoms may range from the above with or without nausea, vomiting, irritability, somnolence, lethargy, poor feeding, respiratory distress, seizures, hypothermia, and bulging fontanels in infants.

Meningitis in infants may not demonstrate neck stiffness. The presence of persistent fever in an infant with predisposing risk factors for meningitis like exposure to someone with HiB meningitis or Neisseria meningitis, recent ear or respiratory infection, travel to endemic areas, neurosurgical procedures penetrating head trauma, asplenia, cortisol excess, absent opsonizing antibody, complement deficiency, HIV infection, basilar skull fracture, bacteremia, and endocarditis should lower the threshold for a spinal tap.

Practice Points

Practice Points in each chapter are helpful hints related to real life situations that have helped practicing providers in obtaining assessment data.

PRACTICE POINT: Oropharyngeal Cancer and Human Papillomavirus (HPV)

HPV has been found to be associated with several types of cancer: cervical, vulvar, vaginal, penile, anal, and oropharyngeal (back of the throat, including the base of the tongue and tonsils). The rates for oropharyngeal cancer have been increasing dramatically since 1984, and HPV-related tumors account for the increasing numbers of annual cases, with a significant rise in younger males. Each year, more than 21,000 HPV-associated cancers occur in women; cervical cancer is the most common. More than 12,000 HPV-associated cancers occur each year in men; oropharyngeal cancers are the most common.

Health Promotion

Each system chapter presents a section on health promotion that is based on the objectives of *Healthy People 2020*. Objectives are discussed related to the relevance and significance of the topic area that relates to the objectives and presents health promotion activities that are essential to achieving the objectives. Health promotion is presented in other chapters as appropriate.

Health Promotion

Traumatic Brain Injuries

A TBI is an insult to the brain, not of a degenerative or congenital nature, but caused by an external physical force that may produce a diminished or altered state of consciousness, resulting in neurological and functional impairment (Dawodu, 2011).

- A major goal of *Healthy People 2020* is to reduce fatal and nonfatal traumatic brain injuries (TBI; U.S. Department of Health and Human Services, 2009); the target goal is 10% improvement.

It is estimated that 1.7 million cases of TBI occur per year and contribute to approximately one-third (30.5%) of all injury related deaths in the United States (Faul, Likang, Wald, & Coronado, 2010). Rates of TBI are highest in the very young (0–4 years old), in adolescents and young adults (15–24 years old), and in the elderly (above 65 years old). TBI is significantly higher in men than women with a 2–2.8:1 ratio and a 3.5:1 ratio in severe TBI. The most common causes of TBI include moving

When the skull is broken due to extreme force or penetration by an object, it is described as a penetrating or open-head injury. Brain injury also results from the penetrating object.

Injuries to the brain are also considered primary or secondary as determined by the time that signs and symptoms appear. Primary injuries are the result of the mechanical force that is applied to the head, and the bouncing of the brain within the skull. Secondary injuries develop hours to days after the initial injury and result from further damage to the neurons of the brain, mediated by neurochemical substances released from damaged cells.

In shaken baby syndrome (SBS), the cause of the injury is due more to the vigorous shaking that occurs rather than a forceful impact to the head. The rapid acceleration and deceleration of the brain against the infant's skull is the primary cause of brain injury. The injury is greatly increased if the shaking ends with the infants head hitting a solid or immovable object (wall or crib) (Cabinum-Foeller, 2011). (SBS is further

Lifespan Considerations

Developmental variations occur over the course of an individual's lifespan and events. Awareness of these variations is important to understand and recognize common age-related alterations or modifications that are related to a particular body system. For this reason, Chapters 15–30 use icons to highlight considerations related to children, pregnant women, and older adults.

spots." The fontanels gradually harden and become smaller until they are closed. The posterior fontanel is usually closed at about 2 months, and the anterior fontanel does not completely close until the child is 2 years old. Ossification and fusing of the sutures is not achieved until brain growth is accomplished, at about 6 years of age, and is not fully complete until adulthood.

Generally no continuing changes occur in the head and neck of the child. The features of the face may change as the child approaches puberty, but there is nothing specific that needs to be assessed. Other changes that accompany puberty affect primarily the skin, which has already been described in Chapter 16.

The Pregnant Woman

No specific changes affect the structure of the head and neck of a pregnant woman. The thyroid gland may demonstrate some physiological changes related to T_3 and T_4 and may increase in size, but not to any degree that can be identified by physical examination. If hyperthyroidism develops, there may be a detectable change in the size of the thyroid gland, a bruit may be heard over the gland, and the characteristic eye manifestations may be present along with weight loss. (These manifestations will be covered in more detail in Chapters 19 and 25.)

Headaches are common during pregnancy, particularly during the first and third trimester (Aegidius, Zwart, Hagen, & Stovner, 2009). Although their exact cause is not known, during the first trimester it is thought to be related to the hormonal fluctuations during pregnancy (MacGregor, 2012). Stress, poor

The Older Adult

There are no identified structural changes that accompany aging. As with children, skin-related changes alter the appearance of the face, but there are no expected changes. There are physiological and anatomic changes of the thyroid gland, but none that can be specifically examined.

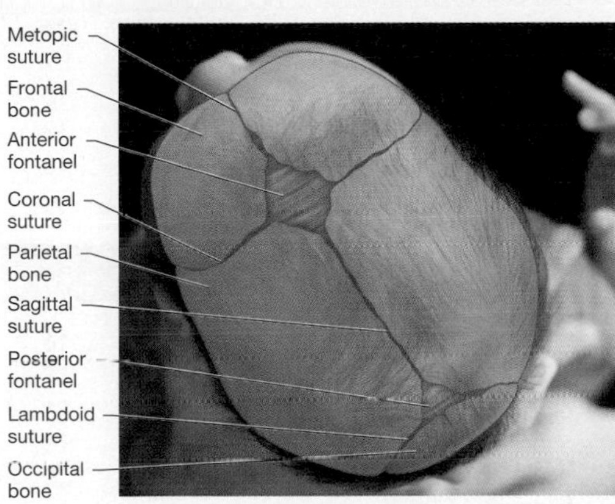

FIGURE 17-6 Superior view of infant's skull identifying sutures and fontanels
Source: Norhazlan/Shutterstock

Electronic Medical Record Documentation

Electronic medical record (EMR) documentation is extensively covered in a separate chapter (Chapter 9) and is also presented and discussed in special sections within Chapters 16–30. Coverage includes both traditional (paper) documentation and electronic medical record (EMR) standards, requirements, benefits, and limitations.

Conditions/Disorders

The conclusion of Chapters 11 and 16–30 present and review the key conditions and disorders that are related to each body system. Each topic includes a brief description of the particular condition, followed by the pathophysiology, and subjective and objective data associated with that condition.

Bell's Palsy

This is a form of unilateral facial paralysis from a dysfunction (neuritis) of cranial nerve VII (facial), causing the inability to control facial muscles on the affected side. The hallmark of this condition is a rapid onset of partial or complete unilateral paralysis that often appears overnight. In rare cases (< 1%), it can occur bilaterally, resulting in total facial paralysis. There appears to be no gender preference, but it is seen more commonly in females between the ages of 10 and 19 and those who are pregnant. In pregnant women, it frequently occurs in the third trimester and those with preeclampsia. In terms of age, those with the highest incidence are adults over 60. The extent of involvement is related to the degree of nerve involvement. The average length of paralysis is 3 weeks and 80%–90% recover without any residual effects.

Pathophysiology

- It is thought that an inflammatory condition leads to swelling of the facial nerve. The nerve travels through the skull in a narrow bone canal beneath the ear. Nerve swelling and compression in the narrow bone canal are thought to lead to nerve inhibition, damage, or death.
- Mounting evidence suggests that herpes simplex I and herpes zoster are the causative agents. These viruses become reactivated from the facial nerve ganglia (Taylor et al., 2011).
- Other etiologies considered are autoimmune, inflammatory, or ischemic causes.
- Brain tumor, stroke, myasthenia gravis, and Lyme disease are possible causes.
- It is the most common acute mononeuropathy and the most common cause of acute facial nerve paralysis (>80%).

Subjective

- Manifestations may include poor closure of the eyelids, decreased tearing, posterior ear pain, and taste disturbances.

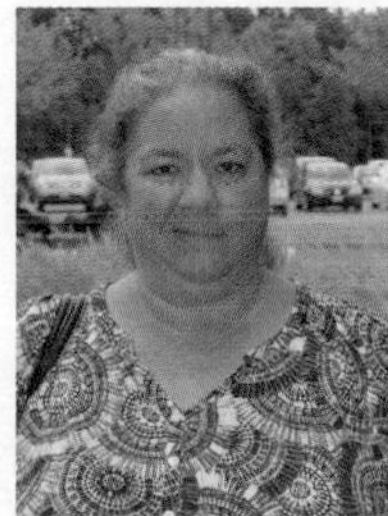

FIGURE 17-28 Bell's palsy

Objective

- Facial paralysis results in drooping of face and asymmetry of facial expressions with movement observed only on the unaffected side.

Review Questions

Each chapter concludes with ten multiple-choice or other type of review question to provide the opportunity for students to test their comprehension of the chapter. The types of questions conform to NCLEX-RN® style and format.

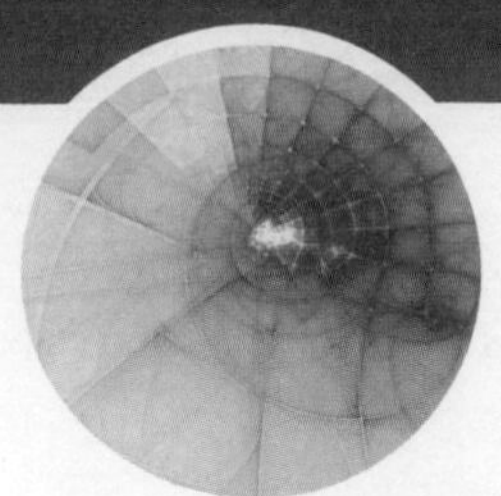

Contents

1 The Foundation and Context of Assessment

I've lain in this bed now for 3 days, and no one is able to tell me what's wrong. I've filled out so many forms and have been poked and prodded everywhere, even some places that I didn't know could be poked. Here comes a new group of doctors; I wonder if they'll tell me anything new.

"Mr. Griffin," she says without looking up, "I'm Doctor Rodriguez and these are my students who will be examining you." *Oh brother, more poking and prodding.* "What brought you into the hospital the other day?" *Do I have to go through this again?* I start telling her about feeling light headed, and then sweating profusely. I also explain about being extremely tired and experiencing some numbness in my right arm.

A few seconds into my explanation, she looks up from the computer and brusquely interrupts me with questions about my personal and family medical history. Typing my answers furiously into her computer, she continues her barrage of questions: What kind of activities do I engage in? Do I smoke? How much exercise do I get? Her tone is painfully polite, but business-like. She makes more eye contact with her computer screen than she does with me, often acknowledging me only with a curt nod.

After her questioning, she leaves and instructs the students to do the exam. They're all polite and look scared. They begin to poke and prod, and I can tell they're not comfortable doing this. I know they're just practicing on me to get more experience. I wish they'd at least introduce themselves and look at me rather than just talking to each other. I wish someone would just tell me what's going on so I wouldn't have to just lie here and be the guinea pig.

LEARNING OUTCOMES

1. Describe the evolution and advancement of assessment within the context of the history of health care provision and practice.
2. Explain the importance of health assessment to health care delivery.
3. Compare and contrast the four levels of assessment within the context of complexity, content, competency, and condition.
4. Describe the critical elements that influence the relationship between patient and health provider.

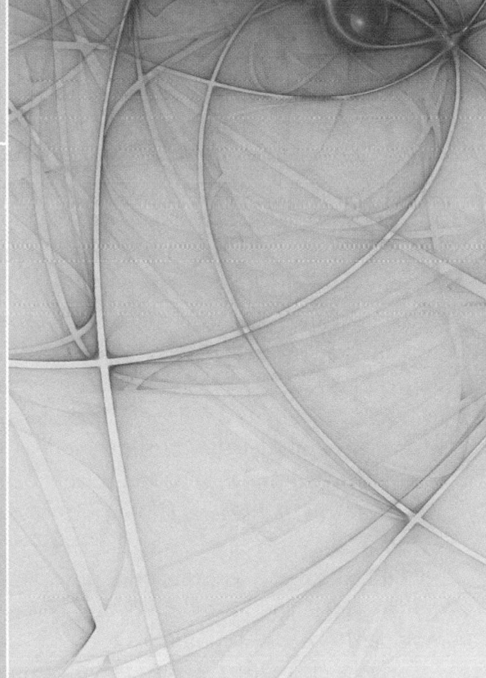

The perception of a provider engaging in personal and respectful relationships with his or her patients is rapidly disappearing. While this component of health care may not be as prevalent as it once was, it still has a significant function in providing quality health care. Opportunities to establish a relationship between the provider and patient may not be as frequent; however, one interaction that promotes this relationship is the health assessment, which consists of a history and physical examination. However, the value of this activity is being questioned and has been referred to as unhelpful, unimportant and not supported by current evidence (Laine, 2002; Mehrotra, Zaslavsky, & Ayanian, 2007; Prochazka, et al., 2005). It has been reported that some providers intentionally leave out the physical exam, believing that the short 15-minute office visit is better spent on talking with the patient or reviewing test results (Knox, 2010). Physicians also assert that some parts of the health assessment are difficult and subjective, so an expensive test might be more reliable than using, say a stethoscope, to listen for any unusual murmur or sound.

While increases in technology have improved health care and provided lifesaving interventions, the opportunity to interact with the patient and establish a relationship should not be dismissed. One reason that is often stated in support of continuing the physical exam is that it provides the opportunity for the "laying on of hands." This action is most likely more symbolic than therapeutic; nevertheless, its meaning and use should not be overlooked. Regardless of such unresolved issues, the consensus on health assessment is that it is a vital process in patient-centered care.

By definition, assessment is the evaluation or estimation of the ability, nature, and quality of an individual or a product. By implication, the end product or outcome of the assessment process is a judgment or a conclusion. In health care practice, assessment includes obtaining relevant and reliable data about a patient and establishing a database so that a comprehensive representation of that individual's health status can be determined. An older, but still relevant and concise definition of health assessment is "a precise, orderly collection of data about the physical, psychological, sociological behavior of the patient" (McCain, 1965).

Health and Patient Assessment

The collection of appropriate and relevant data for purposes of providing health care has been largely shaped by the definition and perception of health or health status. Health and the understanding of health, as well as assessment of a patient's health, have in fact evolved and expanded throughout the history of health care.

Historical Evolution of Assessment

While today's practice of health care is highly dependent on the use of data and a systematic approach to identify disease and its treatment, it has not always been this way. The earliest views of illness and disease, which have persisted since the beginning of civilization, extend back to primitive times when sickness and disease were viewed as punishments from the gods and/or evil spirits for some human activity that displeased them. Because illness was seen as a spiritual form of punishment, the sick sought and obtained treatment from religious figures who were believed to have the power to intervene on their behalf. Thus, any assessment performed was related more to what the person had supposedly done to displease the gods rather than what physiological alterations might be occurring.

Age of Antiquity

In ancient times, knowledge regarding illness and disease accumulated primarily through trial and error, much of which was conducted through the use of plants and herbs for treatment of various ailments. An individual who became proficient in using plants and herbs eventually became known as a "shaman" or "medicine man" whose remedies primarily focused on alleviating symptoms rather than treating the underlying cause. Assessment of the individual was likely practiced, but not in any orderly way.

The earliest recognition of a structure or context contributing to the understanding of a conceptual approach to understanding illness and disease occurred in the 5th century B.C. when Empedocles (492–432 BCE), who along with other Greek philosophers proposed the cosmological theory of four elements or **humors** that composed the structure of matter and were thought to be distributed throughout the body. These elements consisted of (1) fire, (2) air, (3) water, and (4) earth.

Hippocrates (460–370 BCE) accepted this theory and contributed somewhat to its development but he is better remembered for what many consider the "birth of modern medicine." Hippocrates was the first to promote a rational, scientific approach to the diagnosis and treatment of diseases. Hippocrates first advanced the idea that sound medical reasoning was the result of astute observation (of the individual) and assessment of other components related to the individual. He and his followers thus began to record and describe multiple diseases and conditions.

Galen (131–201 CE) studied and commented extensively on the writings of Hippocrates as well as writing his own texts. He is recognized as the founder of the humoral theory of medicine. The early theorists recognized that the four essential elements did not exist in the body but were represented by specific bodily fluids (1) fire (blood), (2) air (yellow bile), (3) water (phlegm), and (4) earth (black bile). The humoral theory was based on the assumption that the proper mixing of these fluids was the secret to health. An increase or decrease in any of the humors resulted in unique patterns of disease.

Galen also became one of the greatest surgeons of the ancient world. He performed many bold surgeries, which included the brain and eye. He also undertook studies of anatomy, which became the foundation for medical education in Medieval Europe.

While the humoral theory for the practice of medicine was widely accepted, no evidence exists that any type of assessment was performed on patients to determine which humor was out of balance. Treatment for the humoral imbalances ranged from using leeches, purgatives, and emetics to using large quantities of alcohol. The curious practice of bloodletting was also periodically performed on individuals to maintain humoral balance. It was believed that bloodletting could release evil spirits from the body and restore the balance of the four humors (Figure 1-1).

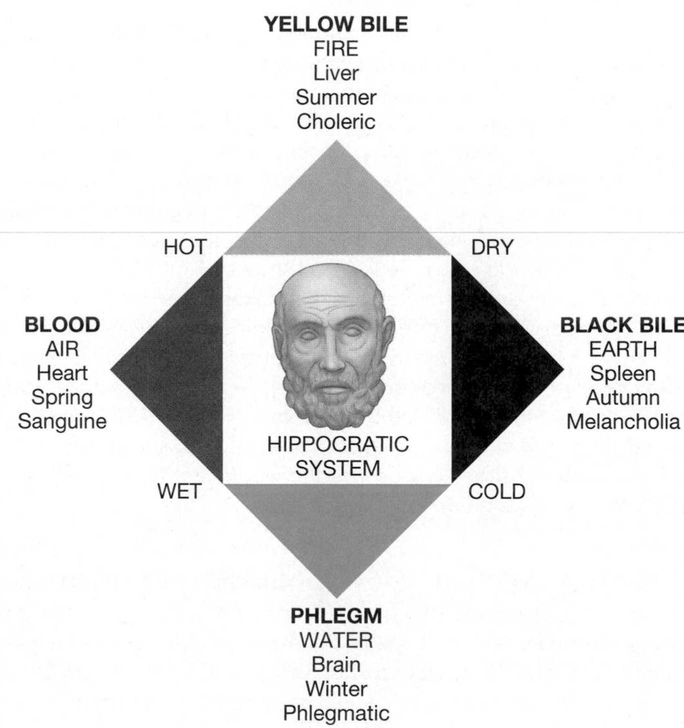

FIGURE 1-1 Theory of Humoral Imbalance

> ***THINK LINK: Did George Washington Bleed to Death?***
> George Washington's death in 1799 is said to have been primarily caused by excessive bloodletting by his physicians. While the practice seems barbaric to modern day health care providers, it was still standard practice at that time. Due to prolonged exposure to cold weather and snow on December 12th, Washington is said to have developed a sore throat that rapidly progressed, subsequently causing severe respiratory problems. He awoke on December 14th with chills and severe dyspnea (Cheatham, 2008). When medicinal mixtures [molasses, vinegar, and butter] were ineffective, Washington—who believed in bloodletting—requested the procedure. Eventually, there were four more episodes of bloodletting, bringing the total amount of blood removed to 126 ounces or 3.75 liters, which is approximately one half of an individual's circulating volume of blood (Vadakan, 2004). While the exact cause of George Washington's death remains uncertain, the amount of blood lost through bloodletting certainly had a significant effect on the outcome.

The theory of humoral imbalance that was practiced in ancient times was not abandoned until much later (1800s) as more empirical evidence began to erode its practice and the beliefs about it.

Along with the Greeks, the Romans also exercised significant influence on the growth and advancement of medical knowledge and practice. They developed many surgical instruments that are still in use today. The Romans were also responsible for advances in cataract surgery.

While much of the credit is given to the Greeks and Romans for the development of medicine, advances in other cultures and areas of the world were also taking place which had a significant influence on the Greeks and Romans. The earliest evidence of systematic medical practice comes from Ancient Egypt and the Babylonian empire. The first known physician, Sekhet-eanach, was from Egypt (Lambert, 2012). Surgery was likewise first performed by Egyptians in 2750 BC, but was primarily limited to treating wounds and broken bones. The earliest known medical text is the *Ebers Papyrus*, an Egyptian textbook that was written around 1500 BC and provides detailed descriptions of examination, diagnosis, treatment, and prognosis of many illnesses and conditions of that time (Figure 1-2).

The greatest Babylonian contribution to medicine was the development of the *Diagnostic Handbook*, written by Esagil-kin-aoli or Borsippa between 1069–1046 BC, which introduced the concepts of diagnosis, prognosis, physical examination, and prescriptions. The *Diagnostic Handbook* contained axioms and assumptions that reflected the modern perspective that examination and inspection of the patient's symptoms facilitates identifying of the patient's condition, its origin and progression, and the probability of recovery. It also contained methods of therapy and etiology and promoted the use of empiricism, logic and rationality in diagnosis, prognosis, and intervention. Other significant medical contributions came from the Indian, Persian, Chinese, Hebrew, and Islamic civilizations and cultures.

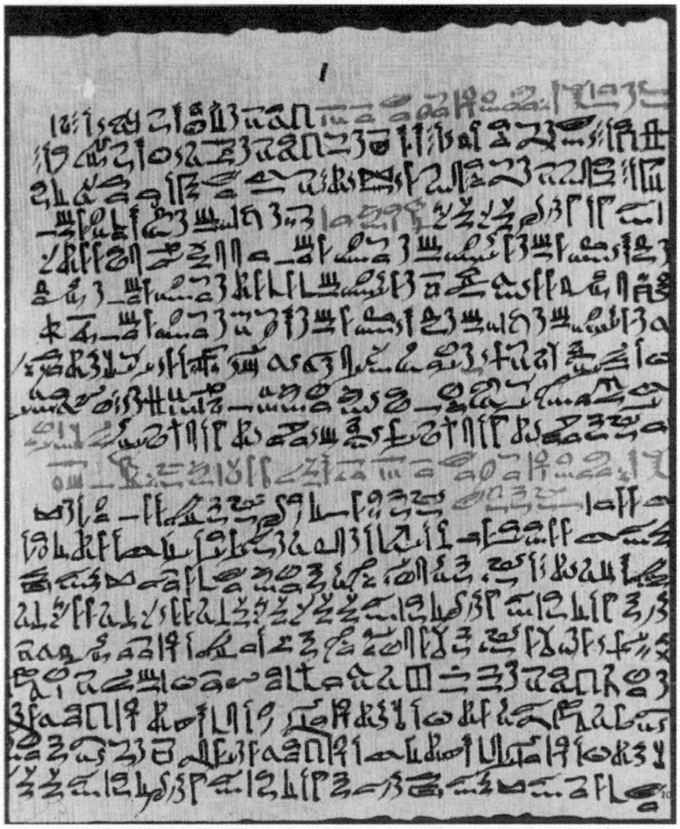

FIGURE 1-2 The *Ebers Papyrus*
Courtesy of the National Library of Medicine

Middle Ages and Renaissance

Historians generally agree that nearly all the advances made in the western world related to medicine and nursing came to a halt when the Roman Empire fell at the start of the Middle Ages (500 CE–1500 CE). Folk practices found their way back into the healing arts, and the practice of medicine became very localized. The eastern half of the Roman Empire however maintained many of the medical advances and passed their knowledge and practices to the Muslims, where it flourished.

The Middle Ages of Europe, which began with the destruction of the Roman Empire, was a period of readjustment, where medieval society was more concerned with keeping peace than nurturing centers of learning. Gradually, Western Europe became more civilized and there was renewed interest in medicine and knowledge. In the 11th century, the medical college of Salerno in Italy was founded, bringing back an organized, professional practice of medicine. Gradually, the body of medical knowledge increased and various treatments and interventions were introduced; however, the identification of specific causes of diseases and conditions remained dormant. Medical practice was still dominated by the ideas of Galen and the theory of the four humors.

During this time, Hildegard of Bingen, a remarkable woman and very productive writer, exercised a strong influence on medical practice (Figure 1-3). While early interest in her work focused on her music, Hildegard also authored several commentaries on natural science and medicine (Sweet, 1999). Her text on medicine (*Causae et curae*) was derived from ancient Greek cosmology of the four elements—air, fire, water, and earth—with their complementary qualities of heat, dryness, moisture, and cold.

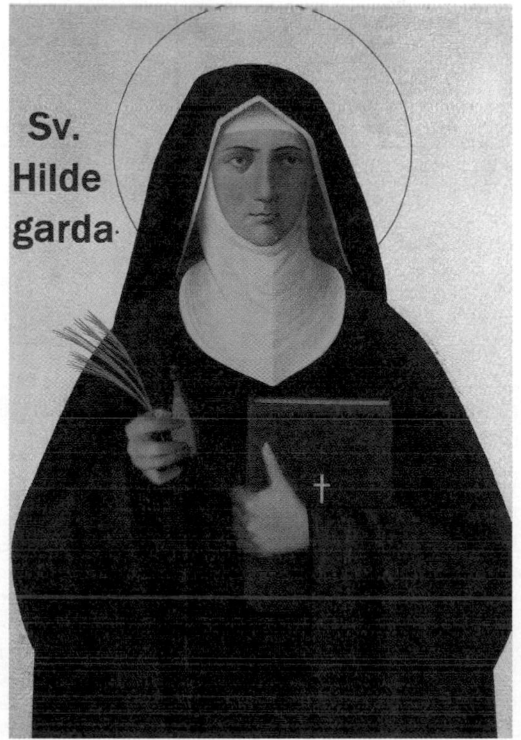

FIGURE 1-3 Hildegard von Bingen
Courtesy Zvonimir Atletic/Shutterstock

It is this balance of the four elements in nature that is reflected in the balance of the four humors of the body (Table 1-1).

Another female physician in the Middle Ages was Jacqueline Felicie de Almania, who practiced in Paris in the 1320s. She was extremely popular and had great success in curing sickness with her own medicines (Elliott, 2005). The medieval practice of medicine was undertaken mostly by lay practitioners and by monks in monasteries who were referred to as **infirmarians** (Sweet, 1999). Monastery infirmaries were also places for bloodletting, and were intended for elderly and sick monks, pilgrims, workers, and the poor from surrounding farm villages. The infirmarians did not necessarily have medical training and, most likely, received instruction from lay practitioners or received hands-on training, passed down from one monk to another. The primary responsibility of the infirmarian was the diagnosis, prognosis, and treatment of diseases. In the 13th century there emerged a new group of individuals who engaged in medical practices but were not considered physicians. These individuals were the barber-surgeons who, along with cutting hair, pulled teeth, performed amputations, and set broken bones (Lambert, 2012). They also performed bloodletting. As individuals of the time were illiterate, barber-surgeons advertised their services (blood and bandages) by placing a red and white pole outside their shops.

Diagnosis depended on the traditional techniques of pulse-taking and tongue inspection and the examination of urine, blood, and stool. Treatment relied on a number of Greco-Roman ideas: the principle of contraries (e.g. "cold and wet" medicines treat "hot and dry" diseases); the principle of repletion/depletion (bleeding, cupping, and purging to remove excess humors); and the principle of energy flow/stagnation (moxibustion and cautery promote the flow of energy) (Sweet, 1999).

Table 1-1 Elements in nature reflected in the balance of four humors

Description	Humor	Organ	Element
Sanguine	Blood	Liver	Air
Choleric	Yellow Bile	Spleen	Fire
Phlegmatic	Phlegm	Lungs	Water
Melancholic	Black Bile	Gall bladder	Earth (land)

***THINK LINK:** Diagnoses of Diabetes Mellitus vs. Diabetes Insipidus*

Most are familiar with the condition known as diabetes in which there is a lack of insulin for the appropriate metabolism of sugars. Another type of diabetes, known as diabetes insipidus, is a lack of anti-diuretic hormone. Both conditions have a common manifestation—excessive urine output. While there was recognition of the two types of diabetes, there was no specific test to differentiate them, so the method that was used was to taste the urine. Urine from an individual that tasted sweet was described as "mellitus," and urine that tasted sour was described as "insipidus." Thus the condition of diabetes mellitus describes an excess of glucose in the urine, not in the blood.

17th–19th Centuries

The onset of the Renaissance led to a renewed interest in medicine. Dissections of cadavers allowed artists and physicians to increase their knowledge of anatomy. In 1628, the English physician William Harvey presented his discovery of the circulatory system and the recognition of the heart as a pump. Another English physician, Thomas Sydenham, is recognized as promoting the importance of careful observation of patients and their symptoms. In 1683, the Dutchman Antonie van Leeuwenhoek was the first to observe bacteria and microorganisms through a microscope. Although microbes were identified, their part in causing diseases was not recognized. In 1761, Leopold Auenbrugger described the technique of percussion, based on the practice of tapping on wine casks to determine the volume of the cask and when to reorder (Verghese et al., 2011). In 1796, Edward Jenner developed the process of vaccination.

During the 1800s, advances in medical practice were slow. There was still no understanding as to the causes of disease. The theory of four humors was still believed although doubt as to its validity began to emerge. In 1819, Rene Laennec discovered the stethoscope when he rolled a sheet of paper into a cone, placed the point in his ear and the base on the patient's chest and heard sounds (Verghese et al., 2011). Laennec made the first stethoscope out of wood and began to correlate what sounds he heard with patient's histories and autopsy results. A major breakthrough occurred in 1847 when Ignaz Semmelweis, a Hungarian doctor, identified simple hand washing as a way to decrease the death rate of women from childbed fever (puerperal sepsis) (Figure 1-4).

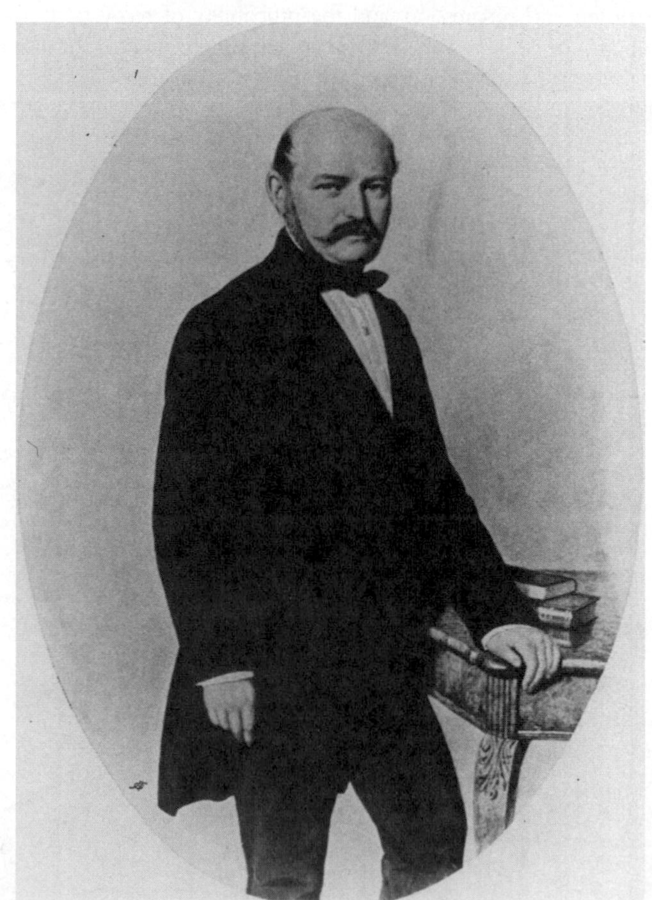

FIGURE 1-4 Ignaz Semmelweis
Courtesy of the National Library of Medicine

In spite of its dramatic effect, hand washing was not incorporated into general practice until Joseph Lister provided evidence in 1867 that increased cleanliness reduced the death rate from infection among hospital patients.

The practice of medicine was significantly altered with the development of the germ theory, which resulted from Louis Pasteur's discovery of microorganisms as a significant cause of diseases (Figure 1-5). In a letter to Pasteur in February 1874, Lister wrote, "Thanks for having, by your brilliant researches, proved to me the truth of the germ theory. You furnished me with the principle upon which alone the antiseptic system can be carried out." (J.H Tiner, 1990, page 111).

The work of Pasteur facilitated the recognition of various microorganisms as the cause of many diseases. Diseases that were related to specific organisms included anthrax, cholera, tuberculosis, rabies, diphtheria, tetanus, pneumonia, typhoid, and leprosy. The use of chloroform as an anesthetic for surgery began as well as the recognition of antiseptics for the prevention of infections.

The 20th century practice of medicine was advanced with the discovery of antibiotics, use of insulin, development of sulfonamides, and vaccine for poliomyelitis. Dialysis for renal failure became a reality with the development of the artificial kidney. Organ transplants also began during the 20th century.

Nursing

Throughout the early periods of medical practice development, the major focus was on a single group of providers so there was no differentiation between physicians and nurses. Even though extended care was often necessary, the recognition of individuals as nurses was not evident because providing care to the sick was naturally expected from female family members and/or friends. As Christianity began spreading throughout the western world, the practice of nursing was eventually associated with it and with the religious orders that were subsequently organized. These new orders were predominantly composed of females. It is, however, unclear as to when the term *nurse* first appeared, or when it was applied to care providers.

The Crusades of the 11th century provided the milieu for the formation of the **Knights of the Hospitaliers**, a group of monks who formed religious and military orders to care for sick and wounded crusaders. As a result of the Hospitaliers' creation and organized care provision, other religious and military orders were formed and hospitals were established throughout Europe.

Eventually, the hospitals that had been founded became overcrowded places that ceased to serve as centers of healing. Instead, they became institutions of death with high mortality rates. The individuals, primarily if not exclusively females, who were recruited to work in these hospitals, often came from the lowest class of citizens as no one else was willing to work under the severe conditions they endured. Care provided was not systematized, nor did formal educational requirements to become such a care provider exist. In fact, the first formal educational training course for nurses was established much later in Kaiserswerth, Germany, in 1836 by German Lutheran Pastor Theodor Fleidner for his Order of Deaconesses.

Florence Nightingale is largely recognized as the founder of professional nursing (Figure 1-6). In 1854, she was appointed to organize a corps of nurses to care for the soldiers fighting in the Crimean War. Nightingale and her nurses went to Scutari as requested and, as a result of their efforts, the mortality rate in hospitals fell from 60% to 1%. The care given focused on providing and maintaining an effective healing environment. This included exposing patients to fresh air and adequate ventilation, promoting cleanliness and healthy eating. It was during this assignment that Nightingale began her efforts to develop care standards for patients and to educate individuals in the art of nursing.

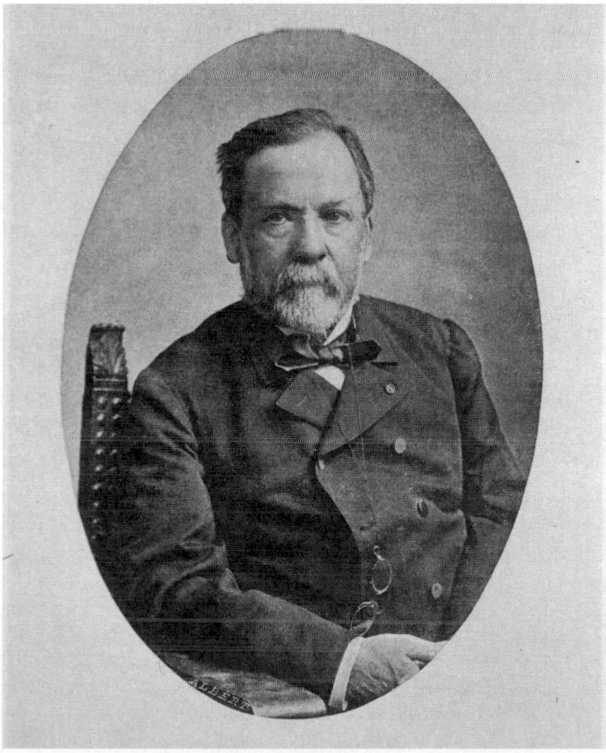

FIGURE 1-5 Louis Pasteur
Courtesy of the National Library of Medicine

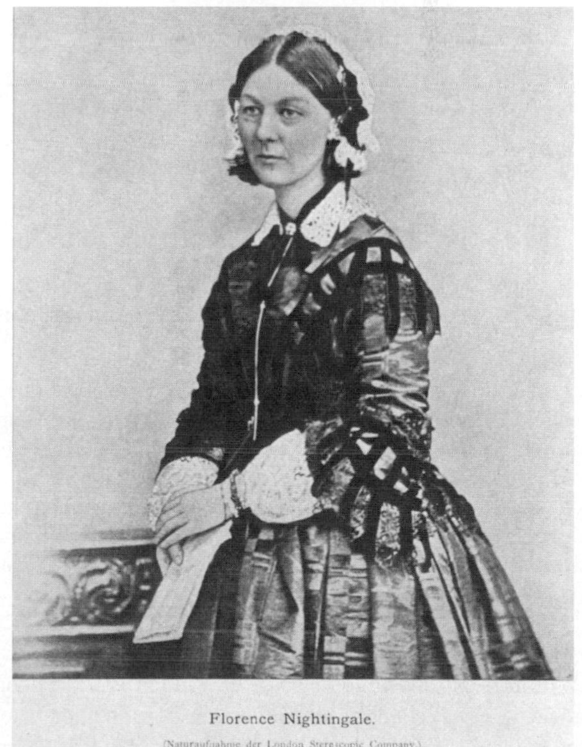

FIGURE 1-6 Florence Nightingale
Courtesy of the National Library of Medicine

In the early stages of developing appropriate nursing care standards, Nightingale actively encouraged nurses to develop their assessment skills. She stressed the importance of accurately assessing sick individuals and other conditions, such as environment, diet, and lighting, which influenced the individual's health status and/or recovery. Traditionally, the role of the nurse had not involved assessment beyond the scope of observation or inspection. Obtaining data from the patient for purposes of problem solving and individualizing care was considered unnecessary for providing quality nursing care.

Modern Times

The beginning of the 20th century brought about the application of the scientific method to research, which in turn, produced rapid advances in understanding illnesses and conditions as well as the identification of newer therapeutic interventions. The discovery of penicillin in the late 1920s initiated a rapid increase in the development of pharmaceuticals to aid in the treatment of disease. Today, as knowledge increases, health assessment plays an increasingly important function in obtaining vital information about the patient and the status of his health.

Throughout the development of medical practice, health has been considered "the absence of disease," and thus the opposite of illness. Up until the beginning of the 20th century, two patient outcomes could be expected—recovery or death. Living with a serious illness was not considered a possibility. Today, however, newer modalities for treatment of illnesses and conditions allow individuals to live healthy and functional lives in the presence of disease, and health assessment now encompasses the collection of data pertaining to a health state that may include certain diseases and conditions.

PRACTICE POINT: Health versus Wellness

On the surface, health and wellness appear to be one and the same. When a person is considered healthy, he or she is thought to be disease-free. Medical treatment has thus traditionally focused on curing an individual's ailment. As medical science advances, however, and better forms of treatment are developed to control certain incurable conditions, more and more individuals are learning how to cope and live with disease. Thus, the concept and definition of health has expanded so that individuals with controllable diseases may also be considered healthy. The contemporary notion of health, therefore, lies in a continuum that ranges from illness to wellness.

Essentially, health refers to the state of our physical being, whether excellent or poor. It depends on a number of factors like heredity, environment, diet, fitness and exercise, sleep, and even emotions. Wellness on the other hand is the conscious decision to assume responsibility for the quality of your life. Viewed in this context, health assessment is what is appears to be: an overall assessment of the individual that includes all states and conditions that can or cannot be cured.

Within health care, the focus of assessment is the individual, or patient who is seeking to remedy or care for a real or potential health problem. While the patient remains the primary source of information, data about his condition is also obtained through various tests and procedures. Within this context, health care is focused on problem solving, decision making and identifying appropriate solutions for the treatment of health problems. Once a problem or problems have been identified, they take the form of a diagnosis. An appropriate diagnosis cannot be formulated without the necessary information, thus assessment is a critical element required for the provision of health care. (Further description and discussion of diagnosis is found in Chapter 3.)

In the United States, traditional health care emphasizes the identification of a specific disease process. Today, alongside this emphasis, there is increasing recognition that health care should also consider the prevention of health problems. As a result, information regarding specific causes of diseases has become increasingly available to help health providers better determine the likelihood of an individual developing a specific disease or condition.

Although the focus of health care may be shifting from identification and treatment to the prevention of specific diseases and conditions, the focus of the assessment does not change. The information required remains the same; what is done with this information may, however, differ within various health care disciplines, such as medicine, nursing, pharmacy, therapy, depending on the discipline and how the data is used within that context. While disciplines may adhere to different methods of thinking and reasoning (e.g., the nursing process, diagnostic reasoning/formulation), the foundation for any and all of these methods is assessment or data collection. Categorization of data may also vary among and within the disciplines, but this does not change how or what data is obtained. What can be done with the data is determined by each discipline's **scope of practice.**

Scope of Practice

In simplest terms, scope of practice is a phrase used to define the procedures, actions, and processes that are permitted by law for a specific profession. The scope of practice of a licensed health care profession is statutorily defined in state laws in the form of a **practice act**. Scopes of practice are continuously evolving, and state legislatures have the authority to approve any adoptions or modifications to any particular scope of practice of a health care profession.

The primary purpose of state regulation through practice acts is to protect the public from inept, dishonest, and unethical practitioners. Regulation helps to assure that licensed individuals are competent to provide services that are appropriate, safe and effective.

While each profession has a specific practice act, these are not mutually exclusive. Health care education and practice have developed in such a way that most professions today share some skills or procedures with other professions. Thus, it is no longer reasonable to expect each profession to have a completely unique scope of practice, exclusive of all others. A major concern within health care today is the overlapping responsibilities and actions of the numerous health care professions. Within this concept of shared practices and responsibilities, therefore, there is need for state legislatures to recognize that certain tasks or services performed by, for instance, physicians, may carry such a considerable risk of harm to the health, safety or well-being of the patient that they should be reserved to doctors, or shared among qualified professions.

Assessment, for instance, may be considered a practice that is not necessarily the sole responsibility of one health care profession. In the course of attending to a patient, all health care practitioners assess a patient's progress and response to services rendered, observing and evaluating his or her physical status. However, it may be important to distinguish between assessment and diagnosis, which is essentially the identification of the cause of signs or symptoms and which should be an act reserved for physicians and other qualified health practitioners.

Since its early inception, the practice of medicine involved obtaining pertinent information from the individuals seeking treatment, formulating a cause for the condition and implementing a specific treatment. The number of possible conclusions that could be reached was based on the available information from the individual and the limited knowledge related to physiology and possible causes of alterations. Even though the knowledge of diseases and their causes may have been faulty by today's knowledge, the process of formulating and identifying a particular disease process and its cause was much the same as the process used today.

Early nursing education did not specifically include the performance of a physical exam within its curriculum. Assessment in nursing has always been presented as data gathering, but that data did not necessarily include physical assessment data, other than vital signs, temperature, and minor deviations from a patient's baseline data. However, with the introduction of hospital critical care units in the 1970s, it became customary, if not essential, to teach nurses how to conduct physical examinations so that they could better monitor patients, provide more accurate and specific information to physicians, and make sound clinical decisions about patient care. Thus, performing physical assessments is now included in the nurse practice acts of most states.

Also in the 1970s, **advanced nursing practice** (ANP) and **nurse practitioners** (NPs) first emerged as patient care grew more complex. The goal of preparing NPs was not necessarily to create competition for doctors, but to train other health care professionals in basic medical diagnosis of common conditions, thus allowing physicians more time to provide care to more complex patient conditions and situations. Up until the late 1980s and early 1990s, NPs were required to be supervised by physicians. Gradually, state nurse practice acts were approved to allow NPs to function independently from physicians; however, the majority of NPs continue to work collaboratively with physician groups in various specialties. Most states also now allow NPs prescriptive privileges upon completion of specific educational requirements.

Today's advanced practice nurse specialists take on responsibilities that range from basic patient care to highly specialized treatments that were once the exclusive domain of physicians. As changes in the provision of health care occur, regulated activities of each profession are likely to change. What will not change is the need for high-quality health care, which is the goal of all health care providers.

With assessment being the essential foundation for health care provision it is essential for providers to have an understanding of each disciplines approach to assessment. As stated previously, the significance and quantity of data needed varies from individual to individual and discipline to discipline.

Typology of Assessment

While all data pertaining to the patient's systems, status and environment is important, a general consensus supports the idea that the extent of a patient assessment or examination varies, depending on various circumstances concerning the patient and what data is required (American Pain Foundation, 2010; Edwards et al. 2001; Nelson-Hogan, 2008; Payne, 2008). Despite this agreement, no established criteria exists to help students or providers determine the depth and amount of data that is important to collect within varying circumstances and/or patient conditions, leaving them perplexed as to what to focus on for clinical practice and judgment.

The provider must often make a decision regarding the depth and amount of data needed. Often, the quantity of data collected is determined by the multiple variables related to the specific setting and the condition of the patient, as well as the amount of time available to perform an assessment and the students/providers proficiency.

To address this issue, this text is based on a typology assessment that is based on four levels, forming a framework designed to help students/providers determine how, when, where, why, and what data may need to be collected. The organization, presentation, and structure of the chapters by types/levels of assessment are not meant to be prescriptive, but rather serve as a conceptual framework to facilitate learning and performing a patient assessment.

Conceptual Framework

A comprehensive assessment involves using a variety of data gathering techniques to collect data about multiple, interrelated aspects of the patient's organ systems, social and emotional status, as well as environmental influences. This process establishes an extensive and reliable data base as the foundation for care provision.

The overall comprehensive patient assessment is conceptualized to occur on **four levels (I, II, II, and IV)**. Each level occurs within a **context** that encompasses the concepts of **competency**, **content**, **complexity,** and **condition** (Table 1-2). Each concept also based on a continuum that spans across the concept.

Table 1-2 Conceptual framework

Context				
Inspection				
Complexity	Level I	Level II	Level III	Level IV
Content				
Condition				
Competency				
Palpation				
Complexity	Level I	Level II	Level III	Level IV
Content				
Condition				
Competency				
Percussion				
Complexity	Level I	Level II	Level III	Level IV
Content				
Condition				
Competency				
Auscultation				
Complexity	Level I	Level II	Level III	Level IV
Content				
Condition				
Competency				

Context—identifies and describes the location where the patient is cared for within the health care organization/system, and where the assessment is performed. The context varies according to the patient's history, condition, pathophysiology, and expected outcomes.

- **Competency** relates to the skill level of the provider that exists on a continuum from least competent to most competent. Competence increases with practice and utilization of assessment skills.
- **Content** identifies and describes the knowledge base of the provider, based on education level, expectations, limitations of a particular discipline and licensure requirements. Content exists on the continuum of basic content to expert content.
- **Complexity** relates to the difficulty of performing or interpreting the results of an assessment technique and exists on a continuum of simple to complex. Complexity can also relate to the patient's condition.
- **Condition** relates to the patient's overall health status and exists on a continuum from a minimal illness to multiple system involvement of an illness.

Each level is considered to be the context encompassing all four concepts. The four levels are not necessarily mutually exclusive but are used as a format for perceiving, practicing, and performing patient assessment.

Level I—the beginning student provider, with minimal competency and knowledge base. Techniques are relatively easy to perform and the patient is in a clinical setting with minor health problems that basically concern one system.

This is the basic bedside exam performed as a daily part of patient care. The patient may be located in a general outpatient setting and may not have a complex condition or complicated care requirements. A simple or complex medical history is taken, depending on the patient's condition. History and physical examination focus on the reason for visit such as cold, UTI, or a sports physical examination. At this stage, the student may be at a beginning or intermediate level, and thus has novice competencies and content related to his or her training and patient's condition. This level requires a basic understanding of the skills and knowledge required in history taking, physical assessment, synthesis, diagnosis and work up of common out-patient conditions. The outpatient however is a setting for savvy clinicians in primary care, oncology, cardiology, orthopedics, and so on. Many clinicians in these various outpatient settings will integrate a higher level clinical assessment.

Level II—requires a more experienced practitioner or an advanced student provider with increased experience, skill and knowledge. Techniques are more involved and advanced and the patient is in a more serious condition with health problems that concern more than one system.

This level places the patient in an inpatient setting where further work up and higher level of care are necessary to return the patient to his or her pre-hospital condition or better yet, much improved from baseline and preferably to previous health and wellness. Inpatient setting gives more time for hospital teams and consultants to help in the synthesis and management of complicated patients needing hospitalization. The process proceeds to a seamless transition to the outpatient setting where the patient is followed up by their primary care provider or specialist.

Level III—requires an advanced and more experienced provider with the knowledge and skills to perform more complex techniques. The patient presents with more severe or immediate health problems that may be one system that is extremely compromised or multiple systems are involved.

At this level, the patient has more complex conditions and care requirements, commonly seen in an emergency room where immediacy of history gathering, physical assessment, synthesis, diagnosis, and actions take place almost simultaneously. The learner here is generally equipped with not only basic pathophysiology but has a compendium of complex case management and ability to make decisions with limited data.

Level IV—requires a master practitioner/provider that is proficient in performance of skills that are complicated or may require more complex thinking skills for interpretation. The patient's condition is also more serious and life threatening.

Because the levels of these exams are not mutually exclusive, the student or provider must still determine the kind and amount of assessment data needed in relation to the patient's condition and care requirements. The four levels are also considered sequential and additive in their contexts, increasing in their scope and demands as well as the time required. While it is not customary to describe or discuss assessment within the scope of these four classifications, the intent here is to assist health care providers to determine and identify what data needs to be obtained within certain circumstances and contexts.

The placement of skills/techniques within the framework presented here is based on "The Stanford 25," which consists of 25 fundamental physical exam skills and their diagnostic benefits (Knox, 2010). Additionally, 30 nursing skills that were commonly used as determined in a survey of practicing RNs (Giddens, 2007) were used to identify level specific examination techniques. Another study surveyed practicing nurses regarding what skills were used "Daily/Weekly, Monthly/Occasionally, and Never" (Secrest, Norwood, & DuMont, 2005) The skills identified in each study were put within a grid to determine similarities and placement of skills within the levels (Table 1-2).

The ability to master the techniques and skills for performing a health assessment depends on the provider and what unique skills each one brings into the process. While the actual assessment techniques may be easy to master and perform, what comprises a successful assessment is determined by the ability to obtain the appropriate information, and processes used to analyze and interpret the patient's data.

Table 1-3 Origins of skills

Giddens (Core Physical Examination Techniques/30)	Secrest (median score indicating use as "Daily/Weekly")	Secrest (median score indicating use as "Monthly/Occasionally")	Secrest (median score indicating use as "Never")	Stanford 25
Inspect overall skin color				Stigmata of liver disease (skin changes)
Evaluate breathing effort				
Assess mental status and level of consciousness				Involuntary movements
Inspect and palpate extremities for edema	LE temperature and edema			
Palpate extremities for temperature	LE for temperature			
Palpate and inspect capillary refill				
Palpate distal pulses for circulation	Radial, brachial artery, LE pulses	Palpate temporal/carotid artery Palpate inguinal nodes Palpate femoral pulse		Blood pressure assessment
Inspect wounds				
Auscultate lung sounds	Breath Sounds			
Auscultate abdomen for bowel sounds	Bowel sounds			
Inspect abdomen	Inspect abdomen		Percuss CVA tenderness	
Auscultate heart sounds	Apical pulse/heart rhythm, rate, and murmurs/auscultate precordial landmarks. Aortic sounds	Auscultate carotid bruit	Auscultate broncophony, egophony, whispered pectoriloquy	PMI (AP)/parasternal heave Cardiac second sounds/splitting
Inspect skin lesions	Inspect skin			
Inspect extremities for skin color and hair growth	LE hair			
Inspect external eyes		Test EOM	Snellen chart Inspect ocular fundus/retinal vessels/ retinal background Red light reflex	Funduscopic Exam
Evaluate Speech				
Palpate abdomen for tenderness and distension	Light abdominal palpation	Percuss abdomen Palpate liver Deep abdominal palpation	Auscultate renal artery Palpate spleen Palpate aorta	Percuss liver Ascites Palpate spleen
Observe ROM of joints	Test ROM	Test neck ROM	Palpate thyroid	Thyroid exam
Inspect chest shape	Inspect chest/chest symmetry/precordium	Palpate precordium for thrills Inspect breasts		
Evaluate face for movement and sensation	Inspect face	Inspect for jugular pulse Test nostril patency Inspect nares	Palpate max/frontal sinus Palpate TMJ Illuminate tender sinus Estimate JVP	Neck veins
Palpate extremities for tenderness				

Continued

Table 1-3 Origins of skills *(continued)*

Giddens (Core Physical Examination Techniques/30)	Secrest (median score indicating use as "Daily/Weekly")	Secrest (median score indicating use as "Monthly/Occasionally")	Secrest (median score indicating use as "Never")	Stanford 25
Assess muscle strength	Handgrips/biceps	Test neck strength against resistance Test triceps/deltoid strength Test hip muscle/ankle/feet strength		Knee Shoulder
Inspect muscles and extremities for size and symmetry	UE/LE symmetry			Hand
Assess hearing on the basis of conversation			Otoscopic exam Hearing tests	
Inspect an examine stool				
Assess gait			Romberg's sign	Common gait abnormalities
PERRLA	Accommodation			Pupillary responses
Glasgow Coma Scale		Test proprioception Test cerebellum; finger to nose RAM DTRs Test Babinski	Test stereognosis, heel to shin, 2-point discrimination	Internal capsule stroke (neurological sign—CNs, muscles, sensation, reflexes, gait) Ankle jerk Cerebellar testing (coordination/gait)
Inspect oral cavity			Grade tonsils Palpate oral cavity	Tongue
Inspect spine				
	Inspect penis, scrotum	Palpate inguinal hernia	Palpate rectum and scrotum	Evaluation of scrotal mass
	Inspect female genitalia			Rectal Exam
		Palpate cervical lymph nodes		
		Palpate tactile fremitus	Percuss diaphragm	
		Palpate chest for lumps/tenderness		
		Percuss lung fields		Percuss lungs
		Test pronator drift		Cervical lymph node assessment
				Bedside ultrasound

Successful Assessments

While assessment often occurs in multiple health care facilities and the scope and level of exam varies, establishing and maintaining a cooperative working relationship with the patient is critically important to achieving success. Such a relationship is established on and sustained through mutual trust. This most fundamental foundation of the patient–provider relationship is also recognized as a part of the healing process.

A significant characteristic of mutual trust is that it is also a two-way process, and that each individual has certain expectations and responsibilities. From the patient's perspective there is the expectation that the provider will exercise professional care, competence, and confidentiality while maintaining patient privacy, autonomy, and individuality and is obligated to be honest and open in providing information requested. From the provider's perspective, there is the expectation that the patient will be truthful when providing information and the obligation to provide appropriate care and maintain confidentiality. The acceptance and recognition of the mutual responsibilities each one has to the other provides assurance that the assessment and care provided will occur in a non judgmental manner. Absent this trust, obtaining the appropriate information will be difficult, and making an accurate assessment will be even more problematic.

In the patient–provider relationship, there may not be mutual approval and acceptance of certain activities and or beliefs of the other. But approval is not a prerequisite to acceptance. Acceptance of others also does not invalidate or negate one's own values and morals.

Even though you may not be aware of it, your behavior and attitudes are present in each and every encounter. When one encounters others with the same values and morals, actions and behaviors do not necessarily have to be scrutinized. However, when one runs into people who have different morals and values, the encounter necessitates an understanding and awareness of what these differences are and how they influence behaviors and attitudes.

Values and Morals

Values are ideals that we believe to be important. **Morals** are a set of guiding principles that help us make choices between right and wrong, or good and bad. Each of us has different values and morals because of who we are, what we choose to stand for and believe in, and the extent to which we allow values and morals to influence the decisions we make.

Morals and values shape the overall culture of certain groups, and facilitate communication between the individuals of each group through language and nonverbal behaviors and actions. Recognizing other's values facilitates greater understanding and allows you to see others as individuals.

While there is the tendency to believe that one's values are right, it is essential to view others' values as different but not necessarily wrong. For a health provider, it is critical to be able to acknowledge that in many instances, patients may make decisions or choices, based on their value systems, which the provider may not necessarily agree with. Indeed, accommodating values in clinical settings is not always simple because patient preferences are so diverse. Understanding the value context of the individual will, however, help the provider appreciate the patient's choices. Understanding the patient's basis for these choices does not mean acceptance of his values, but constitutes respectful recognition that they are important to the patient and may be appropriate for the patient to use.

Values form the basis for an individual's moral development, which is the process of learning what one ought to or ought not to do in certain situations. This is a process that begins in childhood and continues throughout one's lifetime. One's morals are constantly being challenged by changes that occur in society, particularly in the area of technology and what can be accomplished by it; thus, there is a certain amount of relativity to the determination of right or wrong.

Morals are reflected in the laws that are promulgated for the protection of society, but morals and laws do not necessarily correlate directly with each other. The existence of unjust laws, such as those enforcing slavery, for instance, attest to the fact that morality and law do not always agree. Morals encourage the best professional behavior where the law demands only a basic minimum. For example, the law would require providers not to abandon patients they consider undesirable in their practice. Ethical values would obligate a provider to try to work with a patient no matter how disagreeable, until he deems that the patient would be better served by another health professional.

An action by an individual may be legal but not moral, as well as illegal but moral. Laws often change to reflect the changing attitudes and perspectives that accompany moral development. While laws are made to protect individuals, nothing can protect one from another's morals. A moral system is sometimes called a "social contract," and advances the common principle of "the greatest good for the greatest number." This implies that we all uphold our part of the agreement, meaning we obey the moral rules with the expectation that others will also abide by this agreement. Thus, it is only by recognizing others as individuals with their own values and morals that each of us can exist in mutual respect, peace, and dignity.

Morals and values are important elements in the development of personal and professional ethics. Health care providers must recognize the ethical and moral issues inherent in the provider–patient relationship and its effect on health care and our society today.

Ethics

Ethics involves the application of a moral code to the practice of medicine. Everyday, health care professionals make ethical decisions as an integral part of clinical decision making. Ethics has become an intrinsic part of medical practice and continues to shape the contemporary health care professions.

In simple terms, health care ethics try to do the right thing while achieving the best possible outcome for every patient. In a manner of speaking, therefore, ethics is not concerned with determining right or wrong, but in resolving genuine moral dilemmas which arise in health care provision. Ethics thus provides a framework for decision making when there are multiple options, with no real indication of rightness or wrongness. Inherent within ethics and ethical theories is the presence of competing interests. It is these competing interests that need to be identified and evaluated as to which ones are to be considered when applying ethical analysis in practice.

Medical ethics traces its origins to the ancient Greek physician Hippocrates (460–377 BC), who is credited with defining the first ethical standard in medicine: Do no harm. The Hippocratic Oath, written in Ionic Greek, has been considered a rite of passage for practitioners in medicine in many countries and has formed the basis for ethical practice that relates to all providers, regardless of specific discipline. Summarized, the original **Hippocratic Oath** describes the practice of medicine in these terms:

A solemn promise

- of solidarity with educators and other providers.
- of beneficence (to do good or avoid evil) and nonmaleficence (from the Latin *primum non nocere* or "do no harm") towards patients.
- not to assist in suicide or abortion.
- to leave surgery to surgeons.
- not to harm, especially not to seduce patients.
- to maintain confidentiality and never to gossip.

This original content was later modified to many different versions —versions considered by many to be politically and medically correct.

In the application of ethics into practice, the principles of ethics are referred to as obligations or duties. In other words, integrating ethics in all aspects of care and decision making is not a choice; it is a professional duty. The seven primary duties inherent in ethics and

Table 1-4 Obligations of ethical practice

Autonomy	The patient has the right to refuse or choose their treatment (*Voluntas aegroti suprema lex*)
Beneficence	The health provider must act in the best interest of the patient (*Salus aegroti suprema lex*)
Nonmaleficence	The provider must "first, do no harm" (*primum non nocere*)
Utilitarianism	Decisions should promote the good of the largest number of persons
Fidelity	The provider is committed to the concept of accountability
Veracity	The provider has the obligation to full and honest disclosure
Justice	Fairness must be exercised when distributing scarce health resources, and deciding who gets what treatment

ethical practice as they commonly apply to health care discussions are described in the Table 1-4.

Principles such as those shown in Table 1-4 do not give answers about how to handle a particular situation, but provide a useful framework for understanding conflicts.

Autonomy

As commonly understood today, autonomy is the capacity for self-determination and the ability to act and make decisions in the best interest of oneself. Years ago, patients tended to believe, along with their providers, that the health professional always knew best. But the world has changed since that time, and today patients have become much more involved in decisions regarding their care. Recent legal judgments have emphasized that patients who are mentally competent may choose to ignore medical advice and do (or not do) to their own bodies as they wish.

To make an autonomous decision, *the patient must possess all the information* that is needed to make a decision. Withholding information, even at the request of the family, is a violation of autonomy. Additionally, the provider must ensure that the patient has a clear understanding and knowledge regarding the information.

Autonomy, within the context of *health assessment, means allowing the patient to determine what information he will or will not disclose to the provider*. While it is critical that the provider has as much data as possible, it is still the prerogative of the patient to determine what information he chooses to disclose. It is also important for the provider to inform the patient that if any questions arise that he believes to be too sensitive or personal, he is at liberty not to provide answers. However, it is also critical that the patient is made aware of the possibility that failure on his part to disclose information may result in the inability to provide the best possible care or treatment.

Implied in the concept of autonomy is that *the patient is competent to make a self determining decision or choice.* Competency may be difficult to ascertain in certain instances, and is compromised if the patient is a minor or incapable of comprehending the facts of the situation. The definition or process of determining competence does not have universal agreement. There will be times that competence may have to be established by experts.

Beneficence

Beneficence mandates that the *provider work for the good of the patient without regard to personal gain*. It also implies action that is performed for the benefit of the patient. A danger of pursuing beneficence too enthusiastically is that it may interfere with the patient's autonomy. Deciding what is beneficial to the patient can be fraught with difficulty, and poses the temptation for a provider to become paternalistic or even condescending towards the patient in an effort to assure that the "best" is done for him. It involves balancing the benefits against the risks or costs of treatment.

Nonmaleficence

The term *nonmaleficence* derives from the ancient maxim *primum non nocere*, which, translated means "first, do no harm." Nonmaleficence supposes that *the risks of treatment (harm) must be understood in light of the potential benefits*. In health care, treatment may at times involve some degree of harm or pain, but these should not be disproportionate to the benefits intended. Ultimately, the patient must decide whether the potential benefits outweigh the potential harms.

While nonmaleficence is most commonly associated with physical pain, health care providers must be aware of the possibility of a patient experiencing emotional pain also, Emotional or psychological pain is the result of emotional or psychological trauma related to stressful events that shatter one's sense of security and experiencing overwhelming feelings of helplessness and vulnerability (Robinson, Smith, & Segal, 2012). In many instances, patients are subject to emotional trauma when they or a loved one receives a life-threatening diagnosis. While this is unintentional, it is impossible to prevent such a situation or protect a patient from ever experiencing something of this nature.

Utilitarianism

Utilitarianism involves *directing medical resources where they will have the most long-term effect for good.* To a utilitarian, the choice that brings the greatest benefit to the most number of people is the choice that is ethically correct. The distribution of health care services and resources are largely influenced by utilitarianism, where questions arise about which sector of the population receives health care. Another example of the utilitarian approach is the consideration applied to keeping very critically ill patients in intensive care. A hospital's general policy in this regard may be determined by which patients demonstrate profound morbidity, using evidence-based assessment. In practice, however, such ethical problems are much more complex, involving issues about who makes the decision, the right to life and other pressing considerations.

Fidelity

Fidelity means faithfulness, allegiance, or advocacy to the patient. In the context of health care, it implies *meeting the reasonable expectations of the patient.* Reasonable expectations include but are not necessarily limited to the expectation that *the dignity of each individual will be protected and preserved.* It is also reasonable for the patient to expect *competency in the provision of health care.*

The patient likewise has the right to expect that *health care will be provided in line with principles, values, standards, or rules of behavior that guide the health care profession*. These statements are best described in the Code of Ethics of each profession. *Adherence to the policies and procedures of the health care organization* is also a reasonable explanation. That the provider will abide by the scope of practice, as identified and described on his professional license, is also an expectation that is basic to provision of health care.

Lastly, the patient has a reasonable expectation that the *agreements and or conditions of treatment obtained through informed consent or verbal understanding will be honored.*

Veracity

Veracity or conformity to the truth is not strictly confined to health care professionals, but pervades all human relationships and interactions. Being untruthful may take many forms, has many purposes, and leads to many different consequences. For instance, some patients or their families may not want the full truth disclosed to them or, in certain circumstances, a health provider might consider it to be in the patient's best interest not to tell him the truth. Yet the *first application of the principle of veracity relates to informed consent, autonomy and the right of the patient to make decisions based on all available information*. Consideration must also be given to the fact that withholding the truth from a patient can place considerable strain on the provider–patient trust relationship that is important for healing to occur.

Justice

Justice is the most difficult and complex component of all ethics, and is also related to utilitarianism in that *health providers are obligated to treat every patient in the same way, irrespective of age, race, sex, personality, income, or insurance status*. Justice is linked to the need for fair and equitable distribution of resources. Fair and equitable are open to interpretation and may not be perceived in the same way by everyone. Fair and equitable could mean that everyone is given the same amount regardless of need or circumstances; or it may be perceived to be distribution on a "per need" basis and not necessarily for everyone. The health care provider needs to consider three main areas when evaluating justice: fair distribution of scarce resources (distributive justice); competing needs, rights, and obligations (rights-based justice); and respect for morally acceptable laws (legal justice).

The seven principles for ethical conduct may also be exemplified in a code of ethics. A code, such as the one from the American Nurses Association, is more explicit in describing expectations a practicing professional nurse. While the code addresses expectations of a nurse, there is nothing in each section that could not apply to any health care provider or discipline.

Summary

- The earliest form of health care that included some form of systematic assessment was based on the theory of four elements/humors.
- Percussion as an assessment technique was described in 1761, and the stethoscope was invented in 1819.
- Early nursing care was provided by hospitaliers, infirmarians, women who were brought in from off the street.
- Professional nursing came into existence with the work of Florence Nightingale.
- Assessment of the patient provides the foundation for the development of diagnosis and treatment of health conditions.
- Assessment can be placed within the context for four levels with each levels techniques and skills determined by competency, content, complexity, and condition.
- Scope of practice governs what each discipline is allowed to do with patient data that is collected.
- Success at assessment is based on establishing a relationship with a patient that is influenced by values, morals, and ethical principles.

Review Questions

1. The ability of any provider to perform certain procedures in the care of patients is determined and defined by which of the following?
   1. scope of practice
   2. professional organization
   3. employing agency
   4. certification credentials
2. The level of assessment a provider uses for a particular patient's care is determined by which of the following? (Select all that apply.)
   1. context
   2. content
   3. competence
   4. complexity
   5. compensation
3. A patient is brought to the emergency department after a motor vehicle accident in which injuries were sustained. The nurse knows that the assessment required is which of the following?
   1. Level I
   2. Level II
   3. Level III
   4. Level IV
4. When meeting a new patient the provider is committed to establishing the foundation of the provider–patient relationship by working toward the development of which of the following?
   1. competence
   2. trust
   3. skills
   4. a data base

5. The provider must be aware that one's individual values may not be consistent with every patient for whom care is provided. This means that
   1. the ideals that the provider believes to be important may be in conflict with ideals of the patient.
   2. principles that the provider uses to guide decision making may differ from the patient.
   3. the provider and the patient are likely from different cultural backgrounds.
   4. the provider is probably from a different faith tradition than the patient.
6. A provider's practice is guided by specific duties of ethical practice when caring for patients. These duties include which of the following? (Select all that apply.)
   1. justice
   2. competence
   3. autonomy
   4. veracity
   5. awareness
7. The provider is caring for an adult patient who is refusing all treatment for a serious illness. Employing the duty of autonomy, the provider would do which of the following?
   1. Notify the patient's family that the patient is refusing care.
   2. Administer treatments when the patient is sleeping.
   3. Call an administrator to get a court order to treat the patient.
   4. Ensure that the patient is aware of the consequences of refusal.
8. The provider is reviewing a procedure consent with a patient and ensuring that the patient understands the risks of the procedure. This is an example of the ethical principle of which of the following?
   1. veracity
   2. justice
   3. autonomy
   4. nonmaleficence
9. When determining the level of assessment required by a patient situation, the provider views the element of competence as which of the following?
   1. the assessment techniques that would be required
   2. the length of time that the provider has been practicing
   3. the location that the assessment will occur
   4. the education level of the provider
10. The provider is aware that the primary purpose of state regulation of practice for health care providers is to do which of the following?
    1. Provide a database of licensed providers.
    2. Keep records for insurance companies and payers.
    3. Protect the public for incompetent providers.
    4. Develop a source of revenue.

The Individual in Context

2

They arrive and I stir from fitful sleep, pain wracking through my tired body. A troop of unsmiling, white-coated strangers wordlessly pull back my thin blanket, and strip my gown from my shoulders. I don't recognize any of them, and no one tells me their name.

Afraid, I reach out to the nearest one—a woman I presume is a nurse—and ask her to hold my hand. She seems embarrassed, but tentatively takes my hand, as if she's petting a snake. I stare at the cold blank walls, silently enduring this invasion.

Suddenly, one of them digs his hands into my abdomen and asks if I feel any tenderness. *Tenderness*? It's the last thing on my mind as I cringe from his unwanted touch, feeling violated. My anxiety grows by the minute. I close my eyes and pretend that I'm somewhere—anywhere else.

My name is Rosario Guerrero, 53, a widow. I was raised as a traditional Catholic. Up until today, no other man, except my late husband, has touched me beneath my clothes. Because both of my children are overseas, I am alone this morning. My transformation from citizen to hospital patient has become one of the loneliest and frightening experiences of my life.

LEARNING OUTCOMES

1. Describe the purpose and functions of an individual's culture.
2. Discuss the importance of cultural competence.
3. Describe the process of becoming culturally competent.
4. Compare and contrast religion and spirituality.
5. Explicate the basic components of a spiritual assessment.
6. Recognize the stages of growth and development related to various frameworks and the significant life events associated with each one.
7. Differentiate the essential components of a family assessment according to its framework, evolution, and operation.

Each individual is a unique combination of characteristics and attributes. Cultural background, environment, growth and developmental stages, spirituality, family members and characteristics, past experiences and future expectations all contribute to a person's individuality. These attributes also shape a person's views about health, wellness, illness, and health care in general. It is important for the health care provider to have an awareness of these attributes and how they impact patients and their understanding of their illness and recovery. This chapter will present and discuss these attributes as they relate to individuals.

Culture

A definitive definition of culture is almost impossible to come up with. It is a complex entity with each component connected to and influenced by all other components (Spector, 2009). Culture shapes a person's identity and how the person perceives both the world and the immediate environment. The primary purpose of culture is to teach one how to act, think, say, and do; thus it is an integrated system of learned behavior patterns (thoughts, communications, actions, customs, beliefs, values, and institutions) that are characteristic of and represent the members of any given society or group (racial, ethnic, religious, or social). Culture, therefore, is the totality of ways of doing things that are transmitted from generation to generation. Within that context, it may be considered analogous to an inheritance. Unlike a genetic inheritance, which only involves receiving certain physical traits from two individuals, a cultural inheritance comes from multiple sources and involves the transmission of non-physical or behavioral traits. It is impossible for someone to be "acultural," because culture is a component of everything that involves and comprises the individual. On the other hand, it is possible for an individual to become "multi-cultural" when behaviors and activities become a part of an individual that are learned from experiencing or embracing a culture that is dissimilar from one's inherent culture.

Culture is often perceived as a way of identifying and describing differences between individuals and groups. While culture does differentiate one individual from the other, thinking only in terms of differences generally promotes the belief that one culture is right (mine), and one culture is wrong (yours). Within a culture, difference and the experience of being identified as different are often considered negative. Being the same or like another person is valued more than being different. Thus, conformity is expected and rewarded.

Your own culture is basically invisible; you're likely not consciously aware of why or how you do certain things. Learning of culture primarily occurs unconsciously. Awareness and recognition of one's own culture only becomes apparent and problematic when confronted with another culture. When this happens, you may feel anxious and afraid, and realize that one way, your way, of thinking and doing is not necessarily universal.

Within cultures, there are also subcultures, which are groups within the dominant culture that retain or adhere to the characteristics of the culture but develop a unique identity that is not considered a universal attribute. Subcultures often develop around shared interests that may arise from geographic origins or location, religions (belief systems), occupations, political affiliation, age, etc.

Within health care, providers often fail to recognize that the health care environment is a culture (Fox, 2005). This becomes evident when the goals and expectations of Western medicine (biomedicine), with its emphasis on science and technology, conflicts with Eastern medicine and its inclusion of mysticism and traditional healing practices and beliefs. While there is often no scientific foundation for these practices, in many instances, they are successful and contribute to the physical and psychological healing of the individual.

A lack of awareness regarding cultural differences presents impediments in the delivery of health care and is the primary basis for health care disparities among minority and ethnic populations. Differences that contribute to the development of health disparities are often the result of beliefs and values that relate to the following:

- Health, healing, and wellness;
- How illness, disease, and their causes are perceived by both the patient and consumer;
- The behaviors of patients/consumers who are seeking health care and their attitudes toward health care providers;
- The delivery of services by the provider who looks at the world through his or her own limited set of values, which can compromise access for patients from other cultures (U.S. Department of Health and Human Services, 2005).

The disparities gap in health care has gradually increased over the last fifty years as the reasons for migrating to the United States have slowly changed. The late 1800s and early 1900s saw an influx of immigrants from many different countries and cultures. The immigrants tended to shed their cultural heritages, wanting to assimilate as "Americans." America was seen as the land of opportunity, where people could start over. At that time, America was described as a "melting pot," signifying that all the cultural differences seemed to blend together and no one was separated out. There was no cultural identification as an "ethnic American," such as "African American" or "Irish American," everyone was simply American. Understanding and awareness of other cultures was not expected or practiced. Cultural heritage, however, was often recognized by members of the same group getting together for special events and celebrating in ways that preserved their traditions.

In the last decades of the 1900s, immigrants began making a more concerted effort to retain their cultural values and traditions instead of becoming assimilated into the predominant American culture. Many of these groups had been transplanted from their country of origin due to wars and other events that made it unsafe to live there. These individuals and groups, although relieved to escape their own countries, have not necessarily chosen to live in the U.S. and are more likely to try and retain their own cultural practices and values rather than conform to and become a part of a different culture.

This phenomenon can be explained by the concept of Heritage Consistency (Spector, 2009). The "melting pot" of American immigrants consisted of individuals who chose to give up or minimize their cultural heritage and become acculturated, whereas more recent immigrants have chosen to embrace their cultural heritages and not become acculturated.

A consequence of retaining cultural practices and beliefs is a higher incidence of cultural collisions. These collisions often result in misunderstandings, miscommunications, and the formulation of inaccurate assumptions and are often due to a lack of awareness of these differences and their affects (Ondash & Dibble, 2006). This lack of awareness most likely results from a combination of factors that may include the following:

- Lack of knowledge—resulting in an inability to recognize the cultural differences
- Self-protection/denial—leading to an attitude that these differences are not significant, or that our common humanity transcends our differences
- Fear of the unknown or the new—because it is challenging and perhaps intimidating to get to understand something that is new, that does not fit into one's world

- Feeling pressure due to time constraints—which can lead to feeling rushed and unable to look in depth at an individual patient's needs

In an effort to avoid cultural collisions and their negative consequences, health care providers are challenged to become **culturally** and **linguistically competent**.

Cultural Competence

Cultural and linguistic **competence** is best defined as a set of congruent behaviors, attitudes, and policies that come together in a system, agency, or among professionals that enables effective work in cross cultural situations (Office of Minority Health, 2010). "Culture" refers to integrated patterns of human behavior that include the language, thoughts, actions, customs, beliefs, and institutions of racial, ethnic, social, or religious groups. "Competence" implies having the capacity to function effectively as an individual or an organization within the context of the cultural beliefs, practices, and needs presented by patients and their communities.

Cultural and linguistic competency is seen as a way to reduce the disparities gap in health care. While much of health care in the United States is considered "western" or based on empirical science, a growing awareness and use of "eastern" health care practices, which are not primarily science-based now exists. Many of these practices are culturally based and form the perceptions of health and illness for individuals from various cultures. As such, health and health care are cultural constructs, predicated on beliefs about nature, health, disease, and the human body. Both providers and patients each bring their individual, learned cultural patterns of behavior and language to the health care situation, but must transcend them to attain equal access to and quality health care.

THINK LINK: Linguistic Competence

Linguistic competency (LC) is defined as the capacity of an organization and its personnel to communicate effectively, and convey information in a manner that is easily understood by diverse audiences, including individuals' (1) of limited English proficiency, (2) with low-literacy skills or who are not literate, (3) with disabilities, and (4) who are deaf or hard of hearing. It requires organizational and provider capacity to respond effectively to the health and mental health literacy needs of populations served. The capacity for LC is supported by organizational policy, structures, practices, procedures, and dedicated resources (Office of Minority Health, 2010).

Think of cultural competency as existing on a continuum. Terms that are useful to describe a continuum have also been used as meaning the same as cultural competence. Terms that are often used interchangeably with cultural competence include cultural knowledge, cultural awareness, and cultural sensitivity. However, while similar to cultural competence, these terms are also different. No universal agreement exists on whether these terms are different or similar, but it seems reasonable to view them as different, and their separate characteristics suggest that their relationship exists on a continuum.

Cultural Knowledge

Cultural knowledge is recognition of selected characteristics of another culture such as its history, values, belief systems, and the behaviors of its members. While it is often regarded as knowledge of another culture, this term also relates to the recognition and identification of characteristics of one's own culture. Individuals who enter health care professions are also admonished to identify the unique cultural aspects of health and health care.

Cultural Awareness

Cultural awareness recognizes that everyone is shaped by one's cultural background, which influences how individuals perceive the world, self-perception, and relationships with others. Achieving expertise in every culture is not the core requisite of cultural awareness; its purpose is to facilitate exploration of other cultures and how cultural issues can best be addressed.

Cultural awareness is facilitated by asking questions, such as those that focus on understanding the similarities and differences between cultures; how understanding those differences and similarities will help working together; how to better communicate with each other; and why misunderstandings and misperceptions exist between us and our cultures.

Cultural awareness, as a single concept, has also been recognized as existing on four different levels, expanding the concept of cultural awareness on the cultural competence continuum (Quappe & Cantatore, 2005). These four levels have been identified as follows:

1. My way is the only way. **[Parochial stage]**: Cultural knowledge

   In this stage, there is only awareness of one's way of doing things, which is the only way. There is no recognition of cultural differences.

2. I know their way, but my way is better. **[Ethnocentric stage]**: Cultural awareness

   There is awareness of other ways of doing things, but still consider my way as the best. Cultural differences are perceived as problems that cause conflict with the tendency to ignore them or minimize their significance.

3. My way and their way. **[Synergistic stage]**: Cultural sensitivity

   There is awareness of different ways of doing things and the best way depends on the situation. There is also the realization that cultural differences have positive and negative effects and cultural diversity is used to develop new solutions and alternatives.

4. Our way. **[Participatory 3rd culture stage]**: Cultural competence

   Individuals from different cultures unite to create a culture of shared meanings. There is continuous dialogue to create new meanings and new rules to meet the needs of a particular situation.

Cultural Sensitivity

Cultural sensitivity is recognition of the differences and similarities that exist between cultures without designating any value to the differences, such as right or wrong, better or worse, or normal or abnormal. Cultural competence emphasizes the concept of effectively functioning and working within different cultural contexts.

Achieving Cultural Competence

Achieving cultural competence is a personal task that requires discipline, and a structured process. It begins with cultural awareness and the recognition that different is not a negative descriptor. Generally, "different" means that an individual does not fit established expectations and what one is comfortable with. Different does *not* mean unequal, not good enough, or not fitting in. Everyone demonstrates differences from others in some way.

Cultural awareness also requires you to reflect on your own culture and recognize where conflicts exist with other cultures and how those conflicts can be overcome. This requires individuals in all cultures to step outside their cultural limits and acknowledge what positive and negative aspects are present within one's culture. Individuals are culturally aware when they recognize the following:

- We are not all the same.
- Similarities and differences are both important.
- There are multiple ways to reach the same goal and to live life.
- The best way depends on the cultural contingency. Each situation is different and may require a different solution (Quappe & Cantatore, 2005).

Assessing Cultural Competence

An assessment of cultural competence can occur in various ways. It does not necessarily require performing a cultural assessment of a provider; it is essentially how well the health care provider is willing to try to understand the cultural influences and differences that exist in regards to a patient's health status and condition. Specific models for demonstrating cultural competence can be used. Some examples of these include the "LEARN model" (Berlin & Eisenberg, 1983) and Kleinman's "Tool to Elicit Health Beliefs in Clinical Encounters" (Kleinman, Eisenberg, & Good, 1978). Cultural competency may also be demonstrated through cultural care etiquette (Table 2-1).

Achieving cultural competence has largely focused on exposing individuals to all the multiple facets of a specific culture, primarily

Table 2-1 Cultural care manners and conduct

	Time Orientation
Schedules/Appointments	Inform patient when you will be arriving and/or departing.
Promptness	Avoid surprises. Explain your expectations about time. Ask patients from other regions and cultures what they expect.
Inappropriate/Incorrect times	Be aware of the times, meanings, and rituals or practices of patient's ethnic and religious holidays.
	Space
Physical Encounters	Acknowledge from many perspectives, cultural and/or religious customs regarding personal space, gender restrictions for contact and touch with others.
	Communication
Addressing/Acknowledging	Acknowledge the proper manner for recognizing and/or addressing individuals from a specific culture and the ways by which people welcome one another. Recognize when touch, such as an embrace or handshake, is expected and when physical contact is prohibited. Be aware of same gender greeting practices.
Non-verbal Movements/Behaviors	Gestures are not universal in their meanings and/or expressions; what is accepted or sanctioned in one cultural group may be forbidden in another. Smiles may represent friendliness to some, but not to others.
Verbal Communication	Recognize the extent to which an individual is able to communicate in English. Request services of an interpreter when needed. Also recognize that the ability to speak and understand English does indicate that the individual has become acculturated into, or understands the American and/or local cultural beliefs and practices.
Eye Contact	Failure to demonstrate and maintain eye contact may be a sign of respect.
	Social Organization
Celebrations, Holidays, Traditions	Have knowledge of significant dates and why, whether or not to give gifts, and expected rituals at home or religious services. Have knowledge of how events are celebrated, meaning of decorations, colors that may be used for gifts, and traditional or expected rituals at home or religious services.
	Biological Variations
Diet	Recognize what foods can be or are eaten for special events, what foods may be eaten together or are forbidden, what, how, or if eating utensils are used. Are there periods of fasting that are regularly observed?
	Environmental Characteristics
Health Beliefs/Practices	Acknowledge and respect the general health traditions/practices/beliefs for a given patient and validate observations by asking questions.
Attire/Clothing	Have knowledge of any specific dress and grooming requirements. Recognize that certain parts of the body are not to be exposed, particularly to individuals of the opposite gender.
Life Stage	Recognize, but don't assume, that older adults are more likely to embrace traditional beliefs and practices related to health and illness.

through education. The underlying philosophy and overall expectation of teaching cultural competence is that by awareness and understanding of traditional cultural concepts and practices, health disparities will be eliminated and communication will be enhanced. The concept of competence also implies that at some point, an individual will achieve the outcome of being considered competent; however, assessment of achievement of competence elusive and nonspecific (Foster, 2009).

A more comprehensive and descriptive term that goes beyond cultural competence is **cultural humility**. Cultural humility is defined as the following:

> Process that requires humility as individuals continually engage in self-reflection and self-critique as lifelong learners and reflective practitioners, it requires humility in how [providers] bring into check the power imbalances that exist in the dynamics of [provider]–patient communication by using patient-focused interviewing and care, and it is a process that requires humility to develop and maintain mutually respectful and dynamic partnerships with communities. (From "Defining Cultural Humility" by Melanie Tervalon, Jann Murray-Garcia from *The Concepts of Cultural Humility in the Medical Field*. Published by Glax Diversity Council.)

Cultural humility is more reflective of an ongoing process that recognizes fluidity, broadness, and continuous change occurring within cultures. It also implies that an individual, while a member of a particular culture, may not demonstrate all the individual attributes and practices of that particular culture. This does not negate the need to understand and recognize the characteristics, beliefs, and practices of a particular culture, but demonstrates the recognition that cultural manners and customs are learned from the individual, not the members as a whole. Cultural humility also recognizes that cultural behaviors and practices are not universal, but that culture provides its individuals with a compilation of ideas and potential actions that construct a framework that helps in understanding themselves and the overall context of their environment and experiences.

The two major processes associated with cultural humility are self-reflection and self-critique. These processes are not dependent on the provider's knowledge of the patient's cultural beliefs, values, and traditions; but with providers careful consideration to their assumptions and beliefs that are embedded in their own understandings and goals of their encounter with the patient (California Health Advocates, 2012).

Cultural Assessment

There is no specific process to use when doing a cultural assessment. The major goal of a cultural assessment is to identify what cultural values, beliefs, and practices may impact the patient's perception of health and illness, and response to treatment. It is unrealistic to expect that health care providers be cognizant of all the cultural dynamics within all the ethnocultural groups and subgroups that are represented within the United States. It is also imperative that providers avoid using **ethnocentrism** as well as allowing **prejudice** and **stereotyping** to influence cultural assessment and the ability to provide cultural competent care.

Ethnocentrism is the perception and assumption that one's own culture is the best and is the standard by which all other cultures are compared and judged. Recognizing and understanding other cultures does not imply agreement or sanctioning behaviors and actions that may be contrary to one's own culture but helps to suspend judgmental behaviors.

Prejudice exists when a provider is unable to suspend judgment and allows preconceived beliefs and ideas to negatively impact health care provision. It is easy to be prejudiced or have negative opinions about certain groups or individuals without being aware of it. Appearances, such as individuals who are obese or have tattoos, may bring about prejudice. Prejudice is often the result of stereotyping, which is assuming that all individuals who belong to certain groups or demonstrate certain behaviors are all alike. While there may be similarities among individuals, it is inappropriate to expect that all individuals belonging to certain groups are the same.

A cultural assessment is best done by using a generic approach which focuses on the patient rather than the culture. The fundamental principle of cultural assessment is that the patient has the right to cultural beliefs, values, and practices and that these components need to be recognized, respected, and regarded in providing culturally competent care.

The primary effort of the cultural assessment is to determine the significance of the patient's condition or illness related to patient's cultural values, beliefs, and practices. This information can be obtained by formulating questions related to the following:

- Perception of the cause of condition
- Why it started when it did
- Severity of illness/condition; will it have a long/short course
- What treatment should be received; most important results hoped for from treatment
- Main problems experienced from illness/condition
- Greatest fear related to illness/condition

This information can be easily obtained by incorporating related questions throughout the interview rather than as a separate section so that patients don't feel as if their culture or cultural beliefs are being scrutinized.

Spirituality

Intrinsic within cultures is a spiritual context, which helps one to seek answers to many of life's situations and consequences, particularly related to the explanation and examination of purpose and meaning in life. While spirituality may be considered a separate influence within a culture, in many instances, it may be difficult, if not impossible to separate an individual's spiritual beliefs and practices from the values and traditions of his or her culture. While spirituality is often equated with religion or religious beliefs, the context of spirituality is broader than religion. It is not uncommon for an individual to describe oneself as spiritual, but not religious.

Religion and spirituality are both reflected in two related Latin terms: ***religare*** and ***religere***. *Religare* is the Latin term that means "to hold back, bind fast, or tie together." The structure of religious beliefs (doctrine) clearly is related to the meaning of this term. While religion implies a personal belief and acceptance of a set of beliefs, it also has a broader, inclusive aspect to it. Individuals who adhere to the beliefs and tenets of a religion become a part of the larger group that often meets together to express their beliefs. *Religare* can also reflect a nonreligious component, such as when someone is described as engaging in or practicing certain activities like dieting or exercising "religiously." The term provides a specific framework for values, codes of conduct, and rituals.

Religious practices and expressions are commonly tied to a formalized doctrine (dogma) or belief system that recognizes and places God at the core of these beliefs. Some beliefs may be associated with specific demands or requirements that must be met in order for a person to be considered a member of that particular religion. These practices or requirements may be related to, but not necessarily limited to, diet, medical intervention, or prayers. Some examples of these requirements are identified and described in Table 2-2. Of particular significance to health care providers is when religious beliefs may interfere with choices as to whether or not the individual will allow for certain life-saving medical interventions. Religious beliefs and practices are also expressed through rituals or ceremonies, which are often solemn in nature and performed to reinforce one's faith. The importance and practice of these rites and rituals to an individual varies and often increases in importance when experiencing a life-threatening illness or other crises (Table 2-2).

The second Latin term *religere*, is that part of religion that means to reflect, or ponder deeply. This aspect of religion reflects an individual's concern with a relationship to a higher being and the practices and beliefs that influence this relationship. While *religere*

Table 2-2 Texts and spiritual/healing practices of various religions

Religion	Religious Texts	Spiritual/Cultural Healing Practices
Baha'i Faith	The Kitab-i-Iqan (Adquas) Tablets of Baha'u'llah	Prayer
Buddhism	The Tipitaka The Dhammapada	None specific
Christianity		
Protestantism	Holy Bible	Prayer
Catholicism	Holy Bible (Canon of Trent)	Sacrament of sick (Last rites), candles, laying on of hands. Crucifix and Rosary may be present and used in prayers.
Christian Scientist	Holy Bible Science and Health with Key to the Scriptures (Mary Baker Eddy)	Full time healing ministers, Spiritual healing. Organic disease doesn't exist, disease is mental. May refuse or delay treatment; no understanding of signs/symptoms.
Gnosticism	Nag Hammadi library Other Gnostic texts	
Hinduism	Shruti (Vedas, including the Rigveda; also Aranyakas, Brahmanas, Upanishads, Bhagavad Gita, Mahabharata, Ramayana) Pancahtantra	Traditional faith healing practices
Islam	Quran (Kuran, Koran, Qur'an, Coran or al-Qur'an)	Some use of herbal remedies and faith healing Health care providers should be of same gender. Men may desire to maintain daily prayers; may have traditional prayer rug. Dietary restrictions during month of Ramadan Medications with alcohol base may be refused.
Jehovah's Witness	Holy Bible (New World Translation of the Holy Scriptures)	Reading scriptures, no use of blood products
Judaism	Hebrew Bible (Tanakh) The Talmud	Prayers for the sick Orthodox Jews, Kosher dietary practices. Men may wear small skull cap (yarmulke).
Mormonism (LDS)	King James Bible (LDS Edition) Book of Mormon Pearl of Great Price Doctrine and Covenants	Anointing with oil, sealing, prayer, laying on of hands. Coffee, tea, alcohol, and tobacco not used.
New Age	A Course in Miracles Conversations with God Oahspe The Urantia Book Isis Unveiled	
Scientology	Dianetics: The Modern Science of Mental Health	
Sikhism	The Guru Aranth Sahib The Dasven Padshah Da Granth	
Taoism	Tao Te Ching (Dao de jing) Zhuangzi The I Ching	
Unification Church	Divine Principle The Bible as illuminated by more recent revelation	

PRACTICE POINT: *Jehovah's Witnesses, Christian Science, Fundamental Christianity*

Jehovah's Witnesses, Christian Science, and fundamental Christianity are religious groups that have specific practices and beliefs that may interfere with medical interventions. Jehovah's Witnesses refuse to have any blood or blood product transfusions based on their interpretation of certain Bible verses. Members who have willingly accepted blood transfusion are in jeopardy of being dismissed from fellowship. Christian Scientists believe that material matter does not exist and that all that God has made is spiritual. This spiritual reality is the only reality; everything else is an illusion or error. Humans are only experiencing a material existence that will ultimately result in a true spiritual understanding of God and creation. This is their basis for believing that healing occurs through prayer, which for the Christian Scientist, the process of learning more about God's spiritual reality. While prayer is the initial treatment for healing, there is no doctrine that forbids its members for seeking medical treatment. However, Christian Science prayer and medical intervention are not to be used simultaneously. Some congregations associated with fundamental Christianity believe that prayer is the only intervention that is possible. This is different from the Christian Scientist prayer in that this is a prayer to God for healing. The outcome of a specific illness or condition is determined by God and that it is His will whether one is healed or not. Seeking medical intervention for treatment is seen as a lack of faith in God.

may be considered to be a part of religion, it is more reflective of one's spirituality or personal belief than affiliation with a specific religions belief system,

While spiritual beliefs and activities often are expressed and associated with a particular religion or belief system, spirituality is not confined to specific expressions of one's belief in God or a higher power. Spirituality is more individualized and defined by concepts rather than a specific belief structure. Most commonly, these concepts reflect love, compassion, caring, transcendence, and a connection between body, mind, and spirit. Spirituality is also concerned with relationships that exist between God, self, and others. These concepts are also a unique component of many cultures and groups.

Common to these cultural practices or beliefs is the recognition of a supreme or higher authority that is concerned with the well-being of the group and has the power to reward or punish individuals or groups, and a belief in an afterlife. Religious individuals refer to God. Spiritual individuals may refer to God, a god or divine being, or simply a higher authority or supreme being. The higher authorities or supreme beings are often named or described in terms of the elements of nature. Most of these religious beliefs are based on the existence of multiple supreme beings and often recognized as influencing the outcomes of many activities and relationships. These supreme beings are also described as resembling humans, or combinations of humans and animals, or combination of animals.

While religion and spirituality are both concerned with a relationship to a higher or supreme being, some individuals deny the existence of God or any higher power. These individuals are referred to as atheists. Another group of individuals identify themselves as agnostics; they do not deny the existence of God or a supreme being, but there is no relationship or way to establish a relationship between God and humans. The spiritual life of individuals in these groups is concerned about relationships between oneself and others as well as maintaining moral and ethical standards within their lifestyle.

Individuals who are religious and adhere to a specific religious belief system will often have a holy book, symbols, or clothing that are specific to their particular religion that they read, refer to, or wear (see Table 2-2). The Bible is probably the most-commonly recognized religious book and is associated with Christianity; however, other holy books include the Torah for Jews, Koran for Muslims, the 4 Vedas for Hindus. Spiritual individuals may also have a personal book, poetry collection, inspirational writings, or letters that they read to support their beliefs.

Recent practice and studies recognize that a relationship exists between spirituality and health outcomes, although the nature of this relationship remains obscure. The more holistic approach to health care recognizes the relationship that exists between an individual's body, mind, and spirit. Recent studies on spirituality have demonstrated lower levels of depression and an overall better quality of life in individuals who describe themselves as being religious or who participate in religious practices. Religiosity has also been found to be related to decreased morbidity and mortality (Bekelman et al., 2010).

Past practices within health care tended to overlook or ignore an individual's spiritual needs. Recognizing or accommodating an individual's spiritual needs was most likely based on the assumption that an understanding of the individual's religion and its practices or rituals was sufficient to satisfy any spiritual needs. Additionally, any identified need for spiritual support was often referred to a hospital chaplain or the individual's minister, pastor, or rabbi, or other identified spiritual leader. While this may have been appropriate for someone with an identified religion, those who were without a specific religious preference were often not referred to anyone for help or ignored. Additional barriers to addressing spiritual needs include the fear that an individual's religion or practices may be unfamiliar or misunderstood. Or, an individual might be offended by any inquiries into religious practices or beliefs because of the personal and private nature of the subject; or the individual may perceive that the provider would be trying to push or convert them to another religion. A lack of confidence and education into how to assess and/or address spiritual issues and the lack of time are also identified barriers (Tanyi, McKenzie, & Chapek, 2009).

The neglect of addressing spiritual issues is also closely tied to medical advances made and the increased use of technology to treat illnesses and diseases, or at least to prolong life (Puchalski, 2001). While cure is possible for many, it is not possible for everyone. For those with incurable conditions, spirituality is perceived to help with healing rather than curing. Healing, although it has a physiological basis, in the spiritual context is more related to an acceptance of and ability to cope with life-threatening situations when cure is not possible. Healing, in this context, does not necessarily equate to "giving up" but is more in line with acceptance of the inevitable.

Assessing Spirituality

Multiple forms exist to assess an individual's spirituality and many are based on simple four (4) or more letter acronyms. For example, the FICA Spiritual Assessment Tool assesses the following components of a person's spiritual dimension: (1) **F**aith and beliefs, (2) **I**mportance and influence, (3) **C**ommunity, and (4) **A**ddress, or how patient wants to be recognized (Puchalski & Romer, 2000). Although the FICA tool includes specific questions for the patient, the provider may formulate questions as appropriate. It is more important to have a basic understanding of what information is sought in relation to each topic as patients may need interpretation of some terms used or the context for the information sought.

Box 2-1 provides additional examples of acronyms that may be used to assess a patient's spirituality. Using acronyms such as these allows for incorporating spiritual assessment into various conversations that take place between provider and patient. Recognizing the terms that go with the letters of the acronym facilitate doing a spiritual assessment at any time without being dependent on a specific form or format, or within the context of a standardized history.

Growth and Development

Every individual during the course of a lifetime, progresses through specific, cyclical, life stages of growth and development. These stages are important in determining unique, individual characteristics that are related to who and what one is and what one may become.

Box 2-1 Acronyms Used to Assess Spirituality

	HOPE
H	sources of **h**ope
O	**o**rganized religion
P	**p**ersonal practices/beliefs
E	**e**ffects on care/end-of-life issues
	FAITH
F	have **f**aith/importance
A	**a**pplication
I	**i**ntegration into spiritual groups/organization
T	**t**reatment affected by beliefs
H	**h**elp needed for any concerns
	SPIRIT
S	**s**piritual belief system
P	**p**ersonal beliefs/practices
I	**i**ntegrated into spiritual groups/community
R	**r**ituals/restrictions
I	**i**mplications for treatment
T	**t**erminal events expectations
	FACT
F	**f**aith/beliefs
A	**a**ctive, **a**vailable, **a**ccessible, **a**pplicability
C	**c**oping, **c**omfort, **c**onflicts, **c**oncerns
T	**t**reatment

Sources: Data from Anandarajah & Hight, 2001; King, 2002; Maughns, 1996; LaRocca-Pitts, 2008

Within each stage, specific tasks, functions, or goals have been identified that need to be successfully mastered before progressing into another stage. While each stage is associated with certain ages, wide variation exists regarding when individuals pass from one stage to the other, and stages may overlap in successfully mastering developmental tasks.

Growth, as a concept is much easier to observe and follow. Growth is primarily related to increases in body size and the maturation of certain physiological processes that accompany an increase in age. Growth is a quantitative approach to assessment of the individual.

In contrast, development is related to advances or progression in the cognitive, psychological, social, and emotional competencies of life and relationships. Development is a qualitative approach to assessment of the individual. The majority of developmental stages occur during infancy, childhood, and adolescence, thus more attention is directed toward these stages than later stages that occur during one's adult life.

Developmental Frameworks

Multiple developmental frameworks are available to assess growth and development. Because each framework takes a unique perspective on growth and development processes, no single framework currently exists that covers all the unique aspects of growth and development. Common to all frameworks, however, is recognizing the overall process as a series of stages or levels.

Developmental frameworks are often referred to as Ages and Stages frameworks. Specific theorists have identified distinct consecutive stages and what developmental aspect each one focuses on. The four main development frameworks are (1) Piaget's Cognitive Stages, (2) Freud's Psychosexual Stages, (3) Erikson's Psychosocial Stages, and (4) Kohlberg's Moral Judgment Stages. Stages may also be based strictly on an individual's age, which encompasses each of the other stages associated with a specific framework. While experts generally agree on the number of stages, specific age ranges for each differ, however, because there is no strict time determinant for each stage, some variation is not problematic. Box 2-2 illustrates the ages and stages developmental categories.

These stages along with other specific framework stages are in Table 2-3.

Assessing Growth and Development

Assessment of growth and development requires a basic understanding of what physiological, psychological, and emotional components are unique to each stage and what work is essential for an individual to successfully master its requirements.

The stages of infancy through preadolescence require the most task accomplishment of an individual because much of growth and development during these stages involve the maturity of the

Box 2-2 Developmental Stages and Ages

Stage 1: Infancy (birth–1 year)
Stage 2: Toddler–Early childhood (1–3 years)
Stage 3: Preschooler–Early childhood (3–5/6 years)
Stage 4: School-age child (6–10/12 years)
Stage 5: Preadolescent (10 –12/13 years)
Stage 6: Adolescent/Young adult (12/13–19 years)
Stage 7: Early Adult (20–40 years)
Stage 8: Middle adulthood (40–64 years)
Stage 9: Late adulthood (65+ years)

Table 2-3 Comparison of specific framework stages

Stage	Age	Erikson's (Psychosocial)	Piaget's (Cognitive Development)	Freud's Stages (Psychosexual)	Kohlberg (Moral Judgment Stages)
Stage 1	Infancy (birth to 1 year)	Trust vs. mistrust	Sensorimotor	Oral	
Stage 2	Toddler–Early Childhood (1–3 years)	Autonomy vs. Shame/Doubt	Sensorimotor Preoperational	Anal	**Preconventional Level** (Morality stage)
Stage 3	Preschooler–Early Childhood (3–5/6 years)	Initiative vs. Guilt	Preoperational	Phallic	(Individualism, Instrumental, Purpose, and Exchange stage)
Stage 4	School-age child (6–10/12 years)	Industry vs. Inferiority	Preoperational Concrete Operations	Latency	**Conventional Level** (Mutual expectations, Relationships, and Conformity to Moral Norms Stage)
Stage 5	Preadolescent (10–12/13 years)	Identity vs. Role Confusion	Formal Operations	Genital	(Social System and Conscience Stage)
Stage 6	Adolescent/Young Adult (12–13/19 years)	Intimacy vs. Isolation	Formal Operations		**Postconventional Level** (Social Contract or Utility and Individual Rights Stage)
Stage 7	Early Adult (20–40 years)	Generativity vs. **Stagnation**			
Stage 8	Middle Adulthood (40–64 years)				(Universal Ethical Principles Stage)
Stage 9	Late adulthood (65+ years)	Ego Integrity vs. Despair			

neurological system. Previous understanding of the neurological system, primarily the brain, suggested that brain development was complete by early adolescence. However, more recent findings indicate that brain maturation and development continues through young adulthood. The majority of physical growth and maturation also occurs during this time, although it is more sporadic and doesn't occur at the same time in all individuals.

Specific information related to assessment of infants through adolescents is covered in Chapter 10. The remainder of this chapter is primarily devoted to adulthood. A health care provider primarily obtains information about an adult's development through the patient history. No formal assessment tools have been developed for assessing adult development. You must understand developmental tasks and characteristics to be able to ask patients age-appropriate questions as necessary. Carefully listening to an individual's responses and answers will provide important information that is related to mastery and successful completion of developmental tasks.

Early Adulthood

By the time individuals have reached early adulthood, they have completed their growth, and there are no further growth parameters to assess. While linear growth is not possible, medial growth is observed by an increase in the formation and deposition of fat. Metabolic processes begin to slow down, further contributing to excess adipose tissue. The impact of obesity on health is further discussed in Chapter 13.

Developmentally, the early adult needs to establish independence from parents and family and begin to form new relationships and commitments. It is also a time of developing new roles and increasing responsibilities and accountabilities for self in work and social activities and relationships. One's formal education may be complete or may continue, depending on educational goals and/or career requirements. Continuing with one's education may slow down mastery of other developmental tasks, such as achieving independence from parents.

The early adult years are also a time when relationships are expected to progress toward increased intimacy and the choosing of and commitment to a life partner. This also requires the need to learn new roles related to love and cooperation with one's chosen life partner. An early adult may also become a parent during this stage and need to assume this role as well.

It is not unusual for 21st century early adults, particularly females, to delay mastering some of these tasks. An increasing number of females are choosing to enter the workforce and establish a career before seeking to marry and become a parent.

Successful negotiation of this stage results in relationships that are enduring and satisfying. If the young adult is unable to demonstrate emotions or trust others enough to openly express thoughts and feelings, loneliness and isolation from others is likely to occur. Often isolation and loneliness are the catalyst that causes these individuals to engage in high-risk behaviors that may lead to drug and alcohol addiction, sexual promiscuity, or other negative behaviors.

Middle Adulthood

Middle adulthood is the time when a person realizes one's mortality, and that life is half over. Physiologically, the initial signs of aging become apparent. The skin becomes looser, causing the development of lines and wrinkles, particularly around the eyes, mouth, and forehead. The skin beneath the chin and eyes may also begin to sag, causing bags to form under them. The abdomen may begin to develop a pouch due to the loss of skin elasticity and increased fat deposition and the possibility of decreased physical activity.

Hair begins to thin, both in texture and volume, particularly in males who may begin to notice a receding hairline as well as the formation of a bald spot on the posterior portion of the skull. Hair also begins to lose its color, and gray hairs begin to appear.

Physiological systems and activities remain consistent with those of young adulthood with the exception of a slight reduction in respiratory and cardiac function. Somewhere around age 40, the eyes lose their accommodation capability to near vision and reading glasses may become necessary; however, hearing, taste, and touch remain consistent.

Beginning somewhere around the late 40s or early 50s, females will experience symptoms of perimenopause and then menopause. This is due to a decreasing production of estrogen and progesterone, which brings about a decrease and an ultimate cessation in menstruation and an end to reproductive capabilities. Manifestations of menopause start with irregular menstrual cycles as well as hot flashes and mood swings. Reproductive organs begin to atrophy, including a drying out of vaginal mucosa. Males do not experience such an abrupt alteration in reproductive functioning, but do experience a decreased production of testosterone, resulting in decreased production of semen and sperm. Unlike females, males do not experience a cessation in reproductive function and maintain the ability to father a child.

Middle adulthood is also the time when manifestations of chronic conditions may begin to appear, particularly related cardiovascular, endocrine, and musculoskeletal systems. Coronary artery disease and hypertension are common alterations, as well as type 2 diabetes, and arthritis. Females are at high risk for the development of osteoporosis. Diet and exercise are important to prevent the development of these conditions; however, genetics is a significant factor in their cause and onset.

During middle adulthood, individuals often have well-established careers and may experience a sense of achievement and status. Or, this may be a time of career change or starting a career for the first time. Career changes may also require relocation to a new town or state, which involves adjustment. Some middle adults may experience a mid-life crisis, which generally occurs between 40–45 years of age. Personal reflection on one's goals leads to exploration of the meaning of their personal identity, career, and family. Confronting reality may lead to the fact that some life or career goals have not been met. Successful mastering of this task often leads to the realization that one needs to revise earlier goals and develop new perceptions of abilities and expectations.

Middle adulthood is the time when one considers what lasting contribution may be made to the next generation. This is commonly achieved through raising responsible and dependable children or engaging in creating something that will have a significant impact on future generations. While considering what may be passed on to the next generation, it is also a time to begin to anticipate retirement and to plan for future financial, personal, and social stability.

Changes in family structure and dynamics are also a large component of middle adulthood. Many middle adults are concerned with supporting aging parents who have increasing health care and social needs. Realizing and anticipating the eventual loss of parents becomes a challenging task. In some cases, middle adults must change roles with an aging parent, assuming the role of parent and caretaker. Older children may leave home to pursue marriage, careers, or higher education. Preparing for the "empty nest" becomes a major factor to work through. Grown children may also move back home when changes in careers or decreases in income make it difficult to maintain independence. Aging parents may also move in due to the nature of their conditions and health care needs.

This is also the time when significant relationships are nurtured, particular with ones partner and significant others. Empty nesters may have more time to engage in leisure activities and opportunities to nurture and sustain their relationship. During this stage, it also becomes more common to lose significant relationships due to deaths of spouses, friends, and siblings, as well as divorce. Loss of relationships may require the establishment of new relationships with friends or another life partner, which then might require the merger of two family units, which may or may not be successfully achieved.

Generativity is the major task accomplishment for middle adults. The primary activity related to generativity is mentoring and guiding the next generation of individuals to foster their success, survival, and growth. It can be compared to the passing of the torch from one generation to the next. Toward the end of middle adulthood, individuals are concerned with leaving something of themselves behind that can be useful to future generations. This can be something tangible, like books or paintings, or intangible like thoughts, ideas, or ideals. It is also the time to let go of one's creations and endeavors and let others carry them forward.

Failure to master generativity results in **stagnation** of the individual and is the result of failure to master previous developmental tasks. These individuals are unable to identify what is important to pass on to future generations. Severe losses during this time may cause withdrawal and feelings of powerlessness, but they should be temporary and not prevent successful negotiation of this stage.

Late Adulthood

Late adulthood is the time when individuals may be referred to as "aged." Unfortunately, the term aged carries with it significant stereotypes that may cause discrimination. Aged individuals are often perceived to be unhappy, nonproductive, sick, and senile, and a drain on resources. Americans, as a culture, revere youth and beauty over elderly individuals, which is in contrast to many other cultures where the elderly are cherished and revered.

Major advances in health care have allowed individuals to live to an older age. While it used to be uncommon to have individuals live to 100 (centenarians), this population is increasing with survival 3–5 years beyond 100. While many of the elderly are afflicted with forms of dementia requiring them to be institutionalized, many elderly individuals over the age of 80 are alert, active, and contributing members to society. Because of these active and happy elderly individuals, the stereotype of "aged" is disappearing.

Advances in health care have resulted in improved management of chronic health conditions, improving the quality of life of many elderly individuals. While aging is a lifelong process, the rate of its progression is quite variable. In essence, one begins to age from the moment of birth. Initially, aging is viewed as positive, indicating that expected growth and maturation is occurring. Exactly when aging begins to cause a decline in an individual is unknown—some people age rapidly with significant changes, while others age more slowly and demonstrate minimal changes (Figure 2-1).

Physiological process gradually decline with aging, however, they are still capable of functioning appropriately. Specific changes that occur with aging are further identified and described in Chapters 10 and 12.

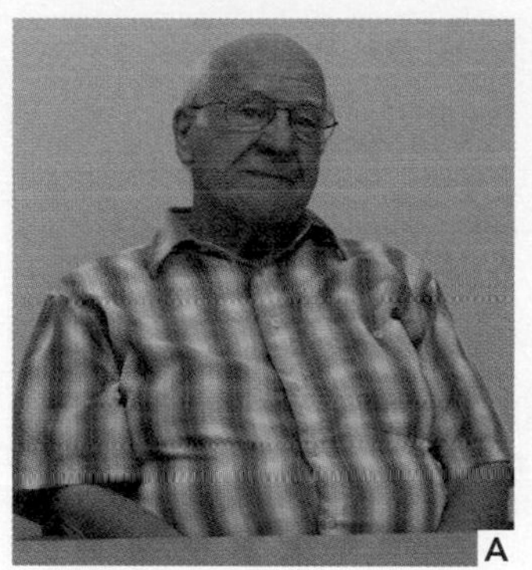

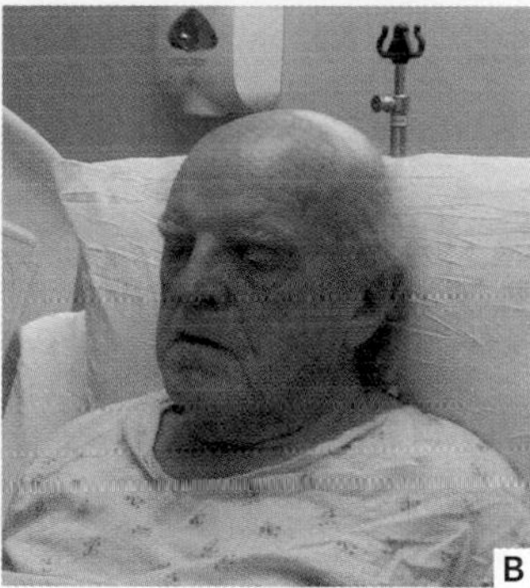

FIGURE 2-1A–B The actual appearance of aging differs by individual

Late adulthood is usually a time when a person has achieved retirement and generally is no longer employed. Some individuals may seek part-time employment to remain busy, satisfy a need to continue to make some contributions, or maintain financial stability. In tenuous financial times, a retired individual may find it necessary to seek some type of employment to provide for basic resources.

While many elderly people view their extra free time as a positive change, in some instances, having a spouse around continuously may put a strain on the relationship. Individuals who live alone may not know how to fill their days, and become lonely and depressed. Older adults may seek ways to avoid this situation, such as developing or engaging in hobbies, community service, and volunteering. These activities are often satisfying and provide a sense of maintaining one's contribution to society and future generations. Multiple opportunities often exist for the older adult to engage in continuing education courses, exploring topics of interest or even pursuing a degree.

Family roles also change and may include a new role as a grandparent. Depending upon location of family members, opportunities to interact with and enjoy the grandchildren may be limited. It is also a possibility that grandparents may assume the role of a parent to a grandchild or children. This requires a significant shift in role responsibilities and may place an excessive burden on the individual or couple, specifically financially and emotionally.

Late adulthood is also the time when one experiences the death of loved ones, including friends, colleagues, siblings, and spouse. This is a reminder of the terminal condition of humans, and the limited amount of time a person has left. Loss of a spouse may mean that the rest of life will continue alone. For elderly spouses who have been together for 50 plus years, it is not uncommon that when one spouse dies, it is not very long before the other one also dies. One last task that is often engaged in is a life review. A life review is an analysis of one's life experiences, considering life's successes and failures from the perspective of age. Successful mastery and completion of this task occurs when one accepts the totality of one's life and feels satisfied with life's choices and outcomes. This provides a sense of contentment and acceptance of the finality of life with integrity and dignity. Failure to accomplish this task leaves the individual with a sense of despair and futility. A person may also feel hopeless, resentment, and afraid to die, or become clinically depressed.

Medical advancement and treatment modalities for many chronic conditions have contributed significantly to increasing the life span for many adults. This had resulted in dividing late adulthood into three categories: young old, old, and old old.

During this last stage, individuals begin to look back over their life and its accomplishments and feel good about who they are and what they accomplished. Looking back, individuals are often able to perceive their past in new and positive ways. Individuals may also have to accept what cannot be changed and come to some type of resolution regarding this. For some, this may not occur until the individual is facing the end of life and is necessary for a peaceful and meaningful death.

Failure to meet the last developmental stage with integrity results in despair. These individuals are unable to feel grateful for their life and are unable to successfully resolve and accept past failures or inadequacies. Their final days or years are full of disappointment and dissatisfaction. Death for these individuals is often not peaceful, but vindictive, filled with turmoil and anger.

Adult Assessment

Assessment of adult developmental stages can be completed by formulating questions related to areas of interest associated with each developmental stage (Table 2-4).

Family

Another contextual component of an individual is membership within a family. Family in its broadest interpretation is simply a collection of or assembly of objects with some common feature or attributes. Family is a widely used term that is used in multiple disciplines and settings; some of these being biology, linguistics, mathematics, chemistry, and physics. The sociological use of family is the most familiar use of the term, which refers to a group of human individuals that have a relationship with each other.

What constitutes a family has changed over the years, but the family unit has been considered the basic social structure within cultures throughout time. The primary function of the family is for socialization of individuals into the values, ideals, and expectations of the predominant culture. The traditional conceptualization of family was based on relationships among individuals that were created by marriage and birth or adoption. This resulted in families that were biologically, genetically, or legally related to each other. Changes in society's values and norms have played a significant part in defining family. Various paradigms, ideologies, and discipline perspectives also determine the composition and configuration of the family and its roles and functions. For all intents and purposes, no single definition of family reflects all of its multiple facets and dimensions. The most universal definition of family is whomever or whatever the individual wants or states it to be.

While the family is not considered the main focus of a patient assessment, recognizing and understanding family dynamics will provide the health care provider with a more definitive picture of the individual. Family dynamics can have an influence on the perception, progression, and resolution of the patient's situation or condition. Family dynamics and interactions can be assessed with various instruments depending on what perspective is taken in regards to family. Regardless of what discipline-specific framework or model is

Table 2-4 Questions/areas of importance for developmental assessment

Young Adult	Middle-Aged Adult	Older Adult
Is the (Young, Middle-Aged, Older) Adult able to:		
Accept physical and emotional self—formation of self-identity/image in adult work which guides decision making? Develop emotional stability? Achieve autonomy/independence from parents both physically and emotionally? Leave home permanently? Experience/express love—physically and emotionally? Engage in intimate relationships with partner? Select an intimate life partner and/or adjust to marriage or partnership? Socialize with individuals and groups? Become a part of a society group and community? Articulate a philosophy regarding life based on one's values? Accept responsibility for providing for self and others? Effectively problem solve life's complications and complexities? Become a parent and rear children?	Engage in health promoting life activities? Adjust to the physical changes of middle age? Achieve satisfaction from supporting and nurturing the growth and development of others? Sustain an enduring and intimate relationship with another? Provide a secure home environment? Gain satisfaction from one's employment or profession? Find satisfaction through work/occupation, civic responsibilities, and family activities? Demonstrate a sense of pride in individual and family achievements and contributions? Participate in supporting and sustaining community growth and development? Launch children into responsible, happy adulthood? Reorient oneself to aging parents? Revitalize marriage? Realign sex roles?	Adapt/accept age changes in physical appearance? Stay physically healthy and adjust to limitations? Acknowledge aging changes that affect relationships and physical functions? Sustain connections with family, relatives, and friends? Find companionship and friendship? Engage in external activities and interests beyond the scope of self and home? Learn to use leisure time pleasurably? Accept transitions that accompany retirement, death, and illnesses? Adjust to revised work roles? Sustain relationships with past friends and establish new relationships with others of own age? Maintain identity and social status? Engage in activities/practices that promote and sustain physical health? Find significance and purpose in the past and accept the imminent death of self and others? Assimilate spiritual/philosophical values into acceptance and understanding of self? Recognize significant achievements and activities that have been successful and meaningful to family and society? Achieve integrity through acceptance of one's life?

used for family assessment, each one is comprised of three essential dimensions: framework or structure, evolution or development, and operation or function.

Structure

The structural aspect of the family framework can be conceptualized as having 3 components: (1) intrinsic structure, (2) extrinsic structure, and (3) milieu.

Intrinsic Structure

Intrinsic structure focuses on the individual family members and the connections between them. Subcategories of intrinsic structure include (1) membership, (2) gender and gender roles, (3) hierarchy, (4) subgroups, (5) limits, and (6) authority.

Family members can be best identified through a genogram. Specific details of a genogram are further discussed in Chapter 5. Once the gender of each individual is established, how gender roles are demonstrated is determined. Values and beliefs related to gender roles vary from family to family, as well as differences related to generational and cultural ideals and perceptions. Norms for gender roles are initially established within the family and then further shaped and determined by cultural and peer expectations.

Hierarchy refers to what position an individual holds within the family. Expectations and behaviors of individuals are often a reflection of one's rank order in the family and how one is treated due to their rank. Future relationships and interactions are also a reflection of this family position. One's position in the family ranking is also considered a determinant of the power structure within the family. In addition to a genogram, an attachment diagram may be developed which identifies and describes relationships that exist within the family (Figure 2-2).

Each family includes subgroups, or smaller units within the family that can be determined by gender, interests, age, work and free time schedules, and position. Subgroups often evolve rather than being created, and function within certain rules and expectations, which may or may not be apparent to family members, either within or outside of the subgroup. Subgroups are generally an accepted or sanctioned component of a family.

Limits exist within families to maintain separate and distinct subsystems. Limits are implemented and supported by rules, tasks, and expectations that differentiate one subsystem from another. Healthy families have subsystems with well-defined limits but are fluid enough to allow communication and connection between them. Limits that are too strict result in detached family members who have minimal effective communication and connection between themselves. Limits that are too ambiguous and permeable result in enmeshed families where separating from family members and achieving individuality is constrained or obstructed. This may increase a sense of acceptance and belonging, but at the cost of one's loss of autonomy.

Extrinsic Structure

Extrinsic structure is the associations and links between family members and external groups, organizations, or individuals. Two dimensions of extrinsic structure affect family dynamics: (1) extended or augmented family and (2) external systems. Extended

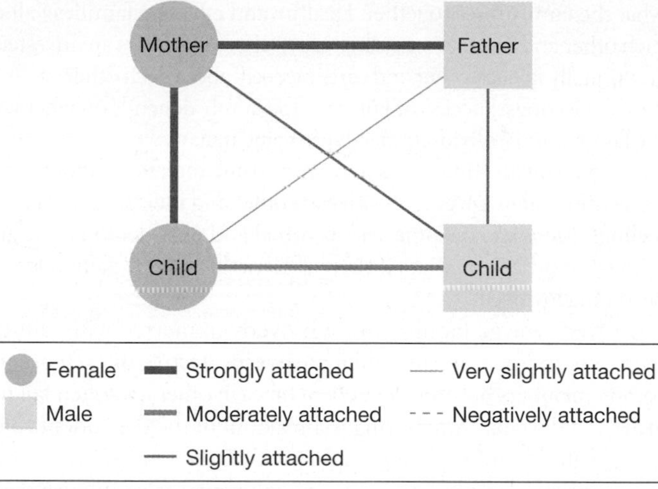

FIGURE 2-2 Attachment diagram

or augmented family members are those who do not reside with or are present within the family's residence. These are generally relatives who maintain contact and interact with the family. The amount and degree of interaction is often dependent upon location and distance between the family and relatives. Contact between them varies from weekly to monthly to yearly. Extrinsic family also includes family members or relatives who may be "cut off" from connection and interaction with family members. This separation and isolation of the family member may be self imposed or mandated by the family.

Augmented family members may also be close friends who are considered part of the family, despite the lack of genetic connection. Legal definitions of family members may conflict with personal (patient) definitions of family, creating tension and delays in decision making regarding provision of care and interventions that affect the outcomes of severe illnesses and other critical health conditions.

Extrinsic systems are other systems that are larger or greater than the family, and that the family interacts with and has an influence on its members. The interaction(s) may be individual or as a group. These systems include but are not necessarily limited to institutions, agencies, and significant others. Examples of these would be schools, churches, recreational and fitness centers, employing agencies, co-workers, friends, neighbors,

Extrinsic systems may be described with the use of another attachment diagram that indentifies the relationships and the degree of attachment and/or stress that accompanies each relationship (Figure 2-3).

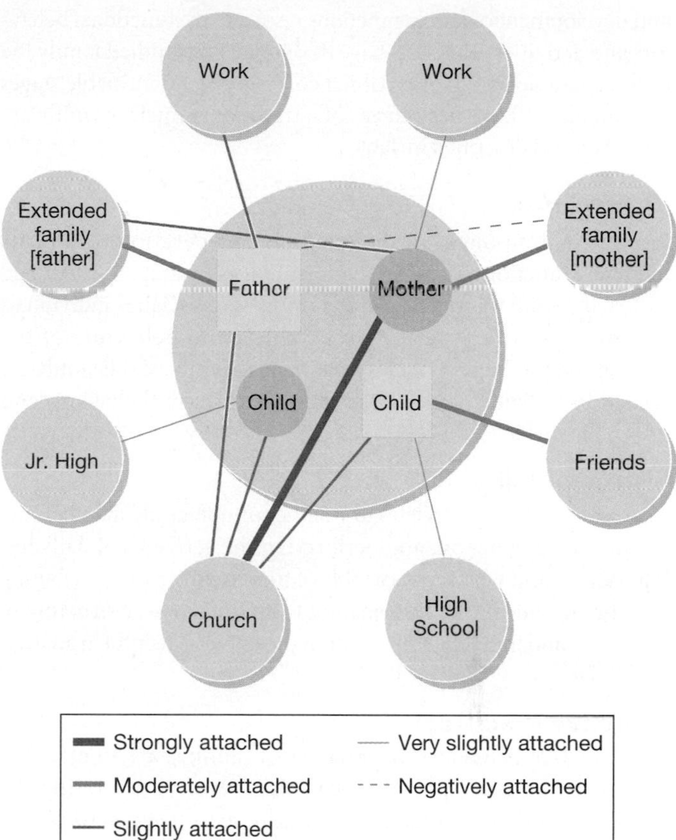

FIGURE 2-3 Relationships of family members to extrinsic systems

Milieu

The milieu of the family is concerned with the relevant background and the interrelated circumstances which determine the overall family's environment or context. The components of the family's milieu includes (1) race, (2) ethnic origin, (3) social status, (4) religious beliefs/practices or spirituality, and (5) external surroundings and/or conditions.

Race and ethnic origin are more than simply the country of one's birth, skin color, and physical characteristics. While these attributes may be used to describe individuals, they may or may not identify with them. More recently, more emphasis has been placed on identification with one's heritage and ethnic background; however, adherence to cultural practices and rituals may not be important to the family.

While no absolute criteria exist to determine one's social status or standing, primary attributes associated with it relate to education, income level, and occupation. These determinants are not absolute and the family may experience a decrease or increase in status depending on any alterations that occur within them. One's social status or standing is also a product of an individual's or family's perception and comparison to other families and individuals.

Religious beliefs, practices, and spirituality have a significant influence on the families, values, and perspective on life in general and specifically health and health care practices. The ethnicity and cultural heritage of the family or family members closely interact with religious and spiritual practices. The absence of any religion or spiritual practices also affects personal values and beliefs.

The external surroundings and conditions include the home, neighborhood, and surrounding community. Significant influences include safety issues within and around the house, and whether the family or individual members feel safe within their neighborhood. Relationships with neighbors also are a significant influence on the family's interaction and satisfaction with the surrounding environment. The presence of any actual or potential extrinsic or intrinsic pollutants also is an important factor contributing to environmental safety and health related issues.

Evolution

Families, like individuals progress through stages of growth and development that are vital to maintaining the health and wellness of the family and its members. The disruption or termination of growth and development of family functions results in dysfunctional behaviors and activities. Theorists have developed and studied family life cycles and associated tasks, which consist of six identifiable stages (Friedman, 1992). These stages of a traditional nuclear family are identified and described in Table 2-5.

Operation

The third component of the family is its operation or how its members function as both individuals and as a group. As identified earlier, the primary function of the family is to socialize individuals (children) in the norms, mores, values, and behaviors of the predominant culture. Other operational activities of the family are related to instrumentality, affective and expressive behaviors, and health care behaviors.

Instrumentality

Instrumental function relates to whether or not family members are capable of carrying out and performing the activities of daily living. Who is and who is not capable of functioning as a contributing member to the family? Information from the intrinsic structure of the family and individual roles within the family is helpful in analysis of this data.

Affective Practices

The affective behaviors or practices of families are to meet the psychosocial needs of individual members by facilitating the formation and development of a healthy self-esteem and a stable personality. It is a measurement of how involved emotionally the members of the family are with each other, not necessarily how or what the family does together. Healthy and effective families value each other and interact empathetically; where members are invested emotionally in each other and care intensely about each other's activities and feelings. Success or failure of the family depends on whether the family's and individual's needs are being met.

Underinvolved families may share some interests but demonstrate minimal involvement with each other and their situations and feelings. Members become self absorbed and only demonstrate an interest in other members if there is something to be gained from becoming involved.

Overinvolved families become overly immersed with family members and matters and often are overprotective of each other. Family members become dependent on each other and often fail to grow and develop. Attempting to break out of the dependent role may create resentment and conflict within the family. Symbiotic involvement is present when overinvolvement is so intense that there are vague and ambiguous limits between two or more members. Symbiotic relationships are least effective because limits are not respected. Without limits, it becomes problematic in identifying or differentiating between parent and child roles.

Expressive Practices

Expressive practices of the family are the communication patterns that are demonstrated within the family. Expressive practices are assessed through (1) emotional communication, (2) verbal communication, (3) nonverbal communication, and (4) circular communication.

Emotional communication is the expression of a broad range and type of emotions and feelings. Emotional communication

Table 2-5 Developmental dimension of families (stages)

Stage 1	Leaving Home	Single, young adult accepting emotional, financial responsibility for self	Differentiates self from family of origin Develops intimate relationships Seeks/begins employment to achieve financial independence
Stage 2	Marriage; Joining Families	Joining of two individuals with three families: his, hers, theirs	Couple identity Realign relationships with families/friends Consider parenthood
Stage 3	Families with Young Children	Adults caretakers of younger generation Increasing responsibilities—dealing with demands of children when finances limited Career development of couple	Adapting to addition of individuals to marital dyad Negotiation of joint child rearing, financial and household responsibilities Realign relationships with extended family to incorporate parenting/grandparenting roles
Stage 4	Families with Adolescents	Rapid biological, emotional and sociocultural changes, often resulting in intense upheaval and transition	Parent/child relationship shifts to allow adolescent to move in/out of system Reevaluate midlife marital/career issues Initial transition to joint caring for aging parents
Stage 5	Families in Transition	Children moving out--> empty nest Children moving back home (not growing up, want same things/lifestyle that parents had/have)	Realignment of marital dyad New relationships—in-laws, grandchildren Coping with death/disabilities of parents Adult–Adult relationship with child(ren)
Stage 6	Families in Later Life		Sustain self/couple functioning during physical/functional decline Middle generation takes more central role Recognition and acceptance of older generation wisdom/experience without overstepping boundaries Adapts/copes with death—own/spouse/significant others Engages in life review

Adapted from: *Family Nursing: Research, Theory, and Practice*, 5th edition by M. R. Friedman, V. R. Bowen, and E. Jones. Copyright © 2003, pp. 107. Reprinted and electronically reproduced by Pearson Education, Inc., Upper Saddle River, New Jersey.

patterns may be determined by member's roles and gender, but individuals should be allowed to freely express their emotions and feelings and perceive that their expression is acceptable and appropriate. Families that demonstrate emotional difficulties often have a limited range and breadth of emotions expressed, or have specific expectations of what is sanctioned and allowed. Specific expectations are often based on inappropriate or incorrect stereotypes.

Verbal communication is an expression of a relationship that is interpreted or understood by the meaning of its verbal content rather than its semantic context. Effective verbal communication is direct with the content is transmitted straight to the recipient. Indirect or displaced communication occurs when the message is transmitted to an inconsequential individual who may or may not redirect the message. Masked verbal communication occurs when the intended message is distorted or obfuscated.

Nonverbal communication is interpreted as messages that are communicated without any verbal expression. Generally, nonverbal communication is assessed through body position, eye contact, touch, gestures, and proximity of one to another. Nonverbal communication is significantly related to culture and should always be assessed within the cultural context of the individual and family. Within families, certain looks, actions often communicate thoughts, feelings, and directions that are interpreted only within the context of one's family. Paraverbal communication accompanies nonverbal messages and provides additional data about the message. Paraverbal messages reflect how the message is delivered related to voice sounds used in communicating the message. Voice sounds relate to tone, inflections, volume, and rate.

Circular communication is reciprocal in nature and is based on the assumption that each person influences the behavior of the other. The influence of one person on another may be positive or negative, depending on the intent of the communication.

Health Care Behaviors

The health care behavior function of a family is related to what beliefs are held by family members related to health problems, their sources, how they should be treated and who should be treating them, as well as what the perceived outcome is. Health beliefs and practices are also related to one's cultural affiliations and beliefs. There may or may not be agreement among the family members as to how health conditions of family members should be viewed. Older family members may be less willing to give up cultural beliefs and practices whereas younger family members are more likely to accept and seek medical treatment.

Decisions related to health care interventions and treatments are dependent on all dimensions and functions of the family. It is important for all members of the health care team to be aware of family dynamics and how health care for members of the family will be and is affected. Issues related to when to initiate or terminate treatment can be sources of extreme stress and disagreements between and among family members. Even if a formal family assessment is not completed, understanding the elements of family function and dynamics will provide the health care provider with the tools and knowledge to make appropriate and meaningful observations of the family dynamics and to use this knowledge to assist family members and others in making appropriate health care decisions.

In addition to families' beliefs and practices related to health behaviors, past experiences with the health care system and providers of health care also have a significant effect on one's health beliefs and practices and willingness to participate in one's health care. Obviously, positive experiences will promote feelings of trust and overall satisfaction with the health care system and the providers associated with it. Conversely, negative experiences will promote feelings of distrust in and possibly betrayal by the health care system and its providers.

While it is unfortunate that negative experiences and outcomes do happen, the patient and/or family members will need help recognizing that even though negative experiences may have occurred, that doesn't mean it will happen again. It is also important for providers to not condone or condemn previous providers who were involved with the negative experience. To do so might create feelings of distrust and the perception of a lack of empathy on the part of the provider. This may also give the impression that the provider does not believe the patient or family members.

Summary

- The overall context of the individual is complex and composed of multiple variables.
- Although congruency may exist among individuals from and within similar situations, conditions, and backgrounds, do not assume that everyone will conform to certain norms and expectations.
- To the extent possible, consider the individual's unique context (cultural, spiritual, developmental, family) and address individual personal and health care needs within an individual framework.
- Understanding the particular attributes of the various dimensions of an individual enables you to assess and address the patient appropriately as an individual.

Review Questions

1. When conducting a health history with a patient of the Jewish faith, the provider expects that the patient's diet may not include pork products. This is an example of the provider's
   1. cultural knowledge.
   2. cultural awareness.
   3. cultural sensitivity.
   4. cultural competence.
2. When asked about religious beliefs during a health history interview the patient seems surprised and asks the provider the purpose of these questions. The provider should explain that this information is important because of which of the following?
   1. It helps providers to understand end-of-life wishes.
   2. Often religion dictates what treatments are acceptable to the patient.
   3. It allows providers the opportunity to incorporate beliefs into care.
   4. It will allow staff to contact the appropriate religious leader in an emergency.
3. The provider uses the genogram to document a patient's family history. By symbolically listing each member of the patient's family the provider is depicting the family's
   1. intrinsic structure.
   2. extrinsic structure.
   3. milieu.
   4. roles.
4. A 35-year-old female tells the provider that she is married and has two children. She does not work outside of the home. The provider has gathered information about which areas of family assessment? (Select all that apply.)
   1. Intrinsic structure
   2. Gender roles
   3. Hierarchy
   4. Authority
   5. Sub-groups
5. The provider is gathering information from a new patient about the family's milieu. Which questions will assist the provider in gathering this information? (Select all that apply.)
   1. "Is that a married name that you are using?"
   2. "Can you tell me what ethnic group you consider yourself to be part of?"
   3. "Do you attend religious services regularly?"
   4. "Do practice any particular religion?"
   5. "Can you tell me about the neighborhood that you and your family live in?"
6. The provider is interviewing a couple who married 6 months earlier and is planning to have a child in the near future. In which stage of family development would the provider place this family?
   1. Stage 1
   2. Stage 2
   3. Stage 3
   4. Stage 4
7. The provider is working with families with young children. When assessing these families the provider is aware that the primary function of family is to do which of the following?
   1. Ensure that appropriate health care is provided.
   2. Meet the economic demands of having children.
   3. Provide educational opportunities for their children.
   4. Socialize children in the norms of the culture.
8. Awareness of the cultural beliefs and attitudes of patients by providers and other providers may contribute to which of the following?
   1. Improved efficiency in care
   2. Standardization of care delivery
   3. Cost savings to the health care institutions
   4. Health disparities among minority populations
9. Providers in a local health care facility are being encouraged to enroll in a sign language course. By encouraging this program the facility is fostering an environment of which of the following?
   1. Linguistic competence
   2. Health promotion
   3. Cultural knowledge
   4. Cultural awareness
10. The provider gathers information about a patient's background, beliefs, and family during an initial assessment because this information
    1. is required by most agencies as a part of the assessment process.
    2. is necessary to the formation of a diagnosis or origin of symptoms.
    3. will assist in the development of the formation of individualized plans of care.
    4. helps to ensure that staff with similar backgrounds will care for the patient.

The Provider in Context

"And are you the one who is responsible for my care?" Mrs. Anna asks very sweetly from her new bed on the ward.

"Well, I'll be your nurse while you're on this unit," I begin, "so I'll be at the bedside a great deal, making sure that you have everything that you need."

"So who will tell me what's going on with my body and how to fix it?"

"Well, the residents will be working with you closely to figure out what your diagnosis is."

A quizzical look comes over her aged face: "A... resident? What's a resident?"

I pause; how should I explain? "You see, a resident is a physician who is still in training. They work with an attending who oversees all major decisions regarding your care."

Now Mrs. Anna is frowning. "Miss, you are very kind, but I don't understand. What is an attending?"

The door swings open and the oncology fellow steps in. *This won't help matters*, I think. "Hi Mrs. Anna, my name is Dr. Penn. I'm one of the oncology fellows."

"So are you the... attending...who I should speak to about my diagnosis?"

"Oh, no, that would be Dr. Sandoval. I'm just consulting on your case from an oncology perspective."

What a hopelessly complex system to the uninitiated—and how disorienting this must feel to patients! "Dr. Penn," I cut in, "would you mind returning in a few minutes?" He steps quietly out of the room and I sit at the foot of Mrs. Anna's bed. "I'm sorry I wasn't clearer about this before. The truth is, you don't have a single provider. Although for some reason we have a bunch of titles for different people, we all work together as a team to help get you better." Mrs. Anna, wringing the edge of her blanket in her hands, looks up with the first glimmer of understanding. Progress!

LEARNING OUTCOMES

1. Summarize the steps in the problem-solving process.
2. Compare and contrast various thinking strategies and their use in problem solving.
3. Characterize attributes of critical thinkers.
4. Compare and contrast clinical decision making with problem solving.
5. Explain the steps of the clinical reasoning process used to formulate a diagnosis.
6. Describe internal and external factors that affect clinical decision making and critical thinking.

The previous chapter focused on unique individual characteristics of the patient and the provider. In addition to individual characteristics that influence the interaction between provider and individual, the context of the provider also includes the activities that characterize and contribute to problem solving, critical thinking, and clinical reasoning. This chapter focuses on the provider and the attributes of these three processes that contribute to and comprise the provider's context.

Context of Provider

The overall purpose and goal of patient assessment is to obtain data that reflects the patient's health care needs and to find ways to respond to those needs for the provision of individualized health care. In most clinical situations, patient's needs are regarded and identified as patient's problems. In some situations, however, patients are concerned with preventing certain health conditions that they may feel at risk for developing. Thus, it is essential for providers to look beyond the restrictions of problem-oriented health care and include the broader perspective of health promotion and disease prevention. While a preventive perspective and approach is important, there is still the need to involve critical-thinking and problem-solving skills in whatever concern or condition a patient may identify and present with. With this in mind, the remainder of the discussion will be primarily related to problem solving as this is the general context of health care provision.

Problem identification is the most significant component and depends on the accuracy and inclusion of critical information by the patient. It is also essential for the provider to keep in mind the possibility that the patient may identify a symptom of an underlying problem instead of the actual problem, emphasizing the importance of a correct problem.

Once the problem (concern) has been identified, a resolution or plan is needed to eliminate or modify the problem. These activities describe the process known as problem solving, thus establishing patient assessment within a problem-solving paradigm. Inherent within the problem-solving process is decision making. The ability to make appropriate decisions to resolve or minimize a problem requires well-developed decision making skills. Crucial to both processes is the ability to think clearly and critically.

Thinking and Problem Solving

Thinking is the quintessential cognitive or mental activity that characterizes humans. It is an "active organized, purposeful mental process that links ideas together by making logical connections among perceptions, beliefs, knowledge, judgments, and feelings" (Wilkinson, 2012, p. 42). Every discovery, accomplishment, and advancement is the result of thought. Every intentional activity originates with thinking. Thinking allows for ordering and interpreting one's environment to make it significant as a representation of one's reality. Thinking is an active cognitive process that functions during our conscious waking hours. Even though there is no conscious awareness of thinking activities, thinking is occurring. Paramount to thinking is acquisition of a vocabulary and language, which are necessary for identification and expression of our thinking and thoughts.

Thinking results in the development and formulation of thoughts. Although we often don't think about the nature of our thinking and thoughts, thoughts can be categorized into various types. More than likely, these types of thoughts have been unconsciously developed and formulated throughout one's life. A conscious awareness of these thoughts is recommended to develop and maximize critical-thinking skills. A taxonomy of these specific thoughts and the nature of the elements that fosters their development are as follows:

- Point of view—frame of reference, perspective, orientation of individual
- Purpose of thinking—the goal or objective of thoughts
- Question at issue—the problem or issue being considered
- Information—the data, facts, observations, or experiences
- Interpretation and Inference—the conclusions or solutions that are formulated
- Concepts—the theories, definition, axioms, laws, principles, and models
- Assumptions—the presuppositions or what is taken for granted
- Implications and consequences (Paul & Elder, 2001, p. 2)

Ironically, the goal of thinking is to create conditions in which thinking is not required. Therefore, thinking begins with a problem, question, or situation, and terminates with a solution or strategy, making it an essential component to problem solving.

Problem solving is the foundation for all scientific disciplines and relies on a systematic approach for consistency in diverse situations. Problem solving within scientific disciplines is frequently referred to as the **scientific method** (Figure 3-1). The scientific method had its origins with the ancient Greeks and their emphasis on developing skills related to thinking about and understanding the world around them. It is safe to say the scientific method is responsible for many innovations and inventions that were developed to solve specific problems.

Approaches to problem solving and applying the scientific method to problem solving have been identified and described in various ways. Problem solving strategies are generally described as occurring by following a certain number of steps that range from four to eight. Regardless of how many steps or activities have been identified or described as techniques for problem solving, the essential methodology follows a logical, sequential core process.

Cognition/Thinking Models

Thinking models are means of engaging in cognitive processes that are conducive for problem solving. Models represent and identify methods for carrying out certain processes or activities and contain tools to assist in problem solving. Tools, within any discipline, are only as good as the individuals who use them and develop the skills to apply them. The artist's paint brush is only a tool, but the difference in how a painting turns out is how the individual artist applies those tools. Two painters may be looking at the same scene, but the actual painting is going to reflect the individual painter's skills. Providers in many aspects are artists who employ various tools in the provision of patient care. The difference between providers is in how they learn and apply those tools. Thinking strategies are considered tools that the provider applies to the process of problem solving. Thinking strategies are represented as components or steps within various frameworks or models and not mutually exclusive.

For all intents and purposes, frameworks or models of problem solving or decision making have emerged from two perspectives—the information-processing model, also called the **hypothetico-deductive model**, and the **intuitive-humanist model** (Banning, 2007). Thinking strategies associated with each model may be used unconsciously, however, cognitive awareness and implementation of the various strategies is important for successful problem solving. One model's strategy may be easier for a provider to use than the others, but limiting or not using the other strategies should be avoided.

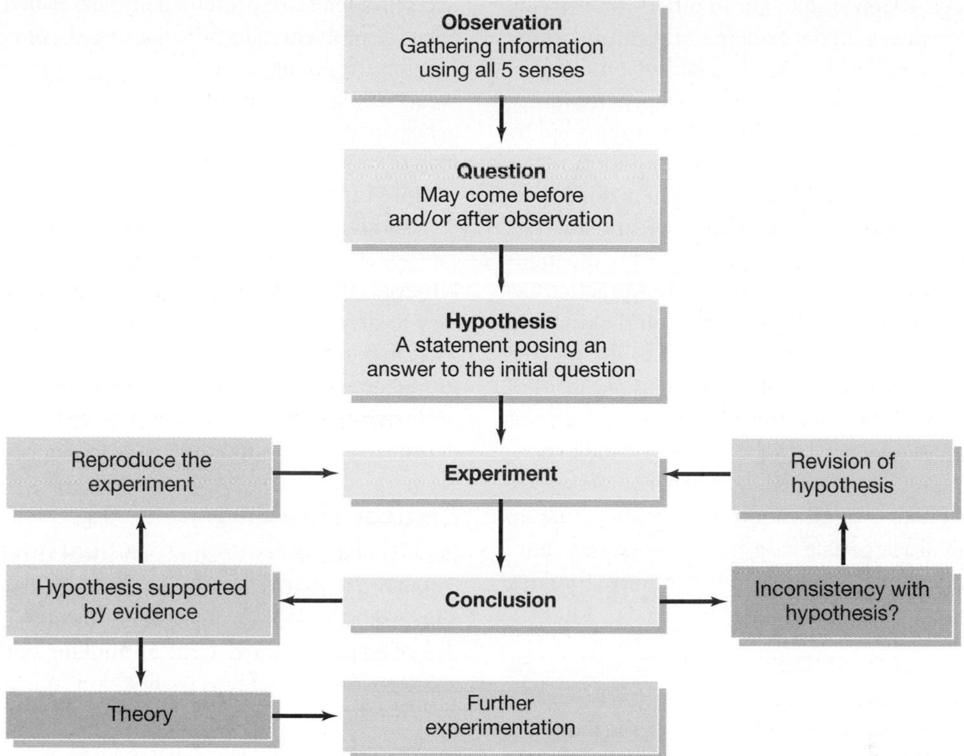

FIGURE 3-1 The Scientific Method

Hypothetico-Deductive Model

Thinking approaches in the hypothetical-deductive model are described as "analytical and are characterized as deductive, slow, rational, rule based, and low in emotional investment" (Croskerry & Norman, 2008, p. S25). Additionally, analytic thinking tends to be logical, linear, focused, objective, provides an explanation, and functions best in conditions that are static with a high degree of predictability, and where time is not limited. The hypothetico-deductive model has commonly been perceived as the superior diagnostic thinking or reasoning process that facilitates the development of evidence-based practice (Crandall & Wears, 2008).

Analytic thinking approaches also encompass **ritualistic thinking**, also characterized as **reflexive thinking**. Ritualistic thinking produces an automatic or habitual response that is often initiated without conscious awareness or extensive deliberations. This strategy is often used when there is a well-defined cause-and-effect relationship. The provider automatically responds to a familiar or previously encountered situation in the same manner without going through a conscious deliberation process. For example, if a patient states, "I need to go to the bathroom," the provider automatically provides a urinal for the patient or assists the patient to the bathroom.

Ritualistic thinking occurs when standard **protocols** or procedures are in place. Protocols are predetermined interventions or treatments that are developed within the health care organization to guide behavior and actions related to specific conditions or situations. They also provide the basis for a certain level of standardized care and decision making. Standardized care is a diagnostic or treatment process that providers should follow for a certain type of patient, illness, or clinical circumstance. Consider a situation in which a diabetic patient with an infection is admitted to a patient care unit in a local hospital. A standard protocol or standard of care has been established that all diabetic patients will have their blood glucose monitored three times a day. Even though the diabetes is not the patient's primary problem, the provider relies on the protocol to provide standardized diabetic care.

Intuitive-Humanistic Model

The second model is the intuitive-humanistic model which is associated with nonanalytical thinking. Nonanalytical thinking approaches are contrary to those associated with analytical thinking. It is connected to patterns and recognition, and is a "decision mode that is dominated by **heuristics**. Heuristics are general decision-making strategies individuals' use that ignore information yet are frequently correct (Gigerenzer & Gaissmaier, 2011). Heuristics are important tools to assist in diagnostic reasoning, particularly in nonanalytical thinking, but should not be so rigidly adhered to so as to inhibit alternative ways of thinking and reasoning. Failure to recognize use of faulty heuristics or incorrect pattern recognition will most likely result in failure to represent the real problem and cause random formulation of hypotheses (Bowen, 2006). Heuristics tend to be used more frequently under conditions of uncertainty (Croskerry & Norman, 2008). Heuristics are also referred to as mental short cuts, maxims, and rules of thumb, [and are] fast, associative, inductive, frugal, and often primed by an affective component" (Croskerry & Norman, 2008). It is also nonlinear, nonfocused, big-picture oriented, based on past experiences, and dynamic.

Nonanalytical thinking or **intuitive thinking** is the primary thinking approach within this model. Intuition may be defined as "a process of arriving at accurate conclusions based on receiving relatively small amounts of knowledge and/or information"

(Billay, Myrick, Luhanga, & Yonge, 2007) or in other words, trying to conceptualize reality when material evidence of reality is lacking or unavailable. Intuition embodies physical sensations such as gut feelings, emotional awareness that embodies premonitions, apprehension, and reassuring feelings, which were supported by feelings of unease, anxiety, or fear (Banning, 2007). Intuition has often instigated investigations that have resulted in major breakthroughs in human perceptions, experimentation, and analysis (Ali, n.d.). While empirical knowledge and evidence are the foundation of scientific disciplines, and evidence-based practice has made significant contributions to clinical decision making and improved patient outcomes, intuition is recognized as also making a significant contribution as an essential component of the art of decision making and clinical practice. Intuitive thinking occurs at the unconscious level and is largely based on personal and experiential knowledge from previous interactions and encounters.

Sorting out which data is significant to the present situation requires the acquisition of a large data base of experience, thus, novice providers should not expect to be able to use intuitive thinking right away.

PRACTICE POINT: Using the Intuitive Method

The provider must exercise caution regarding intuitive methods in order to prevent making a judgment based on inclusive evidence, erroneous information, or personal experiences that inaccurately reflect the patient's situation. Because intuition is subjective in nature, relying on personal experiences may introduce an element of bias into the decision making process and have detrimental effects for both the patient and provider.

Another thinking strategy associated with nonanalytical thinking is **trial and error**. This method relates to **random thinking** (free association of ideas) and requires little or no previous knowledge to formulate solutions. The trial-and-error method of thinking is based on the premise that there is no specific cause-and-effect relationship; the provider must be aware that what may have worked for one patient may not necessarily work in all similar situations. Outcomes are usually not recorded for future situations. Random thinking requires energy, time, guesswork, and choices (selecting methods that work, discarding methods that do not).

Trial-and-error thinking promotes identifying creative solutions for problems without the restrictions imposed by rote performance and the need for factual data. By using random thinking, the provider is encouraged to think creatively or "outside the box." Creative thinking is the product of reasoning and imagination that promotes the generation of new and original solutions based on the premise that there is more than one way to solve a problem (O'Reilly, 1993).

The use of the two recognized models of cognitive operations is now referred to as *dual process theory*. Instead of being perceived as two mutually exclusive processes, thinking is perceived as a combination of the two. Individuals may prefer one model over another and/or only use one model at a time; however, a blending of both models may be the method of choice.

Regardless of one's thinking approaches, the crucial element needed for achieving a successful outcome or solution is the correct identification of the problem. Failure to correctly identify the problem results in faulty thinking and, most likely, obtaining irrelevant data. Problems are presented and described in various ways and often the problem must be "constructed from circumstances that are puzzling, troubling, uncertain, and possibly irrelevant" (Crandall & Wears, 2008). The nature of problems also needs to be determined to help in identifying appropriate thinking strategies. The more common or routine problems generally do not require sophisticated or advanced approaches.

Although the process of problem solving is presented in a linear format, the end result or a desired outcome is not always initially achieved. When this happens, assessment of the process is necessary to determine what additional information may be needed, what may need to be modified, or if new hypotheses need to be formulated (see Figure 3-1). Essential to competence and success in problem solving is the capability to consistently practice and participate in critical thinking.

Critical Thinking

Because of the abstract nature of **critical thinking**, a wide variety of definitions related to its skills and processes exist (Moulton et al., 2007; Shin et al., 2006). The essence of critical-thinking skills can be better described than defined. Critical-thinking skills are described as the ability to think logically, actively seeking out all dimensions of a situation for the purposes of conceptualizing, analyzing, synthesizing, and evaluating information gathered by observation, experience, reflection, reasoning, or communication for the purpose of guiding one's beliefs and actions. It should also be recognized and perceived as a process, a rational act used as a means rather than a result (Shin et al, 2006).

Critical thinking applies to both thinking models and is not confined to any specific thinking strategy. Critical thinking can be regarded as a combination of thinking strategies and types of thoughts. There is no magic formula that can be applied to these two components of critical thinking to ensure competence in critical thinking. Individuals develop their own skills in critical thinking. Combining these two components, in multiple ways, makes it is possible to identify characteristics and attributes that best describe critical thinkers (Box 3-1).

A significant feature that is crucial to develop critical-thinking skills and that is inherent within these characteristics is the ability to engage in **reflective thinking**, or thinking about thinking (Forneris & Peden-McAlpine, 2007). Reflective thinking facilitates examination of one's self for the purpose of developing self-awareness. Reflective thinking is also referred to as **meta-cognition** and requires taking time to deliberate, meditate, and contemplate situations in an unhurried manner so that a conclusion or resolution may be obtained in a reasonable and logical manner (Fletcher & Carruthers, 2012). The reflective approach considers the possibility of "if . . . then" relationships leading to appropriate outcomes. There is increasing recognition that reflective thinking is an essential attribute of competent health care providers (Mann, Gordon, & MacLeod, 2009). There is also the argument that critical reflection is an essential process for evidence based practice (Avis & Freshwater, 2006).

Reflective thinking is presumed to consist of five stages:

- State of doubt, confusion, or uncertainty resulting from difficulty in understanding a situation or solution to a problem;
- Defining the difficulty by purposeful examination of the attributes of the problem (analysis);
- Emergence of a possible explanation or solution to the problem using inductive thinking;

- Generation of alternative ideas and/or hypotheses through deductive reasoning; and
- Test new hypotheses (Mamede & Schmidt, 2004).

The essential outcome of reflective thinking, in addition to developing self-awareness, is to learn from past mistakes through recognition and identification of personal and contextual factors that contributed to the errors. Previous experiences or situations along with current patient information are reviewed to help identify and clarify possible relationships that exist within current or similar situations, producing new data that is integrated into new ways of perceiving and thinking that facilitates the pursuing of meaning, increasing self-awareness as well as sensitivity to the situation (Simpson & Courtney, 2007). Reflection as a process is an opportunity to improve decision making to prevent use of processes that contributed to past errors (Elder et al., 2007). Participating in reflective thinking provides oneself with feedback (Figure 3-2).

Feedback comes from a variety of sources and assists in refining and redefining possible reasons for or solutions to problems or altered health states. A common factor that has been identified as a cause of diagnostic error is the lack of feedback. There is an absence of systematic procedures in place to gauge the effectiveness of diagnostic decisions based on feedback related to outcomes (Schiff, 2008). This lack of feedback has been perpetuated by the perception of diagnosis as a single, one time activity. To remedy this, it is proposed to regard diagnosis as a dynamic, continuous process that requires revision and regenerating potential solutions over time

Box 3-1	Characteristics and Attributes of Critical Thinkers

Critical thinkers have inquiring minds, ask questions, and persist in the need to obtain the greatest amount of information possible so that their data base for decision making and problem solving is adequate.
Critical thinkers have a conscious knowledge of the limits of their knowledge, including an awareness of instances when one's instinctive egocentric thoughts are potentially deceptive, causing the individual to ignore or deny contradictory data. They also do not claim to know more than they actually do.
Critical thinkers evaluate all the aspects of a situation and consider alternative points of view before identifying specific problems and making decisions.
Critical thinkers are independent and not easily persuaded by others beliefs and arguments without carefully analyzing the overall situation and forming their own conclusions based on the data and analysis.
Critical thinkers are nonjudgmental and fair in their approach to the situation and do not make decisions or identify problems based on subjective and arbitrary data and attempt to remove prejudice and bias from their deliberations.
Critical thinkers are also capable of imaginatively putting themselves in the place of others to genuinely understand them. This also implies the ability to reconstruct with reasonable accuracy the viewpoints and reasoning of others and to reason from premises, assumptions, and ideas other than their own.
Critical thinkers have confidence that over time, individual and collective interests will be best served by giving the greatest freedom to reason so that individuals may reach their own conclusion and develop independent thought to formulate rational viewpoints, reach reasonable conclusions, and think coherently and logically.

Sources: Dillon, 2007; Green, 2000; Paul & Elder, 2001

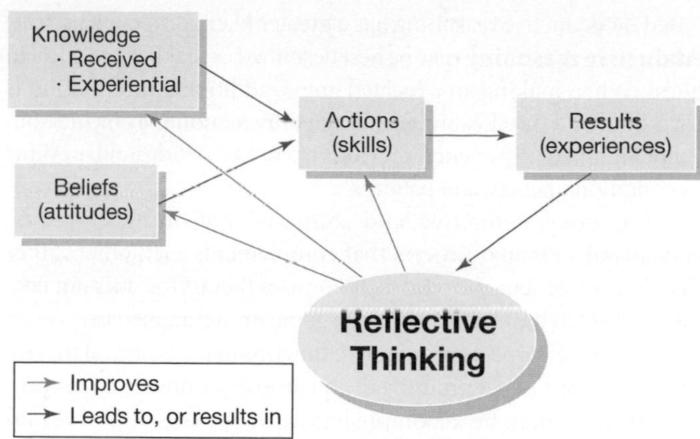

FIGURE 3-2 The Reflective Thinking Process

(Rudolph & Morrison, 2008). Reflective thinking is strengthened through the use of the processes of analysis and synthesis.

Analysis is the process in which a situation or activity is broken down into its component parts and individually examined. Once all of the component parts are identified and examined, the next step is synthesis. **Synthesis** is the process of reassembling the components into a logical and coherent whole so that rational judgments and solutions may be developed specific to the situation and/or health care needs of the patient.

From a problem-solving approach, synthesis is a process used to resolve contradictions and opposing ideas, to develop solutions and actions that promote balance, stability, and coherence, and to relieve any tension or stress from the presence of opposing or competing goals philosophies (Paletz & Peng, 2009). The inclination to consider and to reach logical and purposeful conclusions through synthesis is dependent on the recognition and use of dialectical thinking, as well as being tantamount to a well-developed reasoning ability.

Reasoning

Reasoning is a cognitive process based on principles of logic and is the ability to distinguish between fact (truth) and assumptions (beliefs) so that appropriate conclusions (diagnosis) or decisions may be formulated. Additionally, reasoning provides the basic justification and rationale for taking certain actions (Johnson & Webber, 2005). The ability to reason is a cognitive skill in humans, and is the differentiating characteristic that separates humans from animals. Well-developed critical-thinking skills are the foundation for achieving success at reasoning is demonstrated by the capacity to consciously recognize the need to change beliefs, attitudes, accepted practices, and other restrictions to facilitate autonomy and self-reliance.

Reasoning may be categorized into three types—inductive, deductive, and abductive. **Inductive reasoning** involves generalization, which requires going from specific to general. For example, when a patient who is overweight also reports shortness of breath during activity, it may be reasonable to conclude that all overweight patients will experience shortness of breath (SOB) during activity. This may seem to be a reasonable conclusion, however, there is no assurance that it is in fact true. In contrast, **deductive reasoning** involves going from general to specific. With deductive reasoning, conclusions are reached based on information obtained from a larger group. In this case, observations that many obese individuals also experience SOB make it reasonable to conclude that an obese individual will also experience shortness of breath. A conclusion based on deductive reasoning has a greater likelihood of being true. **Abductive reasoning** may be best described as making an educated guess. When making an educated guess, additional information is used to draw a conclusion. Additional information may include but is not limited to experience, previous encounters with similar events or conditions, beliefs, and patterns.

Inductive, deductive, and abductive reasoning should be considered a circular process that complements each other rather than linear that separates and dichotomizes them. One does not necessarily lead to the other, but may be going on simultaneously.

As with all aspects of cognitive functioning, it is critical to have criteria to assist in determining the quality of reasoning. Assessment of reasoning may be accomplished with the use of **Universal Intellectual Standards** (Paul & Elder, 2001). The nine universal standards are clarity, accuracy, precision, relevance, depth, breadth, logic, significance, and fairness. Table 3-1 provides questions that can be asked for each standard to help the provider gain an understanding of and internalize them.

The quality of reasoning may be determined by applying these universal intellectual standards to the process for the resolution of a problem, issue, or situation. It is crucial that critical thinkers have a thorough knowledge and understanding of these standards. The sequencing of these standards is not linear and not dependent on each other. These standards and their characteristics are not necessarily unique to certain individuals, but innate within everyone; however, they need to be recognized, exercised, and developed so that they become an integral component of thinking and the unconscious elements of reasoning.

As stated previously, reasoning frequently results in recognizing the need for change, which could be internal change (values, beliefs, ideals) or external change (environment, etc.). Either way, this is stressful and presents a significant challenge to many individuals. Change is less stressful and challenging and more likely to occur in individuals who are **open minded**. "Open mindedness is an intellectual virtue that involves a willingness to take relevant evidence and argument into account in forming or revising beliefs and values, especially when there is some reason [one] might resist such evidence and argument, with a view to arriving at true and defensible conclusions" (Hare, 2004, p. 3).

Open mindedness is the basis for divergent thinking. **Divergent thinking** is the ability of the provider to interpret a question or problem in multiple ways, as well as the ability to develop multiple answers to a question or problem (Abbasi, 2011). Divergent thinking is used when relevant data is separated from irrelevant data, pertinent data is analyzed, and various possibilities are explored to reach appropriate conclusions. Open mindedness should not be taken to imply that one's mind should be changed when there is evidence to the contrary. It only implies a willingness to change after carefully examining one's beliefs and values from a differing perspective. An open-minded person may still have firm convictions.

Table 3-1 Universal intellectual standards with application questions

Standard	Questions
Clarity	Are we referring to the same concept/subject? Could you give me an example or illustration? Could I or you express that point in another way?
Accuracy	How could we check on that? How reliable are our sources? How could we verify that?
Precision	Could I or you be more specific? Could I or you provide more details? Could I or you be more exact?
Relevance	How does this logically relate to the problem? How does this affect the question? How does that assist us with the issue?
Depth	What factors or issues make this a difficult problem? What are some of the complexities of this question? What are some of the difficulties we need to deal with?
Breadth	What other perspectives do I or we need to consider? What other points of view do I or we need to consider? What other ways of looking at this do I or we need to consider?
Logic	Does this logically all fit together? Does the conclusion/solution fit with the initial problem? Does the conclusion/solution relate to evidence?
Significance	Is this the most critical problem to consider? Is this the primary idea to focus on? Which of these facts are most important?
Fairness	Do I have a vested interest in this issue? Am I empathically representing the perspective of others? Am I or are we making assumptions that may bias our thinking?

Sources: R. Paul and Elder, L., 2005; Austin, 2012; Boettcher, 2009; Wolfe, N.D.

Clinical Decision Making

Reasoning is an important skill with significant implications for clinical practice. Reasoning used in clinical practice is most commonly identified as **clinical decision making** (Simmons, 2010), **clinical diagnostic reasoning** (Bowen, 2006), or **clinical judgment** (Tanner, 2006). While there may be slight differences in how these terms are defined or described, for all intents and purposes they all encompass the essence of clinical decision making. Clinical decision making is a process in which critical thinking skills and reasoning are applied holistically to patient data for the purposes of identifying specific health-related needs or pathologic problems. Additionally, clinical decision making is also used to identify specific areas for intervention to alleviate the problem, or to assist the patient to cope with a situation when no cure exists or is available. In health care terms, clinical decision making results in some form of a conclusion. In health care clinical decision making results in the formulation of a **diagnosis**, which is identification of the nature of the patient's health or health care needs.

Diagnosis, as a generic descriptor, is not necessarily limited in its use to any specific discipline or profession. A diagnosis simply represents identification of a problem that needs to be addressed in a specific way. A diagnosis may be developed in different ways in various disciplines, but the development of a diagnosis is carried out by many disciplines, those that are health care related and those that are not. For example, a car mechanic diagnoses specific problems within the working structures of the car; a plumber formulates a diagnosis regarding a problem with the pipes and drainage system of a building. In any instance, a diagnosis, or problem identification, must be formulated so that appropriate interventions may be implemented to eliminate or reduce the effects of the disease, injury, or condition.

The purpose and function of diagnosis, however, differs among disciplines. Within health care, a **medical diagnosis** identifies a specific pathological condition that requires specific medical interventions to treat and/or cure it. In contrast, a **nursing diagnosis** identifies areas in which nursing interventions would be appropriate to assist the patient in coping with the pathological condition or health alteration. Nursing diagnoses identify areas in which nurses may intervene independently and may not necessarily be under direct orders from physicians. In areas where both nursing and medical interventions are necessary, **collaborative practice** is appropriate.

Advanced Practice Nurses (APNs/APRNs) receive advanced education to prepare them to make a medical diagnosis regarding the patient's health status. The parameters of their practice and independent diagnostic privileges and treatment modalities are governed by each state's nurse practice act. Other individuals who are educated and legally allowed to medically diagnose patient's conditions are physician assistants (PAs), who work specifically with and are directly responsible to a physician.

Regardless of which health care provider develops a diagnosis, the process remains the same and follows a systematic, methodical approach, which closely mirrors the problem solving process as depicted in Table 3-2.

Problem Identification

The initial step for both processes is the identification of an apparent problem. It is commonly described by the patient in general terms or manifestations most likely related to the problem. An individual who may be experiencing a myocardial infarction is more than likely to describe the problem as chest pain and not specifically state the problem as a myocardial infarction. In the same context, an individual is most likely to describe a problem with an automobile as a symptom, for example, the car won't start rather than the battery is dead. In both situations, the patient and the car owner may have an idea of what the real problem is but don't necessarily have the knowledge, tools, or tests available to confirm the actual problem.

Data Collection

Data collection by the health care provider may occur prior to actually meeting the patient. Data collected at this point may be described as pre-assessment data. Pre-assessment data is obtained by word of mouth and written material.

Table 3-2 Comparison of diagnosis development and problem-solving processes

Problem Solving	Diagnosis Development
Identify the problem	Chief complaint (patient problem)
Collect relevant data from several sources	Data collection (history, physical exam, additional data) Accurate presentation of problem (framing)
Formulate hypothesis	Preliminary diagnosis Synthesis of data (differential diagnoses) Formulation of diagnosis
Plan ways to test hypothesis (diagnosis)	Develop treatment plan (management)
Implement tests	Interventions
Interpret the results	Outcomes

Data that is gathered by word of mouth may come from conversations with other health care personnel who have previously interacted with the patient. It must, however, be remembered that this information may be biased and influenced by prior experiences and interactions that may be positive or negative. Preliminary data may also come from information recorded in the patient's medical record, lab tests, admission records, and from family members.

Following the gathering of pre-assessment data, the provider–patient encounter occurs. This initial interaction with the patient allows the provider to formulate a preliminary analysis of the patient's situation and condition. The preliminary data is obtained by observing the overall presentation of the patient as well as paying attention to other manifestations related to sounds and odors that may or may not be associated with the patient's problem. After the initial encounter, the provider begins the collection of subjective (history) and objective (examination) data. Chapters 4 and 5 detail interviewing techniques and how to gather a health history (subjective data) and perform a physical exam, respectively.

Inherent within the data collection process is the recognition and acquisition of cues and inferences. A **cue** may be defined as identifiable physiological or psychosocial changes experienced by the patient, perceived through history or assessment and understood in relation to a specific body of knowledge and philosophical beliefs (Levett-Jones et al., 2010; Mast, 2007; Roter et al., 2006). Cues in essence relate to and are comparable to nonverbal behaviors which are communicative behaviors that are not expressed linguistically (Mast, 2007; Roter et al., 2006). How the patient answers questions, changes or inflections in the tone of voice, the facial expressions demonstrated during the history may all be considered as cues that can point towards ideas, worries, or expectations the patient has not shared before (Hartnab & Ravesteijn, 2008).

Cues also serve to formulate inferences and influence decision making. **Inferences** are judgments or mini-conclusions based on factual data that go beyond the data to make statements about something not presently known about the relationship between data (Wilkinson, 2012). Making an inference requires transitioning from one proposition or judgment that is considered true to another proposition that is also considered true based on the truthfulness of the original proposition. Inferences may also be derived from **pattern recognition** based on patient cues. Pattern recognition is a method where the provider uses past experience to recognize patterns of clinical characteristics. Over time, there emerges a consistency of clues that are associated with specific disease processes or conditions. The ability to interpret cues, make inferences, and recognize patterns develops over time with practice and experience. It is an essential internal process that cannot necessarily be identified or taught.

PRACTICE POINT: Inferences vs. Assumptions

Inferences are not to be confused with assumptions. Assumptions are something that is taken for granted based on information or something that is previously learned and is believed to be true. Inferences may be based on assumptions as they are believed to be true (Paul & Elder, 2012).

Accurate Presentation of Problem (Framing)

Tantamount to formulating a correct diagnosis is a well-formulated problem or problems. The quantities of data collected as well as its quality are significant determinants of problem identification. Problems must often be "constructed from circumstances that are puzzling, troubling, uncertain, and possibly irrelevant" (Crandall & Wears, 2008). From this data, the provider starts, "almost subconsciously, to frame or contextualize the patient's problem as a clinically meaningful representation (Scott, 2009).

Framing is a cognitive shortcut used to develop or construct a schema or a view point of a situation that reasonably represents the situation or problem (Bednarz, 2012). It is a process of interpreting complex data in a way that allows for the development of a solution. An individual's frames are constructed through his or her experience, values, beliefs, culture, and form the basis for the perception and interpretation of stimuli. Additionally, frames function to help the individual understand and interpret the world and environment, and attribute meaning to one's context. How a problem is represented is significantly influenced by how an individual's frame is developed.

It is essential that the provider develop a meaningful interpretation of patient data to develop an authentic and realistic frame of the patient's problem. This is accomplished through analysis of patient data, progressing through four steps.

Ordering and Arranging Data

Data is initially organized by ordering and arranging the data into logical groups or clusters, either by system or region of the body. This process is also referred to as **classification**, which is an essential process for making sense out of situations or conditions. Initially the beginning or novice provider will consciously have to work on organizing and arranging these data; however, with time, practice, and an increased knowledge base the provider will become experienced and competent, and develop expertise so that this activity will become automatic and require very little conscious effort. The novice provider must also learn to differentiate between cues that are relevant and those that are not (Hoffman, Aitken, & Duffield, 2009).

Assess the Significance of and Prioritize the Clustered Data

Relationships between and within the clusters and data clusters themselves must be determined so that problem(s) may be identified and probable cause(s) may be found. Relationships and connections between data clusters are aided by recognition and interpretation of cues and inferences.

Preliminary Diagnosis/Probable Cause

When data that is characteristic of common or frequent illnesses or conditions, a preliminary diagnosis may be a final one also. However, in many instances, but not all, the data is not characteristic of common disorders and there is a degree of uncertainty about what is actually causing the problem. In such instances, multiple hypotheses may be necessary and formulated. This does not necessarily indicate poor or faulty diagnostic reasoning, but is more likely to be due to inadequate or ambiguous data, or indeterminate relationships or patterns. Providers with less clinical experience and knowledge are more likely to generate multiple diagnoses.

In simplistic terms, the probable origin or cause contributing to the patient's condition can be related to three classifications of altered processes: pathological, pathophysiological, or psychopathological. **Pathological causes** are alterations that affect the structure of the body, bones, muscle, and tissues. Appendicitis and bone fractures would both be considered pathological alterations. **Pathophysiological causes** are alterations in structure as well as function. Hepatitis (inflammation of the liver) causes structural alterations as well as changes to the various functions of the liver. **Psychopathological causes** are alterations in thought and emotions. Anxiety, depression, and bi-polar conditions are examples of these types of alterations.

A fourth category is related to the **patient's human responses** to the altered process(es). This is considered the practice focus of nursing and encompasses multiple dimensions of the individual. These dimensions were fully described in Chapter 1. Broadly speaking, human responses are physiological, psychological, emotional, cultural, and spiritual in nature and are based on the patient data. Manifestations of these responses can be further classified according to specific domains or taxonomy of responses. The North American Nursing Diagnosis Association (NANDA) has developed 13 domains that comprise the nature of human responses (Carpenito-Moyet, 2008) (Box 3-2).

Box 3-2 Thirteen NANDA Domains

1. Activity/Rest
2. Comfort
3. Coping/Stress Tolerance
4. Elimination
5. Growth/Development
6. Health Promotion
7. Life Principles
8. Nutrition
9. Perception/Cognition
10. Role Relationships
11. Safety/Protection
12. Self-perception
13. Sexuality

Synthesis of Data

The overall goal at this step is to assess the data or obtain additional data that permits the provider to accept, reject, or modify any preliminary diagnostic hypotheses that are under consideration. A crucial systematic method of identifying unknowns by comparing and clarifying possible diagnoses is described as **differential diagnosis**. A differential diagnosis is essentially a process of the elimination of improbable diagnoses.

In instances where a presenting sign, symptom, or response may have multiple causes, it is essential to determine what the specific cause is. This may be critical to diagnosing potential life threatening conditions. While intuitive thinking may be a starting point for differentiating, analytical thinking skills are best utilized in differential diagnosis. Relying on intuitive thinking may result in a premature diagnostic conclusion with failure to consider the correct diagnosis (Ely, Graber, & Croskerry, 2011).

The process of differential diagnosis begins with careful symptom analysis. This is discussed in depth in Chapter 6.

A careful analysis of history data is essential to determine if there is the need for additional data. Additional data comes from various sources. Sometimes asking the same question in a different way will get the needed data. For example, data the patient does not consider important may be obtained in this way. Also, do not assume that the patient has provided all the data. It is not unusual for the patient to give as a reason for not initially providing the data "You didn't ask me about that." Past experiences with patients (patterns, heuristics, etc.) with similar data are reviewed and comparisons made for similarities and differences. Additional data is also obtained from consultation with colleagues, review of texts, and Internet resources. Additional tests (body fluid analysis, radiological scans) may also be needed.

Certain conditions or disorders do not have specific standardized criterion or characteristic manifestations that allow for an accurate determination of cause. Conditions and disorders of this type can only be diagnosed by elimination of other probable causes of the health problem. Elimination of diagnoses is identified as **ruling out**.

> *THINK LINK: Ruling Out (Multiple Sclerosis)*
> Multiple sclerosis (MS) is a pathological condition that can only be diagnosed by ruling out other causes. No definitive test or procedure to establish a diagnosis of MS currently exists. MS is a neurological condition that causes the destruction of the myelin covering of nerves, which impedes the conduction of nerve impulses to the muscles. The symptoms can vary depending on which nerves are affected and initial symptoms may be vague and nondescript, and may characterize other neurological conditions. Once all other possible causes for the symptoms and manifestations are ruled out, a diagnosis of MS can be made.

Establish the Diagnosis/Making a Clinical Judgment

The final step is the formulation and identification of a diagnosis. Depending on the discipline, a medical or nursing diagnosis is developed. Every activity thus far has been a process of distilling the data to a point in which a simple or single statement identifies or describes the nature of the patient's health condition and responses. A diagnosis provides direction for the plan of care related to the appropriateness and scope of practice of the respective discipline.

Once the diagnosis has been established it must be validated. Multiple individuals may enter into this activity. First, the patient must be made aware of the diagnosis and/or problem and determine if it explains what the individual may be experiencing. Other health care providers may also be consulted as to whether they agree or disagree with the diagnosis and/or problem and may be asked to confirm the diagnosis based on their experience and expertise. Other types of data, such as laboratory data, x-rays, and scans, may be obtained to confirm the diagnosis.

Another means to validate the diagnosis is to evaluate whether the problem was solved or disappeared after the interventions were implemented. This may take a little longer, but it does confirm that the diagnosis was correct and that appropriate interventions alleviated the situation and/or solved the problem.

While clinical decision making essentially ends with the formulation of a diagnosis, the overall problem solving process does not end. However, for the purposes of this text, formulating a diagnosis will be the terminal step. Developing a plan to test the hypothesis (diagnosis), implementation or interventions are required to appropriately treat the patient, and interpretation or evaluation of the results are essential to providing quality health care.

Diagnostic Errors

Despite critical thinking and using the clinical reasoning process, the possibility of making a diagnostic error always exists. Any health care provider that formulates a diagnosis is capable of making a diagnostic error. One of the difficulties in determining the magnitude of diagnostic errors is there is no valid method to measure errors (Winters, Aswani, & Pronovost, 2011). Autopsies, which have been the standard for determining diagnostic errors, have found that error rates occur at 10%–20% (Scott, 2009). This rate of errors translates into 44,000–98,000 deaths annually attributed to medical errors (Mamede, Schmidt, & Rikers, 2007). This error rate has remained relatively consistent over a number or years.

> *THINK LINK: Human Error*
> The high numbers of deaths related to diagnostic errors is staggering. In most instances, the finger is pointed at the diagnostician as the cause of error, assuming that a human was responsible for the error. While the human is ultimately responsible for making the diagnosis, there are multiple variables that contribute to the context in which the error in diagnosis occurred. Reason (2000) identified two approaches for evaluating errors. A **person approach** focuses on who made the error and efforts to reduce error focus on reducing variability in human behavior. A **systems approach** assumes that humans are fallible and that errors are inevitable, not because of human causes, but as a consequence of system contexts and factors. A systems approach considers human factors as only a part of the error and not the totality of the problem.

Diagnostic Error Categories

Graber, Franklin, and Gordon (2005) developed a taxonomy of diagnostic error categories that was based on three primary types of errors:

- **No fault errors**
  - Masked or unusual presentation of disease
  - Patient-related error (uncooperative, deceptive)
- **System-related errors**
  - Technical failure and equipment problems
  - Organizational flaws
- **Cognitive errors**
  - Faulty knowledge
  - Faulty data gathering
  - Faulty synthesis

No Fault Errors

No fault errors, while they may cause significant errors, are errors in which no known remedial action can be taken to prevent them from reoccurring. To some extent these may also be perceived to be patient-focused errors because they are dependent on the patient's ability to describe the symptoms accurately and cooperate with providers. Withholding information or providing incorrect information may be deliberate on the part of the patient to prevent disclosure of information that may be perceived to be detrimental to the patient's persona or well-being. A significant contribution to no-fault errors is an atypical or masked disease presentation.

System or Process Errors

System or process errors are rather clear cut and generally have remedial processes that exist or need to be developed to eliminate them as a contributing factor to diagnostic errors. A small percentage of system errors have been found to be related to technical and equipment malfunction or failure. Other causes included lack of awareness or knowledge of policies and procedures, or inefficient processes (Graber et al., 2005). The major contributor to diagnostic errors and is increasingly recognized as a preventable factor in medical mishaps is communication breakdown or failures (Singh et al., 2007), which includes inadequate or inefficient teamwork and failure to inform others of significant data.

Cognitive Errors

Cognitive errors are provider-caused errors that need to be identified so that remediating activities can be put in place to reduce or eliminate their impact on diagnosis development. Cognitive errors are primarily related to faulty or inadequate clinical reasoning skills (Scott, 2009) related to knowledge, data, or synthesis.

Faulty knowledge can be primarily attributed to lack of experience or familiarity with a specific condition or disease. Lack of knowledge often facilitates the novice provider to use intuitive-humanistic, nonanalytical thinking. At this point, the novice's knowledge base is inadequate to support hypothetico-deductive, analytical thinking. Unfortunately, the remediation for this type of error is dependent on time and experience, over which the novice provider does not have any control.

Faulty data gathering can have a significant effect on formulating accurate diagnoses. Faulty data gathering may result from incomplete data, inadequate data, and incorrect interpretation of data. Steps to remediate these errors again are somewhat time dependent, allowing the novice provider to gain experience in obtaining data efficiently as well as developing skill in interviewing and history taking. Asking the appropriate questions for symptom analysis is also necessary. The quality of clinical reasoning is only as effective as the quantity and quality of data that the provider has available to analyze and synthesize.

Faulty synthesis may also be perceived to be faulty critical thinking or clinical reasoning. A significant aggregate of cognitive errors that are associated with critical-thinking errors are collectively described as **cognitive dispositions to respond** (CDR), which are correlated with failures in perception, failed heuristics, and biases (Croskerry, 2003). Biases are the most common type of CDRs, predisposing the provider to be overly influenced by certain personal or professional beliefs and attitudes.

Personal biases are most often associated with **egocentric thinking**. Egocentric thinking results from individuals not considering or recognizing other's needs, rights, and points of view. Egocentric thinking also results from individuals not recognizing or accepting the limitations of their own points of view. It is highly unlikely that egocentric thinking is recognized in oneself unless there is a conscious effort to overcome it. Egocentric thinking is also seen as a means of self-preservation by preventing anything from causing one to think differently and possibly make changes. Egocentric thinking may be overcome or eliminated by becoming culturally competent, as described and outlined in Chapter 2.

Professional/**cognitive biases** have more to do with factors that are related to and influence decision making and critical thinking. These may be influenced by personal biases, but not always. A sample of cognitive biases is presented in Table 3-3.

Remediation for faulty synthesis and CDRs is primarily dependent on **reflective thinking** or **meta-cognition**. Reflective thinking could also be perceived to be an analysis of the original frame. As previously discussed reflective thinking is accomplished through reexamining the steps of the critical thinking process and attempting to discern cause and affect errors in thinking. Critical reflection regarding professional practice has been identified as essential for maintaining and improving provider expertise (Mamede et al., 2007).

Table 3-3 Examples of cognitive biases and errors

Cognitive Biases	Error
Availability heuristic	Tendency to conclude diagnoses as more likely if they are more easily retrievable from memory as well as past experience with similar cases
Base rate neglect	Tendency to ignore the true rate of disease and pursue rare but more exotic diagnosis
Representativeness	Tendency to be guided by prototypical features of disease or health state and miss atypical variants
Confirmation bias	Tendency to seek data to confirm, not refute, the hypothesis
Premature closure (anchoring heuristic)	Tendency to stop too soon and not order the critical test or gather the critical information
Attribution	Tendency to attribute symptoms to wrong cause based on negative stereotypes
Affective error	Tendency to prefer what is hoped will happen to the less appealing alternatives; information that fulfills desires is valued too highly
Framing effects	Diagnostic decision making unduly biased by subtle cues and collateral information
Blind obedience	Placing undue reliance on test results or "expert" opinion

Sources: Ely et al, 2011; Hicks et al, 2011; Norman, 2010; Croskerry, 2002

As previously pointed out, a common factor that has been identified as a cause of diagnostic error is an absence of systematic procedures in place to gauge the effectiveness of diagnostic decisions based on feedback related to outcomes (Schiff, 2008). Lack of feedback means that learning has not occurred.

Factors Influencing Critical Thinking and Clinical Reasoning

Diagnostic errors are multivariable in their origin and are somewhat unpredictable in nature. While most diagnostic errors are related to cognitive factors, there are other influences that affect the quality of clinical reasoning. The ability to control any of these factors is dependent on the ability to recognize the existence and presence of any of these factors through reflection and meta-cognition.

Time Constraints

Time constraints are a significant potential barrier to critical thinking. This is especially characteristic of decision making in emergency rooms. Critical-thinking skills are used most advantageously in situations in which time is not important and interventions are not required immediately. When time is limited, heuristics are frequently used; however, they are often inaccurate and demonstrate a high degree of catastrophic failure (Croskerry, 2003).

Experience Level

Obviously the amount of experience the provider has will determine the proficiency in all areas of health care. Students entering health care disciplines will most likely be novices in all areas and for purposes of this text, novices in collection of data.

As with any skill acquisition, practice makes perfect, thus, the more opportunities to practice the skill, the more proficient and expert one will become.

Most skill performance and cognitive processes go through stages of transition in their learning and practice. The most common framework for assessing skill acquisition, learning, and performance is based on a **novice to expert continuum**. The levels between novice and expert vary from three to five, depending on which theorist is used to conceptualize the process.

Individuals in the novice category are beginning to understand and learn specific skills and/or cognitive processes. They are generally unsure of their abilities and follow a well-defined or delineated process. Thinking (or conscious awareness) precedes performance. As they practice, they become more confidant demonstrate qualitative differences as they progress through the intermediate states (Moulton et al, 2007). These intermediate stages represent increasing confidence and competence in the performance of the skills and processes. The intermediate steps may be defined as a singular stage of competence or as three stages: advanced beginner, competence, and proficiency. Eventually one becomes an expert where practice becomes experience-based, integrating intuitive knowing, recognizing how thinking and performance occur simultaneously.

While definitions differentiate between levels, the transition from one level to the next is not well defined; neither is there an accurate or agreed upon definition of expert. Qualitatively, expert performance in diagnostic reasoning has been described as a combination of knowledge based reasoning skills, and an accumulation of experiences with patients that is qualitatively different from that of competent and beginner (practitioners) (Crespo, Torres, & Recio, 2004).

Overconfidence

Overconfidence, or an over estimation of one's perception of accuracy and actual accuracy, has been identified as another frequent cause of diagnostic error (Jolly & Atkinson, 2009). Overconfidence, however, is a universal, innate characteristic of humans, and is often the result of a fear of being perceived as weak and uncertain. There is a stigma associated with lack of confidence and inability to determine the cause of patient's conditions.

A significant diagnostic error associated with overconfidence is premature closure or failure to consider alternative explanations or causes. Premature closure has been found to be the result of faulty or inadequate data synthesis (Graber et al., 2005).

Diagnostic Complexity

Clinical decision making (diagnostic reasoning) is not a well-defined process but a complex process based on scientific reasoning and critical thinking skills; however, it is also an art. The art of clinical decision making relates to the ability to analyze and synthesize the data efficiently and effectively. The range of diagnostic complexity tasks are determined by the quantity of conditions that the patient may have as well as the number of cues related to those conditions.

The simplest diagnostic task is to determine the presence or absence of a condition based on one cue. A child with whooping cough has a distinctive cough, which is characteristic of the condition. There might be other cues that would support a diagnosis of whooping cough, but its presence could be determined by one cue. The most complex diagnostic task would be the presence of two or more conditions with multiple cues. A significant contribution to complexity is **comorbidity**, in which a patient has coexisting health conditions which may or may not be related to the presenting condition. Patients with comorbid conditions present a challenge for diagnostic reasoning as multiple cues are present, making separating and combining the cues a very complex exercise. Also contributing to clinical complexity is the concept of holism and holistic care, which recognizes the integration and adaptation of multiple systems. Such a complex adaptive system may act in ways that are not predictable and whose actions often change the context for other interconnected systems and its actions.

Memory/Recall

Success in critical thinking and clinical reasoning also depends on the ability to recall significant aspects of past experiences and compare those aspects with the present situation is critical in analysis and synthesis of data. Obviously, the greater number of experiences one has gone through increases the amount of information that can be recalled.

Memory is categorized into three components: sensory, short-term, and long term. **Sensory memory** is comprised of information that is acquired through the senses from internal and external environments. For retention of sensory memory, attention to the particular stimulus must be given to them so that it can be classified and sent to working memory for further action.

Relationships between sensory stimuli and experiences need to be recognized so that appropriate actions may be taken. These actions then often regulate reflexive or automated responses.

Short-term memory is concerned with current activities and recent, relevant information. Short-term memory is also referred to as **working memory** (WM), as this is a more accurate description of the activities and time limitations that occur in this component. Working memory is limited in its information storage capacity as well as the length of time information is available. Unless other processing is used to maintain memory, 15–20 seconds is the amount of time that WM is stored.

In contrast, **long-term memory** (LTM) is the section of the memory system that is the repository for information that is held for longer than seconds or minutes. It appears that LTM has an infinite capability for amount and time of storage. The speed at which data from LTM can be recalled varies between individuals. Difficulty in recalling stored memory is frequently identified as forgetfulness. However, forgetting does not represent the actual difficulty; any difficulty encountered with LTM is more likely related to access and retrieval.

Personal Variability

Factors that contribute to the provider's context have to do with temporary intrapersonal factors such as one's physical, mental, and emotional states. Physical alterations, for example fatigue, sleep deprivation, and sleep debt will also affect critical thinking and decision making (Croskerry, 2006). These conditions or situations cause circadian rhythm disruption, which can have detrimental effects on an individual's attempts to solving complex or nonroutine problems (Kuhn, 2002). Pain and/or illness, as well as emotional distress (anxiety, anger, and depression) are also factors affecting the provider's performance level.

Much of assessment is dependent on sensory input and its interpretation. Anything that affects the provider's sensory organs, for example, head cold, allergies, or lost contact, will affect the provider's assessment capabilities.

Nonintrapersonal factors that affect the context include the physical setting and use and familiarity with equipment (diagnostic and computers).

Summary

- Problem solving is the foundation for all scientific disciplines and parallels the steps of scientific method that consists of six steps.
- Two frameworks or models of thinking processes are used for critical thinking and problem solving: the hypothetico-deductive model and the intuitive-humanist model.
- Critical thinkers use different forms of thinking and types of thoughts.
- Critical thinking is essential for decision making and diagnostic/clinical reasoning. Critical-thinking skills are developed and not necessarily taught. They are best developed in situations in which the provider must be disciplined when beginning to look at relationships between data that is obtained and all the environmental influences that affect the patient and the patient's actual health status.
- Clinical decision making is a parallel process to problem solving.
- The process of formulating a diagnosis consists of six essential steps.
- Diagnostic/clinical reasoning is prone to errors that may be the result of human (patient/provider) factors or system (organizational) factors.

Review Questions

1. The provider utilizes reflexive thinking in patient care situations where
   1. creative solutions are needed.
   2. protocols are expected to be followed.
   3. intuitive thinking is impractical.
   4. the purpose or goal of thinking is unclear.
2. The provider separates patient data into subjective and objective data and examines these components. This process of examining the component parts of a situation or condition is called which of the following?
   1. analysis
   2. decomposition
   3. synthesis
   4. comparison
3. A patient in the third trimester of pregnancy reports urinary frequency. The provider tells the patient that "urinary frequency is common in late pregnancy." This response is the result of which type of thinking?
   1. trial and error
   2. intuitive
   3. inductive
   4. egocentric
4. When addressing the needs of a patient with multiple complicated problems, the provider asks, "Which of these problems is most important?" By asking this the provider is addressing which of the following?
   1. depth of the problem
   2. breadth of the problem
   3. significance of the problem
   4. relevance of the problem
5. When making clinical decisions related to patient care, the provider makes these decisions based on processing information that primarily consists of which of the following?
   1. innuendos
   2. hints
   3. tips
   4. cues
6. The provider has asked several colleagues to review a difficult patient situation and offer opinions to be considered before making decisions. In this situation the provider is displaying what intellectual virtue?
   1. open mindedness
   2. communication skills
   3. autonomy
   4. intuition
7. The provider identified that a new patient is at risk for impaired skin integrity due to prolonged immobility. This is an example of which of the following? (Select all that apply.)
   1. medical diagnosis
   2. nursing diagnosis
   3. intervention
   4. evaluation
   5. problem
8. The provider is reviewing preassessment data on a new patient. The type of data that the provider may be reviewing during this process includes which of the following? (Select all that apply.)
   1. operative reports from prior surgeries
   2. most recent laboratory reports
   3. letters from referring providers
   4. objective physical examination data
   5. insurance company authorizations
9. After gathering assessment data the provider concludes that the patient's complaints of a rash are likely due to exposure to a substance to which the patient has a known allergy. The provider would categorize this patient's problem as which of the following?
   1. pathological
   2. pathophysiological
   3. psychopathological
   4. psychosomatic
10. The provider is working with a provider who tends to seek data that will confirm the provider's assumptions about a patient's diagnosis, rather than look at all data.

    This is characteristic of which of the following?
    1. premature closure
    2. affective error
    3. confirmation bias
    4. attribution

4

The Context of Interviewing

We had been taught, over the course of 6 months, how to conduct each part of the interview. There was a recommended order—the chief complaint, history of present illness, past medical history, social history, family history, allergies, and medications. We had practiced this dozens of times with standardized patients from "gelling in" and introduction down to the final handshake. My evaluations always praised my "excellent rapport-building skills" and "unique ability to put the patients at ease." Then why am I so nervous now? Standing against the wall outside of B324, my first real patient's room, my heart races and my hands feel clammy. I just need to follow the routine I've done so many times before, but now I'm at a complete loss. What is the first question I'm supposed to ask? Is it even a question? Maybe I'll just say my name first and shake hands. I look at the piece of paper and pen I'm holding—maybe I'll leave them in my pocket and pull them out when the time is right. OK, stop thinking so much, just go inside!

"*Mr. Leonard!*" I practically shout, hand outstretched, as I bound toward the head of the bed.

Mr. Leonard's eyes spring open and he starts to shake violently under the covers. "*Oh! You half scared me to death!*" I probably should have knocked first. "*Aren't you going to wash your hands? I don't want your hospital germs getting me in worse trouble than I already am,*" he says, turning on his right side and coughing up some mucus. Right, I should have washed my hands first.

"*My apologies, sir, let me ...*" I trail off as Mr. Leonard coughs again heavily and empties more mucus into a cup. "*I'm sorry, sir, I ...*" His coughing grows louder and more abrasive, drowning out my words. In the throes of a short gasp of air, he stammers, "I don't want to talk right now!"

"Okay nice meeting you!" I turn for the door and am back in the hallway in record time. This isn't exactly the standardized patient experience I was expecting, and not at all how I imagined my first day on the clinical unit. It seems that, despite my training and preparation, my skills at the patient interview will be developed slowly, through real situations and struggles.

Interviewing is a clinical skill that is essential to every professional health care provider. Every patient interaction includes some aspect of interviewing, making it a critical component of the overall management of patient care. Interviewing is the primary means for obtaining historical or subjective data.

LEARNING OUTCOMES

1. Summarize the concepts and skills necessary to conduct an effective interview.
2. Compare and contrast therapeutic and nontherapeutic communication techniques.
3. Explain ways to establish rapport and a trusting relationship with the patient.
4. Recognize patient and environmental variables that affect the interview.
5. Formulate various types of questions used in conducting the interview.
6. Explain challenging situations that can occur and how to remain focused during the interview.

Principles of Interviewing

The ability to conduct effective interviews is a skill that is constantly used and refined; it is the primary source of patient information. Each patient is unique with individual health care needs that can only be identified and expressed by each patient. Investing time in the initial interview has long-term benefits for both the patient and the provider. As in all situations, interviewing occurs within a particular context. Successful patient interviews are guided by six basic principles that create an appropriate context for effective interviewing. The interview is effective to the degree that the provider does the following:

1. Allows and promotes freedom of expression by patients
2. Establishes, understands, and communicates the goals for the interview effectively
3. Relates to and accepts the patient unconditionally and without using value judgments
4. Recognizes, examines, encourages, and clarifies mutual thoughts and feelings that may affect care management
5. Assesses patient needs, management goals, and the behavioral responses to care provided consistently
6. Demonstrates and encourages the use of feedback with patients in conveying, implementing, and evaluating care management goals.

Data obtained from the interview is essential for appropriate, individualized care. Patient information obtained throughout the interview can be classified into six types:

1. **Descriptive**—an account of a narration by the patient regarding a happening or event in which the patient was a participant or an observer.
2. **Perception**—an account or explanation of the extent and nature of the information the patient has at a basic level, the amount of information that one has, and in what form it is perceived.
3. **Behaviors**—a determination of what the patient did, what has been done, what will be done or what actions by others have been observed.
4. **Attitudes and beliefs**—the identification of underlying assumptions or premises on which the respondent's comments and judgments are based.
5. **Feelings**—the respondent's account of physical, emotional and other feelings as well as the revelation of these through observation of personal physical reactions during the interview.
6. **Values**—the patients identification of those attributes, possessions, beliefs, actions that are considered good or bad, desirable or undesirable.

The patient interview is a fundamental clinical skill for every health care provider, but is especially critical for primary care disciplines (Beck, Daughtridge, & Sloane, 2002). Frequently, interviewing the patient is the first opportunity the provider has to interact with the patient and begin establishing rapport. Environments and settings where an interview is performed, and the scope of the data needed vary, depending on the condition and needs of the patient (Figure 4-1). The skills required to perform an interview, however, do not change.

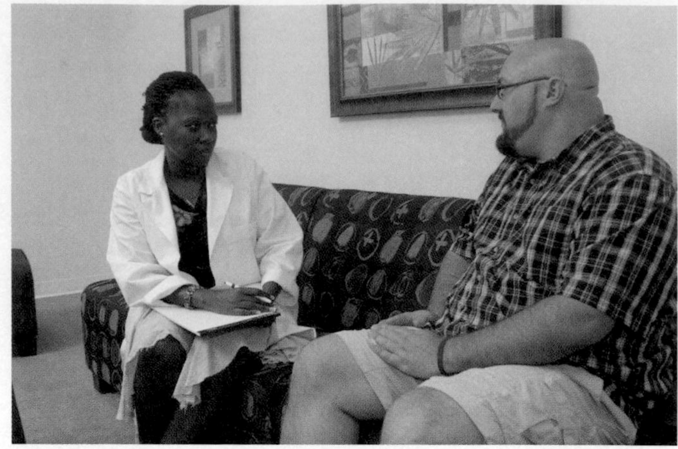

FIGURE 4-1 The patient interview may occur in a variety of settings

Interviewing Concepts

The foundation underlying competency in any skill is based on the recognition and understanding of the specific and unique characteristics and requirements related to implementation of that skill. The development of a provider's competence and skill in interviewing is subject to this same principle. Characteristics that are essential to understanding and implementing dynamic interviewing are (1) objectivity, (2) precision, and (3) reliability/validity (Coulenan & Block, 2006).

Objectivity

Objectivity during the interview is incorporated by eliminating prior personal prejudices, beliefs, and preconceptions or making any judgmental observations. Objectivity requires the provider to recognize these traits and disengage from them.

Objectivity during the interview helps ensure the accuracy and validity of the history data. It is highly unlikely that individuals can remove every bias and preconception; however, the greater one's awareness of these beliefs and attitudes, the greater the probability that they may be suppressed to obtain data that is as accurate and valid as possible.

Inability to remove biases and preconceived ideas prior to and during the interview leads to devaluing certain patient data and/or ignoring other pertinent data. Providers may come to a wrong conclusion regarding the patient's condition(s), resulting in an improper diagnosis. For example, a provider who believes all obese individuals are psychologically maladjusted and is unable to recognize that this stereotype and belief negatively influences the ability to relate to obese patients, might be biased in understanding the patient's responses to interview questions. Data that might contradict one's personal beliefs would most likely be ignored, and additional data that might help determine the specific health care needs of this individual would not be obtained, resulting in data that is inaccurate and invalid.

Precision

Precision refers to how a provider creates detailed descriptions and also removes any ambiguity from the data. Data from the interview must be meaningful and explicit for all members of the health care team. Data obtained during the interview consists of words—words that the patient uses to tell a story that consists of experienced situations and sensations. The patient's descriptions must be detailed enough so that there are similar interpretations of these situations and sensations. Precision is attained through appropriate questioning of the patient to get the pertinent details.

> ***PRACTICE POINT: Transitioning Between Topics***
> The provider should identify when a topic in the health history is going to change. This is also called *bridging*. When going from system to system for example, say to the patient, "I'm now going to ask you some questions about your lungs/heart." This transition sets the context for the next set of questions. Going from one system to another without bridging sets the patient up for providing wrong or inaccurate information. While you have access to the sequence of questions, remember that the patient does not, so to make sure you are both going in the same direction, let the patient know what the journey is going to be.

The provider who fails to be precise in data collection will have ambiguous data that is relatively meaningless. As with failure to be objective, failure in precision results in the inability to draw appropriate conclusions about the patient's health status. For instance, if a patient indicates he is experiencing chest pain, it is critical that the provider obtain further data to provide a detailed, precise description of this symptom so that it is properly identified. Although chest pain may be the initial description, multiple causes exist for chest pain, each with its own unique characteristics. The provider's failure to identify these characteristics properly leads to inappropriate classification of the chest pain and perhaps wrong interventions to alleviate the pain and precipitating causes. Precision in data collection is aided by the ability to analyze a patient's concern or condition. This may be accomplished by performing a symptom analysis. A symptom analysis is done to identify and describe various attributes of the patients expressed concern or condition. (A symptom analysis if further described and discussed in Chapter 5.)

> ***PRACTICE POINT: Quantifying Patient Responses***
> To increase precision in describing data, it is often helpful to give the patient an opportunity to indicate the severity or degree of the symptom or perception on a scale (generally 1–10). A patient's response of "I thought it worked fairly well" to express satisfaction regarding a particular intervention, lacks precision. However, if the patient rated satisfaction as 7 out of 10, the provider has a better way of documenting the satisfaction rather than just indicating "worked fairly well."
>
> There is no gold standard as to what extent 7 varies from 8, but this is still a more precise presentation of the patient data and provides clearer data for other individuals involved in the patient's care. It also provides a comparison number to determine if satisfaction with other interventions may be better or worse than the present satisfaction.

Reliability/Validity

Reliability refers to obtaining comparable results, under similar conditions. In other words, even though different individuals may perform a health history on the same patient, they should elicit the same information from the patient. Reliability is an important factor related to history, but there are intervening variables that may interfere with the accuracy of the data and affect its reliability.

The health history interview is a human interaction between the provider and patient, both with unique characteristics, (Figure 4-2). These characteristics affect each individual's perceptions and interpretations and may significantly influence the overall outcome of the history. Frequently, a patient in a health care organization is interviewed by multiple providers, resulting in different providers obtaining slightly different versions of the patients history. In many instances the slight variations may not be significant, but sometimes this may create feelings of distrust and be a reason for devaluing history data.

Variations in history data directly affect its reliability; however, variations in the history are often due to slight differences in how providers perform the history. No two providers will ask questions in the exact same way, so the patient's answers might vary accordingly. Each provider may also interpret a patient's words or inflections differently, resulting in paying more attention to one aspect of the patient's responses than another provider.

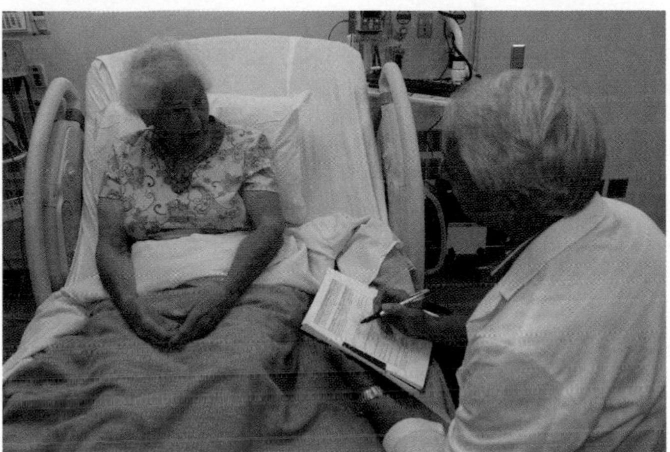

FIGURE 4-2 The patient–provider interview setting

> ***PRACTICE POINT: Notes During the Interview***
> Generally, it is not considered appropriate to take notes during the interview. However, novice providers may feel more comfortable if they can jot down notes during the interview. While some information needs to be written down, such as vital signs, you should not be taking voluminous notes during the interview. Specific information that needs to be documented correctly should be written down. Never use note taking as a crutch in taking a history; it should not take the place of maintaining your focus and attention on the patient. Also inform the patient that you will be taking occasional notes to make sure that you have the data recorded correctly.

The patient's unique characteristics will also influence the reliability of history data. Patients who enter a health care organization with a problem most likely do not have a thorough understanding about the situation. During the initial encounter with the health care provider, the patient may not be aware of all the details of the problem and may present the data in a disorganized and disjointed manner. However, as the result of repetition and refocusing to answer the questions multiple times, the patient recognizes what information is significant. Also, information that the patient may have previously forgotten or considered unnecessary and irrelevant may suddenly be remembered or become significant. As a result, more recent interviewers may obtain further data regarding the patient's condition.

Another characteristic of patient data that is closely aligned with reliability is its **validity** or accuracy. Reliability of data is relatively easy to determine by comparing data obtained from various providers and how well the data correlate with each other. Validity, in contrast, is more difficult to determine. Even though patient data from various sources may correlate well with each other, it may not, however, be accurate.

Patients may engage in self-diagnosis and attempt to hypothesize about the cause and conditions surrounding their symptoms. Information related to symptoms is frequently obtained from friends, family, TV, self-help books, the Internet, as well as cultural and religious beliefs and practices. Patients generally are unable to differentiate accurate information from inaccurate information. With these data and beliefs in mind, patients most likely will come to a wrong conclusion and provide answers that support their beliefs and conclusions. With repeated questioning and attempts to help patients focus on the symptoms, patients' perceptions may change and may result in providing different, more accurate responses than previously given.

Patients may also attempt to figure out what the provider or others want to hear. Someone may have convinced or strongly suggested to the patient that certain manifestations demonstrated by the patient are associated with a certain condition, so the patient's responses reflect this. Some patient's may also fear "letting the provider down" and construct responses accordingly. If the provider suspects that this is happening, remind the patient that it is important to provide data from experiences and sensations that are personally and individually encountered and that you have no preconceived expectations that the patient needs to satisfy.

Therapeutic Communication

Listening to the patient in a manner that promotes openness and honesty is essential to interviewing. History data should give the provider an accurate reflection of who the patient is, what constitutes the overall perception of self, and how one's world is constructed. This open environment exists when the provider uses interviewing skills that demonstrate therapeutic communication, which is characterized through demonstrating respect, empathy, and genuineness.

Respect

Respect is demonstrated by an acceptance of the patient as a unique individual with values, beliefs, attitudes, and practices that define who/what that person is, even though they may differ from the providers. Demonstrating respect does require the provider to suspend one's own attitudes and practices but to look beyond the patient's practices and ideas and suspending critical judgments regarding health care habits.

At times, this presents a difficult challenge to the provider, particularly when some practices and beliefs are contrary to current healthy lifestyle choices, such as smoking, sexual practices, and diet. Respect concentrates on how best to assist patients to overcome their challenges and/or illness without expecting them to adapt in a way that compromises their uniqueness. Suggestions on promoting respect for the patient are outlined in Table 4-1.

Empathy

Empathy is an experience that occurs between two or more individuals and is characterized by the ability to exchange, to enter into, or share in and comprehend the momentary psychological state of another. This sharing of feelings facilitates establishing a trusting relationship. To empathize is to participate in, but not become immersed in the other's issue or problem. Through sharing, there is identification and incorporation of the other's experience that establishes a connectedness between the two. To be empathetic, however, requires that the provider detach from the patient's subjective experience and remain objective. It is the objectivity of empathy that characterizes empathy as a helping function that facilitates resolution of an issue or other problems.

The degree to which one can empathize is largely determined by the similarity between the two individuals and their shared experiences. That does not mean that if the provider has not experienced the exact situation that it is not possible to empathize. Obviously, if the situations are very similar, it is easier to empathize, however, in some instances the provider will need to identify a related experience to empathize. For example, while the provider may not have experienced the loss of a loved one, everyone to

Table 4-1 Suggestions for promoting respect

Step	Suggestion
1	Introduce yourself clearly. Identify your purpose and role.
2	Ask how the patient wishes to be addressed. Don't assume that everyone wants to be addressed by a first name. If you wish to be addressed by a certain title, then also address the patient by an appropriate title (i.e., Mr., Mrs., Miss, Ms.).
3	Consider the patient's comfort during the interview. Check that the patient is comfortable before starting the interview. If the patient appears to be getting tired, determine if the interview should be terminated and continued on at a later time.
4	Make sure that your position is such that you can maintain eye contact with the patient. (This is something that needs to be determined as to its appropriateness related to the patient's cultural beliefs and practices. If in doubt, ask the patient whether this is ok or not. See Table 4-2.)
5	Inform the patient about the conduct of the interview. Make sure that he or she knows what part of the history you will be asking about. This will make the patient feel a part of the history and prevent any surprises and abrupt topic changes.
6	Indicate as best you can that you have heard what the patient has said. Provide the patient with adequate time to respond to the question. Make sure that the patient has finished the response before moving on with the next question. The practice of empathy also is an indication that the provider has heard what the patient stated.

Table 4-2 Dimensions of nonverbal behavior and possible interpretations

Nonverbal Dimension	Behaviors	Possible Interpretation
Eyes	Direct eye contact	Interested, readiness for interpersonal communication; attentive. If prolonged, may be threatening. Sustained eye contact between two individuals of the same gender (usually men) indicates sincerity and a plea to be believed.
	Unwilling or lack of sustained eye contact	Distracted, uncomfortable, or trying to conceal real feelings In some cultures (Asian, Hispanic, Middle Eastern, and Native American) lack of eye contact is considered a demonstration of respect or deference. In many Asian, African, and Latin American cultures, extended eye contact may be taken as an affront or challenge of authority.
	Lowering of eyes—looking down or away	Preoccupation; distraction Muslims often lower their gaze and try not to focus on the opposite gender's features except for the hands and feet. In the Japanese culture, lowering of the eyes is a gesture of respect when speaking to a superior.
	Blinking rapidly, darting	Excessive blinking may indicate anxiety, distress, feeling uncomfortable; or may have something under contact.
	Pupil dilation	Alarm or keen interest
	Tearing	Sadness or happiness
Mouth/Lips	Smile	Positive thought, feeling, or action in context of interview; greeting
	Pursed (tight) lips	Stress (anxiety), determination, anger, hostility
	Biting lip/lower lip quivering	Anger, sadness, anxiety
	Open mouth without speaking	Surprise, suppression of a yawn
Facial Expression	Eye contact with smiles	Happiness, comfortableness
	Eyes strained, furrowed brow, lips pursed	Anger, concern, sadness
	Eyes rigid, mouth rigid [unanimated]	Preoccupation, anxiety fear
Head	Nodding head up and down	Confirmation, agreement, or listening, attending
	Shaking head from side to side	Disagreement or disapproval
	Head hung down, jaw lowered to chest	Sadness, concern
Shoulders	Shrugging	Uncertainty, ambivalence
	Leaning forward	Eagerness; attentiveness, openness to communication
	Slouched stooped, rounded or turned away from a person	Sadness or ambivalence; lack of receptivity to interpersonal communication
Arms and hands	Arms folded across chest	Avoidance of interpersonal exchange or dislike
	Trembling, fidgety hands	Anger or anxiety
	Fists clenching to objects or holding hands tightly	Anxiety or anger
	Arms unfolded—arms and hands gesturing in conversation	Accenting or emphasizing points during conversation; or openness to interpersonal conversation
	Rarely gesturing, hands/arms stiff	Tension or anger
Legs and feet	Crossing/uncrossing legs repeatedly	Anxiety, depression
	Foot tapping	Anxiety; impatience—wanting to make a point
	Legs and feet appear stiff and controlled	Uptightness or anxiety; closed to extensive interpersonal conversation

Continued

Table 4-2 Dimensions of nonverbal behavior and possible interpretations *(continued)*

Nonverbal Dimension	Behaviors	Possible Interpretation
Total Body	Facing other person squarely or facing forward	Openness to interpersonal communication and exchange
	Turning of body orientation at an angle, not directly facing person, or slouching in seat	Less openness to interpersonal conversation
	Rocking back and forth in chair or squirming in seat	Concern, worry, anxiety
	Stiff—sitting erect and rigidly on edge of chair	Tension, anxiety, concern
Distance	Moves away	Indication that personal space has been invaded; increased arousal, discomfort
	Moves closer	Seeking closer interaction, more intimacy
Position in room	Sits behind or next to an object in the room (desk/table)	Seeking protection or more space
	Sits near interviewer without any obstructing objects	Expression of adequate comfort level

some extent has experienced loss. By remembering those feelings associated with the loss, the provider is able to demonstrate empathy toward the patient.

Historically, health care providers were expected to suppress any emotion within the provider-patient relationship; which was to insure objectivity and detachment from the patient (Halpern, 2003). This was not because empathy was perceived to be unimportant, but to prevent any emotional involvement with the patient. There was also the perception that empathy was one dimensional and was only related to emotional connections between individuals.

More recently empathy has been perceived to consist of two types—cognitive empathy and affective empathy (Davis, 2009). Cognitive empathy is the ability of an individual to recognize another individual's emotional state and respond appropriately (Selph et al., 2008). Cognitive empathy is not dependent on an emotional attachment or identification with the other. Affective empathy conversely has an emotional component in that the individual imagines how another is feeling and may temporarily be emotionally attached to another. Affective empathy, because of its emotional context, has been mistaken as sympathy. Empathy is not to be confused with sympathy (Table 4-3).

While similar to empathy, sympathy retains the subjective relationship between the two individuals, rather than allowing an objective approach to the situation. When the individual demonstrates sympathy instead of empathy, there is the immersion of the one with the other and the objective helping ability is lost. It is not wrong to demonstrate sympathy, but to maintain a helping relationship, the difference between the two needs to be recognized.

Empathy is also identified as one of the five core components of emotional intelligence (EI). Emotional intelligence is described as an individual's ability to recognize and monitor one's emotions and those of others for motivating ourselves, and to use that information to guide one's thinking and actions (Goleman, 2001). Emotional intelligence has frequently been identified as essential for successful leadership within the business environment, where adaptability within complex interpersonal contexts and under diverse circumstances is an essential skill. Application of EI within the health care system is just as essential (Ioannidou & Konstantikaki, 2008). Patients' emotional experiences during

Table 4-3 Empathy vs. sympathy

Component	Empathy	Sympathy
Relationship to feelings	"Borrows" patient's feelings	"Takes on" patient's feelings
Sense of identity	Maintains self identity	Loses self-identity
Objectivity	Objective	Subjective
Perception of other's feelings	Accurate perception	Inaccurate perception
Provider's emotional resource	Understanding and support	Condolence and pity

THINK LINK:* *Empathy vs. Sympathy

The following scenario illustrates the difference between empathy and sympathy. Imagine that a person has fallen into a well. A sympathetic person comes along and sees the individual alone in the dark, damp well and thinks that it's not right for the person to be all alone in that state. So the sympathetic person jumps into the well to keep the other person company and share in the miserableness of the situation. An empathetic person comes along and sees the person in the well and also thinks that it's dark and damp down there, and that the person is probably miserable being all alone. Instead of jumping into the well to share the situation, however, the empathetic person finds a rope to help the person get out of the well. While the empathetic person essentially perceived the situation in the same way as the sympathetic person, he chose to help the person get out of the situation. The empathetic person didn't necessarily need to experience being alone down in a well to appreciate what it must be like for that unfortunate individual.

clinical care are significant factors in their satisfaction. Patient satisfaction with clinical care is also influenced by a provider's verbal and nonverbal communication. Research examining the relationship between EI and empathy is minimal at this point, however, EI is recognized as an affective factor that is desired in health care providers (Stratton et al. 2005).

Emotional intelligence is not necessarily an innate characteristic. The ability to demonstrate EI varies from individual to individual, however, it is recognized that there are ways to develop or improve one's EI (Table 4-4).

Genuineness

Genuineness is characterized by being yourself in both your personal and professional demeanor. Genuineness begins with the **introduction** to the patient. When you introduce yourself to the patient, your role as a student must clearly be identified regardless of your specific discipline. How the patient responds to this may vary, but it is important that the patient understands who you are and what you are doing. Being genuine also identifies what you can or cannot do for the patient.

Genuineness also requires establishing and maintaining boundaries that are appropriate to a provider–patient relationship. Maintaining clear boundaries prevents the provider from becoming overly involved with the patient on a personal basis. As the provider and patient become more comfortable with each other, there might be the temptation to engage in more personal disclosure on the part of the provider.

Personal disclosure on the part of the provider is a highly sensitive and controversial subject. Although it is appropriate to express emotions relative to the patient's condition and experiences (empathy), becoming overly involved (sympathy) is to be avoided. There are instances when the patient is interested in you as a person rather than a professional. While disclosing some personal information or expressing emotion may be appropriate, you need to differentiate a professional response from a personal response and determine how much information is necessary to maintain a working relationship with the patient.

More recently, self-disclosure has been promoted for its therapeutic effects (Deering, 1999). Another term that describes self-disclosure is **therapeutic reciprocity**, which is defined as the "mutual, collaborative, probabilistic, instructive, and empowering exchange of feelings, thought, and behaviors between the [health care provider] and patient for the purpose of enhancing the human outcomes of the relationship for all parties concerned" (Marck, 1990). Self-disclosure or therapeutic reciprocity may be used to (1) convey a sense that the provider understands the patient's experiences, (2) enhance trust, (3) decrease loneliness, and (4) decrease role distancing. Critical attributes that are essential to therapeutic reciprocity include compassion, discernment, and trust (Vivaldelli, 2007).

Therapeutic reciprocity also raises ethical issues. When using self-disclosure, it is important to identify the purpose for which it is being used. Self-disclosure should always be focused on meeting the needs of the patient and not the needs of the provider. Interactions with patients must be conducted in a manner that is equitable for all patients. When therapeutic reciprocity is only used with patients with whom the provider shares a sense of similarity, its use is not justified. The ethical use of therapeutic reciprocity is determined to a greater extent by whether providers are able to "connect" with patients who are different or difficult rather than those who are similar to the provider (Olsen, 2007).

This may seem antithetical to demonstrating empathy. Providers must recognize that identification of emotions and your experience with them is not the same as expressing emotion. Feelings and emotions are a part of who we are as people, thus having a warm, caring demeanor is appropriate to prevent the provider from coming across as a cold, uncaring individual who is only interested in obtaining health information from the patient.

Table 4-4 Top 10 suggestions for developing emotional intelligence

Label your feelings rather than labeling people or situations.	"I feel impatient." vs. "This is ridiculous." "I feel hurt and bitter." vs. "You are an insensitive jerk." "I feel afraid." vs. "You are driving like an idiot."
Distinguish between thoughts and feelings.	Thoughts: "I feel like…and I feel as if …& I feel that." Feelings: I feel (feeling word).
Take responsibility for your own feelings.	"I feel jealous." vs. "You are making me jealous."
Use your feelings to help make decisions.	"How will I feel if I do this?" "How will I feel if I don't?"
Show respect for other people's feelings.	Ask: "How will you feel if I do this?" "How will you feel if I don't?"
Feel energized, not angry.	Use what others call "anger" to help feel energized to take productive action.
Validate other individual's feelings.	Show empathy, understanding, and acceptance of other individual's feelings.
Practice getting a positive value from their/your emotions.	Ask yourself: "How do I feel?" and "What would help me feel better?"
Don't advise, command, control, criticize, judge, or lecture others.	Instead, try to just listen with empathy and nonjudgment.
Avoid individuals who invalidate you.	Although this is not always possible, at least try to spend less time with them, or give them no psychological power over you.

The Interview

Interviewing is a goal-directed method of communication—a medium for interaction between the health care provider and patient. Social conversations are not interviews; however, when the provider converses with a patient with a specific goal in mind, interviewing is taking place. Interviewing cannot occur without effective interaction between the provider and patient. Some caveats of interviewing provide the foundation for the verbal component of interaction (Table 4-5).

Purpose

Interviewing in health care is specific to the patient's needs that emerge from the content of the interview. The interview may also offer the opportunity for the provider to supply information to the patient; however, during the interview, this to be kept at a minimum. Identifying patient's educational needs should be noted for later opportunities to provide the appropriate information.

Table 4-5 Caveats of interviewing

1.	An interview is a conversation with a purpose.
2.	Carefully prepare for each interview. A good interviewer listens more than talks. Each of us has two ears and only one mouth for a purpose.
3.	Be natural; be yourself. Do not try to adopt manners of others.
4.	Put person at ease. Your opening comments need not be on the subject of the interview. Establish rapport.
5.	Come to the point as quickly as circumstances permit. Remember the definition of an interview, "A conversation with a purpose." Never lose sight of that purpose, even if the conversation may be temporarily sidetracked.
6.	Hold interview in as favorable setting as possible.
7.	Help patient to understand the implication of factual evidence. Seldom offer advice directly. Never use pressure to get patient to agree with you.
8.	Let patient take lead in making decisions. Don't try to give all the answers in the first 10 minutes; they will probably be wrong. Even if they are right it is better if the patient can be allowed to formulate the decision.
9.	Avoid being placed on the defensive. A patient may dump the problem in your lap as if to say, "Here it is. What do I do now?" Instead of answering questions, reflect the questions back to the patient. This implies that you both recognized what the problem is, and remains the patient's, at all times. The patient should take the leading role in working out the problem, and you helping the patient to arrive at a decision and plan a course of action. Good guidance is stimulating a choice between alternatives.
10.	Respect the personality of the person. Avoid prying, superiority. Help the patient to maintain dignity and respect. Maintain mutual faith and confidence.
11.	Be aware of your limitations. Frankly recognize that some problems must be referred. You cannot know all of the answers all of the time. End the interview with a constructive note. Share with the individual if you plan to return or not.

Setting

The setting for the interview is most commonly a hospital room or a clinic exam room. Depending on the patient's location, the setting could also be in the patient's home during a home visit over the telephone. Any setting outside the home is unfamiliar to the patient. Every patient, as well as every setting, is going to be unique, requiring the provider to adapt to each situation to provide and maintain an environment that is conducive to conducting the interview. Additionally, each interview and setting will be influenced by patient, provider, and environmental variables that may or may not be able to be controlled (see Figure 4-3).

Privacy is an essential quality to provide and maintain for every patient interview situation. The patient is requested to provide personal information, and a sense of privacy helps put the patient at ease and facilitate data gathering. Within a clinic setting, it is easier to maintain privacy as the interview is commonly conducted in a private examining room. In the hospital it is more difficult, particularly in rooms with more than one patient. Drawing the curtains around the bed maintains the patient's sense of privacy. If the patient is ambulatory, it would be appropriate to relocate to a more private area. If there are visitors, they should be asked to leave for the duration of the interview.

The comfort of the patient is also important to the success of the interview. If the patient is experiencing pain or other difficulties, assess the situation to determine if the interview should continue or be postponed until another time. Environmental comfort is also essential. Avoid extremes of temperature, but note that individual requirements vary widely, and the age of the patient also influences temperature accommodations. Remove any other distractions to the extent possible. If the patient is watching TV, request that the TV be turned off. Noise from other sources such as roommate's visitors or TV may be harder to control; however, politely asking to reduce the noise level is appropriate in this situation.

Before beginning the interview, find an appropriate location and a comfortable position that allows for eye contact to be made (depending on the ethnic and cultural practices) as well as maintaining the comfort of the patient. Also make sure that provider and patient are positioned close to each other so that neither the patient nor provider needs to speak louder to be heard. Hospital rooms are not always conducive to do this, but it is important to do as much as possible to attain this.

Interview Structure

The interview may be conceptualized as occurring in three phases: (1) introduction, (2) working phase, and (3) termination.

Introduction

The provider initiates the interview by introducing him/herself and informing to the patient of what to expect. The provider's role in the process should also be identified. For example, the provider may be a student, physician, nurse, physician assistant, nurse practitioner, or any other type of provider. This is not a time for social conversation; however it is important to present oneself as genuinely interested in the patient and comfortable with the process. It is appropriate to start the interview with a general question that does not require the patient to provide any specific information. This is also the time when initial impressions are formed, by both the provider and the patient, thus, the provider needs to be aware of the importance of making a positive first impression.

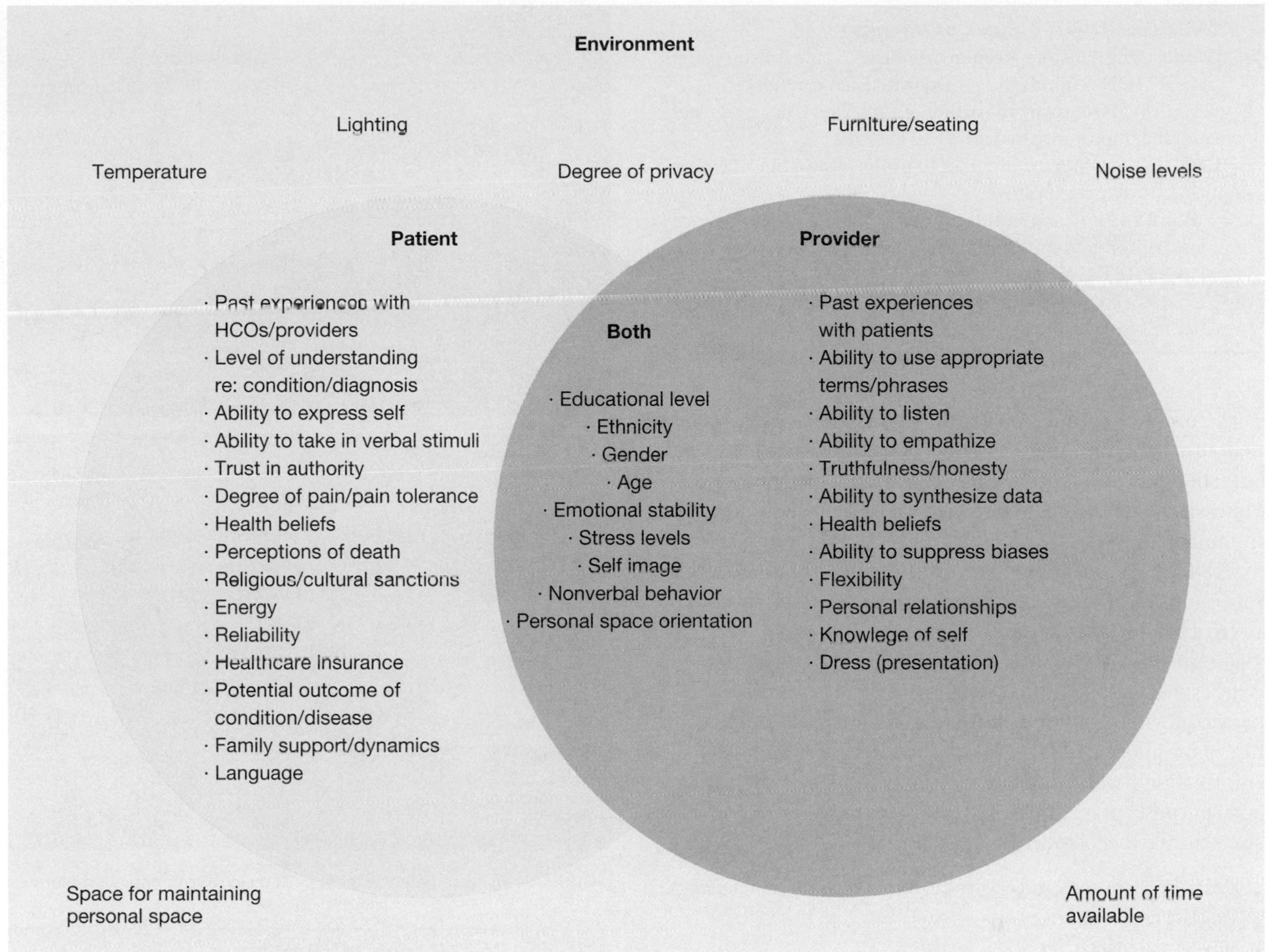

FIGURE 4-3 Variables that affect the context of the patient interview

During the introduction, address the patient by name and establish how the patient wishes to be addressed. Use of first names is discouraged; although, increasingly more individuals are comfortable with the use of their first name. If the provider wishes to be addressed by his or her title and surname, then that should also be identified. It is inappropriate to expect that the patient is comfortable being addressed by the first name but that the provider should be addressed by the title and surname. The patient may be uncomfortable with addressing the provider using only the first name; however, that is the patient's choice.

The amount of time the interview should take should be identified, what type of questions will be asked, and what topics will be covered. It is unlikely that hospitalized patients will only have one health history taken; however, the provider must not assume that the patient will always know what to expect. Erring on the side of providing more information is preferable to erring on the side of assuming the patient knows what to expect.

The first aspect of the patient encounter is no different than any other and often the initial interaction begins with observing the other's physical appearance. Many cues can be obtained from patients just be making astute observations of their appearance. Some diseases and conditions have obvious physical characteristics that accompany them. In other instances, patient's may just "look sick." Experience with ill individuals will increase the provider's ability to identify the characteristics that accompany "looking sick." (More specifics regarding initial observations are covered in Chapter 7 General Appearance.)

PRACTICE POINT: Who's Assessing Whom?

Although most of this chapter is devoted to assessing the patient, the patient is also assessing the examiner and forming opinions. The initial contact with the patient is just as important to the patient as it is to the provider. Initial impressions go a long way to establishing rapport. Provider behavior, the ability to engage the patient in conversation, and showing respect are all attributes of the provider that the patient pays attention to.

Working Phase

The **working phase** comprises the majority of the interview. This is the data-collecting phase when the questions are asked with patient responses. The various types of questions and communication techniques are used extensively in this phase. The working phase is patient focused and structured to be as efficient as possible.

PRACTICE POINT: 5 Rules of Vowels

When performing a history, keep in mind the "5 rules of vowels":

- A = **AUDITION** reminds the provider to listen carefully
- E = **EVALUATION** refers to sorting out relevant from irrelevant data and the importance of data
- I = **INQUIRY** enables the provider to probe into significant areas requiring further clarification
- O = **OBSERVATION** reminds the provider to note the importance of nonverbal communication, regardless of what is said
- U = **UNDERSTANDING** reminds the provider to be aware of the patient's concerns and apprehensions and to allow the provider to be more empathetic and nonjudgmental

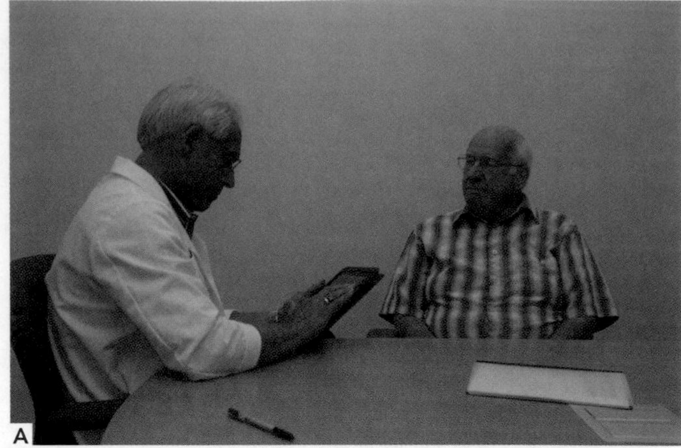

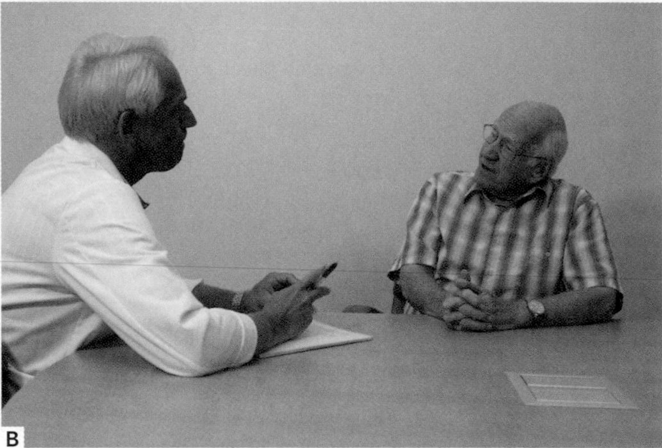

FIGURE 4-4 **a)** Incompetent listener position vs. **b)** competent listener position

Verbal Communication (Asking the Questions) Engaging the patient in an interview implies the use of questions to elicit specific information that is the core and also the most challenging aspect of the interview. Tantamount to interviewing is having well-developed communication skills. Communication is the act of transmitting facts, feelings, and meanings by words, gestures, or other actions from one to another. Communication consists of verbal and nonverbal communication, both of which are important.

The quality of the information received is only as pertinent and specific as the question asked. An effective question encourages the patient to provide the information, but also serves as a guide as to the nature of the information sought. By using the six categories of types of information that is sought (see p. 44), you may develop several general purposes of questions. Use questions to obtain responses or answers that do the following:

1. Describe, elaborate, and clarify perceptions, ideas, and feelings.
2. Validate observations.
3. Substantiate facts.
4. Determine the reliability of information received.
5. Interpret the meaning of a group of facts.
6. Compare information with some predetermined criteria.
7. Formulate solutions based on prior assessment and comparisons.
8. Evaluate the outcome of a plan or action.

Questions can be categorized into two types: **closed ended** and **open ended**. Closed-ended questions, also described as **directed questions**, require limited information or a simple "yes" or "no" as an answer. These are generally used when there is no need for additional data to clarify patient information. Validation of existing data is also an appropriate use of closed-ended questions. A novice interviewer will probably feel more comfortable with closed-ended questions and use them more frequently; however, these are also the least helpful in obtaining useful information.

Open-ended questions provide more information about the patient's experiences and responses to present and past illnesses. Use of open-ended questions also promotes the active participation of patients; however, their use also provides opportunity for patients to wander off topic. When this happens, do not lose sight of the overall goal of the interview and guide the patient back to the interview.

Active (Critical) Listening Although asking questions is an important aspect of the interview process, it is no less important than listening to the patient's responses. When open-ended questions are used, there is more information that the provider needs to pay attention to. By demonstrating active listening, the provider recognizes the importance of the patient data and further encourages patient participation. **Active listening** requires the provider to listen to what is being said, but also how it is being said. Voice inflections, hesitations, voice cracking are all subtleties that may indicate areas of difficulty or stress for the patient (Figure 4-4).

THINK LINK: Hearing vs. Listening

Hearing and listening are both related to auditory stimuli but they differ in how they are used. Hearing is simply the act of perceiving sound and is a physical act, requiring only reception of sound waves. Listening, in contrast, is a mental, conscious activity and effort that requires concentrating on the sound, determine its meaning (interpret) and responding to it.

Table 4-6 Process of listening

Steps	Description
Receive	Stimuli taken in
Select	Focus on the stimuli
Interpret	Meaning attached to stimuli
Understand	Message integrated into a frame of reference
Evaluate	Information judged on its merits
Resolve	Determine what to do with information

Table 4-7 Characteristics of the critical and noncritical listener

Critical Listener	Noncritical Listener
A. Has the following attitudes toward the listening situation:	
Wants to listen	Is indifferent or bored
Finds a personal reason for listening	Is not clear about why he is listening
Is willing to do what is needed in the listening situation	Expects the patient to do all of the work
B. Has the following attitude toward the patients verbal responses:	
Is receptive and open minded	Is suspicious and antagonistic
Is aware of the effect of own prejudices	Is unaware of the effect of his own prejudices
Is willing to hear the patient out to the end	Stops listening at the slightest provocation
Makes understanding the most important objective	Makes agreement or disagreement the most important objective
C. Has the following attitude toward the patient:	
Is friendly and sympathetic	Is indifferent or hostile
Respects the speaker as a person	Is critical or suspicious
D. Prepares to listen in the following ways:	
Tries to learn about the subject	Isn't interested in subject, speaker, or situation
Sits where he can see and hear	Sits where he can avoid listening or leaves first
Tries to eliminate distractions in the environment	Welcomes distractions in his environment
Is ready to take notes when appropriate	Can't decide when and how to take notes
E. Does the following things while listening:	
Relates what the patient is saying to past knowledge and experience	Thinks of other things during his extra thinking time
Looks in the direction of the patient	Doodles, looks out the window, or watches other listeners
Evaluates the speech as heard and understands it	Prejudges the speech on the basis of speaker, subject, or situation
Is attentive, accepting the responsibility as a listener	Fakes attention or expects the speaker to command his attention
Eliminates or quickly adjusts to distractions in himself	Dwells on the inner distractions or creates them
Takes notes suitable for this purpose	Takes the same kind of notes in all situations
Tries to locate the central idea	Listens for facts
Considers relationship between points made by the patient	Is unaware of or unwilling to look for relationships between points
Recognizes the difference between facts and opinions	Confuses facts and opinions
Recognizes the purpose of illustrations and examples used	Is confused and diverted by examples and illustrations
Selects important details for retention	Tries to remember all details
Is aware of implications and inferences in what is verbalized	Is unaware of implications of what is verbalized
Can distinguish relevant from irrelevant material in the speech	Cannot tell which material is relevant and which is irrelevant
Recognizes the effects of emphasis, inflection, rate, volume, gesture, and quality on meaning	Is unaware of influence of factors of delivery on meaning
Interprets what is heard in terms of the speaker's stated or implied purpose	Fails to recognize the patient's purpose
F. Follows up on his listening in the following ways:	
Is able to give an accurate restatement of the main points in the speech	Recalls disconnected points or unimportant details
Asks questions of the speaker if there is an opportunity	Asks no questions and is impatient with those who do
Talks about what has been said with others	Talks about the speaker rather than what is said
Constructs an outline of the speech for his notes	Neither makes an outline nor reviews his notes
Looks for opportunities to refer to what has been said in speaking or writing	Wants to forget the whole affair as quickly as possible

Table 4-8 Therapeutic techniques

Technique	Description	Example
Facilitation	Encourages the patient to say more, either through verbal encouragement or a period of silence that allows for patient reflection and further response.	*"Can you tell me more about this particular experience?"* Phrases such as "uh-huh" and "go on" are also useful as facilitating techniques.
Clarification	Asks for further information to increase the provider's understanding of the patient's response.	*"I'm not sure that I understand what you mean by ________. Can you help me understand what you are saying?"*
Restatement	Repeats the response back to the patient, using different words, to validate the provider's understanding of the response.	*"If I understand you correctly, you are saying that you are experiencing abdominal pain?"* in response to patient stating "bad stomach ache."
Reflection	Repeating the patient's response back to the patient to encourage further elaboration and that the provider is interested in more information.	*"You are saying that you are very anxious about your tests tomorrow?"*
Confrontation	Points out inconsistencies that the provider observes between the patient's responses and the provider's observations or other data about the patient. Confrontation should be used in a way the represents a need to eliminate a misunderstanding or confusion rather than as a derogatory statement.	*"I'm confused. You just said that your pain was not so bad, but previously you indicated that you were really having quite a bit of pain. I'd like to know what you are really experiencing."*
Interpretation	Shares with the patient conclusions that the provider has drawn from the patient's data.	*"From what you have told me, I think you might be experiencing __________."*
Summarizing	Condenses the data obtained to help clarify a sequence of events. This is especially helpful with patients who ramble and do not provide sequential data.	*"OK, Mr. McVay, we've gone through each body system and from your responses it seems that your major concerns are your high blood pressure and headaches. Is that what you think also?"*

Active listening has many attributes that contribute to its overall effectiveness. It is a practice that requires conscious involvement of and implementation of many attributes. While active listening is the term that has been used when referring to focusing on what is being said, as with critical thinking, critical listening implies a multidimensional process. The process of listening is described in Table 4-6, while Table 4-7 provides information on attributes associated with critical and noncritical listeners.

Therapeutic Techniques When using open-ended questions it is essential to also engage in appropriate communication techniques. These **therapeutic techniques** are used to help the patient clarify responses to questions. They are also used to elicit further information from the patient. When patients are asked about sensitive issues, they may be hesitant to provide all the needed information. Therapeutic techniques help to draw the patient out and facilitate provision of further data. They also help to comfort the patient and to establish a caring and helpful relationship. Therapeutic techniques require practice and conscious, thoughtful involvement on the part of the provider. Table 4-8 shows examples of therapeutic techniques.

Nontherapeutic Techniques **Nontherapeutic techniques** are often automatic responses that individuals use during social conversations. They are responses that don't require forethought or the formulation of a response that will be helpful for the other person. The provider's anxiety during the interview or feelings of discomfort during silences makes it easy to revert to nontherapeutic techniques, which effectively cut off the patient and prevent the provider from obtaining meaningful data and often characterize the provider as noncaring and noninvolved. Use of nontherapeutic techniques sends the message that the provider is in control of the interview and will limit what topics and/or terms may be used. When tempted to use these techniques, ask the question "Who is benefiting from this technique—the patient or I?"

Providing False Assurance/Reassurance Providing **false assurance** or **reassurance** is demonstrating optimism, which is often perceived is a positive quality in individuals; however, it is not an appropriate characteristic to use to give another individual false hope. A common response to a situation or condition with a potentially unfavorable outcome is to say, "Oh, I'm sure that everything will be all right and turn out for the good." It is more important to recognize the anxiety or other feelings that the patient is experiencing and providing the opportunity to express and discuss these with the provider. The only reassurance that is appropriate is to indicate that the best care will be provided and that during the interview or other conversations that the health care concerns and feelings are recognized and acknowledged.

Giving Unsolicited Advice Patients come to providers to find out what health issues or conditions may be present and also to learn what interventions might be indicated to treat the condition. In situations like this, it is very tempting for a novice to assume a helper role and provide the patient with possible solutions. When patients ask straightforward questions as to what might be appropriate in treating certain conditions, providing the appropriate information is appropriate. However, the provider needs to be aware of situations when the patient is manipulating the provider into giving advice to help the patient and/or family in decision making. This is an important trap to avoid as this gives the patient a pretext to hold the provider responsible for making the decision rather than the patient.

Abusing Authority Patients frequently look to providers as authority figures and make assumptions that they know what is best. It may be a boost to one's ego when the patient acts in this way, making it tempting to play into this role, However, the relationship between the provider and patient does not parallel a parent (authority)–child (subordinate) relationship and providers should not demonstrate any behaviors that implies such a relationship. Ultimately, the patient must make the appropriate health care choices and decisions, and they should be made without undue influence from providers.

Using Avoidance Language Avoidance language is characterized by the use of euphemisms to avoid reality or hide one's feelings. Providers use avoidance language when they don't want to cause stress or upset the patient regarding unpleasant situations or conditions such as death or cancer. The provider may use the terms growth or mass, or tumor rather than directly stating "cancer." While these terms are not necessarily incorrect, they are less explicit in relationship to the actual condition or cause. This is inappropriately used to protect the provider from having to bring up such issues. It also sends a message that indicates the provider is uncomfortable with discussion of certain topics and/or issues.

THINK LINK: *Avoidance Language*
Avoidance language is often used when referring to death. When a family pet needs to be euthanized, instead of saying "we're going to put Fido to death" it is stated as "we're going to put Fido to sleep," or "we're going to put Fido down." Patient's families also often use avoidance language to "protect" the patient from having to deal with reality. Often, the use of avoidance language prevents any open and frank discussion regarding the real issue and often serves to negatively impact family dynamics by suppressing discussion about one's real feelings and emotions.

Engaging in Distancing Engaging in distancing serves to remove oneself from patients by using impersonal language to addressing the symptom or condition. It is an attempt to remove the messenger from the message. The intent may be to "soften the blow" of reality; however, this may also communicate to the patient that the provider is threatened also.

It is different if the patient does not have an understanding of the condition or symptom that necessitates using terminology that the patient understands; however, distancing should not be used to "soften the truth." It is important to use specific terms to prevent any confusion and misinterpretation by the patient.

Providers also demonstrate distancing when they pay selective attention to expressed problems. This may be due to the provider's inexperience with certain types of problems or just not wanting to be overburdened with multiple problems. Normalizing is another way providers demonstrate distancing, which are attempts to decrease the importance of the patient's problems or symptoms. "Everyone feels like that at some time" or "This isn't anything to worry about" are phrases that normalize and are often used by a provider as a protection from one's own emotional reactions such as anger, fear, or sadness.

Patients may also engage in distancing also by using impersonal terms to put space between a threat and self. For example, instead of identifying or describing a particular symptom as mine, the patient may describe it as a concern of another individual using the third person—he, she, or another acquaintance associated with the patient—my neighbor, my sister, my friend is concerned about a "problem." In this way the patient is not identified or associated with the symptom(s) or condition(s).

Using Professional Jargon Using professional jargon is a very easy trap to fall into. Providers become accustomed to using and communicating in "medicalese." Patients often fail to ask for clarification regarding medical terminology because they don't want to inconvenience the provider or to have to demonstrate their ignorance. This results in the patient providing vague or inaccurate, or insufficient information. Jargon is probably unconsciously used by the provider, but awareness of its use requires constant attention and awareness. At the beginning of the interview the provider should instruct the patient to ask for clarification of any term that is not understood. Giving the patient permission to do this removes any barriers that the patient may perceive to exist; however, it should not sound or appear as condescending.

Using Leading/Biased Questions Biased questioning is characterized by asking questions in a way that requires the patient to choose a response that might be better than another one or will please the provider. The patient may also be unconsciously asking, "How does the provider want me to respond?" rather than just providing the facts. The patient may also feel pressured to live up to the value system of the provider when responding to the question. Leading questions are often used to prevent further questioning or discussion related to topics the provider is uncomfortable with. Often these areas are related to behaviors that are known to be detrimental to the patient's health or perceived to be detrimental Topics such as sexuality, sexual behaviors, drug use, smoking, alcohol consumption are all areas that are somewhat controversial.

An example of a leading question would be "You don't (smoke, drink, use drugs, etc.) do you?" The patient is faced with a dilemma as to how to answer the question. The message implied in the question is that the provider believes that these behaviors are bad. *I don't want the provider to think of me as a bad person so I had better provide the "right" answer, even if it means I have to lie.* This may relieve the provider of addressing the situation, but promotes obtaining inaccurate data and may alienate the patient.

Talking Too Much This behavior hardly needs to be described. Some providers may feel that it is their responsibility to keep the interview going, particularly if the patient takes more time to answer the question. When this occurs, the provider begins to talk to eliminate the silence and reduce anxiety. At times it may be appropriate to help the patient formulate a response but should not be done in a way that prevents the patient from using one's own terms. The primary responsibility of the provider is to concentrate on keeping the interview patient focused rather than to concentrate on keeping the interview moving.

PRACTICE POINT: *Silence*
Most individuals are uncomfortable with silence. It is awkward to sit with someone and not be engaging in verbal communication. Silence, however, can be therapeutic. The patient may need some time to phrase the response accurately or time to pull thoughts together. Also, when discussing emotional topics, such as loss or a potential diagnosis, the patient may need time to let those emotions out, most likely in the form of crying. If the provider is not aware of the usefulness of silence and feels the need to keep the interview going, the provider is not respecting the patient's needs and jeopardizes the patient–provider relationship.

Interrupting Interrupting is characterized by not allowing the patient to complete a thought or sentence. It is common for a provider to anticipate what the patient will say and to cut the patient off with one's prediction of the patient response. It is possible that the anticipated response is not accurate, and again the patient may not want to contradict what the provider has already stated. It is also a technique that may be unconsciously used to keep the interview going.

Use of "Why" Questions Use of "why" questions during a medical interview puts the patient on the defensive and implies that the patient's actions or behaviors need to be explained. Their use also implies that the actions were harmful or not appropriate. This often creates a feeling of guilt in the patient and prevents full disclosure by the patient. How, what, when, and where type questions are appropriate to ask, but not why. The patient may feel obligated to justify some actions or behaviors, but that is the prerogative of the patient and should not be requested by the provider.

Nonverbal Communication (Body Language)

Providers also need to be aware of nonverbal communication which is often referred to as body language (Figure 4-5). While the purpose of interviewing the patient is to obtain verbal responses to specific questions, the patient's body language is also communicating information. Body language consists of body posture, gestures, facial expressions, and eye movements. Just as the provider needs to be engaged in active listening, the provider also needs to be engaged in active observation of the patient for nonverbal cues. While statistics vary, there is a general consensus that the majority of communication occurs through body language.

The provider should compare nonverbal behavior with verbal communication, assessing for congruency between the two. When there is congruency, the two reinforce each other. When there is incongruence, the nonverbal message tends to be a more reliable indicator of the patient's real feelings and attitudes, because there is less conscious control over it. It is important for the provider to remember that nonverbal messages are also being sent to the patient and that the patient is scrutinizing the provider as well.

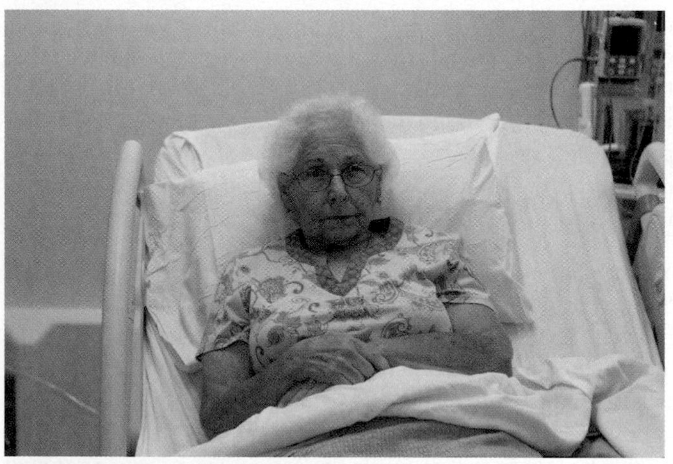

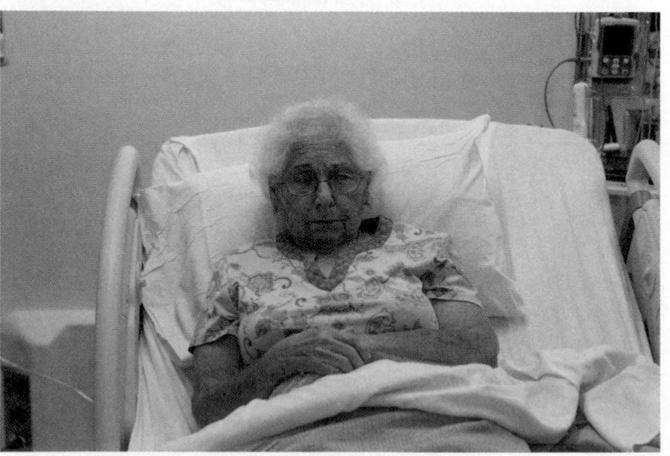

FIGURE 4-5 Examples of nonverbal communication

Termination The **termination** phase brings closure to the interview. This should occur gradually to avoid leaving the patient with a negative impression of the provider. During this phase, the provider gives the patient a chance to ask questions and provide any information that the provider failed to elicit. As the provider becomes more comfortable with interviewing, this time may be used to provide a summary of the data to the patient regarding the provider's initial impressions. This will also provide an opportunity for the development of collaborative health issues related to the health care needs of the patient. This is a skill that takes time to develop and is not necessarily a requirement for each interview.

Potentially Challenging Situations

Every interviewing situation is unique. Both provider and patient possess characteristics and attributes that negatively or positively affect the interview. Recognizing possible challenges that may emerge during interviews will help to prevent or manage them.

Time Constraints

Time is something that frequently gets away from everyone; this is also true when conducting the interview. The provider needs to be cognizant of the time it is taking to conduct the interview and keep the interview within a reasonable time frame. This, however, needs to be balanced with the need of the patient to have adequate time to thoroughly answer the questions. Patients may appreciate the attention and the opportunity to engage in conversation and attempt to keep the interview going. Assertiveness is necessary to keep the interview focused and within the specified time frame. The amount of time is also determined by the type of assessment and the amount of data that needs to be obtained.

Silent (Reticent) Patients

Some patients may be reluctant to talk about themselves or are anxious about the situation. It may take some patients more time to comfortably engage in the interview. Beginning the interview with closed-ended questions will provide opportunities to respond to questions without having to elaborate. As the patient becomes more comfortable with the interview and provider, gradually progressing towards open-ended questions will further engage the patient in the process. The silence of the patient should not be confused with the therapeutic use of silence. Waiting for the patient to initiate or formulate a response may only increase the patient's reluctance and anxiety.

Talkative Patients

Some patients who appreciate the attention and having someone willing to listen may take advantage of this situation and talk about other personal aspects of their histories. They may answer the question and then proceed onto another topic. The challenge for the provider is to keep the patient focused and not continuously wander off the subject. Tactfully interrupting the patient and refocusing on the current question may be all that is needed. Use of closed-ended questions is another strategy that can be used to redirect and refocus the patient. If time permits, allowing 5–10 minutes for the patient to talk freely may be appropriate. During that time, listen carefully as there may be important clues to follow up on when the interview begins or continues.

Personal Questions/Curiosity About Provider

Patients may feel somewhat uncomfortable being the focus of all the attention, so they may feel the need to engage the provider in the conversation by asking personal questions. The patient may perceive that this exchange of information is more of a social conversation and respond and react based on this perception. The provider may feel compelled to respond to such questions. Responses that support the patient and demonstrate empathy are appropriate; however, responses that provide personal data/issues should be avoided. (See previous discussion of Personal Disclosure.)

Displays of Emotion

Discussion of sensitive issues during the interview may initiate intense feelings and reactions in the patient that may precipitate emotional responses during the interview. These are common responses and may be therapeutic for the patient.

Crying

Crying is a natural emotion and usually therapeutic, so avoid any attempts to prevent the patient from doing so. Crying occurs when certain emotions reach a threshold of intensity or when coping ability is ineffective or there are feelings of hopelessness and loss of control (Ryde, Friedrichsen, & Strang, 2006). Recognition that crying is appropriate may be demonstrated by offering the patient tissues and verbally reassuring the patient that it is permissible to cry and appropriate to do so (Figure 4-6). Allowing patient's time to express their feelings and emotions is a critical provider response. This may require the provider to sit quietly in silence. The provider should be comfortable with silence and not give in to the desire to move on to a more comfortable topic. In certain situations, the patient may need more time to recover and postponing the remainder of the interview may be the right thing to do.

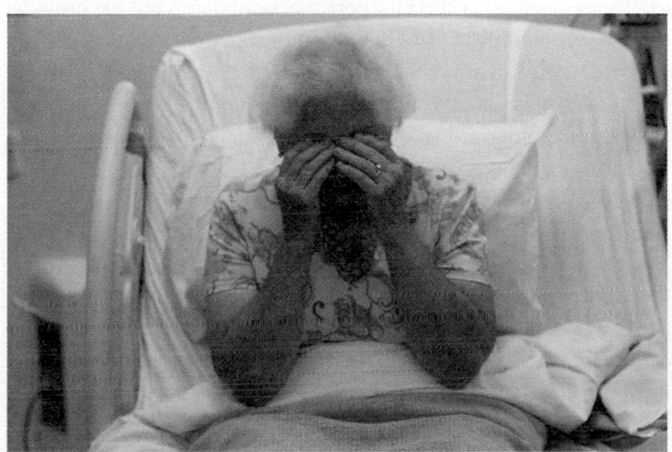

FIGURE 4-6 Patient crying

Perceptions regarding the appropriateness of demonstrating emotions and crying vary. Some individuals may perceive crying to be a sign of weakness and a loss of control. These individuals need assurance and support that it is neither of these and is an appropriate mechanism for release of feelings and emotions. For some patients, crying is a release of tension and a way to relax (Ryde et al., 2006). Perceptions of crying are primarily influenced by gender and cultural norms and expectations. Feelings after a crying episode is also influenced by how common crying is in a person's culture and whether shame is a component of the overall cultural climate. For individuals who have a negative perception of crying, it is important for them to know and understand that expression of emotions is considered confidential information and what occurs during the interview will not be shared with others.

Crying is most often associated with experiences of loss or impending loss; however, it can also be an expression that accompanies joy and happiness. Crying in these situations is primarily the result of an overwhelming emotion that reaches a threshold point and is expressed in crying. It is much easier to respond to the patient that is crying because of happiness rather than crying because of sadness. Even though the reason for crying is totally opposite to crying due to sadness, it may still be perceived by some individuals as inappropriate and a loss of control. Crying due to sadness or due to joy has been described as "an expression for an inner emotional force that was provoked by different factors and caused a change in their balance" (Ryde et al., 2006, p. 55). A release of this inner emotional force is often therapeutic by restoring a sense of balance or control and often has a positive effect on communication.

While crying is most often perceived as a patient response, providers also need to be aware of their own vulnerability toward expressing emotions in the presence of patients. This is especially true if the provider has gone through the same or similar experiences. Sharing in these experiences is the quintessential component of empathy and should not be suppressed. This may be important for the patient and interpreted as a demonstration of caring. Empathetic crying is not necessarily wrong, but the provider needs to maintain an objective perspective throughout the interview. If the provider is unable to maintain this objectivity, it is recommended that the interview be postponed for a while or have another provider continue with the interview.

Anger

Anger is another emotion that the patient may express. Anger that is expressed is not necessarily a personal attack on the interviewer. Anger is often the outward expression of inner feelings of helplessness and/or loss of control. A patient may have difficulty in identifying these inner feelings so they become manifested and expressed as anger. Before moving on with the history, it is best to deal with the anger. A patient who may have a potentially life-threatening diagnosis needs to work through feelings of anger. Recognizing and identifying the feeling of anger with the patient and asking about it often facilitate an open discussion about it.

Dealing with anger during the interview may be uncomfortable and threatening for the provider. Recognizing that it is not a personal attack and that anger is a manifestation of other feelings reduces the perception of threat and enables the provider to help the patient work through those feelings. It is futile to continue with the interview until the issues causing the anger are addressed. Allowing the patient to express anger in a nonthreatening environment and actively listening to the content will help to defuse the situation. Do not attempt to argue with the patient or try to reason from another viewpoint; this only serves to escalate the patient's anger. If the patient does not give any indication of calming down, it is wise to postpone the interview. It may also be necessary to request assistance if the patient becomes a danger to self and/or others.

There may also be times when the provider has feelings of anger that are unrelated to the interviewing situation. These feelings may be unconsciously expressed or demonstrated and are likely to interfere with the interview. While it is often difficult to identify one's own feelings, awareness of nonverbal cues from the patient may be helpful in recognizing one's expression of anger.

Using Touch

The use of touch during the interview should be carefully assessed and used judiciously. Interpretation of touch is closely tied to age, gender, culture, and past experiences. Being comfortable with touching and being touched varies widely within today's diverse cultures. There is no hard and fast rule about when or when not to use touch. Caution should be used when the provider is unsure about how it will be interpreted. If there is any doubt about its use, it is best not to do it. The circumstances and environment for the interview also play a part in determining if touch is appropriate (Figure 4-7).

When used, touch conveys a feeling of compassion and empathy. The provider should be aware of what is desired to be communicated by touch. Even though it might not be meant to be, touch is an invasion of personal body space. This may or may not be acceptable to the patient. Personal body space is often determined by cultural mores and values as well as one's own perception of what might be considered "too close."

Demonstration of Unwanted Behaviors

Patients may not always demonstrate appropriate behaviors during the interview. This may cause the provider distress as well as the premature termination of the interview or obtaining inadequate data. Although these patient behaviors are infrequent, awareness of the possibility and their potential effects is important.

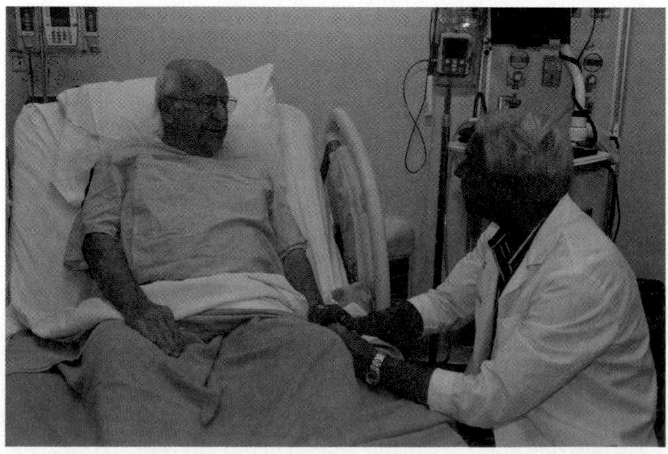

FIGURE 4-7 Demonstration of touch

Seductive Patient

Severe illness or the potential threat of loss of body image can cause patients to question whether they will still be attractive to the opposite gender or whether they will still be able to function sexually. These thoughts and feelings may be expressed through flirtatious behavior and/or sexual aggression. The provider must again be aware that the demonstrated behaviors are only manifestations of underlying fears and anxieties. Some patients may use sexuality as a way to increase perceptions of self-worth or self-esteem. Seduction is not always across genders, nor is it always sexual. Patients may act seductively to "charm" the provider. They may also act that way as a way to maintain some control within a sometimes powerless situation.

The relationship between the provider and the patient is and must always be a professional relationship. The provider's main purpose is to assist the patient in achieving optimal wellness. The initial reaction and feelings to seductive behavior are frequently shock, embarrassment, and possibly anger. Feelings of confusion and disruption are also possible and uncertainty as to how to handle the situation. Although the provider's initial actions and reactions may be the result of instincts, it is important to remain as calm as possible. When responding to the patient, focus on the behavior and not on the patient. It is appropriate to indicate that you are uncomfortable with the patient's behavior or language and that you expect that the behaviors will not be repeated. Although it may be tempting to just ignore the behavior, this is not an effective means of managing the situation. Ignoring it may have the opposite effect and make the patient try harder to gain your attention.

Conversely, there may be patients that the provider finds attractive. While this is not common, there is always the possibility that it may happen. Patients and providers of both genders are vulnerable to such feelings. If this occurs, denial of feelings is not the answer; denial may increase the likelihood of acting on those feelings. If such feelings become evident, acceptance and recognition of them will help to prevent inappropriate behaviors. While it is more than likely that the provider did nothing to encourage feelings of attractiveness in the patient, self-reflection about comments, mannerisms, and clothing will help in assessing whether either of these contributed to the patient's assessment of the situation.

While there is no way to prevent patient encounters such as this, it is better to be prepared for such encounters. Most instances related to seductive behavior have to do with violations of personal boundaries. There are no set criteria for personal boundaries but the provider must clearly identify the boundaries of the provider–patient relationship and when and how they may be breached. Failure to establish set boundaries most likely will result in boundary confusion characterized by ambiguous feelings around sexuality and sexual issues.

Modesty Issues

The seductive patient is most likely to be willing to expose more areas of the body associated with sexuality; many other patients are more concerned with protecting their modesty and not exposing the "private" parts of the body. While it is considered essential to expose these parts during a physical exam, it was not always this way. It wasn't until the mid-19th century that exposure of any part of the body was considered a part of the examination. Thus, on the opposite end of the spectrum, providers need to be aware and concerned about the patient's need for modesty. This is more commonly related to providers and patients of the opposite gender, but there are also patients who may feel the same way with same gender encounters (Bernstein, 2012).

In an effort to overcome any perceived discomfort or embarrassment associated with examining exposed parts, the exam was viewed and treated as a scientific ritual and it was necessary for scientific advancement; providers were also encouraged to develop an objective and dispassionate distance with the patient (Henderson, 2011). In doing so, providers may have reduced their own anxiety and discomfort, but it did nothing to alleviate patient's anxiety and discomfort. Even though the need for examination of these areas of the body remains, the need for the patient to be treated with respect and compassion also remains and will help to maintain the dignity of the patient and the provider and their respect for each other (Henderson, 2011).

Manipulative Patient

As with the seductive patient, the manipulative patient often craves extra attention or is trying to keep some level of control over what is happening. Patients may also feel the need to validate that they are liked and use manipulation as a means to obtain this. Manipulative patients demonstrate impulsive behavior that is focused on getting what they want (Hull & Broquet, 2007). Excessive flattery is often an indication that the patient is being manipulative. The provider needs to be cautious when this occurs; the tendency is to reply in a flattering way to the patient. The provider needs to be aware of this and respond to it in a therapeutic way.

Likewise, the provider may have a need to be liked, and use manipulation on the patient. This is highly unprofessional and must not occur. Hospitalized patients are very vulnerable and can be easily manipulated into doing what the provider wants. Patients may perceive that they have no choice but to do as the provider requests.

However manifested, manipulation is the malicious and intentional taking advantage of the position, needs, unconscious fears or weaknesses of others by someone through cunning and deceptive maneuvers that gratify his or her own wants or desires without any concern, interest or respect for the feelings or emotions of others. Inducing guilt in another individual is a common technique used by manipulative individuals. Often, the manipulative individual will use subtlety to gain control over the individual and situation so that one is not even aware of being manipulated.

Handling the manipulative patient is difficult. Labeling a patient as manipulative will most likely affect how other providers relate to the patient, thus it is imperative to be confident in making that determination. Involving and consulting with other health care providers is an essential step in the process. When working with the patient, it is not helpful to confront them or to give in to their requests. Negotiation is the recommended action to take.

Patients Who Require Adaptations

Occasionally the provider will encounter patients who present with conditions or situations that require some adaptation. To the extent possible, adaptations should make the patient feel as comfortable as possible without drawing undue attention to the accommodation.

Patients Who Do Not Speak English

Migration patterns over the past decade have increased the probability of encountering individuals with limited English proficiency (LEP) (Hudelson, 2005). Individuals with LEP increased from 14 million in 1990 to 21.4 million in 2000 (Gany et al., 2007) and they have less access to health care services putting their health and their communities at risk (Karliner, Jacobs, Chen, & Mutha, 2007). In these instances, it is futile to attempt obtaining a history by using gestures and broken phrases. The history should be obtained through the use of an interpreter who has an excellent command of the English language as well as the ability to interpret medical language correctly (Rosenberg, Leanza, & Seller, 2007). If the interpreter is unable to effectively translate medical questions using accurate terminology, the data obtained is unreliable and most likely inaccurate.

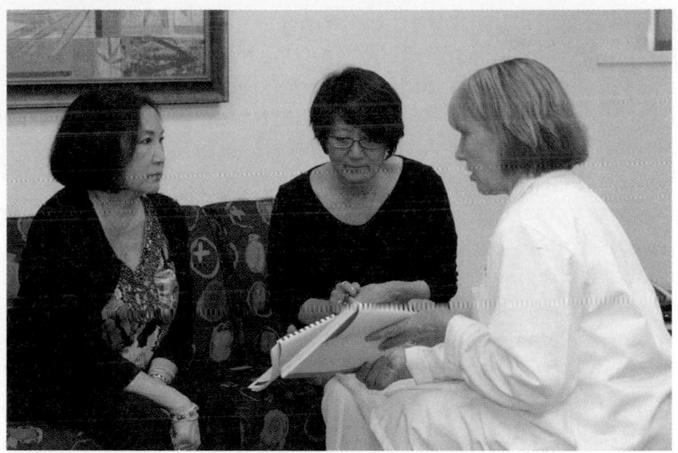

FIGURE 4-8 Patient with interpreter

Ideally, the interpreter should not be a member of the patient's family. This is often tempting to do as it would seem to make the patient more comfortable; however, it might be that the patient does not want family members to be privy to certain information. It is also possible that the family member might have a difficult time asking about sensitive and personal issues (Figure 4-8). Having family members present also violates the patient's confidentiality. If the situation is such that a family member is the only available interpreter, or if there were time constraints, it could be considered acceptable to use the family member. Providers have indicated that working with professional interpreters is preferable as the professional interpreter is less likely to have an agenda and it is easier for the physician to maintain control over the interview (Rosenberg et al., 2007).

Interpreters must understand that their function is to translate everything, not to condense or summarize. To the extent possible, interpreters should make every effort to use the exact terms and words that the patient uses. Interpreters are also responsible for making sure that the patient understands the context of the question. If interpreters try to make the responses more "medical sounding" the details of the patient's condition may be incorrect.

The provider must also make a conscious effort to speak directly to the patient and maintain eye contact with the patient, even though the verbal message is going to the interpreter. The questions should be addressed to the patient as if the patient were to respond. The interpreter should be sitting close enough to the patient so that the provider doesn't have to turn away from the patient every time the interpreter relates the patient information. These behaviors should facilitate building a relationship with the patient; however, physicians have reported that having an interpreter interfered with patient–provider relationships and that the patient was trying harder to build a relationship with the interpreter than the physician (Rosenberg et al., 2007).

Patient with Impaired Hearing

Obtaining a history from a hearing impaired individual is much the same as from an individual who does not speak English. How the patient communicates should be determined so that the appropriate assistance can be obtained (Pacala & Yueh, 2012). Some individuals are very good at lip reading so that the provider only has to make sure that his or her lips are always visible to the patient. Patients who lip read generally do so with speech articulated at a regular pace so it is not necessary to over articulate, slow down, or shout for the patient to read the lips (Smith, 2002). Shouting has a tendency to increase the inflection of the voice into the higher frequency range where hearing impaired adults have greater difficulty understanding speech (Pacala & Yueh, 2012). Keep in mind though; that some medical terms are probably not familiar to the patient, so validating the patient's understanding of these words is essential. If the person uses sign language, an individual fluent in signing should be present.

It may be that the patient is only hard of hearing, which requires the provider to speak slower and in a louder volume. Using a lower voice tone will also help the hearing impaired patient as the high frequency sounds are often the first ones that are lost. Individuals may be hesitant to admit that they have a difficult time hearing. Elimination of extraneous noises also facilitates hearing for these patients. Do not confront the patient unless it is very difficult to get the patient to provide appropriate responses. If all else fails, communicating via hand writing may be the only alternative. This will enable the provider to obtain correct information but most likely will prolong the history taking process. Confirm that the patient has the time and that the provider also has the time to obtain the history in this manner.

Patient with Impaired Vision

With the visually impaired patient, identifying yourself and your approach is important. Instead of offering your hand for a handshake, ask the patient, "May I shake your hand?" so that the patient knows to extend his or her hand. If you need to touch the patient for any reason, indicate your intent to do so or ask permission. If anyone else is in the room or enters the room during the interview, make sure that the patient is made aware of another person's presence. Be aware also that the patient is most likely to be able to tell if and when the provider is not present.

Individuals who are visually impaired are not necessarily hearing impaired. Avoid speaking slower and louder when communicating with the visually impaired.

Developmental Variations

Providers will need to modify their interviewing techniques to meet the developmental stages or capabilities of their patients.

Infants and Children

Interviewing of infants and children is primarily accomplished through interviewing the parents. During an interview, observe the interaction between the infant/child and parent. As the child grows and develops, more involvement with the health history should be encouraged; however, when the child is capable of providing reliable and accurate data is individually determined. Specific information obtained for the infant and child is further detailed in Chapters 5 and 10.

Adolescents

The first decision to make when interviewing adolescents is whether to obtain a pediatric or adult database. There are no specific rules or guidelines to help in making this decision. Either one will need to be modified as the child develops and matures.

The provider also has to decide whether to interview the patient alone or in the presence of a parent. This becomes more significant as the adolescent develops and matures. Confidentiality is important to maintain with the adolescent, therefore, as personal and maturation issues become more important to the patient, interviewing the adolescent privately is necessary. Adolescence is a turbulent, developmental period, thus, the more issues and concerns that can be addressed, and the more correct information that can be provided is of utmost importance for the adolescent's overall health and well-being.

Specific topics and issues that need to be addressed in the adolescent years include home, education, activities, drugs, sexuality, suicide, safety from injury, and violence. More specific information is detailed in Chapters 5 and 10.

Older Adults

The elderly can now be identified as belonging to specific age categories. **Young-old** individuals are between the ages of 65 and 74. **Middle-old** encompasses the ages from 75 and 84, and **old-old** are those above the age of 85. There are no specific adaptations that are needed when interviewing an older adult, however, they may need accommodations related to their vision and hearing.

PRACTICE POINT: Clues/Cues to Identify Hard-of-Hearing (HOH) Patients

Some individuals may not be aware that they are HOH, or deny that fact. Hard of hearing is an indicator of age, and it may be difficult for some to admit that age is "creeping up on them." The loudness of the patient's verbal responses can provide clues and cues as to the hearing ability of the patient. Obviously, a patient request that you "speak louder" is an indicator of difficulty in hearing. This is consistent with a neural hearing loss. Observe whether the patient favors one side (ear) over another. If this occurs, ask the patient if you should move to allow the patient to hear with the preferred ear. Note if the patient appears to be lip reading. The patient may be focusing on your lips, rather than maintaining eye contact.

If the patient is experiencing a conductive hearing loss, he or she may be speaking in a lower volume. This is because in a conductive hearing loss, the voice is heard louder by the individual than during regular conversation. The perception is that the volume is also heard louder by the provider, thus the patient speaks in a lower volume (see Chapter 19).

The elderly may also be described by their functional capabilities. A **functional assessment** should be performed on the elderly patient to determine if he or she is **healthy elderly** or **frail elderly**. The determination of frail versus healthy is determined by evaluation of one's functional abilities against the standard adult performance.

The elderly often have multiple health problems and issues and are frequently on multiple drugs. The elderly often self-medicate and may use alternative and over-the-counter drugs on top of their prescription medications. A thorough medication history is mandatory to evaluate the potential for serious drug interactions.

Summary

- Interviewing a patient is a form of communication and is performed through obtaining a health history.
- Effective interviewing obtains patient data that is based on 6 principles as well as 14 skills and can be assessed relative to its objectivity, precision, reliability, sensitivity/specificity.
- Therapeutic techniques for interviewing are used to help clarify patient's responses as well as eliciting further information from the patient.
- A trusting relationship between a patient and provider is based on respect and the demonstration of empathy.
- Multiple variables, in both the patient and provider, and the environment have an effect on the conduct and outcome of the health history interview.
- Questions are described according to two types—closed ended or open ended.

Review Questions

1. To establish an objective awareness of the patient's experiences and situation, the provider should develop an ability to demonstrate which of the following?
   1. sympathy
   2. empathy
   3. antipathy
   4. apathy
2. To maintain and remain impartial while interviewing a patient for the purpose of health assessment the provider should do which of the following?
   1. Identify with the patient.
   2. Communicate with the patient.
   3. Disregard one's prejudices and biases.
   4. Eliminate ones emotions and feelings.
3. By accepting the patient as a unique individual with values and beliefs, the provider demonstrates which of the following?
   1. approval
   2. admiration
   3. validation
   4. respect
4. While assessing a patient returning from the operating room the provider asks, "Are you experiencing pain right now?" This is an example of what type of communication technique?
   1. closed ended question
   2. clarification
   3. structured response question
   4. interrogatory question
5. During the health assessment interview the provider asks the patient, "You practice safe sex, don't you?" This is an example of what type of communication technique?
   1. closed-ended question
   2. leading question
   3. validation
   4. reflection
6. A provider who successfully engages in therapeutic communication with a patient will demonstrate which of the following?
   1. verbal accuracy
   2. elocution techniques
   3. active listening
   4. appropriate verbosity
7. It is important for the provider to ensure precision is used in data collection about the patient to make sure that the data is which of the following?
   1. more objective
   2. less ambiguous
   3. less subjective
   4. more reproducible
8. When the patient begins to cry during the interview, the provider should do which of the following?
   1. Leave for a couple of minutes to provide privacy.
   2. Change the subject to a less sensitive subject.
   3. Sit quietly until the patient has regained composure.
   4. Move closer to the patient and place his or her hands on the patient.
9. A faculty member is explaining to novice students the difference between the use of empathy and sympathy as communication techniques to use when interviewing patients. When discussing sympathy, the instructor should include which of the following? (Select all that apply.)
   1. assuming the patient's feelings
   2. offering condolence to the patient
   3. providing support to the patient
   4. remaining objective in the situation
   5. losing self-identity
10. When using therapeutic reciprocity, the provider is aware that it should be used with patients for the purpose of which of the following? (Select all that apply.)
    1. relieving stress for the provider
    2. enhancing provider–patient trust
    3. reducing patient loneliness
    4. sharing provider–patient similarities
    5. decreasing distance created by roles

5 Health History

I put away the blood pressure cuff. Thirty-one-year-old Mr. Stanton is new to the clinic, and he has significant hypertension. "188/95," I say aloud, scribbling the numbers on the chart. Now comes my favorite part of the entire encounter—the history. With so many possible explanations for this one finding, it amazes me that an astute health professional can often deduce the cause by history alone. How long has his blood pressure been this high? Does he have symptoms along with the hypertension? Does this run in his family, or is he an outlier? Does he smoke, which would certainly raise his risk index for coronary artery disease? I begin my questioning feeling like Sherlock Holmes stepping onto a fresh crime scene.

After 10 minutes of targeted inquiry, Mr. Stanton had revealed the following: his blood pressure at home was usually in the 120s/80s, but every now and then it would suddenly shoot up to the 180s or 190s systolic. When this happened, he would develop a pounding headache and start sweating. He had palpitations and tremulousness along with these symptoms. He didn't know much of his family history because he was adopted. He was diagnosed with hypothyroidism 4 years ago after "a mass" had to be removed.

Ten minutes of inquiry—using nothing but words, medical knowledge, and a bit of clinical intuition—and I have a leading diagnosis in mind. It is certainly uncommon, and I have never seen a real case before, but the picture fits too perfectly. Could this be a pheochromocytoma? And could this patient have something more, such as a syndrome like multiple endocrine neoplasia? His history of a thyroid tumor and symptoms consistent with paroxysmal catecholamine surges leads me to think so.

LEARNING OUTCOMES

1. Explain the two significant functions of taking the health history.
2. Describe the basic health data parameters for obtaining a health history.
3. Explain the process of doing a symptom analysis using a mnemonic (COLDERRA).
4. Compare and contrast the biomedical (disease; provider centered) model approach with the biopsychosocial (holistic, patient-centered) approach to history taking.
5. Compare and contrast the various frameworks for organizing and clustering data obtained through the health history.
6. Relate developmental variations to adaptations needed for the health history.

The overall assessment of the patient begins with obtaining the patient's health history. The health history is a comprehensive account of the patient's past and present health status. The health history is an indispensable tool to identify actual and potential patient health problems. Although taking an accurate health history does not require mastering a manual skill, the provider must develop the skill of asking questions to obtain appropriate health data and art of working with the patient to develop a relationship (Dwamena, Fortin VI, & Smith, 2005). The most effective and essential skill to acquire in taking a patient's history is the art of listening (Fitzgerald, 2005). Excellence in history taking is experiential and develops through repetition (Anderson, Hansen, Sondergaard, & Bro, 2008).

Functions of the Health History

The primary function of taking the health history (HH) is to provide the patient with an opportunity to relay specific information about a health care concern or problem (Kravitz & Kravitz, 2005). It is a tool to assist the provider in obtaining data that accurately describes the patient and the unique characteristics and structure that comprise the patient's physical, social, psychological, and emotional environment and experiences. Thus, the provider obtains significant insights into the patient's world, which aid and support the planning and provision of care to meet the patient's health care needs. An accurate health history is essential since it provides essential data that is required to make appropriate and accurate clinical judgments.

An accurate health history depends on the patient being a reliable historian. While no specific criteria exist to establish the reliability of the patient, a patient who understands the questions, provides appropriate answers, and appears to be grounded in reality would be considered a reliable historian. Orientation to person, place, and time is another parameter contributes to patient reliability. Infants and children would not be considered reliable, and the parent or guardian who responds to the questions is the individual to be considered as reliable or not. Elderly individuals who demonstrate manifestations of dementia would also be considered unreliable and the individual's care taker is the one considered reliable or not.

The secondary function of the health history is to give the provider the opportunity to establish a meaningful connection with the patient (Kravitz & Kravitz, 2005). In any health care agency, a meaningful relationship that promotes the development of mutual trust and understanding is essential to create a framework for mutual cooperation and successful provision of optimum health care. Obtaining the health history is frequently the provider's first encounter with the patient; therefore, it is imperative that this inter action takes place in a manner that facilitates a positive experience for the patient. Studies have revealed that initially patients provide only superficial clues related to their histories until they sense empathy and will then disclose more personal and anxiety-provoking information (Halpern, 2012). A positive experience facilitates the development of confidence and trust in the provider, increasing the likelihood of obtaining accurate and correct information. Empathy and reflective communication techniques are significant behaviors providers may demonstrate that contribute to patient satisfaction (Pollack et al., 2011).

The health history also guides the provider in the conduct of the physical examination. Information obtained during the health history directs the provider in determining what additional objective information is necessary to validate the health history data and what to focus on during the physical examination.

Obtaining appropriate data also requires excellent communication, interviewing, and active-listening skills. Excellent communication skills also help the patient relax and create a comfortable environment for the patient. Specific information and a discussion on communication skills and how to interview the patient are described in Chapter 4.

The general format of the health history and the categories used for organizing and clustering the data are basically the same for all health care disciplines. The format for a health history provides the rubric for the sequence of the questions and represents the particular health care discipline. The basic categories for data collection that comprise the health history are identified as the following:

Biographical information
Chief concern/complaint
History of present illness (symptom analysis)
Present health
Family health
Physiological parameters (review of systems)
Sociological parameters
Psychological parameters
Developmental parameters

Questions used to elicit information from the patient during the health history should be organized and logically sequenced, assuring a consistent approach to obtaining data. As previously identified in Chapter 1, information obtained through the health history is subjective data indicating that it reflects the patient's perceptions and statements. Subjective data associated with the experience of an unexpected or unique sensation is referred to as a **symptom**. Not all subjective data is considered a symptom, but symptoms can be described only by the patient.

Approaches to the Health History

The approach to taking a health history can be perceived to occur in two complementary formats—**patient-centered interviewing** and **provider-centered interviewing** (Fortin VI, Dwamena, Frankel, & Smith, 2012). Using the patient-centered approach to interviewing has been found to have significant advantages, particularly on improving a patient's health outcomes (Lein & Wills, 2007; Lyles, Dwamena, Lein, & Smith, 2001; Stewart et al., 2000). Other advantages include increased patient and provider satisfaction, and fewer malpractice complaints or suits (Rouf, Chumley, & Dobbie, 2009)

Patient-centered interviewing occurs during the first part of the history. This is the time for allowing the patient to describe what is going on regarding the reason for seeing the provider as well as identifying goals and expected outcomes. Evaluation of expertise in the art of conducting a patient centered interview may be accomplished by assessing the provider's comfortableness with and ability to do the following:

1. Make patient comfortable and set stage for the [interview].
2. Efficiently negotiate the patient's agenda for the [interview].
3. Elicit patient's explanatory model for their illness.
4. Elicit the patient's personal story in an open-ended manner.
5. Elicit the patient's emotional reactions in an open-ended manner.
6. Effectively inform the patient about necessary information.
7. Effectively motivate patient to change unhealthy behaviors.
8. Manage the patient's expressed emotion.
9. Conduct the open-ended, patient-centered aspect of the ... interview effectively.
10. Obtain patient's description in an open-ended manner (Hatem et al., 2007).

At the completion of the patient-centered history, the health history proceeds and becomes provider focused, completing the history taking (Figure 5-1). The patient centered approach to the health history occurs in a sequence of five phases.

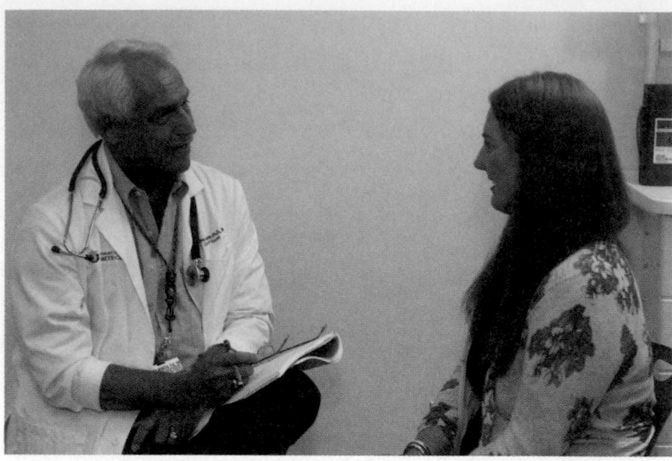

FIGURE 5-1 Beginning the health history

Phase 1: Establish the context for the health history

Greet the patient by name and introduce self

Provide privacy and comfort

Eliminate any distractions and/or barriers to communication (loud TV/radio, visitors, etc.)

Biographical Information Biographical data identifies the patient and provides specific information that differentiates one patient's health record from another. It also assists the provider in identifying potential areas that may influence the patient's health status and any issues that may need clarification for later problem identification and diagnosis. Biographical data consists of the following:

- patient's name
- phone number
- address
- contact person
- gender
- age
- birth date
- birth place
- race
- nationality
- cultural background
- marital status
- names of persons living with the patient
- education
- religion
- occupation

This information may easily be filled out on a self-reporting questionnaire and obtained prior to the health history. Generally, time for taking a health history is limited, thus obtaining biographical data prior to the history is the most efficient use of time. As an opening to the interview, the provider might review some of the biographical data for validation purposes.

Phase 2: Determining chief concern/complaint and establish agenda

- Identify time frame [how long the interview should take]
- Identify specific needs (i.e. tests, lab work, and review previous results)
- Listen to and develop a list of all the patient's issues—reason for appointment/requesting to be seen, expectations, desired outcomes
- Summarize

Chief Complaint/Chief Concern The chief complaint (CC) is a brief statement that identifies the reason a patient is seeking health care. This segment is also referred to as the **patient's story**. In most instances the CC will be related to a specific symptom that the patient is experiencing. At other times, the patient may be healthy and only requesting an examination for health screening or health promotion purposes. In this instance, the reason for seeking health care is related to a patient's health concerns, as there is no problem that needs further analysis. Recently, instead of identifying this as a chief complaint, it is recommended to identify it as a chief concern (Schleifer & Vannatta, 2011).

PRACTICE POINT: Chief Complaint vs. Chief Concern

There is no hard and fast rule as to whether the presenting problem is identified as a chief complaint or chief concern; the meaning of both is well understood among providers. However, when addressing or questioning the patient the term used becomes more significant. Using the term "complaint" may give the patient the impression of being labeled a complainer, which could affect how much information the patient is willing to give. If the patient is worried about being labeled a complainer, a greater likelihood exists that the patient will give less information. Other less problematic phrases or terms that may be used would be "primary reason, major reason, principal purpose, what brings you here."

In patient-centered interviewing, frame the questions in a way that maintains the patient as the primary focus. When eliciting information regarding a certain symptom, instead of focusing on the symptom and asking the question "what did it feel like" change the question to "how did you experience 'the symptom'?" Both questions will obtain the same information, but the first one emphasizes the symptom "it feels like," and the second one emphasizes the patient "how did you?"

When documenting the CC it must be stated in the patient's own words. Examples of patient's chief concerns/complaint are as follows:

"I'm having (I've been having)...

... chest pain all night."

... a burning sensation in my stomach."

... pain in my left leg."

... difficulty breathing for the past few days."

Stating the CC in the patient's terms avoids creating a diagnosis out of the CC and prevents jumping to conclusions. Premature judgment as to what a patient's problem might predispose the provider to making a faulty analysis and improper problem identification because additional data that would allow for a more thorough review was not obtained (Benbassat & Baumal, 2004).

Many patients are routinely exposed to medical language from television advertisements by pharmaceutical companies marketing their products. This may lead the patient to state the CC in medical terms rather than in terms that just describe the symptom (Achkar, 2006). If this is the case, don't necessarily accept the patient's choice of terms as representative of the CC. In some situations, what the patient states about the CC may not have any relation to the actual symptoms. Continue to ask the patient questions to help the patient describe the CC in terms that reflect the symptoms and not their own "diagnosis."

It is not unusual for the patient to have more than one CC (Fortin VI, Dwamena, & Smith, 2012). When this occurs, determining which one is of primary significance is carried out by the patient and provider. It may turn out that the initial concern was not the primary one (Barrier, Li, & Jensen, 2003).

Phase 3: Listening to patient's story/HPI (time for patient to present more details related to chief concern/complaint)

- Initiate patient telling the story—open-ended question/request
- Listen actively while patient's story is told—do not interrupt or break in with your conclusions of questions (Schapira, Tulsky, Buckman, & Pollack, 2008).
- Encourage patient with nonfocused open-ended techniques [silence, nonverbal cues (nodding head, sitting/leaning forward), neutral verbal affirmations (uh-huh, um-hmm)]
- Observe nonverbal cues (facial expressions, body position, and hesitation regarding certain topics, issues, and voice strength).

Whenever a symptom is identified by the patient, a **symptom analysis** is done. A symptom analysis looks at the symptom from its component parts to gain further insight into the symptom and get a more detailed description of the symptom.

A useful mnemonic that may be used to gather data for a symptom analysis is **COLDERRA**. Each letter stands for a specific attribute of a symptom and guides the provider to ask specific questions about the symptom to elicit pertinent data. While listening to the patient describe the chief complaint, identify key information the patient is providing that fits into a category of a symptom analysis. The components of a symptom analysis are as follows:

C = Characteristics This component relates to how the patient is experiencing the symptom. To illustrate, the symptom pain will be used. Ask the patient to describe the symptom as best as possible. Descriptors used by the patient may indicate that it is a burning, throbbing, dull, or aching sensation; or it may be sharp, stabbing, gnawing, or a pressure-type sensation. It is important to help the patient be as precise and as specific as possible: however, be careful not to be too suggestive as to what the patient is experiencing. Patients may perceive that the provider is better able to describe the symptom and may be overly influenced by medical vocabulary or the tendency to want to make a rapid diagnosis.

O = Onset Onset refers to when the patient first noticed the symptom. Ask the patient to identify when the symptom was first noted or experienced. This may also be related to what precipitates the onset of symptoms.

L = Location The location indicates where the symptom is manifested. Ask the patient to identify specifically where on/in the body the symptom is located.

D = Duration Duration refers to the length of time that the symptom has been experienced. Ask the patient to indicate how long the symptom has been present or experienced. If the symptom is episodic, this is then related to the length of time an episode of the symptom lasts. Ask the patient how long each episode lasts.

E = Exacerbation Exacerbation relates to what makes the symptom worse. Ask the patient to identify situations and/or activities that cause the symptom to increase in nature or intensity.

R = Relief Relief refers to what makes the symptom go away or reduces its intensity. Ask the patient what activities, aids, or situations may reduce or relieve the symptom.

R = Radiation Radiation refers to whether the symptom manifestation stays in a particular location or if the pain travels to other parts of the body. Ask the patient whether the symptom, for example, pain, remains in one area of the body or if it is felt in another location of the body.

A = Associated signs/symptoms These are additional or other manifestations that are experienced at the same time as the symptom being analyzed. Ask the patient if there are any other noticeable manifestations that accompany the symptom.

PRACTICE POINT: Risk

Another term or component of the symptom analysis that may be helpful is **risk**. This is not necessarily a component associated with patient responses, but a useful component to keep in mind when listening to patient's responses and noting instances where risk factors for certain diseases or conditions are presented. Such information is also useful for differential diagnosis.

Another descriptor for the symptom analysis is the history of present illness (HPI). While this may imply that a symptom analysis is only done for the chief complaint, it is essential to do a symptom analysis whenever a symptom is identified by the patient. Additional symptoms will most likely be conveyed when the physiological systems are assessed.

COLDERRA is not the only mnemonic device used for symptom analysis. Other mnemonics are identified in Table 5-1, but COLDERRA is the mnemonic method used throughout this text. As you can see,

Table 5-1 Other symptom analysis mnemonics

OPQRST	COLDSPA	OLDCARTS
O – onset	C – character	O – onset
P – precipitating/ palliative factors	O – onset	L – location
Q – quality	L – location	D – duration
R – radiation	D – duration	C – character
S – severity	S – severity	A – aggravating/ associated factors
T – temporal factors	P – pattern	R – relieving factors
	A – associated factors	T – temporal factors
		S – severity

each mnemonic has a slightly different approach to analysis of a symptom, but they all consider the essential qualities needed to analyze a symptom. Regardless of the mnemonic device used for symptom analysis, any one gives the provider with a powerful tool to obtain a more accurate description of the patient's experience.

Once the CC has been determined, move on to establish the agenda. Establishing the agenda provides the opportunity for the patient to communicate the desired expectations related to their health care needs and for the provider to listen to those expressed expectations. Affording the patient the opportunity to establish the agenda reorients the interaction from professional control to patient empowerment (Margalit, Glick, Bengassat, & Cohen, 2004). Despite its importance in providing quality care, physicians frequently fail to request the patient's concerns and expectations, which negatively affect the patient's health outcomes (Bell, Kravitz, Thom, Krupat, & Azari, 2002). It should come as no surprise that when providers understand patient's concerns, patient satisfaction improves as well as adherence to prescribed treatments (Dyche & Swiderski, 2005; Haskard-Zolnierek & DiMatteo, 2009).

Phase 4: Begin more focused interviewing

- Obtain more details if some symptoms not described sufficiently (COLDERRA)
- Validate unclear data
- Explore psychosocial context (feelings, reactions, emotions) of symptoms/experiences

Emotion exploring techniques (Direct—how patient feels; Indirect—how family/others may feel, what patient thinks may be reason/cause of present condition)

Addressing emotion and emotion handling techniques may be facilitated by another acronym, NURS.

Naming/labeling emotion (Identifying/validating emotion experienced/experiencing)

Understanding (empathy) (Stating that there is an understanding of the patient's feelings/emotions)

Respect (Recognition that the patient has had a difficult time, has handled the situation/experience with courage and stamina, or has been through a lot)

Support (Expressing a desire to help the patient) (Smith, 2002)

Phase 5: Move to provider centered aspect of health history

- Complete the remainder of the health history.

The provider centered interview transitions to more focused questions that generally require more specific physiologic information from the patient. At some point, it may be necessary to consider patient centered interviewing techniques. The patient may have provided information related to the chief concern, but at any time during the remainder of the history, other symptoms may be encountered. Depending on the nature of the symptom and its effects on the patient it may be appropriate to obtain the necessary information with a more focused symptom analysis (COLDERRA) rather than the more open ended approach used in the patient centered interview.

Present Health Status

The present health status is a description of the patient's present health from the patient's perspective and whether there have been any changes over the past months or years. If there have been changes noted, determine if the patient is aware of or can identify anything that may have been the cause for the change. For the patient who is ill and presents with specific symptoms, the present health status is definitely influenced by the CC and may be reflected in the patient's perception of health.

PRACTICE POINT: Specificity of Data: Scaling Patient Responses (1–10 scale)

At some points in the HH, the patient is asked to consider the quality of a perception, feeling or emotion related to a specific sensation or experience. When asked how something felt or the severity of the sensation, a typical patient response would be "good," "not so bad," or 'it hurt a lot." These responses do not provide a very good understanding of the patient's real feeling or perception. At times like these, it is helpful to ask the patient to rate or rank the sensation or perception on a scale from 1–10. By doing this, the provider has a more quantitative response from the patient and provides a baseline for future questions related to the patient's specific response. This type of question can be used at any time during the HH when a quantitative response will give more meaning to the data.

Present health data also includes the patient's health practices and goals. Ask the patient to identify what specific practices promote and/or maintain personal health and what personal habits and environmental factors may influence or interfere with the patient's health. Exercise patterns as well as the amount of sedentary activity are identified and explored. The amount of specific substances, i.e. drugs, caffeine, and alcohol ingested, is also identified and recorded. When identifying quantity of ingested substances, precision and specificity must be kept in mind. There may be differing perceptions of how much a "cup of coffee" is and what "one drink" indicates. In these instances, clarify terms so that the data reflects reality.

Other practices related to the patient's health are safety issues and the use of protective devices and their frequency of use. Seatbelts are the most frequently unused safety and protective devices so it is important to determine whether the patient uses them. Driving habits can also expose the patient and others to unsafe conditions. The wide availability of handheld technical devices, driving while texting, or talking on cell phones creates hazardous situations. Recent research has concluded that driving while talking on a cell phone is the equivalent to driving under the influence of alcohol (Strayer, Drews, & Crouch, 2006). Other safety practices that should be explored are use of protective equipment; for example, determine if patients use headgear when bike riding and protective eye wear when engaged in activities that could cause eye injury (woodworking, lawn care, and factory work).

Environmental factors relate to any environmental encounters that pose a health risk. A common concern is one's exposure to toxic agents. This can be due to the location of the patient's home if it is located near factories that emit pollutants into the air and that are then inhaled. Constant exposure to second-hand smoke is another environmental concern. The use of lead-based paint in older homes, and radiation emission from contaminated soil also pose a significant health risks, especially to children.

Another significant environmental factor to consider is noise, which may be present near airports and sometimes an unavoidable factor in the workplace or work environment. Listening to loud music for extended periods of time is also an environmental factor. The patient's use of protective devices against noise needs to be identified.

Feeling safe is another important factor to consider as an environmental issue (Quine & Morrell, 2008). The increasing incidence of violence within our society creates an atmosphere in which patients may no longer feel safe in their surrounding neighborhood. This is especially a concern in the elderly. Fear and insecurity may have a significant influence on a patient's health status by increasing one's anxiety and fear over the safety of self and loved ones.

Feeling safe also affects one's ability or opportunity to engage in physical activity. This is particularly of concern for individuals who would benefit from it, primarily those who are obese (Franzini et al., 2010). Even though there are adequate opportunities for engaging in physical activity, feeling unsafe was detrimental to doing so and significantly influenced individuals decisions as to being or not being physically active.

From a clinical perspective, patients have expressed that feeling safe was an overwhelming need for them, particularly those in intensive care units (Hupcey, 2000). It is counter intuitive to think that patients would feel fearful in an environment that is supposed to facilitate healing and wholeness. From the patient's perspective, constant monitoring and observation, although important to their healing and recovery, they do not promote patients feeling of being safe (Meriläinen, Kyngäs, & Ala-Kokko, 2010).

Past Health Status

The past health status documents historical incidences of the patient's health that may influence the patient's overall current health status. Past health is concerned with multiple topics related to the patient's past experiences with illnesses or other conditions, including childhood illnesses, accidents/injuries, surgeries, hospitalizations, major acute/chronic illnesses, immunizations, allergies, transfusions, medications, and abuse/rape. In many instances, there is overlapping data when responding to inquiries related to one topic provides information needed for another one. Note when this happens and don't repeat the question when that topic is being addressed.

Childhood Illnesses Carefully note childhood diseases, such as measles, mumps, polio, chicken pox, strep throat, scarlet and rheumatic fever, frequent colds, ear infections, and asthma. All of these illnesses have the potential for affecting an adult's health status. If the patient has not had certain diseases, immunization against the disease needs to be verified. (See the following section on immunizations.)

Accidents/Injuries Carefully note the incidence of any major accidents and/or injuries that the patient has experienced. Also determine what the precipitating event was and whether the accident or injury resulted in hospitalization or any complications. A repeated pattern of accidents and injuries should alert the provider to determine whether the patient is exposed to a potentially lethal environment or working conditions. If the patient is an infant or child, the possibility for child abuse needs to be determined. (Assessment for child abuse is covered more fully in Chapter 14.)

Surgeries Surgeries may or may not accompany accidents/injuries, and it should be determined if they are related. Other reasons for surgeries must be noted and the reasons for their occurrence. It should also be noted whether there were any significant complications following any surgery.

Hospitalizations Inquire whether the patient had any hospitalization and for what reason. The previous categories of surgeries and accidents/injuries may account for any hospitalizations; however, there may be other instances that required hospitalization. For females, childbirth is often a reason for being hospitalized, and should be noted.

Major Acute/Chronic Illnesses Inquire whether the patient has experienced any major illnesses that might have an effect on one's health status and whether hospitalization occurred or treatment was on an outpatient basis.

Immunizations Determine whether the patient has received the expected childhood immunizations and whether any boosters have been administered or are required. Commonly administered immunizations include MMR, polio (OPV), and DPT (Table 5-2). Boosters for tetanus and diphtheria are required every 8–10 years. Patients may also have received the hepatitis B vaccine and pediatric patients may also have received the HIB vaccine. Patients in high-risk (elderly, immunocompromised) categories may also have received flu shots and pneumococcal immunizations. The provider should also determine whether the patient has received a TB test and note its results. Certain immunizations that were received in childhood, specifically whooping cough (pertussis) are now being recommended for booster shots in adults.

Allergies It is essential to determine and document any allergies the patient may have to any substance/material, such as drugs, foods (particularly peanuts), soaps, tape, fibers, latex or any other contact agent. The type of reaction the patient experiences must also be described. Reactions can range from a mild rash with itching and runny nose to a full blown anaphylactic shock. In the case of identified drug allergies, determine whether the patient experiences a true reaction or merely irritating side effects (nausea, vomiting). Often patients mistake a drug's side effects with allergic reactions.

Transfusions Determine whether the patient has ever received a blood transfusion. Often, patients who have experienced major surgery may have received a blood transfusion; however, if the patient has not had surgery there are instances when blood may have been administered, for example, severe anemia and hemophiliac emergencies.

Medications Determine what medications the patient is taking, both prescribed and over-the-counter (OTC) medications. Often patients who take multiple OTC medications do not consider that these are actually medications because they have not been prescribed by a physician. An important point to consider is that taking multiple medications, both prescribed and OTC, may have serious consequences for patients—particularly drug interactions and reactions. Often, patients are being treated by multiple specialist providers who prescribe medications without knowing what other medications have been prescribed by other providers.

Herbal supplements also need to be identified. Patients may not consider these substances as medications either because they were most likely bought at a health store and not a drug store. Patients often consider these substances to be natural and therefore are not a drug.

Table 5-2 Adolescent/adult immunizations

Vaccine/Route	Recommended Recipients	Schedule	Contraindications	Precautions
Influenza (inactivated influenza vaccine) IIV IM	All individuals aged 6 months and older (including pregnant women) High risk individuals	1 dose annually Given in fall (October and November)	Severe allergic reaction [e.g., anaphylaxis] after previous dose of any influenza vaccine or to a vaccine component, including egg protein	Moderate or severe acute illness with or without fever History of Guillian-Barré Syndrome within 6 weeks of previous influenza vaccination Individuals who experience only hives with exposure to eggs should receive IIV with additional safety precautions
Influenza (Live attenuated influenza vaccine) LAIV Intranasally	Nonpregnant individuals 49 or younger without high-risk medical conditions	May be given as soon as available	Severe allergic reaction (e.g., anaphylaxis) after previous dose of any influenza vaccine or to a vaccine component, including egg protein Conditions for which the Advisory Committee on Immunization Practices (ACIP) recommends against use, but which are not contraindications in vaccine package insert: immune suppression, certain medical conditions such as asthma, diabetes, heart or kidney disease, and pregnancy	Individuals who have a severe allergy to chicken eggs or who are allergic to any of the nasal-spray vaccine components; Individuals < 2 years/>50 years of age; Individuals with a medical condition/illness: that places them at high risk for complications from influenza (chronic heart or lung disease, such as asthma or reactive airways disease); diabetes or kidney failure; that weaken the immune system or who take medications that can weaken the immune system. Children or adolescents receiving aspirin; Individuals with a history of Guillain-Barré syndrome (a severe paralytic illness, also called GBS) that occurred after receiving influenza vaccine and who are not at risk for severe illness from influenza.
Pneumococcal polysaccharide (PPSV) Pneumococcal conjugate (PCV 13) IM or SC	Individuals 65 years and older Adults younger than 65 years with chronic lung disease, cardiovascular disease, diabetes mellitus, chronic renal failure, nephrotic syndrome, chronic liver disease, alcoholism, immunocompromising conditions, and functional or anatomic asplenia Individuals (19 or older) with chronic diseases or immunocompromising conditions	One time dose—if previous vaccination history unknown One time revaccination 5 years after first dose (19–64 years) with chronic renal failure/ nephrotic syndrome, asplenia, and immunoconmpromising conditions	Severe allergic reaction (e.g., anaphylaxis) after a previous dose or to a vaccine component Severe allergic reaction (e.g., anaphylaxis) after a previous dose or to a vaccine component including to any vaccine containing diphtheria toxoid	Moderate or severe acute illness with or without fever

Continued

Table 5-2 Adolescent/adult immunizations (*continued*)

Vaccine/Route	Recommended Recipients	Schedule	Contraindications	Precautions
Hepatitis B (Hep B) IM	All individuals through 18 years of age Any adult wanting immunity High risk individuals	Three doses—0, 1, 6 month schedule	Severe allergic reaction (e.g., anaphylaxis) after a previous dose or to a vaccine component	Moderate or severe acute illness with or without fever
Hepatitis A (Hep A) IM	Any individual wanting immunity Travel to high risk areas	Two doses with a minimum interval of 6 months between doses	Severe allergic reaction (e.g., anaphylaxis) after a previous dose or to a vaccine component	Moderate or severe acute illness with or without fever
Td, Tdap (Tetanus, diphtheria, pertussis) IM	All adults without a history of a primary series of at least 3 doses of tetanus and diphtheria-toxoid containing vaccine.	Substitute 1 time dose of Tdap for Td booster; then boost with Td every 10 years Booster every 10 years after primary series. Individuals 19–64 may have one time dose of Tdap to replace next Td.	Severe allergic reaction (e.g., anaphylaxis) after a previous dose or to a vaccine component For pertussis-containing vaccines: encephalopathy (e.g., coma, decreased level of consciousness, or prolonged seizures] not attributable to another identifiable cause within 7 days of administration of a previous dose of Tdap or diphtheria and tetanus toxoids and pertussis (DTP) or diphtheria and tetanus toxoids and acellular pertussis (DTaP) vaccine	Moderate or severe acute illness with or without fever History of Guillian-Barré Syndrome within 6 weeks of previous influenza vaccination History of arthritis-type hypersensitivity reactions after a previous dose of tetanus or diphtheria toxoid–containing vaccine; defer vaccination until at least 10 years have elapsed since the last tetanus toxoid–containing vaccine For pertussis-containing vaccines; progressive or unstable neurologic disorder, uncontrolled seizures, or progressive encephalopathy until a treatment regimen has been established and the condition has stabilized
Polio (IVP) IM or SC	Not recommended for those over 18. Unvaccinated adults don't need vaccination unless traveling to certain areas where polio endemic. Vaccinated adults may receive booster if traveling to certain areas.	Refer to AACI recommendations regarding specific situations, schedules and dosing information		Previous anaphylactic reaction of vaccine and any of its components
Varicella (Var Chicken pox) Subcutaneous injection	All adults without evidence of immunity	Two doses needed Second dose 4–8 weeks after first (if second dose delayed), just give second dose.	Severe allergic reaction (e.g., anaphylaxis) after a previous dose or to a vaccine component Known severe immunodeficiency (e.g., from hematologic and solid tumors, receipt of chemotherapy, congenital immunodeficiency or long-term immunosuppressive therapy or patients with human immunodeficiency virus [HIV] infection who are severely immunocompromised) Pregnancy	Recent (within 11 months) receipt of antibody-containing blood product (specific interval depends on product) Moderate or severe acute illness with or without fever Receipt of specific antivirals (i.e., acyclovir, famciclovir, or valacyclovir) 24 hours before vaccination; avoid use of these antiviral drugs for 14 days after vaccination

Continued

Table 5-2 Adolescent/adult immunizations (*continued*)

Vaccine/Route	Recommended Recipients	Schedule	Contraindications	Precautions
Meningococcal Conjugate vaccine (MCV4); Merningococcal polysaccharide vaccine (MPSV4) Intramuscular	Individuals with anatomic or functional asplenia, or persistent complement component deficiencies HIV infected individuals College freshmen [up through 21 years] residing in dormitories	One dose needed. If 1st vaccine was MPSV4— revaccinate every 5 years if still at risk No revaccination after MCV4 unless at increased risk for infection	Severe allergic reaction (e.g., anaphylaxis) after a previous dose or to a vaccine component	Moderate or severe acute illness with or without fever
Polysaccharide vaccine (MPSV4) Subcutaneous injection	Preferred for adults 56 and older			
MMR (measles, mumps, Rubella) Subcutaneous injection	Individuals born in 1957 or later Measles/Mumps component High-risk groups—health care personnel, students entering college, international travelers Rubella component Females of childbearing age who do not have documentation of immunity	One or two doses needed If second dose needed—no sooner than 4 weeks after first dose.	Severe allergic reaction (e.g. anaphylaxis) after a previous dose or to a vaccine component Known severe immunodeficiency (e.g., from hematologic and solid tumors, receipt of chemotherapy, congenital immunodeficiency or long-term immunosuppressive therapy or patients with human immunodeficiency virus [HIV] infection who are severely immunocompromised) Pregnancy	Moderate or severe acute illness with or without fever Recent (within 11 months) receipt of antibody-containing blood product (specific interval depends on product) History of thrombocytopenia or thrombocytopenic purpura Need for tuberculin skin testing
Human papillovirus (HPV) Intramuscular injection	Female (3 doses between 19–26 years) Male (3 doses between 19–21 years; recommended between 22–26 if other risk factors present)	Three doses on 0, 2, 6 month schedule	Severe allergic reaction (e.g., anaphylaxis) after a previous dose or to a vaccine component	Moderate or severe acute illness with or without fever Pregnancy
Zoster (shingles) Subcutaneous injection	Individuals 60 years of age and older	1 dose	Severe allergic reaction (e.g., anaphylaxis) after a previous dose or to a vaccine component Known severe immunodeficiency (e.g., from hematologic and solid tumors, receipt of chemotherapy, or long-term immunosuppressive therapy or patients with HIV infection who are severely immunocompromised) Pregnancy	Moderate or severe acute illness with or without fever Receipt of specific antivirals (e.g., acyclovir, famciclovir, or valacycolovir) 24 hours before vaccination; avoid use of these antiviral drugs for 14 days after vaccination.

ACIP Adult Immunization Work Group. (2013). Advisory committee on immunization practices (ACIP) recommended immunization schedule for adults aged 19 years and older–United States, 2013, Morbidity and *Mortality Weekly Report*, 62, pp. 9–18.

Abuse/Rape This is a very personal area to assess, but it is very important when the long-term consequences that abuse or rape can have on the health of a patient are considered. There may be physiological and psychological consequences associated with the abuse and rape. The holistic approach to patients cannot omit assessing this aspect of the patient's life. (Additional information an assessment of domestic violence is provided in Chapter 14.)

Family History/Health

The incidence of specific illnesses in the immediate and extended family is identified and recorded. The purpose for this inquiry is to assess the potential for genetic predisposition for certain illnesses and conditions. Examples of genetically linked diseases include cardiovascular disease (coronary artery disease, hypertension, and stroke), emphysema (non-smoking related), gout, asthma, alcoholism, mental illness (depression), and certain types of cancers (breast and colon). Other diseases, such as hemophilia, cystic fibrosis, certain anemias (sickle cell, thalassemia), and Tay Sachs disease, are known to be genetically transmitted. Providers should also inquire about family members who may have diabetes mellitus, renal problems, seizures, allergies, obesity, and TB.

Family history is best documented by doing a genogram. The genogram includes three generations, going back to the patient's maternal and paternal grandparents; mother, father, and their siblings; and the patient and siblings. The ages of each individual are identified and the cause of death is recorded along with the age at which the individual died. The specific condition/disease of each patient is also identified.

At this point, the family history is confined to the medical conditions that are present within the immediate and extended family. (Other aspects of family dynamics and interactions are covered in Chapter 2.)

> **PRACTICE POINT: Developing a Genogram**
> A genogram is a visual summary of the patient's family history (patient, spouse, children, parents, and grandparents). Developing a genogram requires that the relationship of family members is done first. This is done by coordinating squares and circles that represent the members of the family with either horizontal or vertical lines. Squares represent males and circles represent females. Horizontal lines represent marriage or the equivalent of, and vertical lines represent offspring. Other aspects of the genogram provide information as to age, health status, physiological conditions, age, and cause of death if known. Most of the symbols used in the genogram are standardized (Figure 5-2); however, there might be some unique symbol that is used in some agencies.

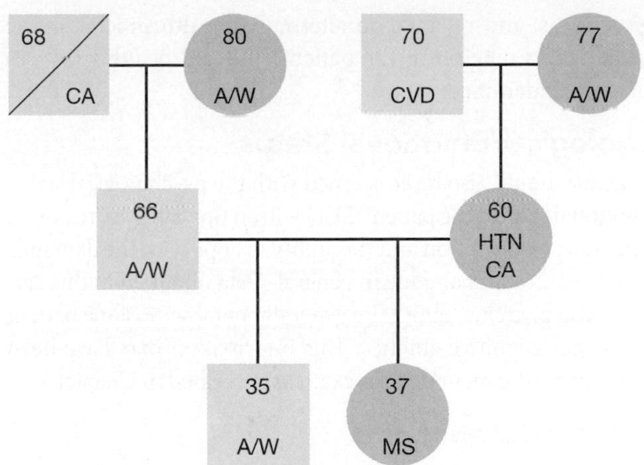

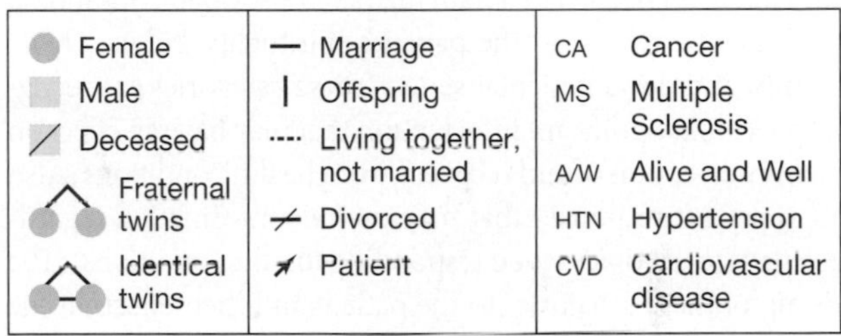

FIGURE 5-2 Key to symbols/abbreviations on genogram

Physiological Status

The provider reviews the physiologic systems of the patient for the presence of any symptoms that may require evaluation and may not have been identified in previous sections of the health history. These systems include the integumentary (skin), neurological, HEENT, respiratory, cardiovascular, gastrointestinal, musculoskeletal, and genitourinary. Questions are posed in such a way as to elicit data related to the functional aspects of each system and to determine the presence or absence of symptoms. If a physiologic system was reviewed extensively under the chief complaint and/or present health, it is not necessary to repeat questions related to that system here. Only information about areas that have not been previously reviewed and need to be addressed are recorded.

> **PRACTICE POINT: Laundry List of Symptoms**
> When assessing the physiological systems, there are usually multiple symptoms associated with each one and that the patient is expected to identify whether any of these symptoms are present or have been experienced. Asking about each symptom and waiting for the patient to reply can become cumbersome and time consuming. The most efficient way to accomplish this is to inform the patient that for each system a list of symptoms will be presented and to indicate which ones are pertinent. While presenting the list of symptoms, do it fast enough to move the history along, but also slow enough that the patient can have enough time to respond.

Sociological Status

The health status of an individual cannot be diagnosed only using physiological data. Data related to other areas of the individual must also be taken into account. The sociological status of an individual is related to the role an individual plays within the family and other organizations, and includes relationships that exist because of specific roles. Other data that relate to a patient's sociological status include economic status, educational level, employment status, and general activities that are undertaken to nurture and maintain roles and relationships.

Within sociological status, also obtain information about values and beliefs. This would be an appropriate section to record health beliefs if they have not been addressed in other areas. Other values and beliefs relate to health practices and the patient's thoughts, ideas, and reliance on alternative health practices. The role of faith and religion in the patient's life and health practices should also be identified.

Psychological/Emotional Status

The provider should also be concerned with the psychological status and emotional state of the patient. Data within this category relates to the patient's self-perception and the ability to cope with the demands of specific health states and life in general. Data obtained in this category can also give clues about the general mental state of the patient and his or her cognitive abilities. This information may have been obtained during the mental status exam as described in Chapter 7.

Additional Categories

As well as these basic categories, other categories may be added to the health history if needed to obtain further holistic data. Additional categories may be related to the patient's spirituality, culture (heritage), family, and developmental status. These categories are recognized as providing significant information that may have an effect on the patient's perception of and recovery from health conditions. Also be alert to patient responses that may provide information regarding these particular topics when responding to other questions. (The relationship of these categories to the patient and their effect on the patient are covered in detail in Chapter 2.)

Organizing Data

Organizing the data follows the format of the health history. The format that is used may vary from discipline to discipline. The traditional approach to formatting and what has been presented here is broadly categorized as the **biomedical model**. This model is primarily used by physicians and provides the foundation for other formats and organizing methods. In this model, each status area is addressed as outlined in the previous section. Physiological data is obtained and organized according to specific body systems, for example, neurological, cardiovascular, and respiratory. Obtaining physiological data in this format is a reason that this approach is also referred to as **review of systems** (ROS) approach.

The medical model approach emphasizes the physiological aspect of the patient, both in terms of obtaining and organizing data and formulating a diagnosis. It is also characterized as an illness or disease approach to obtaining data and treatment of the patient's condition. Eventually, sociological and psychoemotional areas were recognized as factors in causation and treatment of patient's condition; however, the emphasis still remains primarily focused on the patient's physiological data.

Recently there has been a movement toward clustering and organizing data that provides a more holistic or patient-centered approach to the health history. The holistic approach focuses on the totality of a patient, which includes identifying both health and illness parameters. The emphasis is looking at the whole person and integrating all systems to a greater degree, not as separate systems. Within the holistic framework, the **body-mind-spirit** connection is recognized as influencing and maintaining health and coping with disease and is incorporated into treatment goals and interventions. By focusing on the health and the totality of patients, and not just illness and disease, the patient's uniqueness and strengths can be identified, supported, and reinforced.

Nursing models for organizing data tend to be holistic in their approach. A common holistic framework used in obtaining, organizing data, and identifying health care needs is Gordon's Functional Health Patterns (FHP) (2009). Just like the medical model approach, FHP guides the provider in obtaining patient information related to physiological, psychoemotional, sociological, and historical parameters. It is important to recognize that data obtained by using a holistic format is not different

Table 5-3 Comparison of approaches to organizing data

Conceptual Approach vs. System Approach

Concept	Description	Review/Range of Symptoms
Health/ well-being	Recognition of one's state of health and well-being and awareness of appropriate behaviors and activities for health management; inclusive of patient's definition/description of health	Chief concern History of present illness Past medical history Family health history
Nourishment/ Utilization	Behaviors related to adequacy of food and fluid intake concerned with meeting metabolic requirements for sustaining appropriate activity level	GI (ingestion—nutrition, mouth, throat; digestion—abdomen)
Elimination	Behaviors related to excretion of physiological and metabolic waste from the body (bowel, bladder, and skin); inclusive of patient's identification or description of "normal" function	GI (excretion/ bowel habits) GU (urine elimination; male/female genitalia) Skin
Mobility/ performance	Functional behaviors related to ability for purposeful activity and exercise	Respiratory Cardiac Musculoskeletal
Cognizance/ awareness	Behaviors associated with and recognition of external and internal stimuli; inclusive of understanding and comprehension of meaning and interpretation of stimuli	Neurological Head, ear, eyes, nose
Rest/ relaxation/ recreation	Behaviors associated with obtaining an appropriate balance of sleep, leisure, and repose	No specific system associated with this concept
Self-recognition/ self-regulation	Patient's concept and perception of self and behaviors that reflect a positive or negative self-image	Psychological status Sociological status
Connection/ association	Behaviors that reflect awareness of role recognition and acceptance and assumption of those roles	Emotional status Culture Spirituality
Endurance/ patience/ sustainment	Behaviors that reflect skills associated with coping effectiveness and tolerance of stress	
Sustaining/ guiding tenets	Behaviors that reflect individual principles, values, beliefs (including spirituality) and goals that guide patient's choices and/or decisions	
Intimacy/ affection	Behaviors that reflect satisfaction with sexuality related to reproductive capabilities and life stage	Sexuality (gender identify, sexual practices, satisfaction, STIs) Females (obstetrical history)
Regulation	Physiological data that reflects expected parameters associated with growth and development, organ system function, and overall homeostasis	Endocrine, Hematological

from data obtained when using a biomedical format; the difference is related to how the data is clustered and organized.

A holistic approach to obtaining and organizing data from a patient history is more of a conceptual approach rather than a physiological system approach. A conceptual approach is broader in its context and not as restrictive as a system approach. Concepts include physiological systems and parameters and frequently include more than one system resulting in some overlapping of systems. Concepts are also more abstract and can be open to different interpretations so it is important to clarify what physiological parameters are included within a concept. There may also be certain physiological parameters that don't necessarily fit into a concept. In such an instance, don't limit the collection of that data because it doesn't fit, simply record it as additional data or uncategorized data. Uncategorized data could also be considered a concept. Table 5-3 provides a possible framework for collecting and organizing data as well as identifying what physiological systems relate to a particular concept.

Regardless of what format is used to obtain and organize the health history, familiarity with the essential data necessary for a complete health history is of great importance. Although template forms are frequently available in health care settings, familiarity with the process and requisite data to be obtained is essential for the provider. Eventually, an individual approach will become a part of the provider's practice.

Developmental Variations

Frequently the health history needs to be adapted for individuals where specific age or condition related data is needed. The following section focuses on these adaptations. (More specific information related to age and condition-related adaptations is found in Chapters 10, 11, and 12.)

Infants and Children

The health history for infants and children is modified depending on the age of the patient. The modifications will be presented within the medical model /ROS approach. When a holistic approach is used, the data can be obtained within the corresponding functional health pattern category.

Chief Concern/Complaint (CC)

The CC is taken from the parent or other responsible adult. When a child is capable of being a reliable informant, to the extent possible, the child should participate in the history taking.

There may be times when the stated concern is not necessarily the real reason for the visit. If there is reason to believe that there is an underlying concern/reason, explore the real reason. The ability to suspect an underlying reason will take time to develop, but as you gain experience and interact with multiple parents, it becomes easier.

Doing a symptom analysis on an infant or young child presents a challenge. Even though the information will be provided from the parent or adult's perspective, the provider should get as much data about the symptom as possible (Figure 5-3). Parents have an intuitive sense about their children and their behavior. Pay close attention to the parent's observations related to the infant's/child's behavioral changes, which may include indicators of pain, and any alterations in the normal daily activities such as eating, sleeping, and playing. Children are also suggestive, so be aware of anyone, provider or parents, who may be coaching the child to respond in a specific manner.

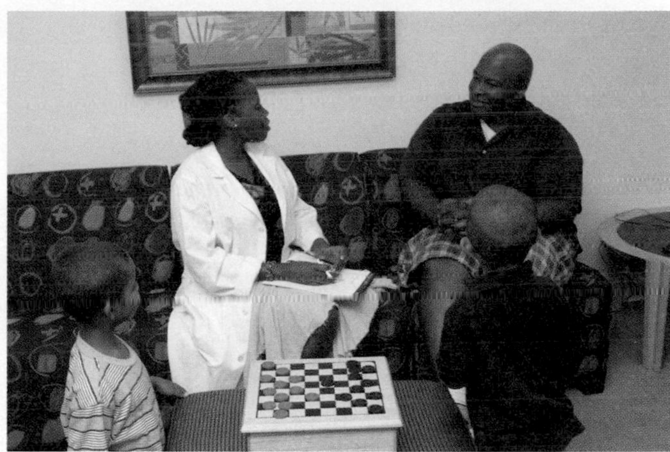

FIGURE 5-3 Interviewing a parent

History of Present Illness (HPI)

The same challenge for symptom analysis can be made for the HPI. Depending on the severity of the illness, assess what impact the condition/illness has had on the family. What is the family's ability to cope and what resources are available.

Past Medical History (PMH)

The PMH of an infant and young child is also concerned with the mother's health during pregnancy and delivery. Questions would include the following:

- What was prenatal care and with what kind of health care practitioner? Frequency of visits? Gestational age at delivery?
- Any complications during pregnancy—bleeding, nausea/vomiting, excess weight gain, high blood pressure, edema, any illnesses/infections?
- Any medications/exposure to toxins/radiation? Use of alcohol, caffeine, cigarettes, street drugs?
- Nutritional status during pregnancy?
- How long/difficult was labor? Vaginal delivery/C-section?
- Anesthetics/analgesics administered? Any complications? APGAR score, birth weight?
- Neonatal status. Length of hospital stay? Complications—bleeding, jaundice, feeding problems? Breast/bottle fed? Appropriate weight gain? Sleeping patterns?

For the older child, less emphasis is placed on the prenatal/neonatal period and more on general childhood activities. Questions would include the following:

- What childhood illnesses—mumps, measles, rubella, chicken pox, ear infections? Recent exposure to illness?
- Any childhood accidents/trauma—auto accidents, falls, fractures, burns, head injuries, ingestion of toxic substances?
- When occurred, treatment, outcome, any long-term effects?
- Any serious or chronic illnesses—meningitis/encephalitis, seizures, respiratory conditions (asthma, pneumonia), allergies, endocrine conditions (DM), renal conditions?
- Age of child when occurred, treatment, any complications or long-term effects?
- Any of the previously identified situations require surgery or hospitalization? Age when occurred, treatment, outcome, reaction to hospitalization?

- Up to date on immunizations?
- Any allergies? To what, what type of reactions?
- What medications taking—prescription, OTC, vitamins?

Developmental History

The developmental history focuses on milestones that the infant/child has achieved or mastered up to this point. Questions would include the following:

- Present height and weight? Gaining weight appropriately?
- Neuromuscular development—when first held head erect when sitting, rollover, sat/walked alone?
- First tooth, first words, first sentences? Toilet trained? Dresses self?
- Does development seem comparable to siblings?
- Gross/fine motor skills appropriate for chronological age?

Family History

The family history is approached in much the same ways as for an adult. A genogram is constructed including the child's siblings, parents, and grandparents. Age of the individuals should be identified if living, or age at death and cause. Any chronic or potential genetic conditions should be identified.

Personal and Social History

The personal and social history focuses on the adjustment of the infant/child to the environment and elements of the environment. Questions would include the following:

- Adjustment to siblings, interaction with family members and other age appropriate individuals?
- History of maladjustment—bedwetting, nail biting, tantrums?
- If in school, how adjusted to school environment, getting along with school mates?
- Home environment—parents married, divorced, separated?
- Income adequate to meet family's needs—transportation, food, shelter?
- Nutritional status—eating appropriate amounts, types of foods? Who prepares food?

Physiological Status/ROS

When obtaining data related to the infant/child's physiological status, additional questions may need to be included.

- Skin—birthmarks, changes in any lesions, diaper rash, eczema?
- HEENT—headaches, dizziness, strabismus, diplopia, able to see board at school, ear aches, otitis media, nasal discharge, cleft palate, frequent sore throats? Dental care—what teeth present, frequency of dental exams, dental hygiene, caries (bottle)?
- Neck—stiffness, limitation of movement?
- Respiratory system—wheezing, difficulty breathing, asthma?
- Cardiovascular—congenital heart problems, murmurs, activity limitations, cyanosis, high blood pressure?
- GI—difficulty with bowel movements, toilet trained, unusual characteristics of stools?
- Renal system—any blood in urine, painful urination, toilet trained, bedwetting?
- Male GU—testicles descended, hypo/epispadius, bulges in scrotum?
- Female GU—vaginal itching, discharge?
- MS—any joint pain/stiffness, limitations in movement, difficulty with gait, able to support self, coordination problems, spinal curvatures?
- Neurological—any numbness, tingling? (Questions in MS system also relate to neurological system.)

Adolescents

Adolescence occurs primarily during the years between 10 and 19. This is a time of rapid growth and development both physically and psychologically. Individuality becomes more important and individuals outside the family become more influential in adolescents lives. Adolescence may be seen as occurring in three stages: early, middle, and late. When each stage occurs is not well defined and varies with each individual.

When taking the health history of the adolescent, it is important to provide time when the adolescent is not in the presence of a parent. Adolescence is a time when experimenting with various activities is most likely to occur and privacy and confidentiality are important to the adolescent. The probability of identifying potential risky behaviors and educating the adolescent on their adverse effects is more likely to happen if the adolescent patient is alone with the provider.

Most of the adaptations for performing a health history on the adolescent focus on the area of psychosocial development.

Physiological changes mostly occur in the reproductive organs as sexual identity and maturity progresses. The adolescent may have many questions and issues about sexuality and maturation; broad areas of concern for the adolescent most likely are related to the following:

- Menstruation—physiology/painful
- Masturbation
- Physical size—too small, too big
- Genital/breast size—too big, too small
- Sexual orientation
- Sexual activity—birth control, pregnancy
- STDs, HIV/AIDS

To initiate the discussion, identify these broad areas of concern and let the adolescent know that it's all right to talk about these issues and that you are comfortable talking about them. Provide the opportunity for discussion by allowing the adolescent to first ask questions. Once the issues and concerns are addressed, ask any question about areas that have not been covered. Keep in mind that the adolescent is probably more comfortable discussing these issues with a provider of the same gender. If this is not possible, reassure the adolescent that you are comfortable with these issues and that you can be trusted. (Sexuality/Sexual history is addressed in Chapter 14.)

The Pregnant Woman

The health history for the pregnant female is modified to the extent that pregnancy is not a disease or pathological condition, but a common occurrence in many females' lives. Each pregnancy may be different; therefore, those unique characteristics need to be recognized, particularly if they cause concern.

The health history for a pregnant female should be adapted to provide the following information (more detail is included in Chapter 11):

- Chief complaint/concern—it is more than likely that the reason for the visit is to document the pregnancy.

- History of present illness—a description of present pregnancy is obtained—last menstrual period (LMP), usual menstrual history (regularity), expected date of delivery (EDD), father of baby.
- Any symptoms—bleeding, spotting, nausea, vomiting, edema
- Obstetric history—information is obtained about previous pregnancies, gravidity/parity, length of pregnancies, weight/gender of infant, type of delivery (spontaneous, C-section). Abortions (spontaneous, elective, therapeutic), length of labor, any complications (pregnancy, labor, delivery, postpartum)
- Menstrual history—additional information includes age at menarche, cycle characteristics, unusual bleeding, and use of contraceptives.
- Gynecologic history—included information regarding last Pap smear, sexual history (age at first intercourse, number of partners, partner orientation, age of partner if a minor). Use of contraceptives, reason for discontinuing and use after pregnancy. Infertility treatments and any use of hormones, particularly diethylstilbestrol (DES). Any history of STDs (dates, types, treatments, complications).
- Past medical history—any exposure to AIDS, TB, hepatitis, or environmental or occupational hazards.
- Family history—any genetic conditions, multiple births, gestational diabetes, preeclampsia/eclampsia, pregnancy induced hypertension (PIH), or congenital anomalies
- Personal and social history—planned pregnancy, if not adoption/abortion, social support available, positive experiences with mothering (mother and mothered), plans for labor, breast feeding, history of abuse
- Physiological status—special attention to reproductive, cardiovascular (obtain baseline BP, prior to pregnancy if possible), pulmonary, and renal systems (baseline function)

The Older Adult

Generally, the format for the health history of the older adult is not that much different than for the adult patient. Some additional questions may be asked that are specific to the older patient. These generally focus on changes associated with the aging process and the functional ability of the patient.

- Chief complaint/concern—may be difficult to determine. Many times symptoms, as they are experienced, are assumed to be related to aging and are not considered significant. Chronology of events may be difficult for the patient to establish and there might also be some confusion and/or memory loss. Sometimes the symptoms experienced are not directly related to the actual cause, for example confusion related to infections.
- Past medical health—it may not be necessary to review the individual's whole past health; going back only 5 to 10 years may be sufficient. It is very important to obtain a medication history for the elderly patient. Nonprescription medications as well as nutritional supplements need to be identified for the possibility of interactions. Many elderly are also on many medications that create problems for them. Frequently, different providers will prescribe a medication without knowing what else the patient may be taking. The problems that the patient is experiencing may be due to all the medications.
- Family history—is not as important in the elderly as in younger individuals.
- Physiological status—primarily changes in the sensory components (eyes, ears) as well as mobility parameters (MS and neurological) are major areas for assessing any alterations.
- Functional assessment—to identify any real or potential difficulties associated with day-to-day activities. A functional assessment should include, but is not necessarily limited to, the following:
  - Mobility—balance, coordination, transferring self, climbing stairs, assist devices
  - Upper extremity strength—grasping small objects, opening jars/medication bottles, ability to reach out or overhead
  - Bathing, dressing, toileting
  - Nutrition—able to feed self, plan/make meals, appetite, money to buy groceries, shopping convenience
  - Environment—any rugs, obstacles, rails
  - Medications—able to take, afford
  - Transportation—public, self, depend on whom?
  - Safety—house locks, environment, neighbors/family close
  - Support systems—friends/family, living arrangements, organizations
  - Health care—access, affordability

Summary

- The functions of the health history are to provide the patient the opportunity to relay significant information about a health concern and to provide the provider the opportunity to establish a relationship with the patient.
- The health history used to obtain data related to the patient's present health status/concern as well as biographical, physiological, psychological, sociological, and emotional states.
- Symptom analysis is done to obtain data related to all the component factors involved in the manifestations of the symptom.
- There are two approaches to obtaining data for the health history—the patient-centered approach and the provider-centered approach.
- Various health disciplines have unique ways of clustering health history data for purposes of clinical decision making.

Review Questions

1. The provider recognizes which of the following statements as true regarding the health history portion of patient assessment?
   1. The health history provides the majority of data needed to make a diagnosis.
   2. The primary focus of the health history is to establish a relationship with the patient.
   3. The health history is obtained after the physical examination.
   4. The health history provides data to identify how the physical exam should proceed.
2. A patient who is being seen for the first time identifies the problem as a bad case of indigestion. The provider would include this information as which of the following?
   1. primary diagnosis
   2. symptom of concern
   3. chief complaint
   4. a diagnosis of heart burn
3. When doing a symptom analysis using COLDERRA, the first question that is generally asked would be which of the following?
   1. "Is this a new or an old symptom?"
   2. "Can you describe what you are feeling?"
   3. How long have you experienced this particular sensation?"
   4. "Are there other family members who have had the same experience?"
4. To include relief measure in the symptom analysis, the provider would include which of the following questions in the patient interview?
   1. "What type of diet are you on?"
   2. "What are your bowel habits?"
   3. "What helps to make the indigestion go away?"
   4. "What medications are you presently taking?"
5. The provider recognizes that primary purpose of doing a family history with each patient is to do which of the following?
   1. Identify exposure to infectious diseases.
   2. Determine if there might be any genetically linked conditions.
   3. Determine the patient's risk for disease.
   4. Identify family members who should be examined by a health care provider.
6. Through using the patient-centered approach to the health history the provider may accomplish which of the following? (Select all that apply.)
   1. improvement of patient outcomes
   2. improvement of patient satisfaction
   3. reduction in provider satisfaction
   4. increase in the time spent with the patient
   5. reduced risk of malpractice complaints
7. The provider recognizes that the portion of the health history that is considered to be provider focused is which of the following?
   1. family history
   2. chief complaint
   3. review of the systems
   4. history of present illness
8. The provider is using a genogram to display a patient's family history. How should the provider denote that the patient's father is deceased when using this tool?
   1. Leave the father off the genogram as it only deals with living relatives.
   2. Write a separate note in the patient's record to note that the father is deceased.
   3. Draw a line through the patient's father on the genogram.
   4. Draw an arrow to the patient's father on the genogram.
9. The provider is planning to organize the data gathered from a patient's health history using Gordon's Functional Health Patterns. Which categories should the provider include? (Select all that apply.)
   1. cognitive/perceptual
   2. neurological
   3. cardiac
   4. exercise/activity
   5. chief concern
10. The provider is conducting a health history interview on a patient who is a young child. What additional information should the provider gather during this interview that would not be included in an adult health history?
    1. immunization history
    2. past medical history
    3. biographical data
    4. maternal health

Clinical Skills of Assessment for Physical Examination

6

Whew, I'm glad that's over! I guess it was supposed to be a physical, but it just seemed like I was poked and prodded, and looked at without any rhyme or reason. This person in a scrub suit comes into my room and tells me that she going to look at a few things and also listen and feel. It seems like every day someone comes into my room to "examine" me—as if I haven't had that done enough. She just seemed so nervous that she couldn't focus on what she was supposed to do. The whole time she was just so disorganized. I would have liked to know what she was going to do or what she was looking for, but all I could hear were mumblings under her breath—I guess she didn't like how the "poking and prodding" was going. It's a good thing that I'm not ticklish, because when she was poking my belly, she barely touched me—it felt more like she was tickling me. I wish she would have asked for some feedback, because if every one of her exams goes like this, I'm not sure I would want her to take care of me again.

LEARNING OUTCOMES

1. Summarize the primary functions of the physical examination.
2. Explain the four clinical skills used in performing a physical exam.
3. Differentiate between various techniques of the clinical skills techniques.
4. Recognize the function and use of the equipment and instruments in the performance a physical exam.
5. Explain Standard Precautions and the procedures necessary to implement them.

The physical examination component of health assessment is directed toward obtaining data that relates to the physiological well-being of the patient. The physical exam is also performed to provide additional information as well as validate information obtained from the history. Physical exam data is considered objective data, indicating that it is obtained through the provider's senses, primarily by seeing, hearing, and feeling selected systems and areas of the patient's body. While these senses are functioning constantly to present to the provider with information about his or her environment, they must be redirected during the course of the examination and skillfully implemented to receive and interpret specific data regarding the patient.

Functions of the Physical Examination

The primary function of the physical examination is to obtain significant data regarding a patient's health status, it is also important for the improvement of the provider–patient relationship and patient safety (Junger et al., 2005). With the increase in use and dependence on technological advances, the significance of clinical skills in performing a physical examination has been questioned (Anderson, Fagan, & Sebastian, 2001). While data obtained from advanced technology is essential, in many instances, there is evidence that technology has not necessarily improved the quality of patient care (Feddock, 2007).

Competency in clinical skills is essential for critical thinking and decision making, which requires analysis and synthesis of all significant obtained data, including data obtained with physical examination clinical skills (Omori, Wong, Antonelli, & Hemmer, 2005). The essence of a skilled physical examination is not an impeccable examination of each organ system, independent of each other; but that providers use their knowledge judiciously to guide the examination in searching for data to facilitate critical thinking and diagnostic reasoning (Garden, 2005).

Learning and mastering the skills and techniques of physical examination requires the student/provider to consciously and critically focus on achieving these skills through repetitive performance of intended cognitive or psychomotor skills. This may also be referred to as "deliberate practice" (Duvivier et al., 2011). It is relatively easy to learn and master the clinical skills of performing the physical exam; what is not so easy is interpretation of data received (Feddock, 2007).

Every day, a person's brain receives, transmits, and recognizes a significant amount of sensory data. The brain unconsciously processes all this data to regulate certain voluntary and involuntary actions and responses; thus an individual is not always aware of all the data received and processed.

Once the student/provider has received data through a specific sensory modality and processed it, the initial step is to determine its significance. In the context of physical examination, this refers primarily to whether the data is an expected or an unexpected representation of the system or area being examined and the context in which the data is obtained. Examination of patients occurs in various contexts and situations, which, for purposes of this text, is described as *levels*.

While the general interpretation is that unexpected data represents a pathological condition or illness, multiple instances exist where the data is unexpected but not necessarily associated with, or a representation of, a pathological condition or illness.

Four clinical skills are used to obtain objective data. These are (1) inspection, (2) palpation, (3) percussion, and (4) auscultation. These clinical skills are incorporated into our everyday activities as health care providers; however, our cognitive awareness of their use is often not recognized.

Inspection

Inspection is assimilation of data through vision or sight. It is easy to think that this is a skill used on a daily basis and may not require any skill development; however, inspection is a disciplined skill of attending to identifying and taking in significant data about the patient. Visual inspection is composed of two levels: looking and observing.

Looking is simply seeing and taking in all aspects of our environment. It is an unconscious activity that is used constantly to assist in identifying objects and individuals within our environment. Looking may be likened to a camera that simply records the data and processes the information to provide a representation or a documentation of the event or object. The significance of visual data is only identified when there is a need to provide meaning to the situation, such as a perceived threat and a need to maintain a safe and protective environment.

Observation, on the other hand, is a conscious effort to study the environment or objects for specific details that require some form of interpretation. Observation also requires recall and inclusion of previous, stored data in order to make comparisons to determine its meaning and significance.

Of the four techniques, observation is the only one that is used continuously throughout the entire examination. Observation begins with the initial patient encounter and provides the majority of information that is obtained through the physical exam. Observation can also be performed at a distance from the patient to prevent an invasion of personal space. Even though observation is constantly used throughout the exam, it may be necessary to take time to concentrate on observing without using any of the other techniques.

Successful observation requires an adequate amount of available light. Direct light may come from direct sources (daylight) or from artificial sources (incandescent). Whatever the source, there needs to be enough light to allow for adequate assessment of skin color(s), texture, and movement without any interference from shadows. In some instances, tangential lighting may be necessary to provide more details related to contour and alterations of the body surface (Figure 6-1).

It is impossible to observe anything that is not exposed to the light. While protection of the patient's modesty is important, it does not eliminate the need for observation of all parts of the body. This may necessitate the moving or manipulation of body parts and drapes to provide adequate exposure for observation.

As with all skills, practice is necessary to develop and refine the ability to perform a task or activity. Conscious awareness of when and how to observe will gradually progress to incorporating it into daily and regular practice.

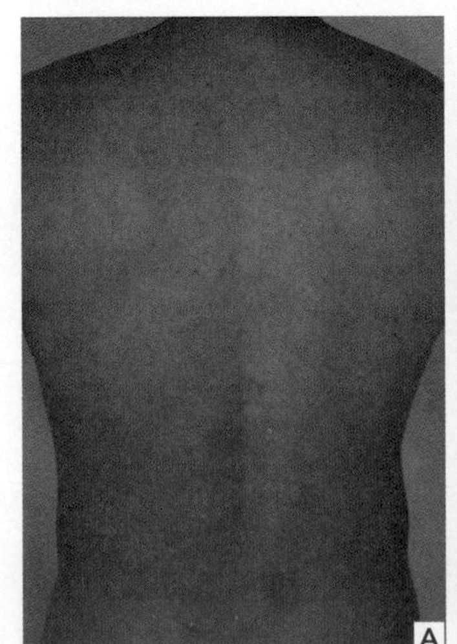

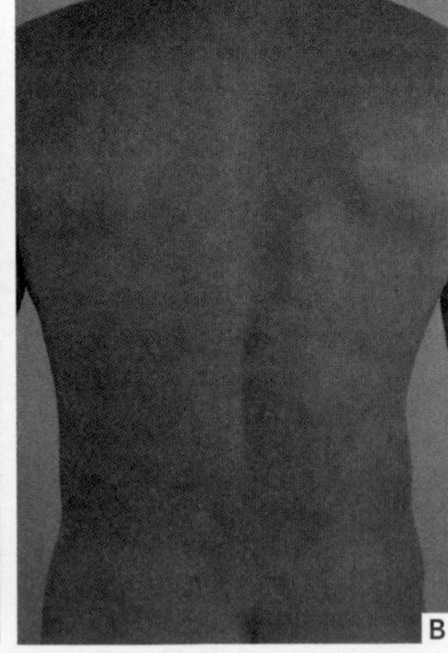

FIGURE 6-1A–B Light sources for assessment: **a)** direct lighting; **b)** indirect lighting

Palpation

Palpation is acquisition of data through tactile sensation. As with observation, taking in and interpreting tactile sensations requires attention to and concentration on the data. Tactile data is primarily obtained through the hands and fingers. It too can be perceived as existing in two components: touching and feeling.

Touch is the placing of the hand and fingers on parts of the body under various circumstances. Touch requires closeness to the patient that invades personal space. A person's comfortableness with touch, both doing and having it done, is frequently influenced by cultural practices, personal characteristics, and the determination of personal space (Table 6-1). Touch also varies by degrees as demonstrated by a light touch to communicate closeness, a firm touch, as in a firm handshake. A firm touch demonstrates assuredness and confidence, which is important to convey to the patient. Even when there may be doubt in regards to how well a technique is performed, do it with confidence. Conversely, touch may also be used to irritate or harm another by tickling and inflicting pain.

Touch is also a means of communication and its use implies a certain amount of closeness experienced by the involved individuals. It frequently is interpreted as a characteristic of affection or support. Touch can be a powerful interaction between individuals and should not be used inappropriately when performing the examination. Touch can also be considered therapeutic, and its use in this manner may be considered as a healing approach.

When performing palpation, inform the patient that it is necessary to use touch to obtain certain data. Touch in this context is referred to as feeling. **Feeling** implies use of touch to discriminate between various characteristics of the underlying tissues and/or organs. Data from feeling related to specific characteristics is best obtained by using various parts of the hand and fingers (Figure 6-2). How this data is obtained will be detailed more specifically for each system.

Palpation is performed as light or deep, depending on the amount of pressure that is required and exerted by the fingers and hand. **Light palpation** goes to a depth of about 1 cm and **deep palpation** goes to a depth of 4 cm (Figure 6-3). The depth of palpation is also determined by how much resistance is present over the area being examined. Light palpation is always performed before deep palpation as deep palpation may produce tenderness or pain, or disrupt tissues or fluids, causing interference with obtaining and interpreting data from light palpation. Deep palpation is primarily used when examining the abdomen as there is no extensive boney framework and muscle to offer any significant resistance to palpation.

Table 6-1 Levels of social distance (proxemics)

Intimate distance (6–8 inches)	Indicates a closer relationship or greater comfort with intimacy between individuals as demonstrated by hugging, whispering, or touching.
Personal distance (1.5–4 feet)	Occurs between family members or close friends. Closeness of relationship demonstrated by how close two individuals stand together when interacting.
Social distance (4–12 feet)	Level of closeness demonstrated with acquaintances. The more acquainted with each other, the closer they stand next to each other.
Public distance (12–25 feet)	Demonstrated in public speaking situations, such as lecturing or making presentations.

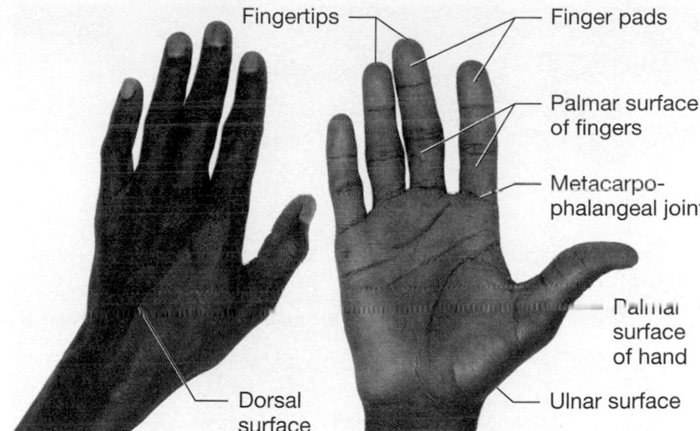

FIGURE 6-2 Various parts of hands are used for specific purposes

Palpation may be accomplished by using either one hand or both. When using one hand, applying pressure and feeling the area is done at the same time. Use of both hands is considered **bimanual**, and again is primarily used for examination of the abdomen (Figure 6-4). When using both hands, one hand is placed over the other with the upper hand applying the pressure and the lower hand doing the feeling. One method is not preferred over the other and depends primarily on the preference of the provider.

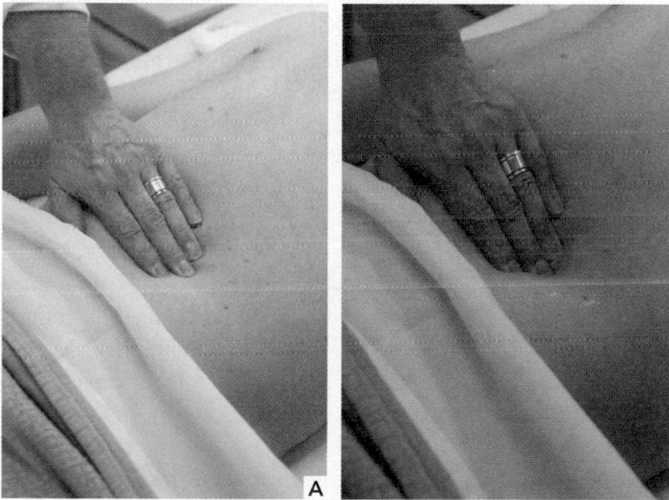

FIGURE 6-3A–B **a)** light palpation; **b)** deep palpation

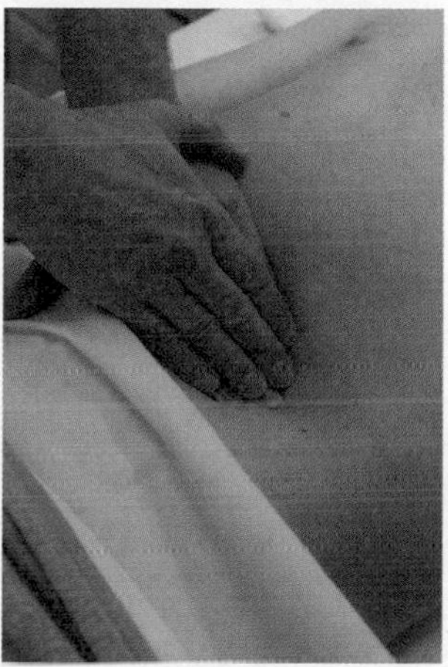

FIGURE 6-4 Bimanual palpation

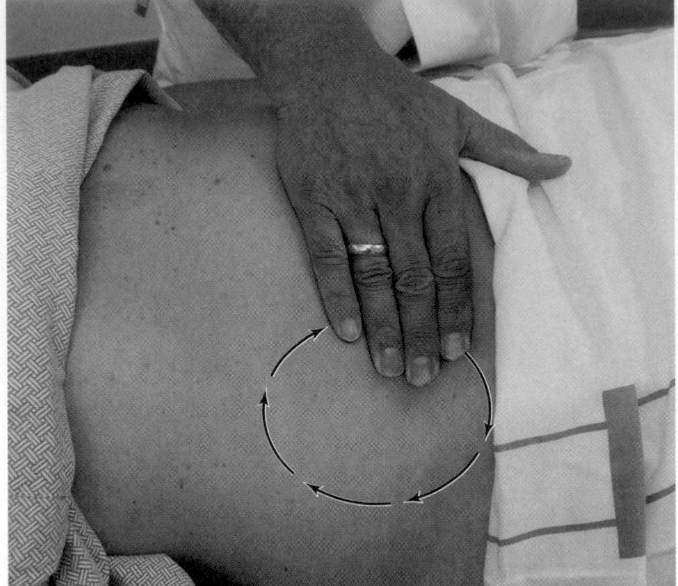

FIGURE 6-5 Moving hands in circular motion

When performing palpation, it is also necessary to move the fingers in a circular motion to increase the possibility of identifying suspicious data. When doing so, the rotary motion of the fingers should be done firmly in a continuous motion (Figure 6-5). A light touch with superficial rotary movements may induce tickling, making it more difficult to accomplish palpation.

It may take a while for the beginning provider to become comfortable with touching and feeling bodies and parts of another individual. Initial attempts at palpation may be done with some hesitation for fear of hurting the patient or touching personal and sensitive areas. Palpation should always be performed by placing the hand firmly on the skin and applying firm pressure, indicating that this is being performed for gathering data and not for taking advantage of the patient. Touching parts of the body that may not need to be examined (depending on the type of exam being performed) is never appropriate and should never be attempted. This sends the wrong message and most likely interferes with the trust a patient places in the provider.

Percussion

Percussion is a technique that requires manual dexterity and skill to perform. The primary purpose of percussion is to produce sounds that can be heard and interpreted. The sensory component involved is the auditory process; the sounds heard are vibrations that are produced by the various structures of the patient's body that are percussed. Percussion is performed by striking or tapping the body surface. While striking may be associated with causing harm or pain, the strikes or taps are only as strong as is necessary to produce the sounds.

Perceiving the auditory signals from percussion also consists of two components: hearing and listening. **Hearing**, like seeing and touching, is something that is constantly occurring. Auditory information comes from a multitude of sources and is often ignored or unconsciously processed. We hear multiple sounds simultaneously but often pay little attention to them.

To appropriately interpret audio data, instead of simply hearing, it is necessary to consciously **listen** and discern the various sources of sound and differentiate between them. Percussion requires the ability to differentiate between various sounds that are produced by the vibrations that occur from striking the body surface. The sounds produced depend on the density of the underlying organs or structures. The density of an organ or tissue is determined by the relative ratio of air to solid material that composes the organ or structure. The greater the amount of solid material, the greater the density, and conversely, the greater the amount of air, the less density there is. The five sounds produced by vibrations from percussion are (1) tympany, (2) hyperresonance, (3) resonance, (4) dullness, and (5) flatness.

For comparison of sounds related to the organs' densities consider that resonance is heard over organs that are comprised of equal amount of air and tissue. Tympany and hyperresonance are heard over organs that have an increased amount of air in them; dullness and flatness are heard over organs that contain an increased amount of tissue. Each of these sounds is heard under expected and unexpected conditions. Expected sounds occur over specific organs or locations on the body. Unexpected sound occurs when certain sounds are heard over specific organs or body locations where they are not expected to be heard and generally indicate some type of pathology. Sounds and their expected locations are identified and described in Table 6-2.

PRACTICE POINT: Fingernails and Temperature

Palpation, when performed properly, is done with short fingernails and warm hands. To appropriately palpate, the fingers are positioned at an angle, so long fingernails prevent proper placement of the fingers as well as poking the skin surface with sharp objects. Palpation is also more comfortable for the patient when the provider's hands are warm. This may be difficult for some providers who have consistently cool hands. Placing cool hands on the patient's abdomen may cause the patient to jerk or tense up. Rubbing the hands together may help to warm the hands, or before palpation is started, inform the patient that your hands are cool and that they will be gently placed on the lower chest or upper arm to condition the patient to the sensation of cool hands. This should prevent any sudden jerking or tensing of the abdominal muscles.

PRACTICE POINT: Mastering Percussion

Percussion requires mastering the technique as well as becoming familiar with the specific tones that it produces. Percussion also requires some coordination in moving the hands together over the percussed area. This requires practice and may be accomplished by percussing various objects or areas. One such activity is to percuss a wall on a horizontal plane to try and locate the studs. The sound will change when going from the space between the studs to where a stud is being percussed. The change in sound is due to the change in density from an air-filled space to a solid-object space. These sounds may not be exactly like the sounds produced by the body, but listening for the change in sounds is important for identifying the exact sound. Another option is to percuss a half-filled gallon bottle of milk or water. Again the sound will change when going from percussing the upper part that is filled with air to the lower portion that is filled with liquid. It's also a good idea to practice on another student or willing person. Knowing where to percuss for expected sounds will also help in identifying its characteristics and its particular tone.

Table 6-2 Percussion sounds

Percussion Tone	Ratio of Air to Tissue	Loudness	Example
Flatness	Air << tissue	Soft	Muscle (Thigh)
Dullness	Air < tissue	Medium	Liver
Resonance	Air = tissue	Loud	Lung
Hyperresonance	Air > tissue	Very Loud	Hyperinflated lung (COPD)
Tympany	Air >> tissue	Loud	Stomach (Gastric Bubble)

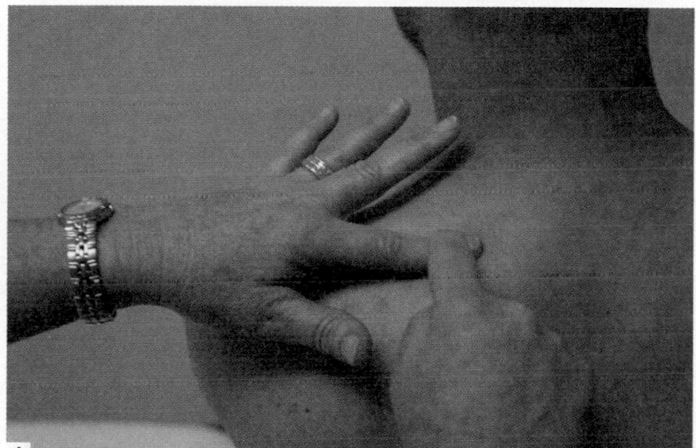

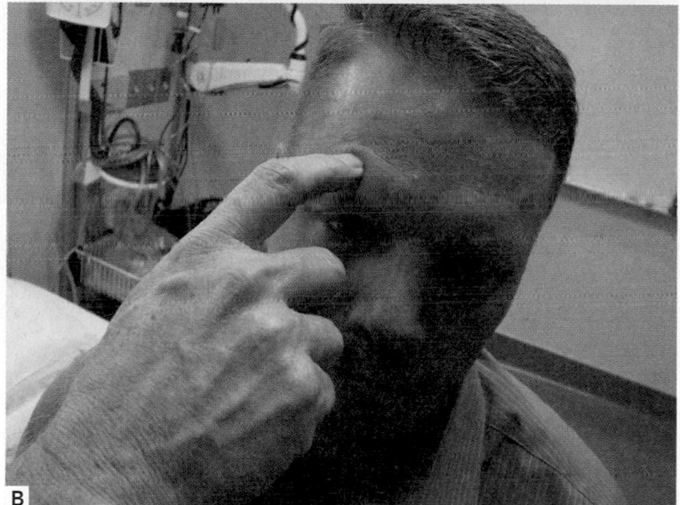

FIGURE 6-6A–B a) Indirect percussion; b) direct percussion

Although percussion is a relative easy technique, it needs to be performed correctly. Percussion can be described as direct or indirect (immediate or mediate). **Direct percussion** is striking the surface of the body directly, whereas **indirect percussion** indicates that there is something between the provider's finger and the body surface (Figure 6-6). During the examination it is the provider's finger of the opposite hand that is the intermediate object.

To perform percussion, begin by placing the distal portion of the middle finger of the nondominate hand over the area to be percussed. This is also referred to as the **plexor** (Figure 6-7a). Only the distal portion of the finger should be in contact with the body surface; if other fingers or parts of the hand are on the surface, there may be interference by absorption of vibrations and decreasing their sounds. The middle finger of the dominant hand will be used to percuss, which is also referred to as the **pleximeter** (Figure 6-7b). With a snap of the wrist, deliver a sharp hit or tap over the interphalangeal joint of the plexor. The downward action of the hit must be from the wrist, not from the forearm or shoulder. Once the tap has been delivered, quickly snap the wrist up to prevent dampening of the sound. The plexor should be tapped 2–3 times to provide adequate time to hear and interpret the sounds produced. Percussion is generally used over a larger surface area so that once a percussion tone has been obtained over one section, move to another and repeat the process. Percussion is performed in a systematic progression from site to site. Specific progression patterns will be identified and described in more detail in various chapters related to the system that is being assessed.

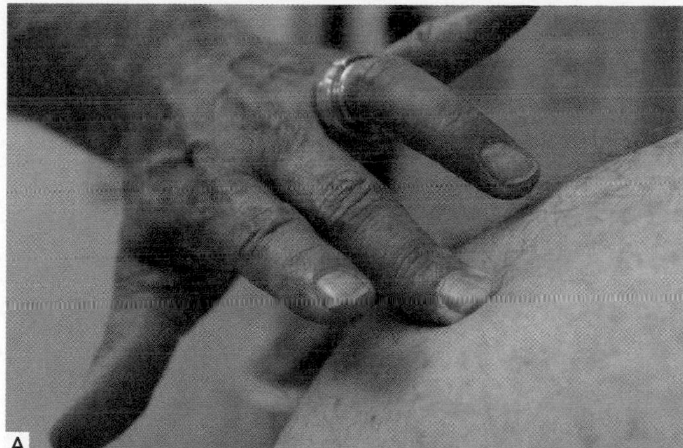

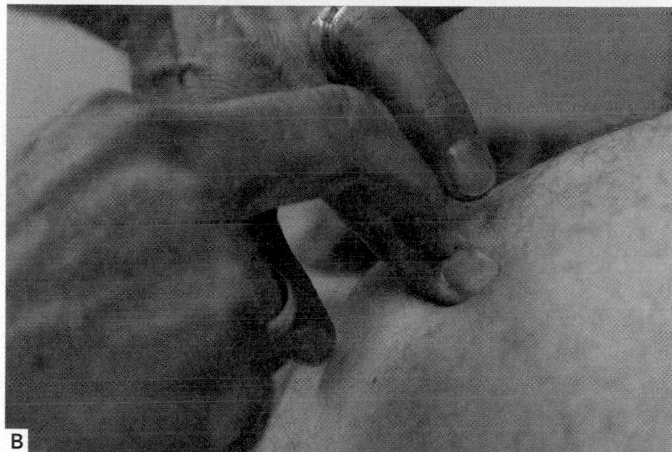

FIGURE 6-7A–B a) Plexor; b) pleximeter

If the sounds produced are not very loud, the tap may need to be stronger or the plexor may need to be placed more firmly on the body surface. Also consider body build and type when evaluating the intensity of the sound. Excess fat and muscle may absorb the

***THINK LINK:** Transmission of Vibrations*

Transmission of vibrations is enhanced when they are going through solid material versus going through air. Thus, when a tissue or organ becomes denser, either through collapse of the tissue or the accumulation of fluid, vibrations will be louder or more intense. To compare or interpret the change of sounds relative to increased density, it is essential to be able to identify what the expected sound is over an area.

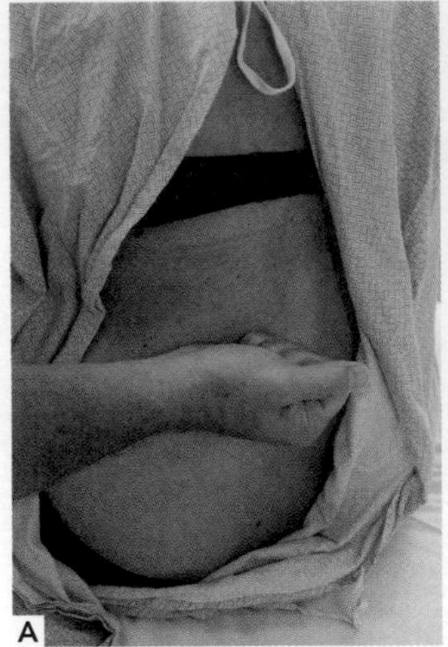

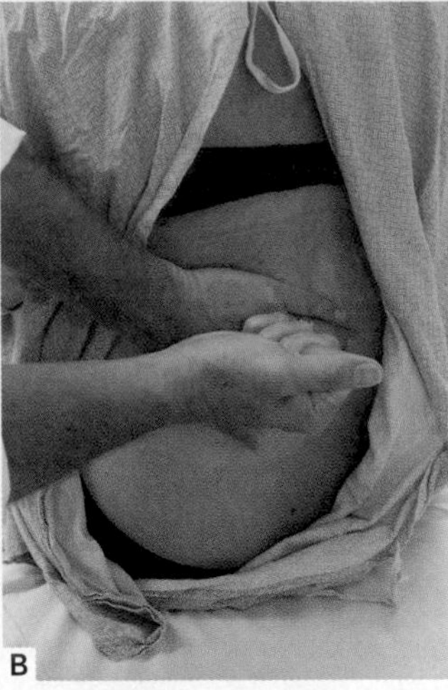

FIGURE 6-8A–B a) Direct and b) indirect fist percussion

vibrations and not transmit them as well to the underlying organs or tissue and back to the surface, causing a diminished intensity.

An additional type of percussion is **fist percussion** (Figure 6-8), which is used more for determining the presence of tenderness or pain of certain organs or locations rather than for producing vibrations. To perform fist percussion, use the ulnar portion of the fist to deliver a firm hit to the area (Figure 6-8a). Again, this may be done directly or indirectly. Indirect percussion is done by placing an open hand over the area and then delivering a firm hit to the hand (Figure 6-8b). Because sound vibrations are not necessary, the whole hand can be placed over the area.

Auscultation

Auscultation is the fourth technique used in physical examination and refers to sounds that are heard through the stethoscope. It is the only technique that is dependent on an additional piece of equipment. Different organs produce different sounds based on their unique characteristics and function, so what sounds are heard depends on which organs are being auscultated. Auscultation of underlying organs validates the presence of expected sounds. As with the other techniques, mastering the skill of placing the stethoscope is easily accomplished; the difficulty is determining where to place it and identifying and differentiating various sounds.

While auscultation is usually not differentiated into direct and indirect, auscultation with a stethoscope is considered an indirect procedure. Before the days of the stethoscope, the provider's ear was placed directly on the body for listening to sounds within. This direct method presented some difficulties in certain situations, particularly when a male was examining a female. The first stethoscope consisted of a hollow tube with one end placed on the body and the other end placed over the provider's ear. This allowed the provider to listen to sounds without being in direct contact with the patient. From this early instrument the modern stethoscope was developed with its unique components.

The specific details related to the components of the stethoscope will be discussed later in this chapter. For now, the characteristics of auscultated sound will be described. During auscultation two pitches of sound may be heard: **low-pitched sounds** and **high-pitched sounds**. The part of the chest piece that is used will help in determining what the pitch of the sounds is expected to be related to what organ(s) is being assessed. High-pitched sounds are produced by the lungs and abdominal organs and are best heard with the diaphragm of the stethoscope. The first two heart sounds are also considered high pitched sounds while murmurs and the third and fourth heart sound are lower pitched and may be best heard with the bell of the chest piece.

Like percussion, auscultation is often performed in a systematic progression. Again, these progression patterns will be identified in later chapters when describing assessment of specific systems and organs. When performing auscultation, certain actions and practices will assist you in becoming comfortable and skilled with the technique. This information is summarized in Table 6-3.

Performing the Exam

The physical exam occurs right after the patient history. In the clinical setting, the patient most likely is already wearing a patient gown. In the office setting, if the patient has not had the opportunity to change clothes and put on a patient gown, have the patient do this prior to starting the exam.

Table 6-3 Success in auscultation

Create a quiet environment	Even if ear pieces placed securely in ear canal, background noise is not eliminated. Turn off or mute TV, radios, and other audio systems.
Place chest piece securely on bare skin	The chest piece of the stethoscope should be in direct contact with the patient's skin without the interference of any articles of clothing. Make sure that the clothing is far enough away to avoid any possibility that it will come in contact with the chest piece. Do not listen to sounds through clothing.
Place ear pieces securely in ear canal	Position the ear pieces so that the sound from the stethoscope is directed toward the tympanic membrane. The ear pieces should have a good seal to block out as much ambient noise as possible.
Be patient	Don't rush auscultation; take time to identify the specific sound, focus on it and allow enough time to fully appreciate it. Closing your eyes may help direct your focus on a specific sound. When multiple sounds are heard, isolate and listen to each sound. It is incorrect to listen and interpret multiple sounds at the same time.
Differentiate characteristics of sound	These characteristics relate to intensity, pitch, duration, and quality. Often these differences are subtle and require a significant amount of practice just listening to various sounds to hear changes that occur. Frequently, you may hear more than one sound, but it is important to focus only on the specific sound being assessed. This will also improve with practice.

Patient Positions for Examination

A thorough physical examination requires that the patient be placed in various positions. The two most used positions are the **seated position** and **supine position**. For patients being examined in the clinical setting, they will most likely be resting in bed in the supine position. Depending on the mobility of the patient, the seated position may also be used. The patient being examined in the office setting will most likely be in the seated position. Along with the positions, appropriate draping in necessary to maintain modesty for the patient. These and other positions in which the patient may be placed are identified and described in Table 6-4.

Table 6-4 Patient positions for exam

Position Name	Type of Examination	
Seated position	Anterior and posterior head and chest	
Fowler's position	Examination of the head, neck, and upper body	90° angle
Semi-Fowler's position	Post-surgical exams; patients with breathing difficulties or lower back injuries	45° angle
Supine position	Examination of the anterior or ventral surface of the body; some x-rays	
Dorsal recumbent position	Examination of the head, neck, chest, and vaginal, rectal, or perineal areas	
Lithotomy position	Vaginal examinations requiring the use of a vaginal speculum; Pap smears	

Continued

Table 6-4 Patient positions for exam (*continued*)

Position Name	Type of Examination
Prone position	Back exams; certain types of surgery. Not used for patients with breathing problems, women in late-term pregnancies, or the elderly
Sims' position	Rectal, perineal, and pelvic exams; rectal temperatures; enemas
Trendelenburg position	Shock or low blood pressure; abdominal surgery
Knee-chest position	Proctologic, rectal, and vaginal exams; sigmoidoscopy procedures
Proctologic (jack-knife) position	Proctologic examinations with a sigmoidoscope

Instruments and Equipment

The four techniques provide the foundation for performing a physical exam; however, at times additional equipment and/or instruments are necessary to supplement the four techniques. Their use during the exam is determined by what procedures need to be done as determined by the scope and data needed from the exam.

Stethoscope

For stethoscopes to function properly and provide transmission of reliable sounds, the parts all need to be working correctly. The most common type of stethoscope used for assessment is the **acoustic stethoscope**. It is composed of three parts: (1) the chest piece, (2) tubing, and (3) ear pieces (Figure 6-9).

The chest piece picks up and transmits the sound and consists of two listening sides—the diaphragm and bell. The diaphragm is a flat circle with rigid material stretched across its base. The diaphragm is

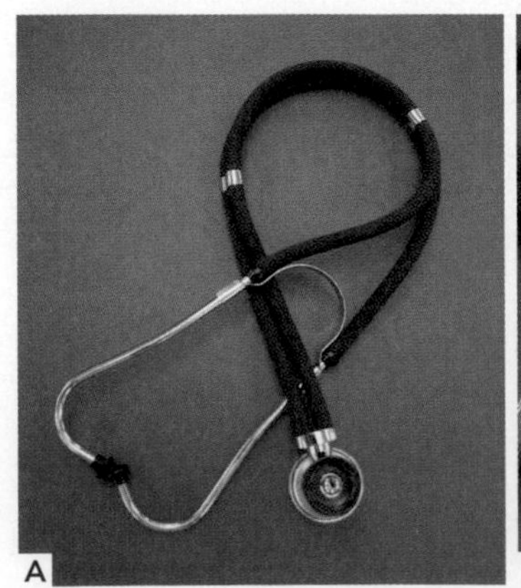

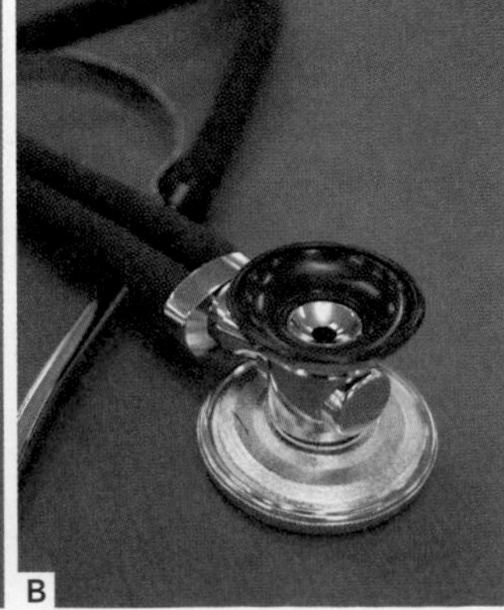

FIGURE 6-9 Stethoscope parts

used to pick up and transmit high-frequency sounds such as breath sounds and the first two heart sounds. The bell of the stethoscope is a concave bowl that is open with no material stretched across it that picks up and transmits low-pitched sounds such as the third and fourth heart sounds as well as murmurs. Both the bell and the diaphragm have an opening at the center that aligns with an opening in the valve that is connected to the tubing. The chest piece rotates around the valve to align the opening of either the bell or diaphragm with the opening in the valve. Chest pieces are also sized for adult or pediatric patients.

If no sounds are heard, check to determine if the sounds are being transmitted by the bell or diaphragm. There should be a visible opening at the bottom of the bell or chest piece indicating that sound is going through. This is easier to see on the bell as there is no covering to obscure the bottom area. Or, the diaphragm can be lightly tapped to determine if the sounds can be heard.

The tubing of the stethoscope usually is determined by personal choice or comfort. Ideally, tubing that is no longer than 12 inches is recommended. The rationale for this is that sound has a shorter distance to travel. However, for tall individuals, shorter tubing requires bending over to a greater extent and may result in sore back muscles. Double tubing is also recommended as each tube goes directly to one ear. A drawback to double tubing is that they tend to rub on each other and may interfere with the actual sounds and/or cause the provider to interpret those sounds as unexpected.

The earpieces must also be properly adjusted and placed correctly in the ears (Figure 6-10). Anatomically, the external ear canal is placed at an angle to the external ear, so for proper listening to occur the ear pieces need to be placed so that the sound is directed toward the tympanic membrane. For this to occur, the earpieces should be pointed toward the nose when placing them into the ear canal. If they are placed in the ear at a 90-degree angle, chances are that the sound will not be transmitted to the tympanic membrane.

When listening with the stethoscope, you will use the two parts of the chest piece differently (Figure 6-12). The diaphragm is placed firmly on the skin and transmits sounds regardless of the pressure placed on it. Sounds that are produced vibrate the diaphragm, which results in acoustic pressure waves that travel through the tubing to the ear pieces. Place the bell placed lightly on

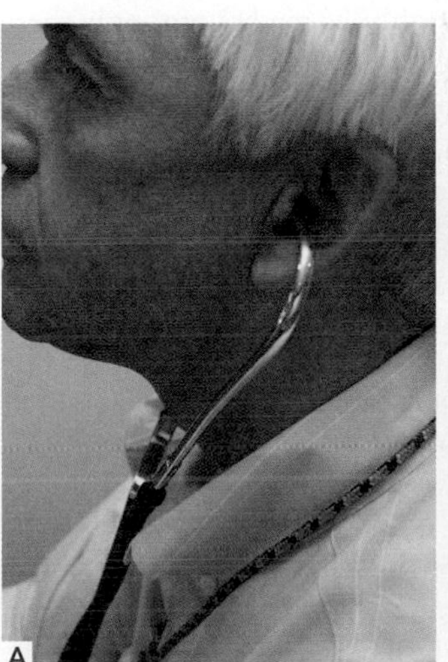

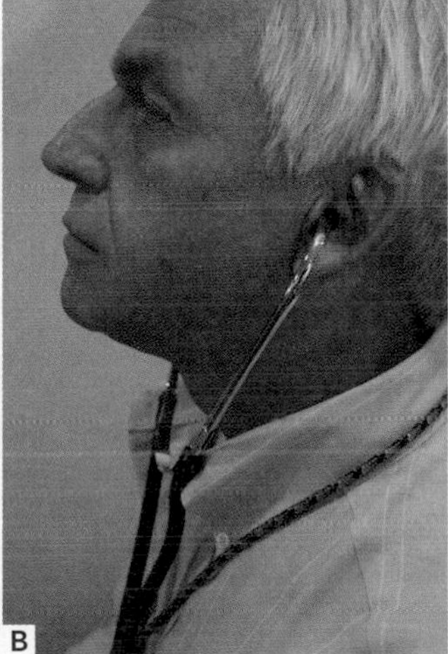

FIGURE 6-10A–B a) Correct and **b)** incorrect placement of earpieces in ear

PRACTICE POINT: Unable to Hear Sounds

When beginning to use the stethoscope, it is not unusual for the student provider to not hear any sounds through the stethoscope. When this occurs, there is most likely a very simple remedy. The first step is to check to make sure that the opening of the chest piece being used is aligned correctly with the opening in the valve. When looking at the opening in the center of the diaphragm of bell, if the openings are aligned, it should appear black (Figure 6-11). If it is not aligned, the closed side of the valve should be visible.

Another way of testing alignment is to gently tap on the diaphragm with the earpieces laced in the ear canal. When the sounds can be heard, the diaphragm opening and the valve opening are aligned.

The other thing to check is to make sure that the earpieces are correctly placed within the ear canal. If the earpieces are not pointing forward, chances are that sounds were not being conducted to the tympanic membrane. Simply remove the ear pieces from the ear canal and twist the earpieces slightly forward.

It also might be possible that there is some type of obstruction either within the earpiece or tubing, or there may be a wax buildup in one or both ears. Removing the obstruction should remedy the problem.

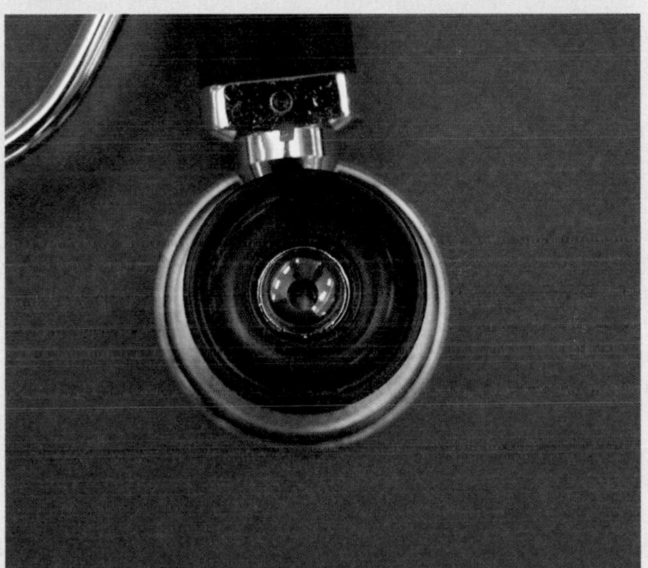

FIGURE 6-11 Alignment of openings in the center of the diaphragm of bell

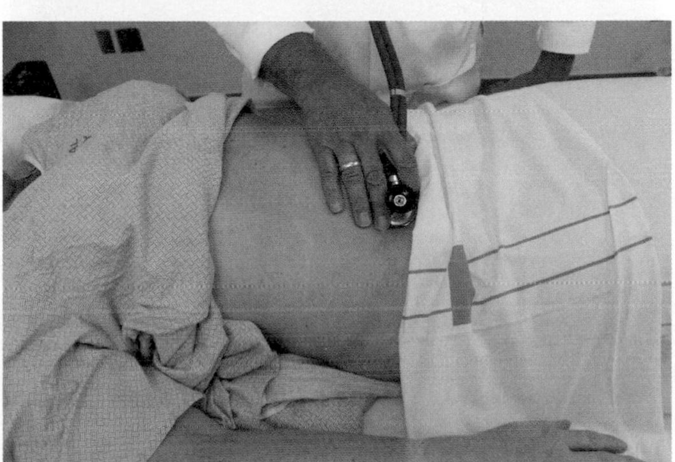

FIGURE 6-12 Use of bell/diaphragm

the skin with just enough pressure to create a seal. This provides the optimum transmission of low-pitched sounds. If too much pressure is placed on the bell, the stretching of the skin creates and acts as a diaphragm, which eliminates the purpose for using the bell. More recently designed stethoscopes only have a bell, which requires that a diaphragm be created by applying increased pressure on the chest piece and stretching the skin.

Another type of stethoscopes that may be used is the **electronic stethoscope** that detects the vibrations on the body surface and then converts them to electrical impulses. These impulses are amplified and then sent to a speaker where they are reconverted to sound waves that come in contact with the ear drum. While supposedly superior to the acoustic stethoscope, a problem associated with electronic stethoscopes is the picking up of ambient sounds as well as amplifying mid-range sounds while reducing the high- and low-frequency range sounds.

Doppler

The **Doppler** is used in instances where sounds are difficult or not able to be heard with a stethoscope. Rather than picking up or detecting vibrations of sounds, a Doppler detects blood flow. A Doppler will have ear pieces connected by tubing that resembles a stethoscope, but will have an ultrasonic component that is placed on the body rather than a chest piece (Figure 6-13). As an ultrasonic device, it requires that transmission gel placed on the skin for the device to work appropriately. Once the gel is in place, the tip of the instrument is positioned directly in the gel.

The Doppler may be useful in many situations; particularly where assessment of blood flow is needed. Systolic blood pressure may be obtained in individuals with weak or difficult to hear Korotkoff sounds. These individuals would be those in shock, infants, or obese. When blood flow to an area or vessel patency needs to be determined, a Doppler is capable of providing this information. It is often used in prenatal assessments to detect fetal heart activity.

Visual Acuity Charts

Visual acuity charts are used to assess the quality of the eye sight of the patient. While various charts may be used to perform this test, all are composed of *optotypes*, or standardized symbols

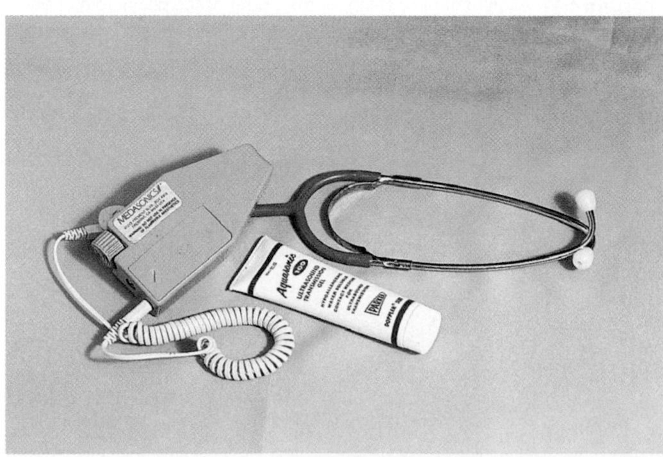

FIGURE 6-13 Doppler stethoscope

> ***PRACTICE POINT: 20/20 = 6/6***
> In countries where measurements are based on the metric system, 20/20 vision is documented as 6/6. Other acuities are documented as ratios with a consistent numerator of 6.

used for testing vision. While the optotypes used vary, each chart contains lines of standardized letters or objects with standardized heights that decrease in size from top to bottom.

Each line is accompanied by a fraction that identifies the visual acuity. Each fraction consists of a numerator that is constant at 20 and a denominator that ranges from 10 to 200. The constant 20 indicates the number of feet that is between the patient and the chart. The denominator is the number of feet away from the chart that an individual with normal eye sight can read the letters or interpret objects. The patient's visual acuity is determined by what line the patient can read/describe correctly.

Expected visual acuity is 20/20; as the denominator increases, the visual acuity of the individual decreases. If the patient can correctly identify the letters of the line that corresponds to 20/40, that is recorded as the patient's visual acuity. When the patient comes to the smallest line that can be correctly interpreted, determine if there are any letters/objects that can be made out in the next line. If there are letters or objects that are correctly identified, then record the visual acuity as 20/40 + # of correct letters (20/40 +3). Examine each eye individually and then test both eyes together. Provide a card or have the patient cover the eye not being tested.

The **Snellen chart** consists of 11 lines of optotypes in block letters of the Arabic alphabet with each line decreasing in height (Figure 6-14). As the lines decrease in size, more letters may be accommodated. Its use is based on the assumption that the patient is capable of identifying letters of the Arabic alphabet. For those patients who are unable to identify letters, there are alternative charts that can be used.

The **Tumbling E chart** consists of lines made up of optotypes of the capital letter "E" that is directed in four different directions (see Figure 6-14). For this test, the patient must simply identify the correct direction of the E—up, down, left, or right. The patient usually does this by extending the 3 middle fingers and pointing them in the direction of the E.

The **HOTV chart** consists of lines made up of only these four letters. The patient is provided with a board that also contains these letters. For the examination, the patient simply has to match the letters on the test board with the letters of each line. The provider may choose to point to the letters in the row as a way to let the patient know which letter to match.

The **LH Symbols (LEA Symbols) chart** consists of four optotypes (square, circle, house, and apple). The LEA symbols are used like the HOTV chart, where the patient matches the object on the chart with the objects on a response card. The LEA symbols chart is tested with the patient at 10 feet away from the chart. Interpretation is the same as for other charts; visual acuity corresponds to the fraction associated with each line.

The **Landolt C chart** (Broken Wheel chart) consists of an optotype that is a ring with a gap, resembling the letter C. The gap is located at various positions (usually left, right, bottom, top and the

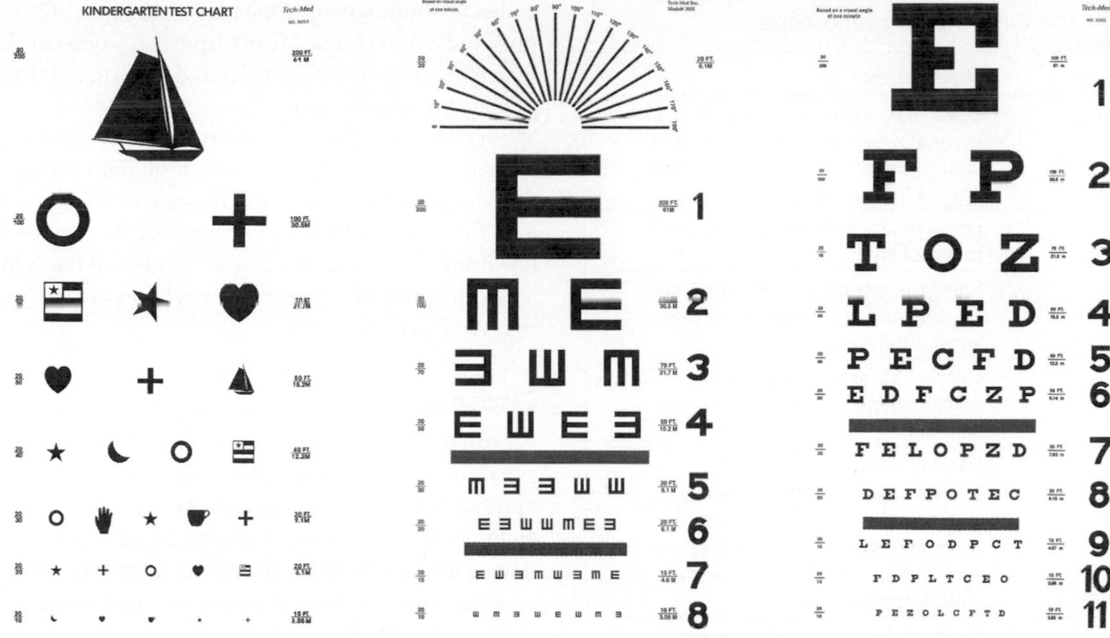

FIGURE 6-14 Examples of different Snellen eye charts

45-degree positions in between). The patient is to identify on which side the gap is. As with other charts, the size of the C and the break are reduced until the subject is no longer able to correctly identify the position of the break.

A **Rosenbaum** or **Jaegar card** may also be used to test for visual acuity (Figure 6 15). The Rosenbaum card is a handheld version of the Snellen chart. Its advantage is that it is portable and only needs to be 14 inches from the patient's eyes. It is used in the same way as the Snellen chart with each line having a corresponding visual acuity fraction. A Jaegar card does not use fractions for visual acuity but uses numbers that correspond to visual acuities fractions.

FIGURE 6-15 Patient reading Jaeger card

Ophthalmoscope

The **ophthalmoscope** is an instrument that allows for the examination of the inner, sensory layer of the eye (retina) and other structures of the interior eye. The ophthalmoscope consists of a head that contains a light source and various lenses and mirrors, and a metal, tubular handle that contains the battery for the light source (Figure 6-16). The head contains an opening (aperture) through which the provider looks. The provider may choose various apertures to look through. These apertures are identified and described in Table 6-5.

Visualization of the interior eye is also facilitated by a series of lenses that are used to bring the area under examination into

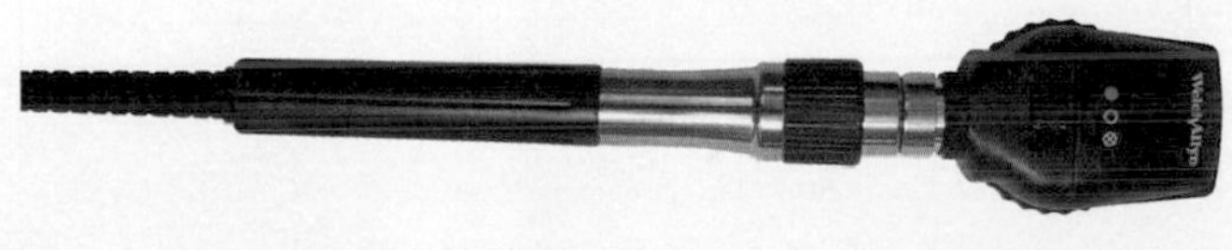

A

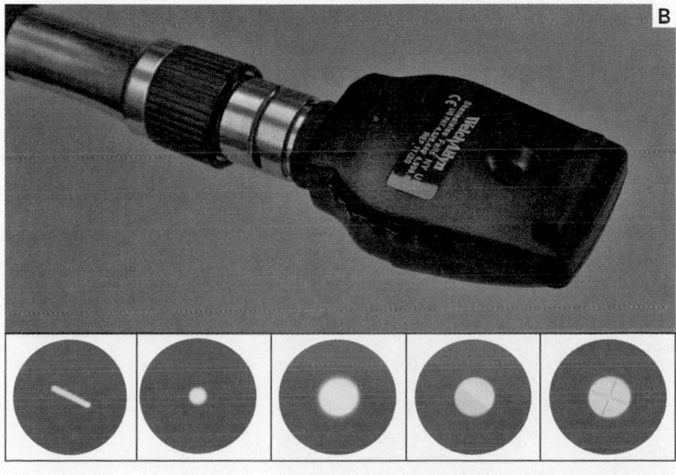

B

FIGURE 6-16A–B a) Ophthalmoscope; b) examples of ophthalmoscope apertures

Table 6-5 Apertures of ophthalmoscope

Apertures	
Slit beam	Used to examine anterior chamber/ cornea of eye. Also used to examine contour of structures/abnormalities in cornea, retina, or lens.
White beam (large/small)	Large beam, most frequently used beam of light
	Small beam—only covers small area of pupil and iris; visualization through small pupil easier
Blue light	Corneal abrasions/ulcers are revealed by examining eye after fluorescein staining.
Red free	Used to visualize the vessels/ hemorrhages in better detail by improving contrast. Retina appears black and white. Vessel caliber and distribution appear more clearly and with better contrast.
Grid pattern	Helps make rough measurements within the eye.
Focusing Wheel	
Red numbers (concave or minus lenses)	Diverges or directs light beams that pass through lens.
Green numbers (convex or plus lenses)	Converges or focuses beams of light to a spot on the opposite side of the lens from the light source.

focus (Figure 6-17). These lenses vary in their diopters (magnification power) and range from ±20 to ±140 bringing objects into focus by converging or diverging light. The diopter number that is being used is displayed in the lens indicator on the front of the head. Rotation of the lens selector disk will change the diopter setting. Red numbers indicate minus lenses (negative numbers) and black numbers indicate plus lenses (positive numbers). The plus and minus lenses function to compensate for myopia or hyperopia in both the provider and patient, but they do not compensate for astigmatism.

The head of the ophthalmoscope is attached to the handle by placing the lower receptacle of the head onto the handle adapter. A firm downward and clockwise rotation of the head while placing it onto the head will lock the two together. To remove the head, push down and turn counterclockwise. To turn on the light source, press down on the on/off button and turn clockwise. The light is turned off by reversing the procedure.

Otoscope

An **otoscope** is a device that illuminates the external auditory canal and ear drum for examination (Figure 6-18). Like the ophthalmoscope, the otoscope head is attached to the handle and turned on in the same manner. One side of the head is cone shaped for insertion into the ear canal and the other side is a window that allows for visualization and slight magnification of the auditory structures.

Prior to insertion of the cone of the otoscope into the auditory canal, place a disposable speculum over the cone. The speculum comes in various sizes, so choose the largest size that will comfortably fit into the auditory canal. In some models, the window slides to the side allowing the provider to insert a cerumen spoon or forceps with the otoscope still in place.

While identified as an instrument for the ear, the otoscope may also be used as a nasal speculum to visualize each nares. When using it this way, use the shortest and widest speculum cover. Most otoscopes also allow for the attachment of a pneumatic tube. This is used to assess fluctuation of the tympanic membrane, primarily when examining children. The pneumatic tube is a short piece of rubber tubing with one end attached to the head of the otoscope and the other end to a hand bulb. Squeezing of the hand bulb produces short puffs of air that strike the tympanic membrane, causing it to move in and out.

Diopter
Diopter number in use
Lens selector disk

FIGURE 6-17 Lenses, diopters, red/green numbers

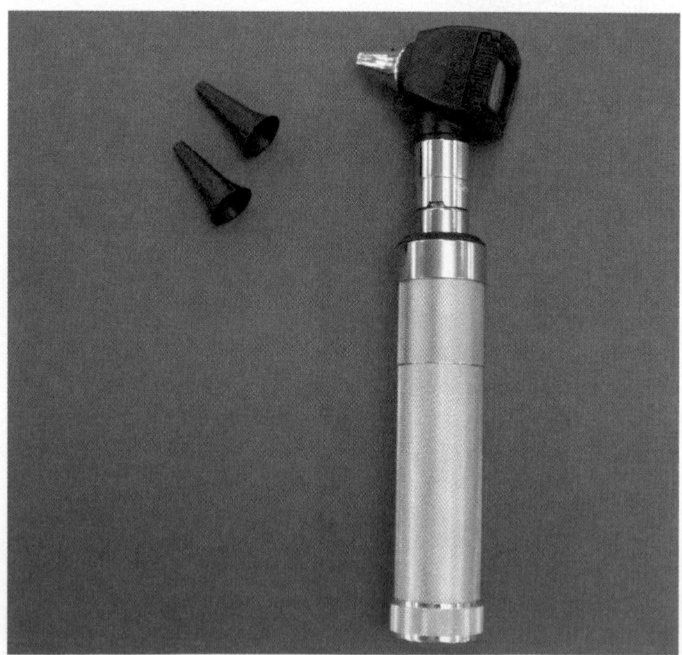

FIGURE 6-18 Otoscope

PRACTICE POINT: Otoscope as Light Source
The otoscope head can be used as a light source if no other source is available. You will need a light source for assessing pupil reaction to light, inspecting the nasal passages, and assessing the mouth and throat.

Nasal Speculum

The **nasal speculum** is used to visualize the lower and middle turbinates of each naris. There is no light source attached to the nasal speculum, so a penlight (or otoscope) must be used to provide adequate lighting for visualization.

The cone of the speculum consists of two blades that separate when the handles are pressed together. Use caution when opening the blades so they do not contact the nasal septum. Before inserting the speculum, tilt the patient's head slightly back to make it easier to look through the opened blades.

Tuning Fork

Tuning forks are Y-shaped instruments used to produce sound for testing auditory function and vibrations for part of the sensory assessment of the neurological exam (Figure 6-19). When set into motion, the vibrations are created that produce a sound wave that is consistent with the number of vibrations per second. The vibrations per second, also known as Hertz, (Hz) are engraved on each fork.

The tuning fork is set into vibrations by hitting the fork on a soft surface or by squeezing the upright prongs together and quickly releasing them. Take care to hold the vibrating fork by its base because anything touching the vibrating prongs will dampen its sound (Figure 6-20).

When using a tuning fork for assessing auditory function, use a fork with a higher frequency (500–1000 Hz) as the volume of speech ranges from 300–3000 Hz. When used during the neurological exam, a lower frequency is best to use as sensitivity to vibrations ranges from 100–00 Hz.

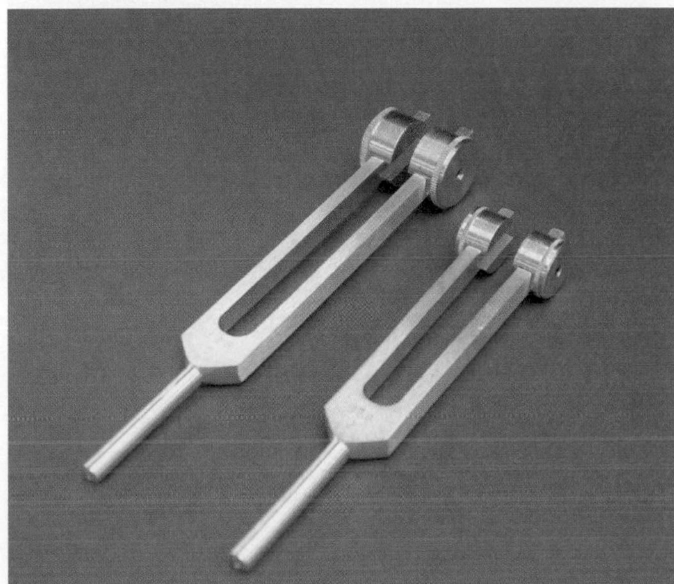

FIGURE 6-19 Tuning forks

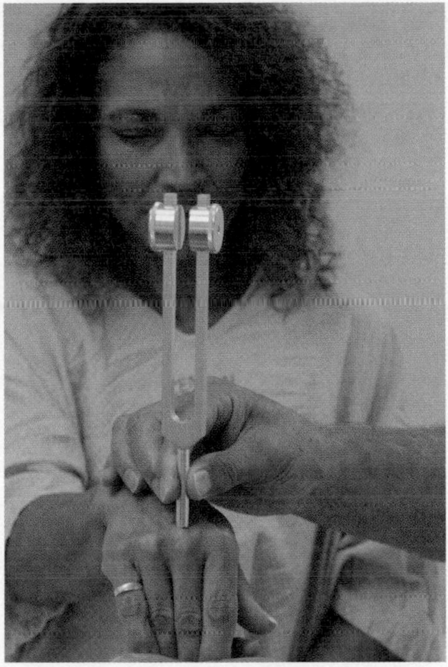

FIGURE 6-20 Holding tuning fork correctly

Reflex Hammer

A **reflex hammer** is used during the neurological exam to assess the deep tendon reflexes (Figure 6-21). The hammer consists of a triangle of hard rubber that is held in place by a metal band that is connected to the handle. The broad side of the hammer is generally used when the tendon is hit directly and the pointed end is generally used when the provider's finger is over the tendon, indirectly striking the tendon by striking the finger.

When using the hammer to strike a tendon, hold it in your hand and use a quick, firm downward snap of your wrist to hit the tendon or your finger. Once the tendon is struck, use another rapid snap of the wrist to bring the hammer back to its original position.

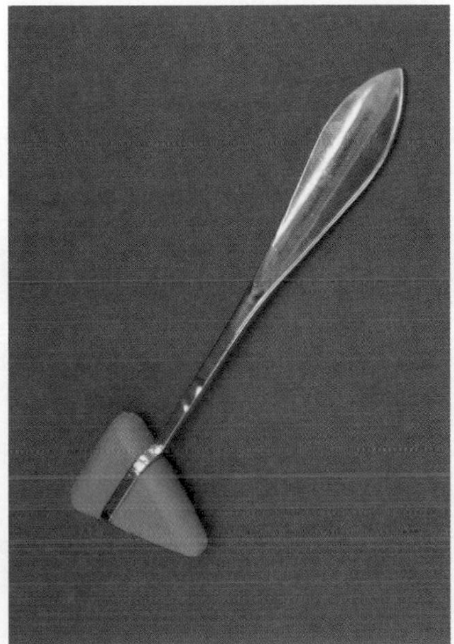

FIGURE 6-21 Reflex hammer

A variant of the reflex hammer is one that has a hard rubber disk for the striking head rather than a triangle. A **neurologic hammer** has a head that is more in the shape of a traditional hammer with a large and small rounded end as the striking surfaces (Figure 6-22).

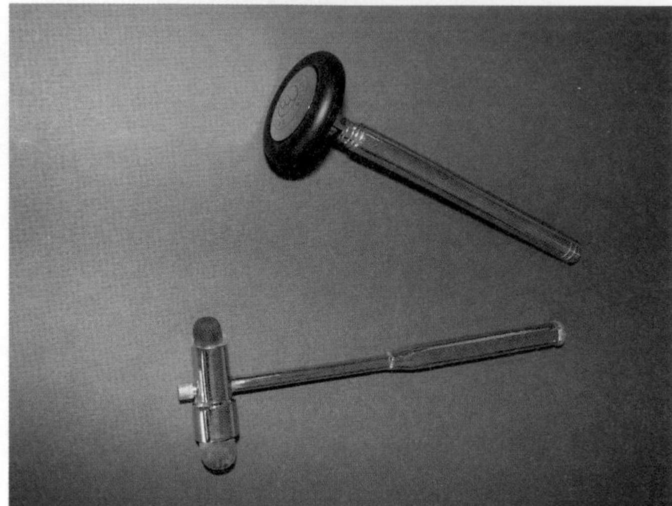

FIGURE 6-22 Neurologic hammer

Tape Measure

A **tape measure** is a measuring tool that is used to determine circumference, diameter, and the length of various lesions and differences in size of various structures and/or body parts (Figure 6-23). It is helpful to have a tape measure that ihs marked in metric and nonmetric distances. The tape measure may be made of paper, which is disposable, or of a material that allows for continuous use. Paper tape measures are stiffer than nondisposable ones and may make it more difficult to obtain accurate measurements. They also may have sharp edges which creates the potential for paper cuts.

Transilluminator

A **transilluminator** is a light source with a strong and narrow beam that is directed to a particular body cavity, helping to differentiate between various substances contained within it (Figure 6-24). Light is transmitted differently through air, fluid, and tissue which is how one is differentiated from the other. A transilluminator may be a specific instrument, or it may be a flashlight or pen light if nothing else is readily available. Be aware of what type of bulb is being used as halogen-type bulbs have to potential for causing skin burns.

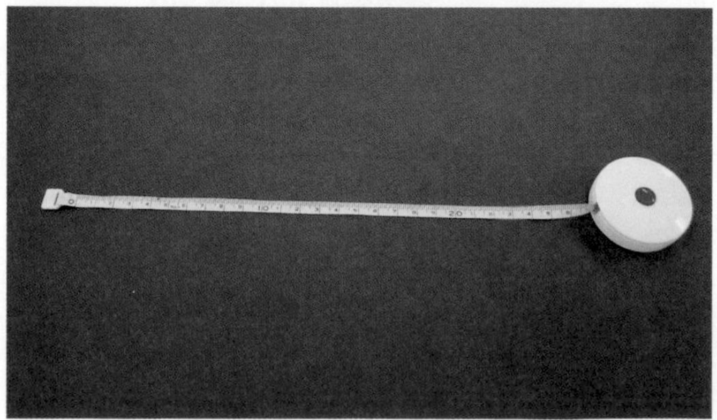

FIGURE 6-23 Tape measure

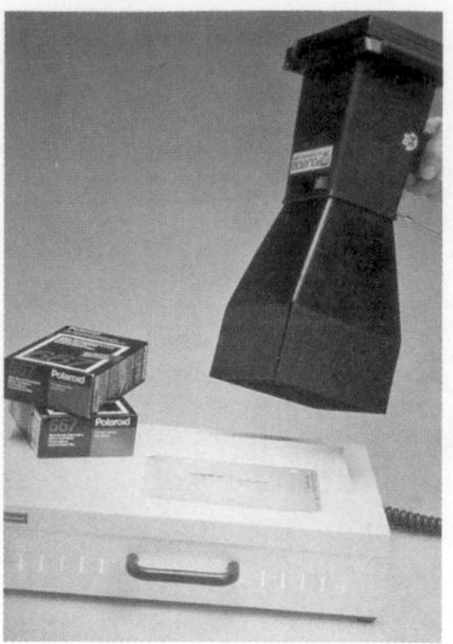

FIGURE 6-24 Transilluminator

When transilluminating, darken the room as much as possible and shine the beam of light directly through or against the area being examined. Observe the red glow that appears through the cavity and note any irregularities/shadows that may appear.

Vaginal Speculum

A **vaginal speculum** consists of two blades and a handle and is used to visualize the vaginal canal and cervix of the female (Figure 6-25). To use the speculum, hold the two blades together as you insert them into the vaginal canal. Once the blades are positioned, spread them apart so that the vaginal walls and cervix can be easily inspected. The lower blade of the speculum is attached to the handle and remains stable; the upper blade is hinged so that when downward pressure is applied the blade opens up increasing the distance between the blades and stretching the vaginal walls,

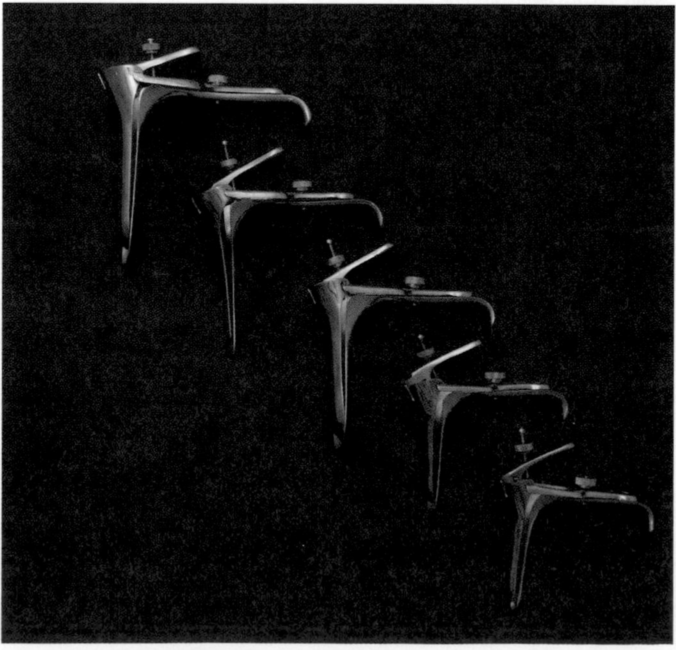

FIGURE 6-25 Vaginal specula

opening up the canal for optimum examination. A thumbscrew maintains the blades in their open position.

There are three types of speculums, and they may be metal or plastic. The Graves speculum comes in a variety of sizes with blades that are 3½ to 5 inches long and ¾ to 1¼ inches wide. The blades are rounded with a slight distance between them when closed. The lower blade is also longer than the top blade due to the longer posterior vaginal wall. The Pederson speculum is similar to the Graves speculum in design and function but with narrower and flatter blades. This type is used for females with small vaginal openings. Pediatric specula are smaller in all dimensions with short, narrow, and flat blades.

Supplementary Instruments and Equipment

In addition to the previously described instruments and equipment, there may be an occasional need for other instruments. The need for more precise measurements often necessitates their use.

Goniometer

A **goniometer** is used when precise measurements of flexion and extension are needed. It consists of two plastic arms that are connected at one end and can rotate on each other (Figure 6-26). The connected end also contains a protractor for accurate measurement of degrees of flexion and extension. When used, the center of the protractor is positioned over the joint and the arms aligned with the long axes of the extremities. The degree of flexion or extension is observed on the protractor and recorded.

Wood's Lamp

A **Wood's lamp** is used if there is a suspicion of the presence of fungi on the skin or skin lesions (Figure 6-27). The light that it emits is essentially a "black light" that causes certain substances to fluoresce. It needs to be used in a dark room or at least a darkened room. The presence of fungi is apparent when there is a yellow-green fluorescence of the skin or lesion.

Dermatoscope

The **dermatoscope** is another instrument that is used in skin assessment. Its primary purpose is to illuminate and magnify a skin lesion for more precise observation of its surface and the subsurface layers and structures of the skin. This function is the result of epiluminescence microscopy (ELM) and digital epiluminescence microscopy (DELM). The dermatoscope is used to confirm a diagnosis or determine which lesions need to be biopsied or removed.

Skinfold Thickness Calipers

Skinfold thickness calipers are used to determine the thickness of the subcutaneous layers of the skin at specific locations of the body (Figure 6-28). The primary purpose of obtaining these measurements is to calculate one's percentage of body fat. These measurements are frequently obtained from individuals who are carrying around excess body fat. While providing more precise information about an individual's percentage of body fat, there are other variables to consider that may cause inaccurate results. An easier method to assess body fat is the body mass index (BMI), which is based on individual's weight and height measurements.

Monofilament

The **monofilament** is an instrument used to determine sensation or sensory loss, particularly on the plantar surface of the foot (Figure 6-29). The instrument consists of a metal bar with a straight wire attached at a 90-degree angle. The wire is designed to bend at 10g of linear pressure.

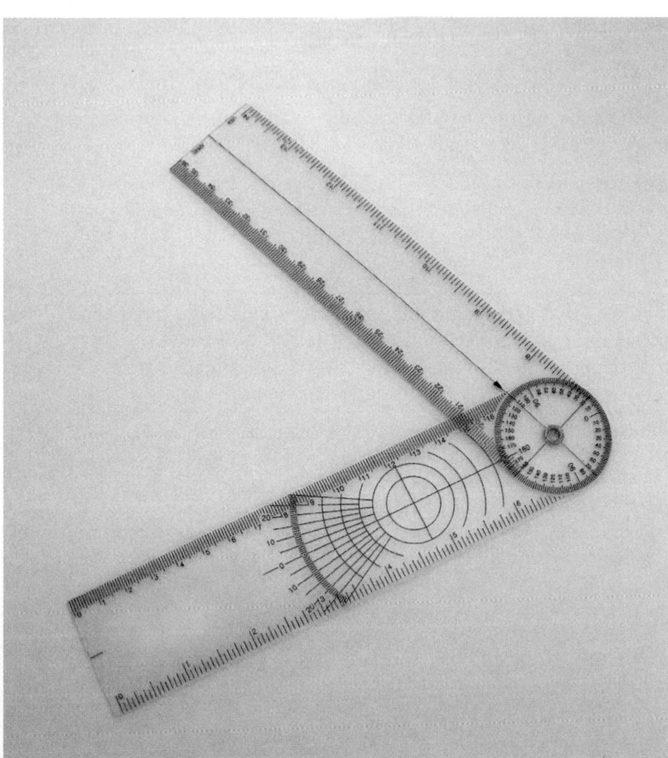

FIGURE 6-26 Goniometer

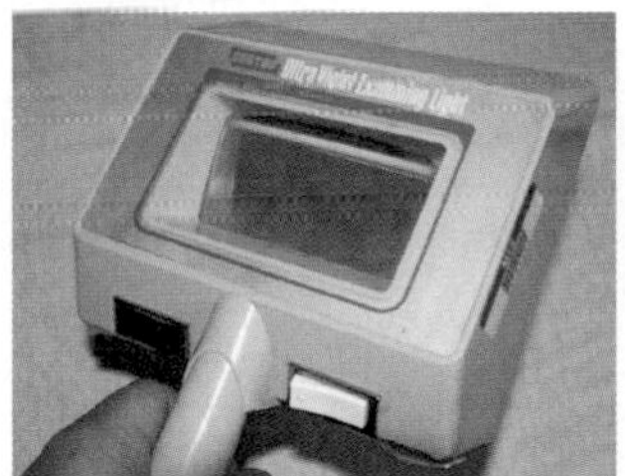

FIGURE 6-27 Wood's lamp

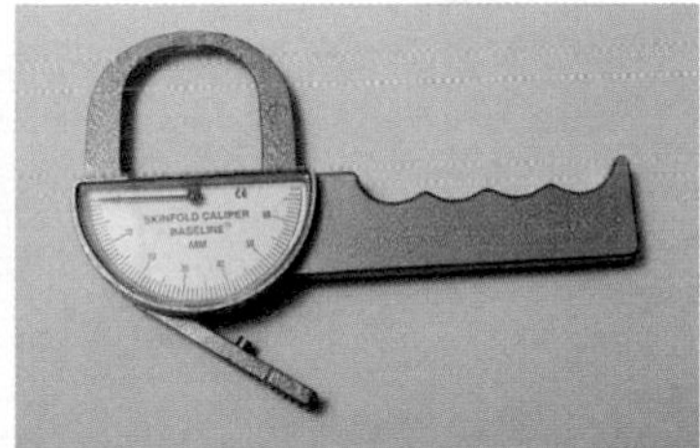

FIGURE 6-28 Skinfold thickness calipers

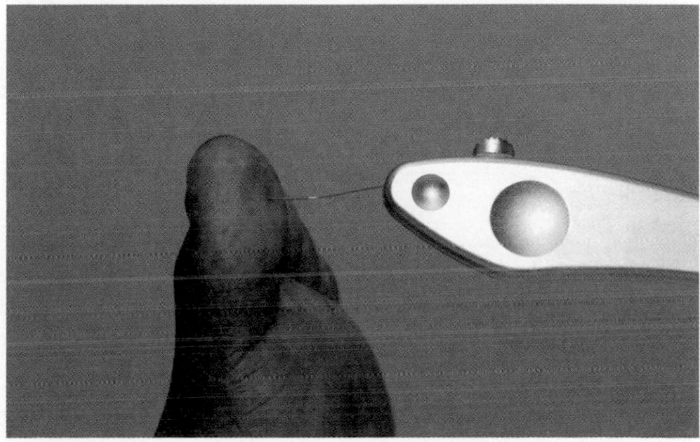

FIGURE 6-29 Placement of monofilament on surface of foot

The monofilament wire is applied to various locations on the skin surface of the foot (Figure 6-29). The patient's eyes should be closed to eliminate visual input as to testing location. Test locations should be random with varying intervals between tests. Apply enough pressure to cause the wire to bend. The patient's failure to feel the end of the monofilament wire on the skin at the point of bending indicates a loss of sensory function on the plantar surface of the foot. Individuals who have lost this sensory input are at risk for serious injury. For example, diabetic patients or others with peripheral neuropathy are at a high risk for this type of sensory loss and should be tested on a routine basis.

Standard Precautions

Standard precautions are implemented to reduce the risk of transmission of microbes through body substances and other known and unknown sources. They represent the essential steps necessary to maintain a basic level of infection control for providers and patients (Table 6-6).

Certain viruses are known to be transmitted via blood and may require additional precautions taken to prevent their transmission (Table 6-7).

In addition to knowing and practicing standard precautions, it is also important for providers to be aware of the degree of risk of exposure associated with medical and/or surgical procedures (Table 6-8).

The earliest set of policies to prevent transmission of infectious agents occurred in 1985, focusing on blood and body precautions, and applying them to all patients, regardless of their infectious status. Prevention of needle-stick injuries was emphasized and the use of masks and eye protection was added to the traditional barriers of gloves and gowns. The use of individual ventilation devices for resuscitation was also introduced. Two years later in 1987, Body Substance Isolation was proposed, which emphasized isolation of all moist and potentially infectious body substances for all patients regardless of infection status. This was accomplished primarily through the use of gloves. From these two sets of policies came Standard Precautions,

Table 6-6 Standard procedures

Factor	Application/Implementation
Hand hygiene	Before gloving and after gloves removed. Hands/other parts of body washed immediately/ thoroughly (40–60 seconds) if contaminated with body fluids, secretions, excretions, contaminated items after all care giving. Providers with cuts, open sores, rashes on hands must wear gloves for all care giving activities/ procedures.
Personal Protective Equipment (PPE)	
Gloves	When in contact with blood, body fluids, excretions, secretions (except sweat), contaminated items; when touching mucous membranes and nonintact skin Always use correct size.
Gown	During procedures and patient care activities or situations where there is potential for exposure to and/or contamination of body fluids, blood draining wounds, or mucous membranes
Resuscitation	Use mouthpiece, resuscitation bag, or other ventilation devices to prevent contact with mouth and oral secretions
Respiratory hygiene/cough etiquette	Instruct symptomatic individuals to cover mouth/nose when sneezing/coughing; use tissues and dispose in no-touch receptacle; wash hands after contamination with respiratory secretions; wear surgical mask if tolerated or maintain spatial separation greater than 3 feet if possible.
Mask, eye protection, face shield	During procedures and patient care activities or situations where there is potential for generation of splashes or sprays of body fluids or blood, primarily when suctioning and endotracheal intubation, or if patient coughing excessively
Environmental Control	
Equipment	Handle contaminated equipment in ways that prevent transfer of microorganisms to others and environment; wear gloves if necessary or visible contamination. Equipment that is shared with other patients must be adequately cleaned/disinfected after each use.
Linen/laundry	Bag linen/laundry at point of use; if contaminated with blood or bodily fluids, wash and dry immediately.
Trash	All contaminated disposable equipment/supplies are bagged in room where it originated.
Needles/sharps	Used needles not recapped, bent, broken, or hand manipulated; if recapping required, insert needle into cap that is lying on a flat surface (one hand scoop). Drop used needles/syringes into puncture resistant container. Replace sharps container when two-thirds filled. Never reach into sharps containers. Never grab at falling instruments.

Table 6-7 Precautions for preventing transmission of blood-borne viruses

Virus	Transmission	Precautions	Immunizations
HAV	Contact (oral/fecal)	Standard Precautions	Health care providers at high risk
		Additional precautions for incontinent patients	
HBV	Blood borne (direct contact with blood or body substances)	Standard precautions	Health care providers. Test for seroconversion 4–8 weeks after third dose of vaccine
HCV	Blood borne (direct contact with blood)	Standard Precautions	No vaccine available
HIV	Blood borne (direct contact with blood or body substances)	Standard precautions Additional precautions may be required in the presence of complicating conditions (e.g., TB)	No vaccine available

Table 6-8 Risk of exposure to blood or body fluids during procedures

High Risk	Moderate Risk	Low Risk
Any submucosal invasion with sharp, hand-held instruments or procedures dealing with sharp pathology and bone spicules, usually in confined spaces or where visibility is poor (orthopedic surgery, trauma, internal cavity surgery)	Minor dental procedures (excluding examination) and routine dental extractions	Interview consultation and dental examination
	Internal and instrument examination and biopsy (endoscopy, vaginal exam, laparoscopy)	Noninvasive examinations or procedures (hearing test), electrocardiography, abdominal ultrasound
	Minor skin surgery	Intact skin palpation (gloves not required) Injections and venipuncture (gloves required)

which are now the basis for the prevention of transmission of infectious agents, and infection.

Standard precautions are based on the presumption that blood, body fluids, excretions (except sweat), nonintact skin, and mucous membranes may be contaminated with transmissible infectious agents (see Table 6-7). Standard precautions are infection prevention practices that apply to all patients, regardless of infection status, in any and all settings where health care is delivered. These practices are hand hygiene; use of gloves, gown, mask, eye protection, or face shield—depending on potential for exposure; and safe injection practices. In addition, any equipment or supplies in the surrounding environment that may have been contaminated with body fluids must be handled or disposed of in a manner that prevents transmission of infectious agents. The extent to which standard precautions are implemented is determined by the nature of the provider–patient interaction and the potential for exposure to blood, secretions, or body fluids. The nature of standard precautions is to protect the patient and provider from each other by putting a barrier in between them.

Additional recommendations to standard precautions (respiratory hygiene/cough etiquette) have been introduced since the outbreak of avian flu (H5N1), swine flu (H1N1), severe acute respiratory syndrome (SARS-CoV) and other flu viral variations. There are also recommendations related to safe injection practices, and the use of masks for the insertion of catheters or injection of material into spinal or epidural spaces via lumbar puncture procedures, such as myelogram, spinal or epidural anesthesia.

Summary

- The primary function of the physical examination is to obtain significant data regarding the patient's health status.
- Physical exam data is obtained through the clinical skills and techniques of inspection, palpation, percussion, and auscultation.
- Various types of equipment are used throughout the physical examination depending on what data is needed.
- Standard precautions are required during provision of care and performance of a physical examination to prevent transmission of blood-borne organisms that cause life-threatening illnesses.

Review Questions

1. The provider has gathered objective information about the patient's skin and is documenting this information as inspection. The provider has gathered this information through the use of which of the following?
   1. sight
   2. hearing
   3. touch
   4. intuition
2. The provider would use deep palpation when performing which part of the physical exam of the patient?
   1. head
   2. abdomen
   3. neurological
   4. respiratory
3. When using the technique of percussion in the examination of a patient the provider is relying on which sense?
   1. sight
   2. hearing
   3. touch
   4. smell
4. The provider is using the technique of percussion over a patient's stomach. The sound that the provider would expect to hear is which of the following?
   1. resonance
   2. hyperresonance
   3. tympany
   4. dullness
5. The provider is using percussion to examine a patient and uses the middle finger of the dominant hand to strike the surface. This finger is referred to as which of the following?
   1. plexor
   2. pleximeter
   3. intermediate object
   4. percussor
6. When preparing to perform a physical assessment of a patient, the provider is aware that which technique will require gathering additional equipment?
   1. inspection
   2. palpation
   3. percussion
   4. auscultation
7. The provider is performing the technique of auscultation when performing a cardiac examination of a patient. The provider should use the bell of the stethoscope to listen for which of the following? (Select all that apply.)
   1. S_1
   2. S_2
   3. S_3
   4. S_4
   5. murmurs
8. The provider may use a Doppler in the examination of a patient when trying to auscultate which of the following? (Select all that apply.)
   1. fetal heart tones
   2. primary pulses
   3. peripheral pulses
   4. blood pressure
   5. breath sounds
9. The provider records a patient's visual acuity as 20/50 after performing an examination with a wall chart. This result means that this patient can read which of the following?
   1. 50 percent of what a person with normal vision can read
   2. 20 lines of a 50 line eye chart
   3. at 20 feet what a person with normal vision can read at 50 feet
   4. at 50 feet what most people can read at 20 feet
10. The provider should use gloves when performing a physical assessment with a patient when which of the following occurs?
    1. the patient is HIV positive
    2. has a known infection
    3. there is a risk of contact with body fluids
    4. if the provider is pregnant

7

General Assessment and the Mental Status Exam

Mary Molewyk Doornbos, PhD, RN

"I can't thank you enough for all that you and your team have done for me." Mr. Price holds my forearm with both his hands and smiles at me. Now two days after his radical prostatectomy, he's in good spirits and healing well.

"You're doing great, Mr. Price," I say. "I'll see you in the morning when I get back to the hospital, okay?" He nods and smiles at me as I turn for the door.

The next morning...

There were five overnight admissions, and I'm pressed for time on my morning rounds. *Mr. Price is in good shape... I can save him for last.* Not the best idea, as it turns out. Just before the team arrives I look in Mr. Price's room, expecting to find him halfway through an omelet while watching the news. Instead he's supine, staring at the ceiling, and muttering gibberish. I rush to his bedside.

"Mr. Price? Can you hear me?" He turns toward me and gives me a blank stare. "Mr. Price, can you tell me your full name?"

"Of course! John Jefferson Price, Junior!" he says, turning his gaze back to the ceiling. *Okay, he knows who he is—that's a good sign.*

"Mr. Price, do you know where you are right now?" He continues to look at the ceiling. "I'm at home right now," he says without blinking, eyes trained on a smoke detector.

"Do you know what year it is?"

"It's 1955..." Suddenly he turns his head back towards me, his brow sharply bent in anger. "Why do you keep asking me silly questions? And how did you get into my house? Are you trying to rob me?" *Not good. He is oriented to himself, but not place or time.* I do my best to assure Mr. Price that I'm there to help him, and remind him of the surgery he just had for his prostate cancer. *What could have caused such a rapid, dramatic shift in his mental status? This was delirium.* I put my hand on Mr. Price's shoulder and scan him from head to toe. He is sweating, shivering slightly, and likely febrile. Looking along the rails of his bed, I see the bag from his Foley catheter dangling over the floor. I look at the urine and see that it is cloudy and dark yellow. *Of course!* He has a urinary tract infection, one of the most common causes of delirium in the elderly population. *That will probably have to be removed and he'll likely be started on antibiotics; and better get a urine sample for urinalysis.* With treatment, I expect to be talking to the present-day Mr. Price again by the end of the day.

LEARNING OUTCOMES

1. Explain the intent and purpose of the general assessment and mental status examination.
2. Summarize the components of the general assessment and mental status examination.
3. Recognize the expected characteristics and manifestations of the components of the general assessment and mental status examination.
4. Explain the relationship between the general assessment and mental status examination.
5. Summarize assessment findings of the general assessment and mental status examination for documentation purposes.

The overall examination begins with a general assessment (GA) and a mental status exam (MSE). While they are identified as separate entities, they are not mutually exclusive; a lot of overlap exists between the two and, to a certain extent, together they may be perceived as one exam. Both are also ongoing throughout the exam. The MSE exam is also considered the initial component of the neurological exam (see Chapter 26), but will be addressed here because there is a direct relationship of the GA to the MSE.

From the initial encounter with the patient to the completion of the exam, the provider is presented with and takes in a continuous flow of information. The ability to process all the information improves with time and practice as well as a concentrated awareness of incoming data. Every aspect of the provider's behavior and scope of observation should be deliberate and directed towards the patient. Paying attention to data obtained during the GA and MSE provides information that may be needed later on in the exam and also helps form an initial impression.

General Assessment

The general assessment is a series of astute, meaningful observations of the patient that provides the initial clinical impression of the patient's general state of health and well-being as well as any outstanding characteristics. While first impressions are not always correct, they are the starting point of the data base for the patient. Incorrect impressions may always be corrected when new or more data is obtained.

The initial patient encounter may occur in a variety of places where health care is provided (Figure 7-1). The GA begins when the provider enters either the exam or patient room, or when the patient arrives at the emergency department. During each of these encounters, the data obtained through observations will also vary depending on the time available and the amount of information needed to initiate treatment. Information obtained through the GA also helps to direct and determine what additional information may be needed to develop a diagnosis and plan.

The overall quality and success of obtaining appropriate and adequate data from the patient depends largely on the attitude of the patient, or the rapport that develops between the provider and patient. Frequently, the initial interview may be their first encounter. The provider's attitude also significantly contributes to developing rapport with the patient. Individuals vary in their ability and skill to develop rapport, but its importance and contribution to success requires the provider to accept responsibility and make a commitment to develop this skill. The patient's attitude may be described as cooperative, uncooperative, hostile, guarded, suspicious or regressed.

Identifying Data

At the start of the general assessment and mental status examination, it is important to gather initial identifying information from the patient. This information helps provide an essential context for the data that is subsequently collected.

Identifying data includes the following:

- Name: What is your full name?
- Note gender (gender identity).
- Age: How old are you? What is the date (month, day, and year) of your birth?
- Race/culture: What country did your ancestors come from? When did your ancestors come to this country?

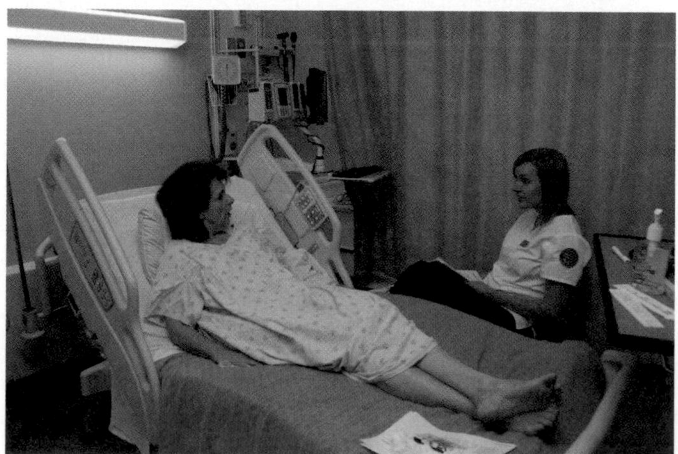

FIGURE 7-1 Provider and patient sitting in patient room

> ***THINK LINK: Gender Identity***
> Gender is primarily considered an either/or attribute of humans. While a majority of individuals may conform to this perception, gender identify is more recently considered to exist on a continuum, ranging from congruence between gender identification with anatomic structures to dissonance between gender identification and anatomic structures. Those in the middle are individuals whose gender identity is comprised of both male and female attributes. The gradations that occur across the continuum are described as **transgender**. Individuals on the far end who experience strong feelings of dissonance between their gender identification and sexual anatomy may experience gender identity disorder (GID) and considered to be **transsexuals.** Transsexuals may go through gender reassignment surgery, but this is not a solution that is chosen by all transsexuals. Transsexuality or GID should be considered a description of a condition or diagnosis and not a label. If there is a question as to whether an individual has some degree of gender identity disorder, it is best to approach the topic in an open and understanding manner that allows the individual to provide information without feeling judged or alienated.

General Presentation

The provider's initial observations of the patient focus on the patient's general presentation. The defining characteristics of the individual, gender, age, and race are often the initial data. Also note whether the patient appears to be the stated age, or appears younger or older; this is called the "apparent age." While everyone ages at different rates, the apparent age may provide clues to underlying problematic conditions.

Physical Appearance and Behavior

The focus of this section is to assess the patient's ability to care for one's self and the motor ability. The motor ability is a component of the musculoskeletal exam and also an essential component of the neurological exam. The initial observations from the GA provide data which may be followed up and refined when these specific systems are examined (see Chapters 26 and 27).

Assessment of Appearance

"Don't judge a book by its cover" is not a consideration for this component of the general appearance assessment. How a patient is dressed and the condition of the clothes as well as body size may provide significant cues related to patient's overall presentation.

Attire relates to how the patient is dressed. Details to note are whether the clothing is clean or soiled, and whether it fits the patient or appears too tight, too small, or too large. Is the patient appropriately dressed given his/her age and lifestyle and does the amount of clothing correlate with the season? Also note if the patient's attire is coordinated and matched or if it appears unusual or bizarre. Also note whether the shoes fit properly and are clean.

Grooming is concerned with the patient's self-care activities and abilities. Observe whether the patient appears neat or unkempt and whether the individual's hair, nails, teeth, and beard are appropriately clean and groomed and whether the hair is clean and healthy looking or greasy and matted. If the patient uses makeup, is it applied appropriately and blended or is it applied in patches with no apparent blending? Is the patient appropriately groomed given his/her age and lifestyle?

Body or breath odor is a reflection of the patient's personal hygiene, but also may indicate the presence of certain pathological conditions. Body odor has a characteristic odor caused by bacterial degradation of body sweat and is usually considered to be a manifestation of poor personal hygiene.

Other odors that may be associated with certain conditions are identified and described in Table 7-1. It is more likely that these particular odors will be present or manifest in patients within health care organizations.

Recording accurate height and weight provides information as to the patient's body build and structure. Comparing these two values with standardized charts allows the provider to determine whether these two values are appropriate to the patient's age. Particularly note any apparent recent weight changes (observe for clothing that is too large or too small).

A significant observation related to the patient's body type is whether it is shaped like an apple or a pear. These two types are determined by location and type of fat distribution (Figure 7-2). **Apple body types** demonstrate fat deposition within the abdomen and are characteristically associated with males. The type of fat is brown fat and associated with cardiovascular disease. **Pear body types** demonstrate fat deposition around the hips and are characteristically associated with females. This type of fat is yellow fat and is not directly related to cardiovascular disease.

Assess an appearance of weight gain to determine whether the gain is from fat deposition or an accumulation of fluid in the tissues (edema). When differentiating fat from fluid, fluid-saturated tissues will demonstrate pitting of the skin and will appear to be stretched and tight, which is due to the skin not having enough time to accommodate the increase in size; fat accumulation will not demonstrate either of these.

While it is often assumed that excessive weight gain is the result of increased caloric intake, weight gain may also occur secondary to certain conditions, the most common one being Cushing's disease or syndrome, which is due to an increase of steroids that causes weight gain. Cushing's may be due to an endocrine disorder (disease) or an increased intake of steroids (syndrome) for medical purposes. The pattern of fat deposition and distribution in Cushing's is different from that of generalized obesity. In Cushing's, the fat is predominately abdominal and face, whereas in generalized obesity, there is body-wide distribution so that the extremities are also increased in size due to fat accumulation (Figure 7-3).

Fat accumulation is a significant manifestation; however, being underweight is also a concern. An unexplained or unplanned weight loss may relate to an underlying condition or disease. Specific diseases or conditions that may cause an unintentional weight loss include poor management of type 1 diabetes mellitus, infections (HIV), hyperthyroidism, and cancer.

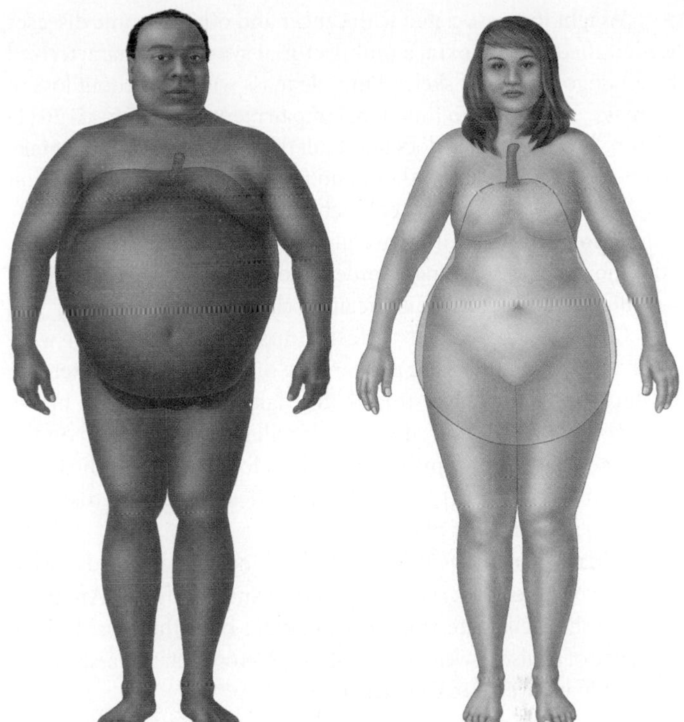

FIGURE 7-2 Apple vs. pear body type

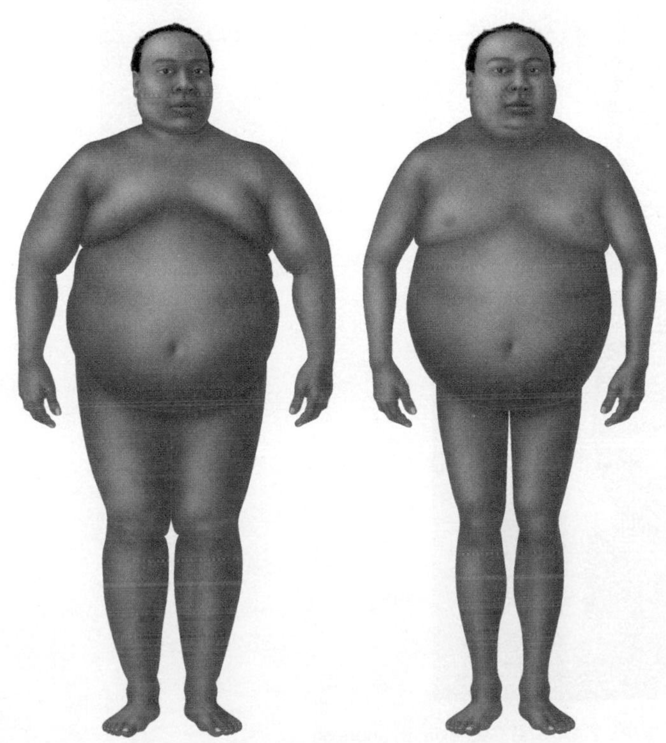

FIGURE 7-3 General fat distribution vs. Cushing's fat distribution

Table 7-1 Odors associated with certain conditions and disorders

Condition	Characteristic Odor
Ketoacidosis (DM)	Fruity odor to breath
Phenylketonuria	Mousey body odor
Maple syrup urine disease	Maple syrup odor to urine
Trimethylaminuria (fish odor syndrome)	Body odor that smells like fish
Liver failure	Ammonia odor to breath (fetor hepaticus)
Alcohol	Sweet odor to breath
High-protein diet (Atkins)	Faint ketone odor to breath
GI disorders (obstruction/bleeding)	Fecal odor to breath/old blood
Poor oral hygiene	Bad breath (halitosis)
Infections	Somewhat organism specific

Weight loss associated with cancer and other chronic diseases is identified as **cachexia**, a multifactorial syndrome characterized by an ongoing loss of skeletal muscle mass with or without loss of fat mass…that leads to functional impairment (Fearon et al., 2011) (Figure 7-4a). Cachexia does not result from decreased caloric intake but decreased protein synthesis and increased protein degradation (Al-Majid & Waters, 2008; Lenk, Schuler, & Adams, 2010).

Anorexia is another weight loss condition; however the condition itself is an eating disorder with concomitant psychological manifestations. In essence, anorexia is self-imposed starvation.

Obvious physical manifestations of an individual with anorexia are the dramatic appearance of thinness, characteristic of starvation, and yellow-tinged, dry, flaky skin along with brittle nails (Figure 7-4b). Fine, downy hair will also be observed on the face, back, legs, and arms in contrast to loss of hair on the head. Frequent vomiting, often seen in anorexics, results in erosion of dental enamel and loss of teeth.

Initial observations also include the skin, but are limited to what is readily visible. Observe the skin color and condition. Are there distinguishing characteristics such as tattoos or birthmarks? Is there evidence of bruises, swelling, or rashes? (A more detailed assessment of the skin is covered in Chapter 16.)

Significance of Findings Related to Appearance

While there are no direct correlations, colorful, eccentric, or bizarre apparel generally suggests mania. In contrast, dirty, unkempt clothing with a disheveled appearance may indicate schizophrenia. Personality traits may be demonstrated by dress and/or accessories related to particular subcultures, body modifications, or clothes that are not associated with the patient's gender. Alcoholism or drug abuse may result in observations of malnutrition, nicotine stains, dental erosions, a rash around the mouth from abusing inhalants, or needle track marks from IV drug injections.

Deterioration in grooming may accompany depression, schizophrenia, substance abuse, or a cognitive disorder such as dementia. Over attention to grooming may be indicative of an obsessive-compulsive personality disorder. Discrepancies from one side of the body to the other may indicate a neurological phenomenon. It is important to recognize that assessments of dress, hygiene, and eye contact have the potential to be affected by the professional provider's cultural bias. Make active attempts to ascertain if you are using culturally bound criteria to evaluate patients relative to these areas.

Facial Expressions

Facial expressions are closely associated with the underlying emotions the patient is experiencing. They are a form of nonverbal communication and are the primary means for conveying social information among humans. They may be a voluntary act, but because of their close association with emotions, they are primarily involuntary.

Facial expressions have been categorized into six primary emotions—anger, fear, surprise, sadness, joy, and disgust (Figure 7-5). While other emotions are expressed, they are likely a variation or combination of the basic six. The facial muscles, which are quite unique in their structure and number, control facial expressions. There are five primary facial muscles that are thought to control the six principle emotions. The total number of facial muscles that are possible is 19, but evidence indicates that not everyone has the same number of facial muscles (Waller, Cray, & Burrows, 2008). Because the facial muscles are flat, difficult to separate from surrounding connective tissue, and attached to each other, changes in facial expression are often very subtle and often represent minute

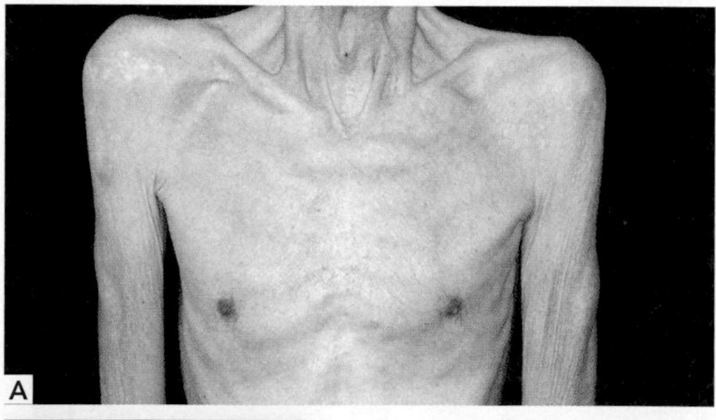

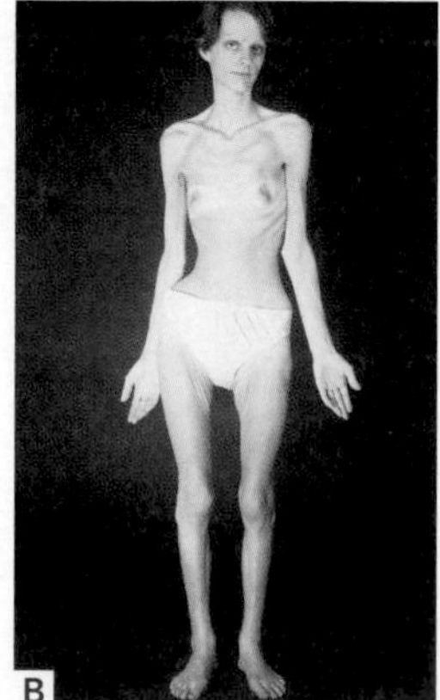

FIGURE 7-4A-B a) Cachexia; b) anorexia

Sources: a. Dr. P Marazzi/Science *Source*; b. Biophoto Associates/Science Source

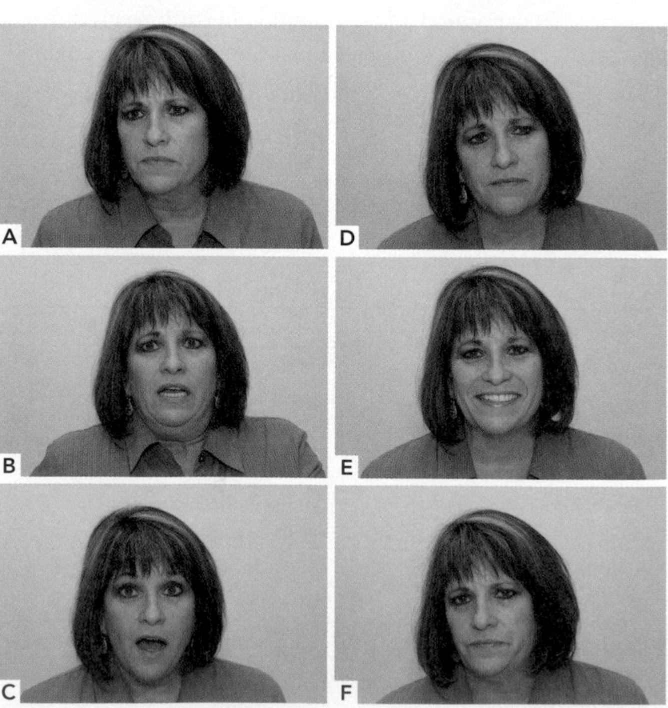

FIGURE 7-5A-F Six facial expressions: a) anger, b) fear, c) surprise, d) sadness, e) joy, and f) disgust

or discrete differences in the proportion and relative position of the facial features (University of Portsmouth, 2008).

The most obvious and immediate cues related to facial expression and overall emotional state comes from the eyes and primarily expressed through eye contact. Maintaining eye contact regulates conversations, demonstrates interest or involvement, and establishes a connection with others. Lack of eye contact is commonly considered a demonstration of inattentiveness or rudeness.

For the general assessment, facial expression is observed throughout the time the provider is with the patient. It is expected that facial expressions will vary according to the content and context of the conversation. It is also expected that the patient will maintain eye contact with the provider when appropriate. The provider must also be aware of cultural differences that exist when assessing eye contact as it may be considered inappropriate or bad in certain cultures (see Chapter 2).

Motor Activity

Assessment of motor activity refers to observation of the patient's overall body movements, which can be demonstrated by the patient's posture, gait, gestures, mannerisms, and general level of activity.

Body Movement

The initial observation of body movement is to note whether it is voluntary or involuntary. Body movements are expected to be voluntary, indicating that the patient has control over and initiates any movement. Movements and actions should also be smooth, deliberate, symmetrical, and coordinated. Also note whether the movement is purposeful or not. Even though movement may be voluntary, if it lacks purpose, then it should be further assessed. Also note if any parts of the patient's body are immobile.

Involuntary body movements occur without patient initiation and are not purposeful in nature. Involuntary movements are referred to as tics, tremors, and convulsions. These movements may be intermittent or constant and are not smooth, deliberate, symmetrical, or coordinated.

Tics Intermittent involuntary body movements are generally identified as **tics**, which are sudden, repetitive, nonrhythmic, motor movements that involve discrete muscle groups, but can also occur as vocalizations. Commonly occurring tics are eye blinking and throat clearing, often observed in individuals who are tense or extremely emotional. Tics may also be quite minimal so as to not be noticed by the provider, and may only be felt by the patient.

Prior to the tic onset, the individual may experience an "urge," which is experienced as a build-up of tension facilitating the need to engage in the tic, relieving or releasing the tension.

There is an element of voluntary response to the urge and initiating the activity so that tics are also considered involuntary or semi-voluntary contributing to their uniqueness and characterization as suppressible, but irresistible (Hawlay, 2011).

Tics are further classified as motor or phonic, simple or complex. Motor tics occur in discrete muscle groups and involve muscle movement. Phonic tics are involuntary sounds produced by moving air through the nose, mouth, or throat.

Simple motor tics are characteristically sudden, brief, meaningless movements and generally involve one muscle group and are easily observed. Motor tic manifestations occur in an endless array of manifestations including eye blinking; head jerking; shoulder shrugging; hand clapping; neck stretching; mouth movements; head, leg, or arm jerking; and facial grimacing. A simple phonic tic may be any sound or noise, commonly manifested as throat clearing, sniffing, or grunting.

Complex motor tics are observed as a cluster of movements that appear to be coordinated, more purposeful, and longer in duration. Manifestations of complex motor tics include pulling at clothes; touching people or objects; **echopraxia**, imitating movements of others; and **copropraxia**, involuntary performance of obscene or forbidden gestures. These activities are common manifestations of Tourette's syndrome.

Tremors **Tremors** are nonintentional rhythmic movements of a body part, which are the result of alternating or irregular synchronous contractions of muscles that have an opposite effect on a joint (Alvarez, 2009). Tremors are the most common of all involuntary movements affecting the hands, arms, head, face, vocal cords, trunk, and legs, with hands the most commonly affected.

Manifestations of tremors include rhythmic shaking of the hands of the affected part, shaky voice, difficulty writing or drawing, problems holding or controlling utensils (eating). They may be triggered or exaggerated by stress or strong emotion, physical exhaustion, or during certain postures or movement. Tremors are most common in middle-aged and older individuals but may occur at any age, with equal distribution among males and females. Tremors may appear occasionally, intermittently, or temporarily.

Tremors are commonly the result of damage to a part of the brain that control muscles throughout the body or particular parts of the body. Damage to the brain can result from neurological disorders, such as multiple sclerosis, stroke, traumatic brain injury, and neurodegenerative diseases (Parkinson's disease). Other causes result from drugs (amphetamines, steroids, psychotropic), or certain conditions (alcohol abuse or withdrawal, mercury poisoning, hyperthyroidism, or liver failure). An **essential tremor**, the most common type, is not associated with any particular condition and is thought to have a genetic origin. The tremor may be mild and nonprogressive in some individuals and in others progressive and involving both sides of the body. The hands are the most commonly involved and may be accompanied by a slight gait disturbance. A **physiological tremor** is common to everyone and has no clinical significance. It is rarely observable and may intensify due to strong emotion (anxiety or fear), physical exhaustion, hypoglycemia, hyperthyroidism, heavy metal poisoning, stimulants, alcohol withdrawal, or fever.

Tremors that are secondary to other conditions may be categorized into the following types: (1) resting (Parkinsonian) tremor, (2) postural (action) tremor, (3) intention (ataxic) tremor, (4) rubral tremor, and (5) dystonic tremor (Table 7-2).

Convulsions The third type of involuntary movement is **convulsions**, which are recurrent major motor seizures that are associated with epilepsy and often referred to as a "seizure."

Table 7-2 Tremors

Tremor	Description	Demonstration
Resting tremor	Coarse rhythmic tremor, often observed in the hands/arms in a resting position.	"Pill rolling" is common description, characteristic of Parkinson's. Deliberate action may decrease its intensity and disappears when limbs in extreme rest, notably during sleep. May start on one side and progress to the other.
Postural tremor	Occurs with any attempt to hold the limbs or trunk in a specific position.	Increases in intensity when limb actively moved (trying to drink from cup). Also disappears when limb fully relaxed.
Intention (ataxic, cerebellar) tremor	Resembles action tremor, but occurs at the end of purposeful movement when fine precise movement needed.	The tremor is an irregular, rhythmic tremor with 2–4 shaky, waving movements per minute.
	When asked to touch the tip of the nose, the individual can initiate the activity but when the finger comes close to the tip and has to touch it, the tremor begins.	Lesions or damage to the cerebellum from stroke, multiple sclerosis, or inherited degenerative disorders. A lesion on one side of the brain produces a tremor on the same side of the body.
Rubral tremor (type of intention tremor)	Characterized by a wing-beating movement of the arms and occurs with a slight movement of the arms or an attempt to maintain a particular posture.	
Dystonic tremor	Movement disorder with sustained involuntary muscle contractions causes twisting and repetitive motions and/or painful and abnormal postures or positions.	Any muscle of body affected by dystonic tremors, most often observed when patient in a particular position or certain movements.

PRACTICE POINT: Tremors and/or Tics

Tremors and tics may not be directly observable during the initial observations made; however, during the examination of the neurological system, they may become apparent when assessing point-to-point testing (finger to nose).

Convulsive movements during a seizure may be categorized as tonic and clonic. The initial brief tonic phase is marked by trunk flexion followed by diffuse extension of the trunk and extremities. The clonic phase features rhythmic flexor contractions of the trunk and limbs, pupillary dilation, elevations of blood pressure and pulse, urinary incontinence, and tongue biting. This is followed by a profound state of depressed consciousness (post-ictal state), which gradually improves over minutes to hours. The disorder may be cryptogenic, familial, or symptomatic (caused by an identified disease process).

Posture

Posture refers to how an individual's body is positioned when standing or sitting and is often considered nonverbal communication. An individual's position provides clues as to the patient's comfort level and/or preparation for certain activities. A specific position or posture may also be assumed to provide protection for a specific part of the body.

While no specific meaning may be ascribed to positions or postures, they may provide clues and cues you can observe. For example, when seated, is the patient sitting erect or slouched in the chair? The comfortableness of the chair and the individual's height relative to the chair height may affect one's position. Generally, a position of comfort in a chair is sitting erect in the center of the chair with perhaps, a slight slouch, creating a curved back with the seat of the individual slightly forward in the chair and only the upper part of the back in contact with the back of the chair. The weight may be slightly shifted to one side or the other so that the individual is sitting slightly off center (Figure 7-6). The arms may be placed on the arms of the chair (if a part of the chair) or placed in the individual's lap. The legs may be stretched out in front of the patient and may or may not be crossed, either at the knee or ankles. The head and neck may be positioned with the face looking slightly downward. A position of comfort also allows the patient to hold the head erect and maintain eye contact with the provider.

Alterations in sitting posture would relate to changes in positions and/or comfort with others and environment. On one extreme is the individual who appears to be in a state of hypervigilance and is constantly scanning the environment and other individuals. This individual would be rigid, sitting erect with a very straight back that is in close contact with the back of the chair. The arms would be

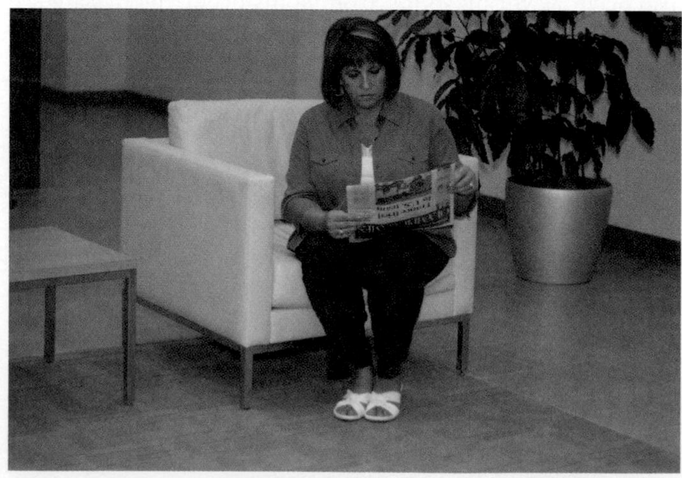

FIGURE 7-6 Position of comfort

positioned with the hands in the lap and the arms in close contact the side of the chest. The feet would be firmly planted on the floor with the knees bent close to 90 degrees. It is unlikely that the legs or ankles would be crossed. The neck would be held erect with the face directed forward (Figure 7-7).

On the other extreme is an individual that appears uninvolved with the environment and rarely looks around. This individual's body might be slouched in a chair with the seat very far forward and his back may appear to be in a straight line, extending from the top of the back of the chair to the edge of the chair. The legs are extended in front of the individual, also in a straight line, and most likely crossed at the ankles. The arms would be folded and held against the anterior chest/abdomen. The neck is flexed so that the chin may be resting on the chest, so looking up or around is quite difficult or impossible. These individuals may be depressed or simply indifferent to the environment or uninvolved with individuals within it. This body language also expresses an unwillingness to cooperate and/or wanting to be left alone (Figure 7-8).

Patients may assume other postures or positions to protect certain areas of the body, most commonly to relieve pain or facilitate breathing. To relieve pain, a patient may choose a position that reduces pressure or weight on the painful site. When you observe an individual in an altered position, determine if this position is due to pain or another reason. Hemiparesis or musculoskeletal alterations may be a factor in these positions.

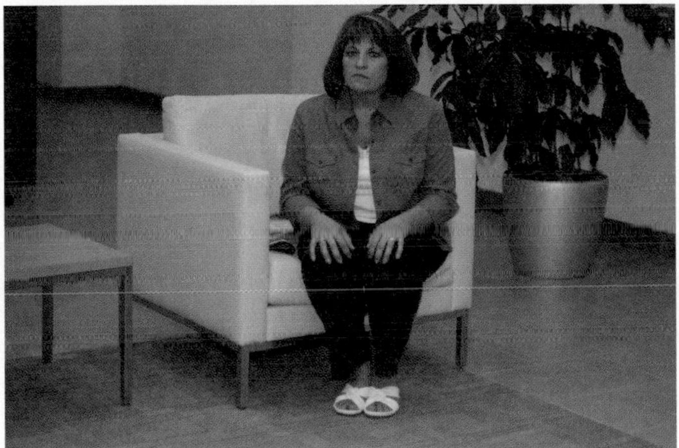

FIGURE 7-7 Position of hypervigilance

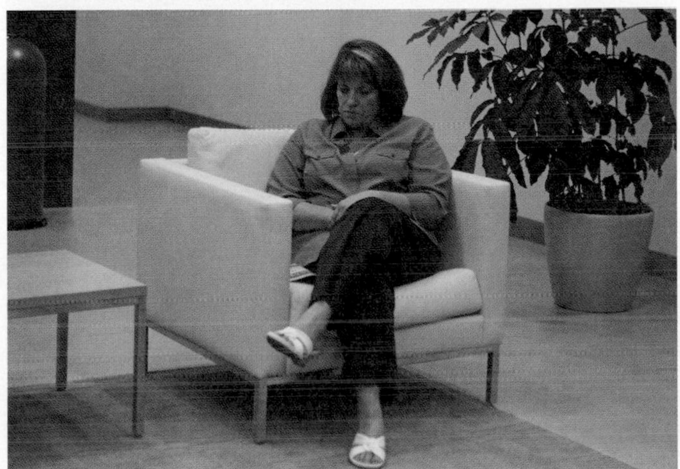

FIGURE 7-8 Position of depression or uninvolvement

Positions to facilitate breathing are assumed to help the muscles of ventilation do their work. Individual with emphysema and COPD are the ones most likely to assume these positions and often use a **tripod position**, seated with their arms folded and supported on a stationary object (overbed stand) or they may be seated with their hands placed on the knees (Figures 7-9 a–b). These positions maximize chest expansion of the thoracic cage, reducing the workload of the ventilatory muscles.

Gait

The final observation of body movement is the patient's gait, which may be observed when the patient enters the room or by asking the patient to walk a certain distance. Gait is described as a series of rhythmical, alternating movements of the trunk and limbs that result in the forward progression of the center of gravity. An individual's gait consists of repetitive cycles of two phases: **swing phase** and **stance phase**. The stance phase is when the weight-bearing extremity is in contact with the ground. The swing phase is when the nonweight-bearing extremity is not in contact with the ground. Each of the phases can be subdivided into four sub-phases (Figure 7-10).

The two phases of gait also determine the individual's **step** and **stride**. Step is the distance between the heel contact of each foot or the advancement of a single foot, whereas stride is the advancement of both feet, or the distance between heel contact of one extremity. Maintaining a gait also depends on two other essential abilities: **equilibrium** and **locomotion**. Equilibrium is the ability

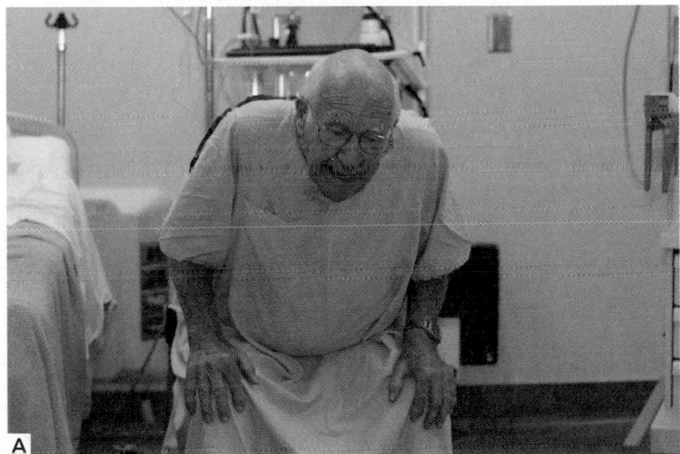

A

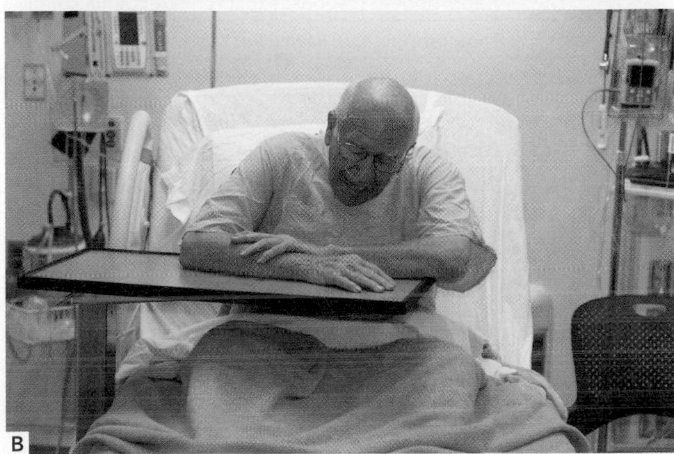

B

FIGURE 7-9A–B Tripod positions

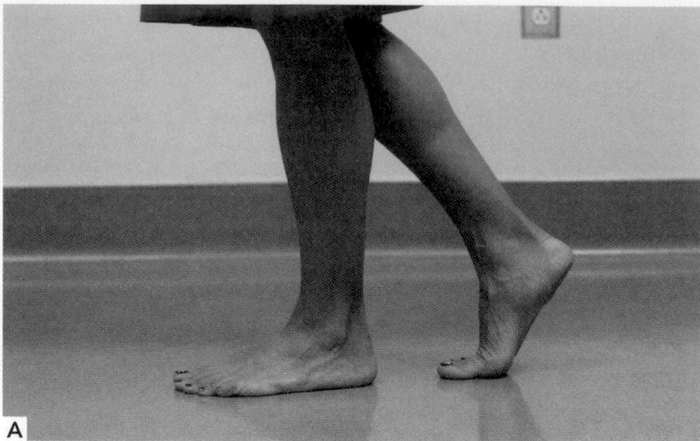

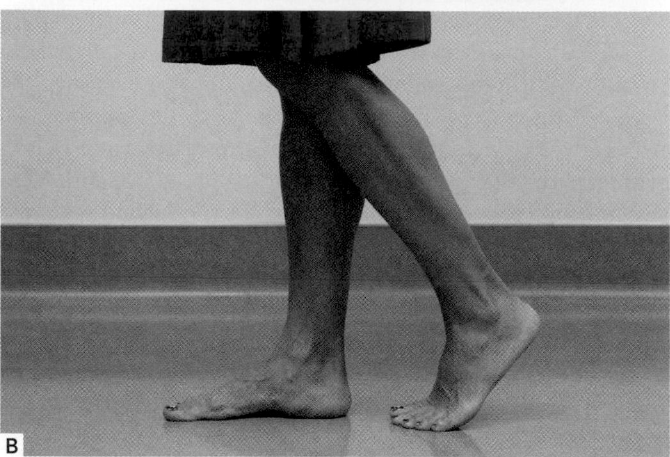

FIGURE 7-10A–B Gait phases

to assume an upright position and maintain balance. Locomotion is the ability to initiate and maintain rhythmic stepping. Additionally, the musculoskeletal system must be intact and the appropriate joints must be functional. The muscles must also demonstrate muscle tone that will be high enough to overcome gravity but low enough to allow movement.

The patient's gait should demonstrate smoothness of movements with a regular cadence or rhythm with 60% of the time spent in the stance phase and 40% of the time in the swing phase. The body and head should be held erect with shoulders and hips remaining level with each stride, and turns should be smooth and easily executed. The length of the stride should be equal with a smooth, rhythmic swaying of the trunk related to the gait phase.

The arms should swing freely and swing in rhythm with the opposite lower extremity. The patient should also be able to walk in a straight line and maintain balance throughout the gait. Any alteration of the gait is commonly observed during the stance phase. An altered gait may be associated with the patient watching the feet while walking, stumbling, shuffling, staggering, and limping; the steps may be uneven and the gait may be lurching, propulsive, spastic, or scissor-like. (Altered gaits related to the components of the two phases are further described and discussed in Chapter 27.)

Significance of Findings Related to Motor Activity

Increased motor activity may be referred to as hyperactivity and is frequently related to anxiety, mania, or use of central nervous system stimulants. Slowed or limited amount of motor activity may be related to depression and referred to as psychomotor retardation. Repetitious motor activity (e.g., hand washing) may be compulsions associated with an obsessive-compulsive disorder. Hand tremors may be associated with Parkinson's disease or a drug-induced phenomenon accompanying the use of anti-psychotic or anti-mania drugs.

Mental Status Examination

The mental status examination is a broad screening tool that is a useful component of the overall assessment. Via observation, interview, and subsequent objective description, it is intended to capture the current psychological and cognitive functioning of the individual. These functions are briefly summarized in Table 7-3. In combination with the findings of the health history, the physical assessment, laboratory results, and information obtained from significant others, it may assist in documenting the mental and emotional health of the patient or may identify specific symptoms that could be indicative of pathology.

The mental status examination has been typically used with psychiatric patients, persons with traumatic brain injuries, and

Table 7-3 Cognitive functions of mental status examination

Cognition	One's ability to understand his or her environment; integrate and process information; and consider, evaluate, and make appropriate responses to internal/external stimuli affected by awareness of surroundings and orientation	
Functions:	**Encompasses/Characteristics:**	**Tested by:**
Basic process that provides foundation for higher level intellectual (executive) abilities		
Attention/ Concentration	Selection of helpful and suppression of distracting stimuli Ability to track a task	• Spell "world" backwards • Listen to digit spans of increasing length and repeat • Listen to string of letters and repeat backwards
Memory	Learning—acquisition of new information Recall—ability to find an bring to consciousness learned information Immediate (seconds) Recent Memory—"current information" (minutes, hours, days) Remote Memory—"old information" (years)	• Immediate: Asking patient to learn a short list of items • Recent: Asking patient about current events • Remote: Asking patient to recall distant information
Language	Word formation Word choice Grammar	• Observation of word formation and content • Oral and written language comprehension • Repetition and naming

Continued

Table 7-3 Cognitive functions of mental status examination *(continued)*

Higher Level (Executive) Abilities		
Cognition	**Encompasses/Characteristics:**	**Tested by:**
Praxis	The ability to perform a skilled movement (motor activity) when the nature of the request is known in the absence of physical disability Activities such as dressing (ADLs)	• Asking patient to copy 2 or 3 dimensional figures or shapes
Calculation	Requires several intact cognitive processes: Knowledge of the table of values Understanding the "meaning" of process Knowledge of symbols Ability to sequence operations	• Performing mathematical operations (verbal and visual)
Reason/ Abstraction	Insight/judgment Ability to manipulate old knowledge Use old knowledge to solve a novel situation Extract principles from a novel situation	• Performance of proverb interpretation • Response to novel situation • Identifying similarities • Identifying appropriate actions

patients with dementia. In addition, it has been commonly used in the general health care setting with patients who become confused or where delirium is suspected. In each situation, the mental status examination can be used to establish a base line level of functioning for the patient as well as to document changes that occur over time.

The mental status examination has become more broadly used in the recent years with an array of patient populations. For example, the mental status examination, as a measure of cognitive function, has been found to be useful in exploring the potential for older adults' participation in primary and secondary health behaviors (Resnick, 2003) the initiation of substance abuse treatment among older adults (Satre, Knight, Dickson-Fuhrmann, & Jarvik, 2004), functional outcomes in hip fracture patients (Feldt & Oh, 2000), older adults' capacity for medication management (Maddigan, Farris, Keating, Wiens, & Johnson, 2003), the impact of exercise on the cognitive decline often associated with diabetes (Colberg, Somma, & Sechrist, 2008), and prognosis assessment for stroke patients at the point of discharge from the hospital (Olai, Omne-Ponten, Borgquist, & Svardsudd, 2007). Clearly the mental status examination can be used in multiple ways in clinical situations and constitutes an essential tool for the professional provider.

Components of the Mental Examination

The components of the mental examination include the following:

Identifying Data	Thought Process
Appearance	Orientation
Motor Activity	Memory
Speech	Level of Concentration
Mood/Affect	General Intellectual Level
Perceptions	Judgment
Thought Content	Insight

Identifying data, appearance, and motor activity have already been described and discussed.

Speech

Speech refers to one's verbal or oral communication. Speech is related to the production of sound and the articulation of vowel and consonant speech sound units. Speech is also the verbal expression of internal thoughts, feelings and perceptions, and external objects. The meaning associated with these expressions is processed within specific areas of the brain.

The mechanical dynamics of speech involve the movement of air from the lungs and through the larynx during exhalation. This production of sound is described as **phonation**. The larynx, which lies between the pharynx and trachea, also contains cartilaginous (vocal) cords that are attached to the muscles of the larynx. Production of the glottal tone occurs primarily in the larynx as air passes through the vocal cords, causing them to vibrate.

The ability to convert sound into words and combining of words is **articulation**. Articulation is dependent upon the function of the larynx and the muscles of the vocal tract that determine the shape and tension of the vocal tract (tongue, cheeks, and mouth) for formation of vowels and consonants of words. The muscles involved with speech production are innervated by 6 of the 12 cranial nerves: trigeminal, facial, glossopharyngeal, vagus, accessory, and hypoglossal.

Assessment of Speech The characteristics of speech are related to quantity, articulation, intonation, as well as patterns. Quantity of speech can be assessed as whether the rate and pace of the individual is slow or rapid. An individual's speech should progress in a manner that allows appropriate articulation of words and representation of thoughts. Expected speech quantity is estimated to be between 150– 175 words per minute. It is not generally assessed that precisely; however, note a paucity of speech—yes/no answers, or minimal word use in responses, lack of additional or supportive information.

Intonation is the variability in sound and pitch that accompanies the production of sound and words. It is expected that variations in the sound and pitch of the individual's speech are present and generally accompany changes in emotions and feelings associated with the topics of the conversation.

Patterns of speech relates to alterations in word formation. Listen for the presence of garbled speech, stuttering, slurring of words, and the presence of an accent. Altered thought processes may also affect the pattern of speech. Also note and listen for the presence of **aphasia**, an acquired speech disorder causing a loss of the ability to produce or comprehend spoken or written language. Note any difficulty related to thinking of specific words or forming words and whether words are used incorrectly.

> ***PRACTICE POINT: Volume and Hearing***
> The volume of the individual's speech may not necessarily indicate a problem with speech but a hearing problem. Types of hearing may be broadly described as conductive or sensori-neural. Louder than expected speech may be indicative of a sensori-neural loss, in contrast to a softer than expected volume may indicate a conductive hearing loss. (These types of hearing loss are further discussed in Chapter 19.)

Also note the presence of **pressured speech** (logorrhea), which is a tendency to speak rapidly and frenziedly, as if motivated by urgency not apparent to the listener. The speech is frequently increased in amount and difficult or impossible to interrupt. It may also be loud and emphatic. Frequently the person talks without any social stimulation and may continue to talk even though no one is listening.

Speech is also assessed as to the correctness and appropriateness of the individual's command of language. Note the connection and flow between words. The choice and use of words is an indicator of the level of education. There might be short pauses in between sentences for the individual to think and formulate additional sentences or responses. Speech is also the primary means for the expression of thoughts, either directly or indirectly. Various alterations in speech patterns are characteristic of thought disorders (Table 7-4).

Significance of Findings Related to Speech An increased quantity of speech that is pressured, loud, and rapid may be indicative of a manic episode of the bipolar illness. A reduction in verbal output coupled with soft, hesitant speech may be a symptom of depression. Slurring of words may be related to substance abuse, while garbled speech may be indicative of a neurological phenomenon. Aphasia may be evidence of dementia or a CVA. Pressured speech is considered one of the first clinical signs of mania. Once again, it is important to be cognizant that an individual's use of speech and language is, to a large extent, determined by his or her culture. This is a significant consideration when assessing this aspect of the mental status examination.

Mood/Affect

Mood refers to a person's self-reported feeling, emotional state, or outlook at a particular moment. Mood encompasses an emotional response or attitude toward something seen, heard, or otherwise experienced. Affect is the patient's observed emotional tone and the visible reactions an individual manifests towards events.

Assessment of the patient's mood includes both the patient and the patient's significant other. This assessment asks questions about the patient's typical mood as well as any recent variations. Box 7-1 gives examples of potential questions.

Affect can be described in terms of range, duration, appropriateness, and intensity. Descriptors used to characterize affect include **expansive/euphoric** (contagious), **euthymic** (normal), **constricted** (limited variation), **blunted** (minimal variation), and **flat** (no variation) (Brannon, 2009). The provider might note a range of emotions from despair to hostility to anxiety to euphoria. In contrast, some patients will exhibit almost no expression as they speak of significant life events; this is called a **flat affect**. Rapid shifting from one affective response to another is called a **labile affect** (Table 7-5).

During the course of the interview, assess for consistency between verbal and nonverbal behavior. Nonverbal indicators of mood might include facial expression, tears, perspiration, flushing, motor activity, respiratory changes, or tremors. It is essential to note any discrepancies between thought content and mood (e.g., giggling at a tragic event), which would indicate an incongruent or inappropriate affect. Intensity of affect may be assessed via the interviewer's subjective quantification of the degree of sadness, anger, anxiety, or other emotions expressed by the patient. It may be useful for the interviewer to rate affect on a scale of 1–10.

Table 7-4 Thought processes expressed through speech

Associative Looseness:	A bizarre organizational thread between ideas that results in a lack of meaningful connections between thoughts, e.g., "My favorite color is red. My sister has auburn colored hair. I get really sunburned whenever I am out in the sun."
Blocking:	A sudden cessation of speech in mid-sentence or mid-thought
Circumlocution:	Round-about expression, substituting a phrase when cannot think of name of object
Circumstantiality:	Excessive, unnecessary, but relevant detail in one's response to a question
Clang Associations:	Use of rhyming words in a nonsensical manner, e.g., Alyssa states, "You are red, fed, head, Ned, Ted, in bed."
Confabulation:	Fabricates events to fill in memory gaps
Echolalia:	Repetition of words that one hears, e.g., The providers states, "You seem very tired today, Julia." Julia replies, "I am very tired today. I am very tired today. I am very tired today."
Flight of Ideas:	An almost continuous flow of rapid conversation in which there are frequent, abrupt changes of topic that may result in incoherence
Neologisms:	The invention of new words that are meaningless to others but have highly symbolic meaning to the author of them, e.g., the client continually speaks of a "washamawhirl."
Perseveration:	Persistent repetition of words or ideas despite apparent efforts to formulate a new response
Tangential:	Presents similarly to circumstantial speech but the client never actually answers the question that was posed
Word Salad:	A jumble of words without any logical connection; "tossed salad" of words, e.g., Jason states, "Hot, raisin, sold, yellow, come, jump...."

Significance of Findings Related to Mood/Affect This series of questions and observations will clearly document symptoms of depression or mania. In addition, evidence of suicidal ideation may be elicited by questions related to the patient's sense of the future and homicidal ideation by questions about interpersonal relationships. Any evidence of suicidal or homicidal ideation should be thoroughly assessed and an appropriate course of action formulated (Chapter 14). Flat and/or inappropriate affect can also be associated with schizophrenia.

Box 7-1 Assessment of Mood

- How would you describe your mood? How would you rate your mood on a scale of 1 to 10?
- How are your spirits?
- How do you feel about ________? (recent life event, i.e., divorce, death)
- Has your mood been fairly stable or has it been changeable?
- Is the patient's mood appropriate to her/his life situation?
- Do you have high or low moods? If so, assess the pattern.
- How do you see your future?

If there is any indication of suicidal ideation, follow up with the questions below: (Further assessment in Chapter 14.)

- Are you having thoughts of suicide?
- Do you have a plan for committing suicide?
- If so, what is your plan for suicide?
- Do you have access to the means that you have identified?
- How do you see your relationships with others?

If there is any indication of homicidal ideation, follow up with the questions below:

- Are you having thoughts of harming another person?
- Do have a plan for harming this person?
- If so, what is your plan?
- Do you have access to the means that you have identified?

Perceptions

Perceptions refer to an awareness derived from sensory processes while a stimulus is present.

Assessment of Perception The mental status examination includes an assessment for the presence or experiencing of **illusions** or **hallucinations**. An illusion is a misinterpretation of actual sensory input. For example, one sees a coat rack in the corner but momentarily misinterprets it as a person lurking in the corner. In contrast, hallucinations are a sensory experience in the absence of sensory input. Thus, hallucinations may involve any of the five senses (Table 7-6).

Auditory hallucinations take on an added dimension when the individual is commanded by the voices to engage in some sort of activity. This type of hallucination is termed a command auditory hallucination, and the activities that the individual feels compelled to engage in are often harmful to self or others. Command auditory hallucinations are extremely dangerous and require thorough assessment of the content, continuous supervision of the patient, and prompt intervention to ensure safety.

PRACTICE POINT: Assessing Alterations in Perception

When assessing for alterations in perceptions, the interviewer should be tactful and diplomatic. For example, consider the following approach: "When people are in situations such as yours they occasionally hear or see peculiar or frightening things. Has this ever happened to you? When?"

Table 7-5 Mood/Affect

Attributes	Descriptors	Characteristics
Expected finding	Euthymia	Appropriate to situation, consistency with mood, congruency with thought content
	Inappropriate affect	Affect clearly discordant with the content of patient's speech
Fluctuations	Even	Unchanging throughout interview
	Labile	Rapid shift of emotions/expressions
Range	Broad, restricted	The palette of a person's facial expression and emotiveness
Intensity	Blunted, flat	Lack of emotional response; no expression of feelings, voice monotone and face immobile
	Animated	Emotional responses visible with facial expressions characteristic of expressed emotion, voice/speech with varying intonation and inflections
Manifestation	Depression	Sad, gloomy, dejected; symptoms may occur with rainy weather, after a holiday, or with an illness; if the situation is temporary, symptoms fade quickly
	Depersonalization (lack of ego boundaries)	Loss of identity, feels estranged, perplexed about own identity and meaning of existence
	Elation	Joy and optimism, overconfidence, increased motor activity, not necessarily pathologic
	Euphoria	Excessive well-being, unusually cheerful or elated, which inappropriate considering mental and physical condition, implies a pathologic mood
	Anxiety	Worried, uneasy, apprehensive, external danger whose source is unknown
	Fear	Worried, uneasy, apprehensive, external danger whose source is known
	Irritability	Annoyed, easily provoked, impatient
	Anger, rage	Furious, loss of control
	Ambivalence	The existence of opposing emotions toward an idea, object, person

Table 7-6 Types of hallucinations

Auditory:	Hearing sounds in the absence of sensory input. For example, a patient hears voices that others do not hear that suggest he is worthless.
Visual:	Seeing things in the absence of sensory input. For example, a patient sees persons in the room that do not exist.
Tactile:	Feeling sensations in the absence of sensory input. For example, a patient is fearful as she feels bugs crawling on her skin when there is no such occurrence.
Gustatory:	Experiencing tastes in the absence of sensory input. For example, a patient reports that he continually tastes blood when there are no physical findings to explain this.
Olfactory:	Experiencing smells in the absence of sensory input. For example, a patient routinely smells "burning flesh" when others do not experience any such olfactory sensation.

In the event that the hallucinations are obvious, it is appropriate to assess them directly and in a matter of fact manner. Questions such as the following may be useful under such circumstances:

Do you ever see or hear things that others do not?
Can you describe what you are seeing?
What are the voices saying to you?
How long have you been hearing the voices?
Are there times when the voices are more intrusive/difficult/prevalent?

Significant Findings Related to Perceptions

Most individuals will experience illusions at various points in time and thus they are of little concern. Hallucinations, on the other hand, are generally indicative of some type of pathology. Auditory hallucinations are the most common type followed by visual hallucinations. These types of hallucinations will accompany schizophrenia. Tactile hallucinations are particularly common during delirium tremors, use of cocaine, and cognitive disorders.

Thought Content

Thought content refers to those ideas that one focuses on during waking hours.

The mental status exam can be helpful in identifying the presence of abnormal thought content. Generally, specific questions are unnecessary if the interviewer simply follows up on the patient's verbal cues and content. For example: "A moment ago you said that you felt as though you were being followed. Could you tell me a bit more about that?" Delusional patients, in particular, often feel compelled to share their thought content. This is another instance in which the significant others of the patient may assist in supplying pertinent data as well. The provider should attempt to ascertain if any of the following are present (Table 7-7).

Table 7-7 Altered thought content

Delusion:	A personal belief that is not based in reality. Common types of delusions include the following: • Grandiose delusion: Belief that one has great fame, power, wealth, or attractiveness. For example, a patient states, "I am the President of the United States and I just enacted the largest tax cut in history." • Paranoid delusion: Excessive suspiciousness, irrational distrust of others, or a belief that others are seeking to harm you or spying on you. For example, "The FBI has bugged my home and is following all of my movements." • Religious delusion: Preoccupation with religious themes. For example, "I know Jesus Christ and his mother Mary well. John the Baptist is a relative of mine as well. Peter, Paul, and Judas were neighbors of mine." • Somatic delusion: Belief that one has some disease, disorder, or disability that is not supported by physical findings. For example, a patient states, "I know that I have cancer of the stomach no matter how much my physician denies it." Or, "My heart stops beating periodically for a period of minutes and then begins again." • Delusion of being controlled: Belief that an outside force is directing one's behavior. For example, "My computer hard drive tells me what my orders are." • Ideas of reference: Belief that external events, objects, or individuals have special significance for the person. For example, "If you listen to the nightly news, you will see that they are regularly talking about my life." • Thought broadcasting: A belief one's thoughts are being disseminated to all. For example, "I know that others are aware of every thought that I am thinking." • Thought insertion: A belief that ideas and thoughts are being introduced into one's brain by outside forces and persons. For example, "There are aliens that continually add thoughts to my head each morning."
Depersonalization:	A sense of being detached from one's body and being an observer of one's own actions. For example, "I feel like I'm outside of myself and watching myself go through the motions of life."
Hypochondriasis:	A preoccupation with bodily functioning and excessive somatic concerns. For example, "I have had numerous problems that the doctors haven't been able to diagnose—shortness of breath, rashes, overall muscle aches, back aches, and diarrhea. It's very frustrating that they don't know what to do about these things."
Obsession:	Recurrent thoughts or impulses that the individual cannot control and finds to be quite distressing. Often the obsession is accompanied by a compulsion, which is a repetitive act that a person feels they must perform to reduce anxiety. For example, a patient may have an obsession related to dirt and germs and then engages in compulsive hand washing 25 times per hour.
Phobia:	An irrational fear that motivates the individual to avoid the stimulus of the fear. For example, a patient may have an irrational fear of close spaces, such as an elevator, which is called claustrophobia.

Significance of Findings Related to Thought Content

Delusions are one of several characteristic symptoms of schizophrenia. They may also be present with dementia. Grandiose delusions are fairly common during manic episodes of the bipolar disorder. Depersonalization is often associated with psychosis as well but occasionally with depression. Hypochondriasis, obsessions, and phobias are generally associated with specific anxiety disorders.

Thought Process

An evaluation of thought processes involves careful listening to the patient's speech during the course of the interview to assess for logical development of thoughts, coherent and relevant responses, and organized and goal directed conversation. See Table 7-7.

Significance of Findings Related to Thought Process

Several of the thought process abnormalities are associated with schizophrenia. Specifically, associative looseness, blocking, clang associations, echolalia, and neologisms. Flight of ideas is a classic symptom of mania. Circumstantiality may indicate a level of paranoia, while perseveration can be associated with psychosis or neurological dysfunction.

Orientation

Orientation refers to a state of awareness or having mental faculties fully intact.

Providers may use a series of specific questions to assess a patient's orientation to person, place, and time efficiently (see Box 7-2). It may be advisable to preface these questions with a statement that will put the patient at ease such as, "I am going to ask you some basic questions that we incorporate into our assessment of all patients. Some of these questions might seem rather self-evident to you."

Box 7-2 Questions to Assess Orientation

Person

What is your name?

Are you married? If so, what is your spouse's name?

Do you have children? Grandchildren? If so, what are their names?

Are you employed? Retired? If so, where do/did you work? What types of work do/did you do?

Place

What city, state do you live in?

Where are we now? (name of clinic/hospital, city, state)?

Time

What is today's date (month, day, year)? (If patient does not know ask him/her to estimate.)

What day of the week is it?

What time of day is it?

What season of the year is it?

PRACTICE POINT: *Oriented X 3 or X 4?*

Orientation may also be expressed and documented as Alert and Oriented X 4. The 4th dimension of orientation generally refers to events or situation, however, no standardization or agreement exists as to what the 4th dimension represents. Assess the 4th dimension by asking the patient to recall recent events or the events that created the situation in which the patient is involved. It primarily assesses short term memory in situations where the patient may have sustained any type of head injury. It is not necessarily assessed in hospitalized patients unless there is a perceived need to have more specific orientation information.

Significance of Findings Related to Orientation

Patients with dementia or delirium will often show symptoms of disorientation. These patients will generally become disoriented to place and/or time prior to being disoriented to person. Patients with schizophrenia may indicate that they are someone else or are somewhere else when questioned about orientation.

Memory

Memory refers to the mental capacity of retaining impressions or of recalling previous experiences. Commonly conceptualized as remembrance, memory is assessed in relationship to remote, recent, immediate, and general grasp recall. Keep in mind that the bulk of the health history requires the patient to demonstrate memory and recall. Unless you have reason to consider the patient an unreliable historian, memory may be assessed by the patient's responses to the health history questions. If a reason exists to suspect that recent or immediate recall is questionable, it would be appropriate to directly assess these types (see Box 7-3).

Box 7-3 Questions to Assess Memory

Remote recall	Recent recall	Immediate recall	General grasp and recall
Events or situations that occurred within a time frame of years ago	Events or situations that occurred in a time frame of weeks or months	Events or situations that occur within a time frame of minutes or hours	Ask the patient to read a brief story and then share the theme of the story and as many pertinent details as possible.
What can you tell me about some of the important past events in your life? (Childhood experiences, educational experiences, marriage, military service, etc.)	What has been happening in your life in the past week?	What did you have for lunch?	
	What events preceded your hospitalization?	Ask the patient to repeat a set of three objects immediately after they are presented and again after 3–4 minutes (e.g., dog, banana, box).	

> ***PRACTICE POINT: Writing Down Words and Objects***
> When giving the patient words or objects for assessment of recall, you also must recall them. To prevent "forgetting" these words/objects, write them down on a sheet of paper. Or, use the same words/objects during each patient examination. Doing this will prevent having to come up with new words/objects for each examination.

Significance of Findings Related to Memory

Memory impairment is a hallmark of dementia. Immediate and recent recall are particularly affected early in the illness while remote recall remains intact for a longer period. It is important to be aware of the phenomenon of **confabulation** relative to patients in early stages of dementia. When a patient with a memory deficit is unable to recall the requested information, he/she will simply create facts or events in an effort to fill in the memory gap. Confabulation functions as a type of coping mechanism for patients whose memory is impaired such that they are unable to recall important pieces of their immediate and recent past. Patients with delirium will also exhibit memory deficits. Anxiety and depression can have a temporary impact on memory—particularly immediate recall. Finally, symptoms related to memory may be found with patients who have a dissociative disorder. **Delirium** and **dementia** are compared and contrasted in Table 7-8.

Level of Concentration

Level of concentration refers to the patient's ability to focus on the task at hand or the ability to pay attention without being distracted by environmental stimuli. The provider should attempt to note the patient's general ability to attend to the interviewer and the questions being asked. Is the patient able to concentrate on the interviewer or is he/she easily distracted by environmental stimuli?

Other strategies to assess the level of concentration include simple repetition and spelling exercises. When using these strategies, it is preferable to share with the patient that you are going to test his or her ability to concentrate. Explain that one's level of concentration may be impacted by various factors such as illness, pain, or anxiety. Patients may be asked to repeat a numerical sequence such as a street address, telephone number, or zip code after having heard it spoken to them slowly and clearly. In addition, patients could be asked to spell a word such as "lunch" or "world" backward.

Significance of Findings Related to Level of Concentration

Patients with mania, depression, delirium, anxiety, and attention deficit/hyperactivity disorder may have difficulties related to concentration.

General Intellectual Level

General intellectual level pertains to the capacity for reasoning, understanding, and comprehension as well as the knowledge of events, circumstances, and information.

Significance of Findings Related to General Intellectual Level

The interpretation of findings related to a patient's general intellectual level has the potential to be culturally bound and thus should be approached cautiously. For example, language, terminology, and familiarity with so-called "common" proverbs may present difficulties for a patient from a culture different than the provider administering the test. It is also imperative that the patient's educational background and the presence of any learning disabilities be taken into account. Factors such as these could inappropriately skew the analysis of the patient's intellectual level.

Obviously, the general intellectual level portion of the mental status examination is significantly impacted by developmental disabilities and dementia. Patients with schizophrenia will also tend to be very concrete in the interpretation of proverbs.

Judgment

Judgment is the ability to make a decision or form an opinion adaptively, constructively, objectively, and wisely, especially in matters affecting action. Generally judgment involves considering a set of facts or circumstances and choosing an appropriate course of action. Judgment may be informally referred to as good sense or discretion.

Judgment can be assessed, in part, by determining if the patient is routinely involved in illegal, dangerous, or destructive activities. In addition, it is common to ask questions relative to what action a person would take in various hypothetical situations (see Box 7-5).

Box 7-4 Questions to Assess General Intellectual Level

<u>General knowledge:</u> Ask patients to name the last five presidents or to name the four largest cities in the United States.

<u>Calculation:</u> Ask patients to do simple calculations such as 18 + 13, 8 × 7, or to serially subtract 7 from 100.

<u>Abstraction:</u> Ask patients to interpret various proverbs or to describe the similarities between two items. For example:

Proverbs

"People who live in glass houses should not throw stones."

"A bird in the hand is better than two in the bush."

"Don't cry over spilled milk."

Similarities

How are a sofa and a chair similar?

How are a candy bar and a doughnut similar?

How are a row boat and a canoe similar?

Evaluate answers in terms of their relevance as well as their degree of concreteness or abstractness. Most patients should be able to give abstract or semi-abstract interpretations. For example, an abstract interpretation of the first proverb would be if you have a particular short-coming it is not wise to criticize others for that same short-coming. An abstract response to the first set of similar items would be that each is a piece of furniture constructed for the purpose of providing seating.

Box 7-5 Questions to Assess Judgment

"What would you do if your house started on fire?"

"What would you do if you saw an automobile accident?"

"What would you do if you found a lost child at the shopping mall?"

"What would you do if you won the lottery?"

The answer to these questions would be assessed in terms of the logic and social appropriateness that is demonstrated in the course of action proposed by the patient. Judgment may be described as impulsive, deliberate, or appropriate.

Table 7-8 Delirium vs. dementia

Delirium	Dementia
Diagnostic features	
Fluctuating consciousness associated with cognitive changes unrelated to preexisting or evolving dementia	Multiple cognitive deficits (impaired memory, and either aphasia, apraxia, or agnosia)
Awareness of environment diminished	Executive functioning impaired (ability to think abstractly, to organize, plan, initiate, sequence, monitor, and stop complex behavior)
Inability to focus, sustain, or shift attention	Impaired function of occupational or social skills, indicative of a decline from previous abilities
Cognitive change may consist of memory impairment, disoriented to time and/or place, or speech alterations such as rambling, pressured and irrelevancy or incoherency	
Complex or simple altered perception which may consist of misinterpretations, illusions, or hallucinations	
Associated Features	
Emotional disturbance: fear, anxiety, irritability, anger, euphoria, apathy	Spatial disorientation, poor judgment/insight, suicidal behavior, slurred speech, anxiety, mood/sleep alterations, vulnerability to physical/psychosocial stressors
Sleep–wake cycle impaired (daytime sleepiness or night time agitation or difficulty in falling asleep)	Progressive, slow and steady destruction of neurons in brain reduces concentration of acetylcholine and other neurotransmitters
Disturbed psychomotor behavior (groping/picking at bedclothes, sudden movements, or lethargy and sluggishness)	
Possible extremes in daytime psychomotor activities	
Onset	
May begin abruptly and rapidly (over hours)	Depends on underlying etiology
Common in children and those over 60	May be sudden (head trauma) or insidious onset that slowly progresses over course of several years.
Course	
Fluctuates with symptoms often worse at night; lucid periods usually in morning	Depends on underlying etiology
	Commonly progressive and stable, and rarely remitting
Duration	
Transient; resolution on few hours to few weeks	May progress to death over several years
	Deterioration may be slowed
Outcome	
Depends on severity; poor prognosis when severe	Generally irreversible
Recovery possible if underlying condition is corrected or self-limiting	Delay in deterioration related to underlying pathology, timely diagnosis, and treatment
If persists, will shift to more stable organic brain syndrome	The more wide spread the structural damage to the brain, the less likely the clinical improvement
May cause death	
Etiologic Factors	
Multifactorial	Primary degenerative dementia (Alzheimer's type)
Systemic infections	Central nervous system infections
Metabolic disorders (hepatic or renal disease, hypoxia, hypercapnia, hypoglycemia, electrolyte imbalance, thiamine deficiency)	Brain trauma
Postoperative states	Viral/prion infection (AIDS, Creutzfeldt-Jakob disease)
Substance intoxication/withdrawal/head trauma	Toxic metabolic disturbance
Lesions of right parietal/occipital lobe	Vascular disease (vascular dementia)
Toxin exposure	Normal pressure hydrocephalus
Anticholinergic effects of medications	Neurologic conditions (Huntington's disease, multiple sclerosis, Parkinson's disease)
	Postanoxic or posthypoglycemic states

Source: Adapted from *Contemporary Psychiatric-Mental Health Nursing*, 3E by C. R. Kneisl & E. Trigoboff. Copyright © 2013, pp. 270. Reprinted and electronically reproduced by permission of Pearson Education, Inc., Upper Saddle River, New Jersey.

Box 7-6 Questions to Assess Insight

"What do you believe is the reason you are here today?"

"How do you interpret this whole situation?"

"Do you believe that you have a problem?"

"What role have others played in your current situation?"

"What suggestions do you have for your treatment?"

It will be particularly important to ascertain the patient's sense of the need for intervention as well as how much responsibility the patient accepts for the current situation. The use of coping mechanisms and ego defense mechanisms (e.g., denial, projection, rationalization) should also be noted.

Significance of Findings Related to Judgment

Judgment may be impaired during a manic episode, in dementia, delirium, schizophrenia, and during instances of intoxication or substance abuse. Further, persons with lesser intellectual ability as measured by a standard IQ test will have greater difficulty with demonstrating appropriate judgment.

Insight

Insight is the apprehending of the true nature of a thing through intuitive understanding.

Significance of Findings Related to Insight

Difficulties relative to insightfulness may be marked with patients having diagnoses such as delirium, dementia, psychosis, eating disorders, substance abuse disorders, or personality disorders. Insight will be more difficult for those with developmental disabilities as well. A variety of other types of patients may have lesser degrees of difficulty with insight and this situation has the potential to impact the therapeutic process.

Response to the Interview

Finally, it is useful to record the patient's response to the interview situation and to the interviewer.

Assessment of the Response to the Interview

Townsend (2009) suggests that the patient's general attitude can be captured by the following categories:

Cooperative/uncooperative: Does the patient refuse to answer questions or willingly respond to them?

Friendly/hostile/defensive: Can the patient be described as sociable, sarcastic, or irritable?

Uninterested/apathetic or attentive/interested: Does the patient exhibit a lack of investment in the interview process? Does the patient actively participate in the assessment?

Guarded/suspicious: Does the patient continuously scan the environment? Does the patient question the motives of the interviewer? Does the patient refuse to answer some of the questions that are posed?

Significance of Findings Related to Response to Interview

An assessment of the patient's response to the interview may provide valuable information about typical responses to new people and situations or perhaps of psychopathology. It will be important to utilize feedback from significant others so as to document similarities or differences between this set of responses and the patient's usual responses.

Modifications for Special Circumstances and Populations

The mental status examination can be a valuable diagnostic tool. Specific adaptations of it may need to be made for children as well as those patients who are nonverbal. Many of the elements requiring observation can be administered as described but modification of the questions for these populations will be necessary. For the nonverbal patient, the questions will need to be "yes" or "no" by means of a gesture. With a child, questions may need to be more focused and concrete and the addition of drawing and/or play may elicit much useful data.

Clearly there may be circumstances that will preclude the administration of the complete exam as described in this chapter. In such cases, the **mini-mental state exam** (MMSE) (Folstein, Folstein, & McHugh, 1975) is the most common instrument and has been widely used since 1975. The MMSE is a 30-point questionnaire that has been used to screen for cognitive impairment, primarily for dementia. It has also been used to follow a progression of changes in cognition, documenting an individual's response to therapy. The MMSE includes only 11 items that focus primarily on the cognitive aspects of mental functioning to the exclusion of items related to mood, thought content, and thought processes.

Scores obtained for the MMSE are used to determine cognitive functioning of the individual and are broken down into the following categories:

25–30 = no cognitive impairment
21–24 = mild cognitive impairment
10–20 = moderate cognitive impairment
<9 = severe cognitive impairment.

Potential Limitations of the Mental Status Examination

In an effort to provide culturally sensitive care to all patients, providers must be aware of the possibility that the mental status examination as outlined may not serve all persons equally well. Parker and Philip (2004) speak to this issue:

> There is a well-documented tendency for cognitive tests to underestimate the abilities of older people in black and minority ethnic groups. This gives rise to a substantially higher risk of a mistaken diagnosis of dementia. Reasons include differences in extent or focus of formal education, lack of familiarity with English, lack of literacy in own first language, and culture-specific factors related to individual test items. (p. 447)

The findings of a study that used MMSE scores adjusted for age and education to screen for dementia with community dwelling elderly black and white women suggested that racial differences may have an impact on the scores independent of age and education. Thus, further research was suggested to better understand the interaction of race and culture on MMSE results (Wood, Giuliano, Bignell, & Pritham, 2006). Similarly, following a pilot study to measure cognitive function in older Mexican American nursing home residents, the researchers concluded that the MMSE may not be an appropriate measure to use to assess cognitive functioning in older Hispanic populations whose educational levels or literacy is low or unknown (Evans, Crogan, & Greenberg, 2008).

VAMC
SLUMS Examination

Questions about this assessment tool? E-mail aging@slu.edu.

Name ______________________ Age ______________________

Is patient alert? ______________________ Level of education ______________________

Department of Veterans Affairs

__/1 (1) **1. What day of the week is it?**

__/1 (1) **2. What is the year?**

__/1 (1) **3. What state are we in?**

3. Please remember these five objects. I will ask you what they are later.

Apple Pen Tie House Car

5. You have $100 and you go to the store and buy a dozen apples for $3 and a tricycle for $20.

(1) **How much did you spend?**

__/3 (2) **How much do you have left?**

6. Please name as many animals as you can in one minute.

__/3 (0) 0–4 animals (1) 5–9 animals (2) 10–14 animals (3) 15+ animals

__/5 **7. What were the five objects I asked you to remember? 1 point for each one correct.**

8. I am going to give you a series of numbers and I would like you to give them to me backwards. For example, if I say 42, you would say 24.

__/2 (0) 87 (1) 649 (1) 8537

9. This is a clock face. Please put in the hour markers and the time at ten minutes to eleven o'clock.

(2) Hour markers okay

__/4 (2) Time correct

__/2 (1) **10. Please place an X in the triangle.**

(1) **Which of the above figures is the largest?**

11. I am going to tell you a story. Please listen carefully because afterwards, I'm going to ask you some questions about it.

Jill was a very successful stockbroker. She made a lot of money on the stock market. She then met Jack, a devastatingly handsome man. She marries him and had three children. They lived in Chicago. She then stopped work and stayed home to bring up her children. When they were teenagers, she went back to work. She and jack lived happily ever after.

(2) **What was the female's name?** (2) **What work did she do?**

__/8 (2) **When did she go back to work?** (2) **What state did she live in?**

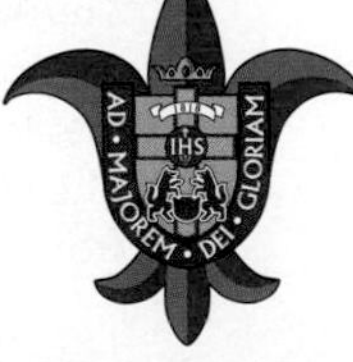

______ **TOTAL SCORE**

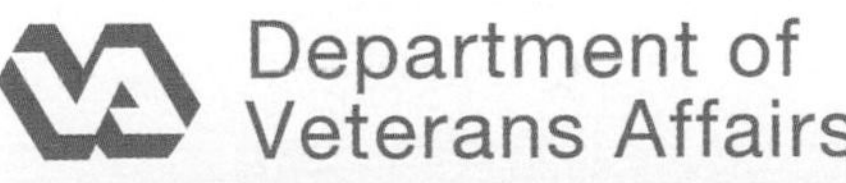

SAINT LOUIS UNIVERSITY

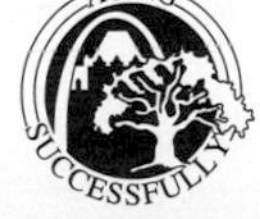

SCORING

High School Education		Less than High School Education
27–30	Normal	25–30
21–26	MNCD*	20–24
1–20	Dementia	1–19

* Mild Neurocognitive Disorder

SH Turiq, N Tumosa, JT Chibnall, HM Perry III, and JE Morley. The Saint Louis University Mental Status (SLUMS) Examination for Detecting Mild Cognitive Impairment and Dementia is more sensitive than the Mini-Mental Status Examination (MMSE) - A pilto study. Jam Geriatri Psych (in press).

FIGURE 7-11 St. Louis University Mental Status (SLUMS) Exam

Source: VAMC SLUMS Examination Assessment Tool. Reproduced by permission of Saint Louis University of Geriatric Medicine.

Beyond age, education, and literacy levels, it is necessary to consider cultural influences relative to issues of eye contact, personal space, standards of grooming and dress, and the understanding of specific proverbs. Thus, there is a need to carefully consider the cultural validity and utility of the mental status examination as well as the briefer MMSE with ethnically diverse populations.

Recently, the MMSE has been found to be limited in its use in differentiating early dementia from subjective memory complaints or related mood disorders (Mitchell, 2009). It has also been determined that the MMSE results in higher incidence of false positives, particularly among older adults who are illiterate and those who come from a low socioeconomic status (Scafuza, Almeida, Vallada, Tasse, & Menezes, 2009).

Other Mental Status Exam Instruments

There are other instruments that can be used in assessing the mental status of a patient. The most recent instrument is the St. Louis University Mental Status (SLUMS) examination (Tariq, Tumosa, Chibnall, Perry III, & Morley, 2006) (Figure 7-11). Both the MMSE and the SLUMS Exam consist of 30 points; however, the SLUMS Exam is scored related to those with or without a high school examination. The SLUMS Exam has also been found to help in the early identification of mild neurocognitive disorder in patients.

Another instrument for detecting early dementia is the AD8, which is a brief reliable and valid informant-based instrument that is able to differentiate individuals with dementia from those without dementia as well as being sensitive to early signs of cognitive impairment (Galvin & Sadowsky, 2012). The AD8 consists of 8 yes/no questions that are based on the early manifestations of Alzheimer's disease, which are as follows:

- Memory losses
- Difficulty in performing ordinary daily tasks
- Language difficulties
- Disorientation (time/place)
- Decreased or diminished judgment/abstract thinking
- Misplacing objects
- Behavior/mood/personality changes
- Decreased initiative (Galvin & Sadowsky, 2012)

These questions are asked of an informant with the total score based on the number of yes responses. Cognitive impairment is likely to be present with a score >1.

An additional dementia screening instrument is the General Practitioners Assessment of Cognition (GPCOG), comprised of a patient cognitive test and informant questionnaire (Brodaty, Kemp, & Low, 2004). Cognitive impairment is considered positive in individuals who score 9 on the patient section; a score between 5 and 8 indicates some impairment but additional information is needed, obtained with the informant interview. This interview consists of 6 yes/no questions for a possible total score of 6. A score of 0–3 from the interview when added to the cognitive test score (5–8) indicates cognitive impairment.

Summary

- The general assessment (GA) is a series of astute, meaningful observations of the patient that provides the initial clinical impression of the patient's general state of health and wellbeing as well as any outstanding characteristics.
- The GA consists of identifying data, general presentation, physical appearance/behavior, facial expressions, and motor activity.
- The mental status examination (MSE) is a robust tool for gathering important assessment data upon which individualized nursing care can be based. The components of the MSE may be assessed by using various instruments. Its utility in a variety of contexts as well as its potential to contribute to desired health care outcomes is evident.
- The MSE is used to assess speech, mood/affect, perceptions, thought content/process, orientation, memory, concentration, intellect, judgment, and insight.
- The GA and MSE are not mutually exclusive and data obtained from the assessments may relate to both.

Review Questions

1. The provider is assessing a patient in the period just following a generalized seizure. The patient is in a state of reduced consciousness. The provider documents this state as which of the following?
   1. an aura
   2. tonic phase
   3. clonic phase
   4. post-ictal phase
2. The provider focuses the assessment on risk for cardiovascular disease if during the general assessment it is noted that the patient has which of the following?
   1. an apple body shape
   2. lost 5 pounds in the last year
   3. a pear body shape
   4. a body mass index in the healthy range

3. The provider begins the general assessment of the patient when which of the following occurs?
   1. the physical examination of the patient begins
   2. after having the patient put on a gown
   3. when first encountering the patient
   4. after all data is gathered

4. During the general assessment the provider notes that the patient is in the tripod position. When interviewing this patient the provider should ask questions about which issue that may relate to this posture?
   1. the patient's respiratory status
   2. A history of back injury
   3. the emotional status of the patient
   4. use of antacids

5. While observing a patient, a constant blinking of the eyes in noted. This movement would be identified and described by the provider as which of the following?
   1. spasm
   2. tremor
   3. spell
   4. tic

6. The provider documents that a patient is experiencing grandiose delusions if the patient states which of the following?
   1. "I am the Pope of the Catholic church."
   2. "Did you hear about me on the 5:00 news last night?"
   3. "My brain is being controlled by Jesus Christ."
   4. "I am the cousin of the Queen of England."

7. A patient whose thought processes are characteristic of neologism would most likely use which of the following terms when talking with the provider?
   1. oratorical
   2. giggilysquat
   3. quibbling
   4. conglomerate

8. The provider is performing a mental status assessment and is about to evaluate the patient's general intellectual level. Which of the following assessments should the provider use? (Select all that apply.)
   1. Ask the patient the name of his first grade teacher.
   2. Ask what the patient ate for breakfast that day.
   3. Ask the patient to state the day of the week.
   4. Ask the patient to perform a simple mathematical calculation.
   5. Ask the patient to explain the saying "A bird in the hand is worth ten in the bush."

9. The provider is collecting data related to the patient's appearance. What information would the provider document as part of this segment of the assessment? (Select all that apply.)
   1. the patient's date of birth
   2. the patient's actual age as it relates to the age he appears
   3. how the patient is dressed
   4. the patient's level of education
   5. color and condition of the patient's skin

10. Facial expressions may include which of the following?
    1. anxiety, fear, disgust
    2. anger, surprise, phobia
    3. surprise, sadness, joy
    4. disgust, euphoria, sadness

8 Vital Signs

It's my second night on the job, and the emergency room is packed. I keep mixing up the stories for two of my patients. Both are men in their mid-40s, presenting with intense 9/10 lower back pain, and requesting pain medication. Both patients had nearly jumped off the table when I palpated their lumbar spine. Neither could recall a recent trauma. Rushing back to the workroom, I review their histories with the attending physician, and am surprised when she tells me to give Dilaudid to one, and Tylenol to the other. Why?

"There are two things you forgot to mention," she begins. "First, one of these patients is well-known to us here in the emergency department. He visits every other day asking for pain medications, and is almost always malingering. Second, his vital signs are entirely normal. However, the other gentleman's heart rate is 125 with a BP of 180/100."

"From the pain, of course," I say. "But it can be from other causes...."

"Let's go see both of these gentlemen, again," she says. "Remember that we unfortunately can't always trust what a patient tells us, but vital signs don't lie."

LEARNING OUTCOMES

1. Summarize the significance of measuring vital signs.
2. Describe the process of thermoregulation and the various types and manifestations of thermal alterations/stress.
3. Explain the relationship between the pulse and stroke volume.
4. Compare and contrast ventilations with respirations.
5. Explain the process of maintaining blood pressure throughout the vascular system.
6. Describe Korotkoff sounds and their relationship to blood pressure readings.
7. Summarize the Gate Theory of pain production and perception.
8. Recognize the four stages of nociceptive pain.
9. Compare and contrast between types of nociceptive pain.
10. Describe various influences on the perception of pain.

Vital signs are measurements of the body's most basic and essential physiological functions. In emergency situations, the vital signs (VS) are the initial and primary measurements used to assess the overall status of an individual's physiological state. Assessing an individual's VS allows for monitoring and detecting changes in the patient's medical condition. When providing information related to a patient's overall status, VS are the initial data that are provided.

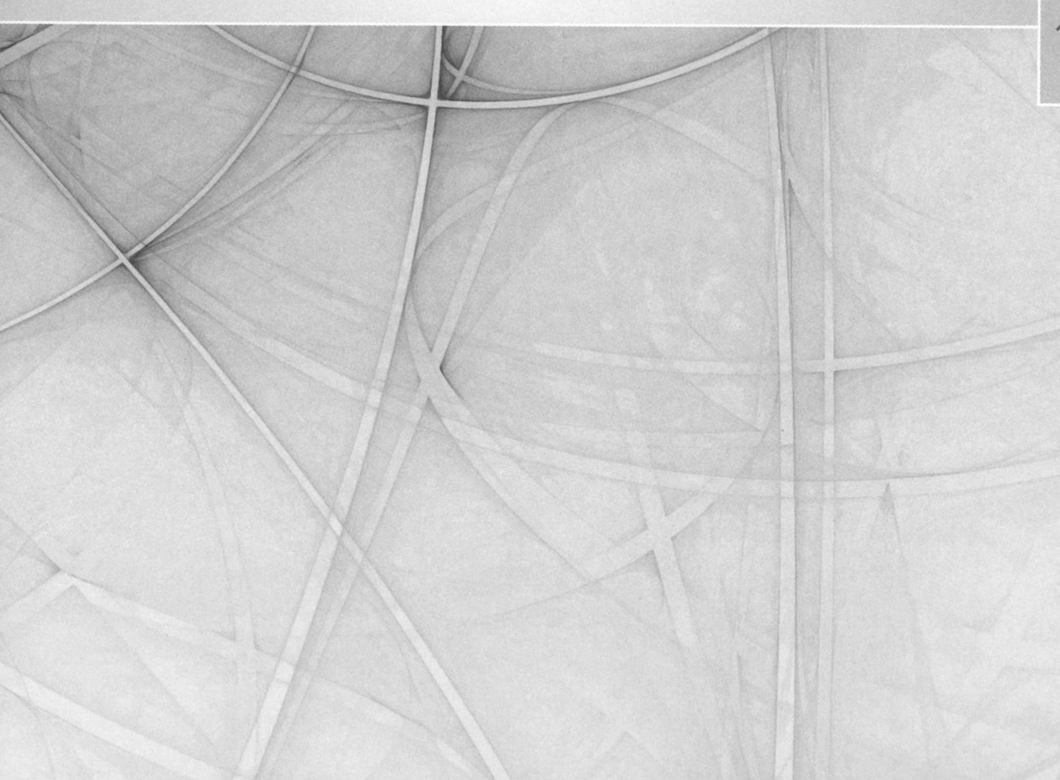

Structure and Function

Vital signs (VS) that have historically been considered the standard measurements of essential physiological information are temperature, pulse, ventilations (respiratory rate), and blood pressure. Pain as the fifth vital sign was first proposed in 1995 by the American Pain Society in recognition of inadequate pain management in patients and since 2001, the Joint Commission has mandated this recognition.

Although the VS data are important by themselves, any changes in any of the parameters are to be correlated with manifestations related to other system data and any data changes. The initial purpose of measuring VS is to establish a baseline from which comparisons may be made to determine any changes. All four vital signs are assessed within a range of results (Table 8-1). Ranges are age determined and any interpretation of results needs to be made in relation to the patient's age.

Table 8-1 Ranges of vital signs parameters

Age	Pulse	Ventilations	Blood Pressure	
			Systolic	Diastolic
Newborn	80–180	30–80		
1 year	80–140	20–40	94–103	49–65
5–8 years	75–120	15–25	103–112	65–70
10 years	50–90	15–25	111–119	73–78
Teenagers	50–90	15–20	120–131	76–81
Adults	60–100	15–20	<120	<80
Older Adults	60–100	15–20	<120	<80

Temperature

Body temperature is a measurement of the body's ability to generate and eliminate heat. Body heat is maintained within relatively narrow limits and is a reflection of one's metabolic rate. Metabolism is the series of chemical reactions that maintains the life of the living organism. These reactions are essential to promote growth and reproduction, maintain structures, and to respond to the environment of the organism. Metabolic reactions produce heat that is then transferred to the surface for removal from the body, depending on the needs of the organism and environmental conditions.

Thermoregulation is the process by which an organism maintains a consistent body temperature or core temperature (CT) through balancing heat production (**thermogenesis**) with heat loss (**thermolysis**); even when environmental conditions are variable. In humans, the mean CT has been considered to be 98.6 degrees F (37 degrees C). The 98.6 degree benchmark was established in the 19th century and was based on the average temperature reading of thousands of individuals. This was done at a time when there was no knowledge of thermoregulation, the influence of hormones and cellular metabolism as well as the effects of physical activity. Additionally, the procedures were nonstandardized and there may have been individuals who were febrile (Sund Levander & Grodzinsky, 2010) Body temperature is now described within a range (97–99) instead of one set-point (Hicks, 2013). Temperatures of the human body vary slightly and increase or decrease depending on internal and external activity. Internal processes include digestion and the female's menstrual cycle. External activity is primarily increased muscular activity associated with exercise or other strenuous activity. Body temperature also varies throughout the day following a diurnal pattern, with higher body temperatures occurring between 10:00 a.m. to 6:00 p.m. and lower temperatures between 11:00 p.m. and 3.00 a.m. (Figure 8-1).

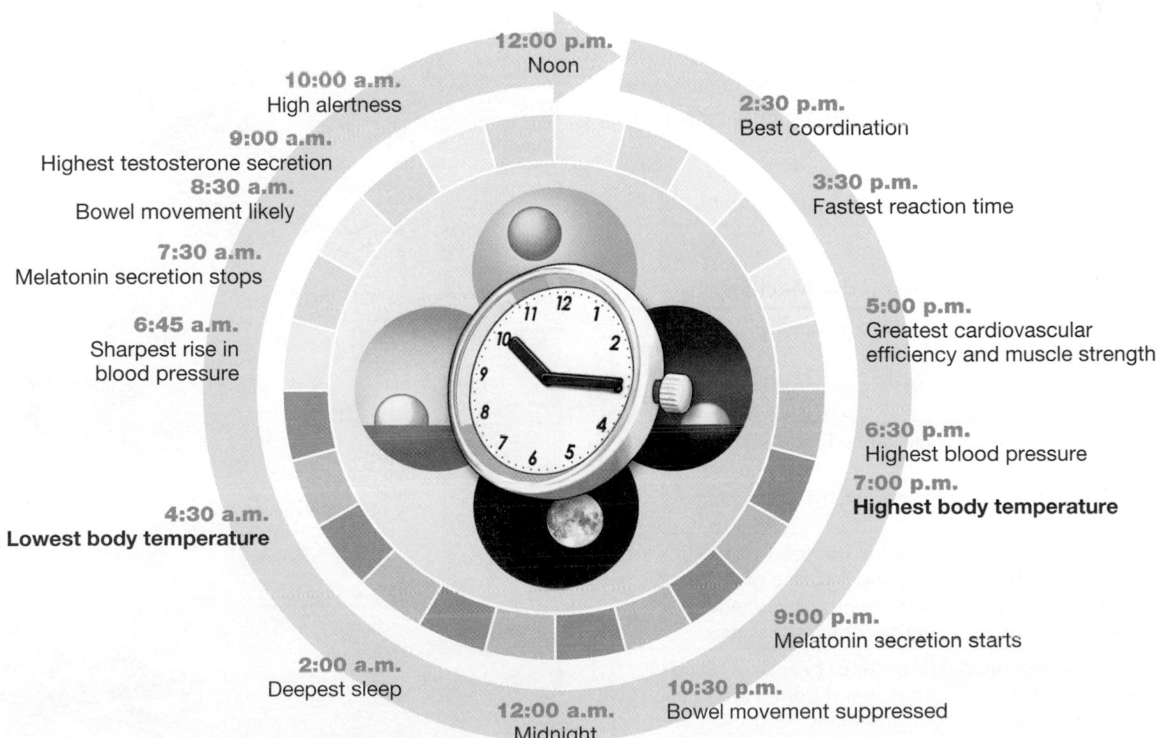

FIGURE 8-1 Variations in body temperature are part of the circadian rhythm

The CT is the temperature at which optimum functioning of the organism occurs. It is also a measure of the internal temperature of the body's internal organs and other parts that are well insulated, as opposed to the skin. The subcutaneous tissue under the skin acts as the body's insulation, and slows down heat exchange.

Core temperature is controlled by the preoptic area (anterior portion) of the hypothalamus, which may be considered the thermostat center (Diaz & Becker, 2010) The hypothalamus receives data from temperature monitoring nerve cells (**thermoreceptors**) in the skin and mucous membranes as well as from internal organs and the hypothalamus itself. Body temperature is continuously monitored by thermoreceptors throughout the body, generating impulses that correspond with the CT.

Thermal regulation and maintaining a consistent CT is a physiologic manifestation of mammals (humans). Organisms that are not able to maintain a consistent body temperature are **thermoconformers**, and have a body temperature that is affected or controlled by the external environment. These organisms are also described as cold blooded.

Most of the heat generated within the body comes from metabolic processes within the liver, heart, brain, and skeletal muscle contractions. To balance heat production, heat loss must take place. The skin is the primary means by which the body's temperature is regulated through heat loss. Heat loss from the skin surface occurs through **evaporative** and non-evaporative processes (Table 8-2).

Evaporative heat loss occurs through sweating, also known as **sensible perspiration**. As the sweat evaporates off the skin, cooling occurs and heat is lost to the environment. **Insensible perspiration** also occurs as water diffuses from the respiratory passages, mucous membranes and skin surfaces.

Non-evaporative cooling mechanisms are radiation, conduction, and convection. **Radiation** is the transfer of heat from the skin surface to the environment in the form of electromagnetic waves. Heat rays are being radiated from the body in all directions. Radiation accounts for 60%–80% of heat exchange at comfortable or low environmental temperatures. **Conduction** is the transfer of heat from the surface of one object to another. Conduction of heat to objects accounts for a minute percentage (3%) of the total heat loss from the body. Conduction to air accounts for about 12% of the body's heat loss. **Convection** is heat loss due to the movement of air. When the body is clothed, there is a layer of warm moist air in contact with the skin. In cool atmospheres, convection currents develop, mixing the air against the skin with fresh air. When exposed to these air currents, the layer of air next to the skin is replaced more rapidly, increasing heat loss by convection. Non-evaporative mechanisms of heat loss become heat gain mechanisms when environmental temperature is greater than body surface temperature (Figure 8-2).

Table 8-2 Heat generation and heat loss mechanisms

Heat Generation Mechanisms	Heat Loss Mechanisms
Muscle metabolism	Sweating, panting
Exercise	
Shivering	
Basal metabolic rate	Decreased cellular metabolism
Thyroxine stimulation	
Sympathetic excitation	
Constriction of blood vessels in the skin because of stimulation of sympathetic centers in the posterior hypothalamus	Dilation of blood vessels in the skin because of inhibition of sympathetic centers in the posterior hypothalamus
Piloerection (hair standing on end). Sympathetic stimulation causes erector pili muscles attached to hair follicles to an upright stance	Transfer of heat from blood to skin and from there to the environment

Thermal Stress

Thermal stress occurs when the body's temperature is above or below the expected body temperature. Body temperature that is maintained within the critical range of degrees F/C is described as **euthermia** or **normothermia**. A temperature above or below the critical range of degrees F/C is describes as **hyperthermia** or **hypothermia**.

Hyperthermia

Hyperthermia is an acute condition that results from the body absorbing more heat that can be dissipated. It occurs most commonly when the body experiences prolonged exposure to high temperatures. The heat regulating processes of the body become overwhelmed and fail, allowing body temperature to rise uncontrollably. Body temperatures above 104 degrees F/40 degrees C are life threatening and require immediate intervention.

Heat related clinical conditions may be categorized into minor and major syndromes. Minor heat syndromes include heat rash, heat cramps, and heat syncope. **Heat rash** (prickly heat) is a skin irritation that results from excessive sweating that occurs in hot, humid weather

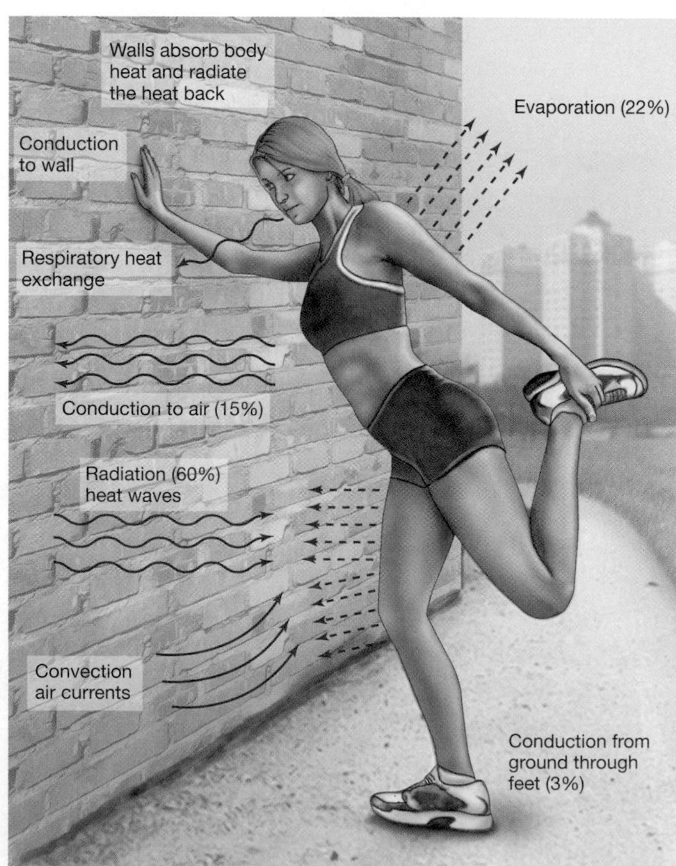

FIGURE 8-2 Methods of cooling: evaporative and non-evaporative

(see Figure 8-3). It is most common in young children, but may occur at any age. Its appearance is like a red cluster of pimples or small blisters.

Heat cramps occur in individuals who have been exercising or engaging in other strenuous activity in high environmental temperatures. Most individuals who develop heat cramps have replaced lost water, but not sodium (salt) resulting in a hyponatremia. Muscle spasms that develop in the arms, legs, or abdomen are characteristic findings. Carpopedal spasms and severe pain may incapacitate hands and feet. Cramping may last from a few minutes to hours. Body temperature is usually not elevated, but the skin may be moist and cool, and sweaty.

Heat syncope is characterized by dizziness or fainting after exposure to high temperatures; primarily after position changes or exercising. Heat syncope may be the result of vasodilatation, volume depletion, and pooling of blood. Like heat cramps, body temperature is not elevated and the skin remains cool but is pale and sweaty. A rapid, weak pulse is also detected commonly.

Major heat syndromes include **heat exhaustion** and **heat stroke**. Heat exhaustion is a non–life-threatening condition characterized by weakness, malaise, nausea, syncope, and other nonspecific symptoms resulting from heat exposure. The primary cause of heat exhaustion is water and electrolyte imbalance from heat exposure that may or may not be accompanied by physical exertion. The body's thermoregulation ability remains functional.

Symptoms are nonspecific and individuals may not associate them with heat exposure. They may include weakness, dizziness, headache and, nausea, with or without vomiting. Patients may also experience syncope, especially after standing for long periods. Individuals appear tired and sweaty and often have an increased heart rate; mental status is generally not impaired. The temperature may be elevated, but rarely exceeds 40 degrees C.

Heat stroke is a life-threatening hyperthermia that is accompanied by systemic inflammation and organ dysfunction. Heat stroke is a manifestation of thermoregulatory failure causing a substantial increase in the core temperature. Death from heat stroke is inevitable if interventions are not initiated when symptoms first appear.

Temperatures often exceed 40 degrees C (104 degrees F), causing changes in one's mental status—confusion, combativeness, and bizarre behavior. The individual also presents with a rapid heart rate and ventilation rate. Release and activation of inflammatory cytokines occurs, and possibly endotoxin from GI flora, resulting in multiple organ dysfunction. Organ dysfunction may develop in the central nervous system, muscles, liver, kidneys, lungs, and heart. The coagulation cascade may be activated, causing disseminated intravascular coagulation. Electrolyte imbalances (hyperkalemia and hypoglycemia) are also present. Due to failure of the thermoregulatory mechanisms, the individual is not sweating and presents with hot, dry, flushed skin.

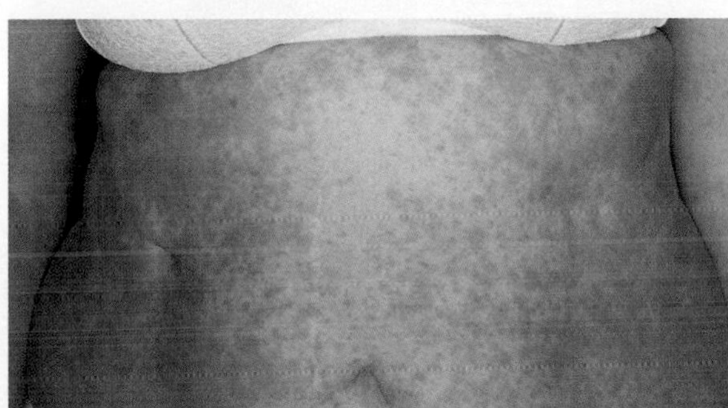

FIGURE 8-3 Heat rash

Source: Science Photo Library/Custom Medical Stock Photo

Heat stroke exists in two variants—classic and exertional. Classic heatstroke develops slowly, over 2–3 days of continuous heat exposure. It is most commonly seen in the elderly during summer heat waves. Additional factors include lack of air conditioning and limited access to fluids.

Exertional heat stroke occurs rapidly in individuals, such as athletes, military recruits, and factory workers, who are healthy and active. Intense activity in a hot, humid environment results in a sudden, enormous heat load that the body is incapable of regulating. In contrast to the individuals with classic heatstroke, the individual with exertional heatstroke will present with sweating.

Mortality from heatstroke is significant, but varies with age, underlying conditions, and the maximum temperature. The two major factors that may determine the outcome are the duration of hyperthermia and promptness in cooling. Approximately 20 percent of survivors have some residual brain damage, in spite of interventions (Knochel, 2010).

Malignant hyperthermia (MH) is unrelated to exposure to excessive heat. MH is a rare, life-threatening, inherited disorder that is initiated by exposure to general anesthetics, particularly volatile anesthetics and succinylcholine, resulting in hypermetabolism of skeletal muscles due to hypercalcemia. It may also be triggered in humans by vigorous exercise and stress, but this is quite rare (Rosenberg, Davis, James, Pollock, & Stowell, 2007). While it is considered to be an intraoperative phenomenon, there are instances where it has occurred postoperatively (Litman, 2013). It is also possible that MH may occur after previous exposure(s) to general anesthetics. Genetically, MH is inherited as an autosomal dominant disorder, thus males and females are affected and only one parent needs to carry the gene. While the gene responsible for MH has been identified, there are over 40 distinct mutations that are responsible for causing MH (Litman, 2013). The number of mutations possible results in incomplete genetic penetrance and variable expressivity leading to inconsistent manifestations and presentation of the condition.

Immediate signs of MH include a rapid rise in body temperature (105 degrees F or higher), muscle rigidity and stiffness, and an increased, irregular heart rate. Testing for MH is expensive and invasive. DNA testing is possible but results are easily confounded by other variables and therefore not reliable. Any previous incidence of MH in family members is cause for suspicion and concern.

THINK LINK:* *Heat and Proteins

To understand what happens to proteins in the presence of excessive heat, consider what happens to the white of an egg when it is exposed to high temperatures. The transformation of a clear, runny liquid to a white, rubbery substance is due to the denaturation (coagulation) of proteins present in the egg white. Once proteins are denatured, reversing the process is impossible. Consider then that the same transformation occurs in the proteins of the body, destroying their composition and make-up, making them incapable of participating in physiological function essential to life. Cellular damage and death are known to occur at temperatures of 40–41 degrees C with extensive denaturing of protein occurring between 40–45 degrees C (Hildebrandt et al., 2002; Lepock, 2003). The effects of protein denaturation result in apoptosis, necrosis, or DNA damage (Hintzsche, Riese, & Stopper, 2012).

Another form of hyperthermia is **fever**, also described as **pyrexia** (Figure 8-4). Unlike other heat related conditions where there is failure to thermoregulate, fever is the result of an increase in the body's regulatory set point. This higher degree resetting requires the body to produce more heat. A fever may be caused by various agents or conditions, but is most frequently associated with some underlying disease or condition. A fever is also considered to be an immune response to neutralize a bacterial or viral invasion. Fever is often accompanied by sickness manifestations, which include lethargy and malaise, anorexia, sleepiness, hyperalgesia, and lack of concentration.

The onset of fever is triggered by pyrogens that initiate the release of **prostaglandin E2** (PGE2), which then acts on the hypothalamus (Huether & Defriez, 2006). The hypothalamus then initiates a systematic response to the rest of the body and stimulates heat production mechanisms to equate to the new temperature level.

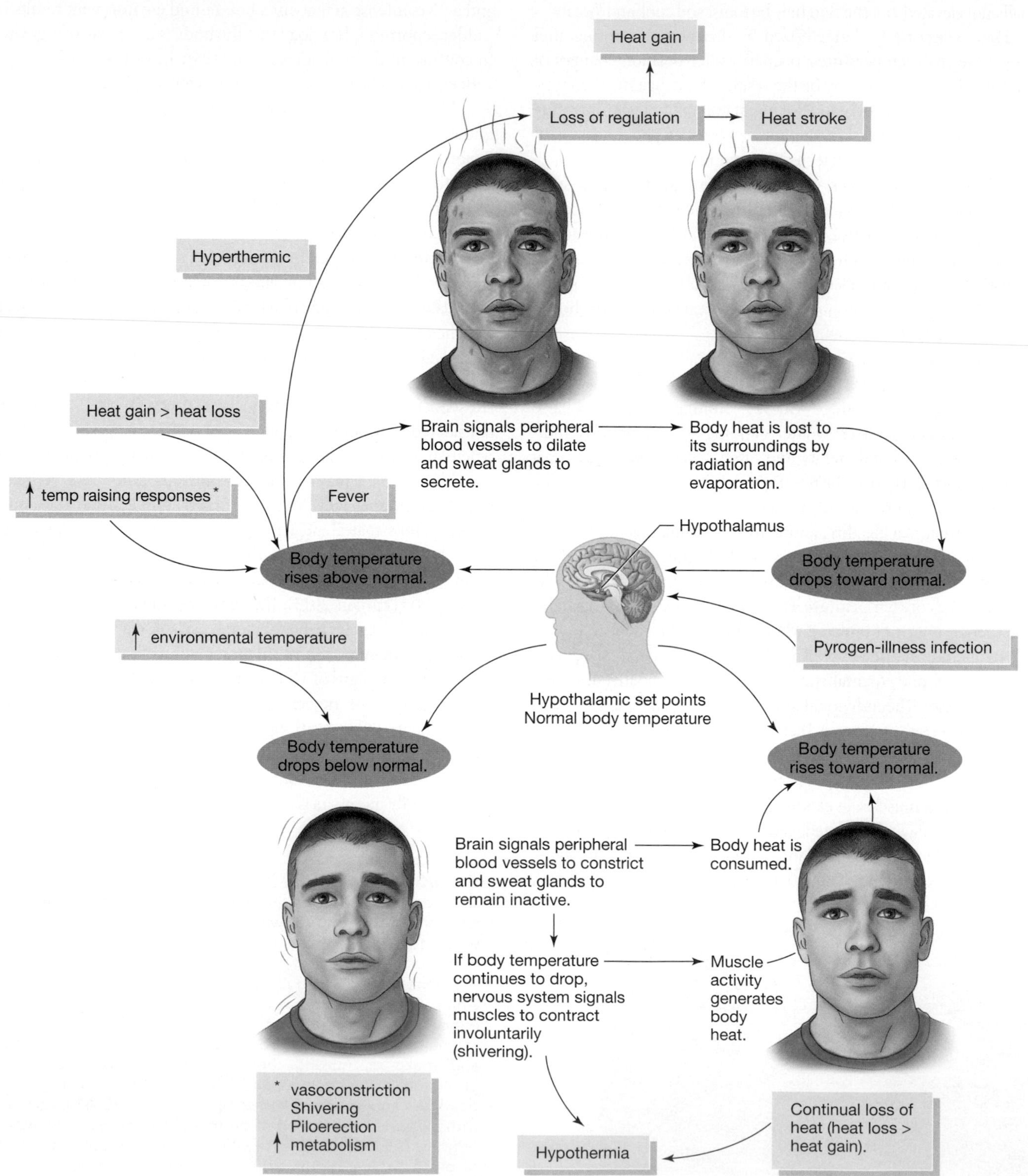

FIGURE 8-4 Thermal regulation

Essentially, all pyrogens are endogenous cytokines that are released from phagocytic cells that act on the hypothalamus to reset the temperature set point. Cytokines consist of interleukins, tumor necrosis factors, macrophage inflammatory proteins, and interferons. These cytokines then bind with endothelial receptors on vessel walls that activate the arachidonic acid pathway, causing the release of PGE2. The increased set point of the temperature will continue as long as PGE2 is present.

A fever is an adaptive response to bacterial or viral induced infections that are associated with certain conditions and disorders. The increase in body temperature kills many microorganisms and produces other effects that create a hostile environment to their growth and reproduction. Essential nutrients for survival (iron, zinc, and copper) are reduced. Switching to a metabolism based on lipolysis and proteolysis eliminates a food source for bacteria. There is also initiation of lysosomol breakdown and auto-destruction of cells, preventing viral infected cells from replicating. Other causes of fever include medicines (antibiotics, narcotics, barbiturates, antihistamines), severe trauma (heart attack, stroke, heat stress, burns), as well as other conditions (arthritis, hyperthyroidism, cancers) (Davis, 2011).

Hyperpyrexia is an extreme elevation of body temperature causing fevers of 41.5 degrees C or higher. This is a medical emergency, and is most likely caused by a serious underlying condition that may result in significant side effects. Intracranial bleeding is the most common cause, but may also accompany sepsis, neuroleptic malignant syndrome, certain drugs, serotonin syndrome, and thyroid storm. Certain infections (chicken pox, measles, enteroviral) may also cause hyperpyrexia.

Localized hyperthermia is present in conditions where there is inflammation. Inflammation increases blood flow to the area, causing the area to feel warm. The area will also demonstrate an increased redness, another result from increased blood flow.

Hypothermia

Hypothermia is opposite of hyperthermia in that the body core temperature drops below what is needed for optimum function of homeostatic metabolic processes. In hypothermia, heat loss exceeds heat production, causing the drop in body core temperature. Hypothermia is present when the core temperature drops below 35.6 degrees C (95 degrees F).

Hypothermia may be classified into 3 types—mild, moderate, and severe. Initial manifestations of hypothermia occur at core temperatures of 34–35 degrees C (93–95 degrees F) and are caused by sympathetic nervous system activity to conserve heat. Shivering, increased heart and ventilation rates, and an increased blood pressure are often present, frequently accompanied by mental confusion. Shivering is an attempt to increase muscle activity to increase heat production.

Moderate hypothermia occurs at core temperatures of 30–34 degrees C (86–93 degrees F) and are characterized by more violent shivering and uncoordinated actions. Movements become slow and labored and the individual may stumble. Mild confusion is also present, although the individual may appear alert. Vasoconstriction increases to help conserve heat and keep internal organs warm, resulting in pale skin with lips, ears, and fingers appearing blue.

Manifestations of severe hypothermia are present at a core temperature of 30–31 degrees C (86–88 degrees F). At this point, manifestations are difficulty in speaking, sluggish thought processes as well as initial symptoms of amnesia. The individual has difficulty with use and coordination of hands, and difficulty with leg coordination results in stumbling and falling.

Below 30 degrees C (86 degrees F) exposed skin appears blue and puffy, coordination and walking are extremely difficult, and the individual becomes incoherent with irrational behavior, and may even become stuporous. Below 28 degrees C, ice crystals form on the inside of cells, causing them to rupture and die (Huether & Defriez, 2006). Cellular metabolism decreases significantly, blood becomes more viscous, and circulation within the microcirculation slows down considerably, increasing blood coagulation. Major organs and systems shut down and begin to fail and the heart and ventilatory rate significantly decrease along with blood pressure. Clinical death precedes brain death due to decreased cellular activity in the brain.

Hypothermia results from exposure to a cold environment. Alcohol consumption is frequently associated with developing hypothermia, but it is also caused by other conditions that increase heat loss, decrease heat production, or alter thermoregulation, such as hypoglycemia (impaired judgment), age (extremely young or old), gender (male), substance abuse, homelessness, and living in cold environments. The probability of developing hypothermia is significantly increased in the presence of alcohol ingestion because alcohol causes vasodilatation which increases blood flow to the extremities, resulting in a feeling of warmth. With more blood circulating to the surface, heat loss is also increased. Additionally, alcohol may cause impaired judgment.

While hypothermia is a measurement related to core temperature, there are also localized, cold related injuries that can result from exposure to cold. These injuries are categorized as occurring with or without freezing of body tissues. Injuries related to nonfreezing of tissues are chilblains, frost nip, and trench foot. **Chilblains** result from chronic exposure to dry, cold temperatures that may not appear until several hours after exposure. Chilblain lesions are inflammatory nodules and bullae that are red or purple appearing areas of swelling that are also itchy and painful. The lesions are most commonly seen on fingers, toes, nose, or ears as well as the pre-tibial area. Chilblains may remain for several days and healing is generally complete after 2–3 weeks. There is usually no long lasting damage but the area may remain sensitive to cold, and they may reoccur.

Trench foot is a more severe injury than chilblains and results from prolonged exposure to wet, cold environmental conditions. Trench foot develops over a period of days and results in pain, numbness/tingling, and swelling of the area. The area may also appear red, blotchy, cyanotic or even black from development of gangrene. The appearance of bullae with open sores may also develop. Amputation may be required when gangrene develops. Recovery takes place over weeks and there may be increased sensitivity to cold as well as residual symptoms.

Frost nip is a superficial cold related injury that is manifest through temporary numbness and tingling. There is no tissue damage and symptoms disappear after rewarming.

Freezing cold related injury is **frost bite** and is the most serious injury (Figure 8-5). The most commonly affected areas are the fingers, toes, nose, and ears, although other areas may be affected, depending on the length of exposure and temperature. Frost bite injuries are due to vasoconstriction and decreased blood flow and the development of intracellular ice crystals.

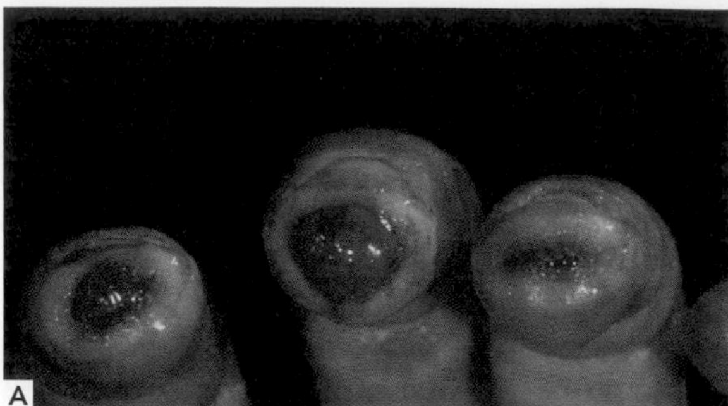

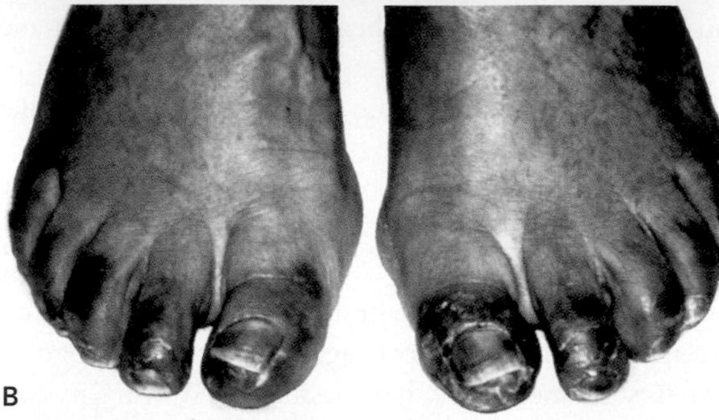

FIGURE 8-5A–B Tissue injuries related to frostbite. **a)** Tissue loss; **b)** gangrene

Sources: a. SIU Biomed Comm/Custom Medical Stock Photo; b. NMSB/Custom Medical Stock Photo

Frostbite injury may be superficial or deep, depending on the depth of injury. Superficial injuries involve the skin and subcutaneous tissue, while deep frostbite injuries extend into the muscle and may involve tendon, nerves, and even bone. Deep injuries result in permanent tissue damage.

Prior to systemic manifestations of hypothermia, there are local alterations that result from prolonged exposure to cold temperatures. Initial manifestations of frostbite include diminished light touch and temperature sensation accompanied by numbness. Pain or a burning sensation may also be experienced leading to the eventual complete loss of sensation. Complete loss of sensation is associated with significant tissue damage. The appearance of the affected skin is pale and waxy with redness appearing after rewarming. With deeper tissue damage, the skin may appear bluish/gray or black. With superficial frostbite, the skin is firm but may be depressed with minimal pressure. With deeper damage, the skin becomes more firm and feels hard to the touch and does not allow depression.

After rewarming, superficial injured tissue becomes edematous with bullae formation (Figure 8-6). There is no permanent damage and full recovery may be expected. Deeper tissue damage may present with hemorrhagic bullae and the skin may take on a purple color. Black, gangrenous tissue will require removal and may include amputation of parts of the affected extremity. Long-term effects of frostbite damage include neuropathic pain, sensory deficits, Raynaud's disease, and arthritis.

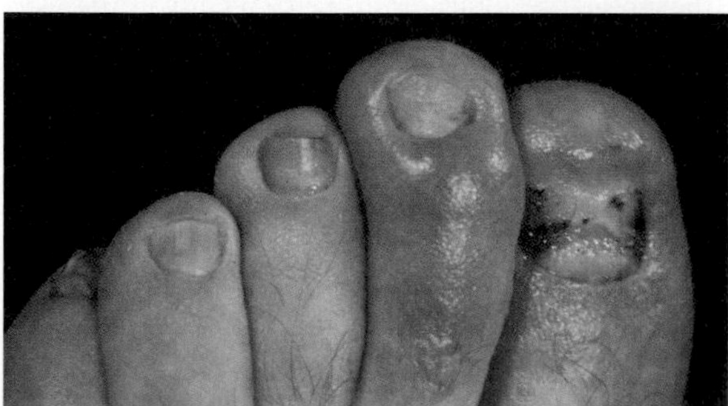

FIGURE 8-6 Tissue changes in the rewarming process

Source: SIU Biomed Comm/Custom Medical Stock Photo

Therapeutic hypothermia is a medical intervention to lower the core temperature in individuals (32–34 degrees C) to prevent or reduce neurologic death due to decreased blood circulation (Nair & Lundbye, 2011). Causes of decreased blood circulation may be due to myocardial infarction or cardiac arrest, and brain infarcts (stroke). Therapeutic hypothermia decreases cellular metabolism, reducing the need for oxygen and providing protection for brain cells and preventing further ischemic damage to other tissues.

Assessing Temperature

The assessment of temperature involves observation, inspection, and palpation.

Observation/Inspection

Body temperature is measured with a thermometer, which can come in various types. The most common thermometers are electronic (digital), ear (tympanic membrane), forehead, disposable, and pacifier. Before taking an oral temperature, determine whether the patient has been smoking, eating, or drinking hot or cold liquids. If any of these have occurred, wait 20–30 minutes before proceeding. If the patient has been engaging in vigorous exercise or has taken a hot bath or shower, wait at least an hour before taking the temperature.

Thermometers While the standard thermometer for many years was the glass, mercury-filled thermometer, they are no longer considered safe for use. The Environmental Protection Agency (EPA) identified mercury as a toxic substance that poses a major threat to the health of the individual and environment should the glass thermometer break and spill the mercury.

Electronic thermometers measure how well electricity is conducted through a wire. An electronic thermometer consists of a probe that is connected to a measuring device with a digital readout; some are a single unit and have the digital readout on a window on the thermometer (Figure 8-7). They are quite accurate when used correctly, and take a temperature within seconds, rather than minutes. Electronic thermometer probes are covered with a disposable sheath for multiple individual uses.

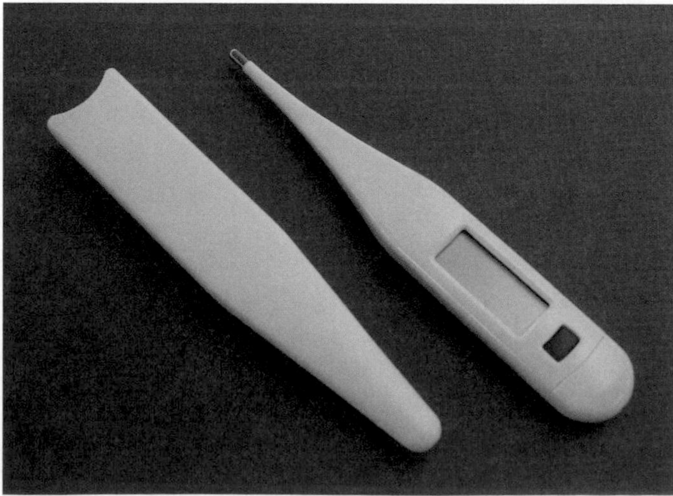

FIGURE 8-7 Electronic thermometer

Ear (tympanic membrane) thermometers use infrared energy to determine body temperature. They are a single unit device that can be held in the palm of one hand and have a cone-shaped appendage that is inserted into the ear (Figure 8-8). Ear thermometers are designed to be used only for tympanic membrane measurement.

Forehead thermometers measure skin temperature to determine body temperature. These thermometers may be a disc that is pressed on the forehead giving a digital readout, or thin strips of plastic with numbers on them.

Disposable thermometers, like forehead thermometers, are thin strips of plastic with colored dots that change color, indicating the temperature. These thermometers may be used orally or rectally and are safe and accurate.

Pacifier thermometers are placed in the infant's mouth and display a digital readout of the temperature. These thermometers may take longer to register and are not as accurate as other types.

Temperatures that are taken with electronic thermometers may be obtained from three primary methods: orally, rectally, and axillary. Orally is the easiest and most convenient method. To obtain an oral temperature, place the covered probe under and to the side of the patient's tongue with the lips closed tightly. Most electronic thermometers emit an audible beep heard when the temperature is recorded.

The rectal temperature is most appropriate for babies and small children and in situations where holding the probe in the mouth might be difficult. This temperature is also the closest to core body temperature, so it is considered more accurate. Before obtaining the rectal temperature, apply a lubricant to the covered probe. For adults, it is easiest to do if the patient is lying on his or her side. Babies and small children may lie on their stomach either across the lap or on a table; however, an older child may be more comfortable in a side-lying position. Spread the buttocks and gently insert the temperature probe into the anal canal sufficiently far enough to place the probe within the canal. The probe should be easy to insert and there should be no resistance to its placement. Hold in place until the temperature is recorded and then remove it. While the covered electronic probe may be used for both oral and rectal temperatures, it is best to keep the electronic devices separate from each other.

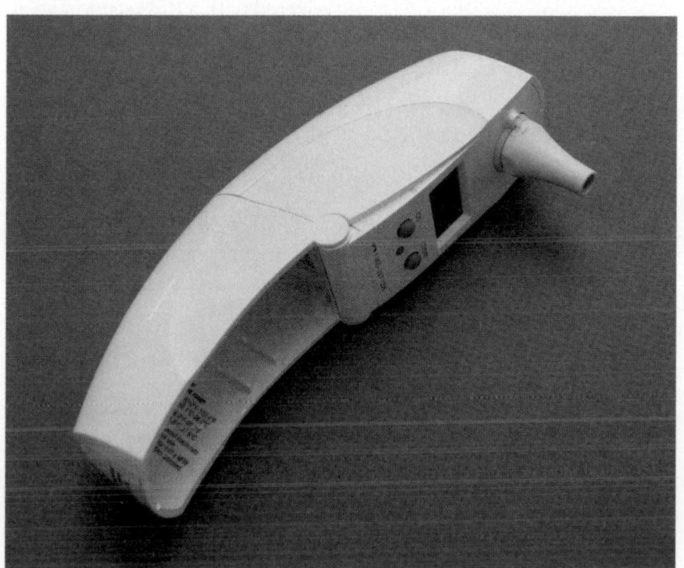

FIGURE 8-8 Tympanic membrane (TM) thermometer

The axillary temperature is taken by placing the tip of the covered probe in the center of the armpit and then pressing the arm against the side to maintain the position of the probe. Leave the probe in place until the temperature is recorded.

The ear/tympanic membrane thermometer's cone appendage is covered with a disposable cone-shaped sheath and inserted into the ear, much like an otoscope. Center the cone tip in the ear and gently push inward with the cone directed toward the tympanic membrane. The thermometer is activated with the press of a button and provides an almost immediate digital readout.

Forehead thermometer strips are pressed against the forehead and the numbers will change color, light up, or provide a digital readout indicating the temperature (Figure 8-9). Forehead thermometers are not as accurate as electronic or ear thermometers. Disposable thermometers are much like electronic thermometer probes and may be used for obtaining oral or rectal temperatures. They are reusable, but only for one individual use.

Palpation

Palpation is used to assess the temperature and moisture of the skin's surface. In the presence of hyperthermia, the skin is going to feel warmer than expected, and in hypothermia, it will feel cooler than expected. In hyperthermia when the body is attempting to cool itself, the skin will be moist from excessive sweating. One exception is when heat stroke is apparent; the thermoregulation mechanisms are nonfunctional, and the skin will be hot and dry. In severe conditions of hypothermia, the skin may feel hard and nonelastic due to ice formation within the underlying cells (freezing).

Peripheral Pulse

The **peripheral pulse** rate is the measurement of the heart rate, or beats per minute. The pulse is created by the forceful ejection of blood from the left ventricle. The force of the ejection creates a pressure wave that causes the arteries to expand to accommodate the pressure and then contract. With each beat of the heart, a pressure wave is created, which can then be felt at various locations on the body and is identified as the *heart rate*.

Palpation

The pulse can only be felt at specific points on the body, and pulse points are identified by their anatomic location. These pulse points are where arteries lie close to the skin surface and are identified as

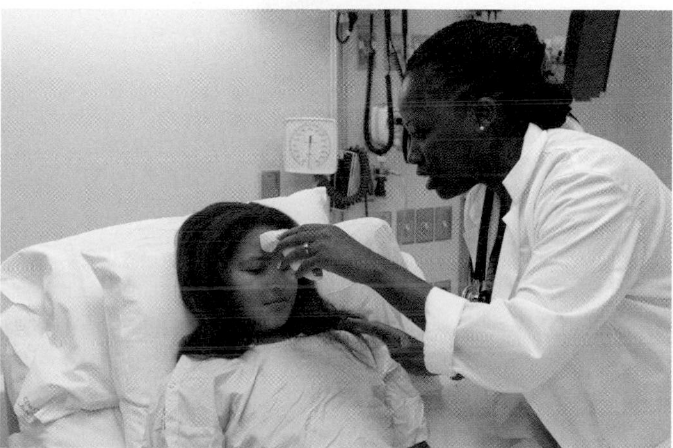

FIGURE 8-9 Taking a temperature using a forehead thermometer

carotid, brachial, radial, femoral, popliteal, posterior tibial, and dorsalis pedis. These locations are identified in Figure 8-10. On some individuals, a temporal pulse may also be present, but its absence or inability to obtain is not significant.

Palpate the pulse by placing two or three fingers over the anatomic site and applying gentle downward pressure against bone or muscle (Figure 8-11). It should not take an excessive amount of pressure to be able to palpate the pulse. The most common and easiest site for obtaining the pulse is the radial pulse, which is over the radial bone on the thumb side of the wrist.

Palpation of the pulse also provides information regarding the pulse's quality and rhythm. Quality is a reflection of the volume of blood that is ejected from the heart and distends the artery, and should be such that the pulse is palpable without exerting undue pressure over the site. Each pulse should also demonstrate the same quality. The rhythm is a reflection of the pulse's regularity. The arterial expansions should be felt as occurring in regular or having equal intervals between expansions.

The radial pulse is generally taken for 60 seconds (1 minute); however, it is also acceptable to count the pulse for 30 seconds and multiply by 2. Note that counting the pulse in this manner is only appropriate when the rate is regular.

Pulse rates vary with age and physical condition. In infants and children, the pulse rate in expected to be 100 or greater per minute. After the age of 6, the pulse rate gradually slows down to the adult range of 60–100 beats per minute. Specific ranges by age were previously identified in Table 8-1.

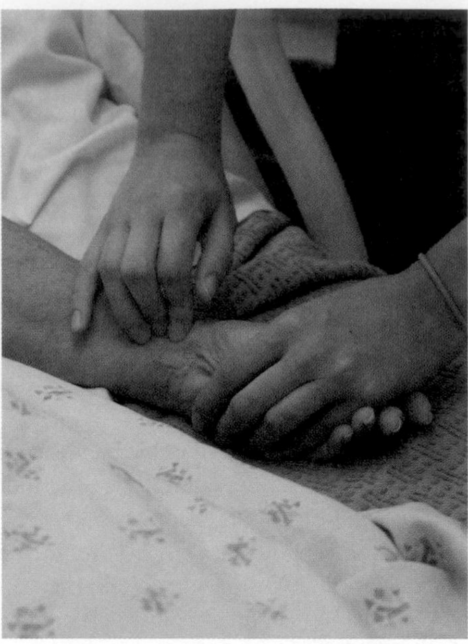

FIGURE 8-11 Applying pressure at pulse point

Apical Pulse

In some situations, it is necessary to obtain an **apical pulse** rate, which is done by listening (auscultating) directly over the heart to obtain the heart rate (Figure 8-12). When listening to the heart for the rate, it is not important to listen in a specific area on the chest; the heart rate can be heard over the entire heart area on the chest. The apical heart rate is often obtained in emergency situations, and if there is an irregular heart rate. (More detailed information regarding the pulse is found in Chapter 24.)

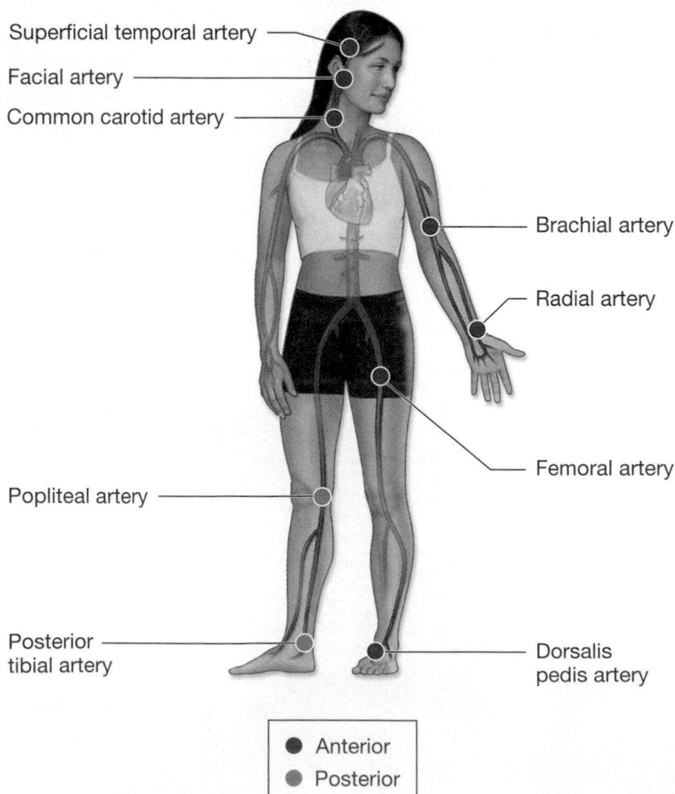

FIGURE 8-10 Pulse point locations

Ventilations

Ventilations are the number of breaths taken within 1 minute. One ventilation cycle consists of 1) inhalation, the inflow of air into the lungs, and 2) exhalation, the outflow of the air out of the lungs.

Ventilations per minute are best observed when the patient is unaware of what is being done because awareness of being observed may cause the patient to alter the breathing pattern (Figure 8-13). Commonly, providers observe ventilations after determining the pulse by leaving their fingers over the radial pulse and observing the individual's ventilatory rate and pattern. If the patient's ventilations are shallow, place his or her arm on the chest so that the rising and falling of the chest may be felt. Count the ventilations for 1 full

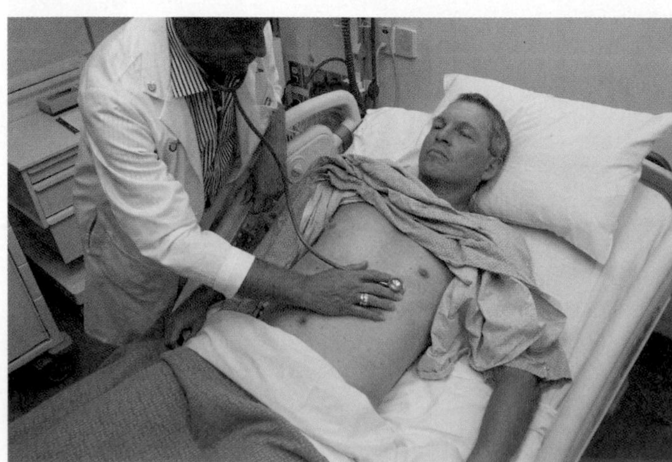

FIGURE 8-12 Apical pulse location

minute because there might be some slight irregularity in the pattern. Like the pulse rate, ventilatory rates vary with age, starting out fast in infants and gradually decreasing to the adult rate. Specific age-related rates were previously identified in Table 8-1. (More detailed information related to assessment of ventilations is discussed in Chapter 23.)

Blood Pressure

The fourth vital sign assessed is blood pressure, the measurement of the pressure that blood flow exerts on the wall of the artery. A blood pressure reading is measured in millimeters of mercury (mmHg) and is described and documented by two readings that are reported as a fraction (132/78). The two measurements recorded are the **systolic pressure** and **diastolic pressure**. The systolic pressure is a measurement of the force exerted against the arterial wall during ventricular contraction and correlates with the pulse wave generated. The diastolic pressure is the force that is exerted during ventricular relaxation or the time period between pulse waves. Because the vascular system is a closed system, a certain amount of pressure is always present and exerted on the arterial walls.

Pressures within the vascular system are also dependent upon two other factors: **cardiac output** (CO) and **peripheral vascular resistance**. CO is the amount of blood ejected from the heart (left ventricle) during one minute. Cardiac output is comprised of stroke volume and heart rate. **Stroke volume** (SV) is the amount of blood ejected from the left ventricle during one ventricular contraction. The heart rate (HR) is the number of beats per minute. Multiplying SV times HR gives the cardiac output. The formula is as follows:

CO = HR (heart rate) × SV (stroke volume)

Peripheral vascular resistance (PVR) is an opposing force that impedes the forward flow of the blood through the vascular system and is determined by three factors: 1) the diameter (radius) of the artery, 2) the length of the artery, and 3) the blood viscosity. PVR is also a reflection of the amount of friction that is present within the blood vessel, consisting of molecules that move against each other (internal friction) as well as moving against the wall of the vessel (external). PVR is not an actual measurement that can be obtained, but can be inferred by blood pressure measurement, thus is primarily associated with the arterial system.

The arteries are muscular in nature and are able to constrict or dilate, which results in a decrease or increase of the diameter. Arterial diameter changes are such that the smaller the diameter of the artery, the greater the friction and the greater resistance and vice versa. Increasing the length of the vessel increases the total area that comes in contact with the blood so that a vessel length of 10 feet will have twice the resistance than a vessel 5 feet in length.

Viscosity of the blood is determined by the amount of solid substances dissolved within it. As the amount of substances increases the concentration of the blood increases, resulting in a fluid (blood) that is denser and slower moving. Increasing the amount of solid substances within the blood also increases the number of particles that move against each other and against the vessel wall, increasing the amount of friction that occurs.

The length of blood vessels remains fairly constant; however, an increase in fatty tissue associated with obesity requires formation of new blood vessels to nourish and support this additional tissue, increasing the length of blood vessels. The diameter of the vessel and the blood viscosity are more likely to change, resulting in blood pressure alterations.

Assessment of Blood Pressure

Blood pressure is measured by indirect or direct methods. More common and non-invasive, the indirect method is obtained with a sphygmomanometer (cuff, tubes, pump, gauge) and a stethoscope (Figure 8-14). The blood pressure cuff consists of a rubber bladder enclosed within a rectangular strip of vinyl material that contains Velcro or clips to allow the cuff to be securely wrapped around an extremity. Two rubber tubes extend from the bladder and are connected to an air pump and a manometer (pressure gauge). Manometers are either a calibrated tube of mercury or a calibrated dial with a moveable hand (Figure 8-15).

The most common site for obtaining a blood pressure is on either upper extremity; however, it may also be obtained on the lower extremities. The deflated cuff is wrapped snugly around the exposed upper arm so that the bottom of the cuff allows for 1–2 inches between the cuff and antecubital fossa. Place the center of the air bladder directly over the brachial artery (Figure 8-16). Next, palpate the antecubital fossa for the brachial artery pulse. Once the pulse is located, a baseline systolic pressure may be obtained. This is obtained by placing 1–2 fingers over the brachial artery pulse and gradually inflate the blood pressure cuff, noting the point at which the pulse in no longer felt. Deflate the cuff and wait 20–30 seconds before obtaining the blood pressure.

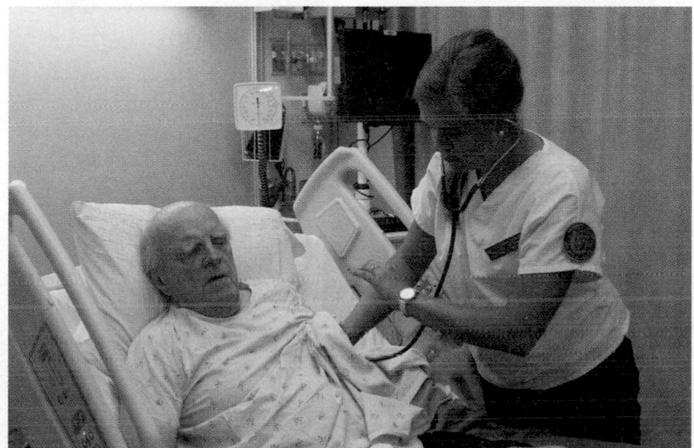

FIGURE 8-13 Observation of patient while taking pulse

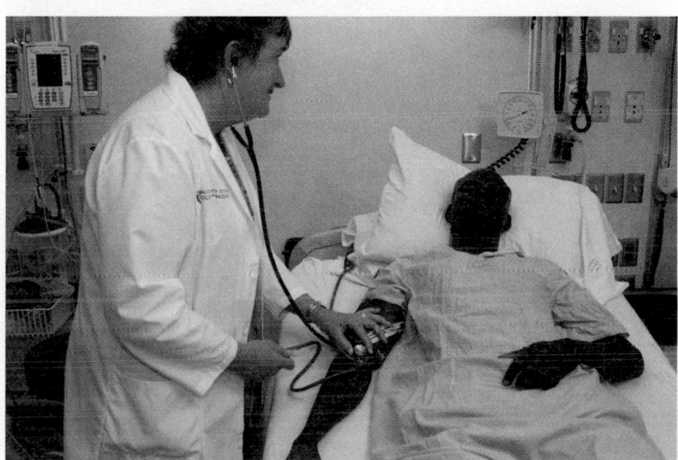

FIGURE 8-14 Indirect measurement of blood pressure (BP)

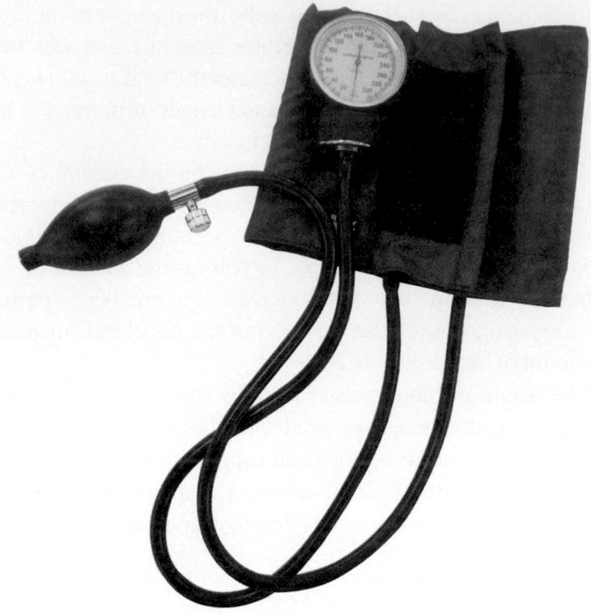

FIGURE 8-15 Manometer (Hg/aneroid)

Begin by placing the diaphragm of the stethoscope over the brachial pulse, holding it in place with the thumb of the opposite hand (Figure 8-17). Begin to inflate the blood pressure cuff to the point that is approximately 30 mmHg above the point where the palpated pulse disappeared. Gradually deflate the cuff (2mmHg/second) and note the needle position where the first sound is heard. This should closely correlate with the point where the pulse disappeared. Continue listening to the sounds and noting where the sound disappears. The point where the sound is first heard is the systolic pressure and the point where it disappears is the diastolic pressure.

The sounds heard during the procedure, called **Korotkoff sounds,** are generated by the flow of blood through the artery that is altered by cuff inflation around the extremity and are heard through five phases (Figure 8-18). Each phase has a distinct sound, but not all sounds may be identifiable in phases 2 and 3. The first Korotkoff sound heard clearly is the systolic pressure (Phase 1). After the first sound, continuous other Korotkoff sounds continue to be heard (Phases 2/3). The point where sound disappears is the last Korotkoff sound (Phase 4),

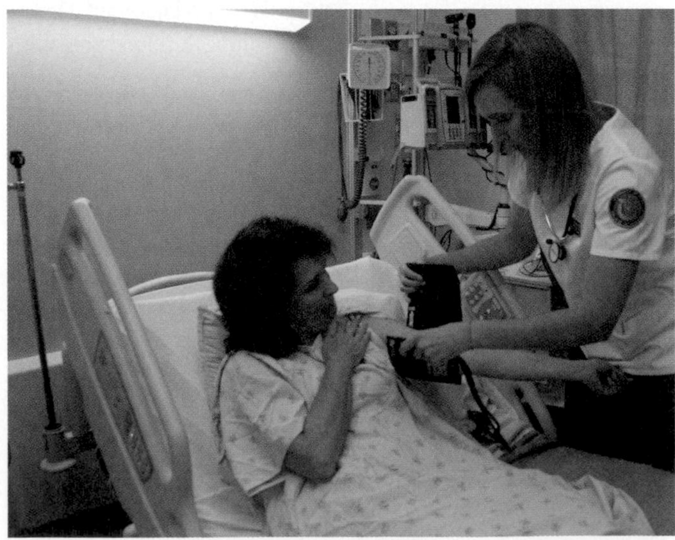

FIGURE 8-16 Placement of blood pressure (BP) cuff

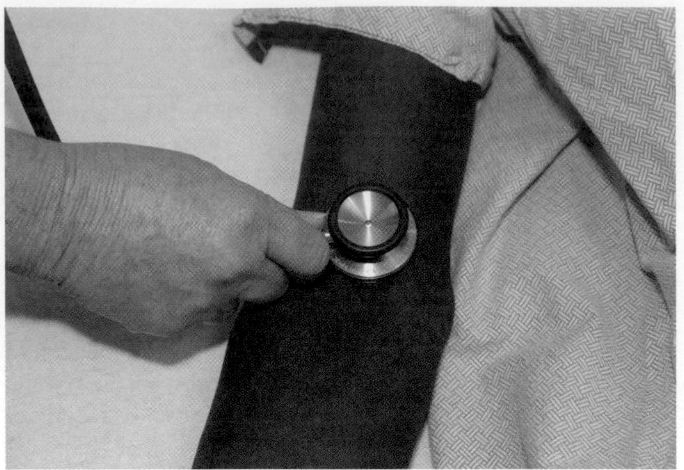

FIGURE 8-17 Diaphragm over brachial artery

followed by the absence of sound (Phase 5). In some individuals, a distinct change or a muffling of the sound, considered the first diastolic sound, occurs close to where the sound disappears. Its point of disappearance is the second diastolic sound. If you hear three audible sounds, record the blood pressure with all three numbers.

In certain patients, you may need to determine the **pulse pressure (PP)** or **mean arterial pressure (MAP)**. The PP is the difference between the systolic pressure reading and the diastolic pressure reading. The MAP is the average pressure that is maintained within the arterial system and reflects the hemodynamic perfusion pressure of the vital organs; it is not just the average of multiple pulse pressure readings or the average of the systolic and diastolic readings. The two phases of the cardiac cycle—systole and diastole—are not equal in time. At a resting heart rate of 60–80, systole occupies one third of the cycle, and diastole occupies two-thirds of the cycle. Equations, shown in Box 8-1, for determining the MAP are based on the duration of these cycles.

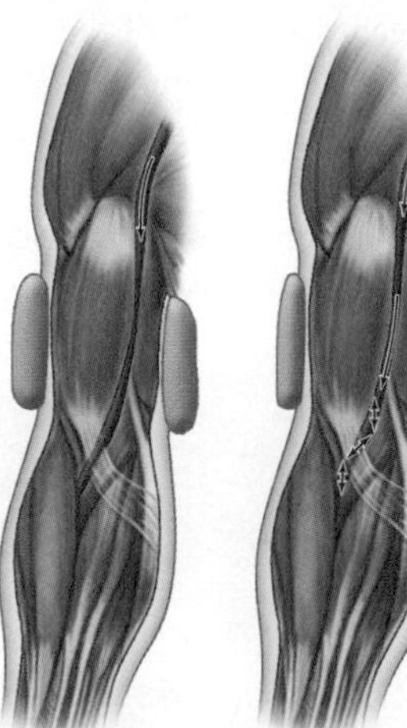
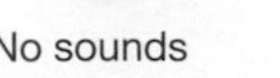
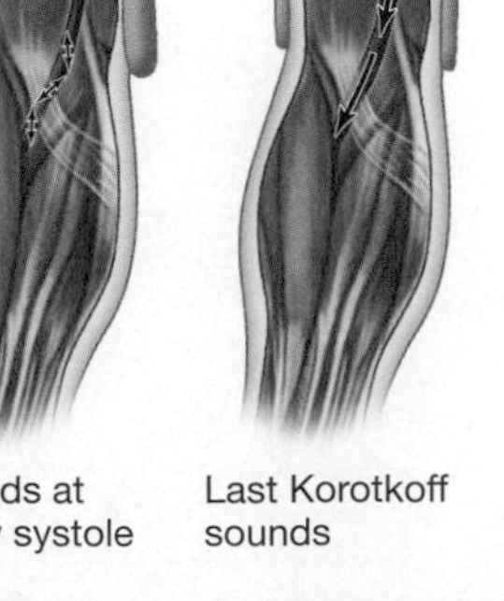
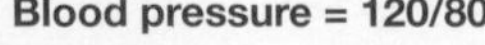

FIGURE 8-18 Korotkoff sounds

When taking a blood pressure, accuracy is of primary importance. While the equipment and procedure are is uncomplicated, many potential errors may cause inaccurate readings (Table 8-3). Blood pressure, like the other vital signs, varies with age and gender; however, in contrast to the others, blood pressure increases with age (see Table 8-1).

The expected blood pressure reading has been 120/80. While this is considered the standard, it is not necessarily the ideal. Some individuals consistently have BP readings that are considerably lower than 120/80. An initial low blood pressure reading needs to be

Box 8-1 MAP Equations

Systolic pressure = 115 Diastolic pressure = 72

MAP = [systolic pressure] × 1/3 + [diastolic pressure] × 2/3
MAP = [115] × 1/3 + [72] × 2/3
MAP = [38] + [47] = 85

MAP = [systolic pressure + 2(diastolic pressure)]/3
MAP = 115 + 2(72)/3 115 + 144 = 259/3
MAP = 86

Table 8-3 Potential errors in measuring blood pressure

Error	Proper Procedure to Prevent Error	Measurement Discrepancy in Systolic/Diastolic Readings Due to Error
Inadequate preparation of the patient	Allow patient to sit quietly for at least 5 minutes	
	Patients should not smoke or drink coffee/tea 30 minutes prior to measurement of BP	6–20 mmHg/XX*
	Patient needs to empty bladder prior to BP measurement.	15/10 mmHg
Problems with equipment and position of equipment, provider, or patient.	Manometers should be calibrated and validated properly and regularly	
	Patient should be properly positioned in chair with back and arm support and feet on the floor	6–10/XX mmHg
	Arm should be supported at the level of the heart, HR and BP tend to be higher if not supported with cuff at heart level; tend to be lower if patient supine and not seated.	1–7/5–11 mmHg
	Patient's feet should be flat on floor, not dangling or crossed.	
	Patient standing with arm unsupported may be position for BP measurement if determining sitting/standing readings.	
Cuff mismatching	Cuff bladder should encircle 80% of patient's arm. Use larger cuffs for overweight individuals and smaller cuffs for pediatrics or small adult.	
	Too small a cuff = higher reading (too small cuff errors are more common than too large cuff errors)	3/3 12/8 mmHg
	Too large a cuff = lower reading	10–20 mmHg
Rounding off numbers	BP numbers should not be rounded to the nearest 5 or 10.	
Deflating cuff too rapidly	This is often why providers round off numbers as the cuff is not deflated slowly enough to determine precise number where sounds are first heard and disappear.	
Incorrect placement of diaphragm	Determine location of brachial pulse prior to placement of diaphragm on antecubital fossa. If location of diaphragm not correct, sounds may not be correctly identified.	
Conversing with each other	Conversation between provider and patient should not take place during procedure. Provider may be distracted and not correctly note appearance and disappearance of sounds	10/10 mmHg
Inadequate exposure of upper arm	Blood pressure measurements should not be taken over clothing. BP cuff should also not be positioned so that rolled up sleeve is not included under the cuff.	5–50 mmHg/XX*
Looking at manometers at an angle	The provider should be positioned so that when looking at the manometers, they are looking straight on. If the provider looks at manometers from an angle, the precise point for systolic and diastolic sounds is not accurate.	
Using wrong arm	It is recommended that the right arm be used when obtaining blood pressure readings.	Primarily for consistency in BP readings

*XX Indicates no diastolic measurements.

evaluated in relationship to other physiological variables and previous blood pressure readings.

Blood pressure may also be obtained by other means. Health care settings are using electronic blood pressure monitors more frequently. These electronic measuring devices are based on the oscillometric method and do not require the use of a stethoscope, but instead use a pressure sensor (transducer) that observes the oscillations of the cuff and converts them electronically to a digital readout. The oscillations are changes that occur in the cuff pressure as a result of oscillations in the blood flow.

Direct measurement of blood pressure requires the placement of an arterial line directly into the lumen of an artery, most commonly the radial artery but other locations are also used. The arterial line is connected to fluid filled tubing that is connected to a pressure sensitive transducer. The pressure of each heartbeat is sensed and measured and converted to a digital readout on a bedside monitor. A wave form is also displayed which gives a visual representation of the arterial pressures (Figure 8-19).

Hypertension

Hypertension is the term that indicates a sustained increase in blood pressure over an individual's mean blood pressure. While an underlying cause exists in about 3% of cases, the majority of cases, called *essential hypertension*, lack a known cause. Hypertension tends to be hereditary, which indicates a genetic component. Other causes include obesity, which is related to the need for the heart to generate a greater pressure to circulate blood throughout the increased body mass, and increased dietary sodium intake, which causes the kidneys to retain excess water to maintain the physiological balance between water and sodium.

Anxiety related to the physical examination, or white coat syndrome, is a minor cause of hypertension. This is a transient manifestation and often, after a few minutes, the increase in blood pressure will disappear.

Hypotension

Hypotension refers to a decreased blood pressure reading that is 30 or greater mmHg below an individual's mean blood pressure. Minor causes of hypotension may be dehydration or a transient drop in peripheral vascular resistance. More severe causes are related to a sustained reduction in peripheral vascular resistance caused by widespread vasodilatation, which is often the case in instances of shock. Massive hemorrhage from trauma or ruptured blood vessels are other life-threatening causes of hypotension. Severe hypotension results in a lack of adequate oxygen delivery to vital organs, causing damage and eventually failure of their physiological function.

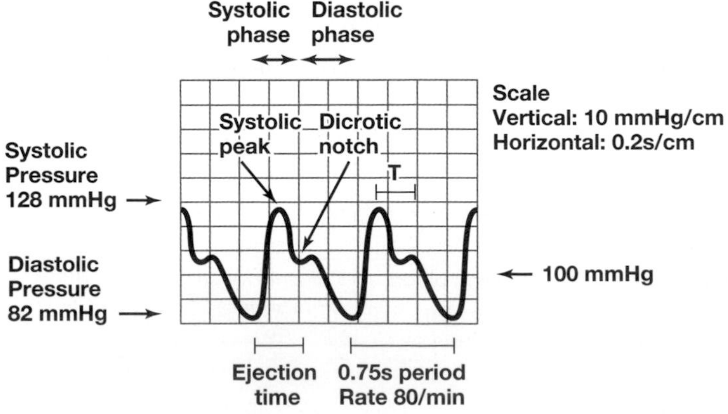

FIGURE 8-19 Waveform of arterial pulse

Pain

Pain is a significant reason for individuals seeking health care, accounting for approximately 80% of symptoms initially identified by patients (Mularski et al., 2006). Since 2001 the Joint Commission has included pain management standards as a requirement for accreditation (Table 8-4). While something frequently avoided, pain, ironically, is essential for survival (Patel, 2010). Its primary function is to warn individuals of impending injury and protect them from further injury or damage. When a person encounters a potentially painful and harmful stimulus, pain triggers a reflex withdrawal from the stimuli or immobilizes a certain area to prevent further harm. Pain serves as a signal indicating the need for medical attention and intervention. Pain also helps individuals recognize what future situations or stimuli to avoid, preventing the reoccurrence of pain.

Pain is an unpleasant sensation; a complex sensory modality associated with actual or potential tissue damage or described in those terms. Pain is universally experienced by everyone at some point during one's lifetime; however the meaning of pain is associated with experiences related to injury very early in life. The experience of pain is subjective and can only be described by the individual. Its manifestations are determined by the individual's report of the perceived sensation. The experience of pain depends on a number of physiological and psychological variables. Pain also has different characteristics, often depending on its location, involved organs, and causes or origins. The characteristics of pain can only be assessed indirectly from the patient's description and physical behaviors (Table 8-5). What causes intense pain in one individual may only cause moderate pain in another because the physical pathology does not directly correlate with the intensity of the pain. Despite the increased attention given to pain and its assessment, the quality of pain management has not significantly improved with as many as 80% of patients undertreated (Gordon et al., 2005; Mularski et al., 2006).

Pain is broadly classified as acute or chronic. While acute or chronic pain itself may not be experienced differently, their physiological mechanisms are different. Acute pain that is not well controlled may progress to chronic pain.

Acute pain has a biological purpose as a warning mechanism to indicate that an illness or injury has taken place. In general, it is localized and time limited, depending on the severity of the illness or injury. The initial response to acute pain is due to stimulation of the sympathetic nervous system and the "fight or flight" symptoms, which

Table 8-4 The Joint Commission standards for pain management

Rights and Ethics	Recognize the right of patients to appropriate assessment and management of pain
Assessment of Persons with Pain	Screen patients for pain during their initial assessment and, when clinically required, during ongoing, periodic reassessments
Education of Persons with Pain	Educate patients suffering from pain and their families about pain management

Source: "Facts about Pain Management" by The Joint Commission. Copyright © 2013 by The Joint Commission. Reproduced by permission of The Joint Commission.

THINK LINK: Pain Insensitivity

Pain is tantamount to survival. Without the sensation of pain, no need would exist for protection from dangerous, life-threatening situations. Individuals who have congenital insensitivity to pain with anhidrosis (CIPA) (Gordon et al., 2005; Mularski et al., 2006) experience no sensation of pain, making them insensitive to injuries and pain, which results in tissue damage and self-mutilating behaviors. Injuries often result in excessive scarring, deformity, infection, and dysfunction with possible amputation of affected extremities. Extremely rare, CIPA is an autosomal recessive condition caused by a mutation or defect in the NTRK1 gene and has no cure (Oliveria, dos Santos, Nogueira, & Mainardes, 2007). Affected individuals often die prematurely because of injuries, fever, of infections.

Anhidrosis, or the inability to sweat, that accompanies CIPA is caused by the lack of innervation to the sweat glands. This makes affected individuals unable to regulate body temperature and prone to overheating in hot weather. Individuals with CIPA may demonstrate intellectual deficiencies, but there are also those who demonstrate average intelligence.

Patient with Hansen's disease (leprosy) also experience pain insensitivity because the organism that causes leprosy (Mycobacterium leprae) invades the nerves and results in the loss of sensation. These individuals are prone to the same complications as those with CIPA. The disfigurement commonly associated with leprosy is actually the result of injuries that occur because of the loss of pain sensation. While leprosy may be curable, the loss of sensation is permanent. Leprosy is rare in the United States and other developed countries; however, it is endemic to other countries, primarily India.

Table 8-5 Physical behaviors of pain

Paralingual vocalizations	Sighs, moans
Facial expressions	Grimacing
Motor activity	Extremely slow movement
Disposition	Irritable
Verbal reports	Questions: "Why did this happen to me?" Requests help with walking
Body postures, gestures	Limping or distorted gait Rubbing or supporting affected area Shifting posture frequently Sitting with rigid posture
Behaviors to reduce pain	Taking medication Using health care system Reduction of tasks or activities Using protective devices (cane, cervical collar)
Functional limitations	Reclining for extended periods of time Moving in guarded or protective manner Stopping to rest when walking

includes increased pulse and ventilations, sweating, dilated pupils, restlessness, and apprehension (Helms & Barone, 2008). Acute pain generally lasts for 3 months or less and recedes with healing.

Chronic pain persists beyond 3 months and essentially serves no useful purpose. More recently is has been suggested that a specific time period cut off is arbitrary and that chronic pain should be considered when it appears that pain persists beyond what should be a reasonable healing time (Singh et al., 2013).

Physiology of Pain

Pain is a complex phenomenon that is not totally understood. The mechanisms and processes involved in pain are essentially the same within each individual; however, the perception of pain varies greatly. Attempts to understand and help in treatment and relief of pain have resulted in the development of multiple theories of pain.

Pain Theories

Proposed theories have attempted to understand the phenomena of pain, yet no complete theory exists to explain all its facets. Proposed by Melzack and Wall, **gate control theory** is the most widely accepted theory of pain (Melzack & Wall, 1965). It supposes that a gating mechanism resides in the dorsal horn of the spinal cord. The gate opens or closes to regulate or modify pain sensations transmitted to the brain.

Within the dorsal horn, thick and thin diameter nerve fibers enter and synapse on **projection (P) cells**. The P cells then transmit signals that go up the **spinothalmic tract** to the brain and to **inhibitory (I) cells**, also within the dorsal horn. The interaction of these cells and pathways determines when and what pain sensations are transmitted to the brain (Figure 8-20).

The gate regulates and modifies pain in relation to the amount of activity within the pain fibers, the amount of activity within other peripheral fibers, and messages sent from the brain (Table 8-6).

The opening and closing of the gate can be summarized as follows:

1. When no input is being received, transmission of impulses to the brain by projector cells is blocked by the inhibitory cells. (Closed Gate)
2. When there is transmission of touch, pressure, and vibration through the thick fibers, both projection and inhibitory cells are stimulated. Transmission of impulses to the brain is blocked by the inhibitory cells. (Closed Gate)
3. When the thin fibers are transmitting a greater amount of stimuli (pain) than the large fibers, or there is only thin fiber stimulation, the inhibitors cells are inactivated. This allows the projection cells to transmit the stimuli up the spinothalmic tract to the brain (thalamus) where it is interpreted as pain. (Open Gate)
4. Descending pathways from the brain then transmit signals to inhibit the projection cells, thus reducing pain perception.

Pain Pathways

The transmission of the pain stimuli from the involved area to the brain is a critical mechanism that initiates the primary reflexive response that protects an individual and prevents further damage. Conveyance of pain requires that the injurious mechanical, thermal, chemical, biological stimuli be converted to electrical impulses (Table 8-7). This conversion occurs within **nociceptors,** specialized primary sensory neuron receptors that are distributed throughout the body tissues, except the brain, and responsible for conducting pain stimuli into the dorsal horn of the spinal cord (Helms & Barone, 2008).

Pain stimuli are transmitted to the spinal cord along two primary sensory, afferent nerve fibers. **A delta (Aδ) fibers** are minimally myelinated axons while the **C fibers** are unmyelinated axons. The myelinated Aδ fiber stimulation causes very localized, short term, and sharp sensations. The Aδ fibers consist of two types, mechanosensitive and mechanothermal. Both fibers respond to mechanical stimuli (pressure/touch) but the mechanothermal also respond to heat.

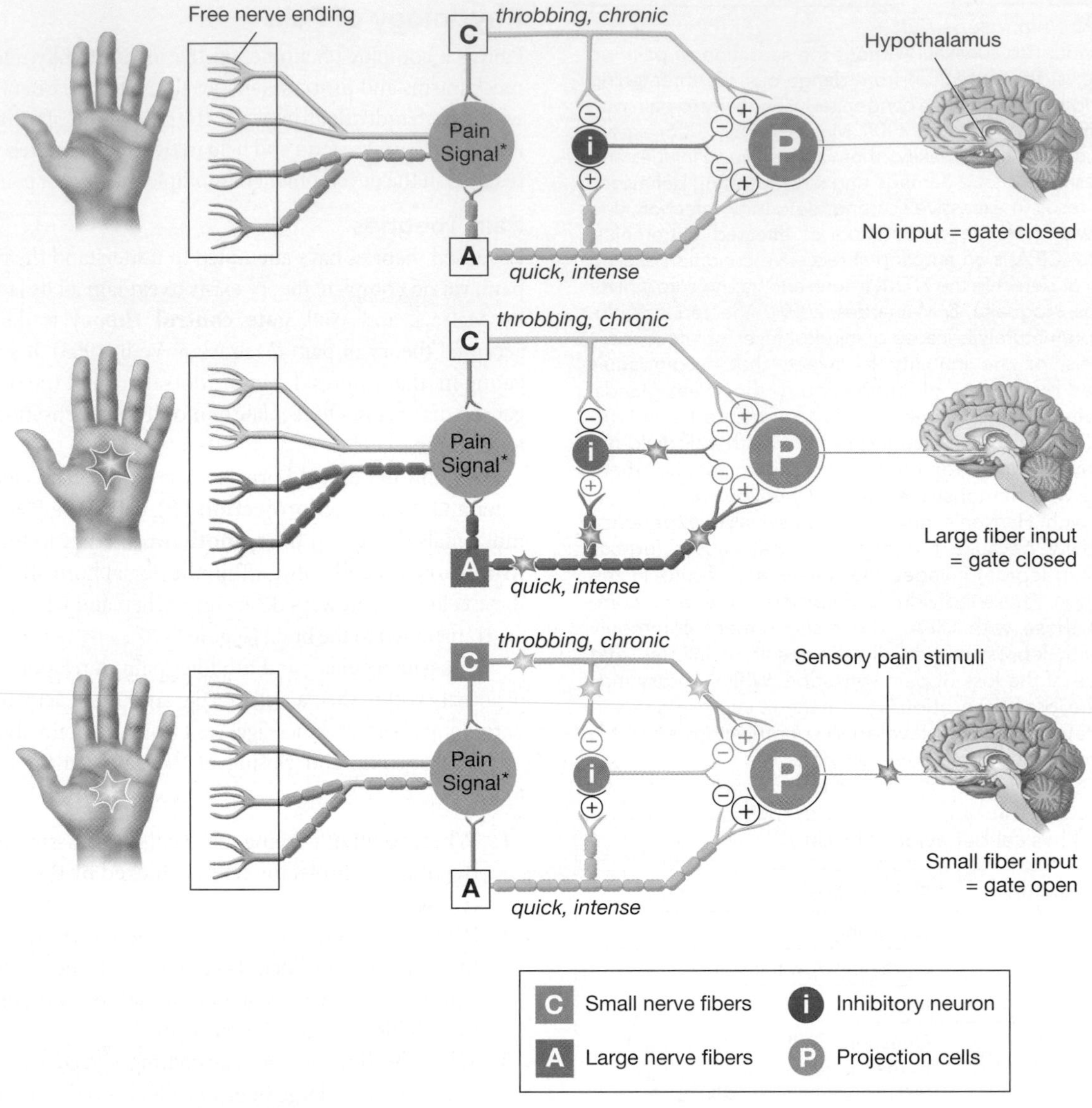

FIGURE 8-20 Gate Theory of Pain

Table 8-6 Gate Regulation/Modulation

Conditions that Open the Gate	Conditions that Close the Gate
Physical Conditions	
Extent of injury	Medications
Inappropriate activity level	Counter stimulation (heat, massage)
Emotional Conditions	
Anxiety/worry	Positive emotions
Tension	Relaxation, rest
Depression	
Mental Conditions	
Focusing on pain	Intense concentration or distraction
Boredom	Involvement and interest in life activities

The unmyelinated C fibers transmit sensations more slowly producing diffuse, aching sensations. The Aδ and C fibers enter the spinal cord through the posterior nerve roots of the dorsal horn and through the track of Lissauer (Figure 8-21). Beyond the tract of Lissaeur is the **substantia gelatinosa** where the nerve fibers synapse with interneurons. The gray matter of the spinal cord is comprised

Table 8-7 Selected chemical substances released with stimuli sufficient to cause tissue damage

Substance	Source
Potassium (K+)	Damaged Cells
Serotonin	Platelets
Bradykinin	Plasma
Prostaglandins	Damaged Cells
Leukotrienes	Damaged Cells
Substance P	Primary Nerve Afferents

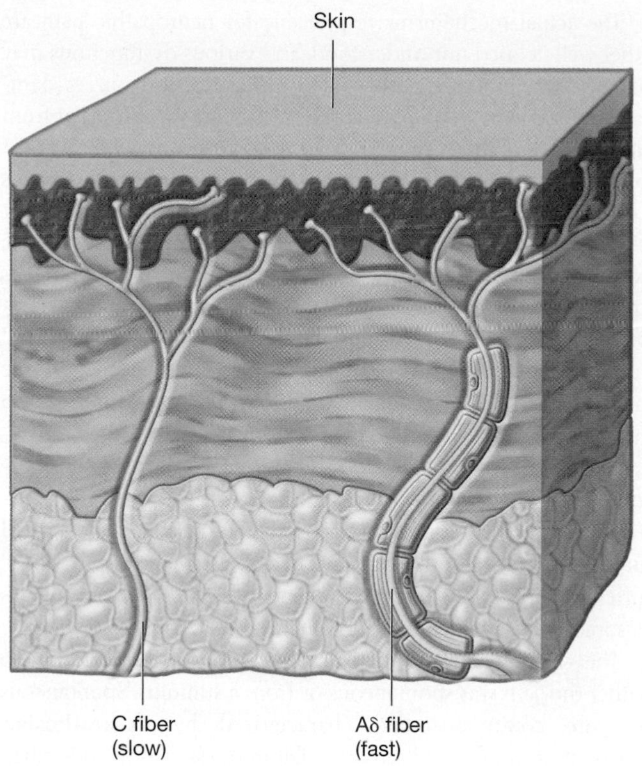

FIGURE 8-21 A delta/C fibers

of sequential, stratified layers of nerve cells (lamina) and the substantia gelatinosa comprises the second layer. The nerve fibers then cross over to the other side of the spinal cord where they ascend to the brain via the anterolateral spinothalmic tract.

Nociceptive Pain

Nociception is the perception of pain that occurs in the presence of irritating/aggravating stimuli (Dubin & Patapoutian, 2010). The most common type of pain, nociceptive pain is acute and self-limiting in nature and disappears after repair and healing occurs. The process of nociceptive pain perception occurs in four stages: (1) transduction, (2) transmission, (3) perception, and (4) modulation (Figure 8-22).

In stage one, **transduction**, the pain signal is transported from the primary source of the pain to the spinal cord following an irritating stimuli that poses a threat to an individual. Stimuli can come from various sources, such as an injury from trauma, chemical, thermal, or physical actions that damage tissues of peripheral, visceral, and somatic structures. The damaged tissues release a variety of detrimental chemical neurotransmitters consisting of substance P, histamine, prostaglandins, serotonin, and bradykinin that initiate an action potential in the form of a pain message that is conducted along the sensory afferent nerves (Aδ) where they enter the dorsal horn of the spinal cord. In the dorsal horn, the nerve fibers synapse with the dorsal horn neurons. The transmission of the pain signal from the nerve fibers to the neurons requires another set of neurotransmitters which consist of P substance, glutamate, and adenosine triphosphate (ATP).

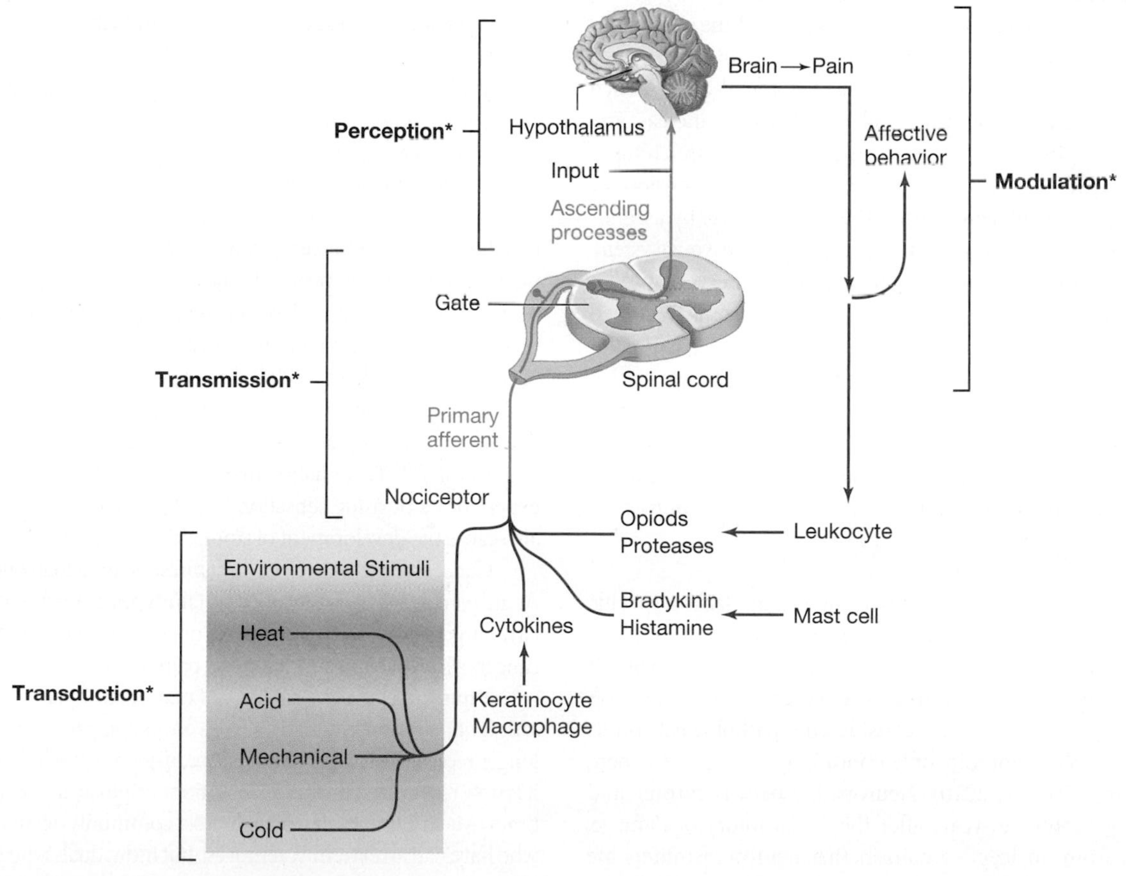

FIGURE 8-22 Four stages of pain perception

Opioid receptors within the synaptic cleft of the dorsal horn are capable of blocking the pain signal from entering the spinothalmic tract. This is accomplished with endogenous or exogenous opioids. If the pain signal is not blocked, it is passed to the spinothalmic tract.

The next stage, **transmission**, involves the transfer of the pain signal from the spinal cord to the brain via the spinothalmic tract terminating in the brainstem and thalamus. Once the pain signal reaches the thalamus, it is distributed to the higher cortical areas of the brain. How this distribution occurs is not well understood at this time.

The third stage, **perception,** is the conscious awareness of the presence and sensation of pain. The emotional response to pain is processed within the limbic system, and the somatosensory areas characterize the sensation. The identification of pain can only occur when the stimuli is interpreted within these higher cortical structures.

The fourth stage, **modulation**, refers to the inhibition or slowing down of the pain signal. The descending tracts from the brainstem to the spinal cord release another group of neurotransmitters that consist of serotonin, norepinephrine, neurotensin, γ-aminobutyric acid (GABA), and endogenous opioids (β-endorphins, enkaphalins, and dynorphins). They produce an analgesic response to the pain signals.

Nociceptive pain primarily comes from two sources and may be referred to as **somatic pain** and **visceral pain**. Somatic pain is primarily caused by injury to some part of the body. It is generally localized to the affected area and goes away when the damage is repaired. This pain is associated with minor wounds and first-degree burns. **Superficial somatic pain** or **cutaneous pain** originates in the skin or superficial tissues; it is sharp, well-defined, and clearly located. **Deep somatic pain** originates in the ligaments, tendons, bones, blood vessels, fasciae and muscles; it is dull, aching and poorly localized. This pain comes from sprained ankles and broken bones.

Visceral pain originates in the larger, abdominal organs, such as the kidney, stomach, intestine, gall bladder, or pancreas and may be caused by direct trauma to the organ or from stretching of the organ or organ capsule due to ischemia, tumor, distension, or severe contractions. Pain signals from these areas travel by ascending nerve fibers as well as fibers of the autonomic nervous system. The transmission of pain signals by the autonomic nervous system accounts for the nausea, vomiting, pallor, and diaphoresis that often accompany visceral pain.

Referred pain is another pain classification, describing pain that is felt or perceived in a specific location that is remote from the actual source of the pain. This occurs when both sites share a common spinal nerve, and the brain is unable to differentiate the specific origin of the pain. Referred pain may originate from somatic or visceral sources.

Neuropathic Pain

Neuropathic pain, in contrast to nociceptive pain, lacks a specific origin nor is it localized to a specific area, or a means of warning and protecting the individual; instead it *is* the source of the pain. It is defined as pain that results from a primary lesion or dysfunction of the somatosensory system and considered a pathological condition rather than the symptom of a condition (Callin & Bennett, 2008; Haanpaa & Treede, 2010). Neuropathic pain is chronic and may persist for months to years after the initial injury or damage. It also differs from nociceptive pain in that neurotransmitters are not involved in the activation and transmission of pain signals; the pain results from neural dysfunction from damage, or pathological alterations within the peripheral or central nervous systems.

The actual mechanisms responsible for neuropathic pain are neither well defined nor understood, and various dysfunctions may lead to its development. It can originate from peripheral sources (damage to peripheral nerve, plexus, dorsal root ganglion, or root) or from central sources (damage to brain or spinal cord). Peripheral causes of neuropathic pain include peripheral sensitization in which neurons become unusually sensitive as a result of a decreased threshold for excitability. They also develop an increased sensitivity to chemical, mechanical, and thermal stimuli activation resulting in spontaneous pathological activity. Conditions associated with peripheral neuropathic pain include herpes zoster infection (post-shingles), HIV related neuropathies, nutritional deficiencies, toxins, and immune related disorders. Diabetic and other peripheral neuropathies are also considered peripheral causes of neuropathic pain.

Central nervous system involvement includes central sensitization in which the neurons of the spinothalamic tract become sensitized and develop the same characteristics of peripheral sensitized neurons. Central neuropathic pain is associated with spinal cord injuries, multiple sclerosis and some types of strokes. Fibromyalgia is also sometimes considered a central neuropathic pain.

The characteristics of neuropathic pain vary depending on whether the pain was spontaneous or from a stimulus. Spontaneous pains are continuous and characterized by **dysaesthesias**, unpleasant or unexpected sensation felt in the skin, often described as burning, tingling, itching, or pins and needles. Aching, gnawing, cramping, or crushing may be descriptions of pain that are deeper in origin. Paroxysmal pains may be described as stabbing, shooting, or like an electric shock; **allodynia** and **hyperalgesia** are two other unexpected responses to pain and are characterized by an unusual and/or intensified pain sensation. Allodynia is pain felt from a stimulus that ordinarily would not initiate a response, such as clothing rubbing on the skin or a cold wind gust. Hyperalgesia is an intensified or exaggerated response to painful stimuli.

Malignant pain is another type of neuropathic pain due to cancer and its destructive invasion of various organs and tissues. Approximately one-third of cancer patients develop some type of cancer-related pain. Tumors invade nearby tissues and organs, exerting pressure on nerves, bones, and blood vessels resulting in pain. Bone pain, from metastasis and neural compression are the two most common causes of chronic pain (Cherny, 2007). Other pain associated with malignancy is due to radiation-induced nerve tissue damage and neuropathies related to paraneoplastic syndromes and chemotherapeutic agents (Chen et al., 2004). Radiation may leave painful scars or the patient may experience a burning sensation after treatments. Chemotherapy may also cause the development of stomatitis (oral ulcers).

Cancer related pain often is manifest as more than one kind of pain. Acute pain may be present after certain types of interventions, particularly surgery. It may also be visceral or somatic in origin. Some types of cancers secrete chemicals that cause pain in the area of the tumor.

Phantom pain is also a type of neuropathic pain in which the sensation of pain or stimuli arises from a missing part of the body that no longer receives messages. Originally considered psychological in nature, it is now recognized that these sensations originate in the spinal cord and brain (Mayo Clinic Staff, 2010). It most commonly occurs in individuals who have had an extremity removed, but individuals who have lost other body parts, such as a breast, eye, penis, or tongue, may also experience it.

Many individuals who have had a limb amputation report the sensation that there is still awareness of the amputated part. This painless

THINK LINK: Paraneoplastic Syndromes
Paraneoplastic syndromes are a group of symptoms that result from substances that are produced by the tumor. The symptoms are often demonstrated in areas that are remote from the tumor itself. In some cases, the immune system is involved. Antibodies (T cells) that are formed to destroy the tumor may cross react with noncancerous cells, causing their destruction. In other instances, physiologically active tumor secretions are the cause. These secretions may be hormones, hormone precursors, enzymes, or cytokines (Santacroce, Diomede, Gagliardi, & Balducci, 2010). In some instances, paraneoplastic syndromes are a precursor to the diagnosis of cancer.

sensation is described as phantom limb sensation; those who were born without limbs or have spinal cord injuries may also experience it. Phantom limb sensation may be described as feelings of cold, warmth, itchiness, or tingling (Mayo Clinic Staff, 2010). Phantom pain is actually pain that originates from the body part that is no longer there and most commonly follows amputation.

While the cause of phantom pain is unknown, it is perceived to originate in the spinal cord and brain; however, specific locations have yet to be identified. Various other factors such as damaged nerve endings, the formation of scar tissue, and the physical memory of pain in the amputated limb are believed to contribute to phantom pain. It is also proposed that the brain region that is responsible for receiving sensations from the amputated limb becomes confused and functions abnormally, resulting in the perception that the limb is still there. Phantom pain is more common in individuals who experienced significant pre-amputation pain than those who had none, and in individuals who had a tumor related amputation rather than a traumatic one (Cherny, 2007).

Pain Assessment

Pain in the United States is estimated to affect more than 76.5 million individuals—more than those affected with diabetes, heart disease, and cancer combined (American Pain Foundation, 2010). While pain is a universal experience, how one experiences pain differs widely depending on age, gender, culture, and pain tolerance. A comprehensive assessment of pain is the foundation of effective pain management (Stevens, Johnston, Taaddio, Gibbins, & Yamada, 2010) and includes data from three dimensions: (1) cognitive (subjective self-reporting of sensation), (2) behavioral (crying, position/posture, facial expressions), and (3) physiological (variability in pulse and blood pressure, oxygen saturation decrease, and increases in metabolic and endocrine processes) (Arif-Rahu, Fisher, & Matsuda, 2012). The most significant dimension of the assessment is the self-reported, subjective, experience, which is the basis for the primary interpretation of pain as "it is what the patient says it is." Even based on that premise, there is still the potential for inadequate pain management; however the primary obstacle is the patient's inability to accurately express the sensation being felt and experienced. This becomes a significant barrier when the patient does not have the cognitive ability to express or communicate the extent of the pain. This is a critical issue in the treatment of pain for infants and small children as well as elderly individuals who are cognitively impaired. Another impediment is that many provider's and patient's pain management decisions are influenced by myths that continue to be perpetuated (Table 8-8).

Infants, Children and Adolescents

Pain in infants is poorly understood and as a result, assessment and treatment of pain in infants has not been adequate (Cignacco et al., 2009). Advances in science and technology, which have increased their survivability, are also the main causes of procedural pain. It is estimated that infants in neonatal intensive care units are subjected to an average of 16 traumatic or invasive procedures a day (Lago et al., 2009).

Historically, ineffective pain management was been based on the belief that infants (neonates) are incapable of and do not experience pains as adults do, as well as the belief that infants do not remember pain (Akuma & Jordan, 2012). There has been gradual recognition and acceptance that infants experience pain, however there are still concerns related to pain management and treatment of infants. Additional beliefs related to infants and pain are included in Table 8-9.

Table 8-8 Myths and truths about pain

Myths	Truths
Signs of pain should be visible in the patient to know the patient is in pain and how much pain.	What patients say about their pain is the best way to know how much and what kind of pain they have. Some patients with severe acute pain and many with chronic pain may not demonstrate any signs of pain.
Using potent medications or prescription pain pills for pain relief can lead to addiction.	Rarely does a person become addicted to potent medications or prescription pain pills when used appropriately for pain relief.
Potent pain medicines are not good and/or cannot be handled by older adult patients.	Pain medication should be based on the patient's medical condition and ability to handle unpleasant side effects, not age. Adjust the initial doses downward for older patients.
The patient's activity level indicates pain severity.	Some patients are able to be active when they are in pain; other patients may be unable to move about.
Individuals with a history of pain throughout a lifetime are able to tolerate pain longer than someone who has not had much pain in life.	There is no evidence that individuals with a history of pain have an increased pain tolerance. Pain tolerance is modified by functions of multiple factors. Genetics, expectations, hormones, stress, and other factors all play roles in pain tolerance. Men and women also experience pain differently. Overall, pain is an individual experience, including the tolerance of it.
A patient's mood (happy, sad, blue, and worried) has no effect on pain.	A patient's emotional state influences pain sensation and its interpretation. Every individual experiences pain differently and what may cause severe pain in one individual may not cause the same severity in another, which is often due to emotional feelings.
The ways customs and religious beliefs of families are not important in management of pain.	Customs and beliefs of individuals and their families can have a great impact on how pain is judged and how the pain will be controlled. Providers need to include these customs and beliefs when deciding how a patient's pain is treated.

Table 8-9 Myths and truth about pain in infants, children and adolescents

Myths	Truths
Infants and Children	
Providers will always know if my baby/child is hurting.	The infant/child is the only person who knows how much pain being experienced. Parents are also good at determining when their infant/child is hurting. Pain is not something a provider can observe, therefore, any information from parents regarding pain is welcome and helpful.
Pain is just part of being in the hospital.	Unfortunately, every bit of pain cannot be eliminated for infants/children who are hospitalized. However, much of it can be controlled to help the infant/child feel better sooner.
If my infant/child gets strong pain medicine, he/she will become addicted to it.	An addict is someone who takes drugs to get "high." Infants who are given pain medications may "get used to it," and adjustments may need to be made by the provider. This is to be expected when an infant/child has been on a medication over time. It is not the same as being addicted to a drug.
The only way to help an infant's/child's pain is with medication.	Providers may use a number of techniques to help your infant/child at stressful time, such as swaddling, positioning, dimmed lights, soft music, sucking on pacifier, and gentle touch. These are very effective ways to control pain in infants/children.
Pain medication will make my child too sleepy or feel "druggy."	Although some pain medications may cause your child to be drowsy, your providers can make changes to help with this common side effect.

It is now recognized that infants are capable of perceiving pain; however how it is experienced and its intensity remain subject to speculation. Evidence exists that around 25–26 weeks' gestation neurophysiological afferent pain pathways reach the cortex, enabling the fetus to experience pain (Ranger, Johnston, & Anand, 2007; Simons & Tibboel, 2006). Data also indicates that while the transmission of pain signals via the ascending pathways are functional, descending inhibitory responses are not as well developed and not so until birth at full term. As a result, premature infants demonstrate a greater sensitivity to pain stimuli and a lowered threshold for excitation which most likely results in these infants feeling pain more severely than older individuals (Badr et al., 2010).

Since the recognition that neonates and infants are capable of experiencing pain, multiple methods for assessing pain in infants and neonates have been developed. Even with assessment tools, however, the ability of providers to recognize and respond to the infant's pain remains an issue because of their inability to verbally express the pain (Ranger et al., 2007). Because infants and small children are unable to provide subjective data related to their pain experience, behavioral and physiological responses to pain have become the foundation for the development of pain assessment tools (Figure 8-23). The most common pain assessment tools that are used with neonates and infants are (1) Premature Infant Pain Profile (PIPP), (2) Neonatal Pain Agitation and Sedation Scale (N-PASS), (3) Neonatal Infant pain Scale (NIPS), and (4) Crying, Requires Oxygen Saturation, Increased Vital Signs, Expression, Sleeplessness (Anand, 2013).

While these tools are helpful, there are issues that affect their usefulness, most significantly that they are not able to capture the subjective data that is needed for identifying its intensity. Another issue with the majority of these measuring instruments is that they have not been tested for reliability and validity (Stevens et al., 2010) and that there are no standardized measurement criteria resulting in variability in the interpretation of behavioral and physiological parameters. It is also questioned as to whether changes in the physiological parameters are specifically due to pain or if there are other causes (Ranger et al., 2007). Additionally, providers may be unaware of available resources to assist in pain assessment or lack knowledge in how to use them (Slater, Canteralla, Franck, & Fitzgerald, 2008). As a result of these issues, pain control and management of infants remains less than ideal (Srouji, Ratnapalan, & Schneeweiss, 2010). While no tool is ideal, there is general consensus that use of them is a good thing with the recommendation that consistent use of an agreed upon tool will optimize its usefulness within a unit or facility.

There is increasing evidence that prolonged exposure to poorly controlled, repetitive painful procedures as a neonate produces long term, significant adverse neurodevelopmental alterations (Gyland, 2012) related to their pain response thresholds (lowered) as well as pain intensity (higher) (Yamada et al., 2008) along with changes in behavioral responses associated with the painful stimuli (Lowery et al., 2007). Evidence also suggests that longer exposure to painful stimuli and a higher number of painful procedures increases neurodevelopmental impairments (Beggs, Currie, Salter, Fitzgerald, & Walker, 2011). These outcomes are particularly influenced by the gestational age of the neonate. Infants less than 27 weeks' gestation are subjected to a greater number of painful procedures and are thus more susceptible to the development of these adverse outcomes.

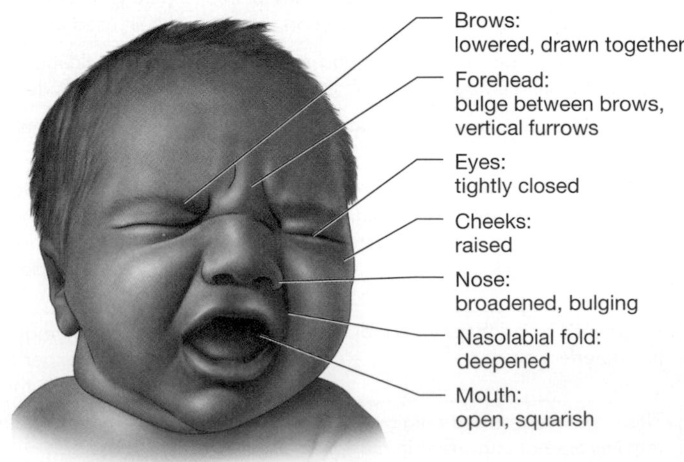

FIGURE 8-23 Behavioral expressions related to pain

While there is no exact age at which a child can be expected to fully self-describe the characteristics associated with the pain sensation, the age of 3 seems to be an appropriate age at which the child is capable of cooperating in describing pain. As the child ages and matures the ability to describe pain becomes more accurate and reliable (Table 8-10).

Pain in the Older Adult

Pain is a common symptom affecting a significant number of elderly adults. It is estimated that 50% of community-dwelling elderly and 75% of residents in long term care facilities experience pain (Weiner, 2007). Like pain in the neonates and infants, pain in the elderly is often unrecognized and undertreated because of misinformation and misunderstanding (Jermyn, Janora, & Surve, 2010). A common misperception relating to pain and the older adult is that pain is associated with aging and it is to be expected as one gets older (Elliott, 2009). Cognitive impairments in the elderly, just as in infants, make it more difficult to assess the subjective nature of the pain (Zwakhalen, Hamers, Abu-Saad, & Berger, 2006). See Table 8-11.

The majority of pain in the elderly is nociceptive and chronic in nature, often caused by ongoing tissue damage or destruction associated with arthritis, osteoporosis, and malignancies. Joints are the most common sites for pain in this population, and musculoskeletal disorders, particularly osteoarthritis and lower back pain (LBP), are the most common cause (Argoff & Carberg, 2005; Jermyn et al., 2010). Chronic pain often has a negative impact on the older adult's functional status, health, and quality of life. Undertreated pain may cause depression, social isolation, cognitive impairment, immobility, and sleep disturbances (Cavalieri, 2007). Individuals with chronic, undertreated pain are also more prone to polypharmacy, which increases the probability for drug interactions. The elderly may also experience neuropathic pain as a result of diabetic neuropathy, post–herpetic neuralgia and trigeminal neuralgia.

A growing body of knowledge indicates that age does affect how various conditions present, particularly related to internal pathological processes (Giamberadino, 2005). Reduced renal excretion and hepatic metabolism, along with pharmacodynamic changes

Table 8-10 Developmental dimensions of pain behaviors and descriptions of pain

Age Group	Understanding of Pain	Behavioral Response	Verbal Description
Early infants (< 6 months)	No apparent understanding of pain; neonates exposed to repeated painful experiences in ICU demonstrate memory of pain (hold their breath) when approached by care providers	Generalized body movements, chin quivering, facial grimacing, poor feeding	Loud crying
Late infants (6–12 months)	Anticipate a painful event such as an immunization with fear; responsive to parental anxiety	Reflex withdrawal to stimulus, facial grimacing, disturbed sleep, irritability, restlessness	Loud crying
Toddlers (1–3 years)	Do not understand what causes pain and why they might have pain; demonstrate fear of painful situations; use common words for pain such as *owie* and *boo-boo*	Localized withdrawal, resistance of entire body aggressive behavior, disturbed sleep	Cries and screams, cannot describe intensity or type of pain
Preschoolers (3–5 years)	Pain is a hurt, have language skills to express pain and skills increase with age; do not relate pain to illness but may relate pain to an injury; often believe pain is punishment; do not understand why a painful procedure will make them feel better or why and injection takes pain away	Active physical resistance, directed aggressive behavior, strikes out physically and verbally when hurts low frustration level	Can identify location and intensity of pain, denies pain, may believe his or her pain is obvious to others
School-age children (6–9 years)	Can understand simple relationships between pain and disease but have no clear understanding of the cause of pain; can understand the need for painful procedures to monitor or treat disease; may associate pain with feeling bad or angry; may recognize psychological pain related to grief and hurt feelings	Passive resistance, clenches fists, holds body rigidly still suffers emotional withdrawal, engages in plea bargaining	Can specify location and intensity of pain and describe its physical characteristics in relation to body parts
Transitional (10–12 years)	Better able to understand the relationship between an event and pain, have a more complex awareness of physical and psychological pain, such as moral dilemmas and mental pain	May pretend comfort to project bravery, may regress with stress and anxiety	Able to describe intensity and location with more characteristics, able to describe psychological pain
Adolescents (13–18 years)	Have a sophisticated understanding of the causes of physical and mental pain; relate to the pain experienced by others; pain has both qualitative and quantitative characteristics	Want to behave in a socially acceptable manner (like adults), show a controlled behavioral response	More sophisticated descriptions as experience is gained; may think nurses are in tune with their thoughts, so they don't need to tell the nurse about their pain

Source: Adapted from *Child Health Nursing: Partnering with Children and Families*, 2E by J. W. Ball, R. C. Bindler, K. J. Cowen. Copyright © 2010, p. 475. Reprinted and electronically reproduced by permission of Pearson Education, Inc., Upper Saddle River, New Jersey.

Table 8-11 Key components for pain assessment

Direct inquiry about the presence of pain	Include use of alternative words to describe pain (ache, discomfort, hurting)
Observation for signs of pain	Individuals with cognitive/communication impairments (unable to verbally express pain)
Description of pain to include	Sensory dimension the nature of pain (sharp, dull, burning) pain location and radiation (patients pointing to site) intensity, using standardized pain assessment scale Affective dimension emotional response to pain (fear, anxiety, depression) Impact (disabling effects of pain at the levels of functional activities [ADLs]) participation (work, social activities, relationships)
Measurement of pain	Standardized scales in format accessible to patient
Cause of pain	Examination and investigation to establish cause

associated with aging, which includes increased sensitivity to some analgesics, particularly opioids, are responsible for an increased risk for adverse reactions (Cavalieri, 2007). Elderly patients with acute visceral pain are highly likely to demonstrate an atypical pattern that suggests a diminished intensity of the pain. Paradoxically, the diminished intensity occurs in the presence of an increase in pathological alterations of the viscera. While it is known that atherosclerosis increases dramatically with increasing age, silent myocardial ischemia and infarction occur more frequently in the elderly (Giamberadino, 2005). Visceral pain related to various malignancies has also been reported. Failure to recognize these manifestations related to pain may be life threatening to elderly patients.

Cultural Influences

Ethnicity has also been found to influence pain tolerance. Many ethnic and minority groups comprise populations that are medically underserved, which gives rise to disparity in treatment and management of pain (Nelson-Hogan, 2008). Cultural beliefs and communication is inherent from birth, and how one lives in and communicates with families have a tremendous influence on how one interprets and expresses concepts of pain (Warne, 2008).

For example, stoicism, fatalism, and reliance on specific and complementary approaches are important for ethnic Chinese individuals, and are cultural factors that have significant implications in the context of symptom treatment. Multiple studies have reported that African Americans report a greater severity of chronic, more pain-related disability, and less control over their pain when compared to a comparable group of white Americans (Baker & Green, 2005). In many ethnic groups, treatment and healing are closely intertwined with spirituality making one's experience, understanding of, and expression of pain more complex (Hastie, Riley, & Fillingim, 2005).

Treatment disparities related to pain experienced by ethnic and minority groups are related to multiple factors; however, the primary cause is due to inadequate assessment of pain (Table 8-12). Recent evidence implies that the most significant variable in the under treatment of pain in minority groups may be due to differences in staff perception of pain intensity in these patients which may be related to myth, lack of empathy, stigma, or explicit discrimination (Lasch, 2002).

Additionally, a discrepancy may exist between the patient's and provider's evaluation of the severity of the pain). With pain being defined as "what the patient states it is," how the patient describes the pain may be different than how the provider interprets the description. Meanings within languages are difficult to determine. It has been found that when determining pain ratings, only providers that shared the same language as the patient were capable of comparable rating the patient's pain (Al-Atiyyat, 2009). Behavioral manifestations of pain may also vary within ethnic groups, making reliance on typical behaviors and expressions as indicators of pain less reliable.

Subjective Data

While objective expressions and mannerisms may provide evidence of pain, its presence can only be subjectively reported. Pain is often a symptom of many conditions, so a precise history of the symptom is essential to its proper identification and treatment.

Pain also has different meanings among individuals. Some may feel they are being punished by God for some past action or behavior and must endure the pain. **Pain tolerance**, or the amount of pain an individual can endure before relief measures are needed, is another factor in assessment. Pain tolerance is not the same as **pain threshold**, which is the minimum stimulus needed to initiate pain perception.

A prevailing belief exists that regular or periodic exposure to pain will condition the individual and increase pain tolerance. This is the basis for desensitizing an individual to allergic stimuli; however, the same cannot be applied to pain. Regular exposure to pain actually sensitizes one to pain, making future pain exposures more painful. Pain synapses that are regularly exposed to repetitive stimuli will increase their responsiveness, responding more vigorously to inevitable exposure to pain stimuli.

Pain tolerance varies widely and is dependent on various individual factors. Evidence has surfaced that genetics is involved. This explanation focuses on the gene that codes for COMT (catachol-o-methyl transferase), an enzyme that metabolizes dopamine. When dopamine is removed from pain receptors in the brain, these receptors are then available to bind with endorphins, leading to pain relief. While this explanation accounts for some aspects of pain tolerance, it does not completely account for differences in pain tolerance.

Psychological influences also play a role particularly emotions, which have been recognized as affecting pain tolerance. Negative emotions such as anxiety, depression, and anger have a negative

Table 8-12 Factors related to pain management disparities for minority patients

Language/interpretation difficulties	Failure to use interpreters. Competent interpreters essential to adequate pain assessment and management. Using tools designed to assess cognitively impaired patients or children unlikely to obtain optimal measurement. Misunderstanding of subtle differences in meaning and interpretation of pain. Pain may be expressed in terms of natural symbols (lightning, trees/roots, spider webs, etc.), which are not like common words used in U.S. (sharp, stabbing, throbbing, aching).
Nonverbal communication interpretation	Nonverbal communication patterns, like language, vary across cultures and are most likely misinterpreted or misunderstood. Failure to clarify or validate nonverbal manifestations on part of providers.
Culturally/linguistically disparate pain assessment tools	Even though translating pain assessment tools into different languages has been done, the translations may convey different impressions or meanings, compromising their validity and usefulness.
Underreporting	The belief that "good" patients don't complain or that pain is inevitable and should stoically endure pain result in unwillingness to admit to having pain or the severity of the pain. Patients who don't have health insurance are more likely to wait to report pain until pain intensity at a "10" before seeking treatment.
Reluctance to use pain medications	Fears and concerns related to opioid use or cultural taboos regarding their use result in patient's adversity to use/request them. Preferences for familiar or culture based remedies also influence their hesitation to use opioids. Genetic differences affect absorption, metabolism, and elimination of drugs causing poor control of pain and/or undesirable side effects. Certain minority groups are more likely to use external coping strategies but less likely to engage in self-care activities, perceiving themselves as having less control over their pain.
Access to pain medications	Patients from ethnic minorities are less likely to have health insurance, limiting their access to medical care, pain management services, and medications. Pharmacies located in poor/minority areas often don't stock opioid medications.
Providers fear of drug abuse	Health care providers often associate certain minority groups as drug seekers or abusers. Fear of drugs being used for these purposes result in inadequate treatment.
Prejudice/discrimination	These attitudes continue to be inherent in American society, adversely affecting minority populations in obtaining adequate and appropriate health care/pain management treatment.

effect on pain, decreasing one's pain tolerance. In contrast, positive emotions have been found to counter balance negative emotions, allowing the individual to have a greater tolerance for the pain and experience less pain.

Gender also appears to have an effect on pain tolerance. Studies have found that males consistently have a higher pain threshold than females. While there is no specific accounting for this result, additional studies did determine that estrogen levels did influence the female's pain tolerance. When estrogen levels were low, females demonstrated a lower pain tolerance and conversely, when estrogen levels were high, females also demonstrated a higher pain tolerance.

The primary focus for assessing pain is to understand your patients as individuals.

THINK LINK:* *Emotive vs. Stoic Responses

Cultural responses to pain may be broadly categorized into two types: stoic and emotive (Table 8-13). While cultural and ethnic similarities may be correlated with either type of pain response, they are not a defining characteristic to be associated with any specific ethnic or cultural group; therefore providers need to be aware of the possibility of stereotyping pain responses related to patient's culture and ethnicity. Within cultures there are often multiple ethnic groups that may vary widely in their practices, beliefs, and mannerism. Individuals from Hispanic, Middle Eastern, and Mediterranean cultures tend to demonstrate expressive responses while those from Northern European and Asian cultures demonstrate stoicism. Cultures that demonstrate stoicism often regard it as honorable and any expression of pain is shameful and inappropriate (Al-Atiyyat, 2009).

Symptom Analysis (COLDERRA)

A comprehensive symptom analysis is critical to identifying the source and cause of the pain as well as appropriate treatment.

In addition to the symptom analysis questions, consider supplementary information that may relate to the pain. You can obtain this from information provided by the patient during the health history interview, or you can ask the patient at the time of the pain assessment. Such supplementary information includes the following:

- Is there a history of pain?
- What is your diagnosis and past medical history (e.g., diabetes, arthritis)?

Table 8-13 Reasons for pain responses

Stoic Response	Emotive Response
• Denial of pain	• Fear of pain
• Desire to be the perfect patient	• A desire for help and fear of not receiving it
• Avoiding loss of control	• Anger
• Avoiding worrying family	• Grief over loss of role and dignity
• Fear of addiction	• Exorcism of pain through the act of crying out
• Fear of overdose and side effects from pain medication	• Experiencing great pain
• Paying the price for past sin and future joys	
• Acceptance of pain	

- Is there a history of surgical operations or medical disorders?
- Has there been any recent trauma?
- Is there a history of heart disease, lung problems, stroke, or hypertension?
- Are you taking any medications (e.g. to reduce the pain; if so, did it help)?
- Do you have any allergies (e.g. to food or medicines)?
- Does the pain hurt on deep inhalation?

Other information may be obtained by observation:

- What is the patient's psychological status (e.g. depression, dementia, anxiety)?
- What is the patient's functional status, including activities of daily living? (Powell, Downing, Ddungu, & Mwangi-Powell, 2010)

Additional Information from the Older Patient A thorough pain assessment in the older patient includes additional questions related to the medication process in the treatment of pain. The additional questions are as follows:

- How are the analgesics administered?
- Does the patient with persistent pain have a separate order for receiving an analgesic on a regular schedule in addition to an as needed medication?
- How often is the patient receiving an as needed medication?
- Are the products being administered properly?
- Are there any problems with acquiring the medication?
- Can the patient/family afford the therapy that has been ordered? (Elliott, 2009)

Pain Assessment Scales

The most significant subjective variable of acute pain assessment is its intensity or magnitude (Jensen et al., 2005). This information is only as meaningful as reported by the patient. While the nature of this data is subjective, attempting to determine its objective quality is

Provider Inquiries	Clinical Reasoning/Logic
Characteristics: How are you experiencing the pain, what does it feel like? What is the intensity of the pain? (1–10 scale) Is it increasing in intensity?	Different types of pain have different characteristics. Nociceptive: Somatic—dull, aching Visceral—cramping squeezing Neuropathic—hot, sharp, shooting, burning, electrical, knifelike, prickling, tingling, dull, ache, cramp, throbbing, stabbing
Onset: Can you identify when you started experiencing the pain. Was/Is there anything that you can identify as bringing the pain on? Sudden or gradual?	Onset of pain may be described as abrupt and sudden, or insidious and gradual. Symptoms may be most severe on waking up in the morning, later in the day, or during the night. It is important to determine whether the patient identifies disturbance in sleep secondary to the pain.
Location: Can you identify where the pain is felt? (Whether it can be specifically located or not also provides information as to what type.)	Nociceptive: Somatic—localized, easy to identify Visceral—generalized, difficult to identify
Duration: How long is the episode of pain? Is it constant/is it intermittent? Cyclical?	Pain is described as acute when present within the first 3–6 months from the onset time and typically has an abrupt start with identifiable associated events. Chronic pain does not resolve within 3–6 months of its initiation and progresses beyond 6 months of duration
Exacerbation: What makes the pain worse, or increased? (Moving, walking sitting, turning, chewing, breathing, defecating, swallowing)	Helps to determine effects of pain on activities of daily living.
Relief: What helps to relieve the pain? Medications? (OTC, opioids, herbs, supplements) Certain activities, positions? Non-pharmacological interventions? (meditation, imaging)	Self-care behaviors vs. medical treatment gives insight into perception of pain and responses to it.
Radiation: Does the pain travel to any other part of the body? If so, where?	Referred pain often originates from a visceral organ. Common manifestations are superficial and deep hyperalgesia, autonomic hyperactivity, tenderness, as well as muscular contractions.
Associated Signs/symptoms: What other manifestations/symptoms do you experience with the pain?	Also helps to determine how pain affects overall functioning.

> ***PRACTICE POINT: Cultural/Ethnic variables related to pain scales***
>
> Most Western cultures have a visual spatial orientation of viewing objects, letters, and writing from left to right corresponding to the written languages. Eastern and cultures have a spatial orientation that goes from right to left, which also corresponds to their written language. Asian symbolic languages are oriented to go from top to bottom. Pain scales have been developed within the Western orientation, making it difficult for individuals from other cultures to correlate their orientation to the pain scales for accurate identification of their pain intensity. If this is the case, the pain scales may need to be adapted to make them meaningful for these individuals.

most helpful in assessing the effectiveness of any treatment. The most common method for determining this is with visual, incremental pain rating scales. Various pain assessment tools have been developed for this purpose.

The simplest and earliest acute pain assessment tool is the **visual analog scale (VAS)**, which is simply a 10 cm straight line with "no pain" on one end and "worst possible pain" on the opposite end (Figure 8-24). The patient is asked to mark on the line where their pain intensity is located. Another form of the VAS is two lines that form a triangle positioned on its side. It may be filled in with a color that starts out as a pastel but progresses to a deep intense color. The patient is asked to rate the pain intensity in the same manner. This may be referred to as a color analog scale (CAS).

Similar to the VAS are the **numerical rating scale (NRS)** instruments. They are similar to the VAS but add numbers on the line. Information is obtained by asking the patient to rate the intensity of pain on a scale from 0–10 (Figure 8-25). Some descriptive terms may be added to help the patient associate the pain with intensity.

Visual Analog Rating Scale

No pain —————————— Worst pain

Directions: Ask the patient to indicate on a 10 cm line where the pain is in relation to the two extremes. Measure from the left-hand side to the mark in centimeters to obtain the rating.

Directions: Ask the patient to indicate on the scale the severity of the pain, with 10 being considered the worst pain imaginable.

Color Rating Scale

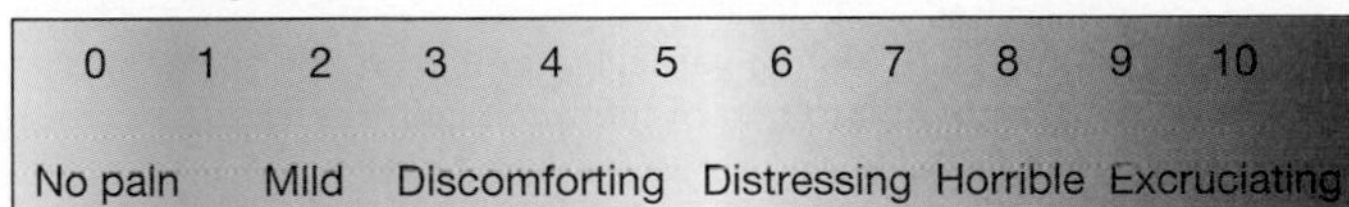

Numeric Rating Scale

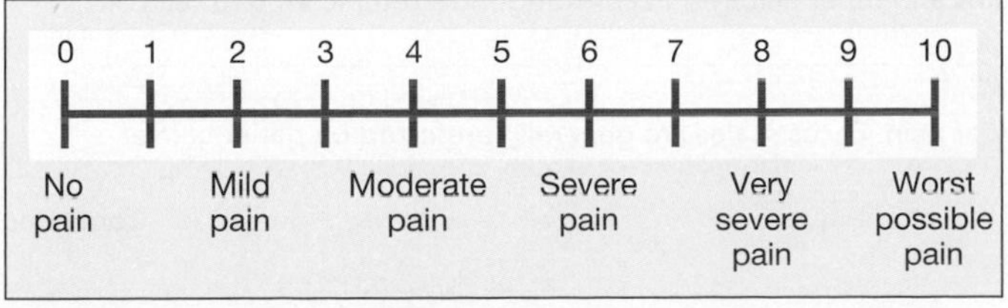

FIGURE 8-24 Visual, color, and numeric analog scales for pain assessment (not drawn to size)

Because these instruments are most useful with adults but not helpful with children, the **Wong-Baker Faces Pain Rating Scale** was developed. Still primarily based on a 0–10 scale, this scale replaces the written or numerical descriptors with six circular faces depicting the range of hurting represented the perception of pain to identify pain intensity. This scale is also helpful to use with patients who have poor language skills because the expressions are universal in their depiction of discomfort, and is most helpful for individuals 3 years of age and older. The "Oucher Scale" is similar to the Wong-Baker scale with the exception that is has photographs of faces depicting varying degrees of pain (Figure 8-25). For both of these tools, the child or adult is asked to pick out the face that best represents how much they hurt. Variations related to gender and ethnic groups may be used to adapt this scale to a particular individual.

The validity of these acute pain assessment instruments is well established, and they have also been found to correlate well with each other.

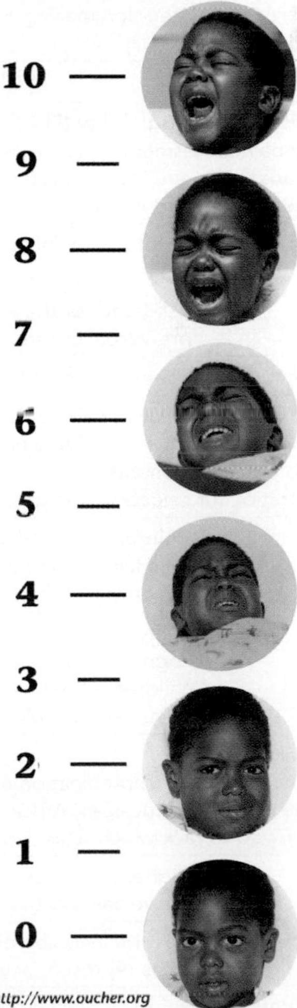

FIGURE 8-25 The Oucher Scale.

Source: The African American version was developed and copyrighted in 1990 by Mary J. Denyes, Ph.D., RN (Wayne State University, Retired) and Antonia M. Villarruel, Ph.D., RN (University of Michigan) USA. Cornelia P. Porter, Ph.D., RN, and Charlotta Marshall, RN, MSN, contributed to the development of this scale. Used with permission.

One important parameter to remember when assessing acute pain is the degree of pain during mobilization (Breivik et al., 2008). While the patient should be comfortable in bed and at rest, patients also require adequate pain control for deep breathing and coughing, required to prevent cardiac and pulmonary complications.

Other tools for assessing acute pain in children or individuals who are cognitively impaired, sedated, or disabled are based on the provider's objective observations rather than patient self-report and include the **FLACC Scale** and **CRIES Scale**. The FLACC (Face, Legs, Activity, Cry, Consolability) rates each of the 5 areas on a scale from 0–2. The FLACC Scale is best for children between the ages of 2–7. The CRIES (Crying, Requires O_2 for SaO_2 <95%, Increased VS, Expression, Sleepless) scale is used on infants up to 6 months of age and is scaled like the FLACC Scale only using different variables. The **COMFORT Scale** is also based on objective variables, and is used on adults who are unable to describe their pain as well as children. Table 8-14 compares the different pain intensity scales.

More sophisticated and longer assessment tools that obtain data related to other variables associated with chronic pain have also been developed. In contrast to acute pain measuring tools, these tools are also concerned with the pain experience over time and how the pain affects other quality of life variables. The **Brief Pain Inventory** is a 32-question assessment of the individual's pain experience and its effect on one's daily routine and activities and quality of life in general. The **McGill Pain Questionnaire** is comprised of groupings of descriptors of pain and requires the individual to rank the descriptors in each group. After this has been done, the provider scores the questionnaire and provides the individual with a pain rating index. More recently, the **PainQuality Assessment Scale** (PQAS) has been developed and differentiates between nociceptive and neuropathic pain (Breivik et al., 2008).

Table 8-14 Comparison of pain intensity scales

Whenever feasible, use a behavioral measurement of pain in conjunction with patient's self-report. If this not possible, then the interpretation of pain behaviors and decision making regarding pain treatment requires careful consideration of the context in which the pain behaviors were observed.	
Children's Pain Intensity Scales < 8 years old	
Face, Legs, Activity, Cry, Consolability (FLACC) Scale An observer-rated pain assessment measurement tool for use with children between the ages of 2 months–7 years or individuals who cannot communicate their pain. Numeric rating scale of 0-10 categorizes no pain, and mild, moderate, and severe pain. The scale has 5 criteria that are each assigned a score of 0, 1 or 2.	
Advantages	Helpful with children unable/unwilling to report pain; quick to use and easily reproducible. Validated for measuring postoperative pain in children with mild to severe cognitive impairment. Validated for the assessment of pain secondary to surgery, trauma, cancer or other painful diseases for all pre-verbal children (including infants). Validated for use with intubated adults in intensive-care units (ICU)
Disadvantages	Usefulness is undemonstrated in newborns, infants, children with special needs, and ventilated pediatric patients
Visual Pain Scale, or Visual Analog Pain Scale Allows patients to self report their level of pain by selecting a point on a line that represents their pain severity. The line may or may not be subdivided into equal increments from 0–10. A common example is a **Pain Thermometer** where the child points to a location on a thermometer illustration (or selects words) that best depicts their hurting.	
Advantages	Helpful with children unable/unwilling to report pain; quick to use and easily reproducible. Demonstrates good sensitivity and validity for most children at age 7 and older. Some pediatric patients find the pain thermometer easier to use than numeric or verbal descriptor (VD) scales.
Disadvantages	Usefulness among different pediatric populations and settings still unproven. May be difficult for use with cognitively/visually impaired patients. VAS does not appear to be a valid measure of pain for many younger (<7) children. Other measures of pain that are better understood by young children may be more valid indicators of pain. Parents' VAS ratings of their children's pain do not reliably reflect the pain reported by children
The OUCHER! Scale A self-report tool consisting of a combination of two separate scales: photographic faces and a 0-100mm vertical numerical rating scale that is available in three versions: Caucasian, African-American and Hispanic. When a child does not fit into one of the three cultures listed, the child should be allowed to pick which scale is preferred.	
Advantages	Higher test-retest reliability than WBFPRS as well as content and construct validity. Generally children at the age of five can use this tool, although some children as young as three are able to use it.
Disadvantages	Despite inclusion of three cultures, lacks females and other cultures. Faces not gender/ethnically neutral. Pain faces represent acute pain, not chronic pain
Faces Pain Scale/Revised (FPS-R) Child selects one of six pictures of line art faces that best depicts severity of pain. Faces scales are generally preferred by patients over analog scales when given a choice.	

Continued

Table 8-14 Comparison of pain intensity scales *(continued)*

Advantages	Has no smiling/tearful faces to confound the affective/sensory component; suitable for use with the most widely used metric (1-10); has a true 0 point and equal interval scales; available in >32 languages. Drawings are essentially ethnic and gender neutral so maybe applicable to broader demographic groups.
Disadvantages	Less preferred than the WBFPRS if available; original FPS had 7 faces and scored 0-6 metric; faces are too subjective and can be confusing; time required to look at the scale is tiring to pediatric patients, especially after surgery.
Wong-Baker FACES Pain Rating Scale (WBFPRS) The scale shows a series of faces ranging from a happy face at 0 ("No hurt") to a crying face at 10 ("Hurts worst"). The patient must choose the face that best describes how they are feeling.	
Advantages	Appropriate for patients with limited verbal or reading skills; simple and quick to use; neutral images are non-specific to gender or ethnicity; offers patients three options for rating pain: facial expressions, numbers, and words. Has been validated for use with patients in pediatric emergency departments
Disadvantages	Occasionally characterized as measuring patient's mood instead of pain level; the sad and crying faces not universally recognized culturally: stoicism may confound cultural interpretation of affect (smiles/tears) with actual pain intensity. Ratings are higher than scales with a neutral (no pain) face [FPS/FPS-R].
Adult Pain Intensity Scales (Unimpaired) Children 8 years and older	
Visual Analogue Scale (VAS) Patient marks the location of pain intensity on a 10 cm straight line. VAS variations may include color gradations (color analog scale) or sideways triangle.	
Advantages	Quick and simple to administer, easy to score and compare with previous ratings; multi-cultural application; widespread validation; considered optimum tool for assessing pain intensity variations. Possible to standardize VAS pain ratings for comparison of pain between different populations. VASs are versatile because they can be used to rate different dimensions of pain on the same scale (intensity and affect/unpleasantness).
Disadvantages	Markedly sensitive to changes in pain intensity may be too abstract for some patients to understand, especially those who have cognitive impairments, altered levels of consciousness post-op, limited visual acuity or manual dexterity, or are ESL speakers. Lacks standardization of terms of the descriptor anchors, length and orientation (vertical/horizontal) of the line.
Numeric Rating Scale (NRS) Patient self-reports pain intensity using a numerical scale of 0-10.	
Advantages	One of the quickest, simplest, and most frequently used instruments to measure pain. Easy to document for comparing with previous ratings; considerable validation; useful to detect treatment outcomes. Easy to instruct patients in correct use. Unlike VAS, can be administered verbally, reducing problems for patients with physical/visual impairments; also allows disabled patients to quantify pain intensity over the phone. Has also been found to be the most responsive scale, and able to detect gender differences in pain intensity.
Disadvantages	Some individuals unable to complete tool if only verbally instructed, decreasing reliability at age extremes, and for nonverbal or cognitively impaired patients. Numbers are too variable from individual to individual.
Verbal Descriptor Scale (VDS) Patient provided with a list of adjectives that describe intensity of pain (no pain, mild pain, moderate pain, severe pain, extreme pain, most intense pain imaginable). Patient responds by identifying applicable adjective. No visual representation of pain intensity.	
Advantages	Quick and simple to use, easily comprehended, well validated and sensitive to treatment effects; intuitively preferred by some patients instead of attempting to express their pain intensity numerically
Disadvantages	Dependence on patient's interpretation/understanding of verbal descriptors in language used to describe pain can be a challenge with different cultures; use problematic among very young/old, the cognitively impaired, and the illiterate, some evidence supports its use with cognitively impaired individuals.
Adult Pain Intensity Scales (Cognitively Impaired)	
Pain Assessment in Advanced Dementia Scale (PAINAD) Provider observes patient for five minutes before scoring a series of 5 behaviors: breathing, negative vocalization, facial expression, body language, and consolability. Scored on a 0-10 scale.	
Advantages	Helpful among adults unable to report pain; it is quick to use and easily reproducible. Patient may be observed during various conditions, such as during a social activity or following administration of pain medication
Disadvantages	Relies upon provider (proxy) to determine indicators of pain, rather than verbal self reporting. Sample size used for development of instrument was small.

Sources: Data from Ferreira-Valente, Pais-Ribeiro, & Jensen, 2011; Garra et al., 2010; Huguet, Stinson, & McGrath, 2010; Kane, Bershadsky, Rockwood, Saleh, & Islam, 2005; Pagé et al., 2012; Powell, Downing, Ddungu, & Mwangi-Powell, 2010; Shields, Cohen, Harbeck-Weber, Powers, & Smith, 2003; Stinson, Kavanagh, Yamada, Gill, & Stevens, 2006; Tomlinson, von Baeyer, Stinson, & Sung, 2010; von Baeyer, 2006; Zwakhalen, Hamers, Abu-Saad, & Berger, 2006

Summary

- Vital signs are measurements of the body's basic and essential physiological functions.
- The human body functions optimally within a narrow range of body (core) temperatures. These temperatures are maintained by thermoregulation within the hypothalamus by balancing heat production with heat loss.
- Thermal stress occurs when the body's core temperature increases or decreases. Hyperthermia results from failure of the thermoregulatory system, resulting in an increased core temperature. Fever (pyrexia) is a form of hyperthermia but results from a resetting of the thermoregulatory set temperature. Hypothermia results from exposure to cold external temperatures causing a greater heat loss than heat production.
- Pulse and ventilations are measurements of the cardiovascular and pulmonary systems with each one functioning within specified parameters that vary with the individual's age.
- Blood pressure is a measurement of the pressures within the vascular system and is a reflection of the work of the heart in maintaining blood circulation.
- Pain is an unpleasant sensory perception to malicious stimuli that functions as a warning for potential tissue damage or harm and is experienced as an acute or chronic condition. Pain travels through sensory pathways that go to the spinal cord and through the spinothalamic tract to the brain. Pain perception is affected by age, culture, and individual characteristics.

Review Questions

1. The provider assesses a patient's temperature and notes that it is elevated. The provider is aware that development of a fever is the result of which of the following?
   1. failure to thermoregulate
   2. an increase in heat production
   3. resetting of the thermoregulatory set point
   4. activation of inflammatory cytokines
2. The provider notes that the patient has a pulse with an irregular rhythm. To accurately assess the patient's peripheral pulse, the provider should do which of the following?
   1. Place the diaphragm of the stethoscope on the patient's chest.
   2. Count the radial pulse for 15 seconds and multiply the result times 4.
   3. Count the radial pulse for 60 seconds.
   4. Put the patient on a cardiac monitor.
3. The best approach for the provider to take to get an accurate count of a patient's ventilation rate is to do which of the following?
   1. Tell the patient to breath normally.
   2. Count ventilations after the pulse has been counted.
   3. Count ventilations only when the patient is asleep.
   4. Count the ventilation rate for 15 seconds and multiply by 4.
4. When recording a patient's mean arterial pressure, the provider is aware that the mean arterial pressure is not necessarily the average obtained of the systolic and diastolic pressures because of which of the following?
   1. Ventricular contraction is greater during systole.
   2. The heart rate needs to be factored in.
   3. Diastole is longer in duration that systole.
   4. Diastolic pressure is actually 10 mmHg less than what is obtained.
5. A patient with consistently high blood pressure readings asks the provider what is causing the high readings. Which potential causes of hypertension should the provider include in this explanation? (Select all that apply.)
   1. family history
   2. obesity
   3. dehydration
   4. dietary factors
   5. anxiety
6. When discussing pain with a group of students caring for postoperative patients the provider explains which stages of pain? (Select all that apply.)
   1. transduction
   2. transmission
   3. perception
   4. control
   5. modulation
7. When taking a history from a new patient, the patient shares with the provider that she had upper back pain during a recent rupture of an ectopic pregnancy. The provider classifies this pain as which of the following?
   1. referred
   2. cutaneous
   3. somatic
   4. visceral
8. The provider working in a clinic that treats primarily older adults is aware that most complaints of pain in this patient population are due to which of the following?
   1. other chronic conditions
   2. medication interactions
   3. acute injury
   4. the normal aging process
9. The provider is assessing the pain level of a patient. It is critical to keep in mind which of the following?
   1. Only objective data should be considered.
   2. Pain can only be perceived by the patient.
   3. The patient's gender is not a factor in this assessment.
   4. Pain relates only to the physical wellness of the patient.
10. Thermal regulation of the body is maintained by which of the following?
    1. evaporation, conduction, and convection
    2. convection, conduction, and transmission
    3. evaporation, radiation, and modulation
    4. conduction, modulation, and transmission

9

Documentation

Katherine A. Sward, PhD, RN

Dr. Lei had warned me about careful documentation before, but feeling perpetually buried under paperwork, language precision had seemed the least of my concerns. I regret that attitude now, sitting in the testimonial booth as an expert witness at the county courthouse. A recent patient on our psychiatry service, Mr. Kim, carried a diagnosis of paranoid schizophrenia, and we believed that he needed to be placed under temporary conservatorship to ensure that he was compliant with his medications. Mr. Kim didn't feel the same way, and requested a hearing.

The patient advocate cross-examining me, Mr. Dansko, is an imposing character, clad in a jet-black suit with a neatly trimmed grey beard. He is holding up printouts of my progress notes in his left hand and gesticulating wildly with his right. "And when you were charting Mr. Kim's status on the day prior to discharge you wrote, and I quote: 'Patient's judgment and insight today are better.' Is this not the case?"

Dr. Lei's voice echoes in my head: "Never write that someone is better; it's an ambiguous term. It could mean that they are improving, or that they are improved." I know what I had meant when I wrote that sentence, but now I have to justify it in court. "Yes, I did write that. But I intended to convey that Mr. Kim's clarity of thought was improved on that day relative to the previous encounter."

My flimsy explanation doesn't hold water and, for better or for worse (in our medical opinion, for worse), Mr. Kim is not placed under conservatorship. I had not anticipated my notes being subjected to this brand of scrutiny, much less an appearance in court. But the lesson is clear enough: document precisely, and say what you mean!

LEARNING OUTCOMES

1. Identify the primary purpose and function of documentation in a health care record.
2. Describe characteristics of health care data and distinguish between poor quality and high quality health care assessment documentation.
3. Analyze the relationship between health care data quality, patient safety, and costs.
4. Critique policies and regulations related to health care records.
5. Summarize reasonable expectations and potential limitations of electronic health records, particularly within the context of documenting assessments.

Quality patient care includes a comprehensive, well-organized history and physical examination, as well as the documentation of that information. Although the format, structure, and process of documentation varies from organization to organization, the need for and the principles of documentation are universal.

Background

Once data have been collected throughout the patient health history and physical examination, passing that information along to other members of the health care team becomes essential. The information is documented in the patient's **health care record**. Also called the medical record or patient chart, these are the documents pertaining to a patient's history, observations and findings, diagnoses, therapies, and status during an episode of health care. This chapter focuses on the records maintained by providers within a hospital or other health care organization (as opposed to **personal health records**, which are maintained by the individual).

Health care records have been kept, in one form or another, since antiquity. By the end of the 19th century, institutional policies began to mandate certain documentation, motivated in part by recognition of lost opportunities for education, research, and communication of best practices. Procedure notes and physical examination findings were among the earliest clinical data recorded; structured forms and graphs were not introduced until early in the 20th century.

As information required in a permanent health record increased, so did the need for a means of managing information (Siegler, 2010). In the second half of the 20th century, computer technology had evolved to the point of playing a significant role in managing information. With the rise in use of technology, the discipline of **informatics** emerged. Informatics is the study of how data, information, and knowledge are collected, classified, stored, and disseminated. The most prominent use of the term, at least in the United States, refers to its use in health care and related disciplines such as biology (Hersh, 2009).

The term *medical informatics* was introduced as an MeSH term in 1987 (DeShazo, LaVallie, & Wolf, 2009), but the adjectives preceding the word "informatics" have evolved across time and in different contexts (Hersh, 2009). The American Medical Informatics Association currently advocates *biomedical informatics (BMI)* as the generic or overarching term, defining BMI as the interdisciplinary scientific field that studies biomedical data, information, and knowledge for scientific inquiry, problem solving, and decision making, motivated by efforts to improve human health (AMIA, 2012a). Interdisciplinary sciences (sometimes called *transdisciplinary sciences*), such as informatics, integrate and synthesize theories and methods across multiple disciplines to develop a common research framework and methodology (Hall et al., 2008; Rebbeck, Pasket, & Sellers, 2010). In addition to *biomedical* informatics, other specific adjectives may refer to an area of emphasis within the field; for example *clinical informatics* (or *medical informatics*) may be used to refer to informatics practice focused on clinical health care whereas *bioinformatics* refers to a focus on biology and genetics. Specific names may also emphasize focus within a clinical discipline, such as *nursing informatics* or *dental informatics* (Hersh, 2009).

The goal of informatics is to improve human health (AMIA, 2012a), including the health of populations, communities, families, and individuals (ANA, 2008). Human health can be improved by optimizing information management and communication (ANA, 2008). Questions of interest to informatics scientists include how to collect and manage the information about a patient, and the most appropriate format for delivering that information to providers and patients. Fundamental issues include how patient data are gathered, how data are accessed and managed in an electronic format, and how to support efficient information retrieval. Informatics is distinguished from computer science and information science by the discipline's primary focus. The primary focus of informatics practice is people and information. **Health information technology** (HIT), sometimes called *information and communications technology (ICT)* when the technology has a strong information exchange or communications component, is seen as simply a tool that can be used to support people and how people can make best use of information (Hersh, 2009). Computers are not the only technology in the informatics arsenal, but they have become an important and ubiquitous aspect of managing health information (Hersh, 2009).

Informatics specialists come from diverse clinical and nonclinical backgrounds (Hersh, 2009). Informatics was recognized as a formal nursing specialty in 1992 (ANA, 2008). In September 2011, clinical informatics was approved as a formal subspecialty for physicians (AMIA, 2012b). Informatics is not just pertinent to those who formally specialize in informatics, though. Informatics competencies, including information literacy and computer and technology knowledge and skills, are increasingly required for all providers, at all levels of health care practice (ANA, 2008). Documentation is intended primarily to support patient care, and secondarily to support research, quality of care monitoring, education, and other clinical purposes. Health care providers are the "end users" of health information systems. For health IT to meet the needs of health care providers, providers at all levels of clinical practice need to be actively involved in the design, selection, implementation, and evaluation of health information systems. Information systems that meet the needs of the users and that fit into users' everyday lives can best be designed with the active involvement of those people for whom those health IT systems are primarily built (Shortliffe & Cimino, 2006).

Purpose and Functions of Health Care Records

The primary purpose of the health care record is to communicate to other members of the health care team the patient's story while receiving care in the health care facility. Managing the large volume of health care data is another important purpose for health care records. Data acquisition, record storage, information presentation, and access to information are part of managing health care data. The patient's health care record can validate the quality of care provided (Monarch, 2007) and provides the evidence supporting reimbursement (billing). Appropriate reimbursement relies upon accurate, comprehensive, and timely generation of billing codes. Coding errors due to inadequate medical documentation can have a significant impact on organizational revenue. A study in Australia (Cheng et al., 2009) showed the most important cause of coding inaccuracies (56% of billing code errors) were due to poor quality documentation. Ease of translating clinical documentation into billing codes has been cited as a crucial characteristic of a high-quality clinical note (Hanson et al., 2012).

The medical record is a legal record of the care given to the patient, thus every health record entry should be approached as if it were going to be held up to legal analysis (Monarch, 2007). Health care records are expected to be accurate and truthful, and are seen as credible evidence in legal proceedings, including professional negligence and malpractice lawsuits, disability determinations, worker's compensation actions, domestic abuse cases, and competency determinations (Austin, 2006). Records need to be kept in a manner that follows legal regulations and accreditation standards, professional practice standards, and standards within the organization (Osborn, Wraa, & Watson, 2010). Examples of documentation standards or policies include requirement for assessment by a registered nurse, specified intervals for reassessment, information from assessments must be used to identify and assign priorities for care needs, and documentation standards for assessment and management of pain (Osborn et al., 2010). Health records document professional accountability. The records need to clearly identify the author—the person who accepts responsibility for the accuracy of data in the record. Documentation of care given by another person, or of clinical information provided by another person, should clearly identify who provided the care and who was the source of the information (AHIMA workgroup, 2005; Harrington et al., 2011).

What is charted has other essential purposes related to how the data are used—what data are entered and the care taken with charting is more than just a matter of good record keeping. The information in a health care record has many other purposes, including the following:

- *Supporting evidence based clinical practice.* Evidence-based practice (EBP, also called *evidence-based medicine* or *EBM*) is the provision of health care based on decisions that make use of the best available scientific evidence in the context of the unique patient, provider, and environment (Hersh, 2009). Best available evidence includes evidence from randomized controlled trials and other research methods including descriptive and qualitative research, as well as incorporation of existing knowledge and scientific principles and information from case reports and expert opinion (Titler, 2008). EBP has been shown to improve health care quality, and EBP guidelines have been created for many conditions such as asthma or diabetes. However, health care knowledge is constantly changing and evolving. As more information is gathered in a specific area, the research evidence must be incorporated into the EBP (Titler, 2008). The massive amount of literature and clinical data that are available can make it difficult for providers to find answers to clinical questions (Geibert, 2006). EBP is dependent on extensive and accurate clinical data, and on methods to support the management and context-sensitive integration of research findings (Hersh, 2009). Electronic health care records (EHRs) are increasingly used to assist providers in this process (Geibert, 2006).
- *Supporting clinical decision making.* Clinical data, information, and knowledge are the cornerstones of health care practice, supporting appropriate decision making and clinical actions (ANA, 2008). Clinical decision support aids aim to interpret scientific knowledge in the context of individual patient-specific information. In today's environment, many of these aids have become computer-based, although paper-based decision aids persist. Whereas EBP guidelines present literature and best practices in a general sense, computer-based **clinical decision support** (CDS) systems are aimed at providing advice and guidance for individual, patient-specific decisions. The explosion of health care knowledge including the interplay between genetics and environmental influences, multiple diagnostic and therapeutic options, time constraints on providers, and regulatory and compliance demands, coupled with the fragmentation of health care services across providers and locations, fuels the need for support with clinical decision making (Greenes, 2007; Osheroff et al., 2007). CDS have become an essential part of health care as a means to avoid errors, optimize quality, and improve the efficiency of health care (Greenes, 2007; Kawamoto et al., 2005). Accurate and reliable clinical documentation is essential for decision support—without high-quality information about the patient's condition providers cannot make good decisions about how to provide care.
- *Planning and implementing quality improvement measures.* Evaluating data across patients can help to evaluate and measure the quality of care provided. Certain quality measures are required as **benchmarks** that allow care to be evaluated across institutions. The Centers for Medicare & Medicaid Services (CMS), for example, requires specific quality measures to be reported by any organization that receives payment from them (CMS, 2011).
- *Providing information for research studies.* Clinical research studies often use data extracted from the health record as a source of information. Data in the health record are used to identify eligible research participants, and clinical data may be used as a primary source of research data. There is increasing use of **knowledge discovery** (so called "data mining") systems that examine health care data to uncover new practice-based evidence and clinical knowledge (Hersh, 2009), using sophisticated linguistic and statistical techniques (Cusack et al., 2012).
- *Education.* The use of case studies has been a long standing tradition in health care education. Data aggregated across multiple records can provide powerful exemplars (Hersh, 2009).
- *Public health surveillance.* Health care documentation is a primary source of information for surveillance and detection of infectious diseases and other public health problems (Hersh, 2009).
- *Policy development, strategic planning.* Quality improvement and benchmarking data reflect the structures, processes, and outcomes of care. These metrics contribute to organizational and national strategic planning and policy development (Hersh, 2009).

Components of Health Care Documentation

Health care documentation serves so many purposes that it must constitute a complete, accurate, and up-to-date record. Any health care record, whether paper or electronic, should reflect each service a patient receives, including radiology, laboratory tests, and medications (Mitre, 2006; Shortliffe & Cimino, 2006). A significant challenge for managing health information is that each of those components may use unique ways of recording information, with different standards for vocabularies, different ways of identifying patients, and other inconsistencies that make it difficult to integrate information (Mitre, 2006).

Major components of electronic health records include, but are not limited to, the following:

- *Administrative components.* Administrative information includes registration and admission/discharge/transfer information that allow patients to be tracked across multiple visits. These systems contain patient identification, chief complaint, employer and payer information, and similar information. Advance directives, living wills, power of attorney for health care decisions, and similar documents may be part of the administrative system (Mitre, 2006).

- *Clinical documentation.* Today's clinical documentation records contain a wide variety of information including physiologic data, problem lists, allergies, and vital signs, in addition to assessments, physical exam findings, and multiple types of clinical progress notes and procedure notes. Medical devices can be integrated into the flow of clinical information, either directly or indirectly (Mitre, 2006).
- *Clinical decision support systems (CDS).* CDS are software components in which clinical observations are linked to databases of health care knowledge in a way that is intended to assist health care professionals with decision making. The extent of decision-making support can range from how information is organized on a page or screen (such as placing the most critical information in a location where it is most likely to be noticed), to simple alerts that point out unexpected test results or reminders for preventive services, to moderately complex drug–drug and drug–allergy checking (which integrate data from multiple locations in the record), to highly complex and interactive "expert" systems that support diagnostic reasoning or that help the provider select between treatment strategies (Greenes, 2007; Mitre, 2006). Although the potential benefits of CDS systems have been widely and consistently documented (Osheroff et al., 2007), the availability of CDS components varies widely between clinical settings and use of CDS in clinical care remains inconsistent (Greenes, 2007; Osheroff et al., 2007). CDS components are most valuable when they are supportive, patient specific, relevant, and provided in a manner that does not interfere with clinical workflow (Greenes, 2007; Kawamoto et al., 2005); the systems should provide specific recommendations rather than just assessments and must be provided at the time and location where decision making is happening (Kawamoto et al., 2005).
- *Computerized provider order entry (CPOE).* CPOE supports electronic ordering for laboratory and radiology tests and procedures, pharmacy orders, and sometimes ancillary orders and other services. CPOE systems range in sophistication from simply supporting the order placement, to systems that incorporate result reporting and CDS components such as order sets (grouping of orders for unique clinical areas or specific problems), alerts, drug–drug and drug–allergy checking, and other mechanisms for supporting decision making around orders (Greenes, 2007; Mitre, 2006).
- *Laboratory system components.* Laboratories typically have internal information systems, serving as a hub for managing findings from laboratory equipment, scheduling, billing, and similar services. Orders and results are communicated between the internal laboratory system and the clinical environment (Mitre, 2006).
- *Radiology system components.* Like laboratory systems, radiology services typically have both internal information systems, and systems to communicate orders and results to and from the clinical environment. Additionally, radiology systems need to manage a large volume of images and video, which is often done by means of a separate picture archiving and communications (PACS) system (Mitre, 2006).
- *Pharmacy system components.* Pharmacy systems tend to be highly automated for internal management and may even include technologies such as specialized robots. Pharmacy interaction in the clinical environment may include barcode medication administration systems, CDS components for drug–drug and drug–allergy checking, and even sophisticated decision support such as assisting with the ordering of appropriate antibiotics (Mitre, 2006; Shortliffe & Cimino, 2006).

Principles of High Quality Health Care Documentation

The health care record communicates information to, and is used by, a wide variety of people in many roles (Monarch, 2007). While the type and format of documentation varies among institutions, specific principles should be followed to assure proper and reliable documentation. Federal and state regulations must be followed, in addition to following the organizations specific policies and procedures for documentation (Harrington et al., 2011).

Confidentiality

Confidentiality is the *sine qua non* of documentation. The health record is the private record of the patient's health condition. Individuals who are caring for the patient need to view information related to the patient's health status. Information can only be shared with other individuals who are authorized to see the information. The Health Insurance Portability and Accountability Act (**HIPAA**) is a U.S. law that was passed in 1996. HIPAA includes two parts. One part protects health insurance coverage for people who become unemployed or who change jobs. The second part deals with standardization of health information systems and appropriate use of health information. Appropriate access to health records is balanced with patient rights' to privacy, confidentiality, and control over their own health information. HIPAA regulations provide clear definitions and implications related to assuring data confidentiality. Failure to comply with HIPAA requirements have severe consequences. Fines as well as criminal penalties can be imposed on the violating institution and the individuals involved (HHS, n.d.). In 2009, the U.S. government passed the HITECH act, which in addition to regulations mandating use of electronic health records, also increased the penalties for HIPAA violations. When HIPAA was first enacted, the maximum penalty for a HIPAA violation was $250,000. Now, the maximum fine is $1.5 million (Monegain, 2009). In general, information may be shared within an institution for purposes of patient care, payment for health care services, or for operational purposes such as quality assessments; or when authorized by the patient (HHS, n.d.).

Legibility

Legible data is essential to communicate effectively and appropriately, and federal regulations require that health care records be legible (Harrington et al., 2011). Illegible writing can cause serious problems from misinterpretation of information. One study, for example, examined case notes written by a variety of health care providers and found that 15% were so illegible that the meaning was unclear (Rodriguez-Vera et al., 2002).

Along with being legible, documentation should include correct spelling. A major issue with legibility is the use of abbreviations. In the past, it was not unusual for individuals and health care organizations to develop their own abbreviations, which presented problems for individuals moving from organization to organization. While abbreviations were used extensively in the past, their use has been widely eliminated to prevent misinterpretation of their meaning. If used at all, documentation should contain only universally known, acceptable abbreviations. Communication problems associated with abbreviations have been linked to errors in provision of health care. The Joint Commission maintains a document restricting the use of abbreviations and symbols in health care records, and requires that organizations maintain a list of approved and disapproved abbreviations (Joint Commission, 2011). Figure 9-1 shows the Joint Commission "Do Not Use" list.

Accuracy

Data accuracy is of critical importance (Harrington et al., 2011). Accurate data are free from error, bias, or assumptions, to the extent possible. Inaccurate data can lead to poor quality decisions and treatment errors, can cause false results for research studies and quality improvement measurement, and can lead health system managers to make incorrect estimates of care provision (Wasserman, 2011). Paper records have been shown to be only moderately accurate, with modest correlations between what is documented in the chart and what actually occurred in clinical care, with highest agreement for tests and medication orders, and lowest for history and physical exam data (Wasserman, 2011). While electronic health records might provide more complete data due to prompts for documentation, there is no guarantee that records will be more accurate simply because of the electronic format. Aspects of data accuracy include correctness, precision, specificity, and completeness.

Correctness

Correct data are a true representation of the patient's health status. Once correct data are obtained, they must also be documented

Official "Do Not Use" List[1]

Do Not Use	*Potential Problem*	Use instead
U, u (unit)	Mistaken for "0" (zero), the number "4" (four) or "cc"	Write "unit"
IU (International Unit)	Mistaken for IV (intravenous) or the number 10 (ten)	Write "International Unit"
Q.D., QD, q.d., qd (daily) Q.O.D., QOD, q.o.d, qod (every other day)	Mistaken for each other Period after the Q mistaken for "I" and the "O" mistaken for "I"	Write "daily" Write "every other day"
Trailing zero (X.0 mg)* Lack of leading zero (.X mg)	Decimal point is missed	Write X mg Write 0.X mg
MS MSO_4 and $MgSO_4$	Can mean morphine sulfate or magnesium sulfate Confused for one another	Write "morphine sulfate" Write "magnesium sulfate"

[1] Applies to all orders and all medication-related documentation that is handwritten (including free-text computer entry) or on pre-printed forms.

***Exception:** A "trailing zero" may be used only where required to demonstrate the level of precision of the value being reported, such as for laboratory results, imaging studies that report size of lesions, or catheter/tube sizes. It may not be used in medication orders or other medication-related documentation.

Additional Abbreviations, Acronyms and Symbols
(For *possible* future inclusion in the Official "Do Not Use" List)

Do Not Use	*Potential Problem*	Use instead
> (greater than) < (less than)	Misinterpreted as the number "7" (seven) or the letter "L" Confused for one another	Write "greater than" Write "less than"
Abbreviations for drug names	Misinterpreted due to similar abbreviations for multiple drugs	Write drug names in full
Apothecary units	Unfamiliar to many practitioners Confused with metric units	Use metric units
@	Mistaken for the number "2" (two)	Write "at"
cc	Mistaken for U (units) when poorly written	Write "mL" or "ml" or "milliliters" ("mL" is prefered)
μg	Mistaken for mg (milligrams) resulting in one thousand-fold overdose	Write "mcg or micrograms"

FIGURE 9-1 The Joint Commission Official Do Not Use List (From "Facts about The Official 'Do Not Use' List" by The Joint Commission. Copyright © 2013 by The Joint Commission. Reproduced by permission of The Joint Commission.)

correctly. It is not uncommon to write down, or enter into an electronic record, unintentional incorrect data. An example is a decimal place error, such as writing that a potassium value is 35 instead of 3.5 (Shortliffe & Cimino, 2006). Hospital policy would direct the next steps for correction or retraction of incorrect information (Harrington, et al., 2011).

Obtaining correct data during a health assessment may require asking some questions that may make the provider or patient uncomfortable, such as questions about sexual practices or drug use. To ensure accuracy, the provider may need to ask for clarification of certain points. It is better to ask the patient for clarification than to guess at what is being said or expressed. It is also important for the provider to be as clear as possible when asking questions, and not to presume that patients will always know how to respond to the questions. Failure to validate understanding of the question can result in unintentional, inaccurate data. Knowing proper physical assessment techniques and terms, and awareness of developmental variations, supports high-quality documentation and in turn supports high-quality decision making.

PRACTICE POINT: Focused Questions

In assessing a patient's history, it is common to ask about medications. A potentially unclear question would be "Do you take any medications?" It may lead to confusion because many patients will interpret this as "medications that a provider ordered and that I am taking now" and will respond accordingly (if they know the answer at all). Most patients will not include medications taken recently (such as antibiotics that were taken last week but now finished), nor will they include over-the-counter medications or herbal remedies in their response. This can cause the provider to overlook drug interactions that might be the cause of the patient's symptoms. A clear and focused approach would be to specifically ask about prescription medications and give a time frame: "What prescription medications have you taken within the past month?" You could then separately ask about OTC medications and herbal remedies, if you suspect a drug interaction as a cause of symptoms.

Precision

Precise data are sufficiently detailed to present a clear, useful description of the patient's health condition. It takes experience and practice to know what level of precision is needed. Precision implies some type of a quantitative response or measure. This is often difficult to do when there are no standardized units of measurement as is often the case with psychosocial concepts like anxiety or pain. Some type of quantitative measure allows the provider to evaluate changes over time (and differences between patients in some cases). For this reason, instruments such as pain scales, sleep inventories, or depression scales may provide valuable information in addition to narrative descriptions. Precision has aspects related to units (e.g., cm or inches for height) and granularity (e.g., measured to the nearest cm or mm), and aspects related to measurement error and variability (Wasserman, 2011). Precision, particularly with psychosocial measures, can be related to the idea of reliability or reproducibility of the measurement (Frank-Stromberg & Olsen, 2004). Some scales have been validated across multiple populations, but even when a validated scale is not available or for concepts such as pain where each patient may interpret the scale differently, quantifying the observation still provides some degree of precision that can be meaningful in describing the patient's condition.

Specificity

Data should be recorded in a manner that represents its nature. More often than not, specificity requires a conscious effort to document appropriately and avoid using generalizations. The most common generalization is "normal." However, definitions of normal are highly variable, and there is seldom an agreed upon gold standard that can be used for comparison. Charting by exception is similar to documenting "normal" in that only things that are found to be abnormal or different from the expected outcome are documented, and only activities that are not completed are noted in the chart. Charting by exception has received several challenges in court, and policies regarding use of normal, within normal limits, and use of charting by exception vary between institutions (NSO, 2012). Other generalized terms include ***fine***, ***usually***, and ***adequate***. Specific data are as detailed and descriptive as is necessary to provide an accurate account of the physical examination and patient's condition. Specific details can be used to determine changes for that particular patient. In some instances, overgeneralizations may be avoided by documenting **pertinent negatives**. Pertinent negative documentation is specifically identifying what is not there.

PRACTICE POINT: Describing IV Insertion Site

A standard assessment of a patient is to document the condition of an IV insertion site. Standard indicators related to the IV site include the presence or absence of redness, swelling, pain, warmth. The ideal situation is that none of these criteria are present; it is common to see documentation that the IV site is normal. More specific documentation, with pertinent negative findings, would be "No redness, warmth, swelling at the IV site, and patient reports no pain at the IV site." This is specific and lets a future reader of this documentation know what criteria were used when assessing this IV site.

Completeness

Documentation should include all the necessary information that is obtained from the history. The patient records should contain sufficient information so that someone reviewing the information would have a clear, detailed representation of what was happening with the patient. It's a common adage regarding health care records that "if it isn't written down, you didn't do it." Negative assessment information (pertinent negatives) can be as important as positive information. Documenting symptoms that are denied by the patient, such as absence of pain, indicates that this information was evaluated.

PRACTICE POINT: "If It Isn't Written Down, It Wasn't Done."

This is an important component of documentation for legal protection of a provider. Unless a witness could validate that an undocumented procedure or intervention was performed, it is very difficult to convince a lawyer or a jury that the expected care activity was completed.

Timeliness is an aspect of completeness. Documentation should be done in a timely manner and timely documentation is required by federal regulations, although local organizational policy is left to interpret what is defined as timely documentation (Harrington et al., 2011). Timeliness is determined by how the data are being used and their context. Many organizations have specific rules about the timing of certain forms of documentation, such as surgical or procedure

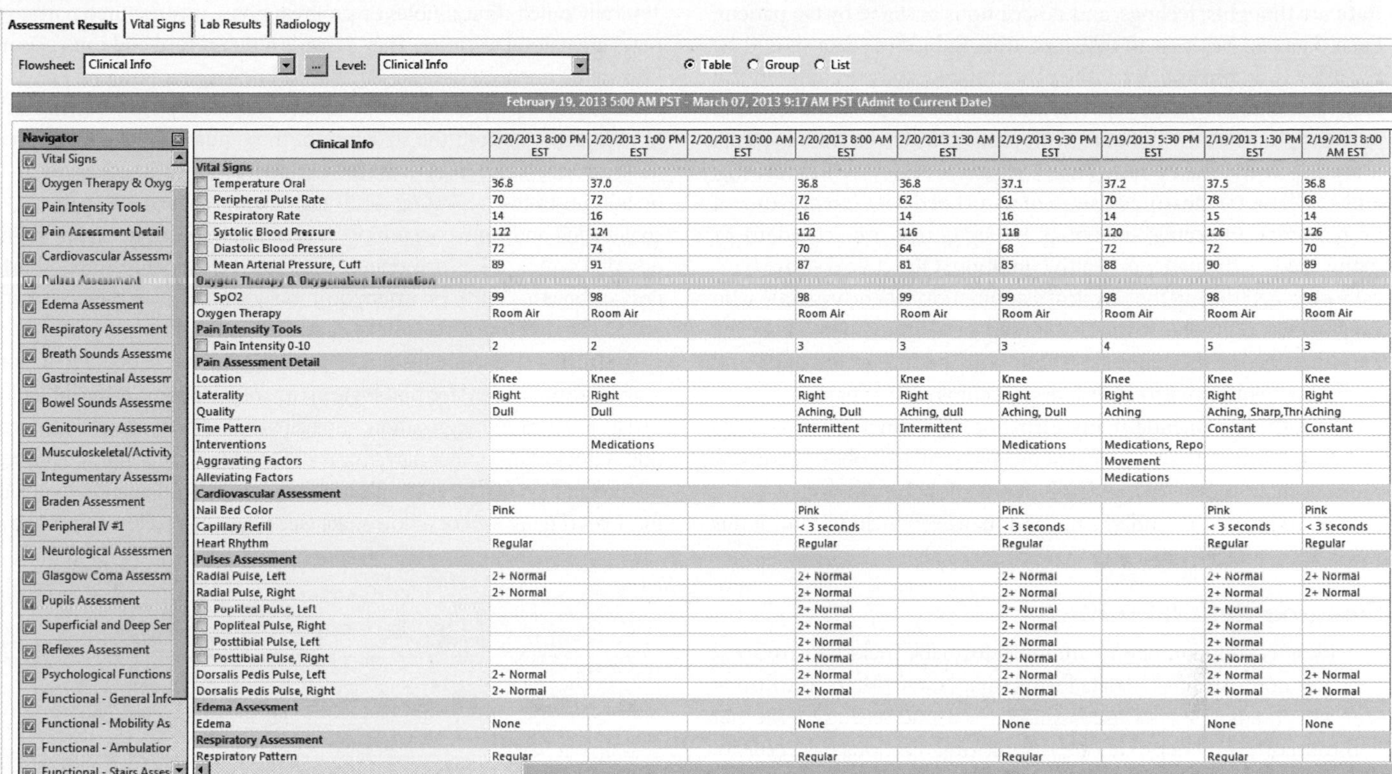

Clinical Info	2/20/2013 8:00 PM EST	2/20/2013 1:00 PM EST	2/20/2013 10:00 AM EST	2/20/2013 8:00 AM EST	2/20/2013 1:30 AM EST	2/19/2013 9:30 PM EST	2/19/2013 5:30 PM EST	2/19/2013 1:30 PM EST	2/19/2013 8:00 AM EST
Vital Signs									
Temperature Oral	36.8	37.0		36.8	36.8	37.1	37.2	37.5	36.8
Peripheral Pulse Rate	70	72		72	62	61	70	78	68
Respiratory Rate	14	16		16	14	16	14	15	14
Systolic Blood Pressure	122	124		122	116	118	120	126	126
Diastolic Blood Pressure	72	74		70	64	68	72	72	70
Mean Arterial Pressure, Cuff	89	91		87	81	85	88	90	89
Oxygen Therapy & Oxygenation Information									
SpO2	99	98		98	99	99	98	98	98
Oxygen Therapy	Room Air	Room Air		Room Air	Room Air	Room Air	Room Air	Room Air	Room Air
Pain Intensity Tools									
Pain Intensity 0-10	2	2		3	3	3	4	5	3
Pain Assessment Detail									
Location	Knee	Knee		Knee	Knee	Knee	Knee	Knee	Knee
Laterality	Right	Right		Right	Right	Right	Right	Right	Right
Quality	Dull	Dull		Aching, Dull	Aching, dull	Aching, Dull	Aching	Aching, Sharp,Thr	Aching
Time Pattern				Intermittent	Intermittent			Constant	Constant
Interventions		Medications				Medications	Medications, Repo		
Aggravating Factors							Movement		
Alleviating Factors							Medications		
Cardiovascular Assessment									
Nail Bed Color	Pink			Pink		Pink		Pink	Pink
Capillary Refill				< 3 seconds		< 3 seconds		< 3 seconds	< 3 seconds
Heart Rhythm	Regular			Regular		Regular		Regular	Regular
Pulses Assessment									
Radial Pulse, Left	2+ Normal			2+ Normal		2+ Normal		2+ Normal	2+ Normal
Radial Pulse, Right	2+ Normal			2+ Normal		2+ Normal		2+ Normal	2+ Normal
Popliteal Pulse, Left				2+ Normal		2+ Normal		2+ Normal	
Popliteal Pulse, Right				2+ Normal		2+ Normal		2+ Normal	
Posttibial Pulse, Left				2+ Normal		2+ Normal		2+ Normal	
Posttibial Pulse, Right				2+ Normal		2+ Normal		2+ Normal	
Dorsalis Pedis Pulse, Left	2+ Normal			2+ Normal		2+ Normal		2+ Normal	2+ Normal
Dorsalis Pedis Pulse, Right	2+ Normal			2+ Normal		2+ Normal		2+ Normal	2+ Normal
Edema Assessment									
Edema	None			None		None		None	None
Respiratory Assessment									
Respiratory Pattern	Regular			Regular		Regular		Regular	

FIGURE 9-2 A flow sheet in an electronic health record

Source: "A Flowsheet in an Electronic Health Record" from *EHR Interface* by Cerner Corporation. Reproduced by permission of Cerner Corporation.

notes. As a rule of thumb, documentation should be completed as near to the time of data collection as possible, so you do not need to rely on your memory. A benefit cited for electronic health records is that such records allow for point of care documentation; however some providers have expressed concerns that documentation in an electronic health record while at the bedside could detract from patient–provider interactions (Cusack et al., 2013).

Conciseness

Concise documentation communicates significant data without excess verbiage. Techniques employed in narrative notes include nonrepetition of introductory phrases, and use of phrases instead of full sentences. Because the subject of the documentation (the patient) is understood, it is appropriate to begin a sentence with a verb. You may often eliminate references to "he" or "she" or references to the patient's name. Flow sheets or checklists, and templates or structured encounter forms can help with conciseness. Flow sheets and checklists are common in paper records, and increasingly seen in electronic health records as well, as shown in Figure 9-2. Free text notes should add to and enhance, rather than duplicate, the information on a flow sheet (Wasserman, 2011).

Reliability

Reliable data are able to be reproduced (Coulehan & Block, 2006). This is easier to achieve in controlled laboratory experiments than with human responses, of course. In health care organizations, reliability might be demonstrated when patients are interviewed by multiple individuals from different disciplines who document the same information. Each individual who interviews the patient may have a slightly different interpretation of the patient's story; however, each interpretation should not be so radically different that they are unrelated to each other. Sometimes valid reasons for differences exist, such as in cases where

- interviewers may hear the same story, but may place emphasis on different aspects.
- interviewers may ask for the same information, but pose the question slightly differently.
- interviewers may explore a different aspect of the patient's response that may cause the patient to recall more or different data.
- patients may emphasize different aspects of their story during subsequent interviews.
- patients may change their stories according to what they perceive to be what the interviewer expects or wants to hear (social desirability).

Characteristics of Health Care Data

Unlike a field such as banking, in which all the data are similar in structure (involving currency and exchange of money or similar assets), a primary characteristic of health care data is **heterogeneity** (nonuniformity). Data come from multiple sources, and many types of health care data exist, including what patients say, what providers observe, and what we record using various devices and monitors.

Just as in evaluating literature, health care data have primary and secondary sources. **Primary data sources** arise directly from a patient encounter and represent the majority of health care data that are documented. Sources that are farther removed from the patient or event (**secondary data sources**) may be more subject to interpretation or bias, and therefore are considered as possibly less accurate. Secondary sources include family members, friends, significant others, and similar sources. Even reports from other health care facilities are sometimes considered secondary sources of data.

Health care data may be subjective or objective. **Subjective data** are thoughts, feelings, and descriptions as stated by the patient. Such data can be open to interpretation. Subjective data should be recorded verbatim as to what the patient stated, and are considered at face value. Subjective data are typically seen in the health history and in descriptions of the patient's symptoms. **Objective data** are data that the provider takes in through the senses (sight, feeling, hearing, and smell) or are measured using some sort of device (an instrument or monitor). Objective data may be signs that are related to or manifested by the patient's health condition. Objective data are typically obtained during the physical examination. There are some who suggest that only objective data should be documented. However, data that record the patient's descriptions can be informative and useful, particularly with subjective symptoms such as pain.

Health data include many forms of data, ranging from words and narrative text, to categorical or ordinal (ordered) observations, to numeric quantities at various levels of precision. Health data may also include structured or coded data, and may even include continuous waveforms, images, or sounds (Wassman, 2011).

Documentation Formats

Providers can document in multiple formats, including free-text narrative notes, structured data forms, images, and others. The format and terminology (words used) varies from one setting to another and from one provider to another. Some organizations have policies specifying a particular format for a given purpose (e.g., a specified format for preoperative notes).

THINK LINK: Subjective and Objective Data

A provider notes the following findings. Which of the following are subjective data? Which are objective?

"Jane Doe is a 25-year-old female presenting with abdominal pain, anxiety, and malaise. Skin is warm and damp, color flushed. Temperature 38.2 C (oral). Abdomen is firm and tender to palpation."

Hint: Subjective data must be reported by the patient. Objective data can be seen or observed by the provider.

Narrative documentation is used in most settings (Figure 9-3). Typically called clinical notes or progress notes, unstructured narrative notes are natural to create. They provide a rich record and can encompass subtle nuances; they are flexible and descriptive accounts of what occurred during a patient's stay (Osborn et al., 2010). However, the lack of uniformity in both the structure of these notes and language used makes it difficult to retrieve data for secondary purposes such as research or administrative reporting, and aggregating data across patients is challenging and time consuming. For example, narrative notes might describe symptoms as orthopnea, dyspnea, difficulty breathing, shortness of breath (SOB), or in any number of other ways (Wasserman, 2011). Handwriting and legibility can be an issue with paper notes.

Structured documentation, especially when that documentation makes use of standard terminologies, is intended to remedy the difficulty in data retrieval and aggregation, and helps ensure that valuable information is not lost in a sea of narrative text. Structured (or semi-structured) documentation can be as simple as a standard documentation template for notes (Figure 9-4) or a flow sheet (see Figure 9-2). Flow sheets allow

1000 RT at bedside to help move pt. back to bed. Servo Control Set on bed & Cares Completed Bag [illegible] as mucous fistula was leaking and getting under Skin looks clean, free of redness/breakdown Pt responds to Stim but doesn't

A

* Final Report *

DELIVERY ROOM REPORT

PROVIDER: ROBYN GELLAR, MD

The patient was complete and pushing for just over three hours. She had adequate epidural anesthesia. Over the last 30 minutes of pushing, thick meconium was noted. The patient was completely exhausted and requested assistance with delivery also. Bladder was straight cathed for a minimal amount of urine. The KIWI cup was applied to the fetal head at the median flexion point. Fetal head position was left occiput anterior, 3+ station. During four contractions over a ten minute period, the fetal head was finally delivered. DeLee suction was done on the perineum with copious amounts of aspirate from the nasopharynx and oropharynx. The remainder of the baby was delivered and handed off to the waiting neonatal team. Viable male, apgars eight and eight , weight 8 pounds, 2 ounces. Placenta delivered intact and spontaneous with a three vessel cord. Estimated blood loss was less than 750 mL. No episiotomy was done. She had a 1+ cm left hymenal laceration that was repaired. She was stable postpartum, and fundus was firm. No complications.

B

FIGURE 9-3A–B Narrative note in a paper chart **(A)** and in an electronic chart **(B)**

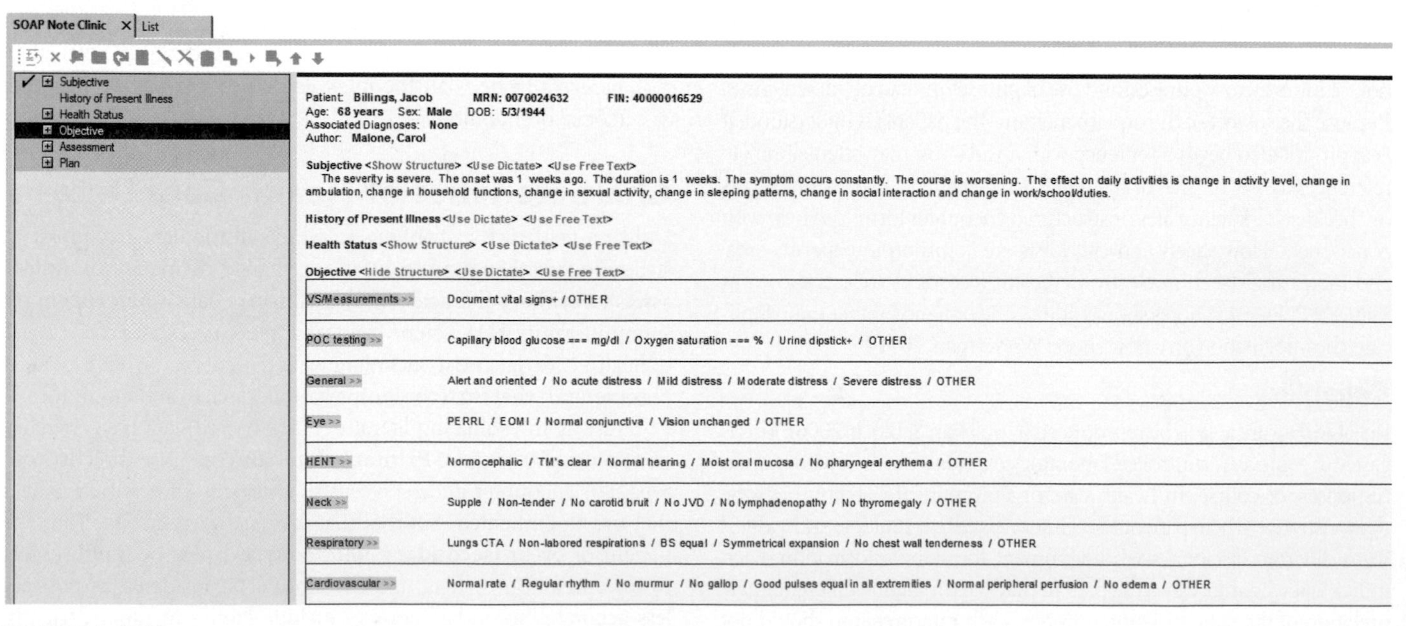

SOAP Note Clinic | List

Subjective
History of Present Illness
Health Status
Objective
Assessment
Plan

Patient: **Billings, Jacob** **MRN: 0070024632** **FIN: 40000016529**
Age: **68 years** Sex: **Male** DOB: **5/3/1944**
Associated Diagnoses: **None**
Author: **Malone, Carol**

Subjective <Show Structure> <Use Dictate> <Use Free Text>
The severity is severe. The onset was 1 weeks ago. The duration is 1 weeks. The symptom occurs constantly. The course is worsening. The effect on daily activities is change in activity level, change in ambulation, change in household functions, change in sexual activity, change in sleeping patterns, change in social interaction and change in work/school/duties.

History of Present Illness <Use Dictate> <Use Free Text>

Health Status <Show Structure> <Use Dictate> <Use Free Text>

Objective <Hide Structure> <Use Dictate> <Use Free Text>

VS/Measurements >>	Document vital signs+ / OTHER
POC testing >>	Capillary blood glucose === mg/dl / Oxygen saturation === % / Urine dipstick+ / OTHER
General >>	Alert and oriented / No acute distress / Mild distress / Moderate distress / Severe distress / OTHER
Eye >>	PERRL / EOMI / Normal conjunctiva / Vision unchanged / OTHER
HENT >>	Normocephalic / TM's clear / Normal hearing / Moist oral mucosa / No pharyngeal erythema / OTHER
Neck >>	Supple / Non-tender / No carotid bruit / No JVD / No lymphadenopathy / No thyromegaly / OTHER
Respiratory >>	Lungs CTA / Non-labored respirations / BS equal / Symmetrical expansion / No chest wall tenderness / OTHER
Cardiovascular >>	Normal rate / Regular rhythm / No murmur / No gallop / Good pulses equal in all extremities / Normal peripheral perfusion / No edema / OTHER

FIGURE 9-4 SOAP note

Source: "SOAP Note" from *EHR Interface* by Cerner Corporation. Reproduced by permission of Cerner Corporation.

for documentation of routine observations, such as vital signs, over time, allowing visualization of trends (Osborn et al., 2010).

Structured documentation could also be detailed in a form with all data represented in standardized/coded terminology (see Figure 9-5). Most often, health care documentation falls somewhere between these two extremes, with portions of the documentation being structured and other documentation in unstructured or semi-structured format (Wasserman, 2011).

Documentation Organizing Strategies

A variety of strategies exist for organizing the information in a health record. Some organizations use a primarily narrative approach, with clinical notes and flow sheets organized chronologically or by categories defined by the type of document (e.g., separate part of the chart for the vital sign flow sheets, intake and output record, physician notes, and nursing notes). A problem-oriented medical record (POMR) may be used in acute and long term settings, in which documentation is organized as baseline data, a problem list, a plan for each problem, narrative progress notes, and a discharge summary (Osborn et al., 2010).

Narrative documentation paints a rich picture but can become lengthy and repetitive. The acronym FACT describes a strategy that uses notes and flow sheets to reduce repetitive documentation. The key elements of a FACT approach are F-Flow sheets for specialized services, A-Assessments that are standardized, C-Concise progress notes that augment flow sheet documentation, and T-Timely entries. The FOCUS system (sometimes called D-A-R system) is an approach to problem-oriented documentation that was designed to highlight the nursing process. FOCUS documentation uses flow sheets to document routine care and monitoring, and notes to augment the flow sheets. Notes are organized by focus area (e.g., a particular concern, nursing diagnosis, or symptom) and contain the data (both subjective and objective), action (plans and actual interventions), and response. Some organizations use charting by exception (CBE) to eliminate repetition, with documentation addressing only abnormal or unexpected findings. A CBE approach to charting should be designed around well-established and explicit guidelines and standards of care, so that the "exception" is sufficiently clear (Osborn et al., 2010).

The lack of structure in a free text narrative note can make it difficult to determine changes in a patient over time, or to aggregate information across patients (Wasserman, 2011). Semi-structured documentation includes a documentation template to organize the data. For example, many organizations use a template called SOAP to organize information: S—Subjective data; O—Objective data; A—Assessment (the patient problem or diagnosis); P—Plan (often with goals or expected outcomes for each specific problem). Variants (SOAPIE, SOAPIER) add additional components to the format: I—Interventions (what was actually done), E—Evaluation of the response to interventions, R—Revision (changes to the plan of care for a given problem). The problem-intervention evaluation (PIE) format is an alternative note template commonly used in settings where condition changes rapidly. Problems are numbered, and interventions and evaluation are labeled with the corresponding problem number (Osborn et al., 2010).

Electronic Health Records

Computers have become ubiquitous in health care as tools used to acquire data and knowledge, and communicate information between people. These tools are useful to help manage information overload, promote efficient and reliable data capture, and to support decision making. Mobile devices (tablet computers, iPads, smart

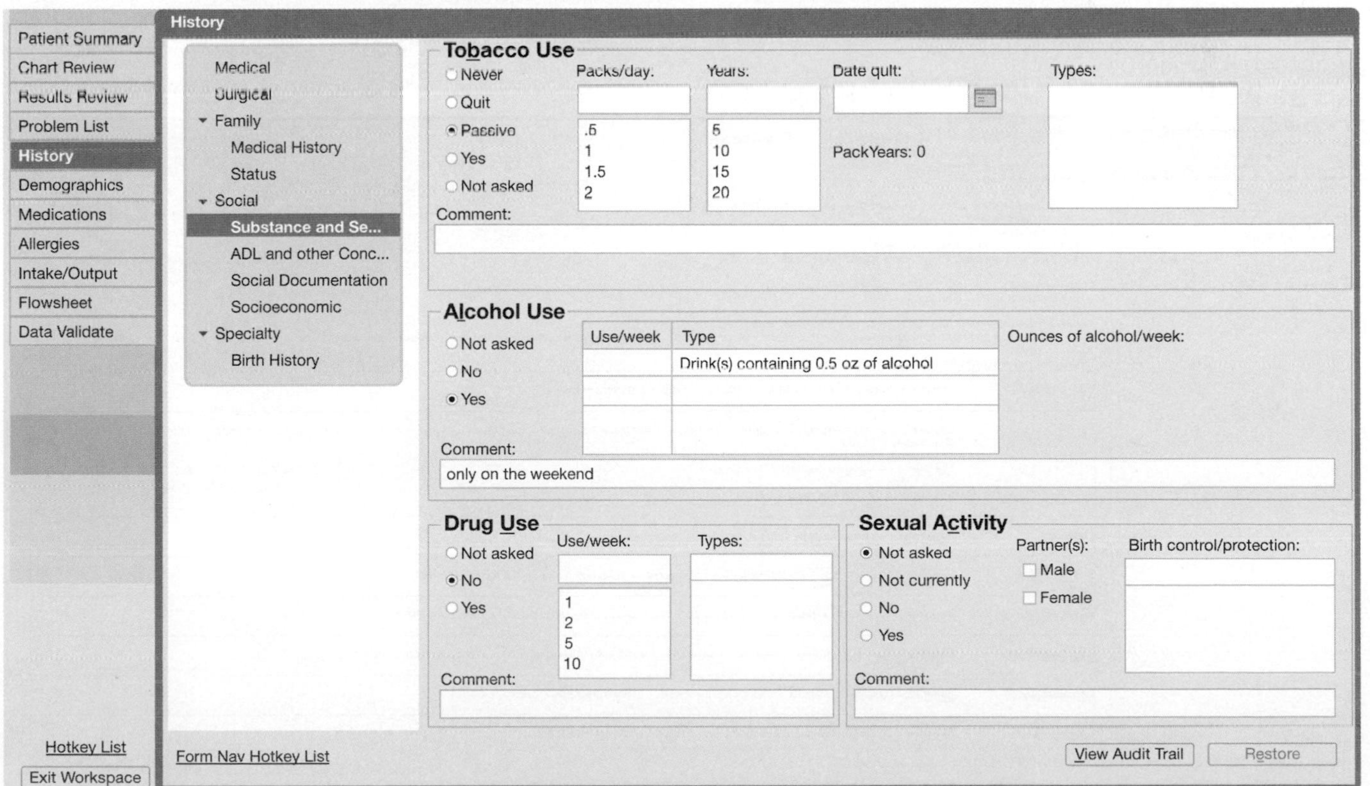

FIGURE 9-5 Structured documentation

Source: From *EHR Interface* by Cerner Corporation. Reproduced by permission of Cerner Corporation.

phones, and the like), patient monitoring systems, IV pumps, medication administration systems, results reporting, ordering systems, and computerized documentation are just a few examples of computers integrated throughout health care processes. Health care documentation is increasingly moving from paper to **electronic health records**. An EHR is a version of the health care record that is maintained within a computer system. The terms *electronic health record (EHR)* and *electronic medical record (EMR)* are sometimes used interchangeably. In other cases, the electronic medical record implies the record within a single institution, whereas electronic health record may refer to a longitudinal record that can include information from multiple institutions.

Despite documented benefits, health care has lagged behind other industries in the use of information technology (Wasserman, 2011). A presidential mandate in 2004 challenged health care organizations to implement electronic health records throughout the U.S. by 2014. Despite broad consensus that use of electronic health records and other forms of health information technology (HIT) should lead to safer, higher-quality, well-coordinated and efficient patient-centered care, the adoption of electronic health records has been sluggish (Cipriano, 2011; Hersh, 2009; Karsh, Weinger, Abbot, & Wears, 2010). The American Recovery and Reinvestment Act (ARRA) of 2009, and the subcomponent referred to as HITECH, augmented the 2004 mandate through financial incentives for "meaningful use" of electronic health records, and financial penalties for organizations failing to make use of EHRs. Health care providers should keep in mind that EHRs are simply a tool, not an all-encompassing solution. It is in how the EHR are used that the real benefits in national health care transformation efforts will be seen (Wasserman, 2011).

General expectations and limitations of electronic health records are discussed in the following sections. Each chapter of this text also contains examples of expectations and limitations specifically relevant to that assessment topic.

Expectations of Electronic Documentation

In a paper record, every page should be marked with the patient's name and ID number. Similarly, electronic records should show the patient's name and ID number on every screen (Figure 9-6). Both paper and electronic records are marked with the date and time, which should be as close as possible to the date and time at which the observation was made or the care occurred.

One way that paper and electronic records differ is in how the records are "signed" or authenticated. Paper records typically use a handwritten signature. Electronic records, on the other hand, use electronic "authentication" (such as a combination of a user name and password) as the "signature" for the provider (Harrington et al., 2011). Documentation is "signed" by attaching an authorized provider's identification to the record. Because electronic authentication is the equivalent of the user's handwritten signature—it is his or her "identity" within the system—each person should have his or her own login information and should protect that login carefully. In many health care organizations, sharing your login information is considered a significant breach of security (AHIMA workgroup, 2005).

When an error is made in a paper health record, typical error correction includes a single line through the entry (making sure the original entry is still legible), indicating "error" and the reason for the error, signature and date of who marked the data in error, and documentation of the correct information. Similar principles should be followed in an electronic health record—the entry should not be deleted, but should be marked as an error (Figure 9-7). The original data should be viewable, the person making the change should be identified, and they should be able to note the reason for the change (AHIMA workgroup, 2005; Harrington et al., 2011).

Electronic health records provide the ability to access and share data appropriately, when and where needed. Because information is more accessible, electronic records can reduce unnecessary orders and tests

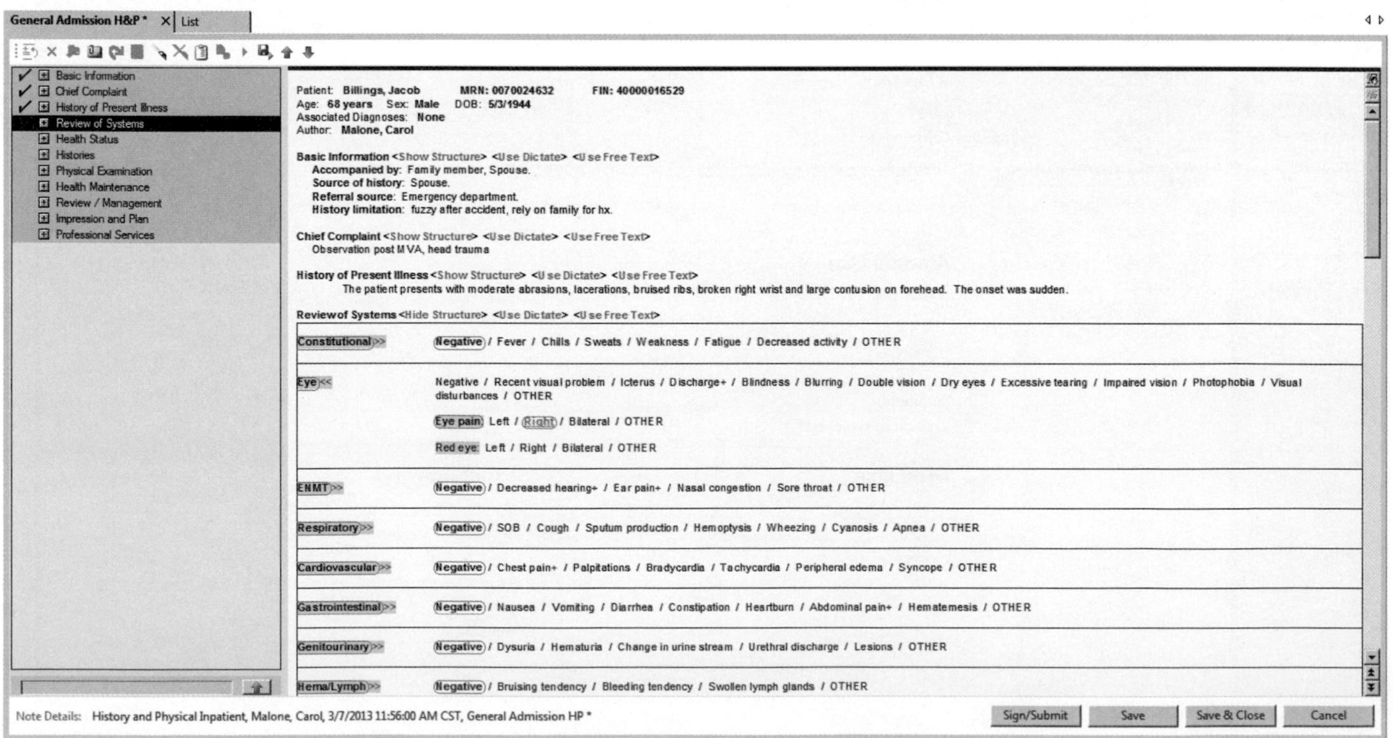

FIGURE 9-6 Every screen in an electronic health record should clearly show the patient's identifying information.

Source: From *EHR Interface* by Cerner Corporation. Reproduced by permission of Cerner Corporation.

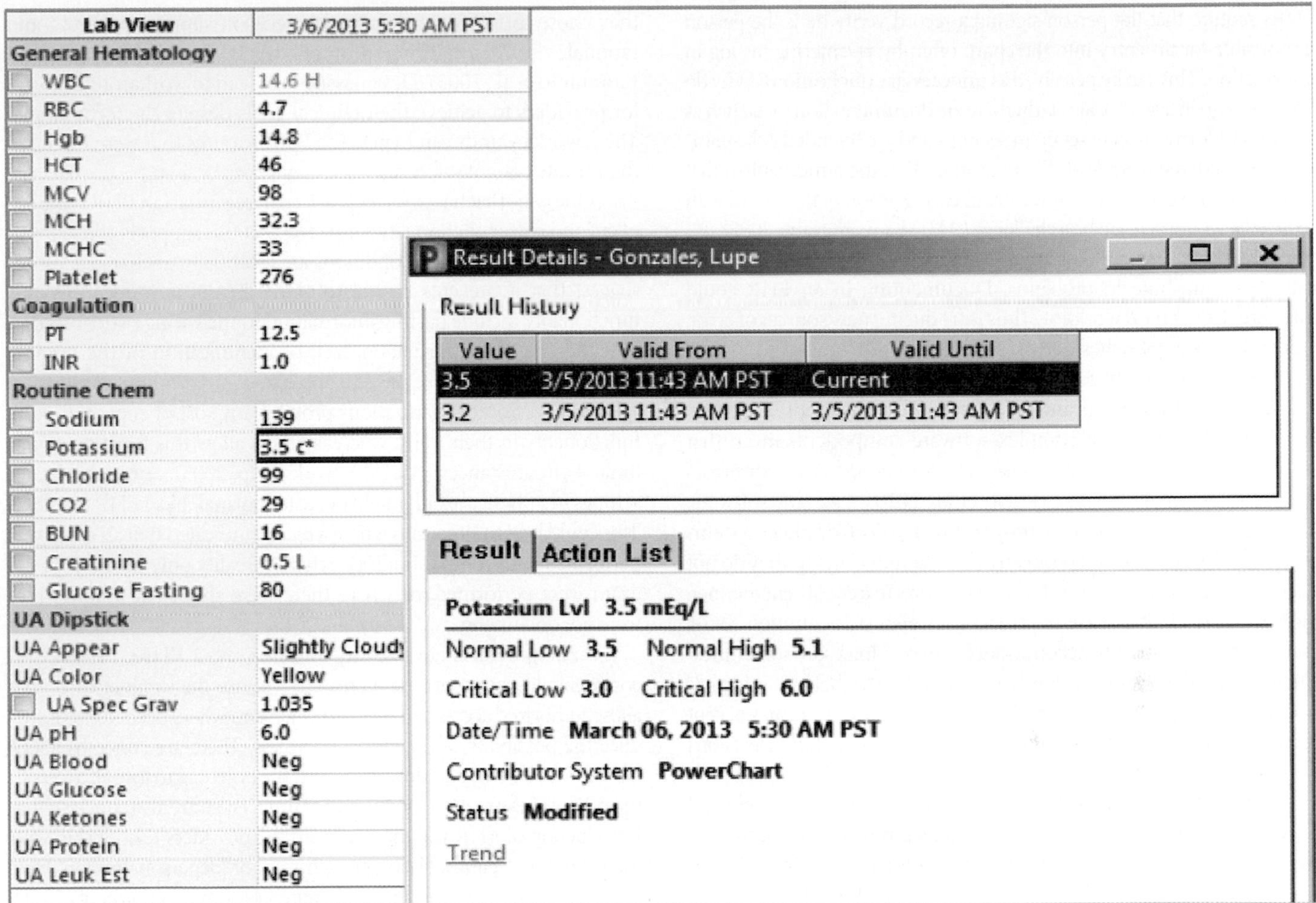

FIGURE 9-7 Electronic charts should allow errors to be corrected, but information should be marked as modified, not deleted.

Source: From *EHR Interface* by Cerner Corporation. Reproduced by permission of Cerner Corporation.

(e.g., duplicate labs). Increased legibility and more complete and comprehensive documentation have been shown to be present with use of electronic health records. Electronic records reflect a chronology of a patient's health care. Many contain the ability to create customized clinical views. Electronic records allow multiple views of the same data, with varying levels of detail and different time chronologies (AHIMA workgroup, 2005). For example, observations of intake and output may occur hourly, with views automatically compressing to 8- or 12-hour "shift views" or daily intake/output balances, perhaps reflected in a chart or graph.

Legibility is one area in which electronic records almost always outperform paper records. Electronic information systems have been shown to reduce medication errors, enhance efficiency, and improve patient safety, both by eliminating problems caused by communication issues and illegible handwriting and through clinical decision support (CDS) functions such as medication error checking (Greenes, 2007; Karsh et al., 2010; Kawamoto et al., 2005). Electronic information systems can facilitate access to health information and thus support evidence-based practice. Electronic records often contain order sets, document templates, and standardized terminologies. These are intended to reduce the use of abbreviations, increase assurance that all readers understand the meaning of terms, and reduce communication errors (AHIMA workgroup, 2005). When an EHR includes clinical decision support (CDS) functions, the knowledge underlying those functions should be evidence based and validated/accepted by the organization (AHIMA workgroup, 2005; Oshcroff et al., 2007).

Limitations of Electronic Documentation

Many health care organizations operate with a minimum number of providers. Shortages in nurses and physicians are compounded with increasing acuity of hospitalized patients. This leaves little time for learning to use new technology such as electronic health records. Software usability factors such as the training needed to learn a system and ease of use are critical influences on the success or failure of an EHR implementation. There is often an initial increase in documentation time when EHR are introduced into an environment, although that tends to resolve as providers become accustomed to the new system (Holroyd-Leduc et al., 2011).

Substantial costs are required to install and maintain an EHR, which can be a significant barrier to their use (Wasserman, 2011). The financing for EHR implementation projects is nontrivial. Initial set up costs are only a fraction of the overall costs for EHR implementation (Lewis, 2012; Wasserman, 2011). Direct costs are compounded by the need to maintain a staff of personnel with specialized expertise (Wasserman, 2011). The majority of health care administrators voice some level of discomfort with the costs of an EHR project and many organizations report that they underestimated the costs, effort, and impact of fully implementing an EHR (Lewis, 2012).

Electronic documentation presents unique authentication issues. While it is technically possible for a computer to keep track of who is logged in to the record and to automatically "sign" documentation based on that login, for professional accountability purposes many

EHRs require that the person signing a record verify he is the person responsible for an entry into the chart, often by re-entering his log in information. This can be perceived as unnecessary duplication ("Why do I need to sign in again?"). Similarly, there are documentation tools such as assessment forms that are set up in sections and are intended to be completed by different people at different times. Finding a mechanism that appropriately balances authentication of each portion of the record with reduced user burden can be a challenge (AHIMA workgroup, 2005).

The same features that are anticipated to make EHR beneficial can also contribute to problems. Documenting in an EHR could interfere with clinical workflow, thus introducing new sources of error. Standardized approaches across patients are anticipated to reduce unnecessary variability. However, because HIT is built by humans it will invariably have errors and failures. Standardized approaches and the interactions between complex software components mean that software errors ("bugs") can cause catastrophic effects, with errors spread across many patients (Karsh et al., 2010). Like any software, EHR can only do what they are programmed to do. Computer systems in general follow rules and perform computations quickly; they do not become tired or distracted and will repeat tasks in a consistent manner. However, they lack a sense of ethics. They also lack common sense, and cannot very readily accommodate "fuzzy" logic or "sometimes" situations. There is a natural tendency for people to "believe" information simply because it comes from a computer, and people may accept recommendations from a computer that are worse than the decisions they would make unaided (Karsh et al., 2010).

Information presentation is known to influence clinical decision making. Design details can affect information availability, perceptions about the importance of information, and in other ways affect clinical decisions and behavior (Karsh et al., 2010). Not all CDS recommendations apply to every patient. Providers should evaluate alerts, reminders, and treatment suggestions based on their knowledge about and analysis of the patient's condition. The record should include the provider's response to decision support—whether they chose to follow or disregard a decision support prompt—and rationale for disregarding prompts (AHIMA workgroup, 2005; Kawamoto et al., 2005). Design issues can lead to workarounds (ways for providers to achieve their clinical goals despite the technology). These workarounds can bypass the EHR features that were intended to promote patient safety and care quality.

One issue that has repeatedly arisen in regards to an EHR is the use of cut and paste functionality. Some feel that this supports efficiency in documenting care when conditions are essentially unchanged; others suggest that it prevents critical thinking. Errors introduced by this functionality include pasting information to the wrong patient record, not updating the information, lack of identification of the original author and date, and use of someone else's words without permission (plagiarism). Some organizations prohibit any sort of copy-and-paste functionality in their EHR, whereas others allow this functionality in limited circumstances (AHIMA workgroup, 2005). Similarly, default settings in a physical exam might be set to "normal" in an EHR template. This could lead to situations where a record indicated that an exam was performed with normal findings, when in reality only portions of the exam were performed, or where there were abnormal findings that were not documented (Wasserman, 2011).

Some providers have voiced concerns about EHRs. Privacy and confidentiality concerns are increased, because the same features that allow authorized access to the record when and where needed also introduce the possibility of unauthorized access. There are concerns about hardware problems and downtime, and the potential to lose all access to the patient's information for a period of time. There are also concerns that introduction of EHR will interfere with the provider's relationship with the patient and family, although such fears of "depersonalization" have not been generally supported in literature (Holroyd-Leduc et al., 2011). The emergence of electronic health records does not mean that paper records are no longer a part of health care documentation. Paper remains useful for certain purposes and likely will continue to persist even in environments that have fully implemented EHRs (Karsh et al., 2010).

Summary

- Documentation is an essential part of clinical practice. The primary purpose of documentation in a health record is communication and supporting clinical decision making. Other purposes include providing the legal record of care, reimbursement, supporting evidence-based practice, and providing information for planning, quality improvement, research, education, and health policy.
- Health care is a complex system with many social and technical influences. Outcomes result from the interaction of people, technology, the environment, organizational culture, and policies that govern health care documentation.
- Electronic health records have advantages and limitations (real and perceived) but are clearly here to stay. With a few notable exceptions, electronic health records are still relatively new. Thus, the anticipated improvements in patient safety, health care quality, and efficiency have not yet been consistently demonstrated.
- Regardless of whether documentation is on paper or in electronic health records, the focus of health care is the interaction between provider and patient. You should be able to document all your observations, and retrieve the information you need to support decision making.
- EHRs are not "the solution" to health care quality issues; they are tools that will only be as good or poor as providers make them. At their best, EHRs can only be as good as the quality of the data entered into them—the quality of the observations and assessments made by health care providers.
- The anticipated benefits of EHR require carefully designed and well-implemented systems that are built in a way that supports clinical needs in a particular context (Karsh et al., 2010). Simply automating an existing paper system may result in a computer system that is easy to learn (because it is familiar) but which may have no effect on the quality of care or the quality of documentation. Health care providers at all levels of expertise must be involved in the development of electronic documentation systems if such systems are to truly reflect clinical practice (Currell & Urquhart, 2003; Shortliffe & Cimino, 2006).

Review Questions

1. Before interviewing the patient the provider asks the patient if anyone outside of providers should be given access to health information. The provider is complying with which of the following?
   1. COBRA regulations
   2. the ANA code of ethics
   3. HIPAA regulations
   4. the Social Security Act
2. When evaluating patient health information the provider would like to focus on information provided by secondary data sources. These sources may include which of the following? (Select all that apply.)
   1. the patient
   2. the patient's children
   3. a neighbor caring for the patient
   4. records from a long term care facility
   5. the vital signs taken by the provider during the physical assessment
3. After completing a health assessment on a new patient, the provider would document which information as subjective data? (Select all that apply.)
   1. symptom alleviating factors
   2. pain scale rating
   3. the presence of an inspiratory wheeze
   4. an oxygen saturation of 99%
   5. skin color
4. The provider enters patient assessment data into a computer system that serves a single hospital. This type of record is referred to as which of the following?
   1. EMR
   2. EHR
   3. HIT
   4. ARRA
5. While documenting information in a patient's paper record the provider makes and error in documentation. Which is the best action for the provider to take?
   1. Obliterate the error with black ink or white tape so the error cannot be detected.
   2. Remove the page from the record and destroy the page by shredding.
   3. Draw a single line through the error and continue with the documentation.
   4. Draw a single line through the error, noting the reason for the change, date, time, and name of the provider.
6. The provider recognizes that the primary purpose of the patient health record is to
   1. document the workload of the providers.
   2. protect providers from liability.
   3. communicate information to providers.
   4. provide the patient with a complete summary of care.
7. The provider is comparing patient fall data between units of a large facility by reviewing the medical records of the patients who fell in a 6-month period. The goal is to develop a fall reduction plan. In this case the medical record is which of the following?
   1. serving as a data source for quality improvement
   2. serving as a tool in clinical decision support
   3. identifying incompetence of providers
   4. measuring the severity of injury to the patient
8. The provider is presenting a patient case in nursing rounds and uses the medical record as a source of information in preparing the presentation. The purpose of the medical record in this situation is which of the following?
   1. policy development
   2. education
   3. research
   4. surveillance
9. The provider recognizes that to protect patient confidentiality, access to the health care record should be limited to which of the following?
   1. hospital employees only
   2. the providers listed as primary providers in the record
   3. the patient's family members
   4. those providing care and authorized to view the record
10. The provider is unable to read the orders written by the patient's physician. The best action for the provider to take is to do which of the following?
    1. Ask a more experienced provider to interpret the orders.
    2. Call the physician and ask that the orders be rewritten in a legible fashion.
    3. Make a guess about what was ordered based on what can be read.
    4. Ask the patient what the physician mentioned during the visit.

10 Infants, Children, and Adolescents

Nancy Pulsipher, MS, RN

It's only my third day in the emergency department, and the waiting room is packed. A new patient was just admitted to room 7, a 17-year-old girl with abdominal pain. *Oh gee!* This is always one of my fears, but it's my responsibility to do a preliminary assessment. As I walk toward the room, I try to remember all the potential causes—*appendicitis, pelvic inflammatory disease, kidney stones, cystitis… don't forget pregnancy!* But then I catch myself—don't jump the gun and try and figure it out before all the data are obtained.

"Hello Julie, my name is Sarah. Do you mind if I call you by your first name? I'm sorry to hear you're not feeling well. What made you come to the ED?" She looks pale and scared as she leans forward in the bed, grasping her lower right abdomen. An emesis basin is close by. "There was a sharp pain that started suddenly 2 hours ago and it wouldn't let up. My stomach got queasy, and I started to vomit and have been vomiting off and on ever since. *Is she pregnant? Although she denies any sexual activity—she further denies vaginal bleeding or discharge, pain with urination, and she's afebrile. I guess that makes kidney stones, cystitis, and PID less likely.*

The attending enters and asks Julie to lay back and relax as much as possible. We both listen for bowel sounds, which are present, but not hyperactive. There is significant tenderness in the RLQ when her abdomen is palpated—but no rebound or guarding. "We'll need to do an ultrasound," the attending says. "There's a small lump that I felt right at the very end pressing on your abdomen.

When we look on the ultrasound monitor and compare the ovaries, the right one is enlarged and rounded with severely diminished blood flow. "This looks like a case of ovarian torsion." The attending explains to Julie that she needs to be taken to surgery quickly to keep from losing the ovary. Julie still looks scared, but a little bit relieved to know that something can be done to help her.

LEARNING OUTCOMES

1. Recognize the differences in the care needs of infants, children, and adolescents during a physical exam.
2. Explain the importance of treating the pediatric patient and the caregiver as the patient unit.
3. Summarize developmentally appropriate approaches to assessing the pediatric patient.
4. Recognize developmentally appropriate and nonthreatening communication techniques used with pediatric patients.
5. Recognize temperamental, cultural, environmental, and emotional contexts as a significant components of the pediatric patient assessment.

Although children appear to be smaller replicas of adults, they are not miniature adults. Children come in multiple sizes, ages, developmental stages, and levels of maturity. Each of these differences presents health care providers with related challenges when caring for the child. The stages and the related patient needs will be presented in this chapter.

Pediatric patients vary from being completely nonverbal or unable to state their needs to being very articulate and definite about what they want or need. Their social skills are also at various levels of sophistication, depending on culture, temperament, and age. Additionally their growth course up to the time they present in a care setting will have an effect on their communication abilities, responses to interactions or procedures, and cooperation with a physical examination. At certain ages most or all pediatric patients will be frightened by anyone who is not the parent or caregiver. At other ages these children need privacy and are less likely to cooperate with parents present during an interview or physical exam. Children between the two extremes show varying gradations of fear and cooperation.

Childhood Characteristics

Pediatric patients span the age range of **newborn** (infancy) through age 18. However, certain aspects of brain, such as the limbic system and prefrontal cortex as well as emotional development extends the upper age limit into the 20s (Wahlstrom, Collins, White, & Luciana, 2010).

While the age span may be relatively short, the changes that occur during this time are extensive and provide the foundation for a successful and fulfilling adulthood. The rapidity of growth and development in children produces substantial changes that reflect age and stage specific achievements. Such extensive changes bring with it a wide variety of variations requiring a great deal of provider flexibility in performing a pediatric examination.

While the goal of assessment of a child is the same as for the adult, the procedures and techniques used are variable and adapted to each child. The provider may need to take advantage of a specific position or time to obtain essential data, even if it is not in the expected sequence of performing an assessment. Certain procedures are also only used on children as they are unique to a specific age or developmental stage. The rapidity of growth and development in children also produces substantial changes that reflect age and stage specific achievements. These changes need to be monitored and assessed.

Many findings during a pediatric physical assessment are only present during childhood. This does not change the importance of what is seen, heard, or felt. Some findings indicate birth defects that need immediate attention if the child is to remain on track for normal development. Other findings require intervention to prevent significant future delays in development or permanent disabilities in adulthood. In the newborn period, some of the findings need urgent attention to prevent sudden death from an unknown cardiac or other physical defect. Providers who are unaware of the importance of these potential situations may miss life-threatening issues, resulting in permanent disability or early preventable death.

A unique characteristic of humans is that their children have an extensive period of "dependency and development," requiring others to satisfy their physical, emotional, and cognitive needs. Within this context, in addition to their parents, their children are vulnerable and dependent on the quality and quantity of social input from multiple sources, including but not necessarily limited to individual, community, organizational, and environmental entities. Their overall health and well-being depends on the actions and behaviors received from groups and individuals associated with these entities and the child's perception of these interactions. Of particular importance is the treatment provided during caregiving.

A child's vulnerability and dependence are also related to his or her variable levels of ability to communicate. Children begin their communication efforts by providing cues and learning how to elicit cues from others and appropriate responses. Those under ages 3 to 4 are not able communicate their health needs to others. Even when they develop their communication abilities, they have a limited vocabulary and have difficulty finding the words to express their feelings or needs. Their social skills are also at various levels of sophistication, depending on culture, temperament, and age.

Additionally, children's maturation progress up to the time they present in a care setting will have an effect on how well they communicate, respond to interactions or procedures, or are able to cooperate during a physical examination. Mothers or other caregivers may recognize cues from their children. Providers are not as likely to recognize individual cues even in children as old as 6 or 7. Some words may hold different meanings for the adult recipient of the child's message.

Each child enters the world with the genetic material to determine many individual and unique characteristics; however, each child essentially enters the world as a clean slate, with few distinct and defining characteristics, but with the potential to be configured into a unique and complex individual. This configuration, which is referred to as development, occurs through processes of progressively more complex interactions between the child and persons, objects, and symbols in his or her proximal environment that occur on a moderately consistent basis over an extended time period (Bronfenbrenner & Morris, 2006). How they are treated and how their needs are met have a significant influence on the outcome of the configuration of the child. Teaching, guiding, loving and supporting within the context of the the family will provide the child with what is needed to grow and mature.

The foundation for the future acquisition and development of appropriate adult behaviors and role function is established during this vulnerable and dependent period. Life begins with only primitive, protective reflexes as well as some basic instincts, inborn characteristics and **temperament**, all of which must be nurtured and strengthened to facilitate development of appropriate, beneficial life skills, and survival strategies. At no other time in an individual's lifetime will the phenomenal amount of learning that takes place during infancy, childhood, and adolescence be repeated.

Each child also develops an individual response to others' actions, expressions, tones of voice, and nonverbal cues. Children can sense others' emotions, especially fear or nervousness; however, they are incapable of processing and reacting to these emotions until further growth and development occurs. They are, though, capable of establishing relationships between their emotions and feelings with situations, which may be positive or negative in their effect on the child.

Recognizing each child's innate characteristics, working with each child's temperament and what each child comes with brings out one's uniqueness. Teaching, guiding, loving, and supporting within the context of the family will provide the child with what is needed to grow and mature. Additionally, stimulation of their senses and building on their reflexes by allowing and encouraging the child to use them will also provide them with valuable life skills.

Childhood Ages and Stages

Growth and development is a dynamic lifelong process that begins in utero and ceases at the moment of death. **Physical development** is readily visible as parents or caregivers observe this progression as each child increases in height and weight and develops specific gender characteristics as the child enters and goes through puberty. The age ranges of pediatric individuals are differentiated by weeks, months, and years (see Table 10-1).

Emotional and cognitive development follows a set sequence of stages. The time span for each stage is variable, being shorter or longer than predicted or estimated based on the child's environment, genetic make-up, mother/infant relationship, and level of stimulation provided within the home environment (or care giving context). Emotional, psychosocial, and cognitive development are less obvious; however, there are specific developmental skills associated with each stage that provides some type of objective measurement of a child's developmental progress. These are often referred to as **developmental milestones**.

Placement of a child within a specific stage is somewhat arbitrary. Differing perspectives are also available to determine which developmental aspect of development relates to the child. The two most common perspectives or frameworks for assessing an individual's developmental progress are Erikson's Psychosocial Stages and Piaget's Cognitive Development Stages (Table 10-2). Erikson's Psychosocial Developmental stages span an individual's entire lifetime, whereas Piaget's Cognitive Developmental stages encompasses the first 14 years of life, or from infancy to adolescence. Even though Erikson's stages include the entire lifespan, the majority of the stages are concerned with infancy through adolescence, reflecting the rapidity of childhood development.

According to Erikson's theory, each stage is also associated with specific developmental tasks/skills that must be successfully accomplished to progress from one stage to the next. Development, however, does not necessarily wait for an individual to accomplish each task successfully. Failure to accomplish each task successfully may have a sustained influence of future task accomplishment and be a cause of psychosocial dysfunction later in life.

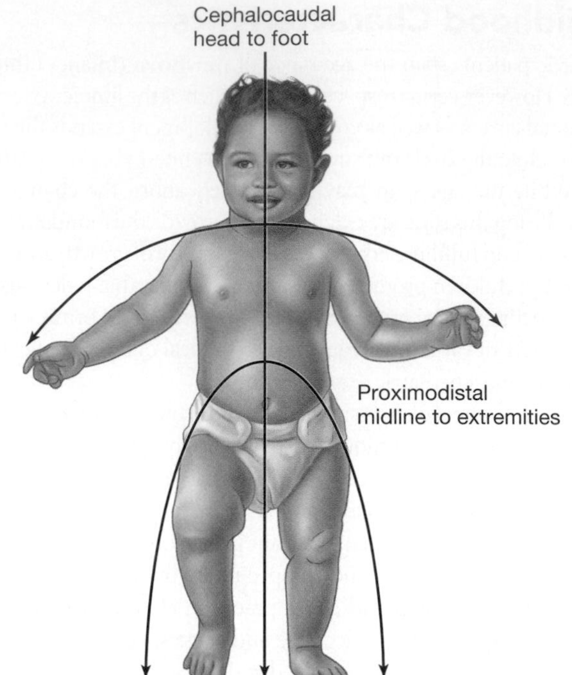

FIGURE 10-1 Patterns and direction of growth

Growth Patterns

Growth occurs in predictable patterns, yet also varies in relationship to genetic influences, environmental conditions, and a variety of other factors, such as serum lead, socioeconomic status (SES) levels, poor social support, later birth order in large family, and access to care, can all contribute to growth delays. The predictable pattern of growth is **cephalocaudal**, or meaning growth begins with the head and progresses downward to the lower body, and **proximodistal**, or progressing from the center of the body and moving to the distal areas (Figure 10-1).

Assessment of physical growth and maturation is also important to determine the existence of any red flags or potential areas for concern. The provider should consider the following as possible red flags that warrant further investigation: slight, minute/unexpected findings, a loss in previously acquired skills, an increase or decrease in muscle tone, and language delays (Hockenberry & Wilson, 2012).

The need for accuracy of growth assessments begins with the newborn. Evaluating growth progression on standardized growth charts should continue throughout childhood and adolescence (Figure 10-2).

Gestational age and history also have an effect on subsequent growth and development and future outcomes and abilities. Delays and questions/concerns related to growth progression and developmental achievements are indicators of alterations in the growing system. The provider can detect potential problems by close monitoring of a pediatric patient's growth curves.

The post-delivery assessment on newborns compares infants' weight in relationship to their gestational age. A wide range of acceptable parameters exist for height, weight, and gestational age. Small for gestational age (SGA) is less than 2,500 grams at birth or below the 10th percentile on the growth chart for age. The head may be proportionate or smaller than the 5th percentile (microcephalic). Fifty percent of SGA infants are below average weight at 3 years of age (see Figure 10-3).

Birth weight reflects intrauterine growth. Poor weight gain early in infancy may indicate failure to thrive, poor feeding habits, malnutrition, neglect and abuse, and cardiac or renal disease.

Large for gestational age (LGA) is greater than two standard deviations above the mean for gestational age or greater than 90th percentile for age on the growth chart (Figure 10-3). The occurrence of LGA may be familial from gestational diabetes, abnormal uterine environment, genetic, or a poorly controlled insulin-dependent mother (Duderstadt, 2006).

Height refers to linear skeletal growth. Measure the height of both infants and toddlers while they are in the recumbent position. Height growth increases come in spurts. Females usually peak and reach their full adult height by age 16, while males potentially continue to grow until ages 18 to 21. Growth ceases when the skeleton is mature. Note that the 2-year-old height is approximately half of the adult height.

Brain growth can be assessed in relationship to head circumference. Measuring a pediatric patient's head circumference is routine during the first 2 years or until closure of fontanels and sutures.

External environmental factors also affect a child's growth. Children take in more air and water per pound of body weight than adults, making them a higher risk for environmental toxins. They also

Table 10-1 Pediatric ages (beginning at birth)

Birth at <37 weeks' gestation	preterm
Birth at 37 weeks to 4 weeks	newborn period
1–6 months	early infancy
6–12 months	late infancy
12 months to about 36 months (1–3 years)	toddler period
3–5 years	preschool age
6–11 years	school age
12–18 years	adolescence

Table 10-2 Developmental theories of Erikson and Piaget

	Erikson (Lifespan Development)				Piaget (Cognitive Development)
Developmental Period	**Stage**	**Competing**	**Characteristics**	**Tasks**	
Infancy; Birth to 1 year of age	Trust/ mistrust	Responsive parenting and nurturing fosters developing a sense of trust. Trust develops as needs are met. Unresponsive, unnurturing, or abusive parenting results in mistrust.	Tolerating frustration in small doses Recognizing mother as distinct from others and self		Sensorimotor state (birth to 2 years)—at birth, responses limited to reflexes; begins to relate to outside events; concerned by sensations and actions that affect him/her directly
Early childhood (toddler); 1–3 years	Autonomy/ shame and doubt	As the child seeks to develop autonomy, the parent must balance the child's exploration with the need to protect the child from harming self.	The toddler seeks to develop a sense of self as well as explore the environment. Trying out own powers of speech Beginning acceptance of reality vs. pleasure principle	1. Differentiating self from others, particularly the mother 2. Tolerating separation from mother or parent 3. Withstanding delayed gratification 4. Controlling bodily functions 5. Acquiring socially acceptable behavior 6. Acquiring verbal communication 7. Interacting with others in a more empathetic way (i.e., understanding another person's emotional state)	Preoperational (2–7 years)—child is still egocentric; thinks everyone sees world as he does
					Preconceptual (2–4 years)—forms general concepts, not capable of reasoning yet
Middle childhood (preschool); 3–5 years	Initiative/ guilt	Child expands relationships beyond parents and environment in the need to develop a sense of self and self-esteem. Parental support, reassurance, and encouragement, while still protecting from harm, brings about positive self-esteem. Punishing or preventing child from self-mastery brings about a sense of failure and guilt.	Development of a strong imagination Development of a conscience Questioning Exploring own body and environment Differentiation of sexes	1. Realizing separateness as an individual 2. Identifying gender roles and functions 3. Developing a sense of initiative 4. Begins to learn acceptable social skills 5. Growing knowledge and use of language for social interaction 6. Developing readiness for school	Perceptual (4–7 years)—capable of some reasoning; but can concentrate on only one aspect of a situation at a time
Late childhood (school age); 6–11 years	Industry/ inferiority	Achievements in this stage produce feelings of confidence, competence, and mastery. Approval of parents, peers, and teachers begins to become important. Parents need to recognize achievements while at the same time helping the child to understand that everyone can't do everything.	Learning to win recognition by producing things Exploring, collecting Learning to relate to own gender	1. Mastering skills needed as an adult 2. Winning approval from other adults and peers 3. Building self-esteem and a positive self-concept 4. Taking a place in a peer group 5. Adopting moral standards	Concrete operations (7–11 years)—reasoning is logical, but limited to own experience; understands cause and effect
Adolescence; 12–18 years	Ego identity/ role confusion	Parents need to balance their wanting to control their child's behavior, etc. with the competing needs of the teenager to find one's own identify apart from family. Parents still need to set boundaries as to what is safe and what is harmful. Expect and accept the teen years to be filled with periods of rebellion, going with the crowd, and a tendency to feel invincible, especially males. Teens are also trying to figure out what and who they are.	Moving toward heterosexuality Selecting vocation Beginning separation from family Integrating personality (altruism, etc.)	1. Searching for one's identity 2. Appreciating one's achievements 3. Growing independent from parents 4. Forming close relationships with peers 5. Developing analytical thinking	Formal operational stage (11–16 years)—acquires ability to develop abstract concepts for him/herself; oriented to problem solving

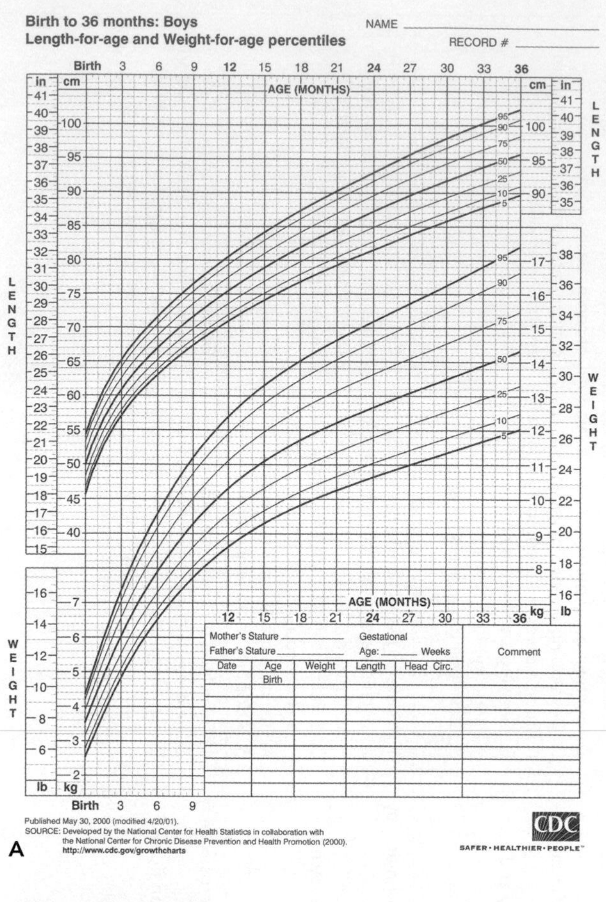

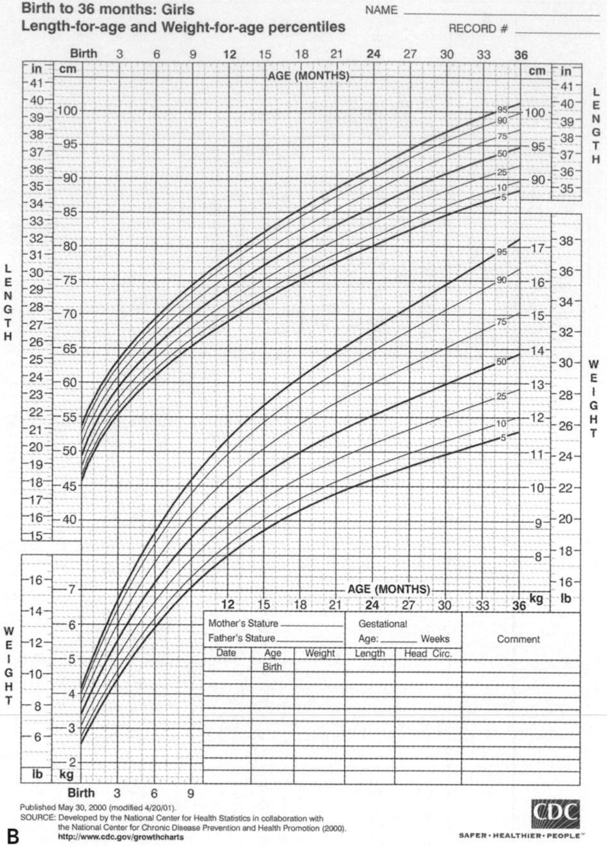

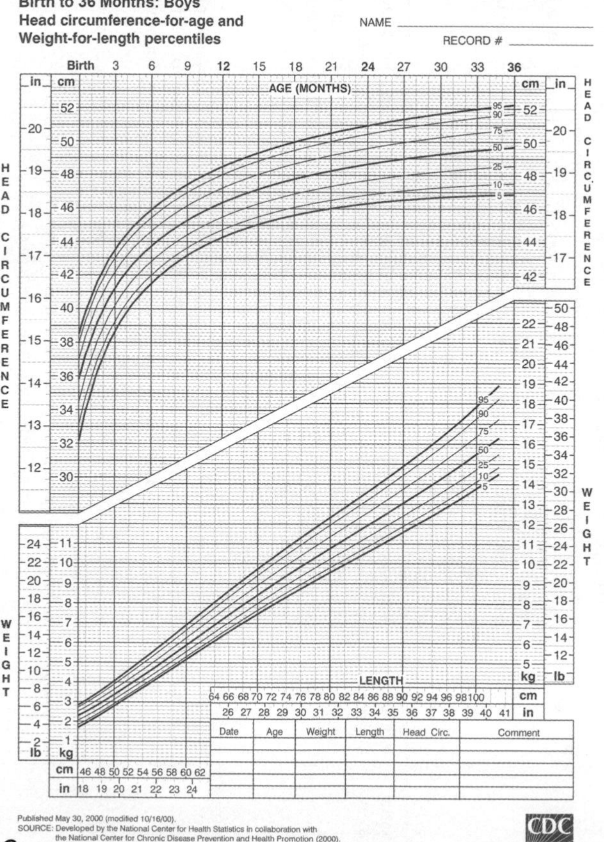

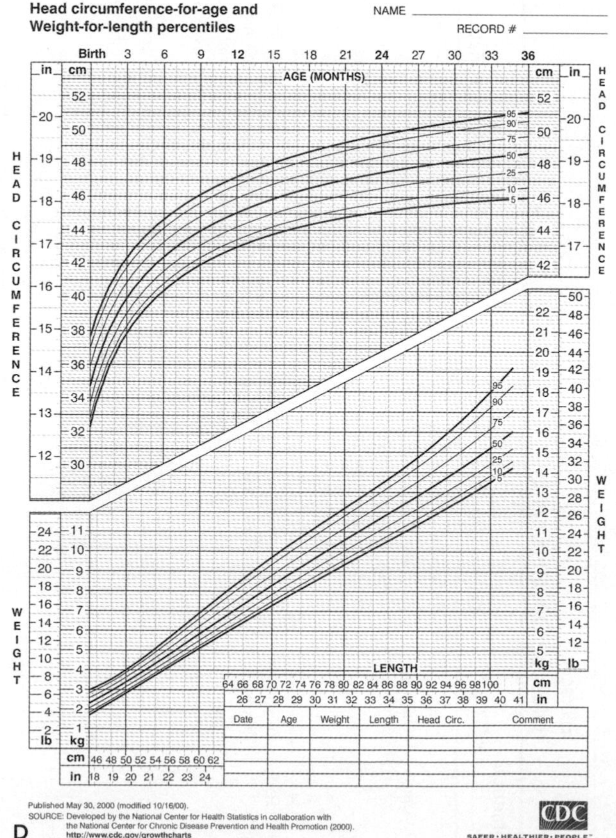

FIGURE 10-2A–D Standardized growth charts

Source: Developed by the National Center for Health Statistics in collaboration with the National Center for Chronic Disease Prevention and Health Promotion http://www.cdc.gov/growthcharts

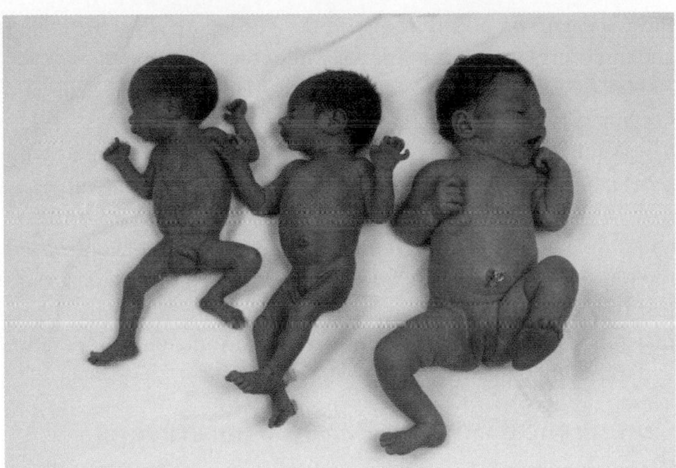

FIGURE 10-3 Examples of infants who are small for gestational age, average, and large for gestational age
Source: Science Photo Library/Custom Medical Stock Photo

absorb substances faster—at a rate of 5:1 over adults. Their respiratory system, gastrointestinal system, and skin are more vulnerable in that they can absorb substances more readily and efficiently than the adult systems. Children also live and play closer to environmental hazards on the ground, which increases the concentration of inhaled toxic substances. The dose-response rate in children for exposure to environmental hazards is more rapid than in adults. All children are at risk for exposure to environmental substances. Different developmental stages have increased risk for some types of exposure (Table 10-3).

Pediatric Assessments

Despite the onset and use of high-tech instruments in health care, expert assessment is still mostly about listening, observing, and thinking critically in a clinical setting. Assessment of the pediatric patient requires the same principles and techniques as those required for an adult assessment; however, adaptability on the part of the provider is essential. While a systematic approach is always preferable, infants and young children do not necessarily cooperate systematically; therefore, the provider may need to adapt certain parts of the exam to when the opportunity presents itself.

Table 10-3 Exposure risk based on developmental stages

Fetal development	Maternal smoking and substance abuse, chemical or biological agents (rubella) may cause congenital defects.
Newborn	Toxicants may be found in breast milk or in the preparation of formula. Additionally, toxicants may come from dermal contacts and parental occupational toxins.
Infant and toddlers	Greater mobility increases risk, hand to mouth, oral exposure, and inhaled from being near to the ground.
Preschool and school age	Toxicants from school, child care settings, and playgrounds.
Adolescents	Occupational hazards, experimentation with drugs, alcohol, and intentional inhalation (gasoline, glue, and tobacco), excess sun (Many Internet resources on common environmental health hazards for children are available).

Communicating with Children

Communication with children primarily occurs during the history taking and should be adapted to the child's age and development; do not presuppose that the child is limited by his or her developmental stage. Take a position that is at the child's eye level and use an approach that is gentle and quiet. Always be truthful when explaining something to a child rather than concealing information for fear of upsetting or frightening the child. Instead, use developmentally appropriate, clear, and simple language.

When appropriate, offer the child choices, avoiding closed, yes/no questions unless you plan to honor the child's "no" response. Provide the child with options regarding when to do a certain procedure such as, "Do you want me to look in your ears or eyes first?" This gives the child a sense of control without giving the option of whether the child will actually let you look in the ears or eyes or not. The child must feel OK and be comfortable with the provider. It often helps to use dolls, puppets, or stuffed animals to communicate information about a procedure before performing it on the child. Avoid analogies, metaphors, and medical jargon; children are very literal. Think about how certain phrases such as "cough your head off" are commonly used by adults, but how frightening this sounds to a child who takes it literally!

Give instructions in a positive manner, avoiding long sentences. When caring for an older child, provide an opportunity to talk with the patient without the presence of parents; privacy and confidentiality are very important to the preadolescent and adolescent and facilitate the establishment of trust between patient and provider.

Infant Communication

Infants are nonverbal; emotions are the language infants use before they acquire speech. Infants react to adult facial expressions and respond to familiar voices by turning towards the person. When adults understand that the infant is communicating through their responses, they can then adjust their own response to meet the specific need the infant is expressing, such as distress or happiness.

Crying is another form of infant communication. Infants communicate by smiling and cooing when they are content and crying when distressed (Hockenberry & Wilson, 2012). Any unpleasant stimuli, external or internal, provoke crying. Hunger, pain, bodily restraint, strangers, loneliness, and cold are a few of these stimuli (Table 10-4). These are the cues that the adult needs to recognize that an infant requires something [intervention] to relieve discomfort or distress. (Perry, Hockenberry, Lowdermilk, & Wilson, 2009).

Early Childhood

When communicating with a toddler or preschool-age child, the provider should focus on the child. Provide explanations regarding what, how, and why things are being done. It is also important to use words that the child will recognize. Remember to be consistent with both terminology and body language. For example, don't smile during a painful procedure.

Play is an important communication technique that may be used with children and is generally considered the "work" of childhood or their "developmental workshop." Play activity is a way the provider can gather a considerable amount of information about the child because it is the child's projection of the inner self. Play activity may also provide a barometer of the child's illness or be used as a

Table 10-4 Infant cries communicate specific needs

Basic cry	Rhythmic in pattern and usually consists of a cry followed by a briefer silence then a shorter whistle that is somewhat higher pitch than the main cry, then another brief rest before the next cry—hunger is part of basic cry need
Angry cry	More excess of air forced through the vocal chords—parents respond differently to this cry
Pain cry	Comes without warning, appears suddenly without preliminary meaning, and may be followed with an extended period of breath holding

therapeutic intervention for the relief of stress and pain. When using play as an assessment technique, make it age-appropriate and consider the energy level of the child so as to avoid making it too exhausting. Stress interferes with healing.

Toddlers are quite vulnerable to the crisis of a serious illness, causing them stress, which is often overwhelming due to their limited ability to cope and insufficient number of coping skills. A serious illness may include hospitalization and separation from caregivers, which may be felt as a loss of control and a threat to their autonomy. The sense of loss of control is often demonstrated through regression of behavior, negativity, and temper tantrums. Regression is an attempt to cope by returning to past patterns of behavior that were successful in previous stages of development. When regression occurs, it is best to ignore it and provide positive reinforcement for maintained developmentally appropriate behaviors.

Preschoolers are egocentric and engage in magical thinking, typical of their age. They may view illness and hospitalization as a punishment for misdeeds or "bad" thoughts. Their thinking is also preoperational, which may make them very fearful of bodily harm, mutilation, castration, and intrusive procedures. Allow them to explore equipment first. Demonstrate procedures on dolls and use nonthreatening words. Children at this age may overestimate their own abilities, and when they lose power, it is very upsetting to them.

School Age

Communication with school-age patients requires an acknowledgement of their fears and encouragement to discuss them. Provide them with privacy and treat their pain effectively. Involve them in the assessment as much as possible by keeping them busy.

School-age children are striving for independence and productivity. Their fears include death, abandonment, permanent injury, boredom, fear of separation from parents and peers, bodily injury, pain, and illness. Patients at this age need privacy and are very anxious about their genital area, enforced dependency, and loss of parental control. They have come to understand disability and death.

Adolescents

Adolescents struggle for independence and liberation. When communicating with such adolescent patients, remember to relate how information about their health may affect their relationships, identity formation, and future plans. Always explain procedures and include details on how the body works (see Figure 10-4). Be honest and mindful of their privacy needs, while considering developmental responses. Adolescents may need help developing coping skills and keeping in touch with their peer group.

Adolescents identify more with their peer group than with their families and find separation from their peers difficult. They may respond with anger and frustration and need information about their conditions. Their main fears include loss of control and separation from peers, loss of identity, enforced dependence, and fear of what illness will do to their independence. Their behaviors may range from being out of control or acting out, to uncooperative and overconfident.

Communication with Parents/Caregivers

When communicating with a patient's parents or caregivers, establish a setting that ensures privacy and confidentiality. It is often helpful to allow the child to play during the parent interview (Figure 10-5). Encourage the parents to talk openly, directing your focus away from the child and on the parent. Use appropriate listening skills and empathy. Be mindful of cultural factors that might influence the parents' responses and reactions.

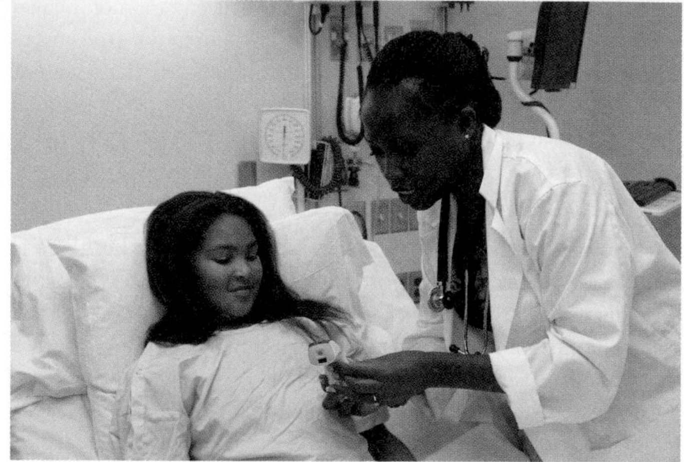

FIGURE 10-4 Explaining details of how equipment works is an important way to gain the trust of an adolescent patient.

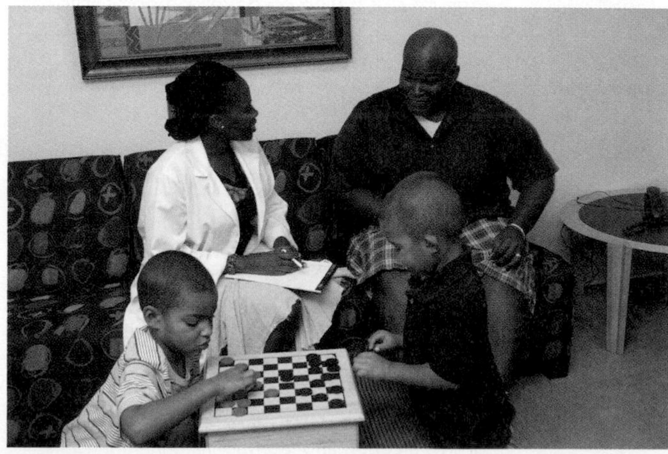

FIGURE 10-5 The provider allows pediatric patients to play nearby while conducting a parent interview.

The provider's respect for and support of the parent–child relationship also reinforces the parent's/caregiver's caring behaviors and elicits needed information regarding this relationship. Important factors/skills/abilities that are needed to foster or create a healthy parent–child relationship include the following:

- Actively listening to family concerns, which helps the provider to understand feelings and values
- Learning what the family expects of the intervention
- Using open-ended questions
- Individualizing care to make it to this child and family; determining the cultural values of the family
- Discussing what the family is doing proactively to support the child
- Eliciting available social supports for the parents; noting involvement of other family members
- Asking about shared family activities—sports, cultural events, religious services
- Confirming and complimenting parental and family strengths

Noting parent–child interactions during an assessment provides a sense of family dynamics, family authority structure, and problem-solving abilities. Observing nonverbal cues and verbalizing what is seen may provide a sense of how engaged the mother/father and child are with each other. Comparing the mother's (parents') affect with the child's demeanor may indicate possible mismatches between what is said and how the child feels.

Child and adolescent cues can show aspects of the "context" of the child's life. A withdrawn or stressed child is showing signs of "strain in the environment." The provider may want to determine if the family needs support or counseling and provide a referral if needed. "Children mirror the emotions of the adults around them. Families in conflict often don't perceive their interactions clearly, or recognize the impact their interactions have on the child" (Duderstadt, 2006).

Family-Centered Care

The entire family is the constant in the child's life; a child cannot be perceived to be a separate entity, apart from the parents placing the pediatric patient within the context of a family and making the family the patient (Duderstadt, 2006). Without this context, assessment behavior is difficult to interpret; therefore, it is important to consider infants and parent(s)/caregivers as the patient. Outside systems must support, respect, encourage, and enhance the family's strength and competence. The needs of all family members must be addressed, as the condition of one family member will affect all family dynamics.

Parents can be a source of comfort to a child during examinations and hospitalizations. An ill child places various degrees of stress on the parents. A nonthreatening illness or condition may only elicit anxiety and minimal fear and a slight disruption to normal family interactions. However, a more serious illness or condition may provoke strong feelings of disbelief, anger, guilt, and depression—especially if the illness is sudden, or there is the possibility of an adverse outcome. It is also common for the parents to experience frustration—especially related to their need for information regarding their child's condition and outcome.

Sibling reactions to an ill child may consist of loneliness, fear, worry, anger, resentment, jealousy, and guilt. Siblings may also feel they somehow caused the illness.

Family-centered care consists of two basic concepts, enabling and empowering. **Enabling** provides opportunities to demonstrate current abilities and competencies and acquire new abilities and competencies as needed; **empowerment** gives back a sense of power and control accomplished by interaction that allows family to maintain or acquire a sense of comfort; behaviors that foster family strengths, abilities, and actions.

Cultural Considerations

Cultural beliefs, values, and practices play a significant role in health care-seeking behavior and impact the delivery and quality of clinical care. Variations among ethnic groups are common; however, variations within ethnic groups can be as wide as those between groups. It is difficult to develop any valid suppositions based on physical characteristics or surname. To the extent possible incorporate cultural practices into patient assessment and care. It is best if a patient assessment can be accomplished in the patient's primary language; however, if this is not possible use an interpreter.

Information that is useful can be obtained by exploring parental beliefs and their impact on the child and assessing cultural values and orientation of the family unit. The provider should also be able to recognize folk illnesses and beliefs, and what influence and impact they have on the child's health in the family and on clinical care. One must also understand personal values and how these may influence care delivery and health outcomes. Care practices should also be adapted to meet the child's health care needs and eliminate health disparities related to race/ethnicity. Cultural competence or cultural humility is essential in providing responsible health care and is also a way to help build honesty and trust in the caring relationship.

Patient Health History

As with an adult assessment, a pediatric assessment begins with the health history. At what age a child can be considered a reliable historian is variable. Components of the health history can be obtained from children as young as 3, however, parental involvement at some points may be needed to validate a child's responses.

Engage the child in the interview process to facilitate assessing their understanding and misconceptions. This offers insight into their social-emotional world. Eye-level encounters are best for young

PRACTICE POINT: Cultural Health Practices and Child Abuse

Some cultural health practices produce bruising of the skin that may be interpreted as evidence of child abuse. When examining children from different cultures it is important to remember that what appears to be abuse is not always the result of abuse. Various health practices of different cultures may produce skin alterations not regularly observed or considered "normal" in the United States or other Western cultures. Some of these practices are identified and described in Table 10-5. While the descriptions make these practices appear abusive, from a cultural perspective they are not.

Table 10-5 Cultural practices

Practice	Technique	Cultural Groups
Cupping (meyboom, banguan/ baguar, badkesh, banki, bahnkes, bekam, buhung, tentusa, kyukaku, gak hoi, Hijamah, kavaa, mihceme)	Heated cup inverted and placed on skin. Suction force created mobilizing blood flow to "draw out" the ailment. Heated air and rim of cup cause circular burns, central ecchymosis, and petechiae.	Middle Eastern, Asian, Latin American, Eastern European
Coining Vietnamese (cao gio) "scratch the wind" Chinese (Gua sha) "scraping bruises" Indonesian/Javanese (kerika/kerokan) "scraping technique"	Oiled skin is rubbed firmly with edge of coin leaving linear red marks, usually on the back. Thought to release illness causing "bad winds" from the body.	Southeast Asian
Spooning (quat sha)	Similar to coining—wet skin rubbed with procelin spoon producing ecchymosis.	Chinese
Moxibustion (acumoxa, auricular mo, moxabustion)	Therapeutic burning of pieces of moxa herb (mugwort) or yarn on the skin leaving small discrete circular burns that may be confused with cigarette burns. Some consider it a form of acupuncture.	Southeast Asian (China, Tibet, Japan, Korea, Vietnam)
Suctioning of fontanelle or pressure on hard palate to cure Caida e mollera	Caida e mollera (sunken/fallen fontanelle) is associated with "bolita" or bump on hard palate or pulling infant off nipple too quickly. In addition to suctioning/pressure, various treatments include the following: poultices of herbs, raw eggs, soap shavings shaving head over fontanel immersion of top of head in water slapping soles of feet or shaking infant vertically while holding upside down	Mexican American

Source: Data from (Boos, 2013; Cao, Li, & Liu, 2012; Ermertcan & Ertan, 2010; Juckett, 2005; Trotter II, 1987)

children. This helps the provider seem more approachable. Make contact when the child is interested. Direct the initial attention to the parent, giving the infant or toddler time to adjust to the provider and the surroundings.

Children are accepting of many different types of interactions and adapt to a person who is at ease and competent at structuring the interview. The child is comfortable when they know what to expect. Talk through each step first to decrease anxiety and help the child be more willing to participate.

- Preschool: Ask about activities, playmates, school or daycare, daily routines, and safety. Teaching or "anticipatory guidance" can happen at the same time, based on the child's responses.
- School age: Interview directly and allow them to participate in their care. Role model for parents how to engage children and teach health and safety issues. This helps children learn the importance of healthy habits.
- Adolescents: Interview separately, after asking parents about any concerns. The adolescent–provider engagement allows the teen an opening for the sharing of personal or sensitive concerns.

Try indirect questioning when the child is reluctant (tell a story and ask how the patient thinks the child may feel, or "some 15-year-olds do . . . do you have friends who do . . .").

Use scenarios—"what would you do if . . ." can engage a younger school age child; "how would you feel if . . ." works for older school-age children; start with less threatening topics and move slowly to more sensitive ones. State expectations clearly—what you need for cooperation or to help the child; do not offer a choice if there is none; avoid yes/no questions; use I messages—"I need you to . . . because I want to help you," etc.; avoid "you." Provide positive role modeling for parents. Preschool or young school-age children can draw pictures for the provider.

Physical Assessment

A major component of the pediatric exam is to use the approach that gains the cooperation of the patient. Children are more variable in their responses to others so it is important to recognize and use different approaches that may be taken.

Follow a "quiet to active" approach to the physical examination, especially with infants and young children. First, do what a child needs to be quiet for (pulse, RR, cardiac and breath sounds, abdominal auscultation for bowel sounds, and blood pressure), and then move from noninvasive assessment to more invasive (inspection of throat and ears [Drutz, 2013]). Vary the approach to suit the temperament and activity level of the child. It is best not to omit parts of the process as something important might be missed.

PRACTICE POINT: Additional Assessment Suggestions

- Focus on parts of the exam that are most pertinent; make as many observations as possible before approaching or touching the child.
- Avoid completely undressing the child (infants may get cold and restless; 3–4-year-olds often are frightened if their clothes are removed.
- Interact with the parents and the child throughout the exam; avoid advance notices of frightening or uncomfortable procedures—best to develop rapport, and then give step-by-step explanations as procedure is done.
- Tell the child what is happening and why, be careful of your word choice—"check" something rather than "take" something, BP cuff "gives hugs," a poke or little pinch rather than a "bee sting," etc., Be truthful—do not say it won't hurt if it will or might—something like "some say this hurts, let me know how you feel about it."

A step-by-step approach to performing a pediatric physical exam is given in Chapter 15. The information presented here is related to approaches that will help in performing a physical exam, not the specific techniques or sequence.

Preterm and Newborn

Perform the assessment in front of the parents. This is a good time for educating the parents and answering their questions. Start with cardiac and respiratory auscultation (quiet approach), while the infant is asleep in parent's arms or on a warmer. Then assess with only a diaper on, under a heat source. Be flexible and adapt the exam to the temperament of the infant. Observe for right and left symmetry, strength, and coordination of movement.

Note overall appearance, skin color, breathing pattern, and alertness level. Repeat observations of concern to determine extent of problem. Keep deviations from the expected in context. Evaluate all unexpected findings objectively—lab tests, vital signs, and diagnostic procedures. Some features can be evaluated subjectively—unusual ear placement or slanted eyes. Look at parents and siblings before determining if a problem exists.

Infant 1–6 Months

Begin with the infant on the parent's lap, on an exam table or bed, with a firm surface for head support. Depending on the patient's comfort, the infant may be moved to the exam table or the entire exam may be done on the parent's lap; if needed, the younger infant can be moved to exam table to finish and to evaluate developmental milestones.

Use a calm, relaxed, and gentle approach. A comfortable parent may decrease anxiety and fear in the child. Before stranger and separation anxiety appear (6–9 months), infants generally enjoy the social interaction of the history and exam. Don't frighten the infant. Do not leave the patient on a table or bedside without the rails being in full up position. Leave the intrusive portions of the exam until the end. To ease the infant during the exam, making repetitive soothing sounds or soothing motions while listening to the heart or lungs has a calming effect. It may also be necessary to pause to allow for feeding, consoling, or changing a diaper.

Older Infant and Toddler

Go slowly, maintaining eye contact. To allay the fear of an older infant, start the history while seated across the room and gradually move closer while talking with the parent. Focus on the parent while slowly showing interest in the child. Smiles and brief eye contacts help relieve the shyness and stranger anxiety that is the norm for this age. Speak to the child before any touching.

Allow the child to touch or play with the equipment to help distract the infant from the examiner and the exam (Figure 10-6). Talking softly and gently, moving slowly, and having the infant in the parent's lap help make the visit more successful. Offer a toy of some kind. The provider can use a doll to show the child what each step is to help calm the toddler. Once an infant sits well, he or she can sit in the parent's lap to start; this helps decrease stranger anxiety. Provide time for the parent to express concerns, needs, and expectations.

Remove clothes slowly, one thing at a time as various areas are examined. Do "quiet things" first, then more active or invasive things. Leave the abdominal and diaper area until last. The child can stay on the parent's lap with the parent and provider sitting knee to knee to support the child. As they get older, make a game of the exam. At the end observe the walking infant or toddler walking around in only a diaper.

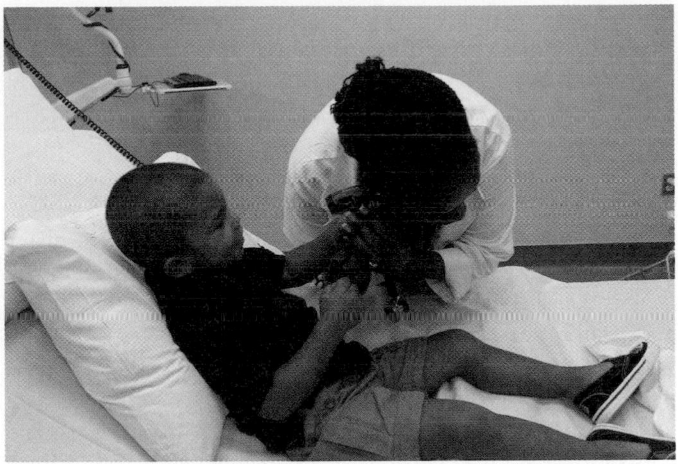

FIGURE 10-6 Allowing a patient to see how equipment works first may decrease his anxiety.

Approach the toddler with a calm, patient, and cheerful manner. Allow the toddler to explore the exam room while provider obtains the history from the parent. Begin the exam on the parent's lap and move to the exam table with the parent helping to position the child. Let the child touch or play with the exam equipment. Start with least intrusive assessments; perform it first on parent or child's stuffed toy to put the toddler at ease. Be sure to praise the child for cooperation. Ask the child to help perform the exam—e.g., push on his tummy then provider puts hand on tummy. If restraint is needed, have the parent assist by holding the child.

Preschool Age

By age 3, children are better able to make eye contact, though they are still shy. They can also separate briefly from parents. Watch the child and listen to interactions. Talk in a slow, even, steady voice. Use the "quiet to active" method. These children like role play, games, and drawing. Use dolls to help alleviate fear and prepare them for what will be done. Modesty starts during this age. Be sure to respect this. It is helpful to let the child handle some of the equipment.

Three-year-old children may be positioned on a parent's lap. Four and five-year-old children are usually comfortable on the exam table by themselves. Go very slowly, patiently, and deliberately in approaching the child. Respect privacy and modesty. Use short, simple explanations. Talk to the child and explain the steps of the exam (Figure 10-6).

Allow the child to make choices. Do not offer a choice when there is not one—avoid yes/no choices. Ask which ear first, for example, and the child will be a willing participant. Gain cooperation by asking for help. Allow the child to feel a sense of control by helping—holding the stethoscope to his chest, for instance. Allow the child to play with the equipment and use games. Give feedback to the child on what you are seeing, and compliment the child when he or she cooperates.

School Age

Talk through each section of the exam. Children at this age like to hear about the body. They are also more independent. Offer them choices, avoiding yes/no choices unless you are prepared to honor the "no." Allow the child to decide who is with them during the exam; respect his or her modesty. You can move head to toe for the assessment, but base your approach on the development level rather than just on the actual age—for all children.

School-age children can think more logically and understand instructions and procedures. They are more willing to cooperate than younger children. Ask them simple questions to build rapport. Communication can provide you with insight into cognitive ability and personality. Acknowledging the child's maturity will gain more cooperation. Tell them what you are doing and why to help the child understand. Patients who are 6–8 years old may not express themselves verbally as well as older children, but they can draw accurately to depict the family or what is wrong with them. Give older children the chance to talk to the provider without the parents in the room. They may find it easier to discuss their pubertal changes without the parents present. Consider their modesty. While younger children may be comfortable in their underwear, older children usually appreciate a gown.

Early, Middle, and Late Adolescence

Development progresses unevenly and can vary widely among the 12- to 18-year-olds. Respect their confidentiality. Ask for parental input first. Interview and examine the adolescent privately away from parents. Avoid power struggles and allow any control that is feasible. Involve them in planning their own health care and habits or choices.

The main reason adolescents seek care is because of an injury or the need for a school or sports physical exam. In forging their identity, they often reject adults' beliefs and values and take risks. When treated as a partner in their health care, some teens are receptive to health care teachings. They are very sensitive and need to be treated with respect, not like little children. Gaining the trust of both the teen and the parents is necessary to ensure that they will provide you with information and allow you to teach them healthy guidelines. Greet the adolescent before greeting the parent. Show interest in the teen. Chat about interests and how things are in general. The visit flows better if there is understanding with the parent and the teen about confidentiality from the beginning.

The teen must understand that the interview will be confidential unless there is a problem that needs to be addressed for health. If there is a medical need, the teen should be informed that the parent must be told. The parent and adolescent should come to an agreement that you will do two interviews, one with the parent and the adolescent and one with the teen alone. This allows the provider to understand how each perceives the other and to be able to stay neutral and open to both parties. Work to understand how the adolescent perceives the problem and the relationships with important people in the teen's life.

The young teen may be timid about sharing concerns, but also may not allow the parent to speak for them. State law determines if the teen can be treated without parental consent. Teens may want to talk about sex and birth control. State laws must be considered in the decision to provide birth control without parental knowledge. Information that is crucial to the health of the adolescent legally needs to be shared with parents because they are legally responsible for the child until age 18.

Report any suspicion of child abuse to the authorities. Try not to overwhelm teens and let them know you are interested in their well-being. Start with talking about their interests. Focus on the needs of the teen and remember that developmental age may not be the same as chronologic or emotional age. Ask nonthreatening questions first—"What do you like to do?" "Tell me about your friend. What is he/she like?" Ask for clarification of abstract phrasing or words if they are unclear. Watch for nonverbal communication. Body language outside the teen's awareness helps you open up the conversations when it is described. Elicit the adolescent's perceptions of the problem. Learn to pause and use silence to allow the teen time to process information and give a response. Asking "What are you thinking?" may encourage a response.

Table 10-6 provides a summary of developmental considerations for the provider when conducting an assessment of a pediatric patient.

Developmental Assessment

A significant component of a pediatric physical exam is to also assess the child's developmental progress. Developmental progress is concerned with acquiring functional skills that will promote independence from adult supervision (Bower, 2010). Children achieve developmental skills at a pace consistent with their genetic capabilities, temperamental style, and environmental opportunities. The care environment strongly affects the development of the child's full potential. Therefore, development is also dependent on having the psychological and physical needs of the child met. The sequence of milestone achievements occurs in an extraordinary consistent pattern within each individual; however, there is wide variability as to the age when successful achievement of tasks and behaviors is attained. Development is all about progress, so any indications of a standstill or regression and loss of previously obtained skills is of significant concern. Early identification of developmental delays or disorders is critical to the health and well-being of the child and families (Council on Children with Disabilities, 2006). Screening for **developmental delays** and behavioral difficulties requires a skilled provider and is one of the most critical aspects of pediatric assessment.

Developmental History

Development encompasses four domains: (1) gross motor, (2) vision and fine motor, (3) hearing, speech and language, and (4) social, emotional, and behavioral (Bower, 2010). Parental concerns about delays in fine and gross motor skills and language are often very accurate. Timely identification and prompt referral for early intervention may prevent the negative consequences of any developmental delay. Developmental assessment begins with observing the level and interaction of the child with parent/caregiver—especially with infants, toddlers, and preschool age.

PRACTICE POINT: Issues that Require Follow-up

Learning disabilities occur in 6–7% of all school-age children in the United States, with disabilities affecting more boys than girls. Attention deficit/hyperactivity disorder (ADHD) occurs in 3–5% of pediatric population, with males having a ratio of 3:1 in the population as compared to females who have a 6:1 ratio. Note that 10%–40% of children with ADHD also have learning disabilities. Autism also causes delays in the development of language skills and social skills, and about 75% of autistic children have cognitive deficits. The myth of immunizations causing autism was debunked recently when the researcher who published the report retracted it.

Table 10-6 Developmental guide for examination of pediatric patients

Infants	Toddlers	Preschoolers	School-Age Children	Adolescents
Discriminating	Apprehensive	Able to respond to directions	Need to "save face"	Hesitant to ask questions
Easily Consoled	Uncomfortable when nude	Able to ask and answer (some) questions	Generally polite and cooperative	Confused with new looks and feelings
Labile, especially when ill	Need security	Understand only what is seen or what is experienced	Not able to understand body functions before age 9	Self-conscious
	Not often distractible	Take words literally	Concerned about privacy	Suspicious of adults
	Curious	Fearful		Idealistic
Approaches	**Approaches**	**Approaches**	**Approaches**	**Approaches**
Examine while held in parent's lap. Do not separate infant from parents.	Friendly, but firm; be flexible—expect active resistance rather than cooperation. Allow child to move around the room.	Gain child's cooperation by seeking his/her help; encourage being an active participant. Compliment on cooperation.	Establish agenda with parent(s). Explain process and procedures simply [what/why]: be prepared for questions	Interview separately from parents. Create an accepting environment.
Approach slowly; avoid abrupt and jerky movements.	Don't offer choices. Encourage physical and verbal activity.	Offer choices between "first or second?" or "now or later?", or "this way or that way?", but avoid "yes" or "no" questions.	Watch for nonverbal cues indicating stress during the exam. Ask simple questions to enhance rapport; if child doesn't participate, return to interview parent(s).	Stress "normality," use "wellness" teaching.
Let infants touch and handle instruments before use. Plan distractions based on developmental stages.	Examine on lap or with parent near; don't separate from parent(s).	Respect child's privacy and modesty. Undress only part being examined.	Examine genital areas last and with matter-of-fact attitude.	Avoid "yes" or "no" questions: Use "tell me about...." Use open-ended questions.
Establish and return steady, friendly gaze.	Plan on having to restrain for ear and sometimes other exams. Explain equipment and procedures. Use toys as icebreakers/distractors.	Give simple explanations. Avoid ambiguous words and phrases.	Use of media to show body parts/function should be used with caution with younger, school-age child.	Respect need for privacy.
Move from noninvasive to invasive; nondistressing to distressing tasks.	Slowly acquaint child with yourself. Keep voice and movements at a steady level.	Allow/encourage imitation of exam techniques—dolls, parent, provider/use games.	Demonstrate how to use equipment.	Assume need for basic information: offer rationale, explanation, and describe findings. Remain objective, don't assume role of parent.
Observe while gaining history/information.	Move from nondistressing to distressing tasks.	No surprises. Talk to child, explain steps of exam.		Avoid use of slang or current teenage fad phrases and words; be careful in using humor.
Relaxed—OK Tense—not OK	Do not offer long lectures—less talk, more action.	Allow child to feel a sense of control.		Reflect and summarize.

Awareness of developmental risk factors can come from complete and accurate prenatal and delivery history. Important information that should be obtained includes the following:

- Mother's age at time of pregnancy
- History of mother's previous pregnancies (gravida, para, miscarriages [gestational age at time])
- Fetal exposure (gestational age) to drugs (prescription/illicit), alcohol, radiation, infections
- Mother's weight gain (excessive associated with preeclampsia/placental insufficiency; poor weight gain associated with fetal growth restriction)
- Reduction/increase in fetal movement
- Results of head ultrasound studies

Important labor and delivery history information includes the following:

- Gestational age when labor occurred (spontaneous/induced)
- Fetal presentation, length of labor, use of vacuum or forceps for delivery
- APGAR scores at 1, 5, and 10 minutes
- Resuscitation of newborn required
- Birth weight, height, head circumference of infant

Developmental Milestones

There are multiple standardized measuring instruments that may be used to determine a child's achievement of developmental milestones (Ringwalt, 2008). These tests are based on cross-sectional observations and analysis of many children to establish norms to which other children may be compared. There are basically two categories of instruments that are presently used: multi-domain screening instruments and social-emotional screening instruments. Each category is further divided into instruments that may be administered by families or other caregivers, and instruments to be administered by professionals (Table 10-7).

Parental concerns and observations are most likely to alert the provider to the possibility of developmental delays and are usually correct in their assessment.

Temperament

Development is also influenced by the child's **temperament**, which may be described as the inborn tendency to respond in a specific way to environmental stimuli or situations. Temperament is defined as "individual characteristics that are assumed to have a biological or genetic basis that determine the individual's affective/emotional, attentional, and motor responses in various circumstances" (Rothbart, 2007), and is stable across the lifespan (Grist & McCord, 2010). Each child is born with a **temperamental bias**, a distinctive constellation of feelings and behaviors that originate in the child's biology and appear early in development. Temperament affects young children's mood and emotions, how they approach and react to situations, their level of fear, frustration, sadness, discomfort, and so on. Temperament also plays a role in subsequent social interactions, responses, and social functioning, as well as playing a significant part in the development of the child's personality.

Infancy is a critical time in which experiences lay the foundation for later competencies. Contributions of individual differences in infant characteristics set the tone and create the conditions around which social interaction and development occur. For example, infants who smile and vocalize in response to social stimulation create an environment different from infants who are likely to fuss or cry in response to some type of stimulation. Infants also differ in threshold for visual and auditory stimulation—one may enjoy a certain level and another might find it aversive. Affective disposition and sensory threshold serve as filters through which sensory and perceptual stimuli are processed and therefore create the environments that infant's experience—the individual differences around which infant cognition and personality develop. Infancy is an important time in which these differences first appear and developmental trajectories begin to set.

> ***PRACTICE POINT: Anticipatory Guidance***
> Health care providers assess emerging issues that a child and family face and give advice that is developmentally consistent, timely, appropriate, and relevant. Parents or caregivers who know what to anticipate developmentally avoid having unrealistic expectations or have appropriate expectations. Part of the role of the care provider is teaching or anticipatory guidance. As a child grows and matures, parents need to have some ideas as to what to expect, based on temperamental and environmental factors. An irritable infant who is also somewhat irregular in eating and sleeping may not be easy to care for. The mother may feel frustrated and dissatisfied with the interactions with her infant if she had other hopes or expectations for how the two would mesh. The mother may need to revise her expectations and approach the infant in a way that the infant feels accepted and loved, thus improving their goodness of fit.

Temperament's Developmental Influence

Differences in temperament can be observed in infants. Some are fussy, sensitive to noises, easily startled and upset, while others are calm and mellow and quickly adapt to regular eating and sleeping routines. These differences continue as children mature. Many 8-year-olds are energetic, intense, and quick responding; others have a deliberate tempo, are reflective, and take time to adjust to new situations, foods, and people. Parents who have several children observe differences in persistence, distractibility, and energy levels, and recognize that one child may be typically outgoing and enthusiastic, while another is shy and "low-key." It is especially important to recognize individual differences in temperament when a child has learning or attention problems, as parents and teachers need to figure out the reasons for a child's behavior.

Temperament influences developmental pathways and outcomes, even in areas believed to be the result of socialization (i.e., conduct problems, empathy, and development of conscience). Temperament develops over time. In the early infant differences in attentional orienting, distress proneness, positive affect, and approach and frustration develop. In the later infant, differences in fearful inhibition to novel or intense stimuli develop, as well as the beginning of effortful control.

While various definitions of temperament have been developed (Chess, Thomas, & Birch, 1968; Keogh, 2003; Kristal, 2005), the definition by Thomas and Chess (1977) is especially appropriate for parents when considering child and family interactions. They defined temperament "as a general term referring to the 'how' of behavior, differing from ability, which focuses on the 'what' and 'how well' of behaving, and from motivation, which explains why one does something" (Keogh, 2003). To explicate temperament, Thomas and Chess also proposed nine constructs that provide the framework for differentiating individual characteristics of temperament (refer to Table 10-8). These constructs were based on their own clinical expertise and research with children and families. Further refinement of these constructs occurred with the definitions developed by Kristal (2005).

From these nine constructs, the following three patterns, or constellations, of child temperament characteristics emerged that influence family relationships and family life.

- "Easy" children are typically adaptable, mild or moderate in activity and intensity, positive in mood, and interested in new experiences. The easy child has regular eating, sleeping, and elimination cycles; positive approach responses to new situations; accepts frustration with little fuss; is in a good mood most of the time; and smiles a lot.
- "Difficult" children tend to be intense, low in adaptability, and negative in mood. The difficult child has irregular eating, sleeping, and elimination cycles; negative approach responses to new situations (frequent and loud crying or throwing tantrums when frustrated); is slow to adapt to change; needs more time to get used to new foods or people; and has problems that center around socialization patterns, and expectations of family, school, and peer groups.

Table 10-7 Developmental milestones

Age	Gross Motor	Fine Motor and Vision	Hearing, Speech and Language	Social, Emotional/ Behavioral	Cortical Functions
6 weeks	Head level with body in ventral suspension	Visually, fixes and follows (midline)	Vocalizes Stills to sounds	Regards faces Smiles	
3–5 months	Holds head at 90 degrees in ventral suspension Rolls over, holds head upright when pulled from supine position	Holds an object placed in hand	Turns to sound Coos	Hand regard, laughs and squeals Reaches out for objects Smiles responsively, gurgles	
6 months	No head lag on pull to sit Sits unsupported In prone, lifts up on forearms	Palmar grasp of objects Transfers objects hand to hand	Babbles Responds to name Imitates sound	Works to reach a toy May finger feed	Awareness of surroundings Interaction with provider (social smile, inquisitiveness, and habituation) Cooing and gurgling
9 months	Crawls Sits steadily unsupported and pivots around	Pincer (finger–thumb) grasp Index finger approach Bangs two cubes together	Jabbers (Two-syllable babble)	Waves bye-bye Plays pat-a-cake, peek-a-boo Indicates wants	Makes non-specific "mama" and "dada" sounds
12 months	Pulls to stand; Cruises; Stands alone (briefly); Walks alone	Puts block in cup; Throws; Drinks from a cup	One or two words	Imitates activities; Plays ball; Object permanence established	
15 months– 18 months	Walks well Walks backwards Runs	Scribbles Builds tower of 2–4 cubes	Points, follows, simple commands 6–12 words	Hugs parents, uses spoon/fork Helps in house Symbolic play	6–8 vocabulary words; Comprehends simple one step commands; Points to 2–3 body parts
2–2 1/2 years	Kicks ball Climbs stairs two feet per step	Tower of 6–8 cubes Circular scribble	Joins 2–3 words; 50% of speech understandable; Dry at night; Knows 5–6 body parts; Identifies two pictures	Removes a garment (sock)	Begins referring to oneself as "I." Knowledge of name/age
3 years	Throws overarm; Stands briefly on one foot; Climbs stairs one foot per step; Pedals tricycle	Tower of nine cubes Copies a circle Cuts with scissors	Talks in sentences Names four pictures	Eats with fork and spoon; Puts on clothing; Names friend; Likely toilet trained	Counts three objects; Understands prepositional concepts; Asks questions; Names three colors (primary)
4 years	Hops on one foot Descends stairs (adult manner) Throws overhand	Cuts across paper with fine scissors	Can tell stories and use compound sentences, prepositions, and plurals	Dresses/undresses self; Brushes teeth; Imitates adult roles; Curious about sex; Nightmare and monster fears; Imaginary friends	Copies a square/cross
5 years	Catches ball with two hands Swings on swing, pumping by self Skips or makes running broad jumps	Prints first name Draws person that has at least 3 parts—head, eyes, nose, mouth, etc.	Asks meaning of words Abstract words are elusive Uses past tense	Complete sphincter control Conformity to peers important Romantic feelings for others	Spells monosyllabic words Counts to 10
6-12 years	Skips with alternating feet Rides bicycle Gains athletic skill; organized sports possible	Prints letters Draws recognizable person with head, body, and limbs	Incomplete sentences decline; Shift from egocentric speech to social speech; Vocabulary expands geometrically (50,000 words by age 12); Adherence to logic	Ties shoes "Rules of game" are key Demonstrating competency is important Sexual feelings not apparent	Copies a diamond Reads polysyllabic words Concepts of division, multiplication, geography, general information like cities, states, large rivers, oceans, etc.

Source: (Data from Bower, 2010; Casey, 2012; Kotagal, 2012)

Table 10-8 Constructs of temperament

Motor Activity	Level of activity/motions during meals, sleeping, playing, bathing etc.
Advance/Retreat	Level of initial acceptance or responsiveness to unique or unusual stimuli
Periodicity	Regularity of maintaining predictability of daily schedule of activities related to sleeping, bathing, eating, etc.
Responsiveness	Amount of stimulation needed to initiate a response to sensory stimuli
Flexibility	Degree of adaptability of child to unique or unusual situations or circumstances
Disposition	Perception or expression of attitudes in general or related to specific encounters/conditions
Reactivity	Level of intensity in response to different or unexpected circumstances
Resolution	Willingness or determination of child to persist with activity to achieve completion in spite of obstacles or barriers
Diversion	Degree or amount of extraneous stimuli needed to distract child away from or interfere with present activity

Source: Data from Chess & Thomas, 1996; Kristal, 2005; Allard & Hunter, 2010; Martin & Fox, 2008

- "Slow-to-warm-up" children are upset by change, are characteristically reluctant and withdraw in new situations, and shy with new people; although given time they adapt slowly and well. The slow-to-warm-up child has negative responses of mild intensity when exposed to new situations, but slowly comes to accept them with repeated exposure; has fairly regular biological routines; problems that vary with other characteristics shown—high activity—problems develop when child has insufficient space, highly rigid schedules, or few constructive activities for motor activity; is persistent—shows problems if attempts to engage in a task were prematurely or abruptly interrupted; is distractible—distressed when asked to work for long periods or beyond capabilities; and is more likely to withdraw (mild intensity) such as clinging to mom, quietly refusing to move or retreating to the corner of the room.

Children with difficult temperament can learn to cope with their sensitivities. If they can't learn, they can become confused, frustrated, and hopeless, and will most likely have to endure constant negative feedback, which creates a vicious cycle of discouragement. They require extra time, guidance, and patience. All children can be raised to be well-adjusted people with positive self-esteem; however, it takes parenting finesse. Effective parents develop attitudes, guidance strategies, and communication skills that work with, rather than against, a child's temperament. Difficult children can learn to be self-controlled, cooperative, and adaptable. Parents and others can be the ones to show the way.

Effortful Control

Temperament is demonstrated by the child's reaction to various forms and types of stimuli and is primarily based on how the stimuli are interpreted. As unique individuals, interpretations are going to vary. Infants and small children often react in a nonspecific manner that often is not congruent with the intensity or nature of the stimuli. For example, anxious and irritable children find negative events more threatening. Effortful control is linked to positive development of coping skills as a way to adapt their temperament to demonstrate contextual appropriate responses and adaptations. Lab and parent reports show effortful control is associated with lower levels of problem behaviors, also found to correlate with and predict low levels of negative emotion, highly committed compliance, high levels of social competence, and conscience.

Effortful control is an important developmental dimension of temperament that is essential for a child to recognize and demonstrate as maturation proceeds. Effortful control is defined as "the ability or efficiency of executive function, to inhibit a dominant response to perform a subdominant response to plan, and to detect errors" (Rothbart & Rueda, 2005). In essence, it is the extent of control the individual has over impulses and emotions. Effortful control includes the abilities to manage attention voluntarily (attentional regulation) and inhibit (inhibitory control) or activate (activational control) behavior as needed to adapt to environmental input, especially when the child does not particularly want to do so (Eisenberg, Spinrad, & Eggum, 2010). Through learning to exercise effortful control, the child learns what is or is not acceptable behavior. For example, the abilities to focus attention when there are distractions, to not interrupt others and sit still during certain functions, to force oneself to do an unpleasant task are aspects of effortful control. These abilities underlie the emergence of **self-regulation**, a major milestone in children's development.

Effortful control is believed to involve executive attention abilities and as part of this has been shown to be involved in the voluntary control of thoughts and feelings, in resolving conflict in regard to discrepant information, correcting errors, and planning new actions.

Temperament also has a role in responses evoked from others. As children age, they are increasingly held responsible for their own behaviors by their socializers. Children who are not well regulated are likely to elicit negative reactions from both peers and adults. In addition, the attentional skills involved in effortful control are likely quite important in learning. Finally, the skills involved in effortful control have an obvious relevance to children's emerging adjustment and social competence.

Genetics play a part in effortful control. Parenting has also been associated with individual differences in effortful control. In general, young children's self-regulation (including behaviors that reflect effortful control) has been positively associated with maternal support and negatively related to a directive and controlling parenting style. Similarly, a secure attachment at 13 months and maternal sensitivity at 22 months predicted effortful control at a later assessment.

Finally, it is clear that effortful control is linked to positive development, even in the first 5 years of life. For example, laboratory or parent report measures of toddlers' and preschoolers' effortful control have been associated with lower levels of problem behaviors, concurrently and at older ages. In addition, young children's effortful control has been found to correlate with, and predict over time, low levels of negative emotion, highly committed compliance, high levels of social competence, and conscience.

Although effortful control has a hereditary basis, it develops rapidly in the first 4 years of life, with marked improvements occurring in the third year. Individual differences in effortful control, although due partly to heredity, are also associated with the quality of mother–child interactions. Warm, supportive parenting, rather than cold, directive parenting, appears to predict higher levels of effortful control. Individual differences in effortful control that emerge during the first 5 years of life have been linked to higher levels of adjustment, social competence, committed compliance, and conscience.

Temperament and Injuries

Failure to learn to regulate emotions is referred to as dysregulation. Dysregulation results in poor judgment on the part of the individual resulting in behaviors that could be considered to be inappropriate or dangerous. Unintentional injuries are a significant cause of pediatric morbidity and mortality (Judy, 2011). Certain temperament traits have been implicated as contributing to high risk of unintentional injuries, which are (1) activity level, (2) impulsivity, and (3) inhibitory control (Schwebel & Gaines, 2007). Of the three, inhibitory control is regarded to be the most consistent and significant trait for predicting high-risk behaviors. A significant result related to these traits is the overestimation of the child's physical abilities and his or her perception of risk and sustaining injuries.

One of the most effective prevention strategies for unintentional injuries is parental or adult physical proximity and supervision (Schwebel & Barton, 2005). Parents and adults who intervene promptly with children when engaging in high-risk activities have children who take fewer risks and experience fewer injuries. Parents and adults who provide physical or verbal intervention when the child begins to act dangerously are thought to cause children to better use self-correcting strategies (Schwebel & Bounds, 2003).

Summary

- A child is not a mini-adult, even though they possess all the physical manifestations and characteristics of the adult. Children come in many shapes and sizes as well as varying abilities and degrees of development and maturity, all of which affects their care needs during a physical examination.
- A child, although a unique individual, is unable to function independently outside the context of a family in meeting one's physical, psychological, emotional needs. As such, a child requires a caregiver who is integral to the survival of the child, forming a relationship with the child that constitutes a patient unit.
- Children at various ages and stages vary in their abilities to understand and comprehend the function of and need for various techniques and procedures associated with a physical examination as well as fully cooperate to allow examination of certain areas of the body. Adaptation in the sequencing of the exam and use of various techniques are needed to engage the child in the exam and elicit their cooperation.
- The ability of a child to communicate appropriately depends on the developmental stage and requires the provider to use appropriate strategies that are nonthreatening and related to the child's abilities and needs.
- Who and what the child is to become is influenced significantly by one's temperament as well as cultural, environmental, and emotional contexts, all of which need to be a part of the pediatric assessment. Recognizing these influences allows the provider to determine if any interventions may need to be implements to maintain or facilitate their positive effects or to implement any changes that maybe needed to reduce any negative influences.

Review Questions

1. The provider is about to perform an abdominal examination on a healthy 3-year-old child. Which of the following statements is true regarding the performance of this examination? (Select all that apply.)
    1. In general the performance of this examination should be similar to that of the adult.
    2. The examination should be performed with the parent or guardian outside of the room.
    3. The examination may need to be altered from the usual order based on the child's response to the process.
    4. The provider should omit the step of palpation of the abdomen in children under age 5.
    5. The abdominal examination is not necessary in a child with no complaints of abdominal pain.
2. When measuring the height of a 12-month-old child, the provider understands that the best way to position the child to obtain this measurement is to do which of the following?
    1. Help the child stand and use the height tool on the scale.
    2. Have the child stand against the wall and mark the height on the wall.
    3. Measure the height while the child is in the parent's lap.
    4. Ask the parent to position the patient on the exam table in a supine position.
3. A provider in a pediatric clinic is about to perform health assessments on a 14-year-old female and her 5-year-old sister. The children are accompanied by both parents. Before beginning the assessment of the 14-year-old, it would be appropriate for the provider to do which of the following?
    1. Ask the parents to leave the room until the interview and examination are complete.
    2. Ask the father to take the younger child to a play area until the interview and examination of the older child are complete.
    3. Ask the family who should be present while the 14-year-old is examined.
    4. Let the family know that part of the interview and examination of the 14-year-old will be conducted privately.
4. A pediatric provider recognizes the importance of family-centered care when asking the following question of a mother during a well-child visit of a 6-month-old?
    1. "Are you still nursing the baby?"
    2. "How often is the baby waking up to feed at night?"
    3. "How are you adjusting to being back at work?"
    4. "Did the baby run a fever after the last vaccine?"

5. During the hospitalization of a 5-year-old child the provider can enable the other members of the child's family by doing which of the following?
   1. limiting visits to the child's immediate family only
   2. completing all care of the child while parents are out of the room
   3. allowing siblings to participate in the child's care as they are able
   4. providing only minimal information about the illness to the family

6. Which statement about involving a child in the health interview is most appropriate?
   1. The parent should be the source of information until the child is an adolescent.
   2. Teens should be interviewed in the presence of the parent.
   3. Pre-schoolers can be participants in the interview by providing information about activities.
   4. Teaching or guidance of parents should occur when the child is out of the room.

7. When preparing to examine a 6-year-old, which approach is best for the provider to take when beginning the examination?
   1. Ask the child if it is oaky for the provider to look in the ears.
   2. Ask the parent if the child has had any pain.
   3. Show the child the equipment to be used.
   4. Tell the child that the examination will not hurt.

8. The provider is about to give an injection to a 5-year-old child. The child asks the provider if it will hurt. Which is the best response for the provider to give the child?
   1. "No, it won't hurt at all."
   2. "Yes, but just for a few minutes."
   3. "It will hurt less if you hold still."
   4. "It will feel like a little pinch."

9. A school nurse in an elementary school in a multi-cultural area should expect which of the following?
   1. Children of African American descent will likely be taller than Caucasian children of the same age.
   2. Asian American children are likely to be taller than other children in their class.
   3. Latino children will be taller than African American children in the school-age years.
   4. Caucasian children will usually be taller and larger than children of all minority groups.

10. The provider is concerned about an 8-year-old child who has been in the emergency department with several playground accidents over the past 3 months. What should the provider include in the child's visit to the clinic? (Select all that apply.)
    1. an assessment of the child's temperament
    2. a discussion of parental discipline and expectations of the child
    3. a depression screening for the child and parents
    4. a complete assessment of the child's nutritional intake
    5. an assessment of fine motor abilities of the child

The Pregnant Woman

11

Linda Bergstrom, RN, CNM, PhD, FACNM
Marianne F. Moore PhD(c), CNM

The whoosh...whoosh of the fetal heart monitor is just as it is supposed to be; the nurse said so. This is their first pregnancy, and the continuous monitoring and attention to labor progression provides the reassurance the Larsons need. Sheila holds her husband's hand, remembering of the times she had raced to her OB provider in a panic with a new and unfamiliar sensation. She had thought her earlier nausea and vomiting was hyperemesis gravidarum because she had read about it online. Her lower abdominal pain had turned out to be round ligament pain; and her shortness of breath had been a natural, physiological symptom of pregnancy. But how was she supposed to know that when she had never been pregnant before?

Despite all of the new changes, she and her husband had survived it all and the time to give birth is here. The last cervical check indicates she is completely dilated and effaced, with the head low in the pelvis. It's time to push!

The next 2 hours feel like an eternity. Sheila is exhausted and her whole body aches. She had refused an epidural, but now regrets that decision. She's sweating profusely, soaking her gown with sweat....

"You're almost there, Sheila, keep trying!" Squeezing her husband's hand, she leans forward pushing with every ounce of her remaining energy. Falling backwards with a cry, she hears another cry that's not her own. She grins, thinking maybe this wasn't so bad after all.

LEARNING OUTCOMES

1. Explain the process of female reproduction related to age, pregnancy, and psychological associated changes and concurrent risk factors.
2. Relate anatomical and physiological body systems to pathophysiological alterations that may be experienced.
3. Describe an appropriate patient history in preparation for examination of the female reproductive system during pregnancy.
4. Describe an examination of the female reproductive system during pregnancy using appropriate techniques and document findings.
5. Explain expected and unexpected findings of an assessment of the female reproductive system during pregnancy.

Pregnancy is a natural, physiological condition that is necessary for the growth and development of a new individual. Most pregnancies occur in early-adult women who are fundamentally healthy, and progress in a typical manner, resulting in a safe, natural birth of a healthy infant. Although pregnancy is a natural, life-sustaining physiological process, it does have the potential for serious complications. Before the 20th century maternal and/or infant death during or soon after birth were not uncommon. The two primary reasons for death associated with birth were infection or hemorrhage. Scientific advances and improved obstetric care and attendance during the 20th century significantly reduced fetal and maternal mortality worldwide. However, in the 21st century mortality rates remain high in developing countries necessitating a call for regional and global initiatives to improve systems and practices.

Assessment of the pregnant female is managed according to three primary goals: 1) forming and developing a relationship between the woman and providers, 2) providing health education for the woman and her family, and 3) surveillance to assure that the pregnancy is proceeding in an expected manner and to recognize actual or potential problems as early as possible. Skilled assessment is critical to achieving appropriate surveillance.

Structure and Function

The female reproductive system is uniquely structured to conceive, develop, and give birth to a new human being. Thus, it is the only organ system that is associated with creation of new life. A detailed description of the female reproductive system is provided in Chapter 30.

In addition to changes of the reproductive system and organs, during pregnancy, a woman's body experiences a number of other system physiological, functional changes related to fetal growth and release of hormones. A more detailed description of system changes is included within Chapters 16–28.

Pregnancy begins with fertilization of an ovum by a sperm (Figure 11-1). After fertilization within the fallopian tube, the zygote (fertilized ovum), over a course of 3–5 days, slowly advances into the uterine cavity where it is implanted by about the 7th day. From the initial solid mass of the blastocyst (embryo), a peripheral layer of cells known as trophoblast separates. The trophoblast attaches the blastocyst (embryo) to the secretory endometrium and starts the complex fetal–maternal circulation that supports the product of conception. Part of the trophoblast becomes the placenta. By the 9th day, the placenta begins to secrete the key pregnancy hormone, human chorionic gonadotropin (HCG).

Indicators of Pregnancy

The initial assessment of the pregnant woman begins when a woman presents with either confirmation of pregnancy or possible symptoms of pregnancy. A woman may suspect that she is pregnant prior to confirmation by a provider. Initial **presumptive symptoms** generally include amenorrhea, fatigue, urinary frequency, breast tenderness, nausea, vomiting, aversion to certain foods, and heightened sense of smell. These are thought to occur as a result of the increased level of hormones.

Anatomic and Physiologic Changes During Pregnancy

Initial physiologic changes occur after fertilization to provide the appropriate environment for the developing pre-embryo. At day 15 the pre-embryo becomes an embryo, and at 9 weeks the embryo becomes a fetus. Pregnancy is marked by a shift of gonadal hormone secretion from the corpus luteum to the placenta, which is considered an endocrine organ with a limited lifespan. Its sole function is synthesizing and secreting proteins and hormones vital to support both maternal and fetal metabolism.

The increased levels of estrogen and progesterone cause the uterus to respond, rapidly increasing in size. Later the increased size is due to the growing fetal body. In early pregnancy, up to about 10 weeks, the uterus may be enlarged irregularly because of the exact site of implantation, called **Piskacek's sign**. Other associated changes in the uterus provide other signs of pregnancy; however, they are not considered as diagnostic.

As the pregnancy progresses, the ovoid shape of the uterus increases, gradually rising out of the pelvis and into the abdominal cavity, placing pressure on and somewhat displacing the digestive organs. Towards the completion of pregnancy, the uterus presses against the diaphragm. Throughout the pregnancy, the uterine muscles increase so that by the end of pregnancy their weight reaches a 10-fold increase.

Symptoms of pregnancy may be present in early pregnancy, but just because a woman feels like she is pregnant, she may not be. There is also an increase in pelvic blood and lymph flow that result in pelvic

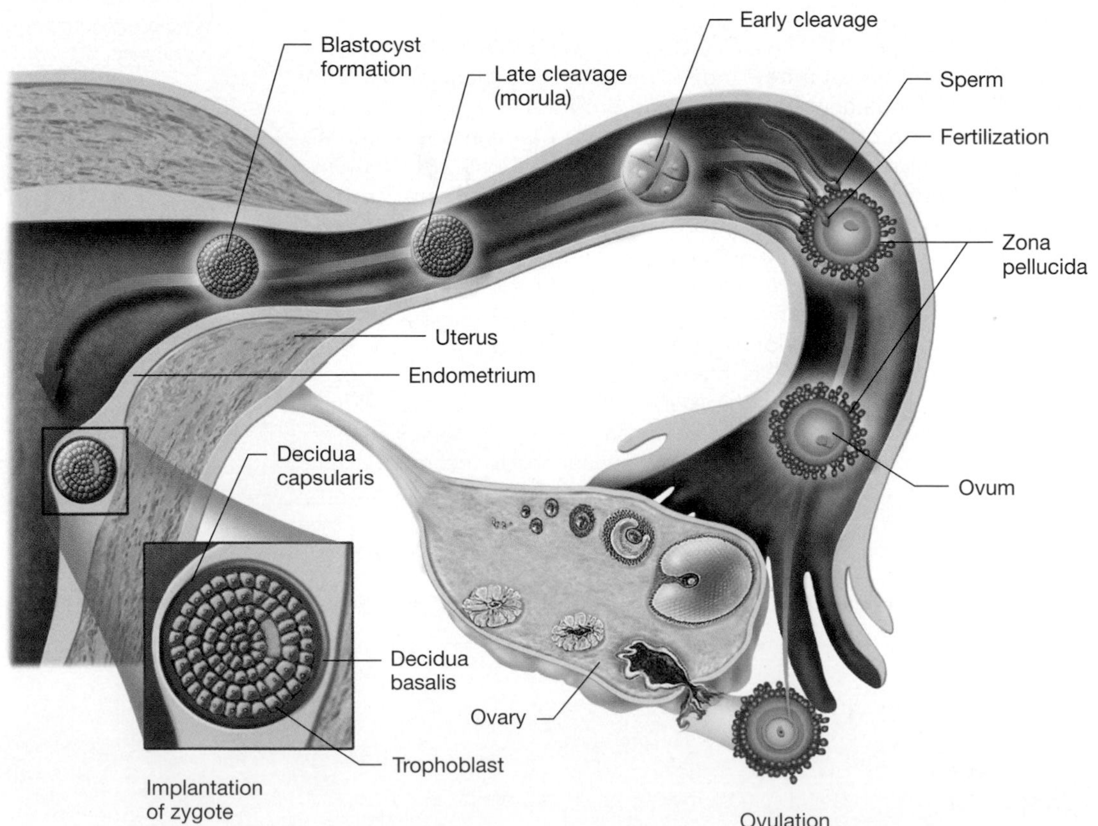

FIGURE 11-1 Pregnancy begins with the fertilization of an ovum by a sperm

edema and congestion. Cervical changes that occur in response to this congestion include a softening (**Goodell's sign**), and blue coloration (**Chadwick's sign**). A mucous plug also develops in the cervical canal. While the uterus is still in the pelvis, softening of the cervical isthmus causes uterine anteflexion, which in turn places pressure on the bladder (**Hegar's sign**).

The vaginal walls thicken secondary to increased connective tissue and smooth muscle hypertrophy. Vaginal secretions increase and become more acidic because of increased lactic acid secretion. The hormones relaxin and progesterone cause all connective tissue to soften and strengthen. Loosening of the pelvic ligaments results in the characteristic "waddle" walk of pregnant women. There is increased mobility of the pelvic bones, which will be useful during labor and birth.

An overall analysis of the stages and progression of pregnancy is presented in Table 11-1.

Specific Tests and Procedures

As part of routine prenatal care, the pregnant patient will undergo a number of tests and procedures throughout her pregnancy.

Pregnancy Tests

A definitive sign of pregnancy is the presence of human chorionic gonadotropin hormone (HCG) in the urine or blood. Chorionic gonadotropin is a glycoprotein produced by the pre-embryo. Production starts around implantation and can be detected in a woman's blood as early as 7 days after ovulation. Plasma levels of HCG rise exponentially, doubling every 48–72 hours reaching its peak at 9–12 weeks and then decline to a stable plateau for the remaining weeks of pregnancy. A woman may have already performed a urine test at home to determine her pregnancy status. Over-the-counter urine and laboratory tests are equally reliable and valid; however, if used too close to a missed period they might produce a false negative. Urine can be collected at any time of day. A serum test is a better test for detecting a very early pregnancy.

Caution in interpreting HCG values should be exercised as some normal pregnancies may have lower HCG levels. An HCG level less than 5 mIU/mL is considered negative and above 25 mIU/mL is considered positive.

Examination for Vaginal Amniotic Fluid

The fetal membranes and the amniotic fluid encased in them have critical functions for protection, growth, and development of the fetus. The fluid environment provides for muscle growth and development by allowing optimum fetal movement. The membranes also provide a barrier to protect the sterile environment from bacterial invasion and contamination.

Unless accompanied by an overlying vaginal infection, amniotic fluid is a watery substance that may be milky or clear and may have solid particles inside, with a characteristic but not unpleasant odor, and is decidedly alkaline. Amniotic fluid surrounds the fetus within the uterus. As it is encased within a membrane within the uterus, it is also sometimes referred to as the bag of waters (BOW). The presence of amniotic fluid can be confirmed visually when the history is clear and the amount is copious and characteristic. A sample of amniotic fluid may be obtained by placing a cotton-tipped swab around or inside the vagina.

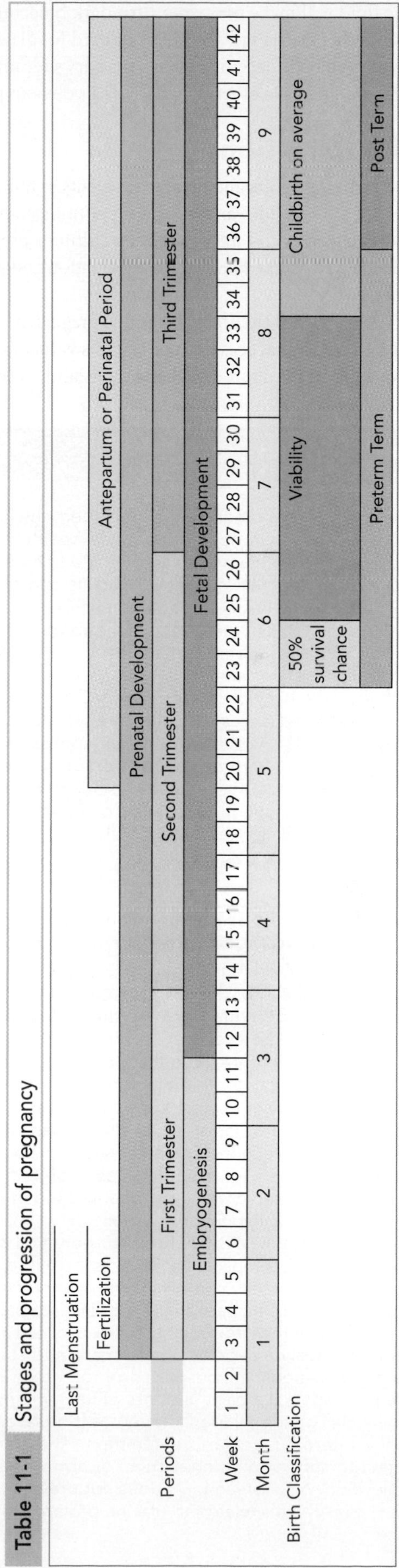

Table 11-1 Stages and progression of pregnancy

Periods	Last Menstruation; Fertilization; Antepartum or Perinatal Period; Prenatal Development; First Trimester; Second Trimester; Third Trimester; Embryogenesis; Fetal Development
Week	1, 2, 3, 4, 5, 6, 7, 8, 9, 10, 11, 12, 13, 14, 15, 16, 17, 18, 19, 20, 21, 22, 23, 24, 25, 26, 27, 28, 29, 30, 31, 32, 33, 34, 35, 36, 37, 38, 39, 40, 41, 42
Month	1, 2, 3, 4, 5, 6, 7, 8, 9
Birth Classification	50% survival chance; Viability; Childbirth on average; Preterm Term; Post Term

Amniotic fluid will make pH paper turn dark blue, but other fluids may also cause this change. The gold standard for diagnosis is observing the characteristic "ferning" pattern on a dry slide under the microscope (Figure 11-2). No other fluid causes this obvious pattern.

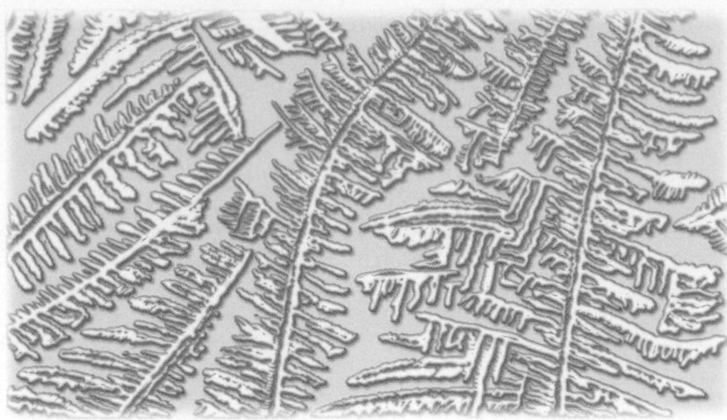

FIGURE 11-2 Ferning of amniotic fluid

Cultural Implications

Pregnancy and birth are significant, pivotal life events in human cultures; however, there are a wide variety of beliefs, attitudes, and practices regarding pregnancy and birth. In many cultures, pregnancy and birth are perceived as a symbol for acts of creation and renewal (Welch & Miller, 2012).

The only near universal cultural belief is that pregnancy is a time of vulnerability. The exact practices that address this vulnerable status vary widely from culture to culture and change constantly with time.

Health Promotion

Around the world, once a pregnancy is confirmed, the health of both the mother and infant becomes a major health care concern. Many factors influence maternal, perinatal, and neonatal mortality. One significant factor is the availability and adequacy of maternal and perinatal care. Those women who do not seek or are unable to take advantage of prenatal care are at high risk for developing significant complications for themselves or the infant. Maternal and infant morbidity and mortality are a measurement of the adequacy of care provided during pregnancy (Table 11-2). Despite advances in health care technology in the U.S., this country is 15th in the world when comparing infant and maternal mortality with other developed countries. As a part of the growing need to meet these health care needs, *Healthy People 2020* has identified specific objectives related to Maternal, Infant, and Child Health (MICH [U.S. Department of Health and Human Services, 2009]).

Cesarean Births

- MICH—07 Reduce cesarean births among low-risk (full-term [37–40 weeks], singleton [one fetus], vertex [head] presentation) women

The rate of Cesarean births has risen steadily worldwide. The total cesarean delivery rate in the U.S. for 2006, 31.1 percent, is the highest level ever reported. WHO and other health-related organizations propose that rates should be in the range of 10%–15%. Reasons for this rapid and steep increase are varied and complex and are related to (1) community standards that disallow even trials of labor (TOL) for women who have had previous Cesarean sections, (2) the ability to schedule and control the time of delivery for the convenience of both woman and provider, and (3) interventions commonly used in modern obstetric practices such as induction of labor.

Cesarean birth is a major abdominal surgery and carries a high risk for developing complications such as increased rates of infection, neonatal pulmonary complications, clotting problems, (thrombosis and emboli), increased risks for placenta previa and accreta, future uterine rupture if trial of labor is opted in future pregnancies, potential damage to other organs and structures, anesthesia complications, increased length of stay, increased costs, more post-operative pain, and loss of function. In subsequent pregnancies abnormal implantation of the placenta secondary to the internal scar is more common. The abdominal scar is subject to separation (dehiscence) or abdominal adhesions may develop. A Cesarean birth does not prevent later-life development of problems related to uterine prolapse or urinary incontinence.

The inherent risks of a major surgery and special risks from Cesarean births are avoided by allowing natural, physiologic labor (or for a trial of labor if the woman has had a previous cesarean section) unless there are definitive medical or obstetrical indications. The risk and benefits should be discussed with the patient.

Table 11-2 Live birth rates and infant mortality

Rates for Selected Countries		
Country	**Birth Rate**	**Infant Mortality Rate**
Afghanistan	37.8	149.2
Argentina	17.5	10.8
Australia	12.3	4.6
Cambodia	25.4	55.5
Canada	10.3	4.9
China	12.3	16.1
Egypt	24.6	25.2
France	12.3	3.3
Germany	8.3	3.5
Ghana	27.6	48.6
India	21.4	7.6
Iraq	28.8	41.7
Japan	7.3	2.8
Mexico	19.1	17.3
Russia	11.1	10.1
Sweden	10.2	2.7
United Kingdom	12.3	4.6
United States	13.8	6.1

Data based on 2011 estimates

Folic Acid Intake

- MICH—14 Increase the proportion of women of childbearing potential with intake of at least 4 mg of folic acid from fortified foods or dietary supplements.
- MICH—15 Reduce the proportion of women and childbearing potential who have low red blood cell folate concentrations.

Health Promotion *continued*

Folic acid is known to be protective against neural tube defects. The neural tube fuses between day 21 and 28, thus, these defects occur very early in the pregnancy. It is imperative that all women of child-bearing age have adequate folic acid levels before becoming pregnant and maintain these levels for at least the first 12 weeks of pregnancy. Daily intake of 4–8 mg is considered adequate and can easily be achieved by both eating high–folic acid foods (oranges, green vegetables, beans) and the use of ordinary multi-vitamins. Grain products (flour, cereals, rice, and pasta) are now supplemented with folic acid in the United States to help achieve this goal. A recent study also suggests that low vitamin B_{12} levels may also contribute to these defects (Pediatrics, March 2009).

Reduce Preterm Births

- MICH—08 Reduce low birth weight (LBW) and very low birth weight (VLBW).
- MICH—09 Reduce preterm births.

Preterm birth (PTB) refers to a delivery that occurs before 37 weeks of gestation. It is the leading cause of neonatal death, and its rate is rising in most developed countries, with the rate in the United States being one of the highest. This may be related to increasing inductions and multiple births. Subclassification is by gestational age or by birth weight. Survival rates of infants have a direct correlation with birth weight and gestational age. Causes of preterm birth remain unknown. Associated risk factors include tobacco and drug use, infectious diseases, fetal abnormalities, history of cervical surgeries, diethylstilbestrol-induced changes in the uterus, polyhydramnios, hemorrhage, pathologic uterine anomalies, traumatic life events, low prepregnancy weight, previous history of preterm birth and multiple gestations. However, about half of all preterm births have no identifiable risk factors.

Multiple gestation pregnancies are a factor associated with preterm birth, which is increasing in the United States secondary to infertility treatment, especially when ovulation-inducing drugs or embryo implantation is used. Another care-related complication is preterm induction of labor. Induction of labor may be necessary if maternal and fetal risks associated with continuation of pregnancy are greater than the risk associated with early delivery. Elective induction is increasing in the United States. While obstetrical reasons for elective induction may exist, some are due to the availability of cervical ripening agents, convenience, and relaxed attitudes toward induction. The Joint Commission issued new perinatal guidelines in 2010 that identified elective delivery between 37–39 weeks as a practice that should decline (Joint Commission, 2012).

A significant factor in meeting these goals is obtaining adequate prenatal care. The goal of prenatal care is to insure the birth of a healthy baby while maintaining parallel health of the mother. Observational studies revealed that prenatal care saves lives. In spite of the known benefit of prenatal care, disparities exist in both developed and undeveloped countries. In the United States, these disparities exist in adolescents, various minority groups, and low-income women.

The traditional model of delivering prenatal care was developed by physicians during the 1920s in an attempt to decrease the incidence and complications of preeclampsia. Over time, the benefits of prenatal care have been recognized; however, evidence of its effectiveness related to health outcomes, health-related behaviors, health care utilization, and health care costs is minimal (Berghella et al., 2011). A major criticism of research in this area is that they are not specific enough in identifying the focus of the research. The model for provision of prenatal care has changed very little since it was first implemented. Newer models of prenatal care, such as care delivered in a group setting (Centering Pregnancy® is one model) (Rising, Kennedy, & Klima, 2004), are being developed; however, research up to this point has not found them to be significantly better the comprehensive routine prenatal care (Benediktsson et al., 2013).

The quality of prenatal care is based on different metrics such as gestational age at which care began and the number of visits. This metric alone doesn't account for any measures of quality of care. Newer indexes such as the optimality index have been developed to address this issue (Low, Seng, & Miller, 2008; Murphy & Fulerton, 2006; Murphy & Fullerton, 2001).

Substance Use or Abuse

- MICH—11 Increase abstinence from alcohol, cigarettes, and illicit drugs among pregnant women.

These substances have the ability to cause permanent damage to the developing fetus, infant, or child. Fetal alcohol syndrome spectrum could be completely eliminated if women abstained from alcohol use during pregnancy. Decreased exposure of infants and children to tobacco would result in better growth, fewer infections, and fewer incidences of pulmonary diseases and asthma. Other outcomes would include saving health care money and resources. Infants born of mothers who use illegal drugs often go through withdrawal and experience physiological and/or neuro-biobehavioral problems that can result in health complications related to feeding, sleeping, movement, interactional capacity, and in general a poor neonatal adaptation process (Jansson & Velez, 2012).

Additionally, because of potential teratogenic fetal effects of drugs, various drug caution should always be exercised when deciding medication options for pregnant women. Many prescription drugs, including large classes like ACE inhibitors and cholesterol-lowering drugs (statins), are contraindicated during pregnancy. All drugs should be used with caution when treating a pregnant woman. Various imaging exams may also be contraindicated or should only be used if benefits clearly outweigh risks. Surgery and anesthesia also have the potential to cause adverse effects on the fetus.

THINK LINK: A Gap Between the Rates of Preterm Births
African American women have twice as many PTB and three to four times earlier PTB than women of other ethnic groups. Although the reasons for disparity in rates remain unknown, risk factors such as socioeconomic factors, education, lack of social support, lack of insurance, smoking, and rates of uterine and vaginal infections have been implicated.

There are no actual food restrictions except alcohol, which is known to have adverse effects upon fetal development or maternal health and excessive intake of vitamin A, which can be teratogenic in doses greater than 10,000 IU/day (1IU=0.3 mcg retinol equivalents). Avoidance of uncooked meat and raw sprouts and unpasteurized dairy products is recommended to prevent foodborne diseases.

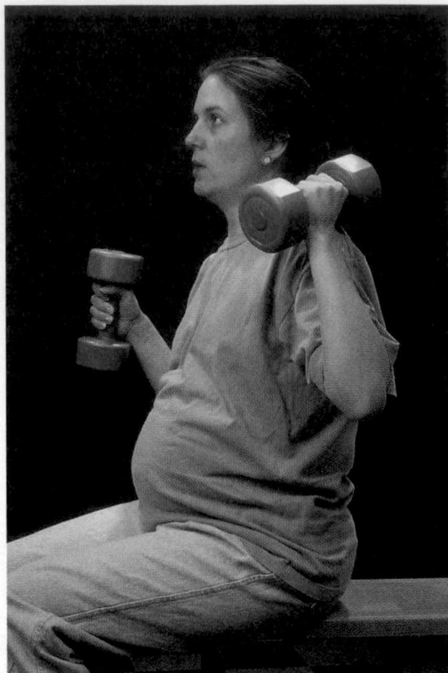

FIGURE 11-3 In the absence of serious complications, pregnant women should remain active
Source: CDC/ James Gathany

In the absence of serious complications like preterm labor, however, almost no common physical activity is known to be harmful as long as the woman has the ability to perform it (Figure 11-3). Pregnant women may lift and carry what they can, for example. They can do any job they have the ability to do; they can drive, walk, and travel in airplanes or boats. If they have been involved in sports and/or athletic competitions and are comfortable in doing so, there are no contraindications for continuing these activities. The general rule is that if a healthy pregnant woman can tolerate and maintain involvement in specific activities, and wants to do so, there are no contraindications to doing so.

Maternal–Infant Assessment

Once a pregnancy has been confirmed, it is imperative that a woman begin receiving prenatal care. The goals of prenatal care are to provide surveillance for early identification of pregnancy complications, to provide an opportunity for health promotion teaching and activities, to treat any medical conditions which may lead to health consequences, and to develop a relationship between the woman and her caregiver.

Pertinent Information

The initial priority is to establish the due date as accurately as possible. All prenatal care decisions will be premised on how far along the woman is in her pregnancy. If the woman is unable to give a reliable last menstrual period (LMP) history, ultrasound examination should be performed as soon as possible to establish the due date.

A due date for a pregnancy does not represent any kind of a contract for when the pregnancy will end. Instead, the date represents the middle day of the 30-day period in which natural labor and birth are most likely to occur. The span of time at which natural labor and birth are considered "normal" is from day one of the 37th week until day seven of the 42nd week. The due date may also be referred to as EDD (estimated date of delivery) or EDB (estimated date of birth). The most common way to determine the due date is to use **Nagele's formula**, which is as follows:

- Establish the first day of the LMP, which represents day 1 of the classic 28-day menstrual cycle.
- Subtract 3 months from the first day of the LMP, and then add 7 days.
- Pay particular attention to dates near the end of the month, and whether the month has 28, 29, 30, or 31 days. This is important to know to establish fetal gestational age related to viability of fetus.

	Month	Day	Year
LMP	4 [April]	3	2012
	−3	+7	+1
EDB	1 [Jan]	10	2013

Gravidity and Parity

Additional information that is usually obtained is **gravidity** and **parity**, which are terms used to provide a concise reproductive history of a woman. Gravidity or gravid refers to the number of pregnancies. Parity or parous refer to number of births. The numbers of these events may be different. A common convention for recording this information is the GTPAL system (Table 11-3). If the older, simpler G-P system is used, the P refers to the parity alone or the number of births at any gestational age past 20 weeks. The birth of multiples is one birth.

> ***THINK LINK: Viability***
> Any birth that happens after 20 weeks, regardless of outcome, is recorded on a birth certificate in the U.S. Demise of a fetus before 20 weeks is not considered the birth of a person in most jurisdictions. Some jurisdictions also require a death certificate for a birth after 20 weeks but before "viability." Due to advances in care for very preterm, low birth weight infants, the age of viability is constantly changing and moving downwards. State laws vary, and definitions about what equals the birth of a person may change in different states in the United States.

Prenatal Assessment

The physical and psychological changes associated with pregnancy are not just unfavorable consequences of an enlarging uterus and hormone alterations, but are modifications that facilitate the transition into motherhood, physically, psychologically, and emotionally (Lothian, 2008). The precise, complex, and deliberate interaction of progesterone, estrogen, and other hormones contribute to the pregnant woman's elevated sensitivity and emotionality, her inclination to be fearful, and an increased concern for the safety of her baby and herself. The providers approach to the examination of the pregnant woman should be based on and guided by the woman's overall perception of and meaning of the pregnancy.

Psychological Changes During Pregnancy

Pregnancy is an experience that is challenging, filled with growth, changes, and fulfillment. A woman's reaction to her pregnancy may be variable, depending on the cause of or reason for the pregnancy. The pregnancy may be planned and anticipated with great joy or it may be unplanned and perceived as an obstacle or a barrier to life's

Table 11-3 The GTPAL system

G	Gravidity or number of pregnancies ever achieved regardless of outcome. Multiple babies in one pregnancy event are recoded as one pregnancy.
T	Term births. Term is generally 37+ weeks. The resulting babies may have been born living or dead. Birth may be by any method.
P	Preterm (before 37 weeks) births that happen after the gestational age of 20 weeks. The resulting babies may have been born living or dead. Birth may be by any method.
A	Abortions, either therapeutic or spontaneous (miscarriages), before 20 weeks. One or more fetuses.
L	Living children at this time. If there are discrepancies in how the various numbers add up, for example, if there was one pregnancy and birth, but two living children or if there are fewer living children than were born, notations about the specific circumstances are usually added (twins, stillbirths, death of a live born child at some later age).

plans. Even if the pregnancy is planned, there are still emotional responses that may be viewed as challenging. It is not uncommon for a woman to initially feel some degree of conflict or lack of readiness related to the pregnancy.

It is likely that the woman will be distressed by feelings of ambivalence and may be cautious in disclosing this information. Providers need to recognize and accept these expressed feelings and to reassure the woman that it is acceptable and an expected emotional response to pregnancy. It is not a reflection on her as a "bad person" or her ability to be a good parent. It is also common for the woman's partner to experience similar emotions and must also supported in accepting them as expected emotions.

Fear and anxiety are also commonly experienced, and demonstrate concern for her health as well as the baby's health. Depending upon the woman's previous experience with pregnancy, there may also be a fear of losing the baby. Previous miscarriages or stillbirths may impact how the woman feels about and

THINK LINK: Expectations of Labor

It is not uncommon for a woman to be concerned about labor and how well she will be able to cope with it. Attendance at childbirth classes is a common preparation for labor and delivery and contributes to a woman's confidence in her ability to maintain a sense of control throughout labor. However, if labor does not go as planned, there is the possibility of the woman feeling that she wasn't able to follow through with her plans and expectations for labor, particularly if this is her first experience. Depending on her ability to accept a change in plans and expectations, as well as the support she receives from her husband and health care staff, she may experience feelings of failure and loss related to control, confidence, and esteem.

responds to this pregnancy. Excessive fear may become debilitating and may aggravate existing pain, discomfort, or distress. It is now recognized that high levels of stress and anxiety put a pregnant woman at a higher risk for the development of complications (Welch & Miller, 2012).

Pregnancy is also a stage in which there are several developmental challenges a woman goes through. While various authors have described specific developmental challenges and tasks, there is no formal standardized identification of the developmental aspects of pregnancy. The developmental component of pregnancy may be summarized as follows:

- Adaptation to and acceptance of the pregnancy and the impact it will have on self and significant relationships (partner/mother)
- Learning to give of oneself on behalf of one's child by acceptance and formulation of, and commitment to the parental role
- Anticipation of events related to labor and delivery
- Adopting coping skills that enable the pregnant woman to face the challenges of the physical, biological, and psychological changes accompanying pregnancy such as loss of self-control, confidence, and self-esteem
- Seeking acceptance of this child by others

Psychological manifestations of pregnancy by trimester are summarized in Table 11-4.

Clinical Context Exemplars

Situation A

Nolanda is a 19-year-old African American woman who presents with a first pregnancy. She is unsure of her LMP because she had recently stopped taking her combined oral contraceptive pill (COC) stating, "I didn't like how it made me feel." She reports a positive pregnancy test at home a week prior. Nolanda lives at home with her supportive mother and one younger sister; her father left years ago and she has two older brothers who are living elsewhere with families of their own. The father of her baby has not been involved since the pregnancy was first discovered. She attends college as a sophomore, and the baby is due in late May, after exams. Her mother is supportive.

1. What other historical information do you need?
2. What examinations and laboratories will you do at this visit?
3. What is the biggest priority of the assessment today?

Situation B

You are the charge nurse on a 12-bed LDRP (labor, delivery, recovery, postpartum) unit. Three patients at term present to the front desk at once, but you only have two LDRP rooms and four surgical rooms. Two patients are primiparas: one has been laboring most of the day (it is afternoon) and the other reports that she thinks her BOW has ruptured, but she is not contracting. The third patient is a G3P2 who is sitting in a wheelchair, who has been contracting since the early afternoon.

1. Who should be placed in the two remaining LDRP rooms?
2. Should the nurse perform a sterile vaginal examination (SVE) on the possible SROM prior to calling the provider? Why or why not?
3. When you assess the labor of the two laboring women, what else would you like to know?

Table 11-4 Psychological issues and physiological responses to pregnancy and childbirth

	First Trimester	Second Trimester	Third Trimester	Third Trimester (Postpartum)
Psychological	Mood swings: Ambivalence–attraction for/against pregnancy, doubt parenting ability, impact of baby on relationships	Mood swings may continue but develops a sense of well-being (adaptation to hormone levels)	Obvious alteration in body image and discomfort (altered self-image from special/beautiful to awkward, unsexy, and large)	Review birth experience
	Also feelings of joy, excitement, anticipation, conflicts, fear, anxiety	Beginning process of attachment (threat of miscarriage passed)	Fear of loss of attractiveness	Acceptance of outcomes of birth experience
		Reality of pregnancy with feeling of initial movements (quickening) of fetus, hearing heartbeat	Fear, anxiety, and vulnerability (increased concern on how good a parent she and her partner will be)	Acceptance of gender, appearance, and behavior of infant
		Focus primarily on needs of self and of fetus	Anticipation of birth and end of pregnancy [planning for labor and delivery]	Choose manner of infant feeding
		Increased interest in sexual activity (fear of pregnancy gone)/sexual fantasies	Preoccupation with birth (increased planning for needs of baby)	Preparation for resuming prepregnancy activities with partner and others
			Concerns for health of self and infant	
			Preparation for child care and alterations in lifestyle	
Physiological (signs/symptoms)	Physical changes and discomforts (nausea, vomiting, fatigue)	Physical changes also validate pregnancy (increased abdominal girth, increased vaginal lubrication)	Enlarging abdomen, edema, striae	
	Amenorrhea			

SUBJECTIVE DATA

The history for the pregnant woman extends beyond the gynecological history including past medical, family, and social histories. There are some aspects of the history that do only pertain to a pregnancy. Other history information that may need to be obtained will be covered in Chapter 30. In addition to information gathered previously related to determining the date for delivery, certain other information is obtained.

History of Present Illness

In spite of the fact that pregnancy is generally supervised by providers, pregnancy is not considered an illness. Illness in the context of pregnancy refers to symptoms that are caused by or related to the pregnancy. The history of present illness (HPI) may take a different presentation or context related to pregnancy. As with other system assessment, any symptom presented should be thoroughly assessed by a symptom analysis (COLDERRA).

Pregnancy can cause a wide variety of discomforts that can be experienced as mild to severe but which do not result in serious complications (Table 11-5). A symptom, such as headache, in a nonpregnant woman would not be a concern within the context of the reproductive system problems but in a pregnant woman it may indicate a serious problem. A pregnant woman may experience challenges related to other body systems that may impact the outcome of pregnancy such as accidents, headaches, diabetes, hypertension, or blood coagulation dysfunction.

Table 11-5 Pregnancy differential diagnosis—symptoms

Amenorrhea	**Endocrine factors:** early menopause; lactation; thyroid, pituitary, adrenal, ovarian dysfunction **Metabolic factors:** malnutrition, anemia, climatic changes, diabetes mellitus, degenerative disorders, long-distance running. **Psychological factors:** emotional shock, fear of pregnancy or STI, intense desire for pregnancy (pseudocyesis) stress **Obliteration** of endometrial cavity by infection or curettage **Systemic disease** (acute or chronic), such as tuberculosis or malignancy **Stress and anxiety:** Stress isn't good for your body, and it can cause you to have delayed ovulation. **Excessive weight loss, or weight gain:** Losing a substantial amount of weight, or gaining too much weight too quickly can cause you to experience menstrual problems, like a missed period or a delayed period. **Contraceptives:** Some women who take certain birth control pills don't have regular periods. **Breastfeeding:** When you breastfeed exclusively, the hormones that are allowing lactation to occur can block ovulation and your regular menstrual cycle. **Eating disorders:** When you have excessively low body weight this can interfere with hormonal functions, which might stop ovulation. **Rigorous Exercise:** Women who participate in activities and sports that require them to undergo rigorous training often experience skipped periods or no periods at all. **Medication:** There are some medications that can disrupt menstrual cycles. **Hormonal imbalance:** When you have hormonal problems, it can change the levels of hormones that your body requires to support ovulation and the menstruation process. **Problems with thyroid** **Uterine scarring**
Nausea/vomiting	**Gastrointestinal disorders** **Acute infections** (encephalitis) **Emotional disorders** such as pseudocyesis or anorexia nervosa
Urinary frequency	**Urinary tract infection** **Cystocele** **Pelvic tumors** **Urethral diverticula** **Emotional tension**
Breast tenderness	**Premenstrual tension** **Chronic cystitis mastitis** **Pseudocyesis** **Hyperestrogenism**
Quickening	**Increased peristalsis** **Flatus** (gas) **Contraction** of abdominal muscle **Shifting** of abdominal contents
	Pregnancy Differential Diagnosis—Signs
Changes in pelvic organs	Increased vascular congestion
Goodell's sign	Estrogen-progestin oral contraceptives
Chadwick's sign	Vulvar, vaginal, cervical hyperemia
Hegar's sign	Excessively soft walls of nonpregnant uterus
Uterine enlargement	Uterine tumors
Braun von Fernwald's sign	Uterine tumors
Enlargement of abdomen	Obesity, ascites, pelvic tumors
Braxton-Hicks contractions	Hematometra, pedunculated submucous, and soft myomas
Uterine soufflé	Large uterine myomas, large ovarian tumors, or any condition with greatly increased uterine blood flow
Pigmentation of skin	Estrogen-progestin oral contraceptives
Chloasma (Melasma)	Melanocyte hormonal stimulation
Linea nigra	Melanocyte hormonal stimulation
Nipples/areola	Melanocyte hormonal stimulation
Abdominal striae	Obesity, pelvic tumor
Ballottement	Uterine tumors/polyps, ascites
Pregnancy tests	Increased pituitary gonadotropins at menopause, choriocarcinoma, hydatidiform mole
Palpation for fetal outline	Uterine myomas

Abdominal/Pelvic Pain

Pelvic pain is a common problem that causes women to seek health care. The provider needs to carefully differentiate pain from the reproductive system from pain caused by the gastrointestinal or genitourinary systems. (Appendicitis is the most common surgical emergency in pregnancy and is often misdiagnosed.) Pain during pregnancy can be from benign causes such as stretching of the round ligaments, or from serious problems such as ectopic pregnancy, infection, or abruptio placenta. Pain can also indicate the onset of labor.

Provider Inquiries	Clinical Reasoning/Logic
Characteristics: Pressure, burning, stabbing, constant, wavelike, does it feel like what you think labor is like?	Sudden, localized, and constant pain is associated with ectopic pregnancy. Crampy, diffuse, abdominal pain, often with vaginal bleeding, characteristic of spontaneous abortion.
Onset: Especially in relationship to the menstrual cycle (before, during, after) or to the week of pregnancy?	Earlier onset during the first half of the pregnancy suggests processes associated with ectopic pregnancy, miscarriage, round ligament stretching and enlarging uterus, whereas later pain part of pregnancy may be related to labor contractions, placental abruption, and uterine rupture.
Location: Is the pain localized or more generalized across the abdomen?	Localization may become a challenge due to the enlarging uterus. Upper abdominal pain suggests diseases like cholecystitis, kidney stones or infection, gastroesophageal reflux disorder (GERD) or peptic ulcer disorder (PUD). Diffuse pain is seen in viral processes, irritable bowel syndrome, lactose intolerance. Pain in front of the pelvic girdle associated with symphysis pubic dysfunction (SPD). May also experience pain in lower back, leg or lower abdominal pain.
Duration: How long does it last? Does it come and go within a short amount of time (a few minutes)?	Persistent backaches and pelvic pressure that comes and goes may indicate the onset of labor. If they occur before 37 weeks, considered preterm labor. Pressure or tightening in the pelvis that is sporadic and not painful is commonly Braxton-Hicks contractions. Progressive pain is worrisome and signals disease processes like appendicitis.
Exacerbation: Any particular activities that make it worse? Especially activities relating to urination, having a bowel movement, or sexual activity?	Women with pain associated with SPD have pain with walking, lifting/carrying objects, rolling in bed, climbing stairs, getting in/out of car, and standing.
Radiation: Does the pain go anywhere else?	Epigastric pain radiating to RLQ suggests appendicitis.

Provider Inquiries	Clinical Reasoning/Logic
Associated signs/symptoms: Especially related to the urinary or digestive systems; bleeding, or vaginal discharge of any kind? Fever, chills, discharge, nausea, vomiting, constipation, diarrhea, melena, hematochezia?	Manifestations associated with pain that are of great significance: • Hemodynamic instability (hypotension, tachycardia, or both) • Syncope or near syncope • Peritoneal signs (rebound tenderness, rigidity, guarding) • Fever chills, and purulent vaginal discharge • Vaginal bleeding
Vaginal Bleeding Vaginal bleeding during pregnancy is common and a source of anxiety for most couples. The cause is almost always due to maternal factors rather than fetal. Gestational age is key as to the etiology for bleeding. Ruling out life-threatening causes of bleeding like ectopic pregnancy is paramount. There are also nonpregnancy-related causes of bleeding such as vaginal lacerations or trauma, vaginal or cervical polyps, STIs, or neoplasms.	
Characteristics: How much? Spotting or does it soak through pads/tampons in a short amount of time? (Asking a woman how many pads/tampons she has used may give misleading information because many women change a pad/tampon long before it is thoroughly soaked) Is it bright red (fresh) or brownish (older)? Clots? How big?	Severe bleeding is seen in spontaneous abortion (miscarriages) or ectopic pregnancy. Although bleeding may be scant in ectopic pregnancy. Bleeding from placenta previa may be varied in amount from scant to profuse.
Onset: In relation to the week of pregnancy or how long ago until coming in for care?	First trimester bleeding suggests ectopic pregnancy, spontaneous abortion, implantation or cervical/vaginal and uterine pathology. In late pregnancy two common serious causes are abruptio placenta or placenta previa.
Location: Certain it is coming from the vagina and not the rectum?	Bleeding found on toilet tissue might come from the rectum in a cause like hemorrhoids, or might originate in the vagina. It might be difficult for a woman to differentiate the two.
Duration: How long has it been going on (minutes to months)?	Persistent heavy bleeding in the first trimester is worrisome for spontaneous abortion. Ectopic pregnancy may present with intermittent bleeding. Placenta previa might begin with small amounts over days.
Exacerbation: Does anything you do make it worse?	Vaginal sexual activity may result in bleeding. This might be benign secondary to normal changes in the cervix, or it might be secondary to cervicitis from an STI. Sexual activity may trigger bleeding from placenta previa.
Relief: Does it stop on its own?	Bleeding from a spontaneous abortion will not stop until the uterus empties; bleeding from other causes, like cervicitis secondary to an STI, often starts and stops on its own.

Provider Inquiries	Clinical Reasoning/Logic
Associated signs/symptoms: Presence of pelvic or abdominal pain: Midline or lateral pelvic pains? Any vaginal discharge other than bleeding? Fever chills? Associated history of PID, prior ectopic pregnancy, presence of IUD device, adnexal surgery and antiphospholipid syndrome, uterine anomaly and parental chromosomal translocation, history of miscarriages, history of IVF?	First trimester vaginal bleeding with midline pain suggests spontaneous abortion, whereas lateral pain makes one suspicious of ectopic pregnancy. Hemodynamic instability and abdominal tenderness suggest ruptured ectopic pregnancy. History serves as clues to etiology of bleeding.
Vaginal Discharge Vaginal discharge can be physiologic and therefore benign, or it can be a symptom of a mild vaginal infection, such as yeast or bacterial vaginosis, or a severe infection such as gonorrhea, or chlamydia. Symptoms during pregnant and nonpregnant state are generally similar. Intense pruritus, burning, irritation, and redness suggest an infection rather than a physiologic phenomenon related to pregnancy, for example, the so-called physiologic leukorrhea, which is associated with oral contraceptive pill (OCP) use, pregnancy, and time of ovulation.	
Characteristics: Color, odor, amount?	In pregnancy, fluid coming from the vagina might be amniotic fluid after premature rupture of the membranes (PROM) or a symptom of an STI. Normal discharge may be yellowish and mildly malodorous but usually not accompanied by severe pruritus or irritation.
Onset: In relationship to the week of pregnancy?	Release of amniotic fluid generally happens in late pregnancy. Discharge from an STI might happen at any time.
Duration: How long ago before seeking care?	If the cause is amniotic fluid secondary to PROM, the risk of infection goes up quickly as time passes. Management may differ depending on how long the membranes have been ruptured.
Relief: Have you done anything to make it better or does it get better on its own?	A woman may try OTC remedies for irritating discharge, but nothing she can do without a prescription is likely to be helpful. If home remedies do solve the problem, it was probably something very benign.
Associated signs/symptom: Itching or skin irritation, symptoms of labor contractions, bleeding, does your partner have anything similar?	Fever, chills, and pain suggest infection. Presence of blisters suggests herpes; other lesions may be secondary to warts. History helps with clues as to etiology.
Edema A pregnant patient may complain of or present with edema or swelling in her face, hands, legs, or feet.	
Characteristics: Where? How much? Pitting? Increasing or decreasing? Bilateral or unilateral? Interfere with any activities?	Edema can be a benign problem of pregnancy related to normal changes in the peripheral vascular system, but edema can also be one of the cardinal symptoms of preeclampsia and other causes like nephritic syndrome or trophoblastic diseases.

Provider Inquiries	Clinical Reasoning/Logic
Onset: Sudden or gradual? When did you first notice it?	Sudden and rapid onset of edema suggest a pathologic process like preeclampsia.
Location: Local to dependent area or is it generalized? Where does it occur (feet, legs, hands, face)?	Edema confined to the feet and ankles or hands alone is not as worrisome as edema that spreads upwards, even into the face.
Duration: Does it come and go at different times of the day or change with activity or rest?	Benign causes of edema tend to come and go with activity and rest. Benign edema is often remedied by rest and elevation of the affected part.
Exacerbation: In relation to time of day, activity, rest or position?	End of the day swelling may be related to postural or gravitational factors.
Relief: Does anything you do make it better? Does it get better on its own or at different times of the day?	As above, a woman can relieve benign edema with simple remedies like rest and elevation.
Radiation: Is it moving up your legs or arms?	Edema that moves up to encompass the entire extremity is worrisome for preeclampsia.
Associated signs/symptoms: Headaches, visual changes, pain in chest or upper abdomen? Pelvic pain? Hypertension, liver function abnormalities, platelet abnormalities, proteinuria? Associated history of hypertension, diabetes, prior history of preeclampsia, prior history or renal diseases?	Any of these accompanying symptoms are suggestive of preeclampsia.

Uterine Contractions

Regular uterine contractions are the sine qua non of labor. Differentiating these from the mild, irregular contractions that occur at any stage of pregnancy may be a challenge. The hallmarks of true labor are contractions increasing in frequency, intensity and duration.

Provider Inquiries	Clinical Reasoning/Logic
Characteristics: Wavelike or constant? How bad? Regular or irregular? **O**nset: How long did contractions begin before seeking care? Week of pregnancy? Certain time of day?	The timing of the onset of regular contractions in relationship to the due date is of critical importance. Preterm labor, which is the most common cause of preterm birth, is determined by gestational age. Contractions that begin after 37 weeks are within the time frame for onset of normal labor. Those that begin before 37 weeks may herald preterm labor and birth. Women can also experience benign, mild, irregular contractions (Braxton-Hicks contractions) throughout the course of pregnancy. (**Braxton-Hicks contractions** may be more noticeable at night or at rest.)
Location: Certain it is the uterus and not the bladder or bowels?	This may be difficult to ascertain.
Duration: How long does it last?	A physiologic uterine contraction will last about a minute or less. A pathologic contraction will last longer and may suggest an emergency like abruptio placentae.
Exacerbation: Anything make it worse?	True uterine contractions will naturally increase in intensity over time no matter what the woman does, but the woman may find that a large variety of things can help her to cope with the contractions.
Relief: Does it come and go on its own? Anything make it better? Does it just stop on its own after awhile?	Braxton-Hicks contractions will go away on their own.
Associated signs/symptoms: Bleeding, vaginal discharge, fetal movement?	Cessation of fetal movement, vaginal bleeding, or fluid from vagina are worrisome accompanying signs of uterine contractions.

Changes in Fetal Movement

Fetal movement typically starts in the second trimester but may occur earlier in parous women. Decreased fetal movement is a common cause of concerns for pregnant women. Frequency of fetal movement is difficult to gauge as it is based on fetal wake–sleep cycles and the woman's perception, which may be variable.

Provider Inquiries	Clinical Reasoning/Logic
Characteristics: What exactly have you noticed? No movement or decreased or increased movement?	Fetuses have normal wake–sleep cycles and can be more or less active at different times of a day. Over time a woman recognizes patterns in how her baby moves inside. It may take some time before she notices that a fetus is not moving as much as before.
Onset: When did you realize that something has changed? Week of pregnancy?	This change of movement can be benign, as may happen in later pregnancy when there is not as much room inside the uterus or could indicate a compromise in fetal health, probably as a result of placental circulatory problems.
Duration: When was the last time you are certain you felt movement?	If it has been several hours (or days) since the woman was certain she felt fetal movement, this is worrisome and may suggest a fetal demise.
Relief: Did you do anything that you think resulted in a change?	It is possible that a woman can make a fetus more active with external stimulation, but if there is absent movement secondary to a demise, there was probably nothing she did that caused the demise. However, she may be worried about this or even feel guilty.
Associated signs/symptoms: Pain, bleeding, discharge?	Accompanying symptoms may suggest serious conditions like abruptio placentae, preterm labor, placenta previa.

Headaches

Headaches can be benign during pregnancy or may be associated with systemic illnesses or preeclampsia especially when they occur after 20 weeks' gestation and in primigravida women. Headaches in pregnancy should be carefully evaluated as they can be the precursor to eclampsia. The work up of headache in pregnancy is similar to nonpregnant women with special attention to blood pressure, gestational age, and protein in the urine.

Provider Inquiries	Clinical Reasoning/Logic
Characteristics: Constant or intermittent? Pounding, stabbing, twisting, squeezing? How bad (pain scale)?	Headaches may be a secondary symptom from high blood pressure.
Onset: When did it begin?	Acute, severe headaches are worrisome.
Location: Forehead, sinuses, neck, all over?	A woman may experience sinus or migraine headaches, which are not related to preeclampsia.
Duration: How long does an episode last?	A headache suggestive of preeclampsia will not go away quickly or easily.
Exacerbation: What makes it worse?	Headaches exacerbated by light, noise, smells are more suggestive of migraines rather than preeclampsia.
Relief: Have you tried anything that made it better? Taken any medication?	A woman cannot usually make a preeclamptic headache go away with things she does herself.
Associated signs/symptoms: Edema or swelling, "feel bad or sick," epigastric pain. Visual changes, hypertension, liver function abnormalities, platelet abnormalities, proteinuria?	Any of these accompanying symptoms are suggestive of preeclampsia.

"Feeling Bad"

A pregnant patient may complain of general symptoms of malaise, feeling sick, ill or "bad," or like she has the flu.

Provider Inquiries	Clinical Reasoning/Logic
Characteristics: Can you describe what you mean by this? How exactly do you feel? Does this make you worried?	Pregnancy-induced hypertension as it progresses to become more serious makes women feel generally sick or ill. Although they may not be able to describe this well, they know something is very wrong. The symptoms are often nonspecific and do not necessarily involve pain. They are probably the result of liver impairment. The woman's symptoms may remind a provider of the complaints of a person with hepatitis or another liver problem.
Onset: When did you first notice it?	This complaint should never be dismissed without thorough evaluation especially in late pregnancy or if there are risk factors for hypertension disorders of pregnancy.
Location: Depends on exact symptoms.	
Duration: How long does it last or has it been going on?	This feeling generally develops slowly over time.
Exacerbation: Anything make it worse?	Symptoms tend to get worse gradually and not in relationship to any particular activities.
Relief: Anything make it better? Especially rest?	Rest may make her symptoms improve but usually there is little she can do to make herself feel better.
Radiation: Depends on exact symptoms but mostly n/a.	
Associated signs/symptoms: Edema or swelling, headache, epigastric pain, visual problems, hypertension, liver function abnormalities, platelet abnormalities, proteinuria?	Any of these accompanying symptoms are suggestive of preeclampsia.

Throat, Upper Abdomen, or Stomach Pain

A pregnant patient may complain of a sore throat or pain in the upper abdomen or stomach.

Provider Inquiries	Clinical Reasoning/Logic
Characteristics: What's your pain like?	Pain in the upper abdomen during pregnancy may be from normal changes of pregnancy such as relaxation of the esophageal sphincter resulting in GERD, but this pain could also be a late symptom of serious preeclampsia. This kind of pain is generally located in the epigastric region and is severe. It is caused by the liver capsule stretching or actually breaking.
Onset: Sudden onset? In relationship to eating or drinking? Day or night time?	GERD generally happens in relation to eating and may occur at night secondary to lying down for sleep. Sudden onset is more suggestive of preeclampsia.
Location: Midline? Mouth, throat, off to one side, all over?	GERD tends to be confined just to the mouth and throat.
Duration: How long does it last?	Pain from preeclampsia generally continues on its own and does not go away.
Exacerbation: What makes it worse?	GERD can be made worse by lying down, by eating certain foods or certain amounts of foods.

Provider Inquiries	Clinical Reasoning/Logic
Relief: What have you tried that makes it better?	Numerous remedies may make GERD symptoms go away. Little can be done to help if the cause is pre-eclampsia
Radiation: Does it seem to move to someplace else or does it seem like it is "growing" in your chest?	GERD is usually felt just in the mouth and throat.
Associated signs/symptoms: Edema or swelling, headache, visual problems, hypertension, liver function abnormalities, platelet abnormalities, proteinuria?	Any of these symptoms are suggestive of preeclampsia.
Visual Changes A pregnant patient may notice changes in her eyes or with her vision.	
Characteristics: Lights, flashes, floaters, diminished in some way, glasses or contact lenses don't work right any more, how bad is it? Does it interfere with activities especially things like driving?	Visual changes may also be a symptom associated with the cerebral edema of pre-eclampsia. It can also be a benign change associated with changes in the shape of the eyeball during pregnancy. In general, woman should NOT get new prescriptions for glasses or contact lenses during pregnancy because mostly likely they will need another new prescription after these benign changes disappear postpartum.
Onset: When did you first notice this? Week of pregnancy?	There are benign changes in eye anatomy that may happen early in pregnancy. Preeclampsia generally happens in late pregnancy.
Associated signs and symptoms: Edema or swelling, headache, epigastric pain, visual problems, hypertension, liver function abnormalities, platelet abnormalities, proteinuria?	Visual changes accompanied by headaches, increased BP and edema suggest preeclampsia. Visual changes may also be associated with diabetes related to blood sugar levels, causing concomitant fluctuations in volume of eye fluids.
Past Medical History Information related to past medical history identifies any conditions that may affect the pregnancy.	
Any history of diabetes (including gestational), thyroid or other endocrine organ disorders?	Endocrine adaptations occur during pregnancy such as insulin resistance due to increased placental secretion of diabetogenic hormones like GH, CRH that drives the release of ACTH and cortisol, HCS and progesterone. Placental hormones affect both glucose and lipid metabolism to ensure that the fetus has adequate supply of nutrients. Excessive increase in BMI during pregnancy is a risk factor for development of gestational diabetes, preeclampsia and preterm birth. Previous gestational diabetes may be a predictive factor for present gestational diabetes.

Provider Inquiries	Clinical Reasoning/Logic
Any problems with excessive bleeding or history of bleeding or clotting diseases? Do you know your blood type and Rh factor? Did you ever get Rhogam in a previous pregnancy?	Bleeding disorders may cause bleeding problems during pregnancy and especially at birth. A woman who has Rh negative blood will need treatment with Rhogam during pregnancy, and possibly after delivery.
History of anemia?	There is physiologic anemia, mild fibrinolysis, neutrophilia mild thrombocytopenia and increased procoagulant factors during pregnancy.
Any heart disease or problems?	There is increased cardiac output, plasma volume and decreased systemic vascular resistance during pregnancy. Pre-existing heart disease may be exacerbated by pregnancy and will always need special consideration during pregnancy.
Conditions like arthritis, multiple sclerosis, other autoimmune disorders?	The outcome of pregnancy is better if autoimmune dysfunction like lupus is in a quiescent stage and when any renal disease is in remission. Autoimmune problems may improve or may worsen during pregnancy. Autoimmune conditions may improve during pregnancy secondary to a generalized mild suppression of the immune system in order that foreign fetal tissue, can develop.
Any hepatitis or liver diseases?	In pregnancy, liver disorders like acute fatty liver, intrahepatic cholestasis, preeclampsia and HELPP syndrome may occur. Pre-existing liver disease may worsen during pregnancy. For example, increased blood volume may worsen a preexisting portal hypertension. Hepatic adenomas are at increased risk for rupture.
Any other diseases or conditions (including psychiatric) for which you are being treated?	Rare problems that affect the bones, such as rickets, may have caused pelvic deformities that may make birth difficult. Injuries to the bony pelvis may also affect birth. Women with spinal cord injuries who have intact female organs can often get pregnant and carry to term, but may have anatomical injuries or motor deficits that make vaginal birth difficult or impossible.
What medications are you taking?	Medications used need to be evaluated for use during pregnancy in light of possible teratogenic possibilities. Whole drug classes are contraindicated in pregnancy. Some medications are particularly contraindicated at different gestational stages like NSAIDs (only safe during second trimester). Any drug continued during pregnancy will need careful consideration (Table 11-6).

Provider Inquiries	Clinical Reasoning/Logic
Any serious injuries to the pelvic area?	C-section increases uterine rupture with trial of labor, abnormal placentation, and adhesions. Because surgical treatment may end up being the method of birth, providers should ask about any problems that happened in previous surgery, like bleeding, embolism, especially problems with anesthesia of any kind. Providers should ask specifically about previous abdominal surgeries of any kind.
Any previous surgery to the genital or abdominal organs? What kind? Why? Have you had your appendix removed? Have you had any previous problems with anesthesia of any kind? Previous C-section? How many?	Providers need to know the pregnant woman's vaccination history or history of experiencing various infectious diseases to help prevent certain birth defects. The only vaccine that can be administered during pregnancy (if indicated) is TDAP and inactivated influenza.
Have you received the complete series of MMR vaccines? Are you vaccinated against varicella and hepatitis B, influenza TDAP (or did you have any of these diseases)? Did you get the vaccination against cervical cancer? Did you take all three injections?	Providers need to know about any history of cancer, especially gynecological cancers. Providers should ask about previous pap test results and any treatments of abnormal results.
Have you had any kind of cancer? Have you had an abnormal pap test? What was done about that?	Past history of Chlamydia may have resulted in scarring of the fallopian tubes, which may result in ectopic pregnancy. Herpes and condylomata infections may cause problems with pregnancy or birth.
Have you ever had any kind of STI? Which one? Was it/is it being treated?	Providers need to know about any present STIs such as HIV infection. Active STIs can be passed to a fetus during the birth process. Reassessment for these infections close to the time of birth is prudent.

Table 11-6 Known teratogens and their effects

Drug (FDA category)	Common Effect	Trimester of greatest danger
Aminoglycosides (C), high doses	VIII cranial nerve damage	unknown
Androgens (X)	Masculinization of female fetus	1st 12 weeks
ACE inhibitors (D)	Renal tubular dysplasia, skull hypoplasia, oligohydramnios, pulmonary hypoplasia	2nd/3rd
Antineoplastics (D) alkylating agents	Growth retardation, cleft palate, microphthalmia, cloudy cornea, agenesis of kidney, cardiac defects	1st–3rd
Antimetabolite agents	Growth retardation, malformation of ear, eye, nose, cleft palate, malformation of extremities, fingers, brain, skull	
Cocaine	Premature birth, abruptio placentae, SIDS, perinatal morbidity growth retardation, in utero stroke, bowel atresia, defects of GU system, heart, limbs, face	
Carbamazepine (C)	Craniofacial abnormalities, growth retardation, neural tube defects, fingernail hypoplasia	1st
Coumadin derivatives (D)	Fetal warfarine syndrome	2nd/3rd
	Optic atrophy, cataracts, mental retardation, microcephaly, microphthalmia, fetal /maternal hemorrhage	
Ethanol (high dose)	Fetal alcohol syndrome	1st

Continued

Table 11-6 Known teratogens and their effects *(continued)*

Drug (FDA category)	Common Effect	Trimester of greatest danger
Iodides, PTU (D)	Goiter, fetal hypothyroidism	3rd
Methimzole	Aplasia cutis	1st
Lithium (D)	Ebstein's anomaly, other cardiac defects	1st
Phentoin [D]	Fetal hydantoin syndrome including heart defect, low nasal bridge, growth retardation, nail hypoplasia, mental retardation	1st
Retinoids (X) (isotretinoin etetinate)	Heart defect, spontaneous abortion, mikcrotia, microcephalus, hydrocephalus, deformity of ears, face limbs, liver, cognitive defects, thymic hypoplasia	1st
Tetracyclines (D)	Weakened fetal bone and tooth enamel dyspolasia, permanent tooth discoloration	2nd/3rd
Thalidomide (X)	Anomalies of ears, teeth, eyes, intestine, limbs, heart kidney, deafness	days 34–50
Valproic acid (D)	Spina bifida, facial anomalies, slow development, microcephaly, CNS and cardiac defects	1st
Vitamin A (X) [>18,000–25,000 IU/day]	Microtia, craniofacial CNS and cardiac anomalies, bowel atresia, limb reductions, urinary tract defects	unknown
NSAID/aspirin	Premature closure of the ductus arteriosus, increase bleeding, increased risk for spontaneous abortion	Third trimester
Glucocorticoids	Increase risk for cleft palate, PROM, intrauterine growth restriction. In the mother, increase risk for hypertension and diabetes, infection and osteoporosis	First trimester for cleft palate

Table 11-7 Sample previous pregnancy chart

	Date	Weeks	Baby info	Weight	Birth type	Problems	Length of labor	Notes
1	Aug 2001	early	n/a	n/a	SAB		n/a	No surgery/in Mexico/FOB #1
2	Nov 2004	on time	M/healthy/Carlos	big	Vag.	none	2 days	In Mexico/no PN care/FOB #1/ breastfed
3	April 2006	39	F/healthy/Andrea	8#7 oz	Vag.	Anemia/PROM/ induction	8 hours	At our clinic & hospital/FOB #2/breastfed
4	Present							FOB #2

History of Past Pregnancies

Pregnancy-related problems and birth defects may reoccur in subsequent pregnancies. To help make appropriate decisions about mode of birth, providers need to know about past birth history and the weight of previous infants.

For each past pregnancy, the provider should make a chart that includes the date of birth, baby's birth weight, method of birth, gestational age at birth, any problems that occurred during pregnancy, birth or postpartum (or lack thereof), whether or not the baby had any health problems that were present at birth or found later that were ascertained to be genetic in origin (see Table 11-7). Each twin or other multiple baby needs its specific information recorded, and it needs to be clear that the pregnancy was multiple. Many providers include baby's sex and name in these charts for social reasons. It may also be useful to record if the various children have the same father or not and if there is any history of genetic conditions known in the father's family of origin. Location of previous births, especially for immigrant women, may also be relevant information. Any miscarriages, therapeutic abortions, or stillbirths should be included in the chart in chronological order. For any kind of pregnancy loss, the following information should be recorded: date, gestational age, if surgery requiring anesthesia was needed, if any secondary problems developed, if it was known that the fetus had genetic abnormalities (and if yes, specific information about the problem).

Provider Inquiries	Clinical Reasoning/Logic

Family History

Information related to family history identifies any conditions in family members that would influence or affect the pregnancy.

Any family history of multiple, naturally achieved pregnancies?

Did your mother or any sisters have any problems in their pregnancies?

Is there any family history of bleeding or blood problems?

Any family history of bleeding/clotting disorders, diabetes, thyroid or other endocrine disorders?

Strong family history of endocrine problems, especially diabetes may be a predictive factor for the development of these kinds of problems. Multiple pregnancies may run in families.

A pregnant woman may be too young to have experienced bleeding problems herself, so family history of bleeding problems may be very important information.

Personal and Social History

Information related to personal and social history identifies what personal habits/behaviors or environmental factors might influence or affect the outcome of the pregnancy.

Tobacco: Use at all? Secondary exposure? If exposure, how much? Ever tried to stop; ever successfully stopped, even for a short time? (Many women are able to quit or cut back their intake considerably during a pregnancy.)

Smoking increases infertility, placental abruption, PROM, low birth weight and placenta previa. Carboxyhemoglobin, cleared slowly from fetal circulation, diminishes tissue oxygenation in the fetus. Nicotine may cause vascular disruption which may contribute to fetal anomalies like cleft lip/palate.

Alcohol: Use at all? How much? How often? Any binge drinking? Ever tried to quit? Want to quit?

Alcohol may cause permanent developmental problems for the fetus; fetal alcohol syndrome, fetal alcohol effects, alcohol related fetal defects termed fetal alcohol spectrum disorder (FASD), still births. Binge drinking effect is worse than daily small intake.

Drugs: All drugs taken including prescription, illegal, over-the-counter, nutritional supplements, and herbal preparations?

A large variety of chemical compounds, including some prescription drugs, are known teratogens.

Nutrition: Usual diet, especially for a pregnant woman. Has nausea or vomiting changed how she eats since she has become pregnant?

Employment/hobbies: Chemical exposures? Long periods of standing? Other physical demands? Excessive heat exposure? At risk for occupational exposure to violence? (e.g. law enforcement or military occupations)

Certain occupations or activities may be related to problems in pregnancy.

Prolonged standing, lifting, and bending exacerbates back pain.

Home neighborhood: Any known exposures to environmental pollutants including agricultural chemicals?

Environmental toxins, radiation, extreme heat, infectious agents, metals, and solvents may put pregnancy and the fetus at risk.

Abuse: Have you ever been hit, kicked, beat up in other ways, been forced to engage in unwanted sexual activities, or experienced psychological ill treatment?

The stress of pregnancy may exacerbate existing marital conflicts and may increase violence.

Partner: Do you want to tell me about your partner? What would you like me to know about him or her? Will she or he be involved in your care? If you had a partner that caused you problems in the past, is there anything I need to know about that situation?

Outcome of pregnancy is highly dependent to emotional support as well. Complicated pregnancy will need support from family and partner.

Further assessment of abuse appears in Chapter 14.

Provider Inquiries	Clinical Reasoning/Logic
Religion/spirituality: Are there any religious or spiritual practices you want me to take into consideration during your care? **Culture:** Is there anything special that you want us to know about that we can consider during your care in order that we can all help you and your baby be safe and grow well? Do you have any special request of us about your care?	Various cultural practices, beliefs and religions factor in planning the care of the mother and fetus.

Developmental Applications

Until the 20th century in developed countries, many societies considered the ideal age for a first pregnancy to be about 15 or 16. This is still true now in many societies around the world. In fact, once a young woman has a fully developed pelvis, she is generally able to achieve a healthy pregnancy and birth. It is very common for a young woman to have a comparatively easy birth followed by a rapid postpartum recovery.

Young age is a risk factor for the development of preeclampsia, but so is old age. Most young women do not develop this problem during pregnancy, but vigilance about it as a possibility is always warranted.

In some more traditional societies, women may experience arranged marriages to older men as a matter of course as soon as they begin menstruation. These young women are able to become pregnant and carry the pregnancy to term, but if their pelvis is not fully developed, they are likely to experience obstructions during labor. If surgical birth is not immediately available, the baby often dies during labor, and the woman may have her pelvic area torn to pieces. Rectovaginal fistulas are common complications after a prolonged labor or failed birth. They are common in areas where access to medical and surgical care is limited. Poverty is an indirect common cause for these fistulas. Rectovaginal fistula contributes to constant foul smelling discharge, which then leads to societal disapproval and failed future child births. Some cultures regard them as divine punishment. Charitable organizations, large and small, local or based in more developed countries, exist specifically to bring needed repair surgery to these women, but the demand for this surgery far outstrips available resources in many places.

In developed countries such as the United States, where adolescents are still regarded as children, not adults, pregnancy results in "emancipation" for consenting to health care. That is, a pregnant teen may consent for herself and her baby to receive health care; she does not need to have a parent sign or give consent for her in order to receive care.

Self-care for wellness is a critically important part of prenatal care, and pregnant teens often have not had to manage this themselves yet, so they may need extra teaching about topics such as healthy nutrition avoidance of alcohol and tobacco. It is not uncommon for teens to have an imbalanced diet; pregnancy can be a good opportunity to teach young women better eating practices.

Young women are just as motivated to help make a healthy baby as anyone. Pregnancy can be a good window of opportunity for them adopt a healthy lifestyle.

As providers plan their patient teaching activities during prenatal care, they should be mindful of normal social and cognitive development of adolescents. For example, pregnancy may be the result of rebellion against parents, and adolescents may think they are invulnerable.

OBJECTIVE DATA

Techniques and procedures discussed may be performed during a regular prenatal exam (**antepartum**) or in an inpatient setting during labor (**intrapartum**) and recovery (**postpartum**).

Inspection:

- General assessment (edema, physical appearance for pain, nutritional status)
- Vital signs
- Ultrasonography
- Contraction stress test (CST)
- Rupture of membranes (ROM)
- Fundal height (PP)
- Amniotic fluid (meconium, ferning)
- Lochia

Palpation:

- Pelvic adequacy (pelvimetry)
- Contraction status
- Cervical dilation/effacement (vaginal exam)
- Reflexes
- Fetal position/presentation (Leopold's maneuver)
- Fetal descent/station

Percussion:

Not usually done but may be better tolerated than deep palpation when a woman presents with abdominal pain

Auscultation:

Blood pressure

Fetal heart rate/tones (FHT)

Inspection: Antepartum Assessment

Inspection Techniques and Expected Findings	Unexpected Findings
Ultrasonography	
The primary focus of the antepartum inspection is fetal health and well-being. Ultrasonography (US) actually generates real time pictures of the fetus in two or three dimensions. It is performed by an educated and certified person in the use of this technology. Certified nurse midwives (CNMs), physician's assistants and physicians usually perform this procedure in their out-patient offices.	
Non-stress Test	
Fetal monitoring performed prior to the onset of contractions is known as a **non-stress test** (NST). This may be done in late pregnancy to assess for fetal well-being in a clinic setting. The test was based on observation that the presence of two or more fetal heart rate accelerations predicted a better perinatal outcome. The advantage of the procedure is that no IV pitocin is used to induce contractions. Drawbacks are the higher false positive and false negative rates.	
The woman rests in a bed in a comfortable position with the head of the bed elevated. She can wear her street clothing, including shoes, and eat, drink, and entertain herself in any way she might like. Apply the fetal heart and uterine contraction sensors and give the patient a special handheld marking device.	
Instruct the patient to press the button on the device each time she perceives fetal movement of any kind. Allow the machine to run for at least 15 minutes, after which the resulting record of the tracing is assessed.	
Various parameters of the tracing may be of interest, but generally the provider is interested in the fetal heart tones (FHT) baseline rate and other characteristics that may be present. In order to be considered a formal non-stress test, naturally occurring accelerations need to be recorded. These accelerations often happen in conjunction with fetal movement, but this is not necessary. A "reactive" NST is desirable, and determined if there are at least 2 episodes of accelerations that go at least 15 beats per minute above baseline over the course of 15–20 minutes.	A "non-reactive" test is one in which these parameters are not achieved within 40 minutes, indicating the need for further assessment with a contraction stress test (CST) or biophysical profile (BPP). For women who have diabetes or are high risk for fetal death, it is recommended that they have NST two times per week after 28 weeks' gestation.
Because fetuses do have sleep–wake cycles, if a NST is begun while the fetus is asleep, it may take more than 15–20 minutes to achieve a reactive NST. The machine can be allowed to run for up to an hour if needed if the FHT tracing looks like the fetus is sleeping. A variety of techniques including acoustic stimulation or gentle, physical pushing of the fetus can be used to wake up an apparently sleeping fetus and to stimulate it to move about. A reactive NST is generally considered a sign of overall fetal health at the time of the test. This result is usually predictive of continued well being for at least 24 more hours.	
Contraction Stress Test (CST)	
Depending on the NST results, a secondary test, **contraction stress test** (CST) may also be indicated. This is seldom performed because it is difficult and expensive. It also requires the insertion of an intravenous catheter and delivery of pitocin to stimulate contractions. CST is done with the idea that uterine contractions transiently restrict O_2 delivery to the fetus and a hypoxic fetus will demonstrate recurrent late decelerations.	Major drawbacks are the contraindications to inducing contractions and the false positive rates.
If naturally occurring uterine contractions are present, an informal CST can also be performed. A negative CST is the desired result. This is the *absence* of late decelerations in the fetal heart rate related to a contraction (hence the word *negative*).	A *positive* CST means that late decelerations were recorded. If deemed necessary by the obstetric provider, contractions can also be induced by manual stimulation of the woman's nipples or with use of the intravenous drug pitocin, but CSTs have fallen out of favor in most settings.
Other antenatal tests are available like amniotic fluid volume, biophysical profile, Doppler velocimetry, uterine artery impedance, and umbilical artery Doppler.	

Inspection: Intrapartum Assessment

Inspection Techniques and Expected Findings	Unexpected Findings
Rupture of Membranes (Intrapartum) Inspection for premature rupture of membranes (PROM) may be done with or without the use of a speculum. (The specific technique for performing a vaginal/speculum exam is fully covered in Chapter 30.) When performing a sterile speculum exam to assess for rupture of membranes, specimens should only be taken for this procedure. First observe for the presence of clear or milky fluid, which usually has a characteristic non offensive smell. Use sterile cotton swabs only. The specimen can come from the vaginal vault or the cervical os. Use one swab to wipe a piece of nitrazine paper to assess the pH of the fluid (the paper will turn dark blue in the presence of basic amniotic fluid; however other kinds of discharge can also cause this pH change like semen, soap in vaginal vault, and some infections) and a second swab to wipe across a dry glass slide. The glass slide is air dried and examined under a microscope. Visualization of "ferning" under the microscope is the gold standard for diagnosing amniotic fluid (refer to Figure 11-2).	PROM is a serious development that is a significant threat to the well-being of the uterine cavity and fetus. When doing the assessment only to evaluate for rupture of membranes in a pregnant woman, use sterile gloves and maintain sterile technique throughout. Thorough inspection and palpation of external structures is unnecessary. Insertion of the speculum may result in copious fluid pouring out of the vagina making further assessment unnecessary.
Amniotic Fluid Prior to or during labor, the fetal membranes (BOW) rupture, causing an immediate release of the amniotic fluid.	
When possible, observe the color of the fluid. It is characteristically clear or pale yellow in color with a slight odor. It also may contain white flecks of vernix caseosa, lanugo, and scalp hair.	Color alterations of the amniotic fluid are of grave concern for the health and survival of the newborn. A significant color change is the appearance of greenish brown fluid. This is indicative of meconium stained amniotic fluid (MSAF).

PRACTICE POINT: Meconium

Meconium is the initial bowel movement of the newborn. It accumulates in the fetus's bowel and is composed of desquamated cells from the intestine and skin, gastrointestinal mucin, lanugo, hair, and fatty material from the vernix caseosa (Fanaroff, 2008). A significant condition associated with MSAF is its aspiration by the fetus. Amniotic fluid is routinely swallowed and inhaled by the fetus with no damage to the developing lungs. In the presence of MSAF, there is a high probability that the newborn has aspirated the contaminated amniotic fluid. Aspiration causes fetal hypoxia and pulmonary dysfunction due to airway obstruction, surfactant alterations, chemical pneumonitis, and pulmonary hypertension (Clark & Clark, 2012). Aspiration of MSAF most likely occurs in utero or just after birth when taking the initial breaths.

Inspection: Intrapartum

Inspection Techniques and Expected Findings	Unexpected Findings

Uterine Contractions

Uterine contractions are commonly assessed with fetal monitoring equipment (Figure 11-4). Fetal monitoring machines have two sensors—one (or more if multiple fetuses) for the FHTs and one to measure the strength and timing of uterine contractions (UCs). As with FHTs contractions can be measured either externally or internally. The external transducer senses changes in uterine position related to muscle contractions at the fundus or top of the uterus. The internal transducer measures changes in internal fluid pressure similar to how a mercury blood pressure manometer works.

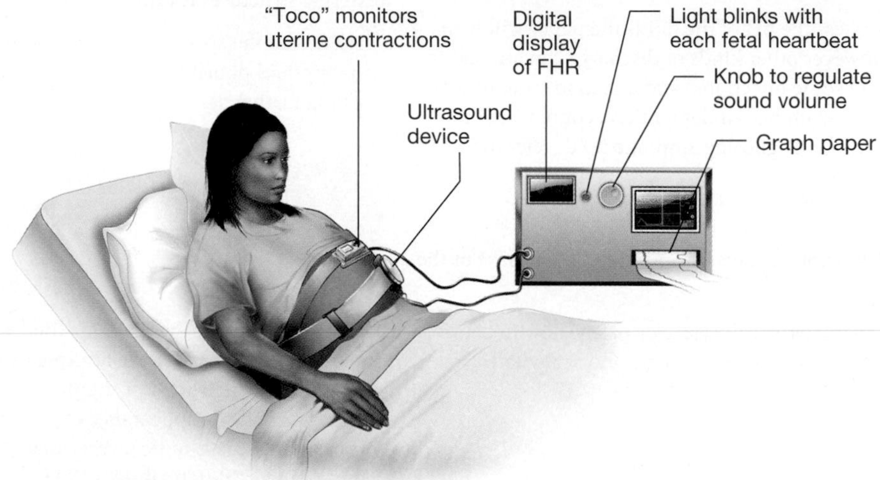

FIGURE 11-4 External monitoring of fetal heart sounds

The external transducer senses changes in uterine muscle contractions at the fundus or top of the uterus. The internal transducer measures changes in internal fluid pressure similar to how a mercury blood pressure manometer works.

Like the internal FHT scalp electrode, the internal pressure sensor requires that the BOW be broken. To use the external transducer, palpate the fundus and apply the dry transducer to that location. It is adjusted until a good signal is achieved and then held in place by the elastic belts or girdle.

An external transducer can be used to assess grossly the beginning, end, and duration of a UC. The strength of a UC can only be judged qualitatively (stronger, weaker, more, less) with external technology. The numbers generated by the machine to indicate strength of contractions when external monitoring is underway are meaningless as units of measure.

Once the internal UC sensor is calibrated, the resulting data reflects accurate changes in internal fluid pressure. Calculations can be performed with the resulting data, and the numbers can be interpreted as numbers (e.g., 10 is twice a big as 20 and 5 is half as much).

PRACTICE POINT: Continuous Fetal Monitoring

During labor, UCs and FHTs can be assessed continuously or intermittently. Continuous monitoring means the sensoring devices are applied and left in place continuously for the duration. Intermittent means the devices can be put on, left for a short while, removed for a while and then replied later for another short interval. For a healthy woman and fetus who are in natural occurring labor at term, continuous monitoring has no known benefit as opposed to intermittent monitoring. The choice of monitoring style is usually one of agency, provider or patient preference and is a matter of controversy within maternity care practice.

PRACTICE POINT: Assessment of the Coping Abilities of a Laboring Woman

Maternity caregivers have long recognized that methods used to assess patients' pain that are the same as those used for the ill and injured (e.g., traditional pain rating scales like the 1–10 scale) are less than optimal in the case of labor pain. Labor pain is pain and *is* severe at least part of the time, but there are important differences between this pain and pain caused by either pathology or injury. Labor pain is physiologic not pathologic. It has a predictable end. It comes and goes during the course of labor. In most labors more time is spent in the pain-free intervals between contractions as opposed to the apex of pain at the height of contractions. In addition, women interpret labor pain differently. Many women do not want to get rid of labor pain; they just want help dealing with it.

Roberts and colleagues (Roberts, Gulliver, Fisher, & Cloyes, 2010) at the University of Utah conceptualized that the most important component to assess is not the level of pain itself but rather how well women are coping with whatever sensation they were experiencing. To that end they developed The Coping with Labor Algorithm tool (Figure 11-5). Using the tool helps caregivers assess how well women are coping with labor pain. The tool is simple to use and meets requirements for accreditation agencies for assessment of the "fifth vital sign" in place of traditional pain rating scales.

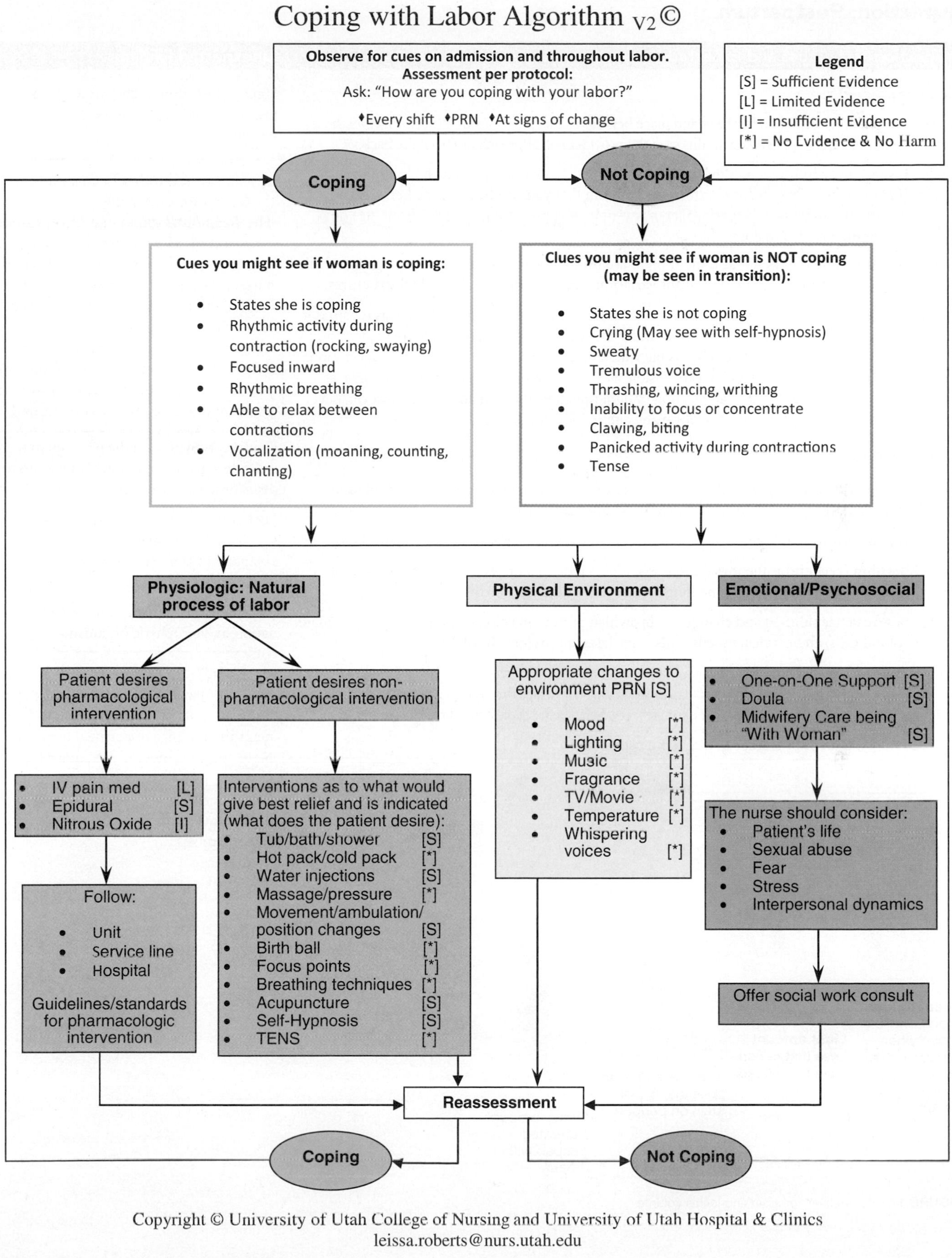

Coping with Labor Algorithm $_{V2}$©

Observe for cues on admission and throughout labor.
Assessment per protocol:
Ask: "How are you coping with your labor?"
♦Every shift ♦PRN ♦At signs of change

Legend
[S] = Sufficient Evidence
[L] = Limited Evidence
[I] = Insufficient Evidence
[*] = No Evidence & No Harm

Coping

Cues you might see if woman is coping:

- States she is coping
- Rhythmic activity during contraction (rocking, swaying)
- Focused inward
- Rhythmic breathing
- Able to relax between contractions
- Vocalization (moaning, counting, chanting)

Not Coping

Clues you might see if woman is NOT coping (may be seen in transition):

- States she is not coping
- Crying (May see with self-hypnosis)
- Sweaty
- Tremulous voice
- Thrashing, wincing, writhing
- Inability to focus or concentrate
- Clawing, biting
- Panicked activity during contractions
- Tense

Physiologic: Natural process of labor

Patient desires pharmacological intervention

- IV pain med [L]
- Epidural [S]
- Nitrous Oxide [I]

Follow:

- Unit
- Service line
- Hospital

Guidelines/standards for pharmacologic intervention

Patient desires non-pharmacological intervention

Interventions as to what would give best relief and is indicated (what does the patient desire):

- Tub/bath/shower [S]
- Hot pack/cold pack [*]
- Water injections [S]
- Massage/pressure [*]
- Movement/ambulation/position changes [S]
- Birth ball [*]
- Focus points [*]
- Breathing techniques [*]
- Acupuncture [S]
- Self-Hypnosis [S]
- TENS [*]

Physical Environment

Appropriate changes to environment PRN [S]

- Mood [*]
- Lighting [*]
- Music [*]
- Fragrance [*]
- TV/Movie [*]
- Temperature [*]
- Whispering voices [*]

Emotional/Psychosocial

- One-on-One Support [S]
- Doula [S]
- Midwifery Care being "With Woman" [S]

The nurse should consider:

- Patient's life
- Sexual abuse
- Fear
- Stress
- Interpersonal dynamics

Offer social work consult

Reassessment

Coping **Not Coping**

leissa.roberts@nurs.utah.edu

FIGURE 11-5 Coping with Labor Algorithm Tool
Source: Adapted from "The Coping With Labor Algorithm: An Alternate Pain Assessment Tool for the Laboring Woman" by L. Roberts, B. Gulliver, J. Fisher, and K. G. Cloyes in *Journal of Midwifery & Women's Health* 55(2):107-116, March-April, 2010. Reproduced by permission of L. Roberts.

Inspection: Postpartum

Inspection Techniques and Expected Findings	Unexpected Findings
Perineum The woman can either lie flat on her back and place her legs in the "frog" position (heels together, knees bent and apart) or can lie on her side. In this case the provider will approach her from the back. Visually inspect any bed protection materials and perineal pads to see how much blood they contain. If approaching from behind, inform the woman that you will be touching her. Gently lift up the upper buttock until the perineal area is visible. If approaching from the front, use one's fingers to separate the labia majora. The perineal area should look not as though there are no significant alterations or variation and all structures should be intact. A non-significant variation would be edema in the labial structures. If an incision (episiotomy) was performed or a laceration occurred during birth and it was repaired in the most common manner (sutures are placed under the top layer of skin and knots are made inside the vagina.), no surgical sutures should be visible with simple inspection. The edges of the laceration/incision should be approximated and may be visible as a very thin red line or may not be visible at all. The area should not be tender to application of light pressure. The woman should, however, have sensation to the area; unless the effects of local anesthesia have not disappeared.	Signs of infection, such as redness or purulent exudate, would be an unexpected finding. ***PRACTICE POINT: The Bartholin's Gland*** The Bartholin's gland can also become obstructed after birth and become enlarged. Usually it is painful due to pressure on surrounding structures. When lanced, the drainage will be viscous but clear. This does not need culture, but a short course of oral cephalosporins is helpful to prevent infection from the procedure. Of course, any cloudy or purulent drainage needs to be cultured.
Discharge (Lochia) In the postpartum period, **lochia** is the vaginal discharge of blood, mucus, and placental tissue. Typically lochia discharge continues for 4 to 6 weeks after childbirth. Lochia progresses through three stages and is described by its contents and color (Figure 11-6). • **Lochia rubra** (cruenta) is the initial discharge and is red in color because it contains a large volume of blood. It typically lasts no longer than 3 to 5 days after birth. • **Lochia serosa** has thinned and changed to brownish or pink in color, containing serous exudate, white blood cells, and cervical mucus. This stage lasts approximately 10 days. • **Lochia alba** (or purulenta) describes lochia once it becomes whitish or yellowish-white in color. It typically begins in the second postpartum week and continues through the 3rd to 6th week after delivery. It's composed primarily of leukocytes, epithelial cells, cholesterol, fat, and mucus. Lochia usually has an odor similar to that of menstrual fluid.	Continuation beyond the 6th week may indicate a genital lesion, which should be determined and treated. Lochia serosa which persists for a few weeks after birth may indicate late postpartum hemorrhaging, and should be determined and treated. Any offensive odor may indicate contamination by saprophytic organisms. ***PRACTICE POINT: REEDA*** The acronym REEDA is a helpful way to remember what to assess for and document the findings of perineal inspection. Note the presence or absence of these factors: **R**= redness **E**=edema **E**=ecchymosis **D**=drainage **A**=approximation

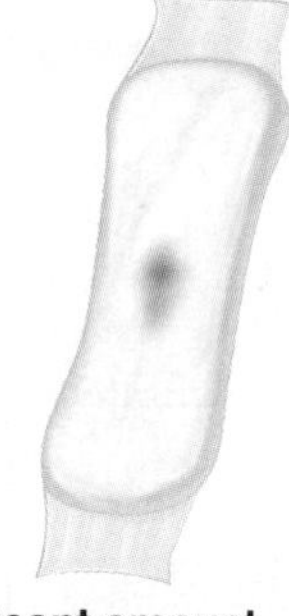

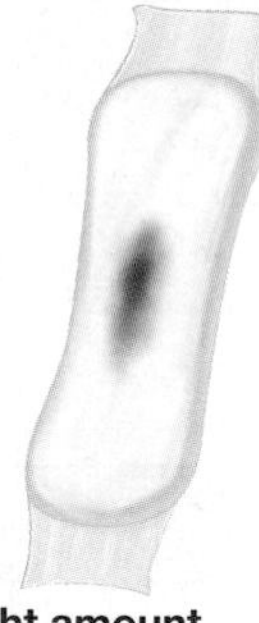

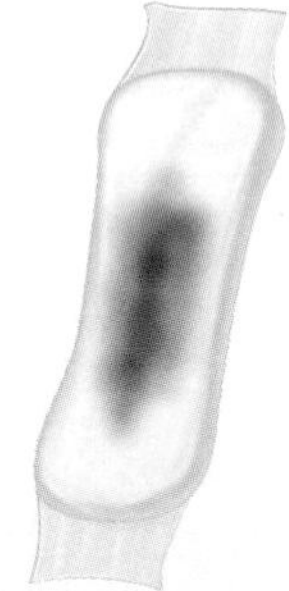

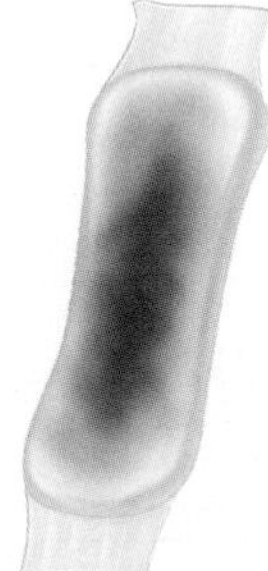

FIGURE 11-6 Guidelines for assessing lochia volume

Palpation: Antepartum/Intrapartum

Palpation Techniques and Expected Findings	Unexpected Findings

Palpation of Fetal Parts (Leopold's maneuvers)

Leopold's maneuvers are used to determine the locations of various parts of the fetal body (Figure 11-7). It cannot be done reliably until after 28 weeks because the fetus is usually too small to palpate until that time. It is not of critical importance until 36 weeks or when the woman is in labor.

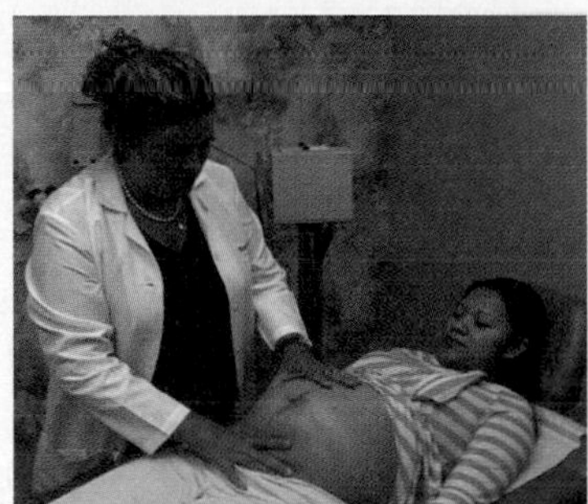

FIGURE 11-7 Provider palpates the head of the fetus

There are four parts to this procedure. The woman should lie mostly flat on her back and bend her knees up slightly. It is very important to accurately determine the presenting part close to the time of labor. Until the fetus runs out of space near the end of pregnancy, the fetus may swim around and be in a variety of positions at any given time. If labor is not imminent or present, the fetal presentation does not matter and may easily change naturally.

Face the woman's head and place both hands on either side of the uterine fundus (Figure 11-8a). Note the part that is found there; the most typical finding would be to find breech (buttocks). This would feel large, firm but irregularly shaped. A head would feel more rounded and more firm; it would also be smaller than a breech. Try to move the part from side to side gently. The breech would not move very much, but a head may bounce away and then back ("balloting" or "ballotable"). If neither a breech nor head can be felt, the fetus is probably in transverse lie.

Remain standing in the same place and slide both hands down the two sides of the uterus (Figure 11-8b). Feel which side (left or right) is large and flat and which side has irregular feeling parts. The flat area is probably the fetal back and the irregular parts are extremities. If the small parts are all over the abdomen and the back cannot be palpated, the fetus is posterior. If the fetus is transverse, the provider should find a head on one side and the breech on the other. The head will feel smaller, more round and firm compared to the breech.

Remain standing in the same position. The third maneuver has a special name, Pawlick's maneuver (Figure 11-8c). Grasp the lower part of the uterus just above the symphysis pubis with the fingers and thumbs of one hand. Encircle the fundus with the second hand, grasping the part that is located there. Try to move the fetus up with gentle pressure. If descent into the pelvis has begun, the fetus will feel fixed in place. If the fetus moves without much effort, it has not begun to descend.

Change positions so you are facing the woman's feet. Place the palms flat on the lower abdomen with fingers pointing towards the woman's feet (Figure 11-8d). Move the fingers down towards the pelvic inlet and try to make the fingers meet in the middle. You should feel two sides of the firm round head. If you can make the fingers meet and feel nothing, descent has not yet begun (and probably the fetus was ballottable in earlier maneuvers). This would also be consistent with transverse lie that should have been previously identified. If the provider cannot get the fingers very far before they are stopped by the two sides, chances are this is a breech, especially if the part found here is not very firm. This finding should be consistent with earlier findings. If the fingers converge but still a small firm part can be felt above the rim, the vertex has descended. This is called "dipping" and the firm part felt above the pelvic rim is a shoulder.

If an abnormal presentation is found at 36 weeks, it may be possible for a midwife or physician to attempt to turn the baby into a cephalic presentation before the onset of labor. If the fetus remains in a non-cephalic position, it may be necessary to schedule a Caesarean birth.

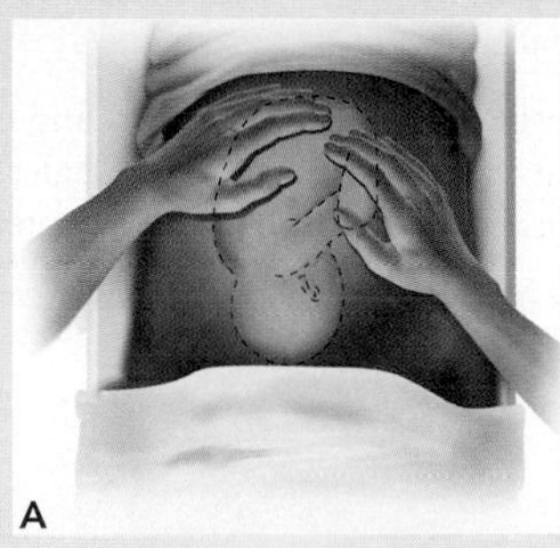

A

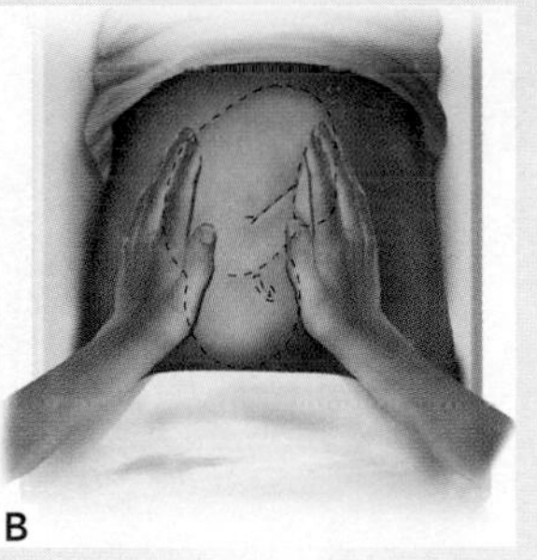

B

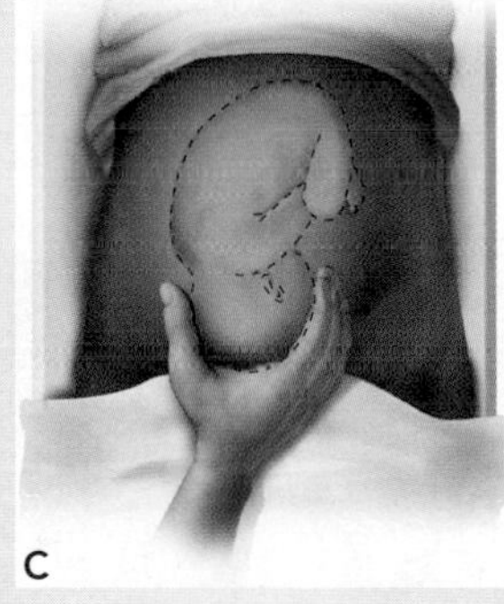

C

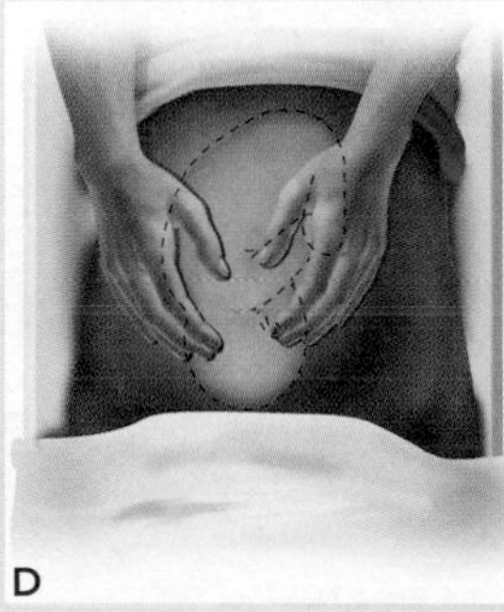

D

FIGURE 11-8A–D Leopold's maneuvers. **a)** first maneuver; **b)** second maneuver; **c)** third maneuver; **d)** fourth maneuver

Palpation Techniques and Expected Findings	Unexpected Findings

Examination of the cervix

Palpation via the vagina to assess for cervical changes (dilation/effacement) and fetal descent in labor (sterile vaginal examination or SVE)

During labor, the cervix is palpated via the vagina for cervical changes and fetal descent in labor (sterile vaginal examination or SVE) (Intrapartum)

Using sterile gloves, the exam can be performed using one or two gloves as preferred by the provider.

Position the woman on the bed or exam table with her knees bent and apart. An alternative position is the "frog" position with the woman's heels together in the middle, the knees bent and apart.

Use sterile lubricant on the index and middle finger of the examining hand. Touch the woman's leg with the non-examining hand and alert her to your entry. Insert the finger by separating the labia, and press downwards to avoid the anterior structures.

As you reach the cervix, feel for size and consistency (Figure 11-9).

PRACTICE POINT: Fetal Location

Vocabulary terms used to describe aspects of the fetal location are as follows:

- Lie: orientation of fetal spine to maternal spine; described as longitudinal, transverse or oblique
- Presentation: fetal part that is entering the pelvis first
- Attitude: position of fetal parts in relationship to each other; described as flexed, straight (military) or extended
- Position: location of presenting fetal part in relationship to maternal pelvis; described as right or left
- Variety: location of fetal back to anterior, lateral, or posterior part of maternal pelvis
- Engagement: location of fetal presenting part to the maternal pelvic inlet

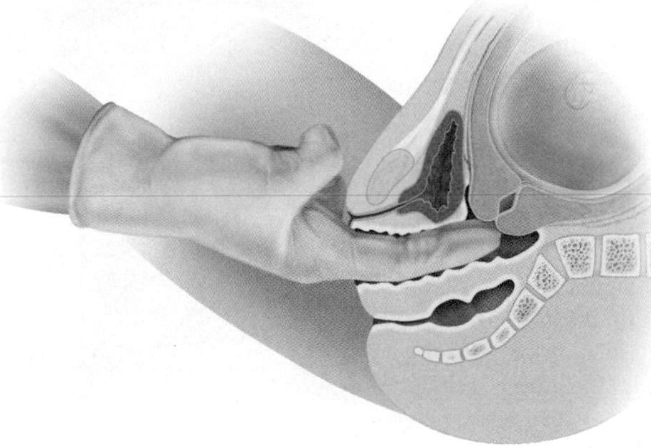

FIGURE 11-9 Gauging cervical dilation

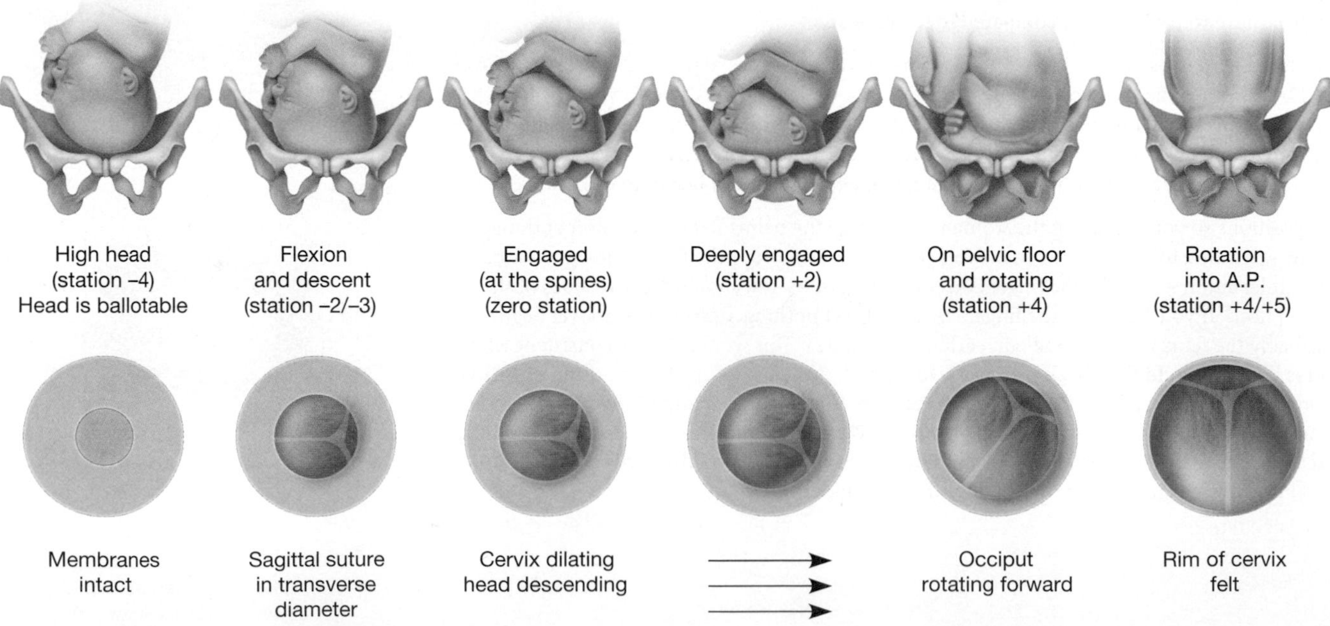

FIGURE 11-10 Guidelines for assessing the dilation of the cervix

Palpation Techniques and Expected Findings

Note these things about the cervix:

Size of the opening is expressed in centimeters. Initially, use of a standardized chart is helpful to realize what the various size openings feel like. For most providers, 1–3 cm will only admit one finger or less. If no fingers are able to be inserted into the opening, this is called "closed." Four to nine centimeters are assessed by noting how far apart two fingers will go. At nine cm the fetal head is usually in the way so that the provider cannot insert both fingers into the opening. However, the provider can still find a whole round cervix by following it around the outside of the fetal head for 360 degrees. If the cervix cannot be found at all, it is completely open or 10 cm (Figure 11-10).

Consistency or thickness of the cervix is known as "effacement." This is expressed as a percentage from 0-100%. There is no objective standard for the various percentages. Low percentages are usually expressed as simply "thick" or "firm." One hundred percent co-occurs with the cervix being completely open.

Fetal Descent

During palpation of the cervix, also palpate for the presentation of the fetus within the birth canal. When palpating, note whether it is a head, the buttocks, or an extremity.

If the presenting part is a head, note what part of the head is felt. Most of the time it will be the top of the head because the provider will feel suture lines, but any part of the face may be felt. If suture lines and fontanels are found, follow them all to discover their location and direction in relationship to the mother's body.

Can the presenting part be moved by tapping it lightly? If you can push the presenting part back up, the part is called "ballotable." If it can barely be felt at all, it can be described as "floating." If the part will not move, it is called "applied" or "well applied."

If the presenting part is applied, locate the ischial spines in the vaginal vault. Form a line in your imagination between the two spines. Form another imaginary line around the widest part of the fetal presenting part. Assess these two lines in relationship to each other. This determines how far the presenting part has descended from the uterus into the vagina and pelvis. It is expressed in centimeters using a negative to positive number system (-5 through 0 to +5).

Unexpected Findings

PRACTICE POINT: Examination of the Bony Pelvis

The major concern related to the pelvis is that it is adequate to allow the passage of the fetus through it. The head of the fetus is the largest body part so if the head is able to make it through the rest of the body will follow. Traditionally there are considered to be four classic kinds of bony pelvises, but in reality there is infinite variety so as to make the categories almost meaningless in clinical practice. There is only one time when the exact contours of a woman's pelvis are meaningful: when she is actually in labor and close to giving birth. A more common measurement is estimating the size of the **pelvic outlet** (Figure 11-11).

Unless a woman has a known pelvic deformity (e.g., from an accident or because she has a past medical history of a disease like rickets), it is generally safe to presume that a woman can give birth vaginally. If true arrest of descent in second stage labor is determined, the provider will likely assess the bony pelvis at that time in order to decide on a clinical management choice (e.g., use of forceps or vacuum extractor versus a Cesarean section). No woman should ever be told in advance of a true diagnosis of a labor abnormality that her pelvis is "too small" to give birth vaginally. This is an excellent way to set up a self-fulfilling prophecy.

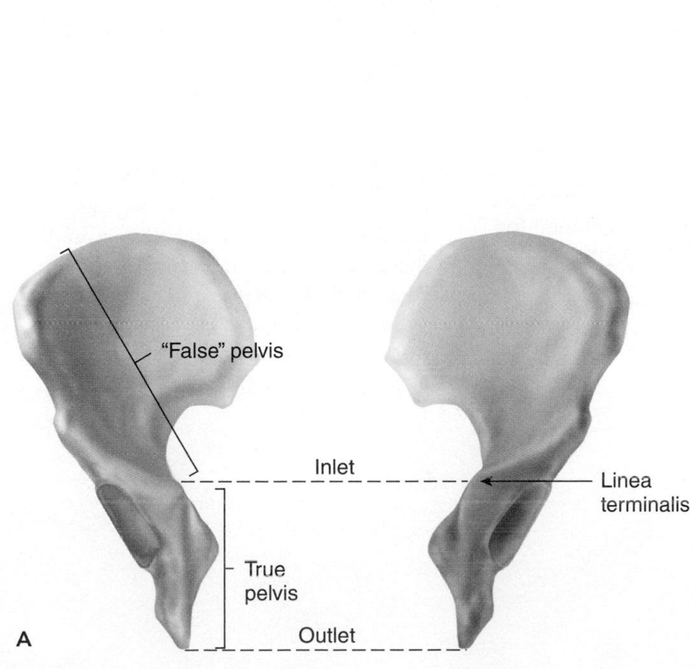

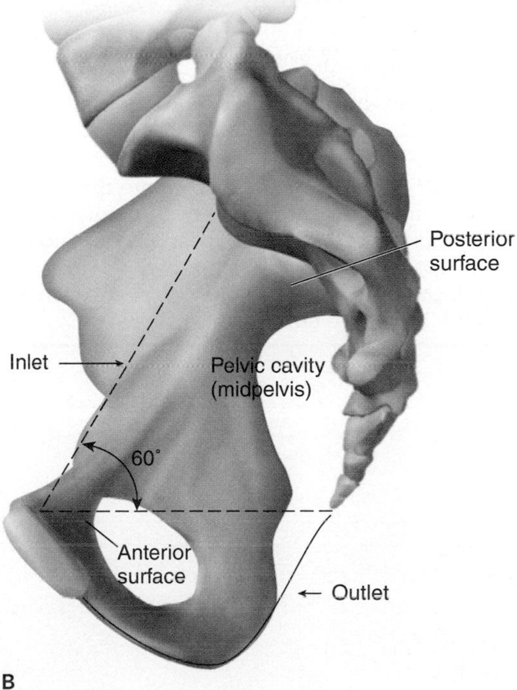

FIGURE 11-11A–B The female pelvis. **a)** false pelvis and **b)** true pelvis

Postpartum

Palpation Techniques and Expected Findings	Unexpected Findings
Uterine Fundus During recovery in the immediate postpartum period, assess the location and characteristics of the now empty uterus regularly. In the immediate recovery period (usually until one hour after birth), palpate the uterine fundus every 15 minutes at least. After that, the frequency becomes agency policy. Commonly the fundus is assessed once every 8–12 hours for the duration of her recovery. Have the woman lie on her back, as flat as possible. Having the head of the bed raised slightly and using head pillows is acceptable as long as the abdomen is mostly flat. After washing your hands, stand at the side of the bed, placing one hand just above the symphysis pubis to help prevent uterine eversion that may result from pressure by the second hand. Either lightly squeeze the bottom of the uterus in between the thumb and forefinger or place the hand on edge, little finger against the skin, and press down. This hand is a "guard" only, ready to exert more pressure later should that be needed. Use the second hand to locate the fundus. Begin higher up in the abdomen beyond the expected location of the fundus. Place the edge of the hand perpendicular to the skin surface with the little finger against the skin. Gradually move the hand down the abdomen removing and replacing the hand in small (about 1 cm) increments, until the fundus is palpated. It should feel like a very firm ball.	Do not press so hard that any pain or discomfort is caused.
Note where the fundus is located in relationship to the umbilicus. Use fingerbreadths as the unit of measure (Figure 11-12). 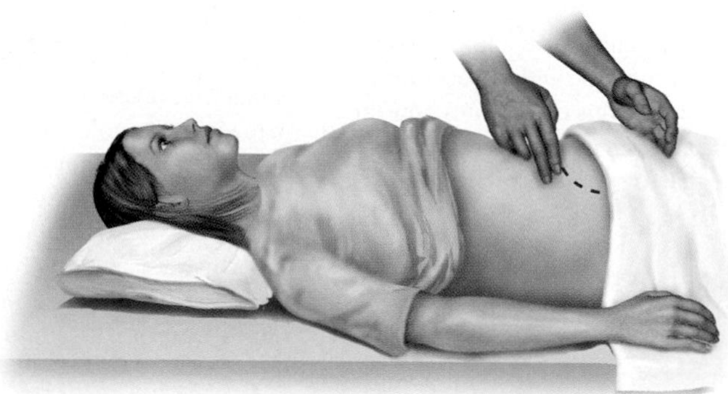 FIGURE 11-12 Measuring the descent of the fundus using fingerbreadths Also note the firmness of the fundus. It should feel and remain very firm. ***THINK LINK: Fingerbreadth*** Most people's fingerbreadth is slightly more than 1 cm. If you know your fingerbreadth is remarkably smaller or larger than this, you may want to actually measure either your fingers or the distance with a tape measure. Commonly the measurement is recorded as at the umbilicus (@u) or some number of fingerbreadths higher (+) or lower (−) than the umbilicus. A common finding on the first postpartum day might be "minus one" or one fingerbreadth below the umbilicus.	If the fundus is not firm, it is described as "boggy." Often with this finding the fundus cannot actually be palpated at all. If the provider cannot locate a firm fundus in the general area of the umbilicus in the immediate postpartum period, aggressive measures are needed as this finding is usually caused by hemorrhaging. First tighten up the guard hand or fingers so they are exerting real downward pressure. Take care not to cause pain, but be firm enough to matter. Then with the examining hand press deeply and firmly downwards. Move the hand in a massaging motion, for example, in a circular motion. This probably will cause great discomfort but shouldn't cause severe pain. Explain to the woman that you are worried about a hemorrhage which is an emergency and that you are doing what is needed in this case. Chances are a great deal of blood will be expelled from the vagina as you are doing this. Continue the pressure and massage until the fundus does begin to feel firm under your hands. If this does not happen within a few seconds, you will need additional help and treatment measures which are beyond the scope of this text.

Auscultation

Auscultation Techniques and Expected Findings	Unexpected Findings
Fetal Heart Tones	
Auscultation of fetal heart tones may be accomplished by using either a fetoscope or Doppler ultrasound technology. Using a fetoscope is much like using a stethoscope, relying on the principles of bone conduction to amplify the sound of the fetal heart (Figure 11-13). An advantage of the fetoscope is that the provider is listening to the actual sound of the fetal heart valves opening and closing, the same as would be heard by using a regular stethoscope on a child, adult or animal. By contrast, the sound heard using Doppler technology is an artificial sound created by the machine based on calculations of the speed of the sound waves sent and received.	The primary disadvantage of using a fetoscope is that only the provider can hear the fetal heart sounds. Women usually do want to hear the sounds of their babies' hearts. The fetoscope cannot hear heart sounds before about 20 weeks of pregnancy, but this feature can make it useful for confirming weeks of pregnancy.
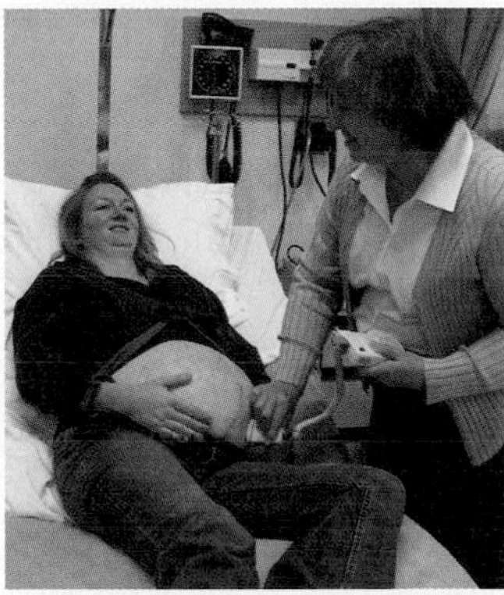 FIGURE 11-13 Using a Doppler device to listen to the fetal heart tones	
Doppler ultrasound can hear fetal heart sounds as early as 8 weeks in some cases, but most commonly first picks up the sounds at 10–12 weeks.	If the sounds cannot be heard at 12 weeks, follow-up examination ultrasound is needed to make sure a viable pregnancy exists.
Locate the fetal back by external palpation. Apply the device being used to assess FHTs to that area.	
Doppler technology requires the application of conduction gel to the part of the device that is applied directly to the maternal skin. Many Doppler devices provide a display of the fetal heart rate, which can simply be recorded. Some models require the provider count the rate. It is essential to differentiate the fetal pulse from the maternal pulse and from the sounds made by blood in the umbilical arteries (funic soufflé). Palpate the maternal radial pulse while listening to the fetal pulse. They should be very different; usually the fetal pulse is about twice the rate of the maternal pulse. It is uncommon to hear funic soufflé, but if present it will sound more like a whistling or whooshing sound; the true fetal heart sound will have an S_1 and an S_2 and sound more like ticking. If there are multiple fetuses, the heart tones will be heard in various places in the maternal abdomen. During labor and delivery and towards the end of pregnancy FHTs can be assessed using a fetal monitor machine. The FHTs can be assessed using an externally placed sensor which uses Doppler technology, or an internally placed sensor which uses the same technology as an EKG to pick up the electroconduction activity of the fetal heart.	Abnormal sounds heard by Doppler devices may or may not be accurate. Such sounds may be real or may be machine artifact. If the same abnormal sound is also heard with a fetoscope, the provider can be assured the sound is valid and therefore requires follow-up care.
Another option for assessing FHTs involves the placement of an internal sensor. Only a provider with specific training performs this procedure. Placement of the sensor is a sterile procedure, and scrupulous technique needs to be followed. The rupture of the membranes must occur for the internal sensor to be used. This might happen spontaneously or may be performed as a procedure.	After the membranes have ruptured, an accession pathway for bacteria from the environment exists, especially after the sensor and its accompanying wire are in place. It is not difficult for the formerly sterile uterine cavity to become infected iatrogenically.
Parameters related FHTs that can be assessed include the following: • Rate, expressed in beats per minute • Variability, or changes in the rate over time • Periodicity or timing of some changes in rate in relationship to accompanying uterine contractions if they are present	

Auscultation Techniques and Expected Findings	Unexpected Findings
External monitoring produces data about the FHT's at the ordinal level. Internal monitoring produces data about the FHTs at the interval level. Therefore externally produced data can be used to make judgments about FHTs that are qualitative (e.g., more, less, higher, lower). Internally produced data can be used to make quantitative assessments (e.g., assessments that are the result of mathematical calculations such as averaging). The vocabulary used to assess FHTs is as follows: • Baseline rate—110–160 bpm is considered a normal baseline rate for a term fetus. The baseline rate can be normal, bradycardic (below 110 bpm) or tachycardic (above 160 bpm). • Variability/Long term variability— oscillations around the baseline (generally about 5–10 bpm) over at least three uterine contraction cycles, if uterine contractions are present. These tend to be 10–15 bpm. • Periodic changes—patterns of change in relationship to uterine contractions when contractions are present. Periodic changes can be characterized by timing —early, variable, or late—and by quality, accelerations or decelerations.	Accelerations need to achieve at least 15 bpm above baseline and to last for at least 15 seconds. No matter when they occur in a contraction cycle they are considered to be either benign or a sign of fetal health. Decelerations, on the other hand, can be just a few bpm (even 1 or 2 below baseline) or very dramatic sudden drops (20+ bpm). They can be very fast (very fast drops with equally fast recovery, patterns that look like spikes) or extended over time. Decelerations that are accompanied by decreased variability are often difficult to see because they are often very subtle, but these kinds of decelerations are the most worrisome, because they can be a sign of compromised fetal oxygenation.
Early decelerations begin at the same time as or very soon after the beginning of a uterine contraction. Generally they occur during the second stage of labor and tend to mirror the contraction. The FHTs return to baseline once the contraction ends. These generally signal a vaso-vagal response of the fetus to the compression of its head experienced during contractions as it descends the birth canal. As long as recovery to baseline occurs, early decelerations are generally not worrisome.	Variables often look more dramatic and are more frequent if the there is little amniotic fluid because of oligohydramnios or if membranes have been ruptured.
Variable decelerations vary; that is about all that can be said of them. They are most common during the second stage of labor. If they are short lasting and recovery to baseline happens quickly, they are less worrisome. They are the result of physical compression to the umbilical cord by some part of the fetus' body and/or the bony pelvis during a contraction. The umbilical cord is composed of sturdy connective tissue which is actually rather difficult to block and keep fully blocked during natural physiologic labor especially if the BOW is intact and the cord has the benefit of fluid in which it can "swim." Because of this, variable decelerations have the "spiky" quality of fast descent followed by equally rapid ascent and recovery.	Late decelerations happen sometime past the apex of a uterine contraction and extend after the contraction ceases. The descent and recovery extend over time and are gradual and smooth. These decelerations are the result of utero-placental insufficiency, or a placenta that is compromised and unable to provide sufficient oxygenation to the fetus. This is a problem that develops over a long time and is very worrisome.

Summary

- Pregnancy is a natural, physiologic event.
- Most pregnant women are young adults who have not yet developed serious health problems in other systems.
- Most pregnancies proceed in a healthy manner and result in the safe natural birth of a healthy infant.
- Both the woman and baby are vulnerable to a variety of uncommon yet serious complications during pregnancy, labor, birth, and the postpartum period.
- Careful assessment is the key to making good care decisions during pregnancy. Sometimes the best care decision during this time is to do nothing except assessment.
- It is as important to be able to recognize expected or healthy findings as it is unexpected ones.

Review Questions

1. The provider is examining a 14-year-old who is 6 weeks pregnant. Because of the patient's age, the provider is concerned that this young mother is at risk for
   1. nutritional problems.
   2. needing a Cesarean birth.
   3. substance abuse during pregnancy.
   4. having a large baby.
2. When entering the examination room of a patient who is 10 weeks pregnant the provider notes that the patient is crying. When asked what is upsetting her, the patient responds that in the last week she feels like she doesn't want to be pregnant and is afraid that she will not be able to love her baby. The best initial action for the provider to take is to
   1. call the father of the baby to provide support for the patient.
   2. request that a social worker come to see the patient.
   3. let the patient know that these feelings are not unusual in early pregnancy.
   4. have the patient see a therapist or counselor to assist in getting these feelings under control.
3. To determine the approximate due date for a patient who is 4 weeks pregnant, which question should the patient be asked?
   1. "When did you last have sexual intercourse?"
   2. "When did you stop using birth control?"
   3. "Have you noticed any nausea in the morning?"
   4. "When did your last period start?"
4. While interviewing a female client, the provider determines that there are many presumptive indicators of pregnancy. Which of the following have likely been revealed by the patient during interview? (Select all that apply.)
   1. pelvic congestion
   2. fatigue
   3. Goodell's sign
   4. Chadwick's sign
   5. breast tenderness
5. During an interview of a patient who is 8 weeks pregnant, the patient indicates that she has had five previous pregnancies; two ended in miscarriage at 12 weeks, and she delivered a set healthy twins by Caesarian delivery at 32 weeks, who are now 7, and delivered two healthy children at 39 and 37 weeks respectively, who are now ages 5 and 3. The nurse would record this information as which of the following?
   1. G=6 T=2 P=1 A=2 L=4
   2. G=5 T=2 P=2 A=2 L=4
   3. G=6 T=2 P=1 A=0 L=4
   4. G=5 T=2 P=2 A=2 L=6
6. The provider is teaching a patient who is 33 weeks pregnant about a non-stress test scheduled for the next day. Which of the following instructions should be included in this instruction? (Select all that apply.)
   1. The patient should be prepared to stay in the hospital for at least 24 hours.
   2. The patient will be made comfortable during the procedure by the use of a sedative medication.
   3. The patient will need to participate in the test by indicating sensations during the test.
   4. An intravenous line will be inserted to administer a drug that will induce contractions.
   5. The test may take as little as 15 minutes, but may require a longer time period to complete.
7. A patient is being admitted to the labor and delivery unit and the provider is about to assess for rupture of the membranes. The provider is aware that the finding that indicates that the membranes have ruptured is fluid that
   1. is thick and gray in color noted on visual inspection of the labia.
   2. produces a fern pattern on microscopic examination.
   3. turns nitrazine paper a greenish brown color.
   4. has an unpleasant acidic odor as it leaves the vaginal canal.
8. The provider preparing to assess fetal heart sounds on a woman who is 12 weeks pregnant. Which of the following describes the correct procedure?
   1. Obtain a Doppler and apply gel right above the symphysis.
   2. Obtain a Doppler and apply gel to the mother's fifth left intercostal space.
   3. Obtain a fetoscope and place the device on the left side of the mother's abdomen.
   4. Obtain a fetoscope and place the device at the uterine fundus.
9. A woman pregnant with her first child is concerned that she has had some light first trimester bleeding. The best initial action for the provider to take is to
   1. ask the patient if she can feel the fetus move.
   2. use a fetoscope to check fetal heart tones.
   3. perform a non-stress test immediately.
   4. ask about the characteristics of the bleeding.
10. When assessing a 14-year-old mother pregnant with her first child at her first prenatal visit, the provider collects which data as a baseline to evaluate the potential development of this pregnancy related problem for which this patient's age puts her at increased risk?
    1. the patient's intake of saturated fats
    2. the date of the patient's last menstrual period
    3. the patient's blood pressure
    4. the patient's medication history

Conditions and Disorders

Ectopic Pregnancy

The embryo implants outside the uterus in an ectopic pregnancy, often in the fallopian tube as scarring may prevent the passage of the fertilized ovum into the uterus.

Pathophysiology

- Suspect in a patient with a late period, vaginal bleeding and abdominal pain.
- Risks include prior history of ectopic pregnancy, tubal surgery or ligation, current IUD use, in utero DES exposure, PID, smoking, multiple sexual partners, and infertility.

Subjective Data

- Severe abdominal pain and bleeding early in the pregnancy (6–8 weeks)
- Pain may refer to shoulder if there is fallopian bleeding.
- Urge to defecate may occur if bleeding on posterior cul-de-sac.
- Lightheadedness if there is rupture.

Objective Data

- Pelvic tenderness usually laterally.
- Cervical or adnexal tenderness; these may be absent if small and unruptured.
- Hypotension and shock if there is rupture.
- Pain usually laterally
- Diagnosis usually made by serial quantitative HCG (normal rise is 66 % every 2 days) and transvaginal US.

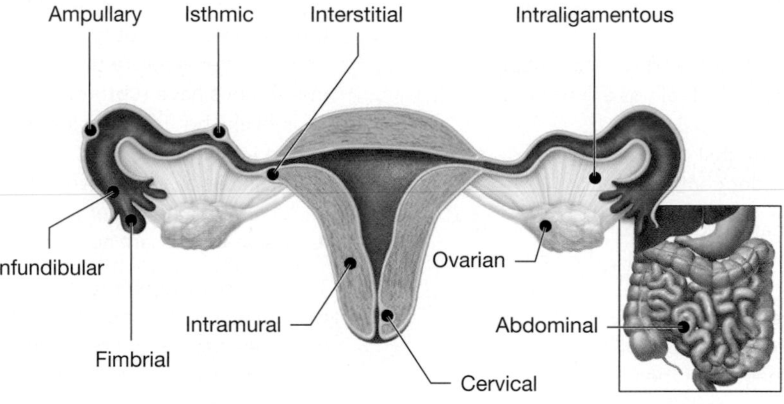

FIGURE 11-14 Implantation sites for an ectopic pregnancy

Multiple Gestation Pregnancies

More than one fetus inside the uterus, due to spontaneous division of fertilized ovum into two or more embryos or release and fertilization of more than one ovum.

Pathophysiology

- May occur naturally or artificially because of infertility treatment.

Subjective Data

- Movement of more than one fetus.

Objective Data

- Usually is found upon early ultrasound examination
- Excessive growth of the uterus
- More than one fetal heartbeat in different locations
- Palpation of different kinds of fetal movement in different places in the uterus

Spontaneous Abortion (Miscarriage)

A naturally occurring termination of a pregnancy prior to 20 weeks' gestation.

Pathophysiology

- Frequently, the causes are unknown and unknowable.
- Most are assumed to result from some kind of genetic abnormality of the embryo/fetus.
- A few cases are secondary to abdominal trauma.

Subjective Data

- Heavy bleeding during early pregnancy
- Abdominal pain and cramping

Objective Data

- Bleeding at least as heavy as a menstrual period or more
- Passage of fetus or fetal tissue
- Open cervix via speculum exam
- Empty uterus on ultrasound examination

Hydatidiform Mole (Molar Pregnancy, Gestational Trophoblastic Disease [GTD])

These are proliferative disorders of trophoblastic cells of the placenta and the result of aberrancy in fertilization. Malignant gestational trophoblastic disease can develop from molar pregnancy. This may be due to activation of oncogenes.

Pathophysiology

- Aberrancy in fertilization where an empty ovum is fertilized by two sperms or single sperm that duplicates (mole).
- Risk factors include advanced maternal age and history of gestational trophoblastic disease.

Subjective Data

- Passage of tissue that look like large, clear colored grapes.
- Never feeling fetal movement.
- Painless vaginal bleeding in the second trimester, often brown colored but sometimes bright red
- More severe nausea than with other pregnancies

Objective Data

- Usually found on ultrasound examination
- Never hearing fetal hearts sounds
- Never palpating fetal movement
- Abnormally high levels on a quantitative HcG test
- Uterus grows larger than would be expected
- Ultrasound—no embryo and no amniotic fluid and the presence of anechoic spaces which correspond to diffuse hydatidiform swelling of the chorionic villi called "moles."

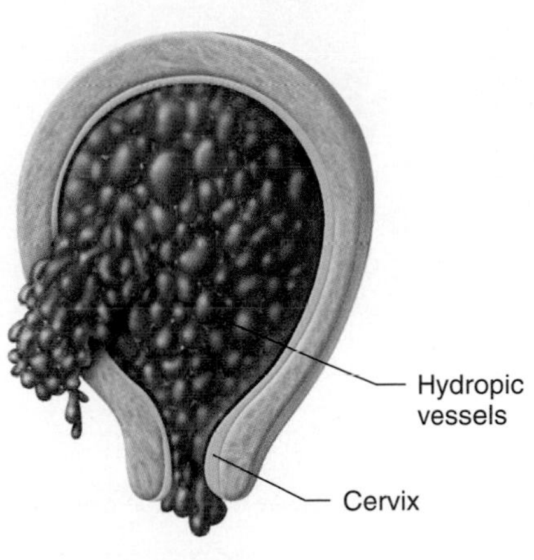

FIGURE 11-15 Hydatiform mole

Placenta Previa

The placenta implants near or proximal to the internal cervical os.

Pathophysiology

- Cause unknown, may be due to suboptimal endometrium in the upper uterine cavity thereby promoting implantation of trophoblast toward the lower uterine wall.
- Risk factors are C-section, previous placenta previa, multiple gestation, multiparity, advanced age, infertility treatment, previous abortion, prior intrauterine procedure, smoking cocaine, male fetus and non white race.
- Early placenta previa may resolve as the lower uterine segment lengthens and uterus enlarges, causing migration of the placenta upward.

Subjective Data

- Painless bright red bleeding in a pregnant woman over 20 weeks' gestation.
- Majority of cases are asymptomatic.
- Some may present with uterine contractions.

Objective Data

- Often found on ultrasound examination.
- If not previously diagnosed, no vaginal examination should be performed until location of placenta is confirmed by transabdominal US first, and then transvaginal US.

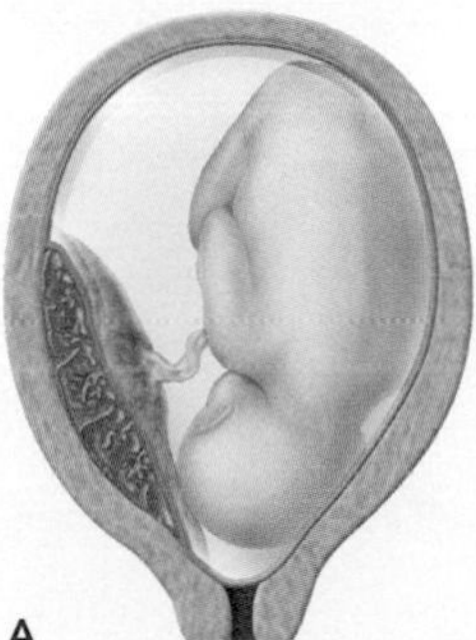

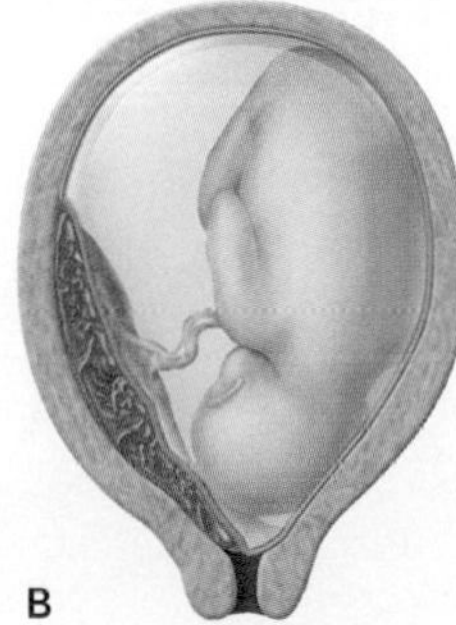

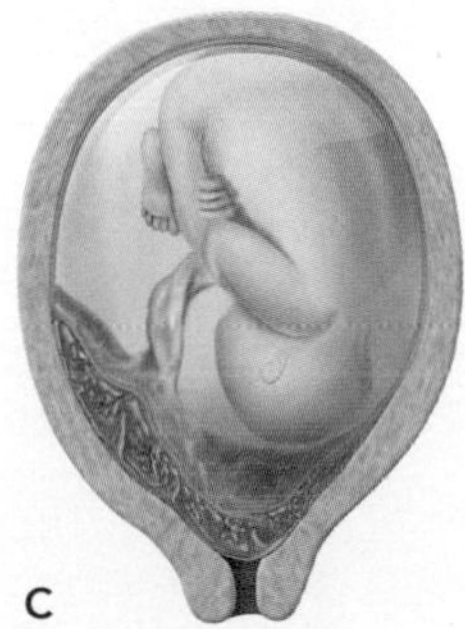

FIGURE 11-16A–C Placenta previa

Abruptio Placentae

Condition where there is partial or total placental detachment prior to delivery.

Pathophysiology

- Usually occurs after 20 weeks' gestation.
- Etiology is rupture of maternal vessels in the decidua basalis where it interfaces with the anchoring villi of the placenta.
- Risk factors are trauma, hypertension, smoking, cocaine, prior abruption.

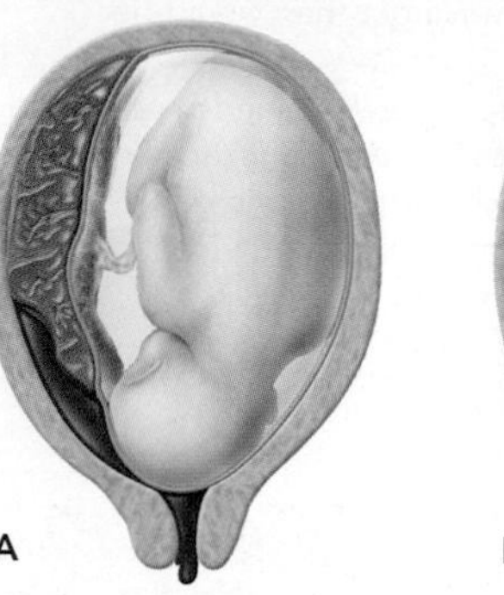

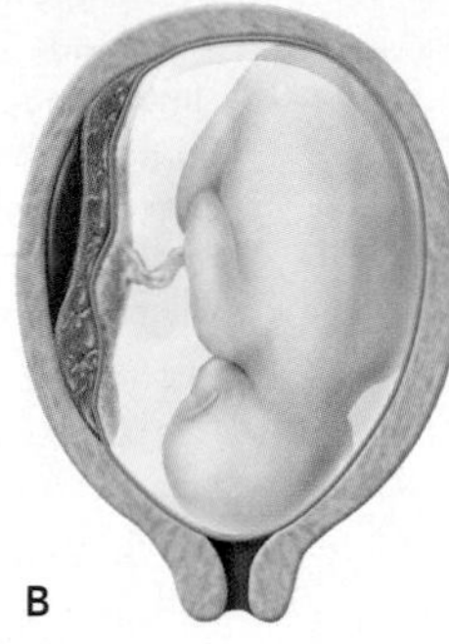

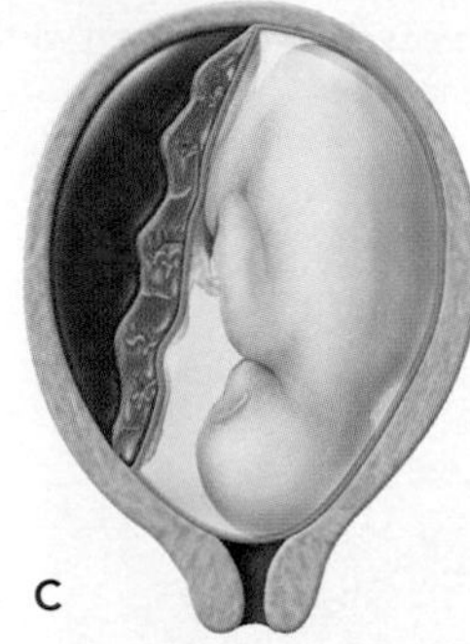

FIGURE 11-17A–C Abruptio placentae

Subjective Data

- Severe abdominal or back pain and bleeding generally after 20 weeks' gestation.

Objective Data

Key findings:

- Abrupt bleeding
- Tenderness usually located on midline of pelvis
- Uterine contractions
- Fetal distress
- Bleeding is common but not always seen (mild or significant)
- High frequency, low amplitude contractions
- Maternal hypotension
- Fetal heart rate abnormalities
- Hypofibrinogenemia <200 or other coagulopathies (increased D dimmer and fibrin split products plus low fibrinogen) or DIC
- Diagnosis is clinical but imaging, laboratory abnormalities, and postpartum pathologic studies can be useful to support the diagnosis.

Gestational Diabetes (GD)

A form of diabetes that emerges during pregnancy and often goes away during the postpartum period.

Pathophysiology

- May represent the first manifestation of DM in a person at risk for diabetes, made worse by the endocrine alteration during pregnancy, combined with increasing BMI, leading to insulin resistance.

Subjective Data

- In a medically managed pregnancy, symptoms of diabetes are rare as women are managed at an earlier stage.
- Factors in the health and pregnancy history such as previous GD, previous LGA infant, family history of DM, or rapid increased in BMI may lead providers to order screening early in pregnancy.

Objective Data

- Diagnosed via glucose challenge test of some sort.
- In the U.S., most women are screened either early in pregnancy based on history or around 24–28 weeks using a 50 gm loading glucose dose for a 1 hour screening test.
- Exact standards for failure of the screening test vary, but if the screening test is failed, then further testing is needed to be diagnostic.

Any of the following values are diagnostic:

- HA1c > or = to 6.5%
- Fasting plasma glucose > or = 126 mg/dl
- Two or more abnormal values on a 100 gm loading dose 3-hour glucose tolerance test

Pregnancy-Induced Hypertension, Preeclampsia, Eclampsia, HELLP Syndrome

This is a continuum of hypertension disorders that arise during pregnancy.

Pathophysiology

- Exact pathophysiology remains unknown, although placenta clearly plays an important role
- Only known cure is delivery of both fetus and placenta.
- Hypertension accompanied with proteinuria are the two cardinal signs.
- Preeclampsia is the early manifestation; eclampsia means at least one grand mal seizure in the absence of other causes has occurred.
- HELLP is the most severe form: H (hemolysis), EL (elevated liver enzymes), LP (low platelets) syndrome. This is often life threatening to the woman and requires tertiary level of care.
- These syndromes place woman at increased risk for renal failure, placental abruption, cerebral hemorrhage, pulmonary edema, hepatic failure, DIC.

Subjective Data

- Headache
- Mild to severe nausea/vomiting
- Gastritis
- Epigastric pain
- Blurred vision or seeing spots
- Large weight gain
- Edema (especially face) or pitting edema (lower extremities) that does not resolve with rest.
- Feeling sick, ill or "bad" or like having the flu
- Dyspnea
- Retrosternal chest pain
- Pulmonary edema
- Altered mental status

Objective Data

- Signs generally do not appear until the second or third trimester.
- Hypertension in someone without pre-existing high blood pressure. Usually must be at least 140 systolic or 90 diastolic on at least two occasions a few hours apart.
- Proteinuria over +1 on ordinary dipstick or more than 300 mg in a 24 hour specimen (usually > 5 gms in 24 hrs).
- Weight gain of > 1.5 kg/ month in the 2nd trimester or > 0.5 kg/ wk in the 3rd trimester
- Hyperreflexia
- Oliguria (<500 ml/24 hours)
- Fetal growth restriction
- Elevated liver enzymes
- Thrombocytopenia (< 100,000 platelets/cubic mL)
- Elevated serum creatinine
- Hemoconcentration
- In HELPP: microangiopathic hemolytic anemia

Premature Rupture of Membranes (PROM), Preterm Premature Rupture of membranes (PPROM)

Spontaneous rupture of membranes before the onset of labor contractions.

Pathophysiology

- PPROM (before 37 weeks) is more dangerous than PROM. This nearly always results in giving birth to a preterm baby.
- Exact mechanism of why this happens remains unknown, many nonspecific risk factors exist.
- Occasionally, can arise secondary to something such as abdominal trauma or intrauterine infection.

Subjective Data

- Fluid coming out of vagina that is usually thin and watery, clear to whitish in color, and contains bits of waxy vernix, has a not unpleasant odor

Objective Data

- Copious amount of obvious amniotic fluid pouring out of the vagina.
- Fluid usually normal in appearance and odor, but can have signs of infection (appearance and odor from pus)
- Observation of similar fluid in vaginal vault when viewed through (sterile) speculum.
- The fluid is alkaline (turns nitrazine paper dark blue)
- Ferning seen under the microscope (diagnostic gold standard)

Premature or Preterm Labor (PTL)

Onset of uterine contractions plus cervical changes after 20 and before 37 weeks. True PTL will inevitably lead to premature birth.

Pathophysiology

- Exact cause remains unknown, and is probably multi-factoral.
- Many nonspecific risk factors, with the most important being a history of previous preterm labor or birth.

Subjective Data

- Abdominal/back and/or pelvic pain of some sort.
- Pain may feel obviously like uterine contractions (wavelike pain that comes and goes) or more like a nonspecific discomfort.
- Possibly slight vaginal bleeding
- Possibly increased vaginal discharge or symptoms of PROM
- Urinary frequency
- Pelvic pressure

Objective Data

- Regular uterine contractions that can be palpated or recorded in a fetal monitoring machine.
- Cervical changes that begin with effacement and become dilatated.
- Contractions and cervical changes need to be present before a diagnosis of labor can be made.

Assessment of Older Adults

Connie Madden, MS, RN
Nanci McLeskey, MCG, MDiv, RN-BC, FNGNA

Mrs. Patil is well known to the emergency department. As her son wheels her up to the registration desk, the charge nurse glances over and sighs. "Looks like they are dropping her off again."

The Patil children, as well intentioned as they may once have been, have all but given up on their mother. "She had another fall at home," her son says. "We wanted to bring her here to make sure that everything is okay." He turns and heads for the door, leaving his aged, severely demented mother alone with the medical staff. The ED nurse and resident are incredulous. "Excuse me, sir, we need you to come back and give us some more information."

"It's the same thing that happened last week. She had another fall and needs to stay here for a few days. My sister usually picks her up from the hospital."

"That shouldn't be a designated role," the nurse whispers to the resident. They wheel Mrs. Patil into an ED bay and begins looking through her previous admissions. Sure enough, she has been here eight times in the past 2 months. Her past history is notable for dementia and numerous supposedly medication-related falls. She desperately needs to be seen by a neurologist and primary care physician to manage her meds, but all of her scheduled outpatient appointments were no-shows. The charge nurse explains, "Her kids would rather treat the hospital like a daycare than take their mother to all of her appointments. It's sad." Mrs. Patil looks up from her wheelchair and gives the three health workers an absent smile.

LEARNING OUTCOMES

1. Identify common changes that occur with aging within each domain of assessment.
2. Distinguish between age-expected age-associated changes and changes that indicate illness.
3. Articulate health promotion and illness prevention strategies for the older adult.
4. Identify the major components of a comprehensive geriatric assessment, which includes listing the domains (various aspects of an older adult) to be assessed and identifying the assessment tools used for each of those domains.
5. Identify sources of appropriate and evidence-based best practice guidelines.
6. Describe appropriate assessment techniques, tools, and screening instruments to address individual needs of the older adult.
7. Recognize the potential difficulties that challenge conducting a comprehensive assessment of an older adult.
8. Explains factors that promote successful assessments of older adults.

The assessment of the older adult requires a multifaceted approach with an overall emphasis on promoting and maintaining wellness and independent function. As people age, change occurs. Age associated change is natural and often predictable. Health care providers eventually will encounter older adults with age-associated changes. Assessment of the older adult, commonly defined as aged 65 or older, requires modification and adaptation in the approach to the individual, management of the environment, and identification of and how to access and use the most appropriate assessment instruments and screening tools.

For health care providers it is essential to recognize an accurate depiction of aging in the 21st century and an understanding of individual age-associated changes that will provide a foundation for an appropriate comprehensive geriatric assessment.

Characteristics of Older Adults

Older adults are identified as the fastest growing age group population. Although the growth rate is expected to stabilize after the last of the baby boomers enter older adulthood, it is estimated that the older adult population will double from 35 million in 2000 to 72 million, comprising 20% of the total U.S. population in 2030 (Federal Interagency Forum on Aging-Related Statistics, 2012). Census Bureau projections indicate that the number of those aged 85 and over may nearly quadruple from 5.5 million to 19 million by 2050. Many older Americans report a variety of chronic health conditions, and more than 37 million of older adults will be managing at least one chronic condition by 2030 (First Consulting Group, 2007). Despite the prevalence of chronic conditions most Americans over age 65 rate their health as good, very good, or excellent. The Older Americans report from the Federal Inter-agency Forum (2012) describes the results of measurement on several key indicators of well-being, which provides an overview of the current status of older Americans. Some selected and general findings of their report are included in Table 12-1.

Table 12-1 Older Americans report

Population	
Number of Older Adults	In 2030 older adults will be 20% of the total population. The oldest-old (> 85) is the fastest growing age group. There are more older woman than older men.
Racial and Ethnic Composition	By 2050 the older population is anticipated to be 58% non-Hispanic white, 20% Hispanic, 12% black, and 9% Asian.
Marital Status	78% of men aged 75–74 are married compared to 56% of women. 58% of men 85 and older are married. Women over 65 are more likely to be widowed than men.
Educational Attainment	80% of older adults had at least a high school diploma. 28% of older men and 18% of older women have a Bachelor's degree.
Living Arrangements	Older men are more likely to live with a spouse. Older black, Asian, and Hispanic women are more likely than non-Hispanic white women to live with relatives other than a spouse.
Older Veterans	Two out of three men over age 65 are veterans. As World War II veterans die the number of veterans will decline.
Economics	
Poverty	Older women are more likely to live in poverty then older men. Older non-Hispanic whites less likely than blacks, Hispanics, and Asians, but 9% of all older people live in poverty.
Income	34% of older adults are in the middle income range; 26% are low income.
Sources of Income	Social Security provides 37% of all older adult income. Social Security provides at least partial income for 88% of older adults.
Health Status	
Life Expectancy	People who live to age 65 live an average of 19.2 more years. Women who live to 85 live an average of 7 years; men 5.9 years.
Mortality	Causes of death (in order of incidence) are heart disease, cancer, chronic respiratory diseases, stroke, Alzheimer's disease, diabetes, flu, pneumonia.
Chronic Conditions	Women have more asthma, arthritis, and hypertension than men. Men have more heart disease, cancer, and diabetes. 21% of older adults have diabetes.
Sensory Impairment and Oral Health	46% of older men and 31% of older women have trouble hearing. 14% of the older population is vision impaired. 33% of older adults are edentulous.
Self-Assessment of Health	76% of older adults rated their health as good, very good, or excellent.
Depressive Symptoms	16% of older women and 11% of older men report depressive symptoms.
Functional Limitations	41% of Medicare enrollees people report a functional limitation; 12% with one or more instrumental activities of daily living (IADLs). 25% percent had difficulty with at least one ADL. Women reported higher levels of functional limitations than men.
Health Risks and Behaviors	
Vaccinations	63% of people aged 65 and received a flu shot in the past. 60% of people aged 65 received a pneumonia vaccination.

Continued

Table 12-1 Older Americans report *(continued)*

Mammography	23% of older women had a mammogram within the past 2 years.
Physical Activity	11% of people aged 65 and report leisure-time exercise. Older men are more likely to exercise than older women.
Obesity	38% of people aged 65 and over are obese.
Cigarette Smoking	10% of older men and 9% of older women smoke. 53% of older men and 29% previously smoked cigarettes.
Use of time	Older adults spend about 25% of their time in leisure activities, and watching TV accounts for half of that time.
Health Care	
Use of Health Care Services	Hospitalization rates are 320 per 1000 Medicare enrollees. The average length of hospital stay is 5.4 days. Skilled nursing facility stay rates are 80 per 1000. There are 14,437 physician visits and consultations and 3,864 home health visits per 1000 Medicare enrollees.
Health Care Expenditures	Low-income individuals incurred higher health care costs than others. Individuals with no chronic conditions had $5,520 health care cost; those with five or more conditions incurred $24,658. Average costs for residents of long-term care facilities were $61,318, compared with only $13,150 among community residents.
Prescription Drugs	Prescription drugs accounted for 16% of health care costs. Average costs per person were $2,834 in 2008.
Sources of Health Insurance	Most Medicare enrollees have a private insurance supplement. About 9% of Medicare enrollees report no supplement.

Source: Adapted From Federal Interagency Forum on Aging-Related Statistics. *Older Americans 2012: Key Indicators of Well-Being.* Washington, DC: Federal Interagency Forum on Aging-Related Statistics.

Theories of Aging

As the study of aging progresses there is increasing awareness that no single theory encompasses the entire aging process. Multiple interactions between biological, psychological, and sociological processes of aging result in infinite variations in how individuals age; in fact, the older adult population is the group that exhibits the widest range of individual characteristics, making identified population norms less useful for prediction of characteristics in the older adult population than in other populations.

These population variations result from not having a single "one size fits all" theory of aging that can explain the wide variation in the older adult population, making it even more important for health care providers to consider the interaction between various theories. Recognition of how theories intersect, potentially either complimenting or confounding each other, increases awareness of the diversity within the aging population resulting in the wide variations of individual biological and psychological characteristics.

Erikson's Developmental Stage Theory and Maslow's Hierarchy of Need Theory are two commonly known and widely recognized examples within the general category of psychological aging theory.

Eric Erickson's Theory

Eric Erickson's theory of the stages of psychosocial development is well known and often used for characterizing and describing an individual's development and progression through eight stages across a life-course. For older adults, Erikson identifies the eighth stage as **Ego Integrity vs. Despair**. Erickson describes this stage as occurring from age 65 through death and is a time when an individual looks back to review his or her life-course from the perspective of a whole lived experience that involved mastering one stage in order to move on to the next. For some older adults, this life-course review includes a sense of integrity that reflects fulfillment resulting from the perception that achievement of goals and accomplishments is a life well lived. For others, a look back on their life may bring about feelings of despair that reflect discontent from a perception of lost opportunities, lack of accomplishment, and unfulfilled potential.

An additional ninth stage was developed by Joan Erickson, who worked closely with her husband, basing this stage on her own observations and notes from Erik's on-going work. In this stage, retrospection becomes more immediately introspective. Questions of autonomy, trust, and identity surface as the older adult attempts to reconcile demands of daily living with transcendence from one existence to another (**gerotranscendance**) (Erikson & Erikson, 1997).

Erickson's theory has had minimal empirical support, but its descriptive framework has been universally used in subsequent research indicating that life review for older adults is an expected and useful process for sorting, categorizing, and extracting meaning from events that occurred during the life-course. Understanding both the process and results of life-course review will assist the health care provider to assess how attitude and values may affect an older individual's approach to health promotion and illness, self-care and prescriptive care, end-of-life decision making, and feelings toward death.

Maslow's Hierarchy of Needs

Maslow's **Hierarchy of Needs** is a commonly used theory that has application to aging by providing a framework that addresses the intersection between motivation and human need (Figure 12-1). This

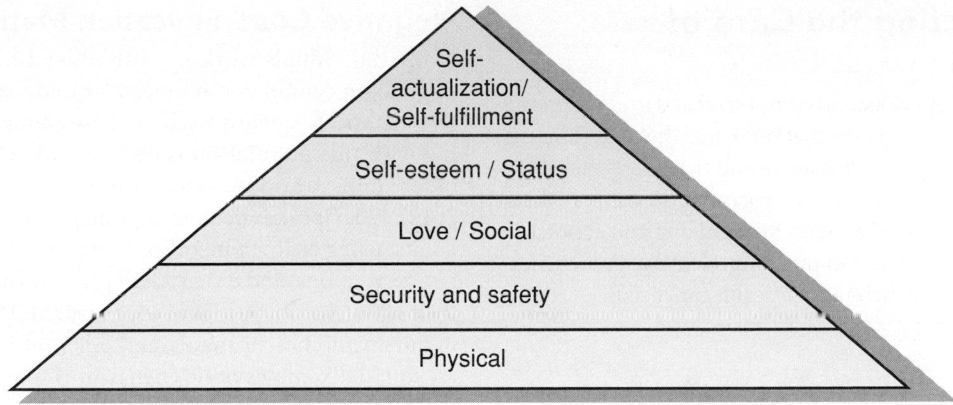

FIGURE 12-1 Maslow's Hierarchy of Needs

Source: From *Motivation and Personality*, 3E by A. H. Maslow, R. D. Frager, and J. Fadiman, 1987. Copyright © 1987. Reprinted and Electronically reproduced by permission of Pearson Education, Inc., Upper Saddle River, New Jersey.

theory ranks bio/psycho/social needs of an individual from the most basic to the most complex. Although this theory posits that lower-level needs take priority over higher level needs, and that higher-level needs can be met only after lower level needs are addressed, it also hypothesizes that individuals are continually striving to achieve higher level needs. For example, although the need for food takes precedence over the need for self-actualization, it is through self-actualization that individuals can attain desirable characteristics such as creativity and independence, and engage in positive and fulfilling interactions.

Maslow's Hierarchy of Needs theory may be helpful to consider as a basic guideline when assessment findings of an older adult indicates needs that are dependent on or conflict with one another. The Hierarchy of Needs may be a particularly effective framework when comparing and prioritizing physiological and psychological needs. For example, consider the needs of an older adult who, although used to living independently alone in his or her own home, is being discharged to a rehabilitation facility from the hospital following knee surgery. Assessment may identify issues of pain, limited mobility, potential fall risk, loss of independence, and sadness to not be going home right away. Using Maslow's Hierarchy of Needs, physiological precedence would take priority in planning individual care, with the understanding that the plan would build to address all levels of need.

A disadvantage of Maslow's Hierarchy of Needs Theory is that many physiological needs are grouped together and may have different levels of immediacy. Careful and thorough assessment is necessary in order to identify those needs that are urgent and/or preventing resolution of other identified needs. Furthermore, although physiologic needs are identified as taking precedence over psychological needs, there are instances when psychological needs are so severe that they interfere with ability to effectively address physiological needs. This reinforces the importance of individualized assessment that is patient centered and built upon a foundation that addresses biological and sociological, as well as psychological domains of the aging process. Table 12-2 provides a brief description of common theories from biological, psychological, and sociological domains that health care providers may find useful to consider when assessing and planning care of an older adult.

Table 12-2 Summary of aging theories

Programmed Theories (Biological)	
Programmed Longevity	Sequential switching on and off of certain genes, with age associated deficits manifested at defined points
Endocrine Theory	Hormonal regulation of the biological clock to control the rate of aging
Immunological Theory	Programmed decline of the immune system leading to increased vulnerability to infectious disease, affecting the outcome of a variety of illnesses
Error Theories (Biological)	
Wear and Tear Theory	Vital parts of organs and cells "wear out" after years of use and become less efficient at repairing malfunctions.
Free Radical Theory	Accumulated oxygen radicals decrease cell function, eventually causing organ failure.
Cross-link Theory	An accumulation of cross-linked proteins that result from glucose-protein binding. The "bound" protein cannot perform normally resulting in age-associated complications.
Psychological Aging Theories	
Erikson's Development Theory	Specific developmental tasks that must be accomplished in stages that build upon each other
Maslow's Hierarchy of Needs	Interdependent levels of human need that motivates individuals to fulfill basic need before moving to more complex needs
Sociological Aging Theories	
Disengagement theory	Older adults and society engage in a reciprocal and mutual withdrawal.
Activity Theory	Continued social involvement results in contentment and life satisfaction.
Continuity Theory	Maintaining and continuing previous values, social ties, relationships, and structures allow individuals to remain "who they are" as they age.

Source: Data from Jin, 2010; Tabloski, 2009

Factors Affecting the Care of Older Adults

Multiple perceptions, behaviors, and attitudes related to aging prevail within cultures and environments that influence the overall beliefs and values that are held concerning aging and the elderly. It is these elements that are used and processed in regards to decision making related to care and treatment of them. Recognizing and appreciating these factors will facilitate a more comprehensive approach to address and understanding their unique health care needs.

Ageism

Current society's perspective and attitudes towards older adults frequently have untoward outcomes. When generalizing one's beliefs for an entire segment of population, we are inclined to hold biases and/or myths towards those individuals. **Ageism** is a term coined by Robert Butler and defined as the systematic stereotyping and discrimination against individuals due to advanced age, similar to racism and sexism (e.g., due to skin color and gender) (Butler, 1989). When attitudes of ageism and belief in aging myths are held by health care providers, they can result in serious consequences, such as preventing adequate communication, and at times get in the way of providing high quality of care. For example, when older adults voice various complaints about their health status to individuals holding ageist beliefs, those complaints are frequently ignored or discounted. (Nelson, 2005; Salzman, 2006). Other consequences include substandard care in influencing policy formation, insurance reimbursement, treatment, rationing services, and frequent exclusion from drug trials, resulting in outcomes of care below par (Bowling, 2007). It was reported in one study where providers provided more information and support to younger patients and not to older patients (Adelman, Greene, & Charon, 1991).

Examples of aging myths related to health status include the beliefs that urinary incontinence, delirium, confusion, and falling are all expected aging changes; an older adult body's reaction to medications is constant; and due to older adults drinking less fluids they are expected to be dehydrated. This is by no means an exhaustive list of aging myths (Mauk, 2008). Unfortunately, aging myths are held by many individuals, and older adults are collectively seen through a negative lens and have been viewed this way for many years.

Elder Abuse

Another consequence of negative beliefs that place less value on older adults than on younger people is the frequent occurrence of elder abuse. An important issue related to elder abuse is that abusive situations often go unnoticed or are disregarded, especially when it comes to the welfare or humanity of an older adult. One reason that this occurs is that health care providers are often not well acquainted with the types of abuse in older adults and therefore do not recognize it when present (Nelson, 2005). Currently, there is increasing elder abuse in the form of neglect, fraud or exploitation, and outright violence, and often is under-reported due to fear of retaliation on the part of the elder (Robinson, deBenedictis, & Segal, 2012). With large numbers of baby boomers now reaching 65 years of age, these negative views are predicted to change. (See Chapter 14 for additional information on elder abuse.)

Negative Communication Methods

Many individuals working with older adults believe that this population cannot communicate or understand well. One negative method frequently used by those communicating and working with this population is **elderspeak**, the manner in which older adults are addressed and/or spoken to (Pioneer Network, 2012). Elderspeak is defined as an altered way of speaking to older adults, using a slow rate of speaking, simplified syntax, vocabulary restrictions, and exaggerated prosody on the assumption that their age makes them cognitively impaired. This has been common in nursing homes, hospitals, and other settings where frail elders are found. Examples of this behavior is someone calling an older adult "sweetie" or "honey," which is frequently interpreted by an older adult as belittling, disrespectful, and condescending (Brown & Draper, 2003).

The use of patronizing communication with older adults is over-accommodation, which is demonstrated by individuals speaking louder, slower, or talking in simpler sentences, which often results in downplaying thoughts or concerns expressed by older individuals.

The third negative communication method is using baby talk that one would use with an infant or toddler (Nelson, 2005). In one study, provider's interactions when working with older adults were found to be condescending, abrupt, and indifferent and they were less likely to agree on main goals, main topics, and primary medical problems at the encounter (Adelman et al., 1991). Older adults view individuals who talk to them this way as less competent, less nurturing, and significantly disrespectful (Ryan, Bourhis, & Knops, 1991).

Lack of Provider Education

Another factor affecting care for older adults is the lack of education by many health care providers in the field of gerontology (the study of the aging process) and geriatric (health care of older adults) medicine (Institute of Medicine, 2008). This situation is caused by either inadequate or lack of gerontology content in academic programs which in turn creates negative attitudes causing individuals not to choose to work in the field of gerontology or geriatric medicine. It is essential that those working with older adults be aware of their attitudes towards older adults and be well educated in the knowledge to care for this segment of the population (Nelson, 2005). All of these issues are of great importance if we are to provide respect, dignity, and person-centered care for this aging population.

Interprofessional Collaboration

Generally and simply, the complexities of care of older adults arise from having lived a long time. While not all care of older adults is physically or medically complex, it is important to remember that there are multiple potential explanations for why complexities are present. Older adults have long life histories with numerous interactions in various types of relationships. They may have values that were formed as adolescents in a generation far removed from the generation of today's health provider. They may have multiple chronic conditions with associated care needs that range from self-management to episodic intervention to total care. Additionally, expected age-associated changes in body systems often result in wide variation of symptoms that are different than common symptoms in younger adult, requiring specialized and relevant assessment tools and intervention approaches. Regardless of the reason, a systematic and collaborative interprofessional approach offers a strategy for ensuring a comprehensive assessment that addresses all aspects of the older adult.

In the 2008 Institute of Medicine Report, *Retooling for an Aging America*, it was recommended to improve care of older adults through a comprehensive assessment of their needs (Institute of Medicine, 2008). Considering the potential for multiple components and levels of complexity, a collaborative approach by an interprofessional geriatric team was needed. Such a team that comprehensively addresses physical, psychological, emotional, and social perspectives is more likely to uncover treatable health problems resulting in better health outcomes than may be achieved by a single discipline assessment, or by those without specific geriatric care knowledge.

An **interprofessional geriatric team** is composed of a variety of providers from various disciplines who collaborate and can address an older adult's status and needs, as well as options and available resources (Figure 12-2). Each team member brings specialized knowledge that contributes to the reciprocal understanding by everyone on the team of the older individual as a whole. Generally, the team is composed of key members that include a geriatric provider, geriatric nurse, geriatric social worker or case manager, and geriatric pharmacist. Frequently an older adult may benefit from further assessment by additional health care providers including a respiratory therapist, occupational therapist, physical therapist, psychologist, and speech-language pathologist. Still other members may include a registered dietitian, optometrist, and clergy. Table 12-3 provides a brief explanation of the role of key and frequent interprofessional geriatric team members in the assessment of an older adult.

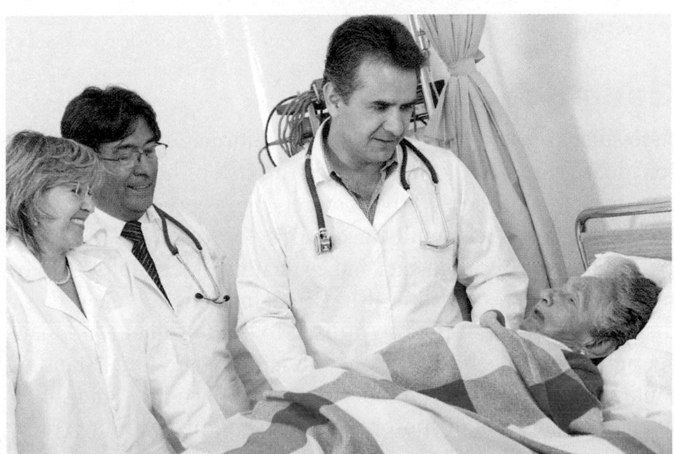

FIGURE 12-2 The members of an interprofessional geriatric team collaborate to address an older adult's status and needs.

Source: Andresr/Shutterstock

Table 12-3 Interprofessional geriatric team members

Profession	Role in Comprehensive Geriatric Assessment
Geriatric Nurse	Assess for optimal functioning in all domains, the need for coordination of care, and prevention/health promotion education.
Geriatric Pharmacist	Assess optimal regimen of medication therapy that includes dose management and issues associated with polypharmacy.
Geriatric Nurse Practitioner	Complete health assessment, including history and physical, assessment of need for coordination of care and prevention/health promotion education.
Geriatric Physician (Gerontologist)	Complete health assessment, including history and physical, assessment of need for coordination of care and prevention/health promotion education.
Geriatric Social Worker	Assess need for various social services and programs, family-support services, and for coordination of medical care.
Occupational Therapist	Assess functional independence and safety in activities of daily living with the older adult and their caregiver(s).
Physical Therapist	Assess disability or mobility limitations and impact on functional ability, potential need for assisting device, and safety education.
Psychologist	Assess affect psychosocial issues, including depression, anxiety, and bereavement and their effect on individual function.
Respiratory Therapist	Assess breathing disorder, effectiveness of treatment, and need for prevention/health promotion education.
Speech-Language Pathologist	Assess communication disorders and management of them, including language-related components associated with cognition.

Age-associated Changes and Approaches

General age-associated appearance and function changes are expected as part of the aging process. While it is important to remember that specific characteristics can vary widely between older adults and still be considered as part of the norm, Table 12-4 provides a brief description of expected assessment findings that will be useful when determining which of those findings may require intervention, referral, or additional follow-up. Specialized assessment and screening tools have been listed in Table 12-5.

Health Status Complexity in Older Adults

Health status complexity is frequently seen in this segment of the population as a result of a number of factors. These factors include geriatric syndromes that often go unrecognized or are inadequately addressed (e.g., functional decline or dementia); age-related and age-associated changes; and various other factors such as diseases, heredity,

Table 12-4 Expected aging function and appearance changes

Face	There is a loss of hair in eyebrows, wrinkles around eyes, atrophy of subcutaneous fat that can make eyes appear sunken and nose and chin more prominent.
Eyes	Benign hyaline deposits cause spots on the retina; corneas may yellow.
Ears	Ear lobes lengthen.
Teeth	Teeth may yellow and have vertical cracks.
Nose	Sense of smell decreases.
Tongue	Sense of taste decreases.
Thorax	More barrel-shaped, loss of intercostal cartilage elasticity resulting in less chest movement/ventilation.
Heart	Systolic murmurs are present in about half of older adults.
Abdomen	Musculature is thinner and subcutaneous fat is thicker. Liver size decreases. Gastrointestinal motility slows.
Musculoskeletal	Decrease in subcutaneous fat increases bony prominences. Shortening of the torso results in more flexed posture. Outward curvature of the spine (Kyphosis).
Neurological	Neuron loss results in less muscle tone and strength. Nerve impulse conduction slows resulting in slower reaction time. Gait is more deliberate and hesitant. Deep tendon reflexes are slowed.
Cognition	Processing slows but intelligence remains the same intelligence. Sensory changes can contribute to processing ability (hearing and vision loss).
Reproductive	Men: Penis size decreases, scrotum hangs lower. Slower and less intense sexual response. Women: Decreased pubic hair, vaginal walls thin, natural lubrication decreases, sensation decreases.

lifestyle, co-existing acute, and chronic conditions. Frequently, these factors interact with one another resulting in complicated and clinically challenging management of these patients' health care needs. Frequently, an older adult comes to a clinic or is a patient in a hospital with nonspecific and seemingly unrelated and/or ordinary common complaints, which are then ignored. This phenomenon reinforces the importance for health care providers caring for older adults to have specialized knowledge in geriatric medicine. When complexity is present, such as **geriatric syndromes**, a comprehensive geriatric assessment is necessary (which will be discussed later in the chapter). Older adults make up 40% of all hospitalized patients (Agency for Healthcare Research and Qualilty, 2008). In the acute setting they are often complicated patients, with greater risk for geriatric syndromes (often multifactorial in nature), and often have multiple organ systems affected (Inouye, Studenski, Tinetti, & Kuchel, 2007).

It is not unusual for older hospitalized patients to suffer from multiple complex medical problems, be on multiple medications, have a vulnerability to iatrogenic (adverse condition resulting from a medical treatment) events, have increased hospital stays (versus younger patients), and be more likely to die in the hospital. Geriatric assessments should be conducted routinely under specific circumstances such as following a hospitalization for an acute illness; when a change of living status is considered; occurrence of an abrupt or significant change in physical, social, or psychological function at annual appointments; or when a second opinion is requested.

Table 12-5 Principles of geriatric assessment

Goal	Promote wellness, independence
Focus	Function, performance (gait, balance, transfers)
Scope	Physical, cognitive, psychological, social domains
Approach	Interprofessional
Efficiency	Ability to perform rapid screens to identify target areas
Success	Maintaining or improving quality of life

Source: From "Principles of Geriatric Assessment" by Thomas M. Gill in ASSESSMENT. GRS Teaching Slides, 2013. Reproduced by permission of the American Geriatrics Society, NY. http://www.geriatricscareonline.org.

Geriatric Syndromes

Geriatric syndromes are defined as health conditions associated with aging and frailty due to a variety of causes, and which do not fall into specific disease categories. Examples of most common syndromes include delirium, falls, incontinence, malnutrition, pressure ulcers, sleep disturbances, infection, poly-pharmacy, depression, and dementia. Frequently these syndromes contribute to adverse and serious outcomes for older patients including increased length of hospital stays, decline in both health and function, and often cause a change in where the patient is being discharged for rehabilitation or a permanent residence (e.g., skilled nursing facility [SNF] or nursing home [NH], and so on). It is essential that health care providers be knowledgeable of these syndromes so that early recognition, assessment, and intervention can be completed when changes occur, avoiding or preventing complications and/or untoward effects. The gold standard for assessing older adults is found in the "How to Try This" series by the Hartford Center for Geriatric (Hartford Institute for Geriatric Nursing, 2012).

Geriatric Assessment

Assessment is a term used for collecting information that is utilized for identifying health problems, or the risk of health problems occurring in older adults. The comprehensive geriatric assessment is designed to further identify medical, psychosocial, and functional capabilities by collecting data and evaluating older adults, thereby maximizing their overall health with aging. Though viewed as a diagnostic process, it is often utilized to both evaluate and manage an older adult's health through describing and understanding multiple issues that are commonly seen in older adults, and subsequent identification of appropriate interventions. Although older and younger patients share similar diseases and chronic conditions, the addition of physiological aging changes, numerous coexisting medical problems, and multiple medications often taken by older adults place them at higher risks for complications. The assessment of an older adult is noticeably different in many aspects from one completed on a younger individual, in that it extends beyond the traditional disease-driven medical evaluation of an individuals' health, evaluating multiple issues, containing greater detail, and requiring more time.

The information collected in the assessment can assist in keeping older adults safe, maintaining their present state of health, preventing situations from becoming worse, and correcting any issues that need to be corrected. By utilizing the assessment tools provided in this chapter we will be in conformity with *Healthy People 2020*'s goal for older adults to improve the health, function, and quality of life for older adults (U.S. Department of Health and Human Services, 2009).

When assessing an older adult it is important to distinguish between expected aging changes versus those changes that are pathological. Performing an assessment is an important component in caring for older adults by providing a baseline for older adult's usual health and social status, and assists in identifying if and when changes may have occurred, and is the foundation for an individualized care plan for an older adult. Evidenced-based tools for screening and assessing are readily available (see Table 12-5), enabling the collection of pertinent data and assisting in determining the health needs of an older adult simply and efficiently. By utilizing the data from a geriatric assessment, health care providers can identity geriatric conditions that need managing and additionally prevent or delay complications. Assessing older adults is not a one-time occurrence, but is a continual process.

Comprehensive Geriatric Assessment

The Comprehensive Geriatric Assessment (CGA) is defined as a multifaceted, interprofessional approach to provide quality of care for older adults, with the goal to promote wellness and independent function and maximize overall health with aging (Rubenstein, 1995). Depending on an older adult's health, there are criteria for identifying appropriate patients for a CGA, excluding patients who are too well or too sick to benefit from this type of assessment (e.g., those with a terminal illness, severe dementia, complete functional dependence, and inevitable nursing home placement). Individuals most likely to benefit from the CGA would be those 85 years and older, individuals with medical comorbidities (e.g., heart failure or cancer), psychosocial problems (e.g., depression or isolation), specific geriatric conditions (e.g., dementia, falls, or functional disability), previous or predicted high health care utilization, and for those considering a change in living situation (e.g., from independent living to assisted living, nursing home or in-home caregivers).

CGA can be conducted in various settings of care such as home, clinic, nursing home, but is more frequently done in the hospital due to the issues related to the time that is required in evaluation, the need for coordination of an interdisciplinary team of various disciplines, and unfortunately due to the lack of reimbursement for various components (e.g., pharmacy, nutrition, outpatient social work, etc.). Conducting this assessment on older adults frequently produces some important outcomes, especially for hospitalized patients, which include improved short-term mortality, better chances of living at home, and improved physical and cognitive functioning (G. I. Ellis & Langhorne, 2005).

Typically the CGA includes multiple dimensions: physical health, placing high value on functional status (Halter et al., 2009), psychological health (cognitive and affective status), social (economic, environmental), and spiritual status, all of which influence an older adult's health. These components are necessary in order to fully understand the health needs of the older adult. There are various evidence-based screening and assessment tools, which guide this systematic and integrated assessment along with clinical skills, judgment, and incorporating the patient's history and physical examination (Olenek, Skowronski, & Schmaltz, 2003).

An older adult's health status is dependent upon influences beyond the appearance of their health condition. The tools utilized in the process examine factors affecting the course of disease and outcome of treatment(s) and from the findings; a coordinated and integrated plan for treatment is developed. Focused areas include functional, physical, mental, emotional, pharmacotherapeutic, and socioeconomic, spiritual, and cultural preferences. Emphasis is placed on quality of life and functional status, prognosis, and outcome that entail a workup of more depth and breadth. Important content areas fostering understanding of individualized aging include focused assessments (cognitive & functioning abilities), geriatric syndromes, sexuality, nutrition, abuse and mistreatment, substance misuse, age-related changes, sensory changes, atypical presentations, oral health, and learning needs. The CGA has been found to lead to improved detection and documentation of geriatric problems (Ellis, Whitehead, Robinson, O'Neill, & Langhorne, 2011).

Influencing Factors on the Comprehensive Geriatric Assessment

By having numerous factors in place prior to and during the actual assessment potentiates the promise of a successful outcome. Those factors include knowledge that a CGA is beneficial for older adults, consideration of certain elements in promoting a successful outcome for the assessment, and awareness of potential barriers.

Benefits Completing a routine comprehensive geriatric assessment on older adults has been shown to have multiple benefits including reduced hospital use and mortality rates, improved mental status, decreased health costs, improved functional ability and overall health outcomes, and lowering hospital readmission rates (Engelhardt, Toseland, Gao, & Banks, 2006). Other positive outcomes have been in identifying individuals with geriatric syndromes, improving the detection and documentation of geriatric problems, and enhancing personal health status by decreasing the potential for or the severity of chronic conditions, encouraging self-efficacy, and empowering individuals in self-care. Research identified that older adults were more likely to be alive in their homes after an emergency visit if the CGA was utilized, and with fewer medical health costs (Ellis, Whitehead, Robinson, et al., 2011).

Successful Outcomes Certain elements have been found necessary for optimal data gathering from a patient and/or caregiver at the time of assessment (Figure 12-3). The environment should be private, with little or no distracting noises (pagers, telephones, etc. off), comfortable seating, and comfortable temperatures. Other components that can add to making this successful are introducing one's self to the patient and family; using patient's last name (upfront, asking how they would like to addressed); sitting directly in front of the individual at eye level; inquiring about hearing or vision problems (deficits); asking questions that are short and simple, allowing sufficient time to answer questions (listen patiently); allowing for questions; being aware of body language (this speaks louder than verbal); and observing minute details (e.g., is the individual having difficultly answering simple questions, are they nervous, and so on).

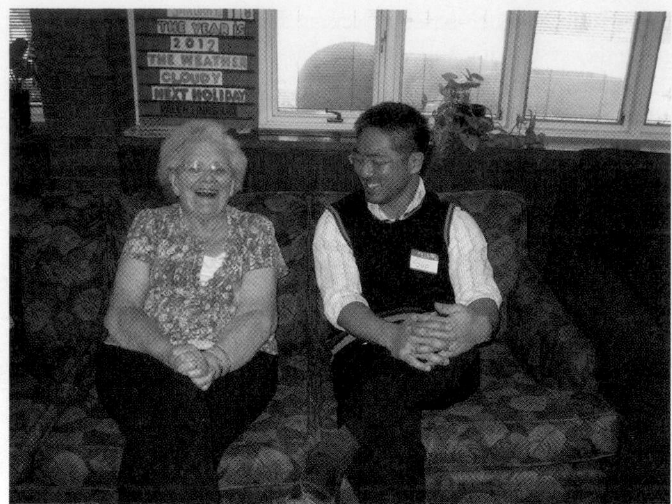

FIGURE 12-3 Choose a comfortable and private environment when gathering data from a patient for optimal results

When assessing an older adult it is essential that one be knowledgeable in expected aging changes for this population. The reliability of the patient as a historian must be assessed, and frequently it may be important and necessary to gather data from multiple sources. Other health care providers can provide valuable information, and most importantly, always include the patient, family members, and caregivers in the process. Other tips for a successful assessment include a proactive approach (e.g., asking them how they are caring for themselves, how they take their medications, and so on), knowing their preferences and needs in order to provide person-centered care, and when possible, baseline care and condition status. When a patient is scheduled for a clinic appointment (especially for an annual check-up) the process can be streamlined with pre-visit questionnaires mailed out prior to the appointment whereby information can be collected (e.g., past medical history, medications, preventive measures and functional status, is someone caring for the patient) and have it brought to the appointment completed by the patient or proxy (i.e., the function or power of somebody authorized to act for another).

Potential Barriers Numerous possible obstacles can be encountered when assessing older adults. Awareness of these potential barriers can enhance the assessment process and may include 1) communication issues affecting ability to speak clearly, understand the spoken word, read, hear, etc., 2) literacy and health literacy levels, 3) under-reporting symptoms believed to be expected aging changes (failing to recognize them as a medical problem), or embarrassment due to the nature of the problem, 4) inaccurate reporting due to vague, nonspecific complaints or multiple complaints, 5) memory problems occurring for various reasons that questions the reliability of the person providing information, 6) lack of time to adequately gather information, and 7) presence of family members or caregivers who may under or overestimate the individual's abilities.

Additionally to consider at the time of assessment is the older adult's health status, energy level, and whether he or she is well or strong enough for an extensive physical or verbal-based assessment. Having a pre-visit questionnaire sent to the patient or caregiver prior to an outpatient visit or scheduled hospitalization can be a time saver in gathering large amounts of information (Lange, 2012).

Components of the Comprehensive Geriatric Assessment

The six essential steps suggested for the CGA to be successful in achieving maximal health and functional benefit include 1) data gathering, 2) discussion of the findings with the interprofessional team, 3) development of a treatment or care plan, 4) implementation of the treatment plan, 5) monitoring patient responses related to the treatment plan, and 6) revising the treatment plan as needed. It is imperative to remember that each older adult is unique and will need an individualized plan of care in order to provide person-centered care, and that engaging the older adult and caregiver(s) as much as possible with education will empower them as part of the team.

Although gathering all this important information may seem an overwhelming task, there are multiple assessment tools (see Table 12-6) available that are simple and time efficient to reduce this burden, especially when initially gathering information.

Step 1: Data Gathering

As with any assessment or examination, the first step focuses on obtaining the appropriate data. While the CGA encompasses six steps, the first step will be the focus of this chapter.

History (General) The initial phase begins with gathering the historical information. This following information forms the basic patient profile and usually includes name, age, sex, birth date, marital status, source of history, and reliability of historian. Additional information is gathered on the patient's past health history, and current health history. Other assessment components include allergies, current medications (prescribed, OTC, home remedies, herbals, and dietary supplements—have the patient bring in a bag that contains all prescribed/unprescribed medications), diet, immunizations, possibility of folk medicine, any necessary medical records, and names and contact information of all involved health care providers. Assessing older adults differs from a standard evaluation by utilizing an interprofessional team to focus on complex problems, functional ability, and quality of life. If there are questions related to accuracy and reliability of the patient, a proxy may be used with consent. If the individual has limited English, an interpreter may be called in. Also inquire about current and/or present issues such as pain, nausea, surgeries, and so forth.

Social History Social history usually follows the initial health history. A strong social support system will frequently determine whether an older adult can remain at home or will need placement in a facility. A social history helps identify who would be available to help the older adult if he or she became ill and/or needed help with activities of daily living. A quick screen for this would be asking the older adult, "Who would be available if you needed to go to the hospital?" Other components of a social assessment include birthplace, residence, education, ethnicity and race, marital status, vocation, hobbies, relationships and support, habits (sleep, ETOH, etc.), spiritual background, current living arrangements, and economic resources to deal with current health issues. Also important is the assessment of utilization or knowledge of community resources currently being used or potentially available. A family health history is also taken along with a review of all of systems (e.g., immediate relatives with cardiac, gastrointestinal issues, etc.).

Caregivers are frequently the essential key to provision of a safe and effective environment for older adults. Caregivers need to be

Table 12-6 Geriatric assessment tools

Domain/Screen/Links	Tools
Functional Status: http://consultgerirn.org/topics/function/want_to_know_more	*Activities of Daily Living (ADLS):* http://consultgerirn.org/uploads/File/trythis/try_this_2.pdf *Independent Activities of Daily Living (IADLS):* http://consultgerirn.org/uploads/File/trythis/try_this_23.pdf
Mobility *Fall Risk screen*: 1. Two or more falls in prior 12 months? 2. Presents with acute fall? 3. Difficulty with walking or balance?	*Hendrick II* (Inpatient): http://consultgerirn.org/uploads/File/trythis/try_this_8.pdf *Timed Up and Go (TUG):* http://www.rehabmeasures.org/PDF%20Library/Timed%20Up%20and%20Go%20Test%20Instructions.pdf *Performance-Oriented Assessment of Gait/Balance (POMA):* http://consultgerirn.org/uploads/File/Tinetti_Assessment_Balance.pdf
Sensory Changes	http://consultgerirn.org/topics/sensory_changes/want_to_know_more
Vision	*Snellen Eye Chart:* http://www.healthcare.uiowa.edu/igec/tools/sensory/snellenChart.pdf
Hearing	*A Brief Hearing Loss Screen:* http://consultgerirn.org/uploads/File/trythis/try_this_12.pdf *Hearing Handicap Inventory for the Elderly(HHIE-S)* http://www.desertsounds.net/Hearing_Handicap_Inventory_for_the_Elderly_Screening_Form.htm *Whisper Test:* http://www.healthcare.uiowa.edu/igec/tools/sensory/whisperedVoice.pdf
Nutrition	*Mini-Nutritional Assessment (MNA):* http://consultgerirn.org/uploads/File/trythis/try_this_9.pdf *DETERMINE:* http://www.hospitalmedicine.org/geriresource/toolbox/pdfs/determine.pdf
Cognition	
Dementia	*Folstein Mini-Mental State Exam (MMSE):* http://enotes.tripod.com/MMSE.pdf *Mini-Cog*: http://consultgerirn.org/uploads/File/trythis/try_this_3.pdf *Brief Evaluation of Executive Dysfunction:* http://consultgerirn.org/uploads/File/trythis/try_this_d3.pdf *The St. Louis University Mental Status Examination (SLUMS)*: http://www.stlouis.va.gov/GRECC/SLUMS_English.pdf *Montreal Cognitive Assessment (MoCA)*: http://www.mocatest.org/pdf_files/test/MoCA-Test-English_7_1.pdf *The Short Blessed*: http://www.regionstrauma.org/downloads/sbt.pdf
Delirium	*Confusion Assessment Measure (CAM)*: http://consultgerirn.org/uploads/File/trythis/try_this_13.pdf
Mood	Depression screen (PHQ-2): Over the last 2 weeks, how often have you been bothered by any of the following problems? 1. During the past month, have you often been bothered by feeling down, depressed, or hopeless? 2. During the past month, have you often been bothered by little interest or pleasure in doing things? Geriatric Depression Scale (GDS): http://consultgerirn.org/uploads/File/trythis/try_this_4.pdf
Medications http://consultgerirn.org/topics/medication/want_to_know_more	*Beers Criteria:* http://consultgerirn.org/uploads/File/trythis/try_this_16_1.pdf
End of Life *Advance Directives:* http://consultgerirn.org/topics/advance_directives/want_to_know_more#item_3	*Living Will* *Durable Power of Attorney* *Instructional or Medical Directive:* *Physicians Orders for Life Sustaining Treatment (POLST):* http://www.ohsu.edu/polst
Pain	*Numeric Rating Scale (NRS) Faces Pain Scale* *Verbal Descriptor Scale (VAS):* http://consultgerirn.org/uploads/File/trythis/try_this_7.pdf
Other **Substance use and Abuse**	ETOH: *SMAST-G:* http://consultgerirn.org/uploads/File/trythis/try_this_17.pdf http://www.nursingcenter.com/pdf.asp?AID=823032 (article)
Sleep http://consultgerirn.org/topics/sleep/want_to_know_more	*Epworth Sleepiness Scale (ESS):* http://consultgerirn.org/uploads/File/trythis/try_this_6_2.pdf Pittsburgh Sleep Quality Index (PSQI) http://consultgerirn.org/uploads/File/trythis/try_this_6_1.pdf
Elder Mistreatment http://consultgerirn.org/topics/elder_mistreatment_and_abuse/want_to_know_more	*Elder Mistreatment Assessment*: http://consultgerirn.org/uploads/File/trythis/try_this_15.pdf
Spirituality	*FICA:* http://consultgerirn.org/uploads/File/trythis/try_this_sp5.pdf
Sexuality	http://consultgerirn.org/topics/sexuality_issues_in_aging/want_to_know_more
Quality of Life (QOL)	One question: Who will help you if......? (e.g., you needed to go to the hospital, you were sick in bed, etc.)

screened periodically for symptoms of depression or burnout, and if present be referred for counseling or support groups. Utilizing the **Modified Caregiver Strain Index** would be helpful if a need is noticed (Onega, 2008). Elder abuse should be considered when completing an assessment, especially when the patient presents with contusions, burns, bite marks, genital or rectal trauma, pressure ulcers, or is malnourished without clinical explanation.

During the intake of the social history, asking a few questions can serve as a brief social support screen. Example question: "Who is available to help you in the event that you get sick or need to go to the hospital?" Early detection of problems of support can benefit planning and finding resource referrals to put in place and keep the individual in the home as long as possible. Assessment of financial situation is especially important for a functionally impaired older adult because there may be state or local benefits available related to his or her income.

Advanced Care Preferences While individuals still have cognitive capacity to make end-of-life decisions, it is important to discuss preferences for specific treatments and interventions. Discussions should include present decisions, such as choosing an appropriate decision maker (i.e., appointing a durable power of attorney, also known as health care proxy) to serve in the individual's place in the event of incapacity, clarifying and articulating one's values over time. Advance directives help guide decision making regarding interventions when an individual is not able to speak for him- or herself and are vital to providing optimal care for this segment of the population.

Living Environment Visiting and conducting an environmental assessment takes time and resources that not all health care professional teams have available. Since this is not always possible, questions for the older adult and his or her family can provide information that will be helpful in putting a care plan in place for being discharged back to the original home setting. Items to be included in the assessment may be stairs, bathing and toileting, medication storage, nutrition and cooking, and financial matters (e.g., enough money for medications, food, etc.).

Culture, Diversity, and Education Diversity in ethnicity in the U.S. population is growing and will be challenging for many of the health care providers, especially in the assessing and care of these individuals. An important aspect of the assessment is to know appropriate ethnic rules of etiquette and taboos for individuals. Valuing a patient's differences is vital in the care of diverse individuals in which inappropriate or irrelevant care can lead to nonadherence and poor outcomes.

In the 2010 Census, just over one-third of the U.S. population reported their race and ethnicity as something other than non-Hispanic white (i.e., "minority"). This group increased from 86.9 million to 111.9 million between 2000 and 2010, representing a growth of 29 percent over the decade (United States Census Bureau, 2012).

Diversity can also include differences in gender roles, family compositions, sexual or religious preferences, educational levels, and socioeconomic status, all of which may require individual appropriate care planning. It is imperative to be somewhat knowledgeable about sociocultural differences so as to modify and adapt assessments and communications to a patient's beliefs and values. It is important to respect patient preferences, especially in promoting trusting relationships that can provide more information about the patient's needs.

Health Literacy

Health literacy is defined as "the degree to which individuals can obtain, process, and understand the basic health information and services they need to make appropriate health decisions." This capacity includes the ability to interpret documents, read, and write. The skills necessary are the ability to read, write, and do basic mathematical computations, and be able to speak and listen effectively in a health care setting (Institute of Medicine, 2006). Health literacy can directly affect one's health outcomes and cost of care (Cutilli, 2007).

It is estimated that 50% of Americans have some trouble with understanding health information and acting upon it (Nielsen-Bohlman, Panzer, & Kindig, 2004). Although in the aging baby boomer population, the literacy level is rising, but a disproportionate number of older adults are still at a basic or below basic literacy level (Kunter, Greenberg, Jin, & Paulsen, 2006). Health care providers need to utilize skills to accommodate individual health literacy levels, such as using good communication skills in assessing an individual's reading ability and preferred written and spoken language, and assessing deficits for vision, hearing, cognition, and readiness for receiving and understanding the information. Additionally, it is very helpful to provide educational materials, encourage questions, supply information in short sentences, and not use acronyms or medical jargon.

Psychological History

Psychological history taking includes assessing both psychological and cognitive function. A large portion of the older adult population with mental illness goes unrecognized and untreated. There is a stigma related to mental illness and older adults generally have a negative attitude about these issues that potentially prevents them from seeking treatment, or causes them to stop treatment prematurely. This assessment component may be complicated by ageism among health care providers who believe mental illness, especially depression, is an expected part of aging, or fail to see treatment as a viable option for older adults.

Signs of depression in this population may include an expression of sadness, hopelessness, helplessness, low self-worth, or feeling of uselessness and that life has no meaning. Mental health issues such as anxiety and depression adversely affect function and physical health in older adults (American Psychological Association, 2005).

The most common mental health conditions among older adults are depression, dementia, and delirium. These conditions are not mutually exclusive and can present major challenges for diagnosing and treating (Arnold, 2004). In the primary care setting 17%–37% of older adults have some type of depression. Not screening, diagnosing, and treating these patients leads to increased risk of poor health outcomes. Quick and simple tools, however, are available to screen these syndromes (see Table 12-6).

Physical Assessment

The physical assessment is the usual sequence in the assessment process following the history and social assessments. In caring for older adults, remember that as one advances in age, the potential for age-associated changes occurs in every system. Despite wide variation regarding when and to what extent changes occur in an individual, by and large, many of the characteristics can be generally expected, described, and considered to be a usual part of aging. Many physical assessment techniques and approaches are the same for both young and older adults, yet older adult specific screening and assessment tools can identify current status and potential health promotion and illness prevention needs in the older adult.

Screenings and assessments should be done on multiple occasions, including when there is a change in health status, on admission and discharge from the hospital, following a hospitalization, and when multiple resources are being utilized in an older adult in the community, nursing home, or any other setting. A wide array of specialized tools and evidence-based protocols are updated regularly and readily accessible for use. The John A. Hartford Foundation Institute for Geriatric Nursing (2013) has developed many assessment and screening tools as part of the "Try This" series, which provides Internet accessible evidence-based geriatric assessment tools that are useful for nurses and other clinicians for ensuring that appropriate care is provided to older adults. Table 12-6 identifies reliable time-efficient tools that are available for use in a variety of settings to evaluate various geriatric domains.

Modification of Assessment Technique and Environment

In addition to the appropriate use of specialized assessment and screening tools, health care providers must be aware of the potential presence of age-associated characteristics that may require some specific modification or accommodation in both the assessment technique and the assessment environment. Table 12-7 identifies some common expected age associated changes and suggestions for potential modification or accommodation of the health providers technique and the environment when assessing the older adult.

Additional Assessment Components

Beyond the physical assessment are numerous areas to explore with older adults, which when addressed, may uncover issues that may be overlooked when the focus is either on the disease or on emergent situations. These areas can often be complex and challenging issues for an older adult, but with assessment and interventions can provide a healthier and higher quality of life. Such components to address include medications, pain, substance abuse, elder mistreatment, spirituality, sleep, and sexuality. Tools for assessing these issues can be found in Table 12-6.

Medications

Older adults, aged 65 and over, are the largest users of prescribed and over-the-counter (OTC) medications in the United States. This is close to 13% of the U.S. population, and they consume approximately one-third of all prescribed and one-half of the OTC medications (Beyth & Short, 2007).

Not only are older adults taking multiple medicines, but frequently the prescriptions are being written by different health care providers, setting them up for drug–drug interactions and adverse drug events (ADE). Medication-related problems are common, costly, and lead to poor outcomes, especially in older adults. Studies have shown that many of the occurrences of adverse drug events are preventable. Addressing the issue of older adults not taking their medications as prescribed may include asking questions that deal with challenges in taking their medications related to enough money to buy medications, or their thinking they didn't need it, and so on.

The 2012 American Geriatric Society (AGS) Beers Criteria has created a list of potentially inappropriate medications for health care providers to be aware of and listing safe pharmacological alternatives. It is to be utilized as a guideline for identifying medications for which the risks of their use in older adults outweigh the benefits. The Beers Criteria are intended for use in all ambulatory and institutional settings of care for populations aged 65 and older in the United States (American Geriatrics Society, 2012).

At each clinic appointment and hospital admission, review prescribed and nonprescribed medications with patients who should be encouraged to bring them to the appointment in their original bottles. Also inquire about any alternative substances that they may be taking (e.g., herbals). An example of a question to ask is "What prescription medications, OTC, vitamins, herbs, or supplements are you taking?" Additionally, ask, "What challenges do you encounter in taking your medications (e.g. finances, making them sick, forgetting when they are to take them, etc.)?"

Pain

Although up to 80% of nursing home residents experience pain regularly, the under-treatment of pain is pervasive. Reasons for this include the belief that pain is an expected part of aging, misconceptions about addiction to pain medications, and a lack of routine treatment.

Persistent pain has been associated with functional impairment, falls, slow rehabilitation, depression, anxiety, decreased socialization, and sleep disturbance, as well as increased health care utilization and costs. In an effort to improve the detection and management of pain, the Joint Commission has mandated the pain screening note pain as "the fifth vital sign." A proactive, consistent approach must be taken to screen for pain and assess older adults for persistent pain (see Chapter 8).

Pain is a common symptom; one study demonstrated that 50% of adults 65 years of age and older answered yes when asked if they had experienced pain in the last 30 days (U.S. Dept. of Health and Human Services, 2009). Still, many individuals hold the myth that pain in older adults is part of the aging process, resulting in either older adults not seeking treatment or health care providers not assessing (McAuliffe, Nay, O'Donnell, & Fetherstonhaugh, 2009) or managing pain properly. Pain for older adults is frequently due to acute or chronic conditions and ranges from 50% to 86% across the all settings.

For optimum functioning and quality of life, it is essential that pain in older adults be managed. Consequences of poor pain assessment and management for older adults can lead to poor sleeping, fatigue, decreased mobility, depression, chronic pain, and a variety of stress-related physical outcomes (e.g., myocardial infarction, respiratory infection, etc.). More than one- half of all inpatient hospital days are occupied by older adults, and more than 9 million surgeries are performed on older adults annually (Rosenthal & Kravic, 2004). Thus, pain is a common experience among older adults in the acute care setting (Herr, 2010). Assessing pain in anyone, but especially older adults, needs to be an individualized approach. When it comes to an individual's pain, "it is what it is" means it is subjective and is what the individual states it is.

A particular challenge in pain assessment and management is in working with individuals who have cognitive impairments, which usually compromise the ability of self-reporting pain. Other

Table 12-7 Common expected age-associated changes

Expected Changes	Assessment and Environment Approach Modification and Adaptation
Hearing Sensorineural (cranial nerve VIII) loss of high-frequency hearing resulting in speech comprehension difficulty Presbyopia is virtually universal. Conductive hearing loss	Talking too loudly usually causes the pitch to rise, which can increase hearing difficulty. Speak in a normal tone at eye level and facing directly toward the older adult. Check carefully for build-up of ear wax or excessive hair, which may block hearing.
Vision Pupil size decreases and the pupillary light reflex may be slowed. The lens may look opaque.	Environment should be well lit during most of the assessment; however, a bright environment can mask glare and contrast sensitivity, so light should be dimmed for visual acuity testing.
Integument Loss of collagen and elasticity and thinning of dermal layer results in fragile skin at risk for injury.	Exam room should be warm and well lit with clear pathways clear so that sharp corners can be avoided. Use care when placing and removing blood pressure cuff and tape. Be sure and avoid causing friction when palpating.
Cardiovascular The left atrium dilates and valves and vascular system in general may stiffen resulting in quieter heart and blood pressure sounds, and increased difficulty palpating peripheral pulses. Orthostatic hypotension commonly occurs (sudden drop in blood pressure when rising to sit or stand).	When assessing heart sounds adjust apical auscultation positioning to the left of where you may hear it in a younger person. Reduce extraneous noise as possible; close door, windows, no overhead music, ask patient to refrain from talking while you are listening. Place stethoscope directly on skin. Use caution when palpating or auscultating the carotid artery to avoid reflexive slowing of heart. Assist patient stand up slowly from a sitting position, and to sit slowly from a lying position.
Pulmonary Changes in chest wall structure result in a more barrel-shaped appearance and can decrease lung expansion. Internally there is a decrease in alveolar number and surface area that can increase risk of hypoxia.	A chair with arms allows the older adult to sit up and lean forward or backward exposing areas of the chest with more stability. A table or desk in front of them offers additional support for their arms. Reduce extraneous noise when auscultating (see Cardiovascular). Have the older adult take only one deep breath at a time and allow time for a couple of normal breaths before the next deep breath request.
Neurologic Gradual loss of neurons result in a decline in short-term memory, ability for new learning, and coordination.	When obtaining a health history, allow time for processing and retrieval of information. Before assessment, if possible arrange for a brown-bag medication assessment (all medications in a brown-bag), and a diet and activity diary to be brought in with patient. Use appropriate patient teaching techniques, (demonstration, teach-back, avoidance of jargon, education to caregivers as needed). Have clear pathways, adequate space for movement, and standby-assistance when assessing balance and coordination.
Musculoskeletal Bone density and strength declines. There is a loss of cartilage and connective tissues in joints; usually more pronounced in weight-bearing joints. Muscles mass declines and ligaments and tendons stiffen.	Examiner movement of joint can cause pain. Allow for periods of rest between assessment activities that require movement to avoid muscle fatigue. Avoid low chairs or seating that would make rising to stand difficult. Have a footstool available for getting on and off of an exam table. When the person is lying down, support the head and neck with a pillow. A pillow under the knees may reduce strain on the lower back.
Genitourinary Female: Epithelium thins and natural vaginal lubrication decreases. The uterus decreases in size and ovaries are not palpable.	Lubricate instruments and gloves adequately for pelvic examination.

Sources: adapted from *Gerontological nursing* by P.A. Tabloski. (2010). Upper Saddle River, NJ: Pearson; and *Health promotion strategies through the life span* by R.B. Murray, J.P. Zentner, and R. Yakimo (2009). Upper Saddle River, NJ, Pearson.

assessment approaches are available under these circumstances, including knowing an underlying cause for pain (e.g., recent surgery, history of arthritis and other previous reports of pain—knee, hip, etc.), observing for pain behaviors (e.g., grimacing, holding or rubbing a body part, etc.), and getting input from the individuals' caregivers (Horgas, Elliott, & Mariske, 2009).

There are a variety of pain scales available for use in older adults, including the Numeric Rating Scale (NRS), Faces Pain Scale-Revised (FPS-R), and the Verbal Descriptor Scale (VAS).

Substance Use and Abuse

It is reported that there is a startling number of baby boomers who are abusing drugs and alcohol and continue this use into their later years, which necessitates this as an essential aspect of an older adult assessment. Alcohol is the most likely substance to be abused by older adults. There are a number of challenging issues related to identification of users in the older population due in part to many similarities of symptoms to those of physical and mental health conditions that frequently affect older adults (Reardon, 2012).

As individuals age they become more vulnerable to the effects of alcohol, which can be complicated by medication use that generally increases with age, and accumulation of comorbidities that affect health status and behavior. The screening of choice is the Short Michigan Alcoholism Screening Instrument–Geriatric Version (SMAST-G), which was developed as the first short-form alcoholism-screening instrument tailored to the needs of older adults.

Elder Mistreatment

According to the National Center on elder abuse, there are no official statistics for total numbers and types of older adult abuse, yet thousands of cases are reported. Elder mistreatment (EM) may include abuse, abandonment, neglect, or exploitation. The Elder Abuse Assessment Instrument (EAI) has been suggested to be the best screening tool. It is a 41-item assessment instrument, separated in seven sections. This assessment does not contain a scoring process, but if the following issues arise, notifying social services is imperative whenever 1) there is any evidence of mistreatment without sufficient clinical explanation, 2) there is a subjective complaint by the elder of EM, and 3) the clinician believes there is high risk or probable abuse, neglect, exploitation, or abandonment. Signs of elder mistreatment and abuse include contusions, burns, bite marks, genital or rectal trauma, pressure ulcers, or malnutrition with no clinical explanation.

Spirituality

Aspects of physical and cognitive dimensions of older adults diminish as one ages, in contrast to the spiritual domain of an individual, which tends to develop and grow even into the later years of life (Figure 12-4). It has also been noted that individuals with dementia have a sense of spirituality and often can recall rituals and details of one's faith or religion. Research demonstrates that religion and spirituality were found to be very important to 72% of those 65- to 74-year-olds and 77% of those 75 years and older (Gallop Poll, 2010). Older adults frequently seek ways to cope and live with end-of-life situations along with aging changes and chronic conditions. Each individual's spirituality will be unique to life's experiences and interpretation of spirituality for oneself. Spirituality is broad term encompassing belief in God, a higher being, or in nature, and has been found to support and enhance one's well-being and overall quality of life (Gaskamp, Sutter, & Meraviglia, 2008). The FICA screening tool is one example of a tool used to perform a spiritual assessment.

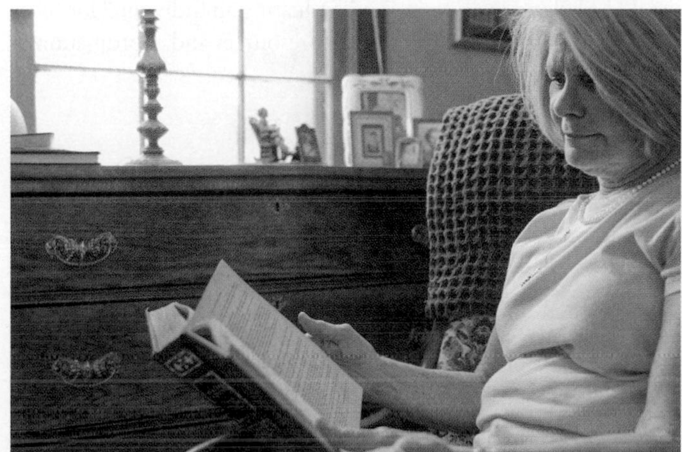

FIGURE 12-4 A person's spirituality may enhance their sense of one's well-being and overall quality of life
Source: CDC/Amanda Mills

Sleep

Although normal aging is accompanied by decreased "deep sleep," sleep efficiency, and increased time awake after sleep onset, these changes should not result in excessive daytime sleepiness. Daytime sleepiness is not only a symptom of sleep disorders but also results in decreased health and functional outcomes in the older adult. Numerous factors can affect nigh-time sleep resulting in excessive sleepiness during the day. This might include psychological disorders, chronic illness symptoms (e.g., pain), medication side effects, environmental factors, and lifestyle preferences. Additionally aging changes and sleep disorders can cause havoc on an older adult's sleep and be exhibited as obstructive sleep apnea, restless leg syndrome, and insomnia. Being hospitalized or admitted to a facility can also add complications in getting sufficient sleep at night for older adults (Boltz, Capezuti, Fulmer, Zwicker, & O'Meara, 2012). The Epworth Sleepiness Scale and the Pittsburgh Sleep Quality Index are examples of tools used to assess sleep quality.

Sexuality

Sexual desires have been generally noted to decrease with age, yet there is evidence (although limited for sexual patterns in later life) that sexual desires, thoughts, and actions continue throughout all decades of life. The ability to assess sexuality in older adults may be complicated by the idea that the topic is taboo and stereotyping and myths held by individuals younger than this population. The health professional should consider that the need for intimacy and sexuality is still prevalent in older adults (Boltz et al., 2012).

Overall Assessment Models

The SPICES and FANCAPES assessments are frequently utilized in hospitals to screen multiple areas related to function and other common conditions in older adults and individuals who are medically vulnerable.

Fulmer Assessment: SPICES

The SPICES assessment is often used for older adults in various settings; it focuses on six common "marker conditions" that include sleep disorders, problems with eating and feeding, incontinence, confusion, evidence of falls, and skin breakdown (Fulmer, 2007).

FANCAPES

Another tool utilized in the hospital is the FANCAPES, which is used for assessing multiple issues in older adults. The letters represent the following:

- F = fluids (hydration and factors contributing to maintaining adequate hydration)
- A = aeration (adequacy of oxygen exchange)
- N = nutrition (physiological, social, economic factors)
- C = communication (communicative ability)
- A = activity (related to ADLs and IADLs)
- P = pain (physical, mental and spiritual)
- E = elimination (bladder and bowel)
- S = socialization (interact, deal with loss)

This tool should be used when there appears to be an actual problem or when something is "wrong" but exact understanding is unclear (Montgomery, Mitty, & Flores, 2008).

Health Promotion and Disease Prevention

Experts posit that early prevention and targeted health promotion can help improve quality of life as people age; however, preventative services are generally underused by and for the older adult population. For health promotion and prevention planning to be successful, the older adult needs to be an integral participant in the process, with opportunity for individual input that is necessary for success implementation of a plan. The health professional must ensure that assessment of individual needs, wishes, and ability is conducted with the understanding that those components will provide a foundation for planning, which is centered on the individual characteristics of the older adult.

Healthy People 2020 identify 10-year national objectives designed to improve the health of all Americans (U.S. Department of Health and Human Services, 2009). Overarching goals include prevention of disease, disability, injury, and premature death for all populations, and promotion of quality of life, which connects foundationally to the specific objective aimed to improve the health, function, and quality of life of older adults. User-friendly and evidence-based resources geared toward both health care providers and individual older adults are accessible on the *Healthy People 2020* Web site.

Exercise

Physical activity is good for all populations and the benefits across all age boundaries with similar results (Figure 12-5). *Healthy People 2020* identifies the benefits specifically for older adults in the prevention of heart disease, stroke, type 2 diabetes, and some types of cancer. Additionally, exercise assists older adults in maintaining muscle and bone health, resulting in the strength, stamina, and balance that allow older adults to remain mobile and independent. Finally, activity and exercise can reduce symptoms of depression. Generally older adults should aim for 2 hours and 30 minutes of moderate aerobic exercise per week, strengthening activities 2 days per week, and balance activities at least 3 times per week (Office of Disease Prevention and Health Promotion, 2012).

Many resources provide recommendations for amount of time and types of exercise that provide the most benefit. Consultation with a physical therapist can be extremely valuable in assessment of an individual's ability and potential when recommending an activity and exercise plan. Healthfinder.gov is a government Web site that has readily accessible information and tools to assist the health professional and individual older adult to learn more about the benefits of and how to incorporate exercise as a part of healthy life.

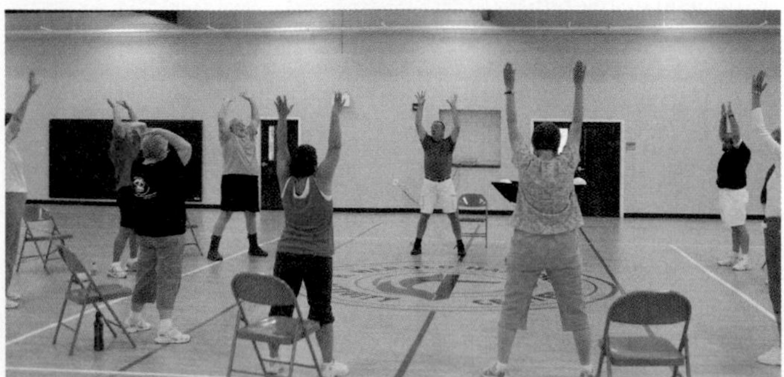

FIGURE 12-5 Regular exercise has important benefits to people of all ages
Source: CDC/Amanda Mills

Nutrition

Older adults often have unique nutritional considerations that result from changes associated with aging; however, just as in all age groups, a balanced diet that incorporates all food groups is recommended. The Academy of Nutrition and Dietetics recommends food intake for older adults that emphasizes fruit, vegetables, whole grains, low-fat items, and protein from lean meat, poultry, fish, beans, and nuts, and is low in saturated and trans fats, cholesterol, salt, and added sugar. This formula should sound familiar to individuals from all age groups who are incorporating a healthy diet; however older adults do have some special nutritional needs that should be considered when promoting healthy eating habits for older adults.

According to the Academy of Nutrition and Dietetics the older adult needs more calcium and vitamin D to promote bone health to maintain functional ability and prevent injury. Foods high in fiber should be encouraged to promote gastrointestinal health and to lower risk of heart disease and type 2 diabetes, and as an aid for weight control. Increasing intake of potassium and lowering intake of sodium can promote better blood pressure, and reduce the risk for high blood pressure and associated complications. Foods that are low in saturated fats, trans fats, and cholesterol can promote healthy cardiovascular function and lower an older adults risk for heart disease (Academy of Nutrition and Dietetics, 2012). Recent evidence indicates that older adults do not get enough vitamin B_{12}, which can result in anemia with associated symptoms of fatigue, weakness, gastrointestinal problems, weight loss, and neurological changes that can affect balance and cognition (National Institutes of Health, 2011). A registered dietitian can conduct a nutritional health screening and assist the older adult in developing a sound nutritional plan for maintaining current health status and avoiding future nutritional risk.

Some risk for poor nutritional status among vulnerable groups of older adults occurs as a result of insufficient financial resources, physical or mental disability, limited mobility, functional dependence, family structure and dynamics, cultural consideration, and lack of knowledge of available resources. An individual may experience any one of these factors singly, or a combination of these and other similar factors. Consultation with a geriatric social worker would be helpful in assessing and evaluating an individual for these risk, and identification of appropriate resources and coordination of access to them.

Immunization

As with all populations, the CDC recommends immunization and re-vaccination as an important strategy for health promotion and illness prevention. All older adults benefit from up-to-date immunization status, but it is particularly important for those older adults who may have increased vulnerability for complications from infections disease due to presence of chronic conditions that already compromise physical health. Some older adults may be at risk because for a variety of reasons they are uncertain about or have limited information about their immunization history. A complete scheduled of recommended immunization and re-vaccination can be accessed on the CDC Web site (Centers for Disease Control and Prevention, 2012a). Prevalence, severity of disease, and increased risk of complications from three particular infectious diseases warrant additional attention.

Influenza

The risk of complications from influenza is much greater for those over age 65 than for those who are younger. Statistics indicate that older adults comprise approximately 90% of seasonal flu deaths each year in the United States (Centers for Disease Control and Prevention, 2012b). It is highly recommended that older adults receive a flu vaccine every year.

Pneumococcal Pneumonia

Older adults are more likely to become ill with pneumonia than younger adults. The potential presence of underlying conditions such as diabetes or any other condition that compromises overall health increase the risk of older adults both in contracting pneumonia and experiencing complications associated with the disease. Pneumonia is most likely to be caused by the pneumococcal bacteria and therefore it is recommended that adults over 65 receive a Pneumovax vaccination, which is effective prevention against most pneumococcal serotypes. (CDC, 2012).

Varicella Zoster (Shingles)

Shingles is a painful skin rash caused by the varicella zoster virus, which is the same virus that causes chicken pox. The varicella zoster virus remains in the nerve cells of the body after having chicken pox, and can reappear years later as shingles. It most commonly happens in older adults, and particularly those who have underlying conditions that compromise their immune system. The pain from shingles can be debilitating, potentially lasting for months or even years, and can scar. It is recommended that adults over age 65 receive the varicella zoster vaccination; definitive history of chicken pox and/or serology testing is not necessary prior to vaccination (CDC, 2012).

Education and Individual Health Behavior Change

Many people believe the old adage "You can't teach an old dog new tricks." While that may be true for dogs (and perhaps even that is not), it certainly is not true for older adults. Many studies have documented that not only do older adults learn but that they also benefit from teaching, as do younger adults (Bastable, 2008). However, just as younger adults have different preferences for learning, so do older adults. For individual teaching to be effective, learning style preference needs to be assessed and acknowledged. Additionally, age-associated changes such as sensory impairments, cognitive process slowing, and any other functional considerations need to be accounted for when planning to teach older adults about their health.

Individual health behavior change for all adults is most likely to be successful when the individual is willing to assume responsibility for the change. This is also true for older adults. In teaching health promotion and illness prevention to older adults it is important to dispel a common myth that age itself means there is limited potential for future improvement (Tabloski, 2010). Because health care providers often interact with an older adult because an event or illness has required intervention, it may be the best time to educate the individual about the potential benefits of health promotion activities and behavior.

Summary

- There is an impending need to appropriately educate adequate numbers of health care professionals to provide effective care to the increasing older adult population.
- The increasing number of older adults seeking health care will increase the need for health care resources.
- Specialized skills and knowledge in the care of older adults will enhance relevance, cost-effectiveness, and quality of health care services.
- Health promotion aging is a strategy for positively addressing real-world daily experiences of older adults.
- Evidence-based assessment tools are readily available and provide a reliable resource for assessment and screening.
- Understanding and accommodating age-associated changes result in relevant assessment findings from which appropriate and efficient care can be planned and implemented.

Review Questions

1. While examining an older adult, the provider notes that the response of the patellar and Achilles reflex responses are present but are slow and muscle strength is somewhat diminished. What should the provider do based on the results of this examination?
   1. Notify the physician about the results.
   2. Document the findings in the record.
   3. Request a physical therapy consult.
   4. Ask the patient about use of drugs.
2. The daughter of an older adult female asks the provider to insert an indwelling urinary catheter in her mother before discharge to deal with her "leaking." What action is appropriate for the provider to take in this situation? (Select all that apply.)
   1. Insert the catheter as requested.
   2. Collect a urine sample from the patient.
   3. Teach the daughter catheter care.
   4. Ask the patient for a history of the problem.
   5. Order necessary supplies for home use.

3. The provider is teaching a group of older adults about the importance of physical activity in maintaining good health. When asked to suggest activities that are recommended for older adults, which would the provider suggest? (Select all that apply.)
   1. Take a brisk walking for 30 minutes, 5 days per week.
   2. Do 60 minutes of weight lifting, 5 days per week.
   3. Enroll in a yoga class 3 days per week.
   4. Run or jog for 30 minutes per week.
   5. Engage in physical activity for a maximum of 90 minutes per week.
4. The provider is completing an assessment of an older adult and asks the patient about his religious affiliation and if he is a member of a church. By asking this question the provider is doing which of the following?
   1. addressing the cognitive domain of assessment
   2. gathering information about emergency notification
   3. obtaining information required by the agency
   4. allowing the patient to provide information on spirituality and beliefs
5. The provider is using the SPICES assessment tool with an older adult. Use of this tool may assist the provider in identifying which of the following?
   1. substance abuse
   2. physical abuse
   3. respiratory problems
   4. incontinence
6. The provider is counseling a patient about the importance of receiving immunizations to prevent illness. Which information that the provider offers to the patient is consistent with current evidence-based practice?
   1. Healthy older adults should only get the vaccine for influenza.
   2. Risk for pneumonia in older adults is increased by the presence of chronic conditions.
   3. The vaccine for shingles is not needed if the patient had chicken pox as a child.
   4. Older adults are not at high risk for contracting the flu, so only those who smoke should receive the vaccine.
7. A new older adult patient tells the provider that he has some difficulty hearing the history questions that the provider is asking. What should the provider include in the assessment of this patient?
   1. an assessment of cranial nerve I
   2. an otoscopic examination
   3. a sound amplifier
   4. the services of an interpreter
8. When assessing the hear sounds of an older adult, the provider should listen for the apical pulse by placing the stethoscope in which location?
   1. 2 ICS left sternal boarder
   2. 3 ICS left sternal boarder
   3. 5 ICS left mid-clavicular line
   4. 5 ICS left anterior axillary line
9. The provider is performing an initial postoperative assessment on an older adult patent with a history of dementia. When assessing the patient for pain the provider should do which of the following?
   1. Request an order for patient controlled analgesia.
   2. Ask the patient's family what the patient usually takes for pain.
   3. Medicate the patient for pain on a routine basis.
   4. Observe the patient for signs of pain and discomfort.
10. The provider is working with an older adult and wishes to ensure that the patient fully understands information about diagnosis and treatment options. What should the provider do for this patient?
   1. Explain the information to the patient's daughter in a phone call.
   2. Tell the patient that there are Web sites with all of the necessary information.
   3. Send the patient some educational material through the mail.
   4. Explain all information in plain language and encourage questions.

Nutrition Assessment

13

Rachael J. Pohle-Krauza, PhD, RDN, LD

Tina's shirt seems exceptionally loose on her slender frame. She says that she's having an amazing time at college—serving on the student council, training with a modern dance team, and getting good grades. I smile back at her, happy she's doing well. However, I cannot stop thinking about how thin she looks. When I saw her 2 years earlier for a routine physical—as far as I remembered—she had looked perfectly healthy.

"It sounds like you have been pretty busy with all those activities, Tina! Have you been finding time for your meals?"

"Well, I usually skip breakfast because I have class at 8 a.m., but I always have celery and carrots to snack on."

I flip through my clinic notes and check her vitals. Her heart rate is 39, her blood pressure 88/47, and her BMI is 16.7.

"Tina, are you at all concerned about your weight?"

"People keep asking me that... ugh—yes! I'd like to lose a few more pounds if possible. I work out three times per day and watch what I eat, so I'm not sure why it's been so hard!"

"Do you mind if I do a quick physical exam?" I take a closer look; her hair appears brittle, the skin on her arms is dry and peeling, and her hands are cold as ice. "Tina, have you lost more than 15 pounds in the past few months?"

"I'd say I lost 20 or so in the past 4 or 5 months. I'm pretty proud!" She looks up at me and smiles, exposing enamel-worn and eroded teeth.

I reach for my stool and sit right in front of Tina. "I'm concerned you may have an eating disorder." Tina purses her lips and shakes her head as her eyes well up with tears. "It's not possible!"

"I want to discuss this with you more," I say calmly. "However, I'm concerned about the instability of your vital signs and would like to admit you to the hospital for treatment."

"It's not possible!" she repeats, slowly hanging her head. My heart feels heavy—this is anorexia nervosa at its worst, and I know that Tina will have a long, harrowing road to recovery.

LEARNING OUTCOMES

1. Explain the ways in which the nutritional status of the population is assessed, including the role of national dietary surveys.
2. Recognize the essential components of a nutrition-focused patient history and a nutrition-oriented physical assessment.
3. Summarize various ways and tools to assess and record current nutrient intake.
4. Explain the use of nutrition-related anthropometry, including stature and waist circumference.
5. Compares various nutrition-related biochemical parameters.
6. Recognizes appropriate assessment parameters to obtain information regarding the general nutrient needs of individual patients.

In recent years, it has become increasingly important to identify diet-related diseases through use of nutritional assessment. Dietary status can exert a great influence on health and can affect growth and development, immune function, and risks of developing diabetes and cancer, and respiratory and heart diseases. It can also affect recovery time when an individual has undergone illness or surgery (USDHHS, 1998; Jensen, 2000; Guzman, 2010; Ludwig, 2011). With our increased ability to alter nutritional conditions, early evaluation of a patient's nutritional status is vital in order to affect health outcomes positively.

Nutritional Assessment of Populations

Assessing the nutritional status of populations is critical to the establishment of baseline information, plan interventions, and progress tracking. In the U.S. population, this process is most typically conducted through the use of national diet and nutrition surveys. Information gathered from these surveys helps to evaluate the quality, quantity, and safety of the food supply, as well as the manner in which food is distributed according to population demographics (such as region, socioeconomic status, and race). Furthermore, national dietary surveys are used to identify nutritional and health problems of the population so that the relationship between diet and disease can be determined. Ultimately, the information these surveys provide is used to establish dietary guidelines, identify priorities for nutrition research, and justify government initiatives such as *Healthy People*, food fortification and labeling standards, and food programs such as Food Stamps or the Child and Adult Care Food Program, as well as the cost-effectiveness of these programs.

National Dietary Surveys

Two major federal entities are responsible for conducting national diet and nutrition surveys. These include the U.S. Department of Health and Human Services (HHS) and the U.S. Department of Agriculture (USDA).

Annually, the National Center for Health Statistics, a subcategory of the Centers for Disease Control and Prevention, conducts the National Health and Nutrition Examination Survey (NHANES). This information provides a cross-section representation of the health and nutrition of the U.S. population that is obtained from a broad range of age groups and racial/ethnic backgrounds. This survey, combines participant interviews (demographic, socioeconomic, dietary, and health-related questions) with a physical examination component (laboratory tests, medical, dental, and physiological measurements). Findings from NHANES are used to determine risk factors for major diseases and disease prevalence (Figure 13-1). In addition, NHANES outcomes provide a basis for national standards for measurement of height, weight, and blood pressure.

The USDA also conducts food intake surveys of individuals within the population. For example, the Continuing Survey of Food Intakes by Individuals (CSFII) was conducted to measure what Americans eat and drink through dietary recalls and food diary records. The USDA subsequently obtained information from the Diet and Health Knowledge Survey (DHKS) as a follow-up to CSFII to further understand factors affecting food choices and obtain information on individuals' knowledge and attitudes about national dietary guidelines. Together, the CSFII and the DHKS, last done in 1994–1998, provided the first national scale survey to link individuals' knowledge and attitudes (DHKS) to individual dietary behaviors (CSFII).

More recently in 2002, in an effort to avoid duplication of service and streamline the assessment process, the DHHS undertook a cooperative effort with the USDA to integrate dietary surveys. Specifically, anthropometric assessment and health history information from NHANES were combined with the data from CSFII, resulting in the *What We Eat in America, NHANES* (WWEIA, NHANES) survey. Data from this effort (available on the USDA Agricultural Research Web site) are released every 2 years, with the first release in 2001–2002 and the most recent in 2009–2010.

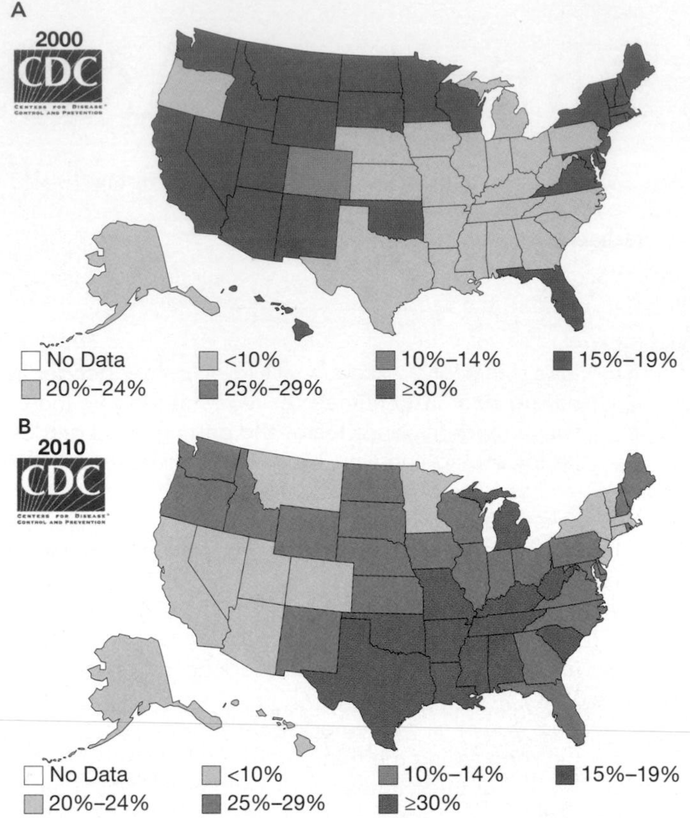

FIGURE 13-1A-B Data from NHANES are used to calculate national health statistics. This example depicts how NHANES data were used to map the change in prevalence of obesity by state between 2000 and 2010.

Healthy People 2020

The *Healthy People* initiative, conducted through the HHS, serves as the foundation for efforts to create a healthier Nation. *Healthy People 2020* is the result of a multiyear process derived from the input of a number of public health entities. The 2020 initiatives have a renewed focus on identifying, measuring, tracking, and reducing health disparities.

One of the major objectives of *Health People 2020* pertains to Nutrition and Weight Status, with the emphasis on promotion of health and chronic disease risk-reduction through the consumption of a healthy diet, and achievement/maintenance of a healthy body weight (U.S. Department of Health and Human Services, 2009;). With strong empirical basis, the Nutrition and Weight Status objectives for *Healthy People 2020* suggest that strategies to change dietary intake and body weight status should address individual behaviors, in addition to policies and environments that support these behaviors in a variety of settings (schools, worksites, health care organizations, and communities). This objective also retains a goal of promoting healthful diets and healthy weight, which encompasses increasing household food security and eliminating hunger. In addition, the objective suggests that Americans with a healthful diet should do the following:

- Consume a variety of nutrient-dense foods within and across the food groups, especially whole grains, fruits, vegetables, low-fat or fat-free milk or milk products, and lean meats and other protein sources.
- Limit the intake of saturated and *trans* fats, cholesterol, added sugars, sodium (salt), and alcohol.

- Limit caloric intake to meet caloric needs.
- Avoid unhealthy weight gain, and those whose weight is too high may also need to lose weight.

Standards for Nutritional Intake

With the increase in nutrition-related chronic disease within the last century, it became apparent that the general U.S. population required a comprehensive set of dietary recommendations. The current nutritional standards, also known as the Dietary Reference Intakes, were developed as a joint effort of the U.S. Food and Nutrition Board and the Canadian Institute of Nutrition and Health. *The Dietary Guidelines for Americans* (http://health.gov/dietaryguidelines) form the basis for the consumer-friendly *MyPlate* food guidance system (Figure 13-2), which was developed to help individuals make more informed, and healthier, food choices.

Dietary Reference Intakes

The **Dietary Reference Intakes (DRIs)**, defined as "reference values that are quantitative estimates of nutrient intakes to be used for planning and assessing diets for apparently healthy people" (Standing Committee on the Scientific Evaluation of Dietary Reference Intakes, 2000) consist of four reference intakes, and also include a recommendation for dietary energy intake (Table 13-1). These references provide recommendations for daily intake of macronutrients (carbohydrate, protein, and fat), micronutrients (vitamins and minerals), total energy (kilocalories), water, fiber, and also provide a standard for physical activity are further discussed in Table 13-17.

A full listing of dietary reference intakes can be found by visiting the Web site for the USDA's National Agricultural Library Food and Nutrition Center.

Table 13-1 The dietary reference intakes

Reference Value	Description
Estimated Average Requirement (EAR)	The average daily nutrient intake level estimated to meet the requirement of half the healthy individuals in a particular life stage and gender group.
Recommended Dietary Allowances (RDA)	The average daily dietary nutrient intake level sufficient to meet the nutrient requirement of nearly all (97%–98%) healthy individuals in a particular life stage and gender group.
Adequate Intake (AI)	The recommended average daily intake level based on observed or experimentally determined approximations or estimates of nutrient intake by a group (or groups) of apparently healthy people that are assumed to be adequate. The AI is used when an RDA cannot be determined.
Tolerable Upper Level Intake (UL)	The highest average daily nutrient intake level that is likely to pose no risk of adverse health effects to almost all individuals in the general population. As intake increases above the UL, the potential risk of adverse effects may increase.

Source: "Definition of Dietary Reference Intakes" from *Standing Committee on the Scientific Evaluation of Dietary Reference Intakes.* Published by National Academy Press, © 2000.

Nutrition Screening and Assessment

U.S. regulatory agencies may require that patients admitted for treatment be screened during their admission for nutritional risks. For example, the Joint Commission standards for nutritional screening state that these are performed when warranted by the patient's needs or condition. The health care organization is responsible for developing criteria that would identify if and when these screenings or more in-depth assessments are needed. When appropriate to the patient's condition, the screenings should be completed within 24 hours after inpatient admission.

The Joint Commission further delineates that nutritional screening is not required for all patients if it has not "been defined by the health care organization's policy, a licensed independent provider with appropriate clinical privileges has determined that it is not necessary in emergency situations, or it is not warranted by the patient's needs or condition" (The Joint Commission, 2011). Thus, the health provider must have a thorough understanding of the health care organization's policies and procedures in this regard.

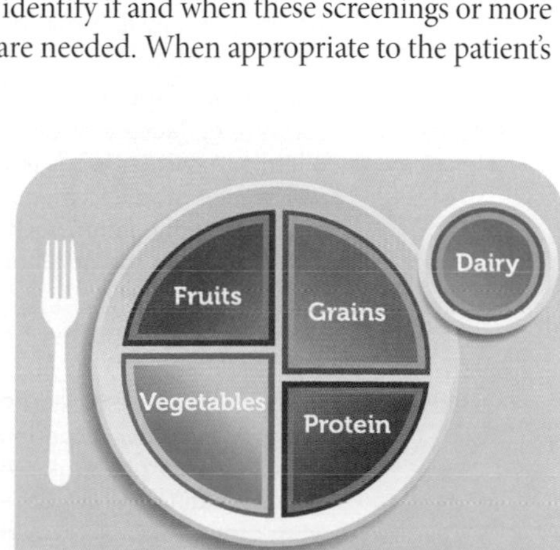

Balancing Calories
- Enjoy your food, but eat less.
- Avoid oversized portions.

Foods to Increase
- Make half your plate fruits and vegetables.
- Make at least half your grains whole grains.
- Switch to fat-free or low-fat (1%) milk.

Foods to Reduce
- Compare sodium in foods like soup, bread, and frozen meals—and choose the foods with lower numbers.
- Drink water instead of sugary drinks.

FIGURE 13-2 MyPlate Food Guidance System
Source: U.S. Department of Agriculture

Assessment of Diet Quality in Individuals

Considering the dietary quality (the degree to which intake matches physiologic need) of specific patients is important, as it greatly influences individual health outcomes. Because nutrient imbalances may exist *before* the patient is admitted to a health care facility (Coates, 1993; Joosten & Hultz, 2008), physiologic and environmental factors affecting *both* usual intake (typical day-to-day intake or intake prior to admission), as well as current intake (i.e., while admitted or during the current treatment period) are equally important to assess.

> **PRACTICE POINT: Obtaining Nutrition-Related Subjective Data**
>
> Subjective data may be obtained through completion of a food diary, which is a comprehensive listing of all foods and beverages consumed each day, over a series of days or weeks (Figure 13-3) or a 24-hour recall, a complete listing of all food and drink consumed in the last 24 hours. In addition, further questions may be asked of the patient (Box 13-1).

Box 13-1 Diet Interview Questions

- How have your eating habits been lately (e.g., prior to admission at home, and also in the hospital)?
- How is your bowel function? When was last bowel movement you had?
- Do you have any problems chewing, swallowing, with mouth pain, nausea, vomiting, diarrhea or constipation?
- Have you sustained any recent weight gains or losses and if so, within what time period?
- What is your ideal (dream) weight? What do you think a practical weight would be for you?
- Do you use and supplements such as multivitamins or herbals?
- Do you have any food allergies?
- What type of diet (if any) do you follow at home? Do you have any type of dietary/food restrictions?
- What is your living situation (e.g., with family, alone), and who prepares meals and does grocery shopping?
- Are you currently employed in or outside of your home?
- What kinds of physical activities do you do on a daily basis?
- Do you have access to a refrigerator, stove, and/or microwave?

Daily Food and Activity Diary

	Monday	Tuesday	Wednesday	Thursday	Friday	Saturday	Sunday
Breakfast							
Lunch							
Dinner							
Total Calories							
Physical Activity							

FIGURE 13-3 Food and activity diary

Patient History

Obtaining appropriate subjective and objective data is an integral component in determining the nutritional status of the patient.

Present and Past Medical History

The patient's present medical history (chief complaint, or reason for seeking medical care) and past medical history should be carefully reviewed, as many factors may affect past and present nutrient intake and energy balance. Table 13-2 lists a number of elements to be included in a nutrition-oriented medical history, as well issues to consider for each.

Table 13-2 Nutritional considerations from the patient history

Patient History	Considerations
Recent weight history	• Unintentional loss (i.e., ≥ 10% of usual weight) within past 6 months may be associated with higher mortality risk and more rapid progression of underlying chronic disease, particularly in elderly patients (Fisher, 1990). Identifying the reasons for unintended weight loss through further inquiry is essential. • Unplanned, rapid weight gain may indicate imbalance of hormones (e.g., thyroid) or issues with fluid retention (edema, such as that seen in congestive heart failure).
Presence/status of chronic disease	• Chronic lung disease and cancer often coexist with malnutrition (Wagner, 2008; Argiles, 2005). • Diabetes or cardiovascular disease often indicate immediate appropriateness for a modified, therapeutic diet.
Psychiatric disorders	• Depression and/or eating disorders (such as anorexia nervosa or binge eating disorder) may cause undesirable weight loss or weight gain.
Previous surgery	• Gastrointestinal surgeries (gastrectomy, bariatric, or intestinal surgeries) may cause early satiety and nutrient malabsorption. • Amputations or surgeries may affect mobility of the upper limbs and impede feeding ability. In this case, the nurse may ask the physician to make a referral to occupational or physical therapy for implementation of assistive feeding devices, or may arrange for the provision of feeding assistance.
Food Allergies/Intolerances	• Patients who are unable to tolerate certain foods (e.g., lactose or gluten intolerant) or are allergic to certain foods (e.g., peanuts, shellfish) will require modified menu items. Providers should identify patients with food allergies or intolerances to the nutrition/dietary department at first opportunity.
Chewing/Swallowing Difficulties	• Edentulous patients may be at risk for decreased nutrient intake and may benefit from soft foods or meals that are soft or ground consistency. • Patients who have experienced neurocognitive deficits (e.g., from stroke, Alzheimer's disease) may have difficulty swallowing, putting them at risk for aspiration. Providers may conduct a bedside swallowing evaluation and/or ask the physician to refer the patient to speech/language pathologist for further evaluation and treatment, as needed.

(*Sources:* Data from Ramsey, 2003; Sitoh, 2000)

Social History

The patient's social history may also have an impact on one's current nutritional status and subsequent health outcomes. A nutrition-oriented social history generally includes questions pertaining to housing situation; socioeconomic and employment status; social support; ability to obtain and prepare foods; religious practices; and the use of tobacco, recreational drugs, and alcohol.

> ***PRACTICE POINT: Alcohol Intake and Nutritional Status***
>
> Alcohol inhibits the breakdown of nutrients and also impairs nutrient absorption by damaging cells in the stomach and gastrointestinal tract, thereby impeding transport of some nutrients into the blood. In addition, deficiencies of some nutrients themselves may perpetuate impaired absorption. For example, inadequacy of the vitamin folic acid causes changes in the cells that line the lumen of the small intestine. These changes cause malabsorption of water and other nutrients involved in fluid and electrolyte balance such as glucose and sodium (Feinman, 1992). Recent research has shown that a large percentage (> 50%) of alcoholics are malnourished (Teixwira et al., 2011) and are often deficient in vitamins A, C, D, E, K, and the B vitamins (Tortora & Derrickson, 2011), and minerals such as calcium, magnesium, iron, and zinc (Marsano, 1989).

Food Availability Food availability data are estimates of the quantity and quality of food supplies moving from production through marketing and consumption on a per capita basis. **Food security** refers to the ability of a person to have access to adequate food for an active, healthy lifestyle at all times. It includes at a minimum 1) foods that are readily available, safe, and nutritionally adequate, and 2) an ability to acquire acceptable foods in ways that are socially acceptable (i.e. without having to commit theft or scavenge and without having to resort to emergency food supplies). Conversely, **food insecurity** refers to limited or uncertain access to safe food, or an inability to acquire food in a socially acceptable way (Committee on National Statistics, 2006). According to the USDA, in 2008, 49.1 million people were living in food insecure households, and of these, 16.7 million were children.

The term "food desert" is used to define low-income communities without ready access to healthy and affordable food (Ver Ploeg et al., 2008). Food deserts are associated with a variety of diet-related health problems, and are most prevalent in low-socioeconomic minority communities in both urban and rural settings (Story et al., 2009). Population-based assessments of dietary intake show that lower income is associated with a poorer diet quality, and that individuals/families with lower income consume fewer fruits and vegetables, a greater proportion of energy from fat, and less fiber compared to higher income individuals (Drewnowski & Spector, 2004; French et al., 2010).

Religious and Cultural Considerations It is also important to consider cultural or religious beliefs and dietary restrictions that may affect food intake and nutritional status of the patient. For instance, persons who are strict vegetarians may require additional protein and/or micronutrients through alternate food sources or commercial supplements. Likewise, those patients who practice Judaism or Islam may have specific dietary restrictions and request alternatives to certain food items (such as pork or shellfish, for example). Table 13-3 summarizes major dietary restrictions for several prominent religious groups. Religious dietary guidelines vary widely even within groups, depending on how closely an individual adheres. Thus, it is always best for the health provider to ask patients what their individual preferences are when conducting a diet interview.

Table 13-3 Religious dietary restrictions

Religious Affiliation	Dietary Restrictions
Hinduism	Most Hindus do not eat beef as cattle are highly respected, and many do not consume any meat or alcohol. Milk and milk products are consumed, but said to be very sacred.
Buddism	The majority of Buddhists are strict vegetarians (vegans), as they believe in abstinence of killing living creatures. They do not drink alcohol, and may also refrain from consumption of onions, garlic, scallions, chives, and leeks, as these are thought to contribute to inappropriate sexual desire or anger.
Judaism	Judaism retains a complex set of dietary laws, known as *kashrut*. In order for a food to be approved for consumption (kosher), an animal must both chew the cud (a digestive process unique to cattle, goats, and sheep) and have a cloven hoof. Birds must have wings, and aquatic organisms must possess both fins and scales. Shellfish, reptiles, and worms found in fruits or vegetables are prohibited. Three hours must be allowed between eating meat and dairy, and utensils and cookware used for dairy and meat-containing foods must be kept separate. Alcohol is permissible; however, wine and grape juice made by non-Jewish persons may not be consumed.
Catholicism	Catholic individuals do not consume meat on Ash Wednesday, Good Friday, and all Fridays in Lent. During these times, fish and animal products such as fat, eggs, dairy, and broth are permissible.
Islam	Muslims do not consume alcohol, pork or pork products, birds of prey, carnivorous animals, or meat and gelatin from non-Halal animals. In order for a slaughter to be considered Halal, the slaughterer must be Muslim, Allah's name must be invoked at the time of slaughter, and the throat, windpipe, and jugular veins must all be cut with a sharp blade.
Mormonism	Mormon persons are discouraged from consuming coffee, tea, alcohol, and large amounts of meat, as caffeine and alcohol are thought to be addictive.

Approximately 2.5% of adults in the United States and 4% of adults in Canada follow vegetarian diets (Mangels, 2003), and there are several common categories of vegetarianism. **Semi-vegetarians** (also called *flexitarians*) eat a mostly vegetarian diet, but may consume meat occasionally. **Lacto-ovo vegetarians** do not eat beef, pork, poultry, fish, shellfish, but do eat eggs and dairy products, while **pescatarians** abstain from eating all meat and animal flesh with the exception of fish. The most restrictive category of vegetarianism, **vegan**, describes individuals who do not eat meat of any kind, dairy, eggs, or foods containing these or other ingredients derived from animal sources. Some vegans also refrain from consuming food items that are derived using animal products in processing, even if the food item itself does not contain the animal product.

Assessment of Current Intake

Knowledge of what the patient is eating while under admission to a facility provides important information about that person's appetite and desire to eat. Patients who exhibit decreased intake of nutrients may have suboptimal health outcomes, and thus require early identification and intervention.

THINK LINK: Tube Feeding in a Patient Undergoing Therapy

The following depicts a case study of a patient who is receiving enteral nutrition, and shows the method for calculating provisions from a tube feeding.

Mr. Smith, a patient at a rehabilitation facility, is receiving a tube feeding via a gastrostomy tube. Based on his estimated nutrient needs, the physician has ordered Jevity 1.5 at 55 mL per hour, continuous. This product contains 1.5 calories per mL. To calculate the total energy that is being provided, first determine to total daily volume (55 mL × 24 hours = 1320 mL), then determine the calories (1320 mL × 1.5 calories/mL = 1980 calories).

Mr. Smith recently started undergoing physical and occupational therapy, each for 1 hour daily. These therapies require that Mr. Smith be temporarily disconnected from his feeding pump. Consider how this might affect his nutrient provisions (2 hours × 55 mL/hour = 110 mL, and 110 mL × 1.5 calories/mL = 165 calories). While 165 calories may not seem like a significant amount, it would result in a weekly deficit of over 1000 calories, meaning that the patient would lose approximately 1/3 of a pound weekly (1 pound is equal to 3500 calories), which over time could result in significant unplanned weight loss.

Nursing staff informed the facility's registered dietitian (RD) of the changes in Mr. Smith's therapy schedule. The RD then reassessed the patient's needs, and made an updated recommendation for a cyclic feeding regimen that would account for the time that the tube feeding would be disconnected (i.e., an increase in the rate for a shorter number of hours), which was subsequently confirmed in a physician's order. Nursing staff then documented the change on the patient's daily flow sheet, and made routine checks of the feeding pump to ensure that the delivery rate and duration were consistent with the updated regimen as ordered.

Anthropometric Assessment

Anthropometry in Greek literally means *the measurement of humans*, and refers to measurement of body weight, size, and proportion. These measurements are all obtained when performing a physical exam, which can also be valuable for evaluation of a patient's nutritional status, and also valuable in measuring the effects of nutritional interventions for trauma, surgery, disease, and malnutrition (Sanchez-Garcia et al., 2007).

Height, Weight, and Body Mass Index

Measurements of height and weight are an integral part of the nutrition assessment and used to calculate body mass index (BMI), an indicator of obesity and underweight. Use of consistent methods to procure these measurements is essential to minimize erroneous variations. Additionally, consistency among staff members responsible for obtaining measurements for specific patients is recommended.

Height

Stature or standing height is an assessment of maximum vertical size. In patients who are able to stand, height should be measured with a fixed stadiometer containing a backboard and a moveable headboard (Figure 13-4). Patients should remove footwear; any hair ornaments, buns, and braids should be removed from the top of the head prior to measurement.

Patients should stand on the platform with the heels of both feet together and the toes pointed slightly outward. Arms should be at sides, legs straight, and shoulders relaxed. Weight is evenly distributed when feet are flat on the floor, and the buttocks, shoulder blades, and back of the head are in contact with the vertical backboard. Direct the patient to look straight ahead, with the head in the Frankfort horizontal plane (when the horizontal line from lower border of the orbit of the eye to the ear canal is parallel to the floor and perpendicular to the vertical backboard). Once correctly positioned, lower the headboard and ask the patient to inhale deeply (allowing the spine to straighten) and stand as tall as possible. Finally, position the headboard firmly on top of the head and record the yielded height.

In nonambulatory patients or those who are unable to stand, stature can be estimated from knee height (see Practice Point). Table 13-4 lists equations that can be used to calculate height using knee height in adults.

PRACTICE POINT: Estimating Stature from Knee Height

Knee height has been shown to be correlated with stature, and as such, can be used to estimate stature (Chumlea, 1994). Knee height should be measured when the patient is lying down on their back, and should be assessed on the left leg (as this is the leg that was used to develop the stature equations in Table 13-6 using a large sliding caliper). The knee should be gently bent so that it is placed at a 90-degree angle. The fixed blade of the caliper should be placed under the heel of the left foot, and the moveable blade placed on the front surface of the left thigh. The shaft of the caliber should be parallel to the fibula outside the lateral malleolus (prominent bone, outside left ankle). The measurement should then be recorded. This process should be repeated twice in order to ensure accuracy of measurement.

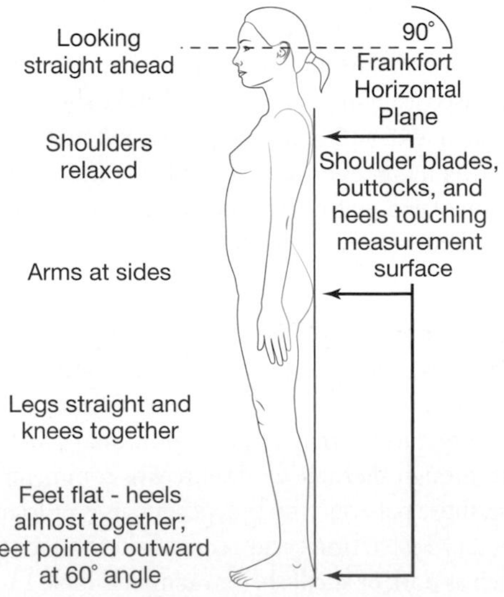

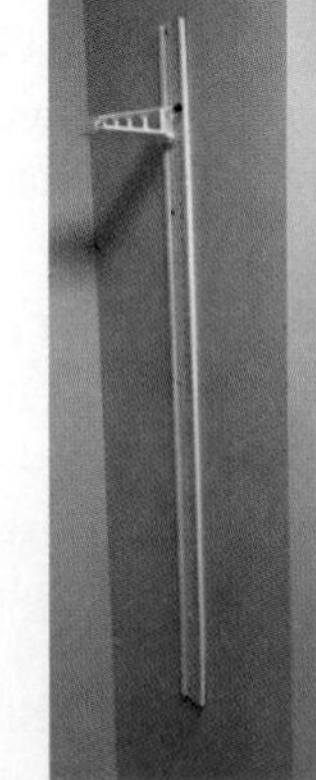

FIGURE 13-4 Stadiometer to measure height

Table 13-4 Stature can be determined in different ways using different bones

White Males	Stature = 71.85 + (1.88 **knee height**)
	64.19 – (0.04 x age) + (2.02 x **knee height**)
	2.32 x **femur** + 65.32 ± 3.94 cm
	2.89 x **humerus** + 78.10 ± 4.57
Black Males	Stature = 73.42 + (1.79 **knee height**)
	79.69 + (1.85 x **knee height**) – (0.14 x age)
	2.10 x **femur** + 72.22 ± 3.91 cm
	2.88 x **humerus** + 74.48 ± 4.23
White Women	Stature = 70.25 + (1.87 **knee height**) (0.06 age)
	84.88 – (0.24 x age) + (1.83 x **knee height**)
	2.47 x **femur** + 54.10 ± 3.72 cm
	3.36 x **humerus** + 57.97 ± 4.45
Black Women	Stature = 68.10 + (1.86 **knee height**) (0.06 age)
	89.58 + (1.61 x **knee height**) – (0.17 x age)
	2.28 x **femur** + 59.76 ± 3.41 cm
	3.08 x **humerus** + 64.67 ± 4.25

Source: Data from Applegate, 2013; Chumlea, Guo, & Steinbaugh, 1994; Nestle Health Science, 2013

Another approach to assessing the height of a bedridden patient is to align the body so that the lower limbs, abdomen, neck, head and shoulders are in a straight line, and then mark on the bed surface the position of the top of the head and base of the heel (Figure 13-5). Once the patient has been transferred to a different area, the distance between the two marks can then be measured with a tape measure. This method is only effective if the patient has no skeletal abnormalities or contractures.

Weight

Scales should be calibrated at least once monthly using manufacturer's instructions for calibration to ensure accuracy. If possible, patients should be weighed in as little clothing as possible (e.g., hospital or dressing gown) and without shoes, and at the same time each day. Feet should be placed in the center of the scale when weight is obtained, and the patient should not hold or lean onto anything as the weight is assessed.

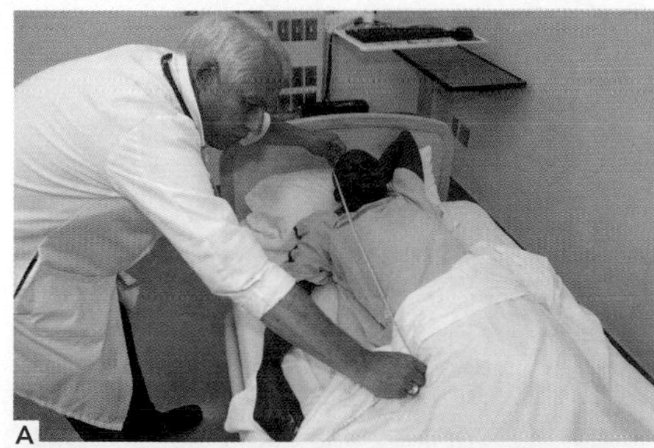

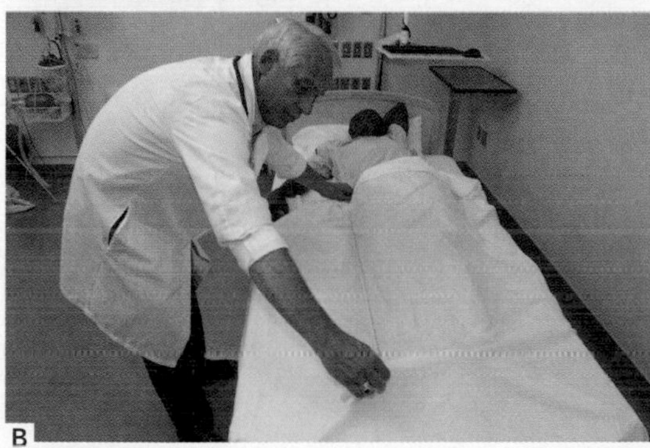

FIGURE 13-5A–B Measuring the height of a bedridden patient

If a prosthetic device is used it should be noted whether or not the device is included in the weight that is obtained. If the patient is nonambulatory and must be weighed in a wheelchair or other assistive device, staff should ensure that the same device is used each time. The device should be weighed separately, and then subtracted from the total weight of the device and the patient together. Always compare weights to the most previous weight obtained, and if a variance of 5 pounds or more is apparent, reweigh the patient to verify results. In addition, research has shown that the weight measurement of an individual may vary (by approximately 3 pounds) depending on the type of scale used (e.g., bed scale versus standing scale or wheelchair scale), and this difference may be even greater in patients with higher bodyweights (Byrd et al., 2011).

Body Mass Index (BMI)

Large-scale population studies (such as NHANES) have shown that mortality risk from heart disease, diabetes, and certain cancers positively correlates with body mass index (BMI), meaning that as BMI increases, so does the risk for these diseases. Other diseases, such as those affecting the digestive and pulmonary systems, also result in increased mortality risk and are characterized by marked weight loss (Flegal, 2005; Figure 13-6). These findings have formed the basis for recommendations that BMI for healthy individuals should fall between 20 kg/m^2 and 25 kg/m^2.

Obesity and overweight are classifications for ranges of weight that are greater than what is generally considered healthy for an individual's given height. These categories also identify ranges of weight that have been demonstrated to increase the likelihood of certain diseases and other health problems. A BMI between 25 and 29.9 is considered overweight, while a BMI of 30 or higher is considered obese. Conversely, a BMI of fewer than 18.5 is typically referred to as underweight, caused primarily by malnutrition stemming from the unavailability of adequate energy from foods. An underweight person may be characterized by anorexia (a lack of appetite for food) because of disease or mental disorder, or by conditions where metabolic needs are in excess of energy intake. Chapter 28 provides more detail about obesity, underweight, and anorexia.

BMI can be easily calculated using height and weight (see Practice Point), or simply assessed using a table such as the one depicted in Figure 13-7.

PRACTICE POINT: Two Methods for Calculating BMI

Method A	Method B
$\text{BMI} = \frac{\text{Weight (in kilograms)}}{[\text{Height (in meters)}]^2}$	$\text{BMI} = \frac{\text{Weight (in pounds)} \times 703}{[\text{Height (in inches)}]^2}$

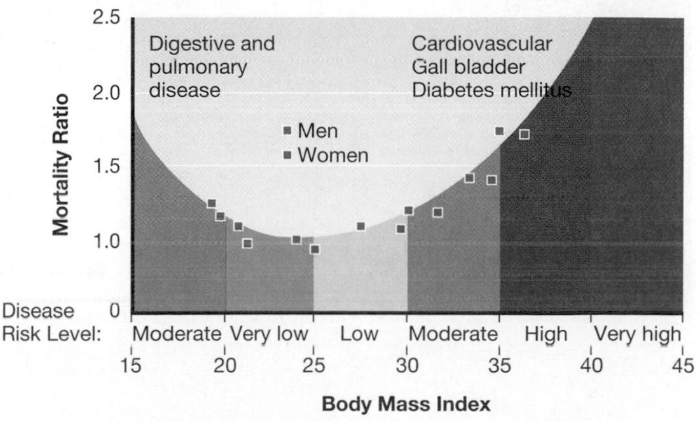

FIGURE 13-6 Weight status and mortality

Body Mass Index Table

	Normal						Overweight					Obese										Extreme Obesity														
BMI	**19**	**20**	**21**	**22**	**23**	**24**	**25**	**26**	**27**	**28**	**29**	**30**	**31**	**32**	**33**	**34**	**35**	**36**	**37**	**38**	**39**	**40**	**41**	**42**	**43**	**44**	**45**	**46**	**47**	**48**	**49**	**50**	**51**	**52**	**53**	**54**
Height (inches)	**Body Weight (pounds)**																																			
58	91	96	100	105	110	115	119	124	129	134	138	143	148	153	158	162	167	172	177	181	186	191	196	201	205	210	215	220	224	229	234	239	244	248	253	258
59	94	99	104	109	114	119	124	128	133	138	143	148	153	158	163	168	173	178	183	188	193	198	203	208	212	217	222	227	232	237	242	247	252	257	262	267
60	97	102	107	112	118	123	128	133	138	143	148	153	158	163	168	174	179	184	189	194	199	204	209	215	220	225	230	235	240	245	250	255	261	266	271	276
61	100	106	111	116	122	127	132	137	143	148	153	158	164	169	174	180	185	190	195	201	206	211	217	222	227	232	238	243	248	254	259	264	269	275	280	285
62	104	109	115	120	126	131	136	142	147	153	158	164	169	175	180	186	191	196	202	207	213	218	224	229	235	240	246	251	256	262	267	273	278	284	289	295
63	107	113	118	124	130	135	141	146	152	158	163	169	175	180	186	191	197	203	208	214	220	225	231	237	242	248	254	259	265	270	278	282	287	293	299	304
64	110	116	122	128	134	140	145	151	157	163	169	174	180	186	192	197	204	209	215	221	227	232	238	244	250	256	262	267	273	279	285	291	296	302	308	314
65	114	120	126	132	138	144	150	156	162	168	174	180	186	192	198	204	210	216	222	228	234	240	246	252	258	264	270	276	282	288	294	300	306	312	318	324
66	118	124	130	136	142	148	155	161	167	173	179	186	192	198	204	210	216	223	229	235	241	247	253	260	266	272	278	284	291	297	303	309	315	322	328	334
67	121	127	134	140	146	153	159	166	172	178	185	191	198	204	211	217	223	230	236	242	249	255	261	268	274	280	287	293	299	306	312	319	325	331	338	344
68	125	131	138	144	151	158	164	171	177	184	190	197	203	210	216	223	230	236	243	249	256	262	269	276	282	289	295	302	308	315	322	328	335	341	348	354
69	128	135	142	149	155	162	169	176	182	189	196	203	209	216	223	230	236	243	250	257	263	270	277	284	291	297	304	311	318	324	331	338	345	351	358	365
70	132	139	146	153	160	167	174	181	188	195	202	209	216	222	229	236	243	250	257	264	271	278	285	292	299	306	313	320	327	334	341	348	355	362	369	376
71	136	143	150	157	165	172	179	186	193	200	208	215	222	229	236	243	250	257	265	272	279	286	293	301	308	315	322	329	338	343	351	358	365	372	379	386
72	140	147	154	162	169	177	184	191	199	206	213	221	228	235	242	250	258	265	272	279	287	294	302	309	316	324	331	338	346	353	361	368	375	383	390	397
73	144	151	159	166	174	182	189	197	204	212	219	227	235	242	250	257	265	272	280	288	295	302	310	318	325	333	340	348	355	363	371	378	386	393	401	408
74	148	155	163	171	179	186	194	202	210	218	225	233	241	249	256	264	272	280	287	295	303	311	319	326	334	342	350	358	365	373	381	389	396	404	412	420
75	152	160	168	176	184	192	200	208	216	224	232	240	248	256	264	272	279	287	295	303	311	319	327	335	343	351	359	367	375	383	391	399	407	415	423	431
76	156	164	172	180	189	197	205	213	221	230	238	246	254	263	271	279	287	295	304	312	320	328	336	344	353	361	369	377	385	394	402	410	418	426	435	443

FIGURE 13-7 Body Mass Index Table

Source: Adapted from Clinical Guidelines on the Identification, Evaluation, and Treatment of Overweight and Obesity in Adults: The Evidence Report.

Waist Circumference

Waist circumference should be measured around the patient's abdomen, above the hipbone (Figure 13-8). To locate the hipbone, palpate the hip area to locate the top of the iliac crest, which is the highest point of the hip bone. Then, place the measuring tape horizontally around the trunk at the level of the iliac crest. Use a wall mirror to check for correct alignment of the measuring tape (especially when measuring overweight patients). The tape measure should be parallel to the floor and held so that it is snug, but does not compress the skin. The measurement should be made at the end of a regular exhalation, and should be repeated a second time to ensure accuracy. Table 13-5 shows the way in which waist circumference and BMI can be used to stratify disease risk.

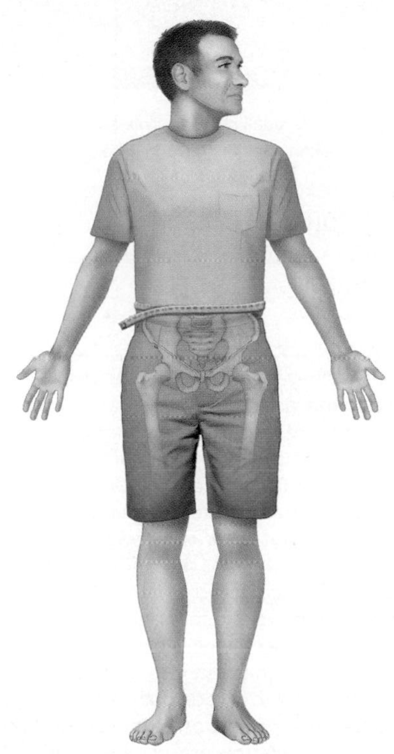

FIGURE 13-8 Waist circumference should be measured around the patient's abdomen, above the hipbone. To locate the hipbone, palpate the hip area to locate the top of the iliac crest.

Skinfold Thickness

Skinfold measurements are a relatively simple and inexpensive way of estimating body composition. In short, once these measurements have been assessed, they can be used in mathematical equations in order to determine an individual's body density, and from that the percentage of body weight from fat mass. Although there are a number of equations that may be used to calculate body density, the most common are generalized for use with adult males and females (Jackson & Pollock, 1978; Jackson, Pollock, & Ward, 1980; Table 13-6). They are considered to be more generalized because they are most accurate in estimating body composition of people with average amounts of body fat. As such, the health provider should be aware that these equations may be less for persons who are very lean or obese. Once body density has been calculated, it can be used in a separate equation to estimate body fat (Siri, 1961; Table 13-6).

Measurements of skinfold thickness are taken at standard anatomical sites around the body, and are usually assessed on the right side for consistency. Depending on the prediction equation used, measurements can be taken at anywhere from three to nine sites, including triceps, biceps, subscapular, thigh, iliac crest, abdomen, chest, calf and/or axilla.

To conduct a skinfold measurement, the tester pinches the skin at the site to raise a double layer of skin and the underlying fat tissue (but not muscle). A specialized caliper (designed for skinfold assessment) is then applied 1 cm below and at right angles to the pinch, and a reading in millimeters is taken. In addition, it is advisable that the mean of two, separate measurements of the same site should be used in the equation. The health provider should be aware that obtaining consistently accurate skinfold measurements requires training and experience. For further information on specific measurement technique, the reader is referred to the NHANES Body Measurements Anthropometry Reference Manual provided by the CDC (www.cdc.gov/nchs/nhanes/nh3rrm.htm).

Nutrition Related Physical Examination

Evaluation of a patient's nutritional status requires the provider to be able to assess and apply information obtained from a number of related sources, including medical, social and dietary history,

Table 13-5 Classification of overweight and obesity by BMI, waist circumference and associated risk from hypertension, type 2 diabetes, and cardiovascular disease

			Disease risk relative to normal weight and waist circumference	
	BMI kg/m²	Obesity Category	Men ≤ 40 inches Women ≤ 30 inches	Men ≥ 40 inches Women ≥ 30 inches
Underweight	< 18.5			
Normal	18.5–24.9			
Overweight	25–29.9		Increased	High
Obesity	30–34.9	1	High	Very High
	35–39.9	2	Very High	Very High
Extreme Obesity	≥ 40	3	Extremely high	Extremely High

Source: Adapted from National Heart, Lung, and Blood Institute (NHLBI), 1998.

Table 13-6 Skinfold thickness and body composition

Estimation of Body Density	
Men[A1]	Body Density = 1.1093800 - 0.0008267*sum + 0.0000016*sum^2 – 0.0002574*age (where sum = summed measurements of chest, abdominal, and thigh skinfold measurements)
Women[A2]	Body Density = 1.0994921 - 0.0009929*sum + 0.0000023*sum^2 – 0.0001392*age (where sum = summed measurements of triceps, suprailiac and thigh skinfold measurements)
Estimation of Body Fat[B]	
Body Fat = (4.95/[Body Density] – 4.50) × 100	

Sources: [A1]Jackson, A.S., Pollock, M.L., 1978; [A2]Jackson, A.S., Pollock, M.L., Ward, A., 1980; [B]Siri, W.E., 1961.

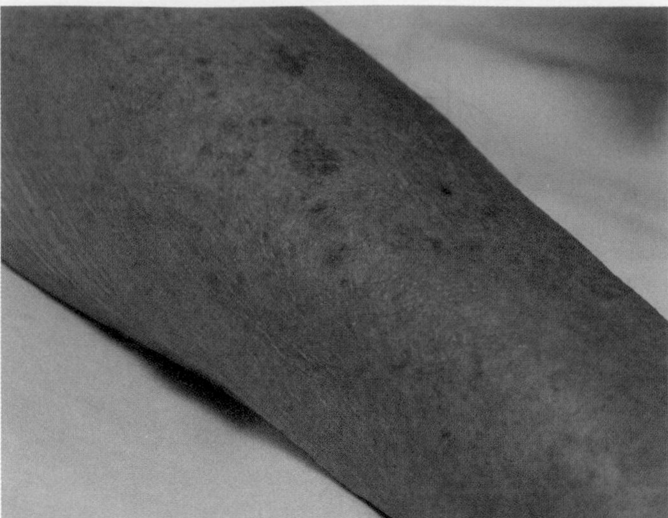

FIGURE 13-9 Petechiae are small red or purple spot on the body caused by a minor hemorrhage (broken capillary blood vessels)

current and historical intake, laboratory data (detailed in a subsequent section), and finally, from the results of physical examination. Review Chapter 6 for a more detailed discussion of assessment techniques. Specific nutrition related findings will be further identified in the system Chapters 16–30.

Vital Signs

Vital signs can provide important insight with regard to several nutrition-related scenarios. Prolonged increases in temperature and respiratory rate may indicate elevated energy and fluid requirements, while chronically high blood pressure may suggest the need for a reduction in dietary sodium intake. Review Chapter 8 for a more detailed discussion of vital sign assessment techniques.

> ***PRACTICE POINT: Estimating Fluid Requirement in a Febrile Patient***
>
> The body loses water around 1.5 liters daily in the form of urine. An additional liter may be excreted through sweating, bowel movements, and breathing, and patients who have an elevated body temperature (i.e., fever or febrile) will have even greater fluid needs. It is recommended that fluid provisions are increased by approximately 12% for every degree (Celsius) that the patient presents with over normal body temperature (Merck Manual, 2010).

Macronutrient/Micronutrient Deficiencies

The exam starts by inspecting the patient's skin for color (pallor, redness, pigmentation), and for the presence of hemorrhagic vascular lesions (petechiae and ecchymosis) (Figure 13-9), as these may indicate nutrient deficiencies. All surfaces of the body should be inspected for pressure sores, particularly in those areas where the bones are close to the skin, such as the ankles, back, elbows, heels, hips, and buttocks. Inspecting the color and healing stage of a pressure ulcer assists in development of the nutritional care plan so that adequate energy, protein, vitamins, and minerals can be provided as needed to accelerate the healing process. The patient's shoulders, triceps, chest, and hands should be inspected to check for loose-fitting skin or loss of fullness, both of which may indicate loss of subcutaneous fat because of **protein-energy malnutrition (PEM)**.

> ***THINK LINK: Protein-Energy Malnutrition***
>
> **Kwashiorkor** and **marasmus** are the most severe kinds of PEM, and may be prominent in certain at-risk populations or in children in developing countries. Kwashiorkor is predominantly a protein deficiency, characterized by normal body weight and skeletal structure. In these patients, hair is dry, brittle, and can be easily plucked without pain. The condition also elicits depletions of serum proteins, such as albumin. Decreased concentrations of these proteins can lead to abnormal fluid distribution, typically seen as edema to the feet and legs and extending into the perineum and upper extremities. In contrast, marasmus patients often exhibit significant loss of body mass and are typically less that 60% of expected/ideal body weight. While this condition imposes losses to both adipose and muscle tissue, serum protein concentration are usually within normal limits, and there is no presence of edema. Here, the body's emaciated condition and compromised health status is also referred to as cachexia.

The condition of the hair and scalp can also indicate suboptimal nutritional status. Hair that is thin, easily pulled out, or dull and lackluster may indicate deficiency of protein, fatty acids, zinc, or iron. It should be noted, however, that more often than not, these characteristics may be attributable to other causes such as chemical bleaching or other cosmetic processing, so it is important to consider the patient's nutrition history.

Fingernails should also be examined, taking into account the shape, color, and angle of the nail and nail bed, as well as the presence of any lesions or abnormal growths. If the nail has a spoon shape to it, otherwise known as **koilynichia**, the patient may have iron deficiency (Figure 13-10). A mottled or overly pale nail bed may signify a deficiency of vitamin A or vitamin C.

Inspect the patient's eyes carefully to note color and texture, as well as the appearance of the sclerae, conjunctiva, and cornea. Eyes that are excessively dry and exhibit foamy accumulations (Bitot's Spots), or those that have ulceration of the cornea (keratomalacia) are often indicative of vitamin A deficiency (Figure 13-11).

The condition of the mouth and oral cavity can also contribute a variety of important information about the patient's nutritional status. The health provider should inspect and palpate the lips, tongue, gums, and mucosa, noting any discolorations, asymmetries, or cracking/fissuring. For example, angular stomatitis, an inflammatory lesion or split at the corner of the mouth, has been associated with deficiencies of riboflavin, iron, and zinc. Pronounced redness of the tongue or atrophy of the taste buds can signify niacin, folate, riboflavin, iron, or vitamin B_{12} deficiency, and a decreased taste sensation has also been associated with deficiencies in zinc.

It is also important to evaluate the condition of the teeth and gums. Spongy or bleeding gums may be secondary to poor vitamin C intake (a condition otherwise known as scurvy). Poor dentition and missing/unfitted dentures can cause food to be improperly chewed and swallowed, leading to inadequate nutrient intake and/or aspiration risk. When conducting an oral examination, the health provider should also perform a general survey of the patient's chewing and swallowing ability, which is especially important for patients who have neurologic deficits because of stroke or other medical conditions (Sitoh, 2000). Many institutions have set protocols for bedside swallowing evaluations, so the health provider should adhere to guidelines set forth by his/her facility. If chewing and/or swallowing function appears to be compromised in any way, or the patient has self-reported difficulty in this regard, then the health provider should recommend further evaluation by a trained speech-language pathologist.

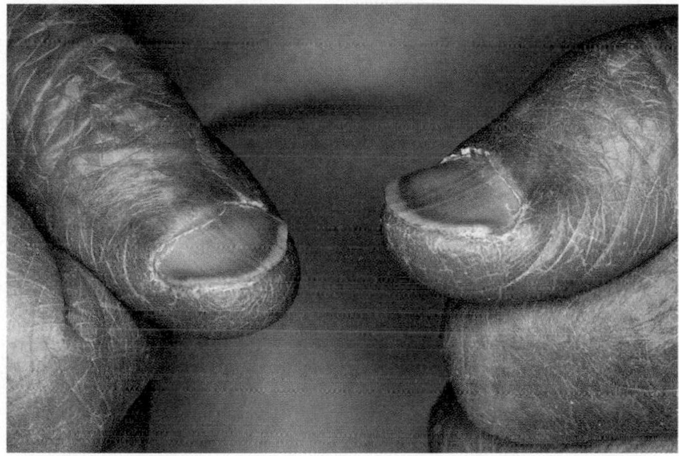

FIGURE 13-10 Iron deficiency may cause koilynichia, or spoon-shaped nails
Source: Wellcome Trust Library/Custom Medical Stock

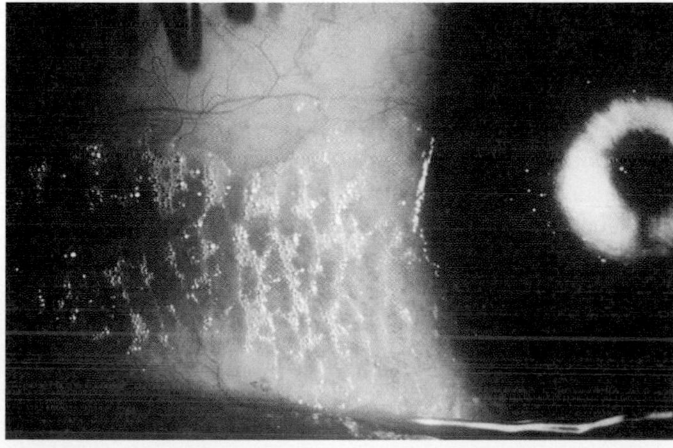

FIGURE 13-11 Bitot's Spots
Source: CDC

Fluid Status

Data from the physical examination can also reveal information about the hydration status of the patient. Combined with findings from laboratory assessments, these data may be helpful in determining underlying etiology. **Underhydration** may be caused by inadequate oral intake or provision from IVs or tube feeding flushes. It may also be attributed to excessive loss from diarrhea or emesis, diaphoresis (perspiration), draining from fistulas, ostomies, wounds or burns, dialysis, paracentesis, or hemorrhage. In contrast, **overhydration** can be caused from excessive oral intake or provision from IVs or flushes, disease processes such as liver failure, renal disease, congestive heart failure, severe hypertension, syndrome of inappropriate antidiuretic hormone; or by interstitial fluid retention caused by poor serum protein status (e.g., hypoalbuminemia). Table 13-7 lists clinical presentations that may occur in the presence of under- or over-hydration. Laboratory indices that are related to fluid status will be discussed further in the next section.

Biochemical Assessment of Nutritional Status

Assessment of nutrition-related laboratory data requires consideration of both the nutritional and non nutritional factors that may affect blood parameters. Interpret laboratory data in the context of dietary history, disease processes and treatment, hydration status and medication usage, as all of these can have a pronounced effect on blood and urine chemistries. The health provider should review the laboratory data in a serial manner, as changes over time are of greater importance than single, static values. Also, since assay methodology may differ widely between laboratories, always use reference values provided by your facility. Finally, it is important to consider effects of treatment/intervention on overall clinical outcome, not on the laboratory value solely, as improvements to the clinical outcome are of greatest importance and remain the ultimate goal. Several of the major nutrition-related laboratory values are provided in the sections that follow. Table 13-8 lists diagnostic tests and reference ranges for a number of select micronutrients.

Electrolyte Assessment

In general, an electrolyte is a chemical that has either a positive (cation) or negative (anion) electrical charge. Physiologic electrolytes (namely, sodium, potassium, calcium, phosphorous, and magnesium) affect the amount of water in the body, the acidity of the blood (pH), muscle action, and a number of other important processes. Table 13-9 lists normative (reference) values for electrolytes.

Table 13-7 Clinical parameters for evaluation of hydration status

	Clinical Finding		
	Vital Sign Abnormality	**Physical Presentation**	**Biochemical (Laboratory) Presentation**
Underhydration	• ↓ blood pressure • ↓ cardiac output • ↓ central venous pressure • ↑ heart rate • ↑ temperature • ↑ vascular resistance	• Input/Intake < Output • Eyes that are sunken into orbit cavity and dry • Skin cool, clammy and pale • Decreased weight • Dry mucous membranes and sticky saliva • Poor skin turgor • Dark urine, oliguria	In the case of dehydration, many laboratory values will be elevated, including the following: • ↑ serum osmolality • ↑ BUN • ↑ sodium • ↑ creatinine • ↑ chloride • ↑ hemoglobin • ↑ hematocrit • ↑ urine-specific gravity
Overhydration	• ↑ blood pressure • ↑ cardiac output • ↑ central venous pressure • ↑ heart rate • ↑ temperature • ↑ vascular resistance	• Input/Intake > Output • Puffy or swollen eyes • Moist skin • Increased weight • Anasarca (generalized edema); edema to the periphery and sacral regions • Shortness of breath, dyspnea • Jugular venous distention	In the case of fluid overload, many laboratory values will be decreased because of the dilutional effects if the excess fluid, for example: • ↑ sodium • ↑ hemoglobin • ↑ hematocrit

Table 13-8 Laboratory tests to determine select micronutrient deficiencies

Deficient Micronutrient	Diagnostic Laboratory Test(s)	Normal Range
Thiamin	Serum Thiamin	1.1–1.6 mg/dL
Vitamin D	25 Hydroxy Vitamin D	50 mg/ml
Zinc	Serum Zinc	67–183 mcg/dL
Vitamin B_{12}	Serum Vitamin B_{12}	200–900 pg/mL
Iron	Hemoglobin Hematocrit Serum Ferritin Serum Iron Total Iron Binding Capacity Serum Transferrin Transferrin Saturation	13.5–18 g/dL (men) 12–15 g/dL (women) 40%–54% (men) 36%–46% (women) 15–445 mcg/L 10– 10 mcg/L 50–150 mcg/dl 240–450 mcg/dL 200–430 mcg/dL 30%–0% (men) 20%–35% (women)
Folate	Serum Folate	3–16 ng/mL

Table 13-9 Normative values for serum electrolytes

Electrolyte	Reference Range
Sodium	135–145 mEq/L
Potassium	3.5–5.0 mEq/L
Calcium (total)	8.5–10.5 mg/dL
Calcium (ionized)	2.0–2.4 mEq/L
Phosphorous	3.0–4.5 mg/dL
Magnesium	1.7–2.2 mg/dL

Sodium

Sodium is the major extra extracellular ion. Abnormally high or low concentrations of sodium indicate a disorder of sodium concentration in the serum (not the total body), and thus are mainly indicative of total body water. **Hypernatremia** is most frequently seen when the patient is dehydrated because of insufficient water intake/provision or excessive output (fistulas, burns, prolonged fever, vomiting, or diarrhea). **Hyponatremia** can occur as a result of overhydration (excessive water intake/provision) or conditions that result in fluid retention (renal disease or congestive heart failure), or excessive sodium loss gastric suctioning (diuretic use, vomiting, diarrhea). In most cases, intervention for hyper- or hyponatremia involves fluid repletion or dieresis, and not sodium replacement.

Potassium

Potassium is the major intracellular cation (at least 95% of the body's potassium is found inside cells), and helps to regulate transmission of nerve impulses, and maintain acid–base and fluid balance. Low concentrations of serum potassium (**hypokalemia**) can be attributed to a wide variety of factors, including use of diuretics (particularly those that are potassium depleting), vomiting, diarrhea, or IV fluid administration without concomitant potassium supplementation. Elevated serum potassium (**hyperkalemia**) is often related to renal failure, as the impaired kidneys are unable to remove excess potassium from the blood. Hyperkalemia can also be caused by inadequate function of the adrenal glands (Addison's disease) or by excessive potassium losses in individuals who have endured severe burns.

Calcium

Over 99% of the body's calcium is found in the skeletal structure (bones) and teeth. Normal concentrations of calcium are tightly regulated by hormones (calcitonin, calcitriol [or bioactive vitamin D] and parathyroid hormone). The large skeletal reserves compensate for reduced calcium intake or gastrointestinal absorption.

Since calcium concentrations can be affected by the patient's albumin status, ionized calcium is the most accurate assessment of true physiologic status. Calcium should also be assessed in the context of serum magnesium and phosphorous concentrations, which should be repeated if low. A number of factors can affect **hypocalcemia** (low serum calcium), some of which include renal failure, vitamin D deficiency, acute pancreatitis, hyperphosphatemia, hypoalbuminemia, hyperparathyroidism, hypomagnesaemia, and usage of certain medications. In contrast, **hypercalcemia** can stem from hyperparathyroidism, medications (thiazide diuretics, lithium, and vitamin A toxicity), malignancies, and immobilization. It can also occur as a result of excess calcitriol [1,25 dihydroxyvitamin D], tuberculosis, sarcoidosis, milk-alkali syndrome (also called Burnett's syndrome, and results from ingestion of large amounts of calcium and absorbable alkali), or after renal transplantation (although all of these are less common causes).

Phosphorous

Phosphorous is the major intracellular anion. Serum phosphorous concentrations, closely linked with those of calcium, are not necessarily a good reflection of true physiologic stores as the majority of phosphorous is found in the skeletal structure and not in the extracellular fluid. Similar to calcium, these stores can act as a buffer to keep serum or intracellular concentrations stable. Low phosphorous concentrations (**hypophosphatemia**) may occur with rickets and osteomalacia (two conditions affecting bone formation), hyperparathyroidism, or chronic antacid use. Antacids contain substances, which bind phosphorous in the gastrointestinal tract, preventing its proper absorption. **Hyperphosphatemia** is most commonly caused by impaired renal excretion, increased phosphorous intake (from phosphate containing laxatives or enemas), hypoparathyroidism or hypothyroidism.

Magnesium

Like calcium and phosphorous, only a very small percentage (< 1%) of magnesium is present in the extracellular fluid. Both hypocalcemia and hypokalemia are associated with magnesium status, and cannot be adequately repleted without concomitant repletion of magnesium. Magnesium depletion (**hypomagnesaemia**) is often apparent in alcoholic patients, those that are critically ill, and in diabetics experiencing osmotic diuresis. Magnesium may also decrease as a result of severe diarrhea, hypoparathyroidism, pancreatitis, Cushing's disease, and excessive diuretic use. Chronic **hypermagnesemia** is often associated with renal failure. Levels may be also be increased by hemolytic anemia, Addison's disease, hyperparathyroidism, and overuse of magnesium-based antacids.

Blood Glucose Assessment

Blood glucose (BG) concentration, commonly referred to as blood sugar level, is the amount of glucose present in the bloodstream at a given time. Under normal physiologic circumstances, the body maintains the BG within a tight range of approximately 70 to 100 mg/dL. The BG is regulated closely by pancreatic hormones glucagon, which stimulates the liver to release glucose into the bloodstream so that BG rises, and insulin, which stimulates cells to take up glucose from the bloodstream, thereby lowering BG (Figure 13-12).

When the BG concentration is persistently above (**hyperglycemia**) or below (**hypoglycemia**) the normal range, it may be indicative of pre-diabetes (glucose intolerance) or diabetes mellitus (DM). DM is a condition characterized by persistent, ongoing hyperglycemia, which may be caused by insufficient insulin production or secretion, or resistance of the cells to the effects of circulating insulin. Both fasting and non-fasting BG concentrations, as well as glycated hemoglobin (Hgb A-1C; a laboratory test that may also be helpful in determining longer-term blood glucose stability) can be used to determine presence of DM, or the physician may order an oral glucose tolerance test (OGTT) to measure the body's ability to metabolize glucose.

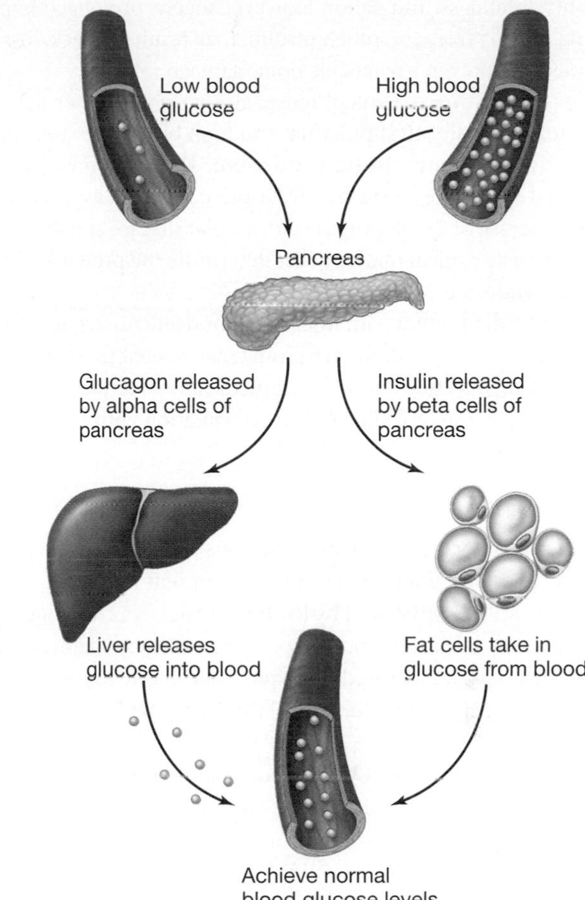

FIGURE 13-12 Blood glucose (BG) is tightly regulated by the hormones glucagon (which increases BG) and glucagon (which decreases BG)

However, it is important to note that there are many reasons (particularly in persons who are acutely ill) that a temporary elevation in BG may present. For example, severe stress, such as that caused by trauma, stroke, heart attack or surgery, or from prolonged receipt of IVs containing large amounts of dextrose, may elevate blood glucose levels. In addition, certain drugs (such as corticosteroids or beta-blockers) can increase or decrease glucose levels.

Long-term hyperglycemia causes damage to the body's microvasculature, which are the smallest vessels of the circulatory system, including capillaries, arterioles, and venules. As such, DM is the root cause of many chronic health problems including impairments to eyesight, compromised kidney function, heart disease, and damaged nerve tissues.

Blood sugar that is too low can also be extremely problematic. Symptoms of transitory hypoglycemia may include a variety of less severe manifestations, such as fatigue, impaired mental functioning, irritability, weakness, and pallor. However severe, prolonged hypoglycemia, usually from too much insulin, may result in shock, loss of consciousness, or even irreversible brain damage.

Elevated fasting plasma glucose, along several other factors (abdominal adiposity, dyslipidemia, and high blood pressure) may be indicative of the **metabolic syndrome**. This syndrome (sometimes called syndrome X) is a constellation of medical disorders that increases the risk of developing cardiovascular disease and diabetes. Table 13-10 lists clinical markers that determine the presence of the metabolic syndrome.

Patients who present with impaired blood glucose regulation or diabetes, and/or the metabolic syndrome may benefit from pharmacologic (insulin injections or oral DM medications) or lifestyle interventions (e.g., therapeutic diet and/or consultation with a registered dietitian and/or exercise physiologist).

Blood Lipid Assessment

A number of factors may increase a person's risk for cardiovascular disease. Cholesterol is a fat like substance present in animal-based foods and it is also synthesized by the body to act as a component of cell membranes, bile acids, and as a precursor for steroid hormones. Most of the body's fat is stored in adipose (fat) tissue in the form of triglycerides. A triglyceride consists of three fatty acids connected to a glycerol.

Cholesterol and triglycerides are fat soluble and must be transported through the bloodstream for storage by lipoproteins. The major lipoproteins that take these substances *to* storage sites are very-low-density lipoprotein (VLDL), and low-density lipoprotein (LDL, sometimes referred to as "bad cholesterol"), while high-density lipoprotein (HDL, sometimes called "good cholesterol") acts as a scavenger to remove excess cholesterol *from* tissues and return it to the liver for reprocessing or conversion to bile.

A number of studies have documented the relationship between total cholesterol and cardiovascular disease, and this association becomes particularly strong as concentrations rise above 200 mg/dL. For example, a study by the National Cholesterol Education Program (2001) showed that men who had cholesterol concentrations above the 90th percentile for this population had four times the risk of coronary heart disease compared with men whose concentrations were below the 10th percentile. LDL and HDL have also been shown to predict cardiovascular risk, and for this reason, providers often use results from the blood lipid profile to stratify risk, plan intervention, and track progress. Table 13-11 lists classifications of total cholesterol, triglycerides, LDL, and HDL. Similar to those who have abnormal blood glucose homeostasis, patients who present with **dyslipidemia** (abnormal blood lipids) may benefit from pharmacologic or lifestyle interventions (e.g., therapeutic diet and/or consultation with a registered dietitian and/or exercise physiologist).

Table 13-10 Clinical indicators of the presence of metabolic syndrome

Clinical Parameter	Defining Value
Fasting Plasma Glucose	≥ 110 mg/dL
Triglycerides	≥ 150 mg/dL
HDL cholesterol	< 40 mg/dL in men < 50 mg/dL in women
Blood pressure	≥ 130 mm Hg systolic ≥ 85 mm Hg diastolic
Abdominal obesity	Waist circumference of > 40 in (> 102 cm) in men and > 35 in (> 88 cm) in women

*A diagnosis of the syndrome can be made when three or more risk factors occur.

Serum Proteins

Providers can use results from serum protein laboratory tests to determine a patient's protein status, and to predict the degree to which they may be at risk for medical complications, and also to track the effectiveness of interventions and a patient's post-treatment progress. Two serum proteins are often used in clinical practice: albumin and prealbumin. Albumin is the most abundant protein in the blood and acts as a carrier for small molecules. It is responsible for maintaining plasma oncotic pressure, which keeps fluid within the vascular space; this is why persons with very low albumin concentrations may develop edema. Concentrations have been shown to indicate decreased physiologic protein status and reduced dietary intake of protein. Low reductions are also associated with increased morbidity and mortality. Albumin correlates well with other measurements of protein status, and is responsive to dietary protein repletion. Normative values for albumin range from 3.5 to 5.0 mg/dL.

Prealbumin (also called transthyretin) acts as binder for the thyroid hormones, and also as a carrier for retinol-binding protein. Like albumin, reduced prealbumin concentrations have been shown to result from poor nutritional status, and to predict morbidity and mortality. The half-life of prealbumin is much less than that

Table 13-11 Classification of blood lipids

	mg/dL
Total Cholesterol	
Desirable	< 200
Borderline High	200–239
High	≥ 240
Triglycerides	
Optimal	< 150
Borderline high	150–199
High	200–499
Very High	≥ 500
LDL Cholesterol	
Optimal	< 100
Near optimal/above optimal	100–129
Borderline high	130–159
High	160–189
Very High	≥ 190
HDL Cholesterol	
Low (undesirable)	< 40
High (desirable)	≥ 60

Source: from the National Cholesterol Education Program, 2001

of albumin, however (only a few days), making prealbumin a more sensitive indicator of the patient's current protein status. Normal prealbumin values should fall in the range of 20–40 mg/dL.

Drug–Nutrient Interactions

A **drug–nutrient interaction** is a reaction between a medication and a nutrient that may adversely affect the action or effect of the drug. Table 13-12 lists a number of drug–nutrient interactions that the health provider may encounter during practice. Additionally, some drugs may cause impairment of nutrient synthesis or absorption. For example, potassium-depleting diuretics (such as those in the thiazide class, Aldoril, Diachlor or loop class, Lasix) often require that the patient receive potassium supplementation for the duration of treatment. The nurse can gain familiarity with these interactions by referencing pharmaceutical manuals such as the *Physician's Desk Reference*.

Assessment of Nutrient Needs

Provision of adequate nutrients for maintenance, healing, and repletion is of great importance for ill patients, as their availability, or lack thereof, can have large impact on morbidity and mortality risk. Therefore, assessment of nutrient needs is a vital step in the patient care process. The following sections describe a number of methods for assessing nutrient needs, and this information should be combined with information obtained from the patient history and physical and biochemical assessment in order to determine the best plan of nutritional care for the patient.

Energy (Calorie) Needs

Scientifically, the term **calorie** refers to a unit that is equal to the amount of heat required to raise the temperature of one kilogram of water by one degree at one atmosphere pressure. In more general

Table 13-12 Select drug–nutrient interactions

Medication	Indication	Drug–Nutrient Interaction
warfarin (Coumadin)	Prevention of blood clot formation	Avoid sudden increases/decreases in intake of foods high in vitamin K as this may counteract anti-clotting effects. Vitamin K-rich foods include kale, spinach, turnip and collard greens, Swiss chard, and large amounts of parsley.
Monoamine Oxidase Inhibitors such as phenelzine (Nardil), tranylcypromine (Parnate), isocarboxazid (Marplan), selegiline (Emsam)	Treatment of depression	Avoid foods high in tyramine (chianti, vermouth, imported beers, aged cheese, smoked, pickled or fermented fish, miso soup, Marmite®, sausage, bologna, pepperoni, and salami) as they may cause hypertensive crisis.
atorvastatin (Lipitor), cerivistatin (Baycol), lovastatin (Mevacor), simvastatin (Zocor)	Antihyperlipidemics	Avoid grapefruit, as it may alter absorption and action of medications.*
ixabepilone (Ixempra) etoposide (Vepesid) temsirolimus (Torisel)	Treatment of cancer	
pimozide (Orap) ziprasidone (Geodon)	Antipsychotic	
ranolazine (Ranexa)	Antianginal	
nifedipine (Procardia)	Antihypertensive	
sildenafil (Viagra, Revatio)	Treatment of erectile dysfunction	
amiodarone (Cordarone)	Management of arrhythmias	
astemizole (Hismanal)	Antihistamine	
budesonide (Entocort)	Treatment of lung disease/ asthma (inhaled steroid)	
buspirone (Buspar)	Depression	
cilostazol (Pletal)	Blood thinner	
colchichine	Treatment of gout	
cyclosporine (Neoral) sirolimus (Rapamune) tacrolimus (Prograf)	Immunosupressant	
eletriptan (Relpax)	Treatment of migraine headaches	
mifepristone (Mifeprex)	Abortefacient	
halofantrine (Halfan) primaquine	Antimalarial	

*This list contains only a select number of drugs that interact with compounds contained in grapefruit. For a complete listing, see Pronsky, 2012.

terms, a kilocalorie is simply a measure of energy expenditure. The calories that are most commonly referred to (i.e., those found in foods or used during exercise) are **kilocalories** (kcal) or 1000 of the calories referred to by the scientific definition. Many sources use the terms calorie and kilocalorie interchangeably, and for the purposes of this text, we will refer to this unit of measurement as a calorie. Daily energy expenditure (i.e., calorie usage) for humans can vary widely from 1600 for highly sedentary individuals to greater than 3000 for those that are very active.

One pound of fat (or adipose tissue) contains 3500 calories. To either gain or lose a pound of fat mass, a person must ingest 3500 calories more or less than the amount that they expend. Likewise, to maintain body weight, a person must consistently ingest the same amount of calories that they expend. Thus, in order to supply adequate provisions for a patient to fulfill energy-balance goals, the ability to determine energy expenditure is very important. There are several ways to accomplish this. One involves direct measurement of expenditure, but this is often impractical because of the cost or equipment it entails, or the discomfort to the patient. There are also a number of mathematical formulas that can be used, and although these provide only an estimate of expenditure, they are fairly accurate when compared to direct measurement.

A method of measuring the exact amount of calories that a patient expends is known as indirect calorimetry. Indirect calorimetry measures number of calories the body burns at rest (or resting energy expenditure). Indirect calorimetry uses measurements of inhaled oxygen and exhaled carbon dioxide, because the amount of oxygen utilized is directly proportional to the amount of energy the patient expends so that the number of calories burned per minute can be determined. While accurate, this method requires special equipment (e.g., a gas analyzer and breathing apparatus). In addition, it can only be performed on patients that are hemodynamically stable, that are able to remain free from movement for a period of time before the test, are cooperative or sedated, and do not have any chest tubes or supplemental oxygen.

There are several formulas that can be used to estimate energy expenditure, depending on the weight status of the patient and the severity of their illness.

Protein

Protein requirements are based on the degree of metabolic stress that the patient is under, his or her current nutritional status, and ability to metabolize protein. **Nitrogen balance** (comparing nitrogen [protein] intake from dietary sources to nitrogen [protein] output from urine, bowel movements, or other physiologic sources) that is positive should be the goal. Table 13-13 lists daily protein requirements for adults, based on medical/physiologic condition.

Dietary Reference Intakes

The dietary reference intakes (DRIs), discussed in the initial sections of this chapter, provide daily intake recommendations. The DRIs for macronutrients (carbohydrate, protein, fiber, and fat) and fluids are listed in Table 13-14.

Table 13-13 Protein requirements for adults

Group/Condition	Range of Protein Requirements
Adult Maintenance	0.8–1.0 gm/kg
Older Adults	1.0 gm/kg
Renal Disease, not on dialysis	0.5–0.8 gm/kg*
Renal Disease, hemodialysis	1–2 gm/kg
Renal Disease, peritoneal dialysis	> 1.2–2.5 gm/kg
Cirrhosis	1.1–1.3 gm/kg
Encephalopathy	0.6–0.8 gm/kg
Cancer	1.0–2.5 gm/kg**
Pulmonary Disease	1.2–1.5 gm/kg
Stroke	1.0–1.25 gm/kg
Critical Illness (burns, sepsis, traumatic brain injury)	1.4–3.0 gm/kg***

* depends on glomerular filtration rate
** varies by type of cancer
*** varies according to severity of illness (burn patients require more protein due to losses through urine and wounds, increased gluconeogenesis, and wound healing

Table 13-14 Dietary reference intakes for macronutrients and fluid

Nutrient	Dietary Reference Intake
Protein	10%–35% of kcal
Carbohydrate	45%–65% of kcal
Fat	20%–35% of kcal
Fiber	Men: 30–38 gm per day Women: 21–25 gm per day
Water/Fluid	30 mL/kcal or minimum of 1500 mL per day

Developmental Applications: Nutrition Assessment of Special Populations

This section discusses considerations that apply to special patient populations, such as infants, children, pregnant women, and older adults, when performing nutritional assessment.

Infants and Children

A child's early years are a particularly critical time for growth and development and the formation of good dietary habits. Nutritional assessment of infants and children requires the expertise of qualified providers, which may require the use of a registered dietician, and requires collaboration with families and child caregivers. It is vital that parents and caregivers provide regular information about an infant or toddler's eating habits, cultural and religious preferences about food, and overall health, particularly for children with health problems or disabilities.

Comprehensive nutritional assessment of an infant or child may include many of the parameters that are evaluated in an adult patient, such as medical history, a physical examinations, laboratory data, height and weight, and dietary/mealtime history. This data is then evaluated to determine a child's current nutritional status. Subsequently, if problems or potential risks are identified, the child's parents and caregivers can work with cooks and health and nutrition providers to develop strategies to address the child's dietary needs.

Childhood nutrition is its own subspecialty, and it is important that the health provider be versed in assessment techniques that are specific to this population. There are a large number of educational resources and assessment tools that are available for use. For example, the U.S. Department of Health and Human Services offers information and resources as part of its *We Can!* (Ways to Enhance Children's Activity & Nutrition) program, a national movement designed to give parents, caregivers, and entire communities a way to help children 8 to 13 years old stay at a healthy weight (www.nhlbi.nih.gov/health/public/heart/obesity/wecan/about-wecan/index.htm).

In addition, childhood growth charts can be downloaded from the Centers for Disease Control and Prevention (www.cdc.gov/growthcharts), and The U.S. Department of Agriculture's Child Care Nutrition Resource System also offers a variety of information on its Web site (www.nal.usda.gov/childcare).

Pregnant and Lactating Women

Nutrition assessment of pregnant women is important for determining prenatal growth and development, and typically includes information regarding the woman's height, weight, prepregnancy weight gain, due date, and dietary patterns. It may also be important to check hemoglobin concentrations to assess for the presence of anemia, as this condition may result in compromised oxygen transport to the developing fetus. Women should consume a well-rounded diet, with adequate food sources of protein, iron, calcium, folate, zinc and fiber, as well as at least 64 ounces of water daily. Energy needs are increased, and the woman should also increase intake by approximately 300 calories each day. The amount of weight a woman should gain during pregnancy depends upon her weight before pregnancy, and should be advised by the physician. Table 13-15 shows guidelines for weight gain during pregnancy. The U.S. Department of Agriculture's (USDA) Food and Nutrition Center (FNIC; http://fnic.nal.usda.gov/) also provides a diverse array of resources on nutrition during pregnancy.

Table 13-15 Guidelines for weight gain during pregnancy

Weight Before Pregnancy	Suggested Weight Gain
Normal Weight (BMI 20–24)	25–35 pounds
Underweight (BMI < 20)	28–40 pounds
Overweight (BMI 25–29)	15–25 pounds
Very Overweight (BMI > 30)	~15 pounds

For lactating women, there are few indicators for nutritional assessment above and beyond those that would be indicated for a normal adult. Instead, the nutritional risk is usually related to the health of the nursing infant (Committee on Nutritional Status During Pregnancy and Lactation, 1991). For women exclusively breastfeeding their infants, energy needs exceed prepregnancy demands by approximately 640 kcal/day during the first 6 months postpartum compared with 300 kcal/day during the last two trimesters of pregnancy, while the demand for some nutrients, such as iron, is considerably less during lactation than during pregnancy. Lactating women are encouraged to eat a healthful, well-balanced diet, and the USDA's FNIC also provides links to numerous resources in this regard (http://fnic.nal.usda.gov/).

Older Adults

Older adults face a unique set of nutrition-related challenges. Malnutrition and/or weight loss (unintended) are common, and can occur for a variety of reasons. For example, reductions in olfactory and taste sensations can lead to a decreased appetite and/or intake. Elderly individuals may feel isolated, experiencing feelings of loneliness or depression, which can hinder normal food consumption patterns. Or, an older person may eat less because of fatigue, or because of chewing difficulties related to altered dentition.

As malnutrition and loss of body weight ensue, older adults often sustain a reduction in muscle mass, which can decrease strength and mobility, and the ability that the person has for self-care. In addition, the poor nutritional status of elderly persons can cause slower recovery from illness, and increased risk of complications, such as infection or poor wound healing. Thus, it is vital that the health provider understand the importance of assessing baseline nutritional status of the elderly patient, and prioritize consumption of nutritious foods.

The National Institute on Aging (part of the U.S. Department of HHS and the National Institutes of Health) provides resources for healthy eating and dietary planning for older adults (www.nia.nih.gov/health/topics/healthy-eating). In addition, the USDA FNIC (http://fnic.nal.usda.gov) has a number of resources on topics of interest to seniors such as healthy eating to reduce risk of disease, and dealing with changes that affect eating (such having to cook for one, or changes in taste).

Summary

- U.S. Department of Health and Human Services (DHHS) and the U.S. Department of Agriculture (USDA) conduct national surveys related to the health and nutrition of the population. Data from these surveys are used to determine risk factors (including those related to nutrition) for major diseases and disease prevalence, and to prioritize public health interventions aimed at reducing associated morbidity and mortality.
- A nutrition-focused patient history is a vital component of nutrition assessment, and contains both objective and subjective data related to the patient's medical and social history, as well as habitual dietary intake.
- Evaluation of nutrient intake should be included in the nutritional assessment, and can be obtained in a variety of ways, such as food diaries, 24-hour recall, oral intake during admission, and provisions from enteral and/or parenteral nutrition support.
- The health provider should conduct a thorough anthropometric assessment of the patient, including height, body weight (with calculation of BMI), and in some cases, measurement of waist circumference and/or skinfold thicknesses.
- A nutrition-oriented physical assessment provides valuable information about the nutritional status of the patient, and should

include visual observation of the patient in order to investigate appearance (inspection), auscultation and percussion, and evaluation of vital signs and other physical sign/symptoms of hydration status and macro/micronutrient deficiency.

- The health provider should include data from biochemical test (such as blood lipids and glucose and electrolyte status) in the nutritional assessment, and consider the nutritional and non-nutritional factors that may affect blood parameters. In addition, the provider should evaluate laboratory data in the context of dietary history, disease processes and treatment, hydration status, and medication usage.
- While the *Dietary Guidelines for Americans* provides general parameters for nutrient needs, assessment of such in individual patients should also be conducted via use of mathematical equations (for example Harris-Benedict or Mifflin St. Jeor) or via indirect calorimetry when available.
- Nutrition assessment techniques for specific populations (e.g., pregnant or lactating women, children, older adults) often mirrors that of the general population; however, the provider should be aware of resources that are available to assess and educate these groups accordingly.

Review Questions

1. The provider understands that when using national diet surveys to assess the nutritional status of patients the purpose of these tools is to do which of the following? (Select all that apply.)
   1. Evaluate food safety.
   2. Identify food distribution patterns.
   3. Establish dietary guidelines.
   4. Enforce food regulations on manufacturers.
   5. Justify government nutrition initiatives.

2. The provider is reviewing the dietary reference intakes with a group of students. In this presentation the provider includes information related to the recommendations for macronutrient intake. These recommendations include those related to which of the following? (Select all that apply.)
   1. protein
   2. calories
   3. vitamins
   4. fat
   5. carbohydrate

3. The provider is concerned that a new patient may be undernourished, particularly in regard to protein and calorie intake. To assess this patient completely the provider should do which of the following?
   1. Ask the patient to complete a 24-hour food intake.
   2. Calculate the patient's body mass index (BMI).
   3. Assess the patient's current intake as well as typical intake of nutrients.
   4. Review the recommendations for daily intake with the patient.

4. The provider notes that records that were sent by another provider about a new patient have notes that the patient is vulnerable to food insecurity. The best action for the provider to take based on this information is to do which of the following?
   1. Refer the patient to a local food bank or other sources of food items.
   2. Enroll the patient in a nutrition education program.
   3. Ask the patient to log intake of all food and fluids for a 7-day period.
   4. Include information on food allergies in the patient's discharge instructions.

5. When assessing a patient with marasmus, the provider would likely note which of the following?
   1. body weight within normal limits
   2. significant edema
   3. normal serum protein values
   4. dry hair that is easily plucked

6. A laboratory report reveals that a patient with congestive heart failure has a sodium level of 130 mEq/L. The provider may anticipate that the physician may order which of the following?
   1. liberal salt allowance for the diet
   2. initiation of an IV to run fluids with sodium chloride
   3. an oral and IV fluid intake restriction
   4. salt tablets to be added to the medication regimen

7. Before administering a dose of an IV diuretic, the provider notes that the patient's most recent serum potassium level is 3.2 mEq/L. The best action for the provider to take is to do which of the following?
   1. Administer the drug as ordered.
   2. Encourage the patient to drink orange juice.
   3. Notify the physician of the potassium level.
   4. Monitor the patient's intake and output.

8. A patient with no history of diabetes mellitus has a fasting blood glucose level reflecting hyperglycemia on 2 consecutive days. The best explanation that the provider can give the patient based on the information that is available?
   1. Tell the patient that the results are likely due to a laboratory error and should be repeated.
   2. Explain that the patient must be diabetic and didn't know it.
   3. Note that blood glucose levels can rise temporarily in response to acute stress.
   4. Tell the patient that the physician will order medications to help control the blood sugar.

9. The provider is working with a patient who has had a recent weight loss and is trying to gain weight. To achieve the goal of a 1 pound per week weight gain, the provider should recommend that the patient add how many calories to the daily intake?
   1. 100
   2. 300
   3. 500
   4. 700

10. A patient with a serum albumin level < 3.5 mg/dL and poor dietary intake of protein is likely to display which symptom?
    1. peripheral edema
    2. red tongue
    3. dehydration
    4. soft gums

High-Risk Assessments

14

The teen clinic van is a massive retrofitted RV with two clinic rooms and a workstation. Today we're stationed in the parking lot behind Bayview High School. After 10 minutes, a student clad in baggy black jeans and a torn white T-shirt strolls slowly towards us.

"Um, is this the health clinic?" he asks, nervously looking behind him.

"Yes it is." I lead him to one of the miniature clinic rooms and close the door. In the close quarters, it's hard to ignore the smell of cigarette smoke.

"So what brings you in today?" I ask.

He shifts nervously on the examination table, briefly making eye contact before looking down at his shoes. "I think I need to find some new friends…."

"Why do you say that?" I say.

"They're a bad influence," he says.

I sense he wants to say more, but I don't want to press him too hard. "I see. Can you tell me more about that?"

"Look, I'm trying to quit smoking. It doesn't feel good for my body, and I'm trying to make the basketball team this year…," I nod empathetically. "…and the friends I have want to smoke all the time. I don't think they'd hang out with me if I quit." This is a critical step for him—I can sense he was uneasy about coming to the clinic in the first place. This isn't a good time to "preach," but is a good opportunity to practice some *motivational interviewing*….

"How do you think you might get off cigarettes given those concerns?" He gives me a surprised look at being asked such a question. "Well…I could tell them I need to be in shape for basketball, and cigarettes make it hard to train."

"That sounds like a good plan. Can you say that to your friends without damaging your relationships?"

"I think so." He smiles, more relaxed. We have built rapport with each other. "Is there something that could help me kick the habit? I smoke two packs a day."

I explained the many options available to him—from gum to pills to the patch. Dr. Koenig reviews the use of nicotine gum while I finish his documentation. He leaves with a 4-week supply of gum and a follow up appointment. I watch him walk confidently back to class, gum in hand, and open for the world to see.

LEARNING OUTCOMES

1. Explicate the need and responsibility for assessment of high risk individuals.
2. Describe the basic information needed for assessment of various high-risk individuals and behaviors.
3. Recognize the characteristics of high-risk individuals based on an individual's history and/or specific behaviors.
4. Explain ways of formulating and asking questions that are less threatening to individuals being assessed for high risk.
5. Identify various tools and instruments that may be used when assessing specific areas of high risk.
6. Recognize physical (objective) manifestations on patient or others that indicate high-risk behaviors are directed towards self or others.

During the history taking component of the assessment, it is often necessary to obtain additional information related to specific activities and behaviors of the patient. These questions primarily relate to topics that are more sensitive in nature, but necessary to determine appropriate interventions and ways to reach the patient. The overall focus is to determine the probability that a behavior or activity has already occurred or may occur in the future and prevention of any future actions or behaviors that may result in negative or life-threatening consequences for the patient or others. As health care providers, the need for specific information outweighs the provider's comfortability in obtaining this data.

Feeling comfortable about asking questions related to the patient's personal activities and thoughts without feeling invasive takes time to develop. When engaging in these assessments, providers must emphasize confidentiality and that this information is necessary to provide comprehensive health care. Some behaviors and practices may be legally questionable, but the patient needs to be assured that this information is not being sought for any legal purposes. While confidentiality is an important concept in regard to sensitive information, all states have statutes that require health care providers to report suspected child abuse and/or neglect. Mandatory reporting of domestic violence is less clear cut and varies among states. Use of weapons or indications that the victim's life may be in danger crosses over into criminal acts that are to be reported.

The primary areas that pertain to high-risk behaviors and activities are addiction (alcohol use, drug use), sexual behavior, abuse (physical and emotional) and self-directed violence.

High-risk behaviors are defined as optional lifestyle choices and activities with uncertain outcomes that place a person at increased risk of sustaining adverse effects that may include a particular condition. Although not limited to any age category, adolescents are more prone to engage in high-risk behaviors (Kianpoor & Bakhshani, 2012), which may have adverse effects on their development or may preclude future successes and progressive development. The overall intent is to prevent high-risk behaviors or limit their effects, but that does not limit the need for assessing adults who have already succumbed to participating in these high-risk activities.

Addiction

Addiction can take many forms and individuals may become addicted to a wide variety of substances or activities. Addiction is a treatable, chronic, relapsing brain disease that results from gradual adaptations of the brain to repeated drug exposure (Contet, Kieffer, & Before, 2004) and characterized by compulsive substance seeking and use behaviors, despite harmful consequences (Feltenstein & See, 2008). Regardless of the addiction, **addictive behaviors** are described as "any activity, substance, object, or behavior that has become the major focus of a person's life to the exclusion of other activities, or that has begun to harm the individual or others physically, mentally, or socially" (Engs, 2003). While chemical addiction is known to cause physical dependence related to the release of specific substances within the brain, psychological dependence is also involved. There may also be a psychological basis for the development of a physical dependency or addiction. Addicted individuals often demonstrate common characteristics in their behavior and are as follows:

1. The person becomes *obsessed* (constantly thinks of) the object, activity, or substance.
2. They will seek it out, or *engage in the behavior even though it is causing harm* (physical problems, poor work or study performance, problems with friends, family fellow workers).
3. The person will *compulsively engage* in the activity, that is, do the activity over and over even if he/she does not want to and find it difficult to stop.
4. Upon cessation of the activity, *withdrawal* symptoms often occur. These can include irritability, craving, restlessness, or depression.
5. The person does not appear to have control as to when, how long, or how much he/she will continue the behavior (*loss of control*). For instance, he drinks six beers when he only wanted one, buys eight pairs of shoes when he only needed one, ate the whole box of cookies, and so on.
6. He/she often *denies problems* resulting from his/her engagement in the behavior, even though others can see the negative effects.
7. Person *hides the behavior* after family or close friends have mentioned their concern (hides food under beds, alcohol bottles in closets, doesn't show spouse credit card bills, etc.).
8. Many individuals with addictive behaviors report a *blackout* for the time they were engaging in the behavior (don't remember how much of what they bought, how much they lost gambling, how many miles they ran on a sore foot, what they did at the party when drinking).
9. *Depression* is common in individuals with addictive behaviors. That is why it is important to make an appointment with a physician to find out what is going on.
10. Individuals with addictive behaviors often have *low self-esteem*, feel anxious if they *do not have control over their environment*, and come from *psychologically or physically abusive families* (From *What are Addictive Behaviors?* by Ruth Clifford Engs. Reproduced by permission of R.C. Engs.).

There are two categories of addiction that are recognized: substance and process. **Substance addictions** primarily involve alcohol and various drugs, both licit and illicit. **Process addictions** include but are not necessarily limited to activities such as eating (food), sex, gambling, work, and shopping (spending) (Garrett, 2009).

The specific mechanisms leading to addiction are not completely understood, resulting in a lack of consistency in how addiction is classified and treated, as well as prevention strategies. Various etiologies and models have been developed in an attempt to understand the underlying determinants. Addiction has been interpreted as a disease, a behavioral/psychological dysfunction, and also to have a genetic basis. A broader approach to understanding addiction is to recognize it as a disorder of brain function like that of any other bodily organ dysfunction that is significantly influenced and affected by multiple personal, environmental, psychological, and physical factors, which may have nothing to do with the addiction itself but may indirectly promote or delay its behavioral expression and also determine ones recovery or remission of addiction (Garrett, 2009).

The neural processes that lead to the development of addictive behaviors are not well understood but evidence suggests it is directly related to the brain's reward system and the action of **neurotransmitters** and **neuropeptides**—dopamine, serotonin, glutamate, gamma-aminobutyric acid (GABA), and endorphins (Koob & Simon, 2009). Of these substances, dopamine is believed to play the primary role (Young, Gobrogge, & Wang, 2011). Dopamine, when released, binds with **mu opioid receptors**, which initiates the reward circuitry producing a "feel good" response or euphoria, often referred to as "a high" (Alcoholism: Clinical & Experimental Research, 2009). The continuous overstimulation and release of dopamine results in a gradual reduction in its production, which then leads to a need for an increased amount of the stimulant to bring about the same "feel good' experience in the individual. This phenomenon is referred to as one's **tolerance threshold**. If this tolerance threshold is exceeded to rapidly or too far, the individual is at risk for an overdose; in the same manner, if the threshold is reduced to rapidly, the individual is as risk for symptoms of withdrawal.

THINK LINK:* *Addiction or Dependence

Dependence is characterized by the development of tolerance and demonstrated by the development of withdrawal symptoms after use of the substance has ended. It may occur with a subset of chemical compounds that are physically or psychologically habit forming. Tolerance is evident when the body becomes less responsive to a specific amount of a substance resulting in the need to increase the amount of the substance to achieve the same effect.

Alcohol Addiction (Alcoholism)

Alcoholism is a chronic condition in which the body becomes dependent on alcohol. Although addiction to other drugs and drug trafficking have been the major focus related to the negative aspects of drug use, alcohol remains the primary drug problem in the United States. It is estimated that more than 10%–23% of alcohol consuming adults in the United States are considered to be alcoholics (Gruber, Roth, & Daley, 2010).

Alcoholic individuals demonstrate an increasing loss of control over drinking—when, how much, or how long one drinks. The individual continues to drink even when there is awareness of problems related to health, relationships, work, or finances. Alcoholism progresses through four stages, each with demonstrations of typical

Table 14-1 Stages of alcoholism

Stage 1	Craving (having a strong need or compulsion to drink) Amount and frequency increases Tolerance to alcohol (the need to increase alcohol intake to experience the same effects) Drinking for emotional escape (mood altering effects of alcohol)
Stage 2	Physical dependence (experiencing physical withdrawal symptoms [nausea. sweating, shaking] when haven't been drinking) Denial/shame (unsuccessful in attempts to stop drinking) Physical symptoms (tremors, migraines, hangovers) Begin to blame others (external factors) Drinking a few drinks before attending social functions Blacking out (not remembering conversations or commitments)
Stage 3	Having legal problems with relationships, employment, finances, or work due to drinking/frequent destructive-violent behavior Loss of interest in activities and hobbies that previously brought pleasure; avoiding family/friends Eye opener (drink when wakes—calm nerves) Feelings of guilt/remorse Gulping drinks, ordering doubles or becoming intentionally intoxicated to feel good or "normal" Unable to drink according to intentions Loss of work/job—all day drinking, need to consume alcohol to function; benders (drunk for days)
Stage 4	Storing alcohol in unusual places at home, work, or in car; need to have alcohol close at hand to get drink when needed (has to drink) DTs with hallucinations

alcoholic behaviors (Table 14-1). The most significant behavior that intersects with each stage is the increasing loss of control, or the inability to limit the amount of alcohol consumed at a given time.

It is possible to demonstrate problems with alcohol but not demonstrate all the symptoms. This is known as **alcohol abuse** meaning that one has a problem with alcohol but is not necessarily dependent on it. More than likely, alcohol abuse will eventually progress to full blown alcoholism.

While anyone may develop alcoholism, there are certain risk factors that are associated with becoming an alcoholic. These are as follows:

- Drinking on a regular basis
- Starting to drink at a young age
- Male (twice as many males are alcoholics)
- Family history (genetic predisposition)
- History of depression or other mental health problems
- Friends/close partners that drink regularly

While alcoholics frequently present with acute intoxication, it is possible for anyone who engages in social drinking to experience acute intoxication. It takes the liver approximately 90 minutes to metabolize one ounce of alcohol. Manifestations of intoxication vary and depend on the individual's **blood alcohol concentration (BAC)**.

Clinical manifestations of acute intoxication are directly related to alcohol's effect on various organs and processes. Multiple metabolic alterations are caused by alcohol intoxication and consist of hypoglycemia, lactic acidosis, hypokalemia, hypomagnesemia, and hypoalbuminemia (Vonghia et al., 2008). Hypotension and hypothermia are related to cardiovascular causes, which include tachycardia, peripheral vasodilatation, and volume depletion. Cardiac atrial and ventricular tachyarrhythmias may also occur alone or with an initial onset of atrial fibrillation.

Decreased ventilatory function and sensitivity predisposes to aspiration of foreign objects. Additionally, decreased ciliary action promotes retention of pulmonary secretions with the potential for the development of bronchitis and pneumonia. Respiratory depression is the primary cause of death from acute alcohol intoxication.

Assessment for Alcoholism

The health history is the most useful component of the individual assessment. Physical manifestations of alcoholism only become apparent when the physiological consequences of alcoholism are recognized. While early recognition and treatment of alcoholism will prevent such consequences, health care providers frequently fail to adequately recognize the existence of alcohol abuse or dependence. Why this occurs is often related to a variety of provider and patient variables. These variables are as follows:

- Patients are in denial that they may have a problem with alcohol. Patients often are able to conceal the amount and frequency of alcohol intake. The gradual onset of the condition and the body's ability to adapt to increasing amounts of alcohol also contribute to the denial of an "alcohol problem." Also, if an alcoholic is confronted, there is often denial of any excess consumption of alcohol.
- Family members also will often deny or minimize any alcohol problems. Unknowingly, they often become enablers and try to protect the family member by covering up or excusing the patient's behaviors and drinking problems.
- Health care providers often have a negative perception of individual with an alcohol problem, perceiving addiction as a character defect that is more of a socioeconomic or psychosocial problem, and not a medical problem. Additionally, alcoholics often have concomitant anti-social (criminal) behaviors and

***THINK LINK:* How Much Blood Alcohol is Required to be Considered Intoxicated?**

Blood Alcohol Concentration/ 100 mL	Social Drinker	Habitual Drinker	Effects at Specific BAC Levels	
0.00–0.05	"Sober"	"Sober"	**0.02–0.03 BAC**: No loss of coordination, slight euphoria and loss of shyness. Depressant effects are not apparent. Mildly relaxed and maybe a little light-headed. Reaction time is slowed down two times.	Most of these people appear clinically normal. Some of them have euphoria. Reaction time is slowed down two times.
			0.04–0.06 BAC: Feeling of well-being, relaxation, lower inhibitions, sensation of warmth. Euphoria. Some minor impairment of reasoning and memory, lowering of caution. Behavior may become exaggerated and emotions intensified (good emotions are better, bad emotions are worse).	
0.06–0.09	Light	"Sober"	**0.07–0.09 BAC**: Slight impairment of balance, speech, vision, reaction time, and hearing. Euphoria; judgment and self-control are reduced, and caution, reason and memory are impaired, .08 is legally impaired and it is illegal to drive at this level. You will probably believe that you are functioning better than you really are.	Loss of inhibitions, self-criticism, concentration and normal judgment. Has an exaggerated self confidence Affected coordination.
0.10–0.15	Moderate	Light	**0.10–0.125 BAC**: Significant impairment of motor coordination and loss of good judgment. Speech may be slurred; balance, vision, reaction time, and hearing will be impaired. Feeling of euphoria.	Reaction time is slowed down four times. Early ataxia, apraxia, and agraphia.
			0.13–0.15 BAC: Gross motor impairment and lack of physical control. Blurred vision and major loss of balance. Euphoria is reduced and dysphoria (anxiety, restlessness) is beginning to appear. Judgment and perception are severely impaired.	Reaction time is slowed down further.
0.16–0.20	Strong	Moderate	**0.16–0.19 BAC**: Dysphoria predominates, nausea may appear. The drinker has the appearance of a "sloppy drunk."	Reaction time is slowed down even further.
0.21–0.25	Strong–Very Strong	Moderate–Strong	**0.20 BAC**: Felling dazed, confused, or otherwise disoriented. May need help to stand or walk. If you injure yourself you may not feel the pain. Some people experience nausea and vomiting at this level. The gag reflex is impaired and you can choke if you do vomit. Blackouts are likely at this level so you may not remember what has happened.	Ataxia, agraphia, apraxia. Coordination severely affected. Emotional instability. Balance disturbances. Apathy and emotional eruptions. Numbness and slowed reaction to pain stimuli. Partial amnesia.
0.26–0.30	Very Strong	Strong–Very Strong	**0.25 BAC**: All mental, physical, and sensory functions are severely impaired. Increased risk of asphyxiation from choking on vomit and of seriously injuring self by falls or other accidents.	Worsening of the above mentioned. Total loss of muscle coordination. Apathy and sometimes stupor. Total loss of orientation; amnesia.
			0.30 BAC: Stupor. You have little comprehension of where you are. You may pass out suddenly and be difficult to awaken.	
0.31–0.40	Stupor–Coma	Very Strong–Stupor	**0.35 BAC:** Coma is possible. This is the level of surgical anesthesia.	Stupor followed by coma. General anesthesia and paresis. Suppression of the vital centers in the brain with cardio respiratory collapse and death.
0.41–0.50	Coma–Death	Coma–Death	**0.40 BAC and up**: Onset of coma, and possible death due to respiratory arrest.	

psychiatric conditions (depression and anxiety), and may be seen as demanding and wasting social resources. They may also be perceived to be weak and incapable of overcoming their condition.

- Health care providers may also be unaware of appropriate screening methods for determining alcohol related problems. Simply inquiring as to "How much do you drink?' is ineffective and only about 50% sensitive in detecting any alcohol problems. There may also be failure to specify the quantity of alcohol taken in. General responses such as two to three drinks per day may mean something totally different to the provider than it does to the patient.

THINK LINK: A Standard Drink

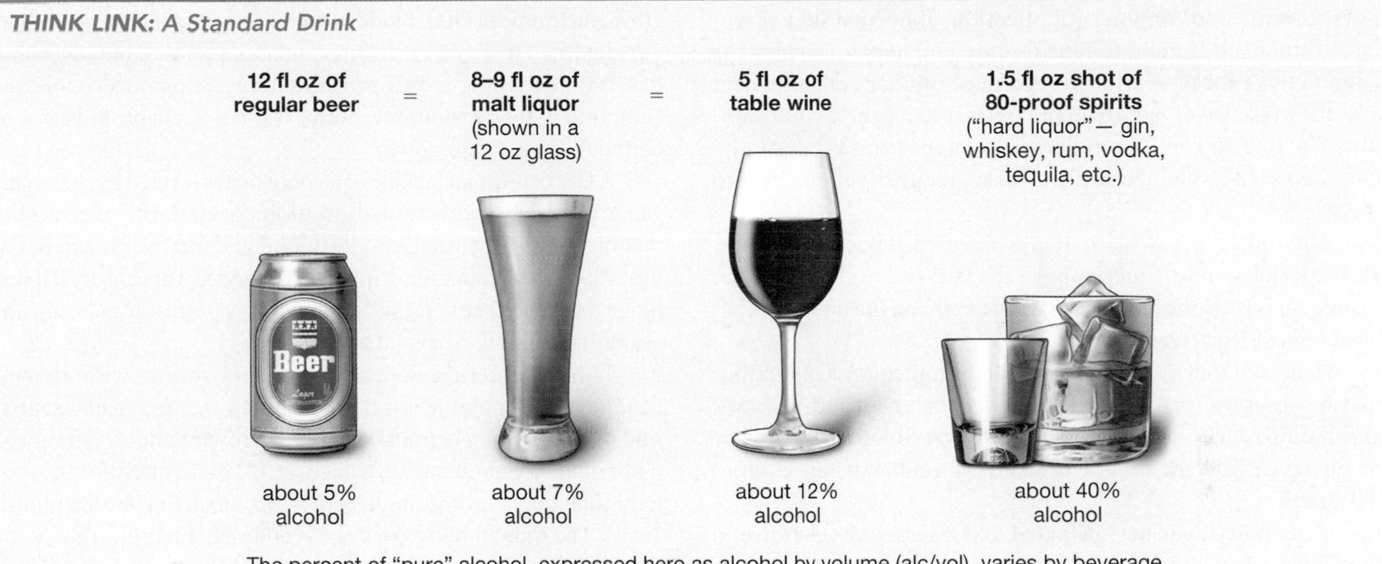
12 fl oz of regular beer
=
8–9 fl oz of malt liquor (shown in a 12 oz glass)
=
5 fl oz of table wine
1.5 fl oz shot of 80-proof spirits ("hard liquor"— gin, whiskey, rum, vodka, tequila, etc.)
Beer
about 5% alcohol
about 7% alcohol
about 12% alcohol
about 40% alcohol
The percent of "pure" alcohol, expressed here as alcohol by volume (alc/vol), varies by beverage.

Source: http://www.niaaa.nih.gov/alcohol-health/overview-alcohol-consumption/standard-drink

Screening patients

Screening for potential alcohol dependence is the primary means to determine who is at risk and what further interventions may be necessary. There are several screening tools that appropriately and effectively identify high-risk individuals. These tools include the **CAGE** questionnaire, the **TACE** questionnaire, the **AUDIT** questionnaire, and the **Michigan Alcoholism Screening Test (MAST)**.

The CAGE questionnaire is a four-question test, making it very easy to incorporate into the overall history of the patient. It is also the best-known and most-studied screening tool for alcoholism. The four questions for the CAGE screening tool are as follows:

1. Have you ever felt the need to **C**ut down on you drinking?
2. Have people **A**nnoyed you by criticizing your drinking?
3. Have you ever felt bad or **G**uilty about your drinking?
4. Have you ever had a drink first thing in the morning (**E**ye opener) to steady your nerves or get rid of a hangover?

Patients who respond with a "yes" to two questions are highly likely to have a drinking problem. The sensitivity of the CAGE questionnaire has been reported to be 75%; however, it has been found to be lower than that, particularly among females and the elderly (Thompson, Lande, & Kalapatapu, 2010).

The TACE questionnaire is similar to the CAGE. It also consists of four questions with the likelihood of alcoholism increasing with every yes response. The TACE questions are as follows:

1. How many drinks does it **T**ake to get you high?
2. Have people **A**nnoyed you by criticizing your drinking?
3. Have you ever felt you ought to **C**ut down on your drinking?
4. Have you ever had a drink first think in the morning to steady your nerves (**E**ye opener)?

The CAGE and TACE screening tools are easy and quick to administer and require only verbal responses from the patient. More involved screening tools have been developed to obtain a broader perspective on the patient's drinking behaviors and patterns, but they are pencil and paper tests that require the patient to take more time to provide answers. These two screening instruments are the Michigan Alcoholism Screening Test (MAST) and the Alcohol Use Disorders Identification Test (AUDIT).

The MAST [Revised] was developed to provide a quantifiable measure of alcohol dependence. It consists of 22 yes/no questions related to alcohol consumption and related behaviors, and can be completed within 15 minutes (Counseling Resource Research Staff, 2013). The test is scored by giving 1 point for each "yes" answer [1 and 4 given 1 point for "no" answer]. Scores of 0-2 indicate no apparent problem, 3-5 indicate early or middle problem drinker, 6 or greater indicate a problem drinker.

The AUDIT was developed to screen for individuals who demonstrate difficulty in alcohol consumption and more specifically to help providers identify individuals who would benefit from decreasing or stop drinking (Table 14-2).

High-risk alcohol behaviors are categorized as (1) hazardous drinking—alcohol consumption that increases the risk of harmful consequences for the user or others, (2) harmful use—alcohol consumption that results in consequences to physical and mental health, and (3) alcohol dependence—a cluster of behavioral, cognitive, and physiological phenomena that may develop after repeated alcohol use (Babor, Higgins-Biddle, Saunders, & Monteiro, 2001). The AUDIT consists of 10 self-report questions and may be administered as an interview or a paper and pencil version. Scores and interpretation of the AUDIT is provided in Table 14-3.

In addition to screening for alcohol use and abuse, it is also important to recognize physical manifestations and laboratory tests that can be useful in screening individuals. Physical manifestations include conjunctival injection, abnormal skin vascularization, hand tremor, tongue tremor, and hepatomegaly. The conjunctiva is observed for the extent of capillary engorgement and the presence of jaundice. In contrast to a pearly white conjunctiva, there is capillary engorgement appearing as burgundy-colored vascular elements as well as a greenish-yellow tinge to the sclera.

Abnormal skin vascularization is observed as fine, reddish blue, wiry arterioles, most commonly on the face and neck. Other skin manifestations are the presence of "goose flesh" on the neck and scattered yellowish patches.

Hand and tongue tremor may be intermittent. A hand tremor may be observed with the arms extended, half bent at the elbows, and hands rotated towards the midline. A tongue tremor may be observed with the tongue protruding a short distance out of the mouth.

Hepatomegaly is best palpated and assessed in relationship to volume (size) and consistency. An increase in volume may be measured by finger breadths below the costal margin. Consistency may be described as firm, hard, or very hard. (Further information is found in Chapter 28.)

Laboratory tests are used to identify biomarkers, which are physiological determinants of alcohol exposure or ingestion, and most likely indicators of an alcohol abuse condition. By themselves, they should not be considered diagnostic, but together with the history, examination, and self-reported behaviors provide data to consider the individual at high risk for alcoholism.

Alcohol biomarkers are categorized as direct or indirect. Indirect biomarkers are used to detect for any toxic effects of alcohol on any organs or physiological chemical processes. These indirect biomarkers and their use are identified and described in Table 14-4.

Direct biomarkers of alcohol are blood levels of alcohol and ethyl glucuronide (EtG). Blood alcohol levels and its interpretations are identified in Table 14-4. Direct measurement of blood alcohol has its limitations as it only provides information on alcohol consumption in the previous few hours; it is not a reliable indicator of chronic alcohol consumption.

EtG is a direct metabolite of alcohol that is formed by the conjugation of ethanol with activated glucuronic acid. Shortly after alcohol ingestion, EtG is detectable in the blood and may be present in the urine up to 5 days after the drinking has stopped, particularly if it was binge drinking. These results make EtG a significant indicator for alcohol consumption beyond a few hours.

Thiamine deficiency is often a comorbidity with alcohol dependency. Thiamine is a B-vitamin (B_1) that plays an essential role in cellular biochemical reactions, growth, and development (Subramanya, Subramanian, & Said, 2010) particularly for the synthesis of brain neurotransmitters (Martin, Singleton, & Stuemhofel, 2004). The human body does not synthesize thiamine, thus, deficiencies of thiamine are primarily due to inadequate dietary intake, a situation frequently associated with alcoholism.

Thiamine deficiency primarily affects the cardiovascular and neurological systems and gives rise to a neurological condition known as **Wernicke Korsakoff syndrome (WKS)**. WKS is comprised of two components: Wernicke's encephalopathy (WE), and Korsakoff's psychosis (KP). Initial manifestations of WE include mental confusion, vomiting, horizontal nystagmus, paralysis of ocular movements, and inability to coordinate movements of lower

Table 14-2 Personnel, settings, and groups considered appropriate for a screening program using the AUDIT

Setting	Target Group	Screening Personnel
Primary care clinic	Medical patients	Nurse, social worker
Emergency department	Accident victims, Intoxicated patients, trauma victims	Physician, nurse, or staff
Physician's room/surgery	Medical patients	General practitioner, family physician or staff
General hospital wards, out-patient clinic	Patients with hypertension, heart disease, gastrointestinal, or neurological disorders	Internist staff
Psychiatric hospital	Psychiatric patients, particularly those who are suicidal	Psychiatrist, staff
Court, jail, prison	DWI offenders, violent criminals	Officers, counselors
Other health-related facilities	Persons demonstrating impaired social or occupational functioning (e.g., marital discord, child neglect, etc.)	Health and human service workers
Military Services	Enlisted men and officers	Medics
Work place Employee assistance program	Workers, especially those having problems with productivity, absenteeism or accidents	Employee assistance staff

Source: From "Box 1" on page 9 from AUDIT: The Alcohol Use Disorders Identification Test, Guidelines for Use in Primary Care, 2nd edition, 2001 by T. F. Babor, J. B. Saunders, M. G. Monteiro, J. C. Higgins-Biddle. Reproduced with permission of the publisher, World Health Organization, Geneva. http://whqlibdoc.who.int/hq/2001/WHO_MSD_MSB_01.6a.pdf. Accessed 06/09/2012.

Table 14-3 The Alcohol Use Disorders Identification Test

Interview Version

Read questions as written. Record answers carefully. Begin the AUDIT by saying, "Now I am going to ask you some questions about your use of alcoholic beverages during this past year." Explain what is meant by "alcoholic beverages" by using local examples of beer, wine, vodka, etc. Code answers in terms of "standard drinks." Place the correct answer number in the box at the right.

1. How often do you have a drink containing alcohol?
   (0) Never (Skip to Qs 9–10)
   (1) Monthly or less
   (2) 2 to 4 times a month
   (3) 2 to 3 times a week
   (4) 4 or more times a week ☐

2. How many drinks containing alcohol do you have on a typical day when you are drinking?
   (0) 1 or 2
   (1) 3 or 4
   (2) 5 or 6
   (3) 7, 8, or 9
   (4) 10 or more ☐

3. How often during the last year have you been unable to remember what happened the night before because you had been drinking?
   (0) Never
   (1) Less than monthly
   (2) Monthly
   (3) Weekly
   (4) Daily or almost daily ☐
   Skip to Questions 9 and 10 if Total Score for Questions 2 and 3 = 0

4. How often during the last year have you found that you were not able to stop drinking once you had started?
   (0) Never
   (1) Less than monthly
   (2) Monthly
   (3) Weekly
   (4) Daily or almost daily ☐

5. How often during the last year have you failed to do what was normally expected from you because of drinking?
   (0) Never
   (1) Less than monthly
   (2) Monthly
   (3) Weekly
   (4) Daily or almost daily ☐
   Record total of specific items here
   If total is greater than recommended cut-off, consult User's Manual.

6. How often during the last year have you needed a first drink in the morning to get yourself going after a heavy drinking session?
   (0) Never
   (1) Less than monthly
   (2) Monthly
   (3) Weekly
   (4) Daily or almost daily ☐

7. How often during the last year have you had a feeling of guilt or remorse after drinking?
   (0) Never
   (1) Less than monthly
   (2) Monthly
   (3) Weekly
   (4) Daily or almost daily ☐

8. How often do you have six or more drinks on one occasion?
   (0) Never
   (1) Less than monthly
   (2) Monthly
   (3) Weekly
   (4) Daily or almost daily ☐

9. Have you or someone else been injured as a result of your drinking?
   (0) No
   (2) Yes, but not in the last year
   (4) Yes, during the last year ☐

10. Has a relative or friend or a doctor or another health worker been concerned about your drinking or suggested you cut down?
   (0) No
   (2) Yes, but not in the last year
   (4) Yes, during the last year ☐

Source: From "Box 4" on page 17 from *AUDIT: The Alcohol Use Disorders Identification Test, Guidelines for Use in Primary Care*, 2nd edition, 2001 by T. F. Babor, J. B. Saunders, M. G. Monteiro, J. C. Higgins-Biddle. Reproduced with permission of the publisher, World Health Organization, Geneva. http://whqlibdoc.who.int/hq/2001/WHO_MSD_MSB_01.6a.pdf. Accessed 06/09/2012.

Table 14-4 Direct biomarkers of alcohol are blood alcohol levels and ethyl glucuronide (EtG)

Biomarker (Indirect)	Type of Drinking Characterized	Sensitivity/Specificity	Used Clinically in U.S.	Comments
Aspartate Amino Transferase (AST, Alanine) Amino Transferase (ALT)	Unknown, but heavy and lasting for several weeks (chronic alcohol abuse)	Moderate/Moderate ALT less sensitive than AST	Yes (best in adults ages 30–60 years of age)	Primarily reflects liver damage that is often related to alcohol
Carbohydrate Deficient Transferrin (CDT)	Heavy alcohol use (at least five drinks per day for approximately 2 weeks)	Moderate/High (equal to or possibly slighter better than GGT—more specific)	Yes (likely less sensitive in women and younger individuals)	Biomarker of resuming heavy drinking after a period of abstinence
Gamma Glutamyl Transferase (GGT)	Chronic alcohol abuse (probably at least five drinks/day for several weeks)	Moderate/Moderate (as screen for heavy drinking)	Yes (best in adults 30–60 years of age)	Probably most common biomarker—reflects liver damage related to alcohol consumption
Mean Corpuscular Volume (MCV)	Unknown, but heavy and lasting for several months (chronic alcohol abuse)	Moderate/Moderate (sensitivity slightly lower GGT as screen for heavy drinking); higher sensitivity in women	Yes (best in adults 30–60 years of age)	Poor biomarker for relapse due to sluggish response to drinking
Biomarker (Direct)	**Type of Drinking Characterized**	**Sensitivity/Specificity**	**Used Clinically in U.S.**	**Comments**
Blood alcohol level (BAC)	Alcohol intake within the past hours (not a good indicator of chronic, excessive alcohol intake)	High/High	Yes	Direct measurement of alcohol level in blood
Ethyl Glucuronide (EtG), ethyl sulfate (EtS)	Possibly as little as one drink; monitoring sobriety/relapse	High/High (direct analysis of nonoxidative alcohol destruction)	New (but promising biomarker)	More research needed (can be detected in urine up to 5 days after binge drinking)
Phosphatidyl ethanol (PEth)	Possibly three to four drinks/day for several days	High/High	New (but promising biomarker)	Linear dose-response relationship with recent drinking levels

extremities (ataxia) (Martin et al., 2004; Nguyen-Khoa, Cope, Busschots, & Vallee, 2010).

An estimated 80%–90% of alcoholics with WE progress to Korsakoff's psychosis, a chronic neuropsychiatric syndrome associated with irreversible brain damage and death. The brain damage (neuronal atrophy) is primarily found in the cerebellum, thalamus, hypothalamus, and brain stem. Manifestations of KP include retrograde and anterograde amnesia. Retrograde amnesia is a loss of memory related to past information whereas anterograde amnesia is a lack of acquisition of recent information. These characteristic memory alterations may also be described as alcohol amnestic disorder (Martin et al., 2004). Once an individual has developed KP, reversal of manifestations related to brain damage is not very successful.

Alcohol Poisoning

Alcohol poisoning is a potentially fatal condition that results from ingesting large amounts of alcohol in a short period of time and in greater amounts than the body can metabolize and eliminate. The most common cause of acute alcohol poisoning is binge drinking, which often occurs in college students at weekend parties. Binge drinking is considered to be rapidly downing five or more drinks for males or 4 or more for females in rapid succession.

Alcohol poisoning is also caused by ingestion of other types of alcohol that may be found in household products. In most instances, ingestion of other alcohols is accidental. The two most common household alcohols are methanol and isopropyl alcohol. Methanol is an ingredient of antifreeze, paints, and solvents. Isopropyl alcohol is rubbing alcohol generally used for its bactericidal properties. Ethanol is also used in cough syrups, mouthwash, and baking flavorings.

Major symptoms of alcohol poisoning consist of the following:

- Confusion or stupor
- Vomiting
- Seizures
- Slow breathing (< eight per minute), or irregular breathing
- Cyanosis of or pale skin
- Hypothermia (low body temperature)
- Unconsciousness (Mayo Clinic Staff, 2010)

Death from alcohol poisoning occurs when the depressant effects of alcohol affect the respiratory center of the brain, causing the individual to pass out and stop breathing. Comatose individuals may also aspirate their own vomit, which contributes to death by causing drowning. Even if the individual survives the acute episode of alcohol poisoning, the potential remains for permanent brain damage.

***THINK LINK:** Risk Factors for Alcohol Poisoning*

	Alcohol Poisoning Risk Factors
Age	Young teens and college students more likely to binge drink; however, the majority of deaths occur in individuals 35–54 years of age.
Gender	Boys/men more likely to have alcohol poisoning; women/girls more vulnerable to effects of alcohol.
Size/weight	Smaller/thinner builds absorb alcohol faster.
Health	Conditions such as heart disease/diabetes make individual more vulnerable to damaging effects of alcohol.
Food consumption	Food in stomach slows absorption of alcohol into bloodstream.
Drug use	Alcohol and drugs (even some prescriptions) don't mix; greatly increase risk for AP.
Type of alcohol	Takes liver 1 hour to metabolize one standard drink; the more one drinks, the faster the accumulation of alcohol in the blood.
Tolerance level	Individuals who drink more often may develop tolerance to alcohol, but this does not completely eliminate risk for AP.
Rate of consumption	The faster one drinks, the greater the risk of AP.
	College Drinking Risk Factors
Division I schools	Students who attend schools with prominent sports teams are more likely to drink.
Geography	Students attending college in Northeast and North Central regions drink more. Students in rural areas also drink more.
Freshman	College students drink more heavily than peers who did not continue education.
Greek presence	Schools with prominent systems have more problem drinking.
Living in dorms	Students who live in dorms have a higher risk of alcohol abuse.

Alcohol Withdrawal

In addition to screening for the presence of alcohol dependency, recognizing the signs and symptoms associated with alcohol withdrawal is also important. Individuals going through withdrawal may present themselves to the emergency department, or it may occur in individuals who are be hospitalized for other reasons and go into withdrawal. Alcohol withdrawal is an emergency situation and early recognition is essential.

Withdrawal signs and symptoms are caused by physical withdrawal and emotional withdrawal. Physical withdrawal occurs primarily with alcohol, opiates, and tranquilizers, whereas emotional withdrawal occurs primarily with cocaine, marijuana, and Ecstasy (methamphetamine). Alcohol withdrawal is the most life-threatening substance withdrawal. The signs and symptoms associated with physical withdrawal make death from alcohol more common than any other substance withdrawal and carries a mortality rate of 20% (McKeown & West, 2010). Manifestations of physical and emotional withdrawal are listed in Table 14-5.

Alcohol withdrawal may occur in four stages: (1) tremulousness, (2) seizures, (3) hallucinations, and (4) delirium tremens. Not everyone will experience all four stages and progression is not necessarily is this particular order.

- *Tremulousness* is characterized by a tremor of the hands or legs. This is particularly observed when the hand is extended and the patient attempts to hold it still. This stage is frequently accompanied by anxiety and restlessness.
- *Seizure* is the second stage and occurs in approximately 25% of individuals experiencing withdrawal. The seizures are frequently generalized with a loss of consciousness and uncontrollable shaking of the body.
- *Hallucinations* also affect about 25 % of individuals going through withdrawal. The most common type of hallucination is visual with the individuals seeing insects or worms crawling over them or on walls. This may be accompanied by a tactile hallucination with the individuals also "feeling" the crawling sensation on their skin. Auditory hallucinations may also occur, but not as frequently as visual and tactile.
- *Delirium tremens* (DTs) is the most dangerous stage of alcohol withdrawal and occurs in approximately 5% of individuals going through withdrawal. Manifestations of DTs may be observed about 48–72 hours after drinking has stopped. The individual remains awake but profoundly confused. Other manifestations of DTs are agitation, delusions, sweating, hallucinations, rapid heart rate, and high blood pressure. This stage is a true emergency and 35% of individuals in stage 4 will die if treatment is not initiated promptly. Even with appropriate intervention, there is still a high mortality rate.

The Clinical Institute Withdrawal of Alcohol Scale Revised (Table 14-6), is an assessment tool that can be used to monitor individuals who are experiencing alcohol withdrawal.

Drug Addiction

Addiction to drugs is much the same as addiction to alcohol. The drug addict demonstrates the same addictive behaviors as the alcoholic and the same processes within the brain create the addiction

Table 14-5 Effects of alcohol on the body of patients with alcohol withdrawal syndrome

System Affected/Cancer Risk	Effect	Mechanism
Central nervous system	Impaired judgment and memory Impaired balance and motor coordination Sleep disturbances Peripheral neuropathy Alcohol-related psychiatric disorders: Dementia Depression Hallucinations Wernicke encephalopathy Korsakoff syndrome	Effects are due to the combination of the direct toxic effects of alcohol on neural tissue, thiamine deficiency, and nutritional deficits.
Cardiovascular	*Beneficial effects* Possible reduction in risk for death due to cardiovascular conditions (one to two drinks per day over long periods) *Deleterious effects* Decreased myocardial contractility Cardiomyopathy Dysrhythmias Mild to moderate hypertension	Beneficial effects occur because alcohol increases levels of high-density lipoprotein and decreases platelet aggregation. Deleterious effects are due to the direct toxic effects of alcohol on cardiac muscle and the vasopressor effects of ethanol.
Hematopoietic	Increased size of red blood cells (mean corpuscular volume) Decreased production of white blood cells Thrombocytopenia	Effects are due to the direct toxic effects of alcohol on bone marrow that cause suppression and malnutrition-related folate deficiency.
Gastrointestinal	Esophageal inflammation Mallory-Weiss lesions Esophageal varices Acute pancreatitis Alcohol-induced hepatitis Cirrhosis	Effects occur because alcohol stimulates an increase in acid production and causes direct damage of the gastric mucosal barrier; cirrhosis occurs as a result of fatty buildup in the liver.
Musculoskeletal	Alcoholic myopathy Lower bone density Increased risk of fractures	Effects on muscle tissue are due to the direct toxic effects of alcohol on muscle tissue. Skeletal effects are due to the direct toxic effects of alcohol on osteoblasts.
Cancer risk	Increased risk for cancer of the following: Breast Esophagus Oral cavity Overall risk of cancer is 10 times greater in persons who are population alcoholic than in the general	Alcohol is not a direct-acting carcinogen but one of its metabolites, acetaldehyde, may act as a tumor promoter. Chronic alcohol use also causes increased degradation of retinol by the liver and results in vitamin A deficiency, which is associated with an increased incidence of cancer.

to drugs as they do to alcohol. In addition to alcohol, common drugs that cause addiction are as follows:

- Opiate and opioid analgesics
  - Morphine and codeine (naturally occurring opiates)
  - Semi-synthetic opioids (heroine, oxycodone, hydrocodone)
  - Synthetic opioids (fentenyl, meperidine, methadone)
- Stimulants
  - Amphetamines/methamphetamines
  - Cocaine
  - Nicotine
- Sedatives and hypnotics (sleep-inducing medications) following
  - Barbiturates
  - Benzodiazapines
  - Quinazolinone sedative/hypnotics

Table 14-6 Clinical institute withdrawal assessment of alcohol scale, revised (CIWA-Ar)

Patient:		Time: (24-hour clock, midnight = 00:00)	
Date:			
Pulse or heart rate, taken for one minute:		Blood pressure:	
Nausea and Vomiting—Ask "Do you feel sick to your stomach? Have you vomited?" Observation.		**Tactile Disturbances**—Ask "Have you any itching pins and needles sensations, any burning, any numbness, or do you feel bugs crawling on or under your skin?" Observation.	
0	no nausea and no vomiting	0	none
1	mild nausea with no vomiting	1	very mild itching, pins and needles, burning or numbness
2		2	mild itching, pins and needles, burning or numbness
3		3	moderate itching, pins and needles, burning or numbness
4	intermittent nausea with dry heaves	4	moderately sever hallucinations
5		5	severe hallucinations
6		6	extremely severe hallucinations
7	constant nausea, frequent dry heaves and vomiting.	7	continuous hallucinations
Tremor—Arms extended and fingers spread apart. Observation.		**Auditory Disturbances**—Ask "Are you more aware of sounds around you? Are they harsh? Do they frighten you? Are you hearing anything that is disturbing to you? Are you hearing things that you know aren't there?" Observation.	
0	no tremor	0	not present
1	not visible, but can be felt fingertip to fingertip	1	very mild harshness or ability to frighten
2		2	mild harshness or ability to frighten
3		3	moderate harshness or ability to frighten
4	moderate, with patient's arms extended	4	moderately severe hallucinations
5		5	severe hallucinations
6		6	extremely severe hallucinations
7	severe, even with arms not extended	7	continuous hallucinations
Paroxysmal Sweats—Observation.		**Headache Fullness in Head**—Ask "Does your head feel different? Does it feel like there is a band around your head?" Do not rate dizziness or lightheadedness. Otherwise, rate severity.	
0	no sweat visible	0	not present
1	barely perceptible sweating, palms moist	1	very mild
2		2	mild
3		3	moderate
4	beads of sweat obvious on forehead	4	moderately severe
5		5	severe
6		6	very severe
7	drenching sweats	7	extremely severe
Agitation—Observation.		**Orientation and Clouding of Sensorium**—Ask "What day is this? Where are you? Who am I?"	
0	normal activity	0	oriented and can do serial additions
1	somewhat more than normal activity	1	cannot do serial additions or is certain about date
2		2	disoriented for date by no more than two calendar days
3		3	disoriented for date by more than two calendar days
4	moderately fidgety and restless	4	disoriented for place and/or person
7	paces back and forth during most of the interview, or constantly thrashes about		
			Total CIWA-Ar Score
	Patients scoring less than 10 do not usually need additional medication for withdrawal		Rater's Initials
			Maximum Possible Score: 67

Source: The CIWA-Ar is not copyrighted and may be reproduced freely. Sullivan, J.T.; Sykora, K.; Schneiderman, J.; Naranjo, C.A.; and Sellers, E.M. Assessment of alcohol withdrawal: The revised Clinical Institute Withdrawal Assessment for Alcohol scale (CIWA-Ar). *British Journal of Addiction, (84)*1989:1353–1357,

Drugs that have a high potential for abuse and addiction are restricted in their availability and use. The Drug Enforcement Agency (DEA) is responsible for restriction guidelines and has identified these drugs by five schedules (Table 14-7).

Not all potentially addicting drugs are placed in a schedule. Nicotine, alcohol, inhalants, and dextromethorphan (cough suppressant) are not scheduled drugs. Caffeine is also considered a drug that can be addictive. Scheduled drugs are manufactured according to strict standards so that variations in the concentration of drug are minimized. Drugs that are "street "manufactured may have wide variations in their concentration, which may lead to accidental overdoses (Table 14-8). Accidental overdoses often result in the death of the user.

Assessment for Drug Use/Abuse

Assessment for drug use/abuse is much the same for alcohol use/abuse. The most reliable indicator is the patient's response to verbal questioning. Denial of a drug problem may also be present in the patient and family members or the patient is trying to hide the behaviors and manifestations of drug abuse/addiction.

During the history taking, additional questions may be necessary to determine the presence of drug abuse/addiction. Screening tools have been developed to obtain the information needed to help identify individuals at risk for abusing drugs or becoming addicted to them. The **CRAFFT** Quiz is a seven-question, yes/no assessment tool designed to identify high-risk individuals. While it is identified as a personal assessment tool, it may also be helpful for the provider to use. The CRAFFT Quiz parallels the CAGE assessment tool for alcoholism. The questions for the CRAFFT Quiz are as follows:

1. Have you used drugs or alcohol in the past 12 months?
2. Have you ever ridden in a CAR driven by someone (including yourself) who was "high" or had been using alcohol or drugs?
3. Do you ever use alcohol or drugs to RELAX, feel better about yourself, or fit in?
4. Do you ever use alcohol or drugs while you are by yourself (ALONE)?
5. Do you ever FORGET things you did while using alcohol or drugs?
6. Does your family or FRIENDS ever tell you that you should cut down on your drinking or drug use?
7. Have you ever gotten in TROUBLE while you were using alcohol or drugs?

The **Drug Abuse Screening Test (DAST)** is another tool that may be used for identifying high-risk individuals. The DAST is a 20-question, yes/no assessment tool that is also described as a "self-test" but does not necessarily exclude it from use during history taking. The DAST test is not to be used for alcohol abuse problems.

Drug delivery systems include taking them orally, by injection (IV mainlining), or by inhalation. Inhalation of drugs may be accomplished by breathing in fumes, gases, or powdered substances. Inhalation also includes smoking. Different methods of taking drugs may result in observable manifestations related to the method.

Specific signs of drug use or abuse may be easily observed during the provider–patient interaction. This interaction may take place in an emergency setting, clinical setting, or public setting. Characteristic manifestations of drug use or abuse are identified in Table 14-9.

Sexuality/Sexual Behavior

Sexuality and sexual behavior are an essential component of an individual's identity and composition and are therefore considered to be an inherent behavior of human function. Even though it is considered a natural and expected function of an individual, there are activities that may be considered to be high-risk behaviors and may have negative or unwanted outcomes. Engaging in sexual activity requires appropriate and responsible decision making; however, it is also possible for individuals to allow emotions and desires to overcome decision-making abilities and make choices to engage in high-risk sexual activity.

Sexual Health

Sexual health encompasses a broad spectrum of components that interact and influence the individual. These components consisting of, but not limited to, include sexual attitudes, sexual desires, sexual behaviors engaged in, sexual preferences, sexual identification, and

Table 14-7 DEA drug schedules

Schedule I	Have the greatest potential for abuse. They have specific storage requirements and are also limited in their production.	Heroine, lysergic acid diethylamide (LSD)
Schedule II	Only available by prescription and are unrefillable. Must be a written order. May result in severe physical or psychological dependence.	Morphine and opium. Meperdine, methadone, oxycodone, fentanyl Stimulants for ADHD: amphetamine, methamphetamine, methylphenidate Others: Cocaine, amobarbital, gluethimide, pentobarbital
Schedule III	Are refillable up to 6 months and may be ordered orally. May result in moderate/low physical dependence or high psychological dependence.	Combination products with less than 15 mg of hydrocodone per dosage unit or not more than 90 mg of codeine per dosage unit. Buprenorphin products.
Schedule IV	Low potential for abuse in proportion to amount of substances.	Alprazolam, clonazaoam, diazepam, lorazepam, midazolam, temazepam, and triazolam
Schedule V	May be available as over the counter. Mostly used for coughing, diarrhea, and pain.	Preparations containing not more than 200 mg of codeine

Table 14-8 Examples of "street" manufactured drugs

Club Drug	Street Name	Action	Effects
Methylenedioxymethamphetamine (MDMA)	Ecstasy, E, X, XTC, Adam, Clarity, Lover's Speed	Amphetamine-based hallucinogenic type of drug taken orally, usually in tablet/capsule form	Increases chances of dehydration, hypertension, heart/kidney failure, increased core body temperature. Long-term effects include confusion, depression, sleep problems, anxiety, paranoia, and loss of memory.
Gamma-hydroxybuterate (GHB) (initially used to treat narcolepsy)	Grievous Bodily Harm, G, Liquid Ecstasy, Georgia Home Boy	CNS depressant that is usually ingested in liquid, powder, tablet, capsule form	Slows heart/breathing rates to dangerous levels Sedative/euphoric effects that begin 10–20 minutes after taking Use with alcohol increases potential harm. Overdose can occur quickly death.
Methamphetamine	Speed, Ice, Chalk, Meth, Crystal, Crank, Fire, Glass	CNS stimulant, in pill, capsule, or powder form that can be snorted, injected, or smoked	Demonstrates signs of agitation, excited speech, lack of appetite, and increased physical activity. Often leads to drastic weight loss, violence, psychotic behavior, paranoia, and possible damage to heart or nervous system.
Ketamine	Special K, K, Vitamin K, Cat Valium	Injectable anesthetic used predominately by veterinarians; available as liquid/powder that can be snorted or smoked, sometimes with marijuana	Impaired attention, leaning/memory function. In larger doses may cause delirium, amnesia, impaired motor function, hypertension, and depression.
PCP	Angel Dust, Hog, Love Boat	Powerful anesthetic used in veterinary medicine	Similar to Ketamine, but stronger.
Rohypnol (not approved for medical use in U.S.)	Roofies, Rophies, Roche, Forget-me-pill	Tasteless/odorless sedative, easily soluble in carbonated beverages; toxic effects aggravated by concurrent use of alcohol	Antegrade amnesia, which makes it popular as "date rape" drug. Can cause decreased blood pressure, drowsiness, visual disturbances, dizziness, and confusion.
Lysergic acid diethylamide (LSD)	Acid, Boomers, Yellow Sunshines	Hallucinogen that causes distortions in sensory perception; usually taken orally as tablet or capsule	Effects often unpredictable, varying on dose, environment, and user. Dilated pupils, higher body core temp, increased heart rate/blood pressure, sweating, dry mouth, and tremors. Can cause numbness, weakness, and nausea. Long-term effects include persistent psychosis and hallucinogenic persisting perception disorder.

Table 14-9 Characteristic manifestations of drug use or abuse

Drug	Symptoms of Withdrawal	Time Frame
Opiates/narcotics (heroine, morphine, codeine)	Mild—runny nose, sweating, yawning, anxiety, and drug cravings Severe—anxiety, insomnia, dilated pupils, increased heart rate/blood pressure, abdominal cramps (nausea, vomiting, and diarrhea), tremors, and bone/muscle pain Individual in recovery from heroine dependence may demonstrate deficits in executive control functions (frontal cortex)	4–10 days
Stimulants (cocaine, amphetamines, methamphetamines)	Excessive tiredness (fatigue), anxiety, intense cravings and depression In some instances may include suicidal ideation and attempts, paranoia, and decreased contact with reality (psychosis)	1–2 weeks
Depressants (barbiturates, benzodiazepines)	Mild—restlessness, anxiety, sleep difficulties, and sweating Serious—hallucinations, tremors, seizures, increased blood pressure/core body temperature	1–4 weeks; 3–5 weeks with tapering

sexual function (Benuto, 2010). The World Health Organization's working definition of sexual health is a

> state of physical, emotional, mental and social well-being in relation to sexuality; it is not merely the absence of disease, dysfunction or infirmity. Sexual health requires a positive and respectful approach to sexuality and sexual relationships, as well as the possibility of having pleasurable and safe sexual experiences, free of coercion discrimination, and violence. For sexual to be attained and maintained, the sexual rights of all persons must be respected, protected, and fulfilled. (World Health Organization, 2002, http://www.who.int/reproductivehealth/topics/sexual_health/sh_definitions/en/, accessed 06/09/2012)

Healthy People 2020 has identified 10 Leading Health Indicators, which are high-priority public health issues in the United States. One of these indicators is "Responsible Sexual Behavior." The specific goal for this indicator is to "promote healthy sexual behaviors, strengthen community capacity, and increase access to quality services to prevent sexually transmitted diseases, and their complications" (U.S. Department of Health and Human Services, 2009).

By acting responsibly, the intended outcomes are to decrease the incidence of unintended and adolescent pregnancies, detect prenatal conditions and STIs early and provide appropriate treatment, decrease infertility rates, and decrease transmission of HIV through detection and treatment. These outcomes maybe achieved through the following objectives:

- Objective FP—1: Increase the proportion of pregnancies that are intended.
- Objective FP—2: Reduce the proportion of females experiencing pregnancy despite use of a reversible contraception.
- Objective FP—7: Increase the proportion of sexually active males/females aged 15–44 years who received reproductive health services.
- Objective FP—9: Increase the proportion of adolescents aged 15–17 years and under who have never had sexual intercourse.
- Objective FP—10: Increase the proportion of sexually active persons aged 15–19 years who use condoms to both effectively prevent pregnancy and provide barrier protection against disease.
- Objective FP—11: Increase the proportion of sexually active persons aged 15–19 years who use condoms and hormonal or intrauterine contraception to both effectively prevent pregnancy and provide barrier protection against disease.

At-Risk Individuals

While anyone has the potential for sexual dysfunction, there are certain individuals who are high risk for experiencing one. As with many problems or dysfunctions, they exist on a continuum of severity and degree of impact on one's optimum functioning.

Adolescents and Teens

Sexuality and teenagers have always been considered a volatile combination. High-risk behaviors are often started during adolescence (Pakpreo, 2005). Unwanted pregnancies among teenage females have remained a consistent concern related to appropriate health care for the teen mother as well as the unborn child. While it is an expected norm that teenagers will refrain from engaging in sexual intimacy, very little is done to help them understand the total ramifications of teenage parenthood. While the frequency of teen pregnancies has been steadily declining, the most recent studies have found that they are on the increase. While teenage sexual activities and behaviors are not approved or sanctioned by society in general, reality provides evidence that they do and will occur, resulting in unplanned and often unwanted pregnancies.

Trends (from 1991 to 2009) in the Youth Risk Behavior Survey indicate that

- rates of sexual activity have decreased (54 to 46 percent).
- rates of sex with more than four persons have decreased (19 to 14 percent).
- rates of condom use at last intercourse increased from 1991 to 2003 (46 to 63 percent) but remained stable from 2003 to 2009 at 61 percent.

Recent statistics on teen pregnancies show that during 2006 and 2007 the birth rate among 14- to 15-year-olds increased by 3% in 2006 and 1% in 2007. The 2006 increase was the first to happen since a 14-year downward trend that began in 1991. Specific causes for this increase are difficult to determine with any specificity.

The most recent statistics reveal that nearly half (48%) of 15- to 19-year-olds have engaged in sex at least once. At age 15, only 13% of teens have experienced a sexual encounter; however by the age of 19, the incidence increases dramatically to 70%. The average age for one's first sexual experience is 17. Even though teens may be putting off sex until they are older, they are also delaying marriage, which increases their risk for unplanned pregnancies and contracting a sexually transmitted infection. The percentages of teens who are sexually experienced vary according to race, ethnicity, and gender.

Overall, non-Hispanic white teens report being more sexually experienced than non-Hispanic black and Hispanic peers. Non-Hispanic black teen males are the most likely to report being sexually experienced. In both non-Hispanic black and Hispanic teens, males are more likely to report being sexually active than females. Within the non-Hispanic white teen population, there is no difference between males and females reporting being sexually experienced.

THINK LINK: Teens and Oral Sex

Sexual activity among teens is not a recent development; it has been occurring for centuries. While in the past many teenagers were married before they turned 16, it is no longer socially acceptable for marriage to take place in the early teen years. Even though early marriages no longer take place, the desire for sexual activity has not diminished.

The teenage birth rate has been declining, but is that an indication that teenagers are less likely to engage in sexual activity? While the decline in birth rate may be an indication that sexual intercourse may be declining, recent studies indicate that oral sex is increasing among teens. Surveys of teens related to oral sex have found that teens consider oral sex to be safer than intercourse and that engaging in oral sex is not actually "having sex." Oral sex is perceived to be less objectionable than intercourse related to one's moral or religious beliefs and values. Female teens also believe that they retain their virginity (technical virgins) if they only engage in oral sex.

Oral sex is also practiced to prevent pregnancy, and is also perceived to be less emotionally damaging than intercourse and believed to protect one against contracting an STI. There is no evidence yet that supports the belief that oral sex is less emotionally damaging, and while the risk of contracting an STI may be less, there still remains the possibility of contracting an STI, particularly HIV, herpes, Chlamydia, and gonorrhea (Cichocki, 2013).

While nearly half of 15- to 19-year-olds report having a sexual experience, the greater majority of those (35%) also report being sexually active, meaning that during the past 3 months they have had sex with one or more individuals. There is no statistical difference between males and females. Differences do exist between race/ethnicity with 37% of Hispanic students and 46% of non-Hispanic black students report being sexually active.

A major factor in addressing the issue is accepting the fact that it occurs and that even "respectable" teens are vulnerable to the hormone surge of puberty. Teens are also less likely to have appropriate education in regards to pregnancy prevention and thus come to rely on multiple myths that continue to circulate. Some of the more common myths are as follows:

- Pregnancy won't occur with the first time; it takes more than one instance for pregnancy to happen.
- Pregnancy won't occur if
  - the male pulls out before ejaculation or doesn't go in all the way.
  - sex takes place while standing up.
  - the female takes the top position.
  - sex occurs in a hot tub or swimming pool.
  - the female does jumping jacks after sex.
  - the female douches, bathes, or urinates immediately after sex.
  - both are virgins.
  - the female doesn't have an orgasm or they (male and female) don't have simultaneous orgasms.
  - the female pushes really hard on her belly button or makes herself cough/sneeze right after sex.
  - the female is on her period or has never had her period.
- Condoms are reusable.
- Plastic wrap may substitute for a condom.

Contraceptive use The most common contraceptives used among teens are condoms and birth control pills (BCP). Overall, statistics indicate a decline in contraceptive use. Use of condoms gradually increased between the years 1991–2005 (46.2% → 62.8%) and then went down slightly to 61.5% in 2007. Use of BCP experienced a more significant decrease going from a high of 20.8% in 1991 to 16% in 2007. During that same time, abortions also decreased in the overall population and among teens.

Along with unwanted pregnancies, sexually active teens place themselves at a higher risk for developing a sexually transmitted infection (STI).

Sexually Transmitted Infections According to the Centers for Disease Control and Prevention, sexually transmitted infections (STIs) continue to be a significant challenge to the public health of the United States. It is estimated that annually 19 million new infections occur, with approximately 50% of them in young adults aged 15–24. In addition to young individuals, females also represent a large population of those affected.

As their identification indicates, sexually transmitted infections are spread and acquired almost exclusively through sexual activity. Failure to recognize and treat STIs contributes significantly to health care costs and often irreversible complications, such as the following:

- Reproductive health, fetal, and perinatal problems
- Cancer
- Aiding and abetting the spread of HIV virus

Chlamydia continues to be the highest reported incidence with approximately 1,100,000 cases identified in 2007. In spite of this large number, even more new cases remain undiagnosed. Often, there are no symptoms that contribute to the large number of unreported cases. Failure to recognize and treat chlamydia affects females more significantly than males. Untreated chlamydia in females may result in pelvic inflammatory disease, which can cause infertility, ectopic pregnancies, and chronic pelvic pain. Males may experience infection of the epididymis and urethra, but rarely have any significant long-term effects. While all ethnic groups are affected, the incidence of chlamydia in disproportionately higher in African American, Native American, and Hispanic females.

The higher incidence of chlamydia in young females necessitates annual screening of sexually active females under age 26. Older females with new or multiple sex partners should also be screened. Failure to screen appropriate individuals is often due to a lack of awareness among providers and/or lack of resources for screening. Including a chlamydia screening with the Pap test has been recommended as a way to increase the percentage of females who have been screened.

Screening and treatment of males is also important to reduce the incidence of chlamydia. Reinfection of diagnosed and treated females by infected males is a significant concern.

Gonorrhea is the second-most frequently reported STI in the United States. Rates of gonorrhea have remained relatively stable over the past 10 years, but are still at too high a level. Similar to chlamydia, gonorrhea is considerably under diagnosed and under reported. Those that are reported represent about one-third of the actual cases. Consequences of untreated gonorrhea are similar to those with chlamydia.

A major concern in treatment of gonorrhea is the development of antibiotic resistance, which has occurred with some antibiotics. Both chlamydia and gonorrhea infection increase the possibility of contracting HIV with the development of AIDS.

While screening for STIs is essential to reducing their incidence, education regarding sexual activity and its consequences is equally essential. Where this occurs is highly controversial. Many parents think that they are the only ones who should talk to their children regarding sex and sexual activity. There are those that also feel that abstinence education is the only type of sex education that is appropriate. It is significant to realize that other countries that have a more open and accepting attitude regarding sexuality and sex activity have lower incidences of STIs and teen pregnancy than the United States.

Older Adults (Individuals with Chronic Disease)

Older adults are at risk for some type of sexual dysfunction for a variety of reasons. It is a common myth that sexual desire and engaging in sexual activity is not important to the older adults (Wilmoth, 2007). While females do lose their ability to become pregnant, males retain their ability to impregnate a female. There are instances where postmenopausal females have become pregnant and have given birth; however, this ability requires medical intervention to allow it to occur.

While older adults are at risk for sexual dysfunction, rarely is the cause directly related to aging. Some conditions become more prevalent as the individual ages (erectile dysfunction, vaginal dryness), but are not necessarily only seen in these individuals. It is also rare that only one individual in the relationship demonstrates a sexual dysfunction. Sexual dysfunctions of couples are often complex, circular, and infrequently expose a clear causal or consequential association (Gregoire, 1999).

A major cause of sexual dysfunction in older adults is the presence of a chronic illness, with either or both individuals affected. With individuals experiencing a longer life, the incidence of chronic illness in older adults is a major condition. Sexual dysfunction in individuals with chronic disease may result from the condition itself or from management and/or treatment of it. Common conditions associated with sexual dysfunction include arthritis, diabetes, heart conditions, and cancer. Additionally, individuals may experience more than one symptom or condition that may interact with each other, resulting in a greater negative effect on the individual. Groups of three of more symptoms that interrelate with each other are identified as *symptom clusters* (Wilmoth, 2007).

Cancer as a chronic disease is the most common condition associated with sexual dysfunction, particularly those that affect the reproductive systems of both genders (Krebs, 2007). Individuals of all ages are susceptible to developing a cancer related sexual dysfunction. Many of these cancers are associated with alterations of body structures, which often lead to issues of self-image, self-esteem, as well as fears for one's life (Krebs, 2008).

Assessing Sexuality and Sexual Behaviors

Assessment of sexuality and sexual behavior is a topic that makes many individuals uncomfortable and may be considered taboo by some (Benuto, 2010). While this is understandable, reckless sexual behavior may have serious if not life-threatening consequences, making it an essential area to be assessed.

A common reason providers identify for avoiding assessing sexual behavior is often a lack of time or a lack of preparation in dealing with these issues. Another reason for avoidance is the assumption that the client is also uncomfortable with the topic so it is best to not embarrass or make the client uncomfortable. Contrary to this assumption is the fact that a large percentage of clients are comfortable with this topic and think that it is important to assess this subject (Nusbaum & Hamilton, 2002).

A major reason for avoiding taking a sexual health history is equating sexuality with sex. While sex and sexual activity are a component of sexuality, it is not the only part. Even if an individual does not engage in sexual activity, he or she still remains a sexual individual. Sexuality is a part of being human, and as such cannot be ignored or not recognized. Sexuality as a broader concept, encompasses gender, gender identify and roles, sexual orientation, eroticism, pleasure, intimacy, and reproduction of the human race (Wilmoth, 2007).

Healthy sexuality has been described and defined as being comprised of eight specific components:

- *Nurturing:* The ability to care for self and to accept caring from others
- *Sensuality:* An awareness of senses (e.g., temperature, texture, color, sound taste, and smell)
- *Sense of self:* The capacity to know and express desires, wants, and areas of discomfort
- *Relationship sexuality:* The ability to sustain warm and caring friendships that are not erotic with both the same and opposite gender
- *Partner sexuality:* A special intimacy with a partner that is clearly erotic
- *Nongenital sexuality:* The exploration of all the ways to be sexual without involving genital contact
- *Genital sexuality:* The ability to abandon self to passion in a temporary surrender of ego and control via genital stimulation
- *Spiritual sexuality:* An extension of the search for meaning and spirituality in a partnership (Marich-Merkin, 2011)

A significant barrier to discussing sexual health is that there is no standard for what is normal. Everyone develops his or her own ideas and attitudes towards what constitutes normal or acceptable sexual behaviors. Thus, the freedom to discuss sexual health issues is hindered by the fear of being judged or labeled as some type of "deviant." Attitudes and opinions related to what is acceptable behavior is frequently influenced by religion as well as social norms and morals. While these sources of influence are significant in socializing one into a culture and society, they can also be a source of misinformation and negative attitudes and perceptions, and may take the form of mandates as to what are acceptable and appropriate.

Just as there are no universal standards or norm for sexual behaviors, there are also no universal standards or norms for how sexuality is expressed. Again, there are social and religious opinions as to how sexuality is expressed, but there is no set standard for correct expression. Maleness and femaleness are expressed in forms of dress, activities, interests, abilities, and so forth. Unfortunately, if individuals do not fit the accepted manner for gender expression, they are often subjected to taunts, bullying, and marginalization, as well as violent threats against their personhood.

While the majority of the health history related to systems is not influenced by an individual's choice or control, there is an element of choice and control in regards to sexual activity and behavior systems. An individual does not have a choice in how the pulmonary system, cardiovascular, or neurological system functions. Much of this activity is unconsciously controlled. It is possible to exert some conscious control under certain conditions, but by default, unconscious mechanisms will take over at some point. A major growth and development milestone is learning how to control certain bodily functions, but it is primarily to delay certain functions or activities.

In contrast, there is very minimal unconscious control over sexual activity and behavior. For the most part, it is a conscious decision as to how and when sexual behavior and activity will occur, as well as expression of one's sexuality. It is this ability to choose that hinders a non-biased or non-prejudiced open discussion related to sexual health. The client may feel judged because of certain choices, and the examiner may feel uncomfortable inquiring about these choices.

A lack of knowledge related to sexual functioning and activity is also a factor in why there is hesitancy to perform a sexual health history. Examiners often indicate that a lack of preparedness and/or lack of knowledge in regard to sexual problems as a significant factor in their avoiding taking a sexual health history (Shell, 2007). Conversely, the patient may feel a lack of knowledge related to sexuality and sexual functioning and not want to risk exposing this deficit.

While the sexual health history is important in identifying primary dysfunction related to sexual activity, behaviors, and expression, the provider must also be aware of secondary sexual dysfunction that may be related to specific disease processes or pharmacological intervention.

Before asking the patient to provide information regarding one's sexual behavior, the patient should be informed as to the need for these questions. Discuss with the patient that while sexual activity is very personal in nature, the intent is not to be voyeuristic, but is as much a part of the individual as all the other topics and systems that are assessed, so questions regarding sex and sexuality should as natural to ask as it is to ask about elimination habits (Nusbaum & Hamilton, 2002). It is important to assure the patient that all of this information is confidential and will only be shared with other members of the health care team. The primary need for this information is to prevent certain consequences (infectious diseases) related to certain sexual behaviors.

How questions are framed and presented to the patient will help in obtaining this information. As with all components of a health history, open-ended questions are the most appropriate in obtaining the appropriate data. The inquiries should also be framed around the concepts of **universality**, **ubiquity**, and **unloading**. Framing questions from this perspective implies that sexual activity and behaviors are not unique or limited to certain individuals and that you as a provider are concerned with what the patient's experience has been. For example, it is not uncommon for young males to experiment or have been asked to engage in male with male sexual activity. To obtain this information, the question may be presented as "It is common for males of your age to consider experimenting with or have been asked to engage in male with male sex; what has been your experience with this?" In this manner, if the patient may have experienced this, he is provided with a situation that allows him to admit that this may be true, but that it doesn't mean that he is a deviant or that he is the only one that this has happened to. It also indicates that the provider is willing to talk about this subject if the patient wants to pursue the issue any further.

Another approach would be to indicate the wide range of experiences regarding certain topics or activities. "Some young males have strong desires to experience male with male sex, some have no desire at all and some have a moderate desire, what has been your experience?"

Due to the personal nature of this topic, it may take the patient a little bit longer to respond to these questions. It may take some time for the patient to muster the courage to respond to the questions. This is a time when the provider needs to be comfortable with silence, allowing the patient as much time as needed to formulate a response. It may be that the patient doesn't how to express experiences or actions. There may be embarrassment at not knowing the appropriate terminology or descriptions. Encourage the patient to put it in his or her own words. Reassure that this information is confidential and will not be judged for "rightness or wrongness," but used only for determining the risk for actual or potential sexual health problems. Also, maintaining eye contact with the patient is a way to demonstrate acceptance and encouragement to proceed with responses to the questions.

Sexual History

When and where the sexual history is done within the comprehensive health history is not important. It would be appropriate to make it a component of the overall initial patient's medical history, or it could be a part of the genito-urinary history. Where ever it is done, approach the topic in a matter-of-fact manner, indicating that this is just another part of the overall history. While it is important to let the patient know what topic the questions will be related to, introduction of each topic allows the provider to introduce the sexual health component in the same manner as each other topic area. It is also tempting to preface the sexual health component with an apology for having to ask these types of questions. This may "excuse" the provider for having to do this, but also sends the message that this is a topic that shouldn't have to be discussed. This sends a message to the patient that the provider really doesn't want to explore this area and discourages the patient from bringing out any concerns or questions.

What questions to ask varies from individual to individual. A standardized form may be available or developed to assist in asking the appropriate questions. These are helpful in assuring that all the appropriate information is obtained. One non-standardized format to assist in developing questions is to use the 5Ps.

1. Past STIs
2. Pregnancy history/plans
3. Partners (how many, gender, frequency)
4. Practices (sexual; oral, anal, toys)
5. Prevention (STIs/HIV; awareness of risk for contracting STIs, how transmitted, ways to prevent?)

To obtain as complete a history as possible keep in mind the following considerations and primary factors for taking a sexual history:

- *Make no assumptions.* Request information related to number and gender of partners, as well as specific sexual practices.
- *Be clear when requesting information about specific activities/behaviors.* While it may be more comfortable for the provider to use medical terms for certain practices, it is highly unlikely that the patient will know what information is being requested. Common terminology is more likely to be understood by the patient. If necessary, practice saying the terms when alone to make it easier to use them for the history.
- *Be tactful and respectful.* It may be necessary to use a translator if there may be a language barrier. It will most likely put the patient at ease in trying to understand and respond to the questions. Make sure that the translator is aware of the nature of the questions and is able to translate appropriately. It will also be helpful if the translator is of the same gender as the patient.
- *Be nonjudgmental.* Recognize the patient's anxieties as well as your own. Also recognize your own biases and assumptions and make a conscious effort to not let them interfere with your questions and responses. Also avoid use of value-laden language. Use the term "partner" rather than spouse, husband or wife, boyfriend or girlfriend. Avoid terms such as "adultery, affair, infidelity," and the like. (Corso et al., 2007).

Violence

Violence is considered the "intentional use of physical force or power, threatened or actual, against oneself, another person, or against a group or community that either results in or has a high likelihood of resulting in injury, death, psychological harm, maldevelopment or deprivation" (Krug, Dahlberg, Mercy, Zwi, & Lozano, 2002). Violence has an adverse effect on the health and welfare of all Americans caused by premature deaths, disability, medical costs, and lost productivity (Corso et al., 2007). Violence is demonstrated in many forms by various individuals.

Abuse

Abuse in its broadest interpretation is the inappropriate use or action on the part of one individual to unfairly or improperly gain some form of benefit, often at the expense of the other individual. It is often aggressive in nature, associated with behavior that is forceful, hostile, or attacking that often physically harms the other individual;

however, not all abuse is physically harmful. Nonphysical abuse often takes the form of psychological or emotional harm, which can be as devastating as physical abuse.

THINK LINK: Rule of Thumb

In colonial America, it was sanctioned for a husband to punish or beat his wife for various indiscretions. The only stipulation was that the stick that was used for administering the punishment could not be any thicker that the husband's thumb. Thus, the common phrase "a rule of thumb" has its origin in an early form of legal administration of violence.

While various forms of abuse have more recently been the focus of awareness through headlines, legislation, and health care, it is not anything new. The overall basis for abuse is the need for one person to have dominance over one or many individuals, which spans throughout history, cultures, and organizations.

Domestic violence is another broad term that is frequently used to identify spousal or partner abuse, and more specifically is referred to as **intimate partner violence**. With this distinction, domestic violence can also include child abuse and elder abuse.

Intimate Partner Violence

Intimate partner violence (IPV) is a significant threat to the health of millions of Americans that is inclusive of individuals within all social strata and socioeconomic status. IPV includes harm or injury that can be physical, sexual, or psychological in nature from a current or previous spouse or partner and occurs in relationships that involve the same or opposite gender. It varies on a continuum of frequency and severity, ranging from one physical encounter to constant severe battering. The Centers for Disease Control (CDC) have described four types of IPV:

- *Physical violence* in the intentional use of physical force with the potential for causing death, disability, injury, or harm.
- *Sexual violence* is divided into three classifications:
  - Use of physical force to compel a person to engage in a sexual act against his/her will, whether or not the act is completed
  - Attempted or completed sex act involving a person who is unable to understand the nature or condition of the act, to decline participation, or to communicate unwillingness to engage in the sexual act
  - Abusive sexual contact
- *Threats of physical or sexual violence* use words, gestures, or weapons to communicate the intent to cause death, disability, injury, or physical harm.
- *Psychological/emotional violence* involves trauma to a victim caused by acts, threats of acts, or coercive tactics. Psychological/emotional abuse can include, but is not limited to humiliating the victim, controlling what the victim can and cannot do, withholding information from the victim, deliberately doing something to make the victim feel diminished or embarrassed, isolating the victim from friends and family, and denying the victim access to money or other basic resources (Centers for Disease Control and Prevention, 2010b).

The abused and the abuser are not easily described or recognized. More often than not, it's the neighbor next door, a high-ranking official in the community or other organization, a well-respected church member, or a variety of other friends and acquaintances. There is also no way to differentiate what characterizes an abuser or the abused.

Factors that contribute to IPV come from a combination of individual, relational, community, and societal conditions. Some of these contributing factors include the following:

Individual:

- Low self-esteem/academic achievement, having few friends, isolated from others, emotional dependence, and insecurity
- Young age and/or aggressive and delinquent behavior as a youth
- Alcohol/drug use/dependence
- Anger, hostility, depression, antisocial/borderline personality traits
- Prior history of being physically abusive, experiencing poor parenting/physical discipline, physical/psychological abuse as a child
- Belief in strict gender roles (male dominance), desire for power/control in relationships
- Low income, unemployed

Relational:

- Relationship conflicts/fights, tension, and other struggles
- Relational instability—divorces/separations
- Dominance/control of the relationship by one partner over the other
- Economic stress
- Unhealthy family relationships and interactions

Community:

- Poverty and associated factors
- Low social resources/support—lack of institutions, relationships, norms that shape a community's social interactions
- Absent or ineffective sanctions against IPV (not willing to get involved or intervene in witnessed violence)

Societal:

- Traditional gender norms/expectations (at home mothers, submissive to husband; working fathers to support family/make decisions) (Centers for Disease Control and Prevention, 2010c)

The common perception of IPV is that of a dominant male abusing a submissive female. Most of the attention paid to and portrayal of IPV in the media perpetuates this image. There is, however, increasing recognition and data to support the fact that there are male victims of IPV within heterosexual relationships.

Effects of IPV

Statistics on IPV and sexual violence vary depending on how each is defined and interpreted. The most recent findings estimate that 18.3% of women and 1.4% of men in the United States report that they have experienced rape at some point in their lives (Black et al., 2011). The types of rape reported were complete or incomplete forced penetration and alcohol- or drug-facilitated completed penetration. The most common perpetrator of IPV was found to be an intimate partner or acquaintance. A small majority of males reported that they were commanded to penetrate someone else. Again, the perpetrator was identified as an intimate partner or acquaintance.

Sexual coercion (unwanted penetration after being pressured in a nonphysical way) was reported by 13% of females and 6% of males. Approximately twice the number of females and males indicated they experienced unwanted sex. A striking difference between males and females is the age at which they were first raped. The majority of females (79.6%) reported their first rape before the age of 25, whereas males (27.8%) reported their first rape occurred at 10 years or younger.

Stalking an individual is also considered a form of sexual violence. While not as prevalent as other forms of sexual violence, 16.2% of females and 5.2% of males reported being victims of stalking to the point where they feared for their own life or that someone close to them would be harmed or killed. Again, the most common perpetrator of stalking of women (66.2%) was a current or former intimate partner; and for males it was an intimate partner (41.4%) or an acquaintance (40%).

The consequences of IPV and sexual violence not only impact the individual but also impact society in terms of costs. Estimated costs in 2003 (updated from 1995 costs) exceeded $8.3 billion. The contributing costs included $460 million for rape, $6.2 billion for physical assault, $461 million for stalking, and 1.2 billion for the value of lives that were lost (Centers for Disease Control and Prevention, 2010a). Individuals who are victims of IPV lose approximately 8 million days of paid work (32,000 full-time jobs) and nearly 5.6 million days of household productivity.

In addition to the social impact, there are serious consequences related to the individual's physical and psychological health. The most serious consequence is the loss of one's life. In 2005, 1510 individuals (329 males, 1181 females) were murdered as a result of IPV. Physical injuries such as scratches, bruises, and welts were reported by 42% of females and 20% of males who were physically attacked since 18 years of age. Most of the reported injuries were minor. More severe physical injuries related to IPV depend on the frequency and severity of the physical attacks and may include bruises, stab wounds, gunshot wounds, internal injuries, head trauma, broken bones, back/pelvic pain, and headaches. Chronic stress has also been found to impact the endocrine and immune system resulting in a variety of conditions which may include fibromyalgia, irritable bowel syndrome, gynecological/gastrointestinal disorders, low-birth-weight babies or perinatal death, sexually transmitted infections including HIV/AIDS, central nervous system disorders, and cardio and peripheral vascular disorders. Children of the couple may also become injured during the physical altercation.

Psychological consequences result from the emotional or psychological abuse that coexists with physical violence. Psychological or emotional abuse may occur without physical violence or abuse, but it is rare for physical abuse or violence to occur without some psychological impact. The psychological consequences may include anxiety/depression, anti-social behaviors, suicidal behaviors (females), low self-esteem, inability to trust/fear of intimacy, symptoms of post-traumatic stress disorder (emotional detachment, sleep disturbances, flashbacks). In addition, female victims are more likely to engage in more high-risk health behaviors such as smoking, alcoholism, drug abuse, and suicide attempts. Victims of abuse are also more likely to experience social isolation.

Assessment of IPV

Multiple standardized forms exist for assessment of IPV and vary in the number of questions that are asked. Regardless of which form an agency may use or one's personal preference for a particular tool, there are some basic areas of concern that should be addressed to assess IPV in any situation.

Actions: "Are you now or have you ever been hit, slapped, kicked, thrown, or attacked by your partner or ex-partner? (If children involved, "Have your children ever witnessed any of these actions against you?" "Have any of these actions been demonstrated against your child/children?") "How often have these events occurred; are they happening more often?"

"Are you now or have you ever been told that you were no good, felt intimidated, threatened, or yelled at by your partner or ex-partner? If threatened, was a weapon or other instrument used? If not threatened, is there easy access to any weapon in the residence?"

"Are you now being or have you ever been forced to engage in sexual activities or sex that you did not want to do? Are there other activities that you are forced to do that you do not want to?"

Safety: "Do you feel safe in your present environment?"

"Do you feel that you (and your children) are in any type of danger?"

"Are you able to go places by yourself or does your partner accompany you at all times?"

"Do you feel safe going home at this time?"

Plan: "Have you ever thought about or attempted to leave your partner?"

"What are your concerns if you would leave your partner?"

"What do you think is keeping you in this relationship?"

"If you don't have a plan, do you think that you could come up with one?" "Are you able to identify some place that you could go to or someone who would be willing to help you?"

While appropriate questions and strategies have been described, there are still instances where there is failure to identify incidences of abuse. Opportunities for meaningful communication related to abuse are often missed due to provider errors, such as questioning the patient in the presence of a third party, failure to acknowledge disclosure of abuse, lack of assessment of safety or level risk, and failure to link the patient with available resources (Rhodes et al., 2007).

In contrast to provider errors, there are also instances of commendable communication efforts in response to disclosure of abuse. These responses consisted of allowing the patient to talk about the experience, determining the safety of the patient and environment, counseling, providing information on law enforcement and legal options, bringing in a social worker, demonstrating empathy and concern, providing helpful opinions, and reinforcing the importance of follow up with referrals (Rhodes et al., 2007).

Childhood Maltreatment

Childhood maltreatment includes all types of abuse and neglect of a child under the age of 18 by a parent, caregiver, or another individual in a custodial role (e.g., clergy, coach, or teacher). Childhood maltreatment is a significant social issue and has been the focus of increasing concern (Teicher, Anderson, & Polcari, 2012).

Recognition of child abuse as abuse and a major social problem is a relatively recent development. Child abuse has existed throughout history; but it wasn't until 1874, when the head of the New York

Society for the Prevention of Cruelty to Animals used its criteria to intervene on behalf of a neglected child, that child abuse was recognized. That same year, the New York Society for the Prevention of Cruelty to Children was founded. Children, however, were still not protected from child labor that required long working hours under harsh conditions.

Child abuse, as defined by federal legislation (The Child Abuse Prevention and Treatment Act) is considered, at a minimum, to be as follows:

- Any recent act or failure to act on the part of a parent or caretaker which results in death, serious physical or emotional harm, sexual abuse or exploitation; or
- An act or failure to act which presents an imminent risk of serious harm

In most instances, these harmful acts are caused by parents or other caregivers, not harm caused by other individuals (acquaintances or strangers).

Each state is given the responsibility for developing its own definition of child abuse within the parameters established by the federal government. In general, there are four recognized categories of childhood maltreatment; however, states are not required to include them as part of their definition. These four categories are as follows:

- *Physical abuse* is willful or non-accidental physical injury inflicted onto the child by a parent, caregiver, or other individual who is given responsibility for the child. Physical abuse may take the form of punching, beating, kicking, biting, shaking, throwing, stabbing, choking, hitting, burning, or otherwise harming the child. Injuries from any of these actions are considered abuse regardless if there was no intent to harm the child (Figure 14-1). Physical discipline (spanking, paddling) is not considered abuse if it was reasonable and caused no bodily harm.
- *Neglect* is the failure to provide for the shelter, safety, supervision, and nutritional needs of the child. Child neglect of any type is generally considered as criminal behavior. Neglect may take the form of physical, educational, or emotional. **Physical neglect** results from refusal or delay in obtaining health care, abandonment, inadequate supervision, expulsion from home, or refusal to permit a runaway to return home. **Educational neglect** results from permission for chronic truancy, failure to enroll a school-age child in school, and failure to attend to special educational needs. **Emotional neglect** results from a significant nonrecognition of a child's need for affection, failure to obtain needed psychological care, spousal abuse or parental substance abuse in presence of a child, and permission for the child to use alcohol or drugs.

  Abandonment is frequently defined as a form of neglect. A child is considered abandoned when the identity of the parents or their location is not known, the child has been deserted and left alone in circumstances that result in harming the child, or the parent/caregiver fails to maintain contact with the child or provide reasonable support during a specified time period.

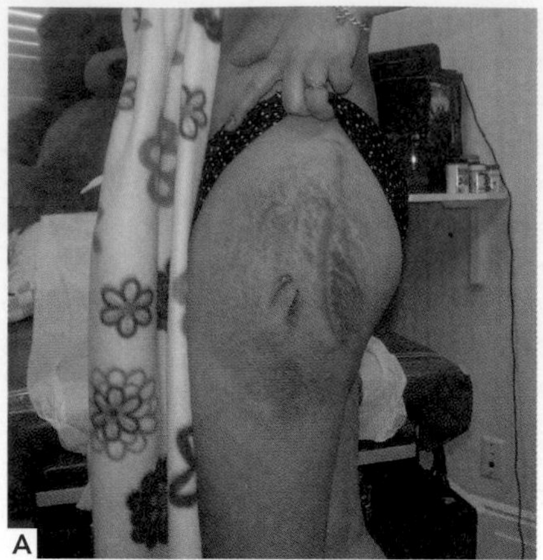

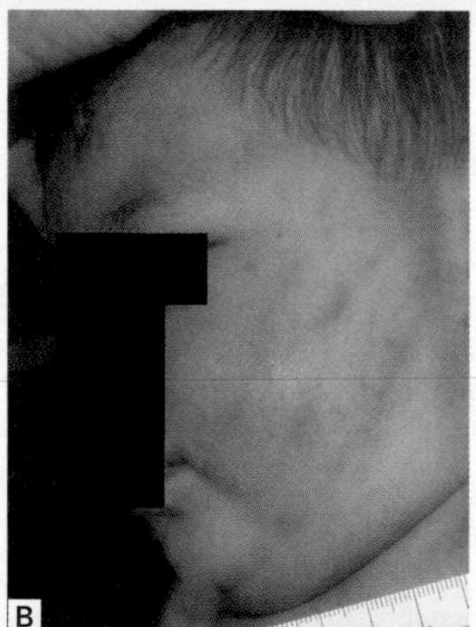

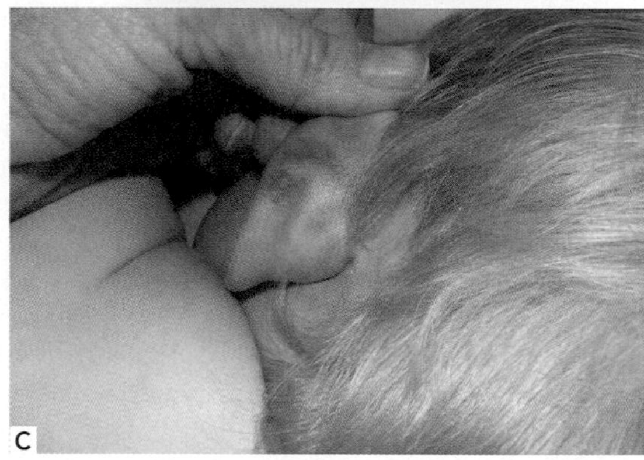

FIGURE 14-1A–C Examples of child abuse
Source: (Photos courtesy of the Center for Safe and Healthy Families at Primary Children's Medical Center, Salt Lake City, UT)

  Substance abuse is also considered a form of neglect in many states. Instances where child abuse or neglect occurs because of substance abuse include the following:

  - Prenatal exposure of a child to harm due to the mother's use of an illegal drug or other substance
  - Manufacture of methamphetamine in the presence of a child
  - Selling, distributing, or giving illegal drugs or alcohol to a child
  - Use of controlled substance by a caregiver that impairs the caregiver's ability to adequately care for that child (Child Welfare Information Gateway, 2008b)

- *Sexual abuse* is involvement of a child in sexual activity for which consent cannot be given, is beyond the child's developmental age, is unable to comprehend, and/or goes against the law or social society taboos. Sexual abuse consists of any activity that exploits a child for one's sexual gratification. Touching a child to express affection or to take care of hygienic needs is considered acceptable—the main difference related to touching activities is whether the individual's intent is to become sexually aroused or to sexually arouse others.

  Sexual abuse encompasses a wide range of activities. Obvious acts of sexual activity with a child are considered abuse. Related behaviors include excessive touching, which may include fondling a child's genitalia, prolonged kissing, cuddling, or French kissing. Looking at a clothed or unclothed child for sexual arousal purposes is also considered abuse. This may also involve taking photographs or filming of a child. Exposing a child to erotic material, which includes excessive nudity, photos, videos/DVDs are also forms of abuse. Collecting or providing pictures, videos/DVDs of children in suggestive poses or naked is illegal and may result in prosecution. Overt interest in or obsession of children, particularly naked or engaged in sexual activity with the intent to become sexually aroused is identified as **pedophilia**. In extreme instances pedophiles will seek out opportunities to engage in sexual relations with children.
- *Emotional abuse* is a form of child abuse; however, it is more difficult to identify and document. Emotional abuse is also referred to as psychological or mental abuse and is characterized by behaviors that may damage or undermine the child's emotional development or sense of self-worth, causing psychological trauma, which may include anxiety, depression, or post-traumatic stress disorder. Behaviors demonstrated by emotional abusers include constant criticism, threats, rejection, degrading, terrorizing, isolating, exploiting, as well as withholding love, support, and guidance. Emotional abuse is also characterized by a sustained repetition of behaviors that creates a climate or environment that remains abusive. A single or sporadic incident does not constitute emotional abuse. Emotional abuse may be demonstrated as a single form of abuse; but frequently is associated with the other forms of abuse.

THINK LINK: Munchausen Syndrome by Proxy

The appearance and demonstration of concern for a child is generally perceived to be an admirable attribute of a caring parent; however, in some instances the care and concern can have deadly effects on a child. Munchausen syndrome by proxy (MSBP) is a disorder in which a caregiver deliberately fabricates or exaggerates a history of symptoms that are not representative of the individual in his or her care. In most instances, the caregiver is the mother who invents symptoms, or creates symptoms, to convince others that her child is ill. In many instances, the child is subjected to unnecessary and often uncomfortable tests and procedures in an effort to determine the cause of the symptoms. The primary motivation for the mother's lying, over concern, and other behaviors is attention seeking for herself by assuming the sick role of the child. It may appear to be antithetical to consider caring, concern, and devotion as a form of child abuse, but at its core, MSBP is deceptive and premeditated, and places the child's life in danger. Some children do die from infections, injuries, or medication overdoses inflicted by the parent/caregiver.

Effects of Child Abuse

The effects of child abuse have immediate and long term ramifications as well as a wide range of manifestations. There are also a wide variety of factors that impact the severity and scope of these effects. The major factors that determine the effects are the type of abuse and the age and developmental stage of the child when the abuse took place. Other factors include the frequency, duration, and severity of the abuse as well as the relationship between the abuser and the child. Some children may also possess certain mitigating characteristics that can protect them from the effects of abuse. This ability to preserve and protect oneself from negative experiences is frequently perceived to be **resilience**. Characteristics of the child that may contribute to resilience include optimism, self-esteem, intelligence, creativity, humor, and independence. These children also are accepted by their peers and have positive influences from teachers, mentors, and other role models (Child Welfare Information Gateway, 2008a).

The immediate effects of physical abuse may be easily observed. Bruises, in varying stages of healing, are present as a result of hitting with a blunt object, slapping, falling, and so forth. Burns may also be observed on the skin. The shape of the burns may indicate what object may have been used to inflict the burns. Cigarette burns are frequently observed. Scars may also be present from previous episodes of abuse. Broken bones are also often caused by abuse, and there may be evidence of healing of previous fractures. Individuals who have experienced neglect and abuse as children often have poor health and are at a higher risk for developing allergies, arthritis, asthma, bronchitis, high blood pressure, and ulcers (Springer, Sheridan, Kuo, & Carnes, 2007).

Head injuries are a severe form of abuse, which may cause extensive brain damage and/or death, and are usually the result of a direct blow to the head, dropping, or throwing a child. Shaking a child vigorously can also cause brain damage and is referred to as **shaken baby syndrome (SBS)**. This type of injury is frequently seen in children less than 2 years of age but may occur in children up to 5 years of age. The average age of victims is between 3 and 8 months of age (Cabinum-Foeller, 2012).

Accurate statistics regarding the incidence of SBS are not available, however, it is estimated that between 1000–1500 infants are victims (MedicineNet, 2012). Of these victims, approximately 25% result in death. Those that survive are often left with blindness, and severe and permanent brain damage resulting in developmental and cognitive delays and impairments.

The damage to the brain in SBS is due to the movement of the brain within the skull. The infant's head is large and heavy in proportion to the rest of the body. The neck muscles are also very weak, allowing the head to flip-flop back and forth quite easily. The brain requires room to grow within the skull, so there is a space between the surface of the brain and the skull bones.

Violent shaking of the infant results in the brain striking the skull bones, causing bruising and often rupturing blood vessels, either on the surface of the brain tissue or internally. Bruising the brain causes it to swell and the ruptured blood vessels cause hemorrhaging in and around the brain. Frequently, there is also rupturing of the retinal blood vessels damaging the retina and bleeding into the eye, which results in blindness. There may also be neck and spinal cord injuries. If the infant's head hits a wall or other object, the sudden impact frequently increases the damage and may result in a skull fracture.

The manifestations of SBS are often not noticed until the swelling of the brain and hemorrhaging cause intracranial pressure to increase, compressing and destroying brain tissue, increasing brain injuries. Early nonspecific signs of SBS include lethargy, irritability, and vomiting. Later manifestations include lethargy, breathing difficulties, and seizures. By the time that SBS is recognized as a cause of these manifestations, it is often too late for interventions to prevent brain damage.

In addition to the immediate physical effects, there is growing awareness of the long term effects of abuse related to psychological, emotional, and behavioral consequences. There is also an increased concern related to the effects of childhood maltreatment on the neurobiological development of the brain. Abuse and/or trauma activate the stress response, which, if prolonged, negatively affects the developing prefrontal cortex, hippocampus, and corpus callosum (Anda et al., 2006; Delima & Vimpani, 2011). Individuals who have experienced childhood maltreatment are at a higher risk for developing depressive disorders with an increased risk for self-directed violence (suicide and self-harming behavior), borderline personality disorder, disassociation, and substance misuse and dependence (addiction) (Delima & Vimpani, 2011).

The acute emotional effects of abuse and neglect include isolation, fear, and a lack of trust, which may result in long term, chronic feelings of low self-esteem, relationship difficulties, and depression. Depression and withdrawal were frequently experienced by children as young as age 3 (Child Welfare Information Gateway, 2008a).

Young adults who have experienced abuse and neglect may also demonstrate poor mental and emotional health. It has been estimated that up to 80% of abused young adults met diagnostic criteria for a psychiatric disorder by the age of 21. Common disorders include depression anxiety, eating disorders, and suicide attempts. Additional psychological and emotional conditions include panic disorder, dissociative disorders, attention-deficit/hyperactivity disorder, anger, post-traumatic stress disorder, and reactive attachment disorder. Individuals with a history of abuse and neglect also demonstrate cognitive difficulties as demonstrated by lower scores on measures of cognitive capacity, language development, and academic performance and achievement.

It is also common for abuse and neglect victims to demonstrate behavioral difficulties, such as delinquency, low academic performance, drug use, and emotional problems. They are also more inclined to demonstrate high-risk sexual behaviors, increasing teen pregnancy and their risk for developing STIs. As teens, they are 11 times more likely to be arrested for juvenile delinquent behaviors, and as adults they are 2.7 times more likely to be arrested for violent and criminal behavior. Drug use and abuse is also demonstrated more frequently in abused and neglected individuals. Drugs used include nicotine, alcohol, and various illicit drugs.

Sadly, approximately one-third of abused and neglected children will ultimately become abusers in some form, repeating a vicious cycle. Others will also become revictimized, becoming victims of rape or involved in physically abusive relationships.

Assessment of Child Abuse/Neglect

Assessment for child abuse is based primarily on observations of behaviors and physical manifestations (Table 14-10).

Elder Abuse

As individuals age, in many instances they lose some of their functional ability to care for themselves and become more dependent on others to meet their care needs. Those with any type of impaired mental capacity often lose their ability to make appropriate decisions regarding some of their care, making them vulnerable to those who are entrusted to make these significant decisions for them. While many caregivers act appropriately on behalf of those whom they care for, there are those individuals who do not and subject the elderly individual to various forms of abuse.

Individuals who are abusive to older adults are not the same type of individuals who are abusive to spouses, partners. or children. These can be individuals without any history of abusive behaviors or having been abused as a child, but in the given circumstances intentionally or unintentionally abuse the elderly. More often than not, these individuals have poor coping abilities for stress, have poor or inadequate support processes in place, are depressed, or are substance abusers (Robinson, de Benedictis, & Segal, 2012).

Elder abuse can occur anywhere the elderly individual resides, but most often in the home where the abusers are more likely to be adult children, grandchildren, or spouses and partners. Institutional settings are also locations where abuse occurs; most commonly these are long-term care facilities. In these settings the care providers may be the perpetrators of the abuse.

Elder abuse is defined as follows:

- *Intentional actions* that cause harm or create a serious risk of harm (whether or not harm is intended) to a vulnerable elder by a caregiver or other person who stands in a trusted relationship to the elder
- *Failure by a caregiver to satisfy the elder's basic needs* or to protect the elder from harm (Sellas & Krouse, 2012)

In addition to this definition, there are several types of elder abuse that have been identified. These are (Sellas & Krouse, 2012, Woolf, 1998):

- *Physical abuse*—any act of violence that causes pain, injury, impairment, or disease, including striking, pushing, force-feeding, and improper use of physical restraints or medication.
- *Emotional or psychological abuse*—intentional infliction of mental harm that causes mental anguish or psychological distress including threats, verbal or nonverbal insults, isolation, humiliation. Some legal definitions require identification of at least 10 episodes of this type of behavior within a single year to constitute abuse.

Table 14-10 Child abuse indicators

Physical Indicators	Behavioral Indicators
Physical Abuse	
Unexplained bruises or injuries	Reports injury by parent or other adult caregiver
Linear bruising, particularly on buttocks, legs, arms, back	Provides difficult to believe explanations for injuries
Injuries where children don't normally have them—face, legs, bottom, or torso	Has difficulty sitting, complains of soreness, or moves uncomfortably
Bruising in various stages of healing at different locations on body	Wears clothing to cover body, particularly when inappropriate to weather
Bruises in shape of object—hand, shoe, iron, stick, belt, etc.	Reports mistreatment of animals at home
Fading bruises or other marks noticeable after and absence from school	Becomes withdrawn, aggressive, or self-destructive
Untreated medical/dental problems	Is bullied or a bully
	Routinely arrives at school or leaves late
	Is overly compliant, overachiever, or overly responsible
	Seems frightened of parents; appears afraid of going home
	Is always watchful/alert—as anticipating something bad to occur
	Has learning problems
	Demonstrates behavior changes just prior to going home from school or when picked up
	Avoids adult contact; cringes or flinches when others get close
Sexual Abuse	
Difficulty walking or sitting	Reports sexual abuse by parent or another adult caregiver
Sudden weight change	Sudden change in behavior or school performance
Frequent somatic complaints, stomachache or headache, sore throat	Inappropriately seductive
Suddenly refuses to change for gym to participate in physical activities	Has sophisticated knowledge or interested in sexual activity and behaviors beyond same-age peers
Sudden negative change in appearance	Perpetrates sexual activity with another child, particularly a younger or more vulnerable child
Frequent urinary or yeast infections not explained by medical condition or treatment	Overly protective of siblings
Becomes pregnant of contracts a STI, particularly if under age fourteen	Avoids a specific person without an obvious reason
Runs away	Talks a lot about an adult
	Threatened by physical contact, closeness
	Comes to school early, leaves late, or doesn't want to go home

- *Financial or material exploitation*—misuse, misappropriation, and/or exploitation of an elderly person's money or material assets for personal gain. Acts such as stealing (money, social security checks, possessions) or coercion (changing a will, assuming power of attorney) constitutes financial abuse.
- *Neglect*—failure of a caretaker to provide for the patient's basic needs. As in the previous examples of abuse, neglect can be physical, emotional, or financial. Physical neglect is failure to provide eyeglasses or dentures, preventive health care, safety precautions, or hygiene. Emotional neglect involves failure to use the resources available to restore or maintain the well-being of the aging adult. **Active neglect** is where the care giver intentionally fails to meet his/her obligations towards the elderly individual. **Passive neglect** is unintentional, frequently due to caregiver overload or lack of information related to appropriate care giving activities.
- *Sexual abuse*—nonconsensual intimate contact or exposure or any similar activity when the patient is incapable of giving consent. Family members, friends, institutional employees, and fellow patents can commit sexual abuse, which can range from exhibitionism to fondling to oral, anal, or vaginal intercourse.
- *Self-neglect*—behavior in which seniors compromise their own health and safety, as when an aging adult refuses needed help with various activities. When the patient is deemed competent, many ethical questions arise regarding the patient's right of autonomy and the physician's oath of beneficence.

- *Abandonment*—the desertion of an elderly person by an individual who has assumed responsibility for providing care for an elder, or by a person with physical custody of an elder.

Neglect and abandonment are the most frequently reported types, accounting for over one-half of the cases or abuse (Robinson et al., 2012).

Assessment of Elder Abuse

While every elderly individual is at risk for maltreatment, identifying its presence may be difficult, especially if there is no physical harm inflicted. Many older adults are reluctant to report any maltreatment as it if often perpetrated by the victim's loved ones. Many face the dilemma of reporting the abuse to friends, family, or police, or continue being abused by someone they depend on or care for deeply. There is also the fear that by reporting the abuse and identifying the perpetrator there may be reprisals that may be worse than the present situation.

Assessment for elder abuse may also include identifying other individuals that may be at risk for engaging in elder abuse behaviors. Individuals who demonstrate the following behaviors are potential elder abusers:

- Use of drugs or alcohol, particularly heavy drinking
- Have high levels of stress
- Lack social support
- Significant emotional or financial dependence on the elder
- Lack of training in caring for elders
- Depression

Effects of Elder Abuse

Physical and sexual abuse will most likely result in injuries that may be easily observed. Some injuries are minor and include cuts, scratches, bruises, and welts. Other injuries are more serious and may result in permanent disabilities as a result of head injuries, broken bones, continuous physical pain, and soreness.

Short-term effects of elder abuse are a threefold increase in mortality as compared to those who are not abused. The exploitation that occurs with the abuse increases the feelings of vulnerability as well as fear and apprehension. Additionally, the elder individual becomes dependent upon those individuals perpetrating the abuse. Financial abuse often leaves the elder individual destitute. Emotional and mental stability may also be threatened.

Self-Directed Violence

Self-directed violence (SDV) encompasses a range of violent behaviors, including acts of fatal and nonfatal suicidal behavior, and non-suicidal intentional self-harm (i.e., behaviors where the intention is not to kill oneself, as in self-mutilation). Though not a behavior, suicidal ideation (i.e., thinking about, considering or planning for suicide) is included in this chapter due to its association with self-directed violent behavior.

Suicide

Suicide is the intentional action of causing one's death. The general perception and belief about suicide is negative, with many religions and Western cultures considering it an offense towards God and a belief in the sanctity of life. It is also considered a serious crime, tantamount to murder. Other cultural views, however, recognize instances or situations in which suicide is viewed as honorable, such as protesting for a cause, participating in resistance, or preserving the honor or safety of others. The majorities of suicides though are often related to personal struggles and despair related to mental disorders (depression), drug and alcohol abuse, and personal stress related to financial or interpersonal difficulties.

Suicide and suicidal behaviors have become a significant public health concern. In 2008, there were 36,035 deaths from suicide and there were 666,000 emergency department visits for nonfatal, self-inflicted injuries (Crosby et al., 2011). Suicide is the second leading cause of death among 25- to 34-year-old individuals and the third leading cause of death of individuals between the ages of 15 to 24 (Fowler, 2012).

Not everyone who attempts suicide is successful. There are more suicide attempts than actual suicides. Suicidal behaviors include suicidal thoughts (ideation), making suicide plans, and suicide attempts. Women are more likely to have suicidal thoughts and attempt suicide. Attempted suicides are often perceived to be pleas for help and the methods chosen are often those that allow for interventions that will save the individual. Poisoning is the most common method used by women. Men are often more successful in their suicide attempts as they frequently chose more immediate and violent methods. Use of a firearm is the most common method used by males.

Suicide Ideation

Suicide ideation is essentially a prelude to a suicide attempt. A majority of individuals who demonstrate suicidal behaviors have a major depressive disorder (DiazGranados et al., 2010). Substance abuse is another risk factor (Raue et al., 2006) as well as negative, significant life events and family events (Horesh, Nachshoni, Wolmer, & Toren, 2009). Compared to individuals in the general population, individuals who attempt or commit suicide experience a greater number of stressors and negative life events. These stressors and events include, but are not limited to, relationship problems, family discord, mental and physical health problems, loss of a significant other, bereavement, imprisonment, and employment-related issues (De Leo & Krysinska, 2008). It has also been reported that urban youth who have experienced bullying as well as those who engaged in bullying are at an increased risk of suicidal ideation and suicide attempts (Hepburn, Azrael, Molnar, & Miller, 2012).

Assessment of Suicide

Suicidal behavior exists on a continuum from thinking about it to actual completion of the act (Table 14-11).

Multiple assessment tools have been developed, however, there does not seem to be uniformity in assessment primarily due to variability in terms related to similar or comparable behavior (Posner, Oquendo, Gould, Stanley, & Davies, 2007). In response to this, the Columbia-Classification Algorithm of Suicidal Assessment was developed, which is capable of differentiating between suicidal ideation and behaviors (Posner et al., 2011). Other tools available include the Modified Scale for Suicidal Ideation (MSSI), which appears to be a reliable and valid instrument to assess suicidal ideation among distressed youth (Pettit et al., 2009), and the Beck Scale for Suicidal Ideation (SSI) (Holi et al., 2005).

Table 14-11 Continuum of suicidal behavior

Suicidal Ideation	Having thoughts about engaging in behaviors that related to harming or killing oneself
Suicide threat (plan)	A threat that is more serious than a casual statement of suicidal intent and that is accompanied by other behavior changes that may indicate a formulation of a specific method for ending one's life These may include mood swings, temper outbursts, a decline in school or work performance, personality changes, sudden or gradual withdrawal from friends, and other significant changes in attitude.
Suicide attempt	A nonfatal, self-inflicted destructive act with explicit or inferred intent to die. The attempt may be thwarted by another person or by circumstances, it may be planned to avoid serious injury, or it may be one in which the out come depends on the circumstances and is not under the individual's control. For example someone who takes a heavy overdose of sleeping pills may or may not be discovered in time.
Suicide	A fatal, self-inflicted destructive act with explicit or inferred intent to die

Source: Adapted from Kneisl, C. R., & Trigoboff, E. Contemporary psychiatric-mental health nursing, 3rd ed. © 2013, pp. 270, 510. Reprinted and electronically reproduced by permission of Pearson Education, Inc., Upper Saddle River, New Jersey.

Regardless of what assessment tool may be used, the overall information that is necessary to obtain is to determine the presence, severity, and duration of suicidal thoughts and feelings. During the medical history component of the interview, a question regarding past or present suicide thoughts or attempts is placed in context and doesn't appear to be anything more than a piece of information that is needed. If the patient's response is positive then more in-depth information should be obtained. While asking every patient about suicide, it is also important for the provider to be aware of what risk factors may be present in the patient's life that may indicate suicidal ideation or intent.

Asking every patient about his or her history related to suicidal thoughts and behaviors is important so that patients who might be a high risk for suicide may be identified. Some of these risk factors may come out during the patient's whole history and should be noted for possible follow-up. Risk factors for suicide are identified in Table 14-12.

Table 14-12 Risk factors for suicide behaviors

- Family History of
  - Suicide
  - Child maltreatment
- Patient history of
  - Previous suicide attempt(s)
  - Mental disorders, particularly depression
  - Alcohol and substance abuse
- Feelings expressed of
  - Hopelessness
  - Isolation (feeling cut off from others)
  - Loss (relational, social, work, or financial)
- Impulsive or aggressive tendencies
- Cultural/religious beliefs (suicide is a dignified solution of a personal dilemma)
- Regional epidemics of suicide (cluster suicides of peers)
- Barriers that prevent or deter access to mental health treatment
- Resistance to pursue treatment due to the stigma related to mental health and substance abuse disorders or to suicidal thoughts
- Easy accessibility to lethal methods (guns, rope, poison)

Source: Adapted from Centers for Disease Control and Prevention. (2009). Injury prevention and control: Suicide prevention.

Effects of Suicide

The major effects of suicide relate to the impact on the emotions and feelings of those who remain and go on living. In addition to the intense feelings of grief that are felt by anyone who experiences a significant loss of a loved one, survivors often also experience feelings of guilt related to not having been able to prevent their loved one from committing suicide. Survivors also are vulnerable to feelings of regret related to any conflicts or problems that may have existed in their relationships with the deceased individual. There are often feelings of regret and guilt that they are alive and that they could have possibly prevented the suicide. Shame is another emotion that is frequently experienced by survivors, which may lead to denial or concealment of the suicide as an attempt to avoid this feeling or having blame placed on them for the suicide. There may also be feelings of isolation and rejection as other family members and friends may avoid the immediate family because they feel uncomfortable with the situation or don't know what to say to them.

There is also a considerable economic burden related to injuries and deaths from self-directed violence as well as exhausting national social and health resources (Crosby, Buckner, & Taylor, 2011). The most recent statistics from the Centers for Disease Control and Prevention set the estimated total cost related to suicide at $26,728,669,000, with the majority of the cost being $26,628,942,000 for work loss (Centers for Disease Control and Prevention, 2012).

Self-Inflicted Violence (Non-suicidal Self-Injury)

Another form of self-directed violence is **self-inflicted violence** (SIV) or non-suicidal self-injury (NSSI), which is deliberately causing harm to oneself without the intent to cause death (Barrocas, Hankin, Young, & Abela, 2012). The most common form of NSSI is cutting, which includes cutting or scratching the skin with a sharp object. Other methods used for NSSI include burning (branding), poisoning, carving words or symbols in the skin, breaking bones, hitting and/or punching self (with hammer or other object), self-piercing/tattooing, head banging, biting, and hair pulling [trichotillomania] (Whitlock, Eckenrode, & Silverman, 2006). In extreme forms, individuals have blinded themselves or amputated their fingers, hands, limbs, feet, or genitalia.

The distinguishing characteristic of NSSI versus suicide is the underlying intent of the behavior, with suicide having the intent to permanently eliminate consciousness (Lofthouse & Yager-Schweller, 2009). Individuals who engage in NSSI often use it as a way to modify consciousness, to relieve or release feelings of deep emotional pain, stress, and anxiety that may be associated with a traumatic event. Frequently these individuals will have a history of physical, emotional, or sexual abuse. There is also the inability to cope with, regulate, express, or understand their emotional state. In addition, they are likely to feel emotionally depleted and NSSI is a way to feel something, even if it is physical pain. Other factors contributing to NSSI behaviors include self-hatred for feeling certain emotions that were considered in appropriate by family or others, or are punishing themselves for being bad and undeserving. These feelings are often embedded within the context of abuse based on the belief that the abuse was their fault or that somehow it was deserved.

While NSSI may be characterized as not having the intent to die, there is mounting evidence that NSSI is a risk factor for suicide as demonstrated by increasing incidence of suicide ideation and behavior (Glenn & Klonsky, 2008). There is also increasing evidence that NSSI frequently co-occurs with eating disorders, primarily bulimia nervosa (Muehlenkamp et al., 2008).

Self-inflicted violence is generally considered to be practiced by teens, but it is not strictly limited to them, and appears to be increasing in frequency among older individuals. The same may be said about the gender distribution in that it has been presumed that NSSI is primarily engaged in by females; however, the findings of various studies bring this into question.

Assessment of Self-Inflicted Violence

Identifying individuals who harm themselves is difficult to do as they frequently have plausible excuses or reasons for covering up this activity. There are, however, certain warning signs that may help to identify individuals who harm themselves. These warning signs include the following:

- Unexplained wounds or scars usually on wrists, arms, thighs, or chest
- Blood stains on clothing, towels, or bedding
- Sharp objects or cutting instruments in individual's belongings
- Frequent "accidents" that are explained away by "being clumsy, prone to accidents"
- Covering up, wearing long sleeves, long pants in hot weather
- Being alone for extended periods of time, particularly in bedroom or bathroom
- Isolation and irritability

Effects of Self-Inflicted Violence

The obvious physical effects of SIV are the presence of scars. Even if cuts are superficial, there will be some form of scarring. Cutting repeatedly in the same area will cause bigger scars to develop. These scars will never disappear; they remain as a constant reminder of this activity. Although not common, there is always the possibility of severing an artery and bleeding to death. Other physical effects of self-harm may include infection, nerve damage, broken bones, hair loss or bald spot, or injury from overdose or poisoning.

There are also personal emotional effects experienced by the individual, although they are often temporary and promote the repeating of the behavior. The emotional effects of SIV may include the following:

- Feeling able to express feelings and emotions that can't be put into words
- Feeling the release of tension that has built up inside
- Promoting a feeling of being in control
- Distraction from overwhelming emotions of difficult life circumstances
- Relief of guilt and punishing oneself
- Feeling alive, or simply feeling something instead of feeling numb (Smith & Segal, 2012)

The other effects are related to one's relationships with others. Individual's reactions to individuals who engage in SIV vary widely. Some may immediately express disgust and disengage from the individual. Others may express shock and are appalled at the behavior and avoid the individual as they don't know how to help the person. Some may be angry as they perceive the individual as manipulative, and some express apprehension about being around this individual. Family members and close friends initially express concern and wanting to help but often become weary and frustrated when the behaviors do not change, eventually withdrawing from the individual. There may also be the feeling of helplessness as most persons are unprepared to intervene or understand this destructive behavior.

Summary

- A high-risk assessment is an important component of the overall assessment in an effort to identify behaviors that place the patient or others in jeopardy of participating in activities/behaviors that may be harmful or injurious.
- To obtain the necessary information regarding high-risk probability, questions related to highly sensitive and personal choices need to be asked.
- Teenagers are more likely to participate in high-risk activities and behaviors. Recognize the characteristics of high-risk individuals based on an individual's history and/or specific behaviors.
- Questions related to sensitive topics may be formulated in such a way as to imply the universality of certain behaviors and experiences so that a patient's behaviors or experiences are not perceived to be unique or unusual.
- Various tools have been developed to assist the provider in assessing high-risk activity and behaviors.
- The presence of bruises or scars that appear to be in various stages of healing, or are patterned are commonly manifestations associated with violent behaviors directed toward the patient (abuse).

Review Questions

1. A student provider is completing the assessment interview for an older adult female. The instructor notes that the student did not ask the patient questions related to alcohol intake or sexual activity. Which is the best approach for the instructor to take?
   1. Ask the questions for the student to complete the history.
   2. Discuss the omission with the group in the post-clinical conference.
   3. Make sure that the student's grade reflects the incomplete assessment.
   4. Discuss the student's reason for omission of the questions privately.
2. The provider is assessing a preschool-age child brought to the clinic by her mother and the mother's partner. The provider notes that the child seems to have regressed developmentally since her last visit, has bruises on her upper arms and back in various stages of healing, and gets visibly upset when the mother's partner tries to assist her to undress. What additional assessment data is the priority for the nurse to gather?
   1. Question the mother about the child's regression.
   2. Note the appearance and location of each bruise.
   3. Ask the child why she is upset during the visit.
   4. Ask the child how she got the bruises.
3. In which of the following situations would the provider initiate a referral to a social service agency to assess an older adult for potential abuse?
   1. An older adult patient is admitted after falling over her grandchild's toy on the staircase.
   2. An older adult tells the nurse that he cannot pay his co-pay because his daughter forgot to cash his pension check.
   3. An older adult patient has lost 10 pounds over the last month and states that he is unable to get to the store.
   4. A homebound older adult patient has developed skin breakdown and tells the nurse that the caregiver has stopped coming to help.
4. A provider in an urgent care center is assessing a teenager brought in by her friends. The provider suspects alcohol poisoning based on physical symptoms of mental confusion; slow, irregular breathing; and pallor. When questioned about the patient's alcohol intake the patient and her friends insist that they have not been drinking. Based on this information the provider should do which of the following first?
   1. Contact the police to report the underaged drinking.
   2. Complete the CAGE questions with the patient.
   3. Draw blood to assess the blood alcohol level of the patient.
   4. Arrange for a referral for substance abuse education.
5. The parent of a college-age student confides in the provider that several empty liquor bottles were found in the back of the closet in her son's room after a weekend that the son was home visiting. The mother told the provider that she questioned her son about drinking, but his response was that "it's not a problem. I have it under control." How should the provider initially respond to the mother? (Select all that apply.)
   1. "If your child is of legal age to drink, there is no reason for concern."
   2. "This is normal behavior in college students and is not cause for concern."
   3. "Denial of problem drinking is very common in those abusing alcohol."
   4. "Hiding alcohol use is a cause for concern because it may indicate an abusive pattern."
   5. "You should have your child evaluated by a psychiatrist as soon as possible."
6. When reviewing the admission assessment data on a new clinic patient, the provider may incorporate the use of a screening tool to assess risk for substance abuse if the following are noted in the assessment?
   1. neurological disorders
   2. use of schedule V substances
   3. use of drugs in the SSRI category
   4. a member of a religious family

7. A student provider is about to do a health history with an older male patient and is concerned about asking questions related to sexuality and sexual function. What principle should the student use in gathering a comprehensive history?
   1. If the patient denies current sexual activity, there is no need to ask for more information.
   2. If the patient is uncomfortable with the questions, discontinue the interview.
   3. Use primarily closed-ended questions for this part of the interview.
   4. Begin by stating that these questions are important to determine the patient's overall health.
8. The provider is completing a health assessment interview with a young woman who admits that she is currently being physically abused by a live-in partner. Which question is a priority for the provider to ask this patient?
   1. "Has your partner hit you?"
   2. "Do you feel safe in your home?"
   3. "Why haven't you left the relationship?"
   4. "Can I contact the police for you?"
9. The provider has administered the CAGE tool to a newly admitted patient. The patient responded "yes" to the first and last questions of the tool. The nurse would interpret this finding to indicate that the patient
   1. is recovering from a substance addiction.
   2. is likely to have a problem with alcohol abuse.
   3. is using prescription medications to get high.
   4. is the child of alcoholic parents.
10. The provider in the emergency department (ED) suspects that a new patient is abusing narcotics. Which tool would be the most appropriate for the provider to incorporate into the assessment that would help to identify this type of substance abuse?
    1. CAGE
    2. CRAFFT
    3. DAST
    4. TACE

The Complete Physical Exam

15

We learned to examine the heart, then the lungs, and then the abdomen. We learned the neurological examination, musculoskeletal, and so on. Although we were taught these components in isolation, one patient made it clear to me that I needed to think of organ systems as being interrelated....

Mr. Cooney was just admitted to Room 442. When I walk in, he's lying on his side with eyes closed, his wife in tears at the bedside. From his history, I know he's 57 and received chemotherapy years ago for Hodgkin's lymphoma. The first thing I notice is his big, protuberant belly.

"He didn't want to come to the hospital," Mrs. Cooney says, "but he was having trouble breathing, his stomach got so big, and now he's out of his mind. I didn't know what else to do!" I try to get Mr. Cooney's attention, but he only briefly opens an eyelid, mumbles something unintelligible, and falls back into his pillow.

"I'm just going to do a brief exam do give me some more information," I say to Mr. Cooney, but again there is no significant response. I take both of his hands and feel his radial pulses—weak and thready, but equal. Placing a flat hand over his heart, I feel his apex beat, but it is faint and over more to the left. When I listen to his heart. I hear a prominent S_3 over the apex, and perhaps even a soft S_4.

When I listen to Mr. Cooney's lungs, and I can hear crackles bilaterally. *No wonder he has difficulty breathing*! Next, I focus my attention on his very distended abdomen; *No bowel sounds*, but when I tap my fingers on the side of his abdomen, I can see a prominent fluid wave—ascites. *It's beginning to come together—everything seems to point to heart failure—but why?*

"Mrs. Cooney," I begin, "During your husband's chemotherapy, do you remember what drugs he received?"

"Well I'm not sure, but I wrote them down, just in case. Here they are."

I look at the list and note that it includes doxorubicin. I think I remember something about doxorubicin causing heart failure, but I had better look it up.

Yup—there it is; doxorubicin can cause dilated cardiomyopathy, which explains the weak pulse, displaced apex beat, crackles, abdominal fluid. This has been a real challenge, but knowing how to get this information and putting it all together gives me a sense of confidence that I can do this!

LEARNING OUTCOMES

1. Summarize the elements of a complete (comprehensive) "head-to-toe" physical examination.
2. Recognize the importance of developing an organized approach to the physical exam.
3. Explain how organ systems are assessed related to a specific area or section of the patient's body.
4. Recognize how the four techniques of the physical exam are integrated for an efficient, complete patient examination.
5. Recognize various adaptations that are made for the physical exam of an infant/child.

The complete (comprehensive) physical exam is a systematic assessment of the physiological systems of the patient. A common reference and approach to this exam is described as a **head-to-toe exam.** As discussed in Chapter 6, the amount of data that is needed varies from patient to patient based on the overall situational context of the exam.

The remaining chapters (16–30) identify and describe the performance and techniques used in the assessment of regions of the patient's body and the underlying system organs that are assessed. For learning purposes, focusing on individual systems allows for application of anatomy and physiology for identification of what needs to be assessed related to specific conditions associated with a specific system. There may be situations where a specific organ system needs to be assessed in greater detail than other systems. Understanding an integrated approach to a head-to-toe physical exam will make it easier to understand how each system fits into a complete physical exam.

Initiating the Exam

A significant purpose for performing a physical exam is to establish a working relationship with the patient. Regardless of where the physical exam takes place, more than likely, this is the first encounter between patient and provider (Figure 15-1). Both the provider and patient bring some anxiety to this encounter. Patients may be anxious about the outcome of the exam and a possible negative diagnosis. They may also feel vulnerable in the sense that they have minimal control over the situation and are expected to do as the provider requests. They will also be expected to expose certain parts of their body to a total stranger and at times, multiple strangers. Symbolically, removing clothing and exposure of intimate, personal areas leaves the patient open to feeling vulnerable and unprotected. A patient experiencing these feelings may try to counter them by becoming somewhat demanding and appear uncooperative. Understanding the source of these behaviors will help the provider respond in a manner that is helpful in minimizing them.

Conversely, the provider/student learning to do the exam is anxious about remembering the right things to do as well as feeling some uncertainty regarding performing the assessment techniques correctly. In these situations, it is appropriate to indicate to the patient that this is a "learning experience" and request his or her patience and understanding. It is also appropriate to convey a sense of confidence, with the understanding that some mistakes may be made.

There is also a significant psychological component to the overall examination. In a figurative sense, the provider is "laying on the hands," which may have a calming and therapeutic effect on the patient. For this reason, when parts of the examination require that the provider's hands be used for collection of certain data, use a calm and deliberative approach. Touch can send a powerful message and should be used appropriately within the context of the exam.

It is the attention to the details and aspects of the examination that constitutes the art of history and physical data gathering. While the argument that modern technology provides better and more accurate data may have validity, there still exists the need for the art within the provision of health care. The "high tech, high touch" connection remains a viable aspect of health care and should not be abandoned. As such, the performance of the physical examination can be adapted to meet the needs and expectations of the patient. For the beginning provider, having a standard, set procedure for the exam can be comforting, but with confidence and experience, knowing when and how to adapt parts of the exam will become easier.

PRACTICE POINT: Who's Examining Whom?

While the focus in the performance of a physical examination is on the provider, the provider must also remember that the patient is also examining the provider. The provider's appearance, demeanor, manners, and mannerisms all communicate messages to the patient that can help or hinder the overall success of the examination. A favorable impression of the provider will help in promoting a helpful and therapeutic relationship.

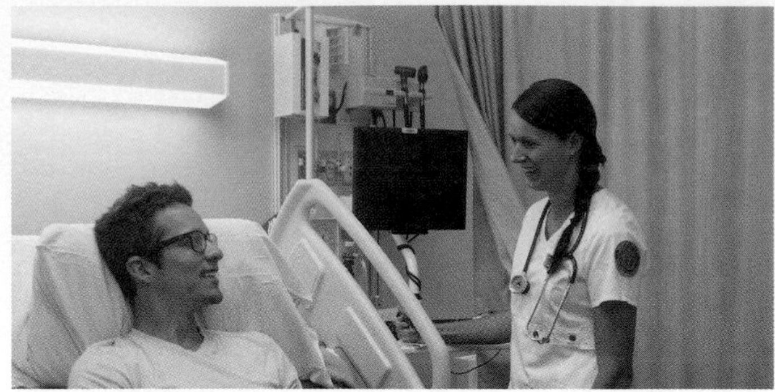

FIGURE 15-1 The physical exam is most likely the first encounter between a patient and a provide

PRACTICE POINT: Recommendations and Reminders

- Respect and understand the patient's culture and practices; don't try and guess what the patient means or indicates.
- Keep the focus and attention on the patient, avoid distractions and interruptions, unless an emergency.
- Recognize and respect the patient's individuality and adapt as much as possible without compromising data collection.
- Pay attention to modesty (for all ages); provide draping as appropriate; when necessary always consider a chaperone.
- Include the patient in the examination; provide explanations as to what is being done and why; also if extra time is needed to confirm findings, assure the patient that this is not an indication that something is wrong.
- Inform patient when there might be some discomfort with a procedure or technique.
- Avoid using a tone of voice that may imply "ordering"; *please* and *thank you* are appropriate to use, but overuse can become tedious and irritating.
- Avoid using the terms *good* and *excellent* after performing a technique because if you forget to say it at some point, the patient may interpret this to mean that there is something wrong or there was a negative finding.
- Pay attention to the patient's body language; observe congruency between absence or presence of pain and facial expressions.

General Assessment

The exam begins with the overall general assessment, which begins as soon as the patient is encountered, but also is continuous throughout the entire exam. Some activities or behaviors may not be readily observable until the patient is asked to do something. Some of the components are also a part of system examinations, allowing the provider to get a head start of some system examinations. Components of the general assessment are identified in Box 15-1.

Box 15-1 Components of General Assessment

Skin color	Facial expressions	Mobility
Dress/posture	Speech (patterns, disorders, language)	Hearing (difficulty, assistive devices)
Stature/build	Musculoskeletal alterations	Vision difficulties
Eye contact	Orientation/mental status	Nutritional status
Ventilation (pulmonary) difficulties	Others present with patient	

Equipment

Prior to the exam, also determine that the appropriate equipment is readily available. Having to constantly interrupt the exam to find needed supplies/equipment wastes time and may require the provider to leave the patient. Box 15-2 lists the typical supplies required to conduct a physical exam.

Box 15-2 Typical Supplies

Cotton balls	Cotton-tipped swabs	Draping material
Examining gloves (right size)	Flashlight/ transilluminator	Gauze squares
Lubricant	Marking pen	Measuring tape/ ruler
Nasal speculum (otoscope)	Odor emitting substances	Ophthalmoscope
Otoscope (pneumatic bulb)	Penlight	Percussion hammer
Sharp/dull articles	Sphygmomanometer	Stethoscope (with bell)
Tasting substances	Thermometer	Tuning forks
Vaginal speculum (female)	Visual acuity screening charts	

Preparatory Steps

Before the physical exam begins, make sure the patient is comfortable and that the room temperature is within a comfortable range. Older adult patients may still feel chilled in a warm room so provide for extra clothing or blankets to keep the patient warm. Also be aware of cultural and/or religious practices that may determine the patient's clothing and exposure.

History

The history precedes the physical examination. Remember that some historical data may also come out during the exam, so even though the provider is concentrating on performing the exam and noting the findings, also listen to what the patient may be saying.

Preliminary Activities

After the history, if not done previously, have the patient empty the bladder. A full bladder can be painful when palpated and if an elderly patient has incontinence issues, pressure on the bladder may cause urine to leak and probably embarrass the patient. Also, have the patient remove as much clothing and needed and put on a gown.

If not done previously, obtain vital sign measurements (temperature, pulse, ventilations), blood pressure (both arms), height and weight and if appropriate calculate body mass index (BMI), and visual acuity (Snellen chart) or other measuring cards.

Performing the Head-to-Toe Assessment

The remainder of the chapter are two tables (Tables 15-1 and 15-2) that provide guidelines for performing a systematic head-to-toe assessment. Each one groups assessment techniques and procedures by body region and provider–patient positioning to make the assessment as efficient as possible and to avoid tiring the patient. The first column describes the procedure used for assessing each body system or region. The second column identifies the expected findings for adults. The third column provides comments related to purpose for the procedure and any special considerations that may need to be taken.

Following the completion of the exam, discuss the results with the patient. If there was the possibility of findings that may be associated with negative outcomes, it is important to inform the patient of the results. Allow time for the patient to ask questions and discuss the implications of the findings. In some instances more data may need to be obtained through further tests or procedures; be honest and forthright regarding this and when the results of the test may be available. It is appropriate to take a positive approach with the patient, but is not appropriate to provide false assurance. Even if there most likely will be a way to turn results into a positive outcome, it is not fair to give the patient false hope.

Table 15-1 Guidelines for a systematic head-to-toe assessment

Procedures	Expected Findings	Comments
Patient seated on exam table/bed, wearing gown; Provider standing in front of patient		
Skin		
The characteristics and manifestations of the skin are assessed throughout the entire exam when specific locations of the body are exposed.		
Note the uniformity/symmetry of skin color.	Uniformity of skin color within the parameters of sun exposure and other natural causes that may affect color. Lesions, if present, may be the result of a specific pathology or simply manifestations of skin characteristics. Note distribution and pattern of any lesions.	Skin color comes in a wide variety of shades that often don't specifically resemble terms used to describe them (pink, olive, ivory, peach); instead of identifying a color, note the uniformity of the distribution of pigment as well as the symmetry. There are some natural causes of shade variations (pink cheeks, pressure spots), so symmetry of these variations needs to be noted.
Palpate skin (dorsal surface of hand) to assess skin temperature.	Uniformity and symmetry of skin temperature within parameters of amount of exposure and ambient temperatures.	Temperature of the skin can vary from location to location depending on the adequacy and competency of the patient's circulatory system, metabolic rate, and exposure to ambient temperatures. In the absence of any pathology, any temperature variations should be equal and symmetrical.
Head and Neck		
It is customary to begin the head-to-toe examination with the head. It is also appropriate to begin the examination with the patient's hands, moving up the upper extremities and then go to the head following the head-to-toe system. The reason for starting at the hands is that the provider starts at a location that doesn't immediately invade the patient's personal space, but gives the patient some time to get used to having another person up close and personal.		
Inspect the patient's head. Note hair color, texture, and distribution. Palpate from the forehead to the posterior triangle of the neck for the posterior cervical lymph nodes.	Symmetrical rounded normocephalic head positioned at midline and erect with no lumps or ridges Even distribution of hair (patterned hair loss) Hair is shiny, smooth Scalp is without any lumps, bumps, or masses	• This technique can detect asymmetry, size changes, enlarged lymph nodes, and tenderness. • Wear gloves for palpation if the patient has scalp lesions. • Inspect and gently palpate the fontanels and sutures in an infant.
Palpate in front of and behind the ears, under the chin, and in the anterior triangle for the anterior cervical lymph nodes using the pads of fingers.	Nonpalpable lymph nodes or small, round, soft, mobile, nontender lymph nodes	• This technique can detect enlarged lymph nodes. • Palpable lymph nodes may be expected/present in a patient younger than age 12.
Palpate the left and then the right carotid artery (Figure 15-2). FIGURE 15-2	Bilateral equality in pulse amplitude and rhythm (+2/3)	• This technique evaluates circulation through the carotid pulse. • Don't palpate both arteries at the same time to avoid occluding blood flow to the brain or possibly causing bradycardia.
Auscultate the carotid arteries.	No bruit heard	• Auscultation in this area can detect a bruit, a sign of turbulent blood flow and significant for the development of a stroke.
Palpate the trachea.	Straight, midline trachea	• This technique evaluates trachea position.
Palpate the suprasternal notch.	Palpable pulsations with an even rhythm	• Palpation in this area allows evaluation of aortic arch pulsations.
Palpate the supraclavicular area.	Nonpalpable lymph nodes	• This technique can detect enlarged lymph nodes.

Continued

Table 15-1 Guidelines for a systematic head-to-toe assessment *(continued)*

Procedures	Expected Findings	Comments
Palpate the thyroid gland, and auscultate for bruits.	Thin, mobile thyroid isthmus; nonpalpable thyroid lobes Thyroid gland rises with swallowing.	• Palpation detects thyroid enlargement, tenderness, or nodules.
Have the patient touch chin to chest and to each shoulder, each ear to the corresponding shoulder, then tip head back as far as possible.	Equal strength and movement of neck muscles Smooth, nonjerky movement of neck	• These maneuvers evaluate range of motion (ROM) in the neck.
Place your hands on the patient's shoulders while the patient shrugs them against resistance. Then place your hand on the patient's left cheek, then the right, and have the patient push against it.	Equal strength and movement of neck muscles	• This procedure checks cranial nerve XI (accessory nerve) functioning and trapezius and sternocleidomastoid muscle strength.
Request/observe the patient smile, frown, wrinkle the forehead, and puff out the cheeks.	Symmetrical facial expressions (smile, frown, and forehead wrinkles, equal puffing out of the cheeks)	• This maneuver evaluates the motor portion of cranial nerve VII (facial nerve). • Symmetry of facial expressions may be observed throughout the entire exam, so a specific point in the exam to do this may be unnecessary.
Occlude one nostril externally with your finger while the patient breathes through the other. Repeat on the other nostril.	Able to inhale freely through each nostril.	• This technique checks the patency of the nasal passages and for septal deviation.
Inspect the internal nostrils using a nasal speculum, penlight, or ophthalmoscope handle with a nasal attachment (Figure 15-3). 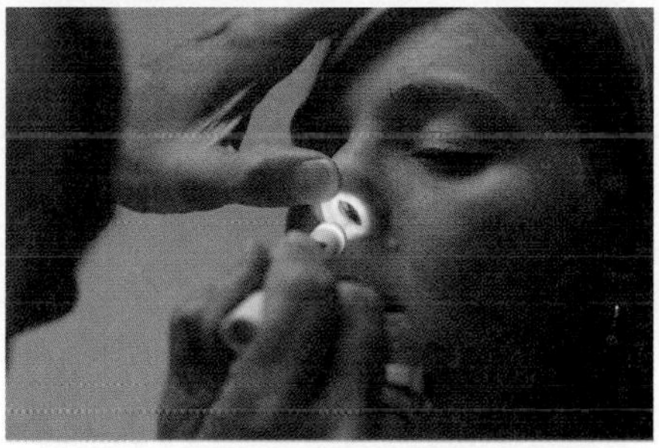 **FIGURE 15-3**	Moist, pink to red nasal mucosa, without deviated septum, lesions, or polyps	• This technique can detect edema, inflammation, and excessive drainage. • Use only a flashlight to inspect an infant's or toddler's nostrils; a nasal speculum is too sharp.
Palpate the nose.	No bumps, lesions, edema, or tenderness; straight (midline) septum	• This technique assesses for structural abnormalities in the nose. • An infant's nose usually is slightly flattened.
Palpate and percuss the frontal and maxillary sinuses. If palpation and percussion elicit tenderness, assess further by transilluminating the sinuses (Figure 15-4). 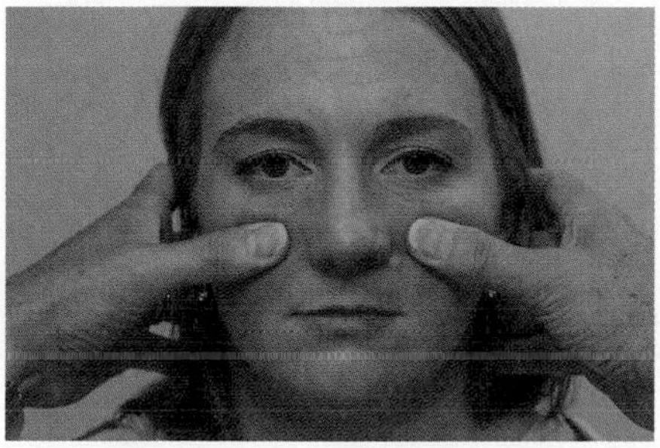 **FIGURE 15-4**	No tenderness on palpation or percussion	• These techniques are used to elicit tenderness, which may indicate sinus congestion or infection. • Transillumination is of limited value and is associated with a high error rate. • In a child under age 8, frontal sinuses commonly are too small to assess.
Palpate the temporomandibular joints as the patient opens and closes the jaws.	Smooth joint movement without pain; correct approximation	• This action assesses the temporomandibular joints and the motor portion of cranial nerve V (trigeminal nerve).

Continued

Table 15-1 Guidelines for a systematic head-to-toe assessment *(continued)*

Procedures	Expected Findings	Comments
Inspect the oral mucosa, gingivae, teeth, and salivary gland openings using a tongue blade and penlight (Figure 15-5). 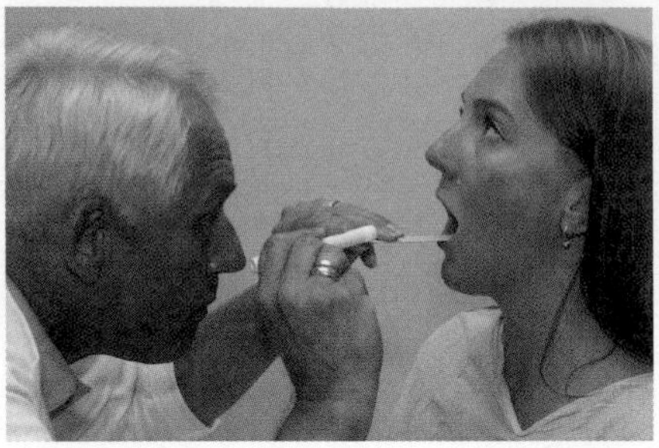 **FIGURE 15-5**	Pink, moist, smooth oral mucosa, without lesions or inflammation; pink, moist slightly irregular gingivae without sponginess or edema; 32 teeth with correct occlusion (alignment) Visible restorations; no cavities	• This technique evaluates the condition of several oral structures. • A child may have up to 20 temporary (baby) teeth. • Slight gingival swelling may be normal during pregnancy.
Observe the tongue and the hard and soft palates.	Pink, slightly rough tongue with a midline depression; pink to light red palates with symmetrical lines Tongue may have white coating and/or fissures.	• Observation provides information about the patient's hydration status and the condition of these oral structures.
Ask the patient to stick out the tongue.	Midline protrusion of tongue without tremors	• This procedure tests cranial nerve XII (hypoglossal nerve).
Ask the patient to say "Ahh" while sticking out tongue. Inspect the visible oral structures.	Simultaneous rise of soft palate and uvula during phonation; pink, midline, cone-shaped uvula; +1 tonsils (both tonsils behind the pillars)	• Phonation ("Ahh'") checks portions of cranial nerves IX and X (glossopharyngeal and vagus nerves). Lowering the tongue aids viewing.
Test the gag reflex using a tongue blade.	Gagging	• Gagging during this procedure indicates that cranial nerves IX and X arc intact.
Place the tongue blade at the side of the tongue while the patient pushes it to the left and right with the tongue.	Equal strength to push tongue blade to left and right	• This action tests cranial nerve XII.
Test the sense of smell by having patient smell a test tube of coffee, chocolate, or another familiar substance/odor (mint, vanilla, orange extract).	Correct identification of odors in both nostrils	• This action tests cranial nerve I (olfactory nerve). • Make sure the patient keeps both eyes closed during the test.
Eyes and Ears		
Perform a visual acuity test using the standard Snellen eye chart or another visual acuity chart, Jaegar card, or newspaper with the patient wearing corrective lenses, if needed.	20/20 vision	• This test assesses the patient's distance vision (central vision), visual acuity, and evaluates cranial nerve II (optic nerve).
Ask the patient to identify the pattern in a specially prepared page of color dots or plates. Test the six cardinal positions of gaze (Figure 15-6).	Correct identification of pattern (numbers/letters) Bilaterally equal, conjugate, parallel eye movement, without nystagmus	• This test assesses the patient's color perception. • This test evaluates the function of each of the six extraocular muscles and tests cranial nerves III, IV, and VI (occulomotor, trochlear, and abducens nerves).
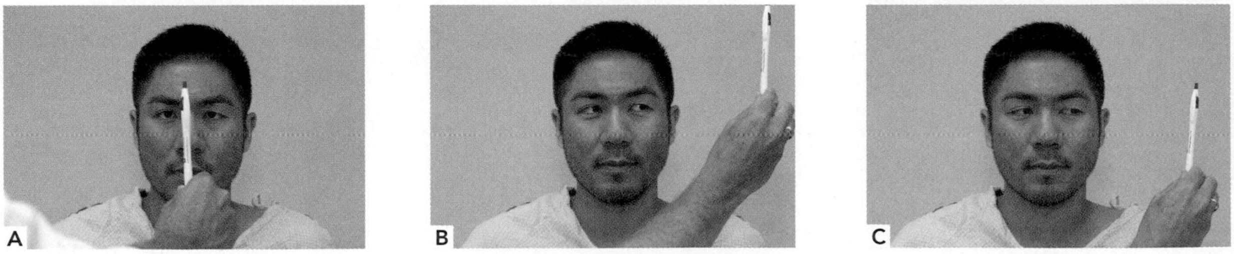 A B C **FIGURE 15-6A–C**		
Inspect the external structures of the eyeball (eyelids, eyelashes, eyebrows, and lacrimal apparatus).	Bright, clear, symmetrical eyes free from nystagmus; eyelids close completely; no lesions, scaling, or inflammation; palpebral fissures equal height; even, symmetrical distribution of eyelashes, eyebrows	• This inspection allows detection of such problems as ptosis, ectropian (outward-turning eyelids), entropion (inward-turning eyelids), and styes.

Continued

Table 15-1 Guidelines for a systematic head-to-toe assessment *(continued)*

Procedures	Expected Findings	Comments
Inspect the conjunctiva and sclera.	Pink palpebral conjunctiva and clear bulbar conjunctiva without swelling, drainage, or hyperemic blood vessels; white, clear sclera	• Inspection detects conjunctivitis and the scleral color changes that may occur with systemic disorders.
Inspect the cornea, iris, and anterior chamber by shining a penlight tangentially across the eye.	Clear, transparent cornea and anterior chamber; illumination of total iris	• This technique assesses the interior chamber depth and the condition of the cornea and iris. • An elderly patient may exhibit a thin, grayish ring in the cornea (called arcus senilis).
Examine the pupils for equality of size, shape, reaction to light, and accommodation.	Pupils equal, round, reactive to light and accommodation (PERRLA), directly and consensually	• Testing the pupillary response to light and accommodation assesses cranial nerves III, IV, and VI.
Observe the red reflex using an ophthalmoscope.	Sharp, distinct orange-red glow through lens	• Presence of the red reflex indicates that the cornea, anterior chamber, and lens are free from opacity and clouding (cataracts). • May have to darken room.
Inspect the ear. Perform an otoscopic examination, if indicated (Figure 15-7). **FIGURE 15-7**	Nearly vertically positioned ears that line up with the outer canthus of eye, match the facial color, are similarly shaped, and are in proportion to the face; no drainage, nodules, or lesions.	• A dark-skinned patient may have darker orange or brown cerumen (ear wax); a fair-skinned patient typically will have yellow cerumen.
Palpate the ear, tragus, and mastoid process.	No pain, swelling, nodules, or lesions	• This assessment technique can detect inflammation or infection. It may also uncover other abnormalities, such as nodules or lesions.
Perform the whispered voice test or watch tick test on one ear at a time.	Whispered voice heard at a distance of 1′ to 2′ (30 to 61 cm); watch-tick heard at a distance of 5″ (13 cm)	• This test provides a gross assessment of hearing cranial nerve VIII (acoustic nerve). • Stand behind or to the side of patient so patient unable to lip read.
Perform Weber's test using a 512 or 1024 hertz (Hz) tuning fork. Place vibrating tuning fork on midline of head.	Tuning fork vibrations heard equally in both ears or in the middle of the head	• This test differentiates conductive from sensorineural hearing loss. • The sound is heard best in the ear with a conductive loss.
Perform the Rinne test using a 512 or 1024 Hz tuning fork. First place vibrating tuning fork on mastoid process until patient no longer hears it. Place tuning fork in front of ear.	Tuning fork vibrations heard in front of the ear for as long as they are heard on the mastoid process	• This test helps differentiate conductive from sensorineural hearing loss.
	Upper Extremities	
Observe the skin and muscle mass of the arms and hands.	Uniform color and texture with no lesions; elastic turgor; bilaterally equal muscle mass	• The skin provides information about hydration and circulation. Muscle mass provides information about injuries or neuromuscular disease.
Ask the patient to extend the arms forward and then rapidly turn the palms up and down.	Steady hands with no tremor or pronator drift; equal, symmetrical, rapid movement.	• This maneuver tests proprioception and cerebellar function.

Continued

Table 15-1 Guidelines for a systematic head-to-toe assessment (*continued*)

Procedures	Expected Findings	Comments
Place your hands on the patient's upturned forearms while the patient pushes up against resistance. Then place your hands under the forearms while the patient pushes down (Figure 15-8). 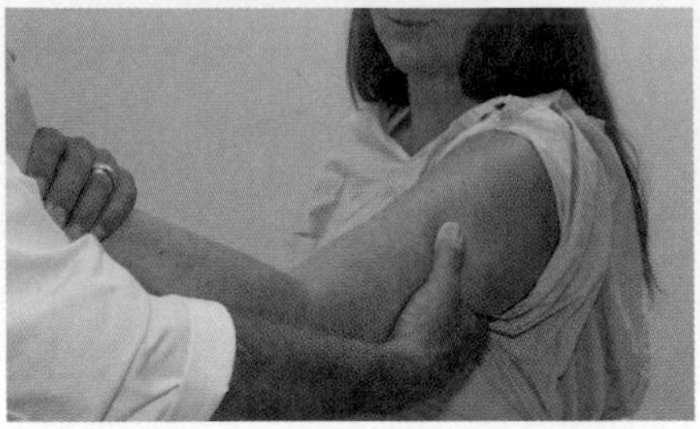 **FIGURE 15-8**	Symmetrical strength and ability to push up and down (overcome) against resistance	• This procedure checks the muscle strength of the arms.
Inspect and palpate the fingers, wrists, and elbow joints.	Smooth, freely movable joints with no swelling, redness or crepitus	• An elderly patient may exhibit osteoarthritic changes.
Palpate the patient's hands to assess skin temperature.	Warm, moist skin with bilaterally even temperature	• Skin temperature assessment provides data about circulation to the area.
Palpate the radial and brachial pulses.	Bilaterally equal rate and rhythm (+2/3).	• Palpation of pulses helps evaluate peripheral vascular status (blood flow to extremities).
Inspect the color, shape, and condition of the patient's fingernails, and test for capillary refill.	Pink nail beds with smooth, rounded nails; brisk (immediate) capillary refill; no clubbing (nail/nail bed angle 160 degrees or <)	• Nail assessment provides data about the integumentary, cardiovascular, and respiratory systems.
Place two fingers in each of the patient's palms while the patient squeezes your fingers.	Bilaterally equal hand strength	• This maneuver tests muscle strength in the hands.
Posterior Thorax		
Provider moves to behind the patient. For males, the gown is pulled down to the waist so that the entire anterior and posterior thorax are exposed. For females, the back is exposed, but the gown covers anterior thorax and breasts.		
Observe the skin, bones, and muscles of the spine, shoulder blades, and back as well as symmetry of expansion and accessory muscle use.	Even skin tone; symmetrical placement of all structures; bilaterally equal shoulder height; symmetrical expansion with inhalation; no accessory muscle use; spine straight, midline; ribs a 45 degree angle	• Observation provides information about lung expansion and accessory muscle use during respiration. It may also detect a deformity that can alter ventilation, such as scoliosis.
Assess the ratio of thoracic anteroposterior to lateral diameter.	Lateral diameter up to twice the anteroposterior diameter (2:1, 5:7)	• This assessment may detect abnormalities, such as an increased anteroposterior diameter (barrel chest may be as low as 1:1). • Anteroposterior diameters vary with age. • Measure an infant's chest circumference at the nipple line.
Palpate down the midline of spine.	Properly aligned spinal processes without lesions or tenderness; firm, symmetrical, evenly spaced muscles	• This technique detects pain in the spine and paraspinous muscles. It also evaluates the muscles' consistency.
Palpate over the posterior thorax.	Smooth surface; no lesions, lumps, or pain	• This technique helps detect musculoskeletal inflammation.
Assess respiratory expansion. Place palm of hands on surface of chest, just below the scapulae and have patient breathe in deeply (Figure 15-9). A B **FIGURE 15-9A–B**	Symmetrical, equal expansion and contraction of the thorax. Each thumb should move an equal distance from the middle of the spine.	• This technique checks for equal expansion of the lungs.

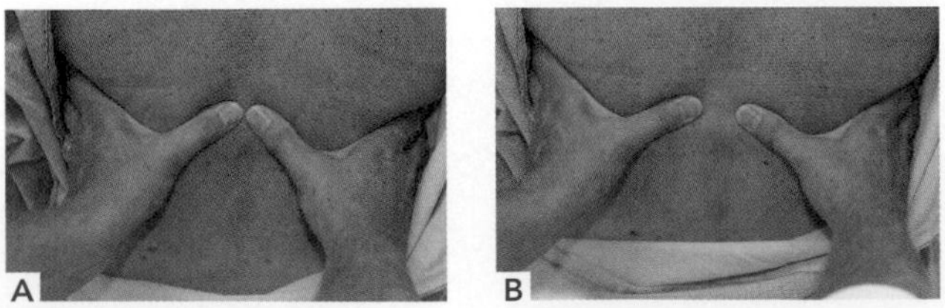

Continued

Table 15-1 Guidelines for a systematic head-to-toe assessment *(continued)*

Procedures	Expected Findings	Comments
Palpate for tactile fremitus as the patient repeats the word "ninety-nine." Place palmar or ulnar aspect of hand on surface of chest, feeling for vibrations as patient phonates.	Equally intense vibrations of both sides of the chest	• Palpation provides information about the content of the lungs; vibrations increase over consolidated or fluid-filled areas and decrease over gas-filled areas.
Percuss over the posterior and lateral lung fields. Down the sides of spine and below scapulae.	Resonant percussion note over the lungs that changes to a dull note at the diaphragm	• This technique helps identify the density of lung tissue and location of the lungs, diaphragm, and other anatomic structures. • Percussion may produce hyperresonant sounds in a patient with chronic obstructive pulmonary disease or an elderly patient because of hyperinflation of lung tissue.
Percuss for diaphragmatic excursion on each side of the posterior thorax. [Resonance to dullness]	Excursion from 1 1/4" to 2 1/4" (3 to 6 cm). Right side excursion may be higher than left side due to the liver, but the distance the diaphragm moves should be the same as on the left.	• This technique evaluates diaphragm movement during respiration.
Auscultate the lungs through the posterior thorax as the patient breathes slowly and deeply through the mouth. Also auscultate lateral areas (Figure 15-10). **FIGURE 15-10**	Bronchovesicular sounds (soft, breezy sounds) between the scapulae; vesicular sounds (soft, swishy sounds about two notes lower than bronchovesicular sounds) in the lung periphery	• Presence of breath sounds documents air flow through tracheobronchial tree. • Lung auscultation helps detect unexpected fluid or mucus accumulation as well as obstructed passages. • Have patient inform you if getting lightheaded. • Auscultate a child's lungs before performing other assessment techniques that may cause crying, which increases the respiratory rate and interferes with clear auscultation. • A child's breath sounds are normally harsher or more bronchial than an adult's due to their smaller chest size.
Anterior Thorax		
Provider moves to front of patient. For males, anterior thorax is already exposed; for females, the gown is lowered to expose the anterior chest.		
Observe the skin, bones, and muscles of the anterior thoracic structure as well as symmetry of expansion and accessory muscle used during ventilation.	Even skin tone; symmetrical placement of all structures; symmetrical costal angle of less than 90 degrees; symmetrical expansion with inhalation; no accessory muscle used.	• Observation provides information about lung expansion and accessory muscle use. • Maintain modesty for female patient. • Anterior thorax assessment not as valuable as posterior assessment. Posterior thorax consists primarily of lower lobes. • Observation may also detect a deformity that can prevent full lung expansion, such as pigeon chest.
Inspect the anterior thorax for lifts, or thrusts. Also note presence of the apical impulse (apex beat).	No lifts, heaves, or thrusts; apical impulse not usually visible	• Apical impulse (apex beat) may be visible in a thin or young patient.
Palpate over the anterior thorax.	Smooth surface; no lesions, lumps, or pain	• This technique helps detect musculoskeletal inflammation.
Assess respiratory expansion. Place open palm of hands at the bottom of the rib cage.	Symmetrical expansion and contraction of the thorax	• This technique checks for equal expansion of the lungs.
Palpate for tactile fremitus as the patient repeats the word "ninety-nine."	Equally intense vibrations of both sides of the chest, with more vibrations in the upper chest than in the lower chest	• Palpation provides information about the content of the lungs.
Percuss over the anterior thorax.	Resonant percussion note over lung fields that changes to a dull note over ribs and other bones	• This technique helps identify the density and location of the lungs, diaphragm, and other anatomic structures. • Percussion is unreliable in an infant because of the infant's small chest size. • Percussion may produce hyperresonant sounds in an elderly patient because of hyperinflation of lung tissue.

Continued

Table 15-1 Guidelines for a systematic head-to-toe assessment (*continued*)

Procedures	Expected Findings	Comments
Auscultate the lungs through the anterior thorax as the patient breathes slowly and deeply through the mouth. Also auscultate lateral areas. *Auscultation should not be performed over a patient's gown or other clothing.*	Bronchovesicular sounds (soft, breezy sounds) between the scapulae; vesicular sounds (soft, swishy sounds about two notes lower than bronchovesicular sounds) in the lung periphery	• Lung auscultation helps detect abnormal fluid or mucus accumulation. • Auscultate a child's lungs before performing other assessment techniques that may cause crying. • Breath sounds are typically harsher or more bronchial in a child.
Inspect the breasts and axillae with the patient's hands resting at the sides of the body, placed on the hips, raised above the head, and leaning forward.	Symmetrical, convex, similar looking breasts with soft, smooth skin and bilaterally similar venous patterns; symmetrical axillae with varying amounts of hair, but no lesions; nipples at same level on chest and of same color	• This technique evaluates the general condition of the breasts and axillae and detects such abnormalities as retraction, dimpling, and flattening. • Expect to see enlarged breasts with darkened nipples and aureole and purplish linear streaks if the patient is pregnant.
Palpate the axillae with the patient's arms resting against the side of the body.	Nonpalpable nodes	• This technique detects nodular enlargements and other abnormalities.
Palpate the breasts and nipples with patient lying supine (Figure 15-11). 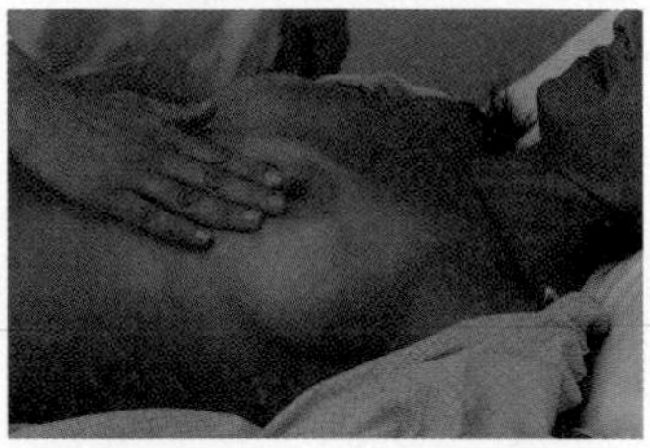 **FIGURE 15-11**	Smooth, relatively elastic tissue without masses, cracks, fissures, areas of induration (hardness), or discharge	• This technique evaluates the consistency and elasticity of the breasts and nipples and may detect nipple discharge. • The premenstrual patient may exhibit breast tenderness, nodularity, and fullness. • A pregnant patient may discharge colostrum from the nipple and may exhibit nodular breasts with prominent venous patterns. • Palpation of the male breast should also be performed, but is not as extensive as palpation of the female breast.
If necessary, put gown back on and assist the patient to a reclining position at a 45-degree angle. The Provider remains on the right side of the patient.		
Inspect the neck for jugular vein distention with patient lying supine at a 45-degree angle (Figure 15-12). 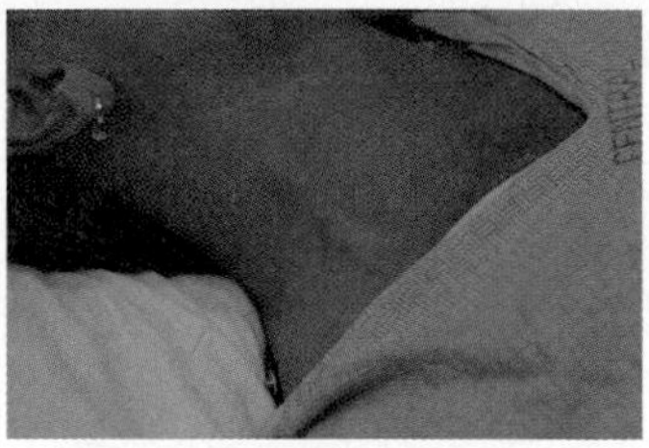 **FIGURE 15-12**	No visible pulsations; or pulsations that are visible in supine position but disappear at 45-degree angle however, venous distension may be observable in some individuals when lying supine but should disappear when elevated to 45 degree angle.	• This technique assesses right-sided heart (atrial) pressure.
Uncover the anterior thorax while keeping the abdomen and lower extremities draped or covered with a blanket.		
Palpate the precordium for the apical impulse.	Apical impulse present in the apical area (fifth intercostal space at the midclavicular line)	• This action evaluates the size and location of the left ventricle.
Auscultate the aortic, pulmonic, Erb's point, tricuspid, and mitral areas for heart sounds (Figure 15-13). 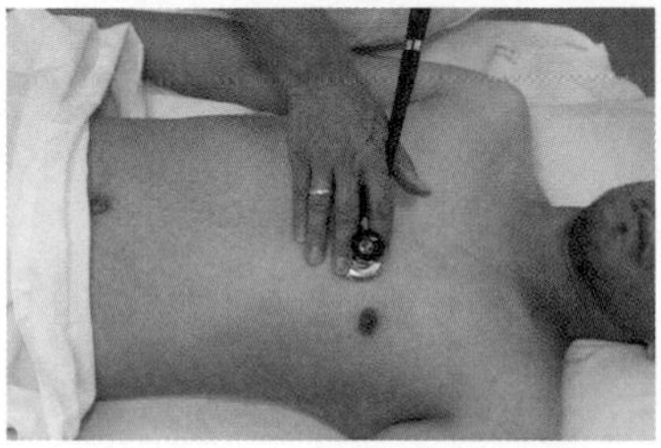 **FIGURE 15-13**	S_1 and S_2 heart sounds with a regular rhythm and an age appropriate rate $S_1 > S_2$ at mitral/tricuspid location $S_2 > S_1$ at aortic/pulmonic location	• Auscultation assesses the heart rate and rhythm and can detect other unexpected heart sounds (splits, murmurs, rubs, S_3/S_4). • A child or a pregnant woman in the third trimester may have functional (innocent) heart murmurs.

Continued

Table 15-1 Guidelines for a systematic head-to-toe assessment *(continued)*

Procedures	Expected Findings	Comments
Lower the back of the exam table/head of bed so the patient is lying supine. If the patient is unable to tolerate lying flat, maintain head elevation at a 30-degree angle. Expose the abdomen from sternal angle to symphysis pubis.		
Abdomen		
Observe the abdominal contour.	Symmetrical flat or rounded contour	• This technique determines whether the abdomen is distended or scaphoid. • An infant or a toddler will have a rounded abdomen (pot belly).
Inspect the abdomen for skin characteristics, symmetry, contour, peristalsis, and pulsations.	Symmetrical contour with no lesions, striae, rash, or visible peristaltic waves	• Inspection can detect an incisional or umbilical hernia.
Auscultate all four quadrants of the abdomen (Figure 15-14). 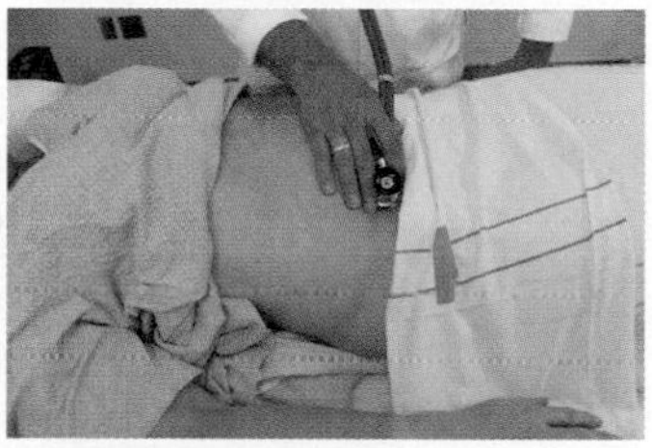 FIGURE 15-14	Bowel sounds present/audible in all four quadrants; no bruits	• Abdominal auscultation can detect unexpected bowel sounds.
Percuss from below the right breast to the inguinal area down the right midclavicular line.	Dull percussion note over the liver; tympanic note over the rest of the abdomen	• Percussion in this area helps evaluate the size of the liver.
Percuss from below the left breast to inguinal area down the left midclavicular line.	Tympanic percussion note	• Percussion that elicits a dull note in this area can detect an enlarged spleen.
Palpate (light/deep palpation) all four abdominal quadrants (Figure 15-15). 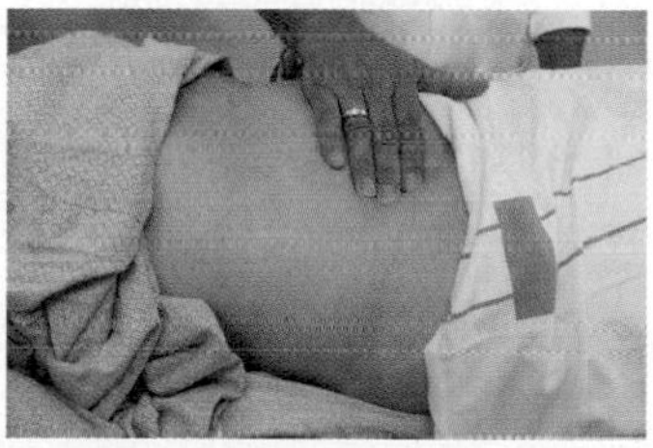 FIGURE 15-15	Nontender organs without masses or pain	• Palpation provides information about the location, size, and condition of the underlying structures.
Palpate for the kidneys on each side abdomen.	Nonpalpable kidneys or solid, firm, smooth kidneys (if palpable)	• This technique evaluates the general condition of the kidneys.
Palpate the liver at the right costal border.	Nonpalpable liver or smooth, firm, nontender liver with a rounded, regular edge (if palpable)	• This technique evaluates the general condition of the liver.
Palpate for the spleen at the left costal border.	Nonpalpable spleen	• This procedure detects splenomegaly (spleen enlargement).
Palpate the femoral pulses in the groin.	Bilaterally equal [+2/3] pulse, rate, with regular rhythm	• Palpation assesses vascular patency.

Continued

Table 15-1 Guidelines for a systematic head-to-toe assessment (*continued*)

Procedures	Expected Findings	Comments
Arrange gown and drape/sheet to cover the abdomen and pubis. Expose the lower extremities.		
Lower Extremities		
Inspect the legs and feet for color, lesions, varicosities, hair growth, nail growth, edema, and muscle mass.	Even skin color; symmetrical hair and nail growth; no lesions, varicosities, or edema; bilaterally equal muscle mass	• Inspection assesses adequate circulatory function.
Test for pitting edema in the pretibial area (Figure 15-16). 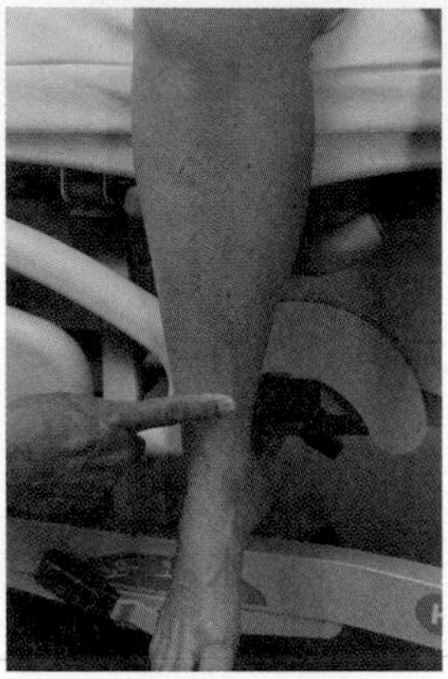 FIGURE 15-16 Palpate for pulses and skin temperature in the posterior tibial, dorsalis pedis, and popliteal areas.	No edema; no pitting. Bilaterally equal pulse rate, rhythm, (+2/3) and skin temperature	• This test assesses for excess interstitial fluid. • Palpation of pulses and temperature in these areas evaluates the patient's peripheral vascular status (blood flow to extremities).
Perform the straight leg test on one leg at a time (have patient flex hip and raise leg).	Painless leg lifting	• This test checks for vertebral disk problems.
Palpate for crepitus as the patient abducts and adducts the hip. Repeat on the opposite leg.	No crepitus; full ROM without pain	• Perform Ortolani's/Barlow's maneuver on an infant to assess hip abduction and adduction.
Ask the patient to raise his thigh against the resistance of your hands. Repeat this procedure on the opposite thigh.	Each thigh lifts easily against (overcome) resistance	• This maneuver tests the motor strength of the upper legs.
Ask the patient to push outward against the resistance of your hands.	Each leg pushes easily against (overcomes) resistance	• This maneuver tests the motor strength of the lower legs.
Ask the patient to pull backward against the resistance of your hands.	Each leg pulls easily against (overcomes) resistance	• This maneuver tests the motor strength of the lower legs.
At this point in the exam, the genitalia and rectal exam may be performed. It is also appropriate to wait until the completion of the physical to do this part of the exam. For the male, it would be done when he is standing.		
The neurological exam may be done with the patient either lying of sitting.		
Nervous System		
Lightly touch the ophthalmic, maxillary, and mandibular areas on each side of the patient's face with cotton tipped applicator (light touch) and a sharp point (light pain).	Correct identification of sensation and location	• This test evaluates the sensory function of cranial nerve V (trigeminal nerve).
Touch the dorsal and palmar surfaces of the arms, hands, and fingers with a cotton-tipped applicator (light touch) and a sharp point (light pain) (Figure 15-17). 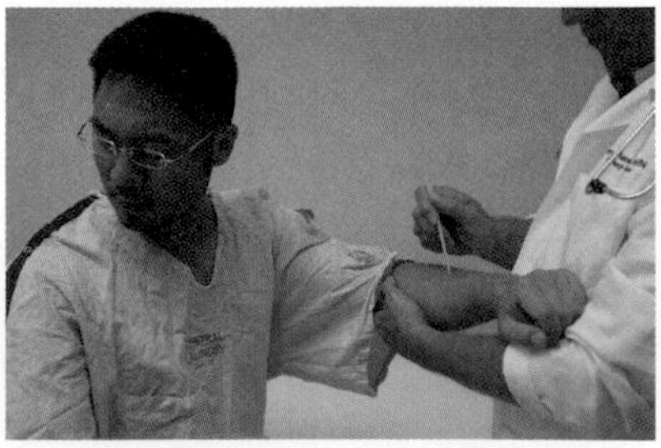 FIGURE 15-17	Correct identification of sensation and location	• This test evaluates the function of the ulnar, radial and medial nerves.

Continued

Table 15-1 Guidelines for a systematic head-to-toe assessment *(continued)*

Procedures	Expected Findings	Comments
Touch several nerve distribution areas on the legs, feet, and toes with a cotton-tipped applicator (light touch) and a sharp point (light pain).	Correct identification of sensation and location	• This test evaluates the function of the dermatome areas randomly.
Elicit brachioradialis deep tendon reflexes (DTR). Place your fingers above the patient's wrist, and tap them with a reflex hammer. Repeat on the other arm.	Flexion of elbow and pronation of forearm Bilaterally equal response	• Reflex arc functioning correctly.
Elicit biceps' DTR. Place your thumb over the antecubital fossa, and tap it with a reflex hammer. Repeat on the other arm.	Contraction of biceps muscle, flexion of forearm. Bilaterally equal response	• Reflex arc functioning correctly.
Elicit the triceps' DTR. Place your thumb over the triceps tendon area, and tap it with the pointed side of a reflex hammer. Repeat on the other arm.	Extension of forearm and contraction of triceps muscle Bilaterally equal response	• Reflex arc functioning correctly.
Elicit the patellar DTR. Tap just below the patella with a reflex hammer. Repeat this procedure on the opposite patella (Figure 15-18). **FIGURE 15-18**	Contraction of quadriceps with extension of lower leg from knee Plantar flexion of foot at ankle Bilaterally equal response	• Reflex arc functioning correctly.
Elicit Achilles DTR. Tap over the Achilles tendon with a reflex hammer. *Provider's opposite hand holds foot in dorsiflexion so that plantar flexion may be observed.*	Plantar flexion of foot at ankle Bilaterally equal response	• Reflex arc functioning correctly
Elicit plantar superficial reflex. Stroke the outer (lateral) edge of the sole of the patient's foot with the end of the reflex hammer handle (or other similar object).	Flexion of great toe, with fanning of other toes Extension of great toe and other toes	• This procedure elicits plantar flexion of all toes. • Expect Babinski's sign in children aged 2 and under.
Ask the patient to demonstrate dorsiflexion by bending both feet upward against provider applied resistance.	Both feet lift easily against resistance	• This procedure tests foot strength and range of motion (ROM).
Ask the patient to demonstrate plantar flexion by bending both feet downward against provider applied resistance.	Both feet push down easily against resistance	• This procedure tests foot strength and ROM.
Using your finger (or other object), trace a one-digit number in the palm of the patient's hand. *Make sure patient's eyes are closed.*	Correct identification of traced number	• This procedure evaluates the patient's tactile discrimination through graphesthesia.
Place a familiar object, such as a key or a coin, in the patient's hand. *Make sure patient's eyes are closed.*	Correct identification of object	• This procedure evaluates the patient's tactile discrimination through stereognosis.
Assist patient to a standing position. Provider moves to examine patient's back.		
Inspect the scapulae, spine, back, and hips as the patient bends forward, backward, and from side to side.	Full ROM, easy flexibility, and no signs of scoliosis or varicosities	• Inspection evaluates the patient's ROM and detects musculoskeletal abnormalities such as scoliosis.
Observe the patient while walking with a regular gait, on the toes, on the heels, and heel to toe.	Steady gait, able to maintain balance, and no signs of muscle weakness or pain in any style of walking	• This technique evaluates the cerebellum and motor system and checks for vertebral disk problems.
Perform the Romberg test. Ask the patient to stand straight with both eyes closed and both arms extended, with hands palms up.	Steady stance with minimal weaving	• This test checks cerebellar functioning and evaluates balance and coordination.

Continued

Table 15-1 Guidelines for a systematic head-to-toe assessment *(continued)*

Procedures	Expected Findings	Comments
While the male patient is standing, the provider sits in a chair to perform the genitalia exam. Have the patient bring the bottom of the gown up as far as needed to expose the genital area.		
Male Genitalia		
Inspect the penis.	Hair distribution pattern in a diamond pattern. Surface skin of shaft of penis is hairless, smooth, without any lesions. In the flaccid state, the penis hangs midline exposing the dorsal surface. The dorsal vein is generally observed. A foreskin may or may not cover the glans penis. Coronal ridge surrounding the lower dorsal portion of the glans that comes to a point on the ventral side of the glans. The meatus centrally located in the center of the glans without any evidence of discharge.	• If foreskin present, it should be retractable and replaced easily. There may also be a white, cheesy substance (smegma) on the surface of the glans when the foreskin is retracted. The glans may also be a darker color (reddish/purple) than the shaft of the penis.
Inspect the scrotum. Palpate the penis and scrotum (Figure 15-19). Compress the shaft of the penis between the thumb and index finger. FIGURE 15-19	The scrotum may also be a darker color and rough appearing due to the presence of rugae. The scrotum may appear to be asymmetrical if it is relaxed and the testicles are freely suspended within it. This is because the left testicle has a longer spermatic cord, thus hangs lower than the right one. The shaft of the penis should feel slightly rubbery in consistency and is easily compressed. It should be free of any lumps and bumps internally. There should also be no pain, tenderness, or any discharge from the meatus. Two oval testicles should be palpated within the scrotum. Their surface should be smooth, firm and rubbery in consistency and tender to slight pressure. The epididymis is also palpated and should be smooth and non-tender. The vas deferens and its accompanying veins and arteries should be present; however it is impossible to differentiate one from the other.	• The scrotum expands and contracts according to temperature changes to maintain optimal temperature for sperm production. • During palpation, move from the base of the penis to the glans, this will bring forward any discharge that may be present due to some infectious process. • A varicocele is an unexpected tortuosity and dilation of the veins accompanying the vas deferens. It is often associated with infertility and feels like a clump of spaghetti within the scrotum.
For the female patient, the genital/speculum exam can be performed prior to standing, or it could be the last procedure depending on the client's preference. If the exam is to be prior to standing, assist the patient into a lithotomy position with appropriate draping. After the standing examination, assist the patient back onto the examining table and then into the lithotomy position.		
Female Genitalia		
Inspect and palpate the external genitalia (pubic hair, labia, clitoris, urethral meatus, vaginal os, perineal, and perianal areas).	Pubic hair pattern an inverted triangle, labia without swelling and easily separated. Urethral meatus superior to vaginal os, below the clitoris, without any vaginal drainage. Labia soft with homogenous texture. Bartholin/Skenes glands without pain, swelling or discharge.	• These procedures assess the external genitalia of females to determine integrity of tissues and whether there are any indicators of STIs. • Lesions present around vaginal os, perineal area may be herpes or other manifestations of organisms causing STIs.
Inspect internal genitalia with vaginal speculum. After insertion of specula, inspect surface tissue of vagina and cervix.	Vaginal mucosa coral pink in color with rugae. Cervix without redness, shape of cervical os depends on whether patient has had previous vaginal delivery. Vagina and cervix without lesions or drainage.	• These procedures assess the integrity of vaginal and cervical tissue, also providing visualization of vaginal surface to determine presence of any lesions that may be associated with STIs.

Continued

Table 15-1 Guidelines for a systematic head-to-toe assessment *(continued)*

Procedures	Expected Findings	Comments
If needed, obtain tissue samples for Pap smear.	There should be no evidence of cellular dysplasia.	• Pap smear provides visualization of cervical cells and the potential or possibility of cervical cancer.
Perform bimanual and rectovaginal exam.		• Bimanual exam assess characteristics of vagina, cervix, uterus, and adnexa. • Rectovaginal exam palpates for status of rectovaginal septum and broad ligaments. • Weakness of rectovaginal septum may facilitate a rectocele or cystocele.
For the rectal exam, the male patient may remain standing after the genitalia exam and position himself leaning over the exam table. For a patient in the hospital, the patient may use the over bed table to lean on. If the patient has remained lying down on the exam table/bed for the genitalia exam, help him to turn on his side into lateral decubitus or knee–chest position. For the female patient, after the genitalia exam and removal of the speculum, help her to turn on her side into a lateral decubitus or knee–chest position.		
Rectal Examination		
If needed, spread the buttocks to expose the perianal region and anus. Inspect condition of surrounding skin.	Perianal skin should be smooth and contiguous and may be slightly darker around the anus. There should be no evidence of inflammation, excoriation, scars, pilonidal dimples, or tufts of hair.	• Ask patient to bear down which will make any fistulas, hemorrhoids, rectal prolapse, and polyps readily visible.
Lubricate the index finger and then press the pad against the opening of the anus. Bearing down by the patient helps to relax the external sphincter. Insert the fingertip into the anal canal.	Sphincter should tighten evenly around finger.	• Inform the patient of the sensation of the need for a bowel movement and assure the patient that this will not happen.
Inform the patient to relax the sphincter and then rotate the finger, palpating the rectal walls and muscle surrounding the anal ring.	Walls should feel smooth without any nodules.	• The palpating finger can only be inserted a distance of about 6–10 cm.
Slowly withdraw the finger and observe for the presence of any fecal material.	Fecal material should be soft and brown.	• Note any evidence of pus or blood. • Tan/gray color suggests obstructive jaundice, black stool associated with upper intestinal bleeding.
For the male patient, before withdrawing finger, palpate the posterior surface of the prostate gland through the anterior rectal wall.		
Prostate Gland Exam		
When rotating the finger around the rectal wall, stop at the anterior side and palpate through it for the prostate gland. Note size, consistency, and mobility.	The gland feels smooth, firm, and slightly mobile, and nontender.	• A soft, boggy prostate is indicative of prostatic hypertrophy, a hard, nodular gland suggests prostate cancer.

The Pediatric Examination

Table 15-2 provides guidelines for performing a systematic pediatric head-to-toe assessment. Two key concepts to keep in mind when performing a physical exam of an infant or child are adaptability and flexibility. Chapter 10 provides information as to how to approach the examination of children. While a consistent routine of sequential steps of examination steps is helpful to "keep on track," with children, the provider must often take advantage of opportunity in obtaining data. Also, remember that children are not just "little adults" so they shouldn't be treated as such. Patience, game playing (hamming it up), and spontaneity are essential in performing successful examinations of children. The more involvement of the child in the exam, the more likely the provider will be successful in obtaining the child's cooperation. There are also some significant alterations that differentiate the adult exam from a child exam, which include the following:

- Gain as much information as possible through observation. Spend some time getting to know the child as you are observing the child at play; a significant amount of information needed related to the neuro-muscular components can be obtained through careful observation. While obtaining the history or other data is an opportune time for these observations. Don't be in too much of a hurry to start the examination, use the preliminary time constructively.
- The location for the exam from around 8 months to 3 years is best performed on the parent's lap. Infants up to 6–8 months will do well on an exam table, but after that, they prefer the security of the parent.
- Keep yourself at the child's level as much as possible. Don't consistently "tower" over the child. This will help in establishing rapport with the child and facilitate a positive interaction.
- Involve the child to the extent possible. Explain procedures and be honest; if there might be some discomfort associated with a technique, let the child know to the extent that the child can understand. This will also help in maintaining your credibility with the child. Also, let the child handle the equipment so there can be familiarity with what is used during the exam.

- Let the child's behavior and activity determine the sequence of the exam. Sometimes giving the child a choice between two viable options is helpful. Asking, "Should I listen to your heart or lungs first?" provides the child with two options, both of which need to be done, but lets the child have some control over the sequence. Key reminders for the sequence of the exam are "least distressing to most distressing," "less invasive to more invasive," as well as "quiet to active."
- Take advantage of opportunities to perform a step out of sequence to get the necessary information. If the child is quiet, take the opportunity to listen to the heart/lungs. Also, use distraction to divert the child's attention to something else, which may quiet the child down enough to allow for what needs to be done.
- Recognize the developmental level of the child so that age appropriate activities and expectations are appropriate.

Table 15-2 Infant/Child assessment

Procedures	Expected Findings	Comments
Vital Signs		
Measurements (height, weight, head circumference); growth measurements (Figure 15-20). FIGURE 15-20	Data that are within standard parameters for specified measurements	• Be aware of cultural aspects of growth and measurement. • Commonly, measurement deviations beyond two standards, or higher than the 95th percentile or lower than the 5th percentile, require further evaluation. • Head circumference should be measured throughout the first 2 years. • *Childhood obesity a major concern. Excessive weight gain during childhood has serious consequences later in life.*
Demonstrate skills: Throwing ball, building blocks, drawing, coloring		
Observe mobility (gait, jumping, hopping, ROM)		
Muscle strength (climbing on parent's lap, sitting on chair, able to get on exam table)		
Child should be sitting on parent's lap/exam table. Child should be undressed except for diaper/underpants (depending on child's age).		
Skin		
Observe skin color/condition. Observe for presence of lesions (birthmarks, hemangiomas, Mongolian spots, nevi).	Uniformity in distribution of pigmentation	• Jaundice in first 24 hours of life most likely due to hemolysis of excess red cells. • Jaundice beyond 2–3 weeks suggests biliary obstruction or liver disease. • Loss of turgor on skin of abdomen, or over calves, is evidence of dehydration. • Scars or injuries (pattern or type) are suggestive of abuse.
Upper Extremities (UEs)		
Assessing extremities first can be done without having to move in closer to the patient. Holding hands or doing some of the coordination activities of the neurological exam facilitates observation of movement or UEs and, observation of characteristics of them.		
UEs inspected for evidence of clubbing, cyanosis, or edema.	UEs of equal length, tone, and mass. Full ROM of joints.	• Acrocyanosis is a common finding in infants.
Note presence of extra digits (polydactyly).		• May occur on own (inherited) or be associated with other syndromes or conditions. • African Americans most common ethnic group with inheritance of extra digit.
Also note the presence of single transverse palmar crease.	Creases that do not go all the way across the palm.	• Single transverse palmar crease associated with Down syndrome.
Palpate brachial/radial pulses.	Plus two quality pulse with regular rhythm and expected rate for age.	• Brachial pulse taken in infants. Older child take radial pulse.

Continued

Table 15-2 Infant/Child assessment *(continued)*

Procedures	Expected Findings	Comments
With older child, do brachial and triceps reflex.	Plus two response.	• Child needs to be old enough to cooperate. • Let child play with reflex hammer to understand that it shouldn't be painful or gently hit a point on the lower extremities so the child also feels the extent of the "hit."
With older child, take BP.	Systolic/diastolic reading within parameters associated with age.	
	Head	
Observe head (size, shape, circumference). Palpate sutures and fontanelles (Figure 15-21). Metopic suture Frontal bone Anterior fontanel Coronal suture Parietal bone Sagittal suture Posterior fontanel Lambdoid suture Occipital bone **FIGURE 15-21** *Source:* Norhazlan/Shutterstock	Uniform in size/shape/symmetry in relation to rest of body. Circumference within expected parameters related to age and size. Sutures are felt as ridges and fontanelles are soft, depressible areas on the infant's head.	• As infant grows, the head size in relation to the rest of the body decreases. • Decreased circumference is suggestive of microcephaly; increased circumference is suggestive of macrocephaly. • Bulging, tense fontanelle often palpated in infants with increased intracranial pressure. • A depressed fontanelle is associated with dehydration.
	Face	
Observe for symmetry of movement, distance between eyes, and altered formation of facial structures (Figure 15-22). 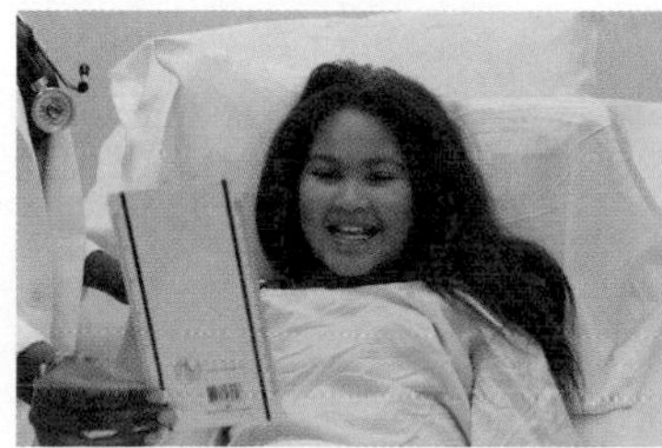 **FIGURE 15-22**	Symmetry of facial movements, external structures appropriately developed and formed, distance between eyes approximately the width of one eye.	• Unique facial deformities/characteristics of certain syndromes. Underdevelopment of upper lip and nasal philtrum are associated with Fetal Alcohol Syndrome.

Continued

Table 15-2 Infant/Child assessment *(continued)*

Procedures	Expected Findings	Comments
	Eyes	
Observe for shape, placement, and palpebral fissures of eyes. Observe for alignment and symmetrical movement.	Eyes positioned in upper third of face, approximately one eye width apart. Corneal light reflex equal in both eyes, without any asymmetrical eye movements.	• Wide set eyes associated with fetal alcohol spectrum syndrome. • Mild strabismus may be noted up to 6 months. • Some infants noted to have epicanthal folds, which may give appearance of strabismus (pseudostrabismus).
Obtain red light reflex.	Red reflection of retina visible through pupil.	• Lack of red light reflection suggestive of congenital cataract, retinoblastoma.
Visual acuity.	Generally unable to test for acuity until child is around 4 years old.	• At 2–4 weeks an infant should follow a light; at 3–4 months, coordinated eye movements should be observed. Eyes converge and infant reaches for object.
	Ears	
Observe ear placement, position, and alignment.	Outer canthus of palpebral fissure should lie up with point where the ear is attached to the skid of the head.	• Low set ears often associated with congenital syndromes associated with decreased mental capacities (Down syndrome).
Observe cues to infant's hearing.	Less than 3 months, loud noises elicit the startle reaction. Beginning at about 4 months, the infant begins to turn head to locate source of sound. Beginning at 6 months, sounds and inflections may be mimicked, also responds to name and other environmental sounds.	
Inspect ear canal and tympanic membrane (TM) with otoscope (Figure 15-23). **FIGURE 15-23**	Ear canal clean, TM pearly gray with visible landmarks.	• The otoscopic exam may need to be done at the very end of the exam as obtaining the cooperation of the child may be a little difficult. • An uncooperative child may have to be restrained by the parent to allow for visualization of the TM.
	Nose	
Observe size and shape of nose, patency with ease of breathing.	An infant's nose is generally flattened. Most of the time, infants are nasal breathers but are capable of switching to mouth breathing if needed.	• Any nasal flaring is indicative of a respiratory problem. • Sinuses are present at birth, but do not develop until much later. • Nasal passages in infant may be obstructed in choanal atresia.
Note any foul-smelling, unilateral discharge from nose; may be due to foreign body in nose.	There should not be any odor or foul smelling discharge from the nose.	• Common among young children.
	Mouth/Throat	
Note the color of the oral mucosa.	Color consistent and uniform. It should also be moist.	
Note presence/condition of any teeth.	Infants may have Epstein's pearls.	• A child should have 20 teeth by 2 1/2 years. • Bottle mouth caries may have significant impact on future teeth decay and caries formation. • Natal teeth are premature primary teeth that are often associated with cleft palate.
Inspect upper palate for presence of clefts.	Palate intact with appropriate arch.	• Characteristic manifestations of cleft lip/palate may be present

Continued

Table 15-2 Infant/Child assessment *(continued)*

Procedures	Expected Findings	Comments
Mouth/Throat		
Observe tonsils for color, size, and surface characteristics.	Tonsils that are the same color as rest of mucosa, not enlarged or moving towards the center of throat.	• Red enlarged, with coating or presence of discharge indicators of inflammation/ infection
Observe tongue for movement and size.	Smooth/even tissue, should be able to touch tongue to upper lip	• Protruding tongue suggests hypothyroidism or Down syndrome.
Neck		
Note position and mobility of neck.	Infant should hold head midline by 2 months and demonstrate head control by 4 months.	• Neck is shortened in infant with under developed muscles. • Thyroid not palpable until after 1 year old. • Congenital torticollis (wry neck) results from bleeding into sternocleidomastoid muscle during stretching from birth.
Palpate lymph nodes (Figure 15-24). 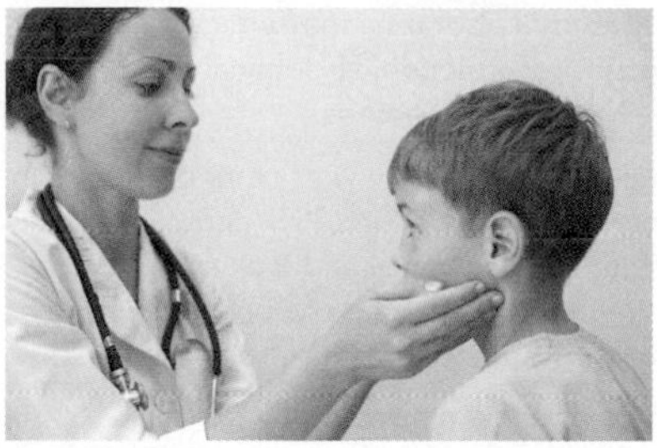 **FIGURE 15-24** *Source:* Pavel L Photo and Video/Shutterstock	Enlarged lymph nodes more likely in children than adults.	• Small, palpable inguinal lymph nodes common in healthy, young child. • Small, mobile, nontender "shotty" nodes common after infection.
Chest		
Observe shape and symmetry of structures and movements.	Symmetrical movement of chest.	• Asymmetric movement indicative of pneumothorax. • Pectus carinatum/excavatum should be noted. Often not serious.
Observe breast development	Breasts of newborns may be engorged. Breast development according to Tanner staging.	• At puberty, note breast development in females. • Gynocomastia may be present in pubertal males. • Widely spaced nipples in female associated with Turner's syndrome. • Estrogen from mother causes the infant's breast tissue to enlarge, there may also be some secretion of milk and is a common finding.
Lungs		
Use appropriate sized stethoscope (bell/diaphragm) when listening to lung sounds (Figure 15-25). 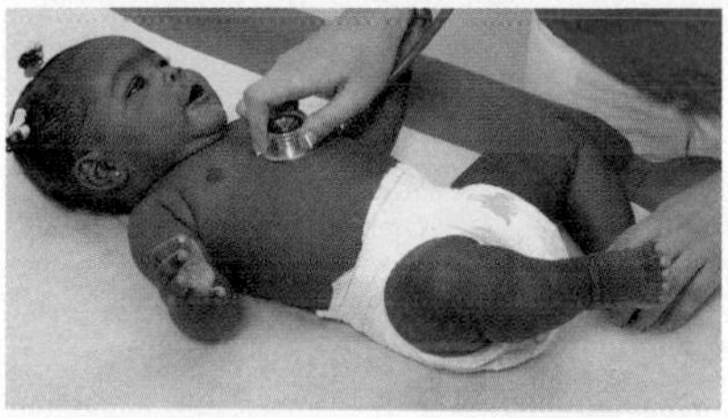 **FIGURE 15-25**	Abdominal breathing more predominant in infants/children.	• Breath sounds more intense in children (bronchovesicular sounds predominate). • Child's breath sounds are typically harsher or more bronchial than an adult's due to smaller chest size.
Observe rate and rhythm	Rate is dependent on age, slowing down as child grows older.	• Not uncommon for infants to demonstrate periodic breathing patterns (pause < 15 seconds).

Continued

Table 15-2 Infant/Child assessment *(continued)*

Procedures	Expected Findings	Comments
Heart		
Location/intensity of apex beat.	In children less than 7 years old, the apex beat is located in the fourth intercostal space, lateral to the mid-clavicular line.	• A right apex beat suggestive of left pneumothorax, left diaphragmatic hernia, or dextrocardia.
Rate/rhythm of heart beat.	Rate is dependent on age, slowing down as child grows older.	• Sinus arrhythmia common in children resulting in slightly irregular heart rhythm.
Note presence of murmurs.	There should not be any sounds that may indicate murmurs.	• Innocent murmur (short, soft, systolic) commonly heard in children.
Abdomen		
Child lying supine on parent's lap, if wearing diaper, loosen it.		
Observe for shape, symmetry, movement.	Infants and children have less developed abdominal muscles so the abdomen is more protuberant and rounded (pot belly).	• A scaphoid abdomen is suggestive of malnutrition or missing abdominal organs as with diaphragmatic hernia or intestinal atresia. • A distended abdomen may indicate an intestinal obstruction, abdominal mass, organomegaly, or ascites.
In newborn infant, observe umbilicus.	Note the presence of any drainage or redness. Should be two arteries and one vein. It is common to observe pulsations in epigastric region of a young infant or thin child.	• Single artery common with other disorders. • If intestinal obstruction of concern, note any visible loops of bowel and look across the abdomen to determine any peristaltic waves visible on surface of abdomen.
Observe for any bulges or protrusions Auscultate for bowel sounds.	A wide bulging above the umbilicus is most likely diastasus rectus due to the rectum abdominus muscles not meeting at the midline. Should be heard every 10–20 seconds.	• A common finding and no functional problems; will resolve or be less noticeable with growth. • There should not be any bruits • A scaphoid abdomen in an infant with respiratory distress may indicate a diaphragmatic hernia.
Palpate for any masses/tenderness (Figure 15-26). 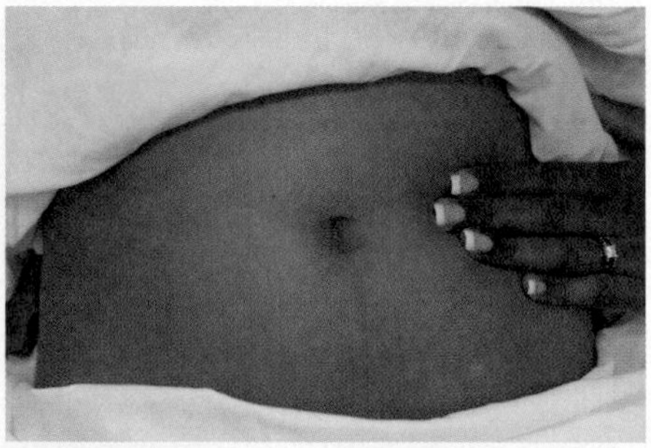 **FIGURE 15-26**	Soft abdomen, without any masses, tenderness, or pain.	• Begin with light palpation and note any facial expression of pain or tenderness. • The liver may be palpated in an infant/toddler about 1–2 cm below the costal margin. Greater than 3 cm suggests hepatomegaly. • Umbilical hernias are common through the second year and will usually disappear spontaneously.
Palpate femoral arteries, inguinal lymph nodes.	Plus two pulse quality. Rate/rhythm in synch with apical heart rate/rhythm.	• A decreased pulse quality of femoral pulses in comparison to brachial pulse quality associated with coarctation of the aorta.

Continued

Table 15-2 Infant/Child assessment *(continued)*

Procedures	Expected Findings	Comments
Lower Extremities (LEs)		
LEs inspected for evidence of clubbing, cyanosis, or edema.	UEs of equal length, tone, and mass. Full ROM of joints.	• Note presence of extra digits. • Note any joint swelling, redness, limitation of movement.
Also inspect for alignment (varus/valgus disorders).		• Inability of dorsiflex and externally rotate foot so that the little toe can be brought in contact with exterior aspect of leg is diagnostic for club foot. • Inability to plantar flex foot properly (at least 45 degrees beyond right angle) is diagnostic for calcaneus deformity.
On infants perform Ortolani's/Barlow's procedure for hip dislocation (Figure 15-27). 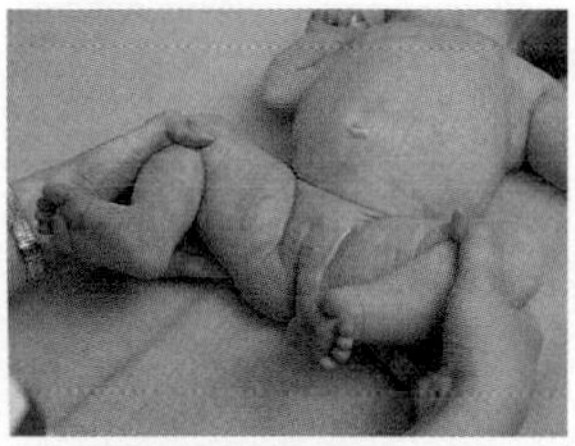 **FIGURE 15-27**	No sounds or movement detected on abduction of hips.	• Presence of "clunk" on abduction of hips characteristic of hip dislocation.
Male Genitalia		
For the male child, returning to a sitting position is preferred for the genitalia examination, particularly for palpation of the scrotum.		
Observe genitalia configuration.	Genitalia should be configured with a penis, scrotum that contains two testes.	• Questionable configuration indicative of unknown gender associated with certain genetic alterations.
Inspect penis for location of metus, if circumcised.	Meatus located at tip of glans penis.	• Meatus located on dorsal or ventral aspect of penis may need surgical intervention. • In infant, foreskin should not be forcibly retracted. Should retract by 4–6 years.
Palpate scrotum for presence of testes. In prepubertal male and during puberty, note development of genitalia and secondary sex characteristics according to Tanner's staging.	Two palpable testes in scrotum. Consistent and expected growth and development of genitalia and secondary sex characteristics.	• Before 12 months of age, testes may need to be "milked" through the inguinal canal. Testes should remain in scrotum by 12 months. • If older child, he should be sitting with knees bent with arms wrapped around them. • A failure to develop or delayed development may be due to endocrine or pituitary gland dysfunction.
Female Genitalia		
Observe genitalia configuration.	Genitalia should be configured with visible labia majora.	• Questionable configuration is indicative of unknown gender associated with certain genetic alterations.
Note any evidence of trauma, injuries to or around genitalia, which may indicate sexual abuse.	Separation of the labia should also reveal a vaginal os and meatus above the vagina.	• Labia may be enlarged in infant due to the presence of maternal hormones. • Constant itching/scratching of the genital area may be related to sexual abuse. • Redness and/or rash may be caused by contact dermatitis from diapers.
The majority of the neurological exam is based on observation during the examination. Depending on how much information has been obtained for the neurological exam throughout the exam, the remainder of the information can be obtained before having the child stand up. The extent of the exam is also dependent on the age and development of the child.		

Continued

Table 15-2 Infant/Child assessment *(continued)*

Procedures	Expected Findings	Comments
Neurological Exam		
Assess cerebral function. Behavior, level of consciousness, intelligence, emotional status, memory, orientation, ability to understand and communicate, auditory–verbal, visual–verbal comprehension. Recognition of objects, speech, writing ability, motor skills.	Age and development stage appropriate responses. By the time the child is 4 years of age, a full neurological exam may be preformed.	• Any lags or deficiencies need to be further evaluated. • Be aware of "soft" indicators of neurological development alterations.
XII Cranial Nerves	Age appropriate responses.	• Pupillary responses and reactions may be difficult to obtain in infants, particularly if they have dark eyes.
Cerebellar function (sitting and standing). Sitting for coordination, standing for balance.	Age appropriate responses.	
Have child stand for the remaining parts of the exam.		
Neurological Exam (Motor, Balance, Gait)		
Observe muscle size, mass, strength, and overall symmetry of posture from front, back, and side.	Muscle mass should be symmetrical with full ROM of all joints.	
Observe muscle movement, gait of child.	Gait and movement should be smooth, coordinated movements. Muscle movement should also be voluntary and purposeful.	• Gower's sign if proximal weakness present (muscular dystrophy).
Observe balance.	Child should maintain balance when walking, running, or standing.	
Inspect spine for alignment (Figure 15-28). **FIGURE 15-28**	Spine should be in straight line with expected curves of spinal segments.	• Infant starts out with C-shaped curve and gradually develops cervical, thoracic, and lumbar curves. • In prepubertal girls, note any lateral curves and any height discrepancies of shoulders and hips, which are indicators of scoliosis.
Neurological Exam (Sensory, Reflexes [DTRs, Superficial, Primitive])		
Gross evaluation of vision and hearing	Child should be able to follow commands, turn head to vocal sounds from provider, locate/visualize a distant object and go to it and pick it up.	• Inability to do any of these indicate possible neurological dysfunction.
Obtain DTRs as appropriate.	Plus two responses	• May be difficult to obtain if child uncooperative. • Triceps and brachioradialis reflex difficult to obtain until about 6 months of age. • May use index finger as reflex hammer in infants.
Primitive reflexes	Indicators of CNS development.	• More concerned if primitive reflexes don't disappear. As the CNS of infant develops, the reflexes go away. Persistence beyond their expected duration associated with CNS alterations or conditions.

Summary

- The comprehensive examination is a systematic, organized assessment of all the organ systems of the body, which are examined in a head-to-toe manner as the provider encounters a specific section of the body.
- An organized, systematic approach to the exam assures that the significant elements of the exam are completed in an efficient and effective format.
- Knowledge of internal anatomic structures and recognition of their locations is essential to appropriately examine them.
- All four examination techniques are used intermittently throughout the examination to obtain accurate organ and system data.
- Examination of a child requires flexibility and patience as the provider may need to alter the sequence of the exam as determined by opportunity and cooperation of infants and children.

Review Questions

1. The provider is performing the general assessment portion of a patient's health assessment. The information gathered during the general assessment would primarily be obtained through which of the following? (Select all that apply.)
   1. interview
   2. inspection
   3. palpation
   4. percussion
   5. auscultation
2. The provider notes that a previous assessment revealed that the patient has a renal bruit. The provider is aware that this finding requires the use of which of the following?
   1. deep palpation
   2. auscultation with a stethoscope
   3. two-handed percussion
   4. inspection
3. The provider is performing a head-to-toe assessment on a male patient with symptoms consistent with prostate enlargement. Which of the following reflect the best approach to the assessment of this patient?
   1. Incorporate the prostate examination into the abdominal examination.
   2. Complete the prostate examination first, and then move on to the rest of the exam.
   3. Leave the prostate examination to be done after the rest of the assessment is completed.
   4. Do the prostate exam at any time that the patient seems ready to have this completed.
4. The provider is examining a patient experiencing difficulty with mobility due to arthritis. To accommodate this, the provider plans to do as much of the examination as possible with the patient in a sitting position. Which systems can the provider assess with the patient sitting? (Select all that apply.)
   1. head and neck
   2. neurological and anterior thorax
   3. cardiac and abdomen
   4. posterior thorax and genital
   5. upper and lower extremities
5. During the examination of the patient's neck, the provider is assessing portions of which systems? (Select all that apply.)
   1. musculoskeletal
   2. neurological
   3. vascular
   4. gastrointestinal
   5. endocrine
6. The provider is to assess a patient whose laboratory results reflect an alteration in renal function. The provider is aware that this system is best assessed during which examination?
   1. genital
   2. rectal
   3. posterior thorax
   4. abdominal
7. When examining the abdomen of a patient with complaints of abdominal pain, the provider would perform which technique after inspection?
   1. light palpation
   2. deep palpation
   3. percussion
   4. auscultation
8. The provider is assessing a patient's deep tendon reflexes (DTRs). The technique primarily used to assess DTRs is which of the following?
   1. inspection
   2. palpation
   3. percussion
   4. auscultation
9. The provider is examining the ears of a 12-month-old child who has been pulling on her right ear. To perform the otoscopic examination, how should the provider position the child?
   1. in a sitting position on the examination table
   2. supine with the head elevated 30 degrees
   3. in the parent or caregivers lap
   4. restrained in an infant seat
10. When assessing the cardiac system of a toddler, the provider identifies which of the following as normal findings for this age group?
    1. a soft systolic murmur
    2. heart rate of 60 beats per minute
    3. apical impulse located on the left at the fifth intercostal space
    4. a bruit over the aortic valve

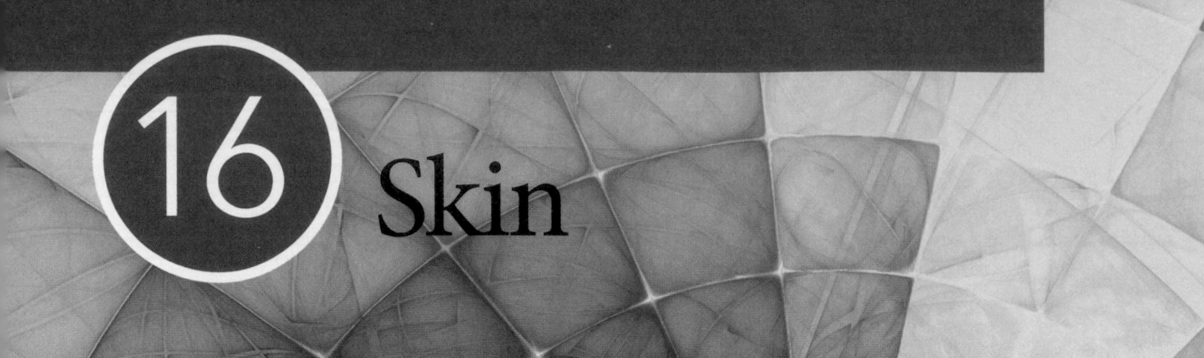

16 Skin

I dip my toes in the water and it is just the right temperature. Throwing my robe to the floor, I take a full step into the tub and slide in up to my neck. I don't feel any pain, and this bath seems no different from any of the hundreds or perhaps thousands of others that I have taken in my life. But I know that isn't true. This time, while the water was running, I added a quarter cup of bleach. I am desperate, and a few of the providers say that this might help.

Psoriasis has come to affect nearly every aspect of my life. Countless roommates have come and gone, all citing a well-conceived pretense when they leave. They don't want to tell me the real reason, that my dreadful, disgusting skin, cracking and flaking, coats the apartment. Whenever I'm brave enough to leave my home, people stare at the red, scaly patches on my arms, legs, face, and scalp. People even ask me to explain my condition in social situations! So, although it's a hot, humid summer, I now cover as much skin as possible whenever I leave the house. Worst of all is the laundry list of therapies—moisturizers, steroids, creams, and botanicals—that have given me false hope. Although some seemed to help at first, all have proven practically useless. I now realize that I shouldn't hold my breath for any remedy, but I find myself doing just that. I submerge my head beneath the water and let the bleach soak in, just for a moment.

LEARNING OUTCOMES

1. Explain the composition and structures within the skin and its appendages.
2. Compare and contrast color alterations of skin and conditions associated with the alterations.
3. Compare and contrast types of skin lesions.
4. Explain age-related skin changes and their significance.
5. Describe nail alterations and conditions associated with the alterations.
6. Differentiate between types of skin cancers.
7. Explain measures that can prevent skin cancer.

The skin, or integumentary system, is essentially a preformed sac that holds an individual together. As an organ, it is often taken for granted, but cosmetically, it receives a lot of attention. The skin's surface is a person's physical presentation to the world and has a significant influence on how one feels about oneself. What makes skin attractive varies from culture to culture. In America, where a youthful appearance is idealized, the desire is to have skin that is as young-looking as possible. In cultures that venerates elders, having older-looking skin is an asset. In some cultures, decorating the skin in various ways contributes to the perception of beauty. Even though the majority of attention to skin is cosmetic, it also is an organ that is physiologically active and often provides information regarding alterations in other organs and systems.

Structure and Function

The skin is the largest organ of the body, which if spread out, would cover an area of 2 square meters and weigh 10–15 pounds. The integumentary system also includes appendages such as the nails and hair, sebaceous and sweat glands, and specialized nerve receptors that are sensitive to cold, heat, pain, and pressure in the external and internal environments (Figure 16-1).

In addition to holding the body together, the skin serves as a protective barrier between the external and internal environments. Externally, it prevents invasion by microorganisms and other foreign substances; internally it provides a mechanical barrier that prevents fluid loss. It also plays a part in protection from the sun's ultraviolet rays through the production of pigment. The skin is also important to temperature regulation and production of vitamin D.

Composition

The skin (integument) is a stratified organ that is composed of two major strata (layers) and substrata that are functionally related to each other (see Figure 16-1). The two main strata are the epidermis and the dermis, which are also described as the **cutaneous membrane**. The epidermis and dermis are situated above a third layer known as the subcutaneous tissue (hypodermis) that consists of loose connective tissue, adipose tissue, and dense connective tissue.

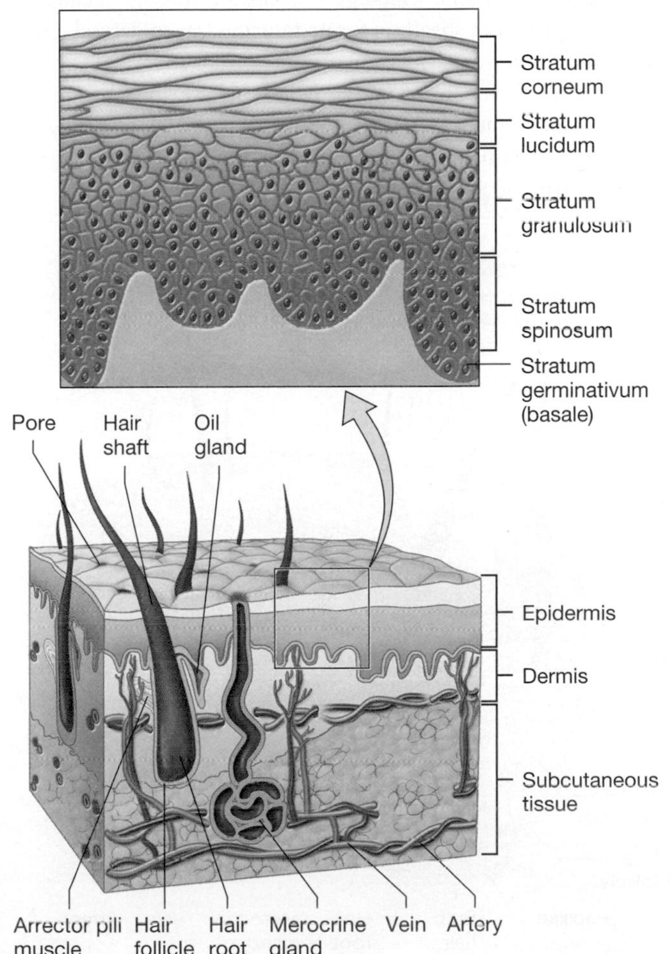

FIGURE 16-1 Anatomical structures of skin

Table 16-1 Layers of the epidermis

Layers of Epidermis	Function
Stratum germinativum (Stratum basale)	Single layer of cells that rests on basement membrane, which separates epidermis from dermis. Continuous cell division with new cells pushing older cells toward the surface.
Stratum spinosum	Spiny prickle cells that interlock to support the skin.
Stratum granulosum	Initiates keratinization that begins the death of epithelial cells.
Stratum lucidum	Protects against ultraviolet rays from sun.
Stratum corneum	Outermost layer that consists of thick rows of dead cells (squames). These cells are filled with keratin, which keeps the skin elastic and prevents lower lying cells from dehydration.

Epidermis

The outermost layer of the skin, the epidermis, is also categorized into thick or thin skin, depending on the thickness of the epidermis and keratin layer. Thick skin is found on the palms of the hands and soles of the feet; thin skin covers the remainder of the body.

The epidermis contains five layers of cells or cell products (Table 16.1). Thick skin contains all five layers; thin skin contains only three or four layers and never contains the stratum lucidum. The epidermal layers also contain four types of cells: **keratinocytes**, which produce keratin; **melanocytes**, which produce melanin, the dark pigment for skin color; **Merkel's cells**, which are probably involved with touch reception; and **Langerhan's cells**, which are associated with the immune system that process antigens.

Dermis

The dermis is the middle layer of skin located between the epidermis and subcutaneous tissue. It is composed of connective tissue that contains a rich supply of capillary networks that nourish the skin. The fine layer of cells between the epidermis and dermis is called the **basement membrane**; it is the glue that attaches the epidermis to the dermis.

The dermis is composed of two sublayers: the papillary dermis and the reticular dermis. The papillary sublayer comprises one-fifth of the dermis and contains the dermal papillae, the contoured ridges that penetrate into the epidermis forming the epidermal ridges (fingerprints). The dermal papillae are also responsible for nourishing the living cells of the epidermis.

The reticular sublayer is composed of avascular, dense irregular connective tissue that is made up of elastin, collagen, and reticulum fibers. These components give the skin strength, resilience, and elasticity. The dermis also contains a dense, complex network of nerve fibers that are sensitive to pain, touch, and temperature. There are also autonomic nerve fibers that innervate blood vessels, glands, and the arrectores pilorum muscles. Other structures of the dermis include sebaceous glands, hair follicles, and sweat glands. The reticular layer also contains **Meissner's and Pacinian corpuscles,** which are concerned with sensory touch perception and deep pressure respectively.

THINK LINK: Lines of Cleavage

The collagen and elastic fibers throughout the body are configured in parallel bundles that are oriented to resist the forces related to various skin movements. The pattern of these bundles creates what are described as lines of cleavage (Figure 16-2). These lines are important to healing and scar formation. Interruptions to the skin caused by cuts or incisions that are parallel to the lines of cleavage will heal with minimal scar formation. In contrast, when the interruption is perpendicular or at right angles to the lines of cleavage, the elastic recoil of the severed fibers pulls the margins of the cut or incision apart, causing increased formation of scar tissue.

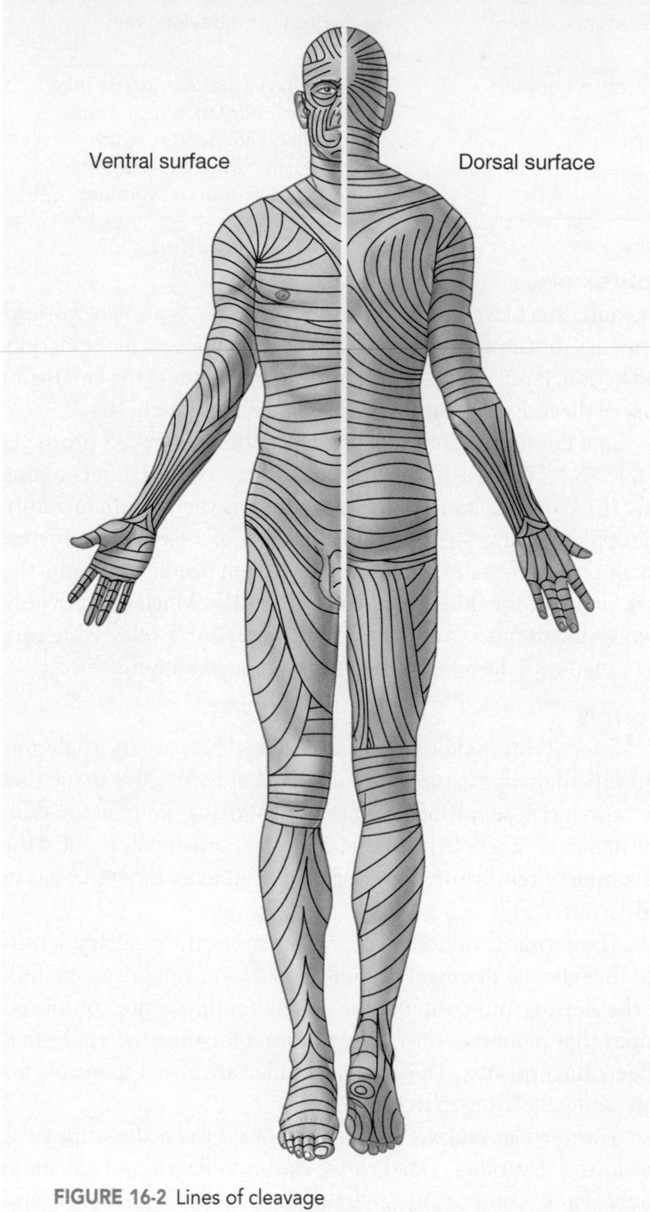

FIGURE 16-2 Lines of cleavage

Subcutaneous Layer (Hypodermis)

The third, or subcutaneous, skin layer is composed of adipose tissue and loose/dense connective tissue. The subcutaneous layer attaches the dermal reticular layer to underlying organs; it also generates heat, provides insulation, acts as a shock absorber, and provides storage for calories.

Skin Color

Skin color depends on the three pigments—melanin, carotene, and oxyhemoglobin—that are present in the skin and the blood. Melanin (brown) is produced by the melanocytes and later transferred as melanosomes to keratinocytes (Martini & Nath, 2009). The number of melanocytes is identical in all individuals. The difference in the amount of pigment produced is genetic. Genetics also determines the number and size of the melanosomes and their distribution within the skin. Melanin production, which is stimulated by sun exposure, functions to protect the skin from ultraviolet radiation and damage. Carotene, a yellow pigment, is stored in subcutaneous fat and also present in heavily keratinized locations, such as a callous, and in yellow vegetables. Most of the carotene in the body comes from the ingestion of these vegetables. The red tones of the skin come from the amount of oxygenated hemoglobin that is circulating.

Skin Appendages (Accessory Structures)

The appendages or accessory structures of the skin consist of hair, fingernails, sweat glands, and sebaceous glands.

Hair Hair, a dead keratinized structure, is formed by the growth of stratum germinativum epidermal cells. These cells grow down into the dermis to become a follicle that is located on papillae of connective tissue and capillaries, which supply it with nourishment (Figure 16-3). The matrix, or lower portion of the follicle, consists of actively proliferating epithelial cells. A hair shaft is produced from these cells in the matrix, which grows outward through a canal or root sheath. The root sheath is formed during the epidermal down growth into the dermis.

Hair growth occurs in the following cycles or phases: anagen (growth), catagen (atrophy), and telogen (resting). Hair is shed when the follicle matrix shrivels. After a period of rest, the follicle forms another matrix and growth occurs again.

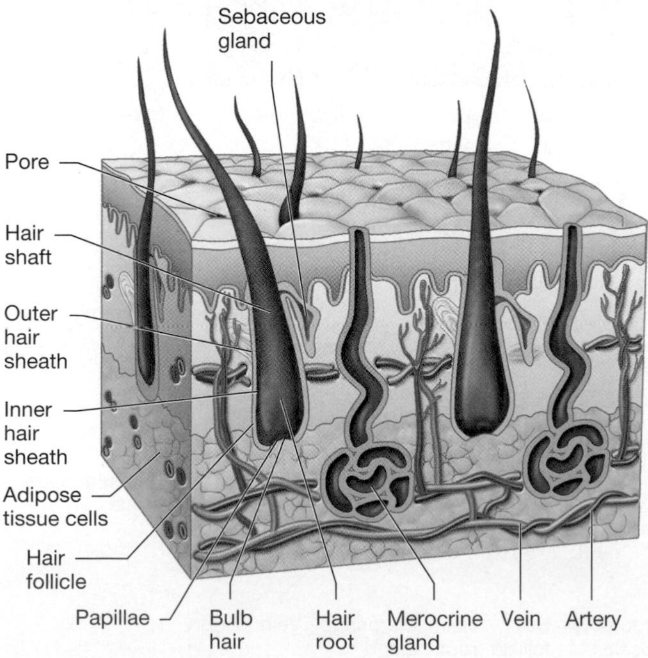

FIGURE 16-3 Anatomy of hair follicle and shaft

Adults have two types of hair: vellus and terminal. **Vellus hair** is short, fine, and nonpigmented peach fuzz type hair covering most of the body. **Terminal hair** is thicker, longer, pigmented, and located over the head and other portions of the body. Certain locations of terminal hair, such as pubic hair, are influenced by hormones and do not appear until puberty. Hair is located over the entire body with the exception of the palms, soles, glans penis, and labia minora.

Nails Nails are hard plates of keratin found on the dorsal aspect of the distal portion of the fingers and toes (Figure 16-4). The **nail plate** is derived from epidermal cells and consists of the proximal **nail matrix**, a fixed middle portion, and the distal free edge. The area under the nail is known as the **nail bed**. Embedded in the posterior nail fold and is the site for nail growth, the matrix is observed as a white, crescent-shaped area, called the lunula. Its margin identifies the point where nail growth stops. The pink color associated with the nails is due to the rich vascular supply to the nail bed. The layer of epithelial cells that cover the nail root is the **eponychium**; the soft tissue surrounding the nail border is known as the **paronychium**.

Sweat Glands Sweat glands belong to a group of glands that secrete their substances into ducts that connect with the external environment. These are exocrine glands, in contrast to endocrine glands, which secrete their substances (hormones) directly into the bloodstream, where they are carried to specific cells, resulting in a specific physiological response.

The two types of sweat glands are merocrine and apocrine. **Merocrine (eccrine) glands** are primarily responsible for body temperature regulation; they open directly to the skin surface and excrete sweat for purposes of cooling by evaporation. Sweat from merocrine glands is composed of water, salt, and other wastes. The approximately 2 to 3 million merocrine glands distributed over the body are capable of secreting 10 liters of sweat per day. Specific locations on the body where merocrine glands are not present are the lip margins, eardrums, nail beds, inner surface of prepuce, labia minora, and glans penis. The merocrine glands are under sympathetic nervous system control.

Apocrine glands are larger than merocrine glands and are located only in specific areas: axillae, nipples, areolae, anogenital area, eyelids, and external ears. They are also found in close association with hair follicles. Apocrine glands become functional during puberty, and when stimulated, they secrete a milky, sticky fluid that contains proteins, carbohydrates, and other substances. These substances are odorless, but when bacteria break them down, a distinct odor, which is known as body odor, is produced.

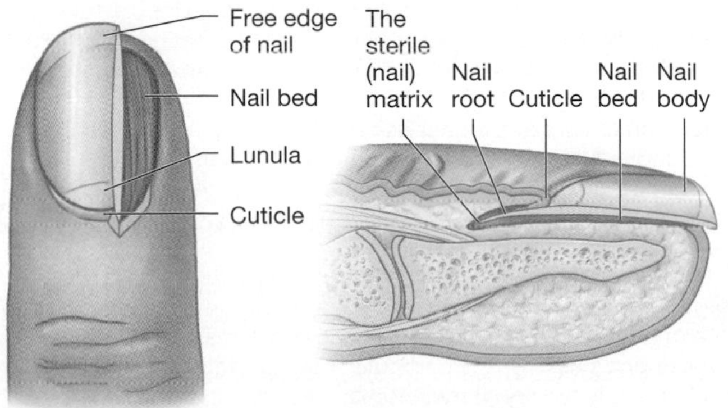

FIGURE 16-4 Anatomical structure of fingernail

Sebaceous Glands The sebaceous glands produce a lipid-rich, oily substance known as sebum. Sebum is discharged directly into the lumen of the hair follicle, where it lubricates the hair shaft and then migrates to the skin surface, where it prevents the skin from drying out. Sebaceous glands are distributed over the entire body, with the largest glands located on the face and upper back. The amount of sebum produced is directly related to hormonal activity, primarily testosterone, and varies throughout the life span.

Developmental Variations

Developmental variations occur over the course of an individual's life span and events. Awareness of these variations is important to understand and recognize common age-related alterations or modifications of the integumentary system.

Infants and Children

The smoother skin of infants and children, as compared to adults, is primarily related to the lack of exposure to environmental variables and the lack of terminal hair. At birth, or shortly thereafter, the infant may experience shedding of the stratum corneum. This may range from mild flakiness to shedding of large sections of keratinized epithelium. The infant may also be covered with **vernix caseosa,** a cheese-like substance of sebum and keratinized epidermis that functions to protect the infant's skin in utero to prevent maceration from amniotic fluid.

The epidermis and dermis are present at birth; however, the subcutaneous layer is poorly developed, thus predisposing infants to hypothermia. The infant's body, particularly the shoulders and back, may be covered with lanugo, a fine silky hair. If present, it is usually lost within 10 to 14 days. The amount of infant head hair varies dramatically, from none to a very thick amount. Most head hair will disappear within 2 to 3 months and be replaced with more permanent hair that usually has a different color and texture.

Merocrine sweat glands begin to function after about 4 weeks. Apocrine glands do not function at this age, resulting in odorless perspiration and skin with a less oily texture than that of adolescents and adults.

Adolescents

On reaching adolescence, appocrine and sebaceous glands become active. Increased appocrine gland activity is associated with increased axillary sweating, which predisposes to the development of body odor. Sebaceous glands respond to increased levels of hormones, causing an increased production of sebum, resulting in an overall oily appearance. Excess sebum also predisposes the adolescent to the development of acne.

The initial appearance of terminal hair occurs primarily in the axillary and pubic areas of both genders, as well as facial hair in the male. The appearance of terminal hair is also a response to increased levels of hormones.

The Pregnant Woman

Pregnancy results in an increased blood flow to the skin, particularly the hands and feet, due to peripheral vasodilation and an increase in numbers of capillaries. This is accompanied by an increase in metabolism, causing overactivity of both the sweat and sebaceous glands. This overactivity plays a significant role in removing the excess heat produced during pregnancy due to the changes in metabolism.

An increase in hormones results in areas of hyperpigmentation, most notably in the nipples and areolae, and vulva; however, scars and nevi may also become darker. These manifestations are generally more evident in women with darker complexion (Tunzi & Gray, 2007). Other areas that may be affected include the abdominal midline and the face. Any existing vascular spiders and/or hemangiomas may enlarge during pregnancy.

Pruritus is also present during pregnancy and may be related to a reoccurrence of an existing alteration or may be considered a pregnancy-specific dermatosis. Pruritus not associated with an underlying skin condition occurs in approximately 20% of pregnant women (Pomeranz, 2013). Specific dermatoses of pregnancy include PUPP (pruritic urticarial papules and plaques of pregnancy), prurigo of pregnancy, intrahepatic cholestasis of pregnancy, pemphigoid gestationis, impetigo herpetiformis, and pruritic folliculitis of pregnancy. Generally, these are not considered risks to pregnancy; however, intrahepatic cholestasis of pregnancy does increase the risk of premature delivery and has been associated with fetal demise, and impetigo herpetiformis has been associated with an increased fetal morbidity (Tunzi & Gray, 2007).

The pregnant woman's skin becomes notably thicker, with fat deposits occurring primarily in the buttocks and hips. These function as maternal reserves later when the woman is nursing. The connective tissue experiences an increased fragility, which may result in its separation, producing stretch marks. These most commonly occur on the abdomen; however, they may also occur on the thighs and breasts.

The Older Adult

In the older adult, sebaceous and sweat gland activity is diminished, resulting in drier skin and less perspiration. The epidermis becomes thin and flat, which gives the skin a parchment appearance, particularly as the vascularity of the dermis decreases. The thinning and flattening of the epidermis result in a decreased barrier function, predisposing older adults to invasion by environmental substances.

A loss of collagen and shrinking of elastic fibers cause the dermis to lose its elasticity, resulting in skin that is wrinkled and creased. A loss of muscle tone contributes to the skin's lax and drooping appearance. A lifetime of sun exposure also contributes to the wrinkled appearance of the skin.

The amount of subcutaneous tissue also decreases in the older adult, particularly in the extremities, making joints and bony prominences appear angular and sharp. The skin depressions of the thoracic, axillary, and supraclavicular areas deepen and take on a more hollow appearance.

Hair changes include a loss of color, change in texture, and decrease in number of hairs. A decrease in melanocytes of the hair matrix results in the graying of hair. The mechanism by which hair turns grey is not well understood but is thought to involve impairment of the melanocyte-keratinocyte functions. At what age this occurs is genetically determined and differs by ethnicity, beginning in the mid-30s for Caucasians, late-30s for Asians, and mid-40s for African Americans (Kaplan et al., 2011). Axillary and pubic hair production declines due to a reduction of androgen hormone. Hair follicle size also changes, resulting in terminal scalp hair transitioning into vellus hair, which may lead to baldness in both genders. This transition to vellus hair is also noted on the hairs of the nares and the tragus of the ear in males. Females may notice the appearance of coarse facial hairs (hirsutism) due to the reduction in estrogen, resulting in a higher androgen/estrogen ratio. Loss of hair from the trunk and extremities is noted in both genders.

Nail growth slows down as a result of decreased peripheral circulation. The toenails frequently become thicker, hard, brittle, and yellowish in appearance. Longitudinal ridges from local trauma at the nail matrix also can occur.

Health Promotion

Skin Cancer

Skin cancer is the most common form of all cancers, accounting for nearly half of all cancers in the United States. Skin cancers comprise three types: basal cell, squamous cell, and melanoma. The most common skin cancers are basal cell and squamous cell carcinomas, which are also described as non-melanoma or keratinocyte cancers. Melanoma is the most severe form of skin cancer, due to its ability to rapidly metastasize throughout the body.

- *The Healthy People 2020* goal related to skin cancer is to reduce the number of melanoma-related cancer deaths to 2.4 per 100,000 (U.S. Department of Health and Human Services, 2009).

Approximately 3.5 million cases of basal and squamous cell skin cancer are found annually in the U.S. The annual rate for skin cancers, primarily melanoma, appears to increase every year by approximately 3%. Melanoma, the most deadly form of skin cancer, accounted for more than 76,250 cases of skin cancer in 2012, comprising only 5% of skin cancers but causing the majority of skin cancer deaths (American Cancer Society, 2012). Total annual deaths in 2011 from skin cancer were approximately 11,980 with 5,750 attributed to melanoma (American Cancer Society, 2011).

Risk Factors

The major risk factor for all types of skin cancer is exposure to ultraviolet (UV) radiation, primarily from the sun. This relates to length of time of exposure as well as distance from the sun. Individuals living at higher elevations are exposed to more intense UV radiation. Artificial sources of UV radiation are just as harmful as UV radiation in sunlight.

Additional sun-related factors for melanoma include skin color and sun burns. Individuals with fair skin that tends to burn rather than tan are at a higher risk for development of melanoma. These individuals tend to have red or blond hair and blue eyes. Having had a severe, blistering sunburn as a child or teen also increases the risk for melanoma. Sunburn in adults also increases the risk for developing melanoma.

A personal or family history of melanoma also increases the risk for a melanoma. Although not always the case, the presence of atypical nevi as well as having more than 50 typical nevi increase one's risk. This is particularly significant if there is a personal or family history of melanoma.

Health Promotion *continued*

Prevention

To prevent the development of skin cancer, the following actions are recommended:

- Avoid sun exposure during the midday (10:00 a.m. to 4:00 p.m.) as much as possible.
- When outside, wear a long-sleeved shirt, long pants, and a hat with a wide brim.
- Avoid UV radiation that is reflected by sand, water, snow, or ice.
- Protect the skin with use of sunscreen lotion. Sunscreens that reflect or absorb or scatter both types of UV (A and B) radiation will help prevent melanoma. Sunscreens with a sun protection factor (SPF) of 30 or greater provide the maximum protection. Sunscreens with a SPF of 12–29 provide moderate protection, and those with an SPF factor of 2–11 provide the least protection.
- Protect the eyes by wearing sunglasses with UV-absorbing lenses that block at least 99% of UVA and UVB radiation.
- Avoid artificial sources of UV radiation (tanning booths and sun lamps).
- Know the ABCs of melanoma (see Table 16-2).

While these ABCs of melanoma are very helpful in identifying a possible melanoma, it has been found that these tips are a challenge for the novice to use (Robinson & Turrisi, 2006). The most consistent parameters that are reported by individuals are a change in size and/or color.

Skin Self-Examination

Screening for skin cancer is an important part of health care. However, many agencies have reported that insufficient evidence exists to recommend for or against routine screening (total-body skin examination) for skin cancer in asymptomatic patients in a primary care setting (Rager, Bridgeford, & Ollila, 2005). Despite this, providers should take advantage of the opportunity to assess the patient's skin during a routine examination.

Providers should also encourage patients to perform monthly skin self-examinations (SSEs). Individuals who engage in monthly SSEs are more likely to present for care at an earlier stage of the cancer and have a 50% lower rate of advanced melanoma, resulting in a significantly reduced mortality rate (63%) from melanoma (Robinson, Fisher, & Turrisi, 2002). Early detection of melanoma is crucial as it is the thickness of the melanoma at time of diagnosis that affects survival (Janda et al., 2006). Performing SSE is enhanced when a partner participates (Robinson, Turrisi, & Stapleton, 2007). It is found that males are more likely to do an SSE when there is a participating partner.

***THINK LINK:** Skin Cancer and UV Radiation*

Ultraviolet radiation is divided into three wavelengths: UVA, UVB, and UVC. UVA rays cause skin damage to cells' DNA and causes skin to age. They are mostly linked to long-term skin damage (wrinkles) and are thought to contribute to skin cancer. UVB rays cause direct damage to DNA and are responsible for sunburns. They are the cause of most skin cancers. UVC rays don't penetrate our atmosphere and so are not present in sunlight (Cancer Reference Information, n.d.).

Table 16-2 The ABCs of melanoma

Asymmetry	One half of the nevus doesn't match the other half.
Border	Border irregularity; the edges are ragged, notched, or blurred; pigment may spread to surrounding skin.
Color	Color is uneven, with various colors (black, brown, tan) present simultaneously; may also be shades or red, blue, grey, pink, or white.

Continued

Table 16-2 The ABCs of melanoma *(continued)*

Diameter	Diameter increases in size to greater than 6 mm (size of an eraser).
Elevation/**E**volution	Recent change from flat lesion to elevated lesion

Source: National Cancer Institute/Larry Meyer (photographer)

TEACHING TIP: Skin Self-Examination Procedure

Instruct patients that the optimum time for an SSE is after a shower or bath in a well-lighted room with both full-length mirror and hand-held mirrors available (Figure 16-5). During the first exam, patients should confirm the location and feel of known birthmarks, moles, or blemishes.

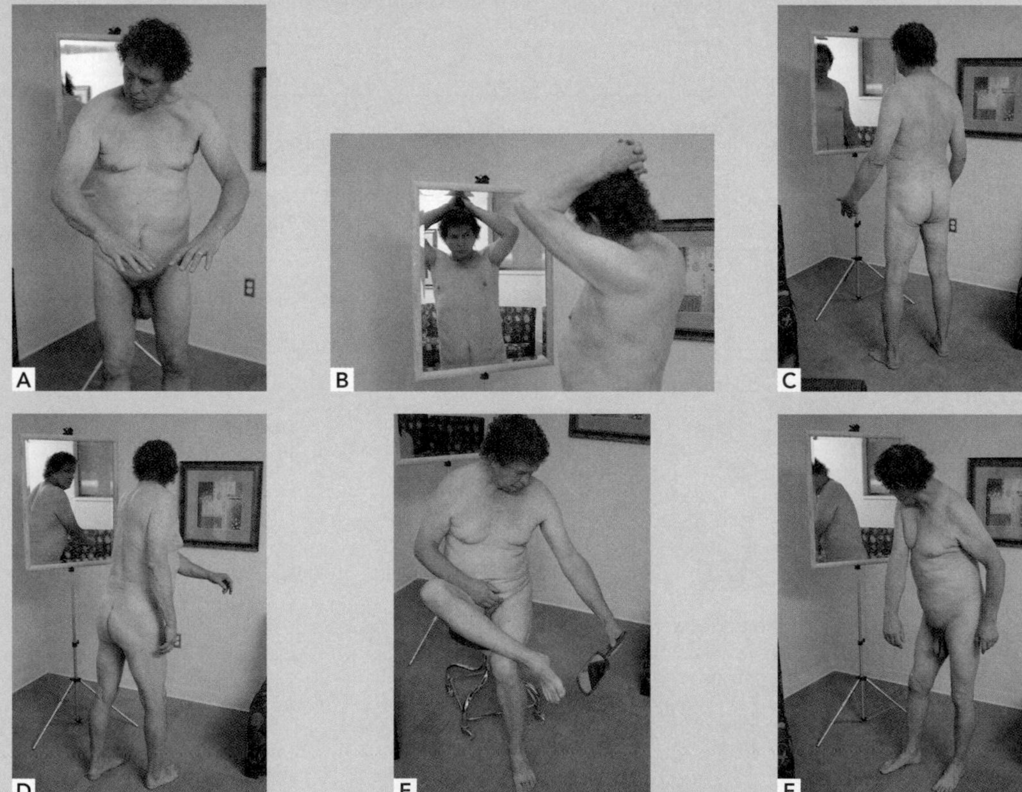

FIGURE 16-5A–F Self-examination of skin

- Check yourself from head to toe. Specific areas that should not be overlooked include the back, scalp, between the buttocks, and the genital area.
  - A new mole (that looks abnormal)
  - A change in the size, shape, color, or texture of a mole
  - A sore that does not heal
- Look at your face, neck, ears, and scalp. A comb or blow dryer may be used to move the hair to facilitate inspection. A partner may be beneficial for this part as this may be a rather difficult area to observe.
- Look at the front and back of your body in the mirror, then raise your arms and look at the right and left side of your body.
- Bend your elbows and inspect carefully your fingernails, palms, forearms, and upper arms.
- Examine the back, front, and sides of your legs. Sit and closely inspect your feet, toenails, soles, and between the toes.

Clinical Context Exemplars

Situation A

You are examining Jess Simmons for complaints of white areas appearing on her hands and forearm. She says, "I want to know what these white patches are." She is worried they might turn into cancer, and she also wonders whether she can prevent more from developing.

1. What would you tell Ms. Simmons that the white patches are most likely to be?
2. How would you respond to Ms. Simmons's question about cancer?
3. What would you tell Ms. Simmons about preventing further white areas from appearing?

Situation B

Thomas Anderson arrives in the office to have a skin lesion evaluated. He wants to know whether the lesion is a melanoma.

1. How would you assess this lesion to determine whether it is a melanoma?
2. What history information would you want to obtain from Mr. Anderson?
3. What manifestations would you be concerned about for other skin cancers?
4. What counsel would you give to Mr. Anderson?

Situation C

During your examination of Mina Rosedale, an older female, she states that she has noticed dark hairs appearing on her upper lip and chin. She asks, "Am I turning into a male?" She wonders what she can do about the new hair growth. She also expresses concern about her hair, stating, "I used to have a full head of thick hair, but now it is becoming thin and seems to be falling out. What can I do to stop this?"

1. How would you respond to Mrs. Rosedale's question?
2. What would you tell Mrs. Rosedale about the hair growth?
3. How would you respond to Mrs. Rosedale's questions about her hair thinning?

Mrs. Rosedale also says, "My skin is also getting wrinkled. Is there anything I can do to prevent this from getting worse?"

4. What would your response be?
5. What other history information would you want to know about Mrs. Rosedale in relation to the skin wrinkling?

SUBJECTIVE DATA

History of Present Illness (CC)

The patient may present to the provider with a variety of concerns that may be directly related to the integumentary system or other systems. Framing the questions will depend on the patient's age, gender, culture, race, emotional or mental status, health practices, and concurrent illnesses. All symptoms presented must be thoroughly assessed with a symptom analysis (COLDERRA).

Pruritus

Pruritus (itching) is an unpleasant sensation that elicits the desire or reflex to scratch and is the most common skin condition, associated with both acute and chronic skin alterations and frequently a significant symptom of other systemic conditions (Garcia-Albea & Limaye, 2012). It may also be related to allergies, age, weather, medications, or insect bites. Recent studies have determined that an itch is similar to pain. Both are unpleasant sensory experiences, but their behavioral response patterns are different. Pain initiates a withdrawal reflex while itch results in a scratch reflex (Ikoma, Steinhoff, Stander, Yosipovitch, & Schmelz, 2006).

Provider Inquiries	Clinical Reasoning/Logic
Characteristics: How experienced? How does area appear? Any noticeable bites, any color changes? Any noticeable changes in skin texture?	Prickling, tingling; intensity 1–10
Onset: When did it start? Anything new related to food, medications, and environment? Known allergies (animals, foods, drugs)? Recent hikes, walks in grassy areas?	Determine if the itching started with anything recently introduced into patient's environment, activities, routine, diet, etc. If itching occurs approximately after 30 minutes of water contact without obvious lesions (aquagenic pruritus), polycythemia vera, myeloproliferative disease, histocyte disorders, and physical urticaria need to be ruled out (Garcia-Albea & Limaye, 2012).

Provider Inquiries	Clinical Reasoning/Logic
Location: Where located? Generalized or localized?	Certain parts of the body are predisposed to itching: ear canals, eyelids, nostrils, perianal and genital areas (Garcia-Albea & Limaye, 2012).
Duration: How long do the episodes of itching last? (Intermittent or continuous? Seasonal?)	Chronic pruritus is an itch that persists for longer than 6 weeks (Yosipovitch & Bernhard, 2013).
Exacerbation: What/when makes itching worse/more intense? • Fluid loss or decreased fluid intake? • Use of ointments (e.g., petroleum, mineral oil)? • Frequent bathing/bathing with hot water for longer than ½ hour? • Use of detergents/bubble baths? • Deodorants/antiperspirants? • Dry environment? • Tight restrictive clothing or clothing made of wool, synthetics, or other harsh fabric? • Emotional stress?	Often reported that itching gets worse at bedtime. Extensive bathing aggravates dry skin, and hot baths cause vasodilation, which further promotes itching. Water, not lipid, regulates the pliability of the epidermis. Some topical agents including talcum powders, perfumed powders, bubble baths, and cornstarch can irritate the skin and cause pruritus. Other common ingredients in over-the-counter lotions and creams that may enhance skin reactions include alcohol and menthol. Residue left by detergents used in laundering clothes and linens, as well as fabric softeners and antistatic products, may aggravate pruritus. Heat increases cutaneous blood flow and may enhance itching. Heat also lowers humidity, and skin loses moisture when the relative humidity is less than 40%.
Relief: What makes itching better or go away? (Creams, lotions, heat/cold, medications [anti-histamines]) How long does relief last? Basic skin care with application of emollient creams or lotions. • Use of mild soaps (for sensitive skin), laundering with mild soaps (e.g., Dreft)? • Limiting bathing to ½ hour daily or every other day • Adding oil at the end of a bath or adding a colloidal oatmeal treatment early to the bath? • Maintenance of a humid environment (e.g., availability/use of humidifiers [stand alone equipment, included in heating/cooling unit]?) • Wearing of loose-fitting clothing and using sheets/blankets made of cotton or other soft fabrics? • Use of distraction, relaxation, positive imagery, or cutaneous stimulation? • Use of oral antihistamines (increased doses at bedtime)? • Use of topical corticosteroids?	Emollients reduce evaporation by forming occlusive and semiocclusive films over the skin surface, encouraging the production of moisture in the layer of epidermis beneath the film (hence, the term *moisturizer*). Tepid baths have an antipruritic effect, possibly resulting from capillary vasoconstriction. Distraction, music therapy, relaxation, and imagery may be useful to relieve symptoms.
Associated signs/symptoms: Any color changes, increased temperature, and other known diseases at present time?	Itching with a rash most often indicates a primary dermatological disorder (Taylor & Zirwas, 2012).

Rashes/Skin Lesions

Rash is one of the top 20 reasons for ER/ED visits in the U.S. (Murphy-Lavoie & LeGros, 2010). The term *rash* has no precise definition and is often related to a wide variety of skin disorders. Most commonly the term is used to describe an eruption or appearance of skin lesions that cover certain areas of the skin.

Provider Inquiries	Clinical Reasoning/Logic
Characteristics: Itching, pain, raised/flat macular/papular, color, temperature changes, bleeding?	Rashes often involve changes in skin color or texture. *Erythematous rash*—diffuse redness of skin due to capillary congestion (Staphylococcal scalded skin syndrome, toxic epidermal necrolysis, toxic shock syndrome, Kawasaki disease, scarlet fever, anaphylaxis) *Maculopapular rash*—combination of macules and papules (lyme disease, Stevens-Johnson syndrome, erythema multiforme, meningococcemia, Rocky Mountain Spotted Fever) *Petechial purpuric rashes*—palpable, raised purpura occurs in asculitid diseases secondary to inflammation/infection (vasculitis); non-palpable purpura in thrombocytopenic conditions (purpura fulminans, disseminated intravascular coagulopathy, thrombotic thrombocytopenia) *Vesiculobullous rash*—diffuse distribution with fever (chicken pox, disseminaterd gonococcal disease, disseminated intravascular coagulopathy), without fever, bullous pemphigoid, pemphigus vulgaris. Localized without fever (contact dermatitis, herpes zoster), with fever (necrotizing fasciitis)
Onset: When was it first noticed? Associated with anything new introduced into patient's diet? Any new foods, medications, known insect bites, seasonal manifestations associated with onset of rash? Environment (exposure to toxins/chemicals, medications)?	Rapid onset related to food/drug allergy, insect bite/sting Atopic dermatitis most often begins in childhood before age 5 and may persist into adulthood. Atopic dermatitis often occurs together with other atopic diseases like hay fever, asthma and allergic conjunctivitis.
Location: Where is rash/lesion located (localized/generalized)? Where did it start?	Localized lesions commonly related to contact or infectious process. Seborrheic dermatitis—located on scalp, forehead, brows, cheeks, and external ears Atopic dermatitis (eczema) may affect any area of the skin, but typically appears on the arms, hands, and feet and behind the knees, in front of the bend of the elbow, and on the ankles, wrists, face, neck and upper chest.
Duration: How long has it been present?	Most deadly rashes progress rapidly. Drug reactions may develop over hours to days.

Provider Inquiries	Clinical Reasoning/Logic
Exacerbation: Anything that makes it worse? Clothing, moisture, heat/cold?	In most patients, symptoms that occur with dermatitis are aggravated by a Staphylococcus aureus infection, dry skin, stress, low humidity and sweating, dust or sand or cigarette smoke. Also, the condition can be worsened by having long and hot baths or showers. The use of solvents, cleaners or detergents and wearing wool fabrics or clothing also may worsen the condition. Viral rashes usually begin centrally and spread peripherally.
Relief: Does anything make it better?	There is no known cure for eczema; however certain treatments, such as drugs (steroids, immunosuppressives), moisturizers, and UV light therapy are recommended to reduce the effects (Bigal et al., 2008).
Associated signs/symptoms	Pruritus accompanying rash is associated with scabies, urticaria, and atopic dermatitis.

Sensitive Skin (Allodynia)

Allodynia is the perception of pain that is caused by usually nonpainful stimuli, such as touch or vibration. Someone with sensitive skin finds touch annoying, uncomfortable, and frequently unbearable. It is often associated with other pain conditions (complex regional pain syndrome, migraines).

Provider Inquiries	Clinical Reasoning/Logic
Characteristics: How do you experience sensitive skin, how does it feel?	Exaggerated type of pain or sensitivity even to non-painful stimuli, such as a breeze. May feel like a crawling on the skin, itchiness, pins and needles, or a burning sensation.
Onset: What typically initiates sensation? Various causes associated with types of sensitivity.	• Tactile or mechanical allodynia is triggered by touch. • Static mechanical allodynia is caused by light touch or pressure. • Dynamic mechanical allodynia occurs when brushing the skin triggers pain. • Thermal allodynia is felt with cold or hot stimuli.
Location: Is the pain localized or generalized?	The pain may be localized or widespread, with intense pain that is usually triggered by stimuli that would not normally elicit pain. In migraine patients, sensitivity to touch on the scalp and abnormal soreness or tenderness of the pericranial muscles were the most common symptom (Mathew, Kailasam, & Seifert, 2004).
Duration: Does the duration of the sensitivity accompany the duration of the migraine?	The duration of the sensitivity is more commonly associated with the severity or intensity of the migraine rather than the duration.
Exacerbation: What makes it worse?	The pain can be provoked by combing or brushing hair, shaving, showering, or wearing glasses or earrings.

Provider Inquiries	Clinical Reasoning/Logic
Radiation: Does the pain radiate?	Allodynia is more progressive in character than radiating. The sensitivity may increase as well as the progression or expansion of the area involved.
Relief: Use of topical pain creams, medications?	Capsaicin, Tiger Balm, Aspercreme, and BioFreeze may work for some individuals. Heat is helpful for some individuals. Topical anesthetic agents may also produce some relief. If allodynia is associated with migraines, treatment for migraine is a priority.
Associated signs/symptoms: Do you suffer from migraines?	Allodynia is more common and more severe in two types of migraine, transformed migraine and episodic migraine, than in other primary headaches. For those with migraine the chance of having allodynia is increased by being female, having frequent headaches, increased body mass index, disability and depression (Bigal et al., 2008).
Skin Changes (Lesions, Hair, Fingernails) Skin changes are most commonly related to color, texture, moles, or a sore (lesion) that does not heal. Changes related to an increase in size or pigmentation, bleeding, pain, itching, chronic irritation of clothing (bras, belts, etc.) or the appearance of new lesions should prompt a high level of suspicion for the development of skin cancer. Changes associated with hair and nails most commonly relate to changes in texture, amount (loss), distribution, color and surface characteristics.	
Characteristics: Describe changes (lesions/moles–appearance/changes, color, size, edges, and texture)	Changes in the skin and appendages often accompany or indicate an underlying disorder or condition. (For changes in lesions associated with melanoma, see Table 16-2.)
Hair (amount, distribution, texture)	Changes in texture of hair are associated with thyroid disorders. Changes in distribution/loss are related to genetics or certain conditions.
Nails (appearance—shape color, brittleness) Any pain, itching, bleeding, exudate?	Changes in fingernails are also associated with specific conditions and alterations.
Onset: When was it first noticed (sudden/gradual onset)? Any exposure to environmental hazards, toxins, medications, individuals with similar conditions, travel?	Onset of a particular change may help to determine or stage the presence of an underlying disorder/condition. Also important to determine any recent travel, changes in environment, new drugs, and relationship to onset.
Location: Where did change occur? Localized or generalized?	Generalized skin color changes are frequently associated with certain systemic conditions. Localized changes are more related to lesions either in their appearance, presence or changes in configuration.
Duration: How long has change been present?	The length of time associated with changes often reflects the onset or initial awareness of change.

Provider Inquiries	Clinical Reasoning/Logic
Exacerbation: Does anything make it more noticeable/sensitive (lotions, temperature [heat/cold], sun exposure)?	Certain drugs or chemicals increase sensitivity to sun. This is considered an allergic or irritant reactions to products mostly, but can also indicate individuals who develop rashes in response to external environmental things, such as plants or foods.
Associated signs/symptoms: Other conditions, fever, relationship to stress/leisure activities? Patient's reaction to change or appearance?	Stress/anxiety over appearance of skin and others' reaction to it.
	Skin lesions associated with vitamin B_{12} deficiency are skin hyperpigmentation, vitiligo, angular stomatitis, and hair changes.

Past Medical History

Information from the past medical history is important to determine if any previous medical condition or situation is a possible cause of present complaint of condition. Depending on how much of a history has been done to determine the patient's present condition (chief concern), some of the information related to past medical history may have already been obtained.

Skin

Provider Inquiries	Clinical Reasoning/Logic
Previous problems: Sensitivities, allergies (skin reactions/disorders)	Information regarding any previous skin conditions will help to determine present condition.
Sun exposure: Tolerance for sun exposure, amount of exposure (burn easily, tan easily), severe sunburns as child?	Information regarding sun exposure identifies risk factors for skin cancer.
Diseases: Cardiac, endocrine, liver, renal? Neuropathies? Migraine history? Shingles? Fibromyalgia? Demyelinating diseases? Midbrain defect?	Information regarding other conditions that can affect skin. Any of these conditions are associated with increased sensitivity of the skin.

Hair

Provider Inquiries	Clinical Reasoning/Logic
Previous problems: Loss, thinning, altered distribution/growth, brittleness, breakage	Information regarding any prior episodes, any pattern to hair loss.
Diseases: Thyroid/liver, severe illnesses, altered nutrition, other skin disorders	Information regarding conditions that can affect the skin.

Nails

Provider Inquiries	Clinical Reasoning/Logic
Previous problems: Injury, infections (bacterial, viral, fungal), artificial nails (how long, any problems)?	Information regarding prior conditions affecting nails.
Systemic disorders: Skin, cardiac, respiratory, endocrine, hematologic? Congenital anomalies? Any other known conditions that may affect the nails?	

Family History

Information regarding any alterations in family members (immediate and distant) may provide clues to possible causes of present condition (chief concern) or the possibility of potential conditions or alterations.

Provider Inquiries	Clinical Reasoning/Logic
Dermatologic diseases/disorders: Any past or current conditions in family members? Skin cancer (type), psoriasis, allergic disorders, infections (bacterial, viral, fungal)?	Information regarding any pattern of diseases/conditions or familial tendency for certain conditions.
Genetic allergic/autoimmune disorders: Asthma, hay fever, Systemic lupus erythematosis?	Information regarding any pattern of diseases/conditions or familial tendency for certain conditions.
Hair patterns: Loss of hair, color alterations?	Information regarding hair loss—genetics or other treatments to hair.

Personal and Social History

Information regarding personal and social activities may provide clues as to cause of present condition or the potential for future alterations or conditions.

Provider Inquiries	Clinical Reasoning/Logic
Skin care habits: How does patient care for skin? **Routine care:** Frequency of bathing/showers (keeping skin clean and odor free)?	Hygiene has to do with the integrity and condition of skin.
Products used: Soaps, lotions, creams, oils? Home remedies? Cosmetics?	Any substances that may be causing condition.
Sun exposure: Patterns and history, use of sunscreen? (Obtain information now if not obtained previously.) Any changes in routine? Skin examination (SSE)? Perform, knowledge of?	Information regarding awareness of skin cancer prevention.
Any piercings or tattoos in past?	Individuals who have had these procedures done are at higher risk for development of hepatitis C.
Hair care habits: Frequency of washing (information regarding cleanliness of hair) Products used (shampoo, rinse, coloring agents, and permanents) (information regarding what substances are used for hair care)? Any changes in routine?	This primarily includes information related to personal care habits and whether practices or any substances used may contribute to skin condition(s).
Nail care habits: Difficulty trimming, cutting? Pattern of cutting? Ingrown nails (information regarding the characteristics of nails and any potential problems)? Biting of nails (information regarding action; does patient do always or only at certain times)?	Nail-biting (onychophagia) is a common stress-relieving habit that often occurs in instances of stress or excitement, as well as in times of boredom or inactivity. It can also be a learned behavior from family members. Nail-biting is the most common of the common "nervous habits" (such as thumb-sucking, nose-picking, hair-twisting or -pulling, tooth-grinding, and picking at skin).
Occupation/Environmental hazard exposure: Chemicals, dyes, toxins, excessive water immersion, plants, sun exposure, and cigarette smoke (information regarding exposure to substances that may affect skin)?	
Drugs: Prescription, recreational, alcohol, cigarette smoking?	Certain drugs can increase sensitivity to sun (see Table 16-3).
Stress: Recent experience (physiologic/psychologic)?	

THINK LINK:* *Smoking and Skin Wrinkles

Individuals who smoke tend to develop wrinkled skin earlier than those who do not smoke. Smokers express a proteolytic enzyme (matrix metalloproteinase) that degrades the collagen matrix in the skin. This enzyme is inhibited by an antiprotease enzyme; however, in smokers, expression of the proteolytic enzyme is greater than that of its inhibitor. Sun damage is also a contributor to premature wrinkling; however, in smokers, early wrinkling was demonstrated in areas that had not been exposed to the sun (Dawson, 2007).

PRACTICE POINT:* *Drugs and Sun

Sun-sensitizing drugs are prescription and over the counter medications that increase the skins susceptibility to reddening and burning from the sun or sun tanning lamps. These drugs are also identified as photosensitizing agents. In addition to sunburn, these drugs may cause blistering, hives, rash, or other skin reactions. These reactions may be described as either photoallergic or phototoxic. Photoallergic reactions result from UV light reacting with the drug or drug ingredient to produce an antigen. Antibodies are then produced by the immune system, so the next time the drug is taken, there is an allergic response. Phototoxic reactions do not involve the immune system. Instead the skin responds as if poisoned, causing symptoms to occur after the drug is ingested the first time. Specific drugs that cause sun sensitivity are listed in Table 16-3.

Table 16-3 Common photosensitive drugs

Drug Used For	Generic Name	Trade Name
Acne	isoretinoin acitretin	Accutane Soriatane
Antibiotics	quinolones cioprofloxacin levofloxacin tetracycline doxycylinne sulfonamides sulfamethoxazole/trimethoprim; cotrimoxazole sulfamethoxazole	 Cipro, Cipro XR, Proquin XR Levaquin Achromycin Vibramycin, Oracea, Adoxa, Atridox Bactrim, Septra Gantanol
Antihistamines	diphenhydramine doxylamine	Benadryl (OTC) Unisom Nightime sleep aid (OTC)
Birth Control	ethinyl estradiol	Alesse, Levulen, Lo/Ovral, Ortho-cept, Ortho-cyclen, Ortho-Novum, Tri-cyclen
Chemotherapy [Cancer]	5-fluroouracil vinblastine dacarbazine	5-FU, Efudex, Carac, Flkuoroplex Velban, Velsar DTIC-Dome
Cardiac	amiodarone nifedipine quinidine diltiazem	Cordarone Procardia Quinaglute, Quinidex Cardizem, Dilacor, Tiazac
Diuretics	furosemide thiazides hydrochlorothiazide	Lasix Hydrodiuril
Diabetes	sulfonureas chlorpopamide glyburide tolazamide tolbutamide	 Diabinese Micronase, DiaBeta, Glynase Tolinase Orinase
Malaria	quinine chloroquine hydroxychloroquine	Quinerva, Quinite, QM–260 Aralen Plaquenil
Pain	Nonsteroidal antiflammatory drugs naproxyn piroxicam ibuprofen	 Naprosyn, Naprelan, Anaprox, Aleve (OTC) Feldene Motrin, Advil (OTC)
Psychatric conditions	phenothiazines chlorpromazine tri-cyclic antidepressants desipramine imiprine haloperidol sertraline ALA or 5-aminolevulinic acid methyl-5-aminolevulinic acid	 Thorazine Norpramin Tofranil Haldol St. John's Wort (OTC) Zoloft Levulan

Developmental Applications

Certain conditions or disorders may be related to certain age groups or situations. Inquiring to obtain age or condition specific information will provide further information for helping to determine causes of the chief concern as identified.

Provider Inquiries	Clinical Reasoning/Logic
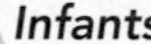 ***Infants***	
Feeding history: Breast/formula, type of formula, new foods introduced, when?	Information regarding any food allergies or intolerances
Diaper history: Type of diapers, cleansing skin routine, use of rubber pants, frequency of change, if washable diapers, how cleaned?	Information to help determine risk for developing diaper rash
Problems with skin rash?	Information regarding maintaining cleanliness of skin and whether practices may contribute to skin conditions
Bathing: Frequency, products used (lotion, oil, soap)? Where is infant bathed?	Information regarding how skin is cared for
Dress/clothing: Type of clothing, washing practices (detergents used)? Amount of clothing (temperature)? Bed clothing, how frequently changed?	Information regarding types of clothing and any potential for skin conditions
Home environment: Temperature/humidity, air conditioning, heating (humidified or drying)?	Information regarding possible causes for drying of skin
Skin: Birthmarks, bruising, rashes, lesions (how occurred)? Habitual movements: Rubbing head against mattress, rug, furniture, and wall?	Any lesions that are congenital or indication of possible physical abuse
 ***Children/Adolescents***	
Eating habits: Types of foods, how much? Junk food (snacks, sodas, candy)?	Information regarding nutrition and possible effects on skin.
Exposure to communicable disease: Measles, chicken pox, scarlet fever? Contagious conditions (Impetigo, lice, scabies)?	Information regarding any possible causes for lesions and possibility of contracting illness.
Immunizations current: MMR, DTaP, polio, chicken pox, HiB, Hepatitis A/B?	Information regarding protection from certain illnesses that may have an effect on skin.
Allergic conditions/disorders: Eczema, urticaria, pruritus, hay fever, asthma, other respiratory disorders?	Information regarding conditions associated with allergies.
Allergies: Food, insects, animals (pets at home)?	Information regarding possible cause of allergies.
Injuries: Frequency of falls, cuts, abrasions (how received?), history of unexplained bruising/injuries?	Information regarding coordination and possible abuse.
Habits/behaviors: Nail biting, manipulation of hair, head banging?	Information regarding habits and possible behavioral problems.
Skin conditions: Acne (when noticed, severity, how treated, how coping)?	Information on condition and if a source of anxiety for patient.
 ***The Pregnant Woman***	
Stage of pregnancy: Weeks gestation or postpartum?	Certain pregnancy dermatoses occur during specific trimesters.
Effect on prepregnancy conditions: Acne (may become more severe), psoriasis (may remit)	Pruritus is a common condition associated with pregnancy.
Hygiene practices: Bathing, lotions, oils, exposure to toxins, irritants? Sun exposure?	Skin care is important during pregnancy; however, there is no known benefit of creams, lotions, or oils used to prevent the appearance of stretch marks.
Any obvious areas of hyperpigmentation?	Areolae, axilla, and genitals most common sites for hyperpigmentation. Facial hyperpigmentation (melasma) a common manifestation and may be cause of concern; however, usually resolves after delivery. Sun exposure may worsen it. Sun exposure may be beneficial for other conditions—psoriasis, pruritic folliculitis.

Provider Inquiries	Clinical Reasoning/Logic
 ***The Older Adult*** **Sensation:** Touch (increased or decreased)?	Information regarding potential for injury if sensation decreased
Pruritus: Frequency, severity, exposure to skin irritants (soap, lotions [with high alcohol content], detergents, medications), type of clothing, humidity?	Information regarding presence of condition and potential causes as well as possible treatments
Healing time: Delayed, increased susceptibility to infections?	Information regarding any changes—potential indicator of cancer
Frequent falls: How often, bruising (cuts, lacerations, abrasions)?	Information regarding potential for injury or breaking the integrity of the skin
Hair loss: Gradual/sudden, pattern of loss?	Information regarding time and location of loss
Other conditions: Diabetes mellitus, peripheral vascular disease, neuropathy?	Information regarding any other conditions that may be contributing to patient's condition or situation

OBJECTIVE DATA

The physical examination of the skin takes place throughout the entire exam when a specific area of the body is uncovered for assessment of underlying structures. The first part of any body-specific section or area assessment begins with the skin. Inspection and palpation are the two techniques used.

Perform the examination in a comfortable environment with adequate illumination. Natural light is preferred if possible. Compare symmetrical areas with each other; there should be consistency in the characteristics of both sides. Also, compare sun-exposed areas with nonexposed areas. The sun produces changes in the skin, and examination of the nonexposed areas gives you a better baseline for the overall condition and characteristics of the patient's skin. If the patient is obese and has areas of skin folds where skin rubs against skin (intertriginous areas), it is essential to assess these areas for any evidence of skin breakdown (Figure 16-6).

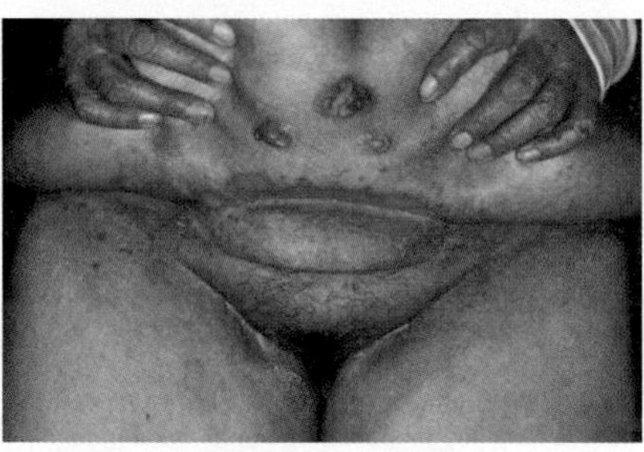

FIGURE 16-6 Intriginous areas of skin
Source: Courtesy of CDC/Dr. Hardin

Using precise terminology is critical; however, at times it may be best to just describe the findings, rather than trying to identify a specific lesion. In most instances, measurements are reported as metric, so familiarity with the metric system is essential.

The complete exam of the skin includes the following:

Inspection

- Integrity (condition, continuity)
- Color: Generalized/localized (uniformity)
- Edema (presence, location, distribution)
- Skin lesions (type, characteristics, pattern, and distribution)
- Hair: Distribution (scalp, facial, body), color, quantity, hygiene
- Fingernails: Shape, contour, color, thickness, cleanliness, capillary refill

Palpation

- Mobility, turgor, temperature, moisture, fingernails, texture
- Edema (pitting)
- Skin lesions
- Scalp/hair—surface characteristics, texture, and quality

Percussion—not performed

Auscultation—not performed

> ***PRACTICE POINT: Lesion Dimensions***
> When establishing the diameter or size of a lesion, it is necessary to have a reference point for comparison, such as some type of metric ruler. However, if one is not available and you know the width of your little finger, you can make an estimation of the diameter. You may also use neurological assessment cards that provide information on pupil size to determine lesion size.

The Level I to Level IV examinations are performed on a continuum, which starts from a basic level and moves to a more comprehensive level based on provider's abilities and knowledge as well as the patient's presentation and location. The examination may start at the outpatient setting and progress to the ED, hospital unit bed, critical care unit, or specialty unit. Frequently all the elements from basic to comprehensive exam are done in one setting such as a primary care setting or clinic.

The condition or illness of the patient is the primary consideration related to the type and amount of data needed to assess the patient's condition, illness, or situation. The arrangement of skills into levels is done for general purposes and is meant to be descriptive rather than prescriptive. The purpose of arranging examination skills into levels is to provide a framework to assist the learner in determining the appropriate data to collect.

Skin, Hair, Nails (Integumentary)

	Level I	Level II	Level III	Level IV
Inspection	Integrity (continuity), thickness	Integrity (controlled trauma)	Integrity (uncontrolled/trauma)	Lesions/Wood's Lamp (fungal infections)
	Color (uniformity) Localized changes	Color (generalized: disease/condition related changes)	Lesions (blanching)	
	Edema (presence, location)	Edema (pitting)		
	Hair (distribution)			
	Nails (configuration/ color)			
	Lesions (vascular)			
	Distribution/ configuration	Lesions (1°/2°)		
Palpation	Mobility and turgor	Fingernails (clubbing)		
	Temperature	Texture		
	Fingernails (CRT)*	Hair (texture)		

*Capillary Refill Time—data obtained from this technique is actually related to the peripheral vascular system, but is included here for convenience.

Inspection: Level I

The Level I assessment is performed on patients with stable conditions that demonstrate minimal pathological alterations. The assessment is performed to gather data associated with the basic expected parameters for each system. The time required to perform a Level I assessment is 10–15 minutes. The patient's condition is expected to remain stable without any drastic, rapid parameter changes.

Inspection Techniques and Expected Findings	Unexpected Findings
Initial inspection for integrity is examination for any breaks or disruptions to the continuity of its surface, which should be intact, smooth, and structurally unified in appearance, without breaks, gaps, or areas of trauma.	The skin surface and/or structure may be altered or disrupted by changes in thickness, trauma/pressure, various conditions, and skin lesions.
Observe for localized changes in skin depth. While the thickness of the skin varies, it is not possible to determine any significant alterations related to its depth.	Calluses (hyperkeratosis) and corns are thick, hardened layers of skin that form to protect an area of skin that is subject to continuous friction and pressure (Figure 16-7). They are most commonly found on weight-bearing locations on the soles of the feet and on the fingers, toes, or hands. They appear as a hardened, raised bump that may be surrounded by a thick, rough area of skin. As they increase in size, they may also become painful, particularly corns. 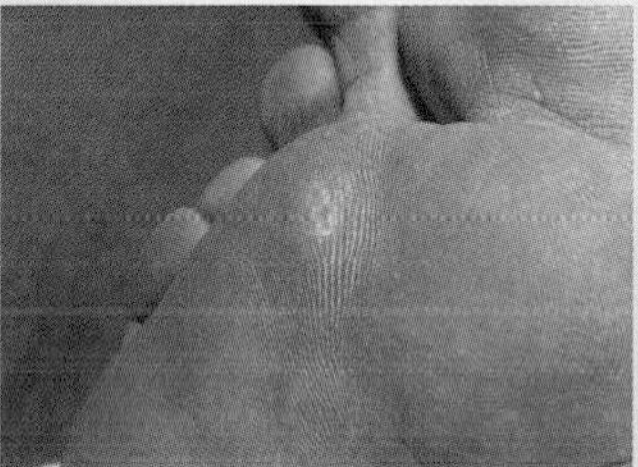 FIGURE 16-7 Callous

Inspection Techniques and Expected Findings

Thoroughly assess patients, especially those at risk, for any signs of skin breakdown. Inspect the skin of these patients for early warning signs of breakdown.

Table 16-4 Traumatic disruptions to the skin

Name/Example	Description
Abrasions (excoriations) 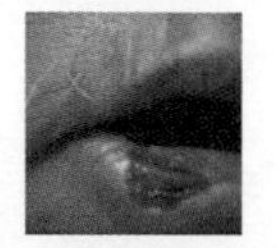 *Source*: Kondor83/Shutterstock	Injury to the superficial layers of the skin (dermis/epidermis) that are produced by friction or scraping the skin across a rough surface. Common causes are falls onto rough surfaces and continuous friction that eventually wears away the upper layers of the skin. May be confined to a small area or may cover a large section of the skin.
Erosions (superficial ulcers) *Source*: DermPics/Science Source	Shallow, scooped out depressions of the epidermis that often appear after the rupture of vesicles, such as chicken pox. They can also be the result of eczema. As there is only a loss of the epidermis, there is generally no bleeding associated with them.
Ulcers 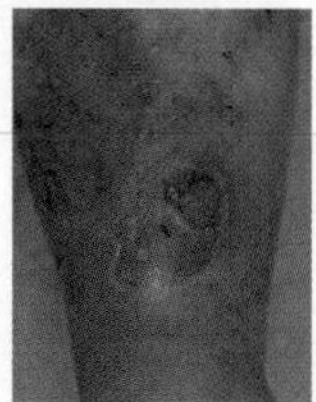 *Source*: Scott Camazine/Science Source	Deep depressions that extend into the dermis and beyond. Pressure ulcers or decubitus ulcers develop in areas where blood flow has been compromised, usually due to increased pressure on an area that exceeds capillary pressure, which reduces or cuts off the blood supply, resulting in ischemia of the underlying tissue (see Table 16-5).

PRACTICE POINT: High Risk Patients

High-risk patients include those with decreased mobility, particularly those on bedrest. The frail skin of the elderly older adult is easily damaged from friction, shear stress, and pressure.

Patients with circulatory problems, both venous and arterial, are also high risk individuals for the development of ulcers. Patients with chronic venous insufficiency are vulnerable to the development of stasis ulcers (Table 16-5). Observe the medial aspect of the lower extremity, just above the ankle, a site where venous stasis ulcers commonly develop. Note that they may develop over any area of the lower extremity and may be observed bilaterally.

Patients with arterial circulation problems may develop arterial (ischemic) ulcers due to tissue damage resulting from decreased or obstructed arterial circulation, causing death of tissue cells.

Assess patient's skin for the presence of neurotrophic (diabetic) ulcers that are the result of nerve damage (neuropathy) from diabetes, which results in decreased sensation of the feet and lower extremities (Figure 16-9).

Skin that is continuously exposed to urine and fecal material is also susceptible to break down. Patients with a poor nutritional status, particularly decreased protein intake, are also at high risk.

FIGURE 16-9 Arterial/diabetic ulcers
Source: Scott Camazine/Science Source Images.

Unexpected Findings

Traumatic disruptions to the continuity of the skin surface may be demonstrated by abrasions (excoriations), erosions, and ulcers (see Table 16-4).

Individuals on bedrest are at high risk for the development of pressure ulcers (see Conditions and Disorders). An early warning sign of skin breakdown is a localized area of redness that blanches (loses color) when pressure is applied.

Venous stasis ulcers result from tissue damage related to fluid leaking into the skin tissue, causing the formation of edema. The area over the damaged tissue gradually erodes away, leaving an open ulcer. The color of the skin where the ulcer develops is often reddish-brown and may be accompanied by a rash, or dry, scaly skin (see Figure 16-8).

The borders of the ulcer are generally irregular and surrounded by edematous, discolored skin. The ulcer's base is commonly red with or without yellow fibrous tissue. If infected, greenish-yellow discharge may be present. Significant amounts of fluid may drain from this type of ulcer.

If there is some external trauma to the skin, the diabetic patient may not be aware of it, and over time the damage to tissue may increase and the tissue may erode away.

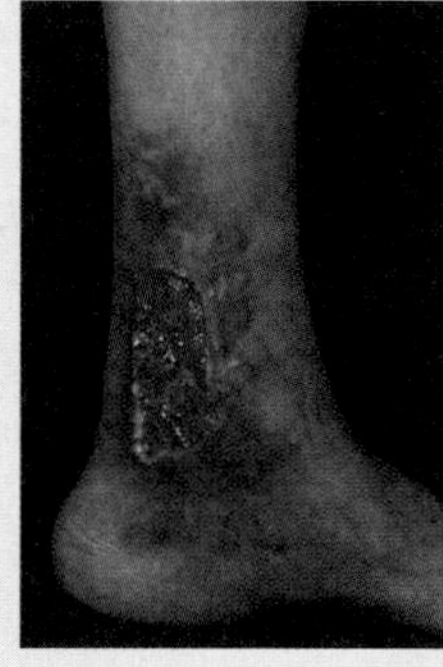

FIGURE 16-8 Venous stasis ulcer
Source: Biophoto Associates, Science Source Photos

THINK LINK: Decubitus (Pressure) Ulcers

Decubitus comes from the Latin term *decumbere*, meaning to lie down. This is more related to the cause of the ulcer rather than describing it. Ulceration occurs in other positions (e.g., sitting) anytime an area of skin is under pressure. The process causing the ulcers follows the same course; thus *pressure sores* or *ulcers* are preferred terms to use.

Table 16-5 Stasis ulcers

Stage	Characteristics
Stage I	Intact skin with pressure related alterations: Temp: warm or cool Consistency: firm or boggy Sensation: pain or itching Color: (light skin) red; (dark skin) red, blue, purple or darker. Will not blanch (turn white) if pressure is applied over reddened skin.
Stage II	Partial-thickness skin loss (epidermis, possibly the dermis, or both). The site presents as an abrasion, ulcer, or blister.
Stage III	Full thickness skin loss; necrosis of subcutaneous tissue (ulcer [crater] present). May extend to, but not into or through, muscle.
Stage IV	Full-thickness skin loss: destruction, necrosis to underlying structures (muscle, bone, or joint capsule); may progress to osteomyelitis. Exposed bone may be visible or palpable.
Unstageable	Unstageable pressure sores are those where tissue at the base of the ulcer is covered by dead skin (slough) that is yellow, tan, green, or brown; or eschar in the wound bed that is tan, brown, or black.

Inspection Techniques and Expected Findings

As you assess the skin surface, concurrently observe the uniformity and homogeneity of the patient's skin color, which should demonstrate evenness in the overall distribution of pigments. Individuals will display a wide variety of skin tones and colors, and the lack of a standardized description for skin color makes it difficult to determine overall skin color (Figure 16-10). Instead of matching the patient's skin to a particular color, it is more practical and meaningful to describe the overall uniformity and distribution of the color or pigment. Assess patients for a uniform "base" color at specific areas of the body. The base color should be present bilaterally and not show a distinct color change. Ethnic and racial characteristics also determine the overall color of the skin and distribution of pigment. In general, color variations should be symmetrical and present as a cohesive variation of skin color.

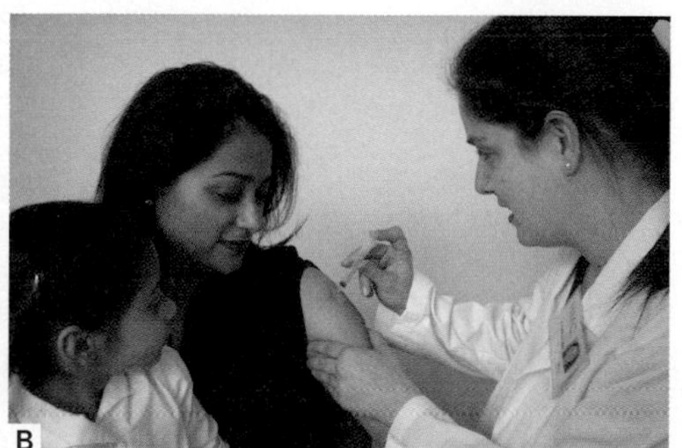

FIGURE 16-10A–B Examples of different skin tones

Sources: a. CDC/Yvonne Green; RN; CNM, MSN, b. CDC/Judy Schmidt/James Gathany

Observe for nonsymmetrical localized skin color changes. A localized change is related to an alteration of one or more components of underlying skin tissue and structures. Localized skin color alterations may be described as **nonvascular** and **vascular.**

Unexpected Findings

Skin color variations may be observed under various circumstances. In warm environments, the skin may become pinker in certain areas as blood flow is increased in an effort to dissipate more heat.

In stressful, embarrassing, or exciting situations, an individual's face may become pinker. In some individuals, joints—particularly knuckles—may demonstrate a darker hue of the underlying skin tone.

Generalized color changes, involving the entire skin, frequently are manifestations of a systematic disorder and are discussed in the Level II exam.

Inspection Techniques and Expected Findings	Unexpected Findings

A freckle is a common nonvascular, nonsignificant, localized color change related to pigment variations. Although a single freckle can be considered a very local color change, a patient may have a wide distribution of freckles throughout the skin. Technically, freckles are classified as skin lesions, or macules; however, a freckle is not considered pathological—it is simply a localized overproduction of melanin (Martini & Nath, 2009). See further discussion of macules in Inspection Level II.

Vitiligo, a non-vascular localized color change, is an acquired pigmentary skin and mucous membrane disorder manifested as hypopigmented or white patches of skin (Figure 16-11).

Patches of vitiligo are areas of the skin where the melanocytes have been destroyed.

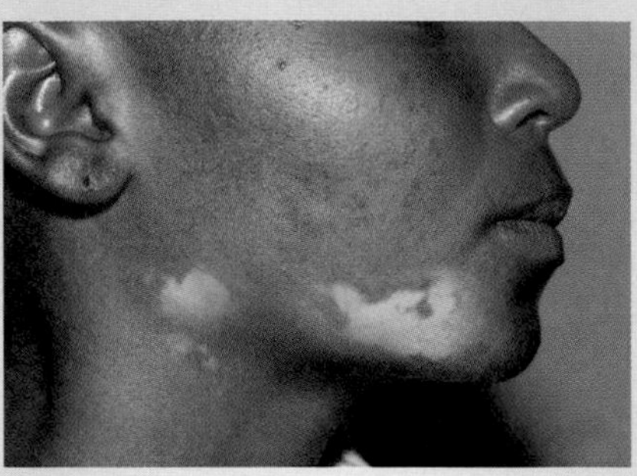

FIGURE 16-11 Vitiligo
Source: John F. Wilson, MD./Science Source Images

A localized color change associated with vascular system involvement is erythema, a localized area of redness due to an increased blood flow to the area (Figure 16-12). It is commonly caused by some degree of external trauma (a significant blow or slap to the skin) that is not severe enough to interrupt the skin's integrity or cause internal damage to the blood vessels, but causes dilation of the underlying arterioles and capillaries, which frequently disappears rapidly, leaving no significant damage to the skin.

Localized erythema is also an indicator of an underlying inflammatory process, with or without accompanying infection that causes blood vessel dilation to increase blood flow to the area. The erythema will remain until the inflammation is gone.

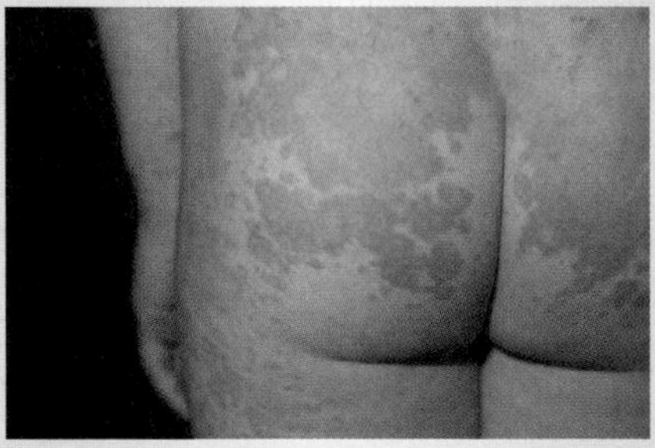

FIGURE 16-12 Erythema migrans
Source: Biophoto Associates/Science Source

Inspect the skin for signs of vascular lesions, which are those that demonstrate color changes caused by an alteration of or damage to blood vessels. Vascular lesions may be described as non-hemorrhagic or hemorrhagic.

Non-hemorrhagic vascular lesions are alterations in blood vessels generally caused by enlargement of and/or an increased visibility of the vessels (capillaries) (Table 16-6). While non-hemorrhagic vascular lesions are not pathological, their presence is not considered an expected finding.

Hemorrhagic lesions result from damage to a blood vessel, causing it to burst open and allow blood to escape into skin tissues. These lesions also demonstrate various color changes as they evolve and heal; such areas may also be referred to as a **bruise**.

Initially, the damaged area is purple with red overtones, becoming darker purple as the blood disappears and healing occurs, with the possible appearance of shades of yellow/green. In most instances, the hemorrhaging is self-limiting, and the color change is localized. Vascular lesions are differentiated from one another by their size and cause (Table 16-7).

Inspection Techniques and Expected Findings	Unexpected Findings
	Ecchymosis (bruise) refers to lesions where hemorrhaging from trauma is the primary cause. If there are other causes, they are identified as petechiae (less than 0.5 cm in diameter) or purpura (larger than 0.5 cm in diameter). Also see Conditions and Disorders.

Table 16-6 Non-hemorrhagic vascular skin lesions

Lesion	Observation (Morphology)	Palpation	Picture
Angioma (Cherry, Spider)	Small, slightly raised red papule that often appear on face, neck, and trunk of body. Spider angioma has small telangectasias radiating from center.	Does not blanch.	*Source*: SPL/CMSP
Venous star	Bluish, spider configuration of linear or irregular shaped radiating legs. No central body.	Does not blanch.	*Source*: Dr. P. Marazzi/Science Source
Telangectasia	Threadlike red lines of permanently dilated capillaries that are visible within the skin.	Blanches with pressure.	
Capillary hemiangioma	Red appearing areas on skin due to dilation of capillaries and malformation of angioblastic tissue. during fetal life. (See section on birthmarks.)	Strawberry/cavernous hemangioma elevated above skin. Spongy feel. Nevus flammeus flat, nonpalpable.	*Source*: CDC

Table 16-7 Hemorrhagic vascular lesions

Lesion	Observation	Palpation	Example
Petchiae	Red-purple color; smaller than 0.5 cm	Smooth, does not blanch.	

Continued

Table 16-7 Hemorrhagic vascular lesions (*continued*)

Lesion	Observation	Palpation	Example
Contusion (bruise)	Bleeding into the dermis, subcutaneous tissues, and internal organs resulting from rupture of blood vessels following impact.	Superficial contusions smooth, not palpable. Area firm and tender to palpation and may demonstrate edema. Deep contusions may cause formation of hematoma that may be palpated.	*Source:* sgm/Shutterstock
Purpura	Red-purple color; greater than 0.5 cm	Smooth, does not blanch	
Ecchymosis	Red-purple color of various sizes	Does not blanch	*Source:* Suzanne Tucker/Shutterstock

Inspection Techniques and Expected Findings

Inspect the skin for the presence of increased fluid within the skin tissues, the most common alteration being edema.

Edema is not necessarily a manifestation of a skin disorder, but may be detected by observation of the skin. Edema has multiple causes, but the overall outcome is the presence of fluid in the interstitial spaces. Like color changes, edema can be localized or generalized.

Assess skin for signs of increased fluid within the outer layers of the skin (maceration). In this condition, the skin becomes vulnerable to infection with bacteria or fungi as well as trauma.

Unexpected Findings

Localized edema accompanies inflammation and also is due to the dilation of the blood vessels, allowing more fluid to leak from the vessels into the interstitial tissues. Edematous skin appears tight and stretched, demonstrating a loss of elasticity and mobility. Skin stretching may accentuate the appearance of the skin's pores (Figure 16-13).

Edematous tissues may also demonstrate pitting, skin indentation that does not return to its original position for a period of time.

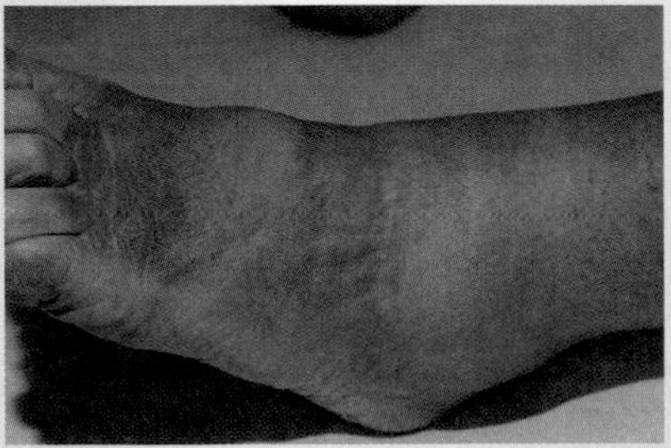

FIGURE 16-13 Edema

Pitting edema (interstitial) is more common than non-pitting (cellular) and is observed in the dependent areas of the body. Unilateral edema causes an obvious difference in size of symmetrical areas and generally has a localized cause.

Inspection Techniques and Expected Findings	Unexpected Findings

Bilateral edema is more characteristic of a centralized cause and will be equally distributed in symmetrical areas. The fluid of edema is located above the vascular and pigmented layers of the skin, which results in the skin being lighter in color in the edematous area.

Macerated skin is skin that has been exposed to excessive moisture and becomes over hydrated (Figure 16-14). In contrast to edema, macerated tissue becomes wrinkled and soft and turns white with degeneration of the tissues.

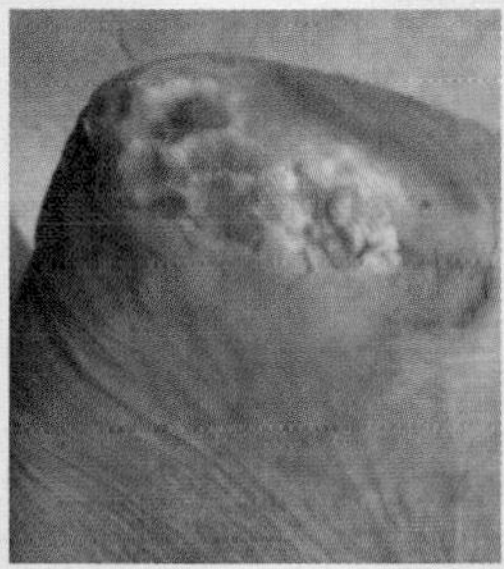

FIGURE 16-14 Maceration

***THINK LINK:** Lesions*

The term *lesions* in relation to the skin is somewhat of a misnomer. Technically, the term *lesion* indicates a pathological alteration associated with a specific condition. Although some skin lesions may be considered pathological, not all fall into that category. However, the term *skin lesion* is uniformly used to identify alterations of the skin.

Continue your observation of the skin to identify the presence of skin lesions, noting their location and patterns.

Observe distribution pattern of lesions.

Observe the arrangement, or appearance of the pattern or configuration of the lesion, which may assume a wide variety of arrangements and demonstrate a variety of specific shapes.

Some lesions are a manifestation of specific conditions or disease processes. In many instances, the appearance of the lesions associated with disease states is similar; however, they may not be specific enough to be considered diagnostic. Some skin lesions were identified previously and described as related to observation of skin integrity.

Various lesion arrangements and shapes are identified and described in Table 16-8.

Table 16-8 Lesion arrangements

Generalized Widely distributed over the skin or in numerous locations simultaneously	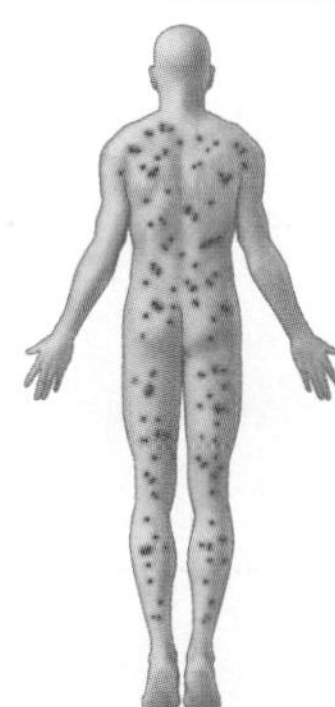

Continued

Table 16-8 Lesion arrangements *(continued)*

Regional Distribution involves a larger area (region) but still remains in a single location	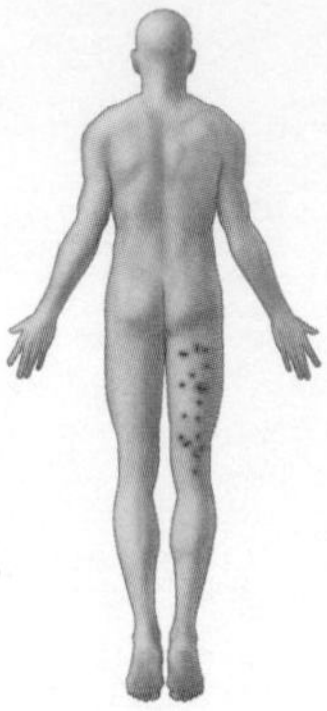
Localized Present in one small area	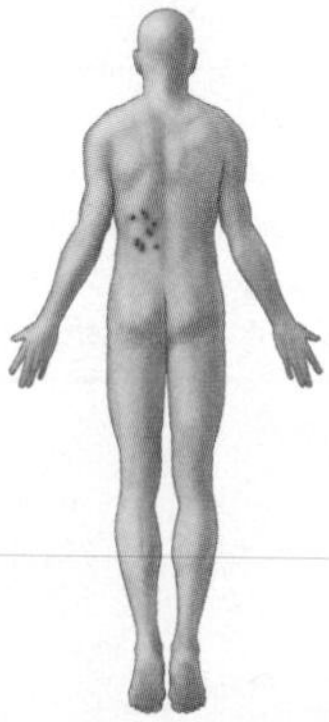

Shape	Arrangement or Pattern	Example
Singular/discrete	Separate from each other	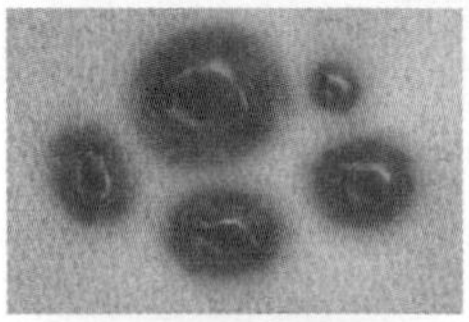
Grouped/clustered (confluent)	Bunched together; they may remain separated from each other or run together	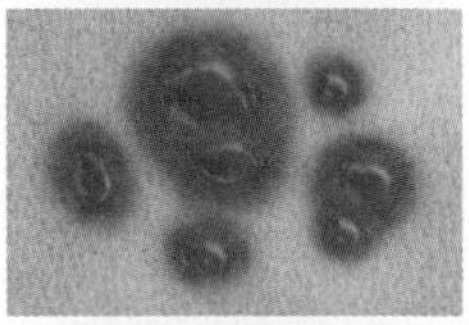
Polycyclic	Arranged in concentric circles or annular lesions that expand and grow together	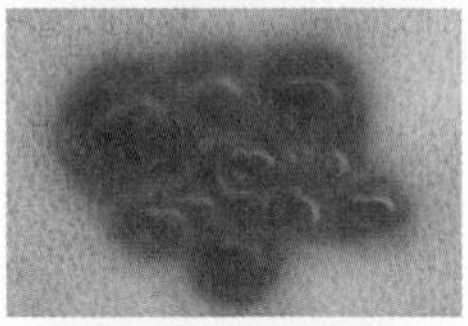
Linear	Arranged in lines	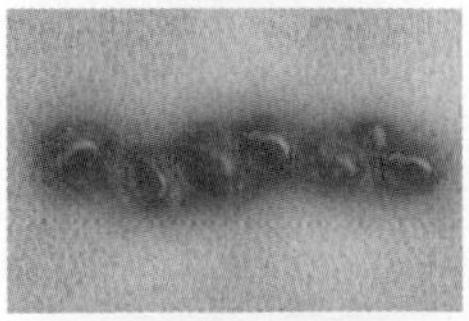
Reticular	Mesh-like or lattice-like in appearance	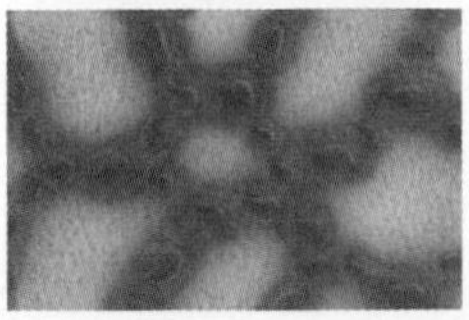

Continued

Table 16-8 Lesion arrangements *(continued)*

Round/oval	Solid-appearing lesion with no central area of lighter color	
Annular	Round lesion with visible center of lighter color	
Target (Iris)	Circle within a circle	
Zosteriform	Linear, but follow a nerve root	

Inspection Techniques and Expected Findings	Unexpected Findings

Hair and Fingernails (Accessory Structures)

Inspect scalp hair for color, distribution, and quantity. You will often make this observation unconsciously. Hair color may be natural or colored with rinses or dyes. Distribution of the hair should be symmetrical.

THINK LINK: ***Hair Loss Myth***
A common myth about baldness is that it is inherited through the mother. In reality, it can be inherited from either or both parents. Genetic inheritance is thought to be an autosomal dominant phenotype in males and an autosomal recessive phenotype in females. Recent studies have refocused on the relative importance of maternal inheritance for androgenetic alopecia (Hilmer et al., 2005).

Alopecia is the absence of scalp hair. Hair loss is either localized or generalized. The most common form of alopecia is androgenetic alopecia (male patterned baldness). Hair loss is generally symmetrical and begins at the front of the head or at the back (Figure 16-15). Hair loss that begins at the back of the head is more likely to lead to baldness.

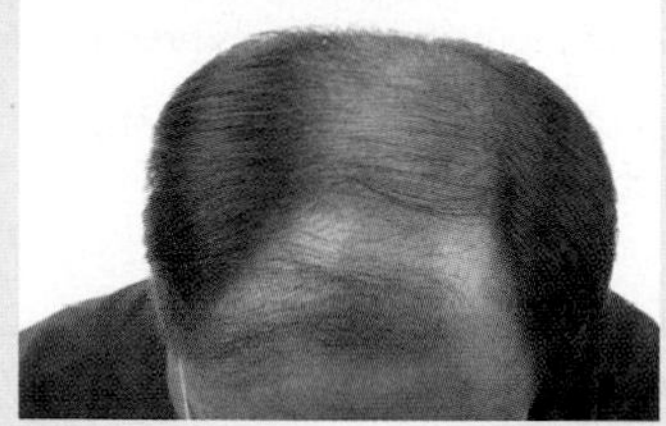

FIGURE 16-15 Male pattern baldness
Source: Gang Liu/Shutterstock

Inspect the patient's body hair for quantity and distribution. Males are more likely to have visible body hair present on the face (cheeks and chin), neck, chest, axillae, back, shoulders, arms, legs, and pubic area. Pubic hair distribution in males is in a triangle with hair extending up to the umbilicus.

Loss or gain of hair may indicate underlying pathology. Loss of hair on the lower extremities indicates poor peripheral perfusion.

Distribution of hair in females is generally limited to arms, legs, axillae, and pubic area. Many females commonly remove the hair on the legs and axillary area. It is not unusual for females also to remove the hair in the pubic area. Female pubic hair distribution is in the shape of an inverted triangle.

Hirsutism, or male-patterned hair growth in females, may be seen in the older adult or may be an indication of an endocrine disorder (see Conditions and Disorders).

Distribution of hair in both genders should be symmetrical.

Inspection Techniques and Expected Findings	Unexpected Findings

While inspecting the hair, also inspect the skin overlying the scalp, which should be very pale to white in color, due to lack of exposure to the sun or other elements. Visible scalp skin, such as areas of baldness, should be consistent in color with the rest of the body. The scalp should be clean and smooth without any evidence of flaking, rashes, redness, or open lesions.

Patchy areas of hair loss accompanied by pustules may indicate tinea capitis, a fungal infection that is highly contagious and transmitted from individual to individual. Infection with parasitic lice is characterized by the presence of white nits (eggs) at the base of the hair shaft (Figure 16-16).

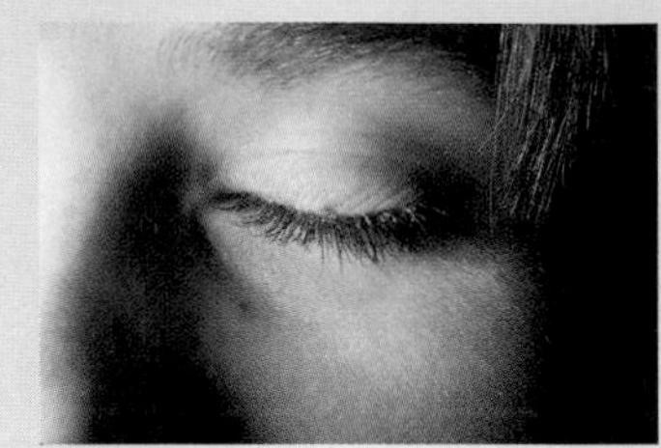

FIGURE 16-16 Nits at the base of the eyelashes
Source: Custom Medical Stock Photo

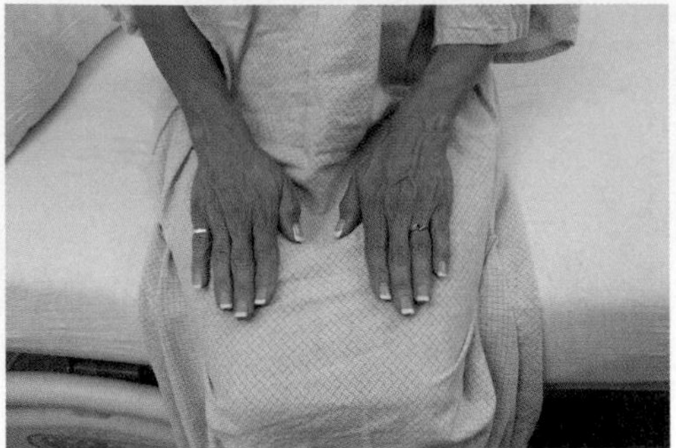

FIGURE 16-17 Inspecting the fingernails for color, shape, and cleanliness

Inspect the nails for cleanliness, color, symmetry, and shape (Figure 16-17).

Initial inspection for cleanliness provides information about the patient's overall perception of self. The nails should be clean with smooth edges with some of the distal portion of the nail extending to or over the tip of the finger. If a female patient has artificial nails, it may be difficult or impossible to determine the condition of the actual fingernail.

Unkempt and dirty nails that have rough and ragged edges due to constant nail biting may indicate in underlying poor self-concept or anxiety disorder.

Nail color changes can occur with the following:

- antimalarial, chemotherapy, and minocycline drugs
- hyperbilirubinemia, malnutrition, Addisons' disease, and Wilson's disease
- pseudomonas infection
- yellow-nail syndrome and onycholysis

The nail edges should be smooth and rounded. Their overall condition is reflective of the care given to them. Some patient's nails are predisposed to splitting or peeling, manifested by the nail splitting into layers at the distal edge of the nail. Patients who have their hands frequently or repeatedly immersed in water are prone to nail peeling.

Nail color should be variations of pink with a white lunula. Individuals with dark skin may have deposits of pigments or bands present in the nail bed.

The nail plate should appear smooth and flat, or slightly convex. Absence of a nail plate (anonychia) may be congenital.

Look across the nail to assess the angle where the nail plate meets the nail bed. This angle should be approximately 160 degrees (Figure 16-18).

An increase in this angle to 180 degrees or more is observed in the presence of clubbing in which the distal portion of the finger assumes a "clubbed" or bulbous appearance.

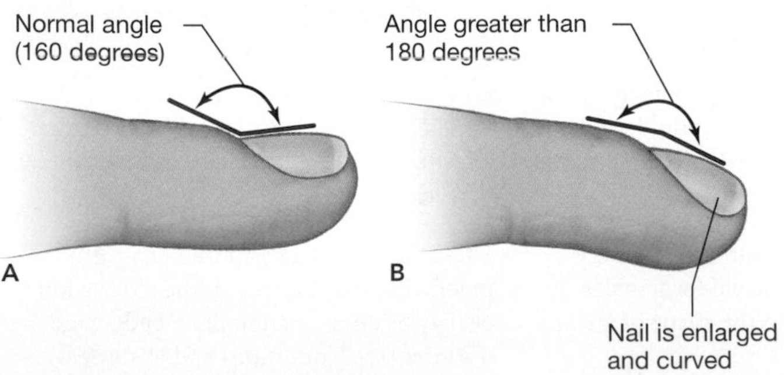

FIGURE 16–18A–B **a)** Normal curvature of a fingernail; **b)** clubbed fingernail

Inspection Techniques and Expected Findings	Unexpected Findings
In addition to observing the angle, perform the Schamroth technique by having the patient place the nail plates of two corresponding fingertips together. In the absence of clubbing, there should be a separation in the shape of a diamond between the two nails (refer to Chapter 24).	In the presence of clubbing there is the loss of this separation.

Inspection: Level II

The Level II Assessment is performed on patients with unstable conditions and who have significant pathological alterations. Data gathered is associated with more depth and/or detail requiring more time, skill, and effort. More than one system is generally involved, and changes in the patient's conditions and assessment parameters have the potential to shift drastically and quickly.

Observe skin integrity in areas where there has been an intentional disruption, resulting in a wound, such as in surgical procedures. Surgical skin interruption is also described as controlled trauma. A surgical wound disrupts all three layers of the skin. Surgical wounds are closed by various materials (sutures, staple, Steri-Strips, and surgical glue) that hold the edges of the wound together to promote optimum healing.

Manifestations of an acute surgical wound should present as closure of the wound with the edges approximated together and held in place. The edges of the wound may appear red as a result of the inflammatory process. There may also be some clear or bloody drainage from the incision site. Clear drainage is serous, bloody drainage is sanguineous; if drainage has both clear and bloody components, it is serosanguineous (Figure 16-19). Drainage may be allowed to exit freely from the wound or drains may be placed to collect excess fluids.

Wounds that have healed present with scar tissue that has formed to close the wound (Figure 16-20). Early scar tissue is red to purple in color and slightly raised. Eventually the color is lost and the tissue may turn to a lighter shade of the surrounding skin. It also becomes thinner and may become slightly sunken below the skin surface. Wounds may be classified into types (Table 16-9).

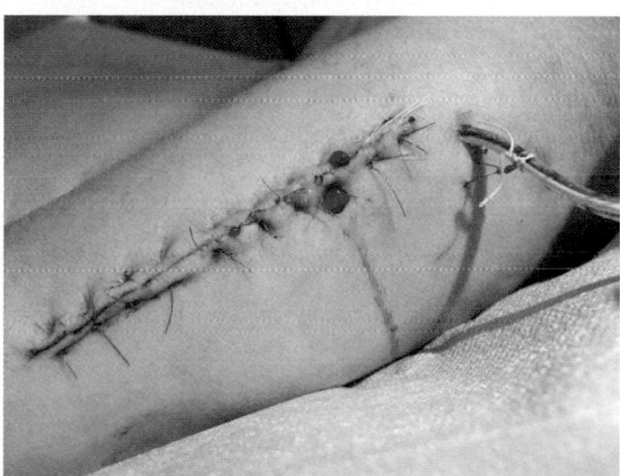

FIGURE 16-19 Surgical wound
Source: rawcaptured/Shutterstock

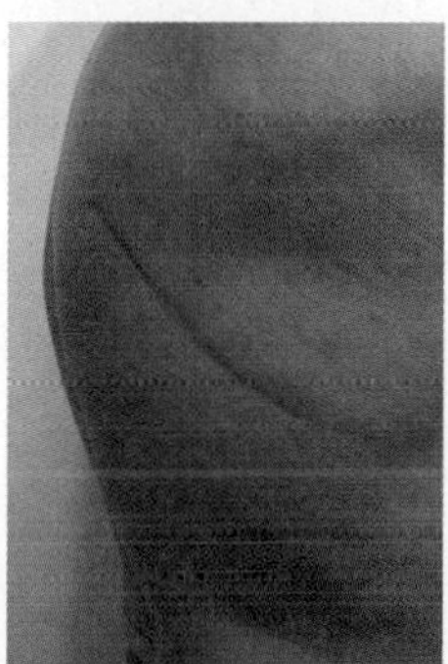

FIGURE 16-20 Scar

Table 16-9 Surgical wound classification

Wound Class Definition	Description	Examples/Procedures
Class I *Clean*	• Non-traumatic, uninfected surgical wounds with no inflammation encountered • No break in technique • Respiratory, gastrointestinal and genitor-urinary tracts not entered • Caesarean section, elective, no pre-rupture of membranes or trial of labor • Clean wounds closed primarily; if necessary, drained with closed drainage	• Vascular procedures • Neurological procedures • Endocrine procedures (thyroidectomy) • Eye surgery • Orthopedic procedures (total hip replacement) • Skin (mastectomy, neck dissection) • Exploratory laparotomy • Miscellaneous procedures (lymph node excision, penile prosthesis • Nonpenetrating blunt trauma
Class II *Clean-contaminated*	• Operative wound clean-contaminated • Gastrointestinal, respiratory or genitor-urinary tracts entered without significant spillage • Procedures involving biliary tract, appendix, vagina, and oropharynx [if no evidence of infection or break in techniques] • Non-traumatic wound with minor break in technique	• Thoracic procedures (bronchoscopy) • GI procedures including: cholecystectomy (any approach), routine appendectomy, small bowel resection, Whipple pancreaticoduodenectomy • GU procedures (transurethral resection of prostate, hysterectomy) • Ear surgery (infected III) • Nose/Oropharynx procedures (infected IV) • GYN procedures (hysterectomy/oophrectomy, Caesarean section, emergency involving pre-rupture of membranes and/or trial of labor) • Any wound open for drainage II (except total hip/knee) • Removing old implants (wires, pins, etc) • Re-operation at the same site
Class III *Contaminated*	• Operative wound with a major break in technique • Open, fresh accidental traumatic wound from clean source • Entrance into the genito-urinary or biliary tracts • Incision encountering acute non-purulent inflammation.	• Open cardiac massage • Gross spillage (bile) from the gastrointestinal tract (during cholecystectomy) • Foreign bodies in a wound (bullets, etc...) • Appendectomy for inflamed appendicitis
Class IV *Dirty-infected*	• Operative wound dirty • Traumatic wound from dirty source • Traumatic wound with delayed treatment • Fecal contamination • Foreign body • Retained devitalized tissue • Operative wound w/acute bacterial inflammation or perforated viscus • Operative wound where clean tissue is transected to gain access to a collection of pus	• Incision and drainage of abscess • Perforated bowel • Wound debridement • Peritonitis

Inspection Techniques and Expected Findings	Unexpected Findings
Observe the skin for generalized color changes. These changes most commonly involve large areas or the entire body and are generally manifestations of a disease process or organ dysfunction located elsewhere in the body. Adequate light is critical to observe any color changes. Daylight is best, but if adequate daylight is unavailable, use overhead fluorescent lighting. In some instances, tangential lighting may help you assess contour, but it is not appropriate for overall skin assessment.	Skin color changes and the condition of the skin are often a reflection of other systemic disorders, so the patient's skin color and color alterations are important to the overall evaluation of the patient (see Table 16-10 and Figure 16-21).

Inspection Techniques and Expected Findings	Unexpected Findings
Pigment alterations are color changes that are due to alterations in the three primary components contributing to the skin's color. An increase in pigment is commonly due to increased sun exposure (tanning) and does not indicate the presence of any disease process. Individuals with light pigmentation demonstrate skin color changes quite readily; however, the darker the skin color, the more difficult it is to determine any significant color change. In these individuals, other structures or locations need to be assessed (Table 16-11).	Nonpigment alterations are changes related to an additional substance in the blood or skin that contributes to the overall color change. An overall appearance of redness is often seen in the presence of a fever. This is due to an increased blood flow to the surface of the skin in an attempt to cool down the body.

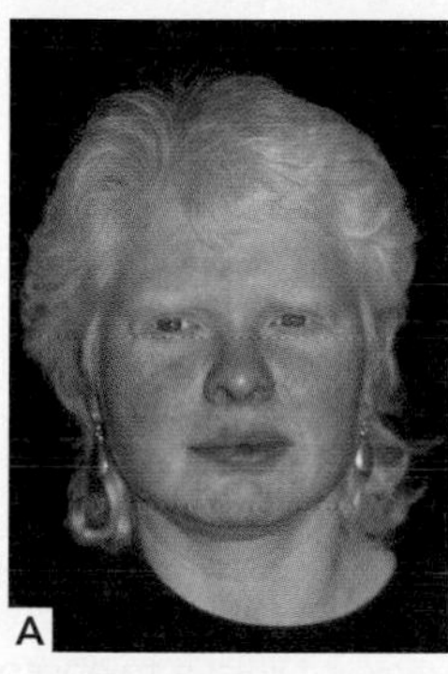

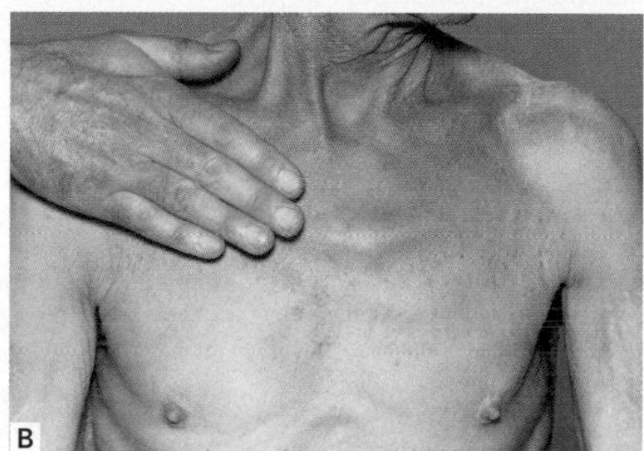

FIGURE 16-21A–B Albinism and jaundice are unexpected pigment-related skin color changes
Source: a. Dr. P. Marazzi/Science Source Images, b. Science Photo Library/Custom Medical Stock Photo

Table 16-10 Color variations of skin color in light and dark-skinned individuals

Clinical Color Manifestations	Common Location	Light Skin	Dark Skin
Blue (Cyanosis)	A pigment-related change due to an increased amount of carbon dioxide in the blood (see Figure 16-30) that combines with hemoglobin to produce deoxyhemoglobin. The blue deoxyhemoglobin thus gives the skin a bluish-gray appearance. Increased carboxyhemoglobin is due to cardiac disease, respiratory disease, cardiac malformations. Cyanosis is caused by localized vasoconstriction, cold, and emotional stress.	Blue-gray mottled skin—more prominent in nail beds, lips, mucous membranes, conjunctiva.	Skin may become darker; ashen-gray color primarily in conjunctiva, oral mucous membranes and nail beds.
Dark Blue/Black (Gangrene)	Tissue death (infarction) to an area that has lost blood flow.	No significant difference related to light or dark skin.	
White (Pallor)	Anemia (low hemoglobin levels); also with decreased tissue perfusion, associated with cardiac/respiratory conditions, shock, or hypotension.	Paleness with loss of red undertones. If skin has natural yellow tone and there may be an increased yellow color.	Black skin appears ashen gray due to loss of red undertones. Brown skin will have more yellow tones.
Loss of melanin, either congenital or acquired.	Congenital loss of pigment due to albinism (see Figure 16-21A). Overall white skin, hair with pink iris. Acquired loss of pigment due to vitiligo, localized patch of lighter to white skin (see Figure 16-11).	Congenital loss of pigment due to albinism. Overall white skin, hair with pink iris. Acquired loss of pigment due to vitiligo, localized patch of lighter to white skin.	Same appearance as for light-skinned individuals.
Yellow/orange (Jaundice)	A deep yellow to orange–appearing skin is a pigment related change that is common in hepatic disorders or other conditions causing a hyperbilirubinemia from an increase in unconjugated bilirubin (see Figure 16-21B). The liver is responsible for conjugating bilirubin for excretion in the urine, but many liver disorders cause a reduction in conjugation, so the excess bilirubin is deposited in the skin.	Increased yellow to orange color of skin; also evident in sclera and oral mucosa.	Difficult to determine. Best observed in sclera and oral mucosa.

Continued

Table 16-10 Color variations of skin color in light and dark-skinned individuals *(continued)*

Clinical Color Manifestations	Common Location	Light Skin	Dark Skin
	A pale, pasty yellow skin is associated with renal failure. Failure of the kidneys to excrete urine results in the accumulation of urinary pigments in the skin. This yellow appearance of the skin is much lighter in color than jaundice. These individuals also have a pale appearance due to an anemia that often accompanies renal failure. Pigment-related color change is caused by an increase in carotene. This is relatively uncommon, but when an individual ingests an overabundance of carrots or other yellow vegetables, the excess carotene is deposited in the skin.		
Red (Erythema; generalized)	Carbon monoxide poisoning (increased carboxyhemoglobin). Carbon monoxide has a stronger affinity to bond with hemoglobin, so oxygen and carbon dioxide are not able to bind to hemoglobin.	Generalized cherry red color to skin; may be more prominent in face and upper torso. Carboxyhemoglobin produces bright red color.	Localized cherry red color in nail beds, lips, and oral mucosa.
Red/purple with shades of yellow or green	Vascular lesions (bruising)—see Table 16-6.	Generally localized to area of bruising. When colors appear depends on age of bruise.	Most likely a deeper bluish or black color. Difficult to observe unless in area of lighter pigmentation.
Increased pigmentation	Increased production of melanin (primarily acquired)	Hyperpigmentation occurs as a result of increased melanin production, resulting in an increased brown coloration to the skin. It may be localized, as in a macule or patch, or as in melasma, which is associated with increased hormone production in pregnancy. Hyperpigmentation may also be generalized, as in ultraviolet exposure or Addison's disease.	Generalized hyperpigmentation is difficult to determine in dark skinned individuals. Localized areas may be observed in some individuals dependent on amount of melanin in base color.

Inspection Techniques and Expected Findings

Inspect the fingernails for changes, as their condition and presentation may provide significant data about the patient.

Unexpected Findings

As color changes may reflect other disease processes, fingernail changes may also be manifestations of some disease process or condition. These alterations are identified and described in Table 16-11.

Table 16-11 Nail alterations with associated conditions

Alteration	Description	Conditions	
Transverse Grooving (Beau's lines)	Temporary disturbance to growth of nail at nail root, causing transverse depressions of the nail plate	Trauma, stress, acute illness (MI, pneumonia, fever) and other diseases (syphilis, peripheral vascular disease, myocarditis, uncontrolled diabetes).	
Koilonychia (Spoon nail)	Lateral elevation of nail plate with central depression	May be congenital without any associated conditions. Onset may occur with iron deficiency anemia, hemochromotosis, Raynaud's disease, SLE, trauma.	

Continued

Table 16-11 Nail alterations with associated conditions *(continued)*

Alteration	Description	Conditions	
Terry's nails	White or light pink nail beds with distal 0.5–3 mm pink band	Cirrhosis, congestive heart failure, diabetes mellitus, cancer, hyperthyroidism, malnutrition, age.	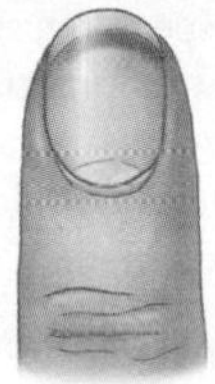
Splinter hemorrhages	Red brown linear streaks	Trauma, psoriasis, idiopathic, subacute bacterial endocarditis.	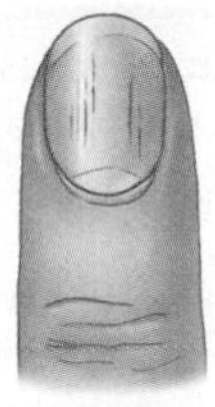
Nail pitting	Sharply defined, ice-pick like depressions on nail plate. May or may not be accompanied with distal detachment of the nail.	Psoriasis; also may occur with alopecia areata, Reiters syndrome, sarcoidosis, pemphigus.	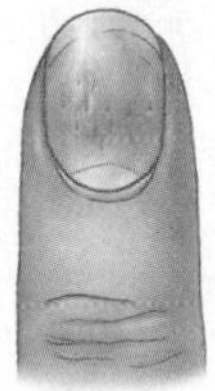
Onycholysis	Separation of nail from nail bed originating at free, distal edge of nail and progressing proximally. Frequently accompanied by yellow discoloration of nail	Psoriasis, trauma, infections (bacterial/viral/fungal), drug reaction (tetracycline) allergic contact dermatitis, maceration, iron deficiency anemia, syphilis.	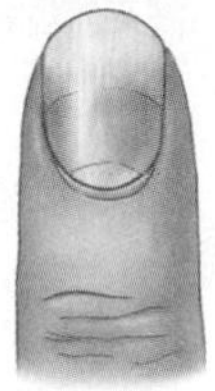
Anonychia (absence of nail)	Congenital absence of nail	Anonychia is a rare anomaly, which may result from a congenital ectodermal defect, ichthyosis, severe infection, severe allergic contact dermatitis, self-inflicted trauma, Raynaud phenomenon, lichen planus, epidermolysis bullosa, or severe exfoliative diseases.	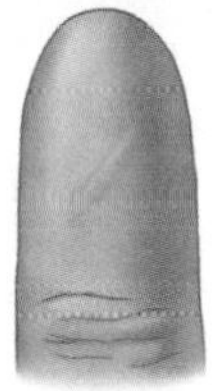
Clubbing (Hippocratic nails)	Soft tissues beneath the proximal nail plate thicken causing sponginess of proximal plate and enlargement of same area giving the distal phalanges of fingers a rounded, bulbous appearance. The angle between nail plate and nail bed increases and becomes greater than 160 degrees.	COPD, other pulmonary conditions, cancers of lung and pleura, cardiovascular disease (congenital heart disease, endocarditis), cirrhosis, thyroid disease	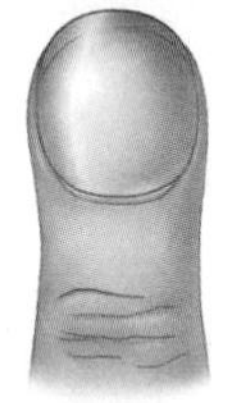
Curved nails	Nails assume a convex curve that resembles clubbing, however, the nail bed-nail plate angle does not increase.	Nonsignificant variation	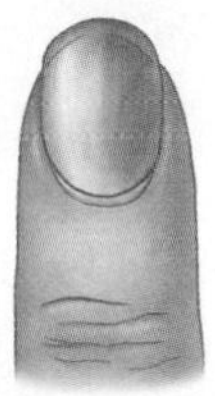
Paronychia	Erythema and swelling of nail folds due to inflammation. Separation of nail plate from cuticle.	Bacterial and viral infections (acute). Repeated exposure to moisture (chronic). Aggressive manicuring and nail biting	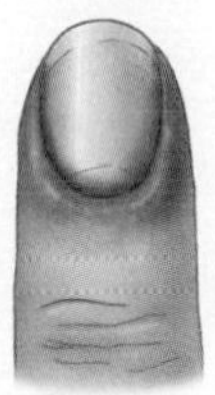

Inspection Techniques and Expected Findings	Unexpected Findings

Assess the skin surface for the presence of primary and/or secondary lesions.

Strictly speaking, skin lesions are classified as vascular, primary, and secondary; however, the criteria that differentiate them are not mutually exclusive. During observation, it is more helpful to describe the unique characteristics of the lesions than to determine their classification. Vascular skin lesions are related to any alterations associated blood vessels and/or capillaries have already been presented.

Primary skin lesions are an initial, spontaneous manifestation of an underlying pathology (Table 16-12).

Secondary skin lesions arise from a change or an evolution of the primary lesion (Table 16-13). Trauma to a primary lesion may also result in a secondary lesion.

Morphology

Morphology of skin lesions is related to their external characteristics. Although all of the previous dimensions of skin lesions relate to their morphology, at this point you will primarily be assessing their external characteristics. Some of these may be observed, but there may also be unique characteristics that need to be palpated.

Characteristics and examples of skin lesions are illustrated in Tables 16-12 and 16-13. For ease in describing skin lesions, inspection and palpation will be discussed together. The lesions will also be identified by their classification. Some lesions have already been discussed but without any reference to their classification. For completeness, they have been placed within their specific classification. Vascular and primary lesions are also grouped according to their morphology, the common attributes that are shared within a group. They are differentiated from each other within their morphological group by either size or contents. Secondary lesions do not have any groups that share a common morphology.

***THINK LINK:* Lesions**

Even though they are defined as associated with pathology, not all causes of skin lesions are pathologic. Although most secondary lesions occur as an evolution of the primary lesion, this should not be considered absolute; there are exceptions.

Table 16-12 Primary skin lesions

Flat, Nonpalpable Lesions				
Macule	Circumscribed, pigmented area, < 1 cm in diameter, of different skin color.	Flat, nonpalpable	Freckle, measles	
Patch	Irregularly shaped, > 1 cm in diameter, circumscribed area of different skin color	Flat, nonpalpable	Vitiligo, Café-au-lait spot	
Palpable, Elevated Solid Masses				
Plaque	Circumscribed area, > 1 cm in diameter	Elevated, flat topped.	Psoriasis, keratoses	
Papule	Circumscribed, pigmented area, < 1 cm in diameter, of different skin color.	Elevated, palpable, firm	Warts, small nevus	

Continued

Table 16-12 Primary skin lesions (*continued*)

		Flat, Nonpalpable Lesions		
Nodule	Same as papule, 1–2 cm in diameter	Elevated, firm, palpable; deeper in dermis	Lipoma	
Tumor	Same as papule, nodule, > 2 cm in diameter. May be same color as skin; may or may not be demarcated.	Elevated, solid, palpable.	Neoplasm, Dermatofibroma	
Wheal	Irregularly shaped area of cutaneous edema, variable diameter, pale pink in color.	Elevated, palpable.	Urticaria (allergic reaction), insect bites	
		Palpable, Elevated, Fluid Filled Masses		
Vesicle	Circumscribed area, filled with fluid, < 1 cm in diameter	Elevated, palpable	Blister, cold sore, chicken pox.	
Bulla	Circumscribed area, filled with fluid, > 1 cm in diameter	Elevated, palpable	Blister, poison ivy, pemphigus.	
Pustule	Similar to vesicle. But filled with purulent fluid	Elevated, palpable	Impetigo, acne; furuncle (boil)—one infected hair follicle, carbuncle—multiple infected hair follicles	
Cyst	Circumscribed, filled with liquid or semisolid material	Elevated, palpable	Sebaceous cyst	

Table 16-13 Secondary skin lesions

Scale	Compact, piled up keratinized epithelial cells; flaky skin	Generally, nonpalpable	Seborrheic dermatitis, post scarlet fever	
Lichenification	Accentuated skin markings	Rough, thickened epidermis from scratching or rubbing	Chronic dermatitis	
Crust	Dried serum, blood, and exudate. Brown, red, black in color.	Slightly elevated, rough	Scab over abrasion, eczema	
Scar	Connective tissue that replaces injured dermis. Shape depends on underlying injury. Dark pink to white in color (depends on age of scar).	New scar is elevated, palpable. Old scar may be atrophic, in which case there would be a slight, smooth indentation of the skin.	Healed wound or surgical incision	
Keloid	Irregularly shaped overgrowth of connective tissue beyond boundaries of wound.	Elevated, palpable	Hypertrophic scar	
Fissure	Linear crack in epidermis into the dermis.	Area may be markedly dry.	Athlete's foot, cheilosis	

Continued

Table 16-13 Secondary skin lesions (*continued*)

Excoriation	Loss of epidermis—dermis may be exposed; linear or dug out traumatized area.	Hollowed out area of epidermis	Abrasion, scratch	
Erosion	Loss of part or all of epidermis, dermis exposed	Post healing, depressed area of epidermis	Post rupture of vesicle or bulla (chicken pox, herpes)	
Ulcer	Loss of epidermis and dermis. May go down to subcutaneous layer and muscle.	Large concave area of lost tissue.	Decubiti, stasis ulcer	
Atrophy	Thinning of skin surface with loss of skin markings; skin becomes translucent. Color depends on age of atrophy—early color reddish purple that eventually turns silvery white (lighter than underlying skin color).	Paper like (parchment) skin	Stretch marks (striae) from pregnancy or obesity; Cushing's syndrome	

Inspection: Level III

The Level III Assessment is performed on patients in urgent situations with significant pathology that may involve one system or many. The assessment may focus on only one system and must be done quickly.

Inspection Techniques and Expected Findings	Unexpected Findings
Assess for skin injuries following blunt trauma, which are produced by an impact with a dull, firm surface or object. Determine the severity of injuries sustained from blunt trauma; this is primarily determined by the amount of kinetic energy transferred to the area and the tissue involved that receives the energy (Table 16-14). The size and weight of the instrument/object and the surface area involved are also factors that determine the degree and type of injury.	Alterations in skin integrity in a Level III exam are related to uncontrolled trauma, most commonly caused by moving vehicle accidents, violence, and burns. Blunt trauma produces various types of skin injuries that disrupt the integrity of the skin's surface, as shown in Table 16-14. (Abrasion, contusion, and laceration have already been described in Table 16-4.) Any of these lesions that are caused by trauma more than likely will be larger in dimensions.

Table 16-14 Types of skin injuries

Name	Description	
Avulsion	A more severe laceration where the soft tissues musculature, and/or bone are torn away from their attachments to other structures.	*Source:* Vladimir Mucibabic/Shutterstock
Fracture	A break, rupture or separation of tissue (most commonly bone) resulting from an impact.	*Source:* Biophoto Associates/Science Source

Inspection Techniques and Expected Findings

Observe for the presence of sharp force injuries produced by pointed or sharp edged objects and causing a relatively well-defined separation of tissues. Identify each injury as a stab, incised, or chop wound (Table 16-15).

Unexpected Findings

Stab wounds are produced when a pointed object directs a force that is perpendicular to the skin surface, allowing it to penetrate the skin surface and underlying tissues. Stab wounds are most often deeper than they are long on the skin surface.

Cut (incised) wounds result when a sharp-edged object produces a force that is directed parallel or tangential to the skin surface. Surgical incisions were described above under conditions of controlled trauma. These wounds are generally longer than they are deep.

Chop wounds are a combination of sharp and blunt force trauma often caused by a heavy object that has a sharp or somewhat sharp edge.

Table 16-15 Blunt force trauma compared with sharp force trauma

	Blunt Force Trauma	Sharp Force Trauma
	Laceration	Incised Wound
Cause	Blunt force trauma	Sharp force trauma
Edges	Ragged/irregular	Cleanly divided
Bruising/Abrasions	Yes	No
Depth	Variable	Can be uniform
Tissue Bridging	Yes	No
Position	Particular bony prominences	Any location
Foreign Bodies	Often contaminated	Usually clean (unless glass)
Hairs	Intact hairs may cross wound	Hairs cleanly divided
Bony Injury	May have associated fractures	Scoring or chipping of bone may occur
Healing	2-degree intention (with extensive scarring)	1-degree intention–good if wound edges approximated Generally leaves fine scarring

Inspection Techniques and Expected Findings	Unexpected Findings

Burns

Assess the skin for a thermal injury. Burns result from exposure to heat or thermal energy from some thermal, chemical, electrical, or radiation source. The energy from the heat source initiates a series of pathophysiological events that result in severe tissue damage or destruction. Thermal burns are caused by exposure to dry heat (flames) or moist heat (steam and hot liquids).

Chemical burns are the result of exposure to either acid or alkaline substances.

Electrical burns are caused by contact with a source of electricity. The extent of tissue damage is related to the type and direction of current and the voltage. Radiation burns result from exposure to ionizing radiation and are most commonly caused by sunlight and radiation therapy.

Document the extent of burn injury as a percentage of the total body surface area (BSA). The severity of tissue damage is related to the depth of tissue damage and surface area of the burn. The depth of tissue damage is classified as superficial, partial thickness (PT), or full thickness (FT) burns (Figure 16-22).

For calculation of the extent of burn injury, measure only partial- and full-thickness burns. Two of the most common methods to determine the extent of burn injury are the "rule of nines" and the Lund and Browder (LB) chart. The "rule of nines" divides the body into five surface areas, assigning a percentage to each that equals nine or an integer of nine (Figure 16-23). The percentage of injury related to each surface area is then estimated and summed. The Lund and Browder assessment chart uses more sections with variable percentages to each, with the added advantage of accounting for the BSA related to age and the degree of injury. Regardless of method, it is critical to be as accurate as possible as initial treatment for deep PT burns and FT burns depends on the extent of damage.

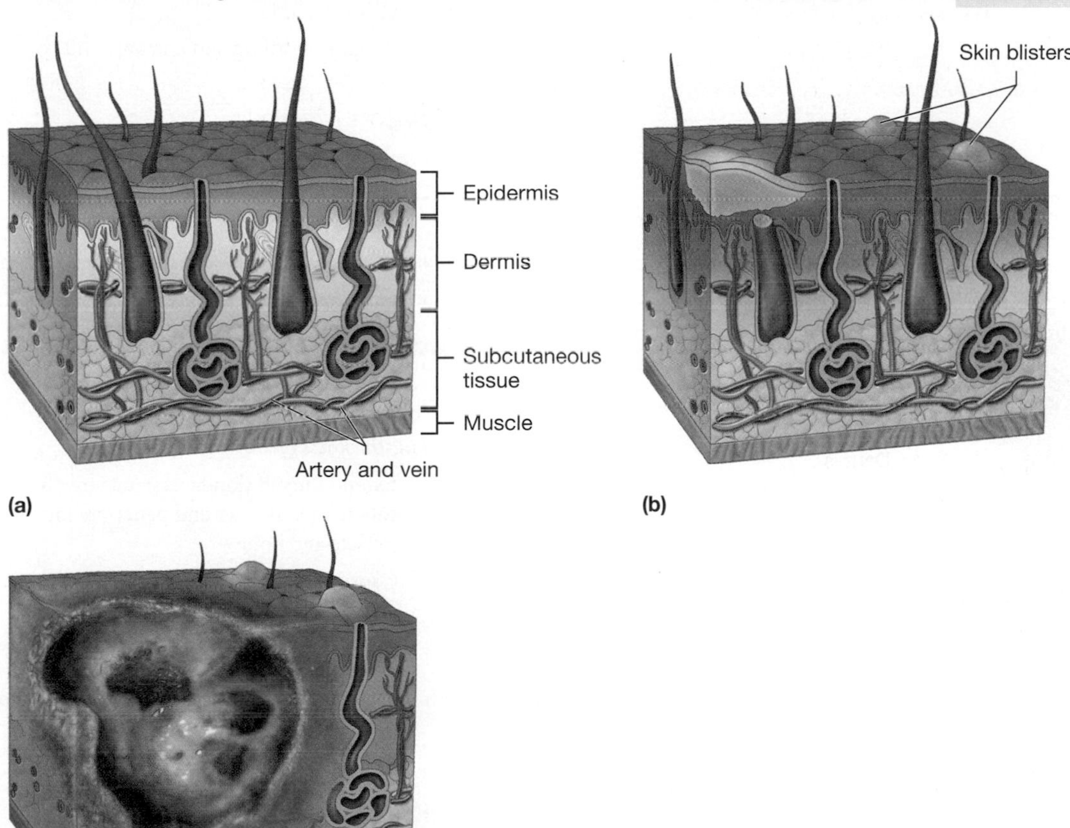

FIGURE 16-22A–C Burn injuries related to tissue depth. **a)** First degree involves top layer of epidermis only; **b)** Second degree involves epidermis and some dermis; **c)** Third degree involves epidermis, dermis, subcutaneous tissue, and some muscle.

Inspection Techniques and Expected Findings

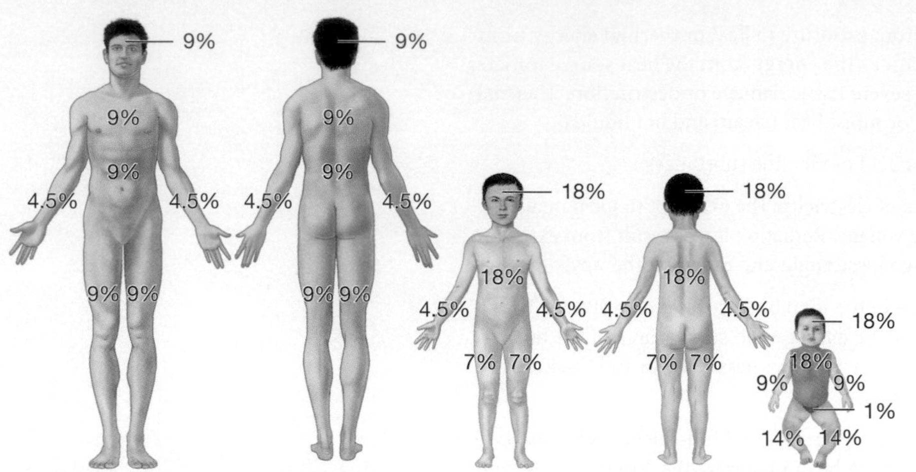

FIGURE 16-23 Estimating the percentage of burns

> ***PRACTICE POINT: Burn Pain***
>
> Deep PT burns are less painful than superficial PT burns but the degree of sensation may vary from area to area. Reduced or absent pain results from the destruction of nerve endings.

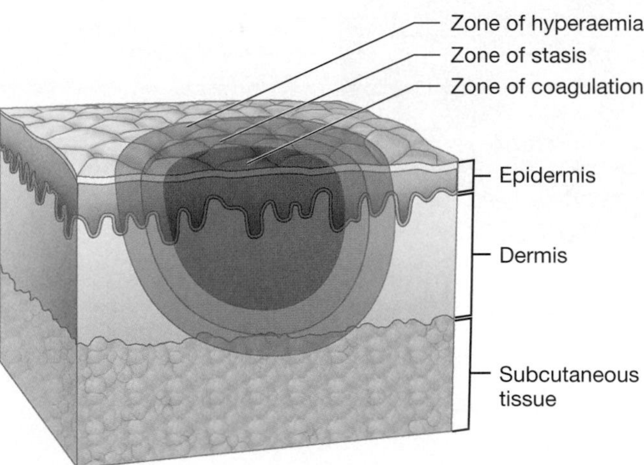

FIGURE 16-24 Zones of burns

Unexpected Findings

Superficial burns:

- Limited to epidermal layer; may be caused by sunburn or a flash injury
- Reddened skin with no damage to the underlying tissues
- No blister formation
- Pain common
- Area blanches upon pressure application

Partial-thickness (PT) burns: Further categorized into superficial or deep partial-thickness burns.

Superficial PT burns:

- Limited to papillae and upper portion of the dermis
- Bright red, with moist glistening appearance and blister formation
- Blanch to pressure, with pain and touch sensations intact.
- Skin is not damaged, and thus able to perform its physiological functions (Wedro, 2011)
- Possible mottling and hairs are still present

Deep PT burns:

- Extend further into the dermis
- Hair follicles, sebaceous, and sweat glands undamaged
- Surface has pale, waxy appearance
- Large, easily ruptured blisters that appear like flat, dry tissue paper
- Diminished capillary refill
- Sensation only to deep pressure

Full-thickness burns:

- Extend into all skin layers; may involve subcutaneous layer and penetrate into muscle and bone
- Caused by extended contact with the source of heat
- Appearance varies, depending on the cause, ranging from pale, waxy, yellow, brown, mottled, charred, or red
- Surface is dry, leathery, and firm to touch
- Pain receptors have been destroyed; therefore the individual has no pain or touch sensation.
- Result in 3 zones of injury that are demonstrated by three concentric circles: (1) zone of coagulation, (2) zone of stasis, and (3) zone of hyperaemia (Figure 16-24) (Hettiaratchy & Dziewulski, 2004).

Inspection: Level IV

The Level IV Assessment is considered a comprehensive exam and includes techniques and skills of advanced prepared providers. Components of the Level IV Exam would be performed whenever the provider would need a complete data base related to a specific system or is the initial examination of the patient and the provider wants a complete data base to establish an overall baseline of each system. In some instances, a provider may wish to obtain more comprehensive data for a hospitalized patient and may use advanced skills and techniques.

In general, there would not be any additional observations or palpation that would need to be made. There might be an increased scrutiny of the various regions of the body for presence of lesions, depending on the presenting condition of the patient. If there is a question regarding the presence of a fungal infection, a Woods lamp is used to confirm its presence (Figure 16-25).

A Wood's lamp is a diagnostic tool used in dermatology by which ultraviolet (UV) light (black light) is directed onto the skin of the patient and observing for the presence of any fluorescence. In skin assessment, the Wood's lamp is used to search for the distinctive color fluorescence of certain dermatophytic fungi such as species of Microsporan (yellow) or corynebacterium (red to orange). UV light is also used to detect the presence and extent of pigmentation loss disorders (vitiligo). It can also be used to diagnose ringworm, corneal scratches, foreign bodies in the eye, blocked tear ducts, acne, tinea versicolor, scabies, alopecia, porphyria, bacterial infections, and other skin conditions.

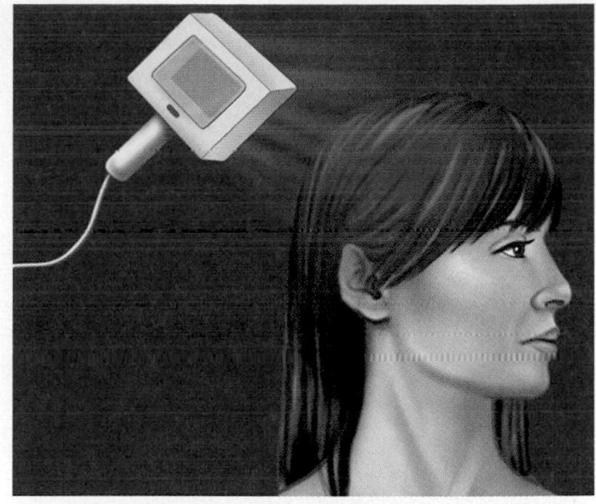

Wood's Lamp Colors	
White Spots	Thick cornea layer, dead cells, and a random horny layer of skin
Blue/White	Normal healthy skin, thin skin, lacking moisture
Light Violet	Dehydrated skin
Brown	Sun damage
Pink/Orange	Oiliness
Bright Fluorescent	Hydrated skin
Yellow/Orange	Comedones

FIGURE 16-25 Wood's lamp

Palpation: Level I

Palpation Techniques and Expected Findings	Unexpected Findings
Perform an initial palpation of the skin to assess for elasticity as observed by the skin's mobility and turgor that reflect the skin's hydration status. Well-hydrated skin is supple and elastic (mobile), moves freely or glides over the underlying muscle and bones, and easily returns to its original position (Figure 16-26).	Decreased mobility is palpated in areas that are edematous. Edematous tissue is expanded with fluid, stretching the skin and causing it to be less elastic and thus less mobile.
Assess turgor by gently pinching a small section of skin between the thumb and first finger, noting how rapidly it returns to its original state. Well-hydrated skin pinches easily and rapidly returns to its original position.	Dehydrated skin and/or skin that has lost its elasticity demonstrate poor turgor by remaining in it's pinched position, known as **tenting**, and slowly returning to its original position. Skin that has lost its elasticity is a result of aging.

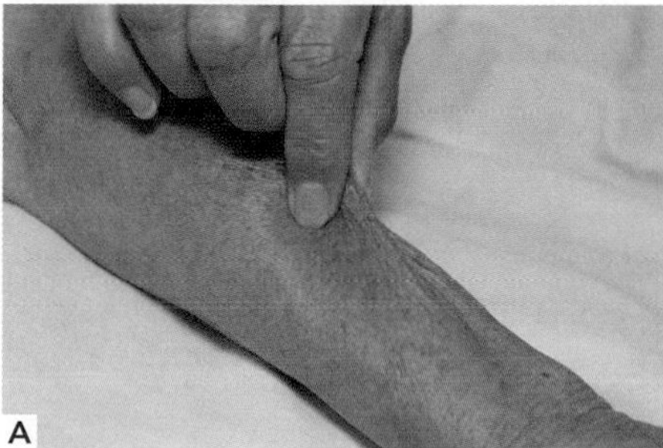
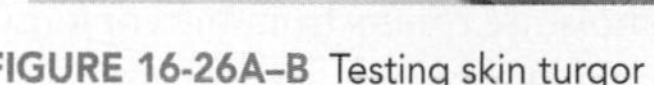
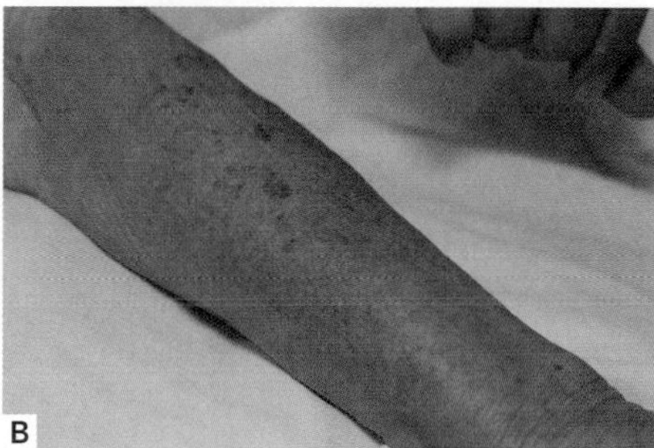

FIGURE 16-26A–B Testing skin turgor

Palpation Techniques and Expected Findings	Unexpected Findings

Skin that has been stretched by edema will also have a characteristic boggy feel after pressure is applied to the area and will frequently leave an indentation (pitting) (Figure 16-27). Edema that pits is classified according to the depth of the indentation. (See Chapter 25 for classification of pitting.) As skin becomes stretched by edema, the skin is tight and not able to be pinched to assess its turgor.

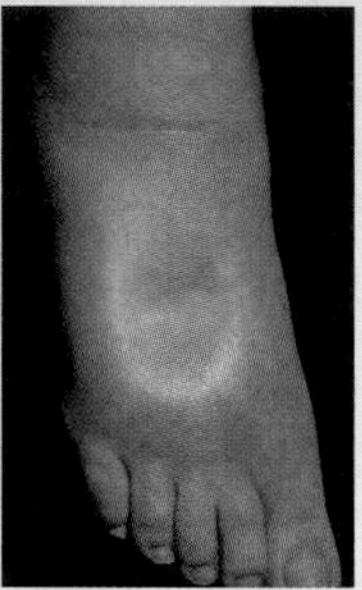

FIGURE 16-27 Pitting edema
Source: SPL/Science Source Images

Palpate the fingernails for capillary refill time (CRT). While this is more of a test related to the adequacy of peripheral circulation, it may be performed with the overall assessment of the nails.

Pinch the nail bed/plate and the tip of the finger between your thumb and index finger until blanching is observed. Immediately release the pinched site and note the time it takes for the return of the original color to the nail bed. This should be less than 3 seconds, indicating adequate tissue circulation and perfusion. (Refer to Chapter 24.)

An increased CRT may be due to peripheral vascular disorders that interfere with circulation and tissue perfusion. It may also be due to vasoconstriction caused by cold external temperatures. Some cyanosis may also be noted in this instance.

Place the back of your hand over an area of skin to assess skin temperature, which ranges from cool to warm.

Notice minor variations in the skin's surface temperature, such as variation in temperature over certain parts of the body (chronic cold hands or cold feet), which should not be of concern if the variations are symmetrical.

Ambient temperature may cause minor variation. For example, in cold weather, the hands and feet may feel cool. This may or may not be accompanied by skin paleness and/or localized distal cyanosis. Assess whether the variations in color and temperature are bilateral.

PRACTICE POINT: Temperature

The patient's internal environment as well as the external environment will affect the temperature findings. Finding appropriate descriptors of skin temperature is difficult, making consistency of temperature a more useful assessment parameter.

The skin temperature is decreased (hypothermia) in states of hypometabolism (hypothyroidism), post anesthesia, and shock. Localized hypothermia may indicate the presence of decreased arterial circulation to an area.

In general, the skin temperature is elevated (hyperthermia) in states of hypermetabolism (hyperthyroidism), after exercise, and in the presence of a fever. Localized hyperthermia may be due to inflammation, trauma, venous circulatory alterations, or sunburn.

Palpation: Level II

Palpate the skin to assess its texture or character and moisture. The skin's surface should feel smooth, soft, and firm, with an even surface. It should also feel soft and supple without evidence of excessive moisture on the surface. Excessive secretion of oil may be characteristic of some individuals, and this is usually evident on the forehead and face.

Skin roughness may be due to excessive dryness or hypothyroidism. The skin may become excessively smooth and velvety to the touch in hyperthyroidism.

Excessive moisture results from the copious perspiration that accompanies increased activity, increased ambient temperature, or excitement.

Palpate the hair for texture, which relates to the thickness of the hair; it may be coarse, medium or fine. Additionally it may be considered kinky, curly, wavy, or straight. Hair should also be shiny, smooth, and resilient.

Hair of an individual with hyper- or hypothyroidism demonstrates characteristic texture. Hair is coarse and brittle in hypothyroidism and smooth and silky in hyperthyroidism. Brittle hair that may fall out in patches is observed in patients with lupus.

Inspection Techniques and Expected Findings	Unexpected Findings
Palpate the skin for the presence of any localized skin elevations (papules, nodules, tumors). These three types of lesions are similar, size being the differentiating factor.	
A common papule is a nevus (plural: *nevi*), commonly referred to as a mole and results from proliferation of dermal and epidermal structures. Nevi appear on most individuals, regardless of primary skin color, and anywhere on the skin. The appearance, color, and number of moles varies by individual (Table 16-16).	Atypical nevi may be characterized as dysplastic, meaning cancerous or precancerous (Table 16-17).
Most nevi are nonsignificant and do not cause any problems.	
Palpation of vascular skin lesions is also performed to assess for the presence of blanching. Blanching is assessed by putting pressure on the lesion and observing for any color change.	When assessing hemorrhagic vascular lesions, blood cells present due to loss of blood into the tissues (hemorrhage) cannot be forced out of the area, thus the lesion will not blanch.
Blanching is performed on vascular lesions. Blanching occurs when red cells are forced out of the area by the pressure and without their red undertones. The area loses color, which generally occurs with non-hemorrhagic vascular lesions.	

Table 16-16 Types of nevi

Type	Features	Characteristics	Comments	
Three Classifications of Nevi (based on location of nevus cells in the skin)				
Junctional	Flat or slightly elevated; uniform pigmentation (dark brown)	Nevus cells at dermo-epidermal junction	Rare at birth; transformation to melanoma rare	
Compound	Slightly elevated; smooth or rough; indistinct border; uniform pigmentation (flesh color to brown)	Nevus cells at dermo-epidermal junction and upper dermis	If white halo around periphery, called a *halo nevus*	*Source*: Biophoto Associates/Science Source
Dermal	Variety of shapes (dome, polypoid, warty, and pedunculated); brown or black—lighter with age	Nevus cells in dermis; may be among fat cells.	Transformation to melanoma rare	*Source*: Biophoto Associates/Science Source
Clinical Variants				
Giant, hairy nevus (congenital)	Present at birth; variable size; may contain coarse hair; uniform pigmentation (brown or black)	Start our flat but become thicker during childhood	At high risk for transformation to melanoma; may occur early in childhood	*Source*: Nathalie Speliers Ufermann/Shutterstock
Blue Nevus	Dark grey-blue-black dermal papule with smooth surface; pigment cell proliferation deep in dermis	Appears in childhood, most commonly on extremities	Possible transformation to melanoma, but not common; sometimes mistaken for melanoma	*Source*: Biophoto Associates/Science Source

Table 16-17 Typical vs. atypical nevi

Feature	Typical Nevi	Atypical Nevi
Distribution/location	Commonly sun-exposed areas above the waist	Anywhere on body mostly on back; also upper/ lower extremities, sun protected areas, breast, scalp, buttock, groin
Numbers	10–40	< 10 – >100 (5%–20%) of adult Caucasians have one small atypical nevus
Age at appearance	None at birth; appear at age 2–6; uniform vertical growth during lifetime; more may appear at puberty	Present as typical nevi ages 2–6; increase in size and number at puberty; increase in numbers through life
Size	Generally < 6 mm	Generally > 5 mm and frequently > 10 mm
Shape	Round/oval with well-defined border that marks where nevi end and surrounding skin begins Consistent macular or papular feature	Irregular borders that may blend into surrounding skin; may have notches Always a macular feature
Color	Consistent tan, brown, or black color Generally, all nevi same color on individual Darker during pregnancy/adolescence; lighter with age	Variable color (brown, black, red, pink) in single nevus Variable colors of nevi on individual
Surface	Starts as flat, smooth spot; becomes elevated but stays smooth	Variable surface characteristics: Smooth and/or scaly, rough, irregular, bumpy feel

Palpation Techniques and Expected Findings

Palpate the fingernails for thickness and adherence to nail bed. Nails should be hard and smooth with uniform thickness.

To assess for adherence, gently pinch the nail between your thumb and forefinger (Figure 16-28). The nail plate should firmly adhere to the nail bed without any movement of the nail plate over the nail bed. The nail base, when palpated, should feel firm.

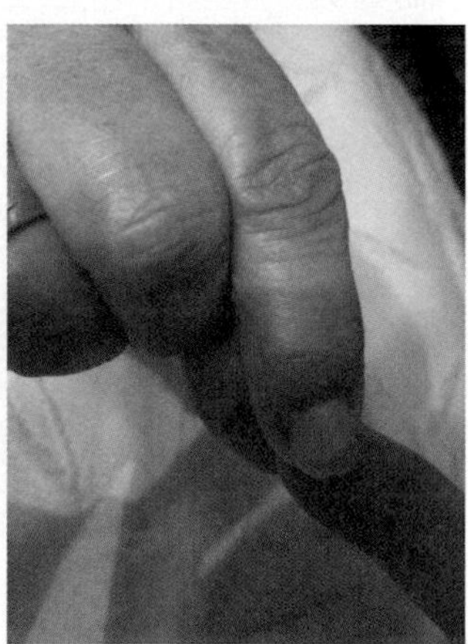

FIGURE 16-28 Assessing the adherence of the nail plate

Unexpected Findings

Thickening of the nail occurs from chronic trauma and fungal infections. Thinning may be caused by inadequate circulation or nutritional deficiencies.

Separation of the nail plate and bed may be caused by psoriasis, trauma, or infection.

A boggy or soft nail base is associated with clubbing.

Palpation: Levels III and IV

Palpation Levels III and IV are generally not used as there is very little related to the skin at these levels that requires palpation. Percussion and auscultation are not used at all with skin as there are no audible sounds that can be or are produced by the skin.

Developmental Applications

Techniques and Expected Findings	Unexpected Findings

Infants and Children

The newborn infant's skin is covered with a cheesy, white substance called the vernix caseosa (Figure 16-29). The infant's skin is initially quite red but later turns the more pinkish color associated with newborns. Skin color is largely determined by the amount of subcutaneous tissue so the less subcutaneous tissue, the more red the infant's skin. Dark-skinned infants are often quite light in appearance and do not demonstrate their expected "darkness" until they are 2 to 3 months old.

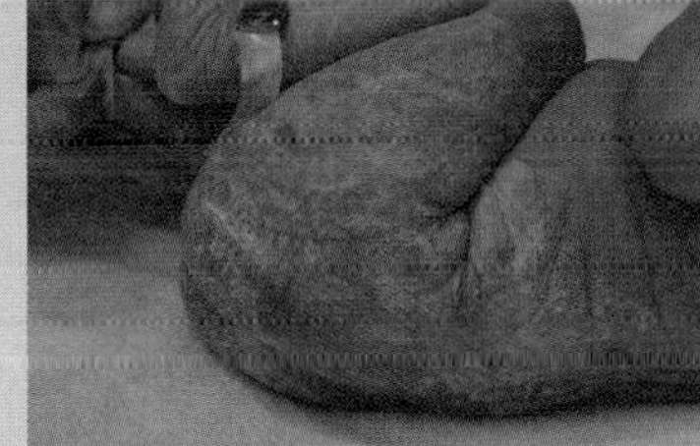

FIGURE 16-29 The skin of the newborn is covered with vernix caseosa, an expected finding
Source: Keith/Custom Medical Stock Photo

Because the infant's merocrine glands are nonfunctional, temperature regulation in the infant is nonexistent, resulting in various nonsignificant color changes. **Acrocyanosis**, cyanosis of the hands and feet may be observed at birth and may continue for a few days if the infant experiences cool ambient temperature (Figure 16-30).

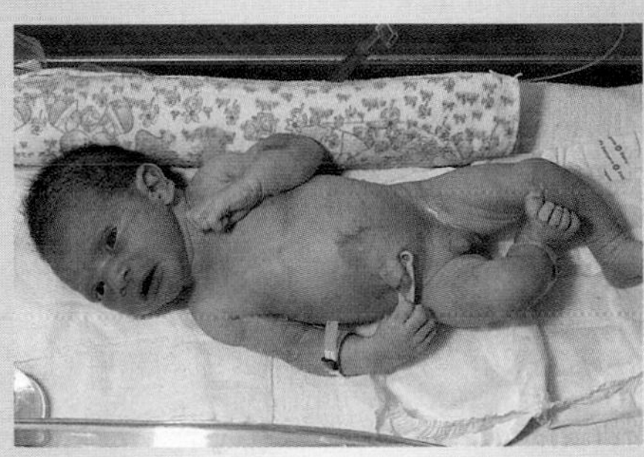

FIGURE 16-30 Acrocyanosis

Cyanosis that persists past a few days and is more apparent in the feet, further evaluation for underlying cardiac defects should be done.

Somewhat along the same lines, **cutis marmorata** (mottling of the skin) is present as a response to changes in ambient temperature.

Harlequin color change refers to one half of the infant demonstrating a greater degree of redness than the other, with a relative distinct line of demarcation at the midline . This condition is self-limiting and doesn't last long.

Infants with dark skin may demonstrate a Mongolian spot (dermal melanosis), an irregular patch of deep blue pigmentation, commonly over the sacral and gluteal area (Figure 16-31). Infants of African, Native American, Asian, or Latin descent are most frequently affected.

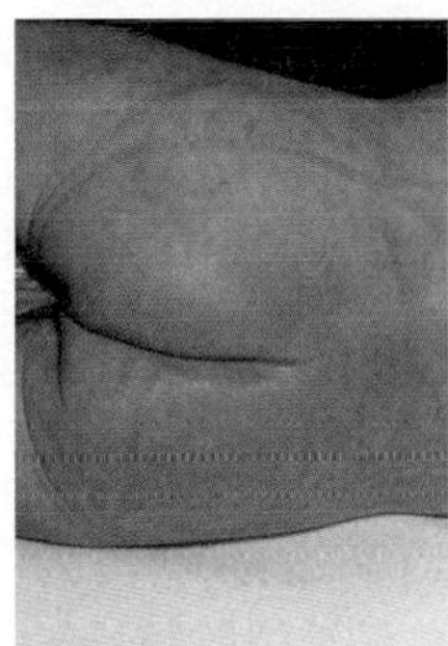

FIGURE 16-31 Mongolian spots
Source: Dr. P. Marazzi/Science Source Images

Jaundice in most instances is physiologic and due to the breakdown of extra red cells. Red cell breakdown releases bilirubin, which is eventually excreted. Physiologic jaundice may start on the first day of life and should disappear by the 8th to 10th day. In rare instances, it may continue for as long as 3 to 4 weeks. Jaundice generally begins on the face and may remain confined to that area or may gradually descend. When assessing the infant for jaundice, remember to inspect the sclera and mucous membranes for color changes. Also, jaundice is easier to detect in natural light.

Jaundice that does not disappear and remains intense is more than likely an indication of an underlying disorder. Increased levels of bilirubin may have a negative effect on the infant's neurological development.

If the jaundice descends below the nipple line, there is cause to be concerned about increasing bilirubin levels.

PRACTICE POINT: Mongolian Spot

Mongolian spots are an accepted skin color change in dark-skinned infants that is nonsignificant. This is especially true when the child is brought in for follow-up appointments. Well-meaning individuals have mistaken the Mongolian spot for evidence of bruising resulting from physical abuse. Once individuals are reported for child abuse, it is very difficult to overcome the suspicions and stereotypes of child abusers.

The infant's skin may demonstrate additional nonsignificant alterations. **Erythema toxicum** is a pink papular rash with superimposed vesicles (Figure 16-32). This generally appears on the chest, back, buttocks, and abdomen. It may first appear at 24–48 hours and disappears within a couple of days. The sebaceous glands of the infant are immature and are easily plugged by sebum producing small, whitish, discrete papules known as **milia**. These are commonly seen within the first 2 to 3 months (Figure 16-33).

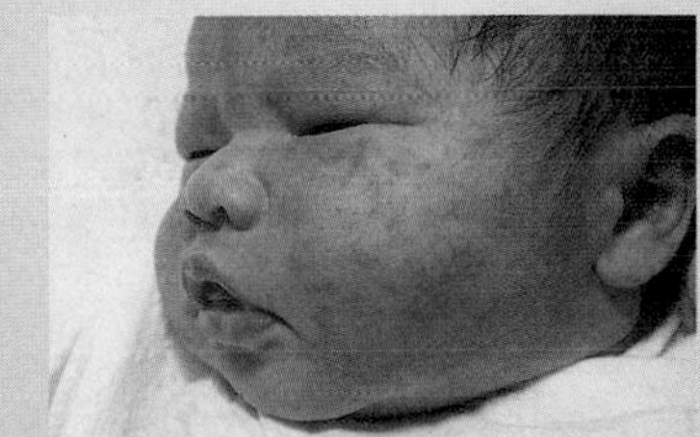

FIGURE 16-32 Erythema toxicams

Techniques and Expected Findings

Inspect the hands and feet of the infant for skin creases. When examining the hands and feet, use flexion to produce the visible lines. The number of creases may be a way of determining the infant's maturity: the greater the numbers of creases, the more mature the infant. There is generally no specific pattern to look for; however, be aware of a single transverse crease on the palm (Figure 16-34).

Previously, this particular crease was identified as a Simian crease, a term which is no longer used as *Simian* is associated with a monkey or an ape. Instead it is referred to as a **single palmar crease**. Inspect the skin for any obvious defects, particularly along the length of the spine and the midline of the head. There should be no obvious openings or protrusions related to skin surface.

THINK LINK: Trichotillomania

Trichotillomania is a traumatic type of self-induced hair loss that results from compulsive twisting or plucking of the hair until it breaks off. The hair loss may occur in round, well-circumscribed patches or diffusely across the scalp that gives an uneven distribution pattern. Other hairy areas, such as eyebrows, eyelashes, or body hair, may be also plucked. Individuals with this disorder often initially seek help from a dermatologist. Trichotillomania is a compulsive behavior that may affect up to 4% of the population. The causes are not clearly understood. Symptoms usually appear before the age of 16. Trichotillomania is generally limited to younger children who frequently outgrow the behavior. The incidence is four times higher in females than males. Most of the time the hair pulling is time-limited to 12 months. Early onset (before age 6) is associated with a better prognosis.

Inspect the skin for any injuries that alter the surface of the skin or disrupt the integrity of the skin. Pay particular attention to injuries that appear to follow a particular pattern or the presence of multiple injuries/bruises that are in various stages of healing.

Unexpected Findings

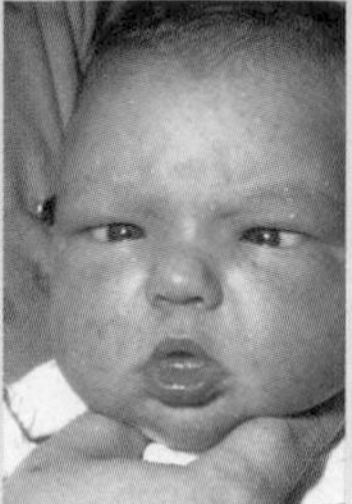

FIGURE 16-33 Milia
Source: Biophoto Associates/Science Source

The single palmar crease is highly suggestive of Down syndrome; however, it is not diagnostic, as it may be observed in other conditions (Figure 16-34).

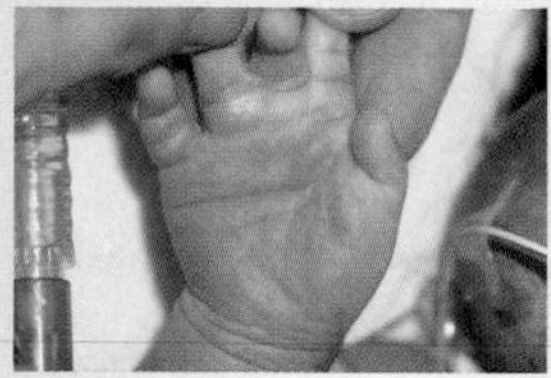

FIGURE 16-34 Single palmar crease
Source: Ralph C. Eagle, Jr./Science Source Images

Any obvious openings or tufts of hair are suggestive of the presence of clefts, tracts, or cysts.

Pattern injuries are bruises or wounds that suggest the type of instrument or object that caused it. These types of injuries are common manifestations of physical child abuse (Figure 16-35). Such objects may be belt buckles, broomsticks, cigarettes, fingers, teeth, or scalding liquids. Scalding liquid burns are frequently well-defined areas, usually on the extremities, resembling a glove or sock. This pattern of burn suggests that that part of the body was immersed in a scalding liquid. Approximately 70% of burns in children are due to scalds—exposure to hot liquids, and a significant number of these are the result of child abuse (Edlich, Drake, & Long III, 2011). Other manifestations of child abuse may be seen as fractures that were not reported or not set appropriately, resulting in deformities. Child abuse is often involved when the child's history does not support the extent or severity of the injury.

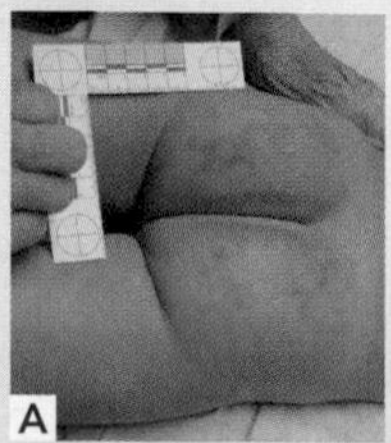

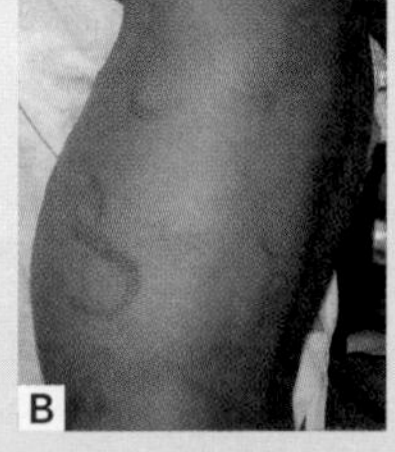

FIGURE 16-35 A-B Abuse patterns
Source: Photos courtesy of the Center for Safe and Healthy Families at Primary Children's Medical Center, Salt Lake City, UT

PRACTICE POINT: Cultural Practices

Certain cultures have health practices or treatments that are demonstrated on the skin that may cause some concern about abuse; however, it is important to recognize the manifestations of these practices and not confuse them with child abuse. These practices or treatments often present in a pattern type arrangement. Two treatments that are often observed in patterns are **coining** and **cupping**, which are used in more traditional cultures. They are also recognized as a form of therapy in alternative medicine practice.

Coining, a type of folk therapy practiced in parts of southeast Asia and Indonesia, is a form of intense massage in which a coin is rubbed vigorously over an area of skin in such a way that red marks are visible on the skin. Most likely, a mild abrasion will accompany the marks. Coining is done to restore balance within the individual.

Cupping is the practice of placing a heated cup on the skin in such a way that an airtight seal is formed. The air inside the cup contracts as it cools, forming a partial vacuum and drawing blood to the area, leaving a series of red rings or circles and possible bruising if the cups are dragged while suctioning. Cupping is done for a variety of conditions, such as arthritis, stomach aches, and bruises. The process is thought to increase blood flow to promote healing or perhaps to draw out any bad energy within the individual.

Although to individuals outside the cultures, coining and cupping may seem to be "abusive," the belief in these practices is real and they will most likely be continued. Before jumping to the conclusion that this is abuse, determine what the marks represent and if the individual or family uses traditional or alternative types of treatments. It is wiser to obtain the necessary data than to jump to wrong conclusions.

Techniques and Expected Findings

Palpate the infant's skin for smoothness, mobility, and turgor. It should feel smooth without any evidence of underlying masses, nodules or tumors. The infant's skin should be supple and resilient, indicating a well hydrated state. The best location for assessing skin turgor on both infants and children is on the abdomen (Figure 16-36). Pinch a section of the skin and observe its return to its original state.

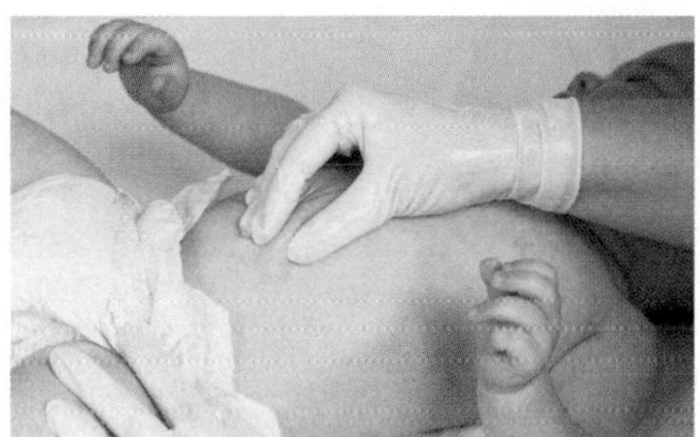

FIGURE 16-36 Assessing skin turgor of a child

As the merocrine glands are nonfunctional in the first month of life, the infant will not demonstrate sweating. In children, excessive sweating or dryness is not necessarily significant. The range of moisture is highly variable in infants and children, thus excessive sweating alone is not indicative of underlying pathology.

The sebaceous glands also become active and result in the adolescent's skin increasing oiliness.

The Pregnant Woman

Various skin alterations are observed in the pregnant female. An increase in pigmentation, to some degree, is seen in all pregnant females, particularly in the areola and nipples, perineum, and axillae. The linea alba, a vertical line that extends from the symphysis pubis to the top of the fundus, may also become hyperpigmented and is identified as the linea nigra (Figure 16-37a). Hyperpigmentation may also be observed on the face as **chloasma** (melasma), and sometimes called the "mask of pregnancy" (Figure 16-37b). Chloasma appears patchy and appears in a symmetrical pattern over the cheeks, bridge of the nose, forehead, and chin. Pigmented nevi and freckles may become darker and larger. There is also the possibility of developing new nevi.

Unexpected Findings

Skin that is lax and demonstrates tenting is an indication of dehydration. As infants have a higher percentage of body water, smaller losses may lead to dehydration. The degree of hydration may be estimated by how long the skin takes to return to its original state (Seidel, Ball, Dains, & Benedict, 2006).

Skin alterations in children, if present, often accompany specific conditions and may be identified according to their characteristics related to skin lesions.

The sebaceous glands become easily plugged, which leads to the development of acne. The presence of acne can be very disturbing to the adolescent and should be taken seriously. The extent of acne is quite variable and in severe cases may become cystic and result in various degrees of scar formation. The lesions associated with acne are identified as comedomes (black heads) and pustules (see Conditions and Disorders).

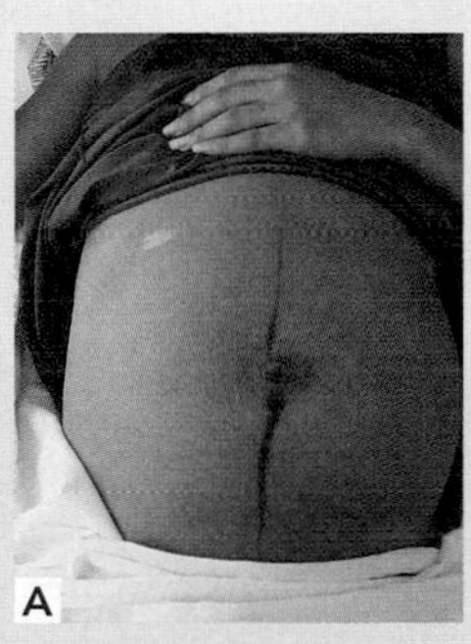

A

Techniques and Expected Findings | **Unexpected Findings**

The palms of the hands may demonstrate palmar erythema, an increased redness with no known cause; it will most likely disappear after delivery.

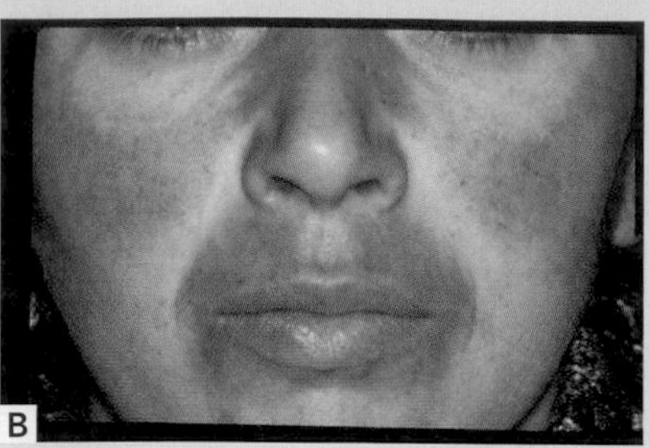

Stretch marks (striae) may also appear over the abdomen, thighs, and breasts. In the initial stage of their appearance they are purplish-pink in color, but as they age they become silvery white and atrophic (Figure 16-37c). Although they never totally disappear, they become less obvious with age.

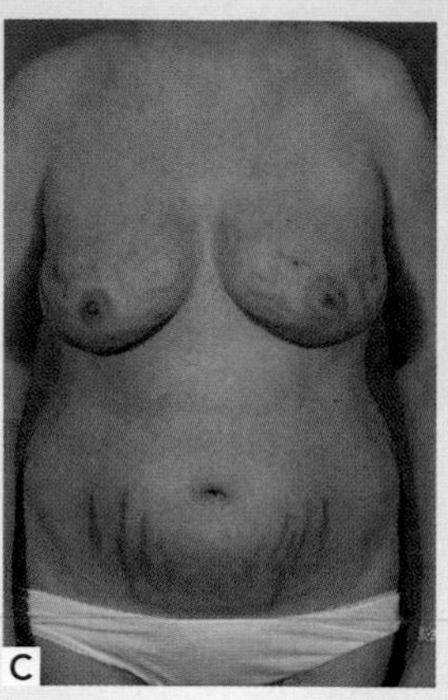

FIGURE 16-37A–C Common skin changes that may occur during pregnancy. **a)** Line nigra **b)** Striae **c)** chloasma

Source: a. George Dodson/Pearson Education; b,c. Science Photo Library/Custom Medical Stock

Other skin manifestations include itching, an increase in telangiectasias, altered hair growth, and cutaneous tags, which are small skin tags that result from epithelial hyperplasia.

Cutaneous tags are most commonly observed on the neck and upper chest. After pregnancy they generally resolve.

Itching may be due to stretching of the skin as well as an increase in bilirubin. There is less hair loss during pregnancy due to an increased growth phase of the hair follicle. After pregnancy, however, hair loss increases but regrowth occurs in 6 to 12 months.

This is generally not a concern unless the itching is accompanied by a rash.

The Older Adult

The skin of the older adult becomes thinner, especially over bony prominences, the dorsal aspect of the hands and feet, forearms and lower legs; it also appears more transparent. This is particularly the case in light-skinned individuals. Areas of hypopigmentation and hyperpigmentation also occur, giving the skin color a less uniform appearance.

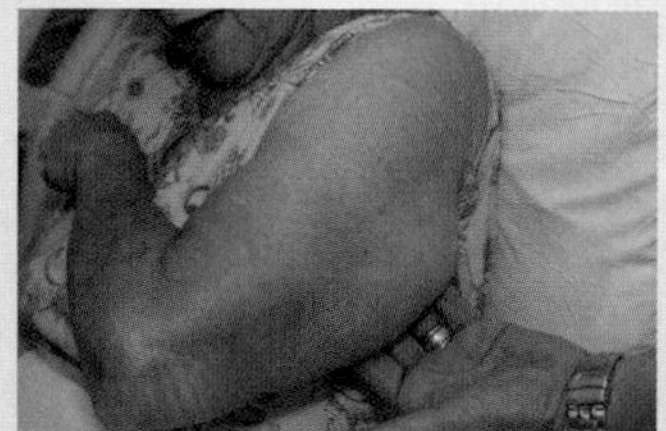

FIGURE 16-38 Skin changes related to aging

A loss of subcutaneous tissue allows the skin to hang more loosely (Figure 16-38). The skin also loses its elasticity, resulting in tenting when pinched. As an expected manifestation of the older adult's skin, tenting is not an appropriate measure of the skin's hydration status. Skin will also show an increase in wrinkling, particularly in sun-exposed areas and the expressive areas of the face. The loss of elasticity also predisposes the skin to droop or sag, particularly under the chin and eyes, and on the ear lobes, breasts, and scrotum. It may also be observed under the upper portion of the arm.

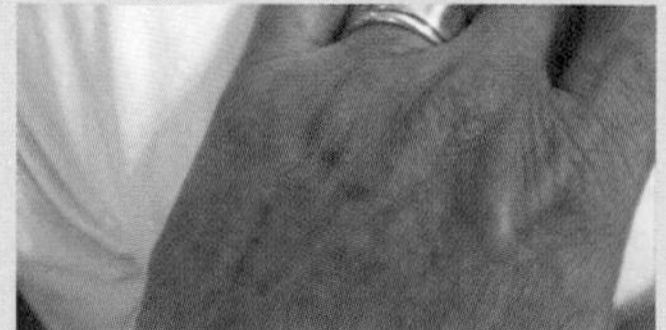

FIGURE 16-39 Lentigines

Inspection Techniques and Expected Findings	Unexpected Findings

The skin of the older adult is prone to the development of various skin lesions, most of which are nonsignificant. These lesions are as follows:

- Lentigines (age or liver spots) may be flat, round, hyperpigmented macules that primarily appear in sun-exposed areas. Small clusters of melanocytes, they appear most commonly on the back of the hands and forearms (Figure 16-39). They are not precancerous and require no treatment.
- Cherry angiomas are tiny, bright red, round papules, most commonly found over the anterior and posterior chest (Figure 16-40). These are present in almost all individuals over 30, generally increase in number with aging, and may eventually turn from red to brown.
- Seborrheic keratoses are raised, thickened areas of hyperpigmentation that appear crusted, scaly, and warty (Figure 16-41). They are most evident on the trunk, but also are present on the face and hands. They develop on both sun-exposed and unexposed skin; they are not considered precancerous.
- Cutaneous tags (acrochordons) result from epidermal hyperplasia that are attached to the skin by stalks (Figure 16-42a). Most common on the upper trunk and neck, they may or may not be pigmented.
- Cutaneous horns are small, horn-shaped, hard projections of keratinized epidermis that appear on the forehead and face (Figure 16-42b). Both cutaneous tags and horns are nonsignificant and not considered precancerous. Their major concern is cosmetic appearance and comfort.
- Sebaceous hyperplasia presents as raised yellow papules with a central depression. They have an increased incidence in males and commonly appear over the forehead, nose, or cheeks.

FIGURE 16-40 Cherry angiomas

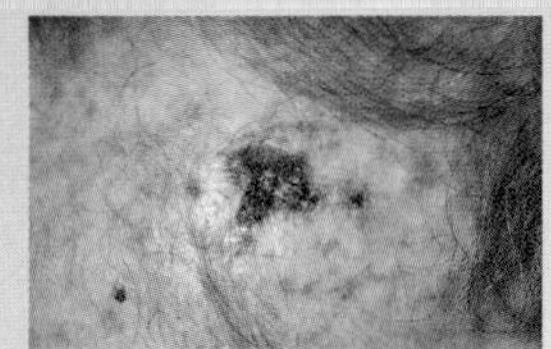

FIGURE 16-41 Seborrheic keratoses
Source: Dr. P. Marazzi/Science Source Images

Less common than seborrheic type, actinic keratoses red-tan scaly plaques that eventually become rough and raised, and may display a whitish scale that adheres to the plaque (see Conditions and Disorders).

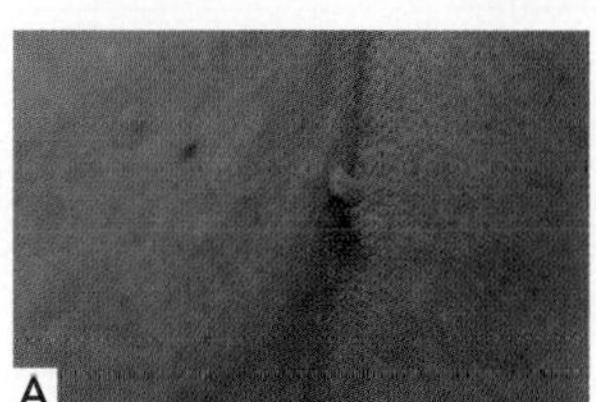

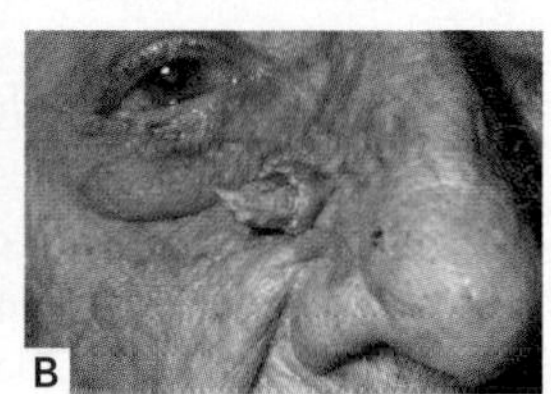

FIGURE 16-42A–B **a)** Cutaneous tags; **b)** cutaneous horns
Source: b. Peter Skinner/Science Source

As the individual ages, the hair loses its pigment and turns various shades of gray. The melanocytes decrease in function, causing the change in hair color. Hair growth also is reduced, with a loss of hair in the axillary and pubic areas. Scalp hair becomes thinner in both genders (Figure 16-43), and males tend to develop coarse nasal and ear hair and females may develop coarse hair on the chin and upper lip. Various degrees of alopecia may be present, and males may develop genetically induced male-patterned baldness that is symmetrical in appearance.

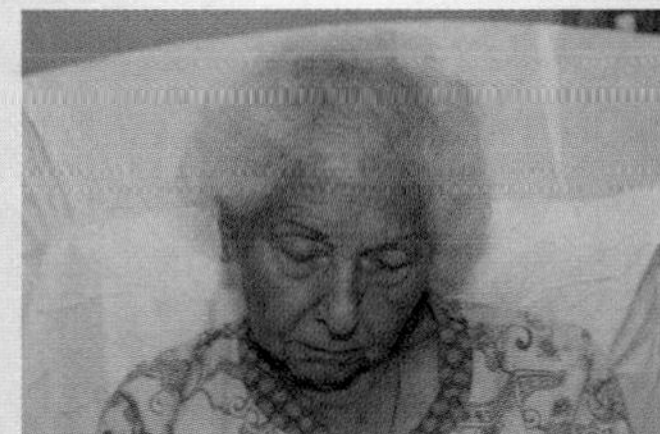

FIGURE 16-43 Thinning hair is a common age-related change

The nails of the older adult have a decreased growth rate and the plates may have longitudinal lines from local injuries to the nail matrix. The nails become brittle and thickened, and may take on a yellow appearance. (Figure 16-44).

The thickening may be due to peripheral vascular disease or infections, primarily fungal in origin. The causal mechanisms for these alterations is not well understood but thought to be related to dysfunctional blood circulation at distal locations or from ultraviolet radiation (Abdullah & Abbas, 2011).

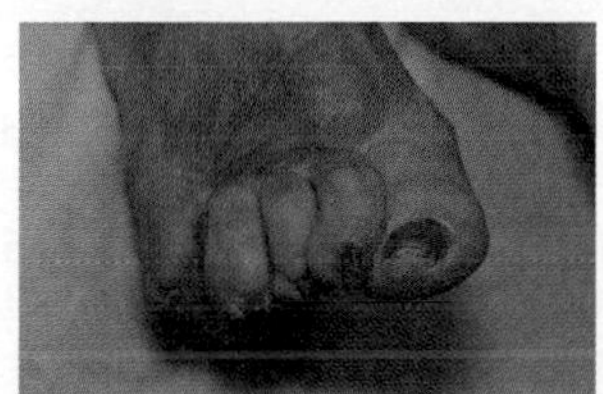

FIGURE 16-44 Nails of the elderly

DOCUMENTATION

General skin—Even, homogeneous distribution of color. Skin is warm, with the exception of hands and feet, and dry. Body hair on arms and scalp evenly distributed. Scars on left knee and right ankle as previously identified.

Head—Scalp uniform whitish color and freely mobile over skull. Hair dark brown in color with wavy consistency and thick feel. Hair shiny, clean, and without any parasites. No lesions, masses noted upon palpation.

Face, neck shoulders, posterior/anterior thorax, abdomen—Color consistent with overall color tones, face and neck lightly tanned. Patch birthmark (reddish purple) 5 cm × 2 cm, asymmetrical on R side of back of neck. Skin warm, dry, smooth, and freely moveable.

Turgor—Skin elastic with immediate return to original position after pinched.

Upper extremities—Consistent color with forearms lightly tanned. Several macules generally scattered over upper portion of both arms. Hair light brown in color and evenly distributed over upper portion of forearms. Turgor of forearms equal bilaterally and demonstrates adequate mobility and elasticity.

Hands—Back of hands consistent color with fingers more pink in color. Hands cool to touch and dry. Fingernails translucent pink with lunula visible. Nail/nail bed angel at 160 degrees with firm nail beds. Nails strong without any evidence of splitting or discolorations/lesions.

Axillae—Hair shaved, hair roots evenly distributed without any evidence of lesions. Skin color lighter that over rest of body.

Lower extremities—Skin color homogeneous in distribution. Two telangiectasias on R leg, over calf on medial aspect. Hair shaved with even distribution of hair roots bilaterally. Scar on left knee, lateral aspect, which curves around knee cap. Linear scar on right ankle, medial aspect, 8 cm in length anterior to malleolus. Temperature warm and evenly distributed with the exception of feet which were cool to touch. No color changes observed.

Electronic Charting

Expectations of Electronic Charting

The provider should be able to document all parts of the integumentary assessment and to record congenital anomalies, as well as birthmarks, tattoos, piercings, or other identifying characteristics in addition to the routine integumentary assessment. The skin/integumentary assessment may involve a separate assessment in the electronic medical record, or may be integrated throughout other assessments.

Objective measurement and description of skin lesions can be challenging. Using precise terminology is necessary. If the electronic charting is done through forms, they should allow adequate flexibility so that the provider can describe issues completely. For example, there is no standardized description for skin color. Rather than attempting to document a particular color, forms should allow you to describe variations on the base color in specific ways or specific areas of the body.

Issues with the skin/integumentary system can be related to many other conditions. You should be able to move readily between the integumentary assessment and related documentation such as environmental exposures, allergy history, or history of communicable diseases, immunizations, or behaviors such as nail biting or eating habits.

Maintaining skin integrity and preventing decubitus ulcers are provider-sensitive patient outcomes. The electronic charting should allow appropriate documentation of assessments, treatments, and outcomes related to this issue. Some electronic charting systems incorporate electronic guidelines or protocols. For example, some systems require that assessments such as the Braden Scale be conducted at prescribed intervals.

The electronic charting may allow the provider to include images and/or diagrams with the charting. This can be helpful in describing lesions and in monitoring changes to skin lesions. If images or diagrams are incorporated, the charting should allow linking textual and pictorial data.

Limitations of Electronic Charting

Some systems may restrict the amount of graphical data that can be used within a record, or may require special permissions to allow the provider to document using graphical data. This happens for two reasons. Graphical data (pictures, diagrams, etc.) create larger files than text, and this can cause issues with server space and communication bandwidth (attempting to store the image can slow down some electronic charting applications). Second, images and other graphics are a common way by which computer viruses are transmitted. Thus, some institutions have concluded that allowing graphical data may increase the security risks of the electronic charting system.

Finally there is a pragmatic issue with graphical data. Creating graphical data and entering such data into the computer can require additional or nonstandard equipment such as cameras, digital pens, and scanners. This both increases the costs of using the electronic charting system and requires the user to learn additional technologies. This can interfere with the provider's workflow and can increase the burden of documenting the skin assessment.

Summary

- The skin is the largest organ of the body that holds the body together as well as protect the inside structures from the outside environment; it also contains sensory receptors, sebaceous and sweat glands, which participate in temperature regulation, as well as melanocytes, which provide skin color and protection from ultraviolet light.
- Accessory organs of the skin include hair and fingernails, which are composed of dead keratinocytes.
- The skin is a significant part of who one is and how one is perceived, so it receives a great amount of attention related to its cosmetic appearance.
- Changes in the skin, particularly color, often reflect and may be the initial indicators of disorders and conditions related to other organ systems.
- Skin lesions are quite common and are often non-pathological; however, they are often associated with other conditions which may have serious consequences.
- Skin cancer (basal cell, squamous cell, melanoma) is the most common type of cancers, most of which are related to sun exposure. Melanoma is the most deadly as it metastasizes throughout the body.
- Skin self-examination is the primary method for prevention and early detection of skin cancers.

Review Questions

1. Shortly after delivery, a new mother asks the provider about the thick, white substance that is on the infant's skin. The provider explains that this substance
   1. prevents excessive heat loss.
   2. protects the skin of the new-born.
   3. is a result of maternal infection.
   4. may be due to injection of drugs by the mother.
2. The provider is discussing the risk for development of melanoma with a patient. The provider should include information on which strategies for risk reduction? (Select all that apply.)
   1. dark-skinned individuals
   2. history of blistering sunburn
   3. a parent with a history of melanoma
   4. presence of 5–10 typical moles
   5. use of lotions with an SPF of 15
3. When performing a skin assessment on a patient the provider notes a nevus on the patient's back. The provider should be concerned that this nevus may be cancerous if the
   1. diameter is 4 mm.
   2. color is brown and uniform.
   3. the border is irregular.
   4. the nevus is flat.
4. The provider used which techniques of examination when examining the skin? (Select all that apply.)
   1. inspection
   2. palpation
   3. direct percussion
   4. indirect percussion
   5. auscultation
5. A parent brings a toddler to the clinic and tells the provider that the child's skin has taken on a yellowish hue and wonders if the child is jaundiced. The provider should begin the assessment by asking the parent about which of the following?
   1. the child's diet
   2. any changes in the child's behavior
   3. if the child has any allergies
   4. any recent skin care routine changes
6. A patient shows the provider several small red-purple areas measuring 7–8 mm in diameter on the lower abdomen. The provider documents that the patient has which of the following?
   1. petechia
   2. purpura
   3. erythema
   4. ecchymosis
7. The provider notes that a new patient has a stage III decubitus ulcer on the sacrum. This staging indicates that
   1. full-thickness skin loss and necrosis of the bone have occurred.
   2. muscle and bone are visible in the ulcer without necrosis.
   3. the skin is intact but reddened.
   4. the skin in the area is firm, but not broken.
8. When assessing for skin changes related to oxygen in the blood in a dark-skinned patient the provider should assess for which of the following?
   1. a bluish hue to the skin of the extremities
   2. a yellowing of the sclera
   3. mottled nail beds
   4. ashen tones to the oral mucous membranes
9. A patient is noted to have a series of skin lesions in a lattice arrangement. The provider would document this finding as which of the following?
   1. a discrete pattern
   2. a linear pattern
   3. a zosteriform pattern
   4. a reticular pattern
10. A patient is seen in the emergency department with several areas of superficial skin burns. To fully assess the burns the provider should do which of the following?
    1. Inspect the entire body any ask the patient about pain level.
    2. Use the rule of nines to assess extend of the burn.
    3. Use the Lund Browder chart to assess the burn area.
    4. Determine the zone of the burn injury.

Conditions and Disorders

SKIN CANCERS

Skin cancer includes basal cell carcinoma, squamous cell carcinoma, and melanoma. It may affect all areas of the body.

Basal Cell Carcinoma (BCC)

BCC accounts for more than 90% of all skin cancers. It has a 90% success rate with treatment and may recur in the same location or at another one. It occurs mainly in fair-skinned patients with a family history of BC carcinoma. Sunlight is a factor in about two-thirds of these cancers and one-third occur in non-sun-exposed areas; thus, the pathogenesis is more complex than UV exposure as *the* cause.

Pathophysiology

- BCC begins in basal cells of lowest layer of epithelium (sun exposed area, light-skinned individuals).
- Rarely metastasizes or causes death, but if untreated, causes significant destruction and disfigurement by invasion of surrounding tissues, so it is still associated with malignancy.
- If not removed, it can become invasive, causing damage by growing into surrounding tissue, particularly when near the eye, ear, or nose.

Subjective Data

- Sore that persists and does not heal; however, superficial basal-cell cancer can present as a red patch-like eczema or may become crusted.
- May cause itching; bleeding when traumatized.
- History of sun exposure (recreational or occupational); sun burns
- Light-skinned

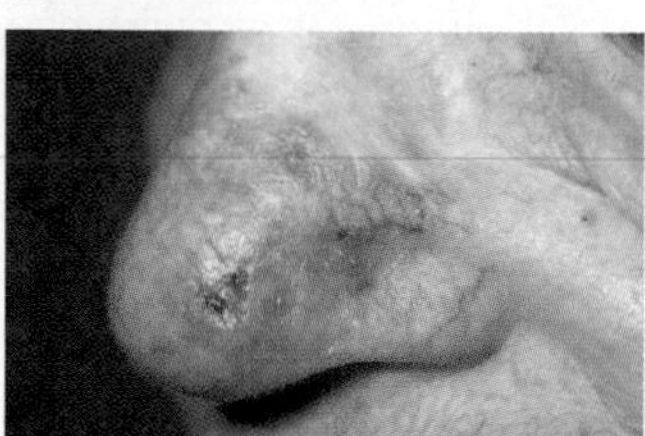

FIGURE 16-45 Basal cell carcinoma
Source: Dr. P. Marazzi/Science Source Images

Objective Data

- Begins as small, dome-shaped shiny, pearly nodule, frequently covered with small, superficial blood vessels (telangiectasias).
- Open sore, may have crusting/bleeding.
- Color may be dark (contains melanin), tan, black, brown, pink/red.

Squamous Cell Carcinoma (SCC)

SCC is a malignancy of the epithelial (squamous) cell, which is the main component of the epidermis. It occurs less frequently than BCC but has a greater tendency to metastasize. Most result from prolonged exposure to UV radiation (sunlight, tanning beds or lamps). Squamous cells also occur in the lining of the digestive tract, lungs, and other locations in the body. SCC occurs as a form of cancer in diverse tissues, such as the lips, mouth, esophagus, urinary bladder, prostate, lung, vagina, and cervix, among others.

Pathophysiology

- Frequently develops from precancerous lesions in sun-exposed parts of the body, such as actinic keratoses.
- Commonly occurs on forehead, cheeks, and back of the hands.
- In addition to sun damage, exposure to arsenic, hydrocarbons, heat, or x-rays may predispose to squamous cell carcinoma; may also develop in scar tissue.

Subjective Data

- Sore that is persistent, and doesn't heal or has increased in size
- Bleeding and crusting may also be present
- History of sun exposure

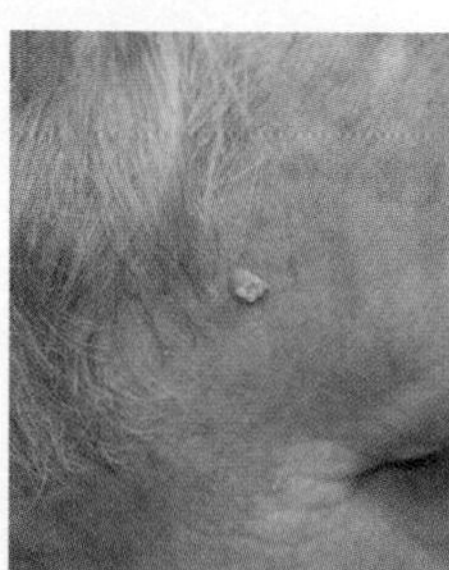

FIGURE 16-46 Squamous cell carcinoma
Source: Kelly Nelson/National Cancer Institute

Objective Data

- Starts out as firm, skin-colored, or red nodules.
- Wart-like growth with central depression that may demonstrate crusting and bleeding.
- Scaly, red patch with irregular borders that my bleed and/or crust.
- May also be open sore with crusting.

Melanoma

Melanoma is a tumor of the melanocytes and one of the deadliest forms of cancer due to its ability to metastasize early, making early detection critical. It can originate in any part of the body that contains melanocytes (i.e., eye, bowel). In its early stages, it is highly curable by surgical removal; however, once it has metastasized, conventional treatments for cancer are used and survival risk becomes greater.

Pathophysiology

- In the earliest stage the melanocytes begin to grow out of control (radial growth phase). It is less than 1 mm thick, and has not reached the blood vessels lower in the skin. It is unlikely that this early-stage cancer will spread to other parts of the body. If detected, it can usually be completely removed with surgery.
- In the invasive radial growth phase, tumor cells begin to grow vertically into epidermis and papillary dermis. Cells acquire invasive potential and are capable of spreading.
- In the vertical growth phase, the tumor attains invasive potential into surrounding tissue and through blood or lymph vessels. Tumor thickness is usually >1 mm (0.04 in), and involves deeper parts of the dermis.
- Lesion thickness is a critical determination as rate of growth is related to its thickness, with thicker lesions having faster growth (Baade et al., 2006).

Subjective Data

- New growth or changes in preexisting mole
- New pigmented lesion with irregularities
- History of dysplastic or atypical nevi
- Family history of melanoma

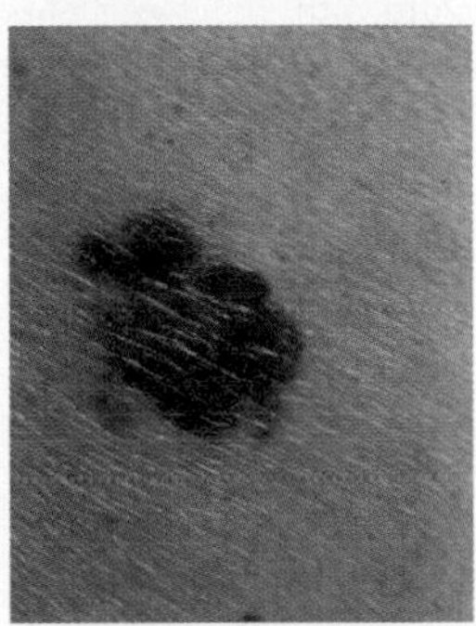

FIGURE 16-47 Melanoma
Source: Courtesy National Cancer Institute/ Larry Meyer

Objective Data

- Approximately 70% of melanomas arise from regular pigmented skin; the other 30% arise from atypical nevi.
- Location of the melanoma differs between genders: in males, melanoma frequently is found on the trunk, head, or neck; in females, it begins on the lower legs. Individuals with dark skin tend to be affected less than those with light or fair skin.

Kaposi's Sarcoma (KS)

KS is a tumor caused by human herpes virus 8 (HHV8, also known as Kaposi's sarcoma-associated herpes virus, KSHV). It is a systemic disease that can present with cutaneous lesions with or without internal involvement. It typically occurs in older males, ages 50–70, of Mediterranean/Eastern European heritage. However, since the 1980s, it is more likely to occur in individuals who are immunosuppressed (associated with HIV infection).

Pathophysiology

- KS is not considered a true sarcoma, (tumor arising from mesenchymal tissue). It arises as a cancer of lymphatic endothelium and forms tumors that are highly vascular, containing abnormally dense and irregular blood vessels, which leak red blood cells into the surrounding tissue and give the tumor its dark color.
- Inflammation around the tumor may produce swelling and pain. KSHV proteins are uniformly detected in KS cancer cells. KS tumors contain cells with an abnormal elongated shape, called *spindle cells.*

Subjective Data

- Pain—if lesions on soles of feet
- GI—dysphagia, nausea, hematemesis (vomiting blood), abdominal pain, blood in stools (melena)
- Pulmonary—cough, dyspnea, coughing up blood (hematemesis), chest pain

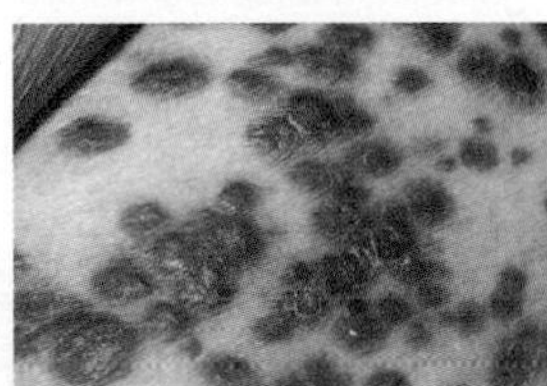

FIGURE 16-48 Kaposi's sarcoma (KS)
Source: Courtesy CDC

Objective Data

- Non-pruritic cutaneous lesions (macular, papular, nodular, or plaque); usually concentrated on lower extremities, head and neck and may also involve skin, oral mucosa, lymph nodes and visceral organs.
- Range in size (several mm to several cm)
  Color—brown, pink, red or violet (difficult to determine in dark skinned individuals)
- Discrete or confluent pattern with linear, symmetric distribution

VASCULAR ANOMALIES (VA)

Vascular anomalies are congenital lesions of abnormal vascular development that are broadly classified as vascular tumors (VT) and vascular malformations (VM) ("Hemangiomas and vascular malformations: Current theory and management," 2012). VT grow by cellular hyperplasia, whereas a vascular malformation represents a localized defect in vascular development. They are more common in Caucasians, and more frequent in females.

Vascular Tumors (Hemangiomas)

Hemangiomas are vascular tumors that are rarely apparent at birth, however, 79%–90% of them appear within the first 4 weeks of life. Tumors that are situated beneath the skin may not appear until 3 to 4 months of age, when the tumor is large enough. They grow rapidly during the first 6 months of life, involute with time and do not necessarily infiltrate but can sometimes become destructive. Considered benign neoplasms unless located where growth may impair vision, hearing, or breathing.

- Infantile hemangiomas are the most common and are benign vascular neoplasms that have a characteristic clinical course manifested by early proliferation that is followed by spontaneous involution (1–6 years).
- Congenital hemangiomas are rare and present at birth, and also less understood.

Pathophysiology

- A VA is a localized defect in blood vessels, primarily an abnormal endothelial proliferation of cutaneous capillaries in the skin that can affect each part of the vasculature (capillaries, arteries, veins, lymphatics or a combination of these). These defects are characterized by an increased number of vessels and vessels that are both enlarged and sinuous.
- If no current or potential complications, hemangiomas not treated, but allowed to go through natural progression with generally no long-term effects or future harmful transformations.

Subjective Data

- None as individuals affected are infants.

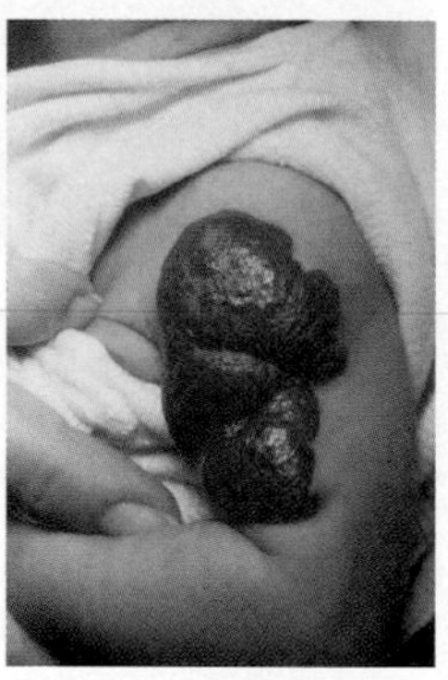

FIGURE 16-49 Hemangioma
Source: Custom Medical Stock Photo

Objective Data

- Deep red, spongy mass that is often raised above the skin and appear almost anywhere on the body, but mostly on face, scalp, back and neck.**Infantile hemangioma** appears during infancy, only one-third present at birth as telangiectatic stain or ecchymotic area.

Nevus Flammeus (Port Wine Stain); Nevus Flammeus Nuchae (Stork bite)

A nevus flammeus is a patch that is caused by a vascular malformation. Unlike hemangiomas, it is present at birth and does not disappear; it remains with the individual for life. It does not fade in color and may get deeper in color with age.

A stork bite is similar to the nevus flammeus, but eventually it becomes lighter and disappears.

Pathophysiology

- Capillary malformation and dilatation of the superficial dermal blood vessels (Antaya, 2007).
- Does not require treatment but pulsed dye laser therapy may lighten it. (McLaughlin, O'Connor, & Ham, 2008)
- Stork bites are apparent on 30% to 50% of newborns and are not associated with any pathology.

Subjective Data

- No significant subjective manifestations except its cosmetic effect.
- If lesion in ophthalmic distribution of trigeminal nerve, may develop glaucoma, which would affect vision.

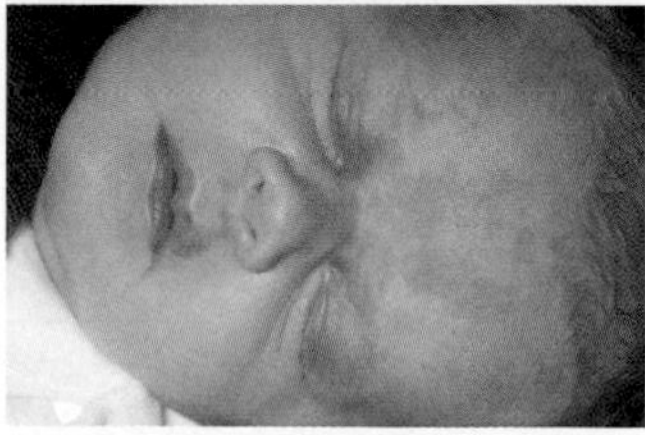

FIGURE 16-50 Stork bites
Source: Dr. P. Marazzi/Science Source Images

Objective Data

- Flat, red-purple lesion that vary in in size.
- Mostly seen on the face.
- Early stains are usually flat and pink in appearance. As the child matures, the color may deepen to a dark red or purplish color. In adulthood, thickening of the lesion or the development of small lumps may occur.
- Stork bites are most commonly seen on the back of the neck, forehead, eyelids, and between the eyebrows.

Pigmented Birthmarks

Other birthmarks that may be observed are pigmented birthmarks that range in color from brown or black to bluish or bluish-gray. Birthmarks in this category include nevi, Mongolian spots (see previous discussion), and café-au-lait spots.

Café-au-Lait Spots

- Usually nonsignificant; however, they are associated with the condition neurofibromatosis, especially if there is a large number of them.

- No significant subjective manifestations, except its cosmetic effect.

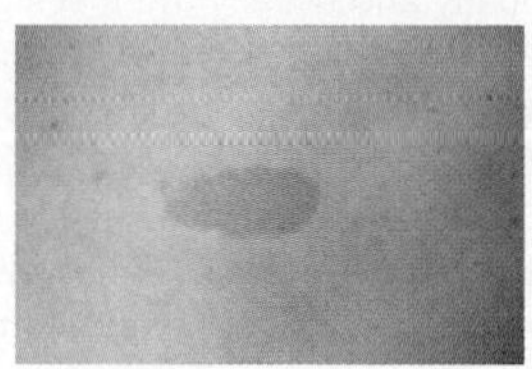

FIGURE 16-51 Café-au-lait spots
Source: Dr. P. Marazzi/Science Source

- Light tan spots that resemble coffee with cream.

INFLAMMATORY AND INFECTIOUS MANIFESTATIONS

Inflammatory skin disorders covers a broad category that includes many conditions ranging in severity, from mild itching to grave medical health complications. These disorders are common in people of all ages and races. They are characterized by irritation and inflammation of the skin.

Eczema

Eczema is a pruritic condition of unknown etiology, often referred to as **atopic dermatitis**. It is a form of chronic skin inflammation and broadly describes a range of persistent skin conditions that primarily relate to dryness and recurring skin rashes characterized by one or more of these symptoms: redness, skin edema, itching, dryness, crusting, flaking, blistering, cracking, oozing, or bleeding. Areas of temporary skin discoloration may appear and are sometimes due to healed injuries. Scratching open a healing lesion may result in scarring and may enlarge the rash. Before a diagnosis of atopic dermatitis can be made, other conditions need to be ruled out: scabies, allergic contact dermatitis, seborrheic dermatitis, cutaneous lymphoma icthyosis, psoriasis, immunodeficiency, and other primary diseases (Kim, 2012).

Pathophysiology

- Poorly understood; two primary hypothesis.
- Primary immune dysfunction with IgE sensitization and a disturbance of the epithelial-barrier.
- Primary effect in epithelial barrier breakdown results in secondary immunologic dysregulation causing inflammation.
- Contact dermatitis is of two types: allergic or atopic.
- Allergic type results from a delayed reaction to an allergen, such as poison ivy or nickel, or an irritant, resulting from direct reaction to a detergent (sodium lauryl sulfate, for example).
- Atopic dermatitis (infantile, flexural, atopic dermatitis) is an allergic disease believed to have a hereditary component and often runs in families whose members also have asthma. Itchy rash is particularly noticeable on head and scalp, neck, inside of elbows, behind knees, and buttocks.

Subjective Data

- Continuous pruritus
- Commonly follows an intermittent course with flare-ups and remissions.

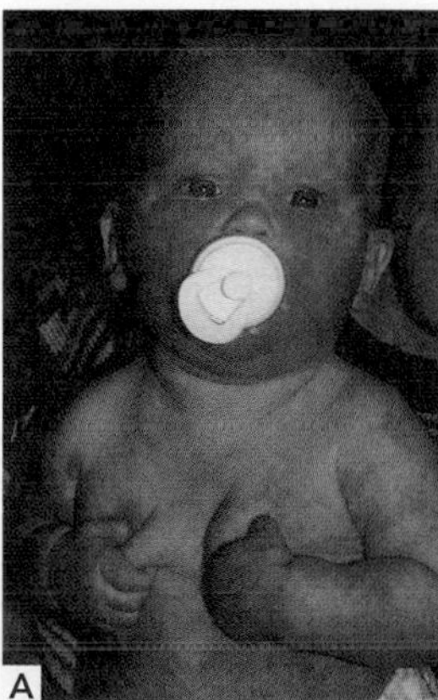

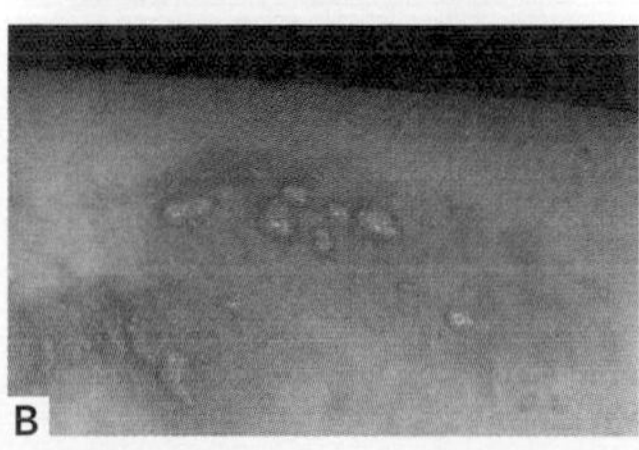

FIGURE 16-52A–B Atopic (eczematous) dermatitis

Objective Data

- Xerosis (dry/flaky skin)
- Lichenification
- Eczematous lesions (redness, itching minute papules and vesicles, weeping/oozing, crusting)
  In children begins in antecubital and popliteal fossa. Later localizes to cheeks, forehead, and scalp.

Seborrheic Dermatitis (SD)

SD is a papulosquamous inflammatory dermatosis with lesions located on the scalp, face, trunk, back, and intertriginous/diaper area due to concentration of sebaceous glands in these areas.

SD has two incidence peaks—infancy and individuals between 40 and 60. In infants SD is known as "cradle cap."

Pathophysiology

- Pathophysiology not completely understood but correlates with proliferation of Malassezia species of fungi (DelRosso & Kim, 2009) with an abnormal immune response (Selden, 2012).
- SD is caused by seborrhea, a pathologic overproduction of sebum, and subsequent infection and inflammation.
- Pathogenesis of SD similar to acne vulgaris.

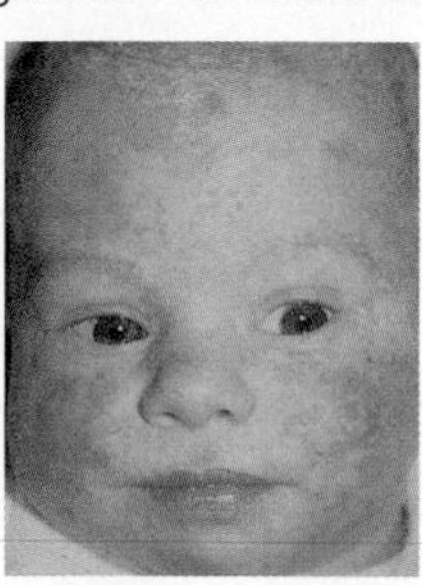

FIGURE 16-53 Seborrheic dermatitis

Subjective Data

- Seborrhoeic dermatitis symptoms appear gradually and usually the first signs are flaky, itching, red skin and scalp.
- Other symptoms include patchy scaling or thick crusts on the scalp, red, greasy skin covered with flaky white or yellow scales, itching, soreness and yellow or white scales that may attach to the hair shaft.
- During active phase may also experience a burning sensation.
- Active state increased in winter and early spring; remissions common in summer.

Objective Data

- Areas of brawny, or greasy scaling over red inflamed skin.
- Lesions range from patchy scaling to widespread, think adherent crusts.
- Most common in hair-bearing areas.
- Hypopigmentation noted in black individuals.
- May develop secondary infection manifested as oozing, crusting with eczematous dermatitis.

Cellulitis

Cellulitis is a localized or diffuse inflammation of connective tissue with severe inflammation of dermal and subcutaneous layers.

Pathophysiology

- Invasion of bacteria normal skin flora or (Streptococcus pyogenes or Staphylococcus aureus) or exogenous bacteria, often occurring where the skin surface has been broken: cracks, cuts, blisters, burns, insect bites, surgical wounds, intravenous drug injection or sites of intravenous catheter insertion.

Subjective Data

- Pain/tenderness
- Swelling
- Warmth
- Skin on the face or lower legs is most commonly affected by this infection, though cellulitis can occur on any part of the body.

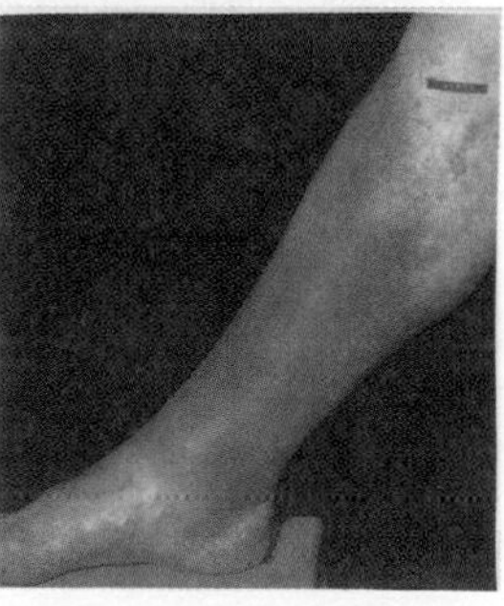

FIGURE 16-54 Cellulitis

Objective Data

- Broad areas of redness
- Red streaking of skin
- Drainage of clear fluid or pus
- Blisters may appear
- Swollen lymph nodes
- Fever

Psoriasis (Plaque)

This common, chronic skin condition manifested by red skin covered with silvery scales and inflammation.

Pathophysiology

- Considered a disorder of the immune system where T cells mistake a normal skin cell for a pathogen and stimulate skin inflammation, causing skin cells to grow faster and pile up on outer surface of skin.
- In plaque psoriasis, skin rapidly accumulates at sites, giving it a silvery-white appearance.
- Genetic transmission.
- Condition induced by: injury, sunlight, strep infections, HIV, drugs (lithium, beta-blockers, antimalarials, NSAIDs) (Motrin, Advil)

Subjective Data

- May have pruritus/burning/soreness
- Swollen and stiff joints
- Flare ups lasting weeks/ months followed by remission

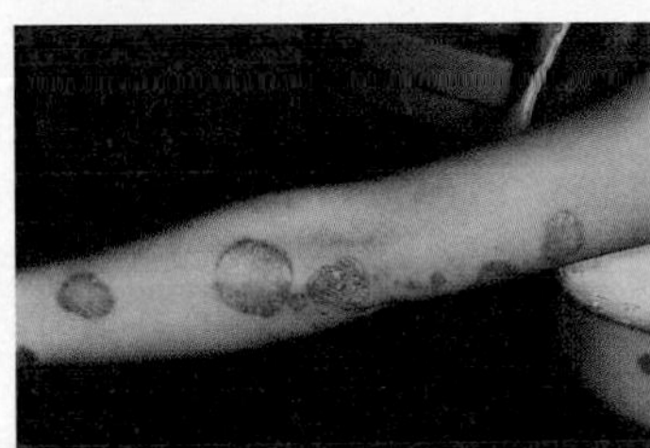

FIGURE 16-55 Psoriasis
Source: Courtesy: CDC/Dr. N.J. Fiumara

Objective Data

- Plaques (salmon colored), raised, scaly areas of skin (knees, elbows, trunk, scalp). Skin can have blue tint when psoriasis on the lower extremities.
- Scales are dry, thin, and silvery white of varying thickness. When scale removed, the skin underneath appears smooth, red, and glossy, usually has small areas that bleed.
- A few to multiple plaques at a time (1 cm to several cm). oval in shape, but may be irregular.
- Plaques tend to appear on symmetrical sides of the body (both knees or both elbows).
- Pitting of nails with discoloration and accumulation of yellow scaly debris, elevating the nail plate.

Rosacea

This is a common, chronic, inflammatory disorder characterized by facial flushing (redness) and diverse clinical manifestations, including telangectasias, coarseness of skin, and an inflammatory papulopustular eruption resembling acne. Common in fair-skinned individuals of European/Celtic heritage, it affects both genders, but is almost three times more common in women, with a peak age of onset between 30 and 60.

Pathophysiology

- Specific cause unknown.
- It is known that something irritates the skin, but rosacea does not seem to be a bacterial infection.
- It tends to affect people who have fair skin or blush easily, and it seems to run in families.
- The National Rosacea Society Expert Committee on the Classification and Staging of Rosacea defined and classified rosacea in into 4 different subtypes (erythematotelangiectatic, papulopustular, phymatous, and ocular) based on specific clinical signs and symptoms (Wilkin et al., 2004).

Subjective Data

- Likely to have a background of facial flushing, commonly occurring in childhood or early teens.
- In adults flushing may be increasingly initiated by hot drinks, heat, emotion, and other causes of rapid body temperature changes, dry skin that may burn or sting.
- Some patients report flushing with alcohol, which is not specific.
- Symptoms usually intermittent but can proceed to permanently flushed skin and associated with development of permanent telangiectasia.
- Some individuals report a gritty quality of eyes and facial edema.

Objective Data

- Variable erythema and telangiectasia noted over cheeks and forehead.
- Inflammatory papules and pustules may be primarily observed over the nose, forehead, and cheeks.
- Noticeable sebaceous glands and in extreme cases, appearance of thickened and deformed nose (rhinophyma).

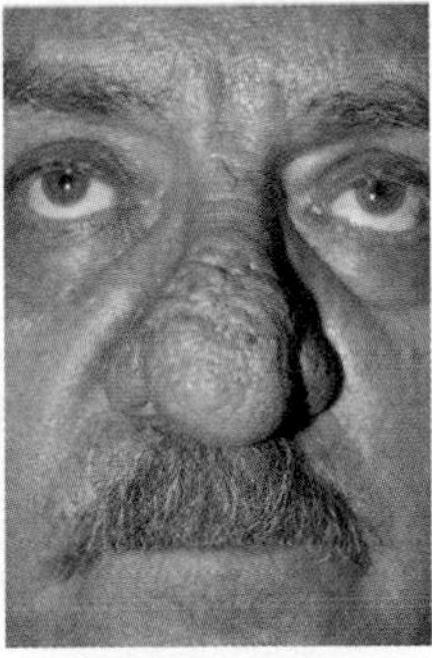

FIGURE 16-56 Rosacea
Source: Dr. Harout Tanielian/Science Source Images

INFLAMMATORY AND INFECTIOUS MANIFESTATIONS (CHILDREN/ADOLESCENTS)

Miliara Rubra (Prickly Heat/Heat Rash)

This occurs when sweat ducts become clogged and the sweat becomes trapped beneath the skin's surface, causing a mild inflammation or rash. Newborns, infants, older adults, and obese individuals are at highest risk for developing heat rash. Heat rash is more common in humid areas as individuals sweat more.

Pathophysiology

- Sweat glands are blocked with excessive sweating so that sweat becomes trapped and can't evaporate.
- Caused by folds of skin touching each other so air is unable to circulate, tight clothing, bundling up in heavy clothing/sheets, use of heavy creams/lotions.
- Infants have immature sweat glands that aren't capable of bringing sweat to surface.

Subjective Data

- Red bumps on skin, itchy/prickly sensation of the skin due to inflammation of superficial skin layers.
- Infants are unable to express sensations—may become fussy.

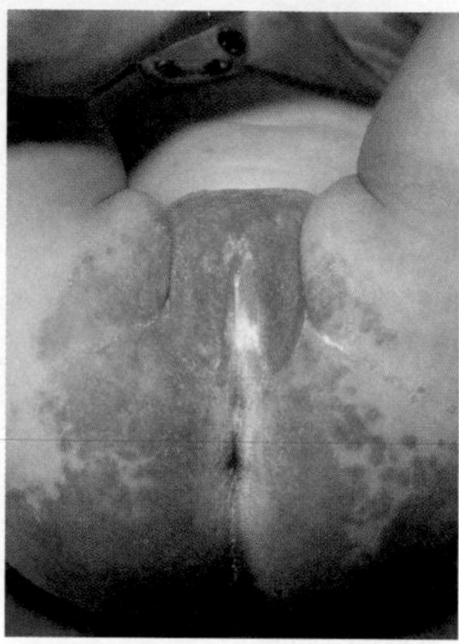

FIGURE 16-57 Miliara rubra (prickly heat/heat rash)
Source: Custom Medical Stock Photo

Objective Data

- If sweat is blocked at most superficial layers of skin, formation of tiny blisters as small beads of sweat occur.
- If sweat blocked in deeper layers of epidermis, area becomes red (erythema) with slightly larger blisters.
- Involved area dry, and can be irritated, itchy, and sore (classic heat rash).
- May develop infection if bacteria have invaded the blocked sweat gland.

Acne Vulgaris

Acne vulgaris (AV) is America's most common skin disease, affecting about 80% of Americans at some time during their lives. Twenty percent will have severe acne, resulting in permanent physical and mental scarring.

Pathophysiology

- Pathogenesis is multifactorial, with genetics having a primary role.
- Develops as result of interplay of four factors: (1) follicular epidermal hyperproliferation with subsequent plugging of the follicle, (2) excess sebum production, (3) the presence and activity of the commensal bacteria *Propionibacterium acnes,* and (4) inflammation.
- Acne scars are the result of inflammation within dermis. Scar is created by the wound trying to heal itself causing formation of too much collagen in one spot.
- Physical acne scars are often referred to as "ice pick" scars due to an indentation in the skin's surface.

Subjective Data

- Local symptoms of AV may include pain or tenderness. Acne can cause negative emotional reactions in affected patients, particularly teens, including depression, anxiety, anger, helplessness, and frustration that result in impaired functional status and decreased quality of life (Fried & Wechsler, 2006).

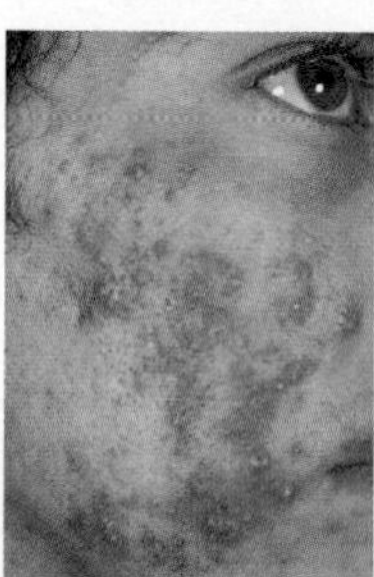

FIGURE 16-58 Acne vulgaris
Source: Biophoto Associates/Science Source Images

Objective Data

- Characterized by noninflammatory, open or closed comedones, inflammatory papules, pustules, and nodules in a sebaceous distribution (e.g., face, upper chest, back).
- AV typically affects areas of skin with densest population of sebaceous follicles (face, upper part of chest, and back).

INFLAMMATORY AND INFECTIOUS DISORDERS (OLDER ADULTS)

Stasis Dermatitis (SD)/Eczema

This is a common inflammatory skin disorder of the lower extremities occurring in patients with chronic venous insufficiency, often in association with varicose veins, dependent chronic edema, hyperpigmentation, and ulcerations. SD is usually the earliest cutaneous manifestation of chronic venous insufficiency with venous hypertension and may be a precursor to more problematic conditions, such as venous leg ulceration and lipodermatosclerosis.

Pathophysiology

- Stasis dermatitis occurs as a direct consequence of venous insufficiency. Disturbed function of the one-way valvular system in the deep venous plexus of the legs results in a backflow of blood from the deep venous system to the superficial venous system, with accompanying venous hypertension.

Subjective Data

- Pruritus is variable but, when present, results in lichenification from chronic scratching.
- May also complain of feeling of fullness or dull aching in lower extremities/ankles.

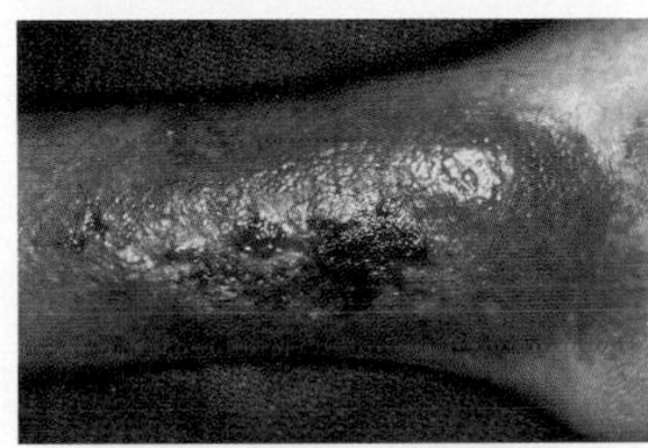

FIGURE 16-59 Stasis dermatitis (SD)/Eczema
Source: CDC

Objective Data

- Stasis dermatitis typically presents with erythematous (mild pink to raging red), scaling, and eczematous patches or plaques, edema, inflammatory and trophic skin changes, hyperpigmentation (hemosiderin deposits), dilated superficial veins on lower extremities.
- The medial ankle is most frequently and severely involved, although the skin changes may extend up to the knee and down to the foot.
- Severe, acute inflammation may result in exudative, weeping patches and plaques.

BACTERIAL INFECTIONS

Humans are natural hosts for many bacterial species that colonize the skin as normal flora. *Staphylococcus aureus* and *Streptococcus pyogenes* are infrequent resident flora, but they account for a wide variety of bacterial infections with exudate. Predisposing factors to infection include minor trauma, preexisting skin disease, poor hygiene, and, rarely, impaired host immunity.

Skin Abscesses: Folliculitis, Carbuncle, Furuncle

- **Abscess**—an accumulation of pus within the dermis and deeper skin tissues.
- **Folliculitis**—caused by damage to hair follicles from friction, an insect bite, blockage of the follicle, shaving, or braids that are too tight and too close to the scalp. Any hair-bearing site can be affected, but the sites most often involved are the face, scalp, thighs, axillae, and inguinal area.
- **Furuncle (boil)**—an infection of the hair follicle in which pus spreads through the dermis into the subcutaneous tissue, with formation of a small abscess.
- **Carbuncle**—an assimilation of multiple, adjacent inflamed follicles into a single inflammatory mass with purulent drainage from multiple follicles.

Pathophysiology

- Presence of inflammatory cells within the wall and ostia of the hair follicle, resulting in a follicular-based pustule.
- Break in integrity of skin allows for bacterial colonization (Staphylococcus aureus) of the hair follicles and can causing local cellulitis and inflammation.

Subjective Data

- Pain, tenderness
- In a severe infection, an individual may experience fever, fatigue, and noticeable swollen lymph nodes.
- Common areas of involvement include the back of the neck, face, axillae, and buttocks.

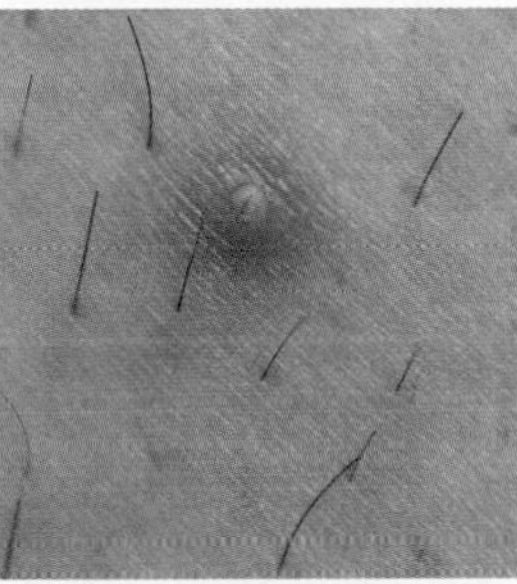

FIGURE 16-60 Furuncle
Source: FCG/Shutterstock

Objective Data

- Multiple small papules/pustules on an erythematous base, penetrated by a central hair, which may not always be visible.
- Manifest as fluctuant and erythematous nodules, frequently surmounted by a pustule and surrounded by a margin of erythematous swelling.
- Spontaneous drainage of purulent material may occur.
- Regional lymphadenopathy may be demonstrated.
- Persistent or recurring lesions may cause scarring and permanent hair loss.

Impetigo

Impetigo is a highly contagious bacterial skin infection most common among pre-school children. Individuals who play close contact sports such as rugby, football and wrestling are also susceptible, regardless of age. Impetigo is not as common in adults. This is a common type of skin infection caused by picking at sores or scratching itchy bites, allowing bacteria causing impetigo to enter the skin.

Pathophysiology

- Caused by two main types of bacteria: *Streptococcus* (non-bullous) and *Staphylococcus* (non-bullous and bullous) organisms, which are common inhabitants of environment and on the surface of most people's skin.

Subjective Data

- Sores are not painful, but may be itchy. Pain, if present, is usually mild.
- Lymph nodes in the affected area may be swollen, but fever is rare.
- Rash that may occur anywhere on the body and but commonly affects the face and other exposed areas.

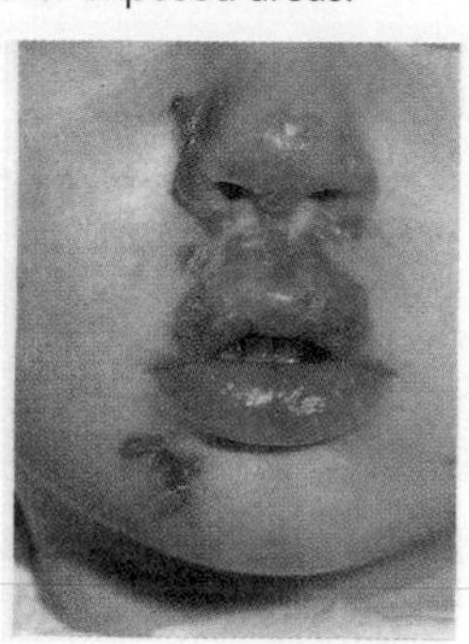

FIGURE 16-61 Impetigo

Objective Data

- Impetigo contagiosa (or nonbullous impetigo), begins as a red sore near the nose or mouth which soon breaks, leaking pus or fluid, and forms a honey-colored scab, followed by a red mark which heals without leaving a scar.
- Bullous impetigo, (mainly children younger than 2 years), involves painless, fluid-filled blisters, mostly on the arms, legs and trunk, surrounded by red and itchy (but not sore) skin.
- The blisters may be large or small. After they break, they form yellow scabs.
- Margins usually fairly well defined.

VIRAL INFECTIONS

There are currently eight identified human herpes viruses. They are ubiquitous and extremely well adapted pathogens. Many infectious diseases associated with viruses can be prevented by vaccines.

Herpes Simplex

The two types of Herpes simplex viruses cause a variety of disease states. Type I—oral/facial infection, Type II—genital infection.

- Herpes simplex virus type 1 (HSV-1), also known as herpes labialis, is the etiologic agent of vesicular lesions of the oral mucosa commonly referred to as "cold sores." HSV-1 can also cause clinical disease in a wide variety of other anatomic locations including the genitalia, liver, lung, eye, and central nervous system. These infections can be severe, particularly in the setting of immunosuppression.
- Although the majority of genital herpes simplex virus (HSV) infections have historically been due to HSV-2, HSV-1 is responsible for an increasing proportion of genital infections.

Pathophysiology

- Inoculation of herpes simplex virus (HSV)-1 at mucosal surfaces or skin sites permits entry of the virus into the epidermis, the dermis, and eventually to sensory and autonomic nerve endings.
- The incubation period of primary genital herpes is 3–7 days (range is 1 day to 3 weeks).
- Once herpes simplex virus (HSV) infection has occurred, the virus lives in a latent state in nerve cell bodies in ganglion neurons and can reactivate. The frequency and severity of reactivation is determined by many factors, including immunodeficiency or stress. Reactivation is more common with HSV-2 than HSV-1.
- Oral/facial (cold sore)—trigeminal ganglia
- Genital—sacral nerve ganglia

Subjective Data

- A prodrome of pain, burning, and tingling at site, followed by the development of vesicles.
- In most patients, fewer than two recurrences manifest each year, but some individuals experience monthly recurrences.
- Fever, headache, malaise, and myalgia (prominent in the first 3–4 days), pain, itching, dysuria, vaginal and urethral discharge.

Objective Data

- Erythematous papules that rapidly develop into tiny, thin-walled, intraepidermal vesicles that become pustular and ulcerate.
- Tender lymphadenopathy

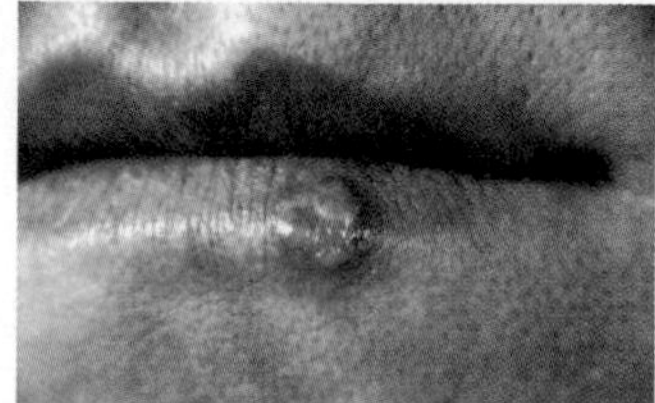

FIGURE 16-62 Herpes simplex
Source: Courtesy CDC/ Dr. Herrmann

Varicella (Chickenpox)

Varicella zoster virus (VZV) is one of eight herpes viruses known to infect humans and vertebrates. It commonly causes chickenpox in children, teens and young adults and herpes zoster (shingles) in adults and rarely in children. This is a highly contagious, self-limited infection that most commonly affects children between 5–10 years of age. Reactivation of the dormant virus results in the characteristic painful dermatomal rash of herpes zoster (shingles), which is often followed by pain in the distribution of the rash (postherpetic neuralgia).

Pathophysiology

- Varicella-zoster virus (VZV) causes chickenpox.
- Average incubation period from viral exposure to onset of symptoms is 12–14 days; with a range of 10–21 days after exposure to the virus.
- Individual contagious from 1–2 days before rash until lesions crust over.
- Following exposure, over 90% of nonimmune individuals will develop chickenpox. VZV is communicable by direct skin-to-skin contact and respiratory droplets (coughing, sneezing) from infected individual.

Subjective Data

- One–two days of fever, sore throat. Lack of appetite and malaise approximately 2 weeks following exposure to HZV.
- Pain occurs in 41% of patients, itching in 27%, and paresthesias in 12%.
- H. Zoster (shingles); Prodromal pain (itching/burning, throbbing, stabbing)
- Pain and sensory loss are the usual symptoms.
- Pain duration is variable but is usually less than 1 month. Pain lasting longer than 1 month is referred to, by definition, as postherpetic neuralgia.

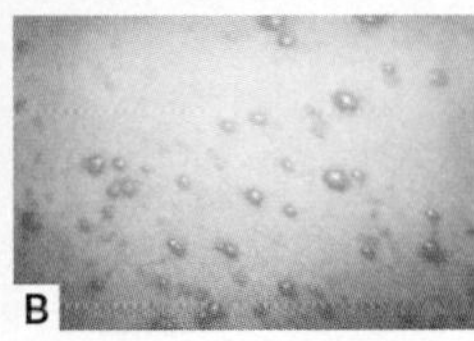

FIGURE 16-63A–B a) Varicella (chickenpox) **b)** Herpes (Varicella zoster, VZV)
Source: CDC; (Courtesy CDC/Joe Miller)

Objective Data

- Within 24 hours of symptoms, characteristic rash develops, starting on the torso spreading distally over next 7 to 10 days to the head, arms, and legs.
- Rash proceeds through predictable course of evolution from red papule ("bug bite" appearance) to blister (vesicle) to pustule and ruptures with scabbing.
- Vesicle/pustular fluids are highly concentrated with infectious virus particles.
- The most common presentation in shingles is a vesicular rash, which most commonly is unilateral, affecting a thoracic or other dermatomes.
- Lesions rarely cause permanent scarring, unless secondary infection develops.

Measles (Rubeola/Rubella)

Measles is an infection of the respiratory system caused by a paramyxovirus. There are two types of measles, although both produce a rash and fever, they are different diseases caused by different viruses.

- Rubeola causes a fever and skin rash in childhood, but can affect other parts of the body; sometimes occurs in adults.
- Rubella is a benign communicable exanthematous disease caused by rubella virus.
- Major complication is a teratogenic effect when pregnant women become infected, especially in the early weeks of gestation. Virus is transmitted to fetus via the placenta and capable of causing serious congenital defects, abortions, and stillbirths.

Pathophysiology

- Rubeola viruses are spread through respiratory route through coughing and sneezing. This is one of the most contagious viruses and can spread rapidly in a susceptible population.
- Classic measles infection in immunocompetent patients consists of the following clinical stages: incubation, prodrome, exanthem, and recovery.
- During the incubation phase virus carried in the respiratory tract before individual demonstrates condition, so can spread the disease without being aware of it.
- Portal of entry of rubella virus is respiratory epithelium of the nasopharynx via aerosolized particles. Approximately 50% of individuals infected with rubella virus are asymptomatic.

Subjective Data

- Prodromal phase begins with the following symptoms:
  - Fever
  - Lethargy
  - Cough
  - Red eyes (conjunctivitis)
  - Runny nose
  - Loss of appetite
- Signs and symptoms usually appear 1–5 days before onset of rash:
- Prodromal symptoms unusual in young children but common in adolescents/adults
- Infection in older children, adolescents, and adults may be complicated by arthralgia, arthritis, and thrombocytopenic purpura
- Eye pain on lateral and upward eye movement

Objective Data

- Exanthem phase–rash 2–4 days after prodromal phase.
- Often starts on face, spreads to trunk, then arms/legs. Usually not itchy, but as it clears, skin may shed (like peeling skin after sunburn).
- Initially small, red bumps that may blend into each other.
- Koplik spots may develop [small, grayish spots on inside of cheek].
- Although rubeola is often a mild disease, and most people recover without problems, rubeola can lead to pneumonia or inflammation of the brain (encephalitis).
- A fine, pink rash that begins on the face and quickly spreads to the trunk and then the arms and legs, before disappearing in the same sequence

- Virus attaches to/invades respiratory epithelium, then spread by blood (primary viremia) to regional and distant lymphatics replicating in the reticuloendothelial system.
- Infected person begins to shed virus from the nasopharynx 3–8 days after exposure; 6–14 days after onset of rash.

- Conjunctivitis
- Sore throat
- Headache
- General body aches
- Low-grade fever
- Chills
- Anorexia
- Nausea
- Tender lymphadenopathy (posterior auricular and suboccipital lymph nodes)

- Forchheimer sign (an enanthem observed in 20% of patients during prodromal period; present in some patients during initial phase of the exanthem; consists of pinpoint or larger petechiae that usually occur on the soft palate)

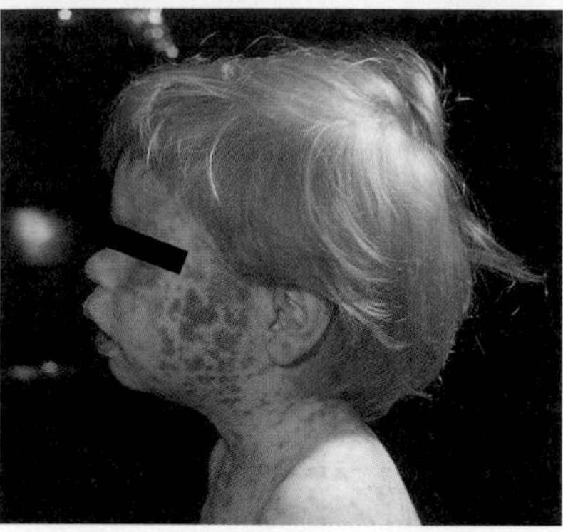

FIGURE 16-64 Rubella (German measles)
Source: CDC

Actinic Keratosis

This is a rough, scaly patch on the skin resulting from years of exposure to the sun. It is most commonly found on areas of skin typically exposed to sun—face, lips, ears, backs of the hands, forearms, scalp, or neck. Considered a precancerous lesion.

An actinic keratosis, also known as solar keratosis, enlarges slowly and usually causes no signs or symptoms other than a patch or small spot on your skin. An actinic keratosis takes years to develop, usually first appearing in older adults.

Pathophysiology

- Begins in the epidermis, which provides a protective layer of skin cells that body continually sheds.
- Skin cells damaged through UV radiation, change the skin's texture and color, causing blotchiness and bumps or lesions.
- The lesions start out as flat scaly areas and later grow into a tough, wartlike area.
- May evolve into squamous cell cancer.

Subjective Data

- Itching or burning in the affected area
- Almost exclusively in Caucasians with greater frequency in males

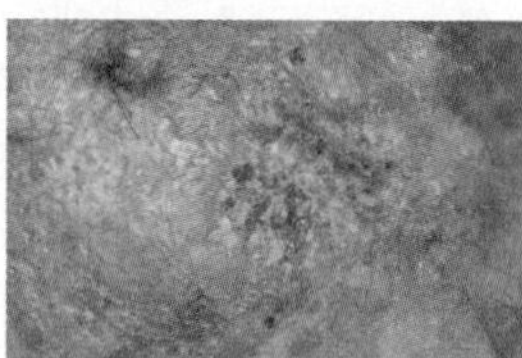

FIGURE 16-65 Actinic keratosis
Source: Biophoto Associates/Science Source

Objective Data

- Rough, dry, or scaly patch of skin, usually less than 1 inch (2.5 centimeters) in diameter
- Flat to slightly raised patch or bump on the top layer of skin
- In some cases, a hard, wartlike surface
- Color ranging from pink to red to brown, or flesh-colored
- May present with cutaneous horn

CONDITIONS AFFECTING ACCESSORY ORGANS (APPENDAGES)

Conditions that affect the accessory appendages of the skin rarely demonstrate manifestations that only pertain to them. Alterations of the nails are primarily associated with other conditions that are reflected in the nails.

Alopecia Areata

This is a recurrent nonscarring, rapidly occurring, patchy hair loss affecting any hair-bearing area and may demonstrate many different patterns. Although medically benign, alopecia areata can cause significant emotional and psychosocial distress in patients and their families. A precipitating factor can be found in 15% of patients such as major life events, febrile illnesses, drugs, pregnancy, trauma, and many other events reported, but no clear relationships appear to exist and most patients do not report a triggering factor.

Pathophysiology

- Exact pathophysiology remains unknown, with the most widely accepted hypothesis being that it is a T-cell–mediated autoimmune condition, most likely to occur in genetically predisposed individuals

Subjective Data

- Alopecia areata is generally asymptomatic, but some patients (14%) experience a burning sensation or pruritus in the affected area.
- Usually localized when first appears.

Objective Data

- Smooth, slightly erythematous (peach color) or normal-colored alopecic patches.
- Hair loss on other hair-bearing areas also favors the diagnosis.

- Rapid onset of total hair loss in a well-defined circular area (Czerkasij, 2007)
- Usually self-limiting and reversible

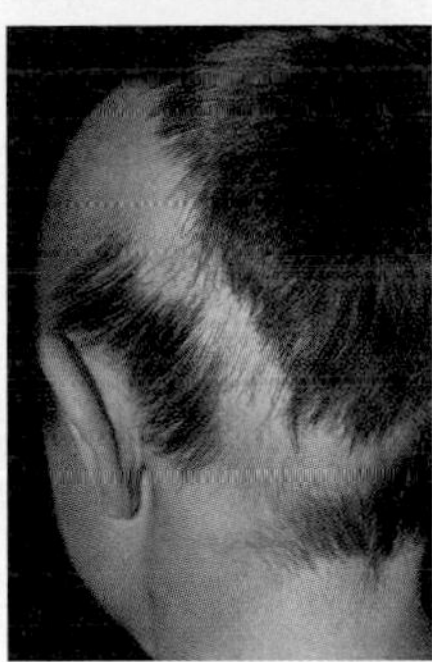

FIGURE 16-66 Alopecia areata
Source: Dr. Harout Tanielian/Science Source Images

- No correlation between the number of patches at onset and subsequent severity.
- Most often affects scalp; however, can affect any hair-bearing area (chin, brow, and extremities).
- More than one area can be affected at once.

- The most common presentation is the appearance of one or many round-to-oval denuded patches.
- No epidermal changes are associated with the hair loss.

Other Forms of Hair Loss

Name	Description
Asymmetrical hair loss	May be due to pathological alterations such as heavy metal poisoning, hypothyroidism, or trichotillomania.
Traction alopecia	Results from hair styles (braids/ponytails) that maintain a consistent pulling force on the hair roots causing them to be pulled out.
Tinea capitis	Hair loss from a fungal infection; more common in school-age children.
Generalized hair loss	May occur after anesthesia, giving birth, stress, or a febrile illness and is identified as Telogen effluvium. When this occurs, the rhythm of hair growth is altered so that more hair growth enters the resting phase, which lasts about 3 months. After 3 months, hair growth resumes.
Androgenetic alopecia	Hair loss that is due to genetic predisposition; it is symmetrical and is commonly referred to as male patterned baldness (see Figure 16-15). Dihydrostestosterone (DHT) plays a key role in male patterned baldness (Mounsey & Reed, 2009). Testosterone is converted to DHT by the enzyme 5-alpha reductase with higher levels of DHT responsible for the hair loss.
Female-pattern alopecia	Females in their 20s and 30s may also manifest adrenal androgen. Characteristically, the hair is gradually lost from the central scalp and not in the typical male pattern.

Hirsutism

This is excessive growth of thick, dark hair in women in locations where women's hair growth usually is minimal or absent. Male-pattern growth of terminal body hair usually occurs in androgen-stimulated locations, such as the face, chest, and areolae. Determination of hirsutism is difficult because hair growth varies among individual women and across ethnic groups. What is considered hirsutism in one culture may be considered typical in another. Dark-haired, darkly pigmented individuals of either gender tend to be more hirsute than blond/fair-skinned persons. This is generally a benign condition and primarily a cosmetic concern. However, when hirsutism is accompanied by masculinizing signs or symptoms, particularly when it occurs well after puberty, it may be a manifestation of a more serious underlying disorder such as an ovarian or adrenal neoplasm.

Pathophysiology

- Associated with abnormally high androgen levels or hair follicles more sensitive to normal androgen levels.
- Increased hair growth often is observed in patients with endocrine disorders characterized by hyperandrogenism, which may be caused by abnormalities of the ovaries or the adrenal glands.

Subjective Data

- Hirsutism exceeding acceptable culturally levels can be as distressing an emotional problem as the loss of scalp hair.
- Onset can take one of several forms. In women with familial hirsutism, it often appears during puberty.

Objective Data

- Excess terminal hair in a masculine pattern; may be difficult to evaluate in women who have blond hair
- This includes the following regions: chest, areolae, linea alba, upper back, lower back, buttocks, inner thighs, external genitalia

- Central overproduction of androgen, increased peripheral conversion of androgen, decreased metabolism, and enhanced receptor binding are proposed mechanisms of hirsutism. For circulating testosterone to exert its stimulatory effects on the hair follicle, it first must be converted into its more potent follicle-active metabolite, dihydrotestosterone by 5-alpha-reductase, within the hair follicle.

- Hirsutism usually develops gradually in patients with polycystic ovary syndrome (PCOS) and congenital adrenal hyperplasia (CAH).
- Also appears abruptly when an androgen-secreting tumor arises.

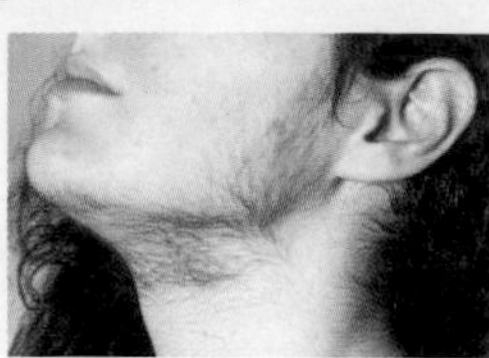

FIGURE 16-67 Hirsutism
Source: John Radcliffe Hospital /Science Source Images

- Other accompanying signs and symptoms may include: acanthosis nigricans, obesity, pelvic mass, virility, acne, alopecia, and signs or symptoms of Cushing's syndrome

Head and Neck

17

Showtime! I spring out of bed, stretching my arms back as far as they will go. As I tiptoe across my cold bathroom tile to the sink, my heart flutters with excitement and anticipation. After 6 years in the business, I've finally landed a lead role and will debut on Broadway tonight! I grin widely as I approach the mirror. What's this? A face with a broken half-smile stares back at me, pearly teeth on the right, pursed lips on the left. In fact, everything on the left side looks unusual—my cheek is sagging, my dimple is barely visible, and when I smile, it accentuates the changes. Sweat appears on my brow; I'm having a stroke! All I can think about is my performance!

"Wow! This is a really classic finding for Bell's palsy! Do you mind if I bring some students in to take a look?" The ER physician turns and strides out of my curtained half-room. I glance at the clock; no one seems to care that I have a show to do in 6 hours. Two young nurses return with the physician. "So, do you think this is central or peripheral in nature?" he asks them. "Could you smile for us and raise your eyebrows?" the first asks me. I comply, feeling like a circus sideshow. "I think it's a peripheral lower motor neuron problem; she can't move her forehead or eyebrows." "Very good!" the physician says, leaving the room with one of the nurses. The second nurse lingers. "My name is Elisa," she says, extending a hand, "I'm sorry that you have to be here on a Saturday afternoon." My eyes well up with tears. "Thanks for saying that.... I'm really stressed out about tonight." Elisa and I talk for the next 20 minutes about my acting career and the importance of tonight's debut, and also about what Bell's palsy is and what I can expect in terms of return of facial function. Although I now understand that I won't be performing tonight, I somehow feel more relaxed. It didn't take much, just a simple expression of empathy and for someone to remember that there is a person behind this face, a person with dreams and aspirations.

LEARNING OUTCOMES

1. Identify anatomic structures of the head and neck.
2. Recognize variations in the manifestations of facial appearances and their relationship to various disorders and conditions.
3. Explain common developmental and lifespan changes in the head and neck and the significance of their findings.
4. Address health promotion issues related to age-associated head and neck injuries.
5. Summarize the techniques used to examine the structures of the head and neck by observation and palpation.
6. Explain documentation of findings using appropriate terms when describing expected and unexpected findings.

Although the head and neck occupy only a small component of the overall body, they contain and protect structures and organs that control and regulate the physiological functions necessary for sustaining life as well as interpreting multiple sensations. The head also contains multiple muscles that permit expression of emotions and feelings, enhancing our communication skills. This chapter focuses on the external sections; special sensory organs will be discussed in the following chapters.

Structure and Function

This section reviews the structure and function of the head and neck separately.

The Head

The internal structures of the head are made up of multiple bones and muscles. The **cranium** is a hemispherical-shaped bony structure that contains the brain and is composed of the **cranial** and **facial bones**. The cranial bones are lined with meninges and encase the brain, protecting it and the special sense organs. Eight cranial bones are identified according to what section of the brain lies underneath, that is, the **frontal**, **parietal (2)**, **occipital**, and **temporal (2) bones** (Figure 17-1). The **sphenoid** and **ethmoid** bones form the floor of the brain case and the orbital (eye) sockets.

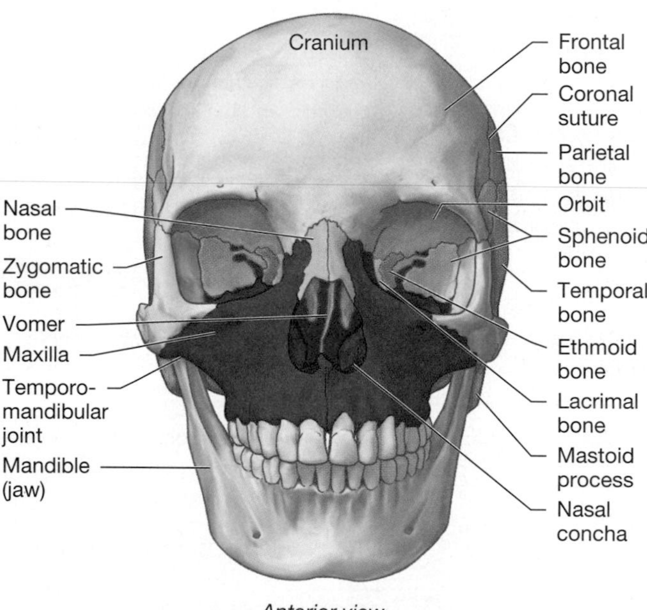

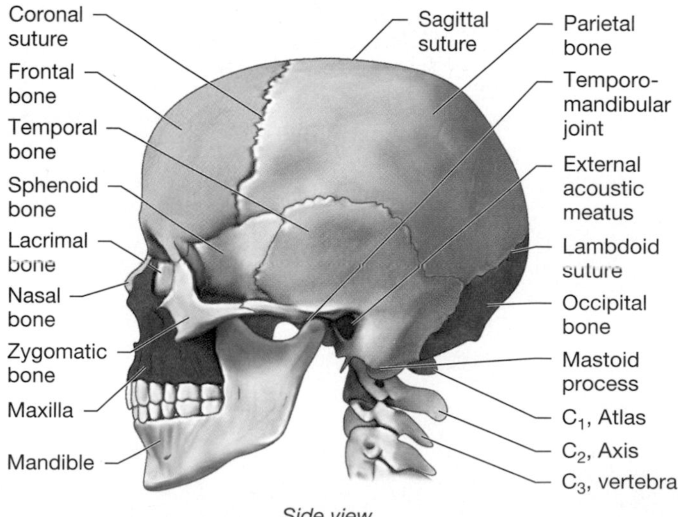

FIGURE 17-1 Anterior and side view of bones of cranium and face

The eight cranial bones are joined together along their edges by immovable joints called **sutures**. Three major sutures transverse the cranium and separate the bones. The **coronal suture** transverses the cranium from ear to ear and separates the anterior and parietal bones. The **sagittal suture** transverses the top of the cranium and separates the two parietal bones. The **lamboidal suture** transverses the posterior cranium, separating the parietal bones from the occipital bones.

The fourteen facial bones consist of paired **nasal**, **zygomatic**, **lacrimal**, **maxillary**, **palatine**, **inferior nasal conchae**, and single **vomer** and **mandible bones**. Like the cranial bones, they are connected by immovable sutures, with one exception, the **mandible**, which articulates with the temporal bone at the **temporomandibular joint (TMJ)**, allowing up and down as well as sideways movement. Various sections or components of the skull are associated with certain facial bones; these are listed and described in Table 17-1.

The face is also composed of muscles, of which the majority are paired, that provide movement necessary to form expressions as well as for chewing and articulation of words (Figure 17-2). The facial muscles are innervated and controlled by cranial nerves V and VII (further discussed in Chapter 26). The superficial temporal artery, the major palpable artery of the face, passes up the side of the face just anterior to the ear, over the temporal muscle and to the forehead.

The bones and muscles also provide the foundation for the formation of other external structures, cavities, and prominences that contribute to the characteristic appearance of the face and provide its landmarks. These structures are the nose, mouth (lips), orbital prominences (eyebrows), eyes (**palpebral fissures**), and ears; all are either midline or equidistant from the midline, providing facial symmetry. Facial movements also cause the formation of creases in the skin that are more visible when certain facial expressions are made. The most prominent crease is the **nasolabial fold**, which appears to the side of the mouth, extending from the lower portion of the nose to the corners of the lips. Although all these components of the face contribute to specific facial characteristics and are observed for symmetry, the nasolabial folds and palpebral fissures are the two identified landmarks used for observation of the face (Figure 17-3).

The Neck

The bones and muscles of the neck include the seven cervical vertebrae and the **sternocleidomastoid** (SCM) and **trapezius muscles**. These bones and muscles work together to provide support and movement for the head and neck.

The first cervical vertebra is the **atlas**, which articulates with the two occipital condyles, projections of the base of the occipital bone located on either side of the foramen magnum. This articulation supports and balances the head. The atlas forms a pivot joint with the second cervical vertebra, the **axis**, which permits turning the head from side to side. The remaining cervical vertebrae are not named and lack special function. The seventh cervical vertebra consists of an extended spinous process known as the **vertebra prominens**. This is a major landmark on the upper back that is used during the examination of the posterior chest.

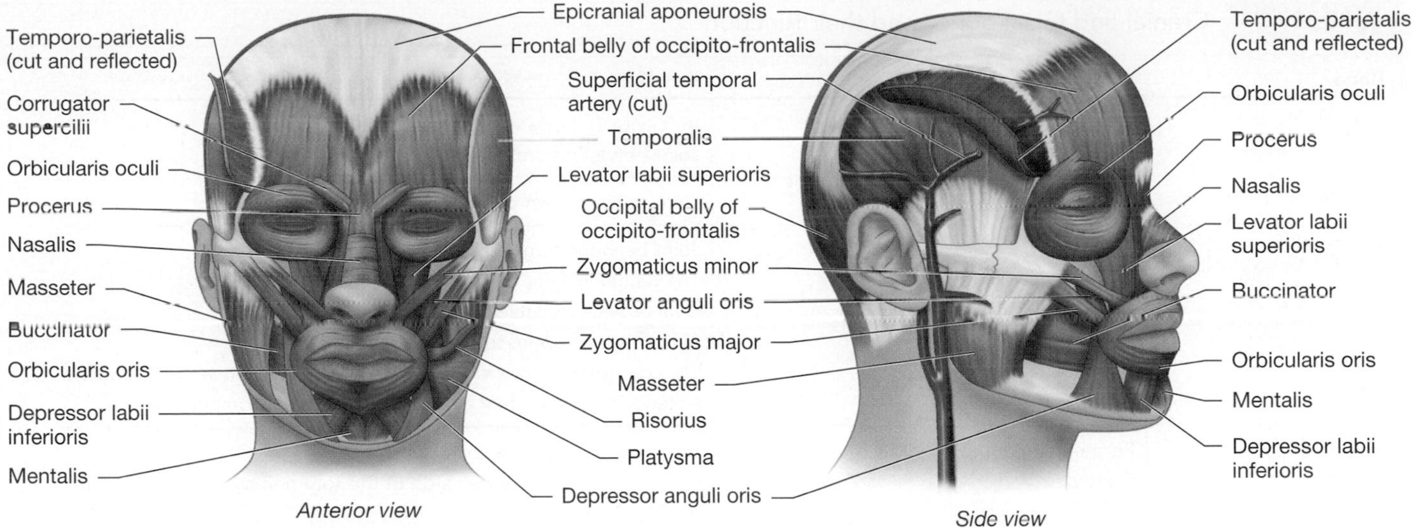

FIGURE 17-2 Muscles of the face

The SCM is attached inferiorly to the upper sternum and the sternal portion of the clavicle, and attached superiorly to the lateral aspect of the mastoid process. The SCM is responsible for elevation of the sternum during inspiration. The inferior attachment of the trapezius muscle is the scapula, the lateral third of the clavicle, and the vertebrae, and is attached superiorly to the occipital prominence (Figure 17-4).

The alignment of these two muscles, along with connecting bones, form two triangles that are used as anatomic landmarks for the neck. The **posterior triangle** is formed by the SCM and trapezius muscle and the clavicle (Figure 17-4). The **anterior triangle** is formed by the medial border of the SCM, the mandible, and the midline of the neck.

The anterior portion of the neck also contains other important structures and blood vessels (Figure 17-5). The structures, in descending order, are the hyoid bone, thyroid cartilage, cricoid cartilage, thyroid gland, and trachea. Located deep in the neck, the common carotid arteries and internal jugular veins run parallel and medially to the SCM. The external jugular veins run diagonally to and cross the SCM. In addition to these structures, the neck contains multiple lymph nodes, which are clustered together into eight groups. (These are further covered in Chapter 21.)

The **hyoid bone** is located just below the mandible. The **thyroid cartilage** is a notched, shieldlike cartilage. This is also known as the larynx and commonly called the "Adams apple," which is frequently more pronounced in males. The notch on the upper portion of the thyroid cartilage is level with the bifurcation of the common carotid arteries. Just below the thyroid cartilage is the **cricoid cartilage**, which is the uppermost ring of tracheal cartilages, essentially marking the beginning of the trachea.

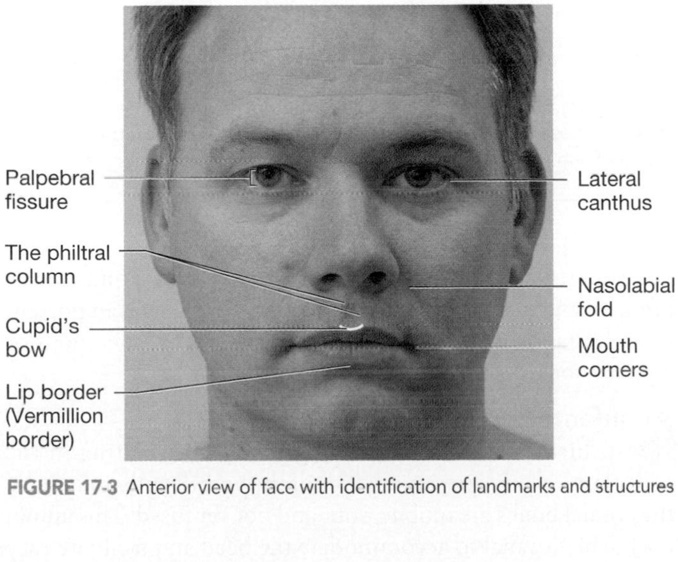

Palpebral fissure
The philtral column
Cupid's bow
Lip border (Vermillion border)
Lateral canthus
Nasolabial fold
Mouth corners

FIGURE 17-3 Anterior view of face with identification of landmarks and structures

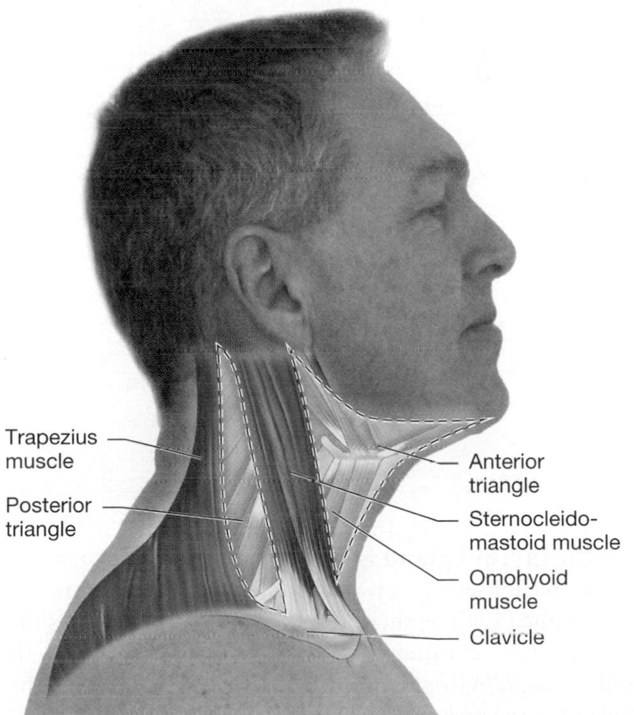

FIGURE 17-4 Side view of head and neck with details of SCM and trapezius muscle and formation of anterior and posterior triangles

Table 17-1 Cranial and facial bones and their function

Bone	Component	Function
Frontal (1)	Frontal Sinus Coronal Suture	Air cavity that opens into nasal cavity Joint between frontal and parietal bones
Parietal (2)	Sagittal Suture	Joint between two parietal bones
Temporal (2)	Squamousal suture External auditory meatus Mastoid process Mastoid sinus Mandibular fossa Zygomatic process	Joint between temporal and parietal bone The tunnel-like ear canal Oval projection behind the ear canal Air cavity that opens into middle ear Oval depression anterior to the ear canal; articulates with mandible Anterior projection that articulates with the zygomatic bone
Occipital (1)	Foramen magnum Condyles Lamboidal suture	Large opening for the spinal cord Oval projections on either side of the foramen magnum; articulate with the atlas Joint between occipital and parietal bones
Sphenoid (1)	Greater wing Sella turcica Sphenoid sinus	Flat, lateral portion between the frontal and temporal bones Central depression the encloses the pituitary gland Air cavity that opens into nasal cavity
Ethmoid (1)	Ethmoid sinus Crista galli Cribiform plate and Olfactory foramina Perpendicular plate Conchae (four are part of ethmoid, two inferior are separate bones)	Air cavity that opens into nasal cavity Superior projection for attachment of meninges On either side of base of crista galli; olfactory nerves pass through foramina Upper part of nasal septum Shelflike projections into nasal cavities that increase surface area of nasal mucosa
Mandible (1)	Body Condyles Sockets	U-shaped portion with lower teeth Oval projections that articulate with the temporal bones Conical depressions that hold roots of lower teeth
Maxilla (2)	Maxillary sinus Palatine process Sockets	Air cavity that opens into nasal cavity Projection that forms anterior part of hard palate Conical depressions that hold roots of upper teeth
Nasal (2)		Forms the bridge of nose
Lacrimal (2)	Lacrimal canal	Opening for nasolacrimal duct to take tears to nasal cavity
Zygomatic (2)		Form point of cheek, articulate with frontal, temporal, and maxillae
Palatine (2)		Forms the posterior of hard palate
Vomer (1)		Lower part of nasal septum
Inferior nasal conchae (2)		Shelf-like projections into nasal cavities that increase surface area of nasal mucosa (The superior and middle conchae are a part of the ethmoid bone.)

Located just below the cricoid cartilage is the thyroid gland. The **thyroid gland** is part of the endocrine system and is responsible for secreting two hormones: triioddthyronine (T_3) and thyroxine (T_4). The thyroid gland comprises two lobes that are connected by an isthmus. The isthmus lies directly below the cricoid cartilage, in front of the trachea. The two lobes of the thyroid gland curve posteriorly around the trachea and are for the most part covered by the SCM, which also serves to protect the gland. In certain individuals, there is an additional structure to the thyroid gland known as the **pyramidal lobe**, which extends upward from the isthmus, just lateral to the midline.

Developmental Variations

Developmental variations occur over the course of an individual's life span and events. Awareness of these variations is important to understand and recognize common age-related alterations or modifications of the head and neck.

Infants and Children

At birth, the brain is the largest organ, resulting in the infant's head representing 25% of the body length. In infants, the cranial bones are mobile, soft, and not yet fused. This allows for the birth canal to accommodate the head and facilitate easy

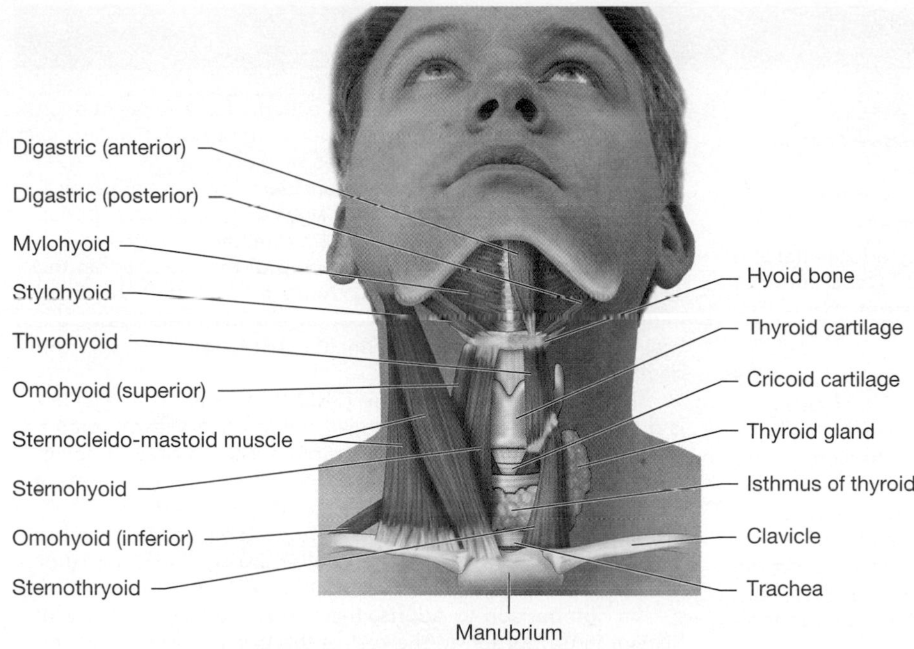

FIGURE 17-5 Anterior/lateral view of neck with internal structures identified

passage of the infant. This also allows for the rapid growth of the brain within the first year of life. The cranial bones are separated by sutures, which will eventually harden and fuse the bones together (Figure 17-6).

In two locations on the infant's skull the sutures are between four bones, leaving open spaces that can be palpated. These two open spaces are known as the **anterior** and **posterior fontanels** or "soft spots." The fontanels gradually harden and become smaller until they are closed. The posterior fontanel is usually closed at about 2 months, and the anterior fontanel does not completely close until the child is 2 years old. Ossification and fusing of the sutures is not achieved until brain growth is accomplished, at about 6 years of age, and is not fully complete until adulthood.

Generally no continuing changes occur in the head and neck of the child. The features of the face may change as the child approaches puberty, but there is nothing specific that needs to be assessed. Other changes that accompany puberty affect primarily the skin, which has already been described in Chapter 16.

The Pregnant Woman

No specific changes affect the structure of the head and neck of a pregnant woman. The thyroid gland may demonstrate some physiological changes related to T_3 and T_4 and may increase in size, but not to any degree that can be identified by physical examination. If hyperthyroidism develops, there may be a detectable change in the size of the thyroid gland, a bruit may be heard over the gland, and the characteristic eye manifestations may be present along with weight loss. (These manifestations will be covered in more detail in Chapters 19 and 25.)

Headaches are common during pregnancy, particularly during the first and third trimester (Aegidius, Zwart, Hagen, & Stovner, 2009). Although their exact cause is not known, during the first trimester it is thought to be related to the hormonal fluctuations during pregnancy (MacGregor, 2012). Stress, poor posture, or visual changes are thought to aggravate them. Additional causes include sleep deprivation, low blood sugar, dehydration, and caffeine withdrawal.

Third trimester headaches are most likely caused by poor posture and tension related to carrying extra weight. Headaches accompanied by high blood pressure are worrisome for preeclampsia and require immediate attention (see Chapter 11).

The Older Adult

There are no identified structural changes that accompany aging. As with children, skin-related changes alter the appearance of the face, but there are no expected changes. There are physiological and anatomic changes of the thyroid gland, but none that can be specifically examined.

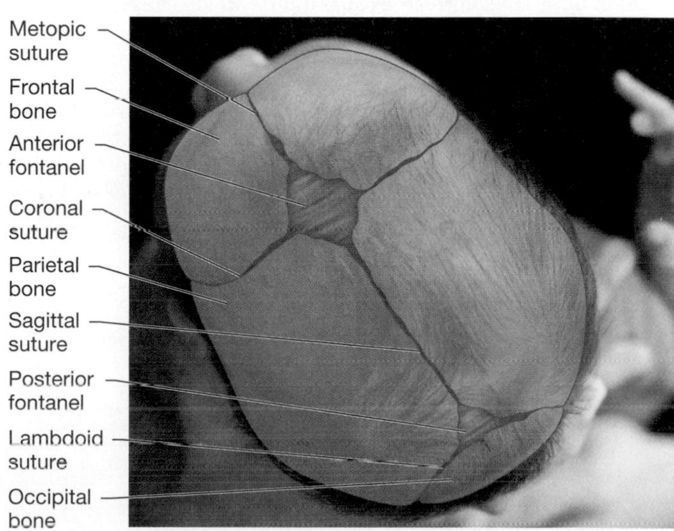

FIGURE 17-6 Superior view of infant's skull identifying sutures and fontanels
Source: Norhazlan/Shutterstock

Health Promotion

Traumatic Brain Injuries

A TBI is an insult to the brain, not of a degenerative or congenital nature, but caused by an external physical force that may produce a diminished or altered state of consciousness, resulting in neurological and functional impairment (Dawodu, 2011).

- A major goal of *Healthy People 2020* is to reduce fatal and nonfatal traumatic brain injuries (TBI; U.S. Department of Health and Human Services, 2009); the target goal is 10% improvement.

It is estimated that 1.7 million cases of TBI occur per year and contribute to approximately one-third (30.5%) of all injury related deaths in the United States (Faul, Likang, Wald, & Coronado, 2010). Rates of TBI are highest in the very young (0–4 years old), in adolescents and young adults (15–24 years old), and in the elderly (above 65 years old). TBI is significantly higher in men than women with a 2–2.8:1 ratio and a 3.5:1 ratio in severe TBI. The most common causes of TBI include moving vehicle accidents (including autos, motorcycles, and bikes), falls (leading cause of TBI in the elderly), violence (including physical abuse), and sports.

The physical force causing the brain injury is of such a nature that the brain moves within the skull. Prognosis is based on clinical severity, mechanism of injury, pathophysiological impact of the injury, age, medical comorbidities, and laboratory results including imaging.

TBI may present as different types. Closed-head injury is when skull integrity is maintained and there is no skull fracture. The most common type is a concussion, which is considered a mild TBI, causing a transitory alteration of the alert state. Individuals often experience full recovery; however, repeated concussions may result in permanent brain damage. A **contusion** is a bruise of the brain associated with bleeding and damage or death to brain tissue. Contusions often occur on the surface of the brain, most commonly of the frontal lobes (Agamanopolis, 2011). The area of impact experiences the initial bruising; however, the force of the impact sends the brain in the opposite direction, hitting the rigid skull on the opposite side. These types of injuries are identified as **coup** (initial bruising) and **contrecoup** (bruising of the opposite side). Severe contusions cause brain tissue swelling resulting in increasing intracranial pressure.

The most serious type of injury and significant cause of death from TBI is **diffuse axonal injury**, which causes the axons of the neurons within the white matter to become stretched and in some instances to be pulled apart and disconnected from each other (Pangilinan Jr., Kellyh, & Hurnyak, 2013). This type of injury results from twisting or torquing of the brain, which stretches, twists, and damages the axons. Most commonly this type of injury results from rapid acceleration and deceleration of the brain, which occurs in moving vehicle accidents and shaken baby syndrome.

When the skull is broken due to extreme force or penetration by an object, it is described as a penetrating or open-head injury. Brain injury also results from the penetrating object.

Injuries to the brain are also considered primary or secondary as determined by the time that signs and symptoms appear. Primary injuries are the result of the mechanical force that is applied to the head, and the bouncing of the brain within the skull. Secondary injuries develop hours to days after the initial injury and result from further damage to the neurons of the brain, mediated by neurochemical substances released from damaged cells.

In shaken baby syndrome (SBS), the cause of the injury is due more to the vigorous shaking that occurs rather than a forceful impact to the head. The rapid acceleration and deceleration of the brain against the infant's skull is the primary cause of brain injury. The injury is greatly increased if the shaking ends with the infants head hitting a solid or immovable object (wall or crib) (Cabinum-Foeller, 2011). (SBS is further discussed in Chapter 14.)

In comparison to adults, the infant's head is larger and heavier in proportion to the rest of the body. Additionally, the neck muscles are weaker, so the shaking is intensified. The brain is also smaller than the skull, so there is more space between the brain and bone, which also adds force to the bouncing of the brain within the cranium. Trauma to the brain results in inflammation and swelling of the of brain tissue, bleeding in the brain, and bleeding in the retinas of the eyes. Unless immediate medical help is received, the victim will most likely sustain significant permanent brain damage.

The major factor in the reduction of traumatic head injuries is prevention. Although not totally preventable, understanding the causes of head injury and taking steps to prevent them from occurring are not excessively expensive and are relatively easy to implement. Actions to prevent head injuries include the following:

- Use of safety equipment such as seat belts, helmets when cycling and skiing, and hardhats when involved in construction or around heavy equipment.
- For cyclists—obey traffic signals; be predictable so that motorists will know what to expect. Also remain visible—reduce cycling during dark hours and wear reflective clothing if cycling during the night.
- Use age-appropriate car seats and boosters for infants and children.
- Always supervise children at play and make sure that their play area is safe.
- Do not drink and drive and do not take rides or travel with anyone who has been or you suspect has been drinking.
- Do not use cell phones or send or receive text messages while driving.

Clinical Context Exemplars

Situation A

A 30-year-old woman with history of migraine headaches comes in with unrelenting, pulsating daily headaches associated with nausea, vomiting, and photophobia. She has been taking Excedrin, Maxalt, Vicodin, and tramadol with no relief.

1. What other history might you ask for?

Situation B

A 14-year-old young woman was brought in by her parents to the emergency department with cold symptoms, fever, and headaches of 12-hour duration. Many of her classmates have the similar symptoms. At the ED, the patient is noted to have fever and a stiff neck, is toxic appearing, and has no focal neurologic findings. An antibiotic was started, CT was done, and lumbar puncture (LP) was performed. The patient became obtunded and died within 10 hours of admission.

1. As you reflect on how you took care of the patient, is there anything that you could have done differently to change the course?
2. What would you predict to be the lumbar puncture results?

Situation C

A 60-year-old man presents with a sudden episode of severe headache, the worst headache in his life.

1. Is there any significance to the age of this patient? Why or why not?
2. How would you differentiate primary headaches from secondary headaches? What questions would you want to ask to help determine which type of headache this might be?
3. What pain characteristics would help you differentiate between the three major primary headache types?

Situation D

A 40-year-old woman noted painful swallowing, ear pain, and 8-pound weight loss in one week, which she attributed to not eating much due to pain when swallowing and stress. She tells you that she just returned from scuba diving to relieve stress and attributes her ear pain to scuba diving.

1. What else will you ask about her history, and what will the focused exam look like?

SUBJECTIVE DATA

History of Present Illness (CC)

The patient may present with specific complaints related to the structures of the head and neck. Framing the questions will depend on the patient's age, gender, culture, race, emotional or mental status, health practices, and concurrent illnesses. All symptoms presented must be thoroughly assessed with a symptom analysis (COLDERRA).

Headache (HA)

Headaches are one of the most common patient concerns. Most benign headaches (75%) fall in the categories of migraine, tension-type headaches, and cluster headaches. These are also known as primary headaches as there is no anatomical or physiological explanation for their presence. Some are attributed to more serious underlying diseases like infection, vascular lesions, neoplasm, and metabolic and systemic diseases. These are known as secondary headaches. It is important not to miss the warning signs of underlying diseases. Benign headaches are more common in women. Red flags in the history include older age of onset (> 50 years); acute onset (thunderclap headache); new onset or significant change from prior headaches; headaches associated with increased or decreased ICP, like Valsalva or bending over or orthostatic change in position; focal neurologic symptoms not associated with aura; signs and symptoms of systemic illness like fever, chills, sweats, and weight loss; and known systemic illness (cancer) or infection (HIV, Cocci). A systematic history is the most important factor in establishing the correct diagnosis of headaches. A comparison of the types of HAs is shown in Table 17-2.

Provider Inquiries	Clinical Reasoning/Logic
Characteristics: What sensations are experienced with headache: throbbing; pounding; boring; dull, nagging, constant pressure; shooting? Severity of pain (1–10)? Any pattern? Recurrence or Frequency of HAs?	Episodic, recurrent, throbbing, pounding moderate to severe headaches are common manifestations of migraine and cluster headaches. Severe headaches are suggestive of subarachnoid hemorrhage, although migraine and clusters can also be moderate to severe.
Onset: Gradual or sudden? Particular time of day? Age of onset?	Sudden onset is characteristic of subarachnoid and intracerebral bleeds. Sudden onset of headaches may be seen in hypertensive emergencies, acute angle closure glaucoma, venous sinus thrombosis or carotid and vertebral artery dissection. Primary headaches

Provider Inquiries	Clinical Reasoning/Logic
	usually begin during childhood or between 20 and 50 years of age. Headaches that begin after age 60 are red flags for secondary headaches associated with temporal arteritis or a mass lesion (Clinch, 2001).
Location: Where is HA felt? Specific location or generalized? One side or both sides? Temporal or jaw pain?	Unilateral headaches suggest migraine; bilateral suggest tension headaches; temporal pain or tenderness or jaw claudication suggest temporal arteritis.
Duration: How long do HAs generally last (hours to days)?	Hours to days are seen in cluster headaches. Tension headaches wax and wane, but may also persist for days.
Exacerbation: What makes HAs worse (light, noise, position, coughing)?	Noise and light aggravates migraines. Bending over or lying position aggravates subarachnoid bleed.
Relief: What have you used to relieve HAs (analgesics—OTC/prescribed)? Effectiveness? Have you done anything to prevent onset if triggers are known?	Rest, sleep, analgesics, and triptans can abort migraine headaches. Triggers, if known, may prevent onset or frequency of migraine.
Radiation: Is HA localized or does it spread to other areas?	
Associated signs/symptoms: What accompanies HA? Are there auras, prodromes, or postdromes? Nausea/vomiting, lightheadedness, visual changes, fever, weakness? Focal neurological signs like papillary asymmetry, visual loss, or holes, ataxia, seizure? Any toxic exposure, other family members' involvement, winter months? Illicit drug use?	Headache plus visual holes suggest glaucoma. Toxic exposure, winter months, and other family members involved suggest carbon monoxide poisoning. Illicit drug abuse like cocaine, sympathomimetics, and methamphetamines increase risk of stroke and intracranial bleed.

Table 17-2 Comparisons of types of headaches

	Primary Headaches			Secondary Headaches		
Type	**Tension**	**Migraine**	**Cluster**	**Hypertensive**	**Temporal Arteritis**	**Subarachnoid hemorrhage**
Characteristics	Pressure, tightness/ constricting Bandlike tightness	Intense, pounding throbbing, pulsating aching pain around one temple	Occur in clusters over period of time (daily for weeks/months)	Generalized, hair band–type pain	Throbbing occurrence of headache Considered a "new headache" Tenderness on sides of scalp when touched	Generally indicates spontaneous or nontraumatic hemorrhaging caused by rupture of cerebral aneurysm or AV malformation
Intensity	Mild to moderate. Increasing intensity	Variable severity	Excruciating—knife/nail being driven into the eye or head			("worst headache in my life") with lateralization to the side of bleed in 30% of cases
Onset/Cause	Adulthood Gradual Onset	Childhood-Adolescence Gradual onset to a rapid crescendo (peaks in 1–2 hours)	20–40 years of age Alcohol, nitroglycerine	Adulthood Uncertain cause	Occurs in older adults, rarely in anyone under 50 Average age of onset is 72 Inflammation or vasculitis involving the temporal artery	Abrupt onset of severe headache

Continued

Table 17-2 Comparisons of types of headaches *(continued)*

	Primary Headaches			Secondary Headaches		
Type	Tension	Migraine	Cluster	Hypertensive	Temporal Arteritis	Subarachnoid hemorrhage
	Adult stresses, anxieties, depression (not necessarily muscle tightness) Low level of endorphin	20% associated with aura				
Location	Bilateral; generalized or localized to back of head/upper neck/temporal frontal area	Majority unilateral; bifrontal or generalized in others	Centered around one or retroorbital eye/unilaterally	Bilateral or occipital	Unilateral/temporal region	Generalized with lateralization
Duration	Variable	Hours to days (4–72 hours)	30 minutes to 3 hours and may last for days Often in early morning hours	Hours	Hours to days	Seconds to minutes
Exacerbation	Continuous muscle tension—driving/keyboarding	Alcohol, foods or stress Daily physical activities Caffeine withdrawal, heat, hypoglycemia, weather change, emotional stress, sleep disturbances, alcohol, neck pain, odors, hormones, smoke, exercise, change in barometric pressure, menstruation, substances like nitrates, MSG	Lying down Alcohol sensitivity	None well identified Increase in blood pressure	Movement of neck and shoulders Chewing	Exertion or physical activity can trigger SAH, anger, caffeine consumption, sexual exertion Risks for SAH are smoking, hypertension, alcohol, genetic risk, sympathomimetic drugs, estrogen deficiency, antithrombotic medications and statins (effects of stains is not well studied)
Relief/treatment	OTC analgesics, relaxation/massage, antidepressants	Sleep, rest Staying quiet, dark room, medications	Moving around Medications	OTC analgesics Antihypertensive medication	Steroids (Prednisone)	Treatment of risk factors and stopping smoking, alcohol, and sympathomimetic drugs.
Associated signs and symptoms	Neck and scalp pain and tenderness	Migraine may occur in four phases: prodromes, aura, headache phase, and postdrome. Prodromes may manifest with euphoria, irritability, craving, depression, yawning, or neck stiffness. Aura may be in the form of visual, motor, verbal, and sensory symptoms and signs (scotomas, visual loss,	Ipsilateral lacrimation and redness of the eye, stuffy nose, rhinorrhea, Horners syndrome (ptosis, miosis and anhidrosis) lid drooping, rhinorrhea with nasal congestion	Sometimes associated with increased BP or uncontrolled BP	Body/joint aches, fever fatigue and sweats anemia In 25% of cases, co-exists with polymyalgia rheumatica If not treated, may lead to blindness	May have brief LOC, seizure, nausea or vomiting, low back pain and meningismus. Some patients may have a warning leak or sentinel headache that precedes the headache by 6–20 days

Continued

Table 17-2 Comparisons of types of headaches (continued)

	Primary Headaches			Secondary Headaches		
Type	Tension	Migraine	Cluster	Hypertensive	Temporal Arteritis	Subarachnoid hemorrhage
		sensory tingling on limbs, dysphasia, or paraphasic errors in speech.) In the postdrome phase, the patient may have headaches with sudden movement of head, fatigue, or exhaustion, and some patients experience euphoria.				

Stiff Neck

Stiff neck is the term referring to an abnormal preferred position of the neck or a normal-appearing position of the neck associated with restricted range of motion. It is a subjective complaint, and when it is supported by a physical finding of restricted ROM on passive movement of the neck especially on flexion, it is called meningismus. Stiffness of the neck may be related to the following:

1. Cervical spine disease: spondylosis, trauma as in acceleration/deceleration injury, whiplash
2. Infection: as in meningitis, retropharyngeal abscess, vertebral osteomylitis
3. Cranial processes: subarachnoid bleed, brain tumors or spinal cord tumors, head and neck tumors like nasopharyngeal carcinoma
4. Dystonia, torticollis, or muscle spasm
5. Rheumatological disorders

Provider Inquiries	Clinical Reasoning/Logic
Characteristics: Unable to move neck at all? Pain with movement, limited movement? Pain continuous or intermittent/cramping? Numbness, tingling, or weakness? Where?	Inability to move the neck is seen in various cervical spine disorders and if accompanied by fever suggests infection or inflammation. If neck pain involves nerves, numbness, tingling, or weakness may be felt in arm, hand, or elsewhere.
Onset: What precipitated onset of stiffness? Any injury, illness—bacterial, viral?	Injury, exertion points toward musculoskeletal component. Illnesses like viral, fungal, or bacterial suggest infection as a cause.
Location: Specific area affected? One side/both sides?	Unilaterality suggests local factors like cervical herniation or spondylosis, and nerve root irritation.
Duration: How long has neck been stiff?	Episodic and intermittent chronic neck pain or stiffness suggests cervical spine disease. Short term, acute neck stiffness along with fever suggests acute infection. Progressive symptoms of more than 6 weeks' duration are significant.

Provider Inquiries	Clinical Reasoning/Logic
Exacerbation: Does anything make it worse (position/movement)? Does it increase with valsalva or any activities that increases intracranial pressure?	Exacerbation with activities that increase intracranial pressure like cough or valsalva suggests intracranial processes.
Relief: Any measures taken to relieve stiffness (medications/alternative therapy)? Effectiveness?	Medications, massage, ice, or heat may improve musculoskeletal or cervical spine disorders.
Radiation: Any radiation pattern to arms, back, shoulders?	Radiation to arms and shoulder suggest cervical spine disorders. Individuals with cervical disorders of various types may have lower extremity and bladder or bowel symptoms, often with minimal neck pain (Devereaux, 2009).
Associated signs/symptoms: Fever, headaches, sweats and fatigue, hip and girdle weakness? History of immunosuppression or cancer? Any arm clumsiness, gait problems, or bladder/bowel problems? Any shocklike pain with flexion of neck (Lhermitte's sign)? History of injury? Rash? Chest pain?	Neck pain with fever, chills, and weight loss in a patient with cancer or immune suppression suggest infection or tumor. Neck stiffness, headache, and fever leads one to suspect meningitis or encephalitis. Neck pain with fever, headache, and fatigue, joint pains, hip and shoulder girdle weakness, and visual loss in an older person suggest temporal arteritis or polymyalgia rheumatic. Lhermitte's sign is seen in cervical compression or herniation or spondylosis and in multiple sclerosis. Rash may be seen in Herpes zoster. Chest pain with radiation to neck suggests cardiac causes. Neck pain with gait instability, clumsiness, and bowel/bladder problems suggest cervical myelopathy.
Thyroid Dysfunction The thyroid gland is a part of the endocrine system; however, the endocrine system is generally not assessed as a separate system. Questions referring to thyroid function are placed here due to its location in the neck. Because hyper- and hypothyroidism have different manifestations, the provider needs to determine if any manifestations of either condition are present. Manifestations of hypothyroidism and hyperthyroidism are shown in Table 17-3. Symptoms seen in thyroid dysfunction are not specific to thyroid and other systemic or organ system involvement by diseases other than thyroid must be ruled out.	
Characteristics: Heat/cold intolerance? Increased energy, hyperactivity, nervousness, lethargy? Swelling in neck? Swallowing difficulties? Any pain? Sleeping difficulties—getting to sleep/waking up?	Thyroid hormone increases basal metabolic rate. In hyperthyroidism, there is increased T_4, increasing basal metabolic rate and leading to tachycardia, arrhythmias Swallowing difficulty seen in subacute thyroiditis as result of inflammation and damage to the thyroid cells. Thyroiditis (Hashimoto, subacute thyroiditis, painless thyroiditis, drug induced, radiation induced, acute suppurative thyroiditis) may be secondary to autoimmune disorders and bacterial or viral infections.

Provider Inquiries	Clinical Reasoning/Logic
Onset: When were changes noted? Were they gradual or sudden?	Most thyroid conditions are gradual, with the exception of acute suppurative/subacute thyroiditis.
Duration: Symptoms generally continuous, so duration is likely to be from time of onset.	Subacute thyroiditis may last from 2 to 8 weeks and may present with hyperthyroidism followed by euthyroidism and hypothyroidism. Graves' ophthalmopathy may or may not get better with treatment of hyperthyroidism.
Exacerbation: Anything noticed to make symptoms worse? Caffeine, alcohol? Medications?	Caffeine may increase adrenergic stimulation and may make tachycardia and hypertension worse. Similarly, alcohol may also increase BP. Medications like selective beta blockers decrease tachycardia and tremors.
Relief: Anything known to make symptoms better? Alternative therapies? Anything avoided? Effectiveness?	Some patients will use alternative treatment like herbs, and it is worthwhile asking what else they are taking besides prescribed medications.
Radiation: Only helpful as thyroid pain may radiate to jaw and ear and may manifest with painful swallowing in subacute thyroiditis.	
Associated signs/symptom: Change in texture of skin/nails/hair, increased prominence of eyes, tachycardia, palpitations, change in elimination patterns? Females—change in menstrual flow/pattern?	Increasing metabolic activity leads to tachycardia, increases peristalsis leading to increased defecation and not necessarily diarrhea, increases reflexes, sweaty palms, and heat intolerance.

Table 17-3 Manifestations of hypothyroidism and hyperthyroidism

System	Hypothyroidism	Hyperthyroidism
	General Characteristics	
Temperature preference	Prefers warm environment (cold intolerant)	Prefers cool environment (heat intolerant)
Weight changes	Gain (growth failure)	Loss (in spite of increased appetite)
Emotional state	Lethargic, fatigued, apathetic	Nervous, easily irritated, energetic, animated
Integumentary		
Skin	Coarse, scaly, dry Carotinemia—yellow hue to skin	Warm, moist (sweating) Swelling of face, hands, and lower extremities
Hair	Coarse, brittle with tendency to break	Fine, with hair loss
Nails	Thick	Thin with tendency to break
Eyes	Periorbital edema, swelling of face	Exophthalmos, conjunctival edema, lid retraction, lid lag, double vision
Neck	May have goiter (in iodine-deficient patients or in goitrous chronic autoimmune thyroiditis) Hoarseness	Swelling (goiter), tenderness over thyroid gland, thyroid nodule. Painless thyroiditis or painful thyroid in subacute or granulomatous thyroiditis
Cardiovascular	Bradycardia Decreased systolic and increased diastolic pressures	Tachycardia, arrhythmias (atrial fibrillation), palpitations Heart failure and edema Increased diastolic and decreased diastolic pressures Hyperdynamic cardiac output with accentuated S_1
Gastrointestinal	Constipation Enlargement of tongue	Increased frequency of bowel movements (not necessarily diarrhea)
Reproductive (female only)	Menorrhagia Delay of puberty	Decreased menstrual flow, amenorrhea
Neuromuscular	Lethargic, no change in muscle strength Delayed relaxation phase on the reflexes Myalgias	Increasing weakness, especially of proximal muscles, tremors Hyperreflexia or brisk reflexes Tremors

Hoarseness/Voice Changes

Hoarseness may be seen in hypothyroidism, or may be from organic causes such as malignancy, infection, sinonasal disease, vocal cord disorders, intubation, irritants, voice fatigue, allergy, reflux, and neurological disorders like Myasthenia Gravis or Parkinson's disease. It may also be from functional causes. Any persistent hoarseness lasting more than two weeks in the absence of an acute upper respiratory tract infection should be investigated.

Provider Inquiries	Clinical Reasoning/Logic
Characteristics: How has voice changed (pitch, tone)?	Hoarseness may be from a variety of etiology mentioned previously.
Onset: When did it first begin? More than few weeks? Is onset in the morning upon arising or in the evening after prolonged use of voice?	More than 2 weeks of hoarseness in the absence of URI needs referral to ENT. Morning hoarseness may be from postnasal drip or reflux.
Duration: Is change constant or intermittent? If intermittent, how long does it last?	Intermittent hoarseness argues against a mass lesion and favors vocal cord fatigue, irritant, reflux, or postnasal drip.
Exacerbation: What makes it worse? Smoking, pollution, acid, allergy, increased use of voice, talking, singing?	The presence of exacerbating factors reduces the risk malignancy.
Relief: What makes it better? Lozenges, rinse, anesthetic sprays? Effectiveness of treatment? Voice rest, relief of allergy or reflux symptoms?	
Associated signs/symptoms: Increased mucus production, sore throat, acid reflux symptoms, postnasal drip, allergic rhinitis or asthma, history of intubation, weight loss, hemoptysis, cough, dyspnea?	Associated symptoms help in defining possible etiology of hoarseness. Symptoms such as hemoptysis, weight loss, cough, stridor, shortness of breath, dysphagia, and odynophagia may signal an underlying malignancy, especially if combined with alcohol use and smoking.

Past Medical History

Past medical history identifies the information needed to determine whether there is any prior incidences/events that may have contributed to the present situation.

Head trauma, closed or open?	May explain headaches and craniofacial injuries and disorders.
Lumbar puncture and brain surgery?	Post-spinal headache may occur. Brain surgery may explain CSF leak, headaches, or neck symptoms.
History of intubation or instrumentation like endoscopy?	Tracheal and endoscopic procedures may cause damage to the oropharynx, larynx, pharynx, vocal cords, arytenoid cartilage, and trachea, causing pain in swallowing and hoarseness.
Radiation treatment to head or neck?	These may lead to cancers of head or neck (thyroid).
History of headaches?	Migraine usually starts during childhood or adolescence, and patient usually presents with history of migraine.
Any surgeries for tumors (head or neck [thyroid])?	May help identify cases of migraine or thyroid disorders.
Is there a history of seizure disorders, Parkinson's, and other neurodegenerative disorders?	Predisposition to falls.
	Chronic daily headaches may be secondary to medication overuse.

Provider Inquiries	Clinical Reasoning/Logic
What medications are taken regularly? Thyroid medicines?	Too many thyroid supplements may explain hyperthyroidism.
Iodine, use or lack thereof?	Excess iodine may result in hyperthyroidism. Iodine deficiency is one of the most common causes of goiter. It is now rare in the United States as a result of widespread distribution of iodine-enriched foods. Iodine deficiency occurs almost exclusively in developing nations.
Lithium?	Lithium may cause hypothyroidism but has been associated with hyperthyroidism as well. Lithium increases intrathyroidal iodine content, inhibits the coupling of iodotyrosine residues to form iodothyronines (thyroxine [T_4] and triiodothyronine [T_3]) [1-3], and inhibits release of T_4 and T_3 (Surks, 2013).
Amiodarone?	Amiodarone contains high levels of iodine. Excess iodine from amiodarone exerts an acute, transient inhibition of iodide organification, but the normal gland escapes this effect due to adaptation of the iodide transport system. In some persons, the thyroid gland is unable to escape the block, and hypothyroidism ensues (Basaria & Cooper, 2005).
Oral contraceptives, tamoxifen, raloxifene, methadone? Androgens, anabolic steroids, and corticosteroids?	Estrogen has a well-known indirect effect on thyroid economy, increasing the thyroxine-binding globulin (TBG), therefore increasing levels of total T_4, not free T_4. TBG binds with thyroxine hormone (T_3/T_4) in circulation. While estrogen administration causes an increase in serum TBG concentration, androgen therapy results in a decrease in this binding protein (Tahboub & Arafah, 2009).
Anti-seizure drugs like phenytoin, phenobarbital, carbamezipine?	Carbamazepin and phenobarbital significantly decrease free thyroxine levels (Uður et al., 2007).
Propranolol?	Propranolol in high doses (above 160 mg/day) also slowly decreases serum triiodothyronine (T_3) concentrations by as much as 30 percent via inhibition of the 5'-monodeiodinase that converts thyroxine (T_4) to T_3 (Ross, 2012).

Family History

Family history provides information regarding family members' illnesses or conditions as potential causes for chief concern or presenting symptoms that may indicate a pattern of presentation associated with transmission of familial/genetic factors predisposing the patient to certain system-related conditions/illnesses. Any of these may indicate a potential or actual cause of head and neck dysfunction.

Provider Inquiries	Clinical Reasoning/Logic
Family history of migraine headaches?	Migraine sufferer usually has associated FH of migraine.
Family history of thyroid disorders?	Information related to possible familial tendencies.
Immune disorders?	Certain thyroid disorder may be caused by autoimmune mechanisms.
Family history of cerebral aneurysm?	A risk factor for cerebral aneurysm.

Personal and Social History

Personal and social history is information related to surroundings and environments that may identify risk factors for certain conditions. These questions can also determine the use of safety measures to prevent head trauma or other factors that may be related to other symptoms or conditions.

Provider Inquiries	Clinical Reasoning/Logic
Place of employment—exposure to chemicals or noxious/strong odors or equipment that places patient at risk for head injury or other head/neck conditions? Use of head protection?	Chemical exposure may cause irritation leading to hoarseness, and strong odors may initiate or aggravate migraine. Traumatic head injuries may occur at place of employment if not wearing protective head gear.
Sports participation—any sports that place patient at risk for possible head injury or other conditions? Use of head protection?	Risk for TBI.
Home—potential hazards (stairs, loose rugs, frequent use of ladders), use of seat belts?	
Stress—tension at work, school, or home that may cause potential problems?	Stress may increase migraine.
Nutritional habits—any recent weight changes, any food intolerances/allergies, consistent diet patterns?	Foods that contain MSG and nitrates may trigger migraine.
Social habits—use of alcohol, drugs? Smoking?	Alcohol, smoking, and sympathomimetics like cocaine and methamphetamines may increase risk for subarachnoid bleed.

Developmental Applications

Certain conditions or disorders may be related to certain age groups or situations. Inquiring to obtain age or condition specific information will provide further information for helping to determine causes of the chief concern as identified.

Infants and Children

Provider Inquiries	Clinical Reasoning/Logic
Prenatal history—mother's use of drugs, alcohol during pregnancy?	Determine risk for fetal alcohol syndrome and drug-related disorders in neonates.
Birth history—birth order, delivery (vaginal or C-section), presentation? Difficult delivery (use of forceps)? Term/preterm?	Determine potential for head injury through the canal or use of forceps that may lead to cephalic abnormalities.
Shape of head—bulging or flattened, molding (estimated time in birth canal), cephalohematoma, caput succedaneum? Condition of fontanels?	Determine potential for any complications related to head/brain.
Head control? Growth/developmental patterns—percentile rankings?	Helps determine if development is proceeding as expected.
Acute illnesses, such as diarrhea, vomiting, fever, irritability, stiff neck?	Helps determine possible causes of stiff neck and headaches.
Congenital anomalies, such as myelomeningocele, encephalocele, microcephaly, hydrocephaly?	Genetic and environmental insults can affect brain development leading to microcephaly. Meningomyelocele may cause brain stem dysfunction leading to swallowing difficulties, vocal cord paresis, and stridor. Strabismus and facial weakness can also occur.

Provider Inquiries	Clinical Reasoning/Logic
Congenital hypothyroidism screening?	Major intervention to prevent manifestations of congenital hypothyroidism.
History of family dysfunction/violence?	Determine potential for physical abuse directed toward infant/child.
The Pregnant Woman	
Stage of pregnancy/postpartum?	Headaches are common in pregnancy and if accompanied by hypertension signal preeclampsia.
Preexisting conditions—hypo/hyperthyroidism? How treated—iodine, antithyroid prescription?	Possible effect on infant.
Use of drugs—hormones?	May increase migraine. Sex hormones also increase TBG, thereby increasing total T_4.
The Older Adult	
Falls are the major source of head injuries in the elderly, so it is important to reduce the risk of falls through prevention.	
Any potential hazards around house that present danger of falling (excess clutter, slippers surfaces, loose rugs)?	Ensuring a safe environment, that is, removing clutter and avoiding slippery surfaces, loose rugs, and unnecessary furniture
Have any recent changes in your medications. If so, have you noticed any difference in mental status, alertness etc.?	Adjustment of medications that interfere with alertness, mental status, blood pressure, and posture balance
Are you engaged in any type of physical activity or other ways to maintain strength? If so, what, how often?	Maintenance of strength and balance through physical activity and physical therapy when appropriate
Are there any safety devices installed around house or other equipment used? If not, do you feel that you need them?	Provision of safety devices like railings, walkers, and wheelchairs should balance; coordination and strengths are compromised
Any dizziness with head, neck movement, assuming upright position from sitting?	Orthostasis can lead to falls.
Any balance/coordination difficulties? Weakness?	Balance and strength are necessary ingredients in maintaining posture.

OBJECTIVE DATA

In terms of sequence, the head and neck exam comes soon after the vital signs and general physical appearance. Most providers perform the cranial nerve examination during the head and neck segment but it may also be covered on the neurological examination. Components of the cardiovascular and pulmonary examination will be covered here as well as in other specific chapters. The primary assessment techniques used are inspection, palpation and auscultation.

Inspection

- Cranium (symmetry and shape)
- Scalp (condition of skin and hair)
- Face (symmetry; color of skin; presence of scars, lesions; inspection of eyes, nose, ears for deformity; swelling; redness)
- Neck (ROM), symmetry and preferred position, inspection for enlarged thyroid gland or nodules
- Jugular venous pulsation, jugular venous distension (cardiovascular exam)
- Carotid pulsation

Palpation

- Cranium (shape)
- Scalp (mobility of scalp, presence of lumps and bumps, swelling and tenderness)
- Face—palpate sinuses-frontal and maxillary, nose, ears for tenderness
- Thyroid gland enlargement, nodules
- Trachea (part of pulmonary exam—palpate for symmetry, deviations, and presence of subcutaneous emphysema)
- Lymph nodes

Arteries (carotid pulsation, temporal artery—cardiovascular exam)

Internal jugular vein

Mastoid

Auscultation

Auscultation of the carotid arteries for bruit

Auscultation of thyroid gland for bruit in hyperthyroid state

Level I to IV Examination

The Level I to Level IV examinations are performed on a continuum, which starts from a basic level and moves to a more comprehensive level based on provider's abilities and knowledge as well as the patient's presentation and location. The examination may start at the outpatient setting and progress to the ED, hospital unit bed, critical care unit, or specialty unit. Frequently all the elements from basic to comprehensive exam are done in one setting, such as a primary care setting or clinic.

The condition or illness of the patient is the primary consideration related to the type and amount of data needed to assess the patient's condition, illness, or situation. The arrangement of skills into levels is done for general purposes and is meant to be descriptive rather than prescriptive. The purpose of arranging examination skills into levels is to provide a framework to assist the learner in determining the appropriate data to collect.

Head/Neck

	Level I	Level II	Level III	Level IV
Inspection	Cranium—size, shape, symmetry	Face (condition characteristics)	Neck/head injuries	Much of what pertains to the Level III exam can be said for the Level IV exam. So much of the head and neck exam relates to other systems that data for the head and neck is obtained through other system assessment.
	Face—structures, appearance, expression*, symmetry*	Neck—jugular venous pulse/ distension*	Glascow Coma Scale	
	Neck—position, symmetry, swelling (thyroid, lymph nodes)	Neck—movement, ROM* active and passive	Meningismus Kernigs also covered in the neurological exam section Brudzinski	
	Scalp (hair distribution)			
Palpation	Cranium—temporal artery pulse*	Trachea*		
	Neck—carotid artery pulse*	Thyroid gland		
		Lymph nodes*		
Auscultation		Carotid*, thyroid bruits		

*may be done with assessment of head and neck but relate to other system assessment

Inspection: Level I

Inspection Techniques and Expected Findings	Unexpected Findings

Head and Cranium

Inspect the patient's cranium for size, shape, and symmetry. The cranium shape has many variations and is influenced by genetics and ethnicity. It should be rounded in appearance, without obvious deformities. No identifiable criteria exist for measurements or proportions to determine or describe its expected appearance. The proportion of head size to body size varies depending on the age of the individual. In the adult, the proportions are generally "eye-balled." The term for the expected shape of the cranium is **normocephalic** (Figure 17-7).

Unexpected findings include **microcephaly**, a cranium size that is smaller than expected, and macrocephaly, a cranium size that is larger than expected. These alterations are further discussed in Conditions and Disorders.

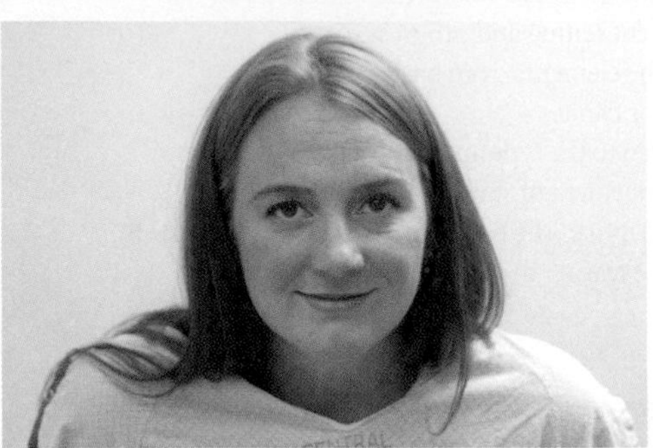

FIGURE 17-7 Frontal view of head and shoulders

If the scalp and hair have not already been inspected and palpated, this is an appropriate place to combine assessments (see Chapter 16). Palpation of the temporomandibular joint may also be done at this time; however, it is a part of the neurological and musculoskeletal exam also (see Chapters 26 and 27).

Symmetry is most commonly assessed by observation, which frequently fails to recognize minor asymmetrical properties of the face (Ercan et al., 2008).

Face

Assess the face for symmetry of shape and movement. Assess symmetry by inspecting structures to the left and right side of the face and inspect midline structures for deformity. It is not unusual for mild asymmetries to exist over the facial midline, and generally these are non-problematic; however, when craniofacial asymmetry becomes functionally or aesthetically problematic, intervention is usually necessary (Kwon, Park, Ryoo, & Lee, 2006).

Facial asymmetry may be congenital or acquired.

The eyes should be approximately one-third of the way down on the face and approximately one eye-width apart from each other (Figure 17-8). They should also be horizontally aligned with each other, which can be assessed by drawing an imaginary straight line through the lateral corners or the eye. The eyes should be on the same plane.

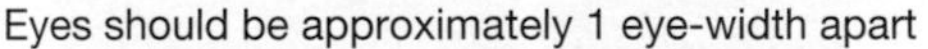

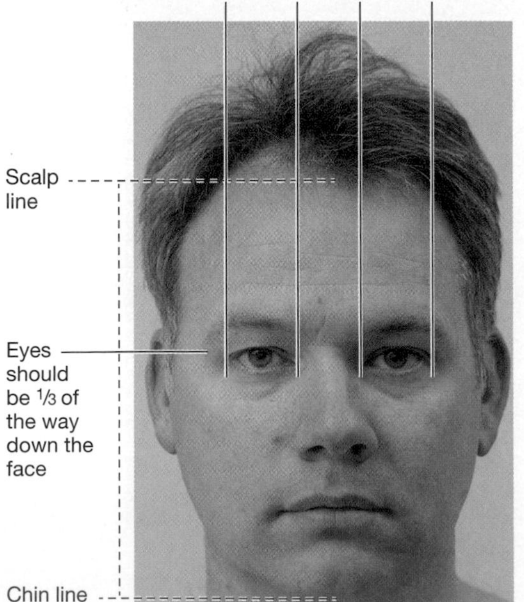

FIGURE 17-8 Close-up of eyes with lines drawn to indicate spacing and alignment

Inspection Techniques and Expected Findings	Unexpected Findings

The nose should be midline with the bridge of the nose equidistant from each eye and the septum in line with the philtrum and notch of the upper lip. The overall shape of the nose should not cause deviation from the midline (Figure 17-9). The skin color of the nose should be consistent with the rest of the body.

The shape of the nose may vary, often due to trauma from a broken nose frequently demonstrated as a deviated septum.

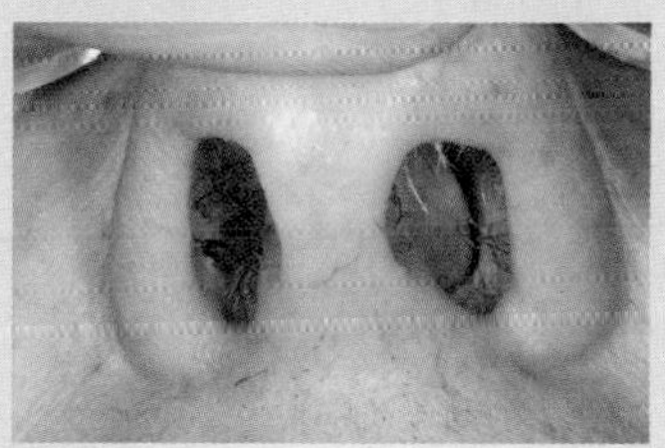

FIGURE 17-9 Deviated septum
Source: Dr. P. Marazzi/Science Source

A red, bulbous-appearing nose may indicate rosacea (see Chapter 16).

A reddened lower portion of the nose may be present during colds or allergies.

The mouth is another midline structure and is made up of the upper and lower lip. The lips of lighter-skinned individuals should be dark pink to light red in color, while those with darker skin often present with a lip color that is a darker shade of the underlying skin color. The width of the mouth is variable, but should be equal on both sides from the midline. The character and appearance of the lips are also related to genetics and ethnicity (Figure 17-10). There should also be symmetry of movement during talking and facial expressions.

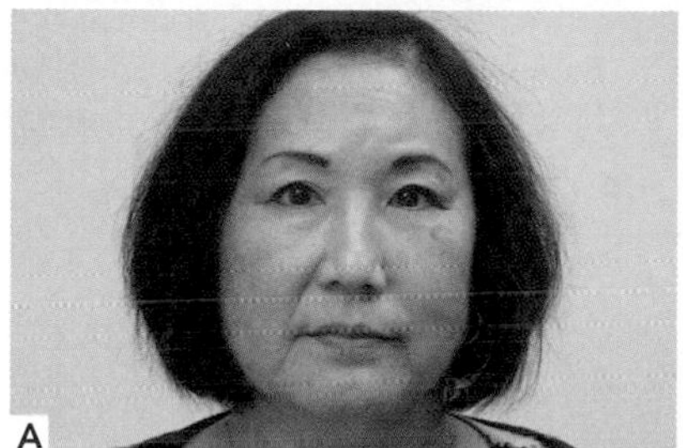

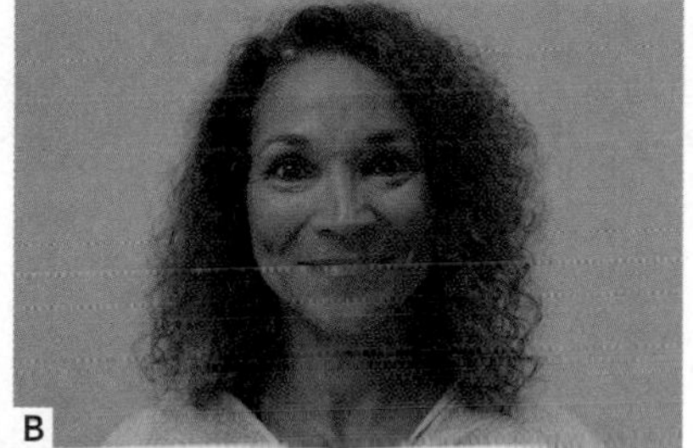

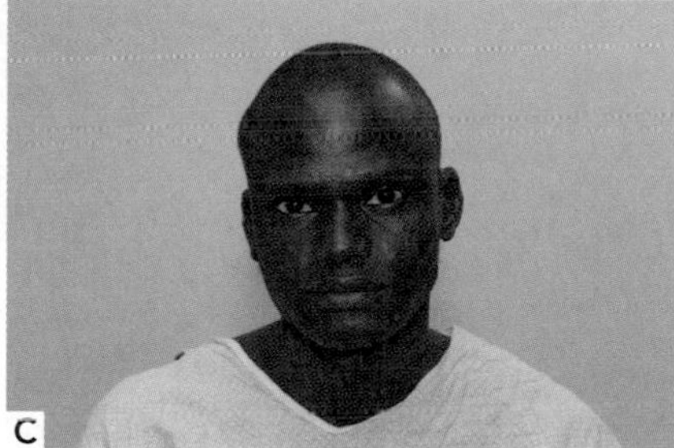

FIGURE 17-10A–C Faces showing ethnic variations

Acquired asymmetry may be a result of dental malocclusion, canting of the occlusal level and dental midline shift. These are corrected by orthognathic surgery.

Congenital causes of mouth asymmetry include cleft lip or palate repair, neurofibromatosis, torticollis, and craniosynostosis.

Acquired causes include TMJ, ankylosis, trauma, radiotherapy, fibrous dysplasia, Romberg's disease, and dental conditions.

The ears are placed symmetrically on the lateral sides of the cranium. Proper position is determined by their relationship to the horizontal alignment of the eyes. Going back to the horizontal line through the corners of the eyes, extend the line laterally to the ear. The top of the ear should be aligned with the horizontal line.

Improper placement of the ears is most commonly related to "low set ears," which indicates that their position is below the horizontal line that extends from the lateral canthus of the eye.

Inspection Techniques and Expected Findings	Unexpected Findings
Other features contributing to facial symmetry are the eyebrows and nasolabial folds. Located above the eyes on the superior portion of the orbital ridge, the eyebrows' shape, position, and movement with facial expressions should be symmetrical.	**Madarosis**, loss of eyebrows and/or eyelashes) is a clinical sign that may be demonstrated in a wide variety of disorders and conditions encompassing local dermatological conditions to complex systemic diseases. (Kumar & Karthikeyan, 2012).
The nasolabial folds may only be visible during facial movement. When present, they should be symmetrically located and demonstrate symmetrical movement.	Nasolabial fold deviation, sagging, or flattening may be the first sign of Bell's palsy. (See Conditions and Disorders.)
Dimples may be present on the cheeks and are frequently bilateral; however, in some instances, they are unilateral. Clefts most commonly appear on the chin and are simply skin indentations. Neither dimples nor clefts are associated with any pathology.	
Cranial nerve assessments associated with the face are CN V and VII. CN V provides mainly sensory interpretation for the face. CN VII also innervates the facial muscles and provides motor messages to them, facilitating muscle movement for various facial expressions. Symmetry of facial movements indicates expected CN VII function (see Chapter 26).	Asymetric facial movements is a characteristic of Bell's Palsy. Other causes of facial nerve paralysis include: trauma, H. zoster, otitis media (acute/chronic), bacterial infections, and noninfectious causes, primarily related to surgery on the face for various reasons.
Neck	
Inspection of the neck should demonstrate placement in the midline, equidistant from the acromioum processes of the shoulders. The neck should be stable enough to support the head without the head wobbling or flopping. The SCM and trapezius muscle should be bilaterally symmetrical without any masses or webbing. The larynx, which connects the pharynx to the trachea, consists of single epiglottic, thyroid, and cricoid cartilages and paired arytenoid, corniculate, and cuneiform cartilages. The hyoid bone, although connected to the larynx, is not considered part of the larynx. The thyroid cartilage (Adam's apple), a midline structure, is an important superficial landmark as to the location of the thyroid gland.	Tremors of the head (titubations of the head), is an equilibrium dysfunction that may be caused by a cerebellar lesion. Obvious swelling or enlargement at the anterior base of the neck may be an indication of thyroid gland enlargement.
Inspection: Level II	
Face	
In addition to symmetry, the overall appearance of the face can provide indicators of underlying conditions. Certain conditions are almost always associated with visible facial alterations. There are a variety of causes for the changes. Congenital disorders often have characteristic facial features, which are discussed in developmental applications (see Disorders and Conditions).	Edema in the cheeks, creating a "moonface," is associated with Cushing's syndrome. Periorbital edema is seen in Nephrotic syndrome. Hyperthyroidism is accompanied by eye changes, causing them to appear "bug eyed," proptosis, prominent stare, lid lag, and Graves' ophthalmopathy. Hypothyroidism may be accompanied by a "lethargic" appearance to the face. Nerve damage to cranial nerve VII causes unilateral facial paralysis (Bell's palsy). Individuals with a terminal illness, most commonly cancer, develop cachexia, which causes a general wasting appearance to the face. A loss of subcutaneous tissue makes the cheeks appear sunken and the nose more prominent.

Inspection Techniques and Expected Findings	Unexpected Findings

Neck

Observe range of motion (ROM) of the neck by having the patient flex, extend, rotate, and laterally turn the head and neck. (Further evaluation of ROM is covered in Chapter 28.) Movement of the neck should be smooth and without any pain, moving both sides equally (Figure 17-11).

Limited ROM—less than expected degrees of rotation. Pain with moving neck, poor posture, trauma (whiplash), spasm (torticollis), musculoskeletal conditions (rheumatoid arthritis, osteoarthritis, osteoporosis, fibromyalgia).

Opisthotonus, which can be seen in TBI, cerebral palsy, tetanus, and meningitis, may be more pronounced in infants. It is a spasm of the entire body in which the entire spine is arched and lifted from the bed, with head and heels supporting the entire body.

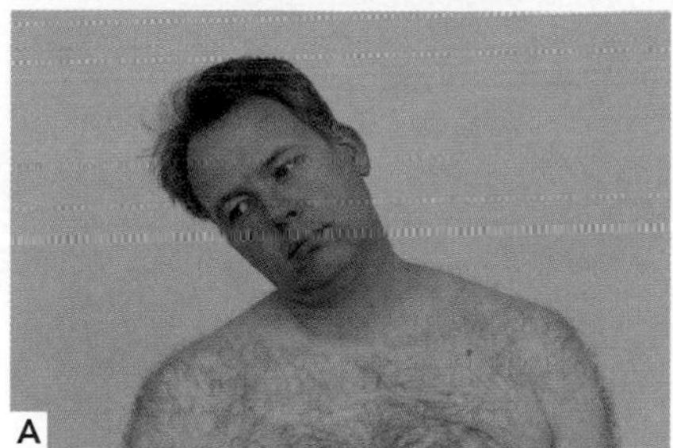

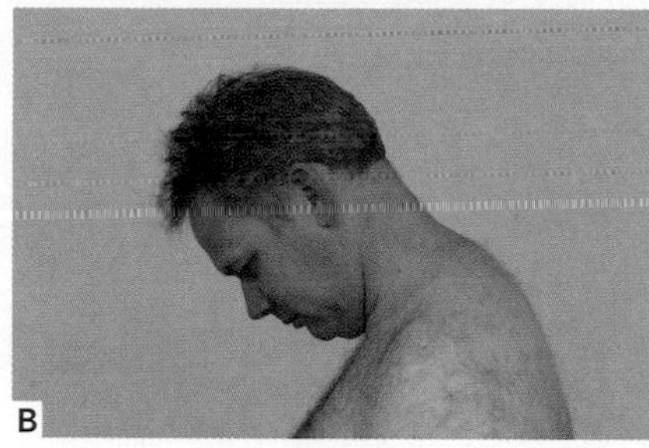

FIGURE 17-11A–B ROM of the neck

Inspection of the neck also provides information regarding the thyroid gland. Begin by having the patient slightly hyperextend the neck (Figure 17-12). Too great hyperextension may make the exam more difficult. Provide the patient with a glass of water and have the patient swallow it. During swallowing, the thyroid gland may be better visualized, allowing for the determination of size, symmetry, and contour. A lateral perspective of the neck may also provide better visualization. During this time it is also possible to observe the neck for any evidence of jugular venous distension (see Chapter 25 for further information).

Swallowing elevates the thyroid gland allowing for better inspection.

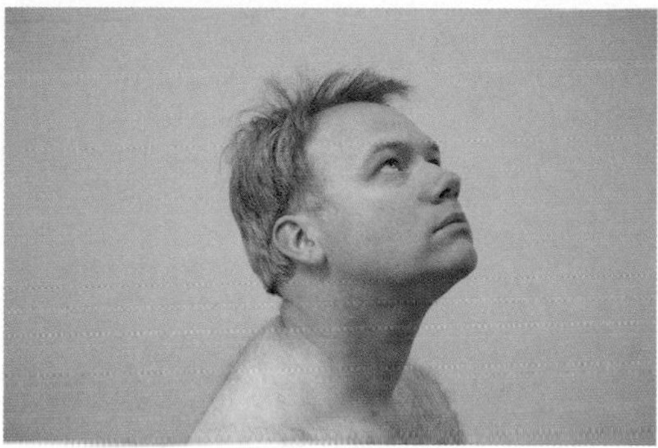

FIGURE 17-12 Frontal photo of neck in slight hyperextension with SCM and trapezius muscles prominent

Inspection: Level III

Much of the Level III exam related to the head and neck is not necessarily performed unless there is specific involvement of the area. An astute provider will note major alterations associated with the head, face, and neck. The ability to note alterations in symmetry or movement will become automatic and will not necessarily be categorized into any specific level of assessment. The details and descriptions of inspection and palpation for Level II exam can be selectively used for the critical exam. The condition of the patient will also determine what elements of the head, face, and neck assessment need to be performed.

THINK LINK: Cushing's Triad

Cushing's triad presence of systemic hypertension, bradycardia, and respiratory depression is a late sign of increased intracranial pressure.

THINK LINK: Meningitis

Patients with meningitis may present with fever, headache, nuchal rigidity [resistance to neck flexion], and altered mental status. However, these symptoms are only present in about 44% of adults with bacterial meningitis and even fewer children. No single sign is pathognomonic, and symptoms may vary and may be nonspecific depending on the host response and age of the patient. Symptoms may range from the above with or without nausea, vomiting, irritability, somnolence, lethargy, poor feeding, respiratory distress, seizures, hypothermia, and bulging fontanels in infants.

Meningitis in infants may not demonstrate neck stiffness. The presence of persistent fever in an infant with predisposing risk factors for meningitis like exposure to someone with HiB meningitis or Neisseria meningitis, recent ear or respiratory infection, travel to endemic areas, neurosurgical procedures penetrating head trauma, asplenia, cortisol excess, absent opsonizing antibody, complement deficiency, HIV infection, basilar skull fracture, bacteremia, and endocarditis should lower the threshold for a spinal tap.

Inspection Techniques and Expected Findings	Unexpected Findings
The most significant component of the critical exam for the head, face, and neck is determining the presence and extent of any head trauma or neck injury. No further assessments of the neck are carried out until it has been determined they can be done without any potential harm to the patient.	Hemodynamic stabilization of patients and cervical spine injury clearance are done simultaneously in head and neck injuries.
Data for emergencies related to head and neck injuries is commonly obtained by using the Glascow Coma Scale (GCS). This instrument gives points (3–15) according to the patient's responses to commands and physical manifestations to determine the severity of head injury. The GCS is described in greater detail in Chapter 26.	Individuals who have experienced mild TBI may demonstrate any of the following: cognitive deficits (reduction in attention, concentration, memory, executive functioning skills); behavioral/emotional changes (irritability, quickness to anger, emotional lability); physical symptoms (nausea/vomiting, dizziness, headache, blurred vision, sleep disturbance fatigue). Individuals who have sustained more severe TBI will most often demonstrate the characteristics of early phase recovery: severely decreased arousal/alertness, no indication or evidence of encoding/storing new information, negligible awareness of self or current situation, marginally purposeful actions, severely limited communication, significant confusion and disorientation. Higher scores correlate with better outcome in TBI patients. **Meningismus** is a term used to describe a constellation of signs and symptoms (triad of neck stiffness or nuchal rigidity, photophobia and headache) commonly used to denote meningeal irritation such as in meningitis and subarachnoid hemorrhage. Meningismus, Kernig and Brudzinski's signs are well described, but none of them are particularly sensitive in detecting meningeal irritation. Individuals with meningitis may present with specific manifestations related to meningeal irritation.

Palpation: Level I

Palpation Techniques and Expected Findings	Unexpected Findings
Head/Cranium Palpate the cranium with a gentle rotary motion for shape and symmetry. Its shape is determined by the bones of the skull and their unique shape. The cranium should be smooth without any palpable bumps, masses, or tenderness. Specific prominences of the skull that can be palpated are the forehead, the lateral edge of the parietal bone, the occipital bone, and the mastoid process. The location of these prominences should be symmetrically located (Figure 17-13).	The sutures between the bones should not be palpable, so the specific bones are not palpable.

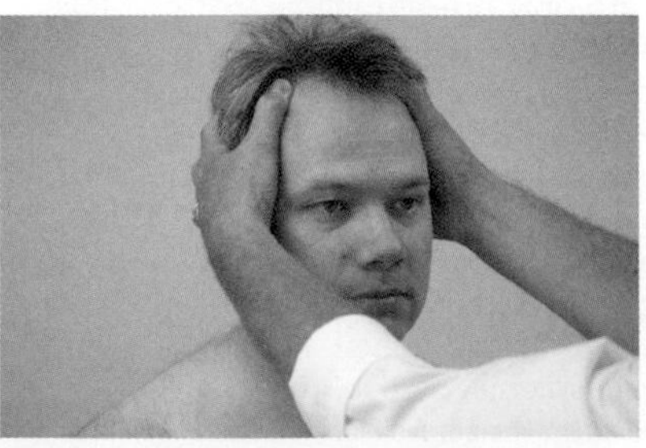

FIGURE 17-13 Palpation the skull

Palpation Techniques and Expected Findings	Unexpected Findings

Palpate the cranium for the presence of the temporal artery pulse. This artery is located above the zygomatic bone midway between the eye and the ear. It is not always palpable, so difficulty or inability to locate the pulse is not considered significant (Figure 17-14).

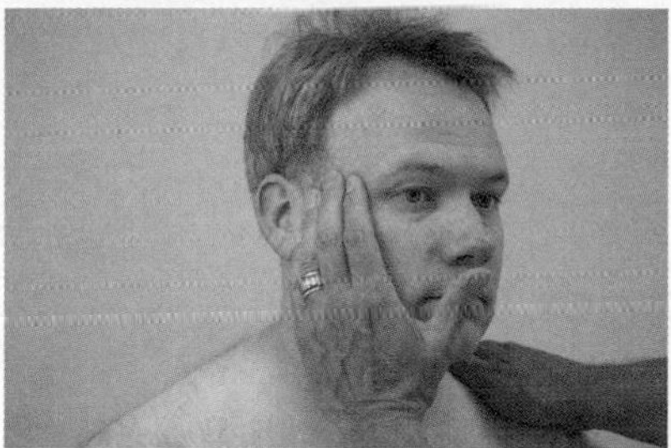

FIGURE 17-14 Palpation of temporal artery

Neck

Initial palpation of the neck is primarily related to other system assessments. Palpate the neck for the presence and quality of the carotid pulse (Figure 17-15). Also palpate it when assessing muscle strength, which is a part of the neurological (CN XI) and musculoskeletal exam.

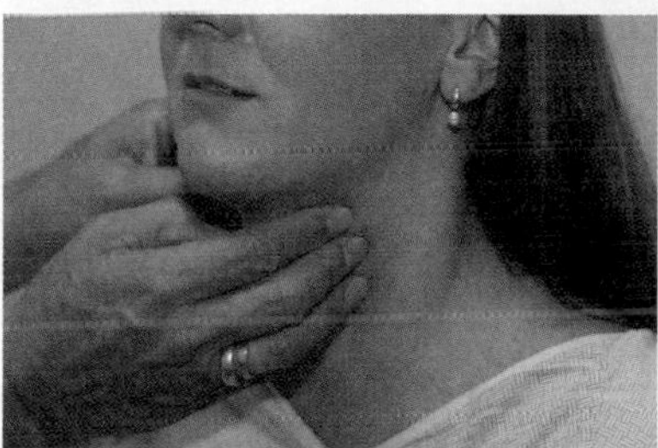

FIGURE 17-15 Palpation of carotid artery

Palpation: Level II

Palpate the neck to assess the trachea, thyroid gland, and lymph nodes. To palpate for the position of the trachea, place your thumbs on each side of the trachea in the lower portion of the neck. (This is also data for assessment of the lungs; see Chapter 23.)

Determine the distance between each thumb and the SCM, which should be equal (Figure 17-16).

An unequal distance or space may be an indication of a mass or other pathology of the neck or chest.

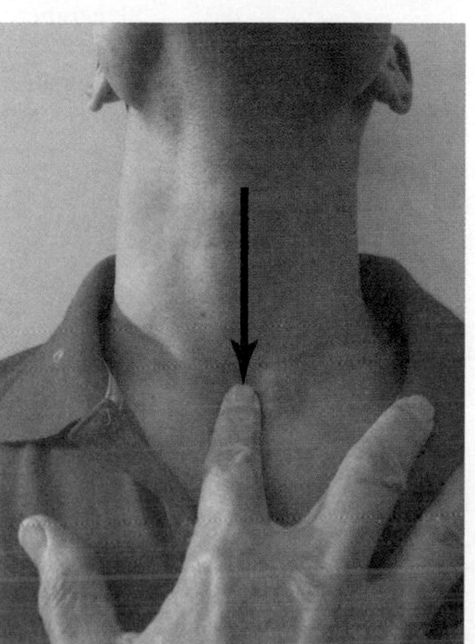

FIGURE 17-16 Palpation of trachea

Palpation Techniques and Expected Findings	Unexpected Findings

Lymph nodes may also be palpated at specific locations on the head and neck (Figure 17-17). (Further information of lymph nodes is provided in Chapter 21.)

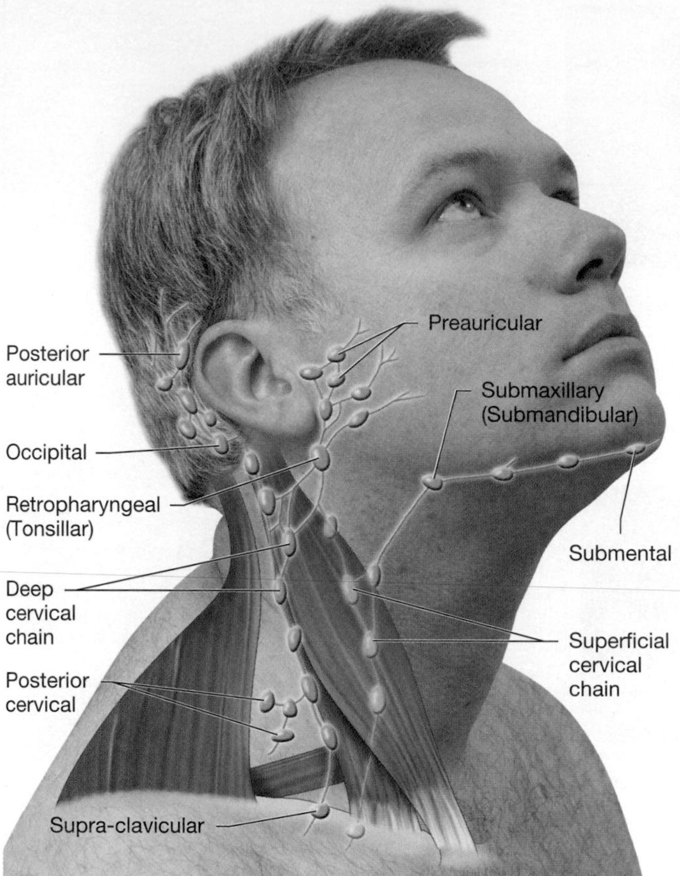

FIGURE 17-17 Location of lymph nodes

Palpate the thyroid gland from either an anterior or a posterior approach; both will provide the same information. Decide which approach works best and use it consistently. The thyroid gland is very soft and spongy. Pressing it from one side may displace it so it can be palpated by the contralateral fingers. It is best palpable on the medial aspect of SCM muscle.

It is also easier to palpate using a light touch; too much pressure may compress the thyroid gland, preventing its complete assessment (see Figure 17-18).

For both approaches, the patient's head should be in the same position. The patient should be sitting with the neck slightly flexed to relax the SCM. Next have the patient turn the neck toward the side that will be examined, further relaxing the muscle. You may also provide the patient with a glass of water for swallowing when requested. It may be easier to have the patient take a sip of water and hold it until requested to swallow.

If examining the patient from the anterior position, first place the ipsilateral thumb over the trachea, approximately 3 cm below the point of the thyroid cartilage. Have the patient swallow the water and try to identify the isthmus of the thyroid gland. Next palpate the lobe of the thyroid gland.

To examine the left lobe, move the right thumb to the side of the neck and gradually move the thumb toward the midline, exerting mild pressure as the thumb is moved. The pressure allows for displacement of the thyroid lobe toward the isthmus so that more of the thyroid gland can be palpated. With the left thumb, palpate the displaced tissue for any nodules. You may ask the patient to swallow again to elevate the tissue as it is palpated. To examine the other side, simply reverse the thumbs and the procedure.

PRACTICE POINT: Thyroid Palpation

Remember, the majority of the thyroid gland is beneath the SCM, so you will only be able to palpate the isthmus and a small portion of the wings.

Palpation Techniques and Expected Findings | **Unexpected Findings**

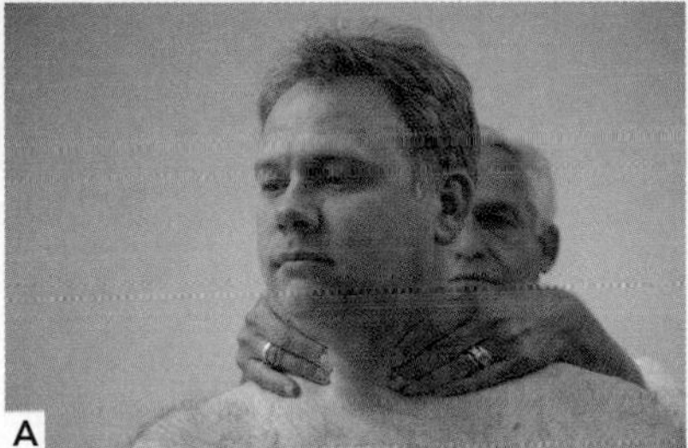

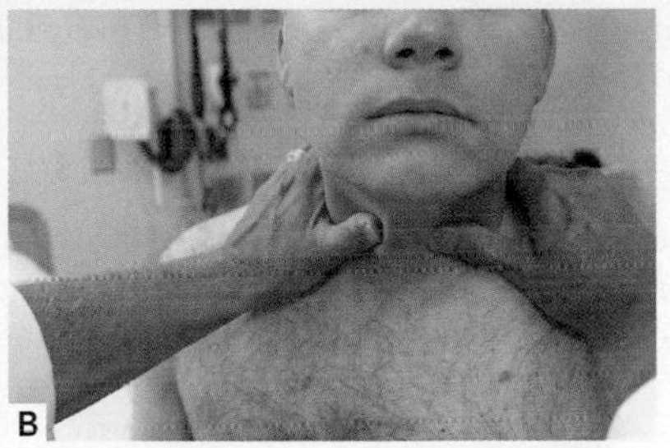

FIGURE 17-18A–B Palpation of thyroid from anterior and posterior approach

For the posterior approach, stand behind the patient and have the patient position the head and neck as previously described. Place two or three fingers just below the cricoid cartilage to identify the isthmus. To examine the right lobe of the thyroid gland, move the right hand to the side of the neck, and with gentle pressure move the fingers forward toward the middle of the neck. With the left hand fingers, gently palpate the thyroid tissue as it is being displaced toward the center. Ask the patient to swallow a sip of water, and as the patient swallows, palpate the thyroid tissue as it is elevated during swallowing.

No additional palpations are required for the cranium and face.

Auscultation: Levels I, II, III

Auscultation Techniques and Expected Findings | **Unexpected Findings**

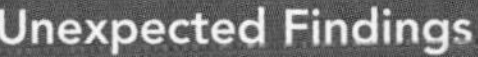

Auscultation of the neck is done to determine the presence of a thyroid bruit, the result of turbulent and accelerated blood flow through the thyroid gland (Figure 17-19). (This is further addressed in Chapter 25.)

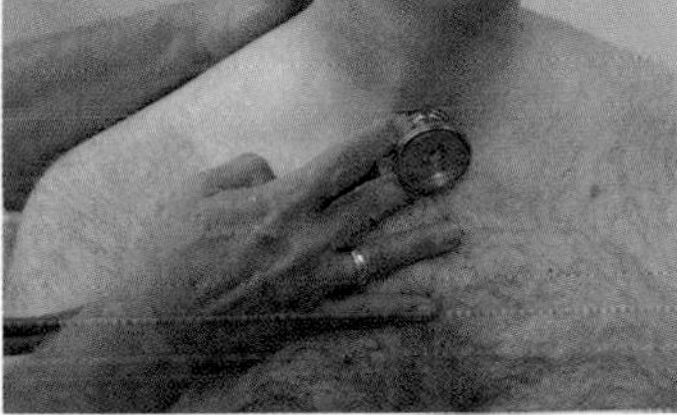

FIGURE 17-19 Auscultation of thyroid bruit

Unexpected Findings: A bruit is an indicator of thyroid hyperplasia. If the thyroid gland is enlarged, it also may be auscultated for the presence of a bruit. This is a blowing sound that corresponds with the heart rate. It is best heard with the bell of a stethoscope.

Developmental Applications

Techniques and Expected Findings | **Unexpected Findings**

Infants and Children

Initially the shape of the infant's head is the result of delivery through the birth canal. During passage through the birth canal, the cranial bones frequently override each other to accommodate the birth canal, resulting in the **molding** (Figure 17-20) of the infant's head. The amount of time that the infant has spent in the mother's pelvis prior to birth also influences the head shape. Infants who are delivered by caesarean section or have a breech presentation may not demonstrate any molding, as the head has traveled through the birth canal. The cranial bones resume their original position approximately 24–36 hours after birth.

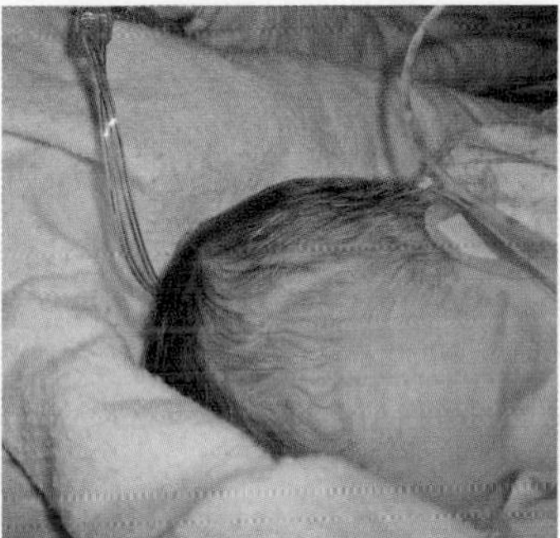

FIGURE 17-20 Molding of infant's head
Source: Courtesy of Jo Engle, RN, MSN, NNP-BC, and Vanessa Howell, RN, MSN

Techniques and Expected Findings

The initial assessment of the infant is the head circumference, frequently referred to as occipital frontal circumference (OFC), A tape measure is used to obtain the head circumference (Figure 17-21). The circumference ranges from 32 to 38 cm with an average of 34 cm.

Obtain the infant's chest circumference and compare it with the head circumference. The chest circumference is 2 cm smaller than the head circumference. During the first 2 years, rapid growth and development of the brain occurs, making the difference between the two measurements consistent until the age of 2 when they become equal. Throughout childhood, the chest circumference continues to grow, eventually reaching a 5–7 cm difference.

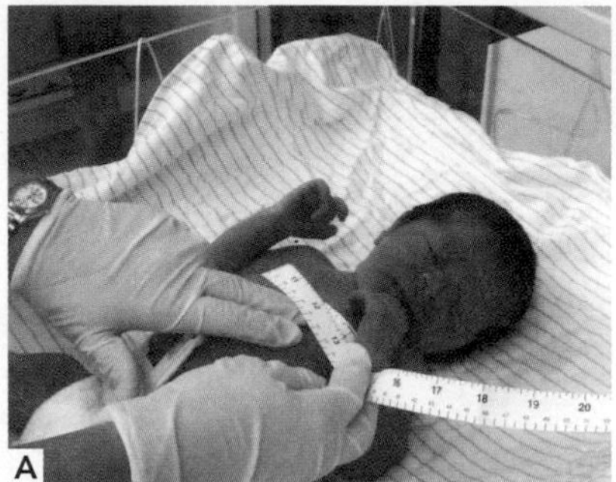

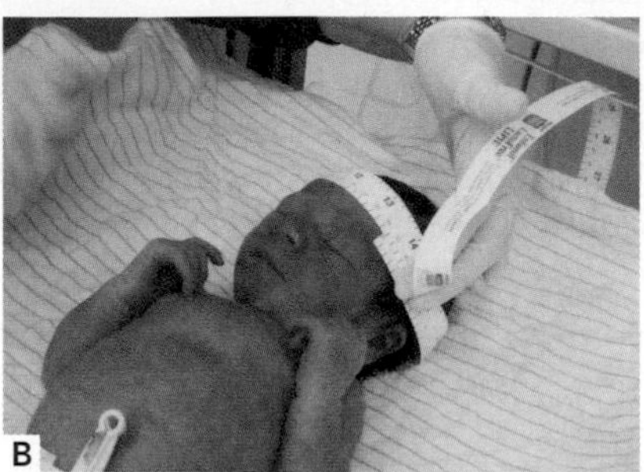

FIGURE 17-21A–B Measurement of chest and occipital-frontal circumference (OFC)
Source: Courtesy of Vanessa Howell, RN, MSN

The infant's head should be symmetrical in appearance. Molding should not alter the symmetry of the cranium.

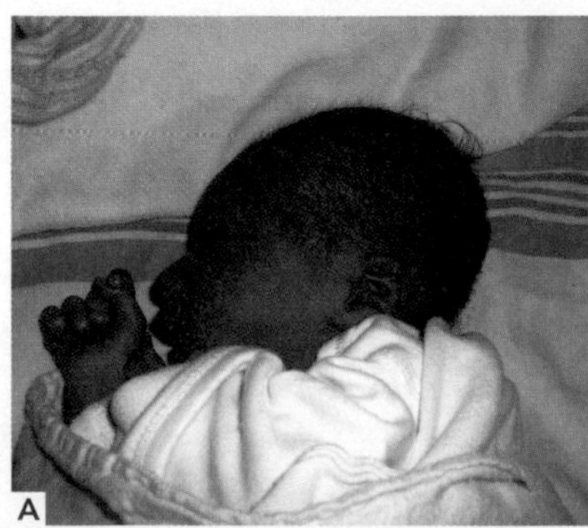

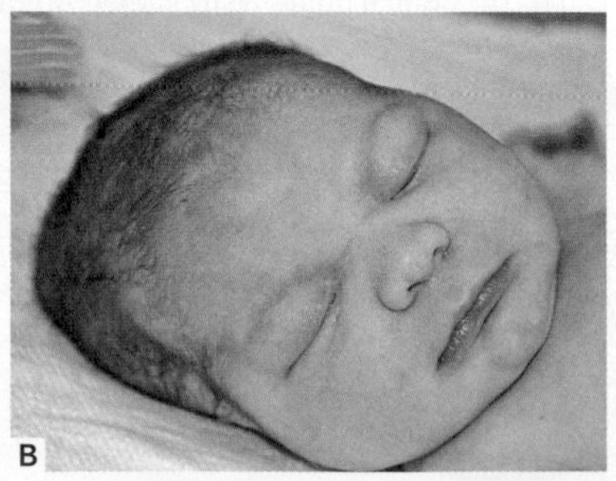

FIGURE 17-23A–B Two unexpected findings: **a)** caput succedaneum; **b)** cephalohematoma
Source B: Courtesy of Jo Engle, RN, MSN, NNP-BC, and Vanessa Howell, RN, MSN

Unexpected Findings

Two conditions that represent altered head size are microcephaly, smaller-than-expected head size, and macrocephaly, larger-than-expected head size. (See Conditions and Disorders.) **Macrocephaly** is a larger-than-expected head size. The most common cause of macrocephaly is **hydrocephalus**.

Anencephaly is a condition in which the brain (cerebrum) fails to develop in utero, resulting in a cranium that is relatively flat due to the absence of any brain tissue. Frequently there is brain stem development so that primary pulmonary and cardiac functions are present.

Hydrocephalus is a condition in which cerebral spinal fluid is unable to be removed from the brain ventricles, causing the ventricles to expand to accommodate the excess fluid (Figure 17-22). As a result of the expanding ventricles, the head also enlarges to accommodate them, causing the head circumference to increase dramatically.

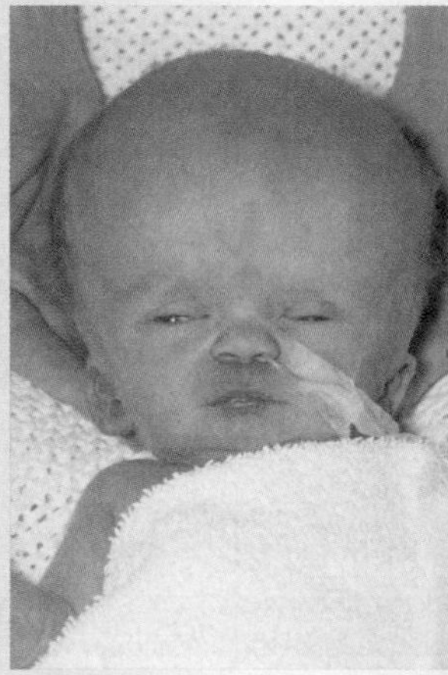

FIGURE 17-22 Macrocephaly (hydrocephalus)
Source: Ansary/Custom Medical Stock Photo

Two conditions that cause asymmetry of the cranium are **caput succedaneum** and **cephalohematoma**, which both result from birth trauma (Figure 17-23). The most common manifestation of birth trauma, caput succedaneum is subcutaneous edema, generally over the presenting part of the head during delivery. The occiput is the most common area involved with the edema crossing the suture lines. The affected area is soft with indistinct margins. The edema usually resolves by itself within the first few days after birth.

Techniques and Expected Findings	Unexpected Findings
	Cephalohematoma is a hemorrhage into the subperiostial space, thus it does not cross suture lines and its margins are well defined. It frequently is observed over the parietal region and may not develop until hours to days after birth. It is self-limiting and liquefies as it ages, disappearing after a few weeks.
The infant's face should be symmetrical with essentially the same features as the adult. Symmetry is easily observed during crying or other facial movements. Inspect the face for any indicators of congenital conditions or any color alterations.	
Assess the infant's head for movement and control. Perform gentle passive range of motion (ROM), turning the infant's head from left to right, flexion, extension, and rotation. The infant's head movements should be smooth without any resistance. After 3 to 4 months of age, the infant's head lag should disappear and the infant is capable of maintaining head control and following a light or small object to assess ROM.	A head tilt or limited ROM may suggest torticollis (wryneck) or SCM injury. (See Conditions and Disorders.)
The infant's neck is short and difficult to observe. It gradually lengthens during the first few years of life. To better observe the infant's neck, support the infant's shoulders and gradually lift the infant, allowing the neck to become extended. There should not be any visible pulsations, edema, distended veins, masses, or webbing.	Webbing, loose fanlike folds, if present may be an indication of Down or Turner syndrome. (See Conditions and Disorders.)
Palpate the infant's cranium to determine the size and tenseness of the anterior and posterior fontanels, which should feel firm with well-defined margins of the cranial bones. They may also feel slightly concave, but there should not be a large indentation.	There might be visible pulsations of the fontanels, but they should not be palpable.
Measure the length and width of the fontanels. The posterior fontanel is triangular shaped and may not be palpable at birth, but if it is it should measure approximately 1 cm. The anterior fontanel is diamond shaped and should not be larger than 4 to 5 cm. It may start out smaller at birth and then enlarge to approximately 2.5 cm by 2.5 cm. The posterior fontanel is expected to close by 1 to 2 months, and the anterior fontanel is expected to close between 9 months and 2 years.	
The cranial bones should feel smooth, firm, and fused, with the exception of the fontanels. A softening of the cranium, known as **craniotabes**, may be palpated along the parietal-occipital suture line, above and behind the ear. If present, a cracking or popping sound is heard, as well as a snapping sensation. There may also be the sensation like pressing on a ping pong ball. This may be considered an expected finding, especially in preterm infants.	Craniotabes is also associated with rickets, osteogenesis imperfecta, congenital syphilis, and hydrocephalus.
Palpate the SCM for strength, tone, and any masses.	A mass in the lower third of the SCM suggests a hematoma.
Palpate the clavicular area for any masses that may be present if the clavicle is fractured. The infant's thyroid gland is difficult to palpate and is generally omitted unless masses of nodules are noted in the neck. Palpation of the thyroid gland in children is basically the same as in adults.	Such fractures may occur during delivery.

Transillumination

Transillumination of an infant's skull is performed if there is suspicion of an intracranial lesion or an increasing head size. Due to the availability of radiographic scans, transillumination is not as frequently performed. To transilluminate the infant's skull, in a darkened room, place a flashlight or penlight firmly against the skull. The light creates a halo effect on the skull around the light. The ring of illumination should be 2 cm or less beyond the rim of the light source in all sections of the head, except the occipital.	If there is illumination beyond these parameters, it is suggestive of an increase in fluid or decreased brain tissue within the skull.

THINK LINK: Bulging Fontanel

Bulging fontanel in infants is neither sensitive nor specific for meningitis. In one review, bulging fontanel was present in only 20% of infants with meningitis and 13% of infants with normal CSF and viral infections other than meningitis.

The Pregnant Woman

The major change of the head and neck in the pregnant woman is the development of a blotchy, brown, hyperpigmentation of the face, known as chloasma (see Chapter 16).

Both thyroid gland activity and hormone production increases during pregnancy, causing a moderate enlargement of the thyroid gland. The increased size results from hyperplasia and increased vascularity. Despite the increased production of thyroid hormones, hyperthyroidism does not typically develop in pregnant women.

Techniques and Expected Findings	Unexpected Findings
 ***The Older Adult*** The faces of the elderly are a reflection of their nutritional status.	The face of the older adult may appear sunken, with loose skin due to the loss of subcutaneous tissue.
The cervical concave curve of the neck becomes accentuated with extension of the head as compensation for the kyphosis of the spine, frequently seen in the elderly. The ROM of the elderly individual's neck may be somewhat limited due to arthritis and degeneration of the spine. Even if there is no limitation or ROM, the motion is often slower and may not be painful, but may result in crepitus.	
Aging effects on the thyroid gland include atrophy and fibrosis of the gland as well as the development of nodules. The major difficulty in diagnosing thyroid dysfunction in older adults is that in most instances, the signs and symptoms that are manifest in the younger client are not present in the elderly. Frequently, the manifestations and characteristics of thyroid dysfunction in the elderly (fatigue, constipation, and cognitive impairment) are the same as those associated with other conditions or are expected aging changes (Mohandas & Gupta, 2003). Additionally, the manifestations may be mistaken for medication side effects, or as evidence of depression or dementia (Rehman et al., 2005).	Thyroid disorders are common in older adults and carry a significant morbidity if not treated (Rehman, Cope, Senseney, & Brezesinski, 2005). The incidence of thyroid disorders increases significantly after the age of 60. In this population, it is estimated that 0.5%–2.3% have hypothyroidism and that 2%–7.4% have overt hyperthyroidism (Mohandas & Gupta, 2003).
Hypothyroidism is frequently insidious in onset. Weight loss is experienced more frequently than weight gain. Thermoregulation in the elderly is less efficient, so many elderly are somewhat cold intolerant, making this classic manifestation less significant. An enlarged, palpable thyroid gland or goiter is uncommon; in fact, palpation of the thyroid in the elderly is more difficult, particularly in elderly females. Posture and skeletal changes associated with aging and osteoporosis change the shape of the neck, making palpation difficult, if not impossible.	Other musculoskeletal manifestations are frequently present in the elderly but not present in younger individuals. These include aches and pains that are not in or around the joints and carpal tunnel syndrome (Goldenberg, 2000).
With hyperthyroidism, the elderly may demonstrate delayed response time as well as a blunted or dull affect. An enlarged thyroid is again, uncommon, occurring in about 20%–40% of those affected. When thyromegaly is present, it is often nodular in the majority of instances. Ocular manifestations (exopthalmos) are also rare due to the lowered incidence of Graves' disease in the elderly. Cardiac involvement is not uncommon and is demonstrated by atrial fibrillation with a low ventricular response rate as well as manifestations of congestive heart failure and angina pectoris (Rehman et al., 2005). Muscle wasting and weakness will often be demonstrated during the musculoskeletal exam. Weight loss is commonly experienced in half of the cases and may exceed 20 pounds.	Apathetic hyperthyroidism may be seen in the elderly. Malignancy is a concern if the thyroid gland demonstrates the presence of nodules that are new or growing, hard or fixed, or single.

DOCUMENTATION

Head: Head erect and positioned on neck at midline without any involuntary movements or tilting. Skull rigid, normocephalic and, covered with dark brown hair that is thick, shiny and clean. Skin moves freely over skull and is intact without lesions or masses with homogenous color.

Face: Facial features symmetrical with symmetrical movement of facial structures when talking and with expressions. Without obvious edema.

Eyes positioned equidistant from midline in upper third of face. Eyebrows are full and even over each eye bilaterally. Eyelids positioned symmetrically over eyeball. Eyelids approximated when closed. Ears positioned on side of head in correct alignment with palpebral fissures. Nose positioned midline with straight septum. Lips appear moist without lesions or cracking.

Neck: Supple without scars, lesions or masses. Trachea midline and elevates with swallowing Thyroid gland felt when individual swallows and is without masses bilaterally. Shoulder shrug/strength equal bilaterally (CN XI).

Electronic Charting

Expectations of Electronic Charting

Like other assessments, you should be able to document all parts of the head and neck assessment including assessment of cranial nerves. Developmental variations should be taken into consideration; for example, documentation of the head and neck assessment for infants and children should include ability to document fontanels. Electronic growth charts should include the ability to chart head circumference, in addition to height and weight charts.

Limitations of Electronic Charting

Limitations for the head and neck assessment are similar to other assessments. Documentation of emotions and communications may require free text, rather than structured charting in some systems.

Summary

- The head (cranium) comprises 8 cranial bones and 14 facial bones that protect the brain and sensory organs and is covered with muscles and skin, which provide support and protection for external structures.
- The external structures of the face (eyes, ears, nose, and mouth) are primarily sensory organs, which are specifically positioned, giving characteristic features of the face.
- The neck, which is centrally positioned between the shoulders, provides support for the head and allows for movement of the cranium (head).
- The neck contains the first 7 cervical vertebrae (through which the spinal cord passes) and the larynx, trachea, and thyroid gland.
- The cranial bones of an infant are not fused, which allows for growth and development of the brain through the first couple of years of life.
- Inspection and palpation are the primary techniques for assessment of the head and neck, which relates to symmetry and recognition of facial alterations that are associated with various conditions and disorders.
- Health promotion issues related to the head and neck are related to the reduction of traumatic brain injuries in all age categories.

Review Questions

1. The provider is caring for a patient with Cushing's syndrome. The provider would expect that the patient's face would appear
    1. rounded with red cheeks.
    2. sunken with prominent cheek bones.
    3. asymmetrical with no movement on one side.
    4. oval with edema around the eyes.
2. When teaching cranial anatomy to a group of students, the provider uses which term when describing the fused joints between the cranial bones?
    1. connections
    2. sutures
    3. links
    4. junctions
3. To assess the symmetry of the nasal labial folds, the provider should ask the patient to do which of the following?
    1. Clench the teeth.
    2. Stick out the tongue.
    3. Smile.
    4. Move the mandible back and forth.
4. When palpating the patient's neck, the provider places the fingers just below the cricoid cartilage to help locate the
    1. carotid artery.
    2. external jugular veins.
    3. lobes of the thyroid gland.
    4. thyroid gland isthmus.
5. When the provider is palpating the right side of the patient's thyroid gland, the patient's head position should be
    1. hyperextended with the chin pointed to the left.
    2. flexed with the chin pointed to the right.
    3. hyperextended with the chin pointed to the right.
    4. flexed with the chin pointed to the left.
6. The provider is teaching a parenting class focused on normal growth and development. When discussing closure of the fontanels of a child's skull, the provider should include which information? (Select all that apply.)
    1. The posterior fontanel is usually closed at about 2 months of age.
    2. The fontanels close when full ossification of the skull has occurred.
    3. The anterior fontanel closes prior to the closure of the posterior fontanel.
    4. Fontanels may not close until adulthood.
    5. The anterior fontanel should be closed by about 2 years of age.
7. The provider is assessing an adult patient with a chief complaint of new onset headaches. The provider would suspect that the client is suffering from migraines because the patient (Select all that apply.)
    1. is a female.
    2. complains of tenderness when the scalp is palpated.
    3. describes the headaches as "throbbing."
    4. states that the location of the pain is in the occipital.
    5. describes an aura before the onset of pain.
8. The provider may suspect that a patient is suffering from hypothyroidism if which assessment finding is noted?
    1. recent weight loss
    2. resting heart rate of 103 beats per minute
    3. thinning hair
    4. dry skin
9. The provider is assessing a patient for symmetry of facial expressions. The function of which cranial nerve is being evaluated?
    1. CN IV
    2. CN V
    3. CN VI
    4. CN VII
10. The provider is preparing to perform an assessment of an older adult patient with a diagnosis of traumatic brain injury. The provider is aware that this patient likely
    1. has a genetic brain condition.
    2. has Alzheimer's type dementia.
    3. suffered an injury.
    4. is having a reaction to medication.

Conditions and Disorders

FACIES

In medical contexts, facies are specific and distinctive facial characteristics that are associated with unique expressions or appearances associated with specific medical conditions. Some facial manifestations are so representative of certain conditions or disorders that they instantly suggest a diagnosis.

Cushing's Syndrome (Disease)

This is a condition in which the manifestations are related to prolonged exposure to increased levels of cortisol.

Pathophysiology

- Cushing's disease refers to a pituitary-dependent endogenous cause of Cushing's syndrome: a tumor (adenoma) in the pituitary gland produces large amounts of ACTH or CRH.
- Cushing's syndrome is caused by exogenous administration of glucocorticoids prescribed by a health care provider to treat other diseases (asthma and rheumatoid arthritis) or in immunosuppression after an organ transplant.
- In rare cases, Cushing's can cause hypercalcemia, which can lead to skin necrosis.

Subjective

- Rapid weight gain, hyperhidrosis (excess sweating).
- Easy bruising and dryness, particularly the hands and other mucous membranes.
- Excess cortisol may cause insomnia, inhibited aromatase, reduced libido, and impotence in men.
- Patients frequently suffer various psychological disturbances, ranging from euphoria to psychosis. Depression and anxiety are also common.

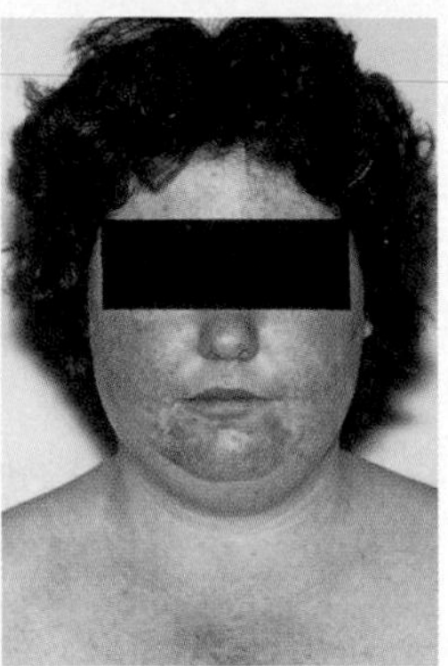

FIGURE 17-24 Cushing's syndrome
Source: John Radcliffe Hospital/Science Source Images

Objective

- Fat deposition of trunk with sparing of the limbs (central obesity), growth of fat pads along the collar bone/back of the neck, and face producing a round face (moon face).
- Skin alterations including telangiectasia; skin thinning resulting in purple or red striae on the trunk, buttocks, arms, legs or breasts; proximal muscle weakness (hips, shoulders).
- Hirsutism, baldness, and/or extremely dry and brittle hair, amenorrhea/oligomenorrhea, and infertility in women due to elevations in androgens.
- Studies have also shown that the resultant amenorrhea is due to hypercortisolism, which feeds back onto the hypothalamus resulting in decreased levels of GnRH release.

Addison's Disease (AD, Chronic Adrenal Insufficiency, Hypocortisolism, and Hypoadrenalism)

This is a rare, chronic endocrine disorder caused by insufficient adrenal gland production of steroid hormones (glucocorticoids and often mineralocorticoids). It is characterized by a number of relatively nonspecific symptoms, such as abdominal pain and weakness, but under certain circumstances, these may progress to Addisonian crisis (adrenal crisis), a medical emergency that may include very low blood pressure and coma. It is a constellation of symptoms indicative of severe adrenal insufficiency, which may result from either previously undiagnosed Addison's disease, a disease process suddenly affecting adrenal function (such as adrenal hemorrhage), or development of another condition (e.g., infection, trauma) in someone known to have Addison's disease. It requires immediate emergency treatment.

Pathophysiology

- Arises from problems with the adrenal gland, (primary adrenal insufficiency), and is unrelated to pituitary gland dysfunction.
- Most frequent cause is destruction of the adrenal gland via autoimmune processes; however, destruction may also be caused by infections, malignancy, certain medications, and trauma. It is also common for the adrenal gland to also stop producing aldosterone.

Subjective

- Symptoms are often nonspecific and may take some time to be recognized.
- Common symptoms: fatigue, lightheadedness upon standing/while upright, muscle weakness, fever, weight loss, difficulty in standing up, anxiety, nausea, vomiting, diarrhea, headache, sweating, changes in mood and personality, and joint and muscle pains.
- Craving for salt or salty foods from urinary losses of sodium.

Objective

- Low blood pressure that decreases with standing (orthostatic hypotension).
- Hyperpigmentation of skin, including areas not exposed to the sun; characteristic sites are skin creases (e.g., of the hands), nipple, and the inside of the cheek (buccal mucosa. Also, old scars may darken.
- Medical conditions, such as type 1 diabetes, thyroid disease (Hashimoto thyroiditis, goiter), and vitiligo often occur together with Addison's. Manifestations of any of these conditions may also occur in the individual with Addison's.

Hypothyroidism

Conditions associated with under production (hypothyroidism) and over production (hyperthyroidism) of thyroid hormone also present with classic facial features. Hypothyroidism is a common endocrine disorder due to a deficiency of thyroid hormone (T_3/T_4). In the United States and other countries in which iodine intake is adequate, autoimmune thyroid disease (Hashimoto disease) is the most common cause of hypothyroidism; worldwide, iodine deficiency remains the foremost cause. Hypothyroidism is not considered to be life threatening unless there is not treatment for it. Advanced, untreated hypothyroidism is referred to as myxedema. At this point, it can be life threatening and may result in death if not treated.

Pathophysiology

- Commonly is a primary process in which thyroid gland is unable to produce sufficient amounts of thyroid hormone.
- Can also be secondary: thyroid gland is normal but receives insufficient stimulation because of low secretion of thyrotropin (i.e., thyroid-stimulating hormone [TSH]) from the pituitary gland.
- Tertiary hypothyroidism, inadequate secretion of thyrotropin-releasing hormone (TRH) from the hypothalamus, leads to insufficient release of TSH, which in turn causes inadequate thyroid stimulation.
- Congenital hypothyroidism, affecting 1/4000 newborns, is due to fetal maldevelopment of the thyroid.

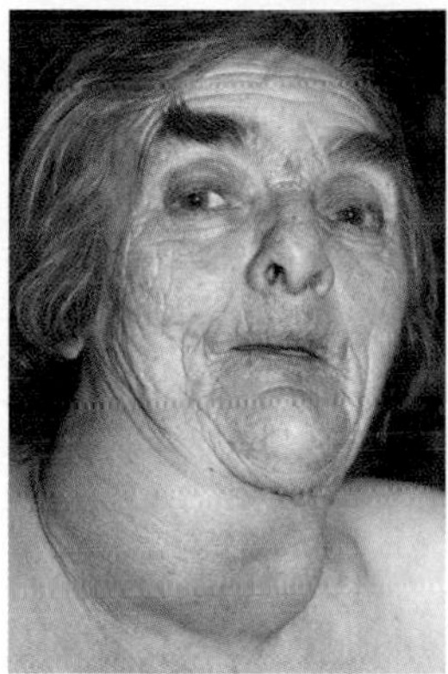

FIGURE 17-25 Face of hypothyroidism
Source: Dr. P. Marazzi/Science Source Images

Subjective

- Decreased appetite
- Cold intolerance
- Dry skin/decreased perspiration/hair loss
- Sleepiness/lethargy
- Muscle pain, joint pain, weakness in the extremities
- Emotional ability, mental impairment, depression
- Forgetfulness, impaired memory, inability to concentrate
- Constipation
- Menstrual disturbances, impaired fertility
- Paresthesias
- Blurred vision/decreased hearing
- Fullness in the throat

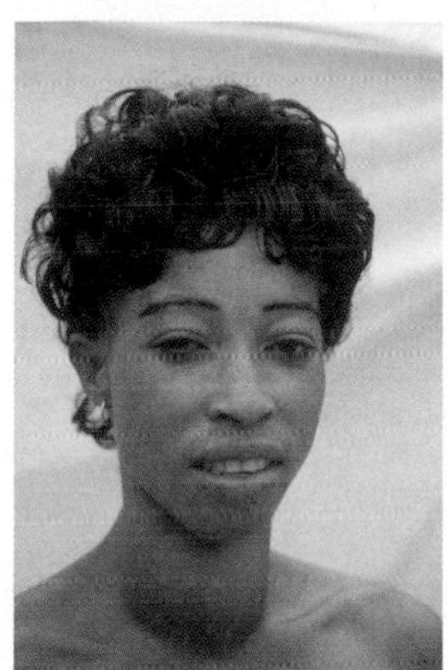

FIGURE 17-26 Goiter
Source: Scott Camazine/Science Source Images

Objective

- Weight gain
- Dull facial expression (less animated), coarse facial features, periorbital puffiness (drooping eyelids), macroglossia
- Slowed speech and movements
- Dry skin
- Pallor
- Coarse, brittle hair/fingernails
- Loss of scalp hair, axillary hair, pubic hair, or a combination
- Goiter (simple or nodular)—only presents as a problem if it gets to large and interferes with breathing/swallowing
- Hoarseness
- Decreased systolic blood pressure and increased diastolic blood pressure
- Bradycardia
- Pericardial effusion
- Nonpitting edema (myxedema)
- Pitting edema of lower extremities
- Hyporeflexia with delayed relaxation, ataxia, or both

PRACTICE POINT: Myxedema

Myxedema coma is a severe form of hypothyroidism that most commonly occurs in individuals with undiagnosed or untreated hypothyroidism who are subjected to an external stress. Features include altered mental status, hypothermia, bradycardia, hypercarbia, hyponatremia. Cardiomegaly, pericardial effusion, cardiogenic shock, and ascites may be present.

Hyperthyroidism

This is a set of disorders that involve excess synthesis and secretion of thyroid hormones by the thyroid gland, resulting in a hypermetabolic condition of thyrotoxicosis. Its most common forms include diffuse toxic goiter (Graves' disease), toxic multinodular goiter (Plummer disease), and toxic adenoma. Graves' disease (50%–60%) is an autoimmune condition in which antibodies stimulate the thyroid gland to grow and enlarge, overproducing thyroid hormone.

Pathophysiology

- Secretion of thyroid hormone (T_3/T_4) is regulated by a complex feedback mechanism by interaction of stimulatory and inhibitory factors. Thyrotropin-releasing hormone (TRH) from hypothalamus stimulates pituitary gland to release TSH, which bind to receptors on thyroid gland releasing thyroid hormones. Elevated levels of T_3/T_4 act on the hypothalamus and decrease TRH secretion and thus the synthesis of TSH.
- Thyroid hormones diffuse into the peripheral circulation, of which 99.9% of T_4 and T_3 is bound to plasma proteins and is inactive. Free T_3 is 20–100 times more biologically active than free T_4.
- Unbound T_3/T_4 results in thyrotoxicosis, which results in an increase in transcription in cellular proteins, causing an increase in the basal metabolic rate.
- Additional manifestations of thyrotoxicosis result from cardiac and respiratory stimulation. Thyroid storm is associated with the extreme manifestations. When thyrotoxicosis transforms into thyroid storm is not well established and is often subjective in nature (Nayak & Burman, 2006).

Subjective

- Nervousness
- Anxiety
- Increased perspiration
- Heat intolerance
- Hyperactivity
- Palpitations

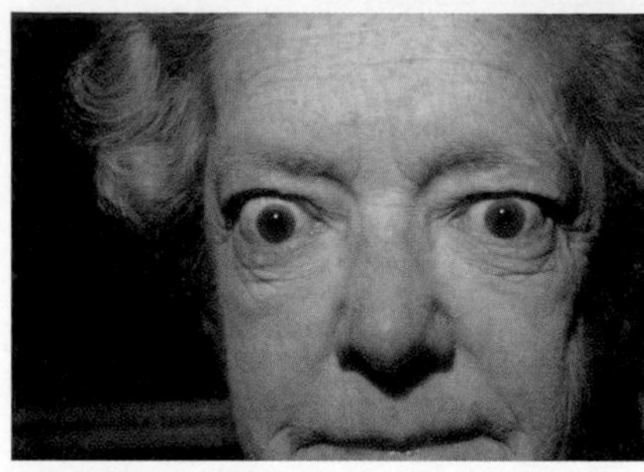

FIGURE 17-27 Exopthalomos
Source: Dr. P. Marazzi

Objective

- Tachycardia or atrial arrhythmia
- Systolic hypertension
- Warm, moist, smooth skin
- Lid lag
- Stare
- Hand tremor
- Muscle weakness
- Weight loss despite increased appetite
- Reduction in menstrual flow or oligomenorrhea
- Appearance of the eyes to "bug out" or protrude from the eye socket (proptosis), giving an over alert appearance and referred to as exopthalmos.

Bell's Palsy

This is a form of unilateral facial paralysis from a dysfunction (neuritis) of cranial nerve VII (facial), causing the inability to control facial muscles on the affected side. The hallmark of this condition is a rapid onset of partial or complete unilateral paralysis that often appears overnight. In rare cases (< 1%), it can occur bilaterally, resulting in total facial paralysis. There appears to be no gender preference, but it is seen more commonly in females between the ages of 10 and 19 and those who are pregnant. In pregnant women, it frequently occurs in the third trimester and those with preeclampsia. In terms of age, those with the highest incidence are adults over 60. The extent of involvement is related to the degree of nerve involvement. The average length of paralysis is 3 weeks and 80%–90% recover without any residual effects.

Pathophysiology

- It is thought that an inflammatory condition leads to swelling of the facial nerve. The nerve travels through the skull in a narrow bone canal beneath the ear. Nerve swelling and compression in the narrow bone canal are thought to lead to nerve inhibition, damage, or death.
- Mounting evidence suggests that herpes simplex I and herpes zoster are the causative agents. These viruses become reactivated from the facial nerve ganglia (Taylor et al., 2011).
- Other etiologies considered are autoimmune, inflammatory, or ischemic causes.
- Brain tumor, stroke, myasthenia gravis, and Lyme disease are possible causes.
- It is the most common acute mononeuropathy and the most common cause of acute facial nerve paralysis (>80%).

Subjective

- Manifestations may include poor closure of the eyelids, decreased tearing, posterior ear pain, and taste disturbances.

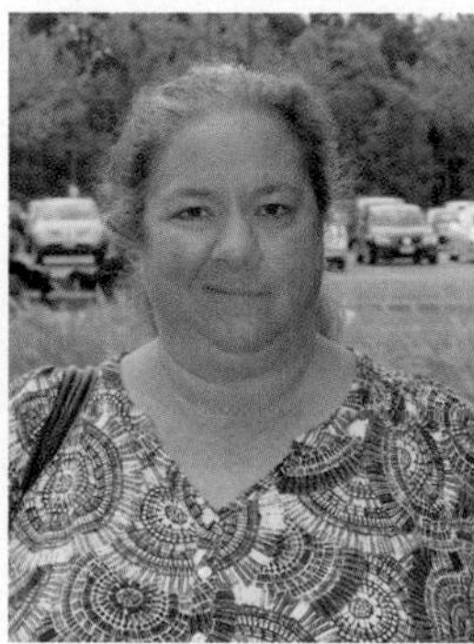

FIGURE 17-28 Bell's palsy

Objective

- Facial paralysis results in drooping of face and asymmetry of facial expressions with movement observed only on the unaffected side.

Nephrotic Syndrome (Facies)

This is a condition in which the glomerulus of the kidneys are being damaged, becoming permeable to protein (albumin). It is not a disease, but a warning that the kidneys are being damaged or destroyed. Without treatment, it may result in kidney failure. It can occur at any age but is most common in children between the ages of 18 months and 8 years.

Pathophysiology

- May be associated with multiple renal conditions that cause damage to the glomerular structures by various mechanisms, which cause a breach of the glomerular filtration barrier.
- Glomerular structural damage is the primary mechanism that may cause proteinuria.
- Albuminuria may occur, or, with greater injury, leakage of all plasma proteins (i.e., proteinuria) may take place.
- Many conditions can cause this glomerular damage, including diabetes, lupus, infection, certain cancers, and some medicines; often the cause is unknown.
- A form of kidney disease called minimal change disease (or "nil disease") causes most of the cases in children, but its cause is unknown.

Subjective

- No noticeable physical symptoms, but when present, they can include shortness of breath caused by fluid buildup in the lungs (pulmonary edema).
- Adults older than 65 may be misdiagnosed with heart failure.
- Children are often thought to have allergies.
- Dry skin.

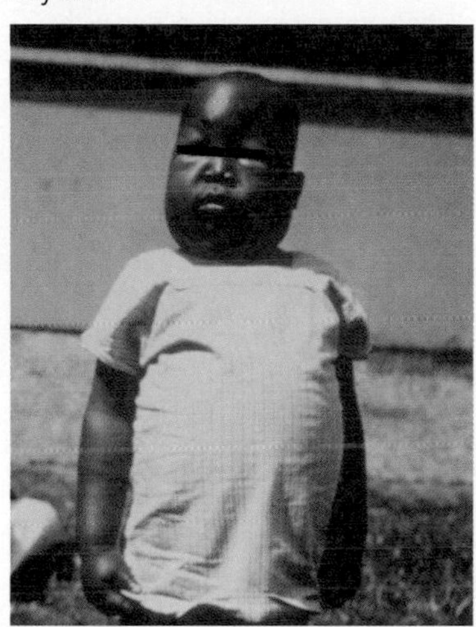

FIGURE 17-29 Face of nephrotic syndrome
Source: CDC/Dr. Myron Schultz

Objective

- Swelling in the tissues around the eyes (periorbital edema) or in the feet or ankles (peripheral edema). This is the most common early symptom of nephrotic syndrome in both children and adults.
- Edema around the eyes may cause the sockets to disappear, giving an overall rounded appearance to the face that is different from the edema of Cushing's syndrome. The skin may also be pale and particularly noticeable on the face.
- Scrotal edema, which may cause testicular torsion.
- Protein in the urine (proteinuria).
- Low protein (albumin) in the blood.
- High cholesterol and triglyceride levels.
- Low blood levels of iron and vitamin D.

Cachexia

Also called wasting syndrome, this is a complex metabolic condition of loss of weight, muscle atrophy, fatigue, weakness, and significant loss of appetite in an individual not actively trying to lose weight. Specifically, it is the loss of body mass that cannot be reversed nutritionally, even if more calories are consumed. All muscles of the body are affected, with the facial appearance of an individual affected most dramatically. It is seen in patients with cancer, AIDS, chronic obstructive lung disease, multiple sclerosis, congestive heart failure, tuberculosis, familial amyloid polyneuropathy, mercury poisoning (acrodynia), and hormonal deficiency. It is a positive risk factor for death, physically weakening patients to a state of immobility from loss of appetite, asthenia, and anemia, and response to standard treatment is usually poor.

Pathophysiology

- The exact mechanism in these diseases that causes cachexia is poorly understood, but there is probably a role for inflammatory cytokines, such as tumor necrosis factor-alpha (nicknamed "cachexin" or "cachectin").
- Malnutrition syndromes are kwashiorkor and marasmus, which don't have an underlying illness; most often symptomatic of severe malnutrition.
- Individuals with eating disorder anorexia nervosa have high plasma levels of ghrelin (also elevated in patients with cancer cachexia).

Subjective

- Weight loss
- Anorexia
- Generalized fatigue (asthenia)

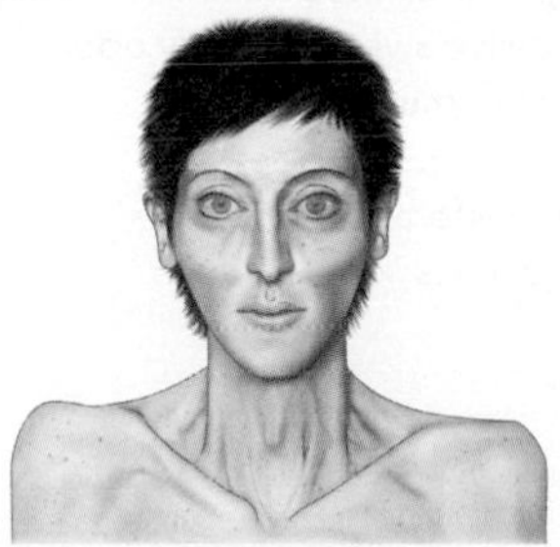

FIGURE 17-30 Cachexia

Objective

- Eyes appear sunken, as well as the cheeks and temporal area.
- Nose becomes more prominent and appears sharp or well defined.
- Skin is also rough and dry.

Systemic Lupus Erythematosus (SLE, Lupus)

SLE is a systemic autoimmune (connective tissue) disease that can affect any part of the body. Parts of the body commonly affected are heart, joints, skin, lungs, blood vessels, liver, kidneys, and nervous system. Its course is unpredictable, alternating with periods of illness (called *flares*) and remission. SLE occurs nine times more often in women, especially those in child-bearing years (15 to 35), and in those of non-European descent. Women with SLE have an increased risk for miscarriage and increased blood pressure (preeclampsia).

Pathophysiology

- The immune system attacks the body's cells by producing antibodies (rogue) against itself, particularly against proteins in the cell nucleus, causing inflammation and tissue damage.
- It is a Type III hypersensitivity reaction in which antibody-immune complexes precipitate and cause a further immune response.
- SLE is triggered by environmental and genetic factors that remain unknown. Other causes may be related to ultraviolet light, viruses, and medications (procainamide, hydralazine).

Subjective

- Common initial and chronic complaints include fever, malaise, joint pains, myalgias, fatigue, weight loss, blood clots, alopecia, and temporary loss of cognitive abilities.
- Because these are commonly associated with other conditions, these symptoms are not diagnostic criteria for SLE.
- When present in conjunction with other manifestations, however, they are considered suggestive.

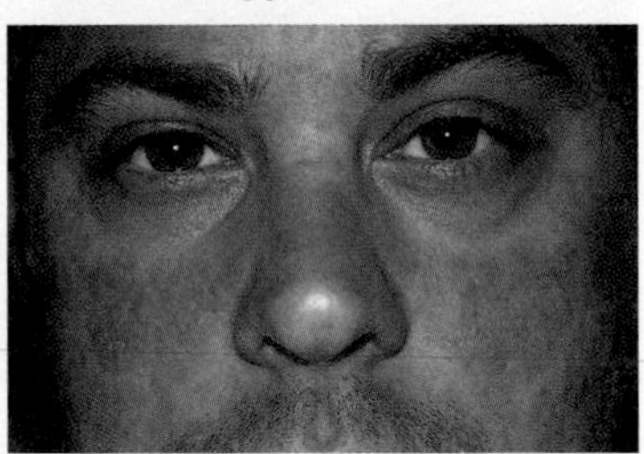

FIGURE 17-31 Butterfly rash of SLE
Source: Science Photo Library/Custom Medical Stock Photo

Objective

- SLE affects many organ systems; however, the signs identified here only relate to dermatological manifestations associated with the head.
- Malar (butterfly) rash is commonly observed.
- Some may exhibit thick, red scaly patches on the skin ("discoid lupus").
- Alopecia occurs in about 45% of individuals with SLE; mouth, ulcers, and lesions on the skin are also possible manifestations.
- Tiny tears in delicate tissue around the eyes can occur after even minimal rubbing.

PRACTICE POINT: SLE

SLE is one of several diseases known as "the great imitators" because it frequently mimics or is mistaken for other conditions. SLE is a classical item in differential diagnosis because SLE symptoms vary widely and come and go unpredictably. Diagnosis can thus be elusive, with some people suffering unexplained symptoms of untreated SLE for years. While there are similarities in manifestations of SLE, there is a high degree of variability related to course or degree of involvement of SLE so that no two cases are exactly alike.

Acromegaly

This is a condition in which there is an overproduction of growth hormone in the adult. Because it is uncommon, the pathogenesis and slow progression of acromegaly makes the disease hard to diagnose in its stages and is frequently missed for years until changes in external features, especially the face, become noticeable. Acromegaly most commonly affects adults in middle age and can result in severe disfigurement, complicating conditions, and premature death if unchecked. It is frequently associated with gigantism.

Pathophysiology

- A variety of disorders may increase the pituitary's GH output, although most commonly it is a GH-producing tumor (pituitary adenoma) derived from a distinct type of cell (somatotrophs).
- During puberty, rapid growth in the length of the bones is due to growth hormone stimulating the epiphysial plate

Subjective

- Individuals may notice that rings no longer fit or shoe size has increased.
- Excessive sweating/body odor
- Fatigue, muscle weakness
- Deeper, husky voice
- Vision alterations
- Headaches

Objective

- Manifestations of this condition result from high level of GH or expanding tumor and are most prominent on the face and hands.
- Soft tissue swelling visibly resulting in enlargement of the hands, feet, nose, lips, and ears, and a general thickening of the skin.

- At some point in the late teens or early twenties, the epiphysial plate fuses so that no more linear growth can occur.
- Growth hormone production after fusion results in lateral bone growth causing the bones to become thicker.

- Difficulty swallowing/enlarged tongue
- Joint pain/limited mobility

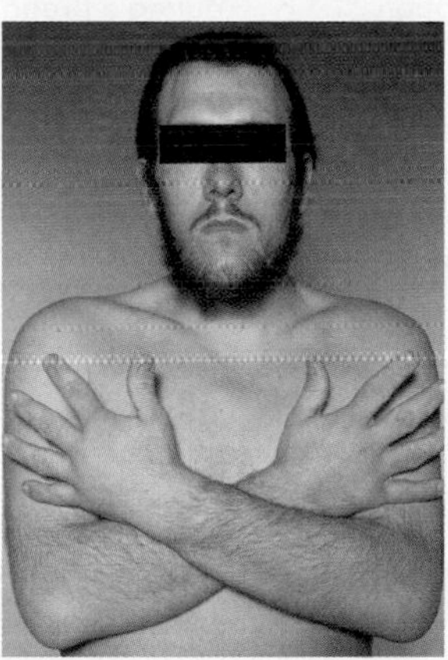

FIGURE 17-32 Acromegaly
Source: John Radcliffe Hospital/Science Source Images

- Soft tissue swelling of internal organs, notably the heart with attendant weakening of its muscularity, and the kidneys, also the vocal cords resulting in a characteristic thick, deep voice and slowing of speech.
- Generalized expansion of the skull at the fontanel and pronounced brow protrusion, often with ocular distension
- Pronounced lower jaw protrusion with attendant macroglossia and teeth gapping
- Possible hirsutism
- Acrochordon (skin tags)
- Carpal tunnel syndrome

Down Syndrome (Trisomy 21)

This is a genetic disorder caused by the presence of all or part of a third copy of chromosome 21. Chromosome 21 is the most commonly affected, but chromosome 17 has also been implicated. It is the most common chromosome abnormality in humans and is typically associated with a delay in cognitive ability (mental retardation), physical growth, and a particular set of facial characteristics. The average IQ of young adults with Down syndrome is around 50 (severe degree of intellectual disability), whereas young adults without the condition typically have an IQ of 100. Down syndrome is characterized by decelerated maturation (neoteny), incomplete morphogenesis (vestigia), and atavisms. Life expectancy for individuals with DS has increased significantly. In the early part of the 20th century, it was not expected that the individual would live much past 10 years.

A pregnancy after age 40 is considered a risk factor for giving birth to a child with DS because older eggs (ova) have a higher risk for improper chromosome separation during meiosis. Between the ages of 35 and 40 the risk increases dramatically from 1 in 400 to 1 in 35.

Pathophysiology

- Trisomy 21 results from a meiotic nondisjunction event in a gamete (i.e., a sperm or egg cell) where chromosome 21 fails to separate (the gamete thus has 24 chromosomes).
- When combined with a normal gamete from the other parent, the embryo now has 47 chromosomes, with three copies of chromosome 21.
- Trisomy 21 is the cause of approximately 95% of observed Down syndromes, with 88% coming from nondisjunction in the maternal gamete and 8% coming from nondisjunction in the paternal gamete.

Subjective

- As DS is diagnosed at birth, there are no specific symptoms stated or needed to make a diagnosis.

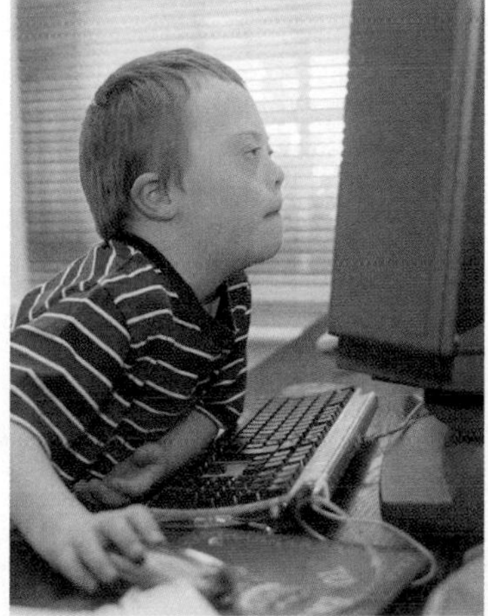

FIGURE 17-33 Down syndrome
Source: Lauren Shear/Science Source Images

Objective

- Manifestations are observed on the face and neck, which are flat and broad, producing a flat nasal bridge and a short neck as well as microgenia (abnormally small chin) and oblique eye fissures of the inner canthus.
- Additionally the tongue may be large and protrude (macroglossia).
- The individual also has small ears that may be unusually shaped and eyes that have an upward slant.
- Growth parameters such as height, weight, and head circumference are smaller in children with DS than in typical individuals of the same age.

Fetal Alcohol Syndrome (FAS)

FAS is a constellation of mental and physical alterations that can develop in a fetus due to high levels of alcohol consumption during pregnancy. Alcohol crosses the placental barrier, causing stunting of fetal growth and/or weight, creating distinctive facial stigmata, damaging neurons and brain structures (resulting in psychological or behavioral problems), and causing other physical damage, with the primary effect being permanent damage to the central nervous system, especially the brain. Prenatal alcohol exposure to developing brain cells and structures at any point during a pregnancy is considered high risk for brain malformation or interruption of development. These cellular alterations result in an array of primary cognitive and functional disabilities (poor memory, attention deficits, impulsive behavior, and poor cause–effect reasoning) as well as secondary disabilities (predispositions to mental health problems and drug addiction).

Pathophysiology

Alcohol places a human fetus at risk:

- The placenta allows free entry of ethanol and toxic metabolites (acetaldehyde) into the fetal circulation. The placental barrier is not a barrier with respect to ethanol.
- The developing fetal nervous system is particularly sensitive to ethanol toxicity, affecting all major processes in the developing central nervous system.
- The fetal liver is incapable of detoxifying ethanol as the ADH and ALDH enzymes are not functioning at this early stage, resulting in fetal exposure to ethanol in the amniotic fluid for periods far longer than the decay time of ethanol in the maternal circulation.
- Essentially, fetal tissues have far less antioxidant protection than adult tissues as they express no significant quantities of ADH or ALDH, and far less antioxidant enzymes.

Subjective

- As FAS is congenital and present at birth, there are no significant symptoms associated with its diagnosis.

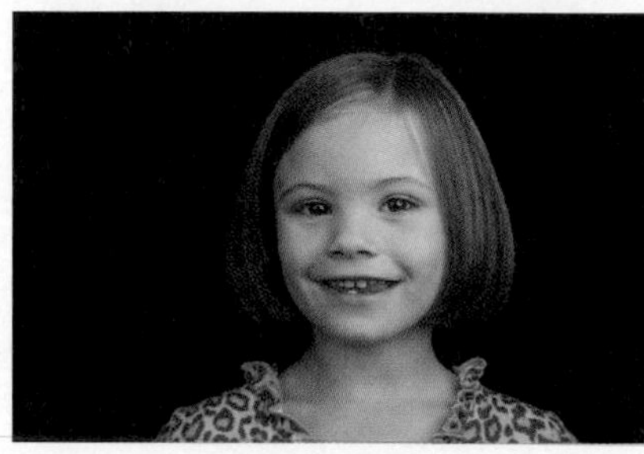

FIGURE 17-34 Fetal alcohol syndrome
Source: Rick's Photography/Shutterstock

Objective

- Characteristic craniofacial abnormalities are often visible in individuals with FAS.
- The presence of FAS facial features indicates brain damage, though brain damage may also exist in their absence.
- FAS facial features are believed to be caused mainly during the 10th and 20th week of gestation.
- Three distinct and diagnostically significant facial features distinguish FAS from other disorders with partially overlapping characteristics.
  - A smooth philtrum—the divot or groove between the nose and upper lip flattens with increased prenatal alcohol exposure.
  - Thin vermilion—the upper lip thins with increased prenatal alcohol exposure.
  - Small palpebral fissures—eye width decreases with increased prenatal alcohol exposure.

Parkinson's Disease

Parkinson's disease is a central nervous system degenerative condition. The motor manifestations of this disease result from the death of dopamine-generating cells in the substantia nigra, a region of the midbrain; the cause of cell death is unknown.

Pathophysiology

- Lack of facial expression is due to muscle rigidity of the facial muscles that results from nerve damage/destruction causing decreased neurotransmitter transmission and communication between muscles and nerves leading to decreased motor function.

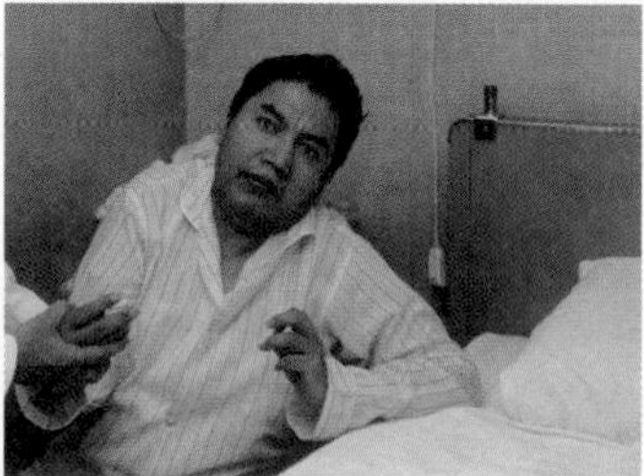

FIGURE 17-35 Face of Parkinsonism
Source: David Leah/Science Source Images

Subjective

Parkinson's disease manifestations vary from person to person. Early manifestations include the following:

- Loss of sense of smell
- Constipation
- REM (sleep) behavior disorder
- Mood disorders
- Orthostatic hypotension
- Loss of automatic movements, such as decreased ability to perform unconscious movements (blinking, smiling, swinging arms when walking, gesturing while talking).
- Speech changes: speaking softly, quickly, slurring or hesitating before talking, monotone speech.
- Writing may appear small and become difficult.

Objective

- **Hypomimia** is demonstrated by a reduced degree of facial expression.
- Motor symptoms often begin on one side of the body and usually remain worse on that side, even after symptoms begin to affect both sides.
- Tremors: shaking in limb or of hand or fingers with back-and-forth rubbing of thumb and forefinger (pill-rolling tremor), hand tremor when at rest.
- Bradykinesia: reduction in ability to move and slow movement, making simple tasks difficult and time-consuming (shorter steps when walking, difficulty getting out of a chair)
- Rigid muscles, including muscle stiffness in any parts of the body, limiting ROM and causing pain.
- Impaired posture and balance; posture becomes stooped or causes balance problems.

Scleroderma

Scleroderma is a rare, chronic, systemic autoimmune dermatological condition that results in tightening and hardening of the skin due to an overproduction of collagen. Connective tissue throughout the body is also affected, causing scarring and hardening of internal organs.

Localized scleroderma affects only the skin, while the systemic type may involve internal organs and blood vessels. Scleroderma is three to four times more common in females than males, occurring most often between 20 and 50 years of age. Localized scleroderma is more common in Caucasians. It is also common in African Americans and Native Americans; however, they often develop the more serious, generalized type.

Diffuse systemic sclerosis/scleroderma is rapidly progressing and affects a large area of the skin and one or more internal organs, frequently the kidneys, esophagus, heart, and lungs. This form can be quite disabling. There are no treatments for scleroderma itself, but individual organ system complications are treated.

Pathophysiology

- The cause is unknown but is considered genetic in origin; the responsible genes have not been identified. May also appear in individual with no family history.
- Arterioles in all organs are affected. Initially, endothelial cells of the arteriole, smooth muscle cells, die off and are replaced by collagen and other fibrous material.
- Inflammatory cells (CD4+ helper T cells) infiltrate the arteriole, causing further damage.

Subjective

- Pulmonary: Two-thirds of all patients report respiratory problems, such as shortness of breath, coughing, and difficulty breathing.
- Esophageal damage makes it difficult to swallow food; acid reflux is common. A sluggish intestine associated with pain and bloating; undigested food can result in diarrhea, weight loss.
- Muscle weakness, joint pain, and stiffness are frequently described.
- Dysphagia may result from collagen deposition in the esophageal submucosa. Dentures or dental prostheses may be difficult to insert or remove.

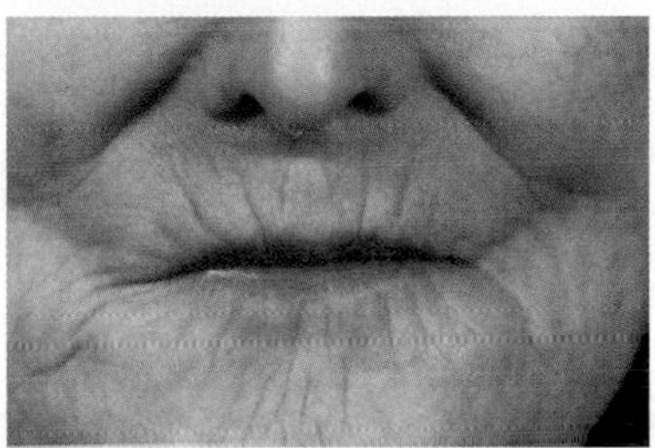

FIGURE 17-36 Face of scleroderma
Source: Wellcome Trust Library/Custom Medical Stock Photo

Objective

- Facial manifestations include skin that appears tight, shiny, and smooth with the possibility of restricted movement. Creases and wrinkles will no longer be visible. Severe tightening may also cause the mouth to appear smaller and narrower.
- Untreated high blood pressure strains the heart; irregular heart rhythm and enlargement of the heart lead to heart failure.
- Scleroderma renal crisis in which malignant hypertension develops and causes acute renal failure was once a common cause of death but is now treatable with ACE inhibitors.
- Alveolitis, pneumonia, and cancer.
- The stomach can develop gastric antral vascular ectasia (GAVE), which occasionally may bleed profusely and cause anemia.
- Carpal tunnel syndrome is common.
- Flat white patches, loss of attached gingival mucosa, gingival recession, and diffuse widening of the periodontal ligament (PDL) space are seen. Inelasticity of the mouth.

HEAD

Conditions and disorders of the head are primarily associated with altered head size, specifically the size of the cranium. Macrocephaly is primarily associated with hydrocephalus and acromegaly (see pages 382 and 390–91).

Microcephaly

Microcephaly is a rare neurological condition in which an infant is born with a smaller than expected head size (cranium). It may or may not be apparent at birth, but it becomes more obvious as the infant grows and is compared to other children of the same age or growth charts. It is usually defined as a head circumference (HC) more than two standard deviations below the mean for age and gender. There is not agreement on the exact number of standard deviations, and there are recommendations that it be three standard deviations below the mean.

Pathophysiology

- Failure of the cranium to enlarge is primarily due to failure of the brain to grow and develop in utero, or it may have just stopped growing.
- Frequently, microcephaly is a manifestation of another syndrome, that is, Down syndrome and other chromosomal alterations and some neurometabolic syndromes. It is also possible for there to be a genetic basis for its cause.

Subjective

- Children with microcephaly may not demonstrate any other symptoms or manifestations and may develop as expected and not have any intelligence deficits.
- When other syndromes are present, developmental delays, particularly with speech/movement and balance/coordination may occur.

Objective

- The primary sign of microcephaly is a head size that is significantly smaller than that of children of the same age and gender.
- Short stature with certain facial characteristics that include enlarged ears and a backward sloping forehead.
- Other manifestations include visual impairment, mental retardation, hyperactivity, and seizures.

- Other conditions that the developing fetus may be exposed to that are known to cause microcephaly include oxygen deficits during fetal development or delivery, exposure to alcohol and other drugs during development, maternal infections (rubella, chicken pox, toxoplasmosis, and cytomegalovirus), and maternal uncontrolled phenylketonuria (PKU).
- Premature closure of the fontanels of the cranium is another cause. Surgery to separate the fused bones will allow for appropriate brain growth and development with no other complications.

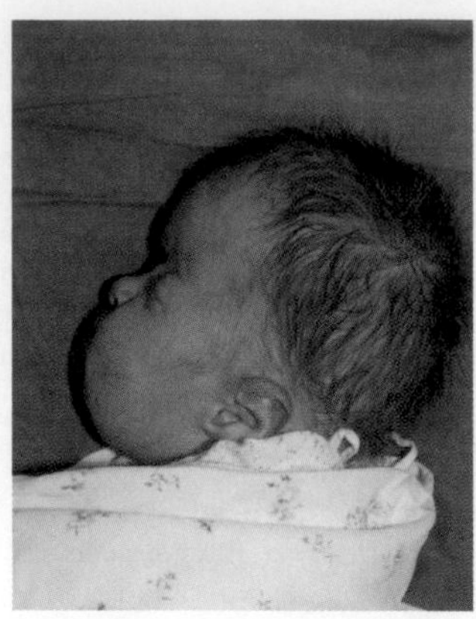

FIGURE 17-37 Microcephaly (craniosysostosis)
Source: Wellcome Trust Library/Custom Medical Stock Photo

NECK

Conditions and disorders of the neck are quite varied and often related to pain associated with cervical spine alterations. Other conditions associated with neck disorders originate with muscles and are described as dystonias.

Torticollis (Wry Neck, Loxia)

Torticollis is a term to describe various conditions related to muscle tone of the head with the neck twisting toward one side, due to flexion, extension, or twisting of the neck muscles beyond their expected position. It may be congenital, caused by an acute situation, or from chronic conditions. It may also occur as a result of an adverse reaction to certain medications. The condition may be easier to treat in infants and children. If it becomes chronic, numbness and tingling may develop due to pressure on the nerve roots in the neck. SCM may increase in size (hypertrophy) from constant stimulation and exercise.

Pathophysiology

- Etiology of congenital muscular torticollis is unclear. Birth trauma or intrauterine malposition is considered the cause of damage to the sternocleidomastoid muscle (SCM).
- Acute torticollis may result from blunt trauma (post-traumatic) to the head and neck or from maintaining an awkward position of the neck for an extended time period (sleeping).
- Acute torticollis is generally self-limiting and resolves in days to weeks. If it develops as a result of medications, stopping them usually resolves the condition.
- After resolution from acute trauma, within days to weeks it may return as a chronic condition.
- The familial type often doesn't appear until between the 3rd to 5th decade of life. If left untreated, it will most likely become permanent.

Subjective

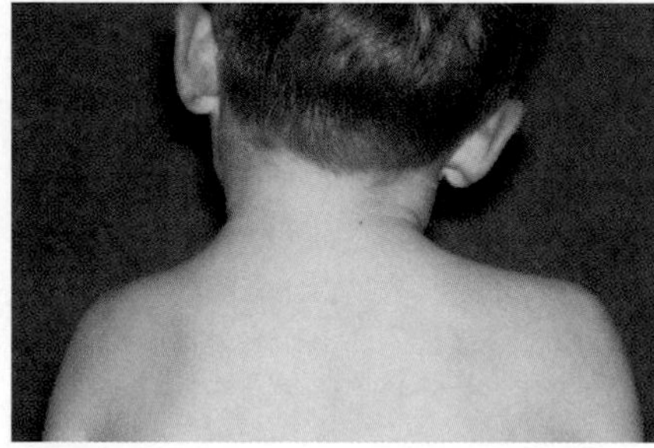

FIGURE 17-38 Tortocollis
Source: National Medical Slide Bank/Custom Medical Stock Photo

Objective

- Shortening or excessive contraction of the SCM limits its range of motion in rotational/lateral bending. The head generally tilts in lateral bending toward the affected muscle, rotated toward the opposite side.
- The type of torticollis can be described according to positions of head and neck as the following:
  - laterocollis: the head is tipped toward the shoulder
  - rotational torticollis: the head rotates along the longitudal axis
  - anterocollis: forward flexion of the head and neck
  - retrocollis: hyperextension of head and neck backward
- A combination of these movements can often be observed.

Neck Webbing (Turner's Syndrome/Noonan's Syndrome)

Neck webbing is characterized by extra folds of skin that extend from the tops of the shoulders to the sides of the neck. While it may be simply a congenital manifestation, its presence may indicate the presence of another condition. Two syndromes that are classically associated with webbed neck are **Turner's syndrome** and **Noonan's syndrome.**

Pathophysiology

- What specifically causes the neck webbing is not known, and it may be removed surgically.
- Noonan's syndrome does not appear to have a genetic alteration as its cause, and there is no other known cause of the syndrome.
- Individuals with Turner's syndrome are always females as it is characterized as having only one sex-determining chromosome (X) or only a partial second chromosome.

Subjective

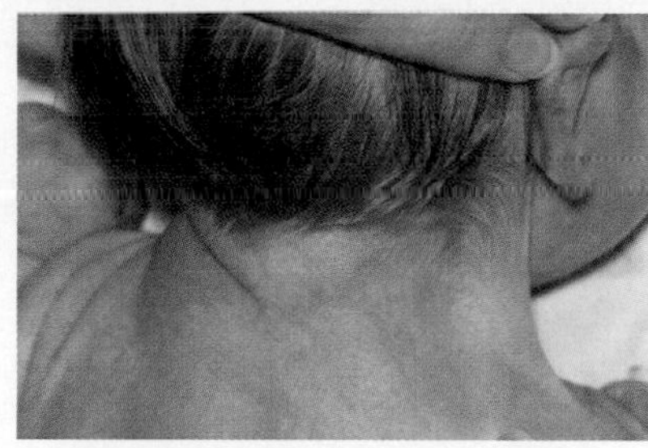

FIGURE 17-39 Neck webbing (Turner's/Noonan's syndrome)
Source: Wellcome Trust Library/Custom Medical Stock Photo

Objective

- While both syndromes demonstrate a webbed neck, other facial manifestations accompany the syndromes.

Noonan's syndrome may demonstrate the following:

- Wide set eyes with an epicanthal fold at the inner border of the eye. Outer eye borders may slant downward, with possible ptosis.
- Ears are frequently low set and rotated backward; may have a thick, fleshy outer border.
- Philtrum is predominant; nose is frequently smaller with an upturned tip.
- Hair is frequently curly or woolly

Turner's syndrome:

- Wide set eyes, low set ears, ptosis of the eyelids.
- Broad chest (*shield chest*), widely spaced nipples.
- Low hairline.

18 The Eye

It isn't fair; I'm only 55 and losing my vision. I've been managing my diabetes well for the past few years. So why am I now going blind? Jerry is terrible when it comes to managing his diabetes, and his eyes are just fine! I feel my way along the wall to the ophthalmologist's office, becoming angrier and angrier. "Good morning!" I glance to my right and see a shadowy form move past, but cannot recognize her features. People on the street are now nothing more than shadows and shapes. How can I live like this?

I somehow find my way into the clinic building and begin climbing the steps to the second floor. Shuffling slowly up to the door, I see a smaller shape moving quickly back and forth in the entryway. The shape is giggling uncontrollably. Damn kids. I reach for the door, hoping the kid will move out of my way. Instead, the kid knocks into my legs and I feel myself falling. "Can't you see that I'm trying to get into this office?" I shout, leaning in close to see the kid's face. The shape takes form—a round, cherubic child looks back at me, one eye tearing up, but the other eye... absent, just a cavernous socket. I recoil. This child, probably no older than 5 or 6, is missing an eye.

I begin to cry. "I...I'm sorry. I didn't know...." The child runs off down the hallway, blurring once more into the limits of my vision. I feel awful, and suddenly I feel deeply fortunate to have had 50 years of outstanding bifocal eyesight. Fumbling for the doorknob, I enter the office, sit down in the chair, and wait quietly for my name to be called.

LEARNING OUTCOMES

1. Describe anatomic structures of the internal and external and their correct position and placement.
2. Explain variations in eye appearances by inspection and their relationship to various pathological and nonpathological conditions.
3. Recognize common lifespan changes in the eyes and the significance of their presence.
4. Explain the techniques used to examine the external and internal structures of the eye by observation and palpation.
5. Summarize documentation of findings using appropriate terms when describing expected and unexpected findings.

As far back as Cicero (106–43 BCE) the eyes have been described as "the interpreter of the mind," which has been reinterpreted in later centuries as the "windows or mirrors to one's soul." And indeed, the eyes seem to be an expression and reflection of the inner emotions of an individual. The eyes seldom betray one's emotions and feelings. The eyes are also major sensory organs responsible for sight. The eyes function to control and maintain sight. Images are received and recorded by the retina, and forwarded to the brain for interpretation, allowing the individual to visually encounter, experience, and control his or her environment. Approximately four-fifths of all the sensory information received by the brain daily comes from the eyes (Lowther & Lindsell, n.d.).

Visual impairment has, therefore, significant impact on an individual's functional status and quality of life.

Structure and Function

The eyes are two global structures that are contained in the orbital cavities of the skull, which only permit the anterior portion to be exposed and visible (Figure 18-1). The eyes function to detect light and convert it into electro-chemical impulses in neurons that are carried to the visual cortex of the brain via the optic nerve where they are perceived as images. The eye is composed of external and internal structures.

External Structures

The external structures of the eye include the eyelid, conjunctiva, lacrimal gland, and the extraocular muscles (Figure 18-2).

Eyelids

The upper and lower eyelids are like curtains that open and close to allow or block visual stimuli from entering the eye, as well as protecting the eye. Composed of skin, conjunctiva, and muscle, the lids also distribute tears over the surface of the eye. The anterior portion of the eye is visible through an opening in the lids called the palpebral fissure. When the eyelids are closed, they should be approximated and totally cover the exposed eyeball. When open, the upper eyelid should cover the upper portion of the iris and the lower lid should be at the level of the lower margin of the iris. The corners of the eye are identified as the canthus; there is a medial and a lateral canthus.

The eyelids contain tarsal plates, or strips of connective tissue that provide shape and structure to the lids. Additionally, they contain meibomian glands, sebaceous glands that lubricate the lids by secreting meibum, an oily substance that prevents evaporation of the eye's tear film.

The eyelashes grow out of hair follicles along the margins of the lids. Eyelashes protect the eye from debris or injury and also provide a sensory function by causing reflexive blinking whenever an object comes near the eye. The eyebrows are positioned on the superior orbital ridge and serve to protect the eye from sweat.

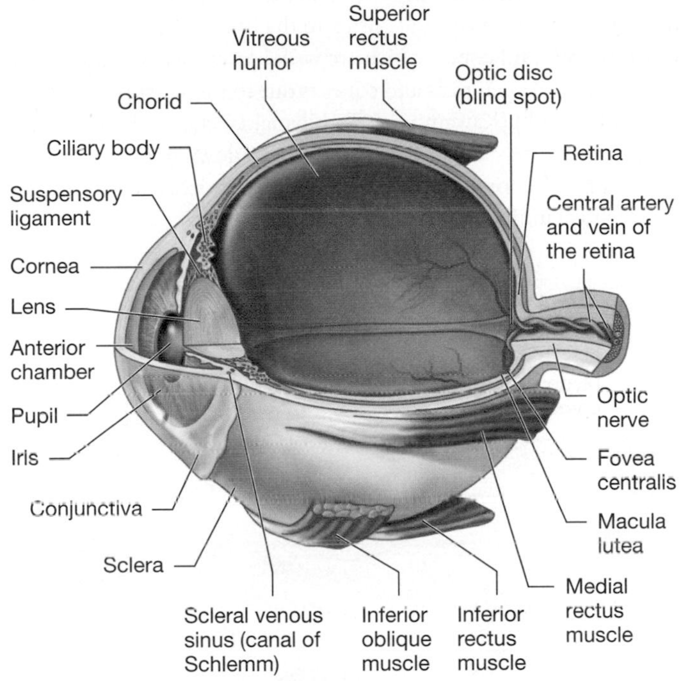

FIGURE 18-1 Anatomy of the human eye

Conjunctiva

The conjunctiva is a transparent membrane that covers the anterior portion of the eye. The palpebral conjunctiva is the lining of the lids and contains multiple small blood vessels. At the superior recess of the lid, it folds back on itself and becomes the bulbar conjunctiva, which lines the anterior, white portion of the eyeball. The bulbar conjunctiva merges with the cornea at the limbus, the external margin of the iris. The cornea is the protective covering of the iris and pupil.

Lacrimal Gland

Located in the upper outer section of the orbit, the lacrimal gland lubricates the conjunctiva and cornea. Its main function is to secrete tears that moisten and cleanse the conjunctiva, washing away any foreign object, such as dust and dirt. The cornea is highly sensitive to irritation and pain and stimulates the production of tears when either occurs.

Tears are drained into the inferior and superior lacrimal puncta that are located at the medial canthus. From the puncta, the tears enter the nasolacrimal ducts and are emptied into the nasolacrimal sac that opens to the inferior meatus of the nose.

Extraocular Muscles

Extraocular movement is executed by the pairing of six ocular muscles so that eye movement is synchronous and parallel, on horizontal and vertical planes with additional oblique movements (Figure 18-3). Synchronous and parallel eye movement is described as conjugate movement. Lateral and horizontal movement is controlled by four rectus (lateral,

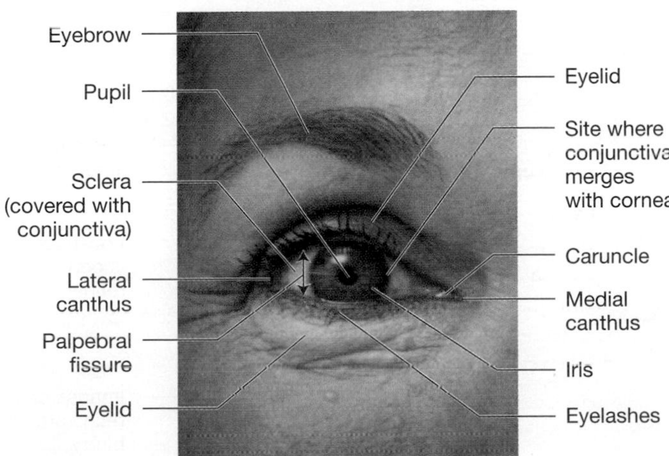

FIGURE 18-2 External structures of the eye

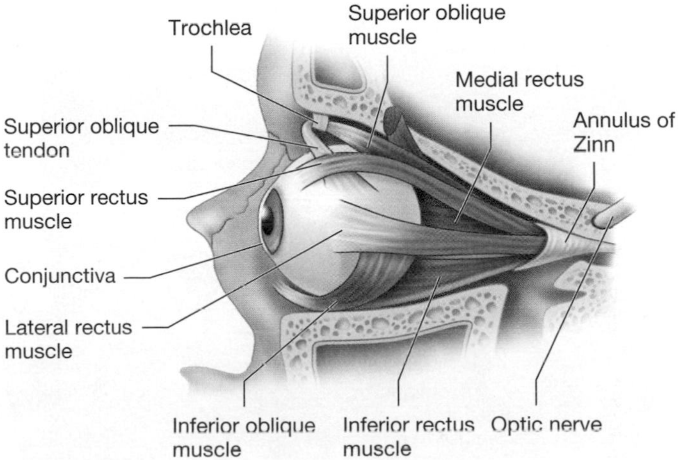

FIGURE 18-3 Extraocular muscles

medial, inferior, superior) muscles and oblique movement by two oblique (inferior, superior) muscles (Figure 18-4). Extraocular muscles are innervated and movements are controlled by three cranial nerves CN III-oculomotor, CN IV-trochlear, and CN VI-abducens.

The extraocular muscles are also responsible for maintaining the position and alignment of the eyeball within the orbital socket. Functional vision requires that the eyeballs be in correct alignment with each other so that the images are recorded on congruent areas of the retinas are seen and recorded single entities.

Internal Structures

The internal structures of the eye are contained in the three layers of the eye, which are the outer layer (sclera), the middle layer (choroids), and the inner coat (retina) (see Figure 18-1).

Sclera

The sclera is the white of the eye and is the supporting structure of the eye. It is dense and avascular. The anterior, transparent portion of the sclera that covers the iris and pupil is the cornea. The cornea, like the lens, refracts light, accounting for about two-thirds of the eye optical power, the degree to which a lens converges or diverges light. Unlike the lens, the cornea's focus is fixed whereas the lens can adjust its curvature, fine tuning the focus for optimum vision. It is densely innervated by sensory nerve fibers from the ophthalmic division of the trigeminal nerve (CN V), which are primary pain receptors.

Choroid Layer

The middle layer of the eyeball is the choroid, which is a darkly pigmented, vascularized portion of the eyeball that nourishes the retina. Anteriorly, the choroid layer is continuous with the ciliary body. The ciliary body is a muscle that is attached to the lens and controls the thickness of the lens. The change in the thickness of the lens is necessary for correct focusing of images on the retina.

The iris is also a component of the choroid layer. The iris is a muscle that is circular and contains the pigment that gives the eyes their distinctive color. The center of the iris is known as the pupil, which is the opening through which light enters the eye. Dilating and contracting of the pupil is the mechanism used by the iris to regulate the amount of light entering the eye.

Positioned directly behind the iris is the lens, a biconvex, crystalline structure that alters its shape so that light entering the eye can be correctly refracted and focused on the retina. The shape of the lens is controlled by the muscles of the ciliary body. Changes in the shape of the eye ball cause refractory errors because of the inability of images to be focused correctly on the retina. Refractory errors are of two broad types: myopia or near sightedness and hyperopia or far sightedness (Figure 18-5).

> ***THINK LINK: Refractory Errors***
>
> Refractory errors are caused by the lens focusing images either in front of the retina (myopia) or behind the retina (hyperopia) and occur because of structural alterations that change the shape of the eyeball. The myopic eyeball is elongated, making the retina further from the lens, making images focused before the light hits the retina. The hyperopic eyeball is too short, bringing the retina closer to the lens, making images focused behind the retina. Refractory errors are corrected with either concave lens (myopia) or convex lens (hyperopia).

Retina

The retina is the innermost layer of the eye and is its functional component. The retina is a sensory network that transforms light impulses into electrical impulses and sends them to the brain via the optic nerve to the visual cortex in the brain. The retina is composed of rods and cones, which are visual receptors. The difference in function between rods and cones is due to the sensitivity of their pigments to light (Kawamura & Tachibanaki, 2008). When light hits the cones and rods, the pigments are broken down to form a protein and vitamin A compound. It is this chemical process that stimulates the electrical impulse that is sent to the brain.

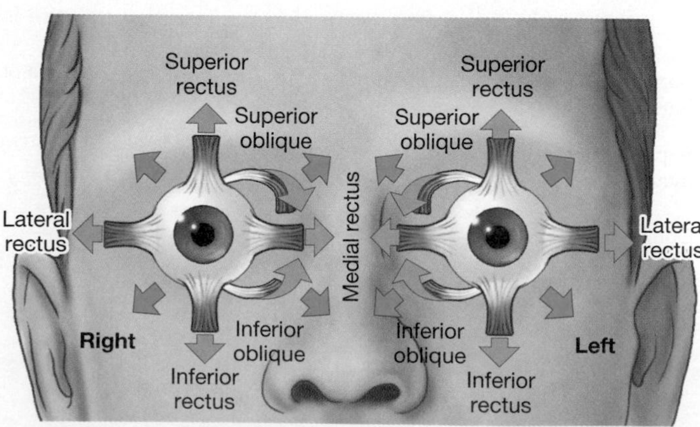

FIGURE 18-4 Eye movements

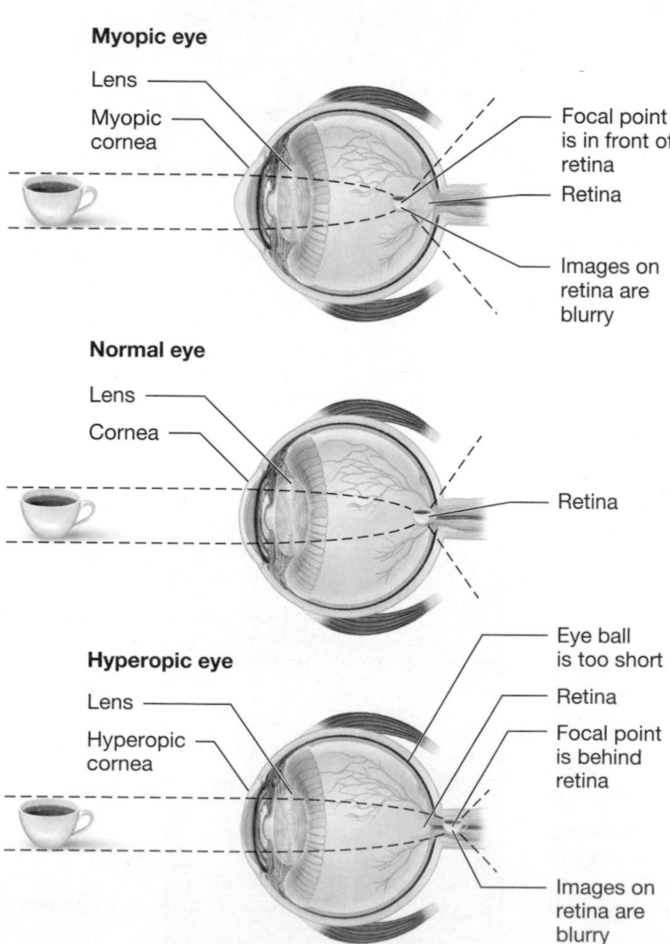

FIGURE 18-5 Refractory errors

The rods contain rhodopsin and function in dim light and provide black and white vision. They are also concerned with peripheral vision. The cones, which contain idopsin, function in bright light and are concerned with central vision as well as providing color to the visual images. There are three different types of cones, differentiated by the color of the wave length that is absorbed: blue, green, and red. Each has a distinct type of opsin, and each responds to a different optimal wavelength. Sensory fibers of the retina converge at the posterior portion of the eyeball to form the optic nerve, which connects the eye to the brain and transmits the visual impulses to the brain. The optic nerve also contains the ophthalmic artery and vein.

The rods and cones are closely aligned with the **retinal pigment epithelium** (RPE), a melanin containing monolayer of hexagonal (cuboidal) cells that is located between the choroid and neural retina and serves as a part of a barrier between the bloodstream and retina (Klimanskaya et al., 2004; Sparrow, Hicks, & Hamel, 2010). This epithelium has multiple, diverse functions that are vital for visual function. It also nourishes the retinal cells as well as regenerates the chemicals used by the rods and cones. It also functions to absorb light so that it will not bounce around to other parts of the retina. Failure of any of these functions may result in retinal degeneration, loss of visual function, and blindness (Strauss, 2005).

Visual Fields

Vision begins with the reflection of light rays off objects within the surrounding environment. The light rays travel through the transparent portions of the eye—the cornea, aqueous humor—to the lens where it is refracted and then continues through the vitreous humor to strike the retina. The retina then transforms the light stimuli into nerve impulses that are transmitted to and transported by the optic nerve to the visual cortex of the occipital lobe for interpretation.

The visual fields are related to the retina and where on the retina the light stimulus is received. The images that are formed from the visual stimuli are upside down and opposite the side of the origin of the visual stimuli. Thus an image that is on the right side of an individual is focused on the left side of the eye and vice versa. The same can be said of images that are superior and inferior, with the retinal images being opposite their site of origin.

For simplicity's sake, the eye and retina will be simply divided in half into a medial and lateral side. Nerve fibers from both sides of the retina converge to form the optic nerve, which exits the eyeball at the posterior aspect. The optic nerve is thus composed of two tracts of fibers—medial and lateral.

The optic nerves travel separately for a while and then converge at the optic chiasm. At the optic chiasm, the lateral nerve fibers stay on their respective left and right sides. The medial fibers, however, cross over (decussate) so that the right medial fibers now merge and travel with the left lateral fibers and the left medial fibers merge and travel with the right lateral fibers.

Each eye has four visual fields—nasal, temporal, superior, and inferior. The nasal visual fields are the same as the medial side of the eye and the temporal visual field is the same as the lateral part of the eye. The two nasal (medial) fields overlap so that the point where each nasal field ends is not well defined. Each visual field is identified by a specific number (angle) of degrees: nasal = 60°, temporal = 90°, superior = 50°, inferior = 70°.

Anatomically the field divides side to side along a vertical axis by the decussation of nasal nerve fibers at the optic chiasm just above the pituitary. The field divides up and down along a horizontal axis by the retinal anatomy of nerve fibers, but this continues posteriorly into the visual cortex.

Compartments of the Eye

The eyeball contains two fluid-filled compartments—the anterior chamber and the vitreous body. The anterior chamber is located directly behind the cornea to the front of the iris and the posterior chamber goes from the iris to the lens, essentially encircling the lens. The anterior chamber, which is approximately 45 degrees (open angle) although it may be around 25 degrees (narrow angle), and the trabecular meshwork are located where the cornea meets the iris. Both chambers are filled with a clear, refractory medium called aqueous humor that is constantly produced by the ciliary body and flows from ciliary processes into the posterior chamber. It then flows through the pupil of the iris into the anterior chamber, where the trabecular meshwork drains aqueous humor via Schlemm's canal into scleral plexuses and general venous blood circulation. Intraocular pressure is maintained by a balance between production and drainage of aqueous humor. Aqueous humor also delivers nutrients to the surrounding tissues and removes any metabolic waste products.

The vitreous body is located behind the lens and occupies the majority of the space within the eyeball. It is filled with a clear, gel-like substance known as vitreous humor. The vitreous body functions to maintain the shape of the eye. It is also a refractory medium that allows transmission of visual impulses to the retina.

Developmental Variations

Developmental variations occur over the course of an individual's lifespan and events. Awareness of these variations is important to understand and recognize common age-related alterations or modifications of the eye.

Infants and Children

Eye formation occurs during the first 8 weeks of gestation. During this time, malformation may occur due to maternal ingestion of drugs or from infections. Vision, however, occurs over a much longer time period and is controlled by the maturation of the nervous system (Table 18-1). The visual system is immature at birth. Visual stimuli are critical for development of unimpaired vision. The brain must receive equally clear, focused images from both eyes for the visual pathways to develop appropriately. Refractive errors, strabismus and cataract if not corrected may lead to amblyopia due to interference with visual development.

Visual acuity at birth is 20/400, and infants will fixate on bright objects, but will be unable to focus. Peripheral vision is present at birth, but central vision, along with the macula, is not fully developed until later. The lacrimal system is not functional at birth, thus the infant will not produce tears until approximately 2–3 months.

Initial eye movement is uncoordinated, however, by 2–3 months the infant begins to demonstrate voluntary control over the eye muscles leading to binocular vision at approximately 9 months. Initial eye color is either brown in dark-skinned infants, or blue in light-skinned infants. More permanent eye color begins to develop at about 3 months of age.

The growth and shape of the eyeball changes throughout childhood as the head and brain grow. The shape of the eyeball begins as hyperopic in the term infant, changing to myopic, and then achieving adult shape and visual acuity by about 6 years of age.

Pupillary reflexes are present at birth. The eyes are symmetrical with pupils that are equal and round, and respond to light. The red light reflex is also present at birth.

Table 18-1 Visual developmental milestones in infants and children

Age	Visual Developmental Levels	Visual Acuity
Birth	Aware of light and dark; eyes closed in bright light Visual fixation can be demonstrated shortly after birth	
Neonatal	Beginning of fixation on near objects (<30 inches)	
2 weeks	Brief fixation on near objects	
4 weeks	Tracts large, moving objects	
6 weeks	Fixation on and tracking of moving objects	
8 weeks	Erratic eye movements when tracking object; beginning convergence	
3 months	Head and eye movement when tracking; improved convergence Noting of bright light and light objects Start of depth perception as well as fusion of images	
4 months	Notices and inspects hands or small objects within distance of 1–2 feet	20/300–200
5 months	Organizing of accommodating convergence reflexes Visually pursues fallen toy Aware of objects greater than 3 feet away	
6 months	Stereopsis and binocular vision develop between age 3–7 months Retrieves small objects Beginning hand–eye coordination Able to maintain fixation on stationary object in the presence of other background motion	20/200–150
7–9 months	Binocular fixation; beginning depth perception	
10–11 months	Greater interest in small objects Tilts head backward to look up	
12–17 months	Differentiates simple geometric shapes (circle/square) Shows interest in pictures Fusion well developed	20/150–100
18–23 months	Convergence well developed Difficulty with distance, peripheral localizing—bumps into objects	
2 years	Accommodation well developed	20/100– 50
3–4 years	Convergence stabilized and steady with improvement in fusion	20/50 –30
4–6 years		20/40– 20

The Pregnant Woman

Physiologic and hormonal alterations during pregnancy may result in changes to the eyes. There may be a mild corneal edema during the third trimester, as well as corneal thickening, producing corneal hypersensitivity along with refractory alterations. Corneal edema results from overall water retention and corneal thickening, all of which disappear after delivery. Fluctuating levels of estrogen are the primary cause of these changes (Spoerl, Zubaty, Raiskup-Wolf, & Pillunat, 2007). Corneal epithelial pigmentation may also be present. Gestational diabetes can cause visual blurring. Diabetic retinopathy, if present, may become significantly worse. The overall effects of corneal changes results in blurred vision. Temporary loss of vision, light sensitivity, blurred vision, auras and flashing lights may be indicators of preeclampsia.

Tears contain an increased amount of lysozyme—producing a greasy sensation. Intraocular pressure also may decrease by as much as 20% (Brown & Sunness, 2006), which is due to progesterone, relaxin, and human chorionic gonadotropin (Datta, Shankar, & Segal, 2010). Due to the number of visual changes accompanying pregnancy, pregnant women may find their contact lenses uncomfortable, be unable to wear them, or choose not to wear them. They may also find their prescription lenses inadequate. Eye changes during pregnancy resolve after delivery, and changing prescriptions during pregnancy is not recommended.

The Older Adult

The most common eye alteration that accompanies aging is the loss of elasticity of the lens and ciliary muscles. As a result, accommodation for near vision is reduced, producing **presbyopia**. Generally, this condition becomes apparent in the 40s, however in some individuals, this may be delayed. The lens may also become cloudy and opaque due to the development of cataracts. Fibers that are formed by the lens become compressed centrally, initiating the development of a cataract. Cataract formation, to some extent, is present by the time one reaches 70 years of age. By the age of 75–85, approximately half of these individuals will have cataracts.

Older adults are also at risk for developing glaucoma, retinopathy (diabetic), and macular degeneration. These conditions are also a significant concern related to health promotion and are further discussed in that section.

Health Promotion

The incidence of visual impairment and blindness resulting from most eye disorders can be decreased with early detection and treatment. A significant factor leading to blindness or other impairments is that most eye disorders do not manifest any symptoms until the vision alteration is irreversible or completely lost. Once vision is lost, it is impossible to restore, thus early intervention with regular vision exams is essential to improving the visual health of the nation. The primary focus areas for health promotion are related to visual screening to prevent visual impairment and prevention of injury.

Vision Screening and Prevention of Impairment

Visual impairment is one of the major causes of disability in the U.S. While no one is immune from developing visual problems, certain groups of individuals are more prone to one type of alteration. The major focus in preventing visual impairment is screening to detect subnormal vision and identification of those at risk for development of impairments. Various groups of individuals are more prone to one type of alteration requiring different screening modalities. Age is a significant factor as more than two thirds of visually impaired individuals are over age 65; however, screening should be started much earlier to prevent future development of impairment.

Objectives of *Healthy People 2020* for the topic area of vision include the following:

- V–1: Increase the proportion of preschool children aged 5 years and under who receive vision screening.
- V–2: Reduce blindness and visual impairment in children and adolescents aged 17 years and under.
- V–5: Reduce visual impairment due to uncorrected refractive error, diabetic retinopathy, glaucoma, cataract, and age-related macular degeneration (AMD).

Since children usually do not complain of visual difficulties, early screening is paramount to prevent irreversible visual loss. Amblyopia is the major visual impairment in children under 5; an estimated 2–4% of preschool children have this condition, which is an alteration in the visual neural pathway of the developing brain. If untreated, it can lead to permanent visual loss in the affected eye. Using existing technology to screen for amblyopia, strabismus, refractive errors, cataract, hyperopia and refractive errors can lead to correction and preservation of vision. Risk factors associated with visual impairments include abnormal light reflex, history of prematurity, metabolic or genetic diseases with ocular implications, unilateral ptosis, asymmetry of vision, acuity worse than 20/40 in a 3–5 year old child and 20/30 in child over 6, and nystagmus. Teens rarely lose their eyesight due to physiological alterations; rather lost vision is primarily due to injury related to sports activities or motor vehicle accidents. Safety is the major issue related to this and is further covered under injury prevention. Diabetic teens require regular eye exams to screen for the development of diabetic retinopathy.

Ethnic differences also contribute to visual impairment distribution. The prevalence of moderate to severe retinopathy is higher for African Americans and Hispanics than non-Hispanic whites. The differences are not accounted for by other factors such as age, duration of diabetes, hypertension or control of blood glucose (Emanuele & Klein et al.). Ethnicity, race, and baseline retinopathy correlates in the veterans affairs diabetes trail (Diabetes Care 2005). Hispanics are three times more likely to develop type 2 diabetes with a greater tendency to develop microvascular complications.

Refractive error blindness is a degree of visual handicap due to the lack proper refractive correction. While not a major problem in the U.S., it is a significant cause of visual impairment throughout the world. While individuals with refractory error blindness may have visual capability, the impairment is significant enough to consider this condition a form of blindness.

Diabetic retinopathy (DR) is the most common and serious complication associated with diabetes, frequently leading to decreased vision and blindness. The longer an individual has diabetes, the higher the risk of developing diabetic retinopathy. After 20 years of diabetes, nearly all type 1 patients will have some retinopathy, and about 50%–80% with type 2 DM (Fraser & D'Amico, 2013). With the increasing number of type 2 diabetes cases, it is expected that there will be more microvascular changes as a result of long standing diabetes. Recent findings suggest that there is a significant increased incidence of acquired color vision impairment in type 2 diabetes patients without diabetic retinopathy, which might be caused by another pathogenesis associated with diabetic retinopathy (Shoji, Sakurai, Sato, Chihara, & Takeuchi, 2011). Chronic hyperglycemia seems to be the major factor contributing to vessel damage.

A **cataract** is a lens opacity that causes partial or total blindness and is the leading cause of blindness in the world. Risk factors include age, smoking, alcohol, UV exposure, diabetes, metabolic syndrome, steroid use, low socio-economic status, and unhealthy lifestyle habits. Acquired cataract may be due to ocular trauma, scleritis, uveitis or radiation. While cataracts could be considered an expected age related condition, regular eye exams are the primary key to early detection and interventions. Other preventative measures include avoiding smoking and second hand smoke, reducing alcohol consumption, protecting eyes from UV exposure, controlling diabetes and other health problems, and eating a healthy diet.

Age-related macular degeneration (AMD) is a chronic eye condition that occurs when the macula of the retina begins to deteriorate (Mayo Clinic Staff, 2007). It is the primary cause of severe vision loss in individuals over the age of 60 and more common in elderly females than males. Central vision is lost, but not peripheral vision; therefore it does not cause total blindness, but does cause legal blindness (20/200); thus, the individual does not become completely disabled or unable to care for self yet can no longer perform activities requiring where fine work nor read small print.

Glaucoma is an optic neuropathy characterized by elevated intraocular pressure that eventually leads to irreversible blindness if untreated. It is the second-leading cause of blindness in the world and more common in older adult males than females. Symptoms of open-angle glaucoma do not appear until late in the disease when central visual loss occurs, putting thousands of individuals at risk for the development of glaucoma and its devastating consequences. It is estimated that there are about 2–3 million individuals with glaucoma and that half of these do not know it (Dahl, 2011). The insidious nature of glaucoma makes awareness and early detection crucial to prevent decreased vision and/or blindness (Table 18-2). Screening for glaucoma is most frequently done by measuring intraocular pressure by tonometry, which measures the pressure by placement of a tonometer directly on the anesthetized eyeball.

Health Promotion *continued*

Injury Prevention

- V–3: Reduce occupational eye injuries.
- V–6: Increase the use of personal protective eyewear in recreational activities and hazardous situations around the home.

Many occupational eye injuries occur because workers are not wearing any eye protection, while others result from wearing improper or poorly fitting eye protection. It is imperative for employers to be sure that employees the wear correct, properly fitting eye and face protection, consistent with work being performed.

Sports and recreational activities account for greater than 40,000 eye injuries annually (Heimmel, 2008); about 90% of these could be prevented with the use of appropriate protective equipment. The two sports most commonly associated with ocular injuries are baseball (ages 5–14 years) and basketball (ages 15–64 years). For protective devices to be effective in preventing eye injuries, they should dissipate a potentially harmful force over a larger area.

Table 18-2 Screening schedule for early detection and prevention of glaucoma

Age	Individuals	Frequency of Examination
20–29	Individuals of African American descent Family history	Every 3–5 years
	Others	At least once
30–39	Individuals of African American descent Family history	Every 2–4 years
	Others	At least twice
40–64	Everyone	With no risk factors, every 3–5 years
65 and older	Everyone	Every 1–2 years

Clinical Context Exemplars

Situation A

The initial assessment of an individual's eyes indicates that the corneal light reflex is not symmetrical.

1. What is the significance of this finding?
2. What concerns would you have in regards to this individual's vision?
3. If this patient was a 3-year-old child, what further assessment would you want to do and why?

The initial assessment of another individual's eyes reveals pupils that are not equal in size.

4. What is the significance of this finding? What are the possible causes of this finding?

Situation B

Another patient has come into the emergency room with pupils that are fixed and dilated.

1. What is the significance of this finding?
2. What is the cause for this finding?

Situation C

A patient has identified that he has trouble seeing things off to his side. Identify the probable cause of this visual field cut that this individual is experiencing.

1. What field cut would one experience? At optic chiasm? Post optic chiasm?
2. Why are the field cuts different?

Situation D

The vision of an elderly patient is described as "blurry in the middle of my eyesight."

1. What is the significance of this finding?
2. What is the probable cause of this visual problem?

Situation E

A 70-year-old man presents with herpetic lesions on tip of his nose.

1. As a clinician, what additional finding will you look for?
2. What will you do next?

SUBJECTIVE DATA

History of Present Illness (CC)

The patient may present with specific concerns related to the structures of the eyes. Framing the questions will depend on the patient's age, gender, culture, race, emotional or mental status, health practices, and concurrent illnesses. All symptoms presented must be thoroughly assessed with a symptom analysis (COLDERRA).

Altered Vision (Blurred, Decreased, Floaters, Blind Spots)

Altered vision may be described by patients in a variety of ways: blurred, decreased, distorted, double vision (diplopia), spots (floaters), glare, hazy/cloudy, nighttime symptoms, and vision issues that occur only with fine print. The provider is therefore responsible for obtaining a detailed history and clarifying the patient's symptoms. Alteration in vision may be due to many causes, such as refractive errors, infection, cataract,macular degeneration, glaucoma, floaters, infection, trauma, inflammation, allergy, and retinopathy (diabetic).

Provider Inquiries	Clinical Reasoning/Logic
Characteristics: Do you have difficulty focusing or experience dry eyes? Describe the visual alteration. Is it unilateral/bilateral, floaters, halos around lights, double vision, blind spots?	Visual disturbances have multiple characteristics; some of these are unique to specific alterations Floaters may be benign or worrisome if they are large, acute and occur as a shower. Dry eye syndrome may cause blurred vision. A halo around lights is associated with acute narrow angle glaucoma. Blind spots (**scotoma**)—loss of visual acuity or fields is seen in glaucoma, optic nerve, or visual pathway alterations and migraine.
Onset: Was the onset of the altered vision sudden or gradual? When did it occur? Was there a known trauma (work environment)?	Sudden showers of floaters signal eye pathologies like retinal detachment or vitreous hemorrhage. Glaucoma may be gradual (open-angle glaucoma) or acute (closed-angle glaucoma).
Location: Adequacy of central or peripheral vision? Are the floaters stationary or do they move? Does it occur in one eye or both?	Certain conditions affect only central vision like (AMD) while others affect the peripheral vision (pituitary adenomas).
Duration: Constant or variable?	Floaters may be constant but may be more pronounced with visual tracking on a white background.
Exacerbation: Is there anything that makes visual alterations worse (position, heat/cold)?	Visual blurring may be worse in diabetics when glucose is high due to increase retinal blood flow and increasing shear stress on the retinal vessels, thereby resulting in vascular leakage and macular edema.
Relief: What measure have you taken to eliminate visual difficulties? Medications (Rx/OTC) effectiveness? Alternative therapies? Prescription lenses?	Closing or covering one eye like in diplopia. Allergic conjunctivitis may be alleviated by some eye medications or OTC medications. Iritis feels better when in a dark room.
Associated signs/symptoms: Do you experience burning/itching; **photophobia** (sensitivity to light), redness, discharge (describe) increased/decreased tearing, dryness?	Burning and itching may be associated with allergic conjunctivitis, light sensitivity is seen in iritis, dry eye syndrome, and corneal abrasions, purulent drainage is seen in bacterial conjunctivitis.

PRACTICE POINT: Floaters

Floaters are visible due to the shadow they cast on the retina. Since they are suspended in vitreous humor, they follow the rapid movements of the eye. These appear as spots, dots, fine wavy lines, spiders, housefly shapes, or cobwebs. Floaters may be benign or a manifestation of an underlying eye disorder. Benign floaters are few in number and have been visualized for a long period. Floaters that appear suddenly (flashers or photopsia), the sudden appearance of small dots (shower of floaters), or the appearance of a "large ring" are indicators of pathology, such as vitreous hemorrhage, posterior vitreous detachment, retinal tears and detachments, and retinopathies. These are significant findings and require immediate medical attention.

Eye Redness

Red eye is a non-specific term that is a common manifestation and a cardinal sign of ocular inflammation caused by dilation of blood vessels of the eye. Its most common cause is conjunctivitis, often referred to as pink eye, but there are multiple other causes and not all eye redness is pink eye. Redness may also be associated with alterations of the eye lids.

Provider Inquiries	Clinical Reasoning/Logic
Characteristics: Is the redness diffuse? Does the eye ache or cause pain? Is the redness bloody (hemorrhagic) appearing? Do you experience itching, watering, discharge? Do you experience increased sensitivity to light (**photophobia**)?	Diffuse redness involving palpebral and bulbar conjunctiva suggest conjunctivitis, which can be bacterial, viral, allergic, toxic or dry–eyes syndrome. Itching is most commonly caused by allergies and also accompanied by watering of the eyes. A purulent discharge is associated with conjunctivitis (often bacterial in origin), or other infectious conditions. Photophobia is associated with corneal abrasion, keratitis, iritis, chemical burns, and scleritis.
Onset: When was redness first noticed? During blunt/or sharp object trauma or with contact lens trauma. Acute or subacute? How many days?	Red eye is usually acute but it may be subacute in allergic or viral conjunctivitis-few days.
Location: Are both eyes affected or just one? Unilateral or bilateral? Is it localized to one area? Eye and eye lid? Does redness surround the iris?	Unilateral presentation in angle closure glaucoma /iritis/corneal abrasion/bacterial conjunctivitis /keratitis. Bilateral in allergic or viral conjunctivitis. Localized as in perilimbal redness in iritis, sectoral redness in episcleritis. Conjunctiva of sclera and eye lids is involved in conjunctivitis.
Duration: How long has redness been present? Constant or worse in a.m. or p.m.?	Allergic conjunctivitis usually lasts during the allergy season. It is worse when a person is exposed to allergens or in the morning.
Exacerbation: What makes it worse? Wearing contact lenses, during allergy season, during viral season? Exposure to light?	Contact lens wearer may be predisposed to trauma or irritation from contact lens. Allergic conjunctivitis is exacerbated during allergy season. Viral conjunctivitis is heightened during viral season.
Relief: What have you attempted to relieve redness or pain? Eye drops, cool packs, closing or opening eyes? Patching eye?	
Associated signs/symptoms: What other symptoms do you have? Pain? Foreign body sensation? Decreased vision? Photophobia? (Patient comes in with hat or sunglasses or patch on eye.) Discharge, excessive tearing, too little tears or dry eyes, is it purulent, mucoid?	Pain accompanies iritis, angle closure glaucoma, keratitis or corneal abrasions. Aching is experienced in episcleritis. Conjunctivitis is not painful. Stye may be painful on the lid margin. Foreign body sensation is a cardinal symptom suggesting a corneal process like in corneal abrasion, foreign body in the cornea or inside the eye. In itching of eyes, it is a component of allergic conjunctivitis. They may also have symptoms of allergic rhinitis -nasal congestion or drainage, itching of nose. In allergic or viral conjunctivitis, sensation is gritty or scratchy.

Provider Inquiries	Clinical Reasoning/Logic
Are you experiencing nasal congestion, sore throat, wheezing, itchy eyes, itchy nose or ears?	Lid and conjunctival process do not give a foreign body sensation. Hemorrhagic appearance with dilated vessels suggest subconjunctival hemorrhage.
	Dry eye syndrome can cause redness of eyes.
	Red eye with diminished vision is worrisome for infectious keratitis, iritis, or angle closure glaucoma.
	Photophobia seen in iritis and bacterial keratitis.
	Crusty morning discharge can be seen in styes, blepharitis and allergic or viral conjunctivitis. Purulent all day drainage is suggestive of bacterial conjunctivitis or keratitis.
	May be seen in viral or allergic conjunctivitis.
Eye Pain (Ophthalmyalgia) Discomfort or pain can be caused by a problem in the eye or structures around it. Eye pain is common, but is rarely a symptom of a serious condition. Most often, the pain resolves on its own, without the need of medicine or treatment. Although eye pain is often accompanied by redness or injection, pain can also occur without redness and may be the initial sign of a vision-threatening condition, a more benign ophthalmologic condition, or a nonophthalmologic condition.	
Characteristics: How are you experiencing the eye pain? Is it burning, throbbing, aching, stabbing, itching, burning?	Pain in the eye may be described as a burning, throbbing, aching, or stabbing sensation in or around the eye. It may also feel like something is stuck in eye.
Irritation, watery eyes, redness?	An eyelash, a piece of dirt or makeup, or having a foreign object in the eye can cause irritation, redness, watery eyes, and pain.
	Dry eye syndrome is a chronic lack of moisture in the eye, often resulting in stinging and burning, red eyes.
Have you/are you experiencing any vision loss?	Eye pain accompanied by vision loss may be a symptom of an emergency medical condition.
Sensitivity to light (photophobia)?	Sensitivity to light is associated with corneal abrasions, uveitis, or foreign body.
Onset: Did the pain occur gradually or did it come on all of a sudden? Exposure to trauma, chemicals, intense light (laser)? Were you hit in the face with any object/material?	A sudden onset of severe deep-seated eye pain could indicate acute angle closure glaucoma. Pain after trauma may indicate damage to the eye.
Location: Do you experience the pain on the surface of the eye or does it seem to be coming from within the eyeball?	**Ocular pain** occurs on the eye's surface and **orbital pain** occurs within the eye. Ocular eye pain might be described as scratching/ itching, burning or shooting pain. It is usually caused by irritation from a foreign object, infection, or trauma.
	Orbital eye pain might be described as throbbing, stabbing, or aching.

Provider Inquiries	Clinical Reasoning/Logic
Does it occur in one eye or both?	Pain in a single eye could be due to trauma. Pain in both the eyes may be due to infection or a systemic disease.
Duration: Is the pain continuous or intermittent?	Pain greater than 2 days warrants further investigation. Patients with intermittent pain around the eyes generally have headache (primary) causes.
Exacerbation: Is there anything that makes the pain worse?	
Radiation: Does the pain radiate?	Generally eye pain does not radiate.
Associated signs/symptoms: Ask the patient about the following: • Decreased vision? • Discharge (clear, or thick and colored)? • Foreign body sensation (feeling that something is in the eye, whether or not anything actually is)? • Headache? • Light sensitivity? • Nausea or vomiting? • Red eye or pinkeye? • Tearing? • Is the eye crusted shut after sleep due to discharge?	Vision loss in addition to eye pain may be a sign of an emergency situation. Other symptoms that need immediate medical attention include: • unusually severe eye pain • eye pain caused by trauma or exposure to a chemical or light • accompanying abdominal pain and vomiting • pain so severe it's impossible to touch the eye • sudden and dramatic vision changes

Past Medical History

Past medical history identifies the information needed to determine whether there are any prior incidences/events that may have contributed to present situation.

Provider Inquiries	Clinical Reasoning/Logic
Trauma to eyes (entire eye or individual part)? When? What caused trauma? How treated, effectiveness of treatment, any long term effects? Eye infections?	Trauma in the past may lead to irregular pupil or opacity of lens.
Eye surgery? What condition treated? What part of eye? LASIK? When performed, how successful, any complications/long term effects?	Surgery on the lenses may show some changes on the pupil.
Contact lens use? History of viral infection like herpes affecting eye, tip of nose?	Contact lens wearers may develop keratitis. Involvement of the nose may affect the eyes.
Chronic conditions that affect eyes/vision (glaucoma, diabetes, atherosclerotic vascular disease, carotid artery disease, hypertension, thyroid disorder, dry eyes as in Sicca or Sjogrens)? Other autoimmune disorders?	These conditions lead to changes in the eyes like decreased acuity, alterations on optic disc. Hypertension may manifest with eye changes like AV nicking or arteriolar narrowing. Diabetic retinopathy and blindness may occur as complications of DM.
Vasculitis like giant cell arteritis? Multiple sclerosis?	Autoimmune disorders are associated with iritis. Vasculitis may cause monocular blindness. Optic neuritis and atrophy are seen in multiple sclerosis and may cause monocular vision loss.
What medications taken/taking (Coumadin, aspirin)?	Medications that may cause hemorrhaging.

Family History

Family history provides information regarding family members' illnesses or conditions as potential causes for chief concern or presenting symptoms. They may indicate a pattern of presentation associated with transmission of familial/genetic factors that predispose the patient to certain system-related conditions/illnesses. Any of these may indicate a potential or actual cause of eye dysfunction.

Provider Inquiries	Clinical Reasoning/Logic
Retinoblastoma (cancer of retina)? Glaucoma, macular degeneration, diabetes, hypertension? Color blindness, retinal detachment, retinitis pigmentosa, cataracts? Visual corrections? Near sightedness, far sightedness, strabismus, ambylopia?	Genetic predisposition is known with these conditions.

Personal and Social History

The following is information related to surroundings and environments that may identify risk factors related to certain conditions. These questions can also determine the use of safety measures to prevent accidents/injuries or other factors that may be related to other symptoms or conditions.

Provider Inquiries	Clinical Reasoning/Logic
Employment/environment: Exposure to gases, toxins, foreign objects, high-speed machinery? Use of protective eye covering at work and during sports activities? Sunglasses outdoors?	Welders and skiers may develop severe **photokeratitis.** High-speed machinery may predispose to foreign-body exposure.
Sports/activities: Engage in sports or activities that have potential for eye damage (racquet ball, cycling, swimming)?	Chemical exposure to eye. Burn injuries. Blunt trauma to the eyeball common in racquetball.
Visual correction: Corrective lenses (glasses or contacts): how long, last exam, vision corrected adequately; care habits for contacts: (cleaning, storage, insertion, removal)? Any changes in regimen? Screening: When was last screening for glaucoma?	Record of annual/biannual assessment Sunglasses protect from foreign bodies and photokeratitis.
Tobacco: Personal use, exposure to second hand smoke?	Tobacco use is a risk factor for glaucoma, cataract, and macular degeneration. Infection with contaminated contact lens solution.

Developmental Applications

Certain conditions or disorders may be related to certain age groups or situations. Inquiring to obtain age or condition specific information will provide further information for helping to determine causes of the chief concern as identified.

Infants and Children

Provider Inquiries	Clinical Reasoning/Logic
Use of oxygen for resuscitation or neonatal care? How long used, what percentage?	Prolonged use of high percentages of oxygen in neonatal period may cause **retinopathy of prematurity.**
Does the infant gaze at mother's face or other objects, blink at bright lights or blink at threatening gestures directed towards face?	Indicates that infant is able to see both friendly and threatening gestures.
Cloudy or white area in pupil (photo or exam), both eyes have symmetrical light reflex?	Cataracts may cause the pupil to appear white like in congenital cataracts, retinopblastoma, congenital rubella, retinopathy of prematurity, congenital **coloboma** (hole or defect of the iris).
Lazy eye or asymmetrical eye movement? When noted, is it constant or intermittent, when does it occur (stress, illness, fatigue). squinting, blinking? Any nystagmus?	Lazy eye or **ambyopia** is a condition when the brain partially or totally ignores visual input from one eye.

Provider Inquiries	Clinical Reasoning/Logic
	Congenital nystagmus may be genetically transmitted as autosomal recessive (AR) or autosomal dominant (AD) or X-linked recessive trait.
Young children: Excessive tearing, rubbing of eyes, styes (hordeolum) frequency; able to reach and grasp small objects?	Excessive tearing may be caused by smoke, pollen and wind but may also be due to a congenital obstruction of the nasolacrimal duct. These may clear by themselves before year 1.
School age: Able to see front of classroom (board) from desk, adequate progression in school? Last visual screening?	Since children usually do not complain of visual difficulties, early screening to detect visual difficulties is paramount to prevent irreversible visual loss. The technology is available digitally to screen for visual disorders like amblyopia, strabismus, refractive errors cataract and hyperopia and refractive errors. Detecting these early can lead to correction and preservation of vision.
The Pregnant Woman	
Any conditions that can induce ocular complications (diabetes, hypertension)?	Diabetes and hypertension are known conditions that are associated with potential damage to the pregnant woman's eyes.
Any symptoms of pregnancy induced hypertension (diplopia, scotomata [area of lost or diminished vision in visual field], blurred vision, amaurosis [loss of sight without any lesion])?	Cases of bitemporal visual defects in pregnancy have been seen due to normal enlargement of the hypophysis (pituitary gland) with subsequent compression of the optic chiasm are reported (Citrik et al., 2008).
The Older Adult	
Any distortion or decrease in central vision?	Cataract, glaucoma, macular degeneration, and diabetic retinopathy are common in the elderly and may manifest with decreased visual acuity.
Do you experience photophobia?	Photophobia is seen in various conditions like migraine, meningitis, or in corneal abrasions or iritis.
Aids to increase vision (lights, magnifiers)?	
Any difficulty getting around house, use of stairs (if in home)?	Decreased visual input may increase risk of falls, and the elderly are particularly vulnerable due to additional conditions of imbalance and weakness.
Excessive tearing; dry eyes?	
Noticed any scleral brown spots?	
Last visual screening (eye exam, glaucoma)? Last time vision corrected?	It is important to assess frequency of visual check to follow changes in intraocular pressure in glaucoma and retinopathy like in diabetes.
How well able to work, read at close distances? Need to use reading glasses?	Eye pain may be seen in glaucoma, retinal detachment.
Eye pain at night (sign of subacute angle closure and symptom of glaucoma).	

OBJECTIVE DATA

In terms of sequence for a head to toe examination, the eye exam is done within the context of the region of the head. The majority of data obtained from the eye exam is also related to the assessment of the cranial nerves for the neurological exam. Most providers perform the cranial nerve examination during the head and neck segment but may also be covered on the neurological examination. The primary assessment techniques used are inspection and palpation.

Inspection

- Periorbital Area
- Position and Placement
- External Structures
  - Overall appearance
  - Eyebrows
  - Eyelids/lashes
  - Eyeball (conjunctiva/sclera, cornea, lens, iris, and pupil)
- Internal Structures (Ophthalmoscope)
  - Red light reflex
  - Retina, Fundus, macula, optic disc, optic cup, and vessels
- Alignment/EOM/Cover-uncover test
- Visual Acuity
- Snellen chart
- Pinhole testing
- Color vision
- Visual Fields

Palpation

- Lacrimal apparatus
- Intraocular pressure

***Percussion** not performed*

***Auscultation** not performed*

The Level I to Level IV examinations are performed on a continuum, which starts from a basic level and moves to a more comprehensive level based on the provider's abilities and knowledge as well as the patient's presentation and location. The examination may start at the outpatient setting and progress to the ED, hospital unit bed, critical care unit, or specialty unit. Frequently all the elements, from basic to comprehensive exam, are done in one setting such as a primary care setting or clinic.

The condition or illness of the patient is the primary consideration related to the type and amount of data needed to assess the patient's condition, illness, or situation. The arrangement of skills into levels is done for general purposes and is meant to be descriptive rather than prescriptive. The purpose of arranging examination skills into levels is to provide a framework to assist the learner in determining the appropriate data to collect.

Eyes

	Level I	Level II	Level III	Level IV
Inspection	Overall appearance (position/placement) Sclera	Eyelids (margins) Blepharitis, hordeolum, dacrocystitis, chalazion	Foreign bodies	Visual Acuity (Snellen chart/Pinhole test) Color blindness
	Pupil size, shape, reaction (CN III)	Accomodation Alignment (EOMs)	Trauma	Iris (anterior chamber)
	Alignment (corneal light reflex)	Lens/Cornea (cataract, red light reflex)	Infections	Fields of vision
	Periorbital area (puffiness, edema)	Iris (shape)		Sclera/conjunctiva (pterygium)
	Eyelids (approximation, ptosis, inversion, eversion) Eyebrows	Internal structures (ophthalmoscope) (retina, fundus, macula, optic disc, optic cup, vessels)		
	Visual acuity (newsprint)			
Palpation				Lacrimal apparatus Intraocular pressure

Inspection: Level I

Inspection Techniques and Expected Findings	Unexpected Findings
Begin the eye exam by observing the periorbital area for any evidence of swelling or edema. In most instances, periorbital edema is non-significant and may be caused by minor alterations such as changes in sleeping habits, excessive salt intake, alcohol and tobacco use, allergies, and aging.	Periorbital edema may accompany other altered health conditions, such as infectious mononucleosis, thyroid dysfunction and nephrotic syndrome. Loss of periorbital fat creates the impression that the eyeballs have recessed, giving the appearance of sunken eyeballs. Other causes are related to inflammatory or infectious disorders.
There may be conjunctival edema.	**Chemosis** or conjunctival edema may be seen in severe vernal (chronic/allergic) conjunctivitis and Grave's disease, angioedema, superior vena cava syndrome. **Enopthalmos** is the posterior displacement of the eyeball within the orbit due to changes in volume within the orbit. It may be caused by weight loss, dehydration, or loss of subcutaneous tissue as in the older adult or in wasting diseases like HIV. It may be congenital or may be acquired as in trauma like blowout fracture of the orbit.
Next observe the eyes' position and symmetry. The eyes should be positioned approximately one third of the way down the face. The linear distance for making this determination is from the scalp line to the chin. The breakdown of this distance into thirds can be easily approximated by placing the thumb and index finger on the bridge of the nose and the scalp line and by moving the fingers down the face to measure the remaining two-thirds. The eyes should also be equidistant from the midline on a horizontal plane. Their spacing, or canthal distance, should be about one eye's width apart from each other.	Eyes that are considered to be wide set would have greater than one eye's width between them. Orbital **hypertelorism** is the term referring to an increased distance between the eyes. It can be seen in a variety of congenital conditions or syndromes like DiGeorge syndrome, LEOPARD syndrome, and craniofacial anomalies as in fetal alcohol syndrome and neurofibromatosis.
Observe the patient's eyelids to check blinking and position. Blinking should occur at a rate of 17 to 26 per minute. It is not necessary to count the number of blinks, but to be aware of significant increases or decreases.	Eye dryness may also increase the rate of blinking.
Bilateral increased blinking occurs during conversation and during situations in which the patient may feel nervous.	Bilateral decreased blinking may be observed in conditions with less dopamine like Parkinson's and increased in conditions with more dopamine as schizophrenia.
The eyelids should be bilaterally positioned over the eyeball so that the upper eyelid covers a portion of the iris. When the lower margin of the upper eyelid covers the iris and a portion of the pupil, it is known as ptosis (droopy lid) (Figure 18-6).	Ptosis is caused by a weakness of the levator muscle of the eyelid, paralysis or lesion of CN III or damage to the superior cervical sympathetic ganglion. Ptosis may be unilateral or bilateral. It may be the result of certain medications or allergies that cause eyelid edema. It may also be seen as a manifestation of headaches. Other conditions include diabetes, hypothyroidism, Pancoast tumor (tumor on apex of the lung) or myasthenia gravis, a condition associated with muscle weakness caused by defective neurotransmission.

Inspection Techniques and Expected Findings	Unexpected Findings

In situations when the upper eyelid does not cover the any portion of iris, the eyes become more prominent, giving the appearance of "bug eyes," This is known as proptosis (Figure 18-7) and may be a nonpathological occurrence. This is frequently observed with hyperthyroidism and identified as exophthalmos.

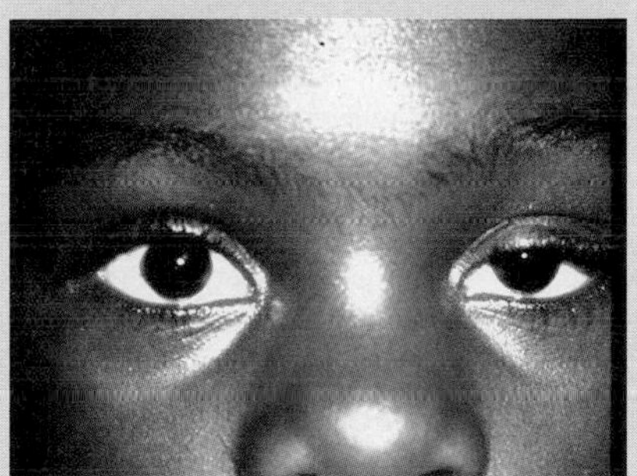

FIGURE 18-6 Ptosis
Source: Courtesy of Randy Carter, OD, The Eye Institute of Utah, Salt Lake City, Utah

Observe for lid lag.

The lower eyelid is positioned so that the upper margin of the eyelid is at the outer border (limbus) lower portion of the iris (Figure 18-8).

Observe for tremors (fasciculations) of the eyelids.

Lagging of the lid movement may be seen.

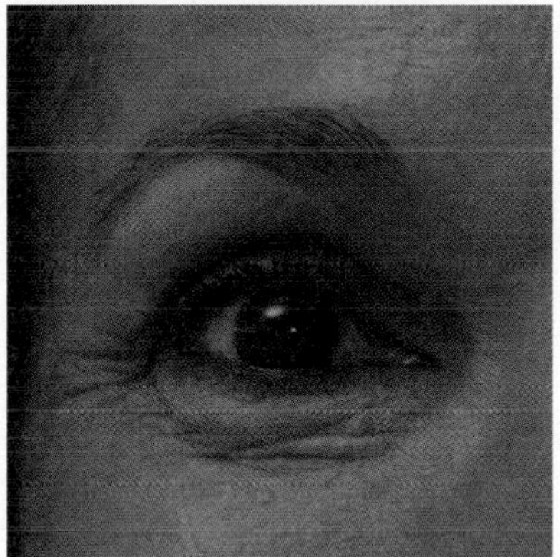

FIGURE 18-8 Lower eyelid at limbus

Fine tremors or fasciculations frequently accompany hyperthyroidism. Lid lag, seen in Graves' disease, refers to the delay in movement of the upper lid relative to the eyeball as patient looks down, thereby exposing the white of the eye on the upper border of the iris.

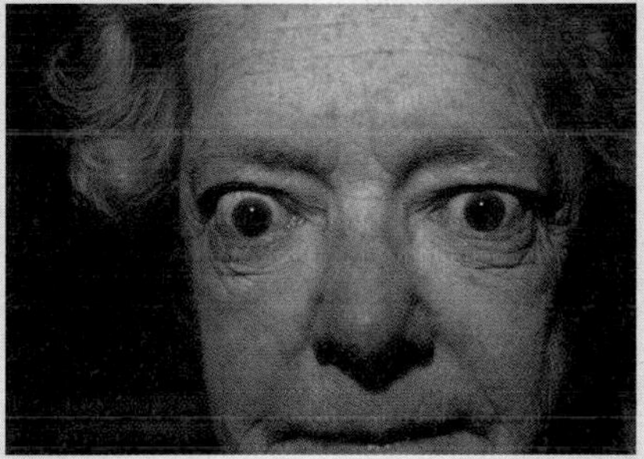

FIGURE 18-7 Exophthalomos
Source: Dr. P. Marazzi

Observe for approximated eyelids; closed eyelids should be approximated or completely cover the exposed portion of the eyeball.

The inability of the eyelids to approximate and cover the eyeball demonstrates lagophthalmos (lid retraction), which frequently accompanies exopthalmos. A major morbidity of this condition is drying of the cornea causing keratopathy, or keratitis. This condition may be seen in Bell's palsy, trauma, CVSA, Guillain–Barré, and Lyme disease.

Inspection Techniques and Expected Findings	Unexpected Findings

Observe the margins of the eyelids for the presence of various alterations. Initial observations are related to the point of contact between the lower eyelid and the eyeball and include the eyelashes.

The margins of the eyelids should be smooth with eyelashes that are curved and directed outward, away from the eyeball.

Alterations would include inversion or eversion.

With inversion, the eyelid turns inward, a condition called entropion (Figure 18-9a). The eyelashes also turn inward and come in contact with the sclera or cornea, causing irritation and possible corneal scratching. The patient often describes the sensation of having a foreign object in the eye. This more commonly affects the lower eyelid.

Eversion (ectropion) is the opposite position of the eyelid and results in the lower eyelid turning outward, exposing the conjunctiva. This condition is characterized by excessive tearing that is not due to an overproduction of tears but because the inferior punctum, which functions to collect tears is also pulled outward, cannot collect the tears (Figure 18-9b).

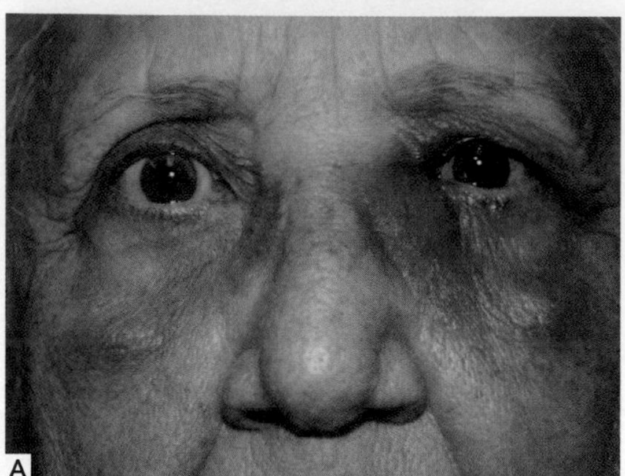

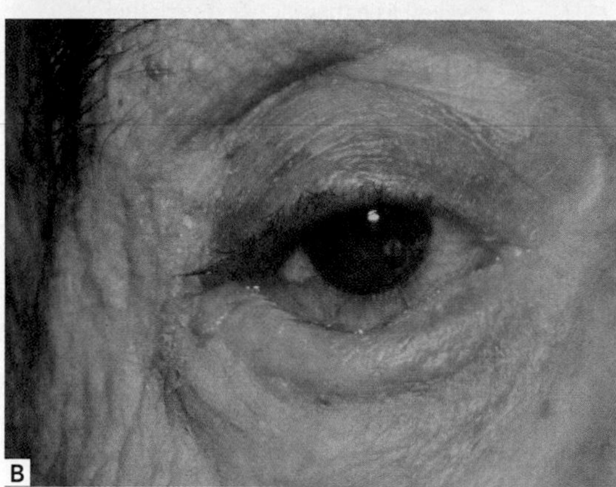

FIGURE 18-9A–B Two unexpected findings are **a)** Entropion; **b)** Ectropion
Source: Courtesy of Randy Carter, OD, The Eye Institute of Utah, Salt Lake City, Utah

Next, assess the pupil's size, shape, and reactivity. The pupil is innervated by CN III, and data about the pupil reflects the functioning of the occulomotor CN. The range of pupil size goes from 2 mm to 10 mm.

The size of the pupil should be equal in both eyes. In approximately 20% of individuals, the pupils are of unequal size, called **anisocoria;** it is not considered pathological if reflexes are present and equal in both sides.

PRACTICE POINT: Pupil Size
Pupil size is a reflection of the amount of light that is needed for correct visual function. The pupil is able to increase or decrease in diameter depending on the amount of light available, so the size of the pupil varies according to the amount of light available.

The expected shape of the pupil is round and equal in shape and size in both eyes.

Anisocoria (unequal pupil) is physiologic in about 20% of people; it is not considered pathological if reflexes are present. New anisocoria should be investigated.

An abnormally large pupil that poorly constricts in a well lit room may be due to trauma to the iris, third cranial nerve palsy, dilating ophthalmic drops, or Adie's pupils.

Inspection Techniques and Expected Findings	Unexpected Findings
	An abnormally small pupils may be from Horner's, iritis, or uveitis. Other alterations of pupil size are identified in Conditions and Disorders. Deviation from the round shape may be due to other pathological conditions like in trauma, inflammation, Argyll Robertson pupils, angle closure glaucoma, surgery or congenital defects like coloboma.
Assess pupil reactivity by observing pupillary action in response to the intensity (luminance) of a light shone directly onto the pupil. Perform your assessment in a slightly darkened room to dilate the pupil. When the pupil has dilated, direct a beam of light onto the pupil and observe the action. The expected response to light is a brisk decrease in size (constriction) of the pupil. There should be an equal response in both pupils. ***PRACTICE POINT: Constriction and Dilation*** Pupillary constriction is described as **miosis** or miotic, while pupil dilation is described as **mydriasis** or mydriatic. Pupillary response is also described as direct or consensual. The pupillary response to direct light is a direct response. A consensual response refers to the pupil in one eye simultaneously constricting when light is applied to the other eye. The pupil receives innervations from CN II and CN III. Stimulation of the sensory (afferent) nerve fibers of CN II in one eye will stimulate the motor (efferent) nerve fibers of CN III in the other eye, thus causing constriction of both pupils (Martini & Nath, 2009).	A sluggish response means constriction was slow. Fixed pupils do not react to light. Pupils that are already constricted to their smallest diameter may or may not be fixed, and would not further constrict. In this situation, darken the room to see if there is any dilation activity. No dilation activity means the pupils are considered fixed. Dilated pupils that do not react to light are described as fixed and dilated. Nonphysiologic dilatation of the pupils is seen in a variety of conditions like CN III pathology (supplies parasympatheric innervation to the iris sphincter muscle causing miosis), trauma, and drugs.
Assess eye alignment by observing the location of the light reflection from any external source on the pupil of the eye. Use the Hirschberg test (corneal light reflex) by observing the location of the light reflection from any external source on the pupil of the eye. The light reflex may be tested directly or indirectly (Figure 18-10). To test directly, shine a light into both eyes from a distance of about 10–12 inches. Note the position of the reflected light on each eye. The position should be in the same spot on each eye. For indirect testing, observe the light reflection from another light source within the patient's environment. 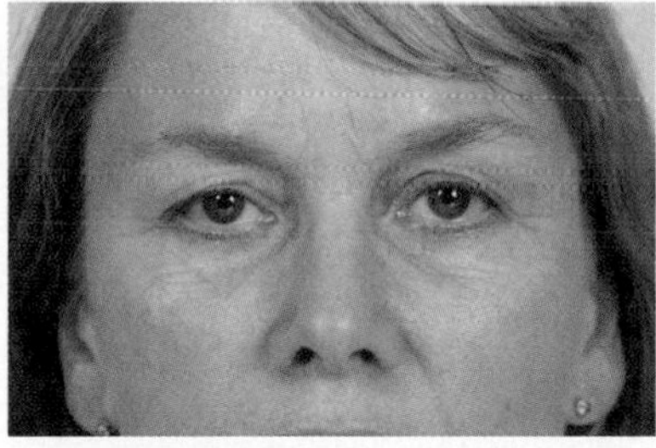 FIGURE 18-10 Hirschberg's/corneal light reflex	Asymmetrical placement of the corneal light reflex indicates that the eyes are not in proper alignment, identified as strabismus, which is generally caused by a weakness or paralysis of eye muscles (see Conditions and Disorders). If strabismus is noted, perform the cover-uncover test. (This is covered in detail in the Infants and Children section).
The iris is a part of the uveal track and is the gateway for the amount of light entering the eye. It is inspected simultaneously with the pupil as the iris actually controls the size and shape of the pupil. It should be flat, round, and with even coloration.	Unexpected findings are altered shapes of the iris and inflammation or infection of the iris (iritis). Iritis (anterior uveitis) may be mistaken for conjunctivitis as it is associated with conjunctival injection. It is usually unilateral, characterized by pain, miosis (small pupil), perilimbal injection (injection close to the sclera-iris junction), blurred vision, and a headache. Iritis is a serious condition that if untreated may lead to glaucoma or blindness. It may be caused by trauma, autoimmune disorders like Reiters syndrome, sarcoidosis, Lyme, ankylosing spondylitis, IBD-inflammatory bowel disease, or infections like TB, toxoplasmosis, syphilis, Lyme disease, and herpes.

Inspection Techniques and Expected Findings	Unexpected Findings

Perform a cursory assessment of visual acuity by having the patient read newsprint from a distance of approximately 14 inches or an arm's length away (Figure 18-11). This provides a gross assessment of the patient's visual ability. It is expected that the patient will be able to read the newsprint. Note whether the patient was wearing corrective lenses or not. If the patient was wearing corrective lenses, it is not necessarily important to test vision without correction.

Unexpected findings would be that the patient is unable to read the newsprint.

While not a significant observation, note the presence and position of the eyebrows, which should be bilateral, with equal distribution of hairs. The eyebrows should also move symmetrically with facial expressions.

Coarse eyebrow hairs along with eyebrows that do not extend beyond the temporal corner of the eye are associated with hypothyroidism.

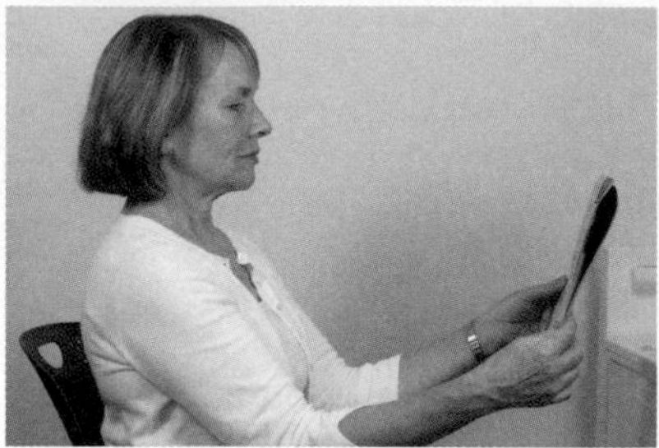

FIGURE 18-11 Newsprint assessment of visual acuity

Inspection: Level II

Sclera, Conjunctiva, Iris

A thorough examination of the sclera and conjunctiva includes manipulation of the eyelids and eyeball to expose areas that are not immediately visible. To perform an initial examination, place your thumbs over the lower orbital ridge bone and gently apply downward pressure so that the conjunctiva of the lower lid is exposed (Figure 18-12). The conjunctiva is transparent and should allow visualization of the color of the lower lids, which is a coral pink with many small vessels visible.

Unexpected findings would be an excessive red conjunctiva, which is associated with conjunctivitis or a pale pink associated with anemia. Bacterial conjunctivitis is usually caused by staphylococcus aureus or streptococcus pneumonia and characterized by conjunctival injection (redness)—unilateral or bilateral with muco-purulent discharge, tearing, burning, and light sensitivity.

Cobblestoning, characterized by giant papillae and papillae along the inner conjunctiva, may be seen in vernal conjunctivitis associated with allergy and atopy.

Subconjunctival hemorrhage is painless contained bleeding manifested by a bright red patch in the sclera that is caused by a rupture of small conjunctival vessels. It may be spontaneous or associated with sneezing, coughing or may be seen in people on aspirin or with high blood pressure. There is no discharge, pain, or visual disturbance. It resolves spontaneously within about a week.

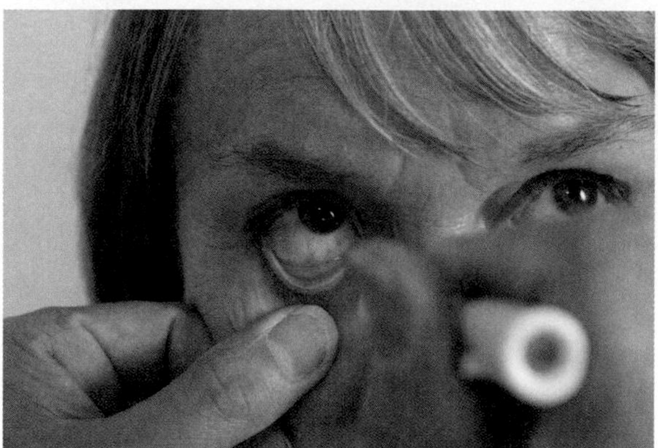

FIGURE 18-12 Exam of lower eyelid and sclera

With the conjunctiva in this position, have the patient look upward to expose the lower portion of the sclera, which should be white, with some visible blood vessels. Common, nonsignificant alterations include a grey-blue sclera in dark-skinned individuals, also described as a "muddy" appearance. In dark-skinned patients the presence of small brown macules on the sclera is also a nonsignificant variant.

An unexpected finding would be a yellow-colored sclera associated with liver disorders.

Blue sclera may be seen in patients on Amiodarone, phenothiazines, malaria drugs and minocyclines, or patients with osteogenesis imperfecta, Marfans, AIDS, Ehlers-Danlos, Turners, psuedoxanthoma elasticum, and other syndromes.

Inspection Techniques and Expected Findings

The upper eyelid conjunctiva is more difficult to inspect and generally is not assessed unless there are unexpected findings of the lower eye lid conjunctiva or there is suspicion of a foreign body.

Begin by having the patient look down to relax the obicularis muscle. Gently grasp the eyelashes and pull the eyelid forward to break the suction between the sclera and conjunctiva. Now that the eye lid is no longer adhered to the sclera, gently pull upward on the eyelashes, everting the eyelid over the cotton tipped swab, exposing the conjunctiva (Figure 18-13). In this position, the conjunctiva can be observed or the foreign body, if there is one, can be safely removed.

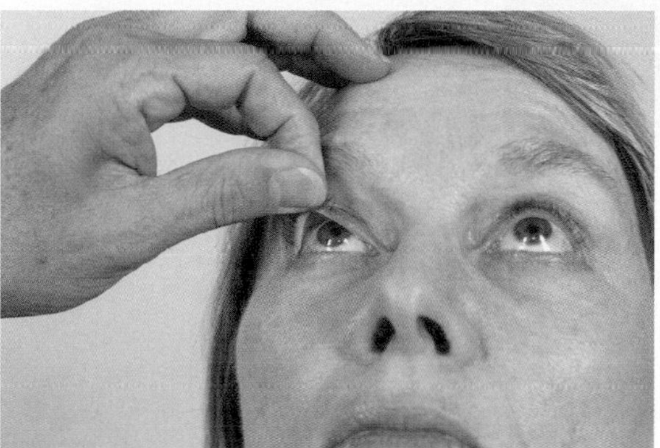

FIGURE 18-13 Examination of upper eyelid

Inspect the margins of the eyelids for any indication of inflammation or infections of eyelids and lacrimal sac.

The lacrimal puncta are small openings on the nasal side of the upper and lower lid that drain tears into the lacrimal duct then finally to the nasolacrimal ducts.

The eyelids may have to be pulled forward to expose the lacrimal puncta.

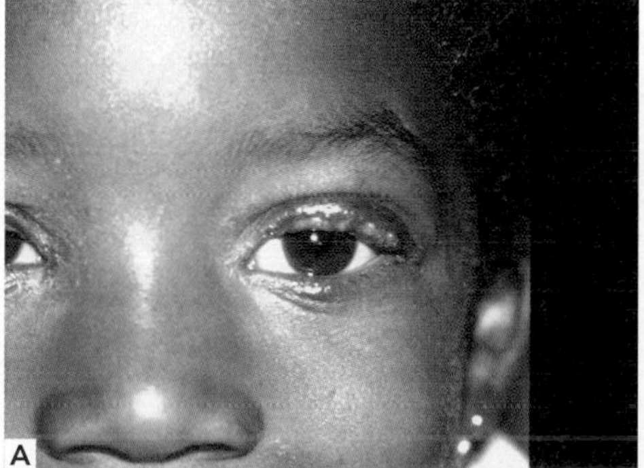

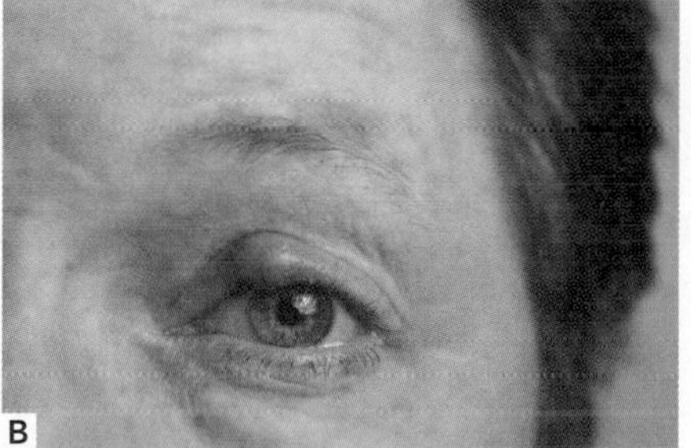

FIGURE 18-15A–B Two unexpected findings: a) blepharitis; b) hordeolum
Source: A Courtesy of Randy Carter, OD, The Eye Institute of Utah, Salt Lake City, Utah

Unexpected Findings

An unexpected finding associated with the conjunctiva is the presence of a pterygium, an overgrowth of conjunctival tissue that spreads from the periphery, commonly the nasal side, toward the cornea (Figure 18-14). Its presence is not associated with any pathological condition, and generally does not cause any problems until it grows over the cornea, interfering with vision. There are no known causes, but they do appear more frequently in patients who are exposed to ultraviolet light, wind, sand, and dust.

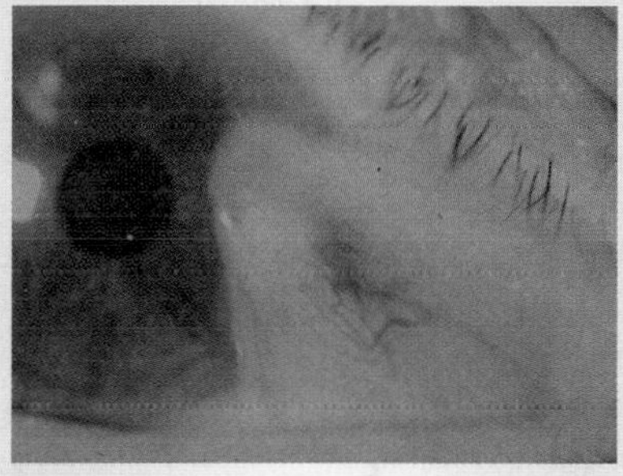

FIGURE 18-14 Pterygium
Source: Courtesy of Randy Carter, OD, The Eye Institute of Utah, Salt Lake City, Utah

Two conditions that may be observed on the eyelids are blepharitis and hordeolum (Figure 18-15). Blepharitis is a chronic inflammation of the eyelid characterized by redness and crusting along the lid margin usually associated with seborrheic dermatitis, rosacea, staphylococcal infection, meibominitis, psoriasis, or parasitic infection.

A hordeolum (stye) is an inflammation or enlargement of a sebaceous gland of the upper or lower lid. Initially, the gland is swollen, red, and inflamed as well as tender. In the advanced stage, it may become a pustule, or furuncle (boil), which may release infectious material that can infect the other eye if untreated.

Dacryocystitis is an infection or inflammation of the nasolacrimal sac, which is commonly caused by obstruction of the nasolacrimal duct (Figure 18-16a).

A chalazion (meibomian gland lipogranuloma) is caused by a blocked meibomian gland (Figure 18-16b). It differs from a hordeolum in that it tends to be subacute or chronic painless nodule or cyst. The cysts usually point to the interior of the lid margin. They can be mistaken for a stye or hordeolum.

Inspection Techniques and Expected Findings	Unexpected Findings

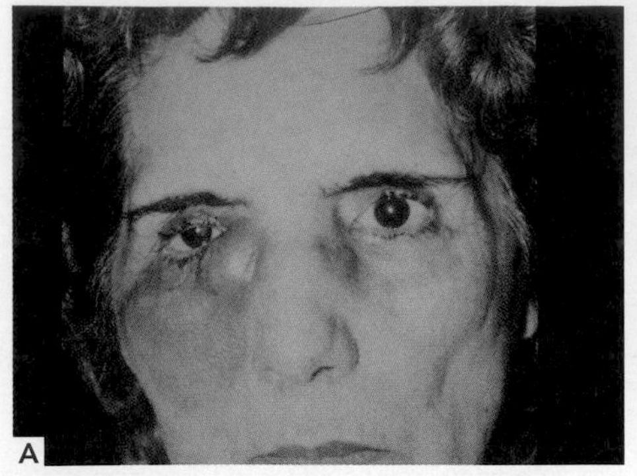
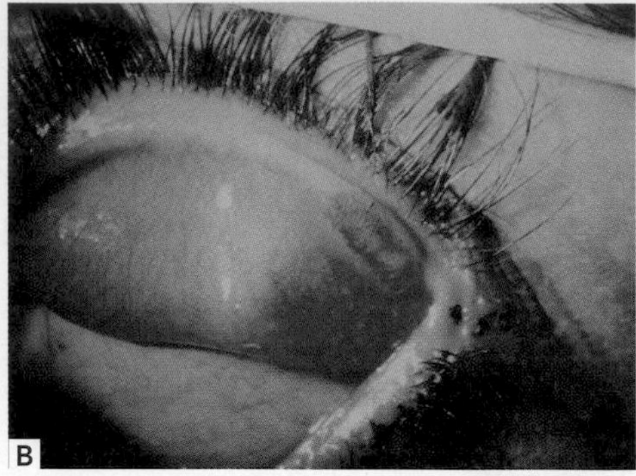

FIGURE 18-16A–B **a)** Dacrocystitis; **b)** Chalazion
Source: Courtesy of Randy Carter, OD, The Eye Institute of Utah, Salt Lake City, Utah

Perform additional assessment of alignment by observing extraocular movements through the six cardinal positions of gaze (Figure 18-17). Extra ocular movements require the coordination of the eye muscles by cranial nerves III, IV, and VI. The occulomotor (III) nerve innervates the superior, inferior, and medial recti as well as the inferior oblique muscles. It also innervates the papillary constrictors and the levator palpebrae superioris muscle. The trochlear (IV) nerve innervates the superior oblique muscle and the abducens (VI) nerve innervates the lateral rectus.

Begin by placing an object at the midpoint of the patient's face, directly in front of the eyes. The object may be your finger, a penlight, reflex hammer, or any other available object. Instruct the patient to move only the eyes and not the head when following the object in your hand. Move your hand in the shape of an "H" by moving horizontally about one foot from the midline. From that point, move the object vertically about one foot up and one foot down from the lateral midpoint. Move back to the starting midpoint and repeat the procedure on the opposite side (Figure 18-17).

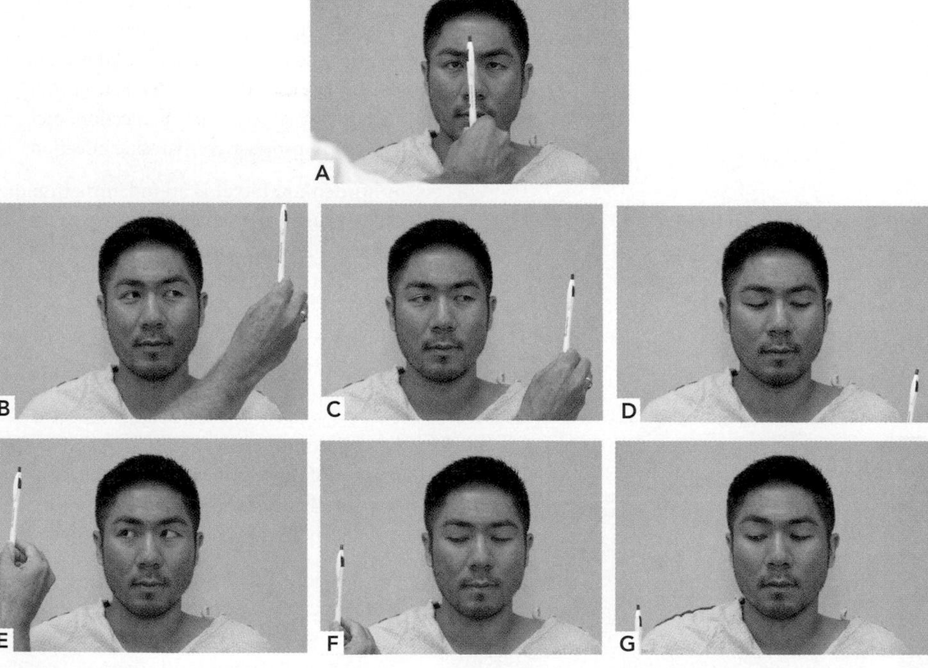

FIGURE 18-17A–G Extra ocular movements

The eyelids may also be swollen due to edema like in nephrotic syndrome, in allergies, infection, fluid retention, thyroid dysfunction, superior vena cava obstruction, trichinosis, excessive crying and sometimes preexisting as an "eyebag" due to excessive suborbicularis oculi fat (see Chapter 17).

Inspection Techniques and Expected Findings

Unexpected Findings

Eye Position	Right Eye	Left Eye	Eye position
center	primary position	primary position	center
up left	Inferior oblique muscle Cranial Nerve III (Oculomotor)	Superior rectus muscle Cranial nerve III (Oculomotor)	up left
left	Medial rectus muscle Cranial Nerve III (Oculomotor)	Lateral rectus muscle Cranial nerve VI (Abducens)	left
down left	Superior oblique muscle Cranial Nerve IV (Trochlear)	Inferior rectus muscle Cranial nerve III (Oculomotor)	down left
up right	Superior rectus muscle Cranial nerve III (Oculomotor)	Inferior oblique muscle Cranial Nerve III (Oculomotor)	up right
right	Lateral rectus muscle Cranial nerve VI (Abducens)	Medial rectus muscle Cranial Nerve III (Oculomotor)	right
down right	Inferior rectus muscle Cranial nerve III (Oculomotor)	Superior oblique muscle Cranial Nerve IV (Trochlear)	down right

The patient's eye movements should be smooth and move symmetrically through the fields of gaze, described as conjugate movement. It is not unusual to observe nystagmus when the eyes are in the extreme lateral gaze.

Observe for evidence of nystagmus, an involuntary, rapid, rhythmic eye movement that may be vertical, horizontal, or rotating. Nystagmus at any other time during the examination is not a routine finding and should be followed up. It may caused by medications like dilantin, alcohol, barbiturates, sedatives, thiamine or B_{12} deficiency, stoke, multiple sclerosis, Meniere's and labyrinthitis, lesions in the midbrain or cerebellum, and benign positional vertigo.

When assessing the pupil for reaction to light, it is often also tested for accommodation. However, during the Level I exam, accommodation is not necessarily assessed. Accommodation refers to the ability of the lens to accommodate when focusing on distant or near objects (Figure 18-18).

To test for accommodation, begin by holding a finger, or another object, approximately 5–6 inches from the patient's nose. Instruct the patient to look at your finger/object and then at another object in the distance. Observe the action of the pupil as the patient alternates focusing on each object. The pupil should constrict as the patient focuses on the close object and should dilate when focusing on the distant object.

Unexpected results would be the inability to accommodate to near or far vision. Presbyopia is the inability to focus on near objects. This is thought to be caused by loss of elasticity of the crystalline lens or loss of power of the ciliary muscle. Early manifestation is difficulty reading fine print especially in suboptimal light conditions. This is corrected by over-the-counter reading glasses.

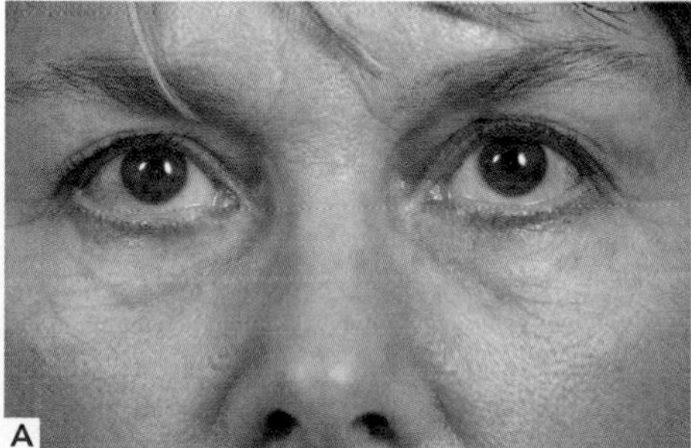

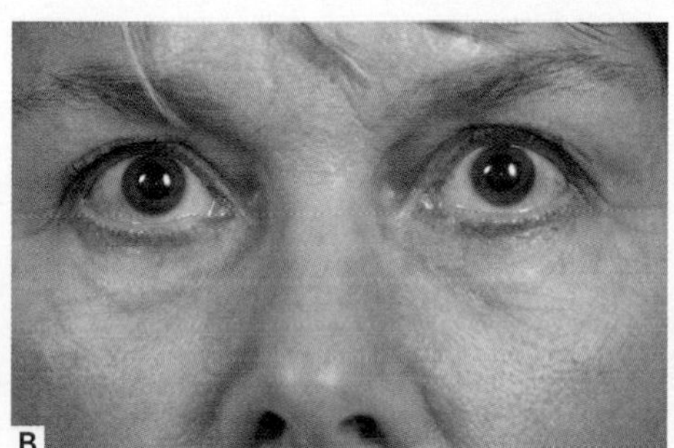

FIGURE 18-18A–B Near and far accommodation: **a)** shows near object; **b)** shows far object.

Inspection Techniques and Expected Findings	Unexpected Findings

Inspect the lens for the presence of any opacities, indicators of cataracts. A cursory assessment of the lens is simply to look directly into the eye.

A more specific assessment of the lens is by obtaining a red light reflex, best accomplished with an ophthalmoscope, looking at the pupil from about 12 inches away. Perform this in a darkened room so that the patient's pupil dilates.

PRACTICE POINT: Ophthalmoscope

When used for this purpose, the ophthalmoscope is only a light source. It is not necessary to change any dial settings.

Begin by turning on the ophthalmoscope and placing the lens of the head in front of either eye. Look directly at the patient's eye until you are in direct alignment with the pupil of the eye. The pupil of the patient's eye should appear red. The red reflection is from light bouncing off the retina, which is red in color. Obtaining this reflex indicates that the lens is clear and allows light to pass through it for accurate interpretation by the retina.

Absent red light reflex may be seen in cataract, retinal detachment, vitreous hemorrhage like in advanced diabetic retinopathy and in retinoblastoma (in infants). Note the presence of any spots or clouding of the lens, which are unexpected findings.

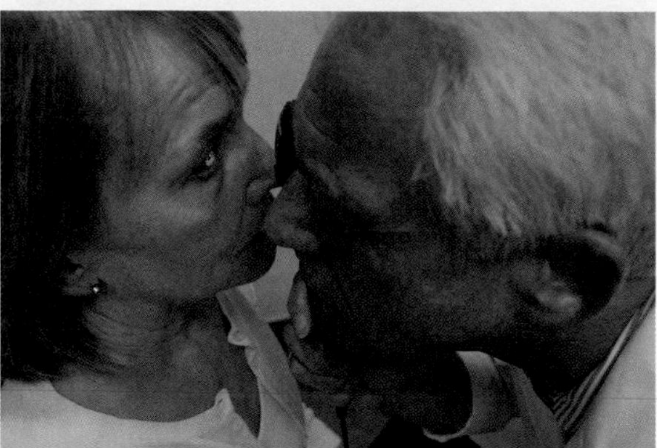

FIGURE 18-19 Red light reflex

THINK LINK: Red Eye

The red light reflex is what is often observed in photos, commonly referred to as red eye. Essentially the same phenomenon occurs when the light from the camera flash passes through the lens and bounces off the retina at the back of the eye, producing the red eye. Individuals who present in the photo with red eye can be assured that they do not have cataracts. Those in the photo who do not present with red eye do not necessarily have cataracts; the angle at which the light hit the lens was most likely not at the correct angle.

Inspection of the internal structures of the eye

Although internal inspection is identified as a component of a Level II examination, it's use is a highly developed skill which would place it at a Level IV. For that reason assessment of the internal structures with an ophthalmoscope is described with Level IV activities.

Inspection: Level III

Much of the eye is surrounded by bone and protected from injury. The small part of the eye that is exposed is vulnerable to injury that may result in devastating consequences.

Perform inspection of the eye to determine if there is any evidence of injury or acute infections of the structures of the eye. Minor injuries may not be visible without the aid of special procedures. A common additional aid is flurosceine dye, which is used to diagnose corneal abrasions, corneal ulcers, and herpetic corneal infections.

Corneal abrasions, scratches on the corneal epithelium, are the most common type of eye injury. They typically present with redness, tearing, photophobia, or a sensation of a foreign body in the eye. They may or may not be visible to initial inspection; however, fluorsceine dye will be taken up by the damaged epithelium and glow green under a blue light. The abrasion is accompanied by intense pain and photophobia due to the fact that the cornea has more nerve endings per surface area than any other part of the body. If the abrasion is caused by an object still in the eye, it must be removed. Abrasions generally heal within 24 hours and do not cause permanent damage.

Inspection Techniques and Expected Findings	Unexpected Findings
	Chemical burns are a very serious injury and can have significant detrimental outcomes. Examples of minor burns are from hairspray and contact lens cleaner. The most serious causes of chemical burns are alkalis, which can produce irreversible visual loss within minutes. Acids produce less severe ocular damage than alkalis. Household cleaning products contain alkalis and may splash into the eyes. Acid burns from exploding car batteries are the most common cause of acid burns. Immediate irrigation of the eyes with water for at least 10 minutes is essential to minimize any damage.
Trauma, either blunt or penetrating, is a major cause of visual loss and/or blindness. Blunt trauma is the most common and can be caused by the eye being struck with a solid object such as a fist, sports equipment (balls, rackets, bats, etc.) or any other solid object. Damage to the eye is caused by the sudden impact that causes compression and indentation of the eyeball.	Sudden blunt impact to the eye leads to rapid increase in intraocular pressure, leading to posterior displacement of the lens-iris diaphragm and rupture of vessels in the iris and ciliary This results in **hyphema**. Blunt trauma may also result in damage to the internal structures of the eye, particularly the retina. There may be hemorrhaging into the retina or the retina may tear and/or become detached. These injuries may not be evident until sometime after the initial trauma, up to years later. Rebleeding from hyphema may lead to glaucoma and vitreous hemorrhage.
Penetrating trauma occurs when the surface of the eye is pierced by a sharp object. In some instances, small, sharp pieces of metal may penetrate the sclera, but not make it into the interior of the eye. Removal of any penetrating object is essential to preventing further damage to either the exterior or interior of the eye.	
Infections of the eye are one of the most frequent reason patients seek emergency medical care. Infection can develop in the eye from irritation, such as getting a small amount of a chemical in the eye. It can also occur after a minor eye injury or a small scratch on the cornea. If untreated, some types of eye infections can damage the eye very quickly.	The most common type is conjunctivitis, otherwise known as pink eye. In broad terms, it is an inflammation of the conjunctiva that may have a variety of causes, including bacteria, viruses, irritations (mechanical, chemical, environmental), allergens, and sexually transmitted diseases. Conjunctivitis presents just as it is described, as a pink eye. Other manifestations include increased tearing, crusting of the eyelid margins, burning/itching, blurred vision, and photophobia. (See Conditions and Disorders.)

Inspection: Level IV

Visual acuity refers to clarity of vision and it is a measure of the spatial resolution of the visual pathway. It is dependent on both sharpness of the retinal focus and the interpretative ability of the visual cortex of the brain. Sharpness of focus is affected by numerous eye structures along the visual axis from tear film, cornea, anterior chamber, pupil, lens, vitreous, and to the retina. The eye is connected to the brain through the optic nerve (CN II). Use the Snellen chart to assess visual acuity. It consists of 11 lines of letters that decrease in size as one goes down the chart (Figure 18-20). If the patient has corrected vision, test both the uncorrected and corrected vision. If time does not permit the testing of both, testing corrected vision will provide information as to the adequacy of the correction or if the patient needs to be referred for additional testing to update the correction.

Inspection Techniques and Expected Findings

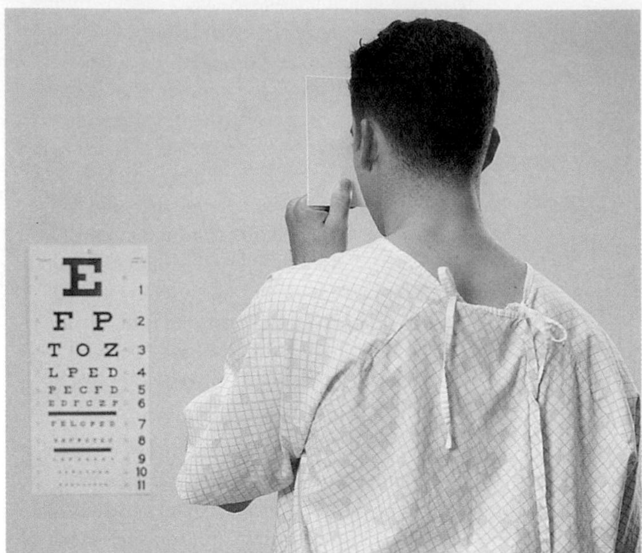

FIGURE 18-20 Assessing distance vision using Snellen chart

Make sure there is plenty of light. Position the patient 20 feet away from the Snellen chart. Have the patient cover one eye, either with a hand or a card, and begin reading the letters in the lines, progressing downward until the letters become too small to recognize and read. Repeat the procedure with the opposite eye.

Document visual acuity as a fraction with the numerator constant at 20. This constant numerator represents the distance between the patient and the Snellen chart. The denominator varies from 10 to 200 and represents the distance at which a normal eye can read the line. Each line is identified with a fraction to indicate the differing distances. The expected result from the visual acuity exam is a reading of 20/20. It is not uncommon, however, for one eye to be better or worse than the other.

PRACTICE POINT: Snellen Exam

Be sure to give the patient enough time to adjust to the changing size of the lines. Make sure not to proceed through the exam too quickly, but don't go so slowly that the patient has time to memorize the letters.

THINK LINK: ***What Does 20/20 Indicate?***

Visual acuity depends upon the accuracy of focusing light on the retina (particularly the macular region), the integrity of the eye's neural elements, and the interpretative ability of the brain. "Normal" visual acuity is frequently considered 20/20. In humans, the maximum acuity of a healthy eye is approximately 20/16 to 20/12, so it is inaccurate to think of 20/20 visual acuity as "perfect" vision. Consider the significance of the 20/20 standard as the lower limit of normal or as a screening cutoff. When used as a screening test, patients who achieve this level need no further assessment.

Visual acuity is also tested for near vision. This is commonly done in patients over age 45 or who complain of difficulty reading. Use a hand-held chart (Jaeger reading card, Snellen card) for this test. Instruct the patient to cover one eye and hold the card approximately 14 inches from the eyes (Figure 18-21). Have the patient start reading the letters in the same way as the Snellen chart, going from large letters to progressively smaller letters until the letters are too small to distinguish. Repeat the procedure with the other eye. Documentation for near vision acuity is the same as with the Snellen chart, with the exception that 14 is used rather than 20 inches.

Unexpected Findings

Unexpected results would be a fraction with a denominator different than 20. A fraction of 20/60 would indicate that the patient sees at 20 feet (numerator is the distance between the individual and the chart) and the denominator here as 60 means that a normal individual can read the same chart from 60 feet away. If the patient is able to read some letters in a line but not all of them, document the acuity as the last line read minus the number of letters the patient missed in the next line, for example, 20/40–2.

Myopia (impaired distance vision) is present when the denominator is greater than the numerator. **Hyperopia** (impaired close vision) is not detected effectively with the Snellen chart (Leone, Mitchell, Morgan et al., 2010).

Vision that cannot be corrected to a minimum of 20/200 is considered legal blindness.

Inspection Techniques and Expected Findings	Unexpected Findings

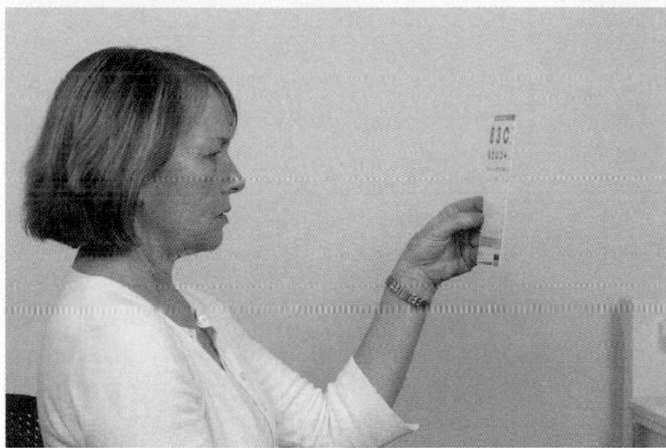

FIGURE 18-21 Jaeger card

The pinhole test is an additional test for visual acuity to differentiate visual defects resulting from refractive errors (myopia, hyperopia, **astigmatism**) from pathological conditions, such as cataracts, optic nerve disease, and so forth (Williams, 2006). Perform pinhole testing by having the patient read the eye chart while looking through a card with a small hole (2 mm) in the center. Such a card can be made by punching a hole in it with the tip of a pencil.

Visual defects that do not improve with pinhole testing can be assumed to result from non-refractive errors of the eye.

Use the Amsler grid to screen for macular degeneration. It consists of horizontal and vertical lines with a dark dot in the center. This measures central vision (Figure 18-22). If patients wear reading glasses or corrective lenses, it is advisable to use them. Expected findings will reveal visualization of the straight lines.

With macular degeneration, the patient will visualize the lines as broken or distorted or the existence of a blind spot. You can also use the grid to monitor changes in vision once they have begun to appear (Sheppared, 2011).

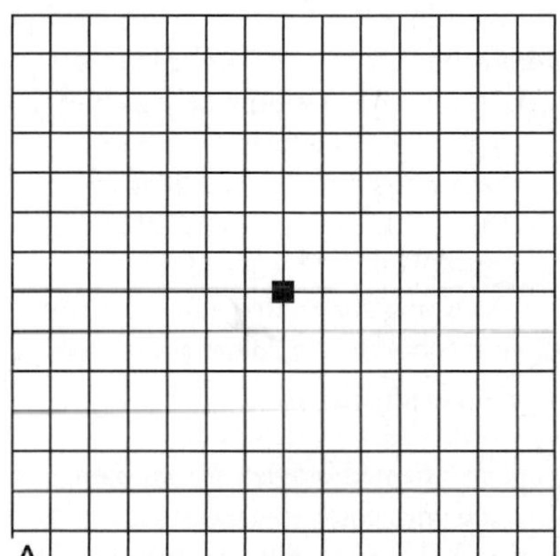

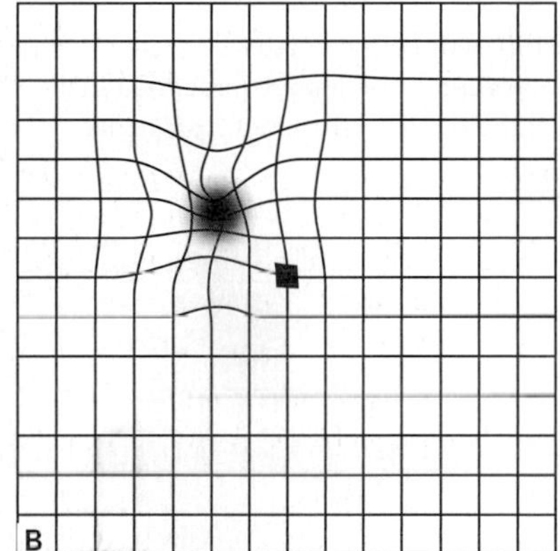

FIGURE 18-22 **a)** Amsler grid; **b)** the same grid viewed by someone with macular degeneration

PRACTICE POINT: Pinhole Testing

Pinhole testing cuts down all extraneous visual input, allowing light to focus only on the fovea. It generally eliminates mild uncorrected refractive errors so that vision improves substantially.

Visual field (VF) testing, while assessing visual parameters, may be considered a neurological rather than ocular test because it assesses the integrity of the optic nerve and its appropriate pathways and divisions.

Standard VF testing in the central 60° (30° radius all around) will find VF deficits from brain tumors, stroke, advanced glaucoma, retinitis pigmentosa, and so on. The only thing it would miss would be a far peripheral retinal detachment that might be found by confrontation. That is so rare that it does not support its use.

If there are any suspicious findings, then obtaining a formal VF on a Humphrey Field Analyzer or similar instrument would be in order. Neurological changes will typically be more evident in the central aspect of the VF. The same is true with ocular abnormalities.

To test visual fields, follow these steps (Figure 18-23):

Always test in a brightly lit room.

Sit 3 to 4 feet from the patient.

Have patient cover one eye with the palm of the hand—no peeking! Instruct the patient to look at your nose and not to move the eye, but to count the fingers as seen. As the patient looks at your nose, the VF is divided into four quadrants. The idea is to check sensitivity in each of those quadrants for neurological purposes.

Present one, two, or five (three and four are too confusing) fingers in each quadrant (one at a time) and ask how many are seen, using any order of quadrants or fingers you desire. Make sure the patient looks at your nose and doesn't glance to the fingers.

Any damage to the optic nerve at any point along its pathway will result in some type of a field cut. The location of the damage and the magnitude of nerve damage determine the extent of the field cut.

Inspection Techniques and Expected Findings	Unexpected Findings

You may also ask the patient to add fingers together by placing your fingers in two quadrants at once. This looks for relative defects where both quadrants "see," but one quandrant is less sensitive and may be ignored by the patient in favor of the better–seeing quadrant.

Next present hands, fingers, or red caps (dilating drop bottle tops) on each side of the vertical meridian and ask if both look the same. This has the same effect looking for relative defects, but is more sensitive. Record results, as the patient would see it, using terms such as "nasal field" or "temporal field" rather than "right" or "left."

Unexpected results would be impaired vision in one or more visual field, unilaterally or bilaterally (Carter, 2007). (See Conditions and Disorders: VF Defects.)

You can observe more than a few pituitary tumors using this technique.

If one finger or red cap is faded in color or shaded as compared to the other, then a defect may exist to that side.

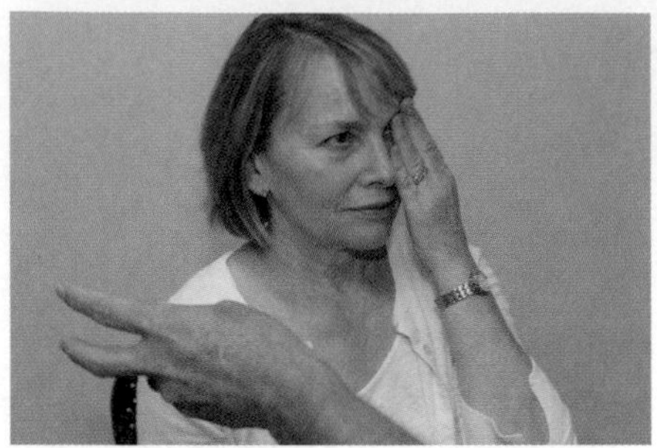

FIGURE 18-23 Testing visual fields

Expected results would be full visual fields in both eyes.

Color Vision Assessment

Test color vision by using pseudoisochromatic plates that have different colored patterns, such as numbers, letters, figures that contain dots that are of various colors and hues that are imbedded in a circle with a background of other colored dots (Figure 18-24). Individuals who are not "color challenged" will be able to identify the various figures within the circles.

Color vision defects are X-linked recessive traits and thus are primarily seen in males. Often referred to as color blindness, these defects are really a deficiency or inability to distinguish between certain colors caused by an absence of specific color absorbing cones. Red and green are the two most common colors associated with color vision deficiency, but yellow and blue may also be involved. There are no specific pathologies or treatment associated with color visual disturbances; however they may lead to learning or safety challenges in cases where distinguishing color is a factor. An individual may also need assistance with color coordinating a wardrobe.

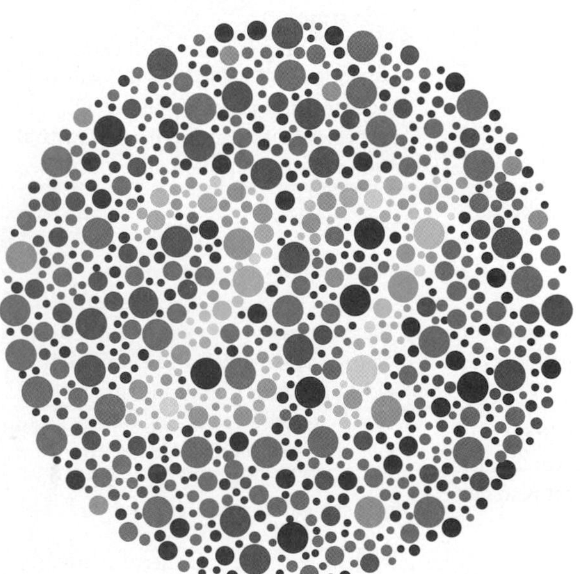

FIGURE 18-24 Color vision plates

Assess the anterior chamber by looking at the distance between the iris and the cornea. The surface shape of the iris is the main determinant of the depth of the chamber.

To assess the anterior chamber, shine a beam of light obliquely across the iris. A flat iris will be fully illuminated and indicates adequate depth of the anterior chamber.

A bulging iris will cause a crescent shadow on the medial side of the iris. This is the iris shape is glaucoma and presents as a shallow chamber.

Inspect the cornea, the transparent part of the sclera, by shining a light into it at an oblique angle. The cornea should be clear without any opacities, cloudiness or irregular reflected light.

If there is a visible light reflection in the cornea, it is most likely due to a corneal abrasion, which can cause severe pain and may cause scarring, interfering with vision.

Inspection Techniques and Expected Findings	Unexpected Findings

PRACTICE POINT: Using Ophthalmoscope

Using the ophthalmoscope requires some practice and coordination. First practice by holding the scope up to your eye and slowly move your head while keeping the lens in front of your eye. Then prac tice using the lens dial by rotating the dial to change the lens. Don't worry about focusing at this point; master your coordination first. Next, practice looking through the lens at various objects throughout the room. Begin with the lens setting at zero. Rotate the lens dial until the object comes into focus. Practice looking at objects at various distances. If you wear glasses, it is best to remove them so that the lens can be as close to your eye as possible. The various lenses of the ophthalmoscope will correct for your visual acuity. If you wear contacts, these can be left in place, but beware if you get too close to the ophthalmoscope lens, your contact may be "blinked" out of your eye. To begin, grasp the handle of the ophthalmoscope so that your index finger is placed on the lens dial to make changing the diopter easier as you examine the eye.

When using the ophthalmoscope, the provider's right eye is used to examine the patient's right eye and the left eye to examine the patient's left eye. For optimum visualization, the opposite eye should be closed. This will take practice and you may find that it is easier to close one eye and keep the other eye open on one side or the other. It's not possible to only use one eye to examine both eyes of the patient. In Figure 18-25, the provider is using his right eye to examine the patient's right eye. If he was to use his right eye to examine the patient's left eye, they would be "nose to nose" and the provider most likely will not be able to get close enough to examine the internal eye.

Next, bring the ophthalmoscope into contact with the eye so that the top of the ophthalmoscope is resting on the eyebrow and the eye is looking through the viewing window. In this position, any movement of the ophthalmoscope will be in concert with your eye. You may place your opposite arm and hand on the patient's shoulders or head to prevent the patient from moving. In this position, you may use your thumb to exert gentle upward pressure on the upper eye lid, which also reminds the patient not to blink.

Start the examination approximately 9–12 inches away from the patient, directing the beam of light onto the pupil. Once the beam of light is shining directly through the pupil, it should appear as red (see earlier discussion of red light reflex).

Focusing on the red light reflex keeps the beam of light in proper alignment for optimum visualization. If the reflex is lost, it is most likely due to movement that occurred. If you lose the reflex, simply locate it again. The presence of the red light reflex indicates that the lens is clear and is capable of transmitting light back to the retina. This is the first observation made. Once the red light reflex has appeared, begin to move in towards the patient, keeping the red light reflex visible.

Inspection: Level IV

Internal Examination (Retina)

Internal examination of the eye requires an ophthalmoscope, which shines a beam of light into the eye through the pupil to allow visualization of the retina. It contains various interchangeable lenses that control the focus you may need to view the inner components.

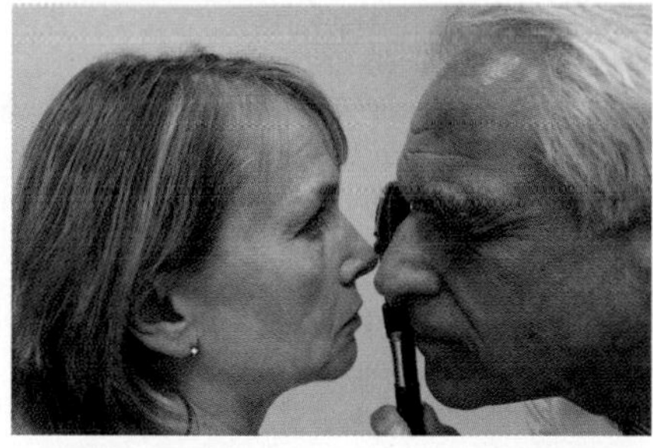

FIGURE 18-25 Examination of eye with ophthalmoscope

Pupil dilation is necessary for an adequate exam of the retina. This may be achieved by dimming the lights in the room; however, if visualization is part of a specific workup, you may dilate the pupil with a mydriatic medication.

Before approaching the patient's eye, instruct the patient to focus on a distant object and to maintain that focus throughout the exam. You must be positioned at eye level with the patient.

Once the red light reflex has appeared, begin to move in toward the patient, keeping the red light reflex visible.

Anything that is present in the lens and interferes with the transmission of light will inhibit the red light reflex. The most common opacity of the lens is a cataract.

Hemorrhage into the vitreous humor is another cause of loss of the red light reflex.

The retina has two major landmarks that can be identified and inspected with the ophthalmoscope: the optic disc and macula.

The first landmark is the optic disk; it is the origin of the optic nerve and located at the back of the retina, slightly off center toward the nasal side of the retina. The optic disc should have well defined margins.

Inspection Techniques and Expected Findings	Unexpected Findings

The second landmark is the macula, the location for central vision and color perception. It is a darker pigmented area on the temporal side of the eye that is less well-defined area than the optic disc. The center of the macula contains the fovea centralis, which appears as a small dot. The macula is composed of only cones and provides the most acute vision when objects are viewed in bright light.

To visualize the retina, place the viewing window of the ophthalmoscope in close proximity to the pupil. You will look through the pupil for retinal details, similar to looking through a keyhole—the closer to the keyhole, the more you can see. As you approach the eye, more details of the retina will begin to come into view. Use the diopters to adjust refraction to bring the retinal structures into focus. What the diopter reading needs to be varies from patient to patient, and practice is the only way to help figure this out. Whether the diopters need to be negative or positive is determined by what refraction is needed to bring the retina into focus.

The retina should appear reddish-pink or yellow-orange, depending on the amount of melanin present as well as the age of the patient (Figure 18-26).

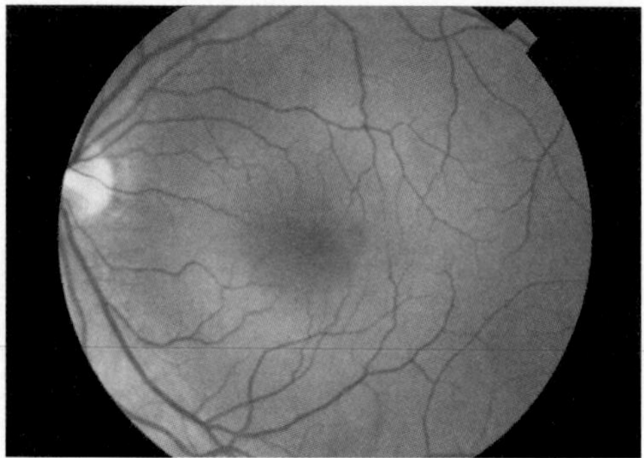

FIGURE 18-26 Retina with expected structures
Source: Kallista Images/CMSP

PRACTICE POINT: Diopter

The "diopter" is the strength of each lens, identified in the small window just below the lens. Positive diopter is identified by black numbers and is used for focusing on points that are nearer to you. Negative diopter strength is identified by red numbers and is used for focusing on distant points. Change the lenses by turning the lens dial clockwise or counterclockwise, depending on the direction of the change needed. To change the beam of light related to its shape and color, adjust the diaphragm dial just below the lens dial.

The closer you can get the ophthalmoscope to the patient's eye, the more you will observe, but only a small portion of the retina will be observable at one time. To better visualize the overall retina, shift the angle of the ophthalmoscope. Remind the patient to keep looking straight ahead; otherwise the retina will also move, making overall observation more difficult.

Your initial view will most likely be of blood vessels in a random segment of the retina. Blood vessels are more visible in the superior and inferior segments of the retina and less so in the medial and temporal segments. The larger, darker vessels are the veins and the smaller, brighter, red vessels are the arteries. You will notice that the arteries and veins branch away from the optic disc in pairs; this configuration helps to locate the disc. To better examine the vessels, follow their point of origin as they branch out distally into the rest of the retina. Their width should gradually decrease as they approach the periphery. The comparison of the width of the arteries to the veins should be in a ratio of 2:3 or 4:5.

Pay attention for any evidence of retinopathies (Table 18-3), particularly in patients with diabetes and hypertension. Diabetic retinopathy (DR) is progressive damage to the eye's retina caused by long-term diabetes. It is a major cause of blindness in diabetics. Individuals with type 1 and type 2 are both at risk for developing DR. DR can be further classified as non-proliferative or proliferative.

The appearance and characteristics of the retinal vessels provide information related to the presence and severity of hypertension. The microcirculation of the retina is more susceptible to hypertensive changes so that they are manifest in the retina early in the course of hypertension. Generalized retinal-arteriolar narrowing and aterio-venous nicking are the initial indicators of retinal damage and are thought to be predictors for developing hypertension in individuals previously considered as normotensive (Wong & Mitchell, 2007).

The arteriole is transparent so that the blood circulating through it can be observed. Light reflects off the arteriole blood, which should be about one fourth of the diameter of the vessel. Pay particular attention to the locations where the blood vessels cross over each other (arteriovenous, or A-V, junction). Crossing should only be observed at a minimum of 2 disc diameters away from the disc. (See Practice Point: Measurement in the Eye). At the AV junction, where the vein crosses beneath the artery, the width of each vessel should be consistent and there should be no space between the arteriole and vein.

This is manifested as a small space between the walls of the two vessels. An evolution of AV nicking is tapering, which is observed as narrowing of the vein before and after crossing the artery. Additionally, banking, a twisting or bending of the veins, may be present. This contributes to a tortuous appearance.

Inspection Techniques and Expected Findings	Unexpected Findings
	In arteriolosclerosis, hypertension causes blockage of the retinal microvasculature leading to microinfarcts (cotton wool spots) and superficial hemorrhages. Thickening of the arteriolar vessel wall results in nicking at the AV junction (AV nicking). Hypertensive retinopathy presents with a "dry" retina (few hemorrhages, rare edema, rare exudate, and multiple cotton wool spots) whereas diabetic retinopathy, in comparison, presents with a "wet" retina (multiple hemorrhage, multiple exudate, extensive edema, and few cotton wool spots) (Sowka, Gerwood, & Kabat, 2009). Changes in the vessels lead to alterations that can be noted along the length of the vessel and at the AV junction (Table 18-4).

Table 18-3 Retinal alterations

Retinal Yellow-White Images	Distinguishing Ophthalmoscopic Appearance	Underlying Cause	Common Related Conditions
Hard exudate	Deep yellow flecks with sharp margins, often circinate	Increased vascular permeability from damaged pre-capillary arterioles, allowing the leakage of serous fluid and lipids into the retina and resulting in thickening of the macula	Any conditions associated with chronic vascular leakage Diabetic retinopathy Hypertensive retinopathy Capillary hemangioma of the retina Choroidal neovascularization Retinal arterial macroaneurysm Radiation changes
Cotton wool spot	Fluffy gray-white; usually near optic disc	Micro-infarcts (focal ischemia) associated with occlusion of precapillary arterioles	Any process that occludes small retinal arterioles: hypertension, diabetes, connective tissue disease, HIV, hypercoagulable conditions
Retinal infiltrate	Yellow white area with fuzzy edges near retinal vessels	Clump of leukocytes (inflammatory cells) sometimes forming granulomas, with micro organisms and dead retinal tissue	Sarcoid; leukemia; infection with candida, CMV, herpes simplex or zoster, lues
Retinal drusen	Scattered clusters of yellow-orange/white specks, often centered around fovea	Debris from dead retinal pigment epithelium	Age-related macular degeneration
Chorioretinal atrophy	Mostly white, often with flecks of black pigment	Both the choroid and retina are damaged, causing them to wither away and stop working	Most common cause of damage is an infection: Toxoplasmosis Toxocara Cytomegalovirus Herpes virus (cold sore chicken pox)
Intraluminal plaque	White/yellow spot frequently located near arterial bifurcations; Hollenhorst plaques are refractile platelet-cholesterol-fibrin yellow flecks. White plaque associated with talc or calcium.	Embolism	Cervical carotid atherostenosis, calcified cardiac valve, IV drug abuse
Myelinated nerve fibers	Feathery white clump usually connected to optic disc	Extension of myelin onto retinal ganglion cell axons	Congenital condition Does not interfere with vision

Table 18-4 Arterial/venous alterations

Retinal changes in hypertensive retinopathy are classified into four groups according to the Keith-Wagner-Barker (KWB) system.

Grade I	Increased light reflex from arterioles Moderate arteriolar narrowing (25%)—seen as silver wiring Focal constriction and vascular tortuosities
Grade II	Grade I changes plus appearance of AV nicking Arterioles reduced by 50%
Grade III	Grade II changes plus appearance of cotton wool spots and flame hemorrhages Arterioles reduced by 66%
Grade IV	Appearance of papilledema Arterioles threadlike or invisible

Sources: Data from Seidel, 2006; Wong & McIntosh, 2005; Hughes, & Moinfar, 2007

Inspection Techniques and Expected Findings

A nonsignificant finding is the presence of myelinated nerve fibers. It is seen on the retina as feathery, white patches that radiate from the optic disc, obliterating the retinal vessels may be seen. This may represent a congenital anomaly and may be mistaken for cotton wool spots.

A few small drusen deposits of fat and cellular debris that accumulate between the retinal pigment epithelium (RPE) and Bruch's membrane in the macular region, are expected to form in the human eye, usually after age 40.

After visualizing the retinal background and blood vessels, return to the origin of the vessels and examine the optic disc, which is the point of origin for the optic nerve. The disc is not centrally located but closer to the medial or nasal portion of the retina.

First examine the shape and margins of the disc. It should be round in appearance, although a more oval shape is not unusual. It also should have well defined margins, particularly in the temporal region, and a more yellow-orange appearance as compared to the rest of the retina. In the center of the optic disc is the physiologic or optic cup, which is the actual point of origin of the blood vessels.

Unexpected Findings

Drusen is also a significant finding associated with dry macular degeneration. They appear as specks of white or yellowish material under the retina and occur in two forms.

Hard drusen are small, solid deposits that apparently are not detrimental when present in small numbers.

Soft drusen are larger with indistinct borders and lift up the RPE as they build up, forcing the two layers apart and causing mild to moderate loss of central vision. Drusen develop long before the abnormal vessels of wet AMD. Retinal alterations are described in Table 18-3.

Cotton wool spots are lesions that appear as soft white spots on the retina. They are caused by microinfarcts of the neural layer of the retina. Hemorrhages appear as red lesions on the retina. Their shape can be rounded or linear.

Papilledema is swelling of the optic disc with anterior bulging of the optic cup caused by increase intracranial pressure (Figure 18-27). It is observed as obliteration or blurring of the disc margins, venous engorgement, loss of venous pulsation, hemorrhages adjacent to the disc, elevation of the optic disc, and Paton's lines, which are radial retinal lines cascading from the optic disc. Papilledema is an indication of increased intracranial pressure as seen in intracerebral bleed, tumors, cerebral venous sinus thrombosis, pseudotumor cerebri, acute high altitude sickness,

Inspection Techniques and Expected Findings	Unexpected Findings

Lyme disease, and malignant hypertension. The increase in intracranial pressure is transmitted to the optic nerve, resulting in swelling of the optic nerve head. If unilateral, it may indicate orbital pathology like optic nerve glioma.

Other alterations associated with the retina are described in Table 18-3.

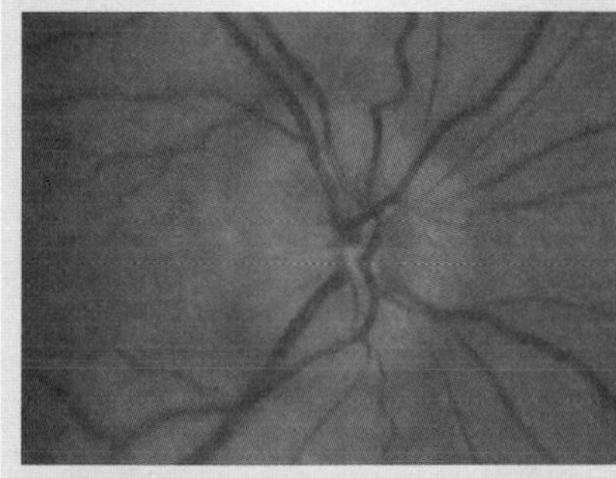

FIGURE 18-27 Papilledema
Source: Courtesy of Randy Carter, OD, The Eye Institute of Utah, Salt Lake City, Utah

PRACTICE POINT: Measurement in the Eye

Providers use specific parameters to describe location, distance, and size on the retina specific parameters that are used. As the visualization of the retina is circular, location is described in relation to the numerals on the face of the clock, for example 3 o'clock position or 10 o'clock position. Size and distance is expressed in terms of disc diameters (DD). The diameter of the optic disc is the standard measurement; thus a lesion on the retina would be described as 3 DD from disc. Size of lesions can also be compared to the disc diameter.

Conclude your inspection with an examination of the macula, also known as the *fovea centralis* or *macula lutea*. This is the area of central vision and is located in the temporal segment approximately 2 disc diameters from the optic disc. It is not a well-defined area, but it does not contain any blood vessels and may be a lighter color than the retina. It is difficult to examine the macula because shining a direct light on the area causes an extreme pupillary constriction. To guarantee the ability to examine the macula, the pupils will need to be dilated with a mydriatic pharmacologic agent.

Palpation: Level IV

Palpation Techniques and Expected Findings	Unexpected Findings

Lacrimal Apparatus

Inspection of the lacrimal apparatus for inflammation (dacrosystitis) has already been discussed. Palpation of the lacrimal apparatus is done to identify or confirm the presence of inflammation (Figure 18-28).

If there is an obvious swelling of the area, there is most likely accompanying tenderness to palpation. If there is redness without swelling, it is most likely to be tender also.

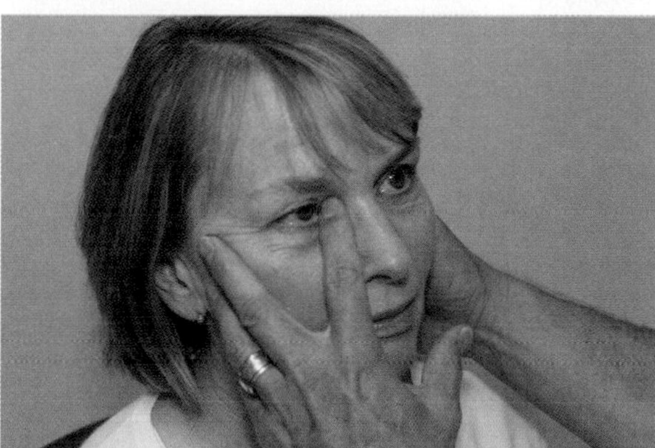

FIGURE 18-28 Palpation of lacrimal gland

To palpate the lacrimal apparatus, place your index finger over the nasolacrimal duct, just inside the orbital rim near the inner canthus, not against the nose. Apply light upward pressure with the finger and note the slight eversion of the lower lid. This allows for visualization of the puncta and if inflamed, or blocked, a back flow of fluid (tears/pus) out of the puncta.

Inflammation of the lacrimal apparatus is relatively rare, but is associated with some conditions.

Palpation Techniques and Expected Findings	Unexpected Findings

Intraocular Pressure

While intraocular pressure can be measured using appropriate equipment, an indirect assessment is to palpate the eyeball to assess for any increased pressure.

The eyeball is generally quite firm, but should allow for a slight indentation when palpated. Have the patient close the eyes and gently place your thumbs over the upper portion of the eyeball and exert mild pressure (Figure 18-29). The eyeball will give slightly.

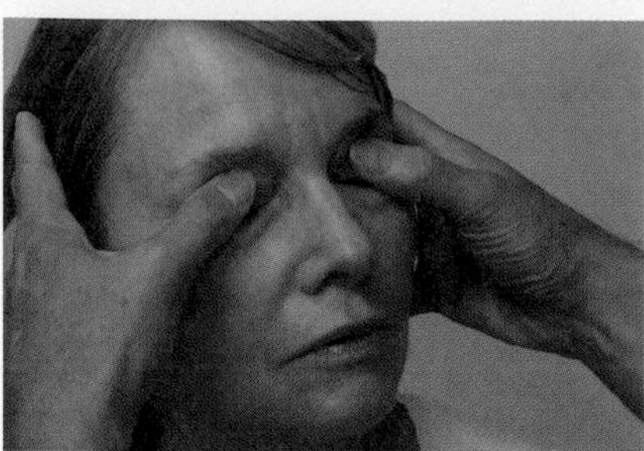

FIGURE 18-29 Palpation of anterior globe

Unexpected Findings: An increase in intraocular pressure is caused by glaucoma, a condition in which fluid in the eye is not properly drained, so that pressure caused by the fluid increases. (See Conditions and Disorders.)

An eye ball that is very firm to hard and does not indent at all is an indication of significantly increased intraocular pressure.

Developmental Applications

Infants and Children

Early detection and treatment of eye disorders in infants and children is essential to prevent permanent visual alterations. Examination of the eyes begins in infancy and should be a part of all well-child visits. Any unexpected findings should prompt referral to an appropriate specialist provider who is educated in treatment of pediatric ophthalmic disorders.

Techniques and Expected Findings	Unexpected Findings

Infant

Initial assessment of the infant's eyes begins with the external structures. The external structures should be symmetrical related to eyebrows, eyelashes, and size. The spacing and distance between the eyes should be as previously described. The palpebral fissures should be horizontal on a plane between the medial and lateral canthus. Infants of Asian parents will demonstrate a slightly upward slant to the plane. The eyelids should completely cover the sclera and cornea. It is common to observe edema of the eyelids, which may be asymmetrical, due to birth, but this is not necessarily significant (Figure 18-30).

Unexpected Findings: Wide set eyes (hypertelorism) are frequently associated with craniofacial defects and some mental retardation conditions (described earlier in this chapter).

Infants with Down syndrome will also demonstrate this upward slant.

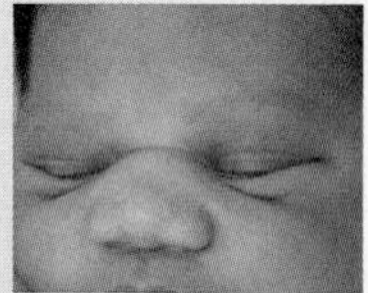

FIGURE 18-30 Edematous eyelids of infant
Source: George Dodson/Lightworks Studio/Pearson Education

Observing the sclera, cornea, and conjunctiva may be difficult in newborns as they seldom open their eyes, especially in bright light. Do not pry the eyes open. Holding or rocking infants into an upright position or holding the infant at arms' length and turning in one direction will also stimulate the eyes to open. If the mother or another individual is present, have her hold the infant upright and observe the infant's eyes from over the mother's shoulder. Make your observation of the eyes quickly because the infant will not keep them open for very long.

The sclera of the newborn often has a blue tint, and also a slight conjunctivitis due to the instillation of medications into the eyes. If present, it should not last for more than 24 hours. The cornea should be clear and transparent. Look for any light reflection on the cornea, which should be symmetrically positioned on each eye. Some asymmetry may be noted in the newborn, but should not persist after 6 months of age. The red light reflex should also be elicited in the newborn. The reflection should be red-orange, just as for the adult, or a light gray in dark pigmented, brown-eyed infants.

Unexpected Findings: Any opacities, dark spots, dull reflex, or absence of a reflex are unexpected results and require further follow-up.

Techniques and Expected Findings	Unexpected Findings

Observe the characteristics of the pupils and iris. The iris is commonly blue or gray in light-skinned infants, brown in dark-skinned infants. The permanent color of the iris is present by 6 to 9 months. The pupils should be round, equal, and reactive to light. Pupil size varies from 2 to 4 mm.

Unequal pupil size may have a sympathetic or parasympathetic cause; however, small differences may be nonsignificant, but should be noted for future comparisons.

Visual acuity assessment in the newborn is primitive. Light perception may be assessed by the blink reflex, which is present when the infant blinks in response to a bright light directed on the pupil. Pupil constriction to light is also an expected response. Subsequent assessment of vision is done by observing the infants ability to fixate upon an object and then the ability to follow the object with the eyes. By 2 weeks the infant should be capable of fixating on an object and begin to follow it. Formal testing of visual acuity with charts or cards does not begin until the infant reaches 3 years of age.

If the eyelids are edematous, initial assessment of vision will need to be delayed.

The initial assessment of visual acuity should also include observation for nystagmus, or spontaneous, involuntary movement of one or both eyes.

The presence of nystagmus in the term infant may be associated with Down syndrome, atrophy of the optic nerve, congenital cataracts, dysfunction of the ocular muscles or nerves, vestibular disorders, and decreased visual acuity (Duderstadt, 2006).

Child

Initial visual acuity testing for the 3-year-old uses Allen cards, which are flash cards containing seven schematic figures: truck, house, birthday cake, bear, telephone, horse, and tree. Before testing begins, be sure that the child is familiar with and can identify each figure; don't use cards the child cannot identify. Begin with the child using both eyes, and stand 1–2 feet away. Have the child identify one or two figures to be certain the child understands what to do. Continue backing up a distance of 2–3 feet while continuing to test the child's ability to identify the figures with each eye and also with both eyes. When a distance is reached at which the child can no longer identify the objects, move forward a few feet to confirm the ability to identify the figures at the shorter distance. Visual acuity is recorded as the furthest distance the child can identify the figures over 30 feet.

Another method for testing visual acuity is the HOTV Test. This test consists of a wall chart that only contains Hs, Os, Vs, and Ts. The child is given another chart that contains a large H, O, V, and T. As the provider points to a letter on the wall chart, the child identifies the same letter on the testing board.

The Tumbling E chart is a version of the Snellen chart, but only consists of the letter E in various positions: pointing up, down, right, or left (Figure 18-31). The size of the letter decreases in size in the same manner as the Snellen chart. As the provider points to each letter, the child is asked to identify its position. This can be done by the child specifically stating *up, down, right,* or *left* if the child is capable of understanding these terms. If the child is not, then have the child point a finger in the same direction as the letter. Once the child becomes literate and can identify the letters of the alphabet, the Snellen chart may be used for visual acuity testing.

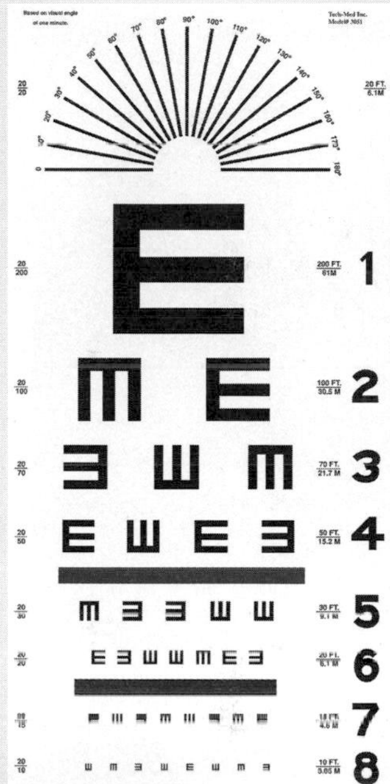

FIGURE 18-31 Tumbling E chart

The funduscopic examination is somewhat difficult to perform on an infant or child. The initial exam consists only of the red light reflex. The first complete funduscopic exam should be done somewhere between 2 and 6 months. At this age, the fundus appears pale with poorly developed blood vessels. There will not be a foveal light reflection due to immaturity of the macula, which is not fully developed until 1 year of age.

Eye examination of the infant through 3 years of age is performed using the previously described procedures. When the child reaches 3 years of age, additional procedures are added or previous procedures are expanded. Decisions to use certain procedures are highly dependent upon the child's developmental stage.

Visual acuity is tested through any of the tests described above. Alignment and mobility are tested to determine the presence of strabismus.

Strabismus is nonbinocular vision or nonalignment of the eyes, which results in double vision and a lack of depth perception. Commonly, these symptoms are not noticed or troubling to the young child. Strabismus that is not diagnosed early enough will ultimately lead to loss of vision in one eye or ambylopia. The brain is unable to process double vision so it shuts down visual stimulation in one eye.

Techniques and Expected Findings	Unexpected Findings

The corneal light reflex is the easiest test to initially determine ocular alignment. Additional testing is done using the simultaneous red reflex test and the cover-uncover test.

Failure of the light reflex to be located in symmetrical positions on each eye is a reason for concern.

The simultaneous red reflex test (Bruckner test) is performed in much the same way when viewing each eye for the red light reflex. Instead of confirming the presence of the red light reflex, visualize the reflex in both eyes simultaneously and compare them with each other related to size, brightness, and color. Each of these should be the same in each eye.

Any movement of the uncovered eye to try to focus on the object indicates that it was originally out of alignment. A medial deviation of the eye is referred to as esotropia; a lateral deviation is referred to as exotropia (Figure 18-33).

The cover-uncover test is used to further evaluate ocular alignment (Figure 18-32). Infants as young as 4 months may have this performed on them. Begin the cover-uncover test by having the infant or child focus on an object. The object does not have to be a far distance away. As the eyes are focusing on the object, occlude one eye, with fingers or a card. Observe the uncovered eye still focusing on the object. An eye in proper alignment will remain focused on the object.

Any movement of the eye indicates poor alignment. In this eye, when covered, the object is no longer focused on the macula. If the eye is out of alignment, this covered eye will move into a relaxed position, referred to as **phoria**. When the eye is uncovered, it will respond by moving to refocus on the object.

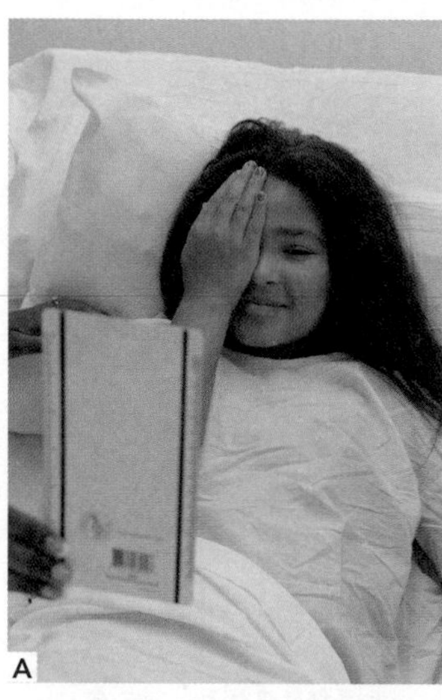

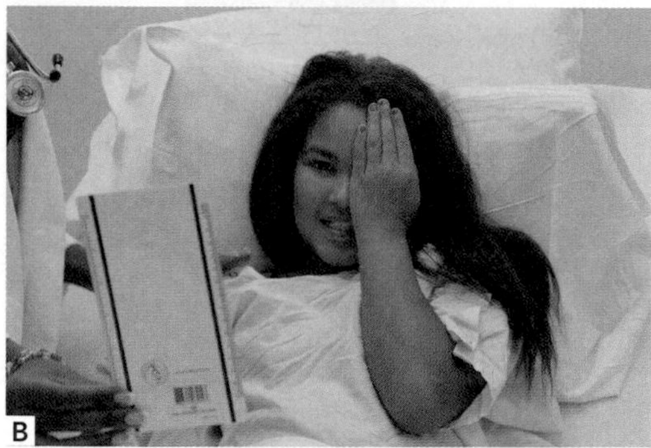

FIGURE 18-32A–B Cover-uncover test

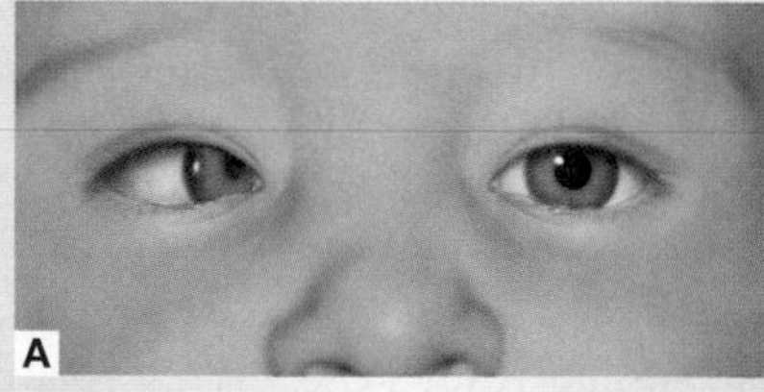

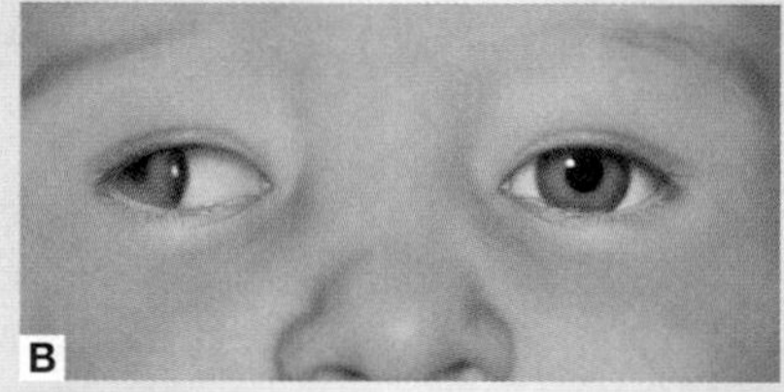

FIGURE 18-33A–B a) Esotropia; b) Exotropia

Next, remove the covering over the other eye. Observe, again for any movement of the eye. A correctly aligned eye will remain in a position of focus on the object.

Techniques and Expected Findings	Unexpected Findings

The Pregnant Woman

There are no specific tests that are performed on the pregnant female. Any minor visual changes that are present should not be treated as having major significance.

Look for visual field defects. These may be disturbing to the patient, but she should be reassured that these will disappear after pregnancy.

If the patient is diabetic, has hypertension, or is preeclamptic, the retina should be completely examined to determine if any major changes have occurred.

Bitemporal hemianopsia may occur due to hypophyseal enlargement, leading to compression of the chiasm.

Retinal vascular changes in preeclampia may occur in pregnancy and may manifest as visual field defects.

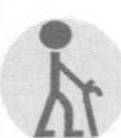

The Older Adult

Visual acuity in the elderly is tested in the same way as the adult.

Presbyopia is a common finding and in the absence of other structural and pathological changes, visual acuity does not change significantly.

Other visual changes that may be present include decreased vision in dim light or darkness and difficulty in color perceptions, especially blues, violets, and greens.

Structures surrounding the eye may manifest various changes. The eyebrows may decrease in numbers of hairs due to loss of hair follicles and may be absent in the outer one-third to one–half of the brow. Hairs that remain are coarse and may begin to grow.

The skin surrounding the eyes becomes lax and loose due to the loss of elastic tissue. The upper eyelids begin to droop and may cover more of the iris. The lower eyelids also become loose and are not approximate with the lower portion of the eyeball (ectropion), exposing the conjunctiva. The puncta also do not drain the tears, so there is also excessive tearing.

Ectropion may cause excessive itching and dryness.

Entropion results in irritation of the sclera and may cause damage to it.

The opposite condition is entropion (discussed previously). The eyes also may appear sunken, due to the loss of periorbital fat. The skin may also develop xanthelasmas, which are creamy yellow plaques that appear on the lids of the inner canthus (Figure 18-34). They begin to appear in the 50s and are more common in females. Their presence is nonsignificant.

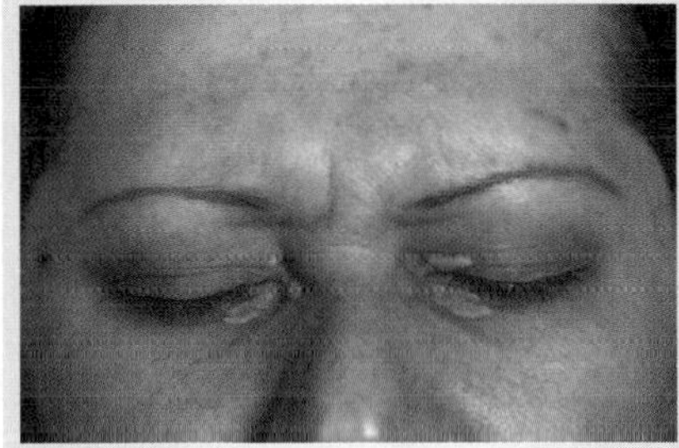

FIGURE 18-34 Xanthelasmas
Source: CMSP

The lacrimal apparatus may reduce the amount of tears produced, which may cause the eyes to appear dry and lose their shine. The patient may also report that the eyes demonstrate a burning sensation.

The sclera may appear less shiny, as described previously. There are no specific changes directly associated with aging. The cornea may appear somewhat cloudy due to deposition of various materials in the aqueous humor. There may be a grey-white circle (arcus senilus) around the cornea at the limbus (Figure 18-35). This is a common age associated alteration and is nonsignificant.

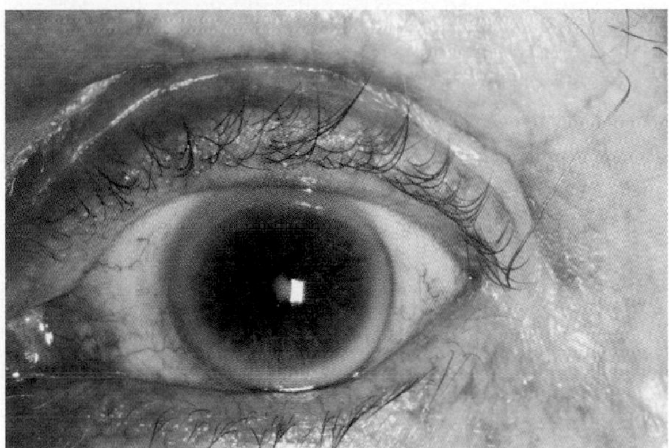

FIGURE 18-35 Arcus senilus is an expected age-related change
Source: E.H. Gill/CMSP

The lens of the eye may demonstrate cloudiness or opacity, indicating the presence of cataracts. This may result in decreased visual acuity as well as decreased vision in the visual fields.

Cataracts that may not be visible to the naked eye will be detected by the inability to obtain the red light reflex.

Techniques and Expected Findings	Unexpected Findings
The iris does not demonstrate any major alterations. There might be some pigmentation changes, but there is no association with any other conditions. The pupil is smaller, but the reason for this is unknown. The light response reflex is also decreased, but presents no difficulties. Patients who are on mitotic medication for glaucoma will demonstrate these pupil changes due to the action of the medication.	Changes in the shape of the iris, bulging toward the cornea, may be demonstrated in the presence of glaucoma. (See previous discussion.)
The retina will demonstrate some changes associated with aging. The rid light reflex is present, but less intense, with the possibility of some evidence of opacities (dark spots). The optic disc may be lighter in color but there should not be any other changes in its characteristics.	Arterial venous nicking is not an expected aging change and should not be present.
The vascular structures of the retina demonstrate age-related changes. The arterioles demonstrate some sclerotic changes, as well as becoming straighter and narrower. The arterioles also appear paler in color (opaque) with an increased visibility of the arteriolar wall light reflex.	
The veins may appear darker in color and larger than the arteries. There will also not be any light reflection.	

DOCUMENTATION

Eyes are positioned equidistant from midline in upper third of face with both pupils symmetrically positioned. Eyebrows are full and even over each eye bilaterally. Upper eyelid covers upper portion of iris but pupils visible bilaterally. Upper and lower eye lids approximated when closed. Outer edges of eyelids without visible areas of swelling or redness. Eye lashes present and curved outward. Eyes are moist and shiny without excessive tearing or discharge. Sclera is white without any significant areas of color change. Conjunctiva are moist and pink. No cloudiness noted of lens. Red light reflex present bilaterally.

Snellen eye chart exam revealed 20/20 in OD (right eye), and 20/15 in OS (left eye)with 20/20 in OU (both eyes), uncorrected. PERRLA** bilaterally (CN II). Consensual response intact. EOM's intact, with conjugate movement; some nystagmus noted in far lateral gaze bilaterally (CN III, IV, VI). Able to identify correct number of fingers in four visual fields at 30°.

Opthalmologic examination. Retina red-orange without any evidence of hemorrhaging or exudates. Arteries and veins without any nicking or crossing changes. Optic disc cream colored with well-defined margins. No cupping of disc. Macula yellow without any lesions.

Electronic Charting

Expectations of Electronic Charting

The entire eye exam should be able to be documented. Accuracy in data entry and an efficient flow of record forms are essential. The system should allow you to chart new exams almost as quickly as you can hand write them. Some electronic records include digital eye exam charts (instead of using a paper eye chart or projector) for testing visual acuity. Graphics of the eye and/or drawing capability should be included and should be integrated with exam notes. If graphics are included, you should be able to draw on or annotate the graphics. Ideally, data from eye examination devices such as autorefractors should be able to be input directly into the medical record (Reing & Wayne, 2006). Digital retinal imaging technology can facilitate and promote surveillance and treatment of conditions such as diabetic retinopathy (Wilson et al., 2005).

Limitations of Electronic Charting

The eye exam is complex, and it can be difficult for structured charting to accommodate all the subtle findings. An obstacle in many electronic charting systems is that many of the clinical observations may need additional free text annotation. Another limitation is that some electronic charting systems may not allow the user to create detailed diagrams in multiple colors (Lobach et al., 2005).

**Documentation for pupil characteristics is the mnemonic PERRLA, which condenses all the information obtained into a very concise abbreviation. The letters of the acronym document that the "Pupils are Equal, Round, and Reactive to Light and Accommodation." This acronym should only be used when expected findings are present and all of the appropriate tests have been performed. If accommodation has not been tested, then the acronym would be PERRL.

Summary

- The eyes are paired sensory organs positioned in the upper third of the face. They function to provide vision for an individual. The eye is considered to have an external and an internal section with only the anterior, external portion visible.
- Changes in the appearance of the external eye may be related to alterations of the structures of the eye, inflammation or infections of the eye, or manifestations of other non-ocular conditions and disorders. Alterations related to the internal eye are assessed with an opthalamoscope.
- Expected age-related changes are associated with a loss of accommodation due to the loss of elasticity of the lens and ciliary muscles, resulting in a reduction in near vision (presbyopia). A common, but not expected, age-related change is the development of a cataract, a clouding of the lens due to compression of fibers within the lens. Aging also puts the older individual at risk for developing glaucoma, retinopathies, macular degeneration, particularly individuals with diabetes and high blood pressure.
- Observation of the eye for possible alterations is aided by use of an opthalamoscope, visual acuity charts, and direct and indirect light sources. Palpation is used to estimate intraocular pressure and pain or tenderness associated with the tear duct.

Review Questions

1. When the provider first meets the patient, observations can be made about which eye structures? (Select all that apply.)
   1. conjunctiva
   2. eye lids
   3. the retina
   4. the posterior chamber
   5. the extraocular muscles

2. Examination of which of the following would require that the provider use an opthalmoscope? (Select all that apply.)
   1. visual acuity
   2. the optic disc
   3. the macula
   4. pupil response
   5. the conjunctiva

3. The provider in a primary care office notices that a patient has had edema around both eyes documented in the record for the last three visits. The appropriate action for the provider to take first is to
   1. document the finding.
   2. test the patient's visual acuity.
   3. discuss the finding with the provider.
   4. ask the patient if he wears glasses.

4. A patient is admitted to the emergency department after several days of vomiting, diarrhea, and fever. The provider notes on additional assessment that the patient's eyes appear sunken and recessed. The provider is aware that this finding will likely improve when
   1. antimicrobial medications are started.
   2. surgery is performed to reverse the problem.
   3. the fever is treated with nonsteroidal medications.
   4. the patient is rehydrated with IV and oral fluids.

5. During a health assessment interview, a patient in her mid-40s tells the provider that she has noticed difficulty in reading recently and is very concerned about this finding. The best initial response for the provider to give the patient is which of the following?
   1. "You should be tested for diabetes."
   2. "This may be due to a bacterial infection."
   3. "You should be sure to tell your eye doctor the next time you visit."
   4. "This is likely due to an age-related change in the lens of your eye."

6. The provider is teaching a class to newly pregnant teens about changes that they may experience during pregnancy. Which of the following should the provider include in this presentation?
   1. Pregnancy usually results in the need to wear glasses for the first time.
   2. Pregnancy causes a significant change in near vision, resulting in prescription change.
   3. Pregnancy related vision changes usually resolve after delivery with no permanent alteration.
   4. Pregnancy causes changes with make the use of contact lenses contraindicated.

7. Which of these techniques would the provider use to examine the pupils of an adult patient?
   1. Turn the examining light away from the patient.
   2. Observe the patient's pupils for reaction when the room lights are dimmed.
   3. Note the degree of pupil constriction when the lights are lowered.
   4. Look for constriction of the left pupil when a light is shone into the right eye.

8. The provider is examining the patient's eyes using an ophthalmoscope. Which of the following reflects that the provider is using the correct technique for this procedure?
   1. The provider holds the instrument in the right hand when examining the patient's right eye.
   2. The provider uses her or his right eye to examine the patient's right eye.
   3. The provider holds the ophthalmoscope 6–8 inches away from the patient's eye.
   4. The provider begins the examination with the ophthalmoscope 1 inch from the patient's eye.

9. The provider is assessing a patient's visual acuity with a Snellen chart. The patient is positioned 20 feet from the chart and can read the line labeled "20/40" with the right eye and "20/100" on the left eye when wearing prescription glasses. How should the provider best note this finding?
   1. Visual acuity within normal limits with correction
   2. Visual acuity 20/70 with correction
   3. Visual acuity R 20/40; L 20/100 with correction, using a Snellen chart
   4. The patient can read the chart when positioned 20 feet away when wearing glasses.

10. Following an examination of the patient's pupils the provider documents "PERRL." This documentation indicates that the pupils were found to be
    1. equal, round, and reactive to light and accommodation.
    2. equal, round, and reactive to light.
    3. equal and reactive on the right and the left.
    4. equal and respond rapidly to light.

Conditions and Disorders

Strabismus

Strabismus (crossed eye) is a disorder in which the two eyes are not aligned in the same direction so that the eyes are not looking at the same object at the same time.

In most children, cause of strabismus unknown. In half or more of the cases it is present at or shortly after birth (congenital strabismus). Strabismus is present in about 4% of children. Other conditions associated with strabismus include cerebral palsy, congenital rubella, hemangioma near the eye during infancy, Noonan or Prader-Willi syndromes, retinopathy of prematurity/retinoblastoma, traumatic brain injury, and trisomy 18.

In adults, strabismus may be caused by botulism, diabetes (acquired paralytic strabismus), Guillain-Barré syndrome, injury to the eye, shellfish poisoning, stroke, traumatic brain injury, and vision loss from any eye disease or injury.

Pathophysiology

- Occurs when the ocular muscles do not work synchronously, resulting in one eye looking at one object, while the other eye moves in a different direction, focusing on a different object.
- Subsequently, two different images are sent to the brain—one from each eye, confusing the brain. In children, the brain may choose to ignore the image from the weaker eye (amblyopia).
- Results more from lack of muscle control rather than muscle weakness.

Subjective Data

- Double vision
- Loss of vision or depth perception

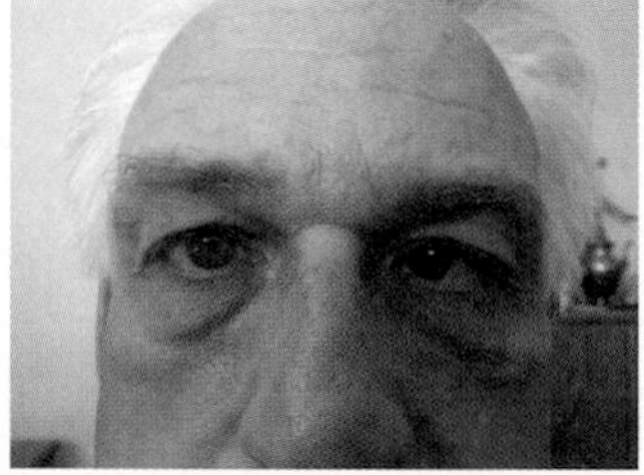

FIGURE 18-36 Strabismus/asymmetrical CLR

Objective Data

- Crossed eyes
- Eyes that do not align in the same direction
- Uncoordinated eye movements (eyes do not move together)

Conjunctivitis

Conjunctivitis (pink eye) is inflammation of the conjunctiva. It is most commonly caused by an infection (viral, but sometimes bacterial), or an allergic reaction. Commonly, conjunctival infections pass from person to person, but can also spread through contaminated objects/water.

Pathophysiology

- Viral conjunctivitis often associated with infection of the upper respiratory tract, a common cold, and/or a sore throat.

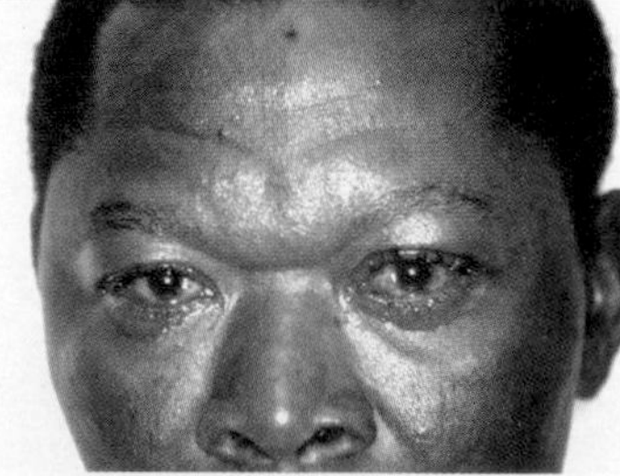

FIGURE 18-37 Conjunctivitis
Source: Courtesy of Randy Carter, OD, The Eye Institute of Utah, Salt Lake City, Utah

Subjective Data

- Conjunctivitis causes relatively nonspecific symptoms.
- Itching (rubbing eyes) is the hallmark symptom of allergic conjunctivitis.
- Other symptoms include history of eczema, or asthma.
- Excessive watering and itching (epiphora).
- Infection usually begins in one eye, but may quickly spread to the other.

Objective Data

- Swelling of conjunctiva (chemosis).
- Pupils should react as expected and visual acuity should not be affected.
- Fine, diffuse pinkness of the conjunctiva, easily mistaken for ciliary injection of iritis.
- A diffuse, less "injected" conjunctivitis (pink rather than red) suggests viral cause, especially if numerous follicles are present on the lower tarsal conjunctiva on biomicroscopy.

- Bacterial (Staphylococci and Streptococci) conjunctivitis causes rapid onset of conjunctival redness (hyperaemia), swelling of the eyelid, and mucopurulent discharge.

- Typically, initial symptoms in one eye, but may spread to the other eye within 2–5 days.
- Purulent discharge (a whitish-yellow, yellow or yellow-brown substance, more commonly known as pus) suggests a bacterial infection.

- Marked grittiness/irritation and a stringy, opaque, greyish or yellowish mucopurulent discharge that may cause the lids to stick together, especially after sleep.
- *Neisseria gonorrhoeae* should be suspected if discharge is thick and copious.

- Chemical eye injury due to an acidic or alkali substance getting in eye.
- Alkalis are typically worse than acidic burns.

- Mild burns will produce conjunctivitis while more severe burns may cause the cornea to turn white.
- Use litmus paper to rule out the diagnosis by verifying that the pH is within the normal range of 7.0–7.2.

Intraocular Hemorrhage (Hemophthalmos, hemophthalmia)

Intraocular hemorrhage means bleeding into the eyeball. It may be the result of physical trauma from direct injury to the eye or medical illness. Severe hemorrhage, particularly when leading to rising pressure inside the eye, may lead to blindness.

Types of intraocular hemorrhage include the following:

- Subconjunctival hemorrhage (under the conjunctiva)
- Hyphema (in the anterior chamber)
- Vitreous hemorrhage (into the vitreous)
- Subretinal hemorrhage (under the retina)
- Submacular hemorrhage (under the macula)

Pathophysiology

- Most subconjunctival hemorrhages (SH) are spontaneous from the conjunctival vessels and appear as a red patch on the sclera.
- Conjunctiva contains nerves and many small blood vessels, which are usually barely visible but become larger and more visible if the eye is inflamed. These blood vessels are somewhat fragile, and their walls may break easily.
- The following can occasionally result in a spontaneous subconjunctival hemorrhage: Sneezing, coughing, straining/vomiting, eye rubbing, trauma, high blood pressure, bleeding disorder, or a medical disorder causing bleeding or inhibiting normal clotting.
- Non-spontaneous—may result from a severe eye infection, trauma to the head or eye, or after eye or eyelid surgery.

Subjective Data

- Often, individual observes a subconjunctival hemorrhage on waking and looking in the mirror.
- Most of the time, no symptoms associated with an SH other than seeing blood over the white part of the eye.
- Most spontaneous SH first noticed by another person noting a red spot on eye.
- Pain with SH is rare.
- When bleeding first occurs, may experience sense of fullness in eye or under the lid.
- As SH resolves, may experience mild eye irritation or merely a sense of awareness of the eye.
- In a spontaneous SH, no blood will escape from eye. If eye wiped with tissue, no blood should be on the tissue.

Objective Data

- The hemorrhage itself is an obvious, sharply outlined, bright red area overlying the sclera. The entire white part of the eye may occasionally be covered by blood.
- The hemorrhage will appear larger within the first 24 hours after its onset and then will slowly decrease in size as the blood is absorbed.
- A subconjunctival hemorrhage (SH) appears as a bright red or dark red patch on the sclera.

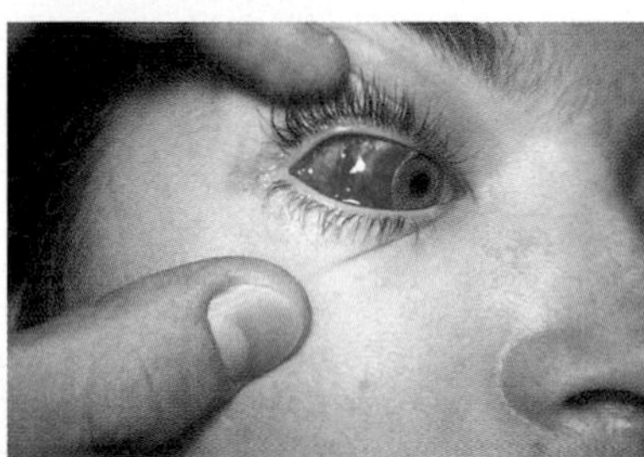

FIGURE 18-38 Intraocular hemmorrhage
Source: Courtesy of Randy Carter, OD, The Eye Institute of Utah, Salt Lake City, Utah

Iritis/Uveitis

This is inflammation of the uveal (middle, pigmented, vascular structures of eye) tract which is comprised of the iris, ciliary body, and choroid. Inflammation occurring in any of these three structures is termed "uveitis." Inflammation may involve any but not necessarily all of these three structures. Severe and permanent visual loss can result from uveitis; additionally, it can lead to other ocular complications, which may produce vision loss, including glaucoma, cataracts, or retinal damage. Early detection/treatment is necessary to reduce the risk of permanent vision loss. Depending upon which structures are inflamed, uveitis may be further subcategorized into one of three main diagnoses that include the following:

- iritis or anterior uveitis (iris and anterior chamber inflamed)
- iridocyclitis or intermediate uveitis (presence of inflammatory cells in vitreous)
- choroiditis or posterior uveitis (retina and choroid inflamed)

Pathophysiology

- May develop following eye trauma or surgery; in association with diseases affecting other organs; or a condition isolated to the eye itself.
- Genetic/infectious mechanisms also a known cause.
- Infectious causes thought to be related to immune reaction directed against foreign molecules/antigens, injuring uveal tract vessels/cells.

Subjective Data

- Depending on which part of eye is inflamed various combinations of symptoms may be present.
  - Redness
  - Light sensitivity
  - Floaters
  - Blurry vision
  - Pain
- Symptoms may appear suddenly, with or without pain. Above symptoms are not strictly associated with uveitis.

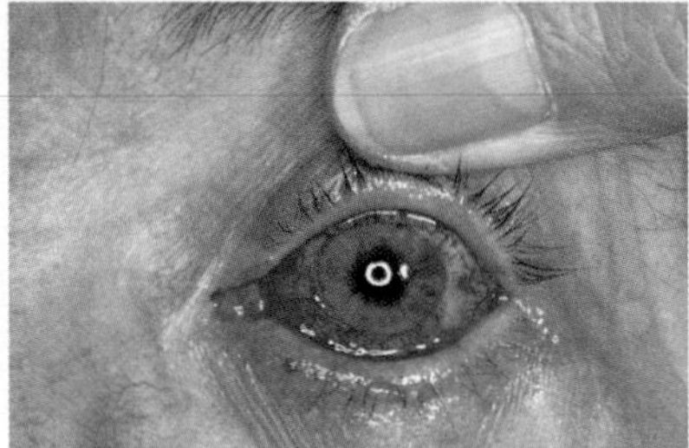

FIGURE 18-39 Iritis (uveitis)
Source: Wellcome Image Library/CMSP

Objective Data

- Dilated ciliary vessels
- Presence of cells and flare in the anterior chamber
- Keratic precipitates (KP) on posterior surface of cornea
- Severe inflammation may give evidence of hypopon (pus in anterior chamber of eye)

Cataract

A cataract is a clouding of the lens of the eye. The lens is usually clear and is composed of encapsulated water and protein. Development of cataracts, common in aging, accounts for approximately 70% of individuals over 75 who develop cataracts. Between 65 and 74 years of age, approximately 50% of the elderly have them (Paine & Randleman, 2007). Most cataracts are bilateral; however, vision may be worse in one eye. They are also more prone to develop in individuals with diabetes and those with a long term use of steroids. They may be apparent in infants and children, due to hereditary causes or maternal infections (German measles) (Paine & Randleman, 2007). Trauma and exposure to UV light, smoke, alcohol, and radiation are also known causes of cataracts.

Pathophysiology

- Clouding of the lens is primarily the result of clumping of protein or accumulation of dead cells within the lens (St. Lukes Eye, 2011). Deposition of these materials within the lens prevents light from reaching the retina leading to decreased and blurry vision.
- Cataracts are generally slow in their development and progression and are not associated with any type of pain.

Subjective Data

- A slow progression results in the insidious onset of decreased and blurred vision.

Other manifestations include the following:

- Increasing difficulty with night vision
- Photophobia
- Brighter light needed for reading and other activities
- Fading or yellowing of colors
- Double vision in one eye

Objective Data

- Clouding of lens resulting in absence of red light reflex
- Decreased visual acuity

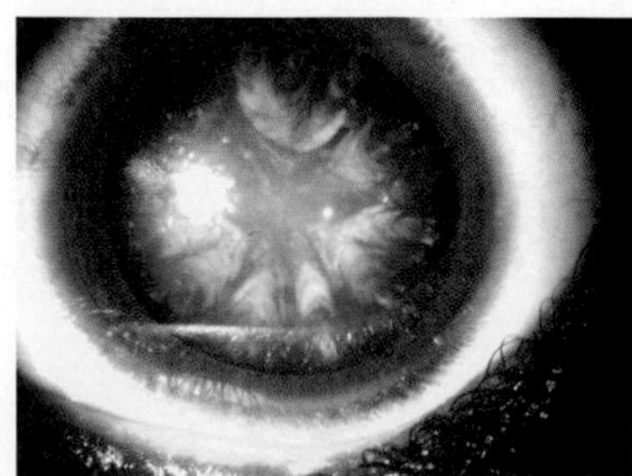

FIGURE 18-40 Cataract
Source: Courtesy of Randy Carter, OD, The Eye Institute of Utah, Salt Lake City, Utah

Diabetic Retinopathy (DR)

DR is the most common and most serious complication associated with diabetes, frequently leading to decreased vision and blindness. The major alteration is damage to the blood vessels that nourish the retina. Increased blood glucose seems to be the major factor contributing to vessel damage. It is estimated that almost 50% of individuals with diabetes have some degree of DR (Mayo Clinic Staff, 2006). It may take 20 years before manifestations of DR become apparent.

Along with early detention and intervention, prevention of DR, or at least delaying any severe symptoms, can be accomplished by maintaining appropriate levels of blood glucose. Individuals who keep control of their blood glucose are more likely to improve their outcomes (Bustos, 2011).

Pathophysiology

- See Table 18-5.
- In initial stage of DR (non-proliferative retinopathy), arteries become weak causing minute hemorrhages of retina.
- Swelling of retina due to edema contributes to decreased vision.
- As DR progresses into the second stage (proliferative retinopathy), there is eventually a decreased delivery of oxygen to the retina causing areas of ischemia to develop.
- To prevent further ischemia, new vessels grow to increase oxygen delivery to retina.
- Other complications may develop—retinal detachment, hemorrhage, cataracts, and glaucoma.

Subjective Data

- Usually no definable symptoms or pain in the early stages of retinopathy.
- Even as the condition progresses, there may not be any indications of visual disturbances.

When present, symptoms of DR may consist of the following:

- Floaters or flashes within visual fields.
- Dark/empty spot in central vision
- Decreased vision or blurred vision. This is frequently variable as it is related to blood sugar levels. Increased blood sugar causes glucose to accumulate in the lens, causing it to swell (Mayo Clinic Staff, 2006). Poor night vision may also be present.

Objective Data

Fundoscopic exam reveals the following:

- Cotton wool spots
- Flame hemorrhages
- Dot-blot hemorrhages

Table 18-5 Stages diabetic retinopathy (DR)

Mild nonproliferative retinopathy	Earliest stage, microaneurysms occur (small areas of balloon-like swelling in the retina's tiny blood vessels).
Moderate nonproliferative retinopathy	As disease progresses, some blood vessels that nourish the retina are blocked.
Severe nonproliferative retinopathy	Many more blood vessels are blocked, depriving several areas of the retina of blood supply, which send signals to body to grow new blood vessels for nourishment.
Proliferative retinopathy	Advanced stage signals sent by retina for nourishment trigger growth of new blood vessels (proliferative retinopathy). New vessels are also fragile and frequently hemorrhage into the retina or vitreous, producing the spots or floaters, as well as decreased vision. If no intervention, bleeding continues as well as development of scar tissue.

Retinopathy of Prematurity (ROP)

Previously identified as retrolental fibroplasia (RLF) this is a condition of the retina associated with prematurely-born infants and who most likely received care in a neonatal intensive care unit (NICU). Thus, all preterm infants are at risk for ROP, with very low birth weight as an additional risk factor. Both oxygen toxicity and relative hypoxia contribute to development of ROP. While there may be other factors that contribute to ROP, the two major risk factors remain to be prematurity and oxygen administration.

Newer methods of titrating oxygen concentrations and oxygen administration have reduced risk of ROP, but it has not been completely eliminated. While oxygen as a risk factor has been addressed, the major risk factor for the prevention of ROP is appropriate and adequate prenatal care to prevent premature birth. Even though there is knowledge of the causes, the incidence of ROP is increasing, most likely due to the increased survival of very low birth weight infants (Chen & Smith, 2006).

Pathophysiology

ROP develops in two phases:

- Phase 1 is caused by premature cessation of blood vessel growth to the edges of the retina.
  - Retinal vascularization begins in utero (fourth month) and is completed just prior to birth.
  - Growth of blood vessels begins at center of optic disc, progressing towards the retinal edge. Premature infants have incomplete vessel growth, leaving a portion of the retina avascular.
  - Increased levels of oxygen in the extrauterine environment and supplemental oxygen produce hyperoxia, causing vascularization to cease. As the infant matures, retina has an increased need for oxygen; however, incomplete vascularization results in retinal tissue hypoxia.
- Phase 2 results from retinal neovascularization initiated by hypoxia which begins at margin between vascular and avascular portions.
  - Eventually, new vessels begin to grow, but their fragility causes hemorrhaging, leading to retinal scarring.
  - Healing scars retract, pulling on retina resulting in detachment and progressing to blindness.

Subjective Data

As ROP occurs in premature infants, subjective data is not relevant.

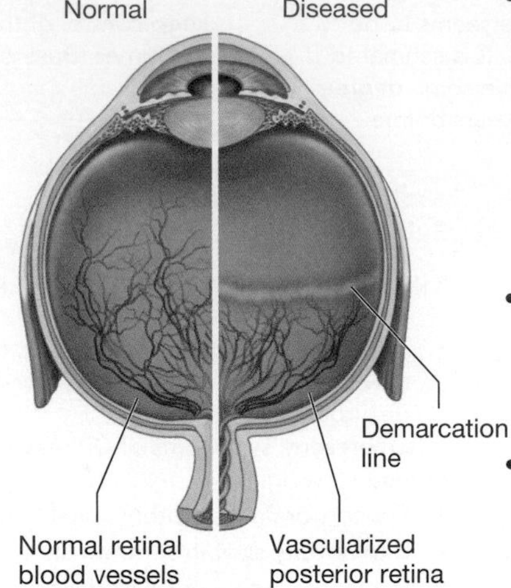

FIGURE 18-41 Retinopathy of prematurity (ROP)

Objective Data

- Diagnosis is based on examination of the retina with ophthalmoscope.
- Stages of ROP defined by the International Classification of Retinopathy of Prematurity (ICROP), based on a number of parameters to describe the disease.
  - Location of the disease into zones (1, 2, and 3),
  - Circumferential extent of the disease based on the clock hours (1–12), and
  - Severity of the disease (stage 1–5)
- Circumferential extent of disease described in segments as the face of a clock with the top of the eye at 12, i.e., stage 1 disease for 3 clock hours from 4 to 7 o'clock
- **Plus disease** may be present at any stage (describes a significant level of vascular dilation and tortuosity observed at the posterior retinal vessels, reflecting increased blood flow through retina).
- **Threshold disease** (50% likelihood of progressing to retinal detachment)
  - Considered present when Stage 3 ROP is present in either Zone I or II, with at least 5 continuous or 8 total clock hours of disease, and presence of Plus disease
  - Progression to Stage 4 (partial retinal detachment), or Stage 5 (total retinal detachment), will result in substantial or total loss of vision for the infant.

Hypertensive Retinopathy (HR)

Hypertensive retinopathy is damage to the retina and retinal circulation due to high blood pressure (i.e., hypertension).

Pathophysiology

- Hypertension leads to a deposition of cholesterol into the tunica intima of medium and large arteries resulting in an overall reduction in the lumen, as well as thickening of the vessel wall.
- Thickening causes arterial wall to lose its transparency; AV nicking may be present at the AV junction.
- Thickened arterial wall occludes the vein as it passes under the artery so that the vein appears to stop just before and after crossing the artery.

Subjective Data

- Most patients are asymptomatic.
- However, symptomatic patients most commonly present with headaches and blurred vision.

Objective Data

Extravascular lesions of the retina include the following:

- Microaneurysms
- Retinal hemorrhages
- Retinal and macular edema
- Retinal lipid deposits
- Cotton-wool spots
- FIPT

Retinal Detachment

RD is the separation of the inner layers of the retina from the underlying layer of support tissue (retinal pigment epithelium/choroid). Initial detachment may be localized; without rapid treatment, entire retina may detach, leading to vision loss and blindness. It is a medical emergency. As the population ages, RDs are becoming more common. It usually occurs in persons aged 40–70 years. However, paintball injuries in young children and teens are becoming increasingly common causes of eye injuries, including traumatic retinal detachments. When the retina becomes detached, bleeding from area blood vessels may cloud the inside of the eye, which is normally filled with vitreous fluid. Central vision becomes severely affected if the macula, the part of the retina responsible for fine vision, becomes detached.

Pathophysiology

- Separation of the sensory retina from the underlying RPE occurs by three basic mechanisms:
  - A hole, tear, or break in the neuronal layer allowing fluid from the vitreous cavity to seep in between and separate sensory and RPE layers (i.e., rhegmatogenous RD)
  - Traction from inflammatory or vascular fibrous membranes on the surface of the retina, which tether to the vitreous
  - Exudation of material into the subretinal space from retinal vessels such as in hypertension, central retinal venous occlusion, vasculitis, or papilledema
- May be associated with congenital malformations, metabolic disorders, trauma (including previous ocular surgery),vascular disease, choroidal tumors, high myopia (>6 diopters) or vitreous disease, or degeneration

Subjective Data

- Painless, but its warning signs and symptoms almost always appear before it occurs or has advanced.
- Initial symptoms commonly include: sensation of a flashing light (photopsia), often accompanied by a shower of floaters and vision loss.
- Over time, patient may report a shadow in peripheral visual field, which may spread to involve entire visual field in a matter of days.
- Vision loss often described as cloudy, irregular, or curtain-like.

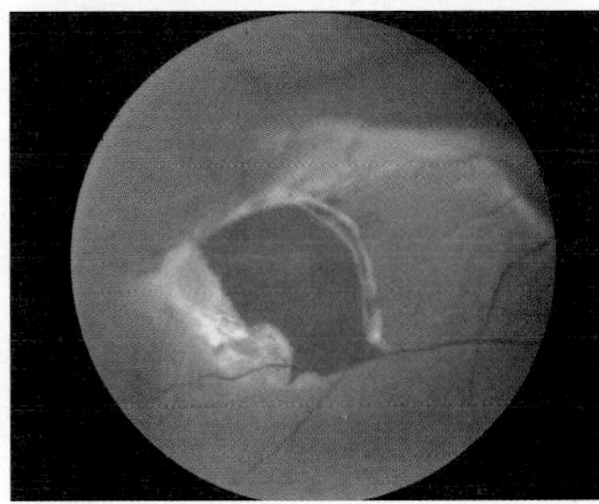

FIGURE 18-42 Retinal detachment
Source: Courtesy of Randy Carter, OD, The Eye Institute of Utah, Salt Lake City, Utah

Objective Data

- Detachment is observed by marked elevation of the retina; appears gray with dark blood vessels that may lie in folds.
- Detached retina may undulate and appear out of focus.
- Shallow detachments are more difficult to detect; comparing the suspected area with an adjacent normal quadrant is helpful to detect any change in retinal transparency.
- A pigmented or nonpigmented line may demarcate the limit of a detachment.

Glaucoma

Glaucoma is a disease in which the optic nerve is damaged in a characteristic pattern from increased intraocular pressure that can permanently damage vision in affected eye(s) and lead to blindness if left untreated. Ocular hypertension refers to individuals with consistently raised intraocular pressure (IOP), but no optic nerve damage. Normal tension or low tension glaucoma refers to individuals with optic nerve damage and associated visual field loss, but normal or low IOP.

Glaucoma caused by increased intraocular pressure is also divided into two categories.

- **Open-angle glaucoma** can also be subdivided into multiple categories. Chronic open-angle glaucoma is the most common type glaucoma in which the drainage mechanism gradually becomes clogged. The exact cause of the blockage is not known; however, it does increase with aging. Other types of open angle glaucoma include normal tension glaucoma, congenital, secondary, pigmentary and exfoliative glaucoma.
- **Acute closed-angle glaucoma** is caused by a blockage of the filtering angle, preventing drainage of aqueous humor. Blockage occurs with dilation of the pupil, which causes the peripheral margin of the iris to close in against its attachment to the cornea, resulting in closure of the filtering angle. Acute closed-angle glaucoma is less common (10%) and is characterized by a sudden increase in intraocular pressure (St. Luke's Cataract and Laser Institute, n.d.).

Pathophysiology

- Underlying cause of open-angle glaucoma is unclear. Increased intraocular pressure is the major risk factor for most glaucomas, and the focus of treatment.
- In open/wide-angle glaucoma, flow is reduced through trabecular mesh-work, due to degeneration/obstruction of trabecular meshwork.
- Loss of aqueous humor absorption leads to increased resistance and thus a chronic, painless buildup of pressure in the eye.
- Exact causes of optic nerve damage from glaucoma is not completely understood, but it involves mechanical compression and/or decreased blood flow of the optic nerve.

Subjective Data

- Acute attack of glaucoma may be accompanied by severe eye pain and headache, and inflamed (red) eye, nausea and vomiting, and blurred vision (Schwartz, 2007).
- Corneal edema is also likely to occur and results in the patient seeing haloes around lights.

Open-angle glaucoma frequently occurs gradually without any specific symptoms. Warning signs that indicate possible nerve damage include the following:

- Unusual trouble adjusting to dark rooms
- Difficulty focusing on near or distant objects
- Squinting or blinking due to unusual sensitivity to light or glare

Objective Data

- Ophthalmoscopy is performed to assess the optic nerve. Cupping of the optic disk is an indicator of increased intraocular pressure (Schwartz, 2007).
- Visual field testing may also be done to determine if there are any field cuts in the peripheral visual fields.

- The many different subtypes of glaucoma can all be considered to be a type of optic neuropathy.

- Change in color of iris
- Red-rimmed, encrusted or swollen lids
- Recurrent pain in or around eyes
- Double vision
- Dark spot at the center of viewing
- Lines and edges appear distorted or wavy
- Excess tearing, "watery eyes"
- Dry eyes with itching or burning;
- Seeing spots, ghostlike images

THINK LINK: Glaucoma

Glaucoma has been called the "silent thief of sight" because the loss of vision often occurs gradually over a long period of time, and symptoms only occur when the disease is quite advanced. Once lost, vision cannot normally be recovered, so treatment is aimed at preventing further loss. Risk factors for developing Glaucoma are identified in Table 18-6.

Table 18-6 Individuals at a higher risk for developing glaucoma

Age	> 45 years of age
History	Family history of glaucoma in parents and siblings
	History of elevated intraocular pressure—there is an association between elevated intraocular pressure and open-angle glaucoma. About 1/6 of patients with open-angle glaucoma will have normal intraocular pressure. Thus although elevated intraocular pressure is associated with open-angle glaucoma, it is neither necessary nor sufficient to diagnose glaucoma and is therefore considered as a risk factor.
	History of eye injury
Race	African American descent—prevalence of open-angle glaucoma is 3 times higher with an age-adjusted rate of blindness that is 6.6 times greater than in whites. Incidence of open-angle glaucoma is also higher in Latinos than in non-Hispanic whites. (Friedman, 2004)
Other possible risk factors	Diabetes, myopia, CV diseases, hypertension, DM, hypothyroidism., steroids, eye injury Nearsightedness (myopia) Use of steroids (cortisone) either in the eye or systematically

Age-related Macular Degeneration (AMD)

AMD is a medical condition that usually affects older adults and results in loss of vision in central portion of visual field (macula) due to damage of retina. It occurs in "dry" and "wet" forms and is a major cause of blindness and visual impairment in older adults (>50 years). The loss of central vision profoundly affects visual functioning. It is quite difficult, for example, to read without central vision. AMD can also make it difficult or impossible to recognize faces, although enough peripheral vision remains to allow other activities of daily life. Macular degeneration by itself will not lead to total blindness. For that matter, only a very small number of people with visual impairment are totally blind. In almost all cases, some vision remains.

Pathophysiology

- The dry (nonexudative) form is due to cellular debris (drusen) accumulating between the retina and choroid, which may cause the retina to become detached.
- Central geographic atrophy results from atrophy of the retinal pigment epithelial layer below the retina, which causes vision loss through loss of photoreceptors (rods and cones) in the central part of the eye.
- The neovascular or exudative "wet" form of AMD causes vision loss due to abnormal blood vessel growth (choroidal neovascularization) in the choriocapillaris, through Bruch's membrane, ultimately leading to leaking of blood and protein below the macula. Bleeding, leaking, and scarring from these blood vessels eventually causes irreversible damage to the photoreceptors and rapid vision loss if left untreated.

Subjective Data

- Blurred vision: Those with nonexudative macular degeneration may be asymptomatic or notice a gradual loss of central vision, whereas those with exudative macular degeneration often notice a rapid onset of vision loss.
- Central scotomas
- Trouble discerning colors, specifically dark from dark and light from light
- Slow recovery of visual function after exposure to bright light
- A loss in contrast sensitivity
- The need for brighter light when reading or doing close work; increasing difficulty adapting to low light levels
- Increasing blurriness of printed words
- A decrease in the intensity or brightness of colors

Objective Data

- Drusen
- Pigmentary alterations
- Exudative changes: hemorrhages in the eye, hard exudates, subretinal/sub-RPE/intraretinal fluid
- Atrophy: incipient and geographic
- Visual acuity drastically decreasing (two levels or more), e.g., 20/20 to 20/80.
- Preferential hyperacuity perimetry changes (for wet AMD). Distorted vision in the form of metamorphopsia in which a grid of straight lines appears wavy and parts of the grid may appear blank. Patients often first notice this when looking at miniblinds in their home.

- The characteristics and manifestations of both types of AMD are outlined in Table 18-7.

- Difficulty recognizing faces
- A gradual increase in the haziness of central or overall vision; crooked central vision
- A blurred or blind spot in the center field of vision
- In advanced AMD, hallucinations of geometric shapes or people

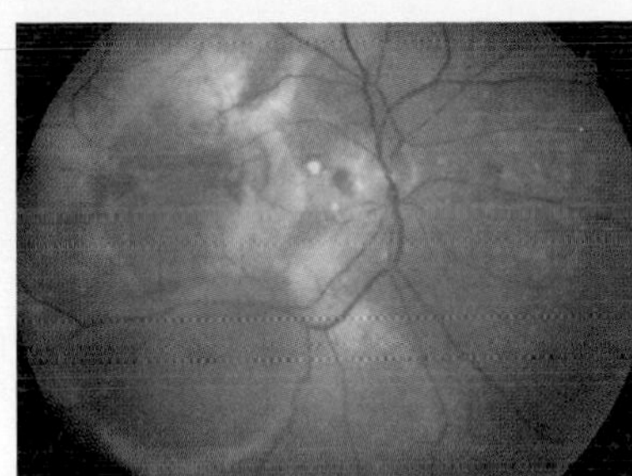

FIGURE 18-43 Macular degeneration
Source: Courtesy of Randy Carter, OD, The Eye Institute of Utah, Salt Lake City, Utah

Table 18-7 Comparison of dry and wet age-related macular degeneration

Type	Dry AMD	Wet AMD
Incidence	90%	10%
Distribution	May only affect one eye (symptoms not manifest until both eyes affected)	May only affect one eye (symptoms not manifest until both eyes affected)
Cause of blindness	10%	90%
Characteristics	Atrophic: Light sensitive cells of macula break down	Neovascular: Growth of new, fragile blood vessels behind retina that leak blood and fluid under macula
Onset	Gradual loss of vision	Rapid progression and loss of vision (20/200)
Conversion	May convert to wet	Starts out as dry AMD
Symptoms	Slightly blurred vision Need for increased illumination Difficulty recognizing faces Blurred spot in central vision	Straight lines appear wavy Rapid loss of central vision Blind spot in central vision
Signs	Drusen Bodies Negative Amsler grid	Drusen Bodies Negative Amsler grid
Risk Factors	Age: most significant Gender: higher incidence in females Smoking: increases risk Family history Elevated cholesterol	Same as dry AMD

Sources: Data from Medicine Net 2002; Mayo Clinic Staff, 2006a; Pons, 2007; Arroyo, 2013

Retinitis pigmentosa (RP)

RP is an inherited group of degenerative eye disorders caused by a genetic defect that causes severe vision impairment and often blindness. The progress of RP is not consistent; some individuals will exhibit symptoms beginning in infancy; symptoms may not appear in others until later in life. Generally, the later the onset, the more progressive the deterioration in sight.

Pathophysiology

- The cells controlling night vision (rods) are most commonly affected; however, in some cases, retinal cone cells are primarily involved.
- Genetic defect causing cell death by apoptosis of rods.

Subjective Data

- Night blindness or nyctalopia
- Tunnel vision (no peripheral vision)
- Peripheral vision (no central vision)
- Latticework vision
- Aversion to glare
- Slow adjustment from dark to light environments and vice versa

Objective Data

- The main sign of the disease is the presence of dark deposits in the retina.

- Course of disease variable but cell death is the final common outcome.

- Blurring of vision
- Poor color separation
- Extreme tiredness

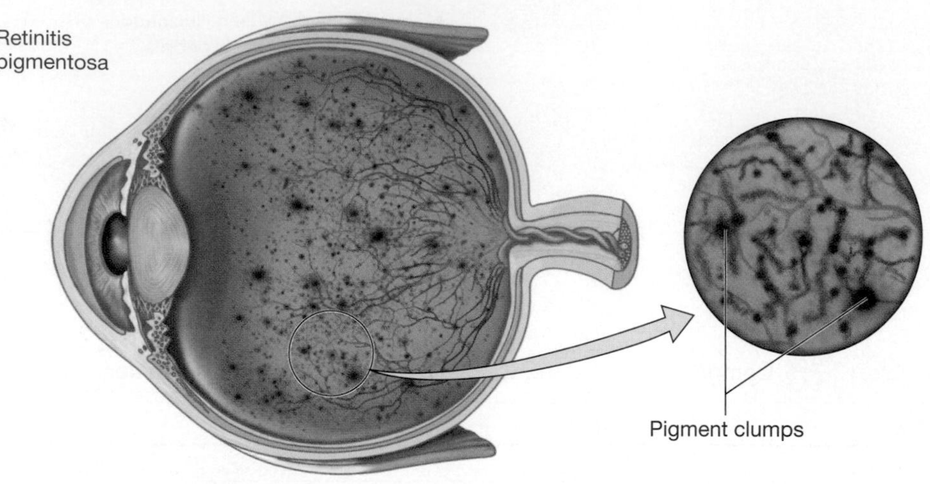

FIGURE 18-44 Retinitis pigmentosa (RP)

Retinoblastoma (Rb)

This is a rapidly developing, rare form of eye cancer that develops from the immature cells of retina, the light-detecting tissue of the eye (1:17,000 live births worldwide) and is the most common malignant tumor of the eye in children (11% in first 12 months). It may occur in one or both (20%–35% of cases) eyes. Approximately 80% of children are diagnosed prior to 3 years of age; diagnosis in children over 6 years of age is extremely rare. If the tumor is restricted to one eye, greater than 95% can be cured. For children with tumors in both eyes, approximately 70%–80% of eyes can be saved, although many of them need radiation therapy. Patients with a hereditary form of retinoblastoma have a genetic predisposition to develop other cancers; they may continue to develop other cancers outside of the eye throughout their lives.

Pathophysiology

- Occurs when nerve cells in the retina develop genetic mutations that cause the cells to continue growing and multiplying to form a tumor
- Retinoblastoma cells can invade further into the eye and nearby structures.
- Can also metastasize to other areas of the body, including the brain and spine

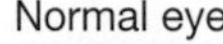

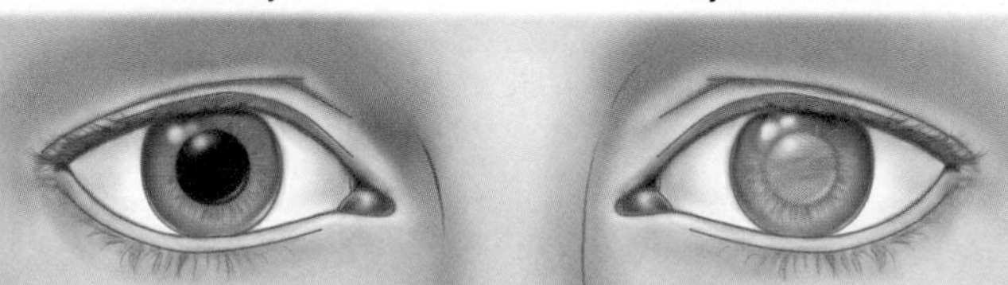

FIGURE 18-45 Retinoblastoma (Rb)

Subjective Data

- If child is old enough, may able to note and report deterioration of eye sight

Objective Data

- A white color in the pupil when light is shone in the eye, called leukocoria (cat's eye reflex)
- Absence of red light reflex
- Eyes that appear to be looking in different directions
- A red and irritated eye with glaucoma
- Eye swelling
- Some children can develop a squint, commonly referred to as "cross-eyed" or "wall-eyed" (strabismus).
- Depending on tumor's position, it may be visible during a simple eye exam with an ophthalmoscope (under anesthesia).

Pupil Alterations

Changes in pupil size can occur as a result of medications, drugs or toxins, which typically affect both pupils equally. Pupil changes caused by medications, drugs or toxins are generally temporary. Neurologic conditions, such as stroke, tumor, or brain injury, also cause changes in pupil size in one or both eyes. Abnormally shaped pupils can occur as a result of abnormalities of prenatal development or injury.

Changes in pupil size and unequal pupil size can occur with serious conditions such as head trauma, brain tumors, stroke, or poisoning.

Pathophysiology

- The basic cause for pupil alterations is an imbalance between sympathetic and parasympathetic control of pupil action.
- Actual causes relate to specific pathologies and the effects they exert on the nervous system.

Subjective Data

- Rarely do pupil alterations have any subjective manifestations independent of the cause.

Objective Data

- Figure 18-46 presents objective data for seven common pupil alterations.

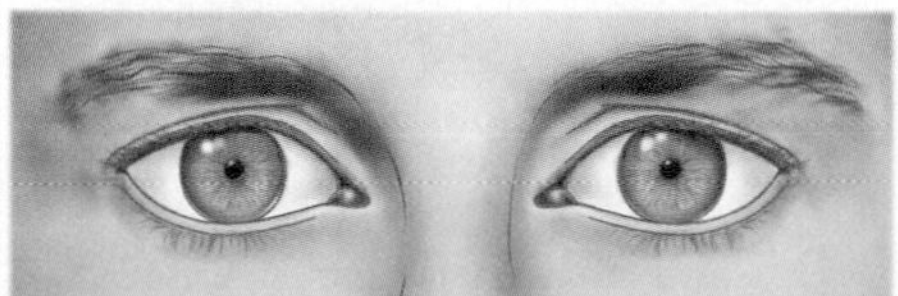

Constricted pupils
Miosis; usually <2 mm in diameter eye drops for glaucoma, drug (opioid) abuse

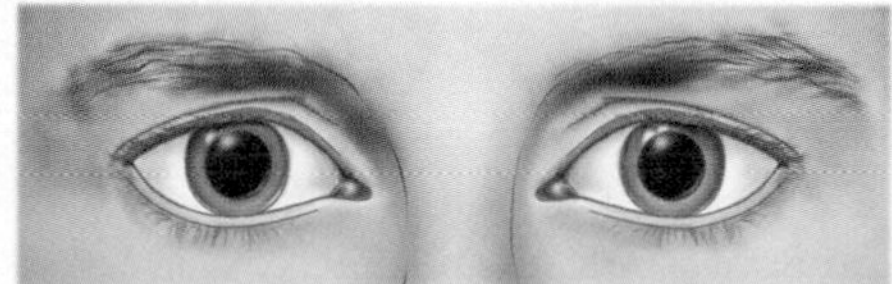

Dilated pupils
Mydriasis; usually >6 mm in diameter, drugs (eye examination)

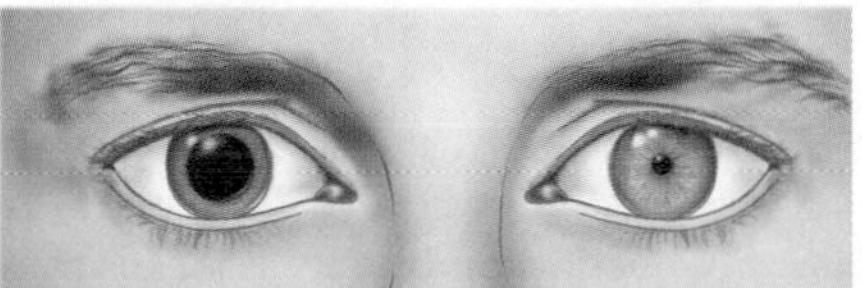

Uneven pupils
Anisocoria (seen in approximately 20% of individuals, but reaction in both eyes); also caused by destruction of sympathetic/parasympathetic pupillary pathway

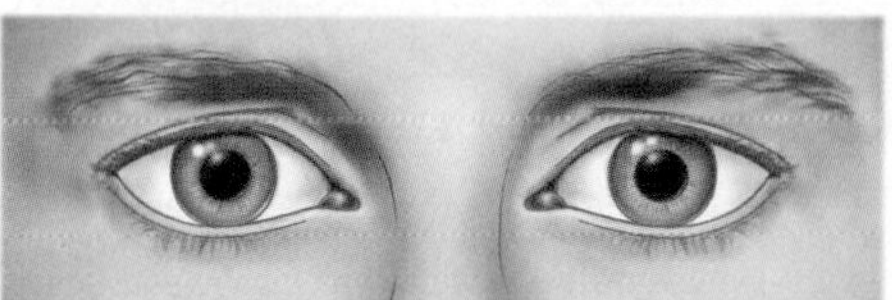

Nonreactive midposition
Failure to constrict with increased light stimulation; retinal degeneration, CN II (Optic) nerve destruction

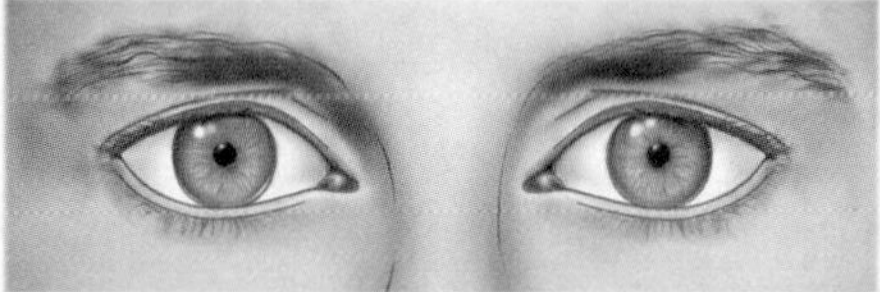

Nonreactive pinpoint
Argyll Robertson pupil
Bilateral, mitotic irregular shaped pupils that fail to constrict with light but do so with convergence

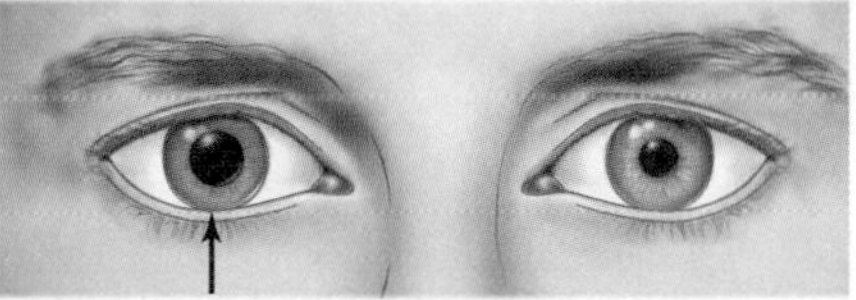

Unilateral fixed and dilated
Adie pupil (tonic pupil)
Affected pupil dilated and reacts slowly or fails to react to light; responds to convergence

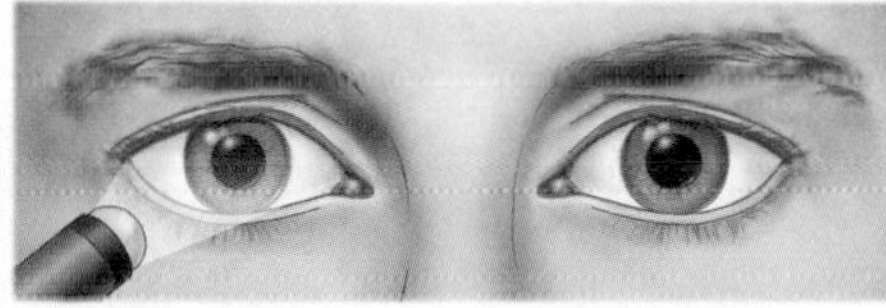

Bilateral dilation
Fixed and dilated (CN III) occulomotor damage from increased intracranial pressure

FIGURE 18-46 Pupil alterations

19 The Ear

"OR 19!" the surgeons wheel Ed Tanner to my bay in the post-anesthesia care unit. His heart rate is a little fast, and although he's still groggy from the anesthesia, I can hear him asking for more pain medication.

I had been reading his history in the record system with great interest. He was a previously healthy 13-year-old, performing well academically and swimming for his middle school. But 2 weeks ago he began complaining of vertigo, headaches, and difficulty hearing on his left side. His mother brought him to the acute care clinic 10 days later and reported that he "wasn't himself" and was speaking gibberish. When the pediatrician looked in his left ear, she reported an "ill-defined white mass behind an intact tympanic membrane." This was a cholesteatoma, a squamous cell mass that had eroded through Ed's skull base to the point of compressing his cerebral cortex.

I administer some fentanyl, and Ed seems to relax. From where I'm standing, the enormous bandage over his left ear looms large. What I find even more interesting than his diagnosis are the physical examinations documented in the records from his annual checkups. In each one, his tympanic membranes are noted to be "intact and non-erythematous," but there is never any mention of a mass. From what I read, congenital cholesteatomas (like the one Ed has) grow over the course of many years, and can be picked up early with careful examination of the middle ear. What a shame that this was not the case for Ed—that his examinations were all interpreted to be normal. I walk around his bed to change the IV drip rate. From this angle, with Ed resting on his bandaged side, he looks totally normal and healthy to me as well.

LEARNING OUTCOMES

1. Describe anatomic structures and characteristics of the external and internal ear as well as their correct position and placement.
2. Explain variations in ear characteristics by inspection and their relationship to various conditions.
3. Recognize common lifespan changes in the function of the ears and the significance of their presence.
4. Explain the techniques used to examine the external and internal structures of the ear by inspection and palpation.
5. Document findings using appropriate terms when describing expected and unexpected findings.

The ear is a paired sensory organ that captures and transmits sound waves to the brain for interpretation. The internal components of the ear are also responsible for facilitating and maintaining balance and equilibrium. Like the eye, the intricate parts of the ear are encased within the bones of the skull for protection. Sound and sight work together to help navigation through life's various positive and negative encounters. Connecting familiar sight and sound sensations with specific experiences helps individuals assimilate cues and clues when assessing new situations to either protect them from danger or facilitate pleasurable experiences.

Structure and Function

The ear is often referred to as having two sections: the internal and external ear. More specifically the structures of the ear are comprised of three sections: the outer, middle and inner ear. The external and outer ear refer to the same section; however, the internal ear is subdivided into two components: the middle and inner ear. The mechanisms for hearing are located within these two components.

External (Outer) Ear

The outer ear is positioned on the lateral side of the head, protruding at a slight angle from the skull and consisting of the auricle (pinna) and external auditory canal. The auricle is composed of cartilage that provids the foundation for its shape and structure and is covered with a layer of skin. The auricle captures and focuses sound waves, localizes sound, and protects the external ear canal. The ear lobe, the lower portion of the auricle, consists of only fatty tissue. The auricle is also composed of other anatomical landmarks that are identified in Figure 19-1. These landmark formations serve as a preamplifier, enhancing the sensitivity to sound. The pinna's shape and position allows sound to bounce off the auricle in different ways to help determine the direction of sound. The forward position of the human auricle allows sound to be heard better from the front than the back.

The external auditory canal is an S-shaped passage or tunnel that extends from the external opening of the ear canal (auditory meatus) to the tympanic membrane (TM) (ear drum) (Figure 19-2). In adults it is approximately 1 inch in length. The walls of the canal consist of cartilage and bone. The outer section of the canal, from the opening to the middle contains cartilage and the inner section, consists of bone. Both sections are covered with a very thin layer of sensitive skin that overlies the cartilage and contains hair follicles surrounded by sebaceous (ceruminous) glands that secrete cerumen (earwax), which lubricates and protects the ear canal. Cerumen has some antibacterial activity that impedes the growth of microorganisms (Martini & Nath, 2009). The auditory canal terminates at the tympanic membrane.

The tympanic membrane (TM) is a triple layered, 0.1mm thick, circular membrane composed of skin, fibrous tissue, and mucous membrane. It is pearl-gray in color and encircled by a dense fibrous ring (annulus) that anchors the membrane in place (Figure 19-2). It is translucent, allowing for restricted visualization of the middle ear. It is also concave in shape and positioned at an oblique angle to the ear canal.

Internal Ear

Middle Ear

The middle ear is an air-filled cavity encased within the temporal bone of the skull. It consists of three small bones (ossicles) that are connected to each other as well as the tympanic membrane and the oval window of the inner ear (see Figure 19-2). These three bones, the malleus (hammer), the incus (anvil), and the stapes (stirrup), are essential to hearing by transmitting vibrations from the tympanic membrane to the oval window. The Eustachian tube is another opening into the middle ear that serves as a cartilaginous and bony passage between the middle ear and the nasopharynx. Its primary function is to equalize the pressure within the middle ear to atmospheric pressure by opening briefly during yawning, sneezing, or swallowing. Equalized pressure is necessary for optimum vibration of the tympanic membrane. The middle ear also amplifies sound via the vibration of the tympanic membrane and ossicles, as well as the difference in size between the TM and the oval window.

Inner Ear

The inner ear is a contained within a bony labyrinth (maze) and has three primary structures: the cochlea, vestibule, and semicircular canals (see Figure 19-2). Unlike the middle ear, it is not encased within a chamber (Elsea, 1996). It contains two fluids: perilymph—which is between the membrane that lines the inner ear (membranous labyrinth) and bone—and endolymph, which fills the membranous structures of the inner ear. The inner ear transmits sound impulses and enables balance and equilibrium.

The cochlea, a coiled, snail-shaped structure, contains the organ of Corti that continues the transmission of sound (see Figure 19-2). The organ of Corti contains stereocilia, minute cells with hairlike projections identified as hair cells that are sound receptors (see Hearing section). The cochlea also contains the oval window, which is where the middle ear bone (stapes) connects to the inner ear.

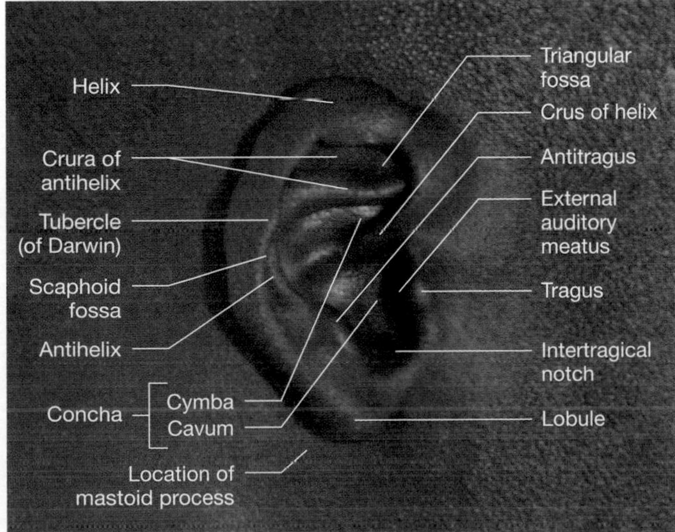

FIGURE 19-1 External ear anatomy

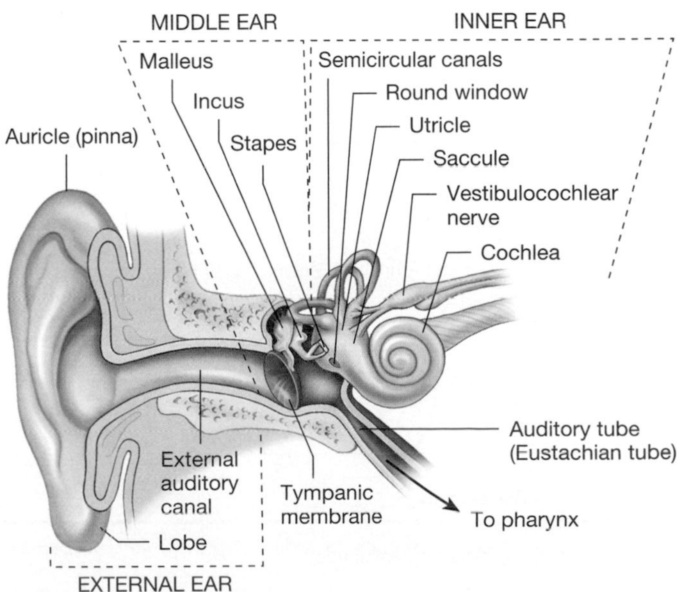

FIGURE 19-2 Auditory canal

Hearing

Hearing is a complex process and is still not completely understood (Harris, 2008). The sense of hearing is the only sensory system that is mechanical (mechanoreceptors) and not chemical (chemoreceptors), making it unique. Hearing begins with vibrations set in motion within the individual's environment. These vibrations send out waves of compressed and expanded air particles that travel at the frequency of the vibrations. The frequency of the vibrations determines the pitch of the sound; the greater the frequencies, the higher the pitch and vice versa. The height of the frequency wave or amplitude determines its loudness; the higher the amplitude, the louder the sound (Figure 19-3).

Six steps are needed for sound to be heard (Figure 19-4). First, sound waves must be detected and directed into auricle. After sound is detected by the auricle, it travels into and through the external ear canal to the tympanic membrane causing the TM to vibrate. The vibrations of the TM are then passed on to the ossicles of the inner ear, which help to amplify the sound.

The three middle ear bones increase the intensity of the vibrations so the cochlear fluid can be vibrated. The vibrations of the TM travel through the malleus and incus to the stapes, which vibrates the oval window, which in turn converts air waves into fluid waves. The tympanic membrane, being larger than the oval window, facilitates considerable amplification of the sound waves (Martini & Nath, 2009).

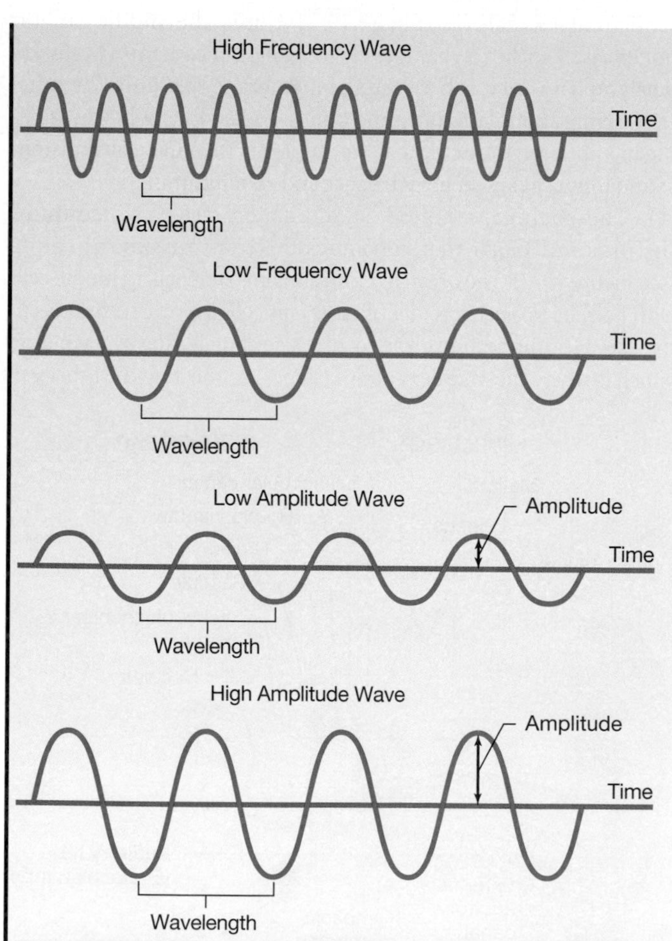

FIGURE 19-3 Pitch, frequency, amplitude

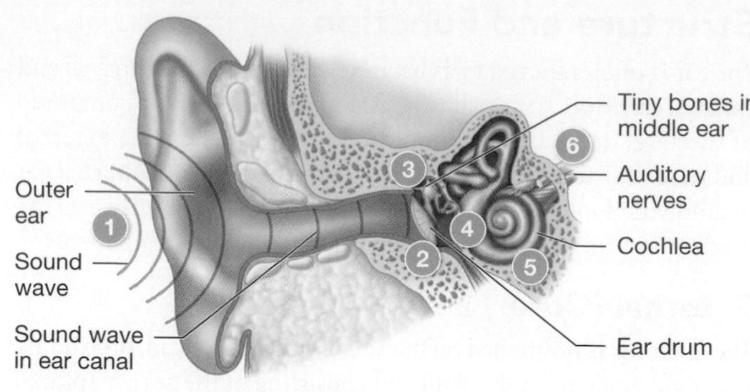

FIGURE 19-4 The steps in the hearing process

The middle ear also filters and buffers the sound waves. Filtering reduces or eliminates extraneous background noise, allowing the individual to focus and concentrate on important sounds. Buffering works to soften the sound, which makes the sound more manageable.

The fluid waves travel through the cochlea where they are converted to electrical impulses, which are transmitted to and interpreted by the brain. The cochlea consists of three tubes that are separated by two sensitive membranes, with the most important being the basilar membrane that stretches along the length of the cochlea.

The stereocilia within the organ of Corti are actually nerve endings from the cochlear branch of CN VIII, which number about 19,000–30,000 and vary in height and flexibility. At the beginning of the cochlea , they are short and stiff, increasing in length and flexibility along the length of the cochlea to the end, where they are taller and more flexible. Height and flexibility allow the hairs to resonate or vibrate at specific sound frequencies, releasing energy that stimulates an action potential that converts the mechanical action to electric impulses. These impulses are carried by CN VIII to the cerebral cortex for interpretation (Gray, 2011). A sound's pitch is determined by where on the organ of Corti the cells are stimulated and the loudness is determined by the number of cells that are stimulated.

Sound Conduction

Conduction of sound occurs through two routes: air and bone. Air conduction occurs by the process that was previously described. It is the most efficient, primary route for hearing.

Bone conduction is considered a backup system and occurs when sound is transmitted by the vibrations of the skull bones. This method bypasses the external ear canal and tympanic membrane and sends vibrations directly to the ossicles of the inner ear. Air conduction and bone conduction occur at the same time, but generally an individual is not aware of bone conduction. Bone conduction predominates when sound vibrations are obstructed in either the external or middle ear; there are multiple reasons why this occurs, some of which may be reversed.

THINK LINK: Voice Pitch and Conduction

When an individual speaks, both bone and air conduction occur. Sound conducted through bone is lower in pitch than sound conducted through air, which makes the sound of one's own voice heard at a lower pitch than what others hear. For this reason, one's own recorded voice, when heard, is higher than the individual expects it to be. This is quite surprising to individuals who are used to hearing their own voice as lower or deeper.

Hearing Loss

Hearing loss is characterized by a decreased sensitivity to sound that results from an alteration along the sound conduction pathway. Although hearing loss and deafness are often used interchangeably, hearing loss is considered to be deterioration in hearing, and deafness is a profound hearing loss (Ruben, 2011). There is no specific identifiable point where one transitions from experiencing a hearing loss to being considered deaf.

Multiple conditions can cause hearing loss, which may or may not be identifiable. There are essentially two types of hearing loss—conductive and sensorineural. A third type, mixed hearing loss, is a combination of conductive and sensorineural hearing loss.

A **conductive hearing loss** results when conduction of sound waves from the air to the fluid filled inner ear is disrupted or prevented. Possible causes include an accumulation of cerumen in the ear canal, infection, fluid in the middle ear (effusion), a perforated or punctured TM, scarring of the TM, fusion of the middle ear bones (otosclerosis), a narrowed ear canal, or middle ear tumors. If any of these causes are treatable or repaired, hearing may be restored.

A **sensorineural hearing loss** results from injury or damage to the auditory nerve or hair cells of the cochlea. The origin may be in the inner ear, the auditory nerve, or within the brain. Sensorineural hearing loss is frequently associated with aging and presents as **presbycusis**, a gradual bilateral hearing loss. Other causes include tumor (acoustic neuroma), viral infections, Meniere's disease, meningitis, cochlear otosclerosis, and exposure to continuous or sudden loud noises, toxic medications, or an inherited condition. Sensorineural hearing loss is considered nonreversible; however, genetic causes of certain forms of congenital hearing loss have been identified and may lead to future interventions (Department of Otolaryngology Head and Neck Surgery, 2007).

Sensorineural hearing loss may be further categorized as either sensory or neural. Sensory loss is associated with abnormalities in the cochlea that result from noise trauma, viral infection, drug toxicity, or Meniere's disease. Neural hearing loss is associated with situations that involve tumors or neurological disorders. Tumors of the auditory nerve (acoustic neuromas) are potentially life threatening, but they are also frequently treatable. Treatment or removal of the tumor, unfortunately, does not restore hearing.

Hearing loss may be partial or total and may develop suddenly or gradually. Initial manifestations relate to difficulty in hearing conversations, particularly with a lot of background noise. The individual may also experience **tinnitus**, a ringing in the ears, or a roaring or hissing sound, which may be present before the awareness of hearing loss (Ruben, 2011). Tinnitus is not a condition but a symptom of some other underlying condition. The most common type of tinnitus is subjective, which is when the sound is only heard by the individual. A more rare type—objective—is when the provider is able to hear the sound during an examination (Cunha & Decicco, 2011).

Hyperacusis, the opposite of a hearing loss, is an increased sensitivity to every day sounds. Other sounds may also be uncomfortable for the individual, particularly sounds with high frequencies. Individuals with hyperacusis have difficulty functioning in everyday environments and may eventually isolate themselves. Hyperacusis frequently develops after exposure to traumatically loud sounds, which can be sudden or cumulative over a period of time.

Balance and Equilibrium

The vestibule and semicircular canals contain specialized sensory receptors for balance and equilibrium that respond to changes in direction and movement of the head through monitoring of gravity, linear acceleration, and rotation (Martini & Nath, 2009).

The vestibule within the inner ear contains two membranous sacs: the utricle and saccule (see Figure 19-2) that are filled with endolymph and contain hair cells that are sensitive to gravity-related changes in the position of the head. Impulses originating from these cells are carried by the vestibular branch of CN VIII to the cerebellum, midbrain, and temporal lobes of the cerebrum. These impulses are interpreted by the cerebellum and midbrain to maintain equilibrium (coordination and balance) at a subconscious level. Conscious awareness of one's position is provided by the cerebrum.

The semicircular canals within the inner ear are fluid-filled membranous ovals that are oriented on three different planes. At the base of each canal is an enlarged section known as the ampulla, which contains more hair cells (Crista galli) that respond to movement. This sensory information is also transmitted to the brain to maintain equilibrium during periods of movement.

Developmental Variations

Developmental variations occur over the course of an individual's life span and events. Awareness of these variations is important to understand and recognize common age-related alterations or modifications of the ear.

Infant and Child

Development of the ear begins around the fourth week of gestation and is basically complete at the end of the first trimester. This is a critical period during which any insult or injury to the fetus may cause permanent hearing impairment. A major concern is maternal rubella, which causes significant damage to the organ of Corti. Prematurity and cytomegalovirus (CMV), which acts like rubella, may also cause hearing impairment. Infections that occur during childhood, otitis media and meningitis, are also responsible for causing hearing loss. Additionally, antibiotics that are needed to treat these conditions may also be responsible for causing damage to the eighth cranial nerve.

Infants who are born with congenital disorders that include craniofacial disorders are more likely to be born with or develop a hearing loss. Down syndrome is the most common cause of a genetically caused hearing loss. This is followed by specific syndromes that include CHARGE, Waardenburg, and Treacher Collins syndromes, all of which are associated with unique physical features or craniofacial disorders (Berke, 2007).

The external auditory canal in infants is shorter and curves upward. The TM is close to adult size but is positioned more horizontally (Figure 19-5). The Eustachian tube of the infant is shorter, wider, and straighter, allowing the influx of nasopharyngeal secretions. As growth occurs during infancy and childhood, the Eustachian tube gradually becomes longer and more curved. The Eustachian tube is surrounded by lymphoid tissue, which increases in size during childhood, increasing the potential for occlusion, making pressure equalization more difficult.

The Pregnant Woman

During pregnancy, there are minimal effects on the ears, however, 5%–30% of pregnant women experience Eustachian tube dysfunction (Funk & Gelbard, 2010). The actual cause is not known but is thought to be related to altered opening pressures caused by a change in surface tension from estrogen acting on prostaglandin E that affects surfactant production (Patel & Levine, 2013). Manifestations include otalgia, autophony, "plugged" ears, hearing loss, and tinnitus. Vertigo and disequilibrium may occur in association with otitis media. Uncomplicated cases usually do not require treatment and spontaneously resolve after delivery.

A sudden sensorineural hearing loss during pregnancy is relatively rare, but it has been associated with toxemia of pregnancy and hypertension. The presumed cause is thought to be due to microemboli that occlude the microcirculation of the cochlea and CN VIII (Funk & Gelbard, 2010). Historically, it was thought that pregnancy exacerbated **otosclerosis** in women who already had it, but this has not been substantiated and is no longer believed.

The Older Adult

Sensorineural hearing gradually decreases with age. Age-related hearing loss is identified as presbycusis and is primarily due to deterioration of the hair cells in the organ of Corti, which begins after the age of 50. Additionally, the capillaries that secrete endolymph, which facilitates sensitization of cochlear hair cells, begin to atrophy, further contributing to hearing loss. Sensorineural hearing impairment begins with the loss of high frequencies and progresses to lower frequency sounds.

Conductive hearing loss also occurs with aging and can be due to a variety of causes. Atrophy of the sebaceous glands of the ear makes cerumen drier, often resulting in impaction and the impedance of sound transmission. This common occurrence is easily reversed. The TM gradually stiffens, particularly in individuals who have had frequent ear infections and have scarring of the TM. Otosclerosis is another cause of hearing loss and is due to fixation of the middle ear bones by the overgrowth and deposition of bone cells along the ossicle chain.

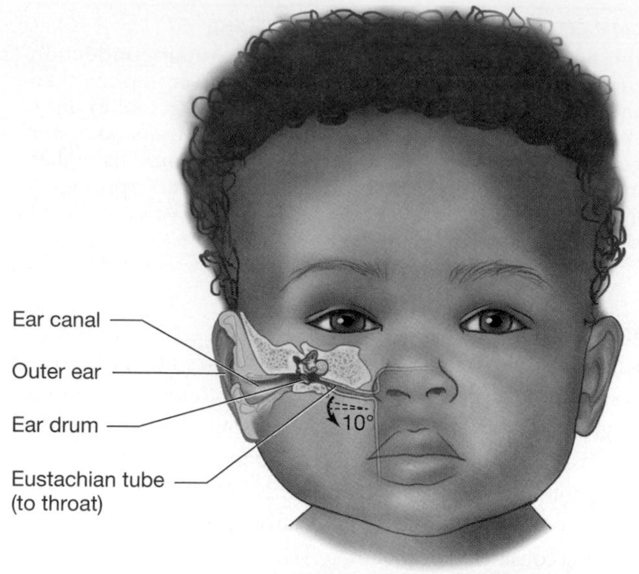

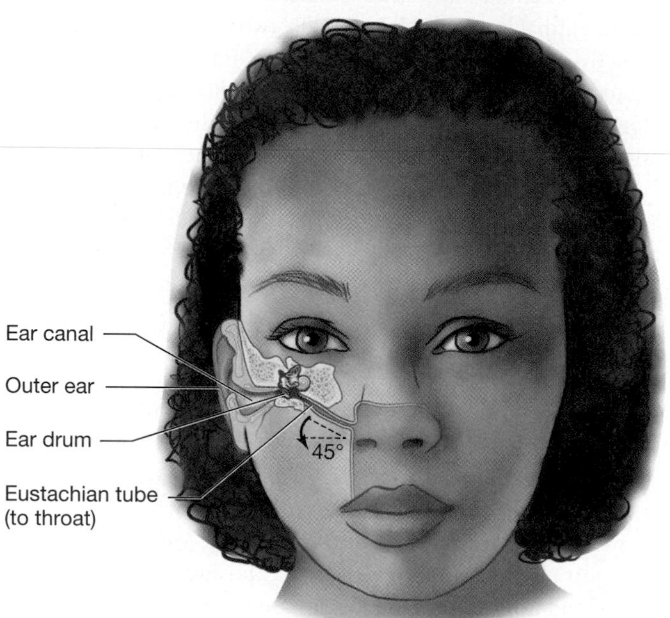

FIGURE 19-5 Comparison of child's and adult's ear canal

Tinnitus is more common in males, particularly those who are 65–74 years of age and experiencing presbycusis (Mayo Clinic Staff, 2011).

Health Promotion

Goals of *Healthy People 2020* related to Hearing and Other Sensory or Communication Disorders (Ear, Nose, and Throat—Voice, Speech, and Language) identifies the need for screening, prevention, early detection, treatment and rehabilitation for optimum hearing health for all ages (U.S. Department of Health and Human Services, 2009).

Hearing Loss

- ENT-VSL—1: Increase the proportion of newborns who are screened for hearing loss by no later than age 1 month, have audiologic evaluation by age 3 months, and are enrolled in appropriate intervention services not later that age 6 months

It is estimated that 28 million individuals in the U.S. are hard of hearing or deaf. Of these, approximately 1.5 million individuals over the age of 3 are bilaterally deaf. Loss of hearing has multiple causes including genetic factors, noise, trauma, ototoxic drugs, and infections. Loss of hearing before the age of 3 has a significant impact on the acquisition and development of language (Delaney & Ruth, 2011a). Language is a primary means of communication; thus the inability to hear speech results in the delay or inability to develop language skills. For this reason, early identification and intervention for hearing impairment is essential for a child's long-term well-being.

Health Promotion *continued*

Unlike vision, hearing in the newborn is fully developed, so the fetus was probably hearing sounds before birth (Graven & Browne, 2008; Hepper & Shahidullah, 1994). Congenital hearing loss is one of the most common anomalies, and occurs in approximately 1–2 infants per 1,000 births (Adcock & Freysdottir, 2013); however these figures do not include hearing loss that develops later in childhood. Approximately one-half of childhood hearing losses are due to genetic causes (Centers for Disease Control and Prevention, 2013).

Recent evidence has demonstrated that prolonged exposure of the fetus to nicotine can result in the development of hearing related cognitive deficits (Ginzel et al., 2007). It is recognized that nicotine appears to damage receptors in the brain that are sensitive to nicotine (Thompson, Levitt, & Stanwood, 2009). The effects of nicotine appear to be present even if the mother used a nicotine patch.

Early hearing screening is recommended for infants before 1 month of age, with optimum screening occurring before discharge from the hospital. (Screening techniques are discussed in Developmental Applications, p. 467. Currently, all 50 states have passed legislation mandating newborn hearing screening (Kibby & Mersch, 2011).

The **whispered voice test** has also been found and used as an effective screening tool for hearing impairment in adults; it may also be used with children (Pirozzo, Papinczak, & Glasziou, 2003). While the whispered voice test appears to be less sensitive in children, its use is not necessarily contraindicated. The major concern related to its use in children was the lack of a standardized protocol.

Otitis Media

- ENT-VSL—2: Decrease otitis media in children and adolescents

Otitis media (OM) is recognized as a cause of hearing loss in children. While a single episode does not place a child at risk, the more episodes of OM, the greater the potential for hearing loss. Recurrent OM is manifest as more than three occurrences within 6 months or four occurrences within 1 year (Natal & Chao, 2011). Chronic OM is the major cause of hearing loss in children (Zamani & Shaw, 2011). The continuous inflammation of the middle ear results in damage to the middle ear bones, interfering with their conduction ability. The fluid also weakens the TM, causing it to collapse and possible attaching itself to the middle ear bones (Perlstein, 2011). If there are no further complications, the TM will heal spontaneously without any hearing deficits. Although rare, OM has been related to incidences of bacteremia and meningitis. Complications are most commonly associated with subacute or chronic OM; however, acute otitis media (AOM) is the most common cause of meningitis (Eaton & Murray, 2011).

Presently, there are no specific preventive measures known to reduce the incidence of OM. Breast feeding decreases the incidence of OM, and elimination of cigarette smoke in the environment is also essential to decrease the incidence (Chanin, 2011). Otitis media with effusion (OME) may precede or predispose the individual to AOM; however, it is a separate condition and should be treated as such.

Hearing Examinations

- ENT-VSL—3: Increase the proportion of persons with hearing impairments who have ever used a hearing aid or assistive listening devices or who have cochlear implants.
- ENT-VSL—4: Increase the proportion of persons who have had a hearing examination on schedule.
- ENT-VSL—5: Increase the number of persons who are referred by their primary care physician or other health care provider for hearing evaluation and treatment.

A hearing aid makes some sounds louder so that a person with hearing loss can listen, communicate, and participate more fully in daily activities and hear more in both quiet and noisy situations. However, only about one out of five people who would benefit from a hearing aid actually uses one.

Recent studies indicate that hearing aid ownership and assistive listening devices (ALD) usage remains low in the older population. Given the significant proportion of older people who self-report and have a measured hearing loss, more could be helped through the increased use of hearing aid and/or ALD technology. Greater efforts are needed to promote the benefits of these technologies and to support their use among older people with hearing loss (Hartley, Rochtchina, Newall, Golding, & Mitchell, 2010).

Hearing Protection

- ENT-VSL—6: Increase the use of hearing protection devices.
- ENT-VSL—7/8: Reduce the proportion of adolescents/adults who have elevated hearing thresholds or audiometric notches, in high frequencies (3, 4, or 6kHz) in both ears, signifying noise-induced hearing loss.

Exposure to loud noises and trauma is the cause of 10 million individuals developing permanent, irreversible hearing loss. An additional 30 million individuals are estimated to be exposed daily to excessive levels of noise that can lead to injury and **noise induced hearing loss** (NIHL) (American Speech-Language-Hearing Association, 2007). Noise-induced hearing loss is the most common occupational condition and the second most self-reported occupational illness or injury (U.S. Department of Health and Human Services, 2000).

Noise is somewhat difficult to define and ranges from unwanted sound to acoustic sounds that can negatively affect the physiological and psychological well-being of an individual. While exposure to noise has been implicated as the cause of hearing loss (Ruben, 2011), there are other significant negative effects that it has on an individual, including the following:

- Increase in blood pressure and ventilations
- Disruption to heart action
- Altered GI function—digestion, upset stomach, ulcers
- Negatively affects developing fetus (causes premature birth)
- Interferes with sleep, even after noise stops
- Augments effects of drugs, alcohol, aging, and carbon monoxide

Noise-induced hearing loss can be caused by a one-time exposure to a sudden increased level of noise, or continuous exposure to increased levels of noise in either work or recreational settings. The extent of NIHL is related to the level of noise, distance from the noise, length of exposure, and individual susceptibility (Table 19-1).

Noises that register above 85 decibels are considered dangerous and a potential cause of damage to hearing (Table 19-1). Noise-induced hearing loss can be easily prevented by protecting the ears from constant exposure. Measures that can be taken for protection from noise include wearing appropriate hearing protectors, reducing exposure time to noise, reducing the volume in personal equipment (headsets, speakers), choosing equipment, appliances, power tools, toys responsibly, or having a hearing test if a concern exists regarding possible damage to hearing.

Tinnitus

ENT-VSL—9/10: Increase the proportion of adults

- bothered by tinnitus in the past 12 months who have seen a doctor, and

Table 19-1 How loud is loud?

Environmental Noise	Decibel Level	OSHA Daily Permissible Noise Level Exposure
Weakest sound heard	0 dB	
Ticking watch	20 dB	
Whisper Quiet Library at 6′	30 dB	
Refrigerator Hum Quiet room	40 dB	
Rainfall	50 dB	
Normal conversation at 3′ Dishwasher Clothes dryer	60–70 dB	
Telephone dial tone Loud singing Washing machine Alarm clock at 2′	80–90 dB	8 (90 dB)
City Traffic (inside car) Train whistle at 500′, Truck Traffic Kitchen blender/Food processor		6 (92 dB)
Jackhammer at 50′ MRI Subway train at 200′ Passing motorcycle	95 dB	4 (95 dB)
Level at which sustained exposure may result in hearing loss		**90–95 dB**
Hand/pneumatic Drill	98 dB	3 (97 dB)
Snowmobile, Motorcycle Blow dryer Subway train	100 dB	2
Power mower at 3′ Chainsaw Snow blower	107 dB	1.5 (102 dB)
Power saw at 3′ Screaming child Maximum output of some MP3 players Model airplane	110 dB	1 (105 dB) 0.5 (110 dB)
Sandblasting Loud Rock Concert Thunderclap	115–20 dB	0.25 or less
Pain begins		**125 dB**
Pneumatic riveter at 4′	125 dB	
Jackhammer Jet engine at 100′	130–140 dB	
Even short term exposure can cause permanent damage-Loudest recommended exposure WITH hearing protection		**140 dB**
Fireworks at 3′	150 dB	
12 Gauge Shotgun Blast	165 dB	
Death of hearing tissue	180 dB	
Loudest sound possible	194 dB	

Health Promotion *continued*

- whom tinnitus is a moderate to severe problem who have tried appropriate treatments.

Tinnitus describes the perception of noise either in one ear, both ears or in the head, when there is no associated external sound. It is not a disease, but a condition that can result from a wide range of underlying causes; however, its most common cause is noise-induced hearing loss. Approximately 20% of the population experience some form of tinnitus. It is not curable, and unless there is a specific cause for it, individuals may not seek treatment from a provider. Any onset of tinnitus should be evaluated by a provider to be certain there is no underlying cause. This is particularly important if the tinnitus is only heard on one side.

Health Promotion *continued*

Balance and Equilibrium

ENT-VSL—11/12/13: Increase the proportion of adults

- with balance or dizziness problems in the past 12 months who had ever seen a health care provider in 2008,
- with moderate to severe balance or dizziness problems who have seen or been referred to a health care specialist for evaluation or treatment, and
- who have tried recommended methods for treating their balance or dizziness problems.

ENT-VSL—14/15: Reduce the proportion of adults with balance and dizziness problems

- who experienced negative or adverse outcomes in the past 12 months, and
- who have fallen in the past 5 years while experiencing symptoms of dizziness, vertigo, or imbalance.

Balance and equilibrium disorders result from alterations within the inner ear. The two most common complaints related to loss of balance and equilibrium are **dizziness** and **vertigo**. Dizziness may often be described as feeling lightheaded or unsteady with the sensation of imbalance or disequilibrium. It is important to determine whether the patient is describing lightheadedness or dizziness. Dizziness is commonly not associated with the perception of turning or spinning; instead, the individual may describe the sensation as rocking or feeling faint.

Vertigo is the sensation of a whirling or rotational motion. With the eyes open, the environment appears to be moving (objective vertigo); with the eyes closed the individual experiences motion (subjective vertigo). It results from a disruption of balance and position senses by the brain of data sent to it from the inner ear. Vertigo may be an unpleasant experience and may limit certain activities; it is rarely a manifestation of a more serious, life-threatening condition. While it may be related to other conditions (inflammation, tumor, and trauma), it is most frequently associated with rapid or unusual position changes of the head (**benign paroxysmal positional vertigo**) (Wedro, 2011).

Vertigo is a common complaint associated with Meniere's disease, which is caused by an alteration of the fluids in the inner ear. The exact cause of Meniere's disease is unknown and most likely results from increased pressure within the endolymphatic system of the inner ear (Balentine, 2011). Usually only one ear is affected; however, in approximately 15% of cases, both ears will be affected. Other manifestations of Meniere's disease are hearing disturbances, tinnitus, and a sensation of fullness or pressure in the ear (Li, 2011).

Clinical Context Exemplars

Situation A

During the history taking, what patient behaviors may indicate a hearing deficiency? What actions could be taken to accommodate a hearing impaired patient?

Situation B

A patient is being worked up for vertigo.

1. What questions would you want to ask to differentiate between subjective and objective vertigo?
2. What might be the cause of the patient's vertigo?

Another patient is being worked up for tinnitus and constant headaches.

1. What might be the relationship between the tinnitus and headaches?
2. What information would you want to obtain regarding this?

Situation C

A new mother, with a history of hearing loss in her family, is concerned about identifying hearing loss in her new infant.

1. What behaviors would you inform the mother to be alert for and why?
2. What is the most significant developmental acquisition that reflects a child's hearing ability?

Situation D

The Weber and Rinne tests are used to assess air conduction and bone conduction. During the Weber test, sound lateralized to the right ear.

1. What information does this provide about the right and left ear?
2. What information would you expect from the Rinne test for each ear?

SUBJECTIVE DATA

History of Present Illness (CC)

The patient may present to the provider with a variety of concerns that may be directly related to the auditory system or other systems. Framing the questions will depend on the patient's age, gender, culture, race, emotional or mental status, health practices, and concurrent illnesses. All symptoms presented must be thoroughly assessed with a symptom analysis (COLDERRA).

Otalgia (Ear Pain/Earache)

Otalgia is a frequent reason for seeking health care. It can be caused by disease in the external, *middle*, or inner ear, but the three are indistinguishable in terms of the pain experienced. It may be caused by several other conditions, such as impacted teeth, sinus disease, inflamed tonsils, infections in the nose and pharynx, throat cancer, and occasionally as a sensory aura that precedes a migraine. Pain that originates within the ear is primary otalgia; pain that originates outside the ear is referred (secondary) otalgia.

Provider Inquiries	Clinical Reasoning/Logic
Characteristics: Describe the ear pain. Is it dull, aching, sharp, stabbing?	
Any discharge (characteristics—bloody, pus, and odor)?	Any discharge suggests infection—may come from canal or ruptured TM.
	External otitis—purulent, sanguineous, or watery
	Otitis media with perforation—purulent
	Otitis media with effusion—no discharge
Onset: When did it start? Sudden or gradual? Any trauma? Recent flight? Exposure to loud noises? Swimming?	Helps to identify any precipitating cause or event
Recent cold/upper respiratory infection? Fever, runny nose?	Otitis externa frequently associated with swimming
	OM frequently follows an upper respiratory infection
Location: Outside of ear? Close to surface or deeper in head? One side or both?	Ear pain may be unilateral or bilateral.
	Pain with OM is often experienced deep in the ear.
Duration: Constant or intermittent?	Pain associated with infection is usually continuous and becomes progressively severe. Intermittent pain is more associated with musculoskeletal conditions.
Exacerbation: Anything that intensifies the pain (changing position, sudden movement, heat/cold, coughing/sneezing)?	In otitis externa, manipulation of auricle elicits pain, not with otitis media
	Pain in AOM is often more severe in the supine position.
Relief: What was tried to alleviate pain? Successful?	Rupture of TM in OM causes a reduction in pain.
Radiation: Localized or does it go to any other area? If so, where?	Pain may be referred to the ear from other locations. In adults, ear pain may be associated with myocardial infarctions.
Associated signs/symptoms: Aural fullness, itching, hearing loss?	Aural fullness, itching and hearing loss may be symptoms of otitis externa.
Fever? Hearing loss?	Slight hearing loss and fever may accompany AOM, OME, or otitis externa.

Acute Hearing (Sensorineural) Loss

Acute hearing loss occurs when sound perception is diminished due to an alteration within the auditory system. In some instances the cause(s) may be identified; however, is some instances the cause is not known.

Provider Inquiries	Clinical Reasoning/Logic
Characteristics: Any particular sounds difficult to hear (high frequencies/low frequencies)?	High frequencies often lost first
Do individuals have to speak louder for you to hear? Difficulty talking on phone?	Difficulty hearing others more often is associated with sensorineural loss.
Do you often hear yourself when talking?	Hearing yourself louder when talking is associated with conductive hearing loss
Does it feel like your ear is blocked or full?	May be another indicator of a conductive hearing loss
Onset: Was the loss sudden or gradual?	By definition sudden sensorineural hearing loss (SSNHL) is an idiopathic hearing loss of at least 30 dB over at least three test frequencies that occur over a 72 hour period (Stachler et al., 2012). Often noted on awakening in morning.

Provider Inquiries	Clinical Reasoning/Logic
Location: One ear or both?	Most instances of SSNHL are unilateral.
Duration: How long have you noticed difficulty in hearing?	Acute hearing loss occurs within 3 days.
Exacerbation: When is hearing worse (noisy environments)?	
Relief: Use of hearing devices? Success?	
Associated signs/symptoms: Tinnitus? Describe it. Any ear pain, ear drainage, fever, focal neurologic symptoms, headache, diplopia, or eye pain/redness?	Tinnitus reported in 90% of patients with SSNHL Possible causes or manifestations of other conditions that may cause SSNHL

PRACTICE POINT: Noise in the Hospital

Noise has been implicated in creating a negative environment for hospitalized patients as well as those who provide care (Buxton et al., 2012; HermanMiller Healthcare, 2006; Mazer, 2012; The Joint Commission, 2013). Noise levels (dB) in hospitals has continuously increased to where they are consistently above the recommended noise level (Stokowski, 2008). While there is the tendency to consider equipment and machines to be the major contributor to noise, conversations between clinicians are also a major source of noise (Beyea, 2007). The more individuals conversing at a time, the greater the contribution to noise. Another major cause for increased noise levels is the material used and layout of hospital units. Square corners and non-sound absorbing surfaces send sound bouncing around (Stokowski, 2008).

In addition to those negative effects mentioned previously, continuous exposure to environmental noise can induce memory alterations, increased agitation, decreased pain tolerance, and feelings of isolation (Mazer, 2005). When any of these manifestations are present, awareness of environmentally generated symptoms is important to consider in maintaining a healing environment for the individual. Simply medicating the individual is often not an appropriate or effective intervention in reducing these manifestations. The most significant impact on the patient as a result of noise is sleep deprivation, which increases patient's anxiety and decreases their confidence in the clinical competence of the care givers (Juang, Lee, Yang, & Chang, 2010). In addition to having a negative impact on patient outcomes, health care providers are at risk of developing some degree of hearing loss.

Vertigo

Vertigo is a category of dizziness causing an individual to experience the sensation or perception of motion, generally due to a dysfunction of the vestibular system of the ear, which is referred to as **peripheral vertigo**, in contrast to **central vertigo**, which is due to an alteration within the brain, usually within the brainstem. When an individual feels as if he or she is moving, it's called **subjective vertigo**; the perception that the surroundings are moving is called **objective vertigo**.

Provider Inquiries	Clinical Reasoning/Logic
Characteristics: To and fro motion or rotary motion? Does it feel like the room is spinning or that you are spinning? Unsteadiness, loss of balance, falling?	Individuals with vertigo feel as though they are spinning around, or the world is spinning around them. Lightheadedness is a feeling that one is about to faint or pass out. Individuals with lightheadedness may feel dizzy, but there is no spinning sensation associated with it. Motor function, gait and coordination are generally intact with peripheral vertigo. Motor function, gait instability and loss of coordination are frequent with central vertigo.

PRACTICE POINT: Vertigo

The unpredictable episodes of vertigo often comprise the most debilitating problem and often force an individual to lie down for several hours, causing a loss of time from work or leisure activities, and possibly causing emotional stress. Vertigo also increases risk of falls, accidents while driving a car or operating heavy machinery, depression or anxiety in dealing with the disease, and permanent hearing loss.

Provider Inquiries	Clinical Reasoning/Logic
Onset: When did sensation begin? Anything noted to initiate sensation?	The onset may be due to a movement or change in position. Sudden onset–peripheral vertigo Gradual onset—central vertigo
Time between stimulus and sensation?	Longer (up to 20 seconds)—peripheral Shorter (up to 5 seconds)—central

Provider Inquiries	Clinical Reasoning/Logic
Duration: Constant sensation or intermittent?	The duration of symptoms can be from seconds to weeks, and symptoms can be constant or intermittent. Intermittent—peripheral vertigo Constant—central vertigo It is important to tell the provider about any recent head trauma or whiplash injury as well as any new medications the affected individual is taking.
Exacerbation: Anything noted to make sensation worse? Is it affected by head movement?	Activity, position changes, reading, bright lights are all possible causes for increasing symptoms of vertigo. Affected—peripheral vertigo Not affected–central vertigo
Relief: Tried anything for relief?	
Associated signs/symptoms: Nausea, vomiting, tinnitus, hearing loss, double vision, sensation of fullness in ear, pain (ear/mastoid), facial weakness, and headache?	These are due to the numerous interconnections within the brainstem: nausea or vomiting, sweating, and/or, abnormal eye movements, headache, hearing loss, tinnitus. Nausea and vomiting more frequent and severe—peripheral vertigo Nausea and vomiting less predictable—central vertigo

Tinnitus

Tinnitus, a subjective sensation of ringing in the ears, is not considered a disease or disorder, but a condition that is associated with a wide variety of underlying causes. In the majority of situations, there is no specific cause. It is a common occurrence (about 30%–35% of individuals) but only about 10%–5% of individuals require medical intervention of treatment.

Provider Inquiries	Clinical Reasoning/Logic
Characteristics: Describe sound (ringing, roaring, pulsing, whooshing, clicking, hissing, crackling, or buzzing)? Pitch? Does the tinnitus occur in rhythm with your heartbeat (pulsatile)?	Tinnitus originates in the individual and is only heard by the individual; thus it cannot be objectively measured by any instrument. Low pitch, rumbling—Meniere's disease High pitch—SN hearing loss Pulsatile tinnitus should be checked immediately.
Onset: When first started? Associated with anything (ototoxic medications [aspirin, antibiotics, diuretics], trauma)? Illnesses?	**Ototoxic** medications identified in Table 19-2. Withdrawal of certain medications (benzodiazepines) may be a cause.

Table 19-2 Ototoxic medications

Analgesics	Antibiotics	Chemotherapy/antiviral drugs	Loop diuretics	Miscellaneous
aspirin	Ciprofloxacin	bleomycin	bumetanide	chloroquine
nonsteroidal anti-inflammatory drugs (ibuprofen, naproxen)	aminoglycosides (Gentamicin, Tobramycin)	interferon	ethacrynic acid	quinine
	chloramphenicol	pegylated interferon-alpha-2b	furosamide	antidepressants
	erythromycin	ciosplatin		varenicline
	tetracycline	metchlorethamine		
	vancomycin	methrotrexate		
	doxycycline	vincristine		

Provider Inquiries	Clinical Reasoning/Logic
	Gradual onset of hearing loss and tinnitus associated with advancing age, usually due to presbycusis. Acute onset associated with loud noise or head trauma. Although rare, pulsatile tinnitus with a sudden onset may develop because of an aneurysm near the ear or due to a sudden onset of very high blood pressure.
Location: One ear, both ears?	Most commonly in one ear, but may affect both. Unilateral tinnitus associated with impacted cerumen, OE, OM. Tinnitus with unilateral sensory hearing loss is characteristic of acoustic neuroma.
Duration: Constant or intermittent? If intermittent, does it occur at same time, follow same pattern?	Continuous tinnitus—SN hearing loss Episodic—Meniere's disease Pulsatile—vascular alteration
Exacerbation: Anything make it worse or sound louder? Louder during the day or at night?	Tinnitus can worsen in some people if they drink alcohol, smoke cigarettes, drink caffeinated beverages, or eat certain foods. During the day, the distractions of activities and sounds may make tinnitus less noticeable. It may seem louder at night or in quieter surroundings. Fatigue and stress may also make tinnitus worse.
Increase in fatigue/stress? Depression?	For reasons not yet entirely clear to researchers, stress and fatigue seem to worsen tinnitus. Because tinnitus (in most cases) is associated with depression, it is important to seek out information related to this.
Relief: What has patient tried for relief? Ask about biofeedback, hypnosis, electrical stimulation, relaxation therapy, counseling, habituation therapies, tinnitus maskers, and sound machines.	Position changes may provide relief. Multiple therapies and home remedies effective in reducing the effects of tinnitus.
If used, have any of these options been effective?	
Associated signs/symptoms: Hearing loss, vertigo, or dizziness? Changes in personality? Difficulty speaking or walking, or any other movement problems?	The presence of vertigo, **otalgia**, otorrhea, or **temporomandibular joint disease** can relate to tinnitus. Changes in personality or movement problems may be signs of a stroke.

Past Medical History

Past medical history provides information as to previous illnesses or conditions that may have an effect on the ears.

Multiple ear infections? Childhood/adulthood? How treated? Effective?	Identifies possible causes for any symptoms
Any surgeries? When? For what?	
Trauma/injuries to ear? When? Severity?	
Medications? What? For what (antibiotics, diuretics, aspirin)?	Certain drugs are known to be ototoxic (see Table 19-2).

Family History

Family history provides information regarding family member's illnesses or conditions as potential causes for chief complaint or presenting symptoms that may indicate a pattern of presentation associated with transmission of familial/genetic factors predisposing the individual to certain system related conditions/illnesses. Any of these may indicate a potential or actual cause of ear dysfunction.

Provider Inquiries	Clinical Reasoning/Logic
Hearing problems/hearing loss? Meniere's disease? Allergies?	Identifies any possible genetic or hereditary causes of symptoms.

Personal and Social History

Personal and social history is information related to surroundings and environments that may identify risk factors related to certain conditions. These questions can also determine the use of safety measures to prevent accidents or injuries to the eyes or other factors that may be related to other symptoms or conditions.

Provider Inquiries	Clinical Reasoning/Logic
Employment/Environment: Exposure to environmental noise (work, home, live near airport, listen to loud music, play in symphony)? Protection worn?	Identifies possible environmental or external causes for symptoms.
Ear cleaning habits/procedures (if needed)?	

PRACTICE POINT: Cleaning of Ears

There is an old saying that "nothing should go in your ears that is smaller than your elbow." The point here is that nothing should be put in the ear that can cause damage to either the external canal or eardrum. A practice of many is to clean the ears with cotton-tipped swabs. While the cotton protects the sharp end of the swab, it also has the potential to push cerumen further into the ear canal, setting the stage for impacted cerumen. Generally, the ears do not require routine cleaning. There are individuals that do overproduce cerumen, which may need to be periodically removed from the ear canal. It is much safer to keep a bulb syringe handy in the shower and irrigate the ear canal with warm water. This easily removes the cerumen plug and causes no damage to the ear canal.

Developmental Applications

Certain conditions or disorders may be related to certain age groups or situations. Inquiring to obtain age or condition specific information will provide further information for helping to determine causes of the chief concern as identified.

Infants and Children

Provider Inquiries	Clinical Reasoning/Logic
Maternal infections (TORCH infections)?	Possible infectious causes for hearing loss
Maternal alcohol/drug use? Treatment with antibiotics (aminoglycosides, salicylates)?	Drugs that are potentially ototoxic
Maternal diabetes, hypertension?	
ABO incompatibility (erythroblastosis fetalis), increased bilirubin?	
Cranio-facial deformities at birth?	Infants with craniofacial deformities at increased risk for chronic OM
Breast feeding?	Reduces risk for OM
Second hand smoke exposure, child care?	Increased risk for otitis media
React appropriately to sound—startle response/change activity? Cooing/babbling sounds?	Helps to assess hearing ability
Speech: First words spoken, pronunciation (clear, understandable), put words together to make sentences?	Assesses appropriate language development
Ear infections—frequency? Pull/tug on ears? Frequent colds/upper respiratory infections/allergies?	
Treated with antibiotics?	Certain antibiotics ototoxic
Ever put anything into ear?	Potential for hearing loss and/or damage to TM
Exposure to loud noises—at home/school?	Increased risk for noise induced hearing loss
Any ringing in ears?	Tinnitus thought to be condition associated with adulthood; however children with hearing loss have high incidence of tinnitus that frequently goes unreported.

Provider Inquiries	Clinical Reasoning/Logic
The Pregnant Woman	
Weeks of pregnancy?	Determine age of fetus and potential for damage to ears
Any known exposure to infectious agents?	Concern for CMV exposure
Immunization status—Rubella? Has child or received vaccination; any boosters?	Protection of fetus from potential infectious agents
Any ringing in the ears?	Tinnitus is a common manifestation of pregnancy and is frequently pulsatile in nature, often synchronous with the pulse of the woman.
The Older Adult	
Any noted hearing loss (interference with activities of daily living)?	Effect a hearing loss has on ability to care for self
Use of hearing devices?	Willingness to use hearing aids

OBJECTIVE DATA

In terms of sequence for a head to toe examination, the ear exam is done within the context of the region of the head. The majority of data obtained from the eye exam is also related to the assessment of the cranial nerves for the neurological exam. Most providers perform the cranial nerve examination during the head and neck segment but may also be covered on the neurological examination. The primary assessment techniques used are inspection and palpation.

Inspection

- Position and placement; attachment
- Size, shape, and symmetry
- Hearing (response to verbal stimuli; whisper test; Weber/Rinne)
- Tympanic membrane
- External auditory canal (color, lesions, discharge, cerumen)
- Balance and coordination

Palpation

- Auricles, tragus, mastoid (tenderness, nodules, swelling)

Percussion *not performed*

Auscultation *not performed*

Level I to IV Examination

The Level I to Level IV examinations are performed on a continuum, which starts from a basic level to a more comprehensive level based on provider's abilities and knowledge as well as the patient's presentation and location. It may start at the outpatient setting, progressing to the ED, hospital unit bed, critical care unit, or specialty unit. Frequently all the elements from basic to comprehensive exam are done in one setting like in a primary care setting or clinic.

The condition/illness of the patient is the primary consideration related to the type and amount of data needed to assess the patient's condition/illness/situation. The arrangement of skills into levels is for general purposes and is meant to be descriptive rather than prescriptive. The purpose of arranging into levels is to provide a framework to assist the learner in determining the appropriate data to collect.

Ears

	Level I	Level II	Level III	Level IV
Inspection	Hearing (response to verbal stimuli; answers questions) Position/ placement Size, shape, symmetry External auditory canal	Angle of attachment (ear/eye alignment) Hearing (whispered voice) Tympanic membrane	TM: trauma/ discharge/perforation	Hearing (Weber/ Rinne) Balance and coordination*
Palpation		Auricle, tragus/mastoid process (tenderness/lesions)		

*The Romberg test is a test of the vestibular component of CN VIII, thus it is a component of the neurological exam.

Inspection: Level I

Inspection Techniques and Expected Findings	Unexpected Findings

Hearing

The initial assessment of the patient's hearing occurs during conversation prior to or during the health history. In the absence of loud or continuous ambient noise, the conscious patient should engage in conversation without having to ask for questions to be repeated or misunderstanding the question. Spontaneous responses should occur when asked by the provider in a moderate level of voice loudness. The provider should not feel as if the loudness of the voice needs to be increased to obtain appropriate responses from the patient.

Observe for clues that indicate hearing difficulty, which are obvious and easily assessed.

If the patient hears better in one ear than the other, the patient will most likely be positioned to favor the good ear or will turn the head to increase hearing.

If the patient seems to be focused on your lips and not maintaining eye contact, the patient is most likely lip-reading.

Asking for questions to be repeated or providing answers that do not relate to the questions are also indicators of hearing difficulties.

Continue the exam with inspection for the presence, position and placement of the ears, which are positioned on the lateral sides of the head with the auricle projecting slightly outward and to the back with an anteroposterior angle of 15–20 degrees (Davison, Bosley, & Sandel IV, 2011) (Figure 19-6). They protrude from the side of the head at approximately 30 degrees (Kelley & Scholes, 2007). The range of size varies, but generally is within 4–10 cm on its vertical axis.

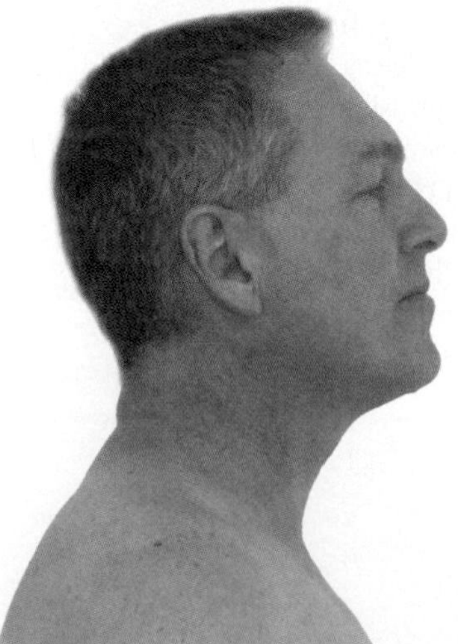

FIGURE 19-6 Auricle-position/placement/alignment

In rare instances one ear may be absent (**aural atresia**) or incompletely formed. This is a congenital defect and frequently accompanies other craniofacial deformities. In most instances the condition is unilateral, with the right ear being more commonly affected than the left. The auricle may be totally absent (**anotia**) or it may be present but small and malformed (**microtia**).

Inspection Techniques and Expected Findings

Unexpected Findings

Observe for the overall size, symmetry, and configuration of the external ear (Figure 19-6). The overall appearance and size should be symmetrical. The skin overlying the ear should be intact with the color the same as the overall skin color.

An auricle smaller than 4 cm would be considered microtia and one that is greater than 10 cm would be macrotia.

It is usually unnecessary to validate the external auricle's landmarks; instead note that characteristics are present bilaterally. The shape, like the size, is difficult to describe other than whether it conforms to expected appearance. Minimal alterations are significant related to the ear's shape (Figure 19-7). A small tubercle (Darwin's tubercle) is a possible, nonsignificant variation. Preauricular pits, located in front of the origination of the auricle, are another nonsignificant variation.

There should be no evidence of lesions, nodules, moles, cysts, or other deformities.

An acquired ear deformity, most commonly from external trauma, may alter auricle shape. Its major cause occurs if the skin is separated from the cartilage by shearing forces or by a hematoma under the skin. If untreated, the cartilage, deprived of its blood supply, dies and begins to contract, resulting in a shriveled up outer ear (Cunha, 2011), called **"cauliflower ear."** Scaling and crusting may accompany eczema, dermatitis, and seborrhea.

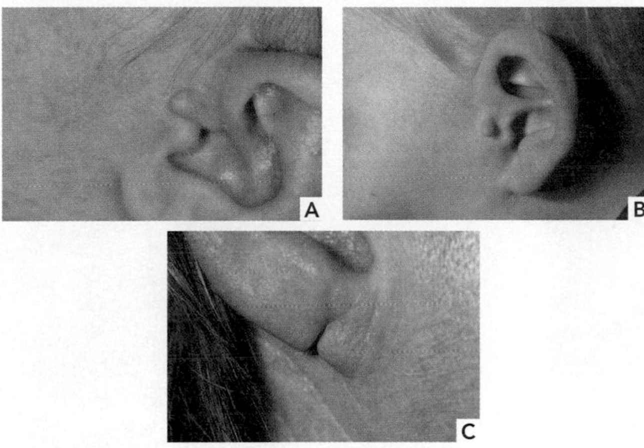

FIGURE 19-7A–C Auricle alterations: a) Accessory auricle ear deformity; b) Auricular appendage; c) Torn earlobe
Source: Dr. P. Marazzi/Science Source Images

Initial observations for the screening exam focus on the external ear opening and ear lobe. Assess the external ear opening for the presence of lesions or discharge.

The characteristics of the discharge have already been described in the previous section. Assess any color changes surrounding the canal opening.

A reddened and swollen external ear canal may be an indication of otitis externa (swimmer's ear). Additionally there may be itching, pain, and possible hearing loss. (See Conditions and Disorders.)

Assess the ear lobe for a diagonal crease across the ear lobe. Ear lobe attachment, or un-attachment, is another nonsignificant variation (Figure 19-8).

PRACTICE POINT: Ear Lobe Crease

This crease's significance remains controversial because it was suggested to be a marker for coronary artery disease, supported by recent studies (Evrengul, 2004). However, this association has also been explained by the increased incidence of both as a result of aging. Despite the lack of a definitive association between CAD and the an ear lobe crease, observing for its presence is an easy assessment that may provide a clue to the patient's condition.

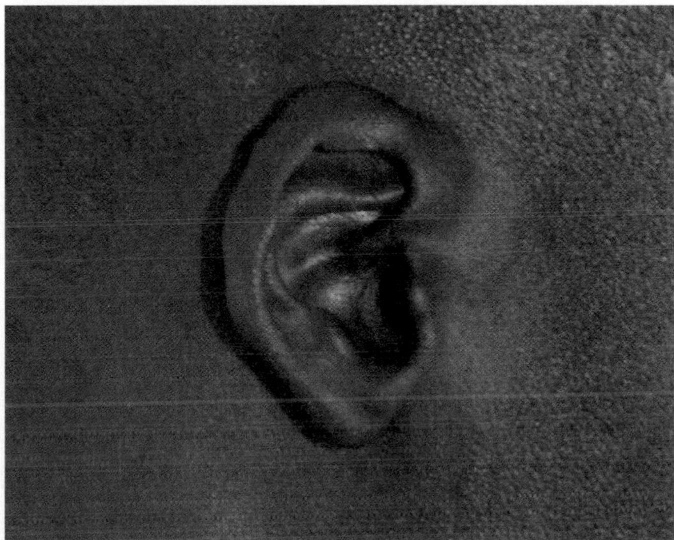

FIGURE 19-8 Ear lobe attachment

Inspection: Level II

Inspection Techniques and Expected Findings	Unexpected Findings

Confirm ear–eye alignment, or the placement of the external ear, by its relationship to the palpebral fissure of the eyes (Figure 19-9). To determine ear placement, extend an imaginary line from the outer canthus of the palpebral fissure on a horizontal plane along the side of the head. The point where the pinna of the ear is attached to the head should be on this line. Or, you may simply observe the ear–eye alignment. The vertical axis of the ear should also not be angled any more than 10 degrees from the overall vertical axis of the side of the head.

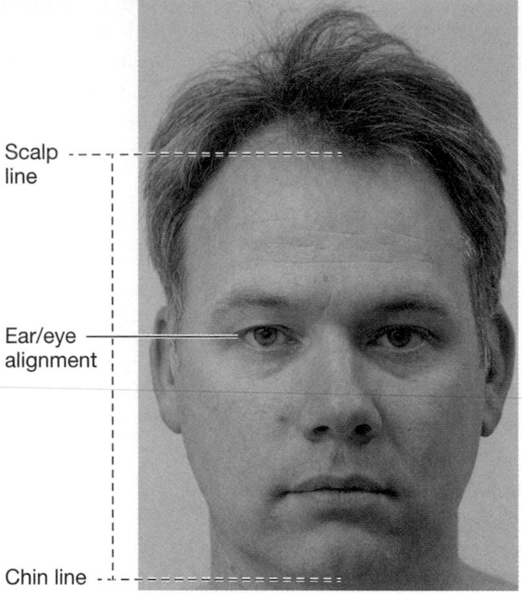

FIGURE 19-9 Ear/eye alignment

Ears that are positioned below the horizontal line are described as **low set ears** (Figure 19-10). This finding is frequently associated with renal disorders or other congenital disorders, often related to those with chromosomal alterations (Down syndrome).

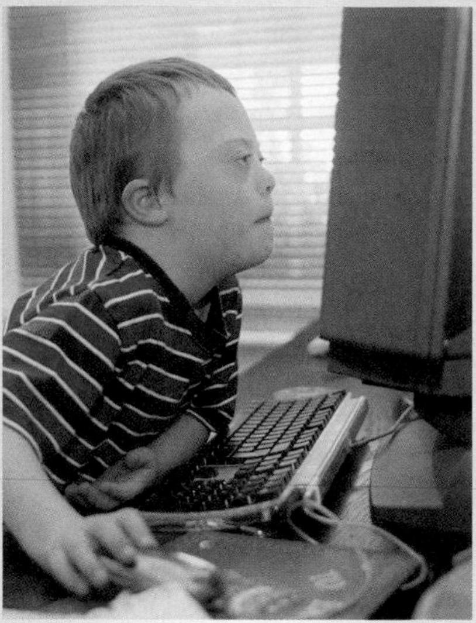

FIGURE 19-10 Low set ears
Source: Lauren Shear/Science Source Images

Use the whispered voice or the ticking watch test to assess hearing for the Level II exam. These are the most basic tests that can be used to screen for hearing loss. For each, test one ear at a time while masking hearing in the other ear. Have the patient place a finger over the tragus of the ear and then push in and out against the ear canal opening in rapid succession.

For the whispered voice test, stand to the side of the patient, approximately 1 to 2 feet away from the ear being tested and out of the patient's line of sight. Instruct the patient to mask the nontested ear as described above by placing one finger on the tragus and exerting enough pressure to close off the external canal while also rotating the finger in a circular motion (Pirozzo, Papinczak, & Glasziou, 2003). Slowly and softly whisper one- and two-syllable words or numbers, asking the patient to repeat them (Figure 19-11). If the patient is unable to repeat any of the words/numbers, repeat the test using a slightly louder whisper (Saunders, 2003). Stop at the level of sound at which the patient can accurately repeat the words/numbers. Repeat the procedure on the opposite ear.

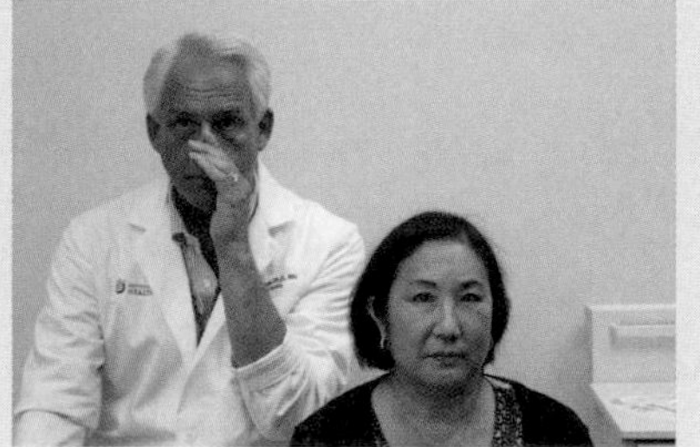

FIGURE 19-11 Whispered voice test

For the ticking watch test, hold a ticking watch one to two inches away from the patient's ear while masking sound in the other ear (Figure 19-12). Ask the patient to identify what is heard.

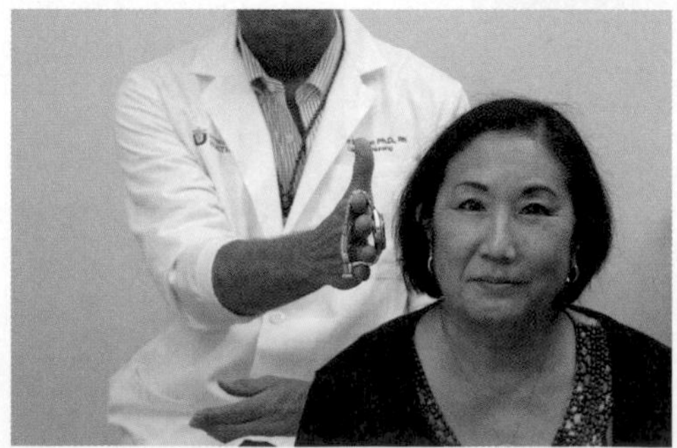

FIGURE 19-12 Ticking watch test

PRACTICE POINT: Ticking Watches

Make sure that the watch has an audible tick by listening to the watch first before using it to test the patient. Newer watches may not have an audible tick or a tick that is very soft.

Inspection Techniques and Expected Findings

Tympanic Membrane Otoscope Examination

Use the otoscope to inspect the external auditory canal and the tympanic membrane. The otoscope's head provides both a light source and slight magnification for observation (Figure 19-13). It also connects to a speculum that is inserted into the auditory canal.

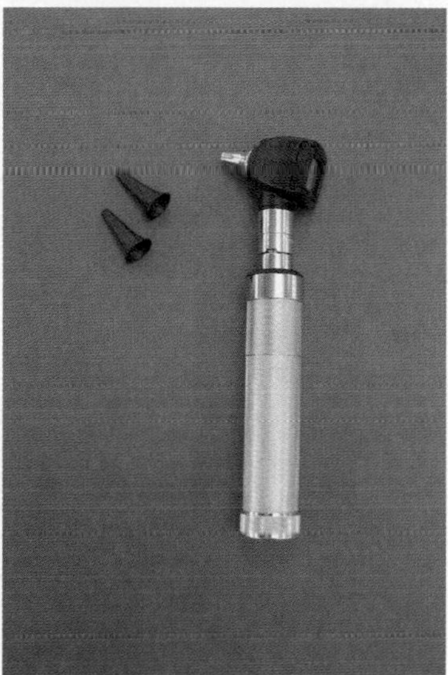

FIGURE 19-13 Otoscope

Use the largest possible speculum on the otoscope that will fit into the ear canal without causing discomfort to the patient. While a smaller speculum may be easier to use and manipulate, it does not provide adequate visualization (Saunders, 2003). Because speculums come in various sizes, access to an appropriately sized speculum is important.

You may move the otoscope slightly to visualize the TM, but keep any movements slow, with minimal manipulation.

To optimize visualization, you may need to slightly straighten the adult ear canal by grasping the pinna with your opposite fingers and gently pulling it upward and slightly toward the back (Figure 19-14). Any straightening should be done before insertion of the speculum.

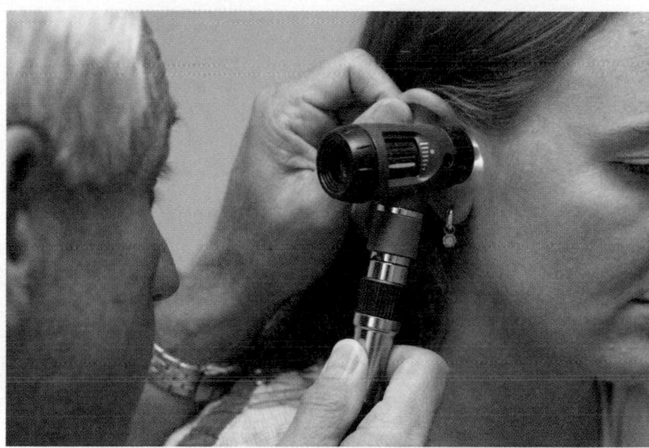

FIGURE 19-14 Holding otoscope and pulling auricle

Unexpected Findings

PRACTICE POINT: Using an Otoscope

Remember three important principles when using an otoscope:

1. Hold the speculum closer to its head than its bottom to prevent your arm or hand movements from transferring into movement of the speculum in the ear canal (Saunders, 2003).
2. Position the patient's head so it is tilted toward the opposite shoulder, allowing you to look downward into the ear.
3. When inserting the speculum, do not place the tip or the sides of the speculum against the sides of the canal or use them to manipulate the ear canal for better visualization. Very little cushioning exists between the skin covering the canal and the bony (cartilaginous) component of the canal. Any pressure exerted against the canal will be quite uncomfortable or painful for the patient.

Inspection Techniques and Expected Findings

Once the speculum is in place, look through the lens to assess the canal's sides, which should be smooth and without visible lesions. In some individuals who are exposed to cold water, small growth of bony swellings (**exotoses**) may be present (Saunders, 2003). Some cerumen may be present; note its amount, color, and characteristics. Its color varies from black/brown to yellow/orange without any odor.

Some individuals overproduce cerumen, which may accumulate in the canal and interfere with observation of the TM. If this is the case, irrigate the ear canal with warm water to remove it. Very dry or hard cerumen may require introduction of a softening agent (mineral oil) into the ear first.

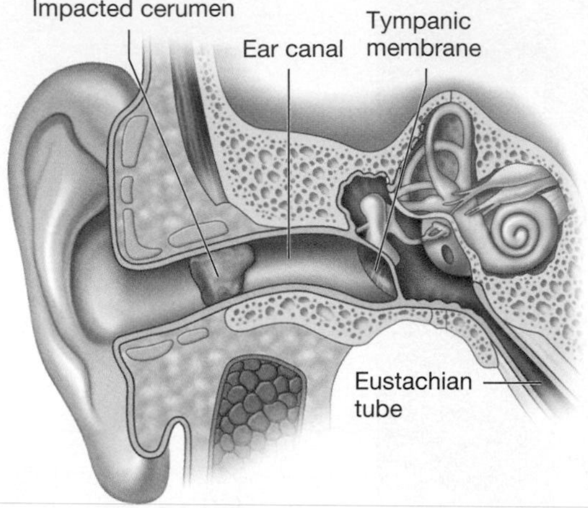

FIGURE 19-15 Impacted cerumen

Following assessment of the ear canal, you may need to insert the speculum a few more mm to inspect the TM for its color, integrity, contour, and landmarks. It should be pearly-gray, translucent and shiny, without any evidence of perforations or tears. It should also appear slightly conical, with a concave shape at the umbo.

TM landmarks are the umbo, malleus, and cone of light. The umbo is close to the center of the TM and is the point where the malleus attaches to it. The manubrium of the malleus may also be visible as a line that is directed from the umbo towards the periphery of the TM (Figure 19-16). The short process of the malleus may also be visible at the end point of the malleus. The cone of light is the other significant landmark, which is actually a reflection of the cone-shaped otoscope light that radiates from the umbo in a continuous pattern towards the periphery. In the right ear it should be at the 5 o'clock position and at 7 o'clock on the left TM.

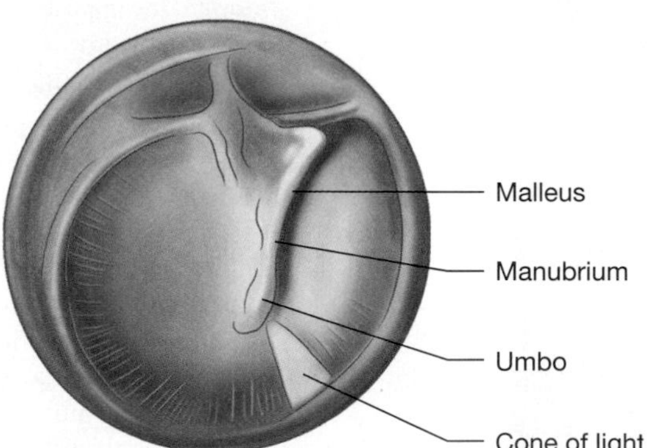

FIGURE 19-16 TM landmarks

You may also assess the mobility of the TM membrane by looking for slight fluctuations when the patient swallows. Or otoscopes that are equipped with pneumatic bulbs are used to assess mobility. With the otoscope in place inside the ear canal, squeeze the bulb to eject a puff of air. As the air hits the TM, there should be an observable movement of the TM.

Unexpected Findings

There is generally cerumen present in the ear canal, but it should not block the ear canal or obstruct visualization of the TM (Figure 19-15). Cerumen is generally not present in the inner one-third of the ear canal. If it is present there, it most likely was pushed there by some other object, such as a cotton tipped swab.

PRACTICE POINT: Ear Irrigation

Irrigation of the ear canal should not be performed in the presence of otitis externa, perforated TM, or myringotomy tubes.

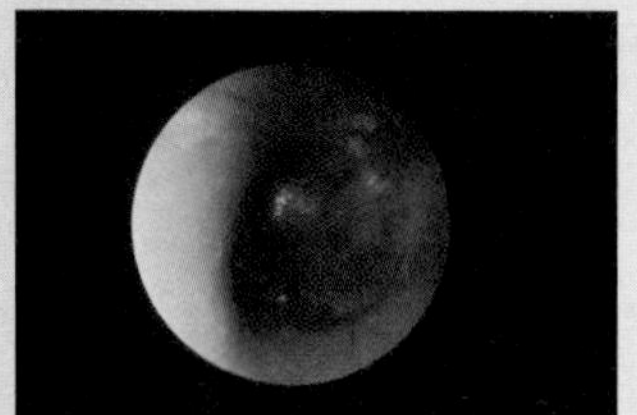

FIGURE 19-17 OM with bulging TM
Source: SIU Biomed Comm/Custom Medical Stock Photo

The contour of the TM may also demonstrate bulging or be retracted. A bulging TM indicates an accumulation of pressure behind the ear drum, within the middle ear, which commonly occurs in the presence of otitis media (Figure 19-17).

A retracted ear drum is present if there is a blocked Eustachian tube, which results in a negative pressure behind the TM, pulling it inward.

A distortion of the cone of light is also observed in changes in the contour of the TM (Figure 19-18). Instead of reflected as a continuous beam of light, it is reflected in multiple areas or does not extend completely from the umbo to the periphery.

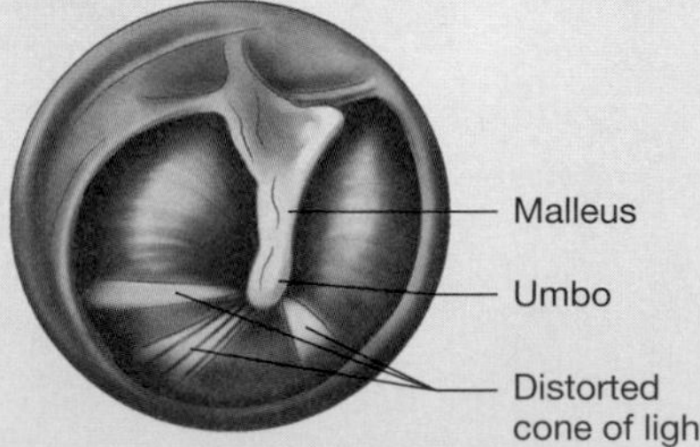

FIGURE 19-18 Distorted cone of light

Inspection: Level III

Inspection Techniques and Expected Findings	Unexpected Findings
Emergency examination and treatment for ear alterations are primarily due to trauma that affects the auricle or tympanic membrane. The external auricle is at high risk for injury due to its exposed and unprotected position along the side of the head (Davison et al., 2011). A laceration, though, may extend into the auditory canal (Malloy & Hollander, 2013).	The most common causes of injuries include bites (human, dog), falls, and moving vehicle accidents. Untreated traumatic auricular or exposure of cartilage after injuries most often end up with infections, erosive chondritis, and necrosis. Loss of auricular cartilage results in notching and replacement of healthy cartilage with fibrocartilage leading to the development of cauliflower ear, both of which cause deformities and are not reversible (Malloy & Hollander, 2013). Trauma to the auricle is also caused by burns and frostbite. Incomplete amputation of the auricle is the most common type of injury. In the majority of instances of traumatic amputation human bites were the most frequent cause (Gault, 2008). Avulsion eternal ear, amputation from tearing away the ear, may result from trauma to the head and neck.
Trauma may also affect the tympanic membrane, which may sustain perforation or ruptured type injuries. Perforation injuries may be due to insertion of pointed instruments into the external ear canal. This may be on purpose or accidental. A ruptured TM may be due to exposure to a rapid change of air pressure or pressure from the buildup of fluid and pressure in the middle ear from otitis media.	Trauma to the TM will be observed as a hole in the TM by examination with the otoscope, with or without drainage. If the rupture has been caused by an inflammation or infection of the middle ear, the ear drum will also appear red. Damage to the ear drum will also most likely cause distortion of the cone of light and may obscure other landmarks on the TM.
In a critical (emergency) situation related to or caused by head trauma (TBI), inspect the ears for any fluid drainage or discharge.	Any discharge from the ear is an unexpected finding. A bloody or clear discharge (cerebrospinal fluid) in the presence of known or suspected head trauma may be indicative of a basilar skull fracture (Turner, Jones, & Handa, 2000). A retroauricular hematoma formation (**battle sign**) is also indicative of a basilar skull fracture. Direct trauma to the ear may result in bleeding into the middle ear (**hemotympanum**), which may also result from retrograde hemorrhage after a nose bleed (epistaxis) (Ghosh, Harrison, & Body, 2006). The tympanic membrane will appear dark blue, purplish, or black. A purulent discharge is suggestive of an infection of the external canal or the presence of a foreign body.

Inspection: Level IV

Inspection Techniques and Expected Findings	Unexpected Findings

The comprehensive exam adds an additional test for hearing related to conduction of sound. Conduction hearing tests use tuning forks (512Hz) and will help to differentiate a sensorineural (air conduction) hearing loss vs. a bone conduction hearing loss. These tests do not help to determine any frequency losses related to hearing (Yoon, 2008).

Both of these tests start with a vibrating tuning fork, which is accomplished by holding the fork by its base and striking it against a relatively hard surface. The base of the hand and the thigh are two areas that can be used for this purpose. An alternate method is to squeeze the two tines of the tuning fork and then rapidly releasing them.

PRACTICE POINT: Holding the Tuning Fork

When holding a vibrating tuning fork, always hold the fork by its base, preferable as low as possible. Any time something touches the vibrating tines of the fork, it decreases the vibrations, diminishing the sound. It may feel awkward at first to hold it this way, but with practice, it will become easier and more comfortable.

The **Weber test** is generally performed first and assesses for the lateralization of sound, or whether sound is heard louder in one ear. After the tuning fork is vibrating, place it on the midline of the patient's head (Figure 19-19). This could be on the forehead or directly on top of the head. Instruct the patient to tell you if the sound is heard equally in both ears or if sound is heard louder in one ear (lateralizes). It is expected that sound is heard equally in both ears. Equality of sound indicates that both air and bone conduction are occurring and that neither is compromised.

THINK LINK: Sound Lateralization

Sound lateralizes to the ear with a conductive hearing loss because the masking effect of air conduction has been lost. In the expected situation, sound is heard by both air conduction and bone conduction, and air conducted sound can mask the bone conducted sound. In the ear that has a bone conduction deficit, the ossicles respond to the direct stimulation of the vibrations and not to any sound that is transmitted by air conduction. Therefore, the ear with a conductive hearing loss does not receive any air conduction sound to mask or dilute bone conduction and sound is lateralized to that ear.

When sound lateralizes to one ear it could either be a conduction hearing loss in that ear or a sensorineural hearing loss in the opposite ear.

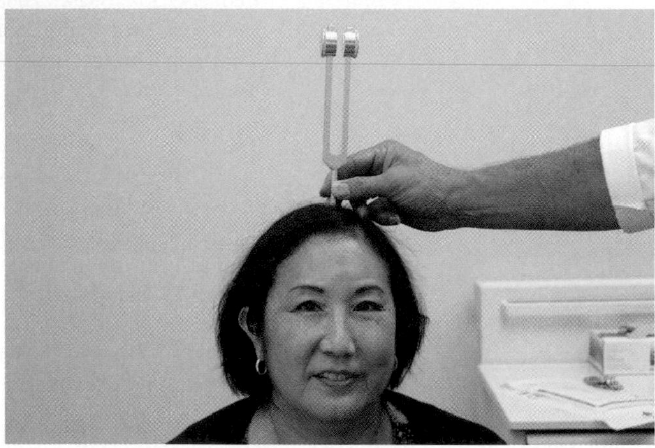

FIGURE 19-19 Weber test

If the patient hears sound equally in both ears, you generally do not need to perform additional tests. However, in the event of sound lateralization (Figure 19-20), it is helpful to perform the Rinne test, which compares air conduction to bone conduction and helps to determine in what ear there is either a deficit of air conduction or bone conduction.

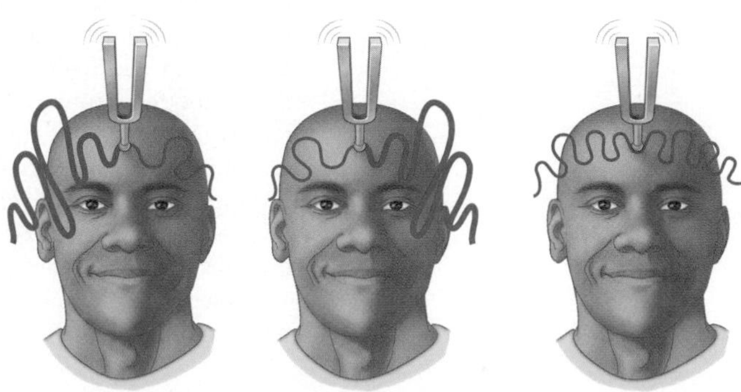

FIGURE 19-20 Lateralization of sound

Inspection Techniques and Expected Findings

Comparison of air conduction to bone conduction has to do with the loudness of sound and the length of time that sound is heard by each conduction type. Air conduction of sound is generally louder and heard twice as long as bone conduction.

Begin the **Rinne test** by vibrating a tuning fork and first placing it on the mastoid process behind the ear, and next placing it in front of the ear canal (Figure 19-21a). Ask the patient if the tone is louder when the stem of the tuning fork is held against the mastoid bone behind the ear or when the tines of the fork are generating an air conducted sound held next to the opening of the ear canal. The expected response is that hearing is heard louder when it is placed outside the ear canal versus behind the ear.

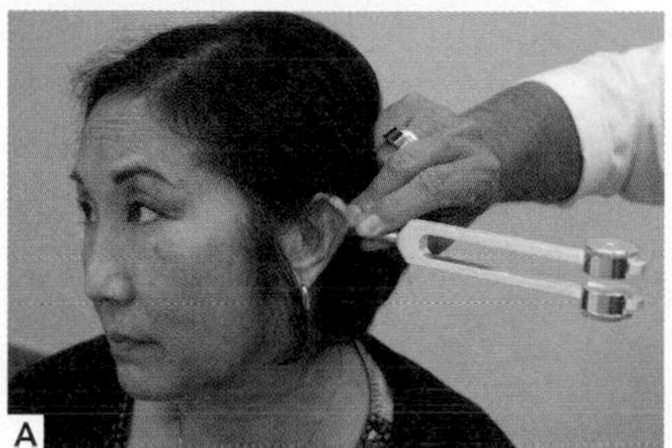

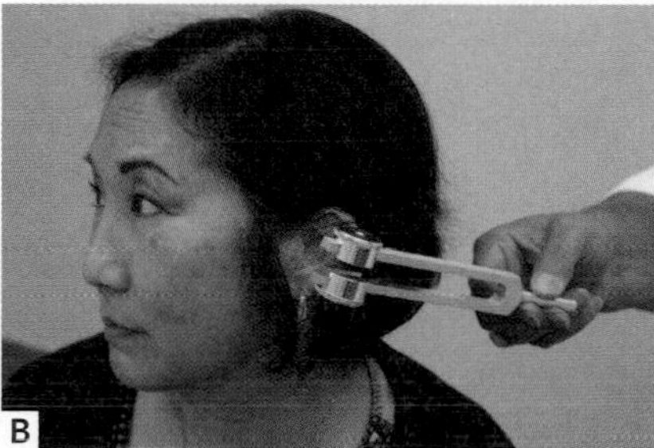

FIGURE 19-21A–B Rinne test

You may also compare the conduction pathways by timing how long the patient hears each type of conduction. Again, vibrate the tuning fork and immediately place it behind one ear on the mastoid process. Begin timing using a watch with a second hand, or begin counting. Have the patient indicate when the sound is no longer heard. Note the length of time and remove the tuning fork from the mastoid process and place it just in front of the auditory canal opening. Do not re-vibrate the tuning fork before placing it in front of the ear. The patient should hear the sound again (by air conduction). Continue timing, instructing the patient to indicate when the sound is again no longer heard. Repeat the procedure on the opposite ear and then compare the times for both ears.

Air conduction should be heard twice as long as bone conduction and can be put into ratio format (AC:BC 2:1). Thus, if the patient heard sound by bone conduction for 8 seconds, the sound should be heard by air conduction by an additional 8 seconds so that bone conduction was 8 seconds and air conduction was 16 seconds.

These hearing tests are screening tests and should not be used for any other purposes than to identify basic hearing deficits (Table 19-3). Any patient with hearing deficits should be referred for a thorough hearing exam from a hearing specialist.

Table 19-3 Interpretation of Weber/Rinne test results

	Weber without lateralization	Weber lateralizes left	Weber lateralizes right
Rinne both ears AC > BC	Expected Bilateral Sensorineural loss	Sensorineural loss in right	Sensorineural loss in left
Rinne left BC > AC		Conductive loss in left	Combined loss: conductive and sensorineural loss in left
Rinne right BC > AC		Combined loss: conductive and sensorineural loss in right	Conductive loss in right
Rinne both ears BC > AC	Conductive loss in both ears	Combined loss in right and conductive loss on left	Combined loss in left and conductive loss on right

Unexpected Findings

PRACTICE POINT: Rinne Test

Remember to explain the procedure before starting. The patient should not have to listen to instructions and at the same time listen to the tuning fork. If for some reason a part of the instructions were omitted, don't start talking to the patient. It is probably best to provide the omitted instructions and start over.

With a conductive loss, the patient will report hearing a louder tone from behind the ear.

With sensorineural hearing loss, the sound will still be heard loudest by air conduction, but is not as loud as the ear without any sensorineural deficit.

If there is a **conductive hearing loss** in one ear (the ear that heard sound louder in the Weber test), bone conduction is equal to or greater than air conduction.

If there is a **sensorineural hearing loss** in one ear, the ratio of air conduction to bone conduction will still be a ratio of 2:1, however, the total length of time that sound is heard will be less than the unaffected ear.

Inspection Techniques and Expected Findings	Unexpected Findings

Equilibrium

The **Romberg test** is used to assess the patient's balance and coordination. Instruct the patient to stand with the feet together, eyes closed, and arms at the side (Figure 19-22). The patient should be able to maintain balance in this position.

If there are alterations of the inner ear, the patient may sway and may lose balance. (Additional tests for balance and coordination are covered in Chapter 27.)

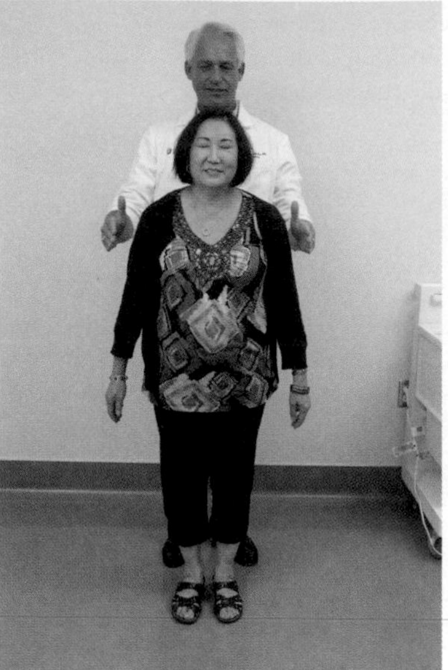

FIGURE 19-22 Romberg test

Palpation: Levels I and II

Palpation of the ear is minimal and could be done in either Level I or II, depending on the presentation and condition of the patient. Without any apparent external alterations or indications of inflammation or tenderness, it would not be necessary to palpate the external ear and surrounding areas.

Palpation Techniques and Expected Findings	Unexpected Findings

Palpate the external ear and the surrounding mastoid area for tenderness, swelling, and nodules (Figure 19-23). The auricle should feel firm and flexible without any nodules or deformities. Gently pull on the auricle, which should cause no pain. The same should be when gently pulling on the ear lobe. Palpation of the mastoid area should not cause pain or tenderness and there should not be any swelling.

Tenderness or pain upon manipulation of the auricle or lobe may be an indication of otitis externa.

If present, tenderness and swelling may indicate mastoiditis or lymphadenitis of the posterior auricular lymph nodes.

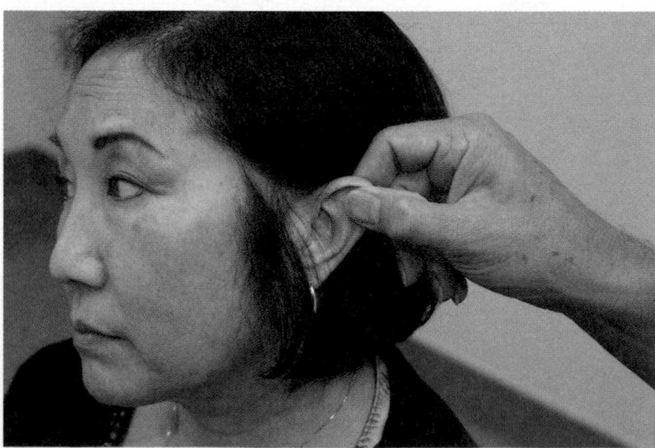

FIGURE 19-23 Palpation of auricle

Developmental Applications

Techniques and Expected Findings	Unexpected Findings

Infants and Children

Assessment of the external ear is much the same in the infant as for the adult. Shape and size should be symmetrical with proper eye-ear alignment and position.

Inspect for the presence of atresia or microtia.

A newborn's auricle is very compliant and should demonstrate instant recoil after bending or flexing of the ear. The auricle of the premature infant is overly compliant and have decreased to absent recoil, depending on the infant's prematurity (Figure 19-24).

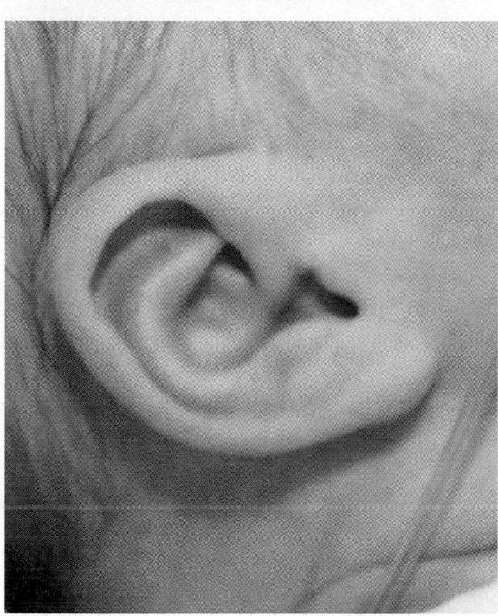

FIGURE 19-24 Infant's ear

Low set ears are associated with frequently occur with other craniofacial deformities or congenital disorders.

Frequently atresia and microtia accompany various heart deformities with a smaller percentage of infants having renal deformities. Microtia, of varying severity, may be present without atresia, but atresia always occurs with microtia. Atresia and microtia occurs in one per 5,000 to 19,000 births, with a higher incidence in Native Americans (Eskimo and Navaho), Hispanic, and Japanese populations (Kelley & Scholes, 2007). Males are also two-and-one-half more times likely to be affected than females. Microtia and atresia are typically unilateral with the right side predominately affected. The cause of microtia and atresia is not known, and it does not appear to be the result of maternal prenatal activities and behaviors or have a genetic basis (Park, 2011). Medications such as thalidomide and isotretinon have been linked to congenital malformations, which includes microtia (Bonilla, 2011).

A benign, congenital anomaly of the ears that is present in infants but does not become a problem until childhood is prominent ear, also known as "**bat ears**." Ears are described as prominent or protruding if the angle between the ear and the side of the head is more than 21–30 degrees (Lin, 2011). The ears may also seem larger, but often it is only that they appear that way. Most often, both ears are affected, but occasionally it may be only present in one. Prominent ears tend to run in families and are more common in males than females. While there is nothing aberrant in regards to the ears function, surgical correction (otoplasty) may be performed for cosmetic purposes.

Infants and children under 3 cannot provide reliable responses to direct conventional hearing assessments, so auditory integrity is assessed through indirect methods. The most basic assessment is to determine the infant's response to a loud noise, such as a hand clap, ringing bell, or loud voice. Infants less than 3 months will demonstrate the startle reflex or other movements in response to the sound. They may also begin to cry or stop breathing for a short period.

Hearing Screening

Screening can also be accomplished with the **auditory brainstem response** (ABR) test. This is not specifically a hearing test but a measurement of electrical activity along the pathway of CN VIII to the midbrain level in response to a click stimulus (Bhattacharyya, 2011). Responses are recorded as waveforms from electrodes placed on the infant's forehead and mastoid processes (Delaney & Ruth, 2011) (Figure 19-25).

Screening tests that indicate no hearing deficits does not mean that there is no further need for routine screening during childhood. Ten percent of hearing losses during childhood become evident after birth. This may be due to chronic otitis media, meningitis, or antibiotics that damage CN VIII.

Techniques and Expected Findings	Unexpected Findings

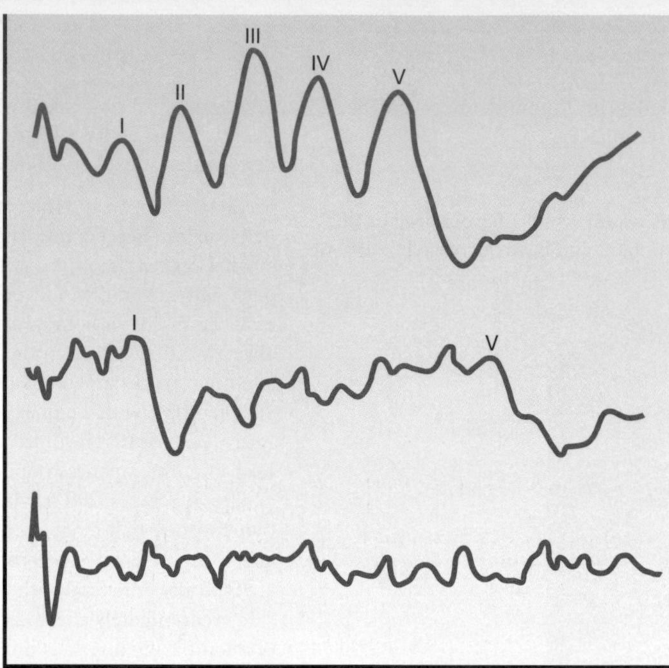

FIGURE 19-25 ABR waveforms

Behaviors observed at home or school that may indicate a hearing deficit include, but are not necessarily limited to the following:

- Inattention to environmental noise or conversations, or greater reactions to movement/facial expressions than sounds
- Puzzled/confused facial expressions
- Frequent requests to have statements/words repeated
- Sound-alike word confusion or difficulty combining words into meaningful sentences
- Development of speech problems (monotonous tone, garbled speech, mispronunciation/ omission of sounds)
- Becomes withdrawn and isolated, disengaging from friends and/or conversations
- Frequent complaints of earaches; pulling on ears and hears better in quiet environments

From 3 to 6 months, the infant's head will turn towards the sound but will not always recognize its location. The infant should start responding to the parent's voice and babbling. The infant also is attracted to and begins to play with sound-producing toys.

From 7 to 12 months the infant begins to respond to his or her name, telephone ringer, and voices of individuals. Infants now respond to softer sounds. Sound recognition and localization also develops and the infant's head will turn 45 degrees toward sounds. Babbling begins as well as the ability to imitate voice sounds. The infant also begins to imitate simple word sounds and understands "no-no" and "bye-bye" correctly as well as using "ma-ma" and "da-da."

During subsequent follow-up/well-child visits, assess hearing by noting appropriate responses to various levels of auditory stimuli. These can be either environmental sounds or verbal sounds from the provider and/or parents.

PRACTICE POINT: Hearing Concerns

It is important to question the parents if they have any concerns regarding the infant's/child's hearing or if they have noticed and behavioral changes that may indicate a hearing deficit.

Auditory processing disorder (APD) affects approximately 5% of school-age children. Children with APD do not lose their sensitivity to hearing, but have a hearing problem that affects their ability to process auditory stimuli appropriately. Essentially, the ears and brain are not coordinated so that the brain cannot recognize and interpret sounds. APD is a complex problem that is often mistaken for other disorders (e.g., AD/HD, autism, dyslexia). There is no known cause; however, head trauma, lead poisoning, and chronic ear infections have been considered as possible reasons.

Symptoms and behaviors of APD are varied with a wide range of severity, and may include the following:

- Easily distracted or bothered by loud or sudden noises
- Upset when in noisy environments
- Improved behavior and/or performance in quiet environments
- Difficulty following directions
- Reading, spelling, writing, or other speech-language difficulties
- Inability to comprehend abstract information
- Difficulty with verbal problem solving (math)
- Disorganized and forgetful
- Difficulty following conversations (Morlet, 2011)

Any of these behaviors should be of concern and are indicators for further investigation.

Techniques and Expected Findings	Unexpected Findings

Middle Ear Assessment

An examination of the TM with an otoscope is also performed on the newborn. A major problem in examining the newborn and infant is gaining their cooperation and keeping/maintaining the head in a stable position.

Depending on the age of the infant, the examination may take place on an examining table or held on the parent's lap. When using the exam table, place the infant in either a supine or prone position. For the prone position, place the infant's arms downward at the side. For the supine position, extend the arms overhead, with the parent keeping them in place.

When assessing the child, if the child is sitting on the parent's lap, have the parent hold the child firmly around the abdomen and legs, securing the head against the parent's chest with the other hand.

The otoscope exam of the infant and child is basically the same as for the adult. Hold the otoscope in such a way that allows the examining hand to rest on the child's head so that any head movement is followed by the provider's hand (Figure 19-26). When inserting the otoscope into the ear canal, it may help to pull down and out on the auricle.

Alterations in the TM membrane in children are most commonly related to frequent episodes of middle ear infections (OM), during which the tympanic membrane often appears red, thickened, or cloudy.

It may also demonstrate bulging, indicating an increased pressure in the middle ear, which may lead to a spontaneous rupture of the TM. When the TM ruptures, foul smelling pus drains from the middle ear. A ruptured TM will eventually heal by scarring. Reoccurring episodes of OM may require the insertion of tubes into the TM to remove drainage from the middle ear and prevent additional TM rupture. When present, these will be observable on the TM during the otoscope examination.

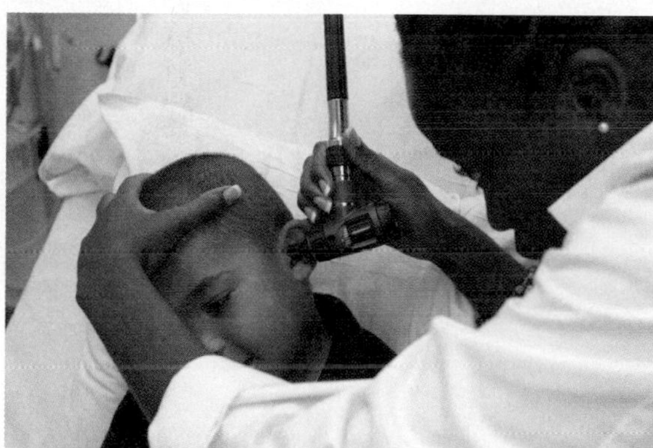

FIGURE 19-26 Otoscope exam of infant/child

The parameters that are assessed in the infant are the same as the adult. Assess the external canal for patency, color, and presence of cerumen. The newborn may still have some vernix in the canals. If present, the examination may be delayed until it is cleared from the canal. Cerumen may also be present in the ear canal. The TM is positioned more horizontally until the newborn is about 4 weeks old, which may make visualization of the TM difficult in the newborn. The TM is also flatter, making the light reflex less direct and more dispersed. The conical shape of the TM does not become apparent until the infant is several months old.

The TM may appear thicker and more opaque as well as grayer. The TM is more vascular after birth, which may give it a reddish appearance. It also may appear redder after the infant has been crying. The mobility of the TM is decreased in the newborn, negating the need for assessment of its mobility. Within the first months of life, the infant's TM matures, gradually manifesting the expected characteristics of the adult TM.

Use ear drum mobility to determine whether a TM may be red from crying or if there may be an otitis media. Assess with a pneumatic otoscope (see previous discussion). If the TM is mobile and demonstrates a flutter, an increase in middle ear pressure due to an infection or inflammation is unlikely.

Immobility and lack of flutter indicates increased pressure in the middle ear, most likely from an otitis media.

It is not uncommon to find foreign objects in the ears of toddlers and preschool children, who frequently place objects in their mouth, nose, and ears. Common objects include small stones, beans, corn, and beads.

If not removed at the time of insertion, they may get stuck and result in an infection and a temporary conductive hearing loss. Children are frequently asymptomatic, with the object only evident at the time of a routine examination.

The Pregnant Woman

No specific hearing parameters are assessed during pregnancy.

As stated previously, a sudden sensorineural hearing loss may occur during pregnancy, but this would be treated as a hearing problem, not as a unique result of pregnancy

Techniques and Expected Findings	Unexpected Findings

The Older Adult

The overall configuration and characteristics of the ear do not change significantly with aging. The ear lobes become more pendulous and wrinkled from a loss of elasticity of the pinna. The ear continues to make cartilage which may cause the pinna to appear larger and more noticeable (Figure 19-27). Coarse, bristly hair also becomes apparent at the entrance to the ear canal and on the tragus.

It is not uncommon for the elderly to develop a conductive hearing loss from impacted cerumen, which is drier due to the loss of sebaceous glands. There may also be an increased amount of keratin in the cerumen, also predisposing the elderly to impacted cerumen.

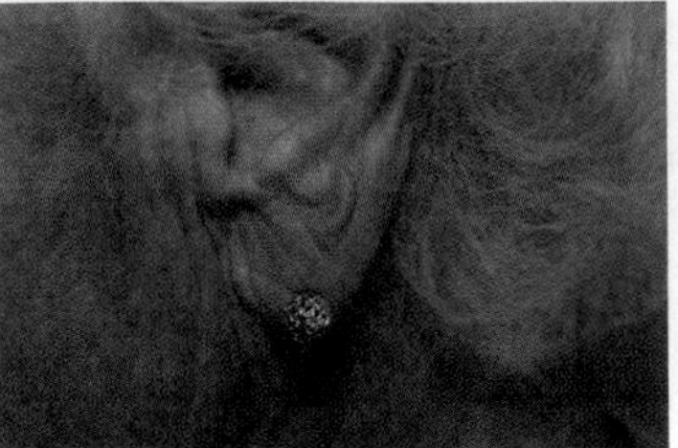

FIGURE 19-27 Elderly ear

The TM should not manifest any significant alterations. The color of the TM may be slightly whiter and more opaque; however, the landmarks should be visible. The TM may be slightly less mobile, but should not be fixed or demonstrate jerky movements.

Hearing loss due to aging is common and is either a sensorineural nearing loss (presbycusis) or a conductive loss caused by otosclerosis.

A loss of high frequency tones is a major manifestation associated with presbycusis. This should become evident with the whispered voice test.

DOCUMENTATION

No reported problems with ear pain or hearing difficulties. Responds to examiner's questions appropriately, without need to have questions repeated. Denies use of hearing devices. States had multiple ear infections as a child with tubes placed in ear drums but has not had any problems as an adult. Did have an ear infection last summer after spending a lot of time in ocean on vacation. Antibiotics cleared up infection without any lasting effects. Does report frequent buildup of wax in R ear that requires irrigation to remove it. Denies any problems with vertigo, dizziness, or tinnitus.

Denies any trauma of injuries to ears. Takes occasional aspirin (2 tablets) or Advil (2 tablets) for occasional headaches. Not more than 3 times per month. No family history of significant hearing loss. Elderly parents gradually became hard of hearing, but seemed to respond to hearing aids. Denies exposure to significant environmental noise. Sometimes teenagers have volume of stereo and TV turned up, but not for extended periods of time. Denies putting anything in ears.

Ears positioned on side of head in correct alignment with palpebral fissures. Pinna is freely moveable and without palpable or visible lesions or masses. No pain upon palpation. Ear canal clean without evidence of redness of drainage. TM clearly visible, pearly gray with umbo and cone of light easily visualized. Cone of light at 5:00 R ear, 7:00 L ear. Some cerumen present in inner ear. Able to repeat words and numbers correctly for whispered voice test. Weber test without lateralization. Rinne test–R ear AC 2X BC (16": 8"), L ear AC 2X BC (15": 7") (CN VIII).

Able to maintain balance with eyes closed and legs/feet positioned next to each other.

Electronic Charting

Expectations of Electronic Charting

The entire ear exam should be documented. Correct terminology should be available for all portions of the exam. Describing the anatomic structures and characteristics and the position and placement of the ears may be best accommodated by a graphical presentation, so drawing capability should be available. Hearing is an important component of the ear exam. You should be able to document a variety of age-appropriate hearing evaluations, from neonatal hearing screenings through the range of informal and formal adult hearing evaluations. You should be able to document occupational (and recreational) noise exposure as part of the hearing screening. There is a strong relationship between hearing impairment and linguistic communication, mood, and social interaction, and you should be able to navigate smoothly between these assessments. Similarly, because of the link between the inner ear and equilibrium, you should be able to smoothly navigate to neurological exams such as assessment of vertigo. In addition to documenting the ear exam, an electronic charting system should ideally contain decision support capabilities. For example, the system should provide an alert warning about drugs that are potentially ototoxic.

Limitations of Electronic Charting

Like the eye exam, a limitation is that some electronic charting systems may not accommodate sufficient graphical capability to create detailed diagrams. In addition, some systems do not accommodate a full range of hearing examination methods.

Summary

- The ears are a paired sensory organ for hearing that are positioned on the lateral sides of the head in alignment with the lateral canthus of the eye.
- The ear consists of an external structure (auricle) and internal structures that facilitate hearing and maintain balance and coordination; the internal structures are the middle ear (ear canal and tympanic membrane) and the inner ear, which contains the three ossicles, organ of Corti, and semi-circular canals.
- Alterations in the ear are often associated with other cranio-facial alterations or are manifestations of other conditions. Absence of an external ear frequently indicates an absence of internal ear structures, resulting in absence of hearing on the affected side. Low-set ears are an alteration that is not always associated with a pathologic or serious condition or disorder.
- Infants are born with their hearing fully developed. Frequent bouts of otitis media can damage the middle ear and result in loss of hearing. As an individual ages, the bones of the middle ear may become less sensitive to sound wave vibrations and cause some level of hearing loss.
- The external ear is inspected for placement, position, and symmetry. The tympanic membrane of the middle ear is inspected with an otoscope. Hearing is tested with a tuning fork to compare bone conduction with air conduction.

Review Questions

1. When examining the ear of a patient the provider is aware that the function of the auricle in hearing is to do which of the following?
   1. Accelerate slow sound waves
   2. Intensify the pitch of the sound
   3. Focus the sound waves
   4. Disperse sound waves
2. The provider is assessing a patient with a probable middle ear infection. An important aspect of the assessment is to visualize the structure that separates the outer from the middle ear. This structure is which of the following?
   1. tragus
   2. tympanic membrane
   3. basilar membrane
   4. oval window
3. A patient is being evaluated for hearing loss and the provider is reviewing the process of sound transmission with the patient. The provider would include that one element of the process is that hair cells have the primary function to do which of the following?
   1. Transmit electrical impulses to CN VIII
   2. Determine the frequency of sound waves
   3. Augment sound
   4. Differentiate air conduction from bone conduction
4. The provider is responsible for teaching the process of hearing to a group of students. The provider should include the pathway for air conduction which is best described by which of the following?
   1. external ear canal, tympanic membrane, ossicles, cochlea
   2. malleus, incus, stapes, utricle, saccule, cochlea
   3. external ear, basilar membrane, ossicles, tympanic membrane, organ of Corti
   4. tympanic membrane, ossicles, semi-circular canals, organ of Corti
5. A patient mentions the complaint that her ears are constantly popping when she travels by airplane. The provider should explain that this is a result of attempts to maintain equilibrium between environmental air and the middle ear by which of the following?
   1. oval window
   2. eustachian tube
   3. vestibular tube
   4. annulus
6. A patient has been told that he has otosclerosis. The provider explains that this diagnosis is associated with which of the following?
   1. conductive hearing loss
   2. tinnitus
   3. vertigo
   4. sensorineural hearing loss
7. The provider is assessing a 2-year-old child for delayed speech development. The parent is concerned that the child may not be hearing commands. When interviewing the parent the provider should focus the assessment on the fact that hearing deficiencies in childhood are most commonly associated with which of the following?
   1. vertigo
   2. presbycusis
   3. microtia
   4. otitis media
8. When inspecting the ears of a patient, the provider should anticipate that the tympanic membrane has the characteristic of which of the following?
   1. immobility
   2. a concave shape
   3. a halo of light
   4. pinkish-red in color
9. The school provider is concerned that a child may have a hearing deficit. To assist in assessing the child's hearing the provider should do which of the following?
   1. Perform a Rhomberg test.
   2. Perform a whispered voice test.
   3. Assess the child's speech.
   4. Observe the child's social behaviors.
   5. Note the frequency of ear infections.
10. The provider is reviewing the bones of transmission of sound through the middle ear with group of students in the audiometry clinic. The provider would include the following when discussing this content?
    1. cochlea
    2. malleus
    3. incus
    4. stapes
    5. pinna

Conditions and Disorders

Otitis Media (OM)

OM is characterized by inflammation and infection of the middle ear, more commonly affecting children than adults. Incidence of OM in children is 50%–65% of those less than 1 year old, and 80%–90% of children less than 3 years old, with a peak incidence in children, 3–18 months old (Donaldson, 2011). OM may manifest as acute (AOM), OM with effusion (OME), and chronic OM with effusion (COME); it is important to differentiate the three conditions. OM is a cause of decreased hearing in children and one of the most frequently cited reasons for seeking care (Perlstein, 2011). It occurs more frequently in children due to their Eustachian tubes being narrower and more horizontal (Waseem & Aslam, 2011).

Pathophysiology

- Acute OM (AOM): characterized by acute onset frequently following an upper respiratory infection (viral or bacterial) that ascends to the middle ear, causing the inflammation and infection. Fluid builds up in the middle ear and becomes trapped behind the eardrum, increasing pressure.
- Otitis media with effusion (OME): characterized by secretion of a thick, sticky noninfectious fluid resembling liquid wax in the middle ear, also referred to as glue, so OME is also known as "**glue ear**."
- Unlike AOM, it is an inflammation of the middle ear without infection.
- Chronic otitis media with effusion (COME) happens when fluid remains in the middle ear for a long time or returns over and over again, even though there is no infection.
- COME makes it harder for children to fight new infections and also can affect their hearing.

Subjective Data

Findings for AOM, OME, and COME all include:

- Pressure causes pain in the ear—commonly called an earache.
- The child may experience a temporary decrease in hearing, but hearing returns after treatment.
- A child with OME may have no symptoms.
- History of repeated incidence of OM

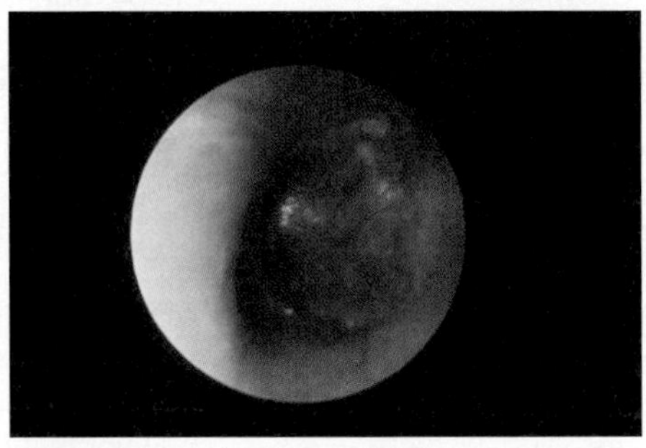

FIGURE 19-28 Otitis media (OM)
Source: SIU Biomed Comm/Custom Medical Stock Photo

Objective Data

- Tugging or pulling at the ear(s)
- Fussiness and crying
- Trouble sleeping
- Fever (especially in infants and younger children)
- Fluid draining from the ear
- Clumsiness or problems with balance
- Trouble hearing or responding to quiet sounds
- The increased pressure can be observed by the bulging of the TM, placing it at risk for spontaneous rupture. When this occurs, there is drainage of a foul-smelling fluid from the middle ear.
- OME will also have visible fluid behind eardrum

Otitis Externa (Swimmer's Ear)

This is an inflammation of the outer ear and ear canal. The thin, immovable skin of the bony ear canal is easily abraded or torn by even minimal physical force.

Pathophysiology

- Acute **otitis externa** is predominantly a microbial or fungal infection with rapid onset that quickly worsens, and becomes very painful and alarming.
- Due to an abundant nerve supply to the ear canal, the pain is often severe enough to interfere with sleep.
- Inflammation of the skin of the ear canal can be secondary to dermatitis (eczema) or with no infection.

Subjective Data

- Pain is the predominant complaint and the only symptom directly related to the severity of acute external otitis.
- Possible ear discharge (otorrhea) and itchiness
- Sufficient swelling and discharge in ear canal may block its opening and cause temporary conductive hearing loss.

Objective Data

- Unlike other ear infections, the pain increases when the outer ear is touched or pulled gently.
- Pushing the tragus typically causes pain in this condition, as to be diagnostic of external otitis on physical examination.
- Inspection reveals a red and swollen canal in well-developed cases.

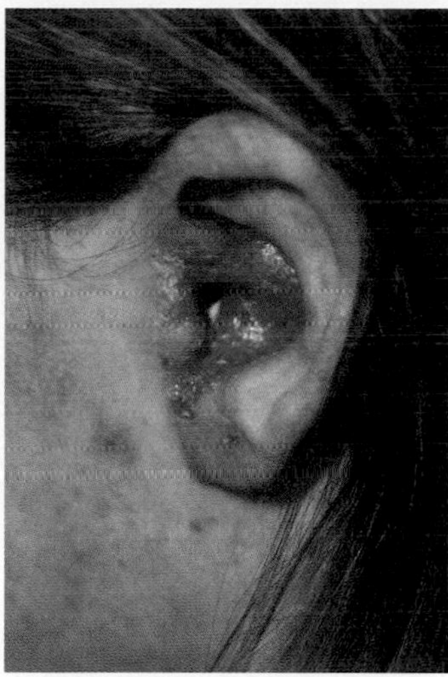

FIGURE 19-29 Otitis externa
Source: Biophoto Associates/Science Source Images

- Pruritus precedes pain in acute inflammation, and is the predominant symptom in chronic disease
- Physical insult to ear canal caused by attempts at self-cleaning, scratching, insertion of small implements in ear (pen caps, hair pins, keys, etc.)
- Prolonged water exposure from swimming or exposure to extreme humidity, which can compromise the protective barrier function of the canal skin

- Ear canal may also appear eczema-like, with scaly shedding of skin.
- It may be difficult to visualize the eardrum with otoscope due to narrowing of ear canal from inflammation and the presence of drainage and debris.

Ménière's Disease

Ménière's Disease is a disorder of the inner ear affecting hearing and balance to various intensities. It is characterized by episodes of vertigo, low-pitched tinnitus, and hearing loss. It usually starts in one ear, but over time it often progresses to involve both ears. A majority (60%–80%) of sufferers recover with or without medical help. Hearing loss usually fluctuates in early stages, becoming more permanent in later stages. Hearing aids and cochlear implants can help remedy damage. Tinnitus can be unpredictable, but patients often adapt to it over time.

Pathophysiology

- While idiopathic, it is thought to be linked to an excess of endolymphatic fluid in the inner ear (*endolymphatic hydrops*), which escapes from the membranous labyrinth and flows into other areas, causing damage. The membranes can become dilated like a balloon when pressure increases and drainage is blocked.
- In some cases, the endolymphatic duct may be obstructed by scar tissue, or narrow from birth; there may be too much fluid secreted by the stria vascularis. Symptoms may appear during a middle ear infection, head trauma, or an upper respiratory tract infection; or as a result of using aspirin, smoking cigarettes, or drinking alcohol.

Subjective Data

Number and intensity of symptoms variable among individuals affected; "classic Ménière's" considered to demonstrate the following four symptoms:

- Rotational vertigo that can be severe, incapacitating, unpredictable, and persist minutes to hours, generally no longer than 24 hours. Prolonged attacks for several days to weeks can severely incapacitate individual, often with increase in volume of tinnitus and temporary, hearing loss. Hearing may improve after attack, but often progressively worsens.
- Unilateral or bilateral hearing loss that is varying and progressive mostly in lower frequencies; sounds can appear tinny or distorted; unusual sensitivity to noise.
- Unilateral or bilateral tinnitus
- A sensation of fullness or pressure in one or both ears

Objective Data

- Vertigo may induce nystagmus, usually in the horizontal plane.
- Sudden, severe attacks of dizziness or vertigo ("drop attacks") can cause person to fall. They are more common later in the disease, but can occur at any time and may be associated with chest pain.
- Headache that is unusual or severe
- Double vision or loss of vision
- Speech impairment
- Leg or arm weakness
- Loss of consciousness
- Falling or difficulty walking
- Numbness or tingling
- Chest pain

Otalgia (Earache)

Primary otalgia is ear pain that originates inside the ear (OE, OM). **Referred otalgia** is ear pain that originates from outside the ear. Otalgia is not always associated with ear disease; it may be caused by other conditions, such as impacted teeth, sinus disease, inflamed tonsils, infections in the nose and pharynx, throat cancer, and occasionally as a sensory aura that precedes a migraine.

Pathophysiology

- The neuroanatomic cause of referred otalgia may come from one of five neural pathways. The general ear region has sensory innervation from four cranial nerves and two spinal segments. Hence, pathology in "non-ear" location innervated by these neural pathways may refer pain to ear via the following:
  - Trigeminal nerve (CN V). Trigeminal neuralgia can cause otalgia (rare). Oral cavity carcinoma can cause referred ear pain via this pathway.
  - Facial nerve (CN VII) coming from teeth, temporomandibular joint (due to its close relation to the ear canal), or the parotid gland.
  - Glossopharyngeal nerve (CN IX), coming from the oropharynx, may be due to pharyngitis, pharyngeal ulceration, tonsillitis, to carcinoma of the oropharynx (base of tongue, soft palate, pharyngeal wall, tonsils).
  - Vagus nerve (CN X), arising from the laryngopharynx (carcinoma of area), or from the esophagus (GERD).
  - Second and third spinal segments, C2 and C3 (Quail, 2005).

Subjective Data

- An earache from a cold can be a sharp, dull, or burning pain ranging from mild to very painful. Even if trapped fluid not infected, still puts pressure on TM, causing it to bulge/throb.

Objective Data

Depending of specific cause, findings from exam may be the following:

- Tender TMJ
- Crepitus/clicking on movement of mandible
- Restricted jaw movement
- Dental caries/abscess
- Gingivitis
- Facial swelling
- Teeth tender on percussion
- Pharyngeal/tonsilar edema
- Exudate
- Decreased neck range of motion
- Tender spinous processes/paraspinal muscles
- Sore throat

Autoimmune Inner Ear Disease (AIED)

First diagnosed in 1979 (Broughton, Meyerhoff, & Cohen, 2004), AIED is a suspected autoimmune disease characterized by rapidly progressive bilateral sensorineural hearing loss that is reversible (Gopen, Keithley, & Harris, 2006). It is a rare disease occurring in less than 1% of the 28 million Americans with a hearing loss.

Pathophysiology

- Thought to be caused by either antibodies or immune cells that cause damage to the inner ear
- There are several autoimmune disorders to which AIED is related: bystander damage, cross-reactions, genetic factors, and drug use (opiate-based painkillers like OxyContin)

Subjective Data

- Sudden hearing loss in one ear progressing rapidly to the second ear that can progress over weeks or months.
- A feeling of fullness in the ear and vertigo
- Tinnitus may also be experienced.

Objective Data

- No specific signs associated with AIED makes it difficult to diagnose; often mistaken for otitis media until hearing loss develops in second ear
- One diagnostic test that is promising is the Western blot immunoassay.

Cholesteatoma

Cholesteatoma is a destructive and expanding growth of keratinizing squamous epithelium in the middle ear and/or mastoid process. The two types are congenital and acquired (Figure 19-30). Acquired cholesteatomas, the more common, are caused by pathological alterations of the ear drum resulting in accumulation of keratin within the middle ear. Congenital abnormalities are less common and grow from birth behind the ear drum, in the form of a keratin-filled cyst.

Pathophysiology

- Keratin-filled cysts that grow medial to the tympanic membrane are due to a birth abnormality, trauma or metaplasia. The following criteria must be met to be considered congenital:

Subjective Data

- The characteristic manifestation of cholesteatoma is ear discharge (constant or intermittent).

Objective Data

- Most common sign of cholesteatoma is drainage and granulation tissue in the ear canal and middle ear.

- Mass medial to the tympanic membrane
- Normal tympanic membrane
- No previous history of ear discharge, perforation or ear surgery
- Congenital cholesteatomas are more frequently found in the anterior side of the ear drum, and a remnant of the epidermoid formation, from which congenital cholesteatoma may originate, has been located in this area.
- More commonly, keratin accumulates in pouch of tympanic membrane that extends into middle ear space.
- May also arise as a result of metaplasia of the middle ear mucosa or implantation following trauma
- The growth expands to fill middle ear space, damaging the ossicles, causing or increasing a conductive hearing loss in affected ear.
- These symptoms also present in other more common conditions (otitis externa), but cholesteatoma is more serious and should not be overlooked.
- Other less common symptoms include: pain, balance disruption, tinnitus, ear ache, headaches and bleeding from the ear, along with facial nerve weakness.
- Balance symptoms in the presence of a cholesteatoma raise the possibility that the cholesteatoma is eroding the balance organs, which form part of the inner ear.
- TM perforation is present in more than 90% of cases. In congenital cholesteatomas the drum often remains intact until middle ear is quite large.
- Frequently, only finding is canal filled with mucous and granulation tissue.
- The patient may have clinical signs of conductive hearing loss. Less frequently there may be signs of imbalance or facial weakness.

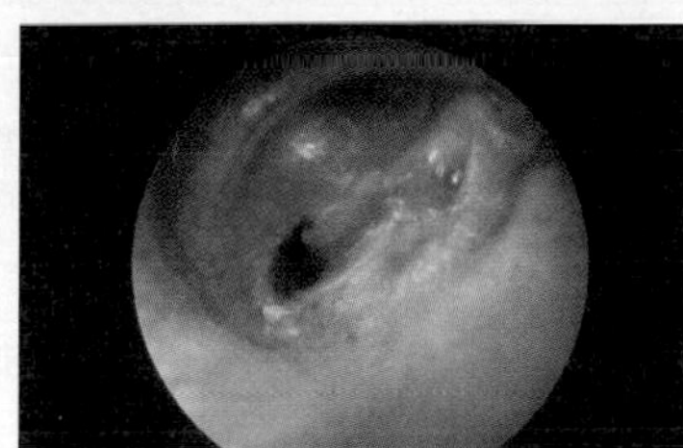

FIGURE 19-30 Cholesteatoma
Source: SIU Biomed Comm/Custom Medical Stock Photo

THINK LINK: Cholesteatoma

When cholesteatoma becomes infected, it may be extremely difficult to eradicate. Because cholesteatoma has no blood supply, systemic antibiotics cannot be delivered to its center. Topical antibiotics surround a cholesteatoma, suppress infection, and penetrate a few millimeters toward its center; however, a large, infected cholesteatoma is resistant to any antimicrobial therapy; otorrhea either persists or recurs, despite frequent and aggressive antibiotic therapy.

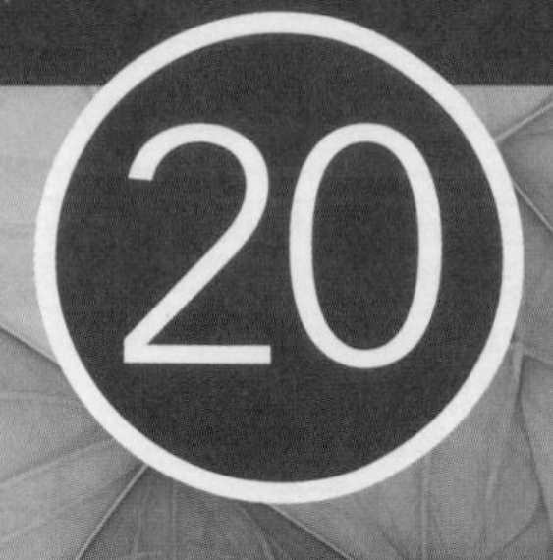

20 Nose, Mouth, Sinuses, and Throat

I review the patient's record before entering his room. Apparently 3-year-old Jack has had a 6-month history of runny nose, congestion, and fevers. A list of diagnoses swirl through my mind, and I already feel overwhelmed. Purulent discharge from the right nostril…MRI confirms acute sinusitis. The most recent note seems to be particularly useful: "Symptoms persist despite antibiotics… follow-up imaging strongly suggests chronic sinusitis." I smirk with a sudden omniscient confidence, and enter his room. Jack is occupied with the buttons on the examination chair, so I ask his foster mother for an update. She says the antibiotics still aren't working, and wants another opinion. I distract Jack with a stuffed monkey before tilting his head back and quickly slipping my otoscope into his right nostril. Just as I suspected—copious pus on an erythematous background. "It looks like it could be chronic sinusitis," I say flatly. "Let me bring in the attending physician for a quick look."

Upon seeing Jack, the first thing Dr. Cox has him do is blow his nose, hard. Greenish pus coats the tissue. "Now lean your head back for me," he says sweetly. Craning his neck just slightly, Dr. Cox eases his otoscope into Jack's nostril and does a slow visual sweep. "Take a look at this," he motions to me. Lining up my eye with his scope, I see, to my utter amazement, what looks like the ashen stub of a cigarette butt. "Do you have something up your nose?" Dr. Cox asks, peering sternly over his glasses at Jack. Jack casually explains that yes, his mother had thrown her cigarette butt away, so he decided to put it up his nose.

I am dumbfounded. None of his three previous physicians had made this diagnosis, and in the barrage of imaging and prescriptions and antibiotics, I had fallen into the same trap! Save Dr. Cox, no one had taken the time to do a thorough physical examination or ask the patient himself, little 3-year-old Jack, who knew exactly what the problem was all along.

LEARNING OUTCOMES

1. Describe the anatomical structures and functions of the nose, mouth, and throat and their correct position and placement.
2. Explain the expected characteristics of the nose, mouth, and throat and their component structures.
3. Recognize variations in appearances by inspection and their relationship to various conditions.
4. Compare and contrast lifespan and developmental changes in the nose, mouth, and throat and their significance.
5. Explain the techniques used to assess the nose, mouth, and throat by observation and palpation.
6. Summarize documentation of findings using appropriate terms when describing expected and unexpected findings.

The nose and the mouth, specifically the lips, along with the eyes, comprise the unique attributes of one's face, giving each of us a distinctive appearance unlike anyone else. As such they also function cosmetically, and significant amounts of money are spent on changing their appearance to enhance one's attractiveness. In addition to their sensory function, they are also involved in the external expression of the gamut of emotions and provide clues as to one's overall mood and affect, facilitating communication between individuals.

Structure and Function

The nose and mouth are the initial passages into the respiratory system and gastrointestinal systems. They merge at the throat, where they then become separated from each other. The mouth serves as a back-up for the nose in situations or conditions where nose breathing is difficult or impossible. The mouth and the nose are also responsible for sensory input through smell and taste. The sinuses and throat are not as involved in any of the above characteristics; however, they help maintain the overall health of the individual. The motor activities of the mouth and throat will be explored to a greater extent in Chapter 26.

Nose

The nose is the external component and first section of the respiratory system. It filters, warms, and humidifies inspired air and serves as a sensory organ for smell. The nose is positioned midline, in the center of the face on its vertical axis (see Figure 20-1). The internal support for the nose is composed of bone and cartilage. The upper one-third of the nose is bone, which is formed by the frontal and maxillary bones of the skull; the lower two-thirds is composed of cartilage and provides flexibility.

The nose is triangular is shape, with its midline extending from the bridge at its top to its lower angle, called the tip. The cartilaginous septum divides the nose in two chambers. The broad base has two oval openings, the **nares (naris)** or nostrils. The nares are separated from each other by the columella, the lower section of the septum. The **ala** is the external rounded portion of the lower nose located where the base attaches to the face.

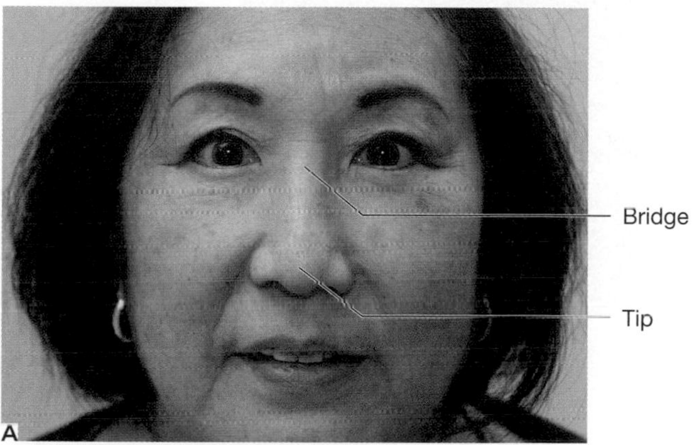

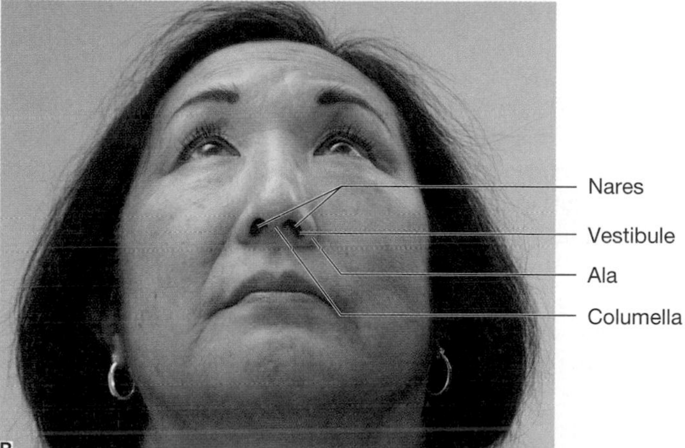

FIGURE 20-1A–B Position of nose/exterior landmarks

The internal chambers of the nose are increased in size. Each naris expands into the vestibule which then expands into each chamber (see Figure 20-2). Each chamber is bordered superiorly by the frontal and sphenoid bone and inferiorly by the hard and soft palates. Posteriorly, the chambers end at the choanae, the openings into the nasopharynx. The inferior, middle, and superior turbinates make up the lateral borders of the nose; they are parallel, bony folds that project into the nasal chambers and increase the nasal chamber's surface to make more blood vessels and mucous membrane available for warming and humidifying the air. Inferior to each turbinate is a meatus, an opening into the nasal chamber, that is identified by the turbinate above it. The meatus provide a means for drainage into the nose. The middle meatus allows drainage from the sinuses; the inferior meatus allows tears to drain from the nasolacrimal duct.

Each chamber is lined with a vascular, ciliated mucous membrane that is covered with mucous secretions. The opening of each naris is also lined with coarse hairs that filter coarse material from the air, whereas the cilia and mucus trap dust, bacteria, and other debris contained in the inspired air. The rich, vascular supply to the membrane provides for humidifying the air as well as warming it; also increasing the redness of the nasal mucosa.

The **Kiesselbach's plexus** is a concentration of small, fragile arteries and veins located at the anterior superior portion of the septum, and is frequently the location for **epistaxis** (nosebleeds). The nose's olfactory function is carried out by sensory receptors located on the cribiform plate, a section of the ethmoid bone. These olfactory receptors merge to form cranial nerve I, which transmits smell sensations to the temporal lobe of the brain for interpretation.

Sinuses

Surrounding the nasal chambers are the paranasal sinuses, four pairs of air-filled cavities located within the bones of the skull that communicate with the nasal chambers (see Figure 20-3). Called the frontal, maxillary, ethmoid, and sphenoid sinuses, each is lined with the same ciliated mucous membrane that lines the nasal cavities. They function to decrease the weight of the skull bones, resonate sound, and provide mucous that drains into the nasal chambers. The openings of the sinuses into the middle meatus are quite small and may become easily obstructed, which can result in inflammation of the sinuses (sinusitis).

Only the maxillary and frontal sinuses can be examined. The frontal sinuses are in the frontal bone, superior to the nasal chambers and medial to the orbital openings. The maxillary sinuses are in the maxillary bone, lateral to the nasal chambers. The other two pairs, the ethmoid and sphenoid sinuses, are deeper and smaller, preventing their examination. The ethmoid sinuses are located behind the frontal sinuses and between the orbits, close to the superior section of the nasal chambers. The sphenoid sinuses are positioned deep in the skull, in the sphenoid bone, which is behind the ethmoid sinuses.

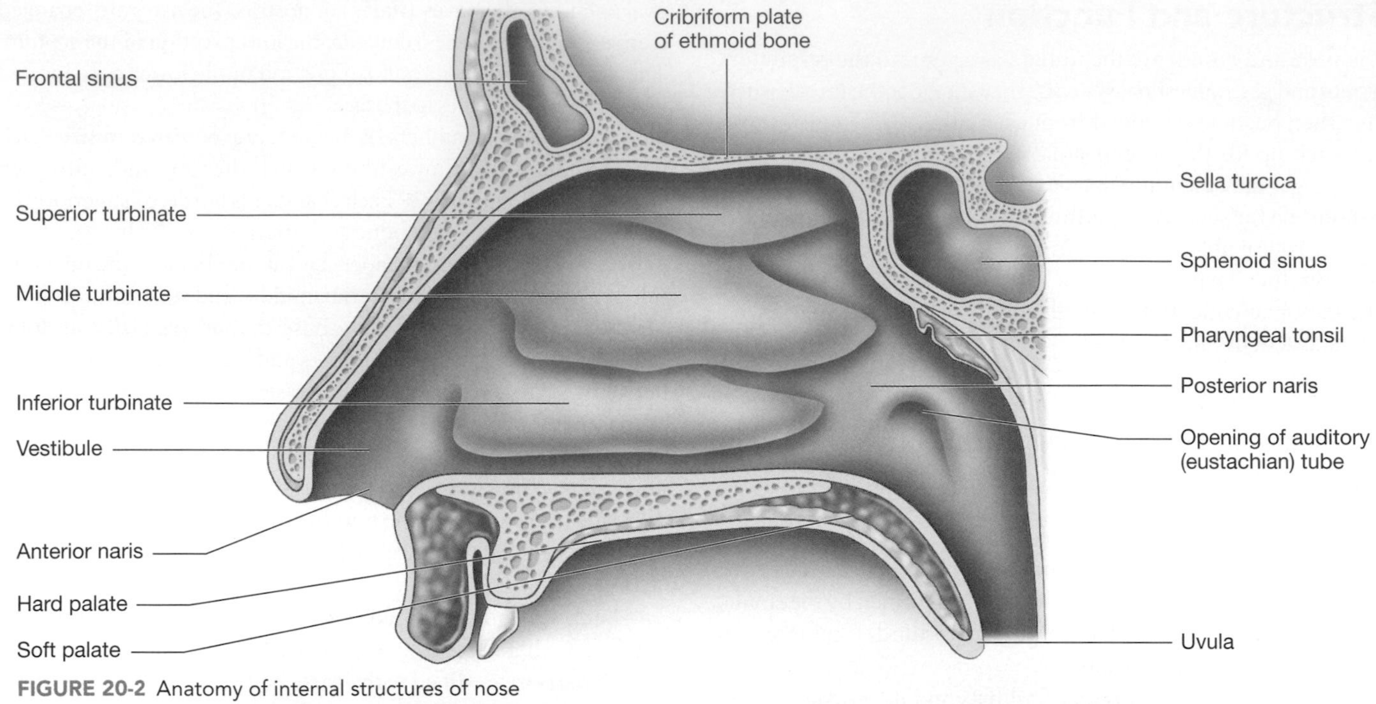

FIGURE 20-2 Anatomy of internal structures of nose

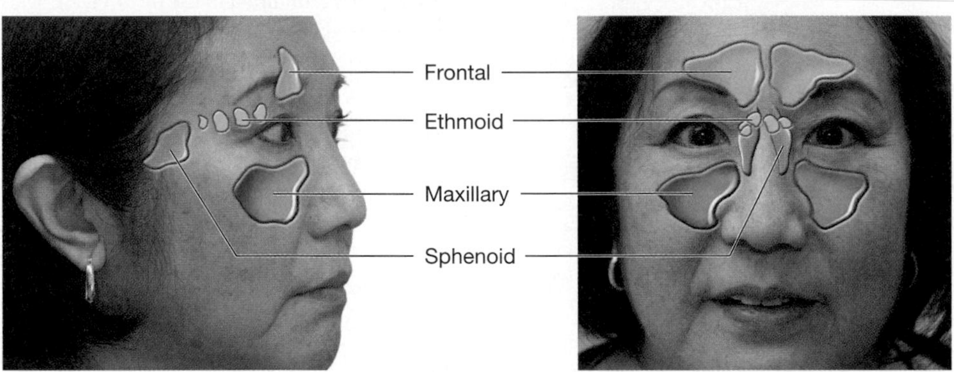

FIGURE 20-3 Anatomy of sinuses (lateral and anterior view)

Mouth and Throat

The mouth (oral cavity) and throat form the beginning segment of the gastrointestinal system; they initiate digestion and swallowing, and provide a passage for solid and liquid food. They also perform a secondary function as a conducting airway to the lungs. In contrast to conducting air, the throat and mouth facilitate expiration of air that is needed for vocal sounds (speech).

The oral cavity connects the external environment to the oropharynx, or the back of the mouth. It is bordered on four sides (see Figure 20-4). The superior (roof) and inferior (floor) borders are the upper palate and the floor of the tongue, and the lateral borders are the cheeks. The lips can be considered an anterior border; however, it is not permanent, as the lips can open and close whenever necessary.

The roof of the mouth is arched and consists of the palate, which is formed by two sections, hard and soft. The larger hard palate is whitish-pink, made of bone, and is the forward section of the palate. The soft palate is the muscular back section and darker in color than the hard palate. The **uvula** is an extension of the soft palate, which hangs down from the middle of the posterior margin of the palate, in line with the anterior pillar.

The cheeks are the sides of the mouth, and composed of skin and muscle that is lined with mucosal membrane, often called oral or buccal mucosa. The space between the buccal mucosa and the outer surface of the gums and teeth may be referred to as the oral vestibule.

The floor of the mouth is comprised of the tongue, underlying muscles, and the mandible, a horseshoe-shaped bone that is covered with soft tissue. The posterior section of the tongue is attached to the back of the oral cavity. The underside of the tongue is attached to the floor of the mouth by the frenulum, a fold of tissue. The tongue is composed of a network of striated muscle, an arrangement that allows the tongue to change its shape and position and aids in chewing, swallowing, teeth cleaning, and speech patterns.

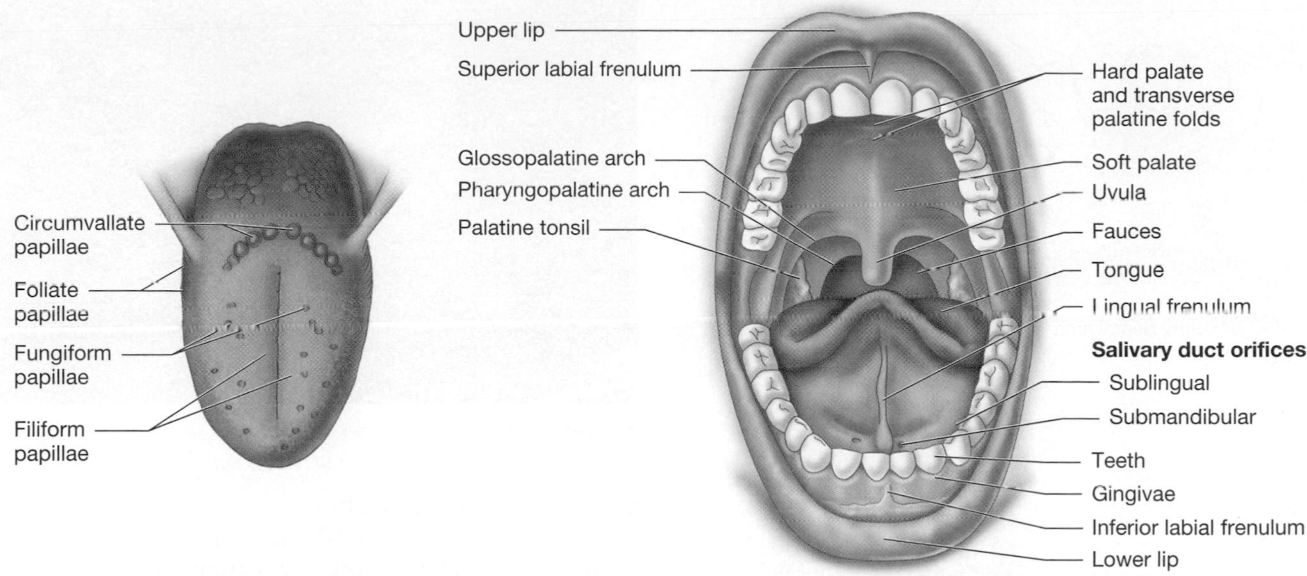

FIGURE 20-4 Anatomy of oral cavity

The tongue is covered with a thick mucous membrane that supports the filiform papillae, rough, bumpy projections on the dorsal aspect (see Figure 20-4). Vallate papillae, which are larger, are located in a "V" position toward the posterior of the tongue. Taste buds, which sense sweet, salt, sour, and bitter sensations, are within the papillae scattered over the tongue's dorsal surface. The tongue's ventral aspect is shiny, with visible blood vessels and folds of thin mucous membrane.

The mouth and throat also contain three pairs of salivary glands—parotid, submandibular, and sublingual—that secrete saliva, a thin, clear fluid that keeps the mouth moist and cleans and protects the mucosa (Figure 20-5). It also moistens food and contains enzymes that initiate the digestive process. The parotid gland is the largest and is located within the cheeks anterior to the ear and extends from the zygomatic arch to the angle of the jaw. Secreted saliva travels from the gland through Stensen's duct to where it opens in the buccal mucosa of the mouth, opposite the second molar. The submandibular gland is located beneath the mandible at the angle of the jaw. Its secreted saliva travels through Wharton's duct, which is positioned upward and forward toward the floor of the mouth. It opens in the mouth on either side of the frenulum. The sublingual gland is the smallest gland and is located in the floor of the mouth underneath the tongue. It excretes saliva through many small openings along the sublingual fold of the ventral side of the tongue.

The mouth also contains upper and lower horseshoe shaped **gingiva** (gums) that are composed of fibrous tissue covered by mucous membrane and are positioned on the floor and roof of the mouth. The gums provide a foundation and support for the teeth by encasing the neck and roots of each tooth. The adult mouth contains 32 permanent teeth; 16 upper and lower, and each consisting of a root, neck, and crown (see Figure 20-6).

The teeth are arranged and aligned to come together appropriately when the mouth is closed, with the maxillary teeth (upper) resting on the mandibular (lower) teeth. Their alignment is referred to as **occlusion** and is important to chewing and speech, as well as appearance, comfort, and health (Nield-Gehrig, 2007; Figure 20-7). **Malocclusion** occurs when there is improper alignment of the upper and lower teeth.

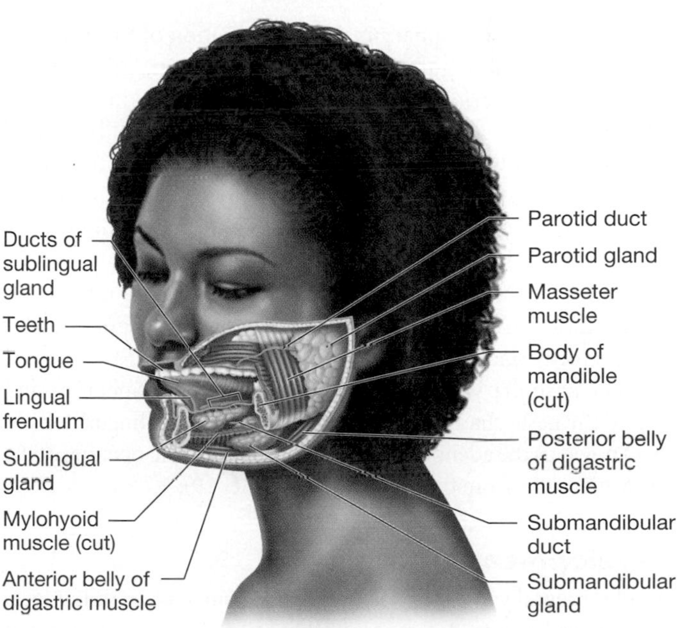

FIGURE 20-5 Anatomy/location of salivary glands

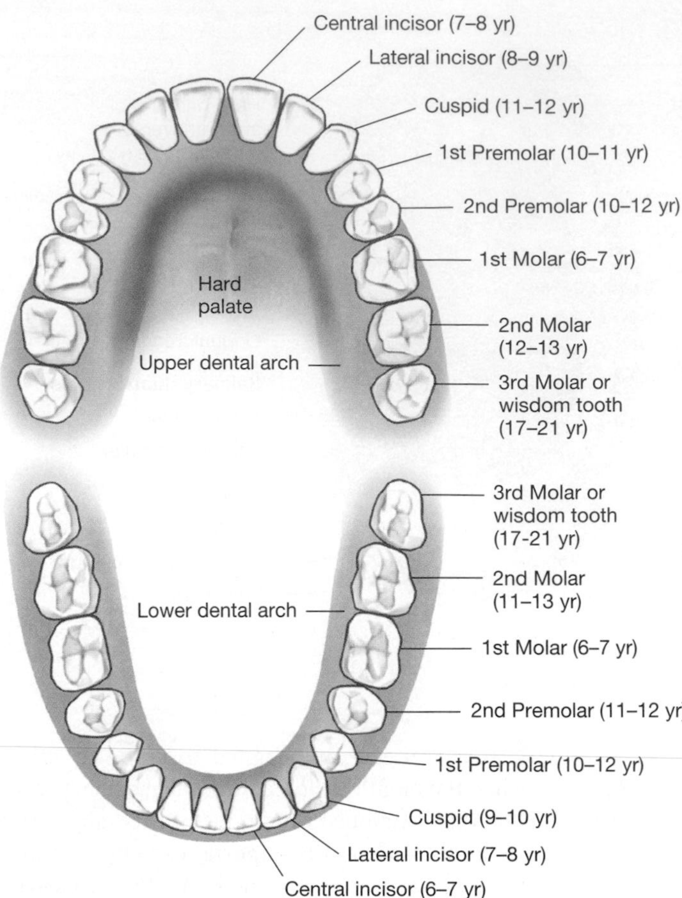

FIGURE 20-6 Permanent teeth

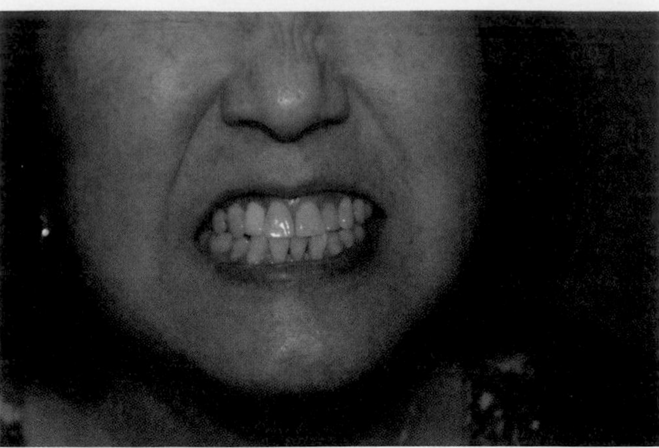

FIGURE 20-7 Occlusion

The throat, or oropharynx, is a continuation of the mouth in the posterior area (Figure 20-8). Two folds of skin, known as the anterior and posterior tonsillar pillars, separate the mouth from the oropharynx. Between the pillars is a grouping of lymphoid tissue known as the palatine tonsils. These are a part of the lymph system and provide protection from invasive microorganisms (see Chapter 21). They primarily function during childhood and may frequently become enlarged and/or inflamed if they become infected. They also contain crypts that trap cellular debris and minute food particles. After puberty, the tonsils become smaller and less functional.

The nasopharynx is the area just behind the oropharynx and behind the nasal chamber. Another set of tonsils, the lingual tonsils, also known as the adenoids, are located here, as is the opening of the Eustachian tube from the middle ear (Chapter 19).

Developmental Variations

Developmental variations occur over the course of an individual's life span and events. Awareness of these variations is important to understand and recognize common age-related alterations or modifications of the mouth, nose, and throat.

Infants and Children

The development of fetal facial structures begins during the fourth to eighth week of gestation. The salivary glands and teeth form between the sixth and eighth week. By the sixth month, the salivary glands begin to produce saliva. Calcification of the primary teeth begins in the fourth week of gestation and continues throughout the first year of life.

The development of the nose begins at the fourth week and is completed by the twelfth week. The palate is formed by fusion of the maxillary prominences during the seventh and eighth week with formation complete by the twelfth week. Incomplete fusion, or failure to fuse, results in a cleft palate.

After birth, salivation increases until the third month and often causes drooling; this continues until the infant masters swallowing. Deciduous (baby) teeth begin to erupt by 6 months; and by 2 years, all 20 teeth should be present (see Figure 20-9). Eruption of the deciduous teeth does not occur until each one is adequately calcified to tolerate chewing.

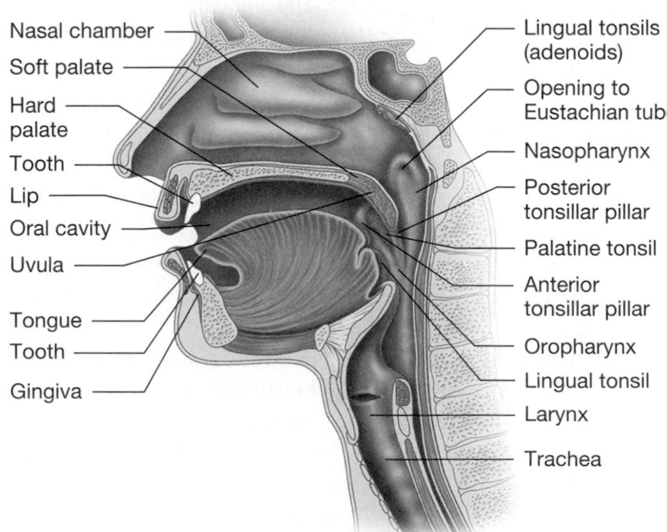

FIGURE 20-8 Anatomy and structures of throat

Deciduous teeth begin to be lost around 6 years of age and by ages 14–15 they are replaced with 32 permanent teeth (see Figure 20-9). Permanent teeth begin their formation in the jaw around 6 months of age. Eventually they exert pressure on the deciduous teeth, causing resorption of their roots. After the roots are gone, the remaining crown is shed, leaving a space for the permanent tooth to occupy. The presence of permanent teeth results in changes in the facial structure and appearance.

The maxillary and ethmoid sinuses are the only sinuses present at birth; however, they are quite small. The maxillary sinuses achieve full size after the permanent teeth are in place, but may not be fully developed until the age of 22–24. The ethmoid sinuses undergo rapid growth between the ages of 6 and 8 and again after puberty, with full development by the age of 12. The sphenoid sinuses do not start growing until after the age of 5, with complete development by the age of 12–15. The frontal sinuses are the last to begin development and start between 4 and 8 years of age. They do not achieve full development until late adolescence. Despite their small size and later development, both the frontal and sphenoid sinuses may become infected during childhood.

The palatine tonsils are generally not visible until the child is around 2 years old. After that time, they can be visualized as extending medially into the oropharynx. They reach their peak growth by 6 years and then begin to decrease in size.

The Pregnant Woman

A frequent complaint of pregnant women is related to increased stuffiness, nose bleeds, fullness in the ears and decreased hearing. These changes are the result of increased vascularity and edema of the upper respiratory tract from elevated estrogen levels. The tympanic membrane and Eustachian tube also become swollen, giving rise to the auditory complaints. The vocal cords may also be affected and cause vocal changes resulting in deepening and/or cracking of the voice. A persistent cough may also develop due to these changes.

Hormonal changes in pregnancy increase the risk of developing oral health problems like gingivitis and periodontitis. Increased levels of progesterone make it easier for certain gingivitis-causing bacteria to grow, as well as make gum tissue more sensitive to plaque, exaggerating the body's response to the toxins (poisons) that result from plaque. If the pregnant woman already has significant gum disease, pregnancy may make it worse. Over 50% of all pregnant women experience the symptoms of pregnancy gingivitis. If not treated properly, pregnancy gingivitis may progress to periodontitis, increasing the risk of premature birth and low birth weight (in addition to tooth loss and gum damage).

The first signs of the disease usually appear during the second month of pregnancy and reach a peak in the eighth month. Signs of pregnancy gingivitis range from redder-looking gums that bleed a little when brushing teeth, to severe swelling and bleeding of gum tissue. The condition normally recedes after birth, unless there are other aggravating factors beyond pregnancy.

THINK LINK:* *Gum Disease and Premature Birth

Major research studies have indicated that there is a link between gum disease and premature birth. One study published in *The Journal of the American Dental Association* found that pregnant women with chronic gum disease were at a greater significant risk to deliver prematurely (before gestational week 37) and underweight babies than were pregnant women with healthy gums. Pregnant women with the most severe periodontal disease delivered the most prematurely. Whether treating gum disease reduces the risk of preterm birth is not yet known (López, Da Silva, Ipinza, & Gutiérrez, 2005).

It has recently been identified that pregnant females with gum disease and high levels of C-reactive protein (CRP) are at a greater risk for developing preeclampsia. The presence of CRP is an indicator of inflammation in the body and when there are other sources of inflammation, the risk is increased (Douglas, 2008).

The Older Adult

The loss of subcutaneous tissue of the face as well as continued cartilage formation makes the nose appear more prominent in some individuals. Nasal hair also becomes more visible as well as coarser and stiffer so that air filtration may not be as effective. There may also be a reduction in the sense of smell caused by the reduction in the number of olfactory nerve fibers. A diminished sense of smell may start around the age of 60 and gradually deteriorate with aging.

Accompanying the loss of smell is the loss of taste due to a loss of papillae on the dorsum of the tongue. The loss of taste begins around the age of 50 and gradually diminishes. There is also a reduction in the production of saliva that also contributes to the loss of taste. There is a wide variation in the degree of sensation loss among individuals as well as the rate of loss.

Other oral cavity changes include changes in the gums, tongue, and soft tissues. Atrophy and thinning of the soft tissue and epithelium lead to an increase in the granular lining on the lips and cheeks. Tongue atrophy causes the loss of the papilliae, and the tongue also becomes more fissured. The gingival tissue loses

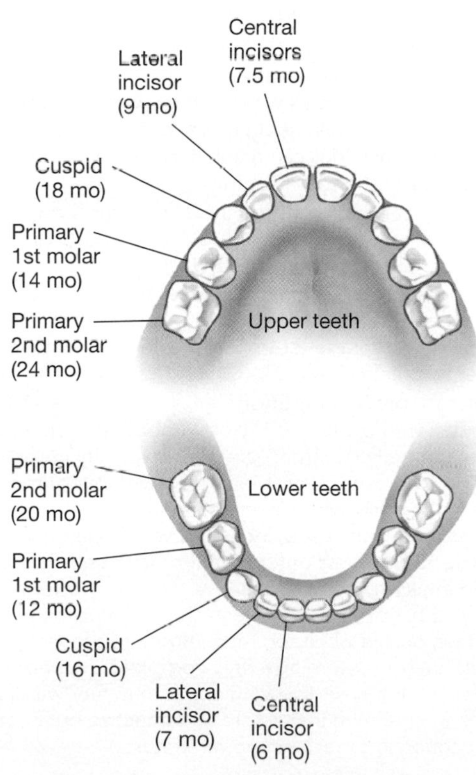

FIGURE 20-9 Eruption pattern of deciduous teeth

elasticity, making it more vulnerable to trauma and causes receding along the margin of the teeth, which may lead to erosion of the teeth.

Other teeth changes may also be present. If the individual has not received appropriate dental care, there may be an increased loss of teeth. There may be some gradual loss of teeth, which can be exacerbated by osteoporosis, but an overall loss is not an expected alteration.

If teeth are lost and the space is not refilled, other teeth may drift, causing a malocclusion, or misalignment of the upper and lower teeth. Malocclusion has been found to affect the chewing efficiency as well as the choice of foods. This has the potential to result in malnutrition as well as gastric alterations (English, Buschang, & Throckmorton, 2002). The adequacy of chewing efficiency is related to the number of teeth missing, which affects the number of tooth surfaces available for mastication. Muscle imbalance also results from malocclusion and may cause muscle spasms, headaches, as well as temporomandibular joint pain and dysfunction.

A major concern for the elderly is the potential for periodontal disease. There is an increased susceptibility to infections in the elderly which leads to a possibility of oral infections that may initiate periodontal problems.

Health Promotion

Oral health is a fundamental and a significant factor of overall health throughout one's lifespan. Oral and craniofacial diseases and conditions cause major hardships and negatively impact the overall quality of health and life for individuals with these conditions. Goals of *Healthy People 2020* related to the topic of Oral Health include the following:

- OH—7, 8, 14: Increase the proportion of low-income children and adolescents, and adults who used the oral health care system, and/or any preventative dental service, in the past 12 months.
- OH—9: Increase the proportion of school-based health centers with an oral health component.
- OH—10: Increase the proportion of local health departments and Federally Qualified Health Centers (FHQCs) that have an oral health component.

Major conditions of concern are **dental caries**, **periodontitis**, **cleft lip**, and **cleft palate**. These conditions are associated with significant physical and psychological distress, which include pain and emotional distress, loss of self-esteem, and difficulty with speaking, chewing, and swallowing.

In addition, there are monetary costs related to increased health care costs and lost productivity due to work and school absences must be taken into account. In extreme cases, they may also be the cause of death. Further contributing to oral health issues are oral and **pharyngeal cancers**. These cancers are most common in older adults, having a significant impact on health care costs and facial alterations related to treatment. They also cause over 8,000 deaths annually.

Dental Caries

- OH—1, 2, 3: Reduce the proportion of children and adolescents who have dental caries in their primary or permanent teeth; reduce the proportion of children, adolescents, and adults with untreated dental decay.
- OH—4: Reduce the proportion of adults who have ever had a permanent tooth extracted because of dental caries or periodontal disease.
- OH—13: Increase the proportion of the U.S. population served by community water systems with optimally fluoridated water.

Dental caries (cavities) are the most common chronic infectious disease/condition, second only to the common cold (Peng, Kazzi, Peng, & Cheng, 2007). Approximately 90% of adults are affected, and in children, it is the most common chronic condition, with an incidence five times that of asthma, which is the second-most chronic condition of childhood (Centers for Disease Control and Prevention, 2005). Despite a noticeable reduction in their overall incidence, it is estimated that by the time children enter the second grade, half of them will have experienced dental caries and 80% will have them by the time they finish high school. Early intervention is important to reverse or prevent the progression of caries.

The major concern with childhood caries is its affect on primary teeth. Factors that appear to influence the development of dental caries are large families, maternal and infant nutrition, and transferring of infectious organisms between caregiver and infant. Poverty is also a significant factor, with fewer than 20% of children on Medicaid receiving at least one annual preventive check-up (Centers for Disease Control and Prevention, 2005). Recent evidence also suggests that a relationship exists between second-hand smoke and the incidence of dental caries (Aligne, Moss, Auinger, & Weitzman, 2003; Slayton, 2012; Hanoika, 2011). The use of inhalers by individuals with asthma as a cause for dental cavities has been determined to not be the case. It appears to be multifactorial and not a cause-and-effect relationship (Maupoime, Shulman, Medina-Solis, & Ladeinde, 2010).

Inappropriate infant feeding practices, such as putting an infant to bed with formula or other sweetened beverages, or pacifiers sweetened with juice, are also considered a significant cause of early childhood caries (London, Laedwig, Ball, & Bindler, 2007). Early childhood caries (ECC), also known as baby bottle caries, baby bottle tooth decay, and bottle rot, is a common bacterial infection characterized by severe decay in the teeth of infants or young children. Its prevalence is epidemic in the U.S.; its rate is highest in minority and rural populations, at times infecting over 70% of the children.

Adults are also subject to caries formation, with an estimated 30% of adults having untreated dental caries. Racial and ethnic minority individuals as well as those with less than a high school education are most likely to have untreated dental caries. Untreated dental caries can result in pain, abscess formation, and eventual loss of the tooth/teeth.

Prevention can be accomplished through individual and community interventions. Individual actions are directed at reducing the amount of bacteria and plaque in the mouth by twice daily brushing and flossing, twice annual dental exams, and teeth cleaning. Brushing with fluoride toothpaste helps strengthen and protect the teeth. Reduction of the intake of sugars and sweets will also help.

Community prevention efforts are primarily carried out by water fluoridation; however, it is not without some controversy. Fluoride is a naturally occurring element, typically in too small a concentration to present a problem; however, over time it does accumulate in the body, which is one of the reasons it works so well to prevent cavities. Conversely, ingesting very large quantities can be quite toxic. Opponents of fluoridation have associated excessive fluoride intake to bone brittleness, cancer, and reproductive problems, and historically, manifestations of fluorosis (staining and brittleness) occurs when too much fluoride is ingested during tooth development (before age 8) is complete. Fluoridation has made it possible for everyone within a community/water district to receive an intervention that is safe and effective but not dependent upon economic or socioeconomic status.

Health Promotion *continued*

Periodontitis

- OH—5: Reduce the proportion of adults aged 45–74 years with moderate or severe periodontitis.

Periodontitis commonly starts out as a **gingivitis**, an inflammation of the gums. Untreated gingivitis ultimately progresses to periodontitis, an infection of the gums, periodontal ligament, or alveolar bone which eventually destroys the tissue that surrounds and supports the teeth. (Grayson, 2005). Ultimately, the erosion of the support for the teeth results in the loss of teeth.

Gingivitis can be reversed if identified early and appropriate oral hygiene (brushing and flossing) is practiced. The presence of gingivitis is generally an indicator of inadequate oral hygiene practices.

Risk factors for the development of periodontal disease include poor dental hygiene, smoking, medications, infections (viral or fungal), poor nutrition, and chronic medical conditions, such as diabetes mellitus. (Carstensen & Fraser, 2006; Torpy, 2006).

Oropharyngeal Cancer

- OH—6: Increase the proportion of oral and pharyngeal cancers detected at the earlier stage.
- C—6: Reduce the oropharyngeal cancer death rate.

The annual incidence of oral cancer pharyngeal cancers (head and neck cancers) is estimated at 35,000 with the majority of cases affecting males (25,000). The annual death rate is estimated to be 7,500 individuals. Oral and pharyngeal cancers encompass cancers of the tongue and floor of the mouth, which are the most common sites for cancer to develop. Less common sites include the lips, salivary glands, gums, and tonsils. The average age of most individuals diagnosed with oral cancers is 62; however, they can be found in individuals less than 55, who up about one-third of the number of cases. At the time of diagnosis, approximately 15% of those diagnosed will already have cancer that has infiltrated adjacent areas. The most common sites are the larynx, esophagus, and lungs.

As with most cancers, effective treatment and long-term survival is dependent on early detection. Detecting oral cancers in stages 0, I, or II is the optimum time as the cancer is less invasive at the site and there is a low risk for metastasis (American Cancer Society, 2007). Previous statistics indicate that only approximately 35% of oral cancers have been detected in Stage I. Risks include tobacco use (in any form), tobacco used in conjunction with alcohol, alcohol use, sun (ultraviolet light) exposure, history of head and neck cancer, human papillomavirus (HPV), and male gender.

Actions to reduce the risk of lip cancer include use of lip balm with sunscreen, wearing a hat with a brim, and not smoking. Early detection for oral and pharyngeal cancers is maximized by awareness of its signs and symptoms. These early symptoms are primarily related to a dysfunction of physiological processes or anatomical alterations. Signs and symptoms of oral cancers are as follows:

- Patches on the inside of the mouth or on the lips. These can be white, red, (or both), are indurated, (firm), and are difficult to remove. Removal of these lesions causes bleeding from the site.
  - White patches (**leukoplakia**) are the most common and may become cancerous
  - Red/white patches (**erythroleukoplakia**)—more likely than white to become cancerous
  - Red patches (**erythroplakia**)—smooth, bright red areas that frequently become cancerous (National Cancer Institute, 2004)
- A sore on the lip that does not heal
- Bleeding in the mouth
- Loose teeth
- Difficulty/pain with swallowing (dysphagia)
- Poor fitting dentures
- A lump in the neck
- An earache (Mayo Clinic Staff, 2006)

These signs and symptoms are not exclusively indicators of oral cancers and may be related to and caused by other conditions. If any of these manifestations are present, they should be investigated as soon as possible.

The primary means for detection of oral and pharyngeal cancers is regular extra oral examination of the head and neck, and intra oral examination of the mouth. Regular, semi-annual dental examinations provide the best opportunity for early cancer detection.

Cleft Palate

- OH—15, 16: Increase the number of states and the District of Columbia that have a system for recording and referring infants and children with cleft lips and cleft palates to craniofacial anomaly rehabilitative teams and craniofacial health surveillance system.

Cleft lip and cleft palate are among the most common congenital birth anomalies, occurring approximately one per 600–700 births (Mayo Clinic Staff, 2008). Because successful treatment for the child with cleft lip or palate requires an interdisciplinary approach, it is essential that proper identification be made early to facilitate appropriate referrals to the interdisciplinary team. This team will work with the parents prior to discharge and supervise the care to prevent complications from occurring (Biavati & Rocha-Worley, 2006). To maintain continuity of care, a comprehensive system to track these infants needs to be in place. Not all states have such a system in place; thus the goal for *Healthy People 2020* is to increase the number of states that have such a system.

PRACTICE POINT: Oropharyngeal Cancer and Human Papillomavirus (HPV)

HPV has been found to be associated with several types of cancer: cervical, vulvar, vaginal, penile, anal, and oropharyngeal (back of the throat, including the base of the tongue and tonsils). The rates for oropharyngeal cancer have been increasing dramatically since 1984, and HPV-related tumors account for the increasing numbers of annual cases, with a significant rise in younger males. Each year, more than 21,000 HPV-associated cancers occur in women; cervical cancer is the most common. More than 12,000 HPV-associated cancers occur each year in men; oropharyngeal cancers are the most common.

Clinical Context Exemplars

Situation A

During the oral assessment of a middle-aged adult, it is noted that there are gaps that are forming between the teeth and gums.

1. What is the significance of this finding?
2. What other manifestations would you assess for?
3. What would you tell the patient regarding your findings and how to arrest the progression of this condition?
4. What is your rationale for providing this information?

Situation B

A 5-year-old child is brought in by his mother, with the mother complaining that there is a constant, foul smelling nasal discharge that has been present for the last 4 days.

1. What information would you want to obtain from the mother?
2. When doing the assessment of the nose, what might you expect to find?
3. What further actions might be appropriate?

Situation C

During the assessment of the throat of an elderly patient, it is noted that there are no visible tonsils.

1. Is this a major concern? Why or why not?
2. What information would you want to obtain from the patient?

This same patient complains of having a dry mouth and is concerned that the absence of tonsils is the cause.

1. What would you tell the patient?
2. What further information would you want to obtain? Why or why not?

SUBJECTIVE DATA

History of Present Illness (CC)

The patient may present to the provider with a variety of concerns that may be directly related to the nose, mouth, or throat or other systems. Framing the questions will depend on the patient's age, gender, culture, race, emotional or mental status, health practices, and concurrent illnesses. All symptoms presented must be thoroughly assessed with a symptom analysis (COLDERRA).

Nasal Discharge (Rhinorrhea)

Rhinorrhea or **rhinorrhoea** commonly referred to as "runny nose," is a condition where the nasal cavity is filled with a significant amount of mucous fluid. This condition occurs relatively frequently and is a common symptom of allergies or certain diseases, such as upper respiratory infections, sinusitis, or allergies. It can also be a side effect of crying, exposure to cold temperatures, cocaine abuse or withdrawal from opioids like methadone.

Provider Inquiries	Clinical Reasoning/Logic
Characteristics: Are you stuffy or congested? Is the discharge watery, purulent, mucoid, bloody?	Excess mucous may accumulate, causing congestion and stuffiness. Characteristics of discharge can help to identify cause—mucoid/watery (allergies, viral/atopic rhinitis), purulent (green—sinusitis, yellow—infection), clear/watery (CSF), bloody (epistaxis), dark/black (mucormycosis/zygomycosis). Blood streaked mucus may be due to frequent or aggressive blowing.
Does it have any odor? Do you have post nasal drip, cough, sore throat? Any blood present?	Excess mucus may run down the back of the throat (postnasal drip) or cause a cough that is usually worse at night. A sore throat may also result from too much mucous drainage.

Provider Inquiries	Clinical Reasoning/Logic
Onset: When did you first notice discharge? Anything noted to bring on discharge?	Recent viral infection/cold or allergies may cause inflammation and lead to increasing nasal discharge. Certain times of year (spring/fall) are associated with pollen, causing allergies. Acute onset suggests bacterial, viral infections, or allergic conditions. Chronic symptoms are seen in chronic sinusitis, nasal polyps, or in perennial allergy. A condition called **vasomotor rhinitis** is high on the list of nonallergy causes. It brings an outpouring of clear, watery discharge from any number of triggers: temperature changes, alcohol, strong odors, airborne irritants, or hot spices. Certain medicines may initiate a nasal drip: NSAIDs (ibuprofen, Aleve, Advil, aspirin, and more), cocaine abuse or withdrawal, and opioid withdrawal, ACE-inhibitors, calcium channel blockers (blood-pressure drugs), and birth-control pills.
Location: Does the drainage occur on both sides of nose or just one side?	Unilateral drainage frequently accompanies acute sinusitis. Bilaterality suggests viral and allergic processes. In cluster headaches, unilateral rhinorrhea and lacrimation may be observed.
Duration: How long have you had discharge? Is it constant or intermittent?	Symptoms should not last more than 3 weeks or more than 10 days in a child under 3 years old. Intermittent or seasonal symptoms may be seen in both allergy and viral infections.
Exacerbation: Anything that makes it worse?	Congestion is often worse when lying down. Environmental exposure like in allergy; exposure to viruses during viral season.
Relief: Anything that makes it better? What remedies have you tried? Are they effective?	Humidifier, antihistamines, drinking extra fluids, sinus irrigations may provide some relief.
Associated signs/symptoms: Any sneezing, nasal congestion, bleeding, itching, watery eyes, mouth breathing, ear pain?	The mucous drainage may plug up the Eustachian tube between the nose and the ear, causing an ear infection and pain. The mucous drip may also plug the sinus passages, causing sinus infection and pain.
Chills or sweating, breathing difficulty, nausea or vomiting, unusual sleepiness, severe headache?	Any of these manifestations are a cause for concern.
Head trauma? Headaches? Migraine?	Head trauma may lead to CSF rhinorrhea. Cluster headache may manifest with unilateral nasal drainage and lacrimation.

Bleeding (Epistaxis)

Epistaxis (nosebleed) can present as an anterior bleed or posterior bleed. Anterior bleeding, which is the most common, is generally self-limiting. Posterior is less common but more likely to lead to persistent bleeding, often necessitating provider attention. Association with hypertension is uncertain. Most patients will have high blood pressure, which may be from the stress of bleeding. It is commonly caused by mucosal irritation or trauma. Patients with genetic diseases like Osler-Weber-Rendu, Von Willebrand disease and other platelet abnormalities may cause epistaxis. Neoplasm, and carotid artery aneurysm have been associated with epistaxis.

Provider Inquiries	Clinical Reasoning/Logic
Characteristics: Is the blood red or brown? Does the blood include clots? Have you experienced oozing or spurting?	Anterior nosebleeds are common and arise from the watershed area known as Keisselbach's plexus. Posterior nosebleed arises commonly from the sphenopalatine artery or carotid artery.
Onset: When did this nosebleed start? When did you first start having nosebleeds? Frequency of nosebleeds? Anything noted that brings on nosebleed (trauma, picking nose, dry air, forceful blowing, allergies, coughing)? Any foreign object placed in nose (primarily related to children)?	Nasal inflammation from rhinosinusitis related to bacterial, viral or allergic origin causes dilation of blood vessels, which may rupture and cause epistaxis. Dry climate dries out nasal membranes, causing them to become irritated. Household heaters during the winter are a frequent cause of nasal dryness.
Location: Does the nosebleed occur on one side or both? Is the blood coming out of nose or going down back of throat?	Anterior hemorrhaging will primarily present in blood draining down the nostril and perhaps also drain into the nasopharynx and oropharynx. Posterior bleeding will most commonly drain to the back of the nose to the oropharynx.
Duration: How long do nose bleeds last?	Most nose bleeds are self-limiting and don't last beyond 12 minutes. They generally stop with pressure like nose pinching. Venous nose bleeds are of short duration; arterial bleeds are of longer duration.
Exacerbation: Anything noted to make them worse? Drugs (snorting cocaine), steroids? Trauma, nose picking, excessive nose blowing? Are you taking any known anticoagulant drugs or prostaglandin inhibitors, such as—ASA, Coumadin, Pradaxa, Plavix, NSAID's, or intranasal steroids?	Inhaled steroid drugs for allergies and sinus congestion are also cause of nose bleeds. Excessive use of aspirin is also a cause of bleeding.
Relief: What remedies are used to stop bleeding? Are they effective?	Applications of ice, pinching bridge of nose, and putting head back are all possible interventions to stop bleeding. Packing of nasal cavity is also useful.
Associated Signs/Symptoms: Coughing, sneezing? Nasal obstruction?	Clots may cause irritative symptoms like sneezing or coughing or obstruction. Nasal neoplasm may present with obstruction and bleeding.

Oral Lesions (With or Without Pain, Burning Mouth Syndrome)

Oral lesions with or without pain may be seen in oral malignancies. They may be due to other causes such as infections with Candida, HIV, cold sores, irritations, trauma, or chemical burns. They may be benign like canker sores.

Burning mouth syndrome (BMS, also termed *glossodynia*, *orodynia*, *burning tongue*, *sore tongue*, *burning tongue syndrome*, *burning mouth*, or *sore mouth*) is the complaint of a burning sensation in the mouth where no underlying dental or medical cause can be identified and no oral signs are found.

Type 1 - Symptoms not present upon waking, and then increase throughout the day
Type 2 - Symptoms upon waking and through the day (most common)
Type 3 - No regular pattern of symptoms

Although BMS can affect anyone, it occurs most commonly in middle-aged or older women.

Provider Inquiries	Clinical Reasoning/Logic
Characteristics: What is appearance of lesion (color, size, open, ulcerated, bleeding or discharge)? How severe the pain? Characteristic of the pain?	The pain of BMS is usually described as burning, scalded, or tingling. The sensation is also described as "discomfort," "tender," "raw," and "annoying" rather than pain or burning. Lesions from oral candidiasis or thrush appear as white pseudomembrane, like a "curdled milk" coating of tongue and cheeks, which reveals an erythematous base when wiped away. Oral cancers appear as a painless white or red patch on the soft tissue of the mouth.
Onset: When was the lesion and/or the pain first noted? Is the pain constant or intermittent? Is this the first time you've had this type of lesion, or have you had previously? When? How frequent?	Onset of BMS pain has no specific timing. It may be gradual but most commonly is spontaneous. Pain is chronic, and rarely spontaneously remits.
Location: Where in mouth is the lesion located (cheeks, gums, tongue)? Do you have lesions any other place on body (genitalia, anus)?	The discomfort from BMS may affect the tongue, gums, lips, inside of cheeks, roof of mouth, or widespread areas of whole mouth. Canker sores are usually inside the mouth, and cold sores are usually on the lips. Malignant sores are usually located on the lateral aspect of the tongue close to the base. Lesions on the genitalia or anus may be associated with STDs. Pain of BMS is generally localized to the mouth or anterior two-thirds of the tongue, and may or may not include the lips, gingival, upper palate, and throat.
Duration: How long does pain last? How long has lesion/pain been there?	Any mouth sores that persist for more than two weeks should be investigated. The burning sensation of BMS often begins in late morning, builds to a peak by evening, and often subsides at night. Some feel constant pain; for others, pain comes and goes.
Exacerbation: Does anything make the lesion/pain worse (food, drink, alcohol)?	Stress, ill-fitting dentures, trauma, and B_{12}/folate deficiency have been implicated to trigger canker sores. These are shallow ulcers in the mouth with surrounding erythema associated with pain. Exacerbating factors for BMS include tension, fatigue, speaking, and hot, acidic, or spicy foods.
Relief: Is there anything relieves the pain? What remedies have you used (mouthwash, saline rinse, OTC analgesics)?	Relieving factors include sleeping, cold, distraction, and alcohol. The pain is often relieved by eating and drinking or when the person's attention is occupied. Pain is not often relived by systemic analgesics, but can sometimes be relieved by topical anesthetics.

Provider Inquiries	Clinical Reasoning/Logic
Associated signs/symptoms: Any changes noted on tongue? Metallic taste? History of tobacco use (smoking, chewing)? Do you wear dentures/appliances (how long worn, how well they fit)?	Xerostomia (dryness) and dysgeusia (altered taste perception) classically accompanies pain. BMS has also been associated with bruxism (teeth grinding), jaw clenching, and tongue thrusting, as well as thirst, headaches, chronic back pain, irritable bowel syndrome, dysmenorrhea, globus pharyngis, anxiety, decreased appetite, depression, and personality disorders.
Sore Throat/Throat Pain (Pharyngitis) Sore throat (pharyngitis) refers to inflammation of the throat that is usually associated with upper respiratory infections (bacterial/viral), GERD, postnasal drip, mouth breathing, infectious mononucleosis, tonsillitis, allergies, inflamed vocal cords, prolonged steroid use, chemical or thermal burns, or instrumentations like intubation and endoscopic gastroduodenoscopy (EGD). Trauma and diphtheria are also possible causes. It is a common manifestation in the outpatient setting and is often accompanied by fever, malaise, cough and nasal congestion.	
Characteristics: Is your throat burning, scratchy? Is the pain associated with swallowing? Is the pain mild, severe?	Allergy may present with scratchy or itching of the throat. Severe pain may be a component of both viral and bacterial pharyngitis, tonsillitis, or peritonsillar abscess or infectious mononucleosis.
Onset: When did it first start? Have you been around individuals with colds, etc.? Acute?	Sudden, severe sore throat with paucity of symptoms of flu like illness favor Group A hemolytic strep. Chronic sore throat with painful swallowing will need to be investigated to rule out invasive infection like Candida esophagitis, HIV, or malignancy.
Location: Is the pain on both sides or one side?	Unilateral sore throat may be due to a peritonsillar abscess, tonsillitis or retropharyngeal abscess. In some cases, dental issues, such as an impacted tooth, may manifest with unilateral throat pain.
Duration: Pain constant or intermittent? How long have you had sore throat?	Acute pharyngitis is characterized by a sudden and rapid onset of symptoms; chronic pharyngitis develops slowly, and possibly lasts for weeks.
Exacerbation: What makes throat more sore (swallowing, certain foods)?	Pain frequently worsens with swallowing. Hot, spicy foods may also worsen pain.
Relief: What remedies have you tried to relieve pain? Effectiveness?	Most patients may already have tried home remedies such as gargling with salt water, anesthetic sprays, Chloraseptic lozenges, apple cider vinegar, and cayenne pepper by the time they present to the provider.
Radiation: Is the pain felt elsewhere, such as the ears and neck?	In some cases, pain may also radiate towards the ears or neck. Pain in the ear may be caused by swelling of the Eustachian tube.

Provider Inquiries	Clinical Reasoning/Logic
Associated signs/symptoms: Do you have redness, swelling of throat, hoarseness, nasal stuffiness, spots on tonsils, fever, chills, drooling, pain with swallowing (odynophagia) or ear pain?	Acute, severe sore throat with absence of cough, presence of fever, lymph node enlargement, tonsillar exudate, palatal petechiae, an occurrence in those younger than 15 years, and an occurrence during winter to spring season favor streptococcal pharyngits (Centor criteria). Muscle aching, aphonia, cough and congestion and other flulike symptoms favor viral infections. Drooling and persistent severe pain in swallowing may be signs of retropharyngeal or peritonsillar abscess. In children, epiglottitis may present with salivary drooling. Odynophagia is present when there is severe inflammation and is a common complaint in Candida esophagitis. Pain in the ear may be caused by swelling of the Eustachian tube, causing blockage that increases pressure on middle ear. Aphonia, hoarseness may accompany viral laryngitis. Persistent hoarseness should be followed up as this is considered a high risk for malignancy.

Sinus/Nasal Congestion (Sinusitis or Rhinosinusitis)

Nasal/sinus congestion is the blockage of the nasal passages and/or paranasal sinuses, usually caused by swollen membranes lining the nose/sinuses. Other causes include structural abnormalities such as deviated septum, small sinus ostia or a concha bullosa, nasal polyps, and prior instances of sinusitis.

Sinusitis refers to inflammation of the paranasal sinuses and may be caused by infections (viral, bacterial, fungal), mucor, autoimmune, or by allergic causes. The most common cause is viral but it is difficult to determine if sinusitis is viral or bacterial in origin; however only about 0.5 to 2% of patients with rhinosinusitis develop bacterial infections. Both smoking and second-hand smoke are associated with rhinosinusitis.

Provider Inquiries	Clinical Reasoning/Logic
Characteristics: Do you experience pain, tenderness, pressure over sinuses? Does the pain increase when bending forward? Do you have runny nose/nasal discharge (if so, characteristics)?	Acute bacterial sinusitis is characterized by nasal congestion, fever, purulent or thick, colored discharge, pain and unilateral sinus tenderness, or pain and **maxillary tooth pain**. Manifestations of chronic sinusitis may additionally include facial pain, headache, night-time coughing, increased symptoms of asthma that were previously minor or controlled, general malaise, thick green/yellow discharge, sensation of facial "fullness" or "tightness" that worsens when bending over, dizziness, and aching teeth.

Provider Inquiries	Clinical Reasoning/Logic
Onset: When did you first notice congestion/pain? Was it after a viral infection? Is onset during a high pollen season? Is the onset of symptoms associated with immune suppressed states like DM, HIV, immunosuppression with drugs?	Acute sinusitis is usually preceded by a previous upper respiratory tract infection, generally of viral origin. The step-up acceleration of symptoms (about 7–10 days of a viral syndrome) suggest acute bacterial sinusitis. Onset may also be in response to particular allergens, particularly various pollens.
Are symptoms acute or chronic?	Acute episodes of sinusitis can also result from fungal invasion seen in patients with diabetes and immune deficiencies (AIDS/transplant patients on immunosuppressive medications) and can be life threatening.
Location: Facial pain over frontal or maxillary sinuses? Do you have tooth pain?	Maxillary pain or pressure in the maxillary (cheek) area, which may also be of dental origin ("odontogenic sinusitis") is caused by periapical or periodontal infection of a maxillary posterior tooth. The inflammatory exudate may erode through the bone into the maxillary sinus.
	Pain or pressure in the frontal sinus cavity (above eyes), and headache suggest frontal sinusitis.
Is the pain behind the eyes (retro–orbital) or between the eyes?	Ethmoid sinusitis pain or pressure is generally located between/behind the eyes
	Sphenoid sinusitis pain or pressure is generally behind the eyes, often refers to the vertex (top of the head).
Duration: How long have you had congestion? Constant or intermittent? How long does each experience last (2–7 days, 4 weeks, 12 weeks)?	Acute viral rhinosinusitis typically lasts for 7 to 10 days and may be complicated by bacterial sinusitis.
	Acute rhinosinusitis is a new infection that may last up to 4 weeks and can be subdivided symptomatically into severe and non-severe.
	Recurrent acute rhinosinusitis consists of four or more separate episodes of acute sinusitis that occur within one year.
	Subacute rhinosinusitis is an infection that lasts between 4 and 12 weeks, and represents a transition between acute and chronic infection.
	Chronic rhinosinusitis occurs when the signs and symptoms last for more than 12 weeks.
	Acute exacerbation of chronic rhinosinusitis occurs when the signs and symptoms of chronic rhinosinusitis exacerbate, but return to baseline after treatment.
Exacerbation: What makes it worse (position, environment)?	Headache/facial pain or dull, constant, or aching pressure often worsen when bending over or lying down—these suggest sinusitis.

Provider Inquiries	Clinical Reasoning/Logic
Relief: What remedies have you used to relieve the symptoms? Have you used any oral or nasal Medications? Have you used any liquids? Home remedies?	Most patients have exhausted home remedies such as sinus rinses, warm compresses, pain medications, and OTC nasal sprays by the time they seek treatment.
Radiation: Does the pain spread and include eye pain, toothache (maxillary)?	Pain often starts on one side of the head and progresses to both sides. Pulpitis may present like maxillary sinusitis.
	See previous discussions.
Associated signs/symptoms: Do you have any other symptoms, such as headache, fever, chills, drainage (purulent or bloody), facial pain, toothache, halitosis, anosmia (loss of sense of smell), malaise, cough, altered consciousness, seizures, or visual problems. Do you have a deviated septum?	Allergy, colds, altered anatomy like deviated septum, immune deficiency, cystic fibrosis, and GERD may increase risks for sinusitis and are known triggers. Purulent rhinorrhea, facial pain/pressure and worsening after 7 days of having a viral process are predictive of bacterial sinusitis.
Sneezing? Lacrimation?	Sneezing, excess productions of watery nasal discharge and watering of the eyes are associated with allergies.

Dental Pain (Toothache)

A toothache (odontalgia or, less frequently, odontalgy) is an aching pain in or around a tooth that is frequently caused by dental caries, pulpitis (inflammation of the pulp), periodontitis, wisdom teeth, cracked tooth, dry socket or tight braces. Non-dental related causes are trigeminal neuralgia or tic douloureux, giant cell arteritis, dry mouth in Sjogrens and SLE, TMJ, maxillary sinusitis, referred pain from MI, and other neuropathies. Sensitivity of the teeth to extreme temperatures may also be interpreted as pain.

Provider Inquiries	Clinical Reasoning/Logic
Characteristics: What is the degree of pain? Is the pain boring, stabbing, burning? Is it associated with eating/chewing (certain foods)? Pressure? Do you notice changes in its severity?	Tooth pain may be sharp, constant, throbbing, "nerve-like" pain. The intensity of aching pain is mild in the beginning but tends to increase after eating or drinking something hot or cold. As the area of inflammation increases, the pain becomes more severe. In some individuals, pain results only when pressure applied to the tooth.
Onset: When first noted? Anything that brings on pain (food/liquid temperature, chewing)?	Toothache symptoms commonly start without any warning.
After dental extraction?	Dry socket syndrome occurs 2 to 3 days after dental extraction.
Location: Is the pain related to a single tooth, generalized area, or TMJ?	Soreness and tenderness may be felt in the gum and jaw area.
Do you feel the pain in other areas?	Pain or swelling may be referred outside the mouth such as the throat, eyes, lips, or cheeks.
Duration: Is the pain constant/intermittent?	Dental pain is generally constant.
Exacerbation: What makes the pain worse (food/liquid temperature, chewing on affected side, types of food)?	The pain often intensifies with additional pressure on the tooth, or if upper and lower teeth touch each other, with chewing food or lying down. Dental pain may also worsen with hot or cold exposure. After a few seconds, once the hot or cold stimulus is removed, the pain usually goes down. If the toothache lasts for longer than 3 minutes, it's likely that the tooth is dying.

Provider Inquiries	Clinical Reasoning/Logic
Relief: What used for relief (medications, mouth washes, avoidance of certain foods)?	OTC pain medications, such as acetaminophen (Tylenol) or ibuprofen (Advil) may be effective. Relief may also be obtained from biting on a cotton ball soaked in oil of cloves. Avoid very cold or hot foods because this may make the pain worse.
Radiation: Does pain go to TMJ?	Toothache pain needs to be differentiated from other sources of pain in the face. Sinusitis, ear or throat pain, or an injury to the temporomandibular joint (TMJ) may be confused with toothache. Pain from a deeper structure (*referred pain*) may be passed along the nerve and be felt in the jaw or tooth. In some instances, it may radiate to the cheek, the ear, or the jaw.
Do you feel any pain in your jaw?	Jaw pain or claudication may be part of the presenting symptom of temporal arteritis.
Do you still have your wisdom teeth?	Wisdom teeth may also be the source of pain. As wisdom teeth (third molars) erupt, they cause inflammation of the gum around the crown, which may become infected. The pain may extend to the jaw and ear. Swelling in the affected area may not allow the jaw to be closed properly. In severe cases, pain in the throat and the floor of the mouth may make it difficult or painful to swallow.
Associated signs/symptoms: Fever, chills, joint pains and weight loss, fatigue, periodontal disease, missing teeth (malocclusion), grinding teeth, mouth odor, lesions? Any bleeding, swelling of gums or elsewhere? Still have wisdom teeth? Other manifestations may include swelling around the tooth, fever or headache, foul-tasting drainage from the infected tooth, pain with chewing, hot or cold sensitivity, bleeding or discharge from around a tooth or gums, and swelling of the jaw.	Infection generally presents with fever, chills, purulent discharge from the infected tooth suggest bacterial infection or abscess. Temporal arteritis is associated with constitutional symptoms like fever, weight loss, fatigue and joint pain.

Altered Taste (Dysgeusia)

Dysgeusia is a distortion of the sense of taste and frequently associated with ageusia (complete lack of taste), and hypogeusia (decreased taste sensitivity). Altered taste or smell may be a primary symptom or secondary symptoms of disease states like respiratory infections, glossitis, Sjogrens, vitamin deficiency, endocrine disease like thyroid and DM, MS, head trauma or medications. Common causes of dysgeusia include chemotherapy like vincristine, asthma treatment with albuterol, zinc deficiency, and various drugs (lithium, antibiotics, ACE inhibitors). Many of the causes for dysgeusia are not fully understood, making idiopathic dysgeusia very common.

Provider Inquiries	Clinical Reasoning/Logic
Characteristics: Any particular tastes affected—sweet, sour, bitter, salty? Any problems with salivation, swallowing, chewing, oral pain, previous ear infections, oral hygiene, or stomach problems? Any problems with smelling?	Alterations in the sense of taste, usually a metallic taste, and sometimes smell are often the only symptoms. Xerostomia (dry mouth syndrome), can precipitate dysgeusia because normal salivary flow and concentration are necessary for taste. Both taste and smell cells work together to produce the sense of taste. In some people with dysgeusia, the sense of smell can also be altered.

Provider Inquiries	Clinical Reasoning/Logic
Onset: Any specific time when first noted?	Altered taste is commonly seen in aging and may relate to inadequate salivary gland secretion or flow (dry mouth syndrome.)
Duration: How long been aware of change?	Duration depends on the cause. If the alteration results from gum disease, dental plaque, a temporary medication, or a short-term condition such as a cold, the dysgeusia should disappear once the cause is removed. If lesions are present in the taste pathway (CN VII & IX and X) or nerves have been damaged, it may be permanent.
Associated signs/symptoms: Did change occur with any other changes/events/experiences? Decreased saliva? Medications? Smoking history?	Dysgeusia is most commonly associated with burning mouth syndrome, medications and decreased saliva.

Past Medical History

Past medical history provides information as to previous illnesses or conditions that may have an effect on the nose, sinuses, mouth, and throat.

Provider Inquiries	Clinical Reasoning/Logic
History of allergies? Allergic to what? (Allergy testing, severity of symptoms) **Chronic conditions:** Cardiovascular disease, hypertension, DM, GERDS, MS, leukemia, asthma, bleeding disorders **Acute conditions:** CVA, nose trauma, mouth trauma, strep infections, frequent sore throats	Prior history of atopic history, allergic rhinitis and asthma can be helpful in determining whether symptoms of nasal congestion is from allergy or other conditions.
Surgeries: Tonsils/adenoids, nose (deviated septum), dental (root canal, tooth extraction)	CVA and head trauma may alter salivary flow and sensation of taste and smell. Bleeding disorders like Von Willebrand disease and other primary or secondary coagulopathies may put a patient at risk for uncontrolled epistaxis.

Family History

Family history provides information regarding family member's illnesses or conditions that may indicate a pattern of presentation associated with transmission of familial/genetic factors predisposing the individual to certain system related conditions/illnesses.

Provider Inquiries	Clinical Reasoning/Logic
Family history of allergies, asthma, cancer, cardiovascular (CV) disease, head and neck cancers, bleeding disorders?	Family history of atopy, CV disease, asthma and cancer are significant contributors to conditions like allergic rhinitis, sinusitis and risk for oral cancers.

Personal and Social History

Personal and social history provides information related to habits, practices and/or environmental influences that may predispose the patient to the development of certain system related conditions/illnesses.

Provider Inquiries	Clinical Reasoning/Logic
Oral Care: Frequency of dental visits, daily brushing, flossing, last visit, childhood cavities/fluoride use? Fluoride in water supply? Drink bottled water?	Bottled water does not have fluoride added so the individual may be missing a significant protection from development of cavities.
History of smoking/tobacco use; alcohol use? Recreational drug use (cocaine)? Sports (mouth/nose protection)?	Smoking or smokeless tobacco use are significantly associated with oral cancers. Alcohol may compound risk of smoking in oral cancers. Inhaling (snorting/sniffing) cocaine is a cause of perforation of the nasal septum.

Developmental Applications

Certain conditions or disorders may be related to certain age groups or situations. Inquiring to obtain age or condition-specific information will provide further information for helping to determine causes of the chief concern as identified.

Provider Inquiries	Clinical Reasoning/Logic
 ***Infants*** Ask the parent or caregiver if the infant has any difficulty breathing? Any difficulty sucking on breast/bottle?	Infants are obligate nose breathers during the first few months of life. Any structural changes, inflammation of nasal passages or obstructions would make it difficult for infants to breathe. Any audible effort to breathe is also an indicator of breathing difficulties. Inability to suck is also an indicator of obstruction. To suck/swallow requires interruption of breathing. If infant is having breathing difficulties, it will expend energy on breathing rather than eating.
Ever notice nasal flaring?	Nasal flaring is another indicator of breathing difficulty.
Pattern of tooth eruption?	Teeth eruption occurs in a sequenced pattern and is an indicator of overall development.
Is the infant bottle- or breastfed? Does the infant get a bottle at bedtime?	Breastfed infants are less likely to need a bottle with them in bed. Having a bottle in bed with infant increases probability of "bottle mouth syndrome." Extended use of bottle also predisposes to middle ear infections.
 ***Children*** Ask the parent, caregiver, or child (if age-appropriate) the following questions:	
Frequent nose bleeds? Difficulty breathing?	In children, hypertrophy of adenoids may be cause of obstruction.
Pushing up nose with palm of hand (allergic salute)?	Indictor of runny nose, often accompanying allergies.
Places objects in nose?	Children commonly like to place objects up their noses, causing obstruction and difficulty breathing. Also may be source of foul odor, if its presence is noted.
Dental habits/care? Regular visits to dentist? Access to fluoride?	Has child been instructed on proper dental care and hygiene? Patterns set in childhood more likely to be continued as adult. Fluoride is known to prevent cavities and can be supplied in drinking water or in tablet form.
Frequent sore throats, inflamed tonsils?	
Difficulty in talking, forming words?	May be caused by ankyloglossia (tongue tied), a condition caused by a shortened lingual frenulum which prevents adequate tongue protrusion. May interfere with breastfeeding and proper word formation.
Teeth eruption? Position? Do they appear to be straight? Any crowding noticed? Still thumb sucking?	
 ***The Pregnant Woman*** Do you have any nasal stuffiness?	Nasal congestion/stuffiness result of increased estrogen levels.
Do you experience nose bleeds?	Nosebleeds also common due to engorged blood vessels.

Provider Inquiries	Clinical Reasoning/Logic
Have you noticed any changes in gums/bleeding?	Gums increase in size from hyperplasia and bleed easily. They will also become softer and a deeper pink in color.
The Older Adult Have you noticed any decrease in smell or taste? Do you find it necessary to add extra salt to food?	Sensory sensitivity decreases with age. Loss of smell may be a safety issue as the elderly may not smell gas leaks or smoke. Increased use of salt or vinegar or lemon may be used to increase flavor of food.
Do you experience dry mouth? What are your current medications, if any?	Dry mouth (xerostomia), a frequent side effect of medications (antidepressants, anticholinergics, antihypertensives, antipsychotics) may lead to dysgeusia.
Have you had a loss of teeth? Do you wear dentures? If so, are you able to care for dentures? Do they fit properly?	Poor oral hygiene may be cause of loss of teeth. Dentures may not be a possibility due to cost. If dentures don't fit properly, will not wear them and may contribute to oral candidiasis and oral lesions. Loss of teeth may interfere with eating properly.

OBJECTIVE DATA

Objective data for the nose, mouth, and throat is obtained through inspection and palpation of the various structures of these tissues and locations. The following is the suggested sequence for the complete examination of the nose, mouth, throat, and sinuses according to the two techniques of data collection, followed by a break down into the taxonomy types of the exam.

Inspection

- Nose
  - General appearance, shape, symmetry, patency
  - Smell (Olfactory sensation; CN)
  - Internal nasal chamber
- Sinuses
  - Transilluminate for opacity
- Mouth/throat (Oropharynx)
  - Lips
  - Teeth/gums
  - Buccal mucosa
  - Tongue
  - Tonsils, pillars, palate, uvula

Palpation

- Nose
  - Patency, tenderness
  - Tongue
  - Teeth/gums
- Sinuses
  - Tenderness
- Mouth

Percussion *not performed*

Auscultation *not performed*

Level I to IV Examination

The Level I to Level IV examinations are performed on a continuum, which starts from a basic level to a more comprehensive level based on provider's abilities and knowledge as well as the patient's presentation and location of the examination. It may start at the outpatient setting progressing to the ED, hospital unit bed, critical care unit, or specialty unit. Frequently all the elements, from basic to comprehensive exam, are done in one setting like in a primary care seting or clinic.

The condition/illness of the patient is the primary consideration related to the type and amount of data needed to assess the patient's /condition/illness/situation. The arrangement of skills into levels is for general purposes and is meant to be descriptive rather than prescriptive. The purpose of arranging into levels is to provide a framework to assist the learner in determining the appropriate data to collect.

Nose, Mouth, Sinuses, and Throat

	Level I	Level II	Level III	Level IV
Inspection	Nose/sinuses Position, shape, symmetry, patency, discharge	Nose/sinuses Mucosa/turbinates, septum	Nose/sinuses Nasal, oral trauma	Nose/sinuses Sinuses: Transillumination
	Mouth–external Lips: color, shape, moisture symmetry, lesions			
	Mouth–internal Buccal mucosa: color, condition, state of hydration, surface characteristics	Mouth–internal Buccal mucosa: Hard palate	Mouth–internal Dental trauma	
	Teeth/gums: presence (number, missing), alignment, color, condition, surface characteristics,			Occlusion Malocclusion
	Tongue: (dorsal) color, surface characteristics (lesions), movement	Tongue–ventral/lateral: characteristics		
	Throat Mucosa: color; surface characteristics (lesions)	Throat Tonsils, pillars, uvula, soft palate color; surface characteristics, size, shape, movement (uvula; CN X)		
Palpation	Nose: patency, tenderness	Sinuses: tenderness		
	Tongue: Tenderness, texture/firmness			
	Teeth/gums: Condition, tenderness, bleeding			

Inspection: Level I

The Level I exam generally does not extensively involve the nose, mouth, and throat unless the patient's hospitalization is directly related to treatment or interventions for any alterations or conditions affecting these structures. Routine data for these structures is limited to what can be observed during the overall assessment.

Inspection Techniques and Expected Findings	Unexpected Findings

Nose/Sinuses

Initial observations are primarily concerned with the nose's placement, overall shape, position, landmark characteristics, and role as a functional unit of the respiratory system.

Any change in nose shape is most likely caused by a history of a broken nose and observed as a deviation or bending of the cartilage ridge from the midline. The severity and frequency of a broken nose determines the degree of deviation. A broken nose may also be the cause of a deviated septum, which is observed on the internal examination of the nose (Figure 20-11).

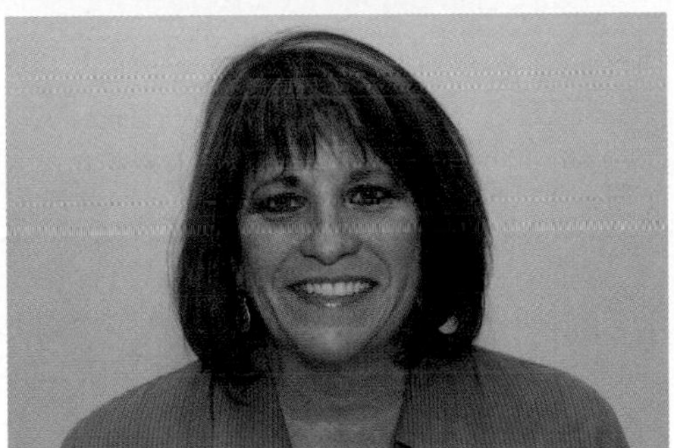

FIGURE 20-10 Anterior view of face, focusing on nose

The overall shape should be triangular, with a symmetrical ridge of cartilage at the midline that forms a straight line from the bridge to the tip. The nose should be in the center of the face in alignment with the ears on the sides of the head (see Figure 20-10). Its color should be consistent with the overall facial coloring, with smooth, intact skin, without any lesions or evidence of trauma. The columella should be midline and aligned with the cartilage ridge. The nares are somewhat oval in shape and positioned laterally on each side of the columella.

Increased redness, papules, and telangiectasis seen in rosacea typically begins on the nose and surrounding region of the face such as the cheeks, forehead and around the eye.

Central cyanosis is typically seen on the nose and lips.

Redness and dryness around the nose may be seen in people with persistent rhinorrhea and allergic rhinitis.

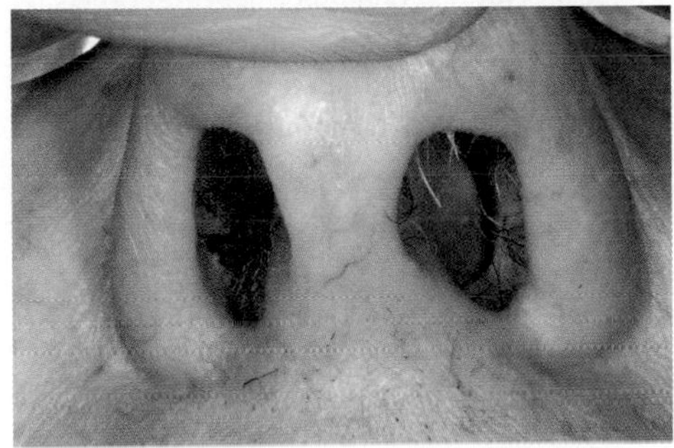

FIGURE 20-11 Deviated septum-external view
Source: Dr. P. Marazzi/Science Source

There should be no evidence of any discharge from the nares or any obstruction.

A bloody discharge may result from trauma or a spontaneous bloody nose.

A watery, clear bilateral discharge accompanied by sneezing, watery eyes, and nasal congestion is associated with allergies.

A unilateral, clear discharge may be cerebral spinal fluid and an indication of head trauma and skull fracture.

Mucoid and purulent discharge frequently accompanies rhinitis and upper respiratory infections.

A thick, unilateral, greenish discharge with a foul odor frequently is an indicator of a foreign body.

Assess patency by observation of the individual's ability to inhale and exhale through the nose.

Investigate obstruction of the nares for possible causes—fracture, bleeding. In severe cases of respiratory difficulty, there may be flaring of the nares (observed in children), which is an indication of respiratory distress.

Note the presence of any body piercing of the nose and nasal septal perforation.

Nasal septal perforation may be seen in cocaine addicts.

In instances of facial trauma, the individual may only be able to breathe through the mouth.

THINK LINK: Nose/Tongue Piercing

The popularity of body piercing as well as its social acceptance is increasing (Carver & Morphis, 2006). As with any procedure that breaks the integrity of the skin, piercing introduces the possibility of infections and other complications. Infections are often localized to the piercing location; however, any infection runs the risk of causing systemic complications. Infectious processes associated with body piercing include abscess formation, osteomyelitis, septic arthritis, acute glomerulonephritis, toxic shock, and endocarditis (Messahel & Musgrove, 2009). Although the incidence is low, transmission of hepatitis B and C virus remains a significant risk factor. Nose piercing carries a greater risk of infection as it is within the "danger triangle of the face" (Messahel & Musgrove, 2009). In addition to the nose, this danger area includes the eyebrows, eyes, and upper lip. The risk involves infection from the danger triangle through the ophthalmic veins, facial veins into the cavernous sinus and brain. The tongue is another popular site for piercing and is also associated with specific complications. Edema formation and hemorrhage may be serious enough to compromise the airway. Aspiration or swallowing of the jewelry is also a risk, but the most frequent complication is chipping or fracturing of teeth (Meltzer, 2005).

Inspection Techniques and Expected Findings	Unexpected Findings

Mouth (External)
Lips

Inspect the lips for color, symmetry, moisture, and swelling. They should be pink to red in color and vertically and horizontally symmetrical, both at rest and with movement (see Figure 20-12). The vermillion border should be well defined without any evidence of cracking, swelling, or lesions.

Vertical lines on the surface of the lips are an expected finding.

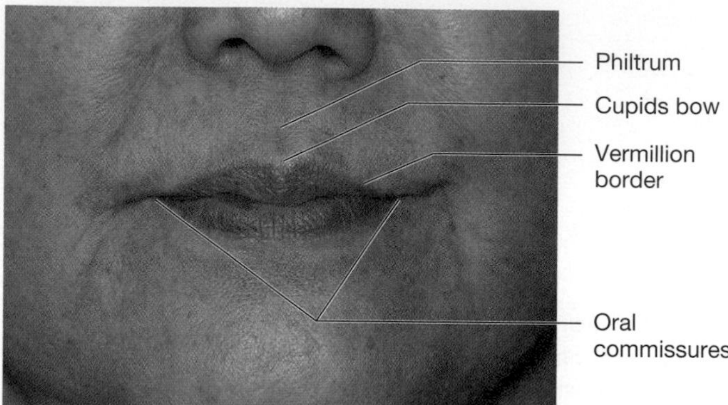

FIGURE 20-12 Lips with expected characteristics

Variation in lip color is dependent on a variety of factors.

Lesions on the lips may result from a variety of sources (Figure 20-13).

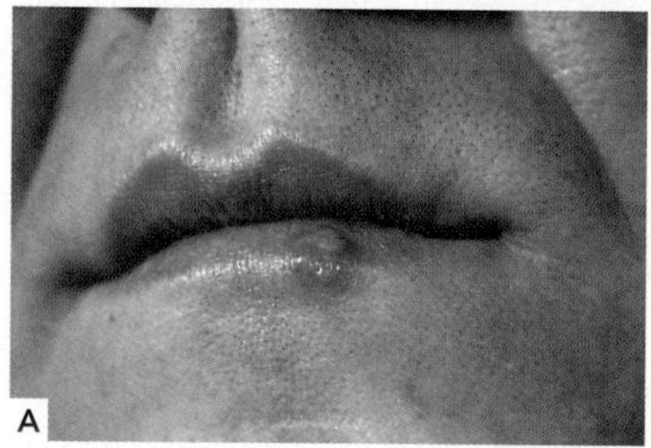

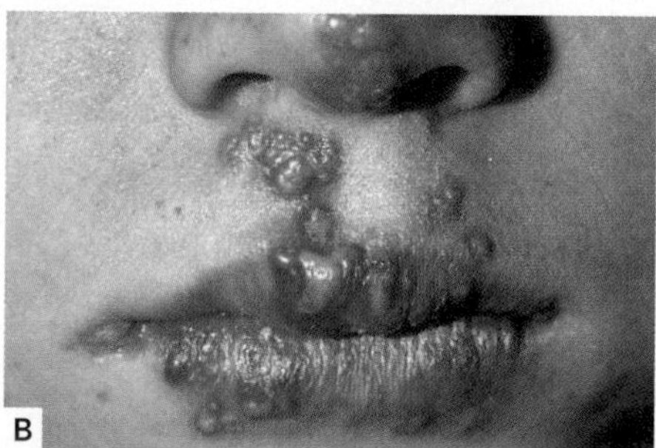

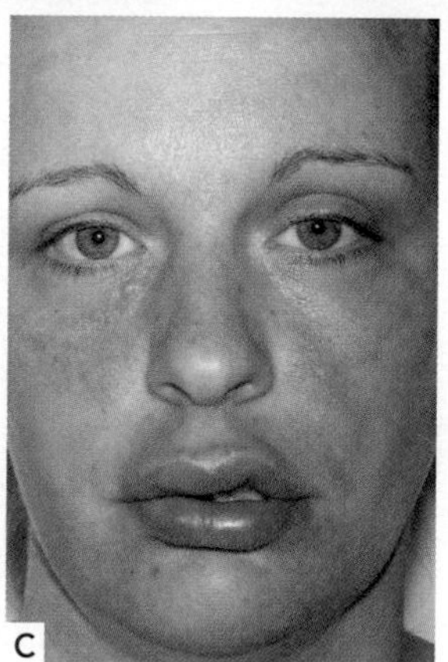

FIGURE 20-13A–C Common alterations of lips **a)** herpes, **b)** shingles, **c)** angioedema
Sources: a. CDC/Dr. Hermann; b, c. Dr. P. Marazzi/Science Source Images

Unexpected Findings

Pale lips are often associated with anemia. Blue-gray lips are associated with cyanosis and may be caused by local or systemic conditions. Circumoral cyanosis is often present due to vasoconstriction in colder temperatures, especially seen in individuals who are swimming in relatively cold water. Cyanosis of the fingertips is often seen also. Lip cyanosis associated with a generalized cyanosis is an indicator of oxygen delivery dysfunction.

Dry, cracked lips (chapped) occur in dehydration and excessive dry and/or cold air.

Herpes simplex viral infections may cause "cold sores" or "fever blisters," manifesting as vesicles or pustules that are usually self-limiting and regress spontaneously.

Cheilosis is a condition where the corners of the lips become cracked (fissures) and sore, and may be caused by extremely dry weather, excessive moisture (excessive salivation), infection from fungi or bacteria, iron deficiency, vitamin B (2 and 6) deficiencies or immunosuppression.

Allergic reactions may angioedema, which may involve the upper or lower lip or both (Figure 20-13).

Cancer or other conditions may also cause lesions.

PRACTICE POINT: Red Lips

The red color or the lips is due to an increased number of dermal papillae and the thinness of the epidermis in this area.

Inspection Techniques and Expected Findings

Mouth (Internal)
Buccal Mucosa

Note the overall condition of the patient's mouth while the patient is talking. Investigate any questionable manifestations (odor, dryness, missing teeth, poor condition of teeth, and tongue color/characteristics) further.

Inspection of the mouth includes the buccal mucosa, the teeth, gums, tongue, and palate. The patient's mouth needs to be open to allow for appropriate visualization of the structures. You will need a light source and a tongue blade to widen areas for inspection and manipulate around parts of the mouth.

Ask the patient to open his or her mouth, and then shine the light on the buccal mucosa (see Figure 20-15). Place the tongue blade in the corner of the mouth to increase the mouth opening and improve visualization, if needed. The mucosa should be pink to pinkish-red in color, moist and without any visible lesions. Inspect the mucosa on both sides of the mouth.

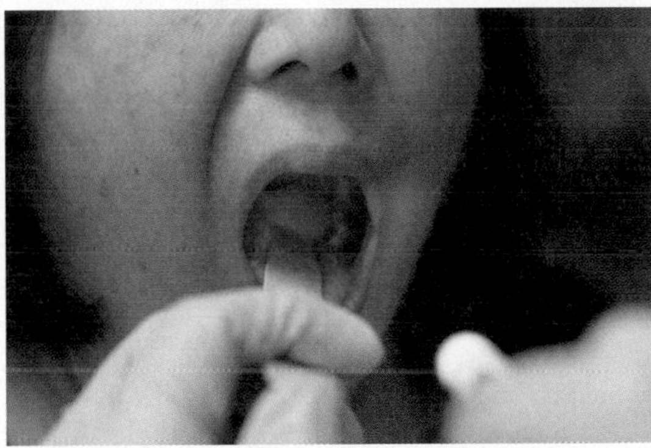

FIGURE 20-15 Inspection of mouth with light and tongue blade

Note the presence of **Fordyce's spots**, small sebaceous gland cysts that appear as yellow/white spots on the buccal mucosa (see Figure 20-16). These lesions are painless and non-significant.

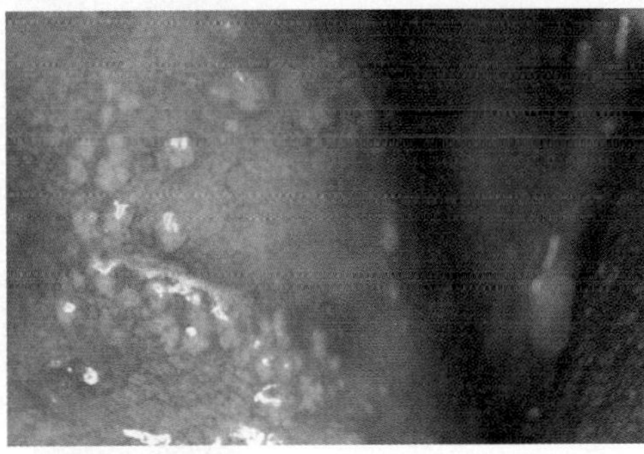

FIGURE 20-16 Fordyce spots
Source: Wellcome Image Library/Custom Medical Stock

Inspect for the presence of Stensen's duct, which should appear as a protrusion that is aligned with the second upper molar. The duct may be whitish-pink or whitish-yellow in color.

> ***PRACTICE POINT: Removal of Dental Appliances***
>
> Remember to ask the patient to remove any dental appliances before examining the mouth. The mucosa of the gums and palate should be identical to the surrounding mucosa, demonstrating that the appliances have a good fit. Any areas of redness, erosion, ulceration or the presence of growths indicate that there may be areas where the appliance causes irritation due to poor fitting. Any of these areas may be precancerous and should be followed. Any lesion that does not resolve within two weeks is suspect for oral cancer. Poor fitting dentures/appliances may also be a cause of poor nutrition as chewing may cause pain.

Unexpected Findings

Buccal mucosa that is deeply pigmented with brownish spots may be a manifestation of a pathologic endocrine disorder (Addison's disease).

Thick, fixed white, red, and combined red and white patches are a major concern as they may represent pre malignant lesions, especially in people with risk factors like tobacco use and family history of oral cancers.

Aphthous stomatitis, or "canker sore," may also be visible on the mucous membranes of the mouth (Figure 20-14). They are painful shallow ulcers with a white-yellow center surrounded by a well defined circle or halo of inflamed, red tissue. Their cause is unknown, but they appear, resolve, and then reappear. Possible triggers are immune reaction, certain foods, dental irritation or trauma, folate, B12, zinc deficiency, emotional stress, and heredity. Stomatitis herpetiformis is a subtype of aphthous stomatitis that resembles herpes simplex, but is not caused by herpes virus.

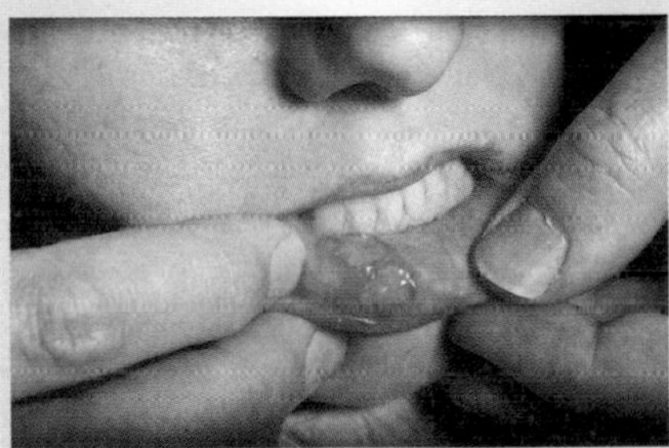

FIGURE 20-14 Apthous stomatitis
Source: CDC/Robert E. Sumpter

Cold sores or herpes simplex are seen on the lips and may be differentiated from canker sores, which are inside the mouth on buccal mucosa or gums.

The opening of Stensen's gland may appear red and puckered in the presence of inflammation or infection like in mumps or blockage with salivary duct stones, leading to **sialadenitis** (inflammation of a salivary gland).

Inspection Techniques and Expected Findings	Unexpected Findings

Teeth/Gums

Although the teeth are primarily assessed during dental visits, you will perform an overall assessment of the teeth during the examination.

Inspect teeth for color, number, and overall condition. Tooth color varies from white to shades of yellow. Teeth should also be straight and evenly spaced without any overlapping. Note any variations in positions as well as any loose, or absent teeth.

Note the number of teeth present and compare to the number expected for the patient's age. Inspect for the presence of any permanent or temporary dental appliances. Observe the condition of the surface of the teeth.

Teeth with smooth surfaces may be the result of excessive grinding of teeth. Inspect for the presence of any cavities as well as the presence of plaque and tartar.

Discoloration of the teeth can be due to excess fluoride (brown) to darker shades of yellow due to smoking, tea, and coffee (Figure 20-17).

The antibiotics tetracycline and doxycycline are known to discolor teeth when given to children whose teeth are still developing (before the age of 8). Mouth rinses and washes containing chlorhexidine and cetylpyridinium chloride can also stain teeth. Antihistamines (like Benadryl), antipsychotic drugs, and anti-hypertensive drugs also cause teeth discoloration.

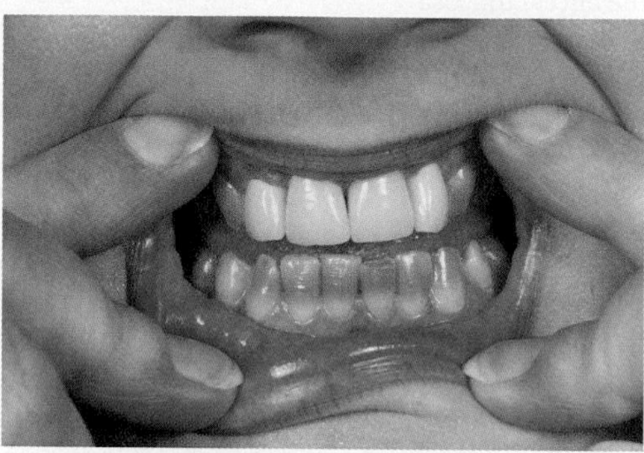

FIGURE 20-17 Teeth stained by tetracycline
Source: Biophoto Associates/Science Source Images

Inspect the gums (gingiva) for color and surface characteristics. They should be pink with evidence of **stippling**, multiple dots distributed over the surface. The margins of the gums with each tooth should be tight and well defined (see Figure 20-18).

The roots of the teeth should not be visible, nor should pockets or crevices exist between the gums and teeth.

Any gingival enlargement (thickening) is often due to hyperplasia (see Figure 20-19). Certain medications (phentoin and cyclosporin) cause this as well as pregnancy and leukemia (acute monomyelocytic).

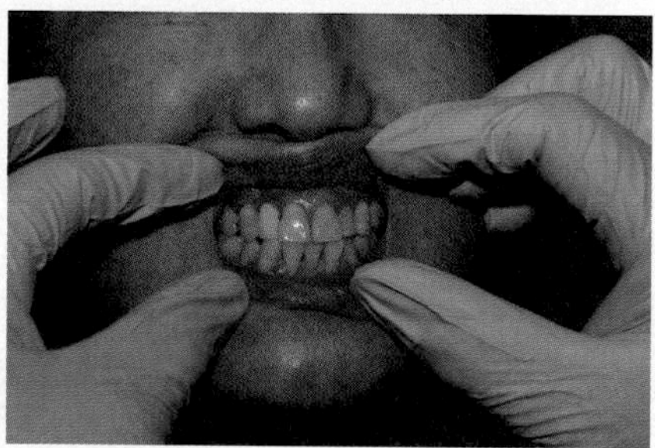

FIGURE 20-18 Inspecting the teeth and gums

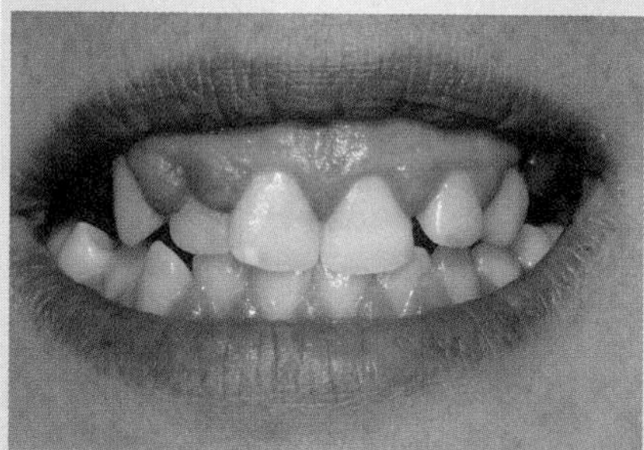

FIGURE 20-19 Gingival hyperplasia
Source: SPL/Science Source Images

THINK LINK: Gingivitis and Coronary Artery Disease
Periodontal disease is frequently the cause of enlarged/thickened gums and its presence may be an indicator of coronary artery disease. Patients with periodontal disease are twice as likely to also have coronary artery disease, most likely caused by increased levels of circulating inflammatory mediators, which are fibrinogen, C-reactive protein, and other cytokines (Mangione, 2008). Note the presence of any lesions, particularly white, raised patches.

Inspection Techniques and Expected Findings	Unexpected Findings

Tongue

Inspect the tongue for color, surface characteristics, and movement. It should appear symmetrical, dark pink, and moist. There might be a thin white coating on the tongue, which is not generally considered a significant finding.

The dorsal surface of the tongue is smooth; however, the presence of papillae gives it a roughened appearance and feel. Small fissures may also be present on the dorsal surface.

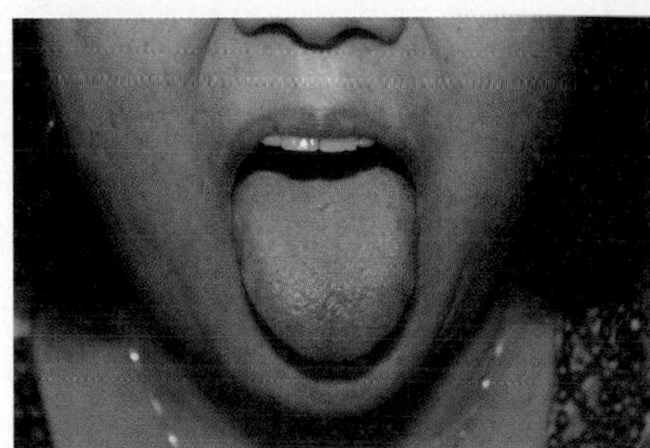

FIGURE 20-20 Tongue (surface characteristics)

The tongue's movement is voluntary and involuntary. Ask the patient to "stick out your tongue" and observe the forward thrust. The tongue should protrude midline without deviation to one side or the other. Ask the patient to move the tongue back and forth from right to left. Again, the movement should be smooth and coordinated. This maneuver also tests the facial (CN VII) and hypoglossal (CN XII) cranial nerves. Details are presented in Chapter 27.

The color of the mucosa of the throat should be the same as the rest of the oral mucosa. It should also be moist and shiny.

Atrophy on one side of the tongue may be due to a neurological disorder.

A beefy red tongue with a smooth surface is characteristic of a vitamin B_6 or B_{12} deficiency.

The patient may also complain of soreness of the tongue.

A hairy tongue, manifested by brown to black elongated papillae, may result from antibiotic therapy (Figure 20-21).

An enlarged tongue is present with mental retardation, hypothyroidism, and acromegaly. A small tongue is seen in malnutrition.

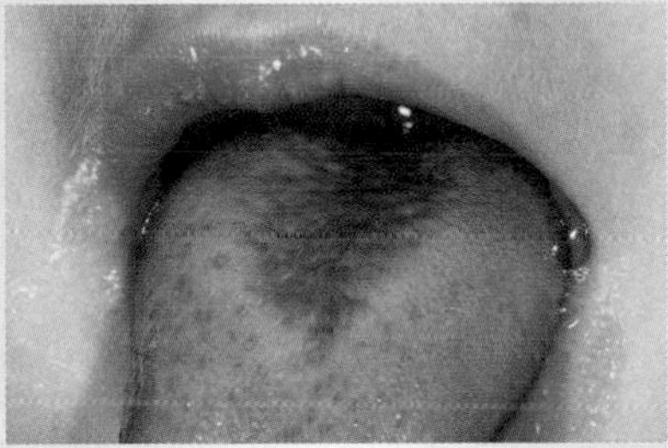

FIGURE 20-21 Black, hairy tongue
Source: Dr. P. Marazzi/Science Source

Throat
Mucosa

The last area to be assessed is the mucosa of the throat for color, and surface characteristics (see Figure 20-22). Visualization may require the use of a tongue blade. Asking the patient to say "ahh" again will slightly enlarge the area and allow for better visualization.

The color of the mucosa of the throat should be the same as the rest of the oral mucosa, and moist and shiny.

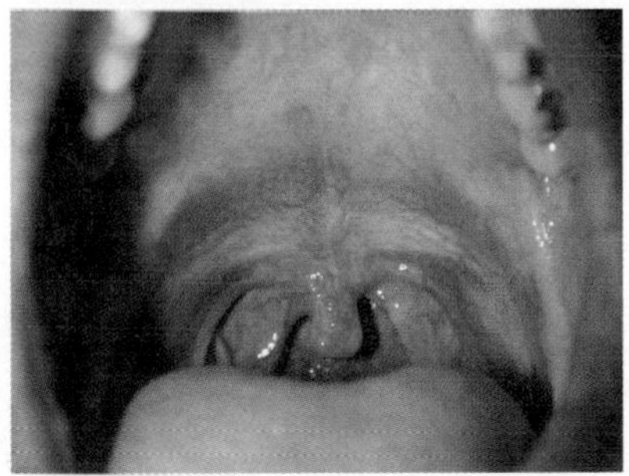

FIGURE 20-22 Visualization of tonsils
Source: Todd A. Bannor/Custom Medical Stock Photo

Inflammation or infection of the tonsils (tonsillitis) will cause the mucosa of the throat to become a deeper red.

Inspection: Level II

For the Level II exam, the internal structures of the nose, mouth, and throat are assessed for their expected characteristics, noting any unexpected findings.

Inspection Techniques and Expected Findings	Unexpected Findings

Nose/Sinuses
Mucosa/Turbinates

Inspection of the internal nasal chamber requires a light source. Use either a nasal speculum with a flashlight, or the otoscope following ear inspection (see Figure 20-23).

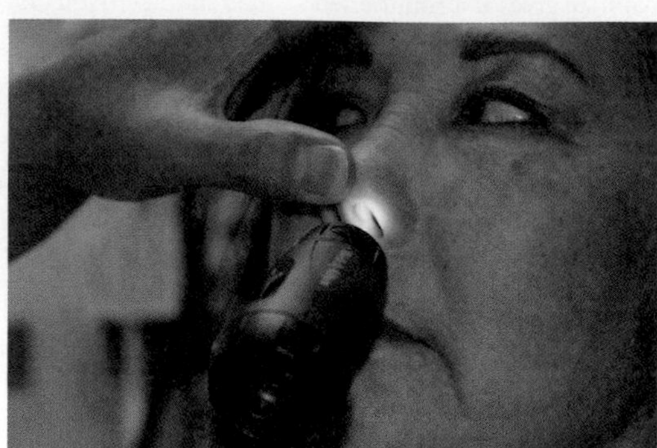

FIGURE 20-23 Inspection with nasal specula, flashlight, and otoscope

Hold the speculum in your palm, using your index finger for stabilization. Use your other hand to hold the light source and/or changing the position of the patient's head.

Gently and slowly, insert the head of the speculum into the patient's naris, avoiding contact with the nasal septum, as touching it can be painful.

Open the speculum on a slightly oblique angle, again, avoiding touching the septum. Once inside the nasal chamber, direct the light source through the speculum into the nasal chamber and inspect the internal tissues and structures of the nose. You may need to tip the patient's head backward to help visualize the turbinates.

The nasal mucosa should be moist and dark pink. The inferior and middle turbinates should be visible and be the same color as the surrounding area (see Figure 20-24).

Pale pink or bluish-gray turbinates that appear boggy and swollen suggest allergies, whereas increased redness of the mucosa is an indicator of inflammation and/or an infection.

Asymmetrical cavities suggest a deviated septum (see Figure 20-11).

Crusting on the anterior portion of the septum may be associated with epistaxis or an indicator of extremely dry climate.

A polyp, a rounded, elongated mass, protruding from the turbinates into the nasal chamber may occasionally be observed (Figure 20-25).

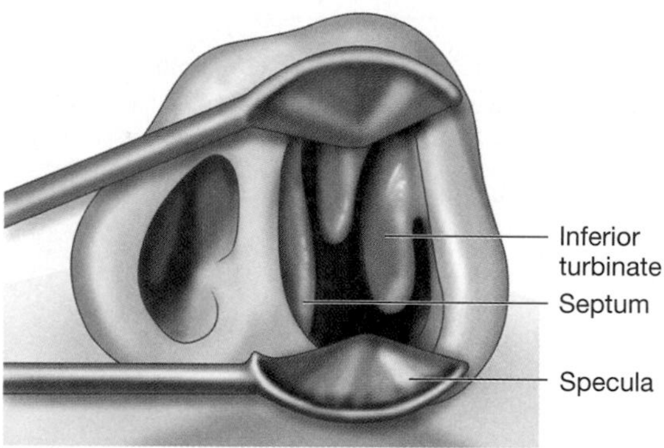

FIGURE 20-24 Internal structures of nose

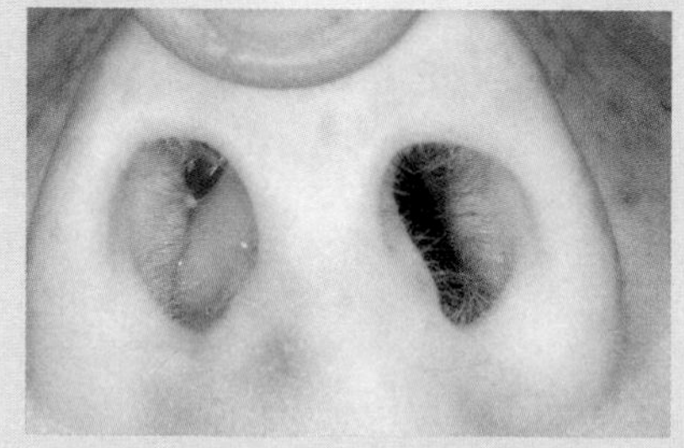

FIGURE 20-25 A nasal polyp is an unexpected finding
Source: Dr. P. Marazzi/Science Source Images

The nasal septum should be straight and midline without any perforations, bleeding, or crusting. The anterior section of the septum should appear thicker than the posterior section. The posterior nasal cavities should appear symmetrical.

Assessment of the sensation of smell via the olfactory nerve (CN I) may be performed here, but is considered a part of the neurological exam. In this exam, the patient is asked to identify and differentiate various smells and odors that are presented. More specific details are described in Chapter 26.

Inspection Techniques and Expected Findings	Unexpected Findings

Mouth (Internal)

Buccal Mucosa

Inspect the hard palate by having the patient tilt the head back, and then directing the light onto the roof of the mouth to visualize it (see Figure 20-26). The hard palate is much lighter in color than the rest of the mouth and somewhat dome-shaped with transverse rugae present. There should be no lesions or nodules present on the surface of the hard palate.

A midline bony ridge protruding from the hard palate is a **torus palatines** (Figure 20-27). This is a benign growth that has no clinical significance.

A nodule that is not midline is suggestive of a tumor.

Other lesions present on the palate or oral cavity are frequently associated with other diseases. A common lesion is that of Kaposi's sarcoma, which is related to HIV infection.

In a small number of individuals, the uvula is split, resulting is a **bifid uvula** (see Figure 20-28). This can be a minor split that occurs at its tip or it could continue upward, almost splitting the uvula into two. A split uvula is nonsignificant and is mostly a cultural variation; however, it may be associated with altered fusion of the soft palate and an indicator of a submucosa cleft.

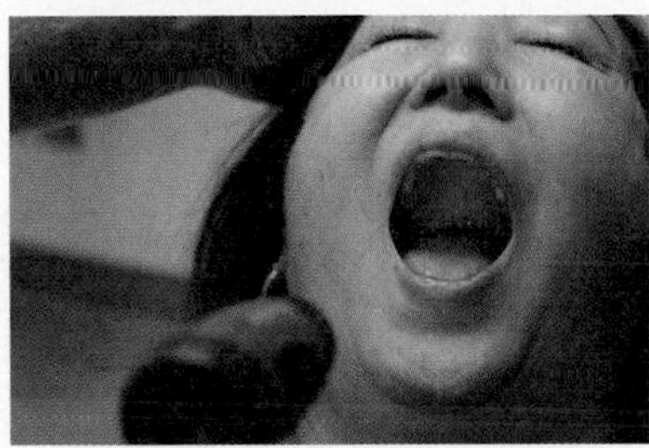

FIGURE 20-26 Visualization of palate

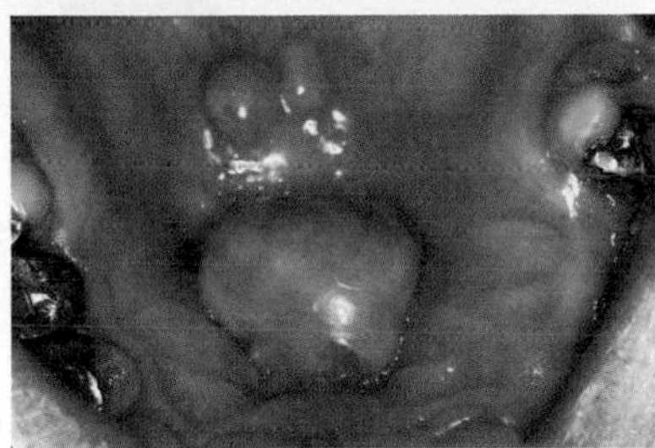

FIGURE 20-27 While unexpected, torus palatines has no clinical significance

Source: E.H. Gill/Custom Medical Stock Photo

The soft palate is pinker, smoother, and a continuation of the hard palate. It is mobile and can be elevated upwards. The uvula is a fleshy, conical shaped projection of the soft palate, hanging downward from the midline (see Figure 20-28).

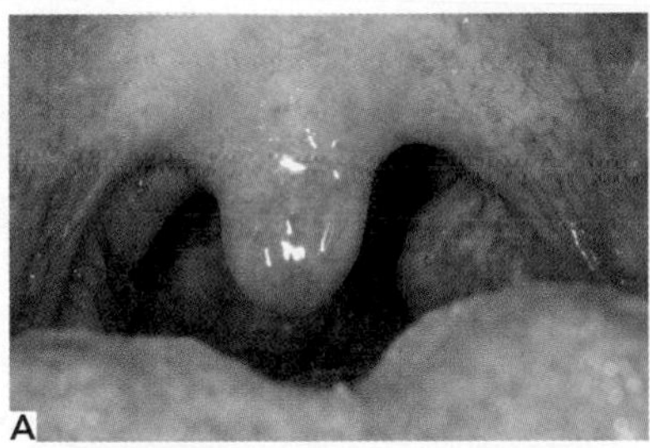

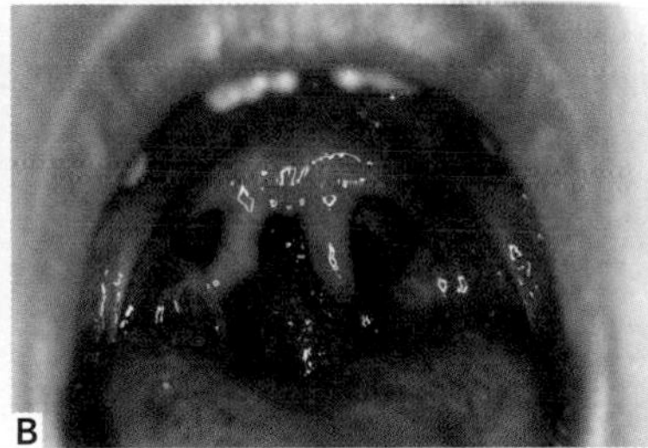

FIGURE 20-28A–B Uvula and split uvula

Sources: a. Dr. P. Marazzi/Science; b. Wellcome Image Library/Custom Medical Stock

Assess elevation of the soft palate by asking the patient to say "ahh," using a tongue depressor, if needed. Place the tongue blade on the posterior aspect of the tongue and press downward. Be careful not to place the tongue blade too far back as this will initiate the gag reflex. As the patient is vocalizing "ahh," observe the movement of the soft palate upwards, which should be symmetrical with the uvula maintaining its midline position.

When the patient is biting down, the trigeminal (CN V) nerve is also being tested. The details of testing CN V are presented in Chapter 26.

Failure of the soft palate to rise symmetrically may be an indicator of vagus (CN X) paralysis. In this instance, the uvula will deviate toward the affected side. Movement of the soft palate and uvula assesses the integrity of the glossopharyngeal (CN IX) and vagus (CN X) cranial nerves. Specific details are presented in Chapter 27.

Inspection Techniques and Expected Findings	Unexpected Findings

Tongue

Assess the ventral surface of the tongue and mouth floor by having the patient touch the roof of the mouth, as far back as possible (Figure 20-29), with the tip of the tongue. The ventral surface should glisten and present a network of small blood vessels. The frenulum is midline and does not prevent the tongue from touching the roof of the mouth.

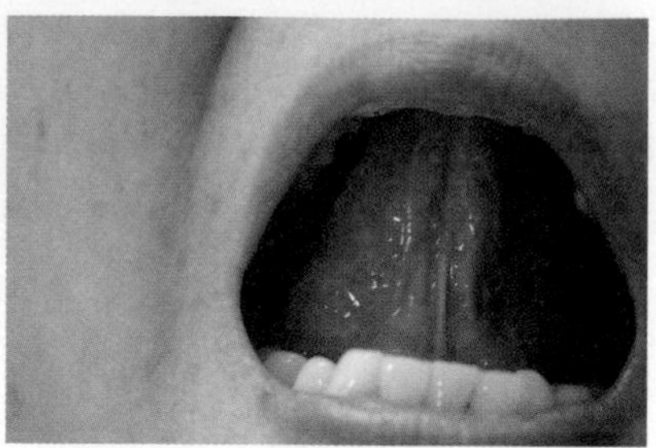

FIGURE 20-29 Asking the patient to touch the top of the mouth with the tongue to check its ventral surface

Inspect the lateral sides of the tongue by having the patient move the tongue side to side, pausing when the tongue is in the extreme side position. If the patient is unable to do this or if closer inspection is needed, place a section of cotton gauze on the dorsal and ventral aspect of the tongue and grasp the tongue between your thumb and index finger (see Figure 20-30). Apply slight pressure with thumb and finger.

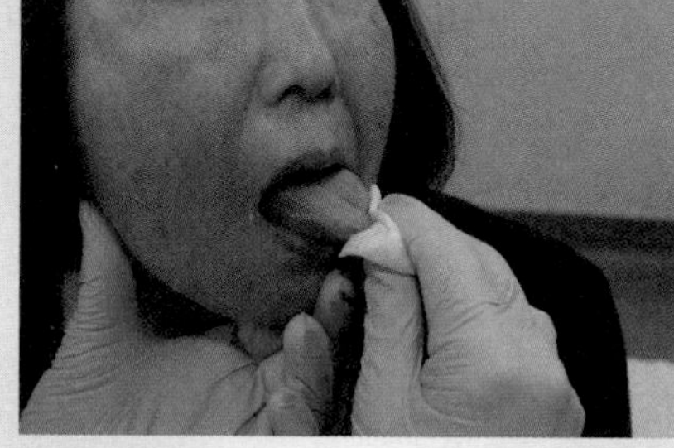

FIGURE 20-30 Provider holding tongue with cotton gauze square showing lateral side of tongue

Throat

The next area to be assessed is the posterior aspect of the throat, which primarily involves the anterior and posterior pillars and the palatine tonsils in between the pillars. These structures are assessed for color, size and surface characteristics.

Tonsils that are inflamed or infected will commonly present as enlarged (+3, +4), due to swelling, and red in color (Figure 20-32).

The size of the tonsils is graded on a +4 scale according to the following criteria (Figure 20-31):

+1 = tonsils visible

+2 = lateral border extends to halfway between the pillars and uvula

+3 = lateral borders extend to touch the uvula

+4 = lateral borders touch each other

Tonsils that are +1 or +2 are observed in healthy individuals. The surface of the tonsil is generally smooth; however, there may be small indentations or crypts visible in some individuals. These crypts may collect food debris or other small particles, but this is usually a nonsignificant finding.

Larger tonsils may be observed in children as lymphoid tissue is enlarged until puberty.

There may or may not be an exudate on the surface of the tonsils in the case of infected tonsils. Crypts that contain food or other particles may be mistaken for exudate that accompanies infected tonsils.

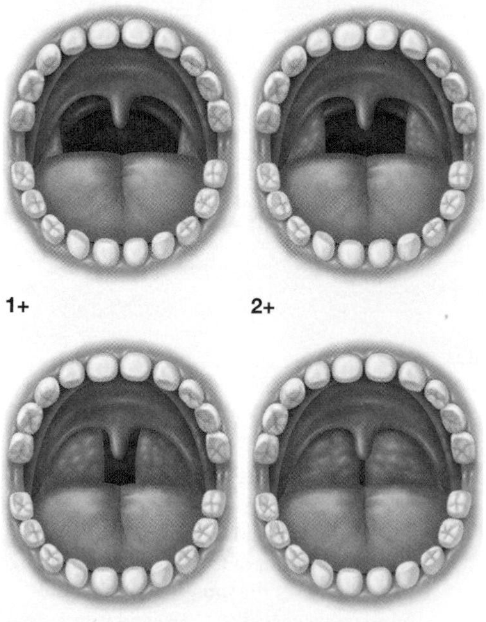

FIGURE 20-31 Grading of the tonsils

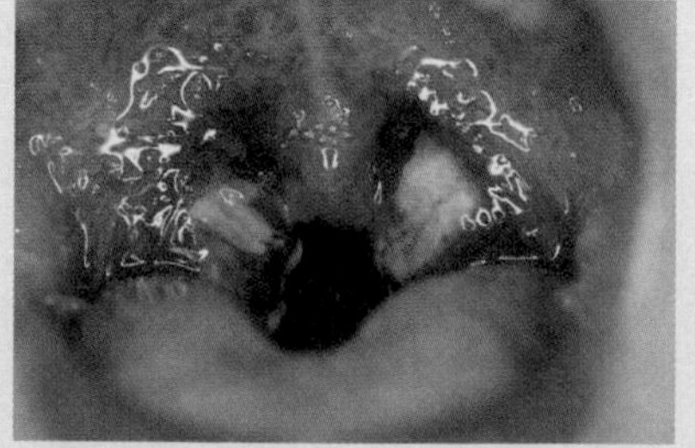

FIGURE 20-32 Inflamed tonsils with exudates
Source: Dr. P. MarazziScience Source Images

Inspection: Level III

Examination of the nose, mouth, sinuses, and throat in emergency situations is primarily related to traumatic injuries. The face is the most exposed portion of the body and most often is also the least protected (Chao, 2011). Facial trauma includes soft tissue damage caused by burns, lacerations, and contusion, as well as fractures of the facial bones, including fractures of the jaw. Symptoms that accompany facial trauma are specific to the injury and commonly consist of pain, swelling, loss of function, and altered shape of the facial structures. The soft tissues of the face are highly vascularized as well as having an abundant nerve supply. Due to the nature of blood vessel and nerve distribution, facial trauma is quite painful, with extensive bleeding. Facial trauma may also involve the eyes and ears; however, these are covered in Chapters 18 and 19.

Inspection Techniques and Expected Findings	Unexpected Findings
Inspection of the mouth is primarily done when there is evidence of facial trauma. Determine sites of active bleeding and note any trauma to the teeth. Inspect for any evidence of broken or lost teeth. If any teeth have been dislodged, determine if they have been located or retrieved as broken teeth can be reimplanted or transplanted. Also determine if there are any loose teeth present in the mouth that need to be removed.	Soft tissue injuries caused by abrasions and lacerations frequently cause extensive bleeding due to the abundant vascular supply to these tissues. Depending on the location and depth of the injuries, cranial nerves V and VII may also be damaged or compromised. Assess for any damage to these nerves. Major causes of facial trauma are accidental and include moving vehicle accidents, industrial accidents, sports injuries, animal bites, and air guns. Facial trauma may also be intentional and is frequently associated with violence caused by assault and battery, domestic violence, and fights. Moving vehicle accidents used to be the primary cause of facial trauma in developed countries; however, that has been replaced with domestic violence as the primary cause. In developing countries, moving vehicle accidents are still the primary cause of facial injuries.
Nasal Trauma Nasal trauma is defined as any injury to the nose or related structures that may result in bleeding, physical deformity, decreased ability to breathe as expected due to obstruction, or an altered sense of smell. The injury may due to internal or external causes.	External injuries are primarily due to blunt force associated with sports injuries, violence (criminal and domestic), abuse, and moving vehicle accidents (bikes, motor cycles, and cars). Causes of external injury frequently, but not always, result in a nasal fracture. The nasal bones are the most frequently fractured bones of the face and are the third most common type of fracture after wrist and collarbone fractures. Although rarely fatal, nasal bone fractures may interfere with breathing and often result in facial deformities. Nasal bones commonly fractured include the nasal, maxilla, lacrimal, and frontal bones. These bones comprise the nasal septal bones as well as those surrounding the eyes. The zygoma (cheekbone) and frontal bone may also be fractured.

Inspection Techniques and Expected Findings	Unexpected Findings

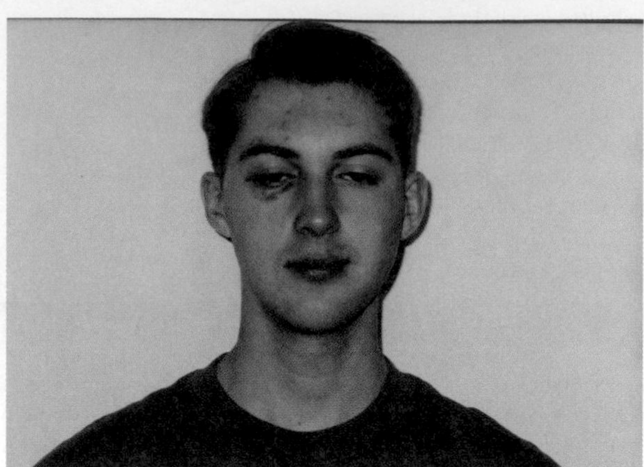

FIGURE 20-33 Hemorrhage around the eyes is an unexpected finding

Direct trauma to the nasal bridge may also cause damage to the cribiform place, which is a section of the base of the skull. This type of damage may result in leakage of cerebrospinal fluid that drains through the nose. Damage to the nasal mucosa may result in formation of scar tissue, which may eventually cause airway obstruction and impairment of the sense of smell. Manifestations of nasal trauma are identified in Table 20-1.

The most common manifestations of nasal trauma include epistaxis, swelling, tenderness of the nasal dorsum, and an obvious nasal deformity. There may also be bruising and bleeding around the eyes (Figure 20-33).

Dental Trauma

Dental trauma is defined as injury to the mouth, including the teeth, lips, gums, tongue, and jawbones. The most frequent type of dental injury is a broken or lost tooth. Causes of dental trauma include those that are associated with nasal trauma, eating hard or hot foods, or drinking hot liquids. A broken tooth frequently has a sharp edge that may cause a laceration of the cheek or tongue. Other soft tissue damage is often caused by falling, hitting or running into a solid or stationary object. Often, individuals may have a sharp or pointed object in the mouth which is pushed against the back of the throat, tongue, or palate. These types of injuries are associated with pain, swelling, and redness, with or without bleeding. A tooth that has been knocked out produces swelling, pain, and bleeding of the socket.

Injury to the tongue is often caused by a fall, seizure, or other types of blunt force.

Tongue lacerations from a fall or seizures occur when it comes between the upper and lower teeth as they clamp down during a seizure or fall. Lacerations that result from a seizure are often observed on the side of the tongue.

A broken jawbone may be suspected if the upper and lower teeth are not aligned appropriately (malocclusion). Additionally, the individual may experience pain in or around the temporomandibular joint as well as a limited ability to open and close the jaw.

Table 20-1 Manifestations of nasal trauma

Type I	Frontal or frontolateral trauma	Injury restricted to soft tissue	Frontal force causes damage ranging from simple fracture of the nasal bones to flattening of the entire nose.
Type IIa	Lateral trauma	Simple, unilateral nondisplaced fracture	Lateral force may depress only one nasal bone; however, with sufficient force, both bones may be displaced. Lateral force can cause severe septal displacement, which can twist or buckle the nose. Septal fragments may interlock, creating further difficulty in reduction.
Type IIb		Simple, bilateral nondisplaced fracture	
Type III	High-velocity trauma	Simple, displaced fracture	
Type IV		Closed comminuted fracture	
Type V		Open, comminuted fracture or complicated fracture	

Inspection: Level IV

There is very little added for a comprehensive examination of the nose, mouth and throat. The procedures and techniques used for the screening exam take minimal time, and all areas and structures assessed are important to cover during a basic examination and do not require advanced skill or training. A Level IV exam may include transillumination of the sinuses and assessment of the teeth for evidence of malocclusion.

Inspection Techniques and Expected Findings	Unexpected Findings

Sinuses

Perform transillumination of the sinuses if there is tenderness noted over the frontal and maxillary sinuses. Do this by shining a light through the sinuses and observing for its passing through the sinuses (see Figure 20-34).

Transillumination is best performed in a darkened room with a transilluminator or a small, bright light. To transilluminate the maxillary sinuses, position the light lateral to the nose, just under the medial aspect of the eye. The light passing through the sinus is observed on the hard palate, inside the patient's mouth. Have the patient open the mouth and look for the light on the hard palate. Perform the procedure on both sides.

To transilluminate the frontal sinuses, position the light against the medial aspect of the supraorbital ridge. Look for a dim red glow just above the eyebrows. Perform the procedure on both sides.

Transmission of light through the sinuses indicates that the sinuses are clear.

Failure to transmit light indicates that the sinuses are congested and filled with secretions. Similar results should be obtained on both sides. Asymmetrical results are significant and may indicate that one sinus is underdeveloped or did not develop.

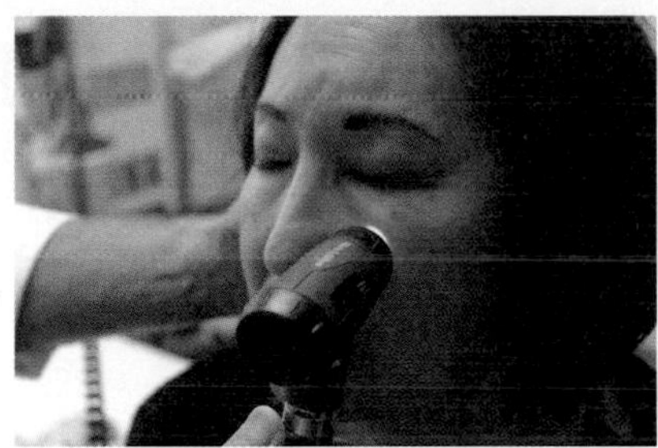

FIGURE 20-34 Transillumination of frontal/maxillary sinuses

Mouth (Internal)

Level IV assessment of the teeth can include a more detailed inspection for the presence of malocclusion. After inspecting the teeth, have the patient bite down and observe the alignment of the teeth. The back teeth should demonstrate the upper teeth are placed directly in the grooves of the lower teeth. In the front, the upper incisors should slightly override the lower incisors.

Malocclusion is classified into three categories (Table 20-2).

If this position of the teeth is not present, there is malocclusion of the teeth (Figure 20-35).

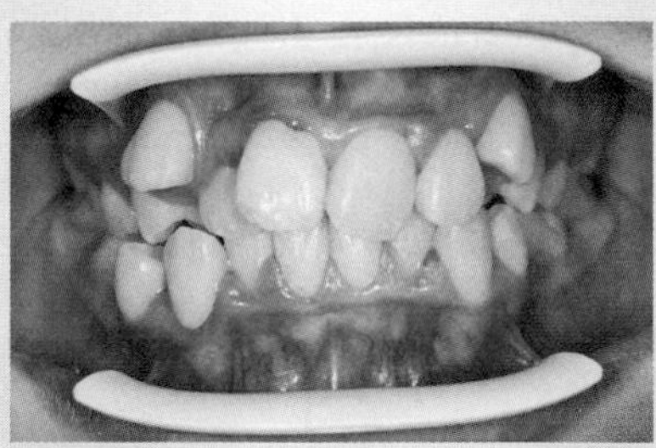

FIGURE 20-35 Malocclusion
Source: botazsolti/Shutterstock

Table 20-2 Classification of malocclusions

Class	Description	Relationship	
		Molar Relation	Canine Relation
Class I	Groove in expected position	The buccal groove of the mandibular first molar is directly in line with the mesiobuccal cusp of maxillary first molar.	The maxillary permanent canine occludes with the distal half of the mandibular canine and the medial half of the mandibular permanent premolar.
Class II, Division 1	Groove is posterior to expected position	The buccal groove of the mandibular first molar is distal to the mesiobuccal cusp of maxillary first molar by at least the width of a premolar.	The distal surface of the mandibular canine is distal to the medial surface of the maxillary canine by at least the width of a premolar.

Continued

Inspection Techniques and Expected Findings	Unexpected Findings

Table 20-2 Classification of malocclusions *(continued)*

Class	Description	Relationship	
	In Class II, Division I all four of the maxillary incisors protrude.		
Class II, Division 2	Groove is posterior to expected position	The buccal groove of the mandibular first molar is distal to the mesiobuccal cusp of maxillary first molar by at least the width of a premolar.	The distal surface of the mandibular canine is distal to the medial surface of the maxillary canine by at least the width of a premolar.
	In Class II, Division 2, both maxillary lateral incisors protrude while both central incisors retrude.		
Class III	Groove is anterior to expected position	The buccal groove of the mandibular first molar is medial to the mesiobuccal cusp of maxillary first molar by at least the width of a premolar.	The distal surface of the mandibular canine is medial to the medial surface of the maxillary canine by at least the width of a premolar.

Palpation: Level I

Palpation Techniques and Expected Findings	Unexpected Findings

Nose

Palpate the bridge and soft tissue of the nose. There should be neither tenderness nor displacement of bone or cartilage, nor any masses. The nose itself should feel firm and pliable. Assess the patency of the nares by gently placing a finger on the side of the nose and applying enough pressure to occlude one side (see Figure 20-36). The patient should still be able to inhale and exhale through the opposite naris. Repeat the procedure on the opposite naris. You may also have the patient perform this.

Unexpected findings would be inability to inhale or exhale through each naris.

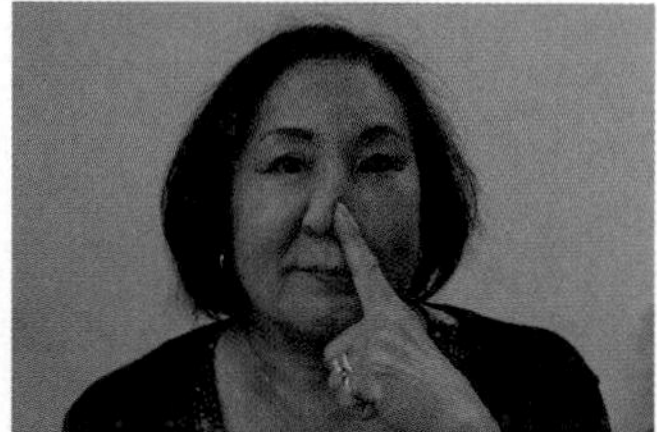

FIGURE 20-36 Assessing patency of nares

Mouth (Internal)

Use palpation to assess the gums, teeth and mucosa surrounding the gums (Figure 20-37). The tongue can also be palpated. The tongue may be palpated for firmness and the presence of any lesions. The tongue is a muscle; therefore, it has a dense texture that gives it a firm feeling. The surface should be smooth without any lesions, nodules, ulcerations, or indurated areas.

Palpate the gums for surface characteristics, particularly for any areas of induration (hardness). The gums and surrounding mucosa should be moist and smooth, without any lumps or hardened areas. The gums should feel firm without any boggy or soft areas.

Soft spongy areas may be an indication of gingival hyperplasia.

The gums should not be tender to palpation nor show any evidence of bleeding or bleeding due to palpation.

If there is any evidence of leukoplakia, palpate for any evidence of induration. Leukoplakia is commonly a firm, indurated lesion that is secured to the underlying tissue and cannot be removed with slight scratching.

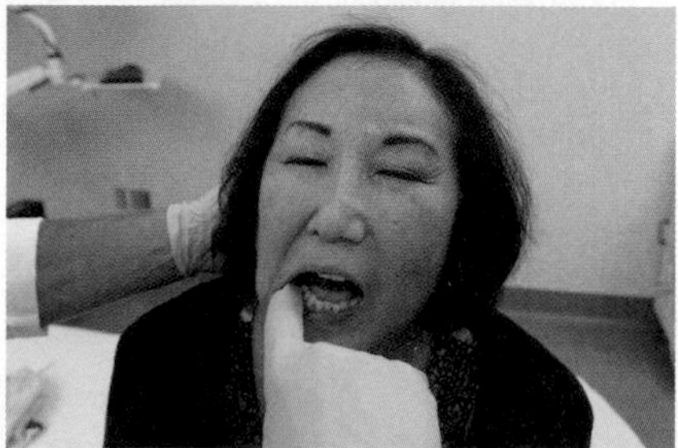

FIGURE 20-37 Palpation of mouth with gloved hand

While palpating the gums, also note any mobility of the teeth. The teeth should be firmly implanted in bone with the gums providing additional structural support.

Gingivitis and periodontal disease may erode the support of the teeth and allow them some movement.

Palpation: Level II

Palpation Techniques and Expected Findings	Unexpected Findings

Sinuses

Palpate the frontal and maxillary sinuses for the presence of tenderness or pain. There should not be any tenderness or pain associated with the pressure.

Unexpected: Any tenderness or pain that is present suggests an infection or obstruction.

Palpate the frontal sinuses by placing the thumbs on the orbital ridge on each side of the nasal bridge and applying upward pressure (see Figure 20-38).

Palpate the maxillary sinuses by placing the thumbs on the zygomatic processes, and again exerting and upward pressure.

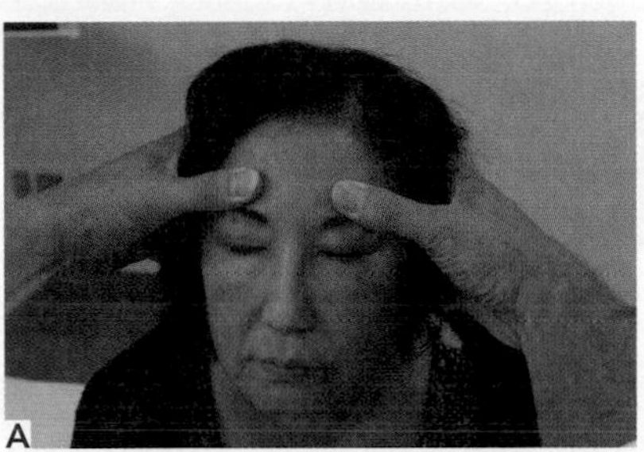
A

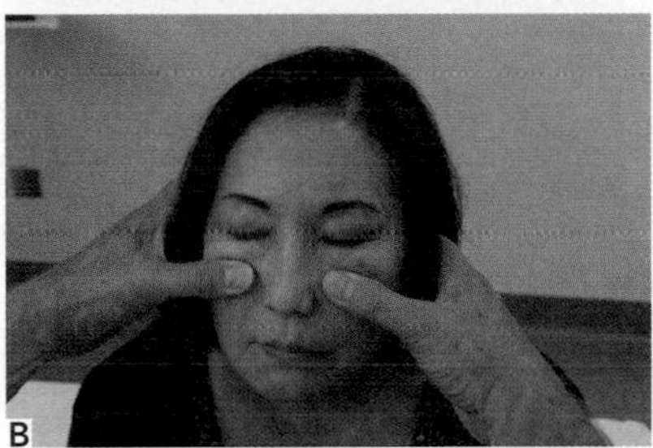
B

FIGURE 20-38A–B Palpation of sinuses

Developmental Applications

Techniques and Expected Findings	Unexpected Findings

Infants and Children

Examination of the nose, mouth and throat of the infant and young child is best done toward the end of a physical examination because this assessment requires the insertion of certain equipment into the nose and oral cavity, which may be perceived as threatening to these patients.

The infant's external nose should be flattened and quite flexible (see Figure 20-39). Determine patency of the nares right after birth.

Unexpected: The nares may be obstructed with amniotic fluid, and should be gently suctioned with a bulb syringe.

If patency is questioned and the infant may be experiencing respiratory distress, the presence of choanal atresia is suspected. This is a condition in which there is membranous or bony plate positioned between the nasal chamber and the oropharynx, obstructing airflow into the lungs.

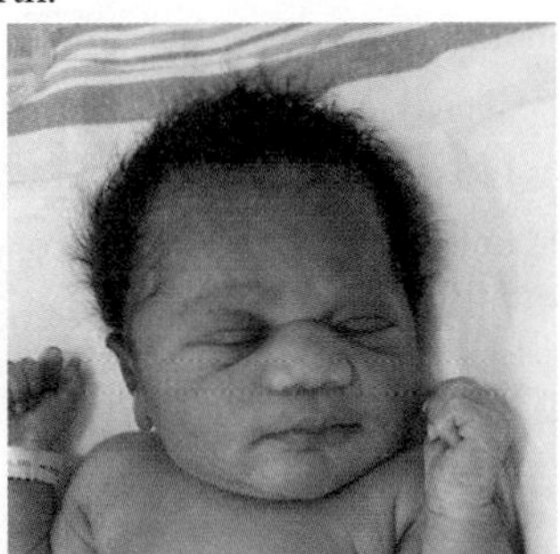

FIGURE 20-39 Infant nose

Passing a small catheter through each nares will determine whether there is choanal atresia.

Unexpected: Failure to pass the catheter indicates obstruction of the nasal passages.

The nasal airway passages of the infant are small, leading to an increased airway resistance. Nose breathing is preferred; however, it has been determined that infants may switch to mouth breathing when necessary (Duderstadt, 2006).

Unexpected: Observe the infant for the presence of nasal flaring, a widening of the nares, which indicates a respiratory distress (see Figure 20-40).

Also observe the nares during feeding, noting any difficulty with breathing, particularly the need to alternate mouth breathing with eating.

Techniques and Expected Findings

In children who experience allergies, observe for the presence of an allergic salute. This presents as a transverse crease across the nose from constant swiping upward with the hand due to constant nasal drainage (see Figure 20-41). Note the presence of any drainage from the nose and its characteristics.

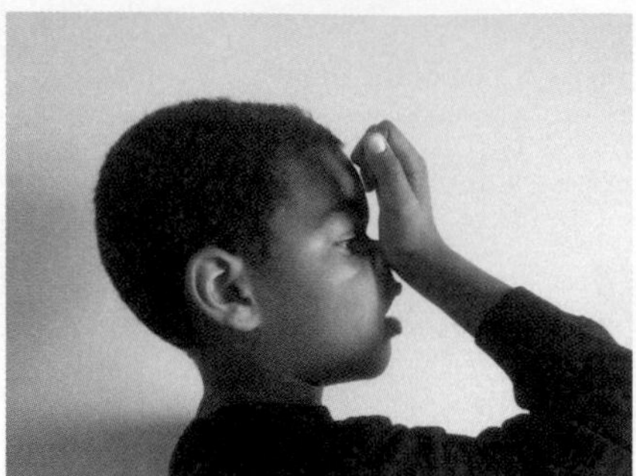

FIGURE 20-41 Allergic salute

Visualization of the nasal chamber may be accomplished with just a light source. While you may use the light from the otoscope, avoid inserting its tip or that of a nasal speculum. Inspection can be accomplished by pushing the tip of the nose upward and shining the light source into the nasal chamber.

The nasal chamber should be free of any blockages caused by foreign objects, polyps, dried nasal secretion, mucus plugs or dried blood. The appearance and characteristics of the nasal chamber are the same as for the adult.

Palpation of the sinuses is performed only on children 8 years and older. The sinuses in children under 8 are limited in their development and too small to actually assess. The area over the sinuses should not be swollen or red in color.

The color and characteristics of the lips and mouth is the same as for the adult.

Saliva secretion does not begin until the infant is 3 months of age and drooling will be present until the infant learns to swallow and control oral secretions. Drooling during teething is also expected.

The mouth of a newborn may present with Epstein's pearls, white pearly papules observed on the hard palate, buccal mucosa and gums. These may be mistaken for erupting teeth, but disappear spontaneously.

Inspect the teeth for number, condition, and pattern of eruption. The number present is related to the infant's or child's age. Note the condition of the teeth. Assess the presence of dental caries and plaque.

Assess the teeth for proper occlusion. Bottle mouth is a serious condition and should be noted.

The tongue should be freely mobile without any lesions or discolorations. The lingual frenulum on the ventral side should permit movement of the tongue past the lips and to the upper palate.

Inspect and palpate the newborn's palate, but after that it is not routinely palpated unless there are lesions, swelling, or erythema. The palate should demonstrate the same characteristics as the adult.

Movement of the soft palate can be observed when the infant is crying and the mouth is open. As with the adult, these movements are also used to assess CNs IX, X, and XII.

Palpate the hard palate to determine if there is a **submucosal cleft** or any other indications of a cleft palate that may not be visible by inspection. While the hard palate is being palpated, it is possible to assess the suck reflex.

If not diagnosed in infancy, it may lead to feeding problems or impaired speech development (Mayo Clinic Staff, 2008).

Unexpected Findings

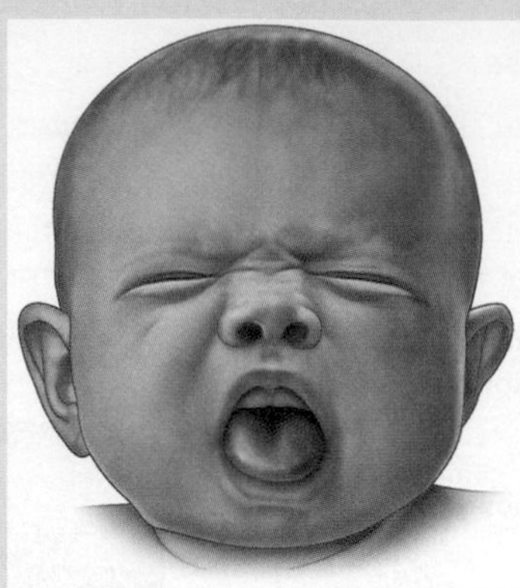

FIGURE 20-40 Nasal flaring in infant indicates respiratory distress

Bilateral drainage usually accompanies allergies and upper respiratory infections.

Drainage due to allergies is generally clear and runny.

Drainage from infections is more mucoid and may be purulent.

Tenderness to palpation is indicative of sinusitis.

Unilateral drainage that is purulent and has a foul odor is often the result of a foreign object in the nose.

Epistaxis may be present and due to irritation/dryness of the nasal mucosa, allergies, or trauma.

If a foreign object is suspected or visualized, have the child attempt to dislodge it by occluding one side of the nose and instructing the child to "blow the nose." If this is not successful, try using small tweezers or a curette. If the object has been lodged in position for an extended period of time, it may be adhered to the nasal wall or septum, making removal difficult (Figure 20-42).

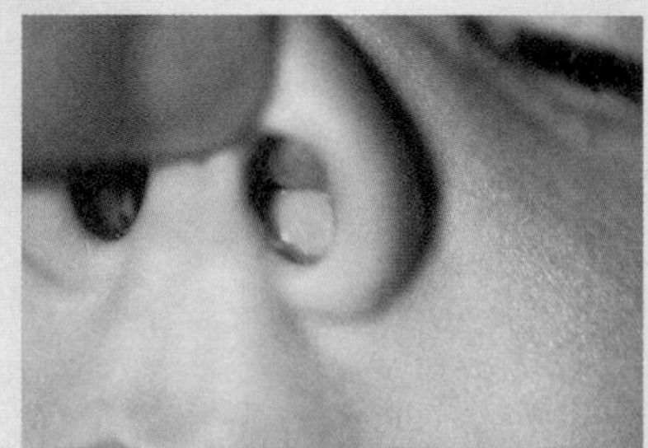

FIGURE 20-42 Foreign object in child's nose
Source: Dr. P. Marazzi/Science Source

Techniques and Expected Findings

Assess the tonsils for color, size, and external characteristics. The tonsils are not visible in the newborn, but gradually enlarge through childhood up to puberty.

The color of the tonsils is the same as the rest of the buccal mucosa, or slightly more pink. The size of the tonsils should be equal and graded on a +4 scale. The surface of the tonsils is smooth, with the possibility of small indentations or crypts.

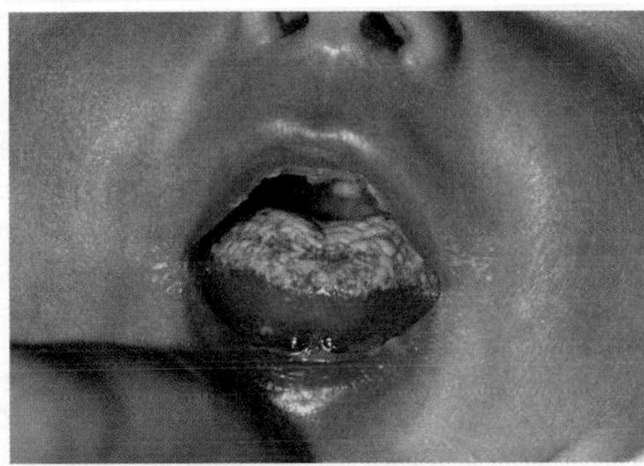

FIGURE 20-43 Thrush is an unexpected finding
Source: Dr. P. Marazzi/Science Source

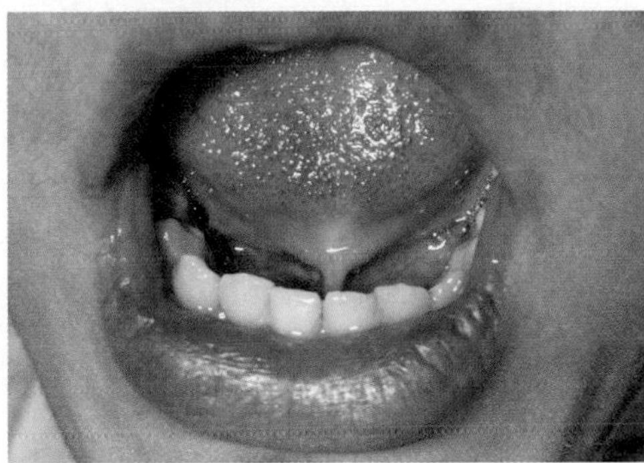

FIGURE 20-44 Anklyoglossia is an unexpected finding
Source: Dr. P. Marazzi/Science Source

Unexpected Findings

Inability to remove the object will require removal by a pediatric otolaryngologist.

Young infants who are nursing or bottle-fed may have a sucking tubercle on the lips which may appear like a blister or callous.

Drooling beyond 15 months may indicate nerve damage and inability to control oral secretions.

White superficial lesions of the mouth are frequently associated with candidiasis, a yeast infection seen in infants and young children. Often referred to as "thrush," this occurs primarily after taking antibiotics or with chronic infections (Figure 20-43). These lesions should not be confused with leukoplakia.

White spots on the primary teeth are areas of decalcification and cavitations, which are an early indicator of dental decay. This is an infectious process of decay caused by the *Streptococcus mutans* and may be transmitted from adult to infant during the first few months of life (Duderstadt, 2006).

Discolored yellow or yellow-brown teeth may be the result of the antibiotic tetracycline. This may be from infant/child use of the drug, or from the mother taking it during the last trimester.

Excessive iron ingestion may cause the teeth to appear green or black. This is reversible with a reduction in the intake of iron.

Bottle mouth is a serious condition and should be noted.

A shortened lingual frenulum (ankyloglossia) may interfere with adequate tongue movement and speech development (Figure 20-44). This condition has also been referred to as "tongue tied."

Macroglossia, an enlarged tongue, is characteristic of infants with hypothyroidism and Down syndrome, and other congenital anomalies.

Note the presence of any **bednar aphthae**, which are the result of sucking. These are small, yellow-white, slightly elevated ulcerated patches that appear on the posterior hard palate on either side of the midline.

Techniques and Expected Findings	Unexpected Findings
	Dark pink to red enlarged tonsils may be present in children with chronic respiratory allergies or viral infection. Bacterial infection is frequently accompanied by a yellow-white exudate that covers the surface of the tonsil and is in the crypts. Tonsillar exudate may also be a manifestation of infectious mononucleosis.
The Pregnant Woman Increased estrogen in the pregnant female results in edema and erythema of the nose and pharynx as well as increased mucus production. There may also be a feeling of sinus congestion and frequent symptoms of a cold. These changes may also result in nosebleeds.	Gingival hypertrophy may also be observed, characterized by swollen, spongy, and red gums that have lost their stippling, making them also appear smooth. The hypertrophy will resolve within two months of delivery.
The Older Adult The nose of the older adult patient often appears more prominent as there is loss of subcutaneous tissue. The nasal mucosa appears less shiny and drier. Bristly hairs also begin to appear in the nasal vestibule, particularly in males. The sense of smell may be diminished, but the ability to differentiate odors should not be affected.	Decreased saliva production affects the self-cleaning characteristics of the mouth, leaving the teeth, tongue and buccal mucosa susceptible to mouth odor, retention of food particles, and poor dental hygiene.
Decreased saliva production may make the lips and mouth drier. The buccal mucosa is thinner and less vascular, giving it a less shiny appearance. If the patient wears dentures, observe for any indications of a poor fit—reddened area, ulcers, etc. The gums appear paler and the stippling may be slightly decreased. There should be no evidence of gingivitis or periodontal disease. The teeth appear somewhat elongated due to exposure of the root surface as bone resorption of the jaw takes place. Note the number of teeth; this will vary depending on the patient's dental hygiene practices and care. The surfaces of the teeth may be slightly worn down, simply due to the age of the patient. If any restorations are evident, note any evidence of deterioration. The tongue may appear more fissured and there may a slight white coating on the tongue. There is a loss of papillae, resulting in a smoother texture of the tongue as well as a diminished sense of taste. Varicosities of the veins on the ventral aspect of the tongue are frequently evident. The tonsils may or may not be visible. If they were removed during childhood, the reason is clear; however, they also may have atrophied to the point where they are difficult to visualize. If they are present, note the surface characteristics and the presence of multiple crypts.	In the majority of cases in which an elderly person complains of severe dry mouth (xerostomia) it is due to medications that they are taking. Many types of medications may cause xerostemia—both non- prescription and prescription drugs, including antihistamines, antihypertensives, antidepressants, pain killers, tranquilizers, and diuretics. Lack of saliva from xerostemia can have significant effects on oral health, such as plaque build-up and the increased risk for gingivitis and periodontal disease. Saliva also bathes the teeth, neutralizes acids, removes bacteria responsible for acid production, and provides a mineral barrier that protects the outer surface of the teeth. Thus a reduction in saliva may lead to increased acid production. Dry mouth can also affect the ability to taste, chew, and swallow. The tongue may also become sensitive and even painful. The oral mucosa may become swollen, red, and painful.

PRACTICE POINT: Elderly Nutrition and Teeth Condition

Any alteration of the teeth may have a significant effect on nutrition. Malocclusion, periodontitis, extensive caries and/or erosion, and missing teeth all affect the ability to chew. Chewing may be painful or simply not effective in breaking down food. Difficulty in chewing will impact the patient's food choices. Assess the patient's ability to take in adequate amounts of nutritional elements. While it may be possible to take in adequate nutritional elements by choosing foods that are easy to chew or that don't have to be chewed, this may not be the case. The ability to taste is also going to affect food choices. If the taste sensation has decreased, food will no longer taste good, thus affecting food choices.

DOCUMENTATION

Upper and lower lips are approximated with equal symmetry. Lip borders well defined and both lips same color. Surface of lips smooth with vertical lines. Without any evidence of lesions, swelling, cracking.

Mucosal lining of mouth intact, shiny, moist, smooth, and coral pink in color. Color evenly distributed without any red or white patches. No areas of swelling or apparent growths. No distinct odors noted.

Gingiva intact, firm to touch, without any evidence of hyperplasia, or pocket formation. 32 teeth present with evidence of dental restorations. Teeth firmly imbedded in gingival, some tartar on central incisors but without any evidence or redness or pocket formation. Teeth of uniform color and no visual evidence of caries formation. Appropriate occlusion of teeth when upper teeth placed over lower teeth.

Tongue dark pink in color with even color distribution. Symmetrical in appearance with midline placement and protrusion. Papillae visible on surface without any areas of smoothness noted. Scattered areas of white coating but no specific white or red lesions noted. Tongue firm to touch. Size of tongue appropriate to size of oral cavity. Ventral surface of tongue/floor of mouth shiny with visible small blood vessels. Lingual frenulum midline and patient able to touch roof of mouth with tip of tongue. Stenson's and Wharton's ducts visible, without any swelling or redness.

Hard and soft palate intact with visual midline ridge. Mucosa firmly attached to bone and hard and firm to touch. Soft palate spongy with uvula midline. Symmetrical elevation with midline elevation of uvula.

Palatine tonsils visible between anterior and posterior pillars. Tonsil size +2. Mucosa intact with even color distribution. Slightly darker in color, but not inflamed. Tonsil surface with some small crypts but no evidence of food in them or any exudate.

Electronic Charting

Expectations of Electronic Charting

You should be able to chart all portions of the nose, mouth, and throat exam, including, when applicable, smell and taste evaluations. The nose, mouth, and throat structures and associated systems are closely linked and you should be able to navigate easily between parts of the exam. The electronic charting should be able to incorporate graphics or images. For example, the presence of patches inside the mouth may be best documented by an image of the lesion.

Among the most well-developed charting systems related to nose, mouth, and throat are records for oral and dental care. Such records need to accommodate radiological technology and digital imaging. Oral/dental findings may reflect overall health, and the charting systems used by dental providers should be compatible with, or at least able to communicate with, the overall electronic health record.

Electronic charting systems should incorporate decision support features that support evidence- based practice. For example, an ideal electronic charting system might alert providers to check for gum disease in pregnant women who have high levels of C-reactive protein, and provide a link to literature showing that pregnant females with gum disease and high levels of C-reactive protein are at a greater risk for developing preeclampsia.

Limitations of Electronic Charting

Forms to document the nose, mouth, and throat examination may be difficult to locate in the electronic record. The components of the exam may be integrated with documentation of respiratory system, gastrointestinal system, or other exams. The components may be split into multiple areas of the chart. Examination of the oral mucosa and teeth, for example, may be isolated into a dental exam form while examination of the nose may be part of a head and neck exam form.

Summary

- The nose is an external triangular structure in the mid-position of the anterior face and functions as an airway to warm and moisten air before it enters the lungs. The mouth is a cavity within the cranium that contains the tongue, teeth, and salivary glands. The opening to the mouth is bordered by the upper and lower lips.
- The throat is the posterior portion of the mouth that begins at the pillars, which contains the tonsils and has connections to the esophagus and trachea. The sinuses are also cavities within the cranium, which function to decrease the weight of the skull bones, resonate sound, and provide mucous that drains into the nasal chambers.
- Variations in structure and function are assessed primarily by inspection and include inflammatory and infections processes, traumatic injuries as well as congenital malformations. Inflammation and infection are associated with pain and discomfort and it may be necessary to remove some structures to prevent further problems. Trauma causes structural damage and if not treated may interfere with breathing.
- An infant's nose, mouth, and throat are fully developed at birth. The sinuses are not fully developed until late childhood. The infant is an obligate nose breather. The infant has no teeth but the deciduous (baby) teeth (20) begin erupting around 6 months of age.
- Permanent teeth begin replacing deciduous teeth around 6 years of age. The development of cavities in permanent teeth is the primary cause for destruction of teeth. Permanent teeth are not physiologically replaced if they are lost or destroyed. The development of periodontal disease is a major concern for the older client.

Review Questions

1. The provider is explaining the structure of the nose to a patient with a recent facial injury. The provider should include in this teaching that the structure and shape of the nose is maintained by which of the following?
   1. cartilage and bone
   2. bone and muscle
   3. cartilage and connective tissue
   4. connective tissue and muscle
2. The provider documents assessment findings from a patient seen in the emergency department and notes that the patient presented with epistaxis. This indicates that the patient had which of the following?
   1. inflamed sinuses
   2. bleeding from the nose
   3. loss of taste
   4. enlarged turbinates
3. The provider notes on inspection of a patient's internal nose enlarged, pale turbinates with thin clear secretions. These findings are consistent with which of the following?
   1. sinusitis
   2. nasal polyps
   3. parotitis
   4. allergies
4. When performing a health assessment on an adult patient the provider uses the technique of transillumination. The provider is aware that transillumination is an appropriate technique to use when
   1. the turbinates are swollen.
   2. the sinuses are tender.
   3. a septum deviation is suspected.
   4. choanal atresia is suspected.
5. During inspection of the mouth of a pregnant female, the provider would expect to find which of the following?
   1. an enlarged tongue with a white coating
   2. tonsils that are +3 with increased redness
   3. hyperplasia of the gums with increased redness
   4. an increase of saliva with hyperplasia of the submandibular gland
6. When inspecting the mouth of a 4-year-old, the provider is aware that an expected finding would be which of the following?
   1. inability to touch the roof of the mouth with the tongue
   2. a split uvula
   3. a bony ridge at the midline of the palate
   4. presence of 20 deciduous teeth
7. Symptoms that would cause the provider to suspect that a patient has an oral cancer would be which of the following? (Select all that apply.)
   1. loose teeth
   2. presence of white patches on the tongue
   3. difficulty swallowing
   4. bloody nose
   5. hyperplasia of the gums
8. When examining the patient the provider examines the Wharton's duct, which is responsible for draining which of the following?
   1. middle turbinates
   2. frontal sinuses
   3. parotid gland
   4. palatine tonsils
9. An older adult patient tells the provider of a loss of appetite and that "food does not taste the same anymore." Keeping expected changes of aging in mind, the provider discusses methods of addressing the problem such as which of the following? (Select all that apply.)
   1. keeping the mouth moist and maintaining hydration
   2. enhancing the flavor of foods with spices and herbs
   3. having a feeding tube surgically inserted
   4. including foods with high saturated fat content in all meals
   5. using an oral antimicrobial rinse to reduce risk of infection
10. When inspecting the throat of a patient the provider notes that the tonsils touch the uvula.This finding is most accurately documented by the provider by noting the tonsils as which of the following?
    1. 1+
    2. 2+
    3. 3+
    4. 4+

Conditions and Disorders

Choanal Atresia (CA)

CA is a congenital disorder where the back of the nasal passage (choana) is blocked, usually by abnormal bony or soft tissue (membranous) due to failed recanalization of the nasal fossae during fetal development that presents as obstruction of one or both posterior nasal cavities. CA occurs in approximately 1 in 7,000–8,000 live births and is the most common abnormality of the nose of newborns. In the majority of cases, it is unilateral and is not associated with any other anomalies. Females are affected twice as frequently as males.

Unilateral CA occurs predominately on the right side. In cases where it is bilateral, it is associated with other congenital anomalies, particularly CHARGE, Treacher-Collins, and Crouzon's syndromes.

Pathophysiology

- The exact cause is unknown but current thought is that is results from persistence of the membrane that develops between the nasal chamber and oropharynx during the seventh week of fetal development.
- There is no precipitating factor that appears to predispose and infant to the development of CA; there is a slightly increased risk with twins.
- The age of the mother as well as the number of pregnancies do not appear to have any effect on the incidence of CA.
- Recent evidence suggests that the antithyroid drugs, carbimazole, and methimazole are responsible for the development of CA in infants whose mothers have taken these drugs during pregnancy (Wolf, Foulds, & Daya, 2006).

Subjective Data

- As a congenital deformity, the infant is unable to identify symptoms.

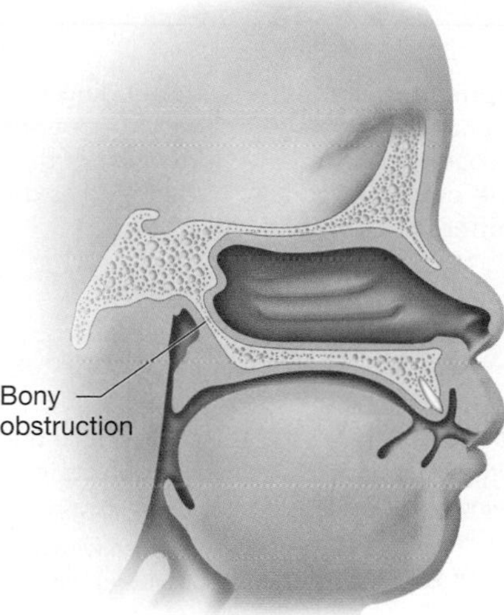

FIGURE 20-45 Choanal atresia (CA)

Objective Data

- Bilateral CA is evident shortly after birth; the infant with CA will demonstrate acute breathing difficulties with cyanosis, and respiratory failure.
- If unilateral, the manifestations are less severe.
- If CA is suspected in a newborn, the diagnosis may be confirmed by the inability to pass a small catheter (6–8F) through the nares into the nasopharynx.

Dental Cavities (Caries)

Tooth decay is a common disorder, second only to the common cold, usually occurring in children and young adults but can affect any person. Tooth decay is a common cause of tooth loss in younger people.

Pathophysiology

- Bacteria in plaque (Streptococcus mutans, lactobacillis, actinomyces) act on sugars/carbohydrates converting them to acids. The pH of the mouth ranges from 6.2 to 7.0. If the oral environment becomes more acidic (< 5 to 6.0), the acids begin to dissolve the minerals of the tooth's surface (calcium and phosphate) producing microscopic lesions on tooth enamel.
- Once all sugars are depleted, acid production ceases; replacement of minerals and repair of tooth begins. Minerals in saliva as well as fluoride are essential to restoration of tooth enamel.
- Failure to remove plaque/ over consumption of sugars reduces the time needed for restoration, allowing the formation of a cavity. The continuous assault of acid on the tooth results in tooth decay.
- Once enamel is breached, decay continues into the softer dentine and tooth pulp, eventually exposing the nerves.

Subjective Data

- A toothache occurs once the decay passes through enamel, the dentinal tubules, which have passages to the nerve of the tooth, and become exposed.
- The pain may worsen with exposure to heat, cold, or sweet foods and drinks.
- Dental caries can also cause bad breath and foul tastes.

Objective Data

- The earliest sign of a new carious lesion is the appearance of a chalky white spot on tooth's surface, indicating an area of demineralization of enamel; called a "microcavity."
- As the lesion continues to demineralize, it can turn brown and will become a cavitation ("cavity").
- A brown, shiny lesion or stain suggests presence of dental caries, but that the demineralization process has stopped.
- A brown spot that is dull in appearance is probably a sign of active caries.

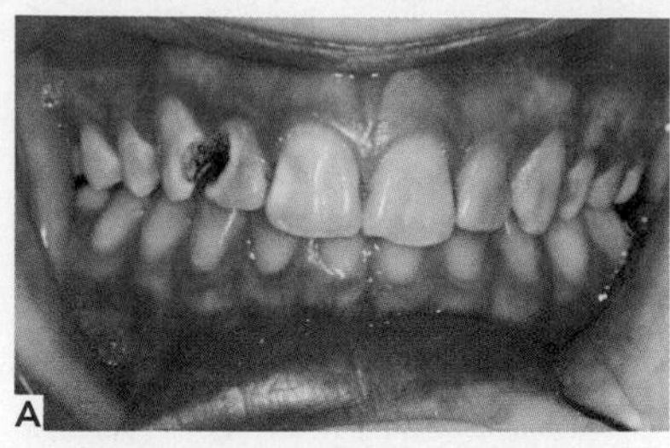

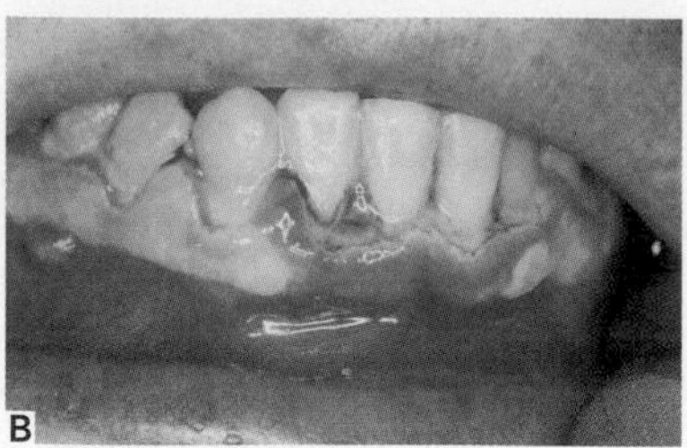

FIGURE 20-46A–B Dental caries and ulcerative gingivitis
Source: Biophoto Associates/Science Source Images

THINK LINK: Dental Caries

The four main criteria necessary for development of caries are a tooth surface (enamel or dentin), caries-causing bacteria, fermentable carbohydrates (such as sucrose), and time. The caries process does not have an inevitable outcome, and different individuals will be susceptible to different degrees depending on the shape of their teeth, oral hygiene habits, and the buffering capacity of their saliva. Because bacteria are involved in the development of dental caries, they may also be identified as dental infections.

Cleft Lip and Cleft Palate

Cleft lip and **cleft palate** (orofacial clefts) are birth defects that occur during fetal development as a result of improper formation/non-fusion of structures that form the mouth, leaving a fissure or opening. Each can occur individually or together. Cleft lip is more common than cleft palate. Isolated orofacial clefts, or clefts that occur with no other birth defects, are one of the most common birth defects in the U.S.

The CDC recently estimated that each year 2,651 babies in the U.S. are born with a cleft palate, and 4,437 babies are born with a cleft lip with or without a cleft palate (Parker et al., 2010).

Pathophysiology

- The exact cause of clefts is unknown. It is thought that there are some genetic contributions as well as environmental factors—drugs (anti-seizure), smoking, viral infections, alcohol, and vitamin B_6 (folic acid) deficiency.
- There may be some familial tendencies for the development of CL and CP; however the risk is less than 10%.
- Gender has a predisposition for each anomaly; males are twice as likely to have cleft lip whereas females are twice as likely to have cleft palate.
- Clefts are more common in infants of Asian and certain Native American groups and are least likely to develop in African American infants (March of Dimes, 2007).

Subjective Data

- It is a congenital deformity in infants.

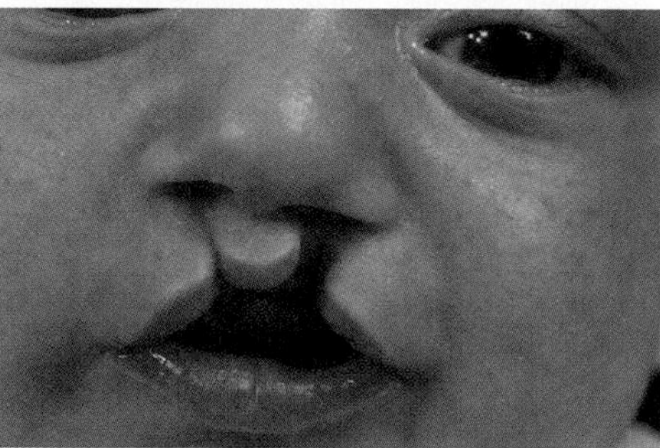

FIGURE 20-47 Cleft lip
Source: Dr. M.A. Ansary/Science Source Images

Objective Data

- Cleft lip and palate have obvious, visible manifestations that are easy to identify immediately after birth.
- There is a vertical gap that exists between the right and left sides of the upper lip, extending to the base of the nose.
- A cleft palate is a gap between the right and left sides of the roof of the mouth and the nasal chamber.
- Submucosal cleft is less common, occurring only in the muscles of the soft palate; concealed by mouth lining, and confirmed by initial palpation of the newborn's mouth.
- If undiagnosed, it may be unknown until feeding problems emerge, or speech development is impaired.

Lymph Glands

21

"This couldn't be... AIDS, could it...?" His voice breaks off as he leans toward me. My patient—Eric Talavera—is a very forthcoming 23-year-old homosexual male, admitted because of a mild fever, fatigue, sore throat, and swollen lymph nodes. Although usually strong willed and optimistic, his anxiety is now palpable. The doctors mentioned that HIV was a distinct possibility given Eric's suggestive sexual history and generalized lymphadenopathy, but I want to be reassuring. "The doctors are still running tests, and there's no use in speculating," I say, switching out the saline bag on his IV pole. "I shouldn't have had unprotected sex." he laments, "What was I thinking?"

"You know, there are lots of things that can cause pharyngitis."

"What's pharyngitis?"

"Sorry, I mean there are many infections that can cause your symptoms, like the sore throat." As a new nurse, I'm still getting used to minimizing medical jargon.

"I see...," he pauses, "...well what do you think is going on?"

I want to excuse myself and page the doctor to speak with him directly, but I know Dr. Fredericks would be busy. I was the one with the patient now, and the one who needed to provide answers and support. But I didn't have any—not yet at least.

"Listen, I know you're concerned, but all we can do is wait for the test results and go from there. If it turns out to be something else, you can consider yourself lucky and make sure to use condoms in the future. In the very least, you have learned something important about safe sex."

"I guess you're right. That helps, thank you." As Eric leans back into his pillow with a heavy sigh, my pager buzzes on my hip. *Re: Talavera—tests confirm infxious mono. Pls tell the pt.* Still looking down at the tiny alphanumeric message, I couldn't help but crack a smile. Giving good news (relatively speaking) always feels good, and I'm eager to be the one to relieve Eric of his burden. Sliding the pager back into its holster, I meet Eric's gaze. "The test results are back...."

LEARNING OUTCOMES

1. Explain the composition and structure of the lymph system.
2. Differentiate between lymph tissue and lymph organs.
3. Compare and contrast manifestations of conditions related to alterations of the lymph system.
4. Explain age-related changes that affect the function and structure of the lymph system.
5. Explain appropriate techniques and maneuvers used for assessment of the lymph system.
6. Identify correct anatomic locations for assessment of lymph system.
7. Summarize documentation findings related to expected and unexpected assessment findings of lymph system.

The lymph glands, along with lymph organs and ducts, are a part of a larger system called the lymphatic system. Much like the neurological system, the lymphatic system is pervasive throughout the entire body and difficult to view as a single, unique system. In other respects, it is also like the cardiovascular system in that it is responsible for circulation of fluid (lymph) throughout the body.

The lymph tissues and organs are a major component of the immune system where they are responsible for **adaptive immune responses**, which is the recognition of foreign substances that pose a threat to the individual and initiating a response to eliminate these foreign invaders. This is in contrast to the **innate immune responses** that rely on intact and functioning physical (skin), mechanical (coughing, sneezing), and chemical (enzymes in saliva, tears, perspiration) protective barriers, as well as the inflammatory process.

Structure and Function

The lymphatic system is a system of nodes, tissues, and organs that are connected by lymph vessels or channels. It circulates lymph and plays a significant role in immunological functions. This system is also responsible for draining interstitial fluid and transportation of dietary fats. **Lymph**, a clear, colorless, alkaline fluid that circulates throughout the body within the lymph vessels is the main component of the lymphatic system. Integral to the lymphatic system are lymphocytes, which are a specific type of white blood cells that are produced in the bone marrow.

Lymph and Lymph Vessels

Lymph originates in the blood as plasma. The pressure within the arterial circulation forces fluid from the blood into the tissues. The majority of this fluid (90%) is reabsorbed across the venous vascular bed; however, the remaining 10% is not reabsorbed and becomes the interstitial fluid, or lymph. Approximately 1 to 2 quarts of lymph circulates through the lymph system and makes up one to three percent of body weight (Lymph Notes, 2007). Lymph removes debris and leftover waste products (dead blood cells, pathogens, cancer cells). It also becomes enriched with dissolved proteins that escape from the intravascular compartment and is absorbed from in between cells.

Lymph vessels originate as lymph capillaries that begin blindly in the intercellular spaces of the soft tissues of the body, just under the skin (see Figure 21-1). They form a meshwork of tiny vessels that branch and interconnect, extending to all tissues. These lymphatic capillaries gradually merge, forming increasingly larger vessels and ending as a lymphatic vessel. The larger lymphatic vessels parallel the venous circulatory network. With the exception of the central nervous system (brain), bone marrow, and placenta, every tissue that is supplied with blood also has lymph circulation.

Movement of the lymph through these capillaries and vessels depends on muscular movement as well as intrathoracic pressure changes that accompany ventilation activity. Smooth muscles in the walls of the vessels also contract sequentially, promoting lymph's forward flow. Lymph vessels contain one-way valves that prevent lymph from flowing back into the tissues.

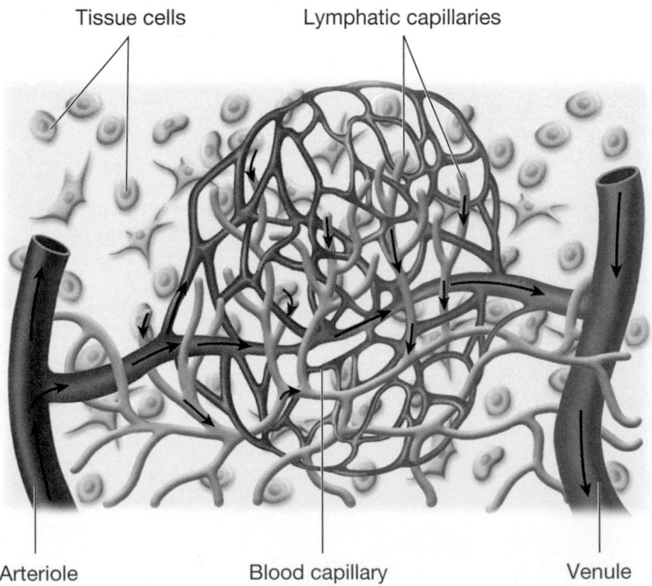

FIGURE 21-1 Lymph circulation (capillaries, vessels)

Lymph is eventually drained into the right lymphatic duct and the thoracic duct (see Figure 21-2). The right lymphatic duct empties into the right subclavian vein and the thoracic duct empties into the left subclavian vein, returning the lymph to the blood.

The small intestine has some unique types of lymphatic vessels, called **lacteals**, that are responsible for absorption and transportation of lipids from the digestive tract (see Figure 21-3).

Lymphoid Tissue

The immunological function of the lymph system occurs primarily in lymphoid tissue and organs. Lymphoid tissue consists mainly of dense aggregates of lymphocytes that are dispersed extensively throughout the body.

Lymphocytes are white blood cells that originate in bone marrow, which then migrate to lymphoid tissues for differentiation and proliferation. The most important lymphocytes are the T and B cells because they are the main participants in the **adaptive immune response**. The B cells differentiate and mature within

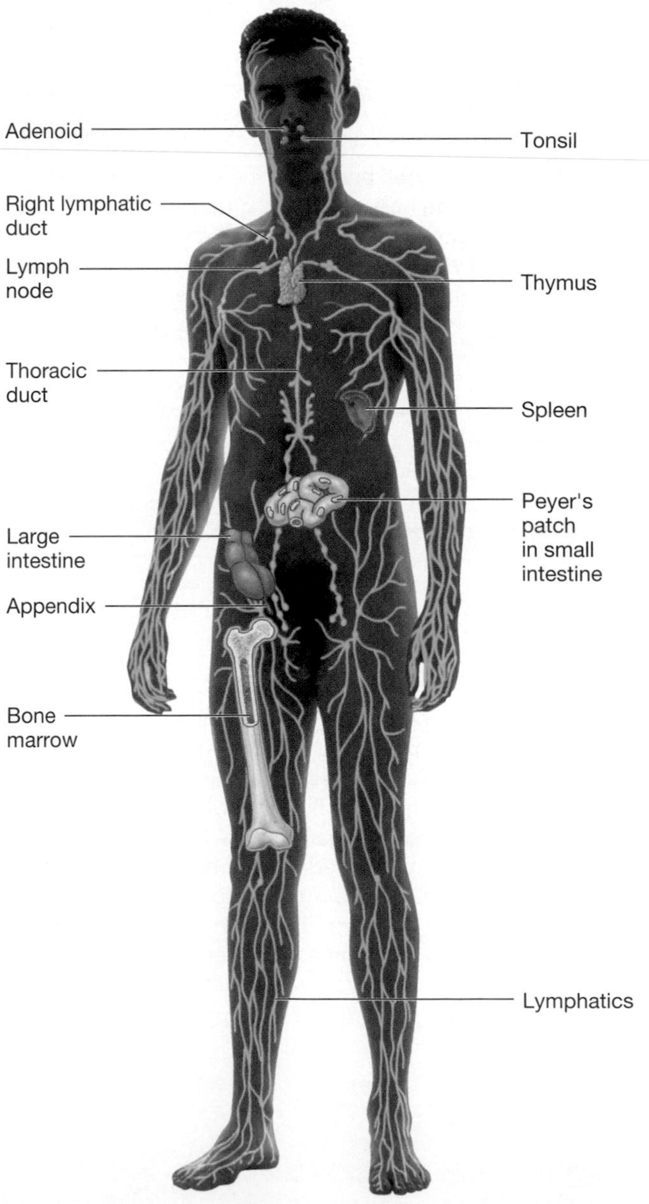

FIGURE 21-2 Drainage of lymph into lymphatic and thoracic ducts

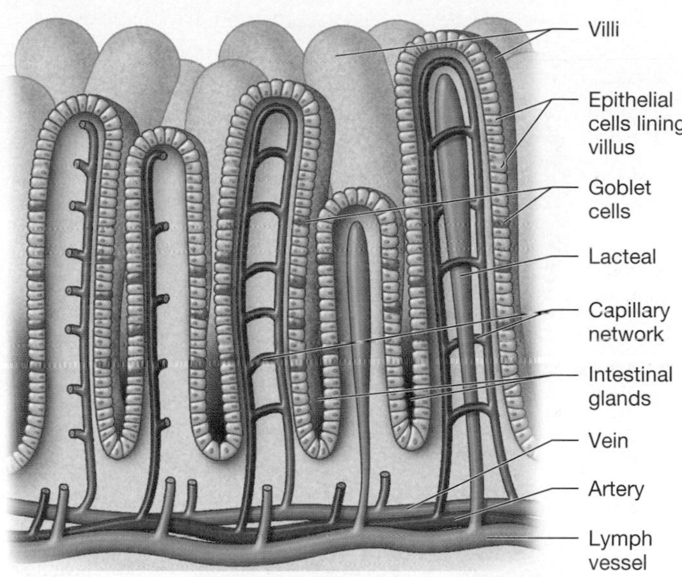

FIGURE 21-3 Lacteals

the bone marrow, and serve the primary function of producing immunoglobulins that participate in the humoral aspect of the adaptive immune response.

The T lymphocytes travel from the bone marrow to the thymus gland where they differentiate into helper T cells (Th cells) and killer T cells (Tk). Helper T cells help both B and Tk cells carry out the immune response. They also recognize antigens and participate in the cellular immune response. Both B and T cells migrate to lymphoid tissue and organs where they remain until they are needed to invoke an immune response.

Lymphoid tissue is comprised of both reticular and lymphatic tissues. Reticular tissue provides the structural matrix and is primarily connective tissue, while lymphatic tissue consists of white cells known as macrophages and lymphocytes. Much of the lymphoid tissue is associated with mucosal epithelium and is located in close proximity to potential portals for the entry of pathogens. These lymphoid tissues are commonly grouped together and described as **mucosal-associated lymphoid tissue (MALT)**. Specific locations for MALT include Peyer's patches within the small intestine, tonsils, adenoids, and the appendix (Grethlein & Perez, 2013). Additional sites for lymphoid tissue include the respiratory and urinary tracts.

The tonsils are aggregations of lymphoid tissue that are situated in the oropharynx and surround the opening to the digestive and respiratory systems. There are two sets of paired tonsils and one single set. The two paired sets are the lingual tonsils and the palatine tonsils and are visible through the mouth in the posterior aspect of the throat. The pharyngeal tonsil (adenoids) is located on the top of the soft palate, just behind the nose, where the nasal passages connect with the throat. The pharyngeal tonsil is not visible through the mouth.

The tonsils and adenoids are strategically located near the entrance to the pulmonary system where they provide surveillance for bacteria and viruses that may be present in inspired air. They also assist in the formation of antibodies to resist and fight present and future infections. This function is important in first few years of life, but becomes less significant as the child ages, most likely after the age of 3. Children who have their tonsils and adenoids removed appear to have no problems with their immune function.

Peyer's patches are aggregates of lymphoid tissue that are scattered throughout the gastrointestinal tract. They are located just under the mucosa throughout the small intestine with the greatest concentration in the ilium and appendix. The lymphoid tissue that is associated with the GI system is analogous to MALT but is referred to as **gut-associated lymphoid tissue (GALT)**.

Lymphoid Organs

The main lymphoid organs are the lymph nodes, thymus, and spleen. They are composed of lymphoid tissue with well-circumscribed borders that are easily differentiated from other surrounding tissue. Lymphoid organs are composed mainly of epithelial cells, or reticular tissue, that contain cells that participate in immune activities.

Lymph Nodes

During the course of lymphatic circulation, lymph vessels pass through specialized lymph tissue identified as lymph nodes. There are approximately 600 to 700 small (1–25 mm), bean-shaped lymph nodes located throughout the human body (see Figure 21-4). They are often in clusters and are identified or described as specific groups, generally in relation to their anatomical location.

Lymph nodes function as a filter to purify the lymph by removing debris, pathogens, and antigens before it is returned to the venous circulation. Lymph nodes contain reticular fibers that trap the debris, macrophages that destroy the pathogens, and dendritic cells that function as antigen presenting cells (APC) that stimulate

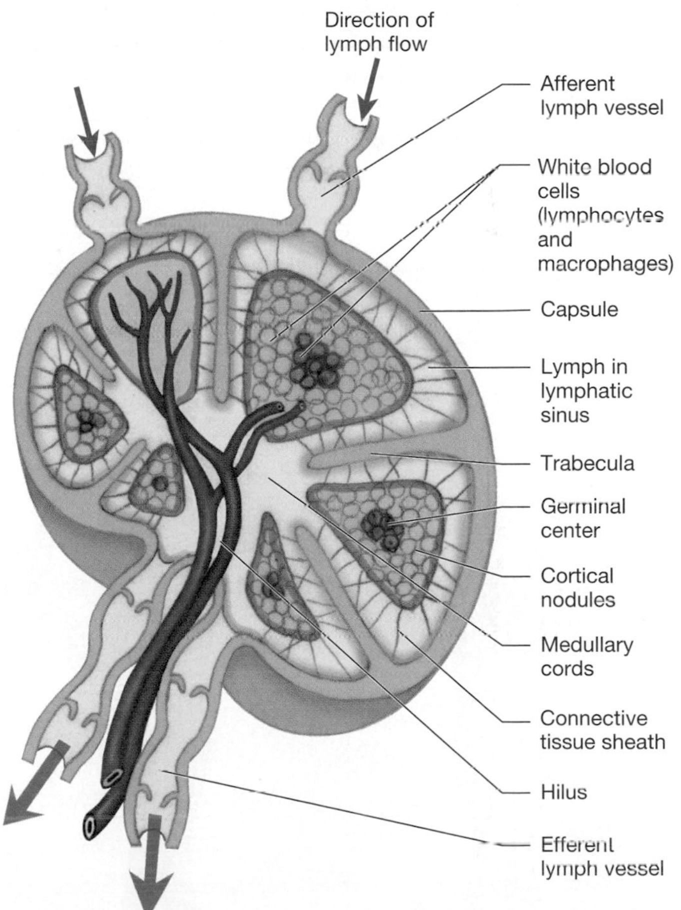

FIGURE 21-4 Lymph node structure

the immune response. Lymph nodes also remove cancerous cells, slowing down the spread of cancer until the lymph node becomes overwhelmed by it.

Lymph nodes are predominately located in the head and neck, axillae, mediastinum, abdomen, and in the extremities along their vascular trunks. Each group drains a particular region of the body (see Figure 21-5).

Head and Neck Lymph Nodes The lymph nodes of the head include the occipital, post-auricular, preauricular, tonsillar, submaxillary, submental. These nodes are located along a chain of lymphatic vessels that begins on the back of the skull, advances toward the back and front of the ear, and then goes down to the mandible and follows the length of the mandible to the point of the chin. The location and drainage of these nodes are identified and described in Figure 21-6.

Cervical (Neck) Lymph Nodes The cervical lymph nodes are located within the anterior and posterior triangles of the neck. The anterior triangle is formed by the medial border of the stermocleidomastoid muscles and the mandible. The posterior triangle is formed by the trapezius and stermocleidomastoid muscles and the clavicle.

Three chains of lymph nodes are positioned in relationship to the triangles (see Figure 21-6). The anterior deep and superficial cervical nodes are a chain of nodes located along the anterior margin of the stermocleidomastoid muscle within the anterior triangle. The posterior cervical and the posterior superficial nodes are two chains of nodes located within the posterior triangle.

Clavicular and Axillary Nodes The clavicular nodes are two groups of lymph nodes that are located above (supraclavicular) and below (subclavicular) the clavicle. They belong to a larger group of lymph nodes that drain the breast area. The axillary nodes are also part of this large group of nodes. The subscapular nodes and anterior axillary nodes are a cluster of nodes that are located within the axillary area. (See Chapter 22 for an illustration of clavicular and axillary lymph nodes.)

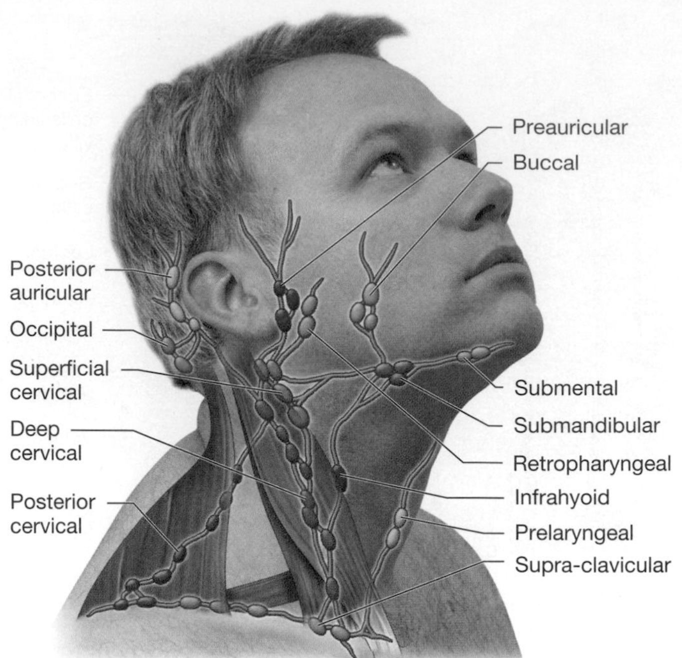

FIGURE 21-6 Location and drainage of head/neck lymph nodes

Epitrochlear Nodes The epitrochlear nodes are a group of nodes that are located on the medial aspect of the arm, superior to the antecubital fossa in the depression between the biceps and brachialis muscles (see Figure 21-7).

Inguinal Lymph Nodes The inguinal lymph nodes include the horizontal (superior) and vertical (inferior) groups of nodes and are located in the groin area (see Figure 21-8). The vertical (superior)

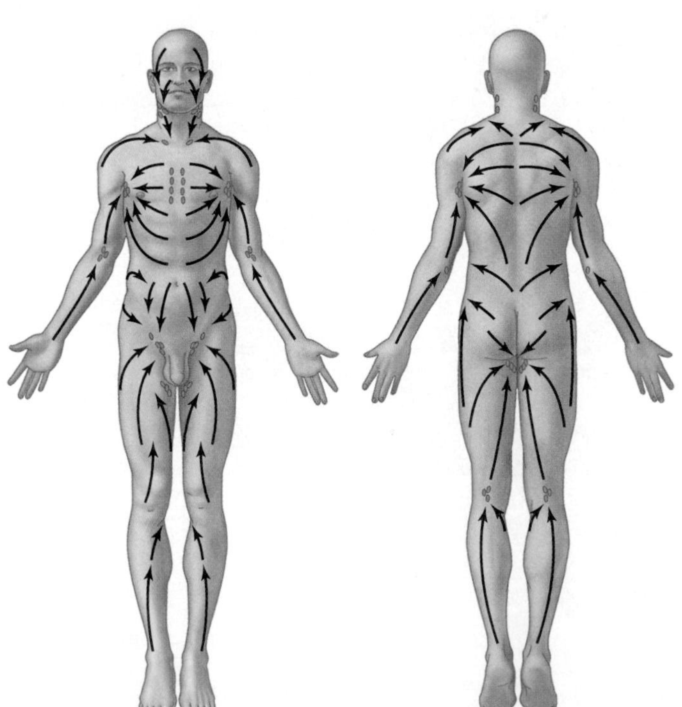

FIGURE 21-5 Regional lymph node drainage

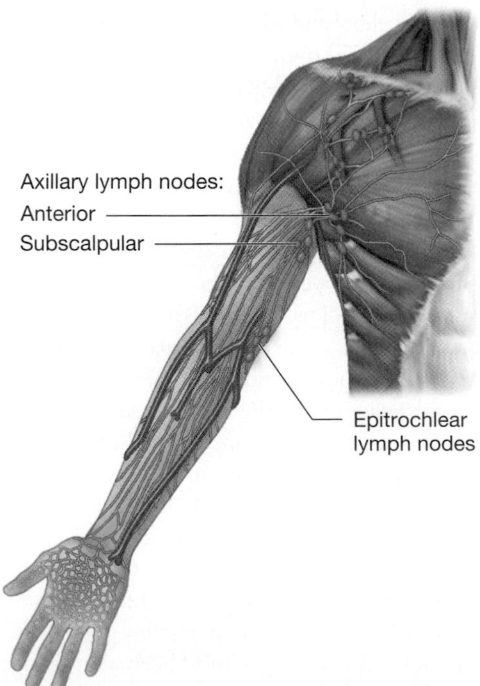

FIGURE 21-7 Axillary and epitrochlear lymph nodes

nodes are located over the inguinal canals, generally in the same area where the femoral pulse may be palpated. The vertical (inferior) nodes are a little deeper and are located on the medial aspect of the thigh, generally at the location where the lower extremity meets the lower section of the abdomen.

Thymus Gland

The **thymus gland** is a major lymph organ that is located in the anterior mediastinum, behind the sternum and upper four costal cartilages (see Figure 21-2). It supplies other lymphoid organs and tissues with T-lymphocytes.

The thymus gland is relatively large at birth and during childhood, reaching its maximum size and weight during puberty, after which time it gradually decreases in size and weight, becoming barely visible in adulthood. It consists of two lobes connected by connective tissue and serves the primary function of providing a site for the maturation of T-cells. Once the T-cells are mature, they migrate to lymphatic tissues. Hormones secreted by the thymus gland, thymosin and thymopoietin, are responsible for differentiation of T-cells.

Spleen

The other major lymphoid organ is the spleen, the largest mass of lymphoid tissue that is positioned in the abdomen between the stomach and diaphragm. In contrast to the lymph node, the spleen also participates in blood circulation. The spleen participates in the immune response, particularly to blood borne pathogens, as well as filtration for removing aged red cells and platelets. It also serves as a reservoir for phagocytes, lymphocytes, and red blood cells, releasing any of these when needed to fight an infection or replace blood that has been lost.

The spleen is composed of lymphoid tissue (white pulp) and venous sinuses (red pulp) (Figure 21-9). The white pulp carries out the immunological function of the spleen, and the red pulp filters out and destroys old, worn out red blood cells. During childhood, the spleen is an important immunologic organ because the other parts of the lymphoid system are not fully developed. The importance of the spleen decreases as an individual ages and is not essential for sustaining life. The spleen is a relatively fragile organ and can be easily damaged or rupture, particularly in instances of trauma.

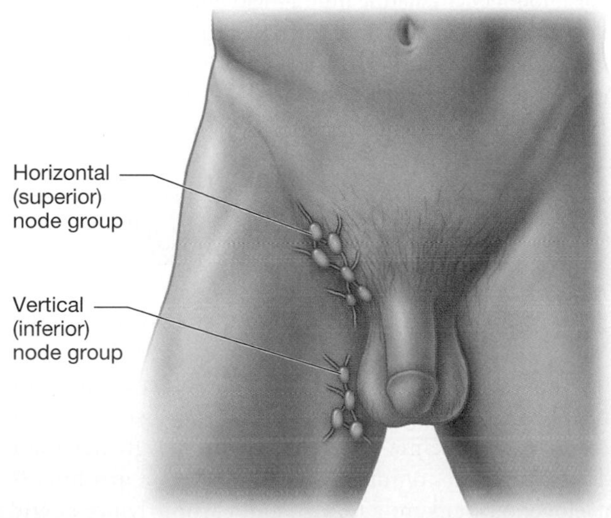

FIGURE 21-8 Inguinal nodes

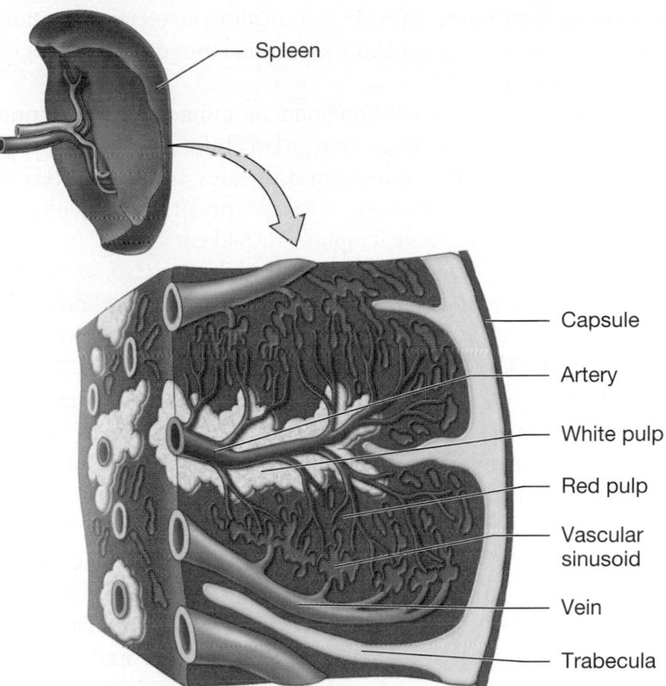

FIGURE 21-9 Structure of spleen

The unique feature of the immune system, the self-recognition of one's self-antigens, permitting the recognition of "non-self" antigens as the stimulus that initiates the immune response. In contrast to this **autoimmunity** is a condition in which the immune system does not recognize self-antigens and initiates an immune response to attack the self-antigens as foreign. The cause of this phenomenon is unknown; however, there are many diseases and conditions that are believed to have an autoimmune connection.

Developmental Variations

Developmental variations occur over the course of an individual's lifespan and events. Awareness of these variations is important to understand and recognize common age related alterations or modifications of the lymph system.

Infants and Children

The lymphatic system develops early in fetal development, with further development and maturation occurring during infancy and throughout childhood into early adolescence. The distribution of lymph nodes in children is the same as for adults.

Lymphoid tissue increases until it reaches its peak in later middle childhood. The volume of lymphatic tissue begins to decrease during adolescence, eventually reaching adult volume. This is most evident in tonsillar tissue. By 6 years of age, the tonsils are approximately adult size, but keep growing until by age 12 they reach their peak size, about twice the adult size. During adolescence, the tonsils begin to decrease in size until they reach adult size. The same can be said of the thymus; however it is an internal organ and thus cannot be directly observed.

The ability to produce antibodies is not fully developed during infancy. Antibodies (immunoglobulins from B cells) from the mother are passed on to the infant, giving them some immediate protection. Breastfeeding is also a way to continue the transmission of antibodies from mother to infant. Vaccinations for certain conditions or diseases may begin at birth with routine immunizations beginning at about 2 months.

Lymphatic cancers, although uncommon during childhood, account for approximately one-third of childhood cancers, with majority of these being leukemias. Males are more likely to develop leukemia than females. The majority of cases of leukemia in childhood are the acute lymphocytic leukemia (ALL) type.

Lymphomas, Hodgkin's and Non-Hodgkin's (NHL), account for significantly fewer incidences of lymphatic cancers in children. The incidence of NHL in children under 5 is approximately 4%, while the incidence for those under 15 is 0.7%.

Infants and children are also vulnerable to congenital immunodeficiencies, with the most severe form being **severe combined immunodeficiency (SCID)**. In this condition, severe T-cell and B-cell dysfunction occurs as a result of genetic mutations in different genes. Most common manifestations are recurrent infections, absent lymphoid tissue, chronic diarrhea and failure to thrive. SCIDs results from a variety of heterogenous genetic conditions, primarily genetic mutations (Bonilla, 2013). Without any treatment, severe infection(s) occur, and the child rarely survives beyond 12 months of age. Acquired immunodeficiencies are relatively rare in children.

Infants may also be born with the HIV virus, making it a congenital disorder that is not caused by genetic alterations, but acquisition of the virus from an HIV infected mother. Early intervention with these infants allows for a greater lifespan than had been previously achieved.

THINK LINK: The Boy in the Bubble

Perhaps the best known case of SCIDS is the "Bubble Boy." David Vetter was born in 1971 with SCIDS. Immediately after birth he was placed in a sterile bubble with the intent to find a cure that would allow him to exit the bubble. However, no back-up plan existed if a cure could not be found. He underwent a bone marrow transplant from his sister, but she harbored the Epstein-Barr virus, and once released in David's body, it caused multiple cancer tumors; he died in 1984.

More recent treatments for SCIDS that have been used include in-utero transplant, pretransplantation therapy, and gene therapy. Gene therapy has been successful in restoring a functional immune system, however; the development of leukemia post-therapy is a major risk (Kugler, 2007).

The Pregnant Woman

No specific considerations relate to the lymphatic system for the pregnant female. As previously identified, maternal antibodies are passed on to the infant through the placenta and later on through breast milk providing temporary immunity for the infant.

What is unique about the immune nature of the lymphatic system during pregnancy is that the mother's immune system does not recognize the developing fetus as foreign material. How this occurs is yet to be completely understood. There are instances where immune problems have caused the spontaneous termination of a pregnancy, but this is quite rare. Although not directly related to pregnancy, in some instances a female may develop antibodies to the male's sperm, resulting in infertility problems where it is extremely difficult for the couple to achieve pregnancy.

PRACTICE POINT: Rh Incompatibility: An Immune Disorder

Rh alloimmunization in pregnancy occurs when an Rh negative mother delivers an Rh positive baby and is exposed to Rh positive RBCS from the infant as a result of transplacental fetomaternal hemorrhage. The most critical time for this occurrence is during delivery. Once exposed to Rh+ antigens from the infant, the mother develops anti-Rh+ antibodies. In subsequent pregnancies, the mothers anti-Rh+ antigens can cross the placenta, attach themselves to the infant's RBCs causing them to be destroyed by the infant's spleen. Infants born to these mothers develop "hemolytic disease" and require an immediate transfusion of blood after delivery. Prevention is administration of anti-D immune globulin to women.

The Older Adult

The lymph nodes of the elderly may decrease in numbers and size. The nodes' characteristics may also change, causing them to feel more fibrotic and fatty. A greater concern for the elderly is a reduction in the function of the immune system.

Older adults are at a greater risk for the development of an infection primarily due to the aging of the immune system or **immunosenescence** (Aspinall, Del Guidice, Effros, Grubeck-Loebenstein, & Sambhara, 2007). Immunosenescence is characterized by a decreased functioning of the immune system resulting in an inappropriate, inefficient, and possibly a detrimental response to infectious agents (Merck Manual of Geriatrics, 2008). Changes occur in both the innate and adaptive immune responses. The primary alterations are due to changes that occur in the T-cells and B-cells.

With the involution of the thymus gland, the amount and concentration of thymic hormones decreases and may be absent in individuals over 60 years of age. What the significance of this is and whether it can be improved with administration of thymic hormones is not known. T-cell alterations are primarily responsible for the age related diminished immune responses. The production of antibodies by B-cells is also affected.

The amount of antibody produced in response to antigens and the overall amount of circulating immunoglobulins also diminishes with aging. The quality of the antibody produced is also diminished, which has significant implications for an elderly individual's response to immunizations. It is unknown whether the decreased function of B-lymphocytes is related to intrinsic alterations or because of T-cell dysfunction.

Malignancies of lymphoid tissues increase in incidence with aging. The incidence of non-Hodgkins lymphoma is approximately 45 cases per 100,000 for individuals between 60 and 64 years of age, and increasing to 112.1 cases per 100,000 between 80 to 84 years of age. The incidence of Hodgkin's lymphoma is much less.

The majority of leukemia cases occur in older adults with more than 50% occurring in individuals over 67 years of age. The incidence of leukemia in adults is 10 times greater than in children. The most common types of leukemia in adults is acute myelogenous leukemia (AML) and chronic lymphocytic leukemia (CLL). The greatest incidence of chronic myelogenous leukemia (CML) is also found in adults.

Health Promotion

Infections and infectious diseases still present significant challenges to the health and well being of individuals worldwide. Despite important advances in knowledge regarding infectious agents and their manifestations, infectious diseases still cause significant morbidity and mortality. Inherent to this circumstance is the emergence of new strains of microorganisms and the reoccurrence of some diseases that were thought to be well controlled (U.S. Department of Health and Human Services, 2009). Concomitant with these concerns is the rapid development of resistance to antimicrobial agents resulting in an increase of acquired infections within health care organizations as well as the community.

Immunization and Infectious Diseases

The goals for *Healthy People 2020* in the topic area of Immunization and infectious diseases (IID) are as follows:

- IID—1 Reduce, eliminate, or maintain elimination of cases of vaccine-preventable diseases.
- IID—5/6 Reduce the number of courses of antibiotics for ear infections for young children and/or prescribed for the sole diagnosis of the common cold.
- IID—7 Achieve and maintain effective vaccination coverage levels for universally recommended vaccines among young children.
- IID—22 Increase the number of public health laboratories monitoring influenza-virus resistance to antiviral agents.
- IID—23/24/25/26 Reduce hepatitis A, chronic hepatitis B virus infections in infants and young children (perinatal infections), hepatitis B and hepatitis C.
- IID—27 Increase the proportion of persons aware they have a hepatitis C infection.
- IID—29 Reduce tuberculosis (TB). (There are actually 32 goals for this topic area.)

The stated goals are those that relate to a broad range of infections or conditions. The total list is of goals appears on the *Health People 2020* Web site.

From the early 1980s until the mid 1990s, infectious disease related deaths increased by 22% (excluding HIV infections). Besides HIV, the leading causes of deaths were from pneumonia and influenza (U.S. Department of Health and Human Services, 2009), which were the fifth leading causes of death in the United States.

International cooperation related to infectious disease control is a significant requirement for control of acquisition and spread of infectious diseases. International travel, importing, and exporting food and other products as well as the indiscriminate use of antibiotics in food sources and humans only increase the potential for worldwide epidemics. In addition, the threat of biological warfare also serves to increase the impact of infectious agents. Public health measures taken or not taken in one area or country also affects the health of local and distant areas and countries.

Vaccines still remain the essential intervention for the prevention of the debilitating and potential fatal manifestations of certain infectious diseases. They have reduced the incidence of certain diseases—polio, rubella, and measles—however, the organisms responsible for them have not disappeared. Under the right circumstances, a significant reduction in vaccinations, they could cause an increase in their incidence and outbreaks of the disease. Vaccinations benefit both the individual and surrounding individuals. When the majority of individuals are vaccinated, they offer protection to those who for various reasons, might not be vaccinated. Those who are not vaccinated are less likely to be exposed to the infectious agent and thus less likely to develop the disease. Vaccinations also provide a significant cost benefit to individuals and families in both direct and indirect costs. In contrast to this savings, infections that are acquired during hospitalizations add significant costs for additional days in the hospital as well as treatment. Hospital acquired infections; particularly those that are antibiotic resistant (methacillin resistant staph aureus [MRSA]) have increased dramatically in recent years. Treatment costs for hospital acquired infections have reached approximately $30.5 billion in the United States (McCaughey, 2006).

A growing trend that is occurring among school-age children, who should be vaccinated, is parents choosing to not have their children immunized. All states provide options for refusal to vaccinate based on medical reasons and/or religious beliefs and practices. A growing number of individuals, however, are refusing vaccinations based on personal beliefs. These beliefs are frequently based on unproved assertions that vaccinations are linked to certain disorders, primarily autism. Much of this information comes from nonmedical or nonprofessional sites on the Internet. The misinformation regarding vaccinations results in parents being more concerned about the risks of the vaccination rather than the risks associated with the disease itself. These unvaccinated children pose a threat to themselves related to contracting the disease as well as to others, those who are also not vaccinated and those who are as there are vaccinated individuals who might contract the disease.

The specific goal of *Healthy People 2020* is to reduce or eliminate indigenous cases of vaccine preventable diseases. Their baseline and target incidences are identified in Table 21-1.

Strategies that are to be used to attain this goal are as follows:

- Improving the quality and quantity of vaccination delivery services
- Minimizing financial burdens for needs persons
- Increasing community participation, education, and partnership
- Improve monitoring of disease and vaccination coverage
- Developing new or improved vaccines and improving vaccine use (U.S. Department of Health and Human Services, 2009)

Vaccination schedules are in Chapter 5.

Table 21-1 Vaccine preventable diseases

Vaccine Preventable Disease	Baseline Data (2008)	Target (2020)
Congenital rubella syndrome (Children < 1 year old)	0	Total elimination
Diphtheria (Individuals < 35)	1	0
Haemophilus influenza type b (Children < 5)	0.27 cases per 100,000 children < 5 years	10% improvement
Hepatitis B (Individuals 2–18 years)	0	Total elimination
Measles (all ages)	30	Projection
Mumps (all ages)	500	Projection
Pertussis (Children < 1)	2,500	10% improvement
Pertussis (adolescents 11–18 years)	2000	Projection
Polio (wild type virus) (Individuals of all ages)	0	Total elimination
Rubella (Individuals of all ages)	10	Projection
Tetanus (Individuals < 35)	14	0
Varicella (Chicken pox) (Individuals of all ages)	100,000	Projection

Source: Data from U.S. Department of Health and Human Services, 2009

Clinical Context Exemplars

Situation A

A 46-year-old female is seen in a clinic for her 3-month post-mastectomy check up. While doing your assessment, she complains that the arm on her surgical side is beginning to enlarge. She doesn't remember anyone informing her that this might happen after surgery and wants to know what is happening.

1. What would you tell her regarding the probable cause of her swelling?
2. What should she be told in regards to the probability that it will eventually go away?
3. What actions and precautions should she be aware of to prevent any complications?

Situation B

A new mother does not want her 6-month-old child to receive any immunizations. Her reason is that her next door neighbor's child developed autism after his MMR vaccination.

1. How would you address this mother's concern related to the risks and benefits of immunizations?
2. The mother decides to have the child receive a vaccination at this visit, but doesn't want the child to have any more. What would you tell this mother?
3. The mother wants to know why vaccinations are necessary if diseases are not longer a threat. What would tell this mother?

Situation C

A 6-year-old child is scheduled for a tonsillectomy. The parents want to know if having the tonsils out now will create problems later in life.

1. What would you tell them?
2. The parents then want to know why there are tonsils and what function do they perform. How would answer their questions?

Situation D

An 18-year-old college student is presenting with a sore throat. After palpating under the mandibular angle, the student wants to know why that area is always palpated first.

1. How would you respond to the question?

SUBJECTIVE DATA

History of Present Illness (CC)

The patient may present to the provider with a variety of concerns that may be directly related to the lymphatic system or other systems. Framing the questions will depend on the patient's age, gender, culture, race, emotional or mental status, health practices, and concurrent illnesses. All symptoms presented must be thoroughly assessed with a symptom analysis (COLDERRA).

Enlarged Lymph Nodes (Lymphadenopathy)

Enlargement of lymph nodes is an indicator of an infection/inflammation in the location of the lymph node related to the drainage patterns of lymph within the affected area. More than likely, the patient is not going to state that there is an "enlarged lymph node" but will probably indicate feeling a "bump, lump, swelling", or other terms associated with an enlarged node. To maintain a subjective interpretation of the symptom, use more generic terms in forming the questions for the symptom analysis.

Provider Inquiries	Clinical Reasoning/Logic
Characteristics: How do the "lumps/bumps" feel? Hard, soft, nodular, tender, warm?	Characteristics of nodes help to determine the cause. Tender, fluctuant cervical nodes suggest strep and staph infections. Hard nodes indicate cancer, firm/rubbery nodes in lymphoma and chronic leukemia, especially in people with risk for cancer like smoking or history of malignancy, favor malignancy. Soft nodes are seen in acute leukemia.
Onset: When were enlarged nodes first noted? Any known infections, trauma, surgery?	Association between enlarged nodes and any infection will help to determine possible underlying cause.
Location: Where are the enlarged nodes located? Do you feel them in just one spot or do you feel them in more than one area?	Lymph nodes (LNs) drain certain areas of body, so specific location of enlargement will help to determine possible source/cause. For example, TB adenitis usually affects the cervical LN and is usually regional and not generalized. Anterior cervical LN usually associated with head and neck infections and systemic infections like EBV, toxoplasmosis, or CMV. Posterior cervical LN usually seen in EBV, TB, lymphoma, head/neck malignancy, and Kikuchi disease. Infectious mononucleosis in contrast with streptococcal pharyngitis typically involves the posterior cervical LN, and inguinal LN groin and may also present with hepatosplenomegaly. Supraclavicular LN always suspicious for malignancy. Axillary LN associated with infection on arms like cat scratch fever, chest and breast.
Duration: How long have nodes been enlarged?	Tender, acute suggest infection, especially if there are physical findings along the same regional lymphatic drainage. In the absence of findings suggestive of infections, malignancy should be suspected.
Exacerbation: Exacerbated by drugs?	Phenytoin is known for causing enlarged lymph nodes. Other drugs include anti-hypertensives, antibiotics (penicillin, cephalosporins, sulfonamides).
Associated signs/symptoms: Fever (persistent), night sweats, weight loss (B symptoms), excessive fatigue, pain, redness, tenderness, warmth, itching?	B symptoms indicate the presence of systemic symptoms, and are a marker of more advanced disease and a negative prognosticator in Hodgkin's lymphoma.

Bleeding

Bleeding and bruising are signs of hemostasis instability. They are frequently associated with platelets deficiency or dysfunction or abnormality in the coagulation cascade as is seen in leukemia or infiltrative diseases of the bone marrow or in conditions that promotes platelet destruction or coagulopathy.

Provider Inquiries	Clinical Reasoning/Logic
Characteristics: Is the bleeding spontaneous? Did it occur a after injury? How much blood was lost? Does it stop easily?	Bleeding that occurs with minor trauma that ordinarily would not initiate bleeding or bleeding that does not stop is highly suspicious for leukemia.
Onset: What precipitates bleeding?	Bleeding with minor trauma or spontaneous bleeding is an unexpected finding.
Location: Where does bleeding most often occur? Bruised area?	Skin, gums, GI, GU, intracerebral bleeding are common locations
Duration: How long does bleeding last? Stops easily?	Excessive bleeding correlates with severe platelet deficiency or severe coagulopathy.
Exacerbation: Anything noted that increases or promotes bleeding episodes?	Trauma, use of aspirin and NSAIDs
Relief: What is used to terminate bleeding episode? Effectiveness?	Most external bleeding stops with direct pressure. Platelet or coagulation factors support may be necessary to relieve the bleeding.
Associated signs/symptoms: Pallor, fainting/dizziness, headache, shortness of breath, chest pain?	Anemia, which leads to poor tissue perfusion, is the end result of excessive bleeding. Signs of poor tissue perfusion are pallor, chest pain, shortness of breath

Swelling of Extremity (Lymphedema)

Lymphedema is the interstitial collection of fluid as a result of disruption of lymphatic flow. Fluid accumulates when the lymphatic flow exceeds the transport capacity of the lymphatic system. A common cause is blockage by tumors, like breast cancer, sarcoma, and lymphoma. It can also be due to genetic or inherited conditions or infection like filariasis. Enlargement of an extremity or area of the body is an indicator of a blockage of lymph drainage from an area. Lymphedema (congenital or inherited) may be primary or secondary, as in malignancy, infiltrative processes, infection or surgical sequelae like axillary LN dissection.

Provider Inquiries	Clinical Reasoning/Logic
Characteristics: What does skin of swollen extremity feel like? Appearance?	Early lymphedema will indent with pressure and remain indented but will feel soft. In late stages, skin will become hard and stiff.
Onset: When was swelling first noted? Previous surgery, trauma, infection, cardiac, renal, or peripheral vascular disorders? Is it gradual or sudden?	Most cases of lymphedema occur after trauma, infection, or surgery. In breast surgery, onset is associated with LN dissection. Lymphedema is usually insidious.
Location: What extremity? Unilateral or bilateral?	In breast surgery it is usually ipsilateral to surgery site, but in pelvic node dissection, lymphedema is usually bilateral.
Duration: Is the swelling intermittent or constant?	Lymphedema is usually constant and progressive.
Exacerbation: What makes it worse? Position changes, heat/cold, use of extremity?	Effect of gravity makes it worse. Placement of extremity in dependent position will be affected by gravity and increase the swelling.
Relief: What makes it better? Position, heat/cold, elevation?	Elevation of extremity, exercise, gentle massage, or elastic support bandages will frequently reduce swelling in early stages. They often lose their effectiveness over time as the condition worsens.
Associated signs/symptoms: Warmth, tightness, heaviness of the extremity, redness, pain, discoloration, ulcerations?	These symptoms frequently accompany lymphedema.

PRACTICE POINT: Night Sweats (nocturnal hyperhidrosis)

Because night sweats have a variety of causes it is imperative to keep in mind other patient history information that may give clues to a specific cause. Other causes of night sweats include the following:

- Menopause: Hot flashes may occur at night causing night sweats in perimenopausal females.
- Idiopathic hyperhidrosis: A condition where the body produces too much sweat without any specific cause.
- Infections: Tuberculosis is commonly associated with night sweats, but it may also be present in other bacterial and parasitic infections, osteomyelitis, and abscesses. AIDS and HIV infection are also causes of night sweats.
- Medications: Antidepressants (all types), niacin (taken for lipid disorders), tamoxifen, nitroglycerine, sildenafil (Viagra).
- Hypoglycemia: Hypoglycemia may occur during night, particularly those on insulin or oral anti-diabetic medications.
- Hormone disorders: Pheochromocytoma, carcinoid syndrome, hyperthyroidism.
- Neurologic conditions: Autonomic dysreflexia, stroke, autonomic neuropathy (Stoppler, 2006).

Night Sweats

Night sweats when accompanied by lymphadenopathy is suspicious for neoplastic or infectious processes.

Provider Inquiries	Clinical Reasoning/Logic
Characteristics: Describe an incident. Drenching sweat, changing sheets, bed clothing?	Night sweats characterized by "drenching" the bed associated with intense hot flashes (Stoppler, 2006). It is important to differentiate sweating due to increased environmental heat or excessive bed clothing or blankets.
Onset: Time of night—constant or variable? Heat wave (hot flash) precede onset?	Hot flashes may occur at night and during the day and should be differentiated from night sweats accompanying neoplastic or infectious processes. A hot flash is a momentary heat sensation and may be accompanied by facial flush and sweats. This is commonly reported during menopause.
Location: Generalized or localized?	A localized warmth and redness of the face and/or trunk is more characteristic of flushing than night sweats.
Duration: How long does it last? How long have they been occurring?	The duration of night sweats per episode is not as significant as is the length of time that the individual has experienced them.
Exacerbation: Anything noted to make sweating increase? Medications or alcohol?	Warm environmental temperature as well as excessive bed clothing/blankets may increase intensity of sweating. Certain medications may cause flushing or sweats.
Relief: What relieves it?	Commonly, night sweats dissipate without any intervention.
Associated signs/symptoms: Fever (subjective/objective), cough, weight loss, fatigue? Any abnormal sensation on chest or abdomen?	Fever when associated with night sweats is generally seen in infection and in malignancies like lymphoma or other neoplasms. Hot flashes are usually accompanied by abnormal sensation on chest, breasts, or abdomen. Even though patient may report feeling warm (subjective), they may not actually have fever (objective).

Past Medical History

Past medical history provides information as to previous illnesses or conditions that may have an effect on the lymphatic system as well as provides information that may help to identify potential causes for chief complaint or other presenting symptoms.

Provider Inquiries	Clinical Reasoning/Logic
Any known exposure to TB; chest x-rays? Any blood transfusion/blood products? Any surgery: Trauma to/removal of lymph nodes; organ transplant? Any chronic illnesses: Cardiac, renal, HIV, cancer, stomach ulcers (*H. pylori*), infectious mononucleosis, Hepatitis C?	Past medical history helps differentiate between neosplastic and infectious diseases. TB may manifest lymphadenopathy and night sweats.
Medications like cholinergics, antidepressants, hormonal agents, hypoglycemic drugs?	Medications may be the cause of fever, sweats, and LN enlargement

Family History

Family history provides information regarding family member's illnesses or conditions as potential causes for chief complaint or presenting symptoms that may indicate a pattern of presentation associated with transmission of familial/genetic factors predisposing the individual to certain system-related conditions/illnesses. Any of these may indicate a potential or actual cause of lymph node dysfunction.

Provider Inquiries	Clinical Reasoning/Logic
Has anyone in your family ever experienced the following: • Malignancies? • Anemia? • Recurrent infections? • Tuberculosis? • Autoimmune disorders?	Genetic predisposition in malignancy and exposures are important component to elicit, i.e., close contact like in TB. Endocrine, diseases like pheochromocytoma, thyroid, and carcinoid may cause sweats and flushes. Autonomic dysfunction may cause sweats.

Personal and Social History

Personal and social history provides information related to habits, practices and/or environmental influences that may predispose the patient to the development of certain system related conditions/illnesses.

Provider Inquiries	Clinical Reasoning/Logic
Any recent travel to high-risk areas for tuberculosis, Epstein-Barr virus, histoplasmosis, coccidiomycosis (Viera, Bond, & Yates, 2003)?	Certain areas of U.S. and the world known to be associated with certain microorganisms that cause specific infections. Parasitic infections like Brucellosis other zoonosis may cause night sweats.
Engaged in high-risk behaviors (unprotected intercourse, IV drug use)?	High-risk behaviors for HIV, endocarditis and other pyogenic infections like abscess and osteomyelitis.
Are your immunizations up to date?	Inadequate immunizations leave the individual susceptible to infectious conditions. Vaccine protection for tetanus, diphtheria, and pertussis (whooping cough) fades with time. Before 2005, only tetanus and diphtheria (Td) were available as a booster shot and was recommended every 10 years for teens and adults. After 2005 pertussis (Tdap) was added for protection against tetanus, diphtheria, and pertussis for pre-teens and older.
Exposure to carcinogenic toxins/agents (radiation, herbicides/insecticides, solvents, hair dye, chemotherapy, anti-immunity drugs)?	Exposure to toxins helps to determine potential causes for lymphoid malignancies.

Developmental Applications

Certain conditions or disorders may be related to certain age groups or situations. Inquiring to obtain age or condition specific information will provide further information to help determine possible cause(s) of the chief concern as identified.

Provider Inquiries	Clinical Reasoning/Logic
Infants and Children	
Immunizations: What immunizations has the child received? Are they up to date?	Determine if child is protected against certain infectious agents. If child not up to immunized, determine reasons for parent not having child immunized.
Has the child had any recent/recurrent infections?	Frequent or recurrent infections may be indicators of immune deficiencies.
The Pregnant Woman	
What is the week of gestation?	Determine age of fetus and potential for damage from infectious agents.
Are your immunizations up to date?	Pregnant women who have never had a dose of Tdap should get one, after the twentieth week of gestation and preferably during the third trimester. If they do not get Tdap during their pregnancy they should get a dose as soon as possible after delivery. Pregnant women who have previously received Tdap and need tetanus or diphtheria vaccine while pregnant should get Td.
Have you had any previous spontaneous abortions?	Frequent spontaneous abortions may indicate immune dysfunction.
Any difficulty getting pregnant?	Difficulty getting pregnant may indicate immune dysfunction.
Previous problems with toxemia?	
Exposure to infectious agents—rubella, CMV?	Rubella and CMV are particularly harmful to the developing fetus.
The Older Adult	
Have you had an recent/recurrent infections? (Frequency?) Related to trauma? Proximity to lymph nodes?	
Have you received a flu shot or immunization for pneumococcal pneumonia?	How well protected against flu and pneumococcus organisms.
How long does it usually take you to recover from infections?	Generally takes older adults longer to recover, extended recovery period may indicate nutritional or immune deficiencies.

OBJECTIVE DATA

The physical examination of the lymphatic system occurs throughout the entire exam whenever a particular region is encountered that is associated with groups of lymph nodes. Examination of the lymphatic system generally consists of inspection and palpation. Division of the lymphatic system into levels is not relevant as there is not a significant continuum of alterations or techniques that necessitates differentiation.

Inspection

- Localized: enlargement, tenderness, warmth
- Tonsils
- Generalized: enlargement, tenderness, warmth
- Tonsils
- Lymph node biopsy

Palpation

- Localized: enlargement, tenderness, redness
- Generalized: enlargement, tenderness, redness
- Spleen (size/enlargement)

***Percussion**—not performed*

***Auscultation**—not performed*

Level I to IV Examination

The Level I to Level IV examinations are performed on a continuum, which starts from a basic level to a more comprehensive level based on provider's abilities and knowledge as well as the patient's presentation and location. It may start at the outpatient setting progressing to the ED, hospital unit bed, critical care unit, or specialty unit. Frequently all the elements from basic to comprehensive exam are done in one setting like in a primary care setting or clinic.

The condition/illness of the patient is the primary consideration related to the type and amount of data needed to assess the patient's /condition/illness/situation. The arrangement of skills into levels is for general purposes and is meant to be descriptive rather than prescriptive. The purpose of arranging into levels is to provide a framework to assist the learner in determining the appropriate data to collect.

Lymph

	Level I	Level II	Level III	Level IV
Inspection	Localized: enlargement, tenderness, warmth	Generalized: enlargement, tenderness, warmth		Lymph node biopsy
	Tonsils*	Tonsils*		
Palpation	Localized: enlargement, tenderness, redness	Generalized: enlargement, tenderness, redness	Spleen (size/ enlargement)	

* Also assessed with another system and may have already been observed.

Inspection: Levels I & II

Inspect each area or region for evidence of lymph node enlargement, swelling, redness, or any red streaks. Additionally, inspect the tonsils for any evidence of enlargement or inflammation/ infection. The tonsils are frequently assessed during the inspection of the mouth and throat (see Chapter 20).

Inspection Techniques and Expected Findings	Unexpected Findings
Observe the lymph nodes (LN) for any evidence of enlargement, redness, edema, and/or the presence of any red streaks.	The lymph nodes that drain a particular area that may be infected or traumatized would also be inspected for any enlargement or evidence of redness.
Pay attention to regional drainage.	Regional—LN in one region suggest local causes and prompt one to look for causes in the area of the LN drainage.

Inspection Techniques and Expected Findings	Unexpected Findings
Distinguish between regional or generalized enlargement.	Generalized LN—LN in two or more non-contiguous regions suggest systemic disease especially if associated with hepatosplenomegaly. Systemic diseases may include HIV, lymphoma, mycobacterial infection, mononucleosis, lupus, and serum sickness from drugs.
Inspect the tonsils primarily for size, color, and any surface lesions or alterations. The specific characteristics of the tonsils have been covered in Chapter 20.	Infected or inflamed tonsils would demonstrate enlargement. As an example, an individual who presents with a sore throat may demonstrate enlarged tonsils.
In most instances, lymph node enlargement is not visible.	An increased redness would probably also have enlarged regional lymph nodes that drain the area, which would be inspected for enlargement as would the tonsils.

THINK LINK: *Red Streaks*
Acute lymphangitis is a potentially serious bacterial infection in the lymphatic vessels, which can rapidly spread to the bloodstream and be fatal. Bacteria that have entered the body through a skin injury gain access to the lymphatic system multiplying so rapidly that the immune system cannot respond quickly enough to halt the infection. The lymphatic vessels becomes inflamed, resulting the characteristic signs of acute lymphangitis which are the wide, red streaks, travelling from the site of infection to the armpit or groin. The affected areas are red, swollen, and painful. Blistering of the affected skin may occur, with the infection spreading through the course of the vessels and causing red streaks.

Inspection: Levels III & IV

Inspection Techniques and Expected Findings	Unexpected Findings
Extensive assessment of the lymph nodes beyond the physical examination—biopsy—is not necessary.	Enlarged lymph nodes accompany a myriad of diseases and conditions, like reaction to infection or malignancy. The absence of regional source of infection may be a source of concern for malignancy especially if nodes are hard, nontender and fixed. Lymphadenopathy that is accompanied by **"B" symptoms** is also highly correlated with lymphomas (Figure 21-10).

THINK LINK: *B Symptoms*
B symptoms refer to systemic symptoms of fever, night sweats, and weight loss often associated with Hodgkin's and non-Hodgkin's lymphoma. Pruritus and fatigue have also been included by some clinicians. The term was derived from Ann Arbor staging of lymphomas which includes Stage I to IV and letters A and B. "A" indicates the absence of systemic symptoms, while B indicates their presence. The presence of B symptoms is a marker for advanced disease and higher histologic grade and a negative prognostic factor in Hodgkin's lymphoma.

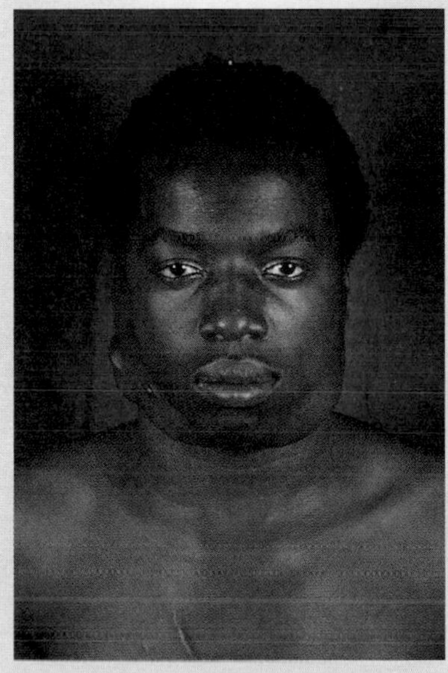

FIGURE 21-10 Localized lymphadenopathy
Source: SPL/Custom Medical Stock Photo

Palpation: Levels I & II

Beginning at the head, you will systematically palpate groups of nodes for their characteristics. There is no specific order for their palpation, but establishing and following a consistent pattern helps to insure that you assess all locations. The pattern used here is only a suggested one; each provider needs to establish a pattern that is best. You should also palpate in between groups of nodes to provide the greatest possibility of palpating over the most lymph nodes.

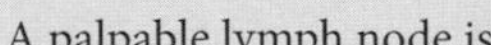

Palpation Techniques and Expected Findings	Unexpected Findings
Palpate the lymph nodes over all locations of known lymph node groups or chains. Because lymph nodes are generally not palpable, you must know expected locations of groups and chains of lymph nodes and anatomic area they drain. This is based on superficial anatomic landmarks.	A palpable lymph node is an unexpected finding and may be seen in infections, trauma, or malignancy. In some thin or healthy individuals, cervical LN and inguinal LN may be palpable and not necessarily evidence of pathology.
Use the pads of your second, third, and fourth fingers, gently placing them over the location of the nodes and applying a gentle pressure with a rotary motion. Palpate for location, consistency, size, and fixation tenderness. The characteristics of nodularity, firmness, tenderness, matted, fixated to deep structures are helpful in defining etiology.	"Shotty" LN is a term used in describing multiple small, nontender, movable LN and is of no diagnostic import. Tender, movable LN suggests infection or inflammation. Nontender, firm, hard, rubbery, fixed LN suggests malignancy. Tenderness of LN associated with redness and recent enlargement is commonly associated with rapid tension in the area as seen in infection. It can be seen in trauma, hemorrhage or malignancy as well.
Palpate for size. Lymph nodes should be less than 1 cm, movable, and soft. LNs are generally larger in adolescents.	Greater than 1 cm is considered pathological.

Head and Neck

The lymph nodes of the head and neck are commonly palpated during the head and neck regional exam when the skull and hair are being palpated. The suggested general order is submental, submandibular, tonsillar, preauricular, post-auricular, occipital, anterior cervical, posterior cervical, supraclavicular and infraclavicular. Beginning at the back of the head, gently palpate the occipital nodes located midway between the occipital ridge and mastoid process (Figure 21-11a). From the occipital nodes, move toward the post-auricular nodes that are located just behind the ear on the mastoid process (Figure 21-11b).	The auricular LNs drain the parietotemporal region of the head, the ear, and mastoid. Any condition like infection and inflammation or malignancy in these areas may be manifested by pathological LN enlargement.

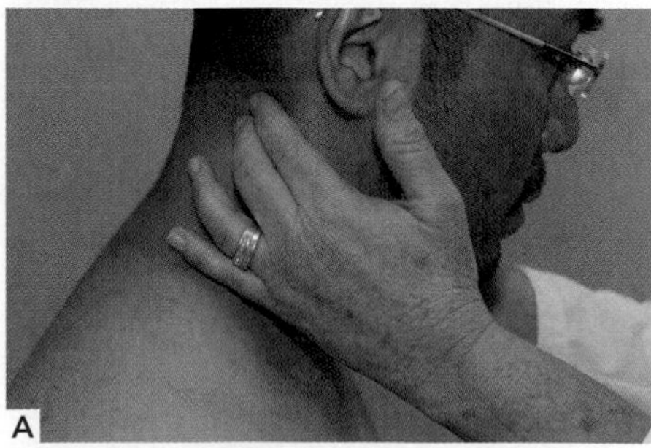

FIGURE 21-11A–B Palpation of head lymph nodes

Palpation Techniques and Expected Findings	Unexpected Findings

Next move your finger pads to the front of the ear to palpate the pre-auricular lymph nodes.

From the front of the ear, move down to the angle of the mandible, palpating the parotid and tonsillar lymph nodes (Figure 21-11c).

From the angle of the mandible, move along the length of the mandible, palpating the submaxillary nodes at the halfway point along the bone and ending at the tip of the mandible where the submental lymph node is located (Figure 21-11d).

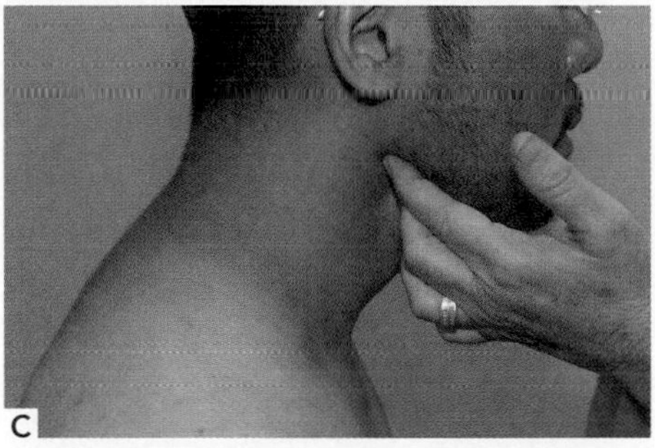

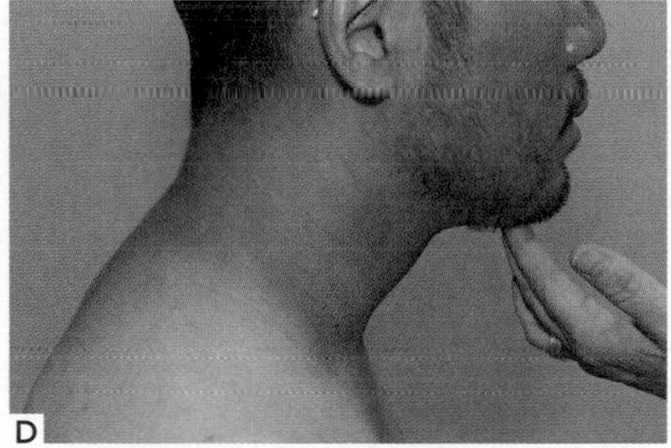

FIGURE 21-11C–D Palpation of head lymph nodes

Next, move on to the neck. Palpate the anterior cervical chain along the anterior border of the sternocleidomastoid muscle (Figure 24-12a).

Palpate the posterior cervical chain along the anterior edge of the trapezius muscle in the posterior triangle. The deep cervical chain is located under the sternocleidomastoid muscle and may be somewhat difficult to palpate, particularly if you use too much pressure. It is best to probe gently around the muscle with the thumb and forefinger.

End palpation of the neck lymph nodes with the supraclavicular nodes, located deep in the angle that is formed by the sternocleidomastoid muscle and the clavicle (Figure 24-12b). To palpate these nodes, instruct the patient to flex the head slightly forward and toward the side that is being examined. You will then hook your left index finger over the clavicle to the lateral side of the sternocleidomastoid muscle, palpating deeply in the area for these nodes.

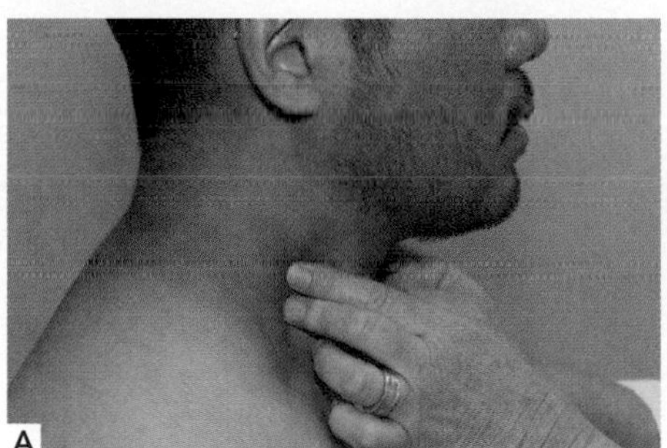

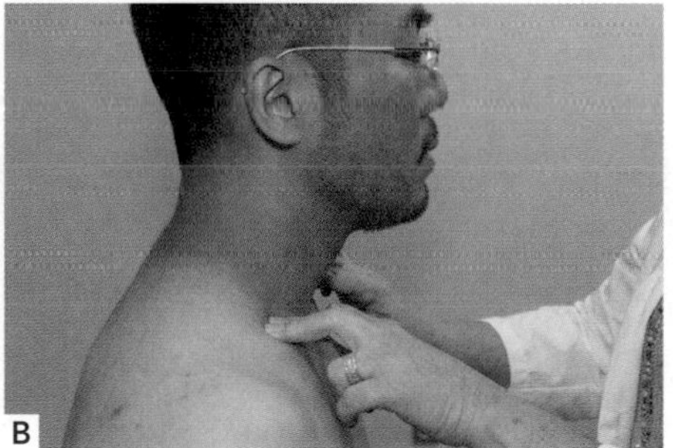

FIGURE 21-12A–B Palpation of neck lymph nodes

Submaxillary, submental, and tonsillar LN enlargement are seen in various orophayngeal infections and malignancy like oral and tongue malignancies.

Anterior cervical LN are often enlarged in head and neck infections, or malignancy and in systemic infections like EBV, CMV and toxoplasmosis.

Posterior cervical LNs are usually seen in infectious mono, TB, AIDS, measles, lymphoma, and head and neck malignancy.

Hard cervical LNs particularly in older adults or smokers suggest malignancy.

Multiple enlarged nontender cervical LN that last weeks to months and are fluctuant or matted associated with fever suggest TB or atypical mycobacterium.

Cervical nodes are often palpable in healthy persons, although palpability decreases with age.

Supraclavicular LNs are high risks for malignancy.

For palpable nodes, note location, size, shape, delimitation (discrete or matted together), mobility, consistency, and tenderness. If nodes are enlarged or tender, assess the areas they drain into for the source of the problem.

- *Acute Infection*—bilateral, nodes enlarged, warm, tender, and firm but freely movable
- *Chronic Inflammation*—nodes are clumped
- *Cancerous Nodes*—nodes are hard, unilateral, nontender, and fixed
- *HIV Infection*—nodes are enlarged, firm, nontender, and mobile; occipital node enlargement is common with HIV infection
- *Virchow's Node*—a single, enlarged, nontender, hard; left supraclavicular node, which may indicate neoplasm in thorax or abdomen.
- *Hodgkin's Lymphoma*—gradual appearance of painless, rubbery, discrete nodes occurs

Palpation Techniques and Expected Findings	Unexpected Findings

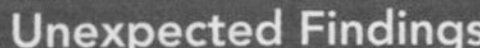

Axilla

The axillary nodes are generally assessed during the examination of the breast, and are palpated in both male and female patients (Figure 21-13). Five groups of lymph nodes are located in the axillary area. (A detailed description of palpation of axillary lymph nodes is provided in Chapter 22.)

The axillary nodes receive drainage from breast tissue and are significant indicators for the presence of breast cancer (see Chapter 22).

Axillary LN receives drainage from the arm, thoracic wall and breast. Malignancy is suspected in the absence of regional signs of infection.

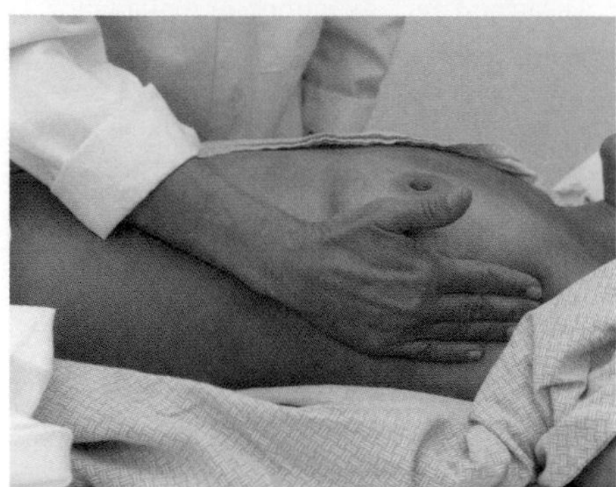

FIGURE 21-13 Palpation of axillary lymph nodes

Epitrochlear Nodes

Palpate the epitrochlear nodes on the medial aspect of the upper extremity in the depression above and posterior to the elbow. The depression is the area between the biceps and brachial muscles. Gently place the pads of the fingers in this area and move in a rotating motion over the area to determine if any nodes are palpable (see Figure 21-14).

Epitrochlear LN are generally not palpable, thus their presence is almost always pathological. They can be enlarged in syphilis, turalemia, sarcoid, lymphoma, and infections of hands and forearm.

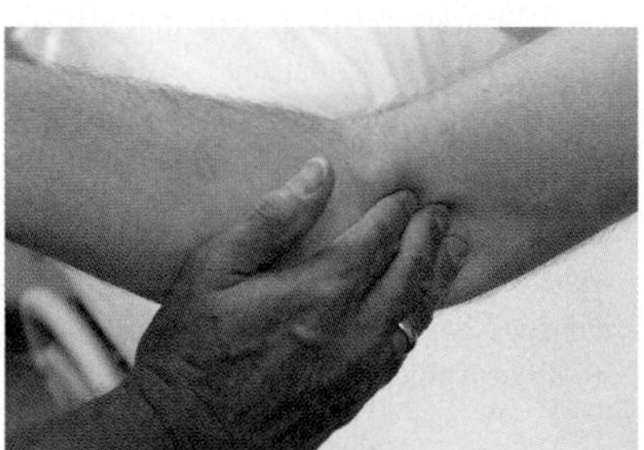

FIGURE 21-14 Palpation of epitrochlear nodes

Inguinal Lymph Nodes

The inguinal lymph nodes are best palpated with the patient in a supine position. They can also be easily assessed when the femoral artery pulse is also palpated.

Palpate the superficial superior inguinal lymph nodes in the fold of skin that is created by the upper thigh and lower portion of the lower abdomen. This also follows the course of the inguinal canals.

Palpate the superficial inferior inguinal lymph nodes on the medial aspect of the upper thigh. These nodes lie in vertical position, so they are palpated as the finger pads are moved downward on the inner thigh (see Figure 21-15).

Inguinal LN are commonly palpable. They can be seen in STI, lower extremity infections, lesions from anus, vulva, and pelvic region.

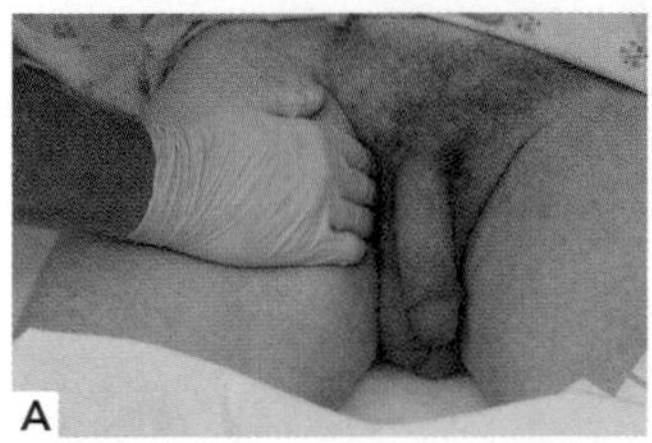

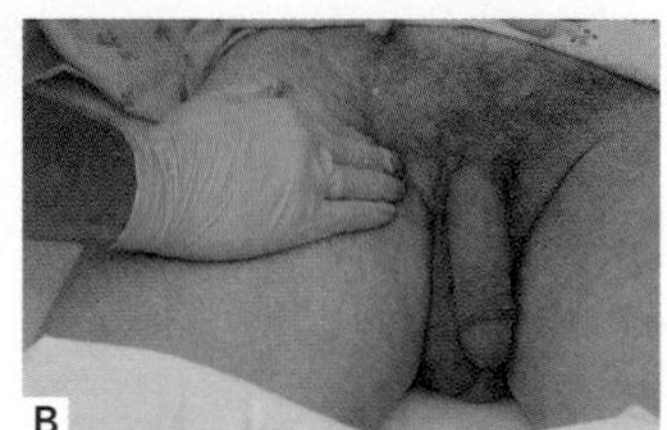

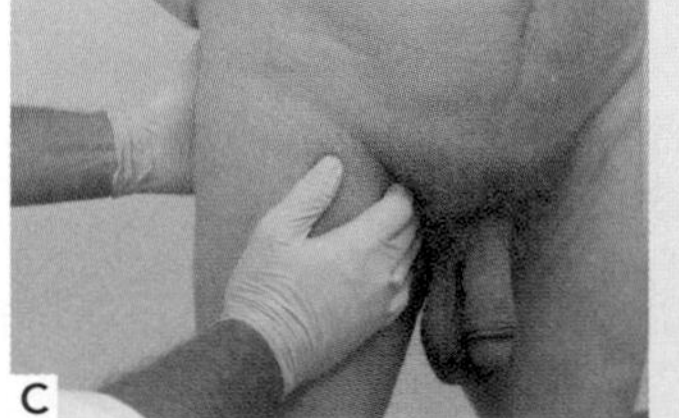

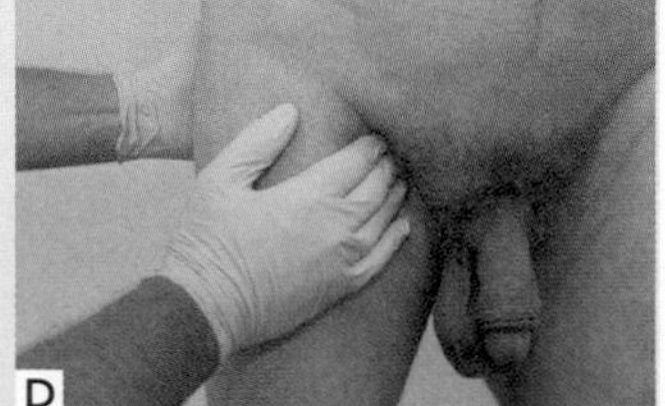

FIGURE 21-15A–D Palpation of inguinal lymph nodes; **a/b)** Patient lying; **c/d)** patient standing

Palpation: Levels III & IV

During the abdominal exam you may palpate the spleen to determine if any enlargement or tenderness exists. The spleen participates in both humoral and cellular immunity. It can be infiltrated in lymphoma and other extramedullary myleoproliferative disorders.

Palpation Techniques and Expected Findings	Unexpected Findings
Spleen The spleen is located on the left side of the abdomen, just under the lower left rib cage (Figure 21-16). In ordinary circumstances, the spleen is not palpable, and the patient does not experience any tenderness. A spleen that is not enlarged or tender is generally not palpable.	An enlarged spleen is palpated as a firm mass that bumps against your hand. For the spleen to be palpable, it must be enlarged (**splenomegaly**) to 3 times its expected size.
When palpating the spleen, you should be on the right side of the patient, reaching across the abdomen, and placing your left hand under the lower left rib cage for support. With this hand, apply pressure upward to lift the spleen toward the surface of the abdomen. Place your right hand below the left costal margin, exerting a small amount of pressure inward. Instruct the patient to take a deep breath and gently palpate for the splenic border (see Figure 21-17). Even when the patient takes in a deep breath, the spleen generally does not descend below the ninth or tenth intercostal space, making it difficult to actually feel the spleen. Spleen can be also percussed at the Traube's space (area overlying the tympanitic gastric bubble on left lower lateral hemithorax).	Unexpected finding is displacement downward of the tympanitic sound in splenomegaly.

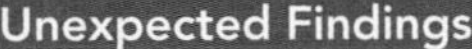

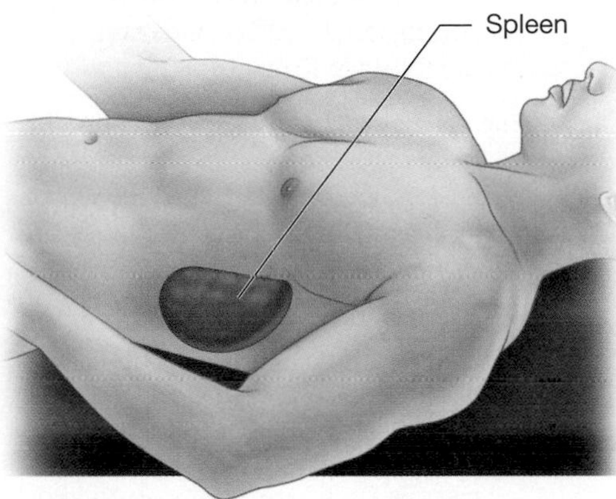

FIGURE 21-16 Location of the spleen

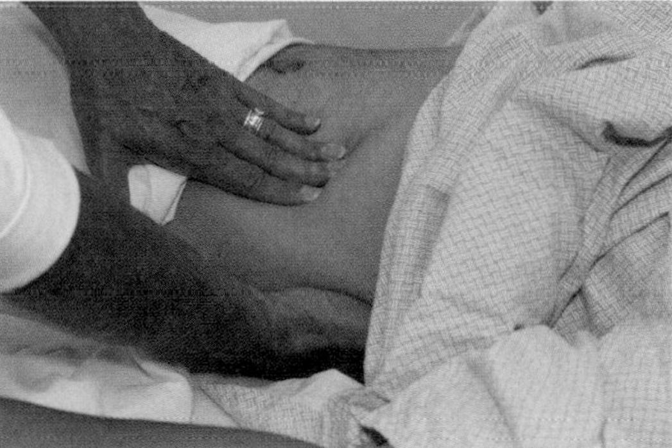

FIGURE 21-17 Palpation of spleen

PRACTICE POINT: Spleen Palpation

The spleen is generally nonpalpable unless there is evidence of trauma, malignancy, and abscess or in liver cirrhosis. But even with trauma, palpation needs to be done gently because this is a relatively fragile organ that may be ruptured if there is evidence of abdominal trauma. Even if the spleen is not ruptured initially, vigorous palpation may cause it to rupture.

Developmental Applications

Techniques and Expected Findings	Unexpected Findings
Infants and Children The lymphoid tissue in the newborn is relatively underdeveloped so that palpable lymph nodes are rarely encountered.	A perinatal infection may cause lymphadenopathy, particularly in the occipital nodes.

Techniques and Expected Findings	Unexpected Findings
Lymphadenopathy is a common clinical presentation throughout childhood due to the increase in and continuing development of lymphoid tissue during the first year and throughout childhood. It is not uncommon to palpate lymph nodes that are less than 3 mm. Small occipital and posterior auricular LN are common in infants but not in older children. Lymph nodes up to 1 cm may be palpable in the cervical and inguinal area, but they are usually nontender, mobile, and smooth on the surface. Along with the lymphadenopathy, enlargement of the tonsils is also frequently encountered. The spleen may also become enlarged, but is generally not a major concern.	Infections are a common occurrence throughout childhood, thus an increased occurrence of infectious or inflammatory lymphadenopathy is expected. Lymphadenopathy as in adults may be caused by infectious and noninfectious causes. In the majority of instances, it occurs as a localized manifestation rather than generalized. The most common sites for enlargement are the inguinal, axillary, and cervical nodes (Nield & Kemat, 2004). Lymph nodes that are hyperplastic and develop in response to viral infections are often described as "**shotty**." These are usually bilaterally small, discrete, mobile, and nontender (Gow, 2008). This descriptive term is in reference to shotgun pellets. In comparison to infectious or inflammatory lymphadenopathy, malignancy-related lymphadenopathy is associated with lymph nodes that are described as firm or rubbery, discrete, nontender, and immobile, or fixed to the skin or underlying structures (Gow, 2008). These characteristics are particularly ominous when accompanied by "B" symptoms—fever, night sweats, fatigue, and weight loss. Other manifestations of malignancy related lymphadenopathy include node enlargement greater than 3 cm, the enlargement has been present for longer than 4 weeks, and the supraclavicular nodes were involved.
The Pregnant Woman There are no specific assessments of lymph tissue and organs for the pregnant female. Toxoplasmosis may be acquired during pregnancy as a result of consuming undercooked meat, contaminated fruits, vegetables, or water, travel to endemic areas, or may present as reinfection (rare).	Toxoplasmosis may manifest with lymphadenopathy with mono-like illness.
The Older Adult Lymph node assessment in the elderly is the same as for the adult. The locations of the lymph nodes are identical. However, the characteristics are similar, but may feel more fibrotic and fatty. An individual's risk for development of cancer is based on many factors; one of them is age.	In the elderly, lymphadenopathy is frequently associated with a malignancy. Specific characteristics may help to identify its cause. Rubbery lymph nodes may indicate lymphoma, hard nodes are frequently associated with a metastatic malignancy, and matted nodes characterize chronic inflammation like TB (Williams, 2007).

Techniques and Expected Findings	Unexpected Findings
	In addition to characteristics, note the extent of involvement, size, and tenderness. The extent of involvement relates to whether the node enlargement is localized (1 chain) or generalized (2 or more chains). Lymph nodes that are greater the 1 cm are also significant as well as any associated tenderness. Tenderness is more characteristic of inflammation.

DOCUMENTATION

Inspection of lymph node groups in specific regions (head, neck, clavicular, epitrochlear, axillary, and inguinal) reveals no visible enlargement. No visible enlargement or evidence of edema noted in upper and lower extremities. No areas of redness or indicators of inflammation/infection distal to node groups. No visible red streaks noted anywhere.

During palpation of node groups in same region, no palpable lymph nodes noted. No tenderness or warmth of area.

Submental lymph nodes palpable, approximately 0.5 cm. Some localized warmth and tenderness noted, node freely moveable with smooth surface. No hardness or unusual consistency.

Electronic Charting

Expectations of Electronic Charting

All portions of the lymphatic system exam should be able to be documented, including immunization status. Ideally the lymphatic system exam findings should be able to be connected to related tests and procedures such as labs, MRI or CT scans, ultrasounds, or lymph node biopsy. Technical developments in radiation oncology have led to image-based treatment planning and increased use of electronic records; electronic charting systems need to accommodate storage, archiving, and retrieval of large volumes of graphical data.

Electronic charting can enhance the ability to communicate information between multiple providers. This is crucial for treatment of conditions that involve the lymphatic system, including tumors, infections, and inflammatory conditions. Electronic registry systems are commonly used to track cancers and to provide data for research; electronic charting systems should be able to generate reports to send to electronic registries. Similarly, electronic charting systems should be able to automatically extract data related to reportable infectious diseases.

Limitations of Electronic Charting

Forms to document examination of the lymphatic system may be difficult to locate in the electronic record. The components of the lymphatic exam may be integrated into the forms for examination of local systems (for example, a tonsil exam may appear within the head and neck documentation). However, many components of the lymphatic system assessment are cellular in nature and not associated with a particular organ system. Some electronic charting systems will not use the term "lymphatic system" but will classify this exam as immunologic. The exam may be grouped with the hematologic or allergic systems.

Summary

- The lymphatic system is composed of lymph fluid, lymph vessels, and lymph glands. The lymph system is parallel to the vascular system and functions to return lymph fluid back to the circulation. It also plays an integral part in immune function.
- The central or primary lymphoid organs are bone marrow that generates lymphocytes from immature progenitor cells as well as where lymphocytes mature into B cells and the thymus gland where lymphocytes mature into T cells.
- Lymphoid tissue is located throughout the body as locations where mature lymphocytes are stored until needed to participate in an immune response. Lymph nodes are masses of lymphatic tissue located along the pathways of lymph circulation. There are various clusters of lymph nodes scattered throughout the body that may be examined. The spleen is an abdominal organ that functions as a reservoir for lymphocytes.
- Conditions and disorders of the lymph system are frequently alterations reflecting other diseases or as a result of damage or removal. Lymphedema is swelling caused by the accumulation of lymph fluid, which may occur if the lymphatic system is damaged or has malformations.
- Lymphadenopathy is swollen/enlarged lymph nodes commonly due to infections, infectious mononucleosis, and cancer, and metastasis of cancerous cells via the lymphatic system.
- Hodgkin's lymphoma is a type of cancer usually resulting from the white blood cells in the body becoming diseased or damaged. Presently, this kind of cancer is easily controlled.
- Lymphoid leukemias and lymphomas are now considered to be tumors of the same type of cell lineage. They are called *leukemia* when in the blood or marrow and *lymphoma* when in lymphatic tissue.

- Immunosenescence refers to the changes that affect the immune system with aging. The consequences of immunosenescence include an increased risk of infections, malignancy, and autoimmune disorders. Malnutrition is relatively common among older adults and can contribute to declining immune function.
- In children the lymphatic system is still developing, thus it is less effective in creating antibodies, resulting in young children more vulnerable to infection. The lymphatic system matures and reaches peak development at around 10–12 years of age then gradually decreasing in size during adolescence.
- Significantly enlarged lymph nodes may be visible, but are commonly examined by palpation at specific sites of node cluster.

Review Questions

1. When teaching a group of students about the lymphatic system the provider would include that lymph consists primarily of which of the following?
   1. plasma and antibodies
   2. red blood cells and protein
   3. interstitial fluid and protein
   4. interstitial fluid and antibodies
2. The provider is caring for a patient with notable lymph node enlargement. When teaching the patient the provider explains that the lymphatic system is primarily associated with which of the following?
   1. fluid and electrolyte balance
   2. innate immunity
   3. acid–base balance
   4. adaptive immunity
3. The provider is aware that the gland associated with the lymph system that functions predominately in pediatric patients is which of the following?
   1. thyroid
   2. thymus
   3. spleen
   4. pineal
4. The provider is assessing a patient with a complaint of painful, tender lymph nodes. The provider knows that this patient most likely has which of the following?
   1. infections
   2. non-Hodgkin's lymphoma
   3. leukemia
   4. night sweats
5. When assessing an elderly patient the provider expects to find lymph nodes that are which of the following?
   1. shotty
   2. tender
   3. fibrotic
   4. mobile
6. The provider is assessing a patient who has sustained an abdominal injury that is affecting the spleen. When explaining that surgical removal of the spleen may be necessary the provider explains that the spleen is a
   1. lymphoid organ that functions in immunity and blood circulation.
   2. gland that shrinks in adult life and secretes hormones.
   3. collection of lymphoid tissue located in the gastrointestinal tract.
   4. part of a grouping of lymphoid tissues commonly referred to as mucosal-associated lymphoid tissue (MALT).
7. When examining the throat of a patient the provider notes enlarged lymphatic tissue in the back of the throat. The provider is aware that this finding is common if this patient is which of the following?
   1. infant
   2. child
   3. young adult
   4. adolescent
8. The provider is to palpate the spleen of a patient. To correctly perform this assessment the provider should do which of the following? (Select all that apply.)
   1. Stand on that patient's right side.
   2. Ask that patient to exhale completely while palpating.
   3. Place the left hand under the patient's left lower rib cage.
   4. Use the right hand to palpate at the costal margin.
   5. Vigorously palpate the splenic boarder.
9. When performing an assessment of a patient's head the provider includes palpation of the lymph nodes including which of the following? (Select all that apply.)
   1. occipital nodes
   2. submental nodes
   3. epitrochlear nodes
   4. tonsillar nodes
   5. inguinal nodes
10. The provider has completed the assessment of a patient's spleen and is to document a normal finding. The provider would document which of the following?
    1. "The spleen is firm on palpation."
    2. "Mild pain and tenderness noted on palpation of the spleen."
    3. "The spleen is nonpalpable."
    4. "The spleen easily palpated at the fifth intercostal space."

Conditions and Disorders

Overall, the lymph system is a rather "behind the scenes" system and not of great concern unless there is some type of alteration that becomes evident.

Lymphedema (Lymphatic Obstruction)

Lymphedema is a condition of localized fluid retention and tissue swelling caused by accumulation of lymph fluid in the interstitial spaces. Tissues with lymphedema are at risk of infection. It may be inherited (primary), the rarer form, or caused by injury to the lymphatic vessels (secondary).

Pathophysiology

Primary lymphedema:

- Exact etiology still unknown.
- Genetically based.
  - Caused by failure of lymphatics to develop properly (congenital [Milroy disease]) or failure of lymph channel valves to function properly (lymphedema praecox [Meige disease]) or lymphedema tarda.
  - Congenital lymphedema presents at birth or within the first year. Lymphedema praecox and tarda are essentially the same, differing in terms of age of onset: praecox manifests before 35 years of age and tarda after 35 years of age.

Acquired lymphedema:

- Due to an injury or some other condition that causes lymphatic dysfunction, such as damage to or removal of lymph nodes from surgery, radiation therapy, infection, or tumor invasion or compression (Revis, 2005).
- Approximately 25%–30% of cases related to breast cancer treatment (surgery, radiation therapy). May also result from other cancers: prostate, uterine, cervical, abdominal, malignant melanoma, as well as from lymphomas.

Parasitic invasion of the lymph system is the most common cause of lymphedema worldwide (Modi, 2007). **Filiarisis** is a parasitic-related infection (Wuchereria bancrofti) that results in massive enlargement of the extremities (**elephantiasis**) (Revis, 2005) (see Figure 21-18).

Subjective Data

- Swelling of part of arm or leg or entire arm or leg, including fingers or toes
- A feeling of heaviness or tightness in arm or leg
- Restricted range of motion in arm/leg
- Aching/discomfort in arm or leg
- Recurring infections in affected limb
- Hardening and thickening of the skin on arm or leg

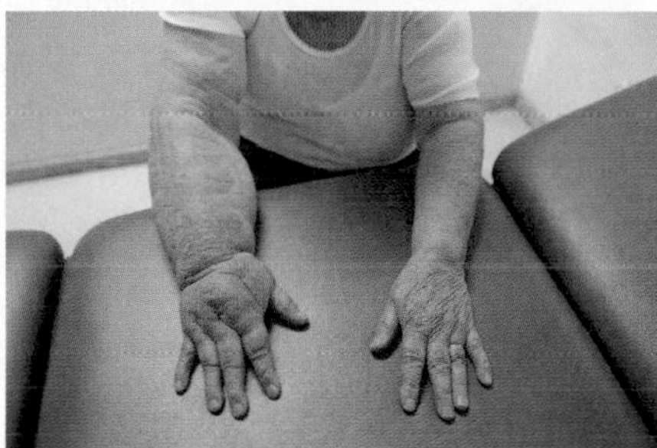

FIGURE 21-18 Lymphedema
Source: Sergio Azenha / Alamy

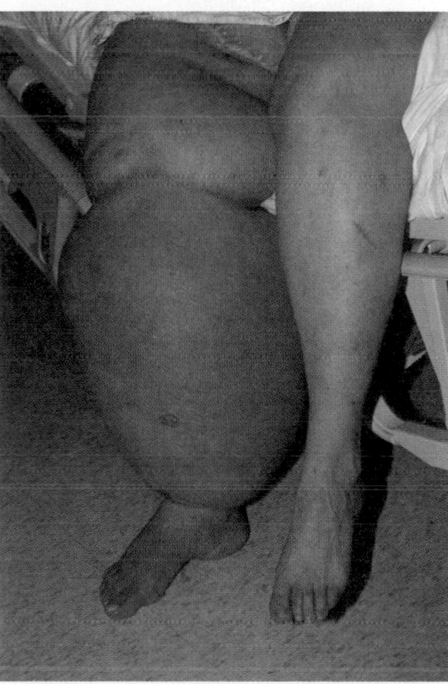

FIGURE 21-19 Filariasis
Source: John Greim/Science Source

Objective Data

- A heavy swollen limb or localized fluid accumulation in other body areas, including the head or neck, discoloration of the skin overlying the lymphedema
- Lymphedema categorized by its severity (usually compared to a healthy extremity):
  - Grade 1 (mild): Involves distal parts (forearm/ hand or lower leg/foot). Circumference differential less than 4 cm; tissue changes not yet present.
  - Grade 2 (moderate): Involves entire limb or corresponding quadrant of the trunk. Circumference differential more than 4 but less than 6 cm. Tissue changes (pitting) apparent.
  - Grade 3a (severe): Present in one limb and associated trunk quadrant. Circumference differential greater than 6 centimeters. Significant skin alterations, (cornification or keratosis, cysts and/or fistulae) present.
  - Grade 3b (massive): Same symptoms as 3a, except two or more extremities affected.
  - Grade 4 (gigantic [elephantiasis]): Affected extremities are huge due to almost complete blockage of the lymph channels. May also affect the head and face.

Splenomegaly (Enlargement or Hypertrophy)

The spleen is about the size of a fist, but a number of conditions can cause an enlarged spleen. It is a soft, spongy organ that performs several critical functions and can be easily damaged. Depending on the underlying cause, the spleen may enlarge to as much as 80 times its regular size. Massive splenomegaly places a heavy burden on the heart and circulatory system and may absorb more than half the cardiac output, whereas under normal circumstances, it absorbs only 5%. The spleen filters out and destroys old and damaged blood cells.

Subjective and objective data are related to exaggerated splenic function as well as the underlying cause of the splenomegaly.

Pathophysiology

- A wide variety of condition are associated with splenomegaly, with many of the mechanisms resulting in exaggerated spleen functions.
  - Immune response hypertrophy (subacute bacterial endocarditis or infectious mononucleosis)
  - RBC destruction hypertrophy (hereditary spherocytosis or thalassemia major)
  - Congestive (splenic vein thrombosis, portal hypertension)
  - Myeloproliferative (chronic myeloid metaplasia)
  - Infiltrative (sarcoidosis and some neoplasms)
  - Neoplastic (chronic lymphocytic leukemia/ lymphomas)

Subjective Data

- Mild, but vague, abdominal pain.
- Pain may be referred to the left shoulder
- Anorexia or a loss of appetite; feeling full without eating or after eating only a small amount (occurs when an enlarged spleen presses on stomach)
- Fatigue, pallor, dyspnea
- Frequent infections
- Easy bleeding, bruising, and/or petechiae (hemolytic process)

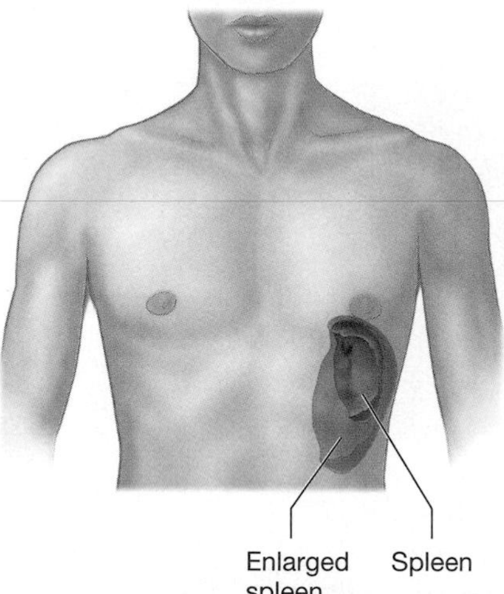

FIGURE 21-20 Splenomegaly

Objective Data

- Palpable left upper quadrant abdominal mass; the enlarged spleen tip can be felt in the left upper quadrant of the abdomen, as it continues to enlarge the tip moves toward the right lower quadrant
- Heart murmur
- Endocarditis or congestive failure
- Bleeding manifestations secondary to thrombocytopenia (petechiae, purpura, ecchymosis)
- Anemia
- Signs of cirrhosis (asterixis, jaundice, telangiectasias, gynecomastia, caput medusa, and ascites)
- Febrile illness (infectious)

PRACTICE POINT: *Enlarged Spleen*

A spleen that is enlarged due to infection often becomes engorged with red cells, leaving it fragile with an increased susceptibility to damage, particularly blunt trauma, and rupture. Spontaneous rupture of the spleen is a grave manifestation that has been known to occur in individuals, particularly males, with infectious mononucleosis.

LYMPHOMAS AND LEUKEMIAS

Lymphomas and leukemias are malignant disorders of components of the lymph system network. While leukemias are technically a hematological malignancy of white cells, it is their immune function that places them in the lymphatic malignancy category. Also, it is the only component of the blood that becomes malignant; there are no malignancies of red cells or platelets.

Lymphoma

Lymphoma is the name for a group of cancers that develop in the lymphatic system. The two main types are **Hodgkin's lymphoma (HL) and non-Hodgkin's lymphoma (NHL)**. Just as cancer represents many different diseases, lymphoma represents many different cancers of lymphocytes—about 35 different subtypes, in fact.

Pathophysiology

- Lymphomas originate with the malignant transformation of a lymphocyte.
- The transformation is the result of an acquired injury to the DNA of a lymphocyte that makes it essentially nonfunctional. This transformed, nonfunctional lymphocyte and all of its descendants have an increased proliferation and survival time.

Subjective Data

- The most common early sign of lymphoma is painless enlargement of one or more lymph nodes, usually the neck or upper chest, but also in the armpit, abdomen, or groin.

Other symptoms of lymphoma may include the following:

- fever without an obvious cause
- persistent cough

Objective Data

- Non-Hodgkin's lymphoma causes lymph nodes to become enlarged. When this occurs in lymph nodes close to the surface of the body they may be seen or felt as lumps under the skin. They may also become hard and nodular, as well as fixed and immobile.
- The exact causes of lymphomas are not confirmed and its diagnosis is dependent up a biopsy of the affected node(s). Caught early enough and treated aggressively, individuals with a lymphoma can experience long term survival.

These malignant cells then accumulate in the lymph nodes producing the masses that cause the node to enlarge.
- Hodgkin's disease is differentiated from NHL by the presence of the **Reed-Sternberg cell,** which is not necessarily a lymphocyte.

- shortness of breath during normal activity
- drenching night sweats
- tiredness or no energy
- unexplained weight loss
- itchy skin
- lymph node pain after drinking alcohol

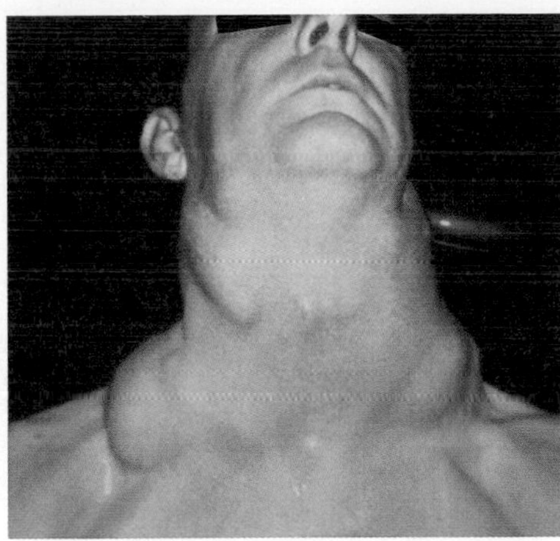

FIGURE 21-21 Enlarged cervical lymph nodes due to Hodgkin's lymphoma
Source: CDC/ Robert E. Sumpter

Leukemia (White Blood)

While the term leukemia technically means "white blood" there is no color change of the blood. Leukemia is a broad term for a group of cancers related to an accumulation of aberrant immature, non-functional white blood cells (blasts) in the blood. There are essentially four types of leukemia based on their progression (acute/chronic) and cell type.

- **Acute leukemia** is a rapidly progressive disease resulting in the accumulation of immature, nonfunctional white cells in the bone marrow and blood. There is also decreased production of red cells and platelets.
- **Chronic leukemia's** have a slower progression accumulation of relatively mature, but still aberrant, white blood cells.
- **Lymphocytic leukemia** affects the lymphocytes, which form lymphoid or lymphatic tissue.
- **Myelogenous leukemia** affects myeloid cells, which give rise to red blood cells, white blood cells and platelet-producing cells.

Pathophysiology

- Caused by the malignant transformation of the DNA of a lymphocyte in the bone marrow.
- These malignant cells accumulate in bone marrow, blood, and other organs, causing them to enlarge and eventually fail.
- The leukemic cells are also nonfunctional, incapable of fighting infection.

Subjective Data

- Symptoms vary, depending on the type of leukemia. Common leukemia signs and symptoms include the following:
  - Fever or chills
  - Persistent fatigue, weakness, dyspnea
  - Frequent infections
  - Weight loss without trying
  - Easy bleeding or bruising
  - Tiny red spots in skin
  - Excessive sweating, especially at night
  - Bone pain or tenderness
  - Headaches

Objective Data

- Anemia (decreased RBC, WBC, platelet counts)
- Petechiae, ecchymosis, purpura
- Pallor
- Swollen lymph nodes, enlarged liver or spleen

IMMUNODEFICIENCIES

Immunodeficiencies are disorders in which some component of the body's immune system is missing or malfunctions. Distinctions between primary or secondary immunodeficiencies are determined as to whether the cause originates in the immune system itself or due to insufficiency of a supporting component of it or an external decreasing factor of it.

Primary Immunodeficiencies (PID)

PIDs are uncommon, chronic, and severe disorders of the immune system in which patients are unable to build up an adequate protective immune response resulting in increased susceptibility to infections (Ballow et al., 2009) that may be fatal. These are genetic in origin; most are diagnosed in children under 1 year, although milder forms may not appear until adulthood.

Pathophysiology

- Aberrancies in the DNA are responsible for many of the defects in primary immunodeficiency.
- The numerous types of primary immunodeficiency disorders can be broadly categorized into six groups based on what part of the immune system that's affected:
  - B cell (antibody) deficiencies (most common)
  - T cell deficiencies
  - Combination B and T cell deficiencies
  - Defective phagocytes
  - Complement deficiencies
  - Unknown (idiopathic)

Subjective Data

- Specific symptoms of a PID depend on the type of defect.
- Generally, the symptoms that result in a diagnosis of an immunodeficiency include recurrent or persistent infections, or developmental delay as resulting from infection.
- Diseases involving the skin, heart, facial development and skeletal system may be present in certain conditions.

Objective Data

- The characteristics of immunodeficiency states range from a deficiency in one type of immunoglobulin to total absence of any immune function.

Secondary Immunodeficiencies (SID)

Also known as **acquired immunodeficiencies,** SIDs result from various immunosuppressive conditions, such as malnutrition, aging and particular medications (e.g., chemotherapy, disease-modifying antirheumatic drugs, immunosuppressive drugs after organ transplants, glucocorticoids).

Pathophysiology

- Many specific diseases indirectly cause immunosuppression, including many cancers, particularly those of the bone marrow and blood cells (leukemia, lymphoma, multiple myeloma), and certain chronic infections.
- Infection with the HIV retrovirus is the most significant acquired immunodeficiency state; it leads to acquired immunodeficiency syndrome (AIDS). HIV directly infects a small number of T helper cells, and also impairs other immune system responses indirectly, making the individual susceptible to life- threatening infections and malignancies.

Subjective Data

- Increased number of infections
- More specific symptoms related to underlying cause(s) of SID

Objective Data

- The infections are types that are mostly demonstrated in immunosuppressed individuals.
- HIV infection will eventually convert to AIDS and ultimately result in the death of the individual from a massive infection or malignancy.

Infectious Mononucleosis (IM)

Frequently called *mono,* this is a common viral infection that is most commonly caused by the Epstein-Barr virus (EBV), and is most frequently diagnosed in teenagers and young adults. Most individuals are exposed to the virus during childhood, when no noticeable or only flulike symptoms occur. Exposure to the virus in early childhood occurs more often in underdeveloped countries resulting in the condition being more common among adolescents and young adults in developed countries. IM may last from weeks to months and generally it resolves without medical intervention. Depending on the intensity, rapidity, and thoroughness of the T-lymphocyte response, malignancy (Hodgkin's disease and non-Hodgkin's lymphoma) may develop if proliferation of EBV-induced B-lymphocyte is uncontrolled. Treatment (rest, fluids, OTC medications) is aimed at easing the symptoms of the illness, which can be done at home.

Pathophysiology

- EBV is transmitted through intimate contact with body secretions, primarily oropharyngeal secretions (saliva). EBV invades the B cells in the oropharyngeal epithelium.

Subjective Data

- The majority of patients with IM are asymptomatic.

Objective Data

- The classic presentation of EBVIM is comprised of the triad of fever, pharyngitis, and lymphadenopathy.

- Circulating B cells disseminate the infection throughout the entire reticular endothelial system (RES), i.e., liver, spleen, and peripheral lymph nodes.
- T-lymphocytes; natural killer (NK) cells and primarily $CD8^+$ cytotoxic T cells control proliferating B lymphocytes infected with EBV.
- A rapid and efficient T cell response results in limiting the primary EBV infection and lifelong suppression of EBV.
- Ineffective T cell response allows for excessive and uncontrolled B cell proliferation, resulting in B-lymphocyte malignancies (e.g., B cell lymphomas).
- The immune response to EBV infection is fever, which occurs because of cytokine release consequent to B-lymphocyte invasion by EBV.
- A proliferation of EBV-infected B lymphocytes leads to lymphocytosis.
- The proliferation of EBV-infected B lymphocytes in the oropharynx leads to pharyngitis.
- The incubation period of IM is 30–60 days, and patients cannot recall close contact with individuals with pharyngitis.
- Virtually all patients report fatigue and prolonged malaise. A sore throat is second only to fatigue and malaise as a presenting symptom.
- Arthralgias and myalgias occur, but are less common than in other viral infectious diseases.
- Nausea and anorexia, without vomiting, are common symptoms.
- Other reported symptoms include cough, eye muscle pain, chest pain, and photophobia.
- Symptoms usually persist for 2 to 3 weeks, but can last for a couple of months.
- Additional early signs include a maculopapular generalized rash, and/or periorbital edema.
- Later physical findings include hepatomegaly, palatal petechiae, jaundice, uvular edema, splenomegaly, and, rarely (1%–2%), findings associated with spontaneous splenic rupture.
- Tonsillar enlargement is common, and massive tonsillar enlargement (kissing tonsils) may be observed and may result in airway obstruction.
- Approximately 90% of adults show serological evidence of previous EBV infection.

22 Breast and Axilla

I wake up like clockwork. Shuffling into Dominic's nursery, I suddenly realize he has not woken up for his middle-of-the-night feeding. He is only 6 months old, and I should be happy that he is starting to sleep through the night, but the thought that one day he won't need me to feed him anymore stirs a sadness in my heart. I settle down in the rocking chair beside his crib and let my mind wander.

I was a brand-new mom when I breastfed him for the first time, and of course I had read every book, taken every class, and exhausted our doctor with questions to prepare for that moment. But like most things in life, nothing could prepare me for the excruciating pain and discomfort I suffered in teaching Dominic to latch onto my breast. After a few weeks of difficulty, however, I found myself loving every minute—it was as if Dominic and I would escape to our own private world. I was everything he needed in order to live, and those moments satisfied me in a way that nothing has since. As I begin to nod off, Dominic lets out a soft wail and I smile to myself. He hasn't outgrown me just yet.

***

Every passing minute in this sterile radiology suite seems to last a century. There is not a single woman here without a furled brow or nervous tremor. It doesn't help that my cousin was diagnosed with breast cancer last week, and the thought that I could be next catapults me into a fit of panic. I pick up a glossy waiting-room magazine, reciting a mantra: "It's not cancer" and flip nervously through the pages. How long does it take to read mammograms? I am only 48. Dominic is only 10, and Liza can't even speak yet. Will she even remember my face once I am gone? How will my parents take the news? How will *I*... cope with breast cancer? The magazine slips from my hands and tumbles to the floor. These wretched breasts are a ticking time bomb, a curse that will send me to an early grave and make orphans of my children.

LEARNING OUTCOMES

1. Correlate knowledge of the breast's structure and function to physical assessment techniques.
2. Explain the development of the breasts and changes that occur during menstrual cycles, reproductive phases, and menopause.
3. Explain the modifiable and nonmodifiable risk factors for breast cancer.
4. Summarize age-related changes that affect the composition, structure, and function of the breasts.
5. Recognize cultural diversity and patient's values during the breast examination.

Breasts in both men and women develop from the same embryological tissues. However, at puberty, female sex hormones, mainly estrogen, initiates further breast development and function, which does not occur in men, due to the higher amount of testosterone. As a result, women's breasts become far more prominent than men's breasts. In the course of a woman's life—from puberty, to pregnancy, lactation, and menopause—her breasts undergo significant transformation in terms of size, shape, structure, and function. This is the result of the complex interplay of hormones, and many other local-growth factors.

Structure and Function

The breasts are paired, cone-shaped mammary glands that prominently occupy the anterior chest wall. They are positioned over the pectoralis major and serratus muscles, spanning from the second rib to the sixth rib longitudinally and between the edge of the sternum and mid-axillary line horizontally (Figure 22-1). Positioned at the apex of each cone is a deeply pigmented nipple that is surrounded by an equally dark pigmented areola, containing sensory nerve endings, sebaceous and apocrine glands.

In mammals, breast development occurs along the **milk lines**, two lines that develop in the embryo, formed by thickenings of the epidermis (the **mammary ridge**) along the ventral surface of both sexes. They extend from the upper limbs to the lower limbs, and are generally not visible in the adult. In most humans only one breast and one nipple arise from each milk line; however, in some individuals more than two nipples develop along the milk lines. The additional nipple is an accessory nipple known as a **supernumerary nipple**. Like other nipples, they are deeply pigmented and sometimes mistakenly diagnosed as moles (Figure 22-2).

The skin covering the breast contains hair follicles as well as sweat and sebaceous glands. The nipples and areola are composed of epithelium with circular and longitudinal smooth muscle fibers, which respond to sensory, tactile, and autonomic stimulation leading to erection. The areolae also contain **Montgomery glands**, which secrete the lubricant for the nipples, opening into the tubercles of Morgagni located around the areola and nipple.

Breast Tissue

The female breast is able to secrete milk used to feed infants, which is produced within the breast tissues. The breast is comprised of three types of tissues: glandular, fibrous, and subcutaneous fat.

The most abundant tissue is glandular, which is arranged into 15–20 lobes that radiate toward the nipple. Each lobe contains lobules, which consist of milk-producing **acini** that drain into the **lactiferous ducts** that terminate at the nipple. Lobule formation and differentiation refer to the transformation from the terminal end buds to the alveolar buds and acini (see Figure 22-3). At birth, glandular breast tissue contains 10-12 primitive ductals that gradually grow and develop into ductal structures terminating with end buds. With the onset of puberty, terminal end buds branch and form new ductals (alveolar buds). This marks the beginning of type 1-4 lobule formation. Type 1 (virginal) lobules consist of 10-11 alveolar buds that have surrounded a terminal duct. Type 2 and 3 lobules are more mature lobules that have formed new alveolar buds. Type 2 lobules are comprised of approximately 47 buds per lobule; Type 3 have approximately 80 buds. Further progression and development into type 4 lobules only occurs during pregnancy when the alveolar buds become acini.

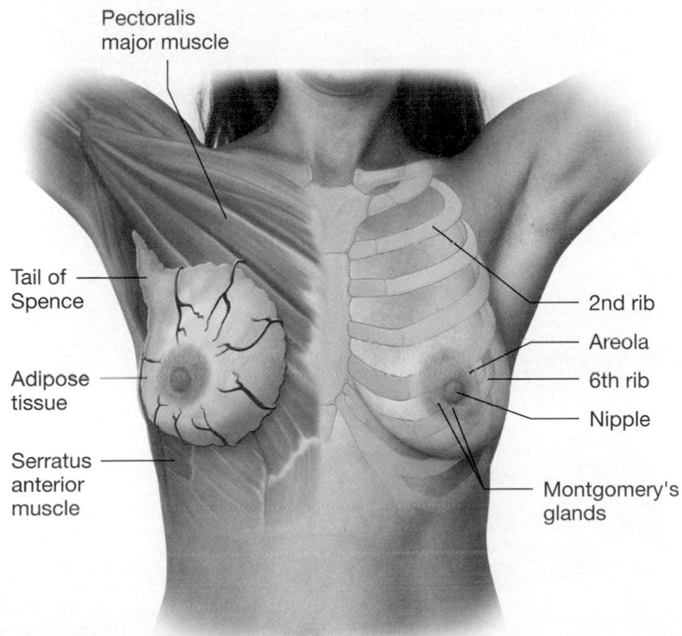

FIGURE 22-1 Superficial landmarks of the chest

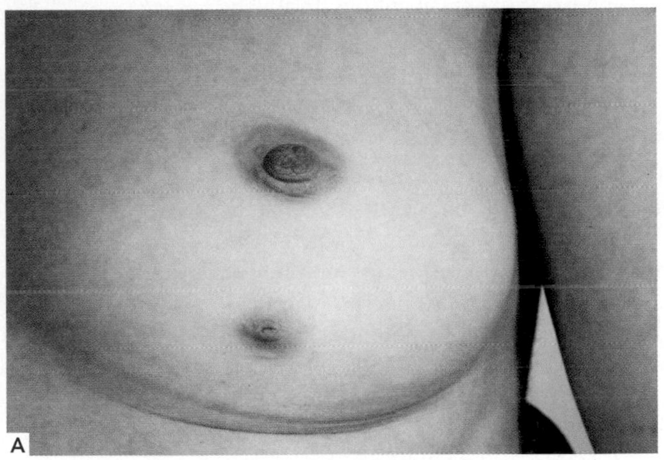

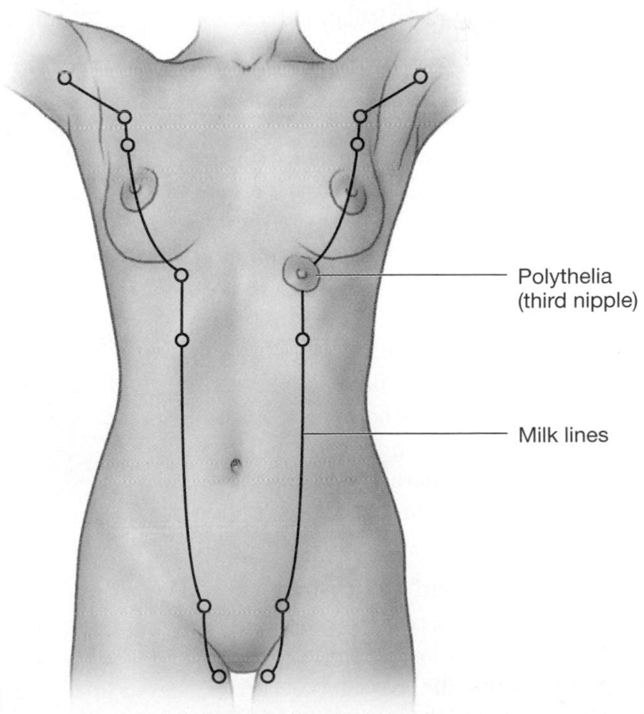

FIGURE 22-2A–B a) Supernumerary nipples; b) Milk lines
Source: a. SPL/Custom Medical Stock Photo

The fibrous tissue provides the supporting matrix to the breast. The Cooper suspensory ligaments extend from the connective tissue layer through the entire breast and attach the breast to the underlying pectoral muscle fascial planes. Subcutaneous and retromammary fat surround the glandular tissue of the breast.

Male Breast

Men and women develop breasts from identical embryological tissues; however, at puberty, female sex hormones, primarily estrogen, promote breast development. Higher amounts of testosterone prevent breast development in males resulting in less prominent breasts, measuring about 2 cm in diameter and appearing like small buttons. In athletic males they may be difficult to distinguish from the well-developed pectoralis muscles.

Breast Lymphatics

The lymphatic drainage of the breast flows in one direction from the superficial to the deep plexus. Approximately 97% of the lymphatics flow to the axillary lymph nodes, and about 3% flow to the internal mammary chain. The axillary lymph nodes are often arbitrarily divided into levels, defined by the borders of the pectoralis minor muscle. The groups of lymph nodes, which are recognized, consist of the following: central axillary, pectoral, brachial, subscapular, lateral, infraclavicular, supraclavicular, and internal (Figure 22-4).

Developmental Variations

Developmental variations occur over the course of an individual's life span and events. Awareness of these variations is important to understand and recognize common age-related alterations or modifications of the breast. The dynamic process of breast development, which actually begins during embryonic life is a result of a complex interaction between systemic hormones (ovarian, pituitary and placental hormones) and local growth factors: epidermal growth factors, fibroblast growth factors and transforming growth factors.

Neonates and Children

At birth, the breast consists of primitive ductal elements that grow steadily until the prepubertal years. The breast in neonates may be enlarged due to the transplacental estrogen transfer from the mother (Figure 22-5). They may secrete a clear or whitish fluid called

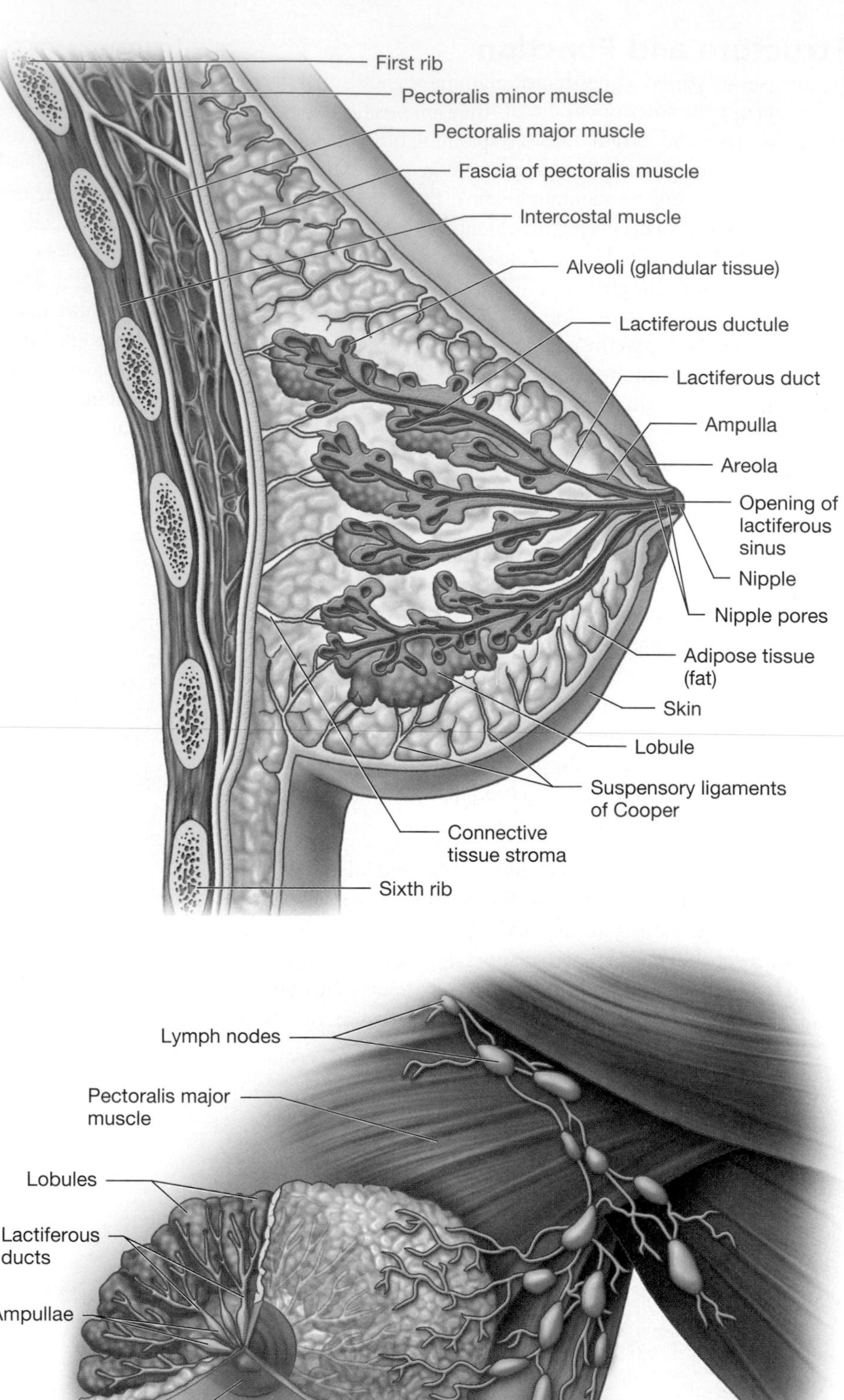

FIGURE 22-3 Cross section of the breast with the tissue component and muscle layer

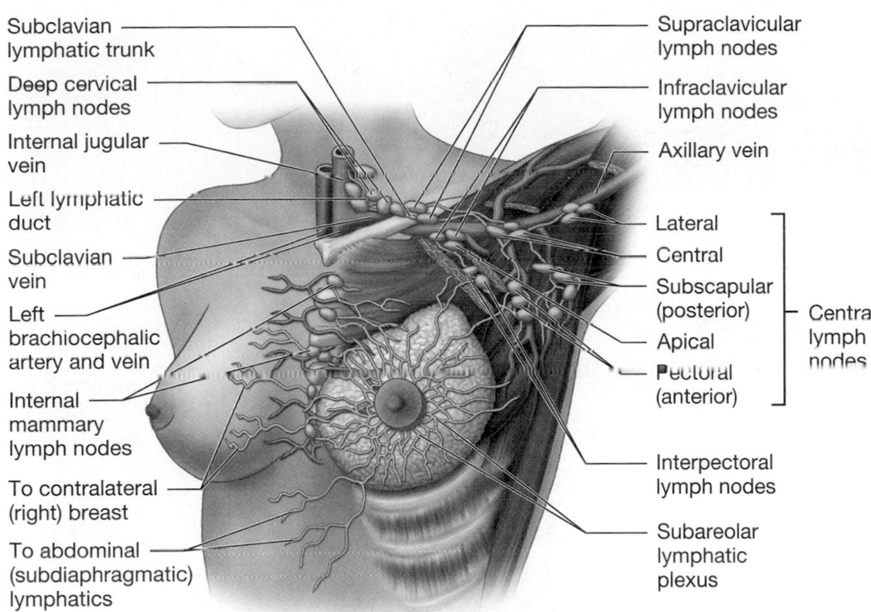

FIGURE 22-4 Axillary and other lymph nodes and lymphatic flow

"witch milk" that disappears in a few days to few weeks coinciding with the decline of the maternal hormones. During prepubertal years, a slow, steady ductal growth with branching occurs; breast changes in boys ceases at this juncture.

Adolescents

With the onset of puberty (10–12 years old), the beginning of female breast development is indicated by the appearance of a bud around the nipple-areolar complex. Breast enlargement begins with a marked increase in the growth and branching of the ducts that is accompanied by an increase in lobule formation, changing the appearance of the breast. This process is under the influence of gonadotropin-releasing hormone (GnRH), which is synthesized and released from the hypothalamus, resulting in the release of follicle stimulating hormone (FSH) and luteinizing hormone (LH) from the anterior pituitary gland. Estrogen and progesterone also play a significant role in breast development by stimulating DNA synthesis and bud formation (Figure 22-6). This is followed by ductile maturation and fatty deposition around the areola. These changes correlate to the increase in estrogen and progesterone.

The external appearance of the breast may initially be asymmetric with nipples displaced lateral to the medial clavicular line between the fourth and fifth intercostal space.

Tanner Stages of Breast Development Breast development from childhood to maturity has been developed and described by Tanner who divided it into 5 stages. These stages are identified and described in Figure 22-7.

> ***THINK LINK: Cultural Variability***
> Variability exists in breast development according to culture. In both Mexican and African Americans, budding may be visible earlier (before 8 years old). Breast size is also believed to be determined by ethnicity. In obese individuals, it may be difficult to delineate excess adipose tissue from breast budding.

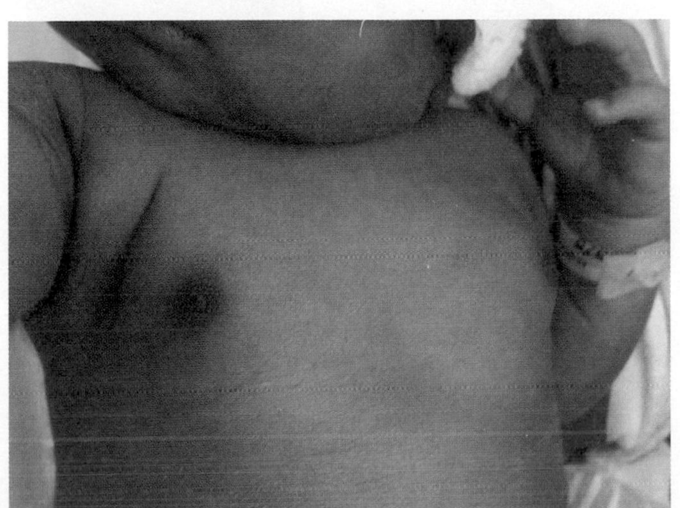

FIGURE 22-5 Infant breast hypertrophy

During menstrual cycles, the breasts undergo a cyclical pattern of change in size, nodularity, and tenderness. They are generally larger and tender a few days before the menstrual cycle, corresponding with the increase in nodularity. They are smaller during the 4th–7th day of the menstrual cycle. These changes follow the follicular and luteal phases of the menstrual cycle.

The Pregnant Woman

Maximal glandular and ductal proliferation and differentiation occur during pregnancy, which may be considered the completion of mammary gland differentiation, due to the influence of progesterone. In response, there is breast and nipple enlargement. Some bluish vascular markings appear on the surface of the skin during this stage in response to the luteal and placental hormones. The changing levels of hormones during pregnancy cause type 2 and 3 lobules to progress to type 4. There is an increase in volume of the breast tissue, ductal sprouting during the first trimester and lobular formation during the second trimester. Late pregnancy is marked by the continuation and enhancement of the secretory activity with accumulation of colostrum.

Increases in pigmentation and size of the nipple and areola occur during pregnancy. Nipples get more erect and Montgomery glands in the areola become more prominent. The differentiation of the secretory cells leads to the increased ability to synthesize and secrete milk. The breast feels more full and nodular and may leak yellow colostrum with squeezing of the nipples after the first trimester.

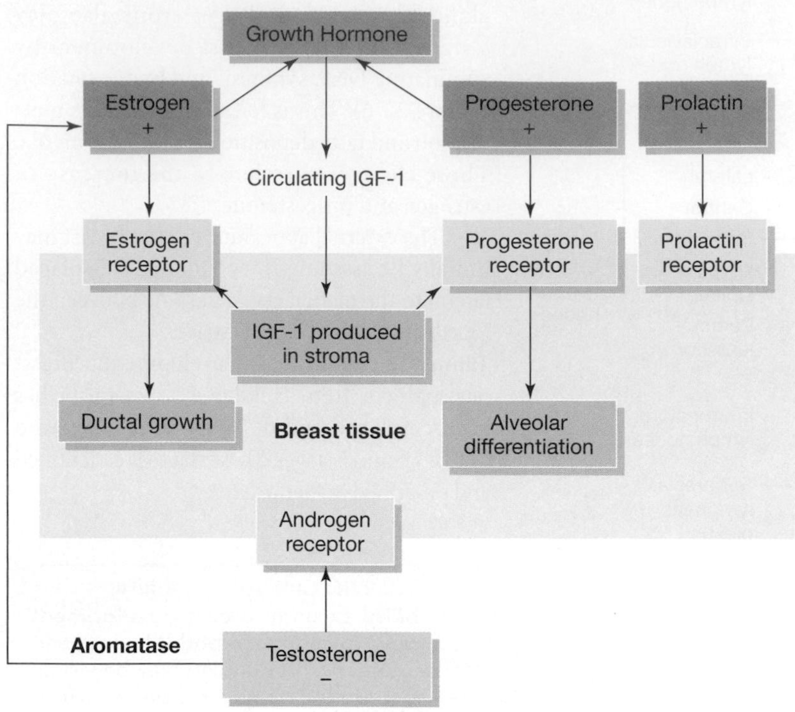

FIGURE 22-6 Hormones affecting development and differentiation of breast tissue.

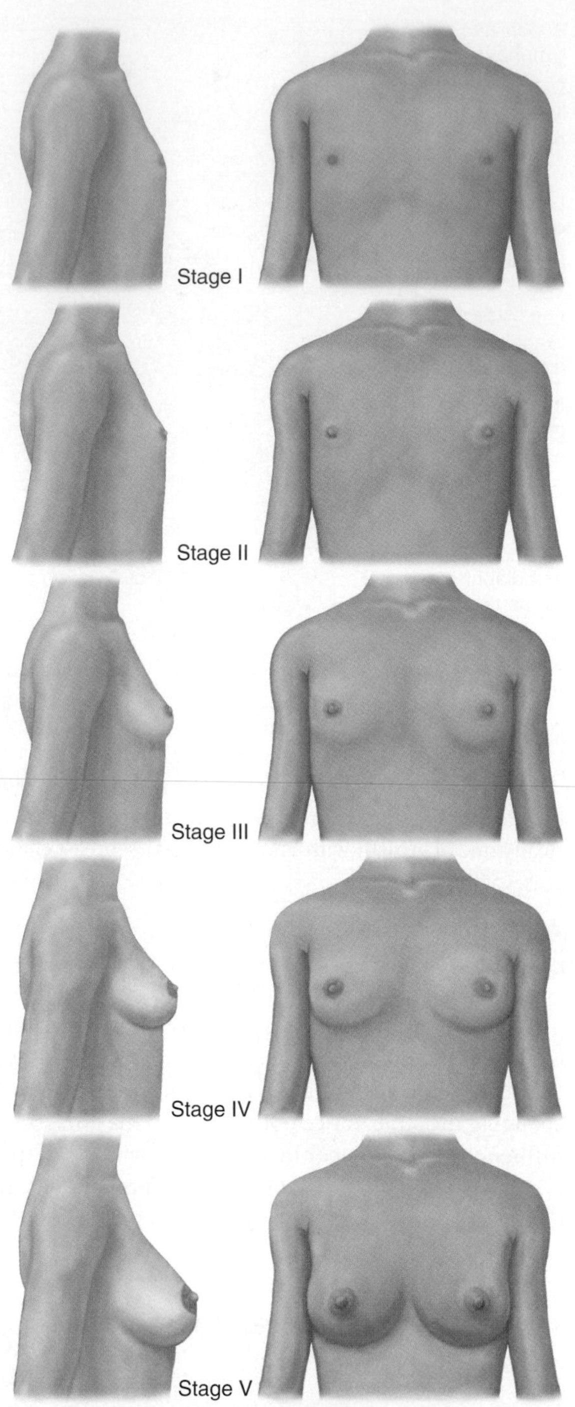

FIGURE 22-7 Tanner's stages of breast development: I, Preadolescent. Only the nipple is raised above the level of the breast, as in the child. II, Budding stage. Areola increased in diameter and surrounding area slightly elevated. III, Breast and areola enlarged. No contour separation. IV, Areola forms a secondary elevation above that of the breast in half of girls. V, Areola is usually part of the general breast contour and is strongly pigmented. Nipple usually projects.

After delivery, colostrum may be expressed from the nipples. Breasts exhibit an increase in size and engorgement and become generally warm, red, shiny, hard, and tender. Milk secretion is stimulated and facilitated by infant sucking. Nipple stimulation and milk removal maintains lactation by stimulation of prolactin release from the anterior pituitary gland and oxytocin from the posterior pituitary. The **"milk let-down" reflex** refers to the neurohormonal stimulation of the nipple triggered by the infant sucking the breast. The breast tenderness improves with frequent breastfeeding; however, there is an increased risk for mastitis and mastodynia (breast tenderness to palpation) at this time.

After lactation, apoptosis (programmed cell death) and tissue remodeling occur as a result of lactogenic hormone withdrawal. This leads to regression, or involution, of the glandular elements.

The Older Woman

Menopause is characterized by atrophy of the glandular elements, with a decline in number of type 2 and 3 lobules and the predominance of type 1 lobules (fat). This is due to ovarian follicular atresia with resulting deficiency of estrogen and progesterone. The fibrous stromal support decreases, which reduces breast size and causes sagging and diminished firmness.

Health Promotion

In 2008, breast cancer accounted for about 23% of the total cancer cases worldwide and currently remains the leading cause of cancer in women, second only to lung cancer as the cause of cancer deaths in women.

Around the world, breast cancer is the most common cancer and is the leading cause of cancer death among women In the United States, a woman has a 1 in 8 lifetime risk of developing breast cancer.

Breast Cancer

The goals of *Healthy People 2020* related to the topic of (breast) cancer are the following:

- C–03 Reduce breast cancer death rate in women.
- C–11 Reduce late-stage female breast cancer.
- C–17 Increase the proportion of women who receive breast cancer screening based on the most recent guidelines (U.S. Department of Health and Human Services, 2009).

Breast cancer is predominantly a disease of women, although it does occur in males. Women generally consider breast cancer more of a health threat than cardiovascular diseases, despite the fact that CV diseases rank as the leading cause of death in both men and women. A woman's chances of developing breast cancer increases with age.

It is recognized that gene mutations, or genes BRCA1 and BRCA2, may be responsible for some breast cancers, but account for only about 5–10 percent of the total numbers. These same genes are also known to increase the risk for ovarian cancer.

Breast Cancer Screening The exact cause of breast cancer remains unclear. Reduction in the numbers of breast cancers necessitates increasing awareness of modifiable and nonmodifiable risk factors, as well as promoting and encouraging participation in breast cancer screening. Approaches to breast cancer screening should incorporate a discussion of individual's values and breast cancer risk analysis derived from history and use of available risk prediction tools. Breast cancer risk prediction tools are used to determine best screening strategies or preventive therapy. The BCRAT (Breast Cancer Risk Assessment Tool, also called the Gail model) takes into account race, ethnicity, age, and history of breast biopsy. The most common screening modalities are clinical breast examination (CBE), self-breast examination (SBE), and mammography (imaging studies). In addition, digital mammography or MRI may be used in certain situations.

In 2009, the United States Preventive Services Task Force (USPSTF) caused a national outcry when they recommended that women aged 40–49 no longer receive routine mammography screening. In response, they adapted their recommendation for screening on women younger than 50 years to read The decision to start regular, biennial screening mammography before age 50 should be an individual one and take the patient's context and values into account regarding specific benefits and harms.

Breast examinations, performed by either a provider or individual have also come under scrutiny relative to their effectiveness in detecting early cancer. SBE has not been shown to improve mortality from breast cancer and consistency of the clinical examination has been challenged with trade-offs as to the provider's time, cost of visit and the work-up of false-positive results. While the benefits of these examinations are questionable, there is no harm in encouraging women to continue the practice. Despite the fact that the revised recommendations were based on evidence, there are still instances where BSE has detected cancerous breast lumps and allowed treatment to be initiated early and preventing the cancer from spreading. Thus, many providers still educate patients, and patients welcome the education as an important component for promotion of breast awareness and health participation (Nelson et al., 2009). Table 22-1 provides the most recent recommendations for screening for breast cancer from multiple cancer associated organizations.

Women who test positive for BRCA1 and 2 are at increased risk for breast and ovarian cancers. Genetic consultation is available to initiate early/intensified surveillance and help them make prevention choices such as chemoprophylaxis or prophylactic mastectomy.

Table 22-1 Breast cancer screening recommendations for women at average risk

American Cancer Society	National Cancer Institute	National Comprehensive Cancer network	U.S. Preventive Services Task Force	Sloan Kettering Cancer Center	American Association of Family Practice	CDC
Mammography						
Every year beginning at age 40	Every 1–2 years beginning at age 40	Every year beginning at age 40	Informed decision making with a health care provider ages 40–49 Every 2 years ages 50–74 Insufficient evidence to assess the additional benefits/harms in women over 75	Every year beginning at age 40	Individualized before age 50 Every 2 years for women ages 50–74. Insufficient evidence for women over 75	Every 2 years beginning at age 50

Continued

Table 22-1 Breast cancer screening recommendations for women at average risk *(continued)*

American Cancer Society	National Cancer Institute	National Comprehensive Cancer network	U.S. Preventive Services Task Force	Sloan Kettering Cancer Center	American Association of Family Practice	CDC
Clinical Breast Exam						
Every 3 years ages 20–39	No specific recommendation	Every 1–3 years ages 25–39	Not enough evidence to recommend for or against	Every year beginning at age 25	Insufficient evidence for or against for women ages 40 and older	No specific recommendation
Every year beginning at age 40		Every year beginning at age 40				
Breast Self-Examination						
Option for women starting in their 20s			Recommends against teaching BSE	Monthly beginning at age 20 (optional). Awareness of breast changes		No specific recommendation
MRI/Digital Mammography						
			Not enough evidence to recommend for or against	Detected more cancers in women under 50, with dense breasts, not yet in menopause	Not enough evidence to recommend for or against	

Clinical Context Exemplars

Situation A

Mrs. Jones is a 49-year-old woman who presents with a palpable breast mass with some discoloration of the skin. She felt this about a month after she tripped and landed on her chest. She did not think much of this as she related the findings to the injury. It is now 2 months after the injury, and she is concerned with the persistent lump.

1. What questions might you ask the patient and why?
2. What observations are important to make during a physical examination?

Situation B

Miss Smith is a 25-year-old woman who palpated a breast mass. She is quite alarmed and in your office demanding an urgent mammogram. Mrs. A is a 60-year-old with diabetes, COPD, history of MI, and dementia who was brought in for annual exam. Her family asked you if screening for breast cancer is warranted. In another examination room is Mrs. B, an 80-year-old woman with mild osteoporosis, exercises regularly with no symptoms except for mild joint pains, and asked you for a screening mammogram.

1. What additional information is needed to determine each woman's need for a mammogram?
2. What evidence might be presented to each woman or family members to help them determine the need for a mammogram?

Situation C

Mr. Ribbs is a 16-year-old young adolescent who presents with breast enlargement. He stopped participating in sports because he was growing increasingly embarrassed by their prominence.

1. What questions might you ask this patient? What is important on the physical examination of this patient?
2. Would this scenario be different if Mr. Ribbs was a 55-year-old man? If so, why?

Situation D

Mr. Frack is a 59-year-old man who is being admitted for a mastectomy for breast cancer. He's somewhat embarrassed that he has a "woman's disease" and doesn't want anyone to know what he's in the hospital for. During his work-up he wants to know why this happened to him, a male, and how much longer he has to live.

1. What would be the most appropriate approach to take to help Mr. Frack understand his situation?
2. Is there any additional information you might need that would be helpful to facilitate his understanding of his condition?
3. What information would you want to provide him to help him in coping with his situation?

SUBJECTIVE DATA

History of Present Illness (CC)

The patient may present to the provider with a variety of concerns that may be directly related to the breast or other systems. Framing the questions will depend on the patient's age, gender, culture, race, emotional or mental status, health practices, and concurrent illnesses. All symptoms presented must be thoroughly assessed with a symptom analysis (COLDERRA).

Breast Mass

A palpable breast mass is a common presentation in women seeking health care and in most instances, it is benign. However, any suspicious findings should be thoroughly examined until a malignancy can be ruled out. It is also important to recognize that in over 50% of the time, women present with a self-discovered breast mass that cannot be palpated by a provider. Thus, vigilance in ruling out a malignancy is these situations must be maintained. Failure to determine the presence of a malignant mass can have devastating consequences for the woman.

Provider Inquiries	Clinical Reasoning/Logic
Characteristics: Do you notice changes in breast size that coincide with menstrual cycles? Changes in shape? More than one mass?	Changes in size of mass based on the luteal/follicular phases of the menstrual cycle are related to physiological changes suggesting benign breast disease. During the follicular phase, breast lumps and tenderness lumps tend to get better, and the opposite is true during the luteal phase. Shape: Irregular, stellate shape lesions are worrisome for cancer. Fibroadenomas and cysts are generally round and well defined.
Onset: When was it first felt-self breast exam or by accident? How often is self breast exam performed? Are you familiar with characteristics of your own breast? In what position when found—supine, standing, other?	Cancer in younger women tends to grow faster than in older women. Younger women tend to have benign disease Age of onset: 18–30, 31–50, > 50 Risk for breast cancer increases with age. The evaluation will likely be different if a woman rarely performs SBE and not familiar with her breast characteristics than with a woman who regularly performs SBE and can determine differences with baseline characteristics.
Location: Which quadrant? One side or both?	Single lesion in one breast may suggest fibroadenoma or a malignant lesion. Bilaterality suggests benign breast disease.
Duration: How long have you had the mass or masses or lumps?	
Relief: Has the mass resolved or downsized after menstrual period?	Lumps that come and go with menstrual cycles suggest benign breast disease.
Risk: Ask the patient about possible modifiable and nonmodifiable risks that might contribute to breast cancer. See Table 22-2.	Reproductive history is important in determining risk, i.e., early menarche, late menopause, late pregnancy suggest prolonged estrogen exposure thereby increasing risks for breast cancer. Hormonal exposure in utero (Hoover et al., 2011; Verloop, van Leeuwen, Helmerhorst, van Boven, & Rookus, 2010) Personal and family history of breast cancer, gene mutation and other breast cancer syndromes increase one's risk. Protective factors include longer breast feeding, increased parity, exercise, reduced postmenopausal body mass index, oophorectomy before 35 years, aspirin once a week.

Provider Inquiries	Clinical Reasoning/Logic
	Women who have been exposed to DES during fetal development are at a greater risk for developing breast cancer (Hoover et al., 2011).
Associated signs/symptoms: Do you have a history of any breast pain, skin changes retraction, dimpling, discharge, sores, change in size and shape?	Pain does not usually accompany breast cancer with some exception-involvement of nerve plexus or deeper structures like bone. Skin changes such as dimpling, retraction, and peau d'orange suggest malignancy. **Peau d'orange** is an orange-peel appearance of the skin due to edema from lymphatic obstruction (refer to Figure 22-11). A bloody discharge is an indication of malignancy.

Table 22-2 Nonmodifiable and modifiable risk factors for breast cancer

	Nonmodifiable Risk Factors
Age	Risk increases with aging. A woman is 100 more times likely to develop breast cancer in her 60s than in her 20s.
Gender	More women than men develop breast cancer. Breast cancer is about 100 times less common among men than among women. For men, the lifetime risk of getting breast cancer is about 1 in 1000. The number of breast cancer cases in men relative to the population has been fairly stable over the last 30 years.
Genetics	Women with an inherited BRCA1 or BRAC2 mutation have a 35% to 85% chance of developing breast cancer during their lifetimes. Males with the mutation have a greater risk for prostate and breast cancer. NBR2 is a gene located near the breast. NBR2 and its relationship to breast cancer has been explored, but no definitive cause and effect has been determined.
Personal history of breast cancer	Cancer in one breast increases risk of developing a new cancer in the other breast. Women who have been diagnosed with ovarian, uterine, or bowel cancer have a higher risk of future development of breast cancer.
Family history of breast cancer	Having one first-degree relative (mother, sister, or daughter) with breast cancer approximately doubles a woman's risk, and having two first-degree relatives increases her risk fivefold. The risk for a woman with a brother who has breast cancer increases by 30% than for a sister.
Previous breast biopsies	Atypical hyperplasia or lobular cancer in situ (LCIS) substantially increases breast cancer risk. Fibrocystic changes without proliferative breast disease do not affect breast cancer risk.
Race/Ethnicity	White women are at higher risk than other racial/ethnic groups. Morbidity increases with improving economic conditions while mortality is related to lower socioeconomic status. In U.S., black women are less likely to be diagnosed with breast cancer but are more likely to die from it. Even after diagnosis, fewer black women seek treatment than white women. Black women under 45 years old more commonly develop breast cancer. In the U.S., BRCA mutations occur more frequently in Jewish women of Eastern Europe descent than in other racial/ethnic groups. Asian, Hispanic, and Native American women have lower morbidity and mortality of breast cancer.
Previous breast radiation	Radiation therapy to the chest area as treatment for another cancer (Hodgkin's disease/non-Hodgkin's lymphoma) significantly increases risk for breast cancer. Risk is highest in women who were treated in adolescence; radiation after age 40 does not significantly increase risk.
Onset of menstruation	Menarche before age 12 or menopause after age 55 slightly increases risk.
Breast density	Breast tissue may be dense or fatty. Older women whose mammograms show more dense tissue are at increased risk.
Diethylstilbesterol (DES) therapy	Women who received DES in the 1940s through the 1960s during their pregnancies have a slightly increased risk.
	Modifiable Risk Factors
Childbirth	Nulliparity or late age at birth of first child (after 30) is associated with an increased risk.
Hormone therapy	Use of combined estrogen/progesterone hormone replacement therapy after menpause (more than 4 years of use) increases risk.
Alcohol	Risk increases with amount of alcohol consumed. Alcohol increases the levels of estrogen.
Diet	Obesity is associated with an increased risk, especially for women after menopause. Having more fat tissue can increase estrogen levels and increase the likelihood of developing breast cancer. No specific dietary fats have been identified for increasing risk.
Physical activity	Women who are physically inactive throughout life may have an increased risk of breast cancer.
Smoking	There is some evidence that smoking is linked to breast cancer; however, a direct link has not been established. This is also true for second-hand smoke.

Table 22-3 Characteristics of breast alterations

	Breast cancer	Fibroadenoma	Benign Breast Disease	Trauma
Age	30–90, risk increases as one gets older	15–25 but can occur up to 55 Decrease in size with menopause	30–50, regresses with the onset of menopause	Any age
Skin changes	Peau d'orange may be seen near the areolar/nipple region, retraction of skin, dimpling, nipple deviation, nipple retraction or breast shape irregularity may be seen	None	None	Bruise or resolving bruise, abrasion at the site of trauma Findings resolve over time
Growth characteristic	Constant growth, cancer in younger women grow rapidly	Rapid and constant growth	Increase or decrease rapidly related to the menstrual cycle	Increase relating to time of trauma due to initial bruising
Shape	Irregular, stellate	Round, lobular or disclike	Round, lobular for cysts. Ropelike and lumpy for fibrocystic breast, variable in trauma	Variable; depends on initial bruise and age of bruise and if organized bruise or not. Variable; depends on sites of trauma
Consistency	Firm, rock hard, stony	Usually firm and rubbery	Soft for cyst; firm rubbery, elastic for fibrocystic breast disease	Organized bruise may be fixed or mobile
Demarcation	Poorly defined, less well demarcated	Well demarcated	Well demarcated and usually bilateral	
Mobility	Fixed	Quite mobile and slippery	Mobile for cysts	
Number	Single	Usually single	Multiple	Single
Tenderness	Usually painless, although may be tender. In general, pain does not accompany breast cancer.	None	Generally tender; cyclical tenderness is maximal prior to the menstrual periods and gets better after a woman's period.	
History	May have personal or FH of breast cancer risk, BRCA 1 or 2 mutation, Post menopausal hormone replacement therapy (HRT), DES use, environmental exposure to carcinogens, nulliparity, early menarche, late menopause, smoking, increase BMI, increase bone density, alcohol use, nullipara, (see risk factors for breast cancer)		History of lump prominence before the periods and decreases with onset of menstruation With history of trauma (in the trauma section)	

Breast Pain/Tenderness

Breast pain is the most common breast condition prompting a visit to a care provider. The frequency of breast cancer in women presenting with breast pain ranges from 1.2% to 6.7%. However, breast pain was the only presenting symptom in up to 15% of women with newly diagnosed cancer (Smith, Pruthi, & Fitzpatrick, 2004). Breast pain can also occur in males but is rarely associated with breast cancer. Some of the causes of male breast pain include running/jogging, infection, cysts, adenoma and alcoholism with liver damage.

Provider Inquiries	Clinical Reasoning/Logic
Characteristics: What type of breast pain are you experiencing? Is it sharp or dull? How severe is the pain?	Pain characteristics, such as a sharp, with dermatomal distribution, suggest Herpes zoster.

Provider Inquiries	Clinical Reasoning/Logic
	Involvement of nerve plexus, intercostal, mammary nerves, lung and bone from deep invasion by breast cancer or metastasis may cause pain. Type of pain may be described as sharp, pleuritic, or dull. Dull pressure or heaviness of the chest suggests cardiac manifestations.
	Breast tenderness in males may be associated with gynecomastia and frequently associated with puberty.
Onset: Is this the first time the breast pain or tenderness has occurred or have you experienced it previously? Is it cyclical or noncyclical in onset?	New onset of pain is seen in herpes zoster, trauma, infection, or recent deeper invasion from cancer or metastasis.
	Breast pain related to hormonal fluctuation suggests physiologic, benign conditions.
	Noncyclical breast pain may be due to large breasts, mastitis, inflammatory breast disease, ductal ecstasias, breast surgery, and medications.
Location: Does the pain or tenderness occur in on one breast or both? Is it local or regional, deep or superficial? Where in the breast is it located?	Bilateral pain suggests benign breast disease related to cyclical changes in women. This is associated with ovulation caused by glandular proliferation as a result of the influence of estrogen on the ductal elements and progesterone on the stoma.
	On the contrary, local/regional pain suggests processes like trauma, infection (herpes zoster, ductal occlusion with localized cellulitis or mastitis) or malignancy.
Is the pain or tenderness outside the breast?	Extra mammary breast pain may be related to cardiac, pulmonary, musculoskeletal, spinal, and esophageal etiologies.
	Gynecomastia is most commonly bilateral but may also present unilaterally.
Duration: How long does the pain last? Is the pain cyclic or continuous in nature? Does it come and go?	Pain related to cycles suggests benign breast disease. Pain resolves usually at onset of menstruation.
Exacerbation: What makes the pain worse? Activity, exercise, menstrual period, lactation breathing, coughing, change in position of chest?	Relationship with activity like movement of the chest wall or breathing suggests chest wall, musculoskeletal, or pleuritic pain from pulmonary etiology. Cardiac pain may mimic breast pain and is generally associated with increased activity.
	Lactational mastitis is a localized, painful inflammation of the breast, which occurs after giving birth and generally associated with pain, redness of the breast, fever, and malaise. It is common in the first month after giving birth. It is related to poor milk drainage and prolonged breast ductal engorgement.
Radiation: Does the pain radiate to any other location (arm, jaw, neck, back)?	Ischemic cardiac pain may mimic breast pain with radiation to axilla or neck.

Provider Inquiries	Clinical Reasoning/Logic
Relief: What makes the pain better or go away? Is it relieved by onset of menstrual period? Is it relieved by rest, medications (what; how many), position change, or complementary therapies? Breastfeeding?	Ischemic cardiac pain usually gets better with rest or nitroglycerine. Fibrocystic breast pain may continue until onset of menstruation.
Risk: History of trauma, hormone therapy, other medications, history of breast cancer diagnosis, history of surgery?	Recent history of trauma increases the chance that changes are from the injury. Hormone therapy may increase fibrocystic breast pain. History of breast cancer may be a red flag for metastatic or regional invasion or recurrence.
Associated Signs/Symptoms: Do you experience nipple discharge, swelling, asymmetry, change in contour, dimpling, crusting, ulcerations, mass, fever, redness?	Pain does not usually accompany breast cancer with some exceptions—involvement of nerve plexus or deeper structures like bone. Fever suggest infection or inflammation. Redness and fluctuance during lactation suggest infection, or abscess. Paget's disease may present with pain, tenderness, drainage, peau d' orange, crusting, and ulcerations around the nipple. Lymphedema suggests lymphatic flow obstruction from tumor or may be a result of lymph node dissection.
Breast or Nipple Discharge Breast or nipple discharge is one of the most common breast complaints. As many as 50%–80% of premenopausal women can express more than one drop of fluid from their breasts. Most nipple discharges are benign in nature. Concerns are papillomas, ductal carcinoma in situ, or ductal carcinomas. Papillomas are generally benign, but may harbor atypia or ductal carcinoma in situ. It is important to differentiate benign from the high-risk conditions. Although rare, nipple discharge occurs in males. It is not unusual for boys going through puberty to experience a milky discharge; however, nipple discharge in older males is associated with a high probability of breast cancer.	
Characteristics: Is the discharge clear, or contain mucus or blood? Is it a milky color?	Bloody drainage is suspicious for malignancy. Although, it can be seen in pregnancy during second or third trimester. Milky, straw-colored, clear, brown, or gray-colored discharge are seen in benign conditions; whitish-yellow, yellow, or green color indicative of infection. Males may experience the same types of discharge, however, any type of discharge in males needs to be evaluated medically.
Onset: When did it start? Did its onset have any relationship with the menstrual cycles, pregnancy, lactation? Does it occur with pressure, squeezing or stimulation, or is it spontaneous, triggered by trauma?	Spontaneous discharge is worrisome for cancer or other pathological causes. Breast stimulation from tight brassiere, self-manipulation or by partner, other traumatic injuries to the chest wall, surgery like thoracotomy are the most common causes of **hyperprolactinemia** and **galactorrhea**, which is defined as nonpathologic, milky nipple discharge unrelated to nursing or pregnancy.
Location: Is the discharge unilateral, uniductal, multiductal, or bilateral?	Bilaterality and multiductal origin of discharge suggest benign breast disease or physiologic galactorrhea, which may be related to endocrine causes or tumors, or medications (dopamine inhibitors).

Provider Inquiries	Clinical Reasoning/Logic
	Uniductal, unilateral drainage suggests a pathological cause like **papilloma** (benign papillary tumor), which can harbor DCIS or atypia or other malignancy.
Duration: How long does the discharge last? Is it cyclic or continuous in nature? Does it come and go?	Persistence suggests worrisome causes. Milk secretions may last 6 months or more after cessation of breastfeeding.
Exacerbation: What makes the drainage worse? Pressure to nipple? Is it spontaneous?	Benign nipple discharge is usually provoked by trauma or manipulation by self or partner, tight brassiere, or trauma. Suspicious etiologies should be considered if drainage is spontaneous.
Relief: Have you tried a draining procedure? If so, was it effective?	Breast pumping or breastfeeding relieve lactational mastitis and help sustain breast engorgement and milk supply.
Risk: History of breast cancer diagnosis, history of mass, lymph nodes, other risks for breast cancer?	Presence of risk factors for breast cancer increases the likelihood that a uniductal, unilateral nipple drainage is neoplastic.
Associated signs/symptoms: History of lactation, pregnancy, any pain, skin changes retraction, dimpling, discharge, sores or excoriations, change in size and shape, testicular atrophy, visual symptoms or changes, history of eczema, mass, pain, asymmetry, lymph node involvement, local infection?	Secretory function of the breast occurs in pregnancy and postpartum period and milk secretions may last for 6 months or more after cessation of breastfeeding. Drainage from eczema needs to be ruled out by careful examination of the skin. Hypogonadism suggests etiology like Klinefelter's and testicular neoplasm. Presence of mass increases risk for cancer. Skin infection or deeper infection may be manifested by discharge. Bitemporal field loss on physical examination suggests chiasmal compression from a pituitary adenoma.
Enlarged Breasts (Macromastia/Gynecomastia) In females, hypertrophy of the breast (macromastia and gigantomastia) is a rare medical condition of the breast connective tissues. Breast hypertrophy is a benign *progressive* enlargement, which can occur in both breasts (bilateral) or only in one breast (unilateral). In males, swelling of the breast tissue in boys or men is described as gynecomastia, and is defined as breast tissue from 0.5 to 1 cm in puberty and >2 cm in adult.	
Characteristics: Increase in breast tissue/weight? Pain or tenderness?	The indication is a breast weight that exceeds approximately 3% of the total body weight. The enlargement can cause muscular discomfort and over-stretching of the skin envelope, which can lead in some cases to ulceration. Gynecomastia may have accompanying sensitivity or mild tenderness but pain is usually minimal.

Provider Inquiries	Clinical Reasoning/Logic
Any skin changes or discharge from nipple?	Presence of skin changes and nipple discharge is worrisome for malignancy.
Is the enlargement concentric (uniform) or eccentric (nonuniform)?	Eccentric enlargement is worrisome especially if accompanied by a mass.
Onset: Did any particular event or condition seem to initiate enlargement?	Breast hypertrophy is classified in one of five ways: as either pubertal (virginal hypertrophy), gestational (gravid macromastia), in adult women without any obvious cause, associated with penicillamine therapy, and associated with extreme obesity. In adolescent gynecomastia, it may occur 6 months after the development of secondary sex characteristic with peak around Tanner stage 3–4. Gynecomastia before puberty or more than 6 months after puberty are red flags. Another peak incidence in 50–80 years of age.
Have you experienced recent weight gain? Have you started any new medications?	Obesity may also present like pseudogynecomastia, which is breast enlargement consisting of adipose rather than glandular tissue.
Location: Are both breasts affected equally, or one more than the other?	Hypertrophy of the breast can affect the breasts equally, but usually affects one breast more than the other, thereby causing asymmetry, when one breast is larger than the other. Gynecomastia that is bilateral suggests a benign disorder. One-third of all adolescent patients with gynecomastia may be unilateral.
Duration: How long have you noticed larger breasts?	Gynecomastia of more than 18 months without resolution is worrisome especially if distribution is eccentric.
Exacerbation: Is there anything that you have noticed that makes enlargement greater? Have you recently gained any weight or started weight lifting?	Weight gain or hypertrophy of pectoralis muscles from weight training may accentuate gynecomastia.
Relief: Is there anything the you have noticed that reduces enlargement?	Weight-reduction regimen for the over-weight woman can alleviate some of the excessive size and volume of her abnormally enlarged breasts. Discontinuation of offending medication may improve the gynecomastia, weight loss may do the same for pseudogynecomastia.
Associated signs/symptoms: History of any pain, mass, skin changes, use of medications, signs of androgen deficiency like hypogonadism, any secondary characteristics at puberty? List of drugs from antibiotics, PPI or H_1 blockers, anti-androgens, alkylating agents, brigs of abuse like alcohol, amphetamines, heroin, marijuana, methadone, hormones, anabolic steroids, psychoactive drugs list. Genetic history of BRCA 1 and 2 mutation?	In females, secondary effects of the enlarged breasts may include such manifestations as shoulder-notching by the brassière strap from the breast weight, kyphosis (excessive, backward curvature of the thoracic region of the spinal column), skin irritation, and skin rash affecting the breast crease.

THINK LINK: Male Breast Cancer

Breast cancer is about 100 times less common among men than among women. The lifetime risk of getting breast cancer for men is about 1 in 1000. The number of breast cancer cases in men relative to the population has been fairly stable over the last 30 years. The American Cancer Society estimates for that for 2013 approximatley:

- 2240 new cases of invasive breast cancer will be diagnosed among men.
- 410 men will die from breast cancer.

It was once thought that the prognosis for men with breast cancer was worse than that for women, but recent studies have not supported this thinking. Men and women with the same stage of breast cancer have a relatively similar outlook for survival.

Breast cancer in men is generally detected by clinical symptoms like mass, pain, nipple changes or discharge, or enlargement of the breast. Male breast cancer accounts for about 1% of all breast cancers. There is a tendency for delay in diagnosis due to decreased awareness and lack of screening procedures. The stage at diagnosis is crucial for improved survival. Risk factors include family history, Jewish ancestry, obesity, chest wall irradiation, having never been married, gynecomastia, and Klinefelter's.

Past Medical History

Past medical history provides information as to previous illnesses or conditions that may have an effect on the breast as well as provides information that may help to identify potential causes for chief complaint or other presenting symptoms.

Provider Inquiries	Clinical Reasoning/Logic
Menarche: When did it start, problems associated with?	The earlier the onset, the higher the risk.
Current menstrual cycles/regularity? Pregnancy/Parity—OB history (age of first live birth) Lactation? Trauma?	Older age of pregnancy and breastfeeding are associated with increased risk. Nulliparous women have higher risk for breast cancer. Increasing risk of breast cancer directly related to length of time exposed to ovarian hormones.
Menopause?	A late onset of menopause is associated with higher risk for breast cancer.
Medications—hormones or medication implicated in gynecomastia	Increased bone density, which may be related to estrogen exposure, has been associated with increased risk.
History of biopsy or abnormal imaging?	Certain pathology findings like atypical ductal hyperplasia and lobular cancer in situ have been associated with risk for invasive breast cancer.
Personal history of breast cancer?	Personal history of breast cancer with in-situ lesions, the 10-year risk of developing cancer on the contralateral abreast is about 5%.
Last imaging and where and what findings?	Higher breast density on imaging, which has been associated with ovarian hormone exposure, has been shown to increase risk as well.
Ionizing radiation to chest and neck?	Exposure to ionizing radiation during childhood/adolescence (nuclear testing, radiation therapy) increases risk for breast cancer. Radiation exposure risk proportionally related to radiation dose, years of exposure and age of exposure.

Family History

Family history provides information regarding family member's illnesses or conditions as potential causes for chief complaint or presenting symptoms that may indicate a pattern of presentation associated with transmission of familial/genetic factors predisposing the individual to certain system related conditions/illnesses. Any of these may indicate a potential or actual cause of a breast disorder.

Provider Inquiries	Purpose
Family history of breast cancer or other cancers—breast, ovarian cancer on both sides of the family and first-degree relatives?	Multiple first-degree relatives with premenopausal breast cancer confer a lifetime risk as high as 50%.
Presence of genetic mutation in the family BRCA 1 and 2?	Most of the risk from genetic mutation is related to BRCA 1/BRCA 2 mutation.

Personal and Social History

Personal and social history provides information related to habits, practices, and/or environmental influences that may predispose the patient to the development of certain system related conditions/illnesses.

Provider Inquiries	Purpose
Tobacco/smoking habits, alcohol use?	There is association between smoking and breast cancer risk.
	Weight gain and vigorous weight lifting with pectoralis hypertrophy are common presentation in men with breast enlargement. Higher body mass index (BMI), increased weight, or postmenopausal weight gain.
Environmental toxins, medications estrogens, DES use? Usual weight? Recent weight gain?	Exogenous estrogen exposure in posthysterectomy patients and use in postmenopausal women or high-serum estrogen on postmenopausal women.
Nutritional status? High fat intake?	Dietary factors such as high fat and red meat intake, alcohol consumption.

OBJECTIVE DATA

Although recent data challenges the value of the clinical breast examination (CBE), it is still considered an essential component of a standard physical examination. Performance of the breast examination requires standardization as to technique and timing of frequency with relevance to patient's presentation. It addresses the patient's concerns when he or she presents with breast symptoms and is also an adjunct to the various breast imaging procedures. It also serves to assess the patient's readiness to learn the self-breast examination. There are differences in recommendations among providers and organizations as to its frequency and utility.

The major elements of the breast examination are inspection and palpation. Preparation includes explanation of the examination to the patient, ensuring privacy and comfort, and discussion of findings. It is important to be courteous, gentle, and reassuring. The examination may have to be repeated if findings are felt to be related to the patient's menstrual cycle. Provider's variability exists as to the preferred method of palpation. It is important to be systematic and consistent. Washing and warming the provider's hands help ensure the patient's comfort.

Level I to IV Examination

The Level I to Level IV examinations are performed in a continuum, which start from a basic level to a more comprehensive level based on the provider's abilities, patient's presentation, and location of the examination. The examination may start at the outpatient setting progressing to the ED, hospital unit bed, ICU, or specialty unit. Frequently all the elements from basic to the comprehensive exam are done in one setting like in a primary care setting, or the ED.

The condition/illness of the patient is the primary consideration related to the type and amount of data needed to assess the patient's /condition/ illness/situation. The arrangement of skills into levels is for general purposes and is meant to be descriptive rather than prescriptive. The purpose of arranging into levels is to provide a framework to assist the learner in determining the appropriate data to collect.

Inspection

External breast (symmetry, nipple/areola, skin dimpling, retraction, color)

Ultrasound and mammography results

Palpation

Internal breast (consistency, texture, size, masses)

Percussion*—not performed*

Auscultation*—not performed*

Breast and Lymph Nodes

	Level I	Level II	Level III	Level IV
Inspection	Breast (external): symmetry, nipple/areola, skin (dimpling, retraction, color)		Ultrasound and mammogram results.	
Palpation	Breast (internal): Consistency, texture, size, masses Axillae/lymph nodes			

Inspection: Levels I and II

Inspection is done with the patient sitting and then assuming four different positions: 1) at rest with arms at sides, 2) arms over the shoulders, 3) palms pressed against hips or palms against each to contract the pectoralis muscle, and 4) leaning forward. Positioning and tensing of the pectoralis muscles may help elicit findings like retraction, dimpling, and asymmetry. Squeezing palms against each other or against hips enhances pectoralis contraction thus eliciting fibrous band contraction against the underlying fascia and may be seen as retraction or dimpling.

For assessment and documentation purposes, the breast is divided into four quadrants by visualizing a vertical and horizontal line that bisects at the nipple. In the upper outer quadrant, breast tissue extends into the axilla as the tail of Spence (Figure 22-8).

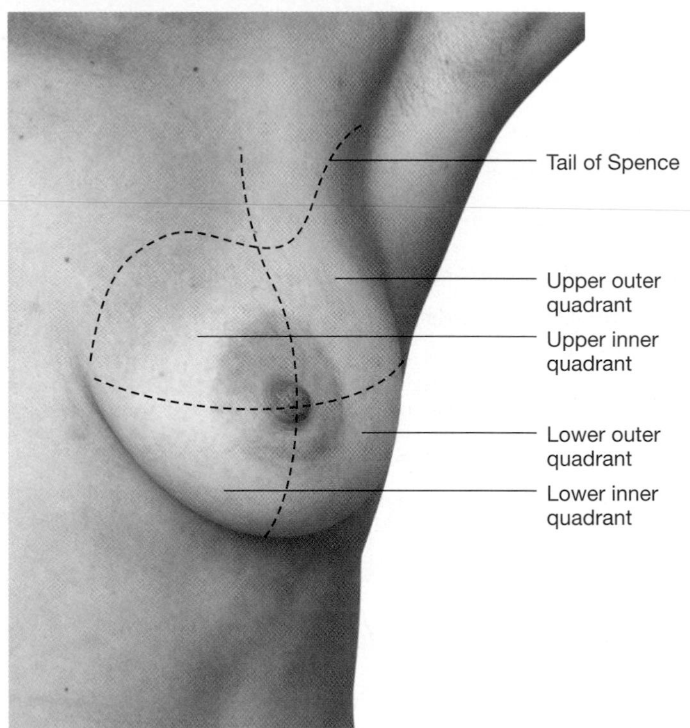

FIGURE 22-8 Quadrants of the breast

Inspection Techniques and Expected Findings	Unexpected Findings

Female

Inspection may be performed in sitting or supine position. Drop the gown to the patient's waist to expose both breasts. Inspect the breasts for symmetry and contour, and for the presence of any alterations of the nipple, areola, and skin surface (Figure 22-9).

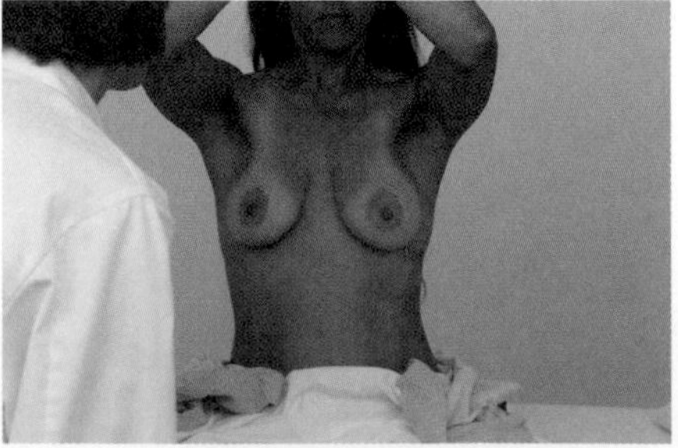

FIGURE 22-9 Inspection of the breasts

Inspection Techniques and Expected Findings	Unexpected Findings
The breasts should be symmetrical in shape, contour, and size; however it is not unusual for one breast to be slightly larger than the other. If this is apparent, most likely the larger breast is on the dominant side of the patient (Figure 22-10). Size may be related to cyclical changes or reproductive phases (pregnancy, lactation or in adolescents, phases of sexual maturity). Changes in contour, retraction, or prominence may be observed differently while in supine position.	Significant asymmetry is an unexpected finding. A large mass may disrupt the contour of the breast. Compare sides.

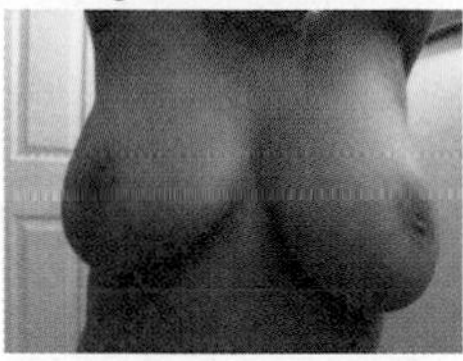

FIGURE 22-10 Breasts of unequal size are not unusual

Inspection Techniques and Expected Findings	Unexpected Findings
The skin surface should be smooth without any indentations, visible lumps or bumps, dimpling, retraction, or rough appearing areas. The color should be symmetrically equal and most likely will be lighter in color because of lack of sun exposure. Milk engorgement may be seen as enlargement of the breasts with **venous prominence** and striae, or stretch marks (Figure 22-12).	The skin surface is altered by the presence of dimpling or retraction of the skin, either with the breast at rest or during changes in position. Another skin change is the presence of peau d'orange, which is characterized as skin that resembles or appears like the rind of the orange (Figure 22-11).

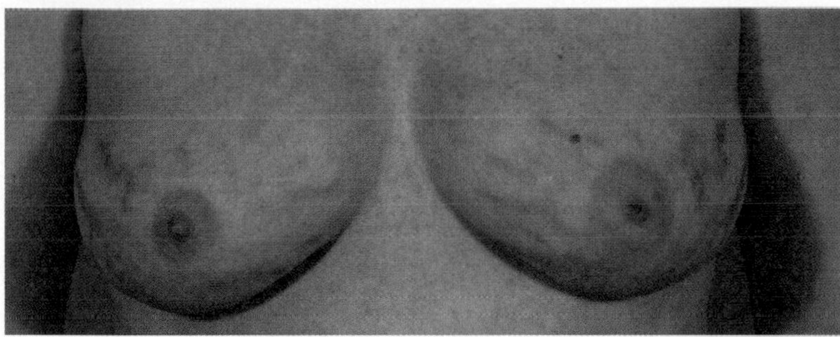

FIGURE 22-12 Striae may be present and may be due to loss of weight or postnursing
Source: Science Photo LibraryCustom Medical Stock Photo

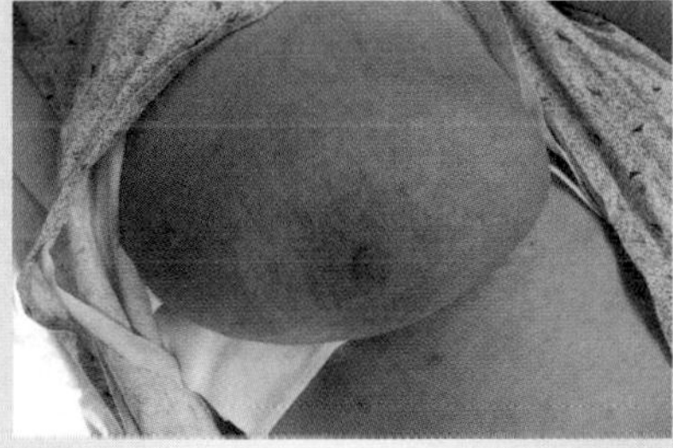

FIGURE 22-11 Peau d'orange
Source: B. Slaven/Custom Medical Stock Photo

The presence of edema or redness is also a possible alteration.

Blisters like in Herpes zoster may cause breast pain with dermatomal distribution. May also represent trauma or burns, abuse.

Redness or erythema may be seen in inflammation (lactational mastitis) or infection (cellulitis or Paget's disease).

Prominent venous patterns may be seen in malignancy, lactation, mastitis, and other disorders like liver disease.

Inspection Techniques and Expected Findings	Unexpected Findings
The nipple should be everted and surrounded by the areola. The nipple and areola are darker in color than the surrounding skin and should be of equal size and coloring. The areola may have some small papules which are Montgomery tubercles (see Figure 22-13). Long-standing nipple inversion can be a nonsignificant variant.	Recent **nipple inversion**, crusting, or asymmetry with inflammation suggest worrisome changes of cancer like Paget's disease or cellulitis or mastitis (see Figure 22-14). Also note areolae that are asymmetrical or different in pigmentation.

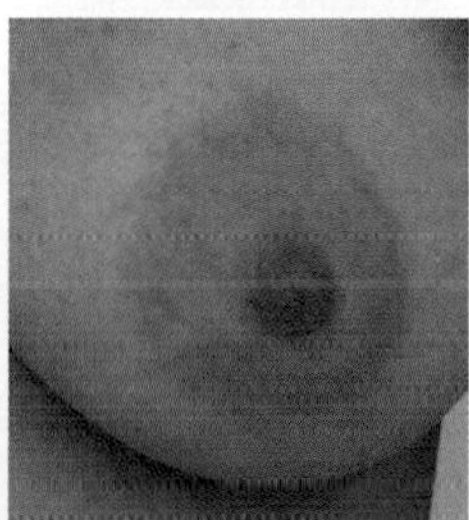

FIGURE 22-13 Close up of nipple

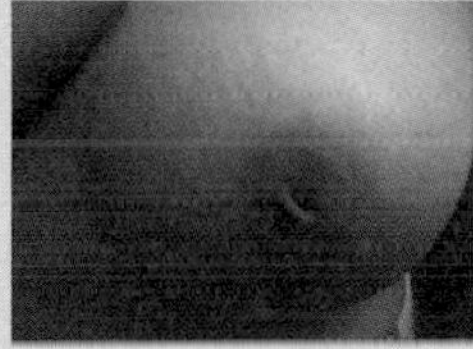

FIGURE 22-14 Nipple inversion

Inspection Techniques and Expected Findings	Unexpected Findings

The nipples should be pointing in the same direction, specifically both pointing outward or inward. There should also be no evidence of any discharge from the nipple.

Note nipples that point in opposite directions (both to the right or left). Note any discharge; serous, bloody, or purulent discharge is particularly ominous.

Observe the breasts for any changes that may become visible during the position changes that the patient goes through. The visible characteristics of the breast should remain the same as when the breasts are at rest. When the patient is leaning over, the breasts should retain their symmetry and hang equally (Figure 22-15).

Dimpling or retraction of the skin may occur during position changes. If a mass in present, it interferes with the mobility of the breast, restricting its movement and causing the skin over the mass to dimple or retract.

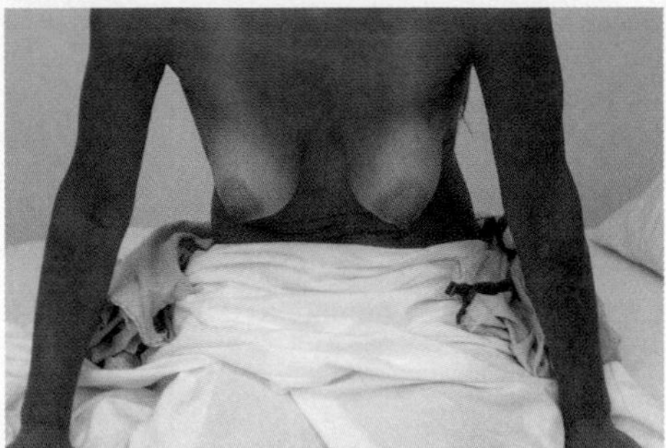

FIGURE 22-15 Observe breast symmetry when patient changes her position

Male

Inspect the nipple/areolar complex for enlargement and drainage or ulcerations. Other than the nipple and areola, the male breast is much less prominent than the female. Inspection of the male breast does not require the patient to move through various position changes (see Figure 22-16).

Symmetrical enlargement may be due to muscle development, especially of the pectoralis muscles; however, the form and shape of this type of enlargement is not due to any hormonal influence.

FIGURE 22-16 Close up of male nipple

Pseudogynecomastia is the enlargement of the breast in men due to adipose tissue with no glandular prominence. It is not due to any hormonal activity (see Figure 22-17).

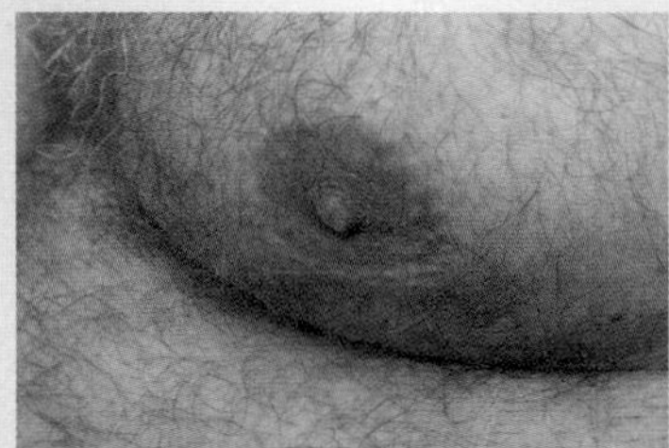

FIGURE 22-17 Pseudogynecomastia
Source: Larry Dunstan/ Science Source

Inspection: Levels III and IV

Inspection at this level is interpretation of imaging results obtained through ultrasound and mammography. Mammography is used as a diagnostic and a screening tool through the process of using low-energy x-rays to create images of the human breast for examination and analysis. It is used for the early detection of breast cancer, typically through detection of characteristic masses and/or microcalcifications. Ultrasound is typically used for further evaluation of masses found on mammography or palpable masses not seen on mammograms. MRIs are useful for further assessment of inconclusive results as well as for screening pre-surgical evaluation in patients with known breast cancer to detect any additional lesions that might change the surgical approach.

Imaging results should present as typical breast tissue without any visible indicators of a mass. The density of the breast tissue is a consideration when interpreting any results. The more dense the breast tissue, the greater the difficulty in visualizing a mass.

Unexpected findings would be images that presented as indicators for the presence of a mass.

Palpation: Levels I and II

Palpation Techniques and Expected Findings	Unexpected Findings

Palpation is better performed with the patient in a supine position except for the lymph node examination where sitting may be a better choice. Position the patient on her/his back with the neck supported with a pillow. The wrist of the side being examined is supinated and resting on forehead or back of the head, and shoulder pressed firmly against the examination table. This position optimally flattens the breast, exposing the medial portion of the breast (Figure 22-18). Findings may need to be confirmed in both sitting and supine positions.

Palpation Techniques and Expected Findings	Unexpected Findings

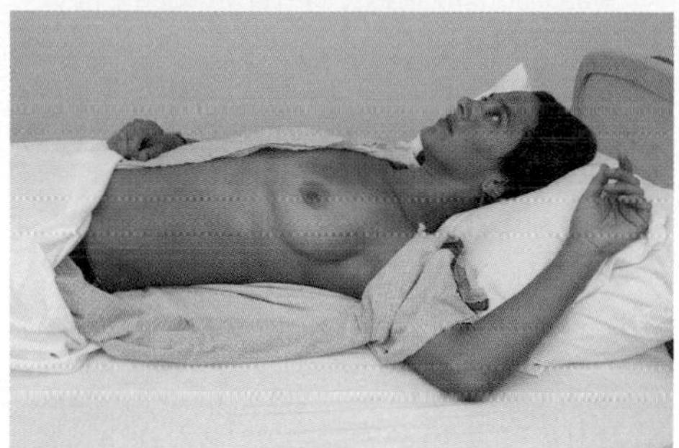

FIGURE 22-18 Position for breast palpation

Palpation utilizes variable pressures (superficial and deep), using partly flexed index, middle, and ring finger pads (Figure 22-19). Use a systematic approach to cover an area on the chest vertically from clavicle to the inframammary fold and horizontally from the sternum to the posterior axillary line. The breast and lymph nodes, including the tail of Spence, are included within this area.

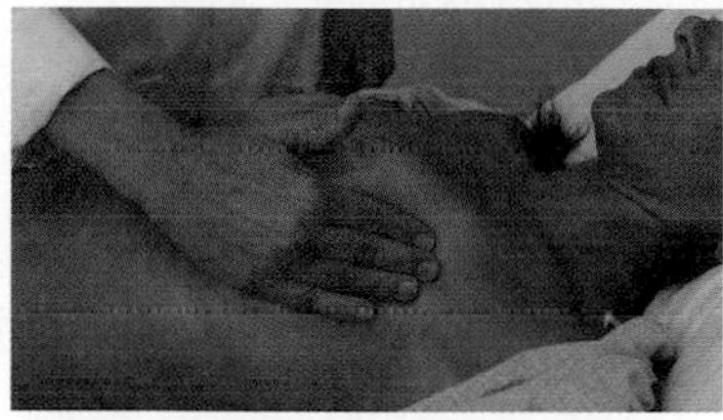

FIGURE 22-19 Palpation using partly flexed index, middle, and ring finger pads

Palpating in a circular motion is recommended as one goes back and forth covering the entire breast area. For large breasts, you may need to increase the pressure exerted.

Various approaches may be used for palpating the breast tissue, including horizontal, vertical, and concentric circles, and wagon wheel (see Figure 22-20). The horizontal/vertical approach follows a vertical or horizontal pattern over the breast tissue. Concentric circles means working from the areola to the edges of the breast tissue in a circular pattern. For the wagon wheel approach, the provider begins palpating from the edge of the areola and going in a straight line to the outer edges of the breast tissue.

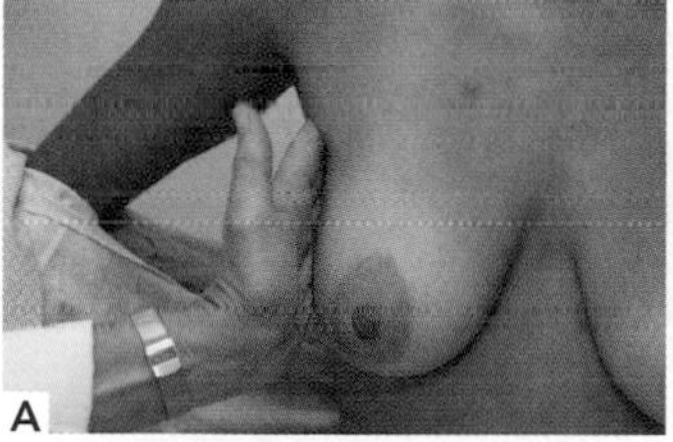

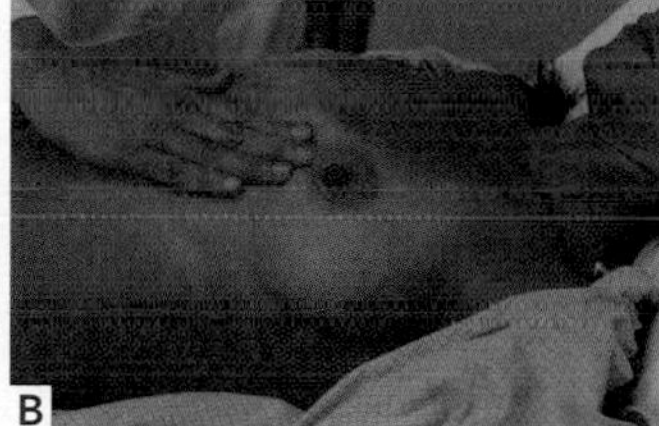

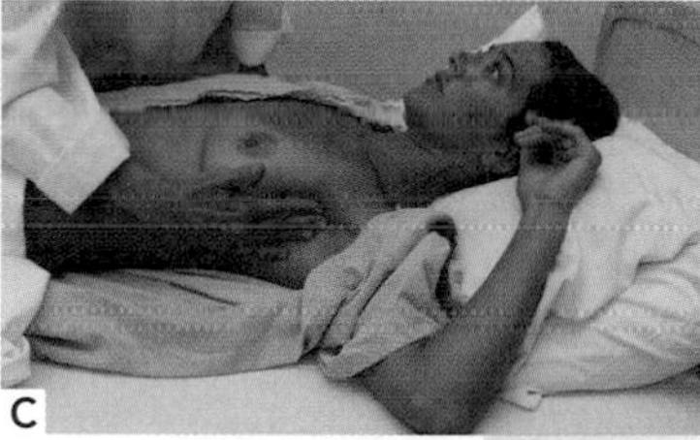

FIGURE 22-20A–C Various breast palpation techniques

Providers may also use a two-handed technique: one hand acts as a support as the other palpates (see Figure 22-21). This technique is generally used for large, pendulous breasts.

Palpate breast tissue for consistency, nodularity, firmness, and tenderness. Glandular tissue feels firm and somewhat nodular. Fat tissue is soft.

Unexpected Findings: The changes in breast tissue are most commonly felt in the upper, outer sections of the breast.

Physiologic consistency varies according to glandular/fat tissue ratio and is dependent on phases of menstrual cycle with increase nodularity during before menstruation. The density of breast tissue will also determine the breasts consistency and feel.

Tenderness is associated with the menstrual cycle. Breasts are generally tender before menstruation.

Unexpected Findings: Fibrocystic breast condition is manifest by lumpiness and occasional discomfort. The glandular tissue is primarily involved, which turns fibrotic producing a cobblestone like texture to the breast. The lumps of fibrocystic breasts are generally freely moveable, have smooth rounded borders with a rubbery texture.

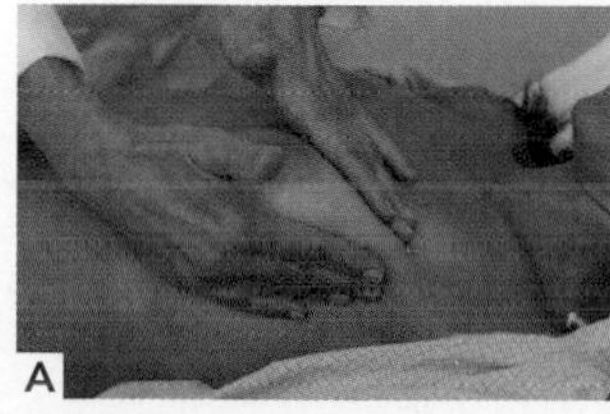

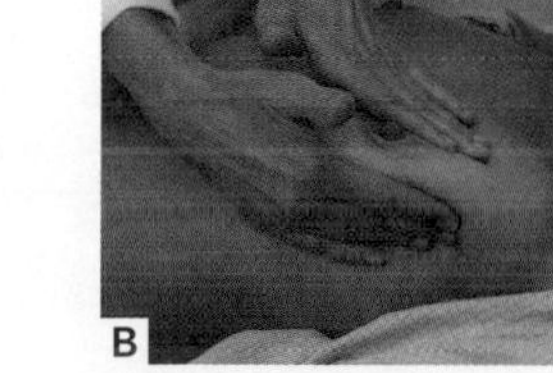

FIGURE 22-21A–B Two-handed technique

Palpation Techniques and Expected Findings	Unexpected Findings

Eighty percent of breast lumps turn out to be benign.

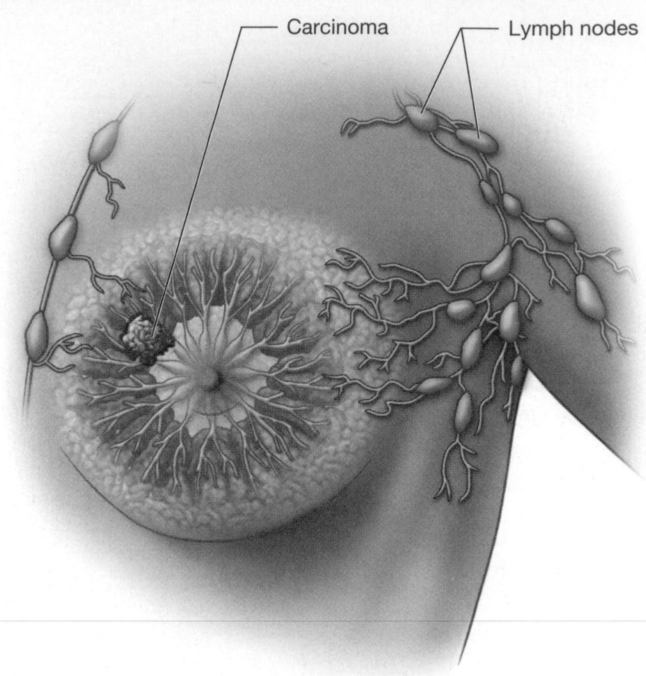

FIGURE 22-22 Breast carcinoma

Occasionally breast cancer may be tender.

Characteristics of lumps that could indicate malignancy are described in Table 22-3 (see page 553) (Figure 22-22). Briefly, concerns over malignancy are when the lump/mass is

- New—any new/recent change identified in breast tissue is cause for concern.
- Irregular in shape/contour—most malignant masses are irregular in shape and do not have a well-rounded and smooth surface. It is also difficult to determine its borders.
- Hard—malignant masses are commonly hard to the touch.
- Non-mobile—malignant masses generally attach themselves to the underlying tissue, making them fixed and nonmoveable.
- Nontender—malignant masses are generally painless.

Palpate the nipple for elasticity, presence of nodules, or mass (see Figure 22-23). If patient is presenting with discharge, compress the areola with index finger to determine site of the ductal involvement. Note color and consistency of discharge taking into account the reproductive cycles.

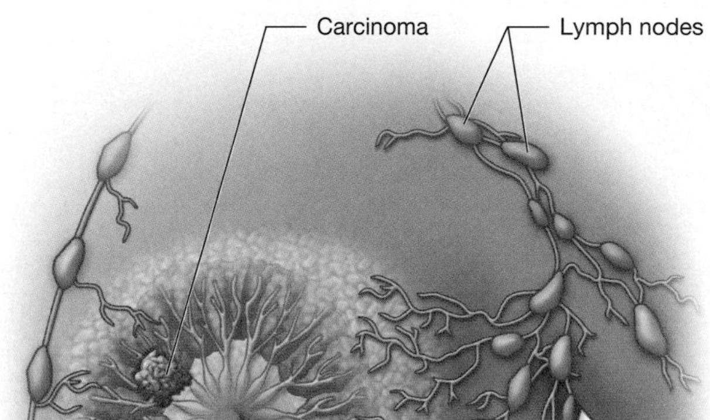

FIGURE 22-23 Nipple palpation

Milky discharge unrelated to pregnancy and lactation may trigger one to look for etiology like pituitary disorders, thyroid disorders, drug use, such as dopamine agonists and psychotropics.

Spontaneous bloody discharge from one breast and 1–2 ducts may be indication of ductal papilloma (Paget's disease) or ductal carcinoma.

Multiductal involvement with non-sanguineous, rusty, serous, brown, black discharge may just need observation and reassurance depending on patient's level of anxiety and risks.

Tenderness, nodularity, and inflammatory changes outside the postoperative period suggest recurrence of breast cancer.

Axillae are best assessed with the patient in a sitting position. Palpate lymph nodes (central axillary lymph nodes are palpable), look for presence of tenderness, note size of lymph node and firmness (see Figure 22-24).

For the right axilla, use left hand and press superiorly aiming for the central axillary and lateral lymph nodes close to the humeral head.

With apposed thumb and rest of the fingers, palpate the medial border of the pectoralis muscle for the anterior axillary lymph nodes.

For the subscapular lymph nodes, stand behind the patient and with apposed thumb and fingers, feel inside the posterior axillary fold.

PRACTICE POINT: Breast Augmentation

The CBE may be challenging in patients who have had breast augmentation. Palpate for nodularity, presence of mass, and differentiate from scar tissue; palpate chest wall with extra attention to axillary and clavicular LN.

Palpation Techniques and Expected Findings	Unexpected Findings
Then palpate the infraclavicular and supraclavicular lymph.	
Most axillary lymph nodes are not palpable.	Clinically palpable lymph nodes are important in staging and are regarded as negative prognostic indicators.

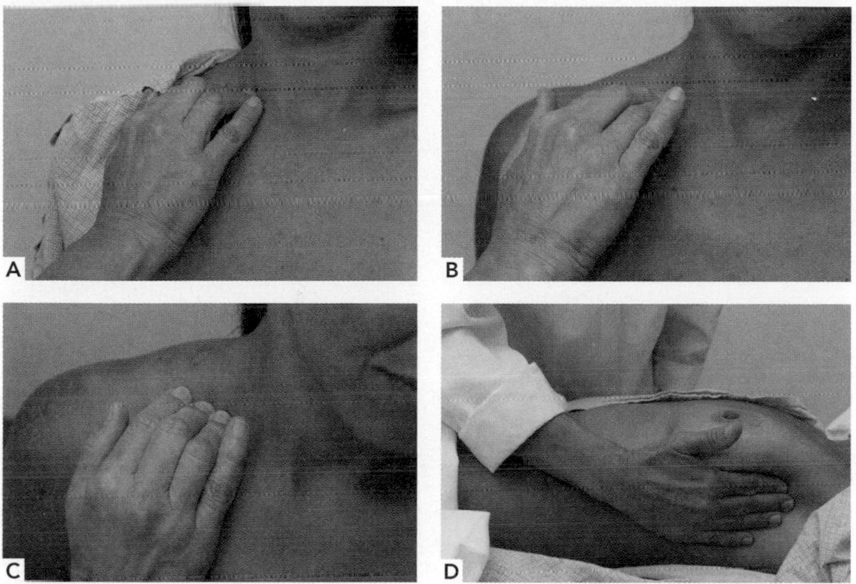

FIGURE 22-24A–D Palpation of axillae/lymph nodes and subscapular lymph nodes

Whether or not to teach the patient self-breast examination is a provider-dependent decision. Although the benefit/harm ratio is low and has not been shown to reduce mortality, it may be a self-driven tool for women to improve breast awareness and encourage self-participation in their care. The steps are similar to the CBE and may be done upright in front of a mirror, in the shower or supine in bed (Figure 22-25). The woman is relaxed, look for symmetry and skin changes and then proceed to palpating each breast while hand is resting behind the occiput. The examining fingers will proceed to palpate either in a vertical strip, back-and-forth motion or concentric manner from the outside border of the breast toward the nipple. Then cover the outer, upper quadrant toward the axilla, and the area toward the infraclavicular region.

Although self-breast examination (SBE) has not been shown to decrease mortality in breast cancer, many clinicians and patients alike believe in its utility. This decision is left to the individual patient or provider.

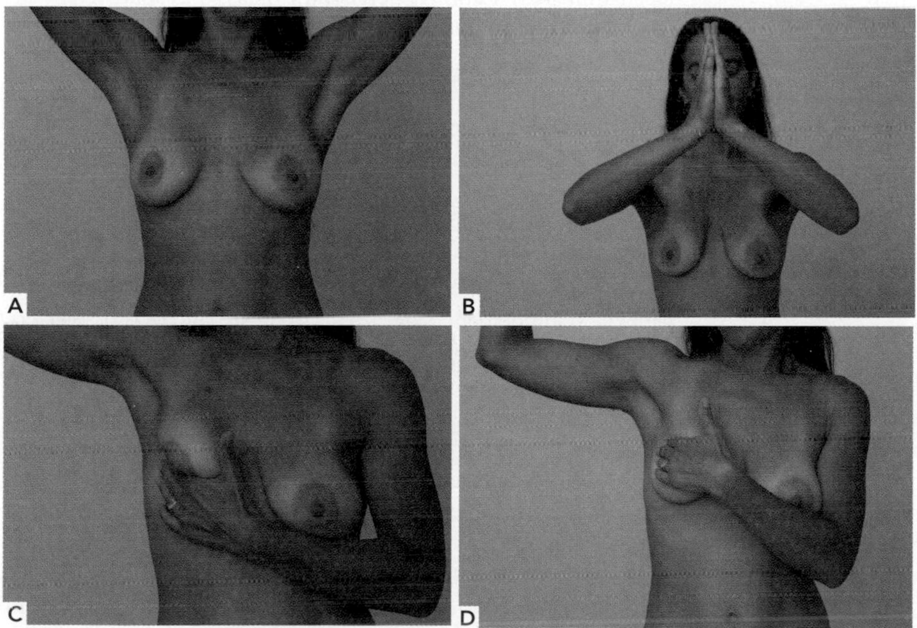

FIGURE 22-25A–D Self-breast examination

Developmental Applications

Techniques and Expected Findings	Unexpected Findings
Infants and Children Neonates and infants require only inspection. Neonates may have mildly enlarged breast and "witch milk" the first few weeks of life.	This could be explained by the influence of maternal estrogen.
Adolescents Telarche, the term for female breast development, starts at puberty and continues through adolescence. This begins as breast bud to full breast formation (refer to Tanner stages, Figure 22-7).	In males, gynecomastia may be seen during puberty or adolescence. Micromastia, or breast hypoplasia, describes the postpubertal underdevelopment of a woman's breast tissue. Agenesis is involution of the breast.
The Pregnant Woman Observation is similar to the adult exam but it is during this period that changes secondary to pregnancy and lactation are seen.	
The Older Adult Atrophy of the breast may start about 40 and continues. The breast tissue becomes less glandular and is slowly replaced by fat tissue.	Risk for breast cancer increases. Biopsy scars, postmastectomy changes, and breast augmentation may be changes that one can see during this period.

DOCUMENTATION

Documentation of findings and discussion, which transpired with the patient, are important to record.

Breast exam: Revealed breast asymmetry with left breast slightly larger than the right. Consistent shape and contour bilaterally in all position changes and movement. No nipple deviation.

Left breast: Contour consistent with expected shape, skin smooth, without dimpling, peau d' orange, redness, or other lesions. no nipple retraction, or discharge. Palpation, revealed nodular texture, with a nontender, mobile, well-delineated 1.2-cm round mass at 3 o'clock, 4 cm from the nipple. No fixation to the skin or chest wall. No palpable lymph nodes.

Right breast with similar nodularity and no dominant mass and no palpable lymph nodes.

Electronic Charting

Expectations of Electronic Charting

You should be able to document all parts of the breast and axilla exam in complete detail, for both male and female patients. Ideally, forms, templates, and prompts should accommodate developmental stages (e.g., prompting for Tanner stages for breast development in age-appropriate patients). Breast cancer is directly related to reproductive factors, environmental factors, and health habits and the electronic charting should allow you to move fluidly between those assessments.

An important aspect of the breast exam is breast cancer prevention and detection. The most common screening for breast cancer is the mammogram. Practices with electronic documentation systems have been shown to provide more mammograms and other preventive services for women than those using paper documentation systems (Tundia et al., 2012). Currently, mammography is primarily captured as digital x-ray images; this is one of the most advanced technologies available for breast cancer screening. In 2011, 3D mammography (also called *tomosynthesis*), in which multiple images create thin cross-sectional views of the breast, was approved by the FDA (FDA, 2013). Electronic charting systems should allow the clinician to view not the mammography report, and may have links to view the actual images (which, like other radiology tests, are typically stored in a separate specialized imaging database).

Electronic charting systems may be enhanced with links to tools such as the breast cancer risk prediction tool or other forms of decision support. Systems may allow clinicians to search across patients to identify which patients have received preventive screenings and which are due for screenings, and some systems can automatically generate reminder letters or e-mails to those patients who have not received screening.

Electronic charting systems have become increasingly essential for managing the vast amount of health care information, which now also may include genetic information. Unlike common laboratory tests like a CBC, genetic tests differ dramatically in their nature and complexity. Clinicians vary in their experience with genetic test information; electronic systems are capable of providing customized views of the results. Although there is legislation protecting individuals from discrimination in health care coverage and employment based on genetic test results, privacy concerns can still play a strong role in a patient's decision to have genetic testing done. Systems should strictly control access to genetic test information, balancing the clinicians need for the information and the confidentiality wishes of the patient and their family. Most electronic health records have built-in mechanisms to filter content based on who is viewing the record, what information is being viewed, and on patient preferences (Ronquillo, 2012).

Patient education and counseling are integrally linked to genetic testing and counseling. Electronic charting systems provide a means through which patients can received focused, targeted educational materials, as well as links to resources such as the Genetics Home Reference, an NLM supported Web site providing consumer-friendly information about genetic testing and genetic-related conditions.

Limitations of Electronic Charting

Cancer prevention guidelines change as more information is learned. Advanced electronic health record functions such as preventive screening reminders are only useful if they provide accurate reminders, so the systems must be updated whenever a change is made to the guidelines. In addition, there is still limited ability to communicate between electronic charting systems in different organizations, so one organization's EHR will likely be "unaware" of screenings done at other organizations, and thus automatically generated screening reminders may be sent to patients who are not, in actuality, due for a screening test.

The use of electronic charting has a positive impact on provision of preventive health care for women, and the more sophisticated the system, the greater the influence. Despite this, the use of advanced electronic charting systems in obstetrics and gynecology has been limited, especially compared to specialties such as cardiology; a recent study showed less than 20% of practices had even basic systems, and just a small fraction had advanced systems that supported sophisticated care (Tundia et al., 2012). On the other hand, advanced reminder systems may not be as important for screenings such as mammograms, because there is high awareness of the need and relatively low cost for the testing.

Summary

- Breast changes occur throughout life.
- The important functions of the breast include sexual identity, personal image and well-being, lactation, and psychosexual function.
- Advances have been made in all of these realms, especially in breast cancer diagnosis, treatment with improved survival, and quality of life.
- Early detection of cancer saves thousands of lives each year. Resources abound for both men and women to help in the decision-making process.

Review Questions

1. The provider is interviewing a patient who is concerned about her risk for developing breast cancer. Which of the following noted in the patient's history increase the risk for breast cancer? (Select all that apply.)
   1. first menstrual period at age 15
   2. mother had breast cancer
   3. the patient is 55 years old.
   4. negative smoking history
   5. has no natural children
2. A 60-year-old woman with history of Hodgkin's lymphoma presents to the provider with a breast mass. Which part of her history is a concern related to breast cancer risk?
   1. She enjoys a glass of wine with dinner.
   2. She received radiation therapy to her chest as a child.
   3. Her husband's mother died of breast cancer.
   4. Her BMI is 25.
3. The provider is examining the breasts of a postmenopausal woman. When performing this exam the nurse should keep in mind which of the following?
   1. Differences noted from the premenopausal state are due to the absence of the lactogenic hormone.
   2. An increase in estrogen and progesterone levels are prevalent during this time in life.
   3. Fibrous tissue that supports the breast in younger women is replaced by adipose tissue.
   4. During menopause, there is marked glandular hypertrophy noted in the breast tissue.
4. When performing a breast exam the provider includes an examination of the lateral nodes by ensuring that the examination includes palpation of the patient's
   1. upper arm.
   2. axilla.
   3. neck.
   4. intercostal spaces.
5. The provider is performing an assessment of a 12-year-old female and notes that areola of the form a mound above the level of the breast. Using the Tanner scale the provider would document that the patient is at which stage of breast development?
   1. stage 2
   2. stage 3
   3. stage 4
   4. stage 5
6. All of the following findings are noted on a premenopausal, 6-month postpartum, female patient's breast examination. Which would the provider discuss with the provider as a cause for concern? (Select all that apply.)
   1. pendulous breasts
   2. asymmetry of breast
   3. lumpy breasts prior to her period
   4. galactorrhea after breast feeding cessation
   5. crusty irritation and bloody drainage around the nipple and areola

7. The provider is developing a health promotion plan for a premenopausal female. When discussing the need for breast cancer screening, the nurse uses the recommendations of the American Cancer Society and includes the following in the plan for this patient: (Select all that apply.)
   1. clinical breast exam annually until age 70
   2. breast self-exam education including the benefits and limitations
   3. mammography every 1–2 years beginning at age 40
   4. magnetic resonance imaging for screening by age 40
   5. genetic testing before determining the need for screening
8. The provider is preparing to palpate the breast tissue of a female client. How should the patient be positioned to optimize the examination?
   1. Sitting with arms at the sides
   2. Sitting with hands on the hips
   3. Standing and bending at the waist
   4. Supine with the arm behind the head
9. The school provider notes that an 8-year-old female has begun to develop breasts. Before discussing this development with the child's parents the nurse may want to do which of the following? (Select all that apply.)
   1. Determine the ethnicity of the child.
   2. Measure the child's height and weight.
   3. Ask the child if the development is of concern.
   4. Find out if there is a history of early development in the family.
   5. Enlist the help of a counselor.
10. To determine the need for early breast cancer screening in a 29-year-old patient, the provider should include which question in the health history interview?
   1. "Do you examine your breasts?"
   2. "Do you plan to have children?"
   3. "Is there a history of breast cancer in your family?"
   4. "Do you smoke?"

Conditions and Disorders

Mammary Duct Ectasia

This is a benign self-limiting breast disorder that is usually asymptomatic and need no treatment unless periductal mastitis or infection occurs. It is a source of anxiety for women especially when it is accompanied by nipple discharge which may be thick and bloody. It is not a risk for breast cancer.

Pathophysiology

- Occurs when the lactiferous ducts beneath the areola or nipple become dilated, blocked or clogged.
- It is common as a woman gets older. It is postulated to be caused by secretory stasis.

Subjective Data

- Breast pain
- Swelling
- Nipple changes

Objective Data

- Nipple discharge
- Tenderness to palpation
- Swelling or redness
- Nipple retraction or inversion

Lactational Mastitis

This is a localized, unilateral, tender inflammation of the breast occurring during the breastfeeding stage. Risk factors include history of mastitis, severe prolonged unilateral breast engorgement, poor milk drainage, nipple excoriations, and cracking.

Pathophysiology

- Breast engorgement, swelling, and clogging lead to cracks, wider pores on the areola thereby allowing organisms to gain access causing infection.
- Infections are commonly caused by *staphylococcus aureus*, Group A and B, corynebacterium.

Subjective Data

- Breast pain and swelling
- Myalgias
- Fever, chills malaise, flulike illness

Objective Data

- Erythema, hardness, and swelling of the breast
- Breast tenderness
- Fever
- Reactive lumphadenopathy

Galactorrhea

Galactorrhea is milk production outside the lactation phase.

Pathophysiology

- Elevated levels of prolactin, hypothalamic pituitary disorder.
- Common etiology prolactin secreting pituitary tumors, hypothalamic-pituitary disorders, pregnancy, amenorrhea
- Systemic causes are thyroid dysfunction, Cushing's, medications (antidepressants, neuroleptics, estrogen, H_2-blockers), marijuana, amphetamines, opiates
- Local causes include sucking, nipple stimulation, and exercise.

Subjective Data

- Spontaneous, bilateral nipple discharge
- Discharge may be milky or serous

Objective Data

- Presence of discharge either spontaneous or provoked

Intraductal Papilloma

This is a benign tumor involving the subareolar ducts which produce nipple discharge. It may have to be excised to rule out malignancy.

Pathophysiology

- Epithelial hyperplasia leading to a wart-like tumor involving the lactiferous ducts.

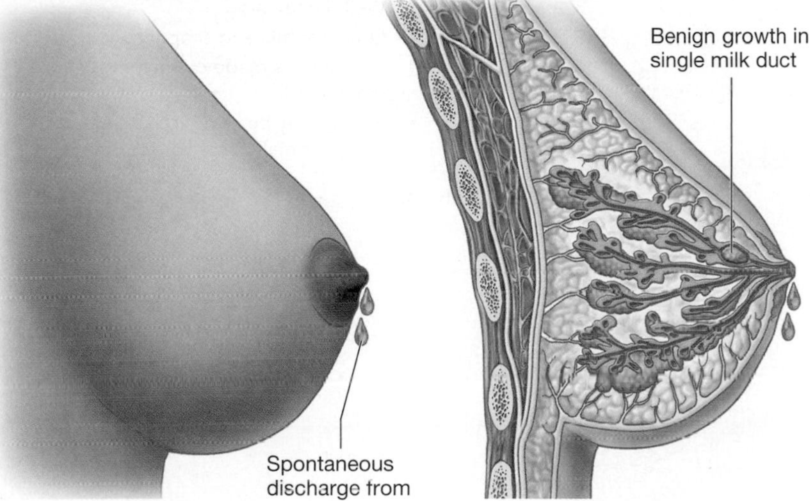

FIGURE 22-26 Intraductal papilloma

Subjective Data

- Unilateral serous or bloody discharge from the nipple

Objective Data

- Presence of discharge either spontaneous or provoked, coming from a single duct, may have an associated mass behind the nipple.
- Serous or bloody discharge.

Paget's Disease of the Nipple

Paget's disease is a skin manifestation of ductal carcinoma.

Pathophysiology

- Uncommon type of cancer that forms in or around the nipple.
- It is almost always associated with underlying breast cancer.

Subjective Data

- Tingling
- Itching
- Irritation
- Paresthesias

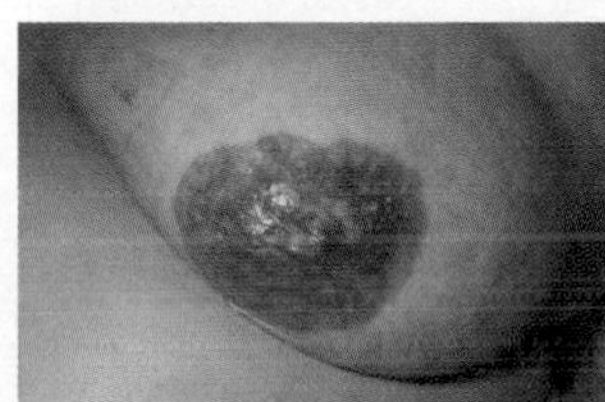

FIGURE 22-27 Paget's disease of the nipple
Source: SPL/CMSP

Objective Data

- Skin changes—excoriations, redness, crusty, scaly patch on nipple, areola, and surrounding skin.
- Looks like eczema.

Benign (Fibrocystic) Breast Disease

This is a term encompassing a group of benign conditions of the breast, occurring in about 80% of women.

Pathophysiology

- Changes are often related to cyclic changes in maturation and involution of the breast glandular tissue.
- Regresses with the onset of menopause.
- Growth increases or decreases rapidly related to the menstrual cycle.

Subjective Data

- Breasts generally tender, with cyclical tenderness maximal prior to the menstrual periods and gets better after a woman's period.
- History of lump prominence before the periods and decreases with onset of menstruation.
- History of breast trauma.

Objective Data

- Ages 30–50
- Cysts are mobile, soft, round, lobular
- Fibrocystic breast disease: firm, rubbery, ropelike and lumpy
- Well demarcated and usually bilateral

Fibroadenoma

Fibroadenoma is the most common benign neoplasm of the breast. While they are usually single, about 10%–15% of women have several lumps and may affect both breasts.

Pathophysiology

- Consist of glandular epithelium and is frequently accompanied by increase in fibrous connective tissue.
- They may increase in size during pregnancy.

Subjective Data

- No report of pain
- Single moveable mass in breast

Objective Data

- Round, lobular or disclike
- Usually firm and rubbery
- Well demarcated
- Quite mobile and slippery
- Diagnosis is made by mammogram or ultrasound
- Biopsy may be done if there are concerns for malignancy or for diagnosis

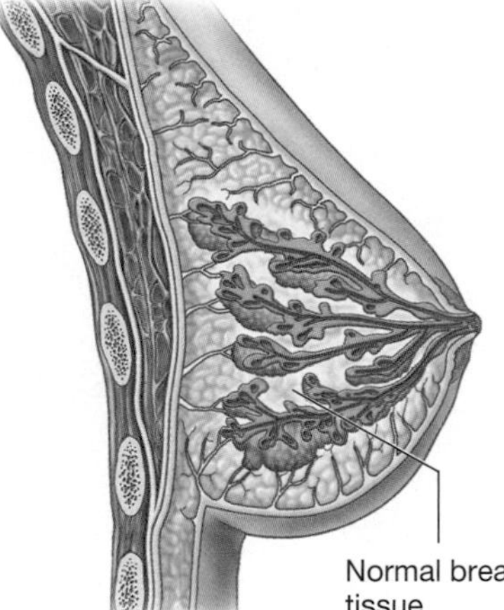

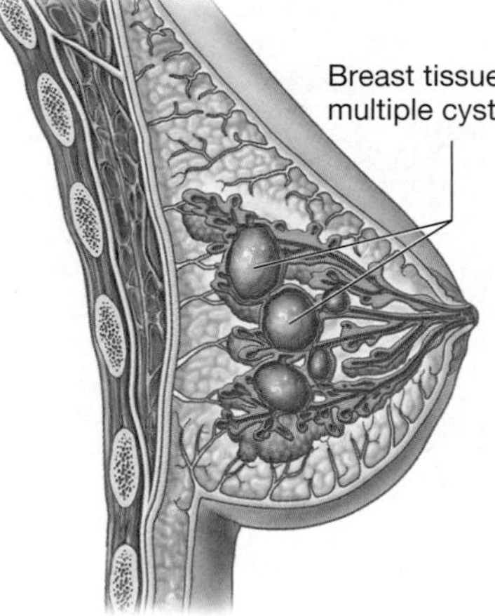

FIGURE 22-28A–B **a)** Normal breast tissue **b)** Fibroadenoma with single cyst and multiple cysts

Gynecomastia

Gynocomastia refers to enlargement of breast tissue in men, and is defined as breast tissue from 0.5 to 1 cm in puberty and >2 cm in adult. It should be differentiated from fat in obese individuals. Fat tissue is less firm when compared to the breast tissue, which feels more granular. The prevalence of gynecomastia increases between the ages of 50 and 80. At least one in four men is affected during this time. Pseudo-gynecomastia refers to enlargement of the breast from adipose tissue. Adolescent males may develop gynecomastia and transient subareolar masses, which may be self-limiting. In most cases, the swollen breast tissue will go away without treatment within 6 months to 2 years. If associated with Klinefelter's, it puts men at increased risk for breast cancer. Genetic mutation increases risk for breast cancer in patients with gynecomastia.

Pathophysiology	Subjective Data	Objective Data
• Attributed to an imbalance of estrogenic and androgenic effects on the breast, resulting in an increased or unopposed estrogen action on the breast tissues. • Conversion of testosterone to estrogen may be another etiologic mechanism. • **Leptin,** a hormone made by adipocytes that acts centrally to control body weight, has been implicated in gynecomastia. • The cause of primary gynecomastia is unknown, but in the majority of instances, it is secondary to other conditions or various medications. • In pathologic states, it is associated with androgen deficiency, testicular tumors, chronic kidney disease and liver disease.	Mostly asymptomatic • Tenderness/pain (rare); if present, commonly associated with breast cancer.	• In pseudogynecomastia, when one presses the breast with thumb and index finger, no resistance is felt until the nipple is reached. Breast enlargement here, is due to adipose tissue. • In true gynecomastia, a ridge of glandular tissue will be felt that is symmetrical to the nipple-areolar complex

Table 22-4 Risk factors for gynecomastia

Medications	Street Drugs	Conditions
Anti-androgens used to treat prostate enlargement or cancer and some other conditions. Examples include flutamide, finasteride (Proscar) and spironolactone (Aldactone).	Alcohol	Hypogonadism. Any of the conditions that interfere with normal testosterone production, such as Klinefelter's syndrome or pituitary insufficiency, can be associated with gynecomastia.
Anabolic steroids and androgens	Amphetamines	Aging. Hormone changes that occur with normal aging can cause gynecomastia, especially in men who are overweight
Highly active antiretroviral therapy (HAART), used in the treatment of HIV positive men. Efavirenz (Sustiva) is more commonly associated with gynecomastia than are other HIV medications.	Marijuana	Tumors. Some tumors, such as those involving the testes, adrenal glands or pituitary gland, can produce hormones that alter the male-female hormone balance.
Anti-anxiety medications, such as diazepam (Valium).	Heroin	Hyperthyroidism. In this condition, the thyroid gland produces too much of the hormone thyroxine.
Tricyclic antidepressants.	Methadone	Kidney failure. About half the people being treated with regular hemodialysis experience gynecomastia due to hormonal changes
Antibiotics.		Liver failure and cirrhosis. Hormonal fluctuations related to liver problems as well as medications taken for cirrhosis are associated with gynecomastia.
Ulcer medications (cimetidine)		Malnutrition and starvation. When body is deprived of adequate nutrition, testosterone levels drop, but estrogen levels remain constant, causing a hormonal imbalance. Gynecomastia can also occur once normal nutrition resumes.
Heart medications, such as digoxin (Lanoxin) and calcium channel blockers.		
Cancer treatment (chemotherapy).		
Herbal products, such as plant oils (tea tree or lavender) used in shampoos, soaps or lotions have been associated with gynecomastia.		

23 Lungs

I shuffle off the field taking quick, shallow breaths. Thank God practice is over. My friends seem to be just fine—they are running around laughing and still taking shots with the soccer ball. As I get into my car for the long drive home, I think to myself that I probably won't finish out the season.

Years later, I find myself in bed with a wave of panic coming over me. It's only 9 o'clock and I'm already wheezing. These days every little thing in the environment seems to be a trigger, and I pray that it won't be another attack. After a few minutes of labored breathing I sit straight up in anticipation. Although it is dark, I can see my silhouette in the mirror across from the bed. "Moon face" really doesn't do justice to the transformative effects of long-term steroids. My wheezing is all I can hear now, and each breath feels like it could be my last. Dropping to the floor, I quickly scan the room. Gone are the soccer balls, tennis rackets, and running shoes. In their stead I find nebulizer machines, inhalers, and peak flow meters. As I desperately puff my way back to baseline, I think of how much I loathe my unshakeable bond to these medications. But then again, where would I be without them? Probably 6 feet under, not breathing at all.

The pulmonary system, also referred to as the *respiratory system* or *ventilator system*, is the biological system that imports atmospheric gases into the lung tissues where gas exchange occurs. In humans and other mammals, the pulmonary system is comprised of airways, lungs, respiratory units, and the respiratory muscles. Molecules of oxygen and carbon dioxide are passively exchanged, by diffusion, between the gaseous external environment and the blood. This exchange process occurs in the alveolar region of the lungs.

LEARNING OUTCOMES

1. Correlate knowledge of the pulmonary system anatomy and physiology to physical assessment techniques.
2. Relate the significant anatomic structures of the lungs and other pulmonary structures to the external thoracic landmarks.
3. Explain expected and unexpected thoracic configurations related to size, shape, symmetry, and movement and anatomic alterations.
4. Explain and differentiate between the mechanical and physiological events of pulmonary ventilation and respiration.
5. Recognize expected and unexpected characteristics of ventilatory patterns and the significance associated with their presence.
6. Identify, describe, and differentiate breath and other pulmonary sounds based on their characteristics demonstrated during ventilation and vocalizations.

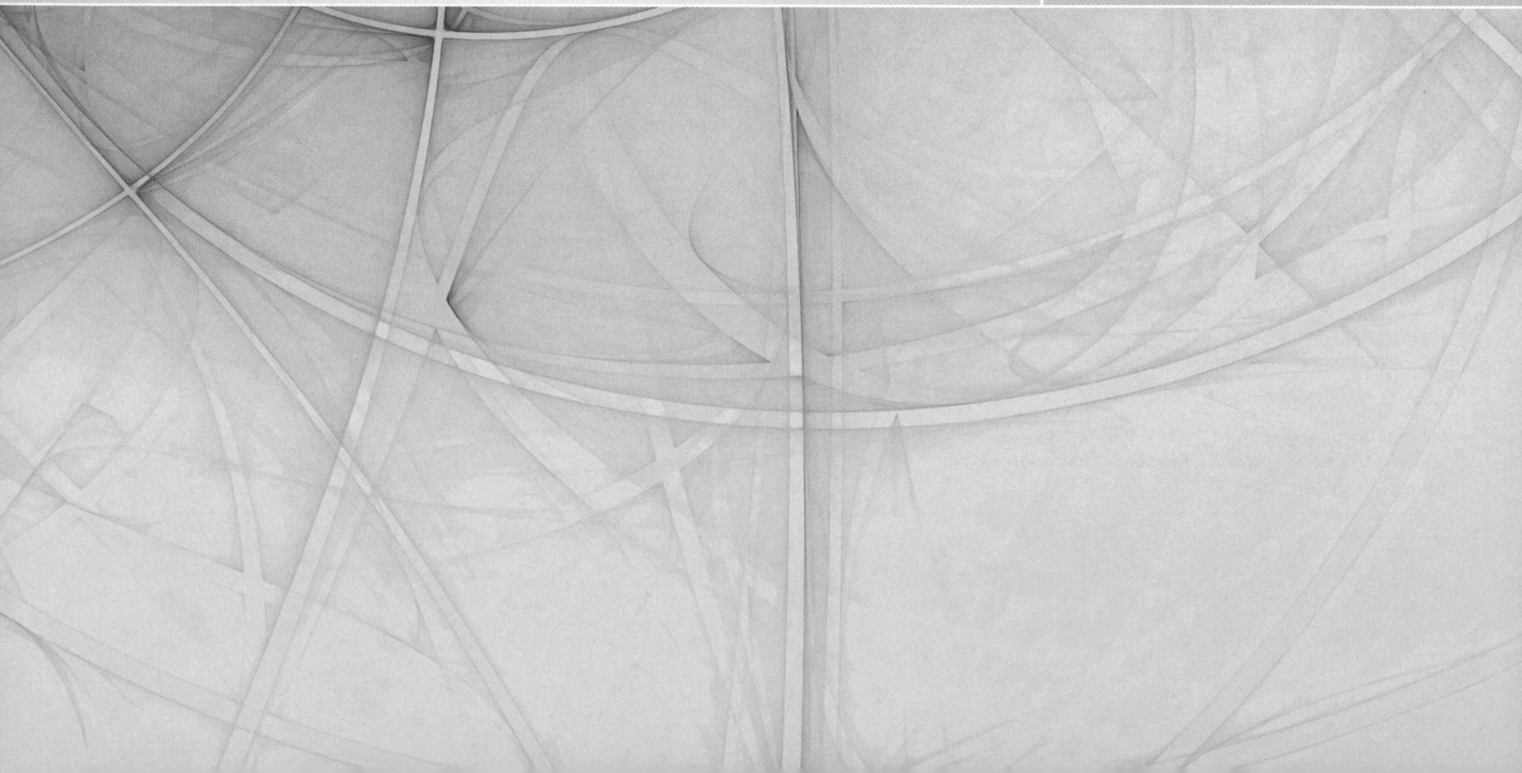

Structure and Function

The lungs, which comprise the primary working structures of the pulmonary system, work together with the heart to maintain oxygen delivery to tissues and organs as well as eliminate carbon dioxide. The work and function of the lungs is dependent on the processes of ventilation and respiration. To maintain lung function, the nervous system exerts involuntary control over ventilation, much like the heart rate; however, unlike the heart, there are times when the individual exerts voluntary control.

Thorax

The thorax consists of an exterior and interior component. The exterior thorax includes the bony structure known as the thoracic or chest cage, which is composed of the manubrium, sternum, xiphoid process, and the costal cartilages anteriorly (Figure 23-1). The lateral bones are the 12 pairs of ribs, and posteriorly, the12 thoracic vertebrae. The thoracic bones are attached to groups of intercostal muscles, which expand and contract during breathing. The primary function of the thoracic cage is to protect the organs within the interior compartment and to provide movement of the chest.

The interior thorax is composed of the mediastinum and the right and left pleural cavities (Figure 23-2). The mediastinum, which is in the middle of the interior compartment, contains the heart, great vessels, esophagus, and trachea; the left and right pleural cavities contain the lungs. The lungs are paired, cone-shaped organs that are anatomically similar to each other, but not exactly symmetrical. The divisions of the lungs and their proximity to other organs are the determining factors causing their dissimilarities. The interior thoracic cage is separated from the abdominal cavity by a muscular membrane, the diaphragm. While these diameters are identified and recognized, there is no standardized way to obtain their actual measurements.

The interior thorax is also described in relation to its two diameters, called the anterior posterior (AP) diameter and the transverse (lateral) diameter (Figure 23-3). These diameters are compared to each other when assessing the configuration of the thorax.

Each pleural cavity is lined with a double-layered serous membrane (pleura) that also overlies each lung. The parietal membrane lines the pleural cavity, whereas the visceral membrane adheres to the external surface of each lung. Between the pleural layers is a lubricating substance that allows the membranes to slide over each other with a minimum of friction. The volume of the intrapleural lubricant is maintained at a constant level by

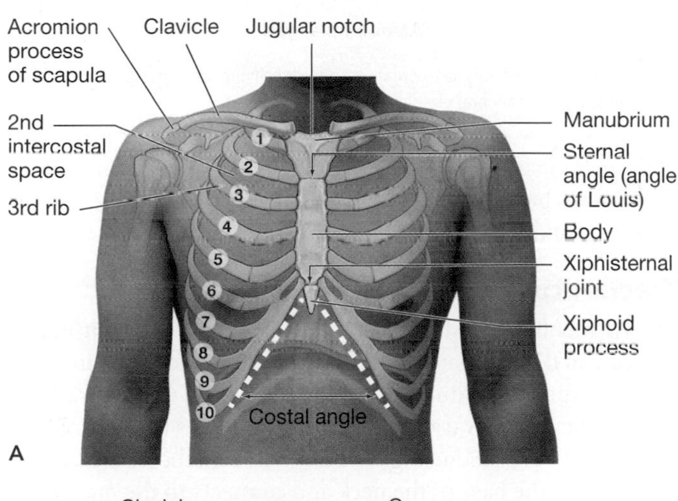

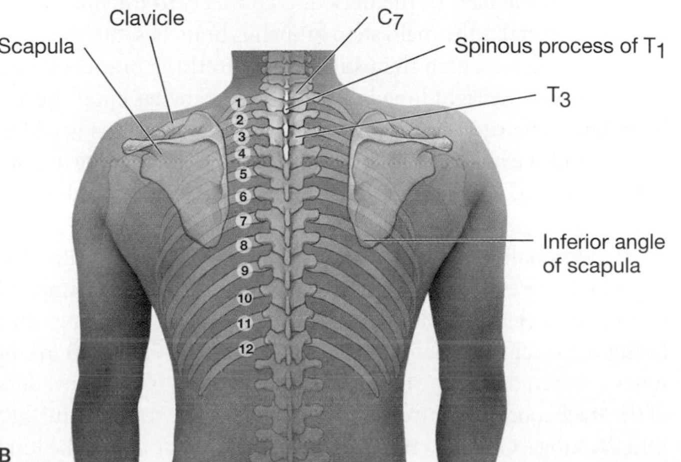

FIGURE 23-1A–B Anterior posterior structures of thoracic cage (rib cage/lungs)

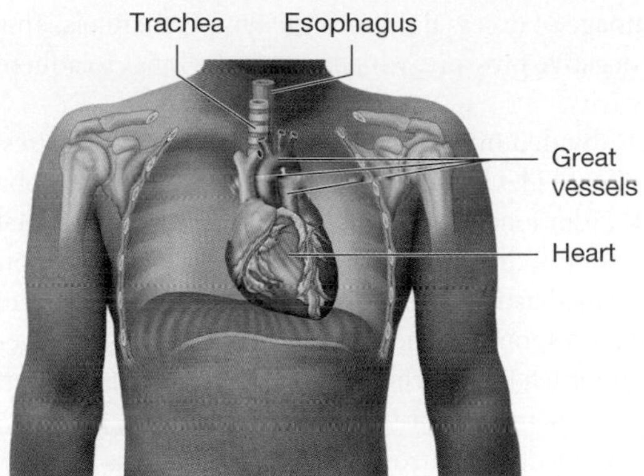

FIGURE 23-2 Interior/internal structures of thorax (mediastinum/pleural cavities)

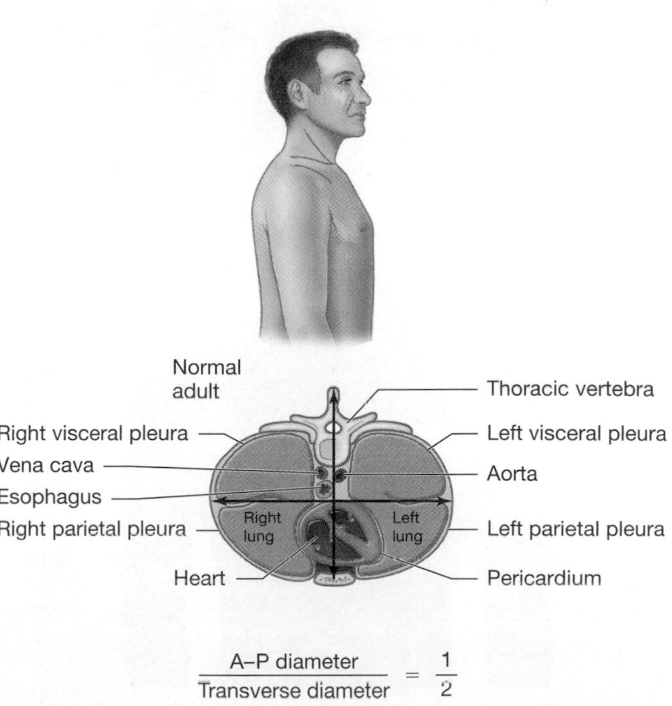

FIGURE 23-3 Cross section of thorax identifying diameters and pleural cavity

continuous drainage of excess fluid into the lymph channels. This creates a slight negative pressure, which causes the lungs to adhere to the thoracic cavity.

Each lung is divided into lobes that are separated by fissures. The oblique fissure divides each lung into an upper and lower lobe (see Figure 23-4). Additionally, the right lung has another horizontal fissure that creates a middle lobe. The heart, which is positioned on the left side of the mediastinum, anatomically occupies the space in the left lung that corresponds to the right middle lobe. This arrangement accounts for the left lung having only two lobes and also the left lung being narrower than the right.

The upper, rounded, and narrow portion of the lung is the apex (*apices* is the plural), and the lower, wider, and flatter portion of the lung is the base. The apices extend approximately four cm above the first rib into the base of the neck. Posteriorly, the apices may rise to the level of T_1. The lower borders of the lung are positioned on the diaphragm at the level of T_9 and may expand downward to T_{12} with inspiration.

Each lung has two separate blood circulation systems—the pulmonary and bronchial systems (Figure 23-5). The pulmonary circulation is a high-flow, low-pressure system that primarily participates in the exchange of oxygen and carbon dioxide within the alveoli, but also provides nutrients and oxygen to the alveoli. The bronchial circulation is a high-pressure, low-flow system that branches off of the thoracic aorta into bronchial arteries that perfuse the conducting airways, bringing oxygen and other nutrients to the lung's cells. The bronchial system is a part of the systemic circulation rather than the pulmonary circulation. However, venous drainage of the bronchial system empties into the pulmonary veins of the pulmonary circulation, adding a small amount of unoxygenated venous blood to the freshly oxygenated blood of the pulmonary circulation.

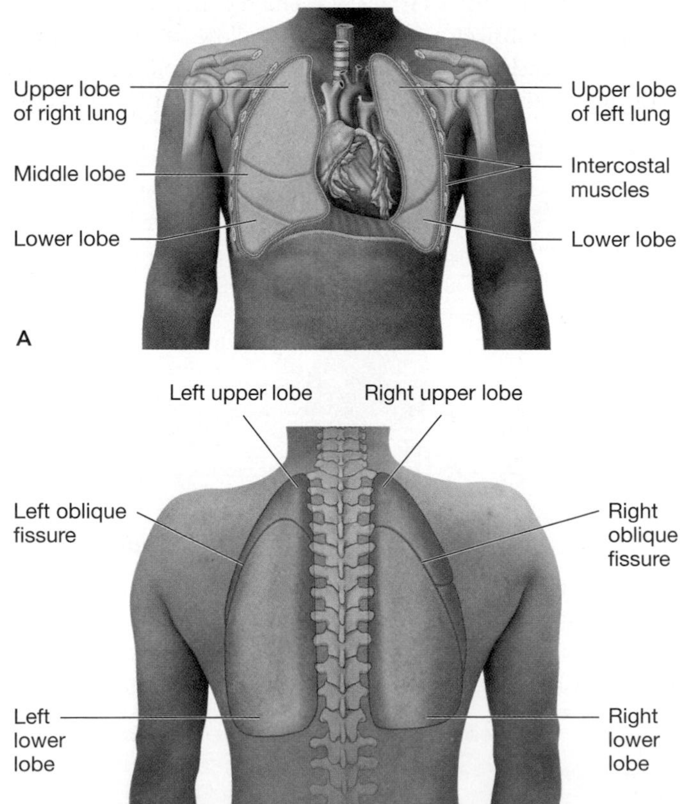

FIGURE 23-4A–B Lung lobes in relation to external chest

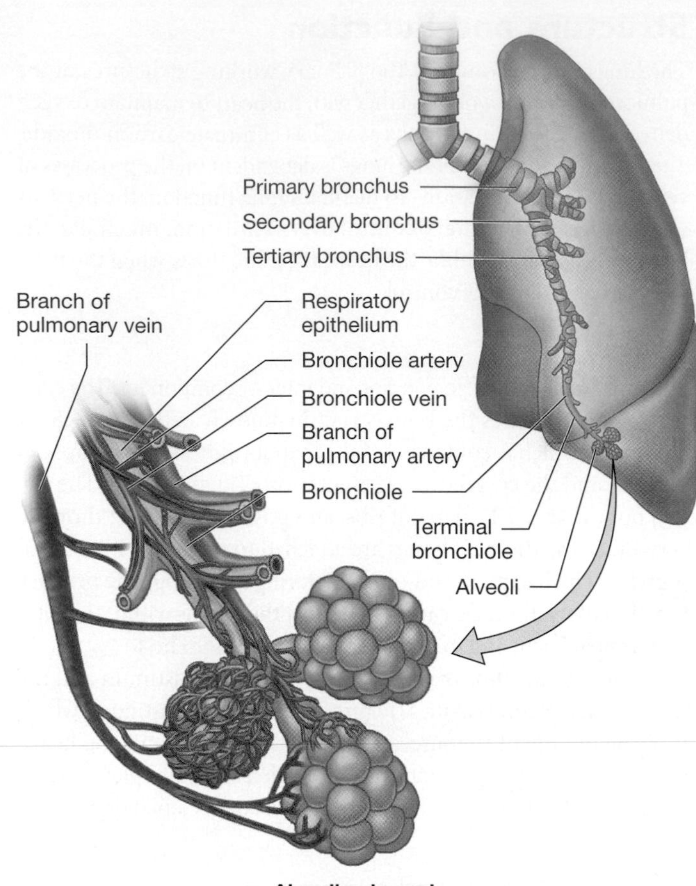

FIGURE 23-5 Pulmonary bronchial system identifying branching of bronchi to bronchioles and bronchial circulation

Tracheobronchial Tree

The tracheobronchial tree is a series of tubes that continually decrease in diameter and are responsible for conducting inspired air to the functional unit of the lung (Figure 23-6). The tracheobronchial tree also warms, filters, and humidifies the inspired air. Functionally, the conducting system begins with the trachea, which is located in the base of the neck and connects to the main stem bronchus. Initially, the main stem bronchus branches into the right and left bronchi, which then subdivide into three branches; one branch enters the right lung lobes and two branches enter the left lung lobes. The right branch of the main stem bronchus is wider, shorter, and at a more vertical position than the left, making it more vulnerable to aspiration of foreign bodies, particularly in children under age 5.

Additionally, the trachea and bronchi are lined with cilia that serve to remove foreign substances and debris that may be trapped by mucus, a clear, viscous substance produced by the lungs and lining the tracheobronchial tree. Approximately 75 to 100 mL of mucus is secreted by the bronchi every day. Mucus traps invaders of the tracheobronchial tree to prevent them from traveling further into the lungs. Ciliary action transports the mucus out of the lung to the conducting bronchioles and bronchi where it can be expelled

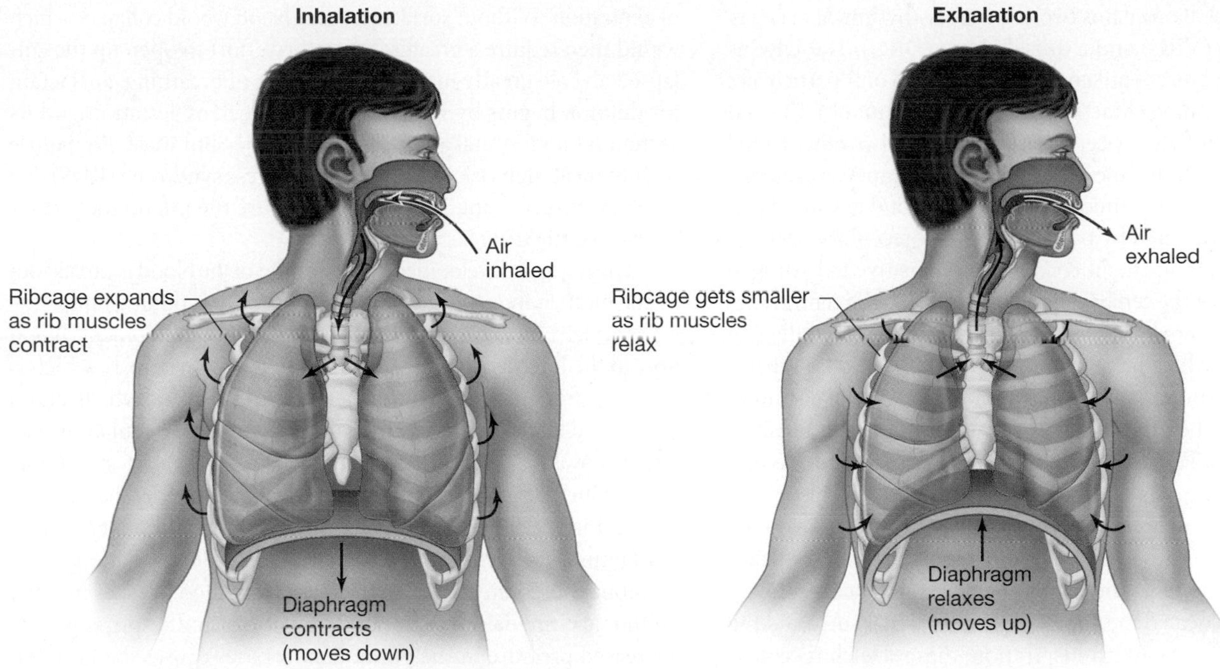

FIGURE 23-6 Two phases of ventilation

with a cough. As a conducting pathway for air, the trachea and bronchi do not participate in any gas exchange; thus, any air that remains in the conducting units is not useful. As a nonfunctional respiratory unit the trachea and conducting bronchioles are considered as "dead space."

After entering the lobes of the lung, the bronchi continue to branch and divide into terminal bronchioles and eventually to respiratory bronchioles that terminate in a respiratory unit or acinus, composed of a respiratory bronchiole, alveolar ducts, alveolar sacs, and alveoli. Each respiratory bronchiole communicates with only one acinus. The functional units of the lung, the alveoli exchange oxygen and carbon dioxide (see Figure 23-6). They are clustered like grapes around each alveolar duct, an arrangement that creates millions of intra-alveolar septa, greatly increasing the surface area within each lung for gas exchange. This creates a total alveolar surface area that is roughly equivalent to that of a tennis court.

Ventilation and Respiration

The physiological functions of the lungs are carried out through the processes of ventilation and respiration. Ventilation is the process of transporting air in and out of the lungs, whereas respiration is the actual exchange of gases (oxygen and carbon dioxide) at the alveoli. Ventilations produce specific breathing patterns and generally reflect physiological demands for oxygen delivery and carbon dioxide elimination.

Ventilations are divided into inspiration (inhalation) and expiration (exhalation). Inspiration is the process of bringing air into the lungs and requires active control. During inspiration, the chest cavity size increases due to muscle activity of the diaphragm and the intercostal muscles that increase the vertical and anteroposterior diameter of the chest. The vertical expansion is caused by contraction of the diaphragm; anteroposterior expansion is caused by the contraction of the intercostal muscles, which raise the ribs and lift the sternum. The increased size of the thorax creates negative intrathoracic pressure relative to atmospheric pressure, creating a vacuum that causes air to rush into the lungs and fill the alveoli. During times of respiratory distress or compromise, accessory muscles may be used to generate an increased inspiratory effort. These muscles include the sternocleidomastoid and trapezius muscles.

Expiration is passive and caused by the relaxation of the muscles used during inspiration. As the muscles relax, the thoracic cavity begins to shrink, which creates positive intrathoracic pressure and forces air out of the lungs. After a brief rest the cycle repeats and continues. In certain situations, expiration is actively controlled, for example, with singers who learn to control the muscles so that expiration is used to create sound. Holding one's breath during swimming or other activities is also active control of expiration.

The two phases of ventilation make up one ventilatory cycle. Under ordinary conditions, control of ventilation is involuntary and mediated by the respiratory centers in the brain stem (pons and

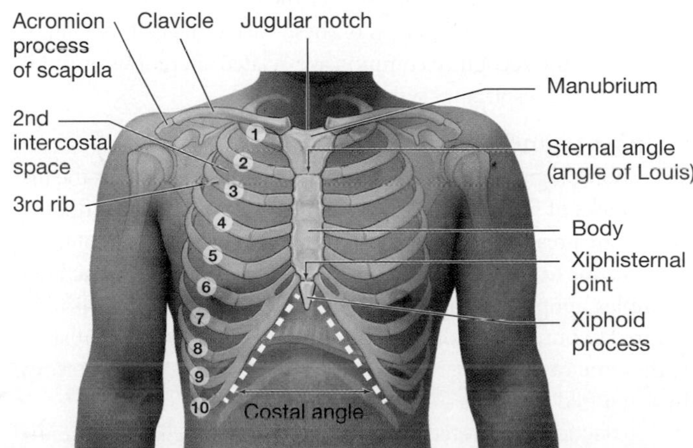

FIGURE 23-7 Sternomanubrial angle (Angle of Louis), the suprasternal notch, and ICSs

medulla). The medulla contains two respiratory rhythmicity centers —a ventral group (VRG) and a dorsal group (DRG). The DRG is operational within every ventilatory cycle. The VRG only participates during forced breathing (Martini, 2011). The output of DRG and VRG respiratory rhythmicity centers is mediated by two other paired nuclei located in the pons—the apneustic and pneumotaxic centers.

The apneustic and pneumotaxic centers respond to stimuli that is picked up and delivered by two sets of chemoreceptors—central and peripheral. Central chemoreceptors are sensitive to hydrogen ion concentration of the cerebral spinal fluid (CSF). The central chemoreceptors are located on the ventral surface of the medulla and are bathed in CSF, which has a carbon dioxide concentration that is equal to arterial carbon dioxide concentration. Peripheral chemoreceptors, located in the carotid bodies and aortic bodies are sensitive to arterial PaO_2 and $PaCO_2$. Information from these locations is carried to the medulla via CN IX (carotid) and CN X (aortic).

Additionally, ventilations are regulated by stretch reflexes known as Hering-Breuer reflexes The Hering-Breuer reflex has an inflation and deflation component. The inflation reflex is initiated by stretch receptors that are located in the smooth muscles that surround the large and small airways. With inspiration, these stretch receptors are stimulated and begin to send sensory impulses to the apneustic center by way of the vagus nerve. These impulses are believed to be inhibitory, thus terminating inspiration. There also is the deflation reflex, which has the opposite effect and initiates inspiration. The location of these receptors and their stimulus are unknown, but impulses are known to be transmitted by the vagus nerve to the brain stem (Kubin, Alheid, Zuperku, & McCrimmon, 2006).

Respiration, in contrast to ventilation, is the actual diffusion or exchange of O_2 and CO_2 through the capillaries that surround the alveoli. Air that is inhaled into the lungs is oxygenated, having a higher concentration of O_2 than the blood. This oxygen differential promotes O_2 diffusion into the blood where it attaches itself to a molecule of hemoglobin, which transports O_2 to peripheral cells. By contrast, inhaled air has a lower concentration of carbon dioxide, thus facilitating the diffusion of CO_2 from the blood into the air. Through the process of expiration, the carbon dioxide is removed from the body. Removal of excess carbon dioxide is also a compensatory pulmonary response to acidosis.

Developmental Variations

Developmental variations occur over the course of an individual's life span and events. Awareness of these variations is important to understand and recognize common age-related alterations or modifications of the respiratory system.

Infants and Children

Embryologically, primitive lung buds are present within the first 5 weeks of fetal life. By 16 weeks, adult numbers of conducting airways are present. At 32 weeks, the lungs are capable of maintaining inflation due to adequate amounts of surfactant present. Surfactant is a complex lipoprotein that lowers surface tension of the alveoli and is required to prevent alveolar collapse and maintain alveolar inflation. At the time of birth, there are millions of alveoli ready to perform their required function.

Surfactant is secreted by pulmonary type II cells and essential to maintaining alveolar expansion so respiration (gas exchange) can occur. It functions by reducing surface tension at the gas/liquid interface in alveoli, preventing the alveoli from collapsing at the end of expiration. Without surfactant, the alveoli would collapse, which would then require a greater inspiratory effort to open up the collapsed alveoli, greatly increasing the work of breathing. Surfactant production begins by the 20th to 23rd week of gestation and its secretion into the fetal airways begins by the 30th week. Premature infants are at high risk for respiratory distress syndrome (RDS) due to a lack of surfactant. The more premature the infant, the greater the risk for RDS.

During fetal development, oxygenation of the blood is carried out by the mother, thus the fetus has no need for functioning lungs. The lungs remain collapsed during the 9 months of development. Blood flow to the lungs is diverted through the ductus arteriosis, which is a conduit from the pulmonary artery to the aorta, and which allows right-sided blood to go directly into the peripheral circulation. The foramen ovale, an opening between the right and left atria, also shunts blood from the right side of the heart to the left side. (See Chapter 24.)

At birth, with the infant's first breath, the pulmonary system must immediately start functioning. With initial lung inflation, intrapulmonary pressure is rapidly decreased and blood rushes into the pulmonary circulation to initiate ventilations and respiration. The decreased pressure in the pulmonary arteries causes the foramen ovale to close. The ductus arteriosis, which diverts blood to bypass pulmonary circulation, contracts and closes within hours of birth. At that point, pulmonary circulation becomes separate from systemic circulation.

Throughout childhood, pulmonary development is continuous. There is an increase in the diameter and length of the airways; the alveoli also increase in size and numbers until adolescence when the adult number of 300 million is reached.

Ventilation rate in infants and children is more rapid than in adults. A newborn's ventilatory rate ranges from 30 to 60 per minute. At 1 to 2 years it ranges from 40 to 60. From 3 to 5 years in continues to decrease with the range being 20 to 30. It is not until the child reaches the age of 10 and beyond that the ventilatory rates fall within the adult range of 12 to 20.

The respiratory function of maintaining O_2/CO_2 balance is the same for both children and adults; however, because of anatomic and physiological characteristics, infants and children differ in their responses to respiratory infections. Some of the responses and manifestations are identified in Table 23.1 (Muscari, 2005).

The chest wall of the infant and young child is relatively thin, making the bony thoracic structures more prominent. Additionally, the structures are more cartilaginous, thus more pliable. The xiphoid process is frequently more prominent and more moveable.

The Pregnant Woman

The enlarging uterus and an increased level of circulating estrogen are primary factors that affect the pregnant woman's pulmonary system. The enlarging uterus elevates the diaphragm, which decreases the vertical diameter of the thoracic cavity. However, there is a compensatory increase in horizontal diameter, which may increase the chest circumference by 6 cm. Increased levels of estrogen relax the thoracic ligaments, allowing for this increased horizontal diameter. This increased diameter causes an increase in the costal angle as well as flaring of the rib cage.

Even though the diaphragm is elevated, it also becomes more moveable, which effectively increases the tidal volume needed to accommodate the increased demand for oxygen by the fetus. The increased tidal volume is the result of the increase in progesterone,

Table 23-1 Respiratory response of infants

Infant/Child Characteristics	Infant/Child Response
Infants are obligatory nose breathers up to 4 months of age	Poor tolerance of nasal congestion
Shorter, broader, a greater horizontal position of Eustachian tubes	Increased susceptibility to ear infections
Smaller airway diameters	Increased severity of respiratory symptoms
Fever, vomiting, and diarrhea	Total body response to respiratory tract infections
Primarily abdominal breathers	Chest muscles are less developed making use of accessory muscles necessary when in respiratory distress.

which decreases airway resistance allowing for increases in the minute ventilation and alveolar ventilation. Ventilations do not necessarily increase; however, due to the increased oxygenation needs and the increased tidal volume, the woman may experience an increased awareness (air hunger) of the need to breathe. This may be interpreted as dyspnea and may create some apprehension, but structurally and physiologically, nothing is wrong.

The pregnant woman may also experience nasal congestion and upper respiratory tract infections secondary to capillary engorgement and swelling of the mucosa of the nose, oropharynx, larynx, and trachea. This is often referred to as rhinitis of pregnancy and is thought to be due to estrogen and placental growth hormone (Hegewald & Crapo, 2011).

The Older Adult

As individuals age, the costal cartilages of the ribs become calcified making the thoracic cage less mobile and stiff. Muscles of ventilation begin to lose their strength after age 50 and continue to decline into the 70s. Additionally, and more significant, the lungs lose their elasticity, resulting in a stiffer, more rigid organ that becomes more difficult to inflate.

The increased rigidity of the thoracic structures and the lungs contributes to the development of a barrel chest. The loss of elasticity in the lungs causes air to be retained in the alveoli, further contributing to the barrel chest. This is demonstrated by a decreased vital capacity and an increased residual volume. Skeletal alterations that also occur in the spine, particularly in females, accentuates the dorsal curve of the thoracic spine, increasing the anteroposterior diameter of the chest.

Additionally, a gradual loss of intra-alveolar septa causes a decrease in the number of alveoli, resulting in a loss of total surface area available for respiration. These changes, along with the loss of elasticity, result in decreased ventilation of the lower lobes. Mucus membranes tend to become drier making it more difficult to get rid of mucus, resulting in its retention. The elderly, therefore, are at increased risk for developing pulmonary complications, for example, atelectasis and pneumonia, particularly postoperatively.

Health Promotion

Healthy People 2020's goals focus on promoting respiratory health through better prevention, detection, treatment and education efforts for two respiratory diseases (RD), asthma, and chronic obstructive disease as well as the reduction of illness, disability, and death related to tobacco use (TU) and second-hand smoke exposure primarily through tobacco cessation efforts. The *Healthy People 2020* objectives have also been expanded to include a number of tobacco use objectives focusing on increased tobacco cessation counseling in health care settings (U.S. Department of Health and Human Services, 2009).

Asthma

- RD–1/2/3 Reduce asthma hospitalizations, hospital emergency department visits, and deaths.
- RD–4/5 Reduce activity limitations among persons with current asthma. Reduce the proportion of persons with asthma who miss school or work days.
- RD–6/7 Increase the proportion of persons with current asthma who receive formal patient education and appropriate asthma care according to National Asthma Education and Prevention Program (NAEPP) guidelines.
- RD–8 Increase the numbers of States, Territories and the District of Columbia with a comprehensive asthma surveillance system for tracking asthma cases, illness, and disability at the State level.

Asthma and chronic pulmonary obstructive disease (COPD) are significant public health concerns. Currently, asthma affects 25.9 million individuals, which includes 7 million children. Greater than one-half of individuals with asthma experience at least one incidence of worsening of asthma symptoms (asthma attack) annually, resulting in 1.7 million emergency department visits and approximately 450,000 hospital admissions. The overall annual economic impact of asthma includes direct costs from hospital admissions and indirect costs related to lost school and work days amounting to greater than $56 billion.

Asthma disparities are also a continuing problem. Individuals from urban and socioeconomic communities are consistently bearing a greater amount of the asthma burden. Racial and ethnic groups are also disproportionately burdened with the prevalence of asthma. In comparison to the overall population, African American and Puerto Rican populations are at a greater risk to have asthma, have a greater severity of asthma, and a greater than average rate of hospitalizations, emergency department visits, and deaths.

Asthma is not preventable but asthma deaths are; however, in the U.S. greater than 3000 deaths occur annually. Daily, preventive therapy can avert the occurrence of symptoms and symptom worsening (attack), allowing individuals with asthma to experience an active life.

Chronic Obstructive Pulmonary Disease (COPD)

- RD–9 Reduce activity limitations among adults with chronic obstructive pulmonary disease.
- RD–10/11/12 Reduce hospitalizations, emergency department visits, and deaths from chronic obstructive pulmonary disease among adults.
- RD–13 Increase the proportion of adults with abnormal lung function whose underlying obstructive disease has been diagnosed.

Health Promotion *continued*

COPD describes a group of conditions that cause airflow restriction and breathing-related problems. The primary disorders comprising COPD are emphysema, chronic bronchitis, and in some cases asthma. In many instances, an individual's lungs demonstrate the presence of both emphysema and bronchitis. COPD develops slowly; worsening over time and limits one's ability to engage in routine activities. Severe COPD often prevents one from participating in even basic activities like walking, cooking, or taking care of one's self.

COPD is a major cause of disability and in 2011, chronic lower respiratory disorders, primarily COPD, were the third leading cause of death in the United States. Fifteen million Americans report that they have been diagnosed with COPD. Greater than 50% of adults with decreased pulmonary function were not aware that they had COPD; thus, actual numbers may be higher.

Tobacco Use

- TU–1/2/3 Reduce tobacco use by adults/adolescents. Reduce the initiation of tobacco use among children, adolescents, and young adults.
- TU–4/5/6 Increase smoking cessation attempts and smoking cessation success by adult smokers and during pregnancy.

Tobacco smoke is the significant factor in the development and progression of COPD in the U.S., although exposure to air pollutants in the home and workplace, genetic factors, and respiratory infections also contribute to its development. In contrast, in the developing world, indoor air quality is considered to contribute a larger role in the development and progression of COPD than it does in the United States.

Smoking remains the leading cause of preventable death in the United States and places a heavy economic burden on health care expenditures (Centers for Disease Control and Prevention (CDC), 2002). The most recent statistics from the CDC estimate that 440,000 deaths per year are caused by cigarette smoking (CDC, 2013). This also represents an additional loss of 5.5 million years of potential life and a loss of 92 billion dollars of productivity annually. The three leading causes of direct smoke-related deaths are: (1) cancer, (2) chronic obstructive pulmonary disease, and (3) ischemic heart disease. Indirect smoking-related deaths can be attributed to (1) smoking during pregnancy, (2) second-hand smoke, and (3) smoking-attributable fires. Smoking during pregnancy causes 910 infant deaths annually, second-hand smoke is associated with 38,111 deaths annually, and smoking-attributable fires results in 918 deaths annually. Although the largest effect of smoking is demonstrated in the pulmonary system, smoking is a major contributor to cardiovascular disorders, particularly coronary artery disease (myocardial infarction and cerebral vascular accidents) as well as peripheral vascular disorders.

Cessation of smoking is the only intervention that reduces the risk of smoking-related pathology. Even though an individual has quit smoking, the damage already done does not necessarily disappear. The major obstacle to quitting smoking is the addictive nature of nicotine. Although nicotine may not be considered a harmful substance, the delivery method contributes to its lethal consequences. Along with inhaling the nicotine, the inhaled smoke contains irritants, oxidants, free radicals, carcinogens, and numerous other toxins. Inhalation of smoke is contradictory to human behavior and survival. In contrast, laboratory animals cannot be taught or manipulated into mimicking humans and inhaling smoke into the lung. Smokeless tobacco can be as detrimental to one's health and is as addictive as smoking. Oral cancers are the major concern with smokeless tobacco.

In spite of the preponderance of evidence regarding the use of tobacco, especially cigarette smoking, as a major health issue, lung cancer is still one of the leading causes of death in the United States. Ironically, it is one of the most preventable cancers. Other pulmonary disorders that are attributable to cigarette smoking include chronic obstructive pulmonary disease (COPD) and emphysema.

Environmental toxins are also recognized as a significant cause of lung cancer. They include asbestos, radon, and other radioactive and volatile carcinogens that may be encountered in the workplace. Exposure to coal dust, while not a primary cause of lung cancer can cause pneumoconiosis, a condition as fatal as lung cancer.

Although no direct relationship has been demonstrated between genetics and lung cancer, it cannot be ruled out as a possible factor as a predisposition to lung cancer. In many instances it is more likely to be an interaction between genetic factors and environmental factor.

Lung cancer used to be considered a male-dominated condition; however, lung cancer in males is decreasing while lung cancer in females is increasing. Lung cancer deaths in females are greater than deaths from breast cancer and ovarian cancer (Thun et al., 2013).

The only recognized prevention behavior for lung cancer is to never start smoking or stop the use of tobacco. For those who are addicted, cessation treatment is available and quite successful in individuals who are motivated to quit. Most cessation treatments include nicotine that is delivered in a form other than inhalation. This form of treatment allows for the gradual reduction of nicotine so that withdrawal is not as rapid and the individual has time to adapt to the lowered levels of nicotine.

In the 2009 Global Adult Tobacco Survey, 26.5% of adults who had ever smoked had been able to quit. However, most untreated smokers will relapse within the first 8 days after quitting (CDC, 2008). The CDC's Morbidity and Mortality (CDC, 2008) reports that most smokers who attempt to quit do not use recommended cessation methods and only 4%–7% of untreated adult smokers are likely to successfully quit.

- TU–8 Increase comprehensive Medicaid insurance coverage of evidence-based treatment for nicotine dependency in States and the District of Columbia.
- TU–9 Increase tobacco screening in health care settings.
- TU–10 Increase tobacco cessation counseling in office-based ambulatory settings.

Health care provider responsibilities in health promotion include assessing and identifying tobacco users and counseling them regarding cessation. When assessing the individual's social habits, it may be beneficial to ask about use of tobacco rather than limiting the options to only smoking.

In 2008, the United States Department of Health and Human Services (DHSS) collaborated with the Agency for Healthcare and Research Quality (AHRQ), CDC, National Cancer Institute (NCI), National Heart, Lung, and Blood Institute (NHLBI), National Institute on Drug Abuse (NIDA), Robert Wood Johnson Foundation, American Legacy Foundation, and University of Wisconsin School of Medicine and Public Health's Center for Tobacco Research and Intervention convened and developed a clinical practice guideline (CPG) called Treating Tobacco Use and Dependence. The primary recommendation stated that at each or nearly all office visits, providers, regardless of practice specialty or patient's chief complaint, inquire about smoking status of all smoking patients, advise, and in addition to pharmacologic therapy, offer brief counseling regarding cessation (DHHS, 2008).

Health Promotion *continued*

Social and Environmental Changes include the following:

- TU–11: Reduce the proportion of nonsmokers exposed to second-hand smoke.
- TU–12: Increase the proportion of persons covered by indoor worksite policies that prohibit smoking.
- TU–13: Establish laws in States, District of Columbia, Territories, and Tribes on smoke-free indoor air that prohibit smoking in public places and worksites.

It is now universally accepted that second-hand smoke is as dangerous to individuals as actually smoking. This is particularly significant to nonsmoking individuals who have close contact or live with an individual that smokes. Children and the elderly are particularly susceptible to this situation. Even though they do not directly inhale the smoke, once it is exhaled by the smoker, it is available to be inhaled by those in close proximity. Because of the dangers of second-hand smoke, it is also becoming more acceptable to prohibit smoking in public buildings and environments.

Clinical Context Exemplars

Situation A

A 72-year-old male who is going to have a pacemaker inserted and who also presents with a history of COPD is admitted to the unit.

1. What observable alterations of his chest would you expect to be present? Why?
2. During your exam you note that there is a decreased tactile fremitus bilaterally, the presence of hyperresonance, and decreased breath sounds. Would you consider these parameters to be consistent with his history? Why?
3. You have determined that this patient could benefit from "pursed lip" breathing. What would you instruct the patient to do and why he should learn to do this?
4. During pulmonary function testing the patient was found to have a prolonged FEV1. What is the significance of this result and why do you think it is associated with obstructive disorders?

Situation B

A 23-year-old male is admitted to the unit with a diagnosis of pneumonia. During your examination, bronchial breath sounds are auscultated in the peripheral lung fields.

1. What is the significance of hearing these sounds here?
2. During percussion of his lung fields, what sound would you expect to obtain?

Situation C

A 17-year-old male and a 68-year-old female both have structural alterations of their thoracic cavities. The 17-year-old has pectus excavatum and the 68-year-old has kyphoscoliosis.

1. Who would you expect to be having more difficulty with ventilations? Why?
2. What is the cause of their structural alterations?

Situation D

A 15-year-old female is being treated in the ED for an acute attack of asthma. She is demonstrating difficulty with her ventilations with audible wheezing and use of accessory muscles.

1. What would you expect to observe in relation to her ventilatory activity?
2. What is happening to cause these manifestations? What breath sounds would you expect to auscultate? Why?
3. Describe the procedure for auscultating her lung fields and why you would be doing it this way?

SUBJECTIVE DATA

History of Present Illness (CC)

The patient may present with specific concerns related to the respiratory system or other systems. Framing the questions will depend on the patient's age, gender, culture, race, emotional or mental status, health practices, and concurrent illnesses. All symptoms presented must be thoroughly assessed with a symptom analysis (COLDERRA).

Cough

In the absence of disease or pathology, a cough is an involuntary, reflexive, functional defense mechanism that maintains an open airway by protecting the lungs from invasion of foreign bodies and the accumulation of excessive secretions. It is a coordinated, forced expiration against a closed glottis. Initially, there is a deep inspiration followed by closure of the glottis. Contraction of the chest, abdominal, and pelvic muscles creates positive pressure within the lungs that forces the glottis to open. Once the glottis is open, there is a forceful expiration that expels air, secretions, and any foreign objects. A persistent cough is frequently an early indicator of pulmonary dysfunction. A cough may be considered as acute or chronic. Further differentiation of coughs is presented in Table 23-2.

Provider Inquiries	Clinical Reasoning/Logic
Characteristics: How would you describe your cough—hacking, dry, moist, productive/nonproductive, barking, hoarse, congested?	A productive cough produces phlegm or mucus (sputum). The mucus may have drained down the back of the throat from the nose or sinuses or may have come up from the lungs. A nonproductive cough is dry and does not produce sputum. A dry, hacking cough may develop toward the end of a cold or after exposure to an irritant, such as dust or smoke. Table 22-2 presents various descriptors that may be used to characterize a cough. Often the type of cough or its description may help in the diagnosis of a respiratory problem.
Onset: When did the cough start (gradual/sudden), any particular time of day (morning, afternoon, evening), is there a consistent pattern? Recent exposure to individual with URI?	Acute coughs begin suddenly and usually last no more than 2 to 3 weeks and are the kind most frequently associated with pulmonary infections (viral) and allergies.
Are you currently taking any medications?	Certain medicines can cause a chronic cough. Examples of these medicines are ACE inhibitors and beta blockers.
Any significant stress? Unidentified onset?	Stress may be the cause of coughing—disappears at night. There is a category of cough that has no identifiable cause and has been referred to as "habit cough, tic cough, or psychogenic cough" (Ramanuja & Kelkar, 2009). Intentional cough has been described as deliberate cough for attention or personal gain and occurs only in the presence of individuals (Farzan, 1997).
Duration: How long have you had the cough? How long does coughing spell last?	Upper respiratory infections are frequently associated with a cough and usually disappear after 2 to 3 weeks. A subacute cough lasts 3 to 8 weeks. This type of cough remains even after a cold or other respiratory infection is over. Chronic coughs last longer than 8 weeks and can be caused by asthma, allergies, COPD, GERD, smoking, throat disorders, such as croup in young children, and some medicines. A persistent cough requires further investigation. Paroxysms of coughing ending in a "whoop" are a manifestation of pertussis (whooping cough).
Exacerbation: What makes cough worse (activity, exposure to cold, position, time of day)?	A cough that becomes worse when recumbent or is precipitated by coffee, tea, caffeine, chocolate, alcohol, or exercise is often due to gastroesophageal reflux, but may also be due to allergies, paroxysmal nocturnal dyspnea, asthma, and breathing hot, dry air. These types of cough may also become worse at night.

Provider Inquiries	Clinical Reasoning/Logic
Relief: What makes cough better? What treatments have you tried (OTC medications, humidity, position, rest)? Are they successful?	Coughs related to allergies often improve with antihistamines and/or nasal steroids. Smokers who give up smoking lose their cough in as little as 1 month after quitting (Seller, 2007).
Associated signs/symptoms: Pain with coughing, SOB, sputum production (characteristics), fatigue, cough up blood?	Runny nose, sore throat, and/or generalized aches/pains most likely have an infectious cause. Episodic wheezing or SOB is associated with asthma. Heartburn or sour taste is associated with gastroesophageal reflux.

Table 23-2 Manifestations of coughs

Descriptions/Type	Characteristics	Associated with
Dry	Cough without production of sputum	Early Congestive Heart Failure Allergies HIV Compression of TB Tree (tumor) Inhalation of irritant/foreign object Viral infections Interstitial lung diseases Pleural effusion Rx Drugs: ACE Inhibitors
Dry, progressing to moist (productive)	Cough that is initially dry but becomes productive of sputum as condition worsens	Atypical and mycoplasma pneumonia Legionnaires' disease Pulmonary embolism (PE)/edema Lung abscess Asthma Silicosis Emphysema (late)
Moist (congested) chronic productive	Cough accompanied by sputum production	Bacterial infection (pneumonia) Inflammation (COPD) Smoking Bronchiectasis Lung abscess Asthma Fungal infections TB
Brassy or hoarse	A non-productive, high-pitched "metallic" cough, often heard in children with acute bacterial or viral laryngotracheitis, often accompanied by inspiratory stridor and respiratory distress	Laryngitis Laryngeal paralysis Laryngotracheal bronchitis Pressure on recurrent laryngeal nerve Mediastinal tumor Aortic aneurysm Left atrial enlargement
Barking	Seal-like sound	Croup Laryngeotracheal Bronchitis
Whooping	Inspiratory whoop at the end of a paroxysm of coughing	Pertussis
Morning	Occurs in early morning, generally when arising from recumbent position	COPD Smoking
Evening	Occurs in late afternoon or early evening	Bronchial asthma Postnasal drip Sinusitis
Weak/debilitated	Inability to generate forceful expiration	Postoperative Generalized weakness Advanced age
Psychogenic (habit/tic cough)	Chronic, dry, cough that doesn't seem to improve May occur several times an hour or minutes	Emotional or psychological problems (may be used to attract attention)

Sputum Production

Sputum may or may not be associated with a cough. Unique properties of a cough frequently will help to identify the underlying pulmonary condition. Sputum production in the presence of a cough does not necessarily indicate the presence of infection.

Provider Inquiries	Clinical Reasoning/Logic
Characteristics: Color (yellow, green, pink, red, white clear), consistency (thick, thin, sticky, frothy)?	See Table 23-3: Types of Sputum.
Onset: When was coughing first noted?	Activity induced asthma causes sputum production and productive cough. In small children, inhalation of a foreign object may be the cause of cough. Exposure to hot, dry air may precipitate coughing in some individuals.
Duration: How long has cough been productive? Episodes of coughing?	A cough associated with pneumonia may start out as a dry cough with subsequent sputum production.
Exacerbation: Anything make sputum worse/different?	Smokers cough (chronic bronchitis) is worse in the morning right after getting up.
Relief: Anything reduce sputum production?	Nothing is specifically associated with reduction in sputum production except to eliminate the underlying condition causing cough.
Associated signs/symptoms: Notice anything else that accompanies sputum production?	Frothy, blood tinged sputum is associated with heart failure.

Table 23-3 Types of sputum

Descriptors (Color)	Characteristics	Associated with
Clear (mucoid)	Sputum that is without any foreign material/clear, white; thin to thick in consistency	Colds Allergies Viral infection Asthma
Mucopurulent	Clear to yellowish, thick	Chronic bronchitis Cystic fibrosis Pneumonia (blood streaked)
Purulent (yellow-green)	Mucus mixed with foreign material from infectious agent. Often accompanied by foul odor that also may provide clues as to infectious agent. Thick in consistency. May separate into layers if left standing.	Bacterial infection Aspiration pneumonia Bronchiectasis Lung abscess
Bloody	Sputum that has definitive streaks of blood or coughing up frank blood	PE (blood may be clotted) TB Pulmonary hemorrhage (carcinoma) (Always question as to whether blood might be swallowed due to nose bleed.)
Rust colored	Yellow-green sputum mixed with blood	Pneumococcal pneumonia TB
Pink tinged/frothy	Mucus that contains white bubbles (air) with small amounts of blood	CHF Pulmonary edema

Shortness of Breath/Dyspnea

Shortness of breath (SOB) and dyspnea are also major symptoms associated with pulmonary dysfunction. The sensation of breathlessness, or dyspnea, is clinically important when a patient recognizes it as abnormal (Shiber & Santana, 2006). Dyspnea, as defined by the American Thoracic Society is: "A subjective experience of breathing discomfort that consists of qualitatively distinct sensations that vary in intensity" (Karnani, Reisfield, & Wilson, 2005). While dyspnea is primarily considered a pulmonary manifestation, other systems and processes are frequently involved (Schwartzstein, 2013).

Provider Inquiries	Clinical Reasoning/Logic
Characteristics: Does SOB occur with inspiration or expiration? What activity associated with SOB, any particular time of day, sleep position?	**Dyspnea** is a subjective experience of difficult or labored breathing. The patient's description of the symptom may be "shortness of breath, can't get enough air, or my chest feels tight" (Karnani et al., 2005). Breathing frequently becomes labored and there may be evidence of retractions. Manifestations of dyspnea frequently accompany compromise of cardiac or pulmonary function. The intensity and severity of dyspnea increases with the severity of the underlying condition. Chest tightness/constriction is associated with bronchoconstriction, and interstitial edema. Increased work/effort of breathing is associated with airway obstruction, neuromuscular disease, or decreased compliance. Air hunger, or the need/urge to breathe is associated with an increased drive to breathe. Rapid, shallow breathing is associated with reduced compliance. Suffocating/smothering are signs of alveolar edema. Heavy breathing or an increased rate is associated with [inadequate oxygen delivery to muscles] (Schwartzstein, 2013).
Onset: What brings on SOB (activity, sleeping, eating, food, pollen, allergies)?	**Paroxysmal nocturnal dyspnea (PND)** is the experience of dyspnea after a period of sleep (1–2 hours). Frequently, it is the sensation of dyspnea that wakes the patient from sleep. PND is frequently an early indicator of congestive heart failure.
Duration: How long does episode last? How long have you been experiencing dyspnea?	Chronic dyspnea is dyspnea that has lasted longer than 1 month.
Exacerbation: What makes episode worse (activity, position)?	**Orthopnea** is the experience of dyspnea or SOB when one assumes a recumbent or prone position. It is frequently described as one or two pillow orthopnea, indicating that the patient needs to lie on one or two pillows to be able to breathe effectively without dyspnea or SOB. **Platypnea** is the opposite of orthopnea and is the experience of dyspnea in the upright position with relief obtained when sitting or lying down. It is an extremely rare condition in which there is a right to left shunt between the atria. Unoxygenated blood does not get circulated to the lungs which then cause hypoxemia and dyspnea in an effort to increase blood oxygen levels. The most common cause of platypnea is an atrial septal defect, often a patent foramen ovale (PFO).
Dyspnea is often brought on by exertion or overexertion and considered an expected outcome.	Dyspnea that occurs at rest or during exertion that is less than expected, is considered pathological and a symptom of a disease state (Shiber & Santana, 2006).

Provider Inquiries	Clinical Reasoning/Logic
Relief: What makes episode better (stop activity, OTC medication, breathing techniques)? Successful?	
Associated signs/symptoms: Pain, cyanosis?	Dyspnea can manifest itself in different ways.

Chest Pain

Chest pain is often thought of to be cardiac in origin, however that is not always the case. There are multiple etiologies of chest pain, with pulmonary causes being one. Any complaint of chest pain needs to be appropriately analyzed to determine the probable cause and to rule out cardiac chest pain. (See Chapter 24.) Pulmonary causes of chest pain may be related to pulmonary vessels, lung parenchyma, airways or pleural tissue (Meisel & Cottrell, 2013). In primary care, approximately 80% of cases of individuals with chest pain are related to benign causes and approximately 50% of these cases are due to musculoskeletal chest pain (Stochkendahl & Christensen, 2010).

Provider Inquiries	Clinical Reasoning/Logic
Characteristics: Differentiate from chest pain of cardiac origin. Timing with ventilations (felt on inhalation, exhalation or both)?	Pulmonary chest pain may be stabbing, sharp, knifelike, or sticking in character (commonly used to describe pleuritic pain and rarely used to describe cardiac pain). Pleuritic chest pain is also associated with pulmonary embolism. Dull, achy, burning pain is associated with pulmonary hypertension.
Onset: When did it begin; what brings it on?	Ischemic pain is often gradual in onset, brought on by some type of activity, and increases in intensity over time. An abrupt onset of pain is more common with pneumothorax, pulmonary embolism, or aortic dissection, with the greatest intensity at the beginning. Some causes of chest pain related to costochondritis, (chest wall syndrome, a musculoskeletal condition), may include: a blow to the chest, heavy lifting, strenuous exercise, and severe coughing. Costochondritis has also been linked to specific conditions, such as osteoarthritis, rheumatoid arthritis and ankylosing spondylitis.
Location: Where is it located?	Location of chest pain may not be all that helpful with the exception of pain on the sides that is exacerbated by inspiration is most likely pleural in origin. Chest pain of cardiac origin is more diffused and often unable to be localized. Costochondritis is associated with pain or tenderness to palpation that usually occurs on the sides (most commonly the left) of the sternum; affects multiple ribs.
Duration: How long does it last; how long have you had it? Continuous or intermittent?	Pain that lasts for only a few seconds or is constant over weeks in not due to ischemia. Costochondritis is often self-limited. It can be a recurring condition that can appear to have little or no signs of onset. It is also considered persistent and prolonged, lasting hours/days.

Provider Inquiries	Clinical Reasoning/Logic
Exacerbation: Anything that makes it worse?	Costochondritis pain often worsens with coughing, deep breathing, or physical activity. If pain is exacerbated or reproduced with pressure applied over the painful area, it is most likely musculoskeletal in origin and not cardiac (Seller, 2007). Pleuritic pain is made worse by breathing and may be increased by lying down.
Relief: Anything that relieves it—heat, rest, position, medication; effective?	Pain relieved by nitroglycerine and/or rest is most likely cardiac in origin. Pain relieved by antacids is most likely related to esophageal reflux. Pain relieved by "splinting" of chest wall is most likely musculoskeletal in origin. Pain made worse by swallowing is associated with esophageal origin.
Radiation: Does the pain travel anywhere? Left/right arm, jaw?	Pain that radiates down the left arm or up to the jaw is commonly a manifestation of cardiac pain. Radiation to the right arm also related to cardiac pain.
Associated signs/symptoms: Shallow breathing, fever, unequal chest expansion, cough, anxiety, air hunger?	Dyspnea—concurrent with chest pain associated with cardiac ischemia or pulmonary pathology. Cough, hoarseness, or wheezing may be related to gastroesophageal reflux.

Hemoptysis

Hemoptysis is the coughing up of blood or bloody sputum. Patients may confuse hemoptysis with hematemesis, which is vomiting up blood. Pseudohemoptysis is bleeding that originates in the nasopharynx (epistaxis) and is subsequently coughed up.

Provider Inquiries	Clinical Reasoning/Logic
Characteristics: What color is the sputum? Is sputum mostly colored or streaked with blood? Is sputum pink/frothy?	Bright red sputum most commonly from respiratory tract; dark red, coffee-colored blood generally from GI tract. Blood streaked sputum indicator of upper respiratory infection. Pink, frothy sputum a mixture of blood, air, and sputum in the alveoli; associated with pneumonia and pulmonary edema related to congestive heart failure.
Sensation of post-nasal drip, bleeding from nares without coughing?	Suggestive of pseudohemoptysis
	Hemoptysis is frequently associated with other conditions/diseases. Hemoptysis is rarely an initial manifestation.
Onset: When did you first notice the bloody sputum? Is there a history of any other illness or condition (COPD, cystic fibrosis, bronchiectasis, heart disease, CHF)?	In adults, bronchitis, bronchogenic carcinoma, and pneumonia are the most common causes; in children, foreign body aspiration and lower respiratory tract infection are most common (Bidwell & Pachner, 2005).
Use of drugs (cocaine, anticoagulants)?	Use of cocaine is associated with pulmonary diffuse alveolar hemorrhage. Anticoagulants reduce clotting ability, predisposing patient to bleeding.
Associated with menses?	Catamenial hemoptysis that is recurrent and coincides with menstrual cycle is due to intrathoracic endometriosis (Weinberger, 2013).

Provider Inquiries	Clinical Reasoning/Logic
Exposure to environmental substances (asbestos, arsenic, chromium, ethers, or nitrogen dioxide (in hockey players)?	Specfic environmental substances are known to increase risk for hemoptysis.
Duration: How long does coughing spell last? Previous episodes?	Sporadic recurrences of mild hemoptysis is common in smokers with chronic bronchitis with onset of acute bronchitis.
Exacerbation: Have you noticed anything that makes it worse or may precipitate its occurrence?	Not of great significance.
Relief: Have you noted anything that has decreased its occurrence?	Cough suppressants may help if due to throat irritation from violent coughing.
Associated signs/symptoms: What else have you experienced that accompanies coughing up blood? Dyspnea? Fever, sputum production? Night sweats, weight loss, fatigue? Chest pain, dyspnea? Leg pain/swelling? Hematuria? Bloody nasal discharge?	Dyspnea may accompany pulmonary infections (pulmonary infections are the primary cause of hemoptysis). Fever and sputum production are associated with pneumonia. Night sweats, weight loss, and fatigue may me associated with cancer or TB. Chest pain or dyspnea may be associated with pneumonia or pulmonary embolism (PE). Leg pain or swelling may also be related to PE. Hematuria may be related to Goodpasture's syndrome. Bloody nasal discharge may be a sign of Wegener's granulomatosis.

PRACTICE POINT: Hemoptysis

Coughing up blood (hemoptysis) should be differentiated from vomiting blood (hematemesis).

Characteristics	Hemoptysis	Hematemesis
Precipitating event	Coughing	Nausea and vomiting
History	Probable history of cardiopulmonary symptoms	Probable history of GI symptoms
Appearance	Frothy	Not frothy
Color	Bright red	Dark red, brown, or "coffee grounds"
Manifestations	Mixed with sputum	Mixed with food
Associated symptoms	Dyspnea	Nausea

Past Medical History

Information related to past medical history identifies any conditions that may affect or cause present pulmonary condition or symptoms.

Provider Inquiries	Clinical Reasoning/Logic
Trauma, surgery (thoracic, nasal, tracheal), hospitalizations for pulmonary conditions? When? What were the outcomes?	Any of these occurrences in the patient's past history may affect present symptoms or condition.
Use of oxygen/ventilation assistive devices?	The need for these are indicative of some type of pulmonary pathology.
Chronic conditions: Pulmonary COPD, bronchiectasis, TB, emphysema, cystic fibrosis, asthma? Nonpulmonary (cardiac, DM, cancer, hematological)?	The presence of any of these disorders will affect patient's present condition or situation.
Testing: Allergies, pulmonary function, TB, chest x-ray?	Data from these tests will help determine present condition or the need for further testing.
Immunizations: Flu, pneumococcal?	Regular immunizations prevent contracting adverse pulmonary conditions.
Medications: Prescribed/OTC?	Medications used will help to determine if any impact on present situation or condition

Family History

Family History provides information regarding family member's illnesses or conditions as potential causes for chief complaint or presenting symptoms that may indicate a pattern of presentation associated with transmission of familial/genetic factors predisposing the individual to certain system related conditions/illnesses. Any of these may indicate a potential or actual cause of pulmonary dysfunction.

Provider Inquiries	Clinical Reasoning/Logic
Ask the patient about a family history of any of the following: Tuberculosis? Cystic fibrosis? Emphysema? Allergies, asthma, dermatitis? Cancer? Bronchiectasis/bronchitis?	Data related to pulmonary conditions of family members will help to determine possible cause or affect on present condition/situation.

Personal and Social History

Personal and social history provides information related to habits, practices and/or environmental influences that may predispose the patient to the development of certain system related conditions/illnesses.

Provider Inquiries	Clinical Reasoning/Logic
Employment/Environment: Type of work, environmental hazards (allergens, toxins, chemicals, animals, vapors, dust, air quality)?	Pathology of the lung may be caused by inhalation of substances that damage tissue. Well-known inhalants are asbestos and coal dust.
Tobacco use: Type (cigar, cigarette, chewing), pack years (packs per day x years), age when started, efforts to quit (successful or not), how long without smoking, exposure to secondary smoke?	Tobacco use known to cause lung pathology
Hobbies: Pigeons, parrots; model building/woodworking—exposure to glue?	"Pigeon breeders' disease", a hypersensitivity pneumonitis, is an uncommon occupational hazard associated with exposure to pigeons and parakeets caused by inhalation of antigenic substances in the birds' excreta. It may also be associated with inhalation of other organic agents (mushrooms, epoxy resin, maple bark, wheat weevil farming, cheese). Initial symptoms include chills, fever, and cough with SOB. Removing the cause may resolve symptoms; continuous exposure, however, may progress to diffuse lung fibrosis. Treatment is with steroids (Kamanger, 2013).
Exposure to respiratory pathogens: Flu, TB?	Identification of possible causes of pulmonary conditions
Travel: Regional (SW—coccidiomycosis; SE/MW U.S.—hisotplasmosis; Africa, Caribbean—HIV, Asia/Orient—SARS, bird flu)? **Nutritional Status:** Obesity (interfere with breathing)	Certain types of fungi are endemic in particular areas of the U.S. and individuals who travel to these areas may possibly develop a fungal pulmonary infection. Fungi spores that inhabit the soil are inhaled when dust and dirt are blown around.
Alcohol/Drug use: Marijuana in particular?	Marijuana smoke is a lung irritant and frequent smokers of marijuana have many of the same respiratory problems as those experienced by smokers of tobacco.
Exercise Tolerance: Able to perform activities?	Individuals should be able to engage in activities without experiencing any respiratory difficulty, unless the activities are above the type the individual usually engages in. See Think Link on p. 588

Provider Inquiries | **Clinical Reasoning/Logic**

THINK LINK: Pickwickian Syndrome (Obesity Hypoventilation Syndrome)

Obese individuals have the potential to develop Obesity Hypoventilation Syndrome (OHS), commonly referred to as *Pickwickian Syndrome*, which gets its name from the red-faced, fat character in Charles Dickens's *The Pickwick Papers*. OHS may affect both children and adults and infrequently non-obese individuals. An individual has OHS when the BMI is ≥ 30 kg/m[2] and has alveolar hypoventilation ($PaCO_2$) > 45 mmHg that cannot be attributed to other conditions. The most common symptom is sleep apnea. Additional symptoms include prolonged drowsiness, twitching, cyanosis, periodic breathing, secondary polycythemia, and right-sided heart failure.

The actual origin and development is not well understood but is most likely the interactions of other obesity related conditions (obstructive sleep apnea, increased work of breathing, respiratory muscle impairment, decreased central ventilatory drive and reduced effects of neurohumoral modulators (e.g. leptin) (Suratt, 2013). Physiological complications include hypertension, arrhythmias, low O_2 and high CO_2 levels in the blood, and peripheral edema. Psychological manifestations (anxiety, hallucinations, irritability, and irrational behavior) may also be demonstrated. Treatment is directed toward weight loss. If sleep apnea persists, use of positive pressure air flow at night may be necessary (Cataletto & Hertz 2013)

Developmental Applications

Certain conditions or disorders may be related to certain age groups or situations. Inquiring to obtain age or condition specific information will provide further information for helping to determine causes of the chief concern as identified.

Infants and Children

Prematurity/Low birth weight: Did your infant experience any pulmonary difficulties (ventilatory assistance—how long)? Respiratory distress syndrome/use of surfactant; bronchopulmonary dysplasia?

Cough/difficulty breathing of sudden onset? Recurrent cough?

Frequent/severe colds; respiratory infections? Previous RSV?

Identifies any problems associated with pregnancy, delivery, and early development and maturity that may influence or cause present pulmonary conditions or symptoms. Familial and environmental influences are also identified.

Recurrent viral bronchitis most common in pre-school age children and most common cause of a persistent cough in children of all ages.

Respiratory Syncytial Virus—especially children under 2.

Family history of allergies: Food (age when new foods introduced/breast fed)?

Exposure to second-hand smoke?

Difficulty feeding/eating (cyanosis, minimal weight gain, perspiration, coughing/choking)?

Episodes of apnea: Frequency (monitored); history of SIDS?

The Pregnant Woman

Have you experienced any: difficulty breathing due to enlarging uterus (multiple fetuses, polyhydramnios)?

Exercise/activity tolerance (changes)?

Exposure to respiratory infections: Flu, pneumonia, (immunizations—yearly)?

Questions help identify any pulmonary problems or difficulties associated with pregnancy that may affect the mother or outcomes of pregnancy.

The Older Adult

Have you experienced any:

Exposure to respiratory infections: Flu, pneumonia, (immunizations—yearly)?

Exposure to environmental hazards: Smog, toxins, chemicals, second-hand smoke (effect on respiratory efforts/infections)?

Identifies any factors related to personal or environmental influences on pulmonary function and pulmonary conditions.

With aging, protective mechanisms also decrease. The cough reflex is less sensitive and may not trigger as readily, and the cough is generally less forceful. The cilia that line the airway are decreased and are also less able to move mucus up and out of the airway. In addition, the nose and breathing passages are drier and secrete less IgA, an antibody that protects against viruses, making the elderly are more susceptible to lung infections, particularly pneumonia and chronic bronchitis.

Provider Inquiries	Clinical Reasoning/Logic
Interference with ADLs/activities related to respiratory difficulties (cough/dyspnea; fatigue)?	Reduced pulmonary functional reserve. At rest: no change; with exertion: Dyspnea, decreased exercise tolerance.
Weight changes: Difficulty with eating (choking, swallowing, SOB)?	Weight loss in the older adult is a worrisome clinical sign and has been associated with mortality. Although lean body mass may decline because of normal physiological changes, when associated with age a loss of more than 4% per year is an independent predictor of mortality. Decreased oral intake may occur slowly in progressive chronic diseases such as Parkinson's disease, COPD, or Alzheimer disease. Elderly smokers who are symptomatic but who do not fulfill the COPD diagnostic criteria have nutritional deficits related to insufficient energy intake that are similar to those seen in COPD patients (Yasushi et al., 2011).

OBJECTIVE DATA

The examination of the pulmonary system (thorax and lungs) includes all four examination techniques: inspection, palpation, percussion, and auscultation. It is best to examine this system with the patient in the sitting position. Remember that both the anterior and posterior aspect of the pulmonary system must be examined; thus, you might want to perform this exam at a point where a switch from anterior to posterior or vice versa can be done. This may take a while to remember, but it will save steps in the process of the exam. Once a systematic approach is developed, it is important to maintain a sequence of events to guarantee a complete examination.

A comfortable ambient temperature is important, as the patient will be undraped for an extended period of time. Appropriate draping is necessary when examining the female patient, but modesty must not take priority over performing a thorough and complete examination. When necessary, breast tissue may be moved or displaced by the health care provider, or the patient may be asked to do this.

A quiet environment is essential, particularly in clinical areas, as the health care provider will be listening for subtle changes in sounds during percussion and auscultation. Adequate overhead lighting is necessary for direct observation and tangential lighting is needed to highlight subtle changes that may be difficult to detect with direct lighting.

Surface Anatomy and Landmarks of the Thorax

Before beginning the physical examination, the provider must know anatomically which portion of the lung is being assessed during the exam. This allows for identification of the location for any unexpected findings.

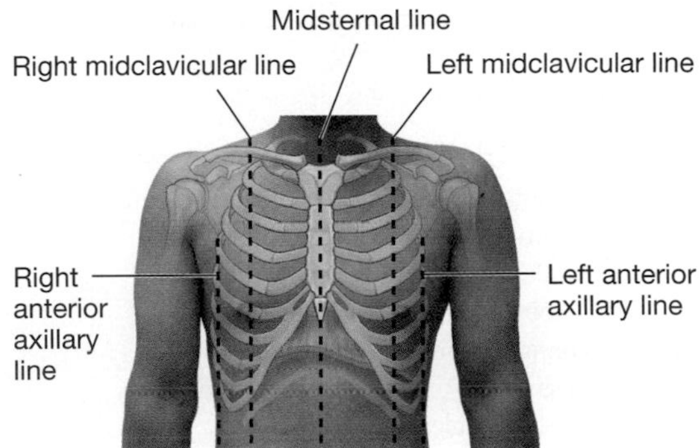

FIGURE 23-8 Anterior reference lines on chest wall

Anterior Thorax

Anteriorly, the predominant portions of the lungs are the upper lobes, as well as the right middle lobe and the lower portions of the lower lobes (see Figure 23-4). The lower portions of the lower lobes are positioned laterally approximately at the sixth intercostal space (ICS). The landmarks of the anterior chest include the suprasternal notch, sternum, sternomanubrial angle, which is also known as the Angle of Louis and the costal angle (Figure 23-8).

The suprasternal notch is located at the top of the sternum and is felt as a U-shaped depression in the bone. The sternum, which is also called the breast bone, is actually made up of three bones—the manubrium, the body, and the xiphoid process. The sternomanubrial angle is the point on the sternum where the manubrium is connected to the body of the sternum. This is an important landmark, as this junction is continuous with the second rib, which is helpful in identifying intercostal spaces. The intercostal spaces are considered horizontal lines to aid in identifying areas on the chest wall. The ICS just below the second rib is the second ICS. The other ICSs are identified in the same manner. The remaining ICSs may be identified by counting down from the second rib and identifying the corresponding ICS.

The costal angle is formed by joining of the right and left costal margins at the tip of the xiphoid process. This angle is usually 90°; however, in instances where the chest enlarges, the angle may increase.

Other important reference points on the anterior thorax are vertical lines that further help to locate underlying findings. On the anterior chest, these lines are the midsternal and midclavicular lines (see Figure 23-8). The midsternal line is a vertical line that goes through the middle of the sternum that divides the anterior thorax into right and left. The midclavicular lines are two (right and left) vertical lines that bisect the clavicle at its midpoint between the sternoclavicular and acromioclavicular joints. This line is also just medial to the nipples.

Posterior Thorax

Posteriorly, the lower lobes comprise the majority of the lung, although small portions of the upper lobes (apices) comprise the uppermost posterior portion of the lungs.

The posterior landmarks are the vertebrae prominens and the spinous processes (see Figure 23-1b). The vertebrae prominens is the spinous process of C_7 and is felt at the base of the neck when the head is flexed. If two vertebrae are felt, the upper one is C_7 and the lower one is T_1.

Having located the vertebrae prominens, it is possible to count down the spinous processes of the vertebra. The attachment of the ribs corresponds with the thoracic vertebrae, however, it is only possible to palpate down to T_4 with any specificity.

The posterior thorax reference lines include the midspinal and the midscapular lines.

The midspinal (vertebral) line divides the posterior chest into right and left sides. The midspinal line is a parallel line to the midsternal line.

The midscapular lines are vertical lines that pass through the scapula at the inferior angle. It is important that the arms are resting at the side of the body to correctly identify this line. When the arms are extended, the scapula moves, dislocating the inferior angle of the scapula. The midscapular lines are parallel lines to the midclavicular lines.

Right Lateral Thorax

The right lateral portion of the lung is composed of the upper, middle, and lower lobes. Approximately half of the anatomical surface of the right thorax is composed of the upper lobe and the other half is shared by the middle and upper lobes. The lateral landmarks are the anterior, mid, and posterior axillary lines (Figure 23-9).

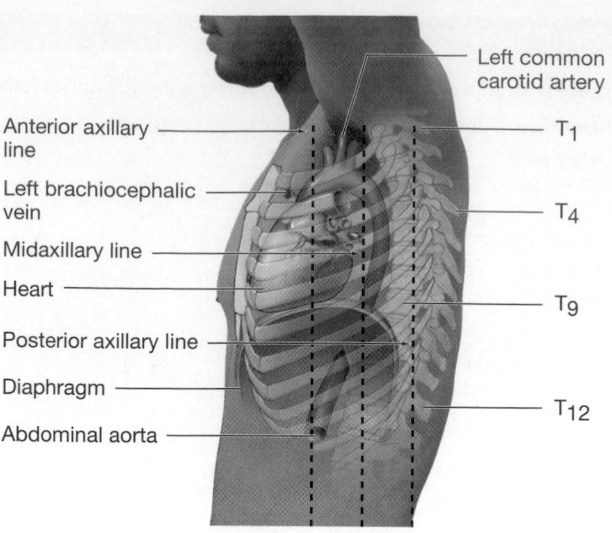

FIGURE 23-9 Lateral reference lines on lateral chest

The midaxillary lines runs down the middle of the axilla and divides the thorax into posterior and anterior sections. The anterior axillary line extends from the anterior axillary fold down the side and the posterior axillary line extends from the posterior axillary fold down the side.

Left Lateral Thorax

The left lateral portion of the lungs is composed of the upper and lower lobes. Approximately half of each lobe is present. The left lateral landmarks are the same and parallel those on the right side.

The physical examination of the pulmonary system occurs during the examination of the chest and often done concurrently with the cardiac exam. All four levels are described; however, for all intents and purposes, the majority of data needed is obtained within the first two levels. The difference between Level I and Level II is basically that the data associated with Level II represents the presence of lung pathology of some sort.

Inspection

Ventilations (rate, rhythm, pattern)
- Effort (spontaneous, assisted, controlled, failure)
- Oxygen saturation
- Position, aids to facilitate breathing
- Audible sounds (stridor, wheezing)
- Chest configuration (anterior and posterior)
- Size and shape, AP: lateral diameter, symmetry, costoveterbral angle, angle of ribs
- Chest movement (thoracic expansion)
- Symmetry, bulging, retractions, use of accessory muscles
- Color/clubbing
- CO_2 blood level (blood chemistry series)
- ABGs

Palpation

- Thoracic muscles/skeleton, trachea position
- Thoracic expansion, symmetry
- Crepitus, vibrations
- Tactile fremitus

Percussion Direct or Indirect

- Percussion tone
- Diaphragmatic excursion

Auscultation

- Air flow
- Bronchial, bronchovesicular, vesicular
- Adventitious sounds (crackles, wheezes, rubs)
- Vocal resonance

Level I to IV Examination

The Level I to Level IV examinations are performed on a continuum, which starts from a basic level to a more comprehensive level based on provider's abilities and knowledge as well as the patient's presentation and location. It may start at the outpatient setting progressing to the ED, hospital unit bed, critical care unit, or specialty unit. Frequently all the elements from basic to comprehensive exam are done in one setting like in a primary care setting or clinic.

The condition/illness of the patient is the primary consideration related to the type and amount of data needed to assess the patient's/condition/illness/situation. The arrangement of skills into levels is for general purposes and is meant to be descriptive rather than prescriptive. The purpose of arranging into levels is to provide a framework to assist the learner in determining the appropriate data to collect.

Lungs (Anterior/Posterior/Lateral)

	Level I	Level II	Level III	Level IV
Inspection	Ventilatory effort (rate/rhythm) Symmetry of chest movement Extrathoracic findings—skin/lips color, fingernails Position Oxygenation (oxygen saturation)	Ventilatory effort (position/posture; equipment to facilitate ventilations). Controlled ventilations Configuration/AP: lateral diameter/structural alterations Oxygenation (arterial blood gases)	Ventilatory effort/rate Blunt trauma Use of accessory muscles	Pulmonary function tests
Palpation	Fingernail beds	Thoracic Expansion Trachea—midline Crepitus	Fremitus	
Percussion		Pulmonary percussion tones Diaphragmatic excursion		
Auscultation	Breath sounds (airflow to both lungs)	Breath sounds; adventitious sounds	Voice sounds: Bronchophony Egophony Whispered pectoriloquy	

Inspection: Level I

Inspection Techniques and Expected Findings	Unexpected Findings
Initial observation of the patient's ventilatory effort, rate, rhythm, and pattern should not be obvious patient awareness of this may initiate a self-conscious response, that may produce erroneous data. Effort is the patient's ability to initiate ventilations and maintain continuous ventilations. The patient should be able to initiate ventilations with ease in any position and not depend on any posture, position, or maneuvers to assist with either component of the ventilatory cycle. Ventilations should be voluntary and spontaneous, quiet, smooth, rhythmic and inconspicuous. In everyday situations and environments, one is not aware of one's own or other's ventilatory effort.	Anything that creates a conscious awareness of the patient's ventilatory effort or any evidence of distress is an indicator that something is wrong.

Inspection Techniques and Expected Findings

The ventilatory rate for an adult varies from 12 to 20 per minute. Ventilations are approximately one-fourth of the patient's heart rate.

Observe the rhythm and pattern of ventilations and chest movement. The expected rhythm and pattern should be ventilations that occur in regular cycles with equal bilateral chest expansion. Ventilation data that is within the stated parameters for effort, rate, rhythm, and pattern are described as **eupnea**.

Depending on the patient's physical status and condition, slight variations in rate may be observed but are not necessarily considered unexpected.

Bradypnea may be observed in well-conditioned athletes or individuals who may be resting or asleep when demands for oxygen are not exceeded. **Tachypnea** is frequently observed after exercise, or in individuals who are at higher elevations.

Unexpected Findings

Any altered regularity or patterns of ventilation are unexpected and should be documented. Their presence may give clues to underlying conditions. Examples of altered breathing patterns related to rate and pattern are described in Table 23-4.

Paradoxical breathing is observed as asynchronous movement of the thoracic cage and the abdomen. It is manifested by drawing in of the thorax and abdominal protrusion on inspiration and the opposite movement during expiration demonstrating a "see-saw" ventilatory pattern. It is caused by the transmission of negative intrathoracic pressure to the abdomen by a weakened, poorly functioning diaphragm. This often accompanies obstructive airway disease or occurs during sleep when the upper airway may become obstructed.

Table 23-4 Altered patterns of ventilation

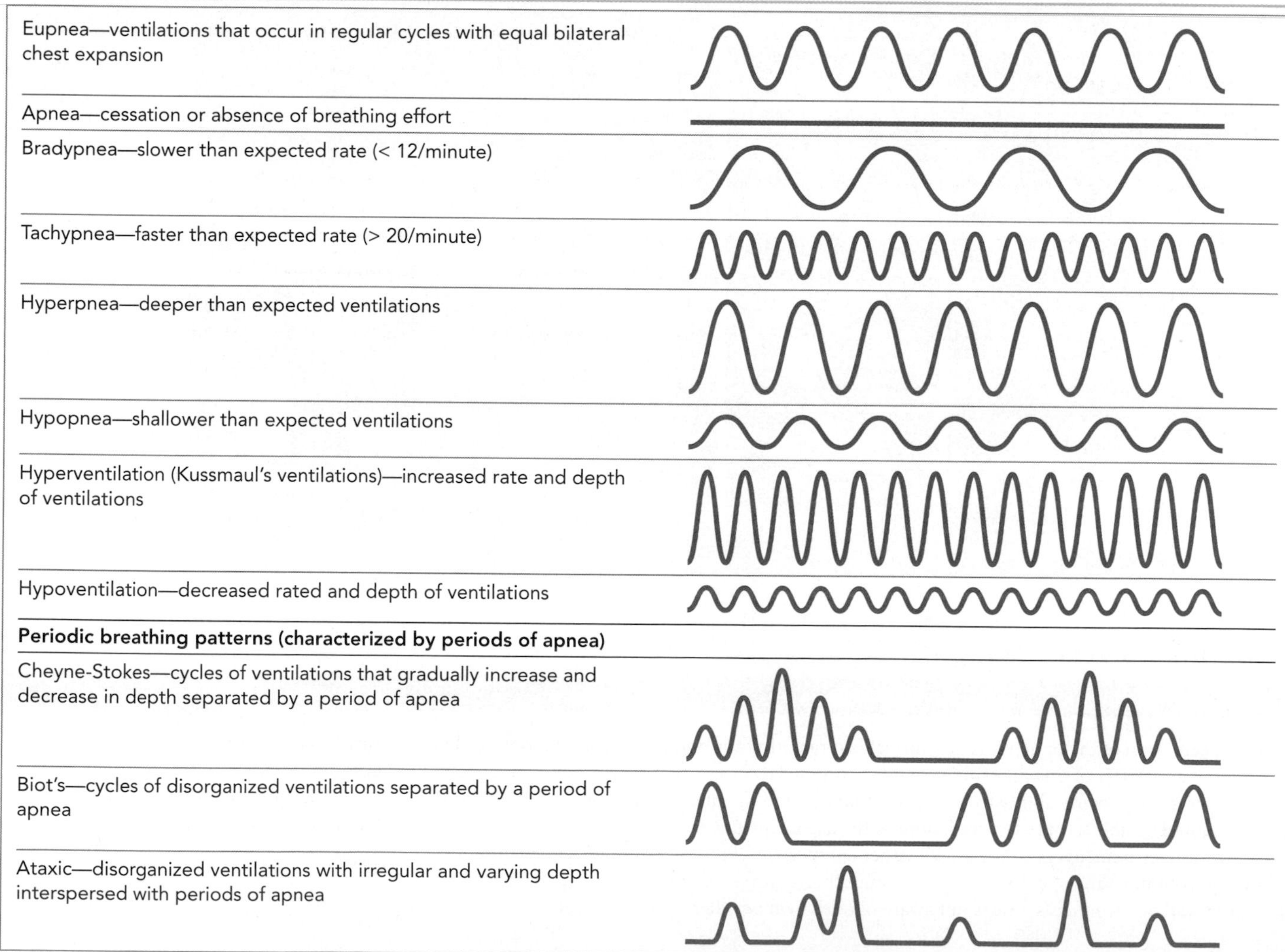

Pattern
Eupnea—ventilations that occur in regular cycles with equal bilateral chest expansion
Apnea—cessation or absence of breathing effort
Bradypnea—slower than expected rate (< 12/minute)
Tachypnea—faster than expected rate (> 20/minute)
Hyperpnea—deeper than expected ventilations
Hypopnea—shallower than expected ventilations
Hyperventilation (Kussmaul's ventilations)—increased rate and depth of ventilations
Hypoventilation—decreased rated and depth of ventilations
Periodic breathing patterns (characterized by periods of apnea)
Cheyne-Stokes—cycles of ventilations that gradually increase and decrease in depth separated by a period of apnea
Biot's—cycles of disorganized ventilations separated by a period of apnea
Ataxic—disorganized ventilations with irregular and varying depth interspersed with periods of apnea

Inspection Techniques and Expected Findings	Unexpected Findings
Additional observations related to pulmonary function may be categorized as extrathoracic findings, as they are observed away from the thoracic region. Inspect the overall skin color, lips and fingers for evidence of adequate oxygenation. Adequate oxygenation is demonstrated by a skin color that demonstrates consistent pigmentation, without any areas of altered, blue-gray coloration. Inspect the shape of the fingernails. Adequate oxygenation is demonstrated by fingernails that are translucent and pink and adhered to the fingernail bed at an angle of 160 degrees and finger tips that are not misshapen or demonstrate altered blue-gray coloration. (See Chapter 16.)	A blue coloration added to the patient's overall skin color (cyanosis) is evidence of poor oxygenation of the tissues due to an increase in carbaminohemoglobin (hemoglobin saturated with CO_2 instead of O_2). Cyanosis may be present in the lips and fingers. The fingers may also display clubbing. Cardiac or pulmonary disorders, COPD, and cystic fibrosis are the most common pulmonary causes of clubbing, and congenital heart disease is a common cardiac cause. (See Chapter 24.)
Also observe the nose for any evidence of air hunger.	Instances of air hunger are frequently accompanied by nasal flaring or a widening of the nares during inspiration. This is common in infants who are experiencing breathing difficulties as they are obligate nose breathers.
Observe the patient's chest for symmetry and symmetrical expansion during inspiration. The chest should appear symmetrical with equal muscle development on both sides. Chest expansion during inspiration should be smooth, bilaterally equal, and symmetrical.	Chest expansion that is asymmetrical, unequal, or that is interrupted or stopped before complete expansion are unexpected findings.

PRACTICE POINT: Thoracic or Diaphragmatic Breathers

The muscles that are primarily used to expand the chest influence the type of breathing characteristic of individuals. Commonly, individuals are categorized as either thoracic or diaphragmatic (abdominal) breathers. Thoracic breathers use primarily the intercostal muscles, whereas diaphragmatic breathers use primarily the diaphragm and abdominal muscles. As a general rule, females are thoracic breathers and males are diaphragmatic breathers.

Observe the ribs for their position and the specific angles they create. When observing the lateral sides of the thorax, the ribs can be described as positioned at a 45-degree angle (Figure 23-10). Again, there is no precise way to measure this angle so it is visualized and estimated. Configuration alterations of the thorax are observed at the sternum and ribs.

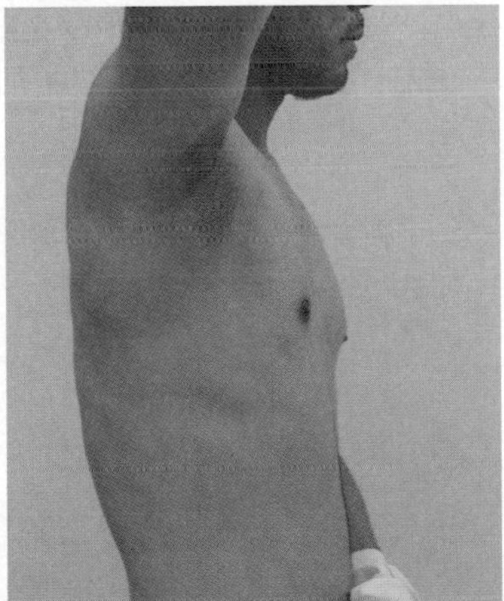

FIGURE 23-10 Ribs at 45-degree angle

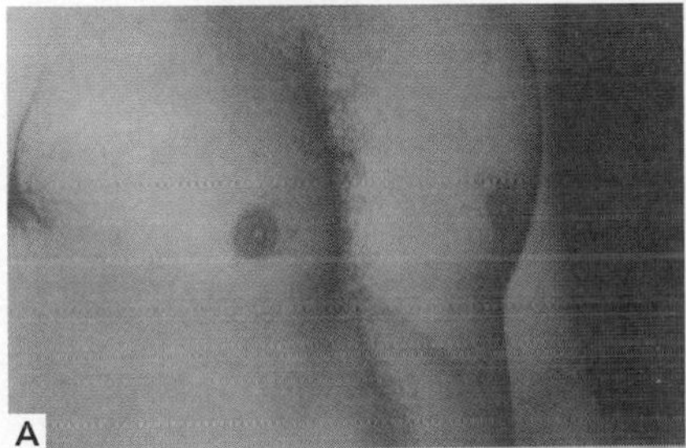

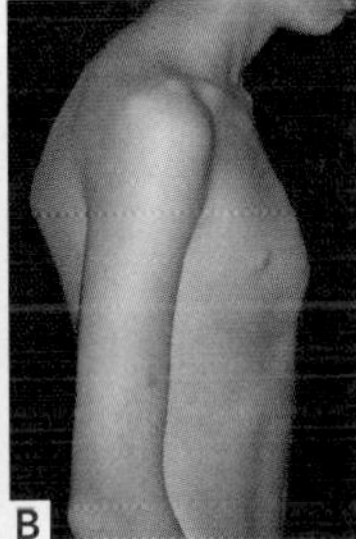

FIGURE 23-11A–B Chest cage alterations **a)** Pectus excavatum; **b)** pectus carinatum

Source: b. Dr. P. Marazzi/Science Photo Library

Sternal alterations are pectus carinatum (pigeon chest) and pectus excavatum (funnel chest) (Figure 23-11).

Pectus carinatum is a protrusion of the sternum, increasing the AP diameter.

Pectus excavatum is a more severe alteration that manifests as a depression or an inward curve on the anterior chest wall. It is thought to be caused by abnormal growth of the bone and cartilage of the ribs and sternum. No specific mechanism has been identified for the overgrowth of the bone and cartilage but it is known to be associated with Marfan's and Poland syndromes (Hebra, 2005). Manifestations range from mild to severe; severe alterations require surgical intervention to correct. In severe cases, chest expansion is restricted, thus decreasing the amount of air transported into the lungs, which severely limits the amount of oxygen available for respiration. Males are more commonly affected and symptoms may not be significant until the rapid growth associated with puberty.

Inspection Techniques and Expected Findings	Unexpected Findings

THINK LINK: Adolescence and Body Image Related to PE/PC

While pectus carinatum and excavatum may not cause significant pathological symptoms or problems, they can cause problems with an individual's body image, particularly in adolescence. Anything that may make the teen appear "different" from others creates anxiety over "acceptance" by others. These individuals may also experience a decreased exercise tolerance and dyspnea with exertion. This is particularly important to male teens who wish to participate in sports activities. When the alteration is minimal there may not be severe distress and or any pulmonary or cardiac problems. During puberty and its accompanying growth spurt, the condition may become worse, creating pulmonary and cardiac symptomatology. A certain number of individuals with severe abnormalities may require surgery, which is optimally done after the age of 6. Children have softer cartilage and more flexible bones, which make for more successful outcomes, particularly cosmetically. Surgery is not performed strictly for cosmetic reasons, thus those with mild to moderate abnormalities, most likely will need to live with and adapt to the condition (Hebra, 2005).

Observe for alterations related to ribs. The costal angle, which is formed by the seventh ribs where they attach to the sternum, should be approximately 90 degrees or less.

Alterations related to ribs are more a result of pulmonary conditions rather than a cause of it. Individuals with COPD eventually develop a barrel chest in which the AP diameter approaches that of the transverse diameter so that the ratio may be 1:1 (Figure 23-12). As the AP diameter increases, the ribs become elevated to the point where they become positioned at a 90-degree angle, rather than a 45-degree angle. An increase in the AP diameter also increases the costal angle to greater than 90 degrees and, when present, is another indicator of barrel chest.

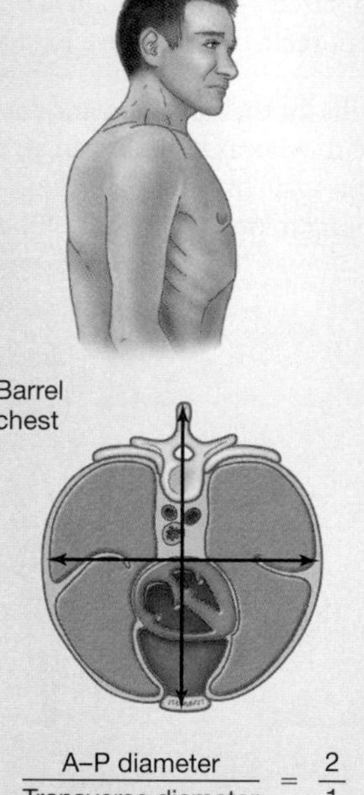

FIGURE 23-12 Barrel chest

Observe the quality of oxygenation of blood observed and oxygen saturation. (See Chapter 5.)

Oxygen saturation parameters are dependent on elevation and barometric pressure.

Unexpected findings would be oxygen saturation below expected parameters.

Inspection Techniques and Expected Findings

Inflammatory and infectious processes within the lungs often produce sputum, a combination of mucus, cellular debris, blood, or microorganisms.

Unexpected Findings

An increase in sputum is an indicator of an inflammatory or infectious process occurring in the lungs. The by-products of these processes combine with the mucus, producing sputum. Table 23-3 presents the various descriptors that may be used to characterize sputum. Each may be associated with specific conditions and pathological alterations (refer to Table 23-3, p. 582).

Inspection: Level II

Additional observations related to ventilatory efforts are the patient's need for increased effort and if any specific positions/posture or any maneuvers are required to facilitate ventilations. Even though muscles are required to perform the work of ventilation, their work and involvement are not evident. Observations of ventilatory effort indicate that ventilatory effort is still spontaneous, but additional maneuvers may be required to facilitate it. In such patients, the effort to breathe and the use of additional muscles for ventilation is more obvious.

Observe if the patient uses specific positions or postures or any maneuvers to facilitate ventilations.

Table 23-5 Restrictive and obstructive pulmonary disorders

	Restrictive Lung Disease**	Obstructive Lung Disease
Disorders	Pneumonia Pulmonary Fibrosis Plural Effusion Pleurisy Structural alterations	Chronic Bronchitis Emphysema Asthma Cystic Fibrosis
Breathing Difficulty	Inspiration	Expiration
Anatomy affected	Lung tissue/thorax	Airways
Pathophysiology	⊠ Lung/thoracic compliance	⊠ Airway resistance
Pathology	Airways consolidated	Airways collapse
Pulmonary Function	⊠ Lung volumes/capacities	⊠ Airway flow rates
Forced Vital Capacity	Decreased	Decreased/normal
Forced Expiratory Volume in One second	Decreased/normal	Decreased/normal
FEV 1/FEV Ratio	Normal/increased	Decreased
Total Lung Capacity	Decreased	Normal/increased
Residual Volume	Normal	Increased

**Restrictive disorders are of two types:
Intrinsic restrictive disorders—alterations in the lung tissue
Extrinsic restrictive disorders—alterations outside the anatomical boundaries of lungs (sternal, rib, spinal alterations)

Whenever ventilations require increased effort, ventilations become labored and the work of breathing increases. Specific pulmonary disorders that affect ventilation may be broadly categorized as restrictive or obstructive (Table 23-5). Restrictive disorders interfere with the ability to expand the lungs to allow air to enter the lungs. Obstructive disorders interfere with the ability of the lungs to deflate and expel air out of the lungs.

Inspection Techniques and Expected Findings	Unexpected Findings

In restrictive and obstructive conditions, accessory muscles become involved in facilitating ventilations.

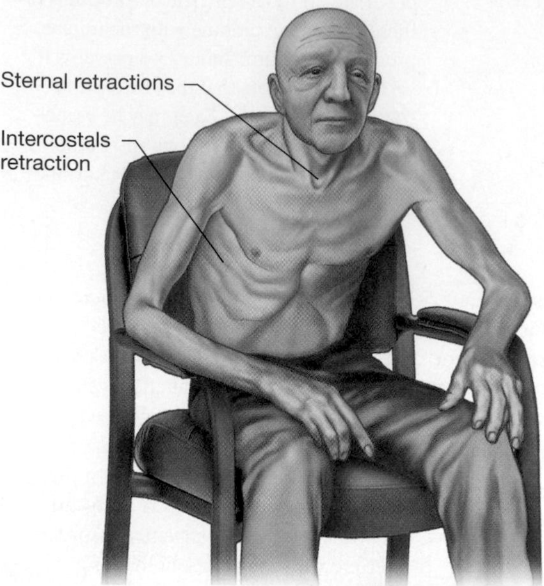

FIGURE 23-13 Retractions in the intercostal spaces are an unexpected finding.

Evidence of accessory muscle use is often observed as retractions, as indentations of the intercostal spaces during inspiration, and usually associated with obstruction (Figure 23-13). In an effort to overcome the obstruction, the muscles pull back during inspiration, increasing intrathoracic pressure.

In more severe obstruction, retractions may also be observed around the sternum, in the clavicular spaces, and the costal margins. Generally, the higher the obstruction within the bronchial tree, the greater the degree of retractions. Unilateral retractions may be observed in the event of foreign body obstruction of the bronchi. Conditions such as asthma and bronchiolitis may cause lower chest retractions.

When increased ventilatory effort is due to a mechanical or functional obstruction of the higher conducting airways (trachea or glottis), it may be accompanied by stridor. It is most commonly heard during inspiration, but may occur during expiration also. It is most common in children, because of their smaller airways, but may be present in adults if the obstruction is severe enough. Stridor is characterized as loud, raspy, and noisy breathing that is audible without a stethoscope.

In addition to internal causes of increased ventilatory effort, structural alterations may also contribute to the need for increased ventilatory effort. As the ribs are connected to the spine, any alteration of the spine will also result in rib alterations. Severe deformities may eventually interfere with ventilatory effort.

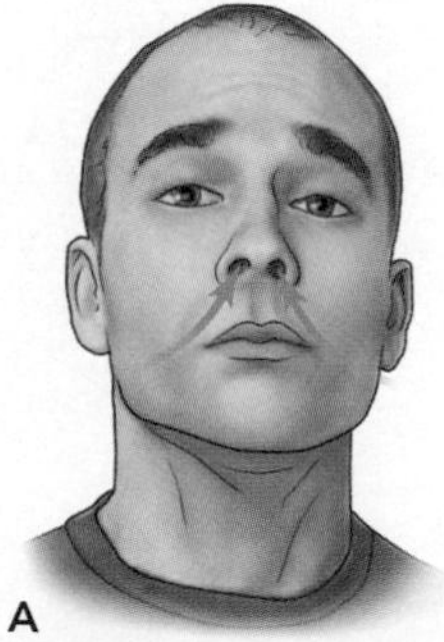
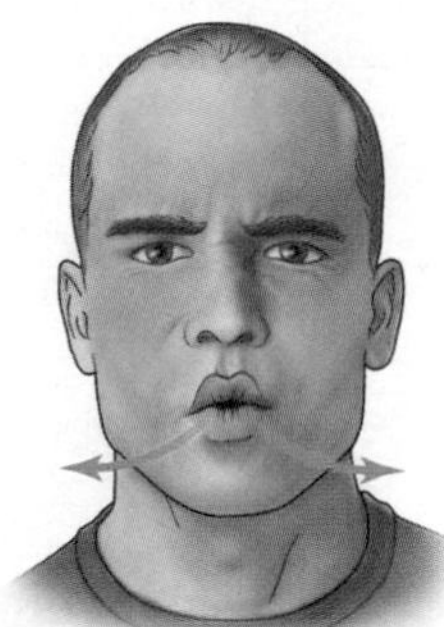

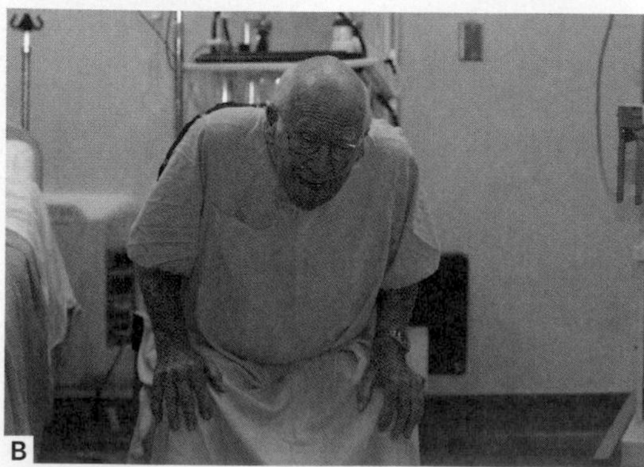

FIGURE 23-14A–B **a)** Pursed lip breathing; **b)** individual who is assuming a tripod position to facilitate breathing

Observable structural alterations result from spinal deviations, which include accentuated thoracic (kyphosis), lumbar (lordosis) curves, or a lateral curvature of the spine (scoliosis). (For further information on these alterations see Chapter 27.)

Individuals experiencing an altered or increased ventilatory effort will most often maintain an upright position to facilitate contraction of the diaphragm. Individuals with chronic obstructive pulmonary disorders will often assume the "tripod position" by leaning forward with the arms supported by the knees, a chair, or bed. This provides leverage that aids the rectus abdominis, intercostal, and accessory neck muscles in facilitating expiration when there is the need to exhale actively (Figure 23-14).

Additionally, the patient may purse the upper and lower lips to create a narrowed opening during expiration (pursed-lipped breathing). This maneuver maintains end-expiratory positive pressure in the lungs, preventing the alveoli from collapsing and aiding the patient in exhalation.

Inspection Techniques and Expected Findings	Unexpected Findings

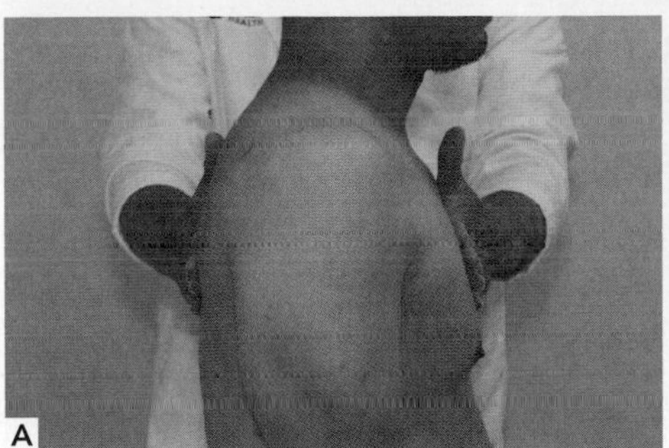

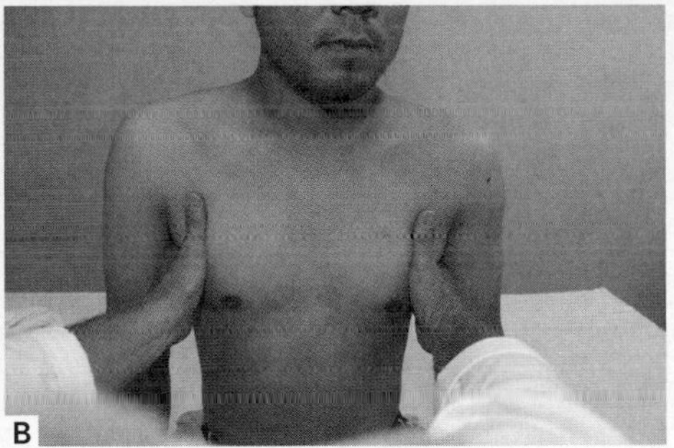

FIGURE 23-15A–B Measuring AP/lateral diameters

Inspect the chest for size, shape, and symmetry. The overall configuration of the chest is determined by the shape of the skeletal structures of the thorax. The shape of the thoracic cavity is oval, which consists of two diameters: anterior-posterior diameter (AP) and lateral or transverse. Initial inspection is to compare the AP diameter to the lateral diameter. This is generally estimated as there is no specific way or formula to actually measure the diameters (Figure 23-15). The ratio of the two diameters is 1:2, with the lateral diameter approximately twice the AP diameter.

Another indicator of increased respiratory effort and difficulty is the number of words that a patient is able to articulate between breaths.

As word formation and speech occurs with expiration, individuals with obstructive lung disease will frequently demonstrate a reduced number of articulated words during expiration. This may be considered a variant of staccato speech in which there are pauses between words. While the patient in respiratory distress may not pause between each word, the fewer words articulated with each breath, the greater the degree of distress.

Observe for the use of any forms of supplemental oxygen or ventilatory support to maintain adequate oxygenation. Supplemental oxygen is often needed in conditions where individuals are no longer able to maintain spontaneous ventilations, or ventilatory effort becomes severely compromised, such as pneumonia or in instances where there is a pneumothorax or atelectasis of a significant amount of lung tissue. It often becomes necessary to provide ventilatory assistance.

Assistance may be supplemental oxygen or controlled/mechanical ventilation. Controlled ventilation is generally used in instances when ventilatory effort is inadequate to oxygenate the blood, along with retention of carbon dioxide. The patient is intubated with an endotracheal (ET) tube, which is inserted through the mouth into the trachea (Figure 23-16). The ET tube is connected to a mechanical ventilator which is set to deliver a certain number of ventilations per minute at a specified tidal volume at a percentage of oxygen that will correct and maintain adequate oxygenation.

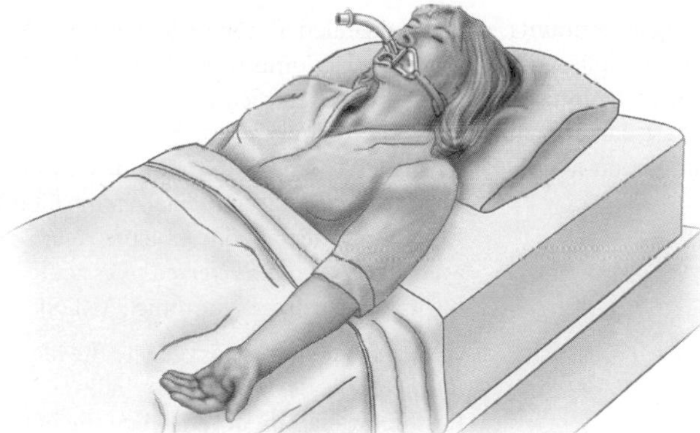

FIGURE 23-16 Intubated patient

Adequate oxygenation is determined by analysis of arterial blood gasses (ABG) that measure the degree of gas exchange in the alveoli as well as the acid–base balance (Table 23-6). Oxygenation is determined by measuring PaO_2 and the SaO_2. About 97% of oxygen in the blood is bound to hemoglobin so the oxygen measured by ABGs is oxygen that is dissolved in arterial blood. The expected value of the PaO_2 is dependent on barometric pressure, which varies depending on what elevation the patient resides at. At sea level, the range of PaO_2 is 80–100 mmHg and decreases in value as the elevation increases. The SaO_2 is the measurement of the percentage of hemoglobin that is saturated with oxygen. The SaO_2 is a constant amount so it is not affected by barometric pressure changes at different elevations.

There is an inverse ratio between hydrogen ion concentration and pH. As the hydrogen ions increase, the blood becomes more acidic and the pH becomes lower. As the hydrogen ions decrease, the blood becomes more alkaline and the pH increases.

Inspection Techniques and Expected Findings	Unexpected Findings

Table 23-6 Arterial blood gas (ABG) values

pH	7.35–7.45	acidity or alkalinity of blood (acidosis vs. alkalosis)
pO_2	80–100 mmHg	partial pressure of dissolved oxygen in blood (arterial)
pCO_2	35–45 mm Hg	partial pressure of dissolved carbon dioxide in blood (arterial)
HCO_3	22–26 mEq/L	metabolic contribution to acid–base balance
BE	-2 to +2	deviation of bicarbonate concentration from baseline (0)
O_2 Sat	96%–98%	percentage of hemoglobin that is saturated with oxygen

The other measurements obtained with ABGs are concerned with and represent acid–base balance. The pH is a measurement of the hydrogen ion concentration in the blood. The pH of the blood is maintained within very narrow limits and wide variations have significant effects on physiological processes that maintain life.

The pH of the blood is also directly related to the pCO_2, or the dissolved carbon dioxide in the blood. In contrast to the PaO_2, the amount of carbon dioxide in the blood results from cellular metabolism so is more constant than PaO_2. The last measurement is the bicarbonate (HCO_3) level. Bicarbonate acts in opposition to $PaCO_2$ to maintain the pH within its specified parameters.

Like the hydrogen ion concentration, when the $PaCO_2$ is high, the pH goes down, and when the $PaCO_2$ is low, the pH goes up.

A low level of HCO_3 is associated with a high level of $PaCO_2$ and a lower pH, whereas a high level of HCO_3 is associated with a lower level of $PaCO_2$ and a higher pH.

Inspection: Level III

Ventilatory effort of individuals within this level is spontaneous but is extremely altered and increased, becoming very labored and rapid. Labored breathing is described as the physical presentation of respiratory distress.

While dyspnea is a subjective experience that may not be observed, labored breathing is easily recognized and obvious. Labored breathing may sometimes be referred to as "air hunger." All the individual's physical resources and efforts are required to breathe and maintain ventilation.

Respiratory distress may be broadly defined as any lung condition that prevents adequate amounts of oxygen to enter the lungs resulting in inadequate oxygenation of the blood. It has multiple causes, with the most common ones being aspiration of stomach contents into the lungs, chemical inhalation, pneumonia, septic shock, and trauma. Respiratory distress caused by any of these damages the alveolar capillary membrane, precipitating the inflammatory process and the accumulation of fluid within the alveoli leading to pulmonary edema.

The fluid-filled alveoli no longer function as respiratory units of the lung so that the individual's increased ventilatory effort is a response to increase the amount of oxygenated air as well as eliminate carbon dioxide that has accumulated in the blood. Respiratory distress due to acutely damaged alveoli is often referred to as acute respiratory distress syndrome (ARDS).

Failure to adequately oxygenate the blood ultimately leads to respiratory failure. Respiratory failure occurs when the pO_2 level in the blood is <50 mmHg and pCO_2 is >50 mmHg as confirmed by ABGs.

Severe respiratory distress is often a major manifestation of traumatic thoracic injuries. Lung trauma is a leading cause of thoracic injuries (Mancini, 2013) contributing to approximately 25% of trauma related deaths and another 25% of total deaths. Automobile accidents are the leading cause of thoracic trauma. Thoracic trauma may be the result of blunt trauma or penetrating trauma. Blunt trauma occurs when the thorax remains intact. Approximately 90% of thoracic injuries are related to blunt trauma.

Blunt trauma results either direct impact or deceleration. A direct impact to the thorax directly transfers the energy from the impact to the chest wall and thoracic organs, causing crush and shear injuries, causing massive tissue injuries and bone (rib) fractures. If a significant amount of pressure is also involved, the intrathoracic pressure increases and may result in the rupture of gas or fluid-filled organs.

Inspection Techniques and Expected Findings	Unexpected Findings
	Injuries resulting from deceleration occur when the forward motion of the thorax stops abruptly and the intrathoracic organs continue to move forward until they collide with the thoracic wall. This causes a second impact, further contributing to tissue damage. Fractured ribs may also damage underlying lung tissue which may cause bruising of the lung or puncture the pleura. Penetrating traumatic injuries result in breaking the integrity of the thorax. There is usually a direct mechanical force that comes into contact with the chest wall. Knives and projectiles are the two most common causes of penetrating lung trauma. Tissue damage is due to stretching and crushing forces and is primarily confined to the path of penetration. Injury severity is determined by the organ that is penetrated and how vital it is. A more significant determinant of injury is the velocity with which the projectile penetrates the underlying tissues. Knife wounds are considered low velocity penetrating projectiles and are confined to the area of penetration. Bullets, by comparison, are high velocity penetrating projectiles. They also cause damage to the tissues adjacent to the path of penetration. Tissue damage is the result of cavitation and shock waves that cause outward extension of the tissues, enlarging the area of damage.
Depending on the cause, manifestations of respiratory distress from thoracic injuries include unequal chest expansion, decreased chest expansion, flail chest, chest pain. These result from direct injury or other complications, impairing lung tissue and ultimately resulting in compromised oxygen delivery and exchange.	Unequal chest expansion is observed with marked atelectasis or pneumonia in which there is significant consolidation of lung tissue. The consolidated lung tissue does not expand during inspiration, so that it does not expand as much as the unaffected lung, resulting in unequal expansion. Pain from thoracic trauma, with or without fractured ribs also limits expansion of the affected side. Fractured ribs will cause pain and possible pneumothorax, a common complication associated with thoracic trauma. (See Conditions and Disorders.) A hemothorax is a collection and accumulation of blood within the pleural space, frequently caused by damage to a major blood vessel along the path of penetration, causing bleeding into the pleural space. (See Conditions and Disorders.)

Inspection Techniques and Expected Findings

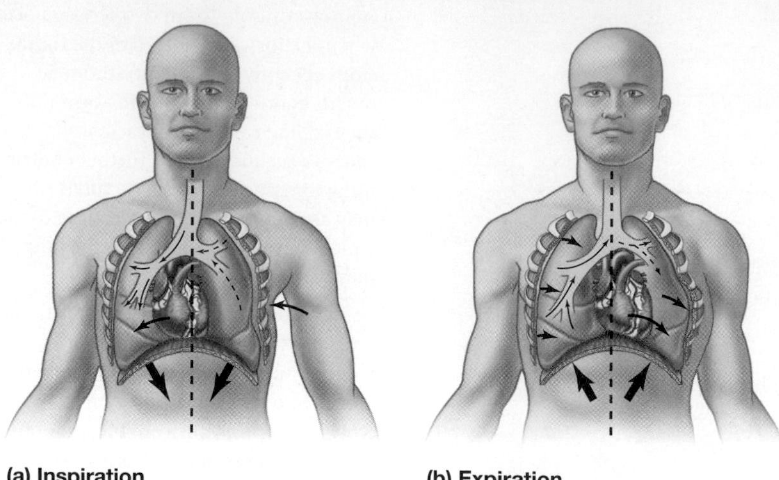

FIGURE 23-17A–B Flail chest

Inspection: Level IV

Pulmonary function tests (PFTs) provide quantitative data regarding the work of the lungs that gives an indication of how much of the air exchanged can be used and how easily it can be moved in and out. They are performed via spirometry, which measures both volume and flow in relation to time, and assists in diagnosing obstructive and restrictive disorders early in the course of the condition.

Capacities and volumes are measured as the parameters for pulmonary function. The most significant clinical parameters are the forced vital capacity (FVC) and the forced expiratory volume in one second (FEV1). FVC is the maximum amount of gas that can be displaced from the lung during a forced expiration. FEV1 is the maximum amount of air that can be exhaled from the lung in one second. Other volumes and capacities measured are identified and described in Figure 23-18.

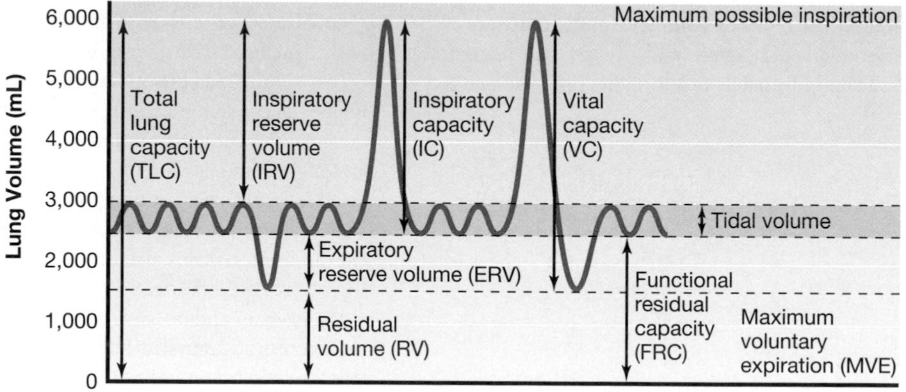

FIGURE 23-18 Identifying capacities and volumes related to pulmonary function tests TLC: volume in lungs at maximal inflation; TV: volume of air inhaled/exhaled during quiet breathing; RV: volume of air remaining in lungs after maximal exhalation; VC: volume of air exhaled after deepest inhalation; ERV: maximum amount of air exhaled after quiet exhalation

Unexpected Findings

Flail chest is a life-threatening condition that results from fractures of the ribs causing detachment from the chest wall (Figure 23-17). The involved ribs are fractured at two or more locations, occurring in 2–3 ribs. Its most conspicuous manifestation is paradoxical chest expansion. Paradoxical movement is observed as opposite movement of the chest so that when the unaffected side is expanding with inspiration, the affected side moves inward and vice versa. During inspiration, the negative pressure that draws air into the lungs also pulls the flail chest wall inward. During expiration, positive pressure expels the air out, decreasing the size of the chest cavity. The flail side, because it has lost the stability provided by the ribs, expands outward.

PRACTICE POINT: Capacities and volumes

Capacities are measurements of total amounts and are comprised of 2 or more volumes added together. Volumes are measurements of amounts of a single unit or action. For example 1 cup is a capacity, but it can be comprised of various volumes like 2 1/2 cups, 4 1/4 cups, etc. Capacity is relatively stable or fixed, whereas volumes can vary but can't exceed the capacity.

Unexpected findings would be PFT measurements that were not within the expected parameters associated with volumes and capacities. A prolonged FEV1 is a classic PFT alteration associated with obstructive pulmonary conditions.

Palpation: Level I

Palpation Techniques and Expected Findings	Unexpected Findings
Level I palpation is palpation of the fingernail bed for evidence of clubbing. Palpation should demonstrate a firm nail bed that is adhered to the nail plate.	The nail bed of a clubbed finger is short and spongy.

Palpation: Level II

Palpation begins with the provider palpating the thoracic muscles and skeleton, feeling for any pulsations, areas of tenderness, superficial lumps, or masses. Overall, there should be none of these present.

Presence of pulsations, tenderness, lumps, or masses are all unexpected findings.

Palpate thoracic expansion to determine symmetry and equality of chest movement with ventilations. This also confirms observation of thoracic expansion (Figure 23-19). With the patient in a sitting position, place your hands on the posterior thorax with the thumbs located at the level of tenth rib in line with the spinal processes. It may be helpful to pinch the skin lightly between your thumbs creating a crease over the spine. During inspiration, observe the movement of the thumbs. They should both move an equal distance away from the spine. Do not place the hands so tightly on the chest that they impair inspiration, giving erroneous results.

To palpate expansion anteriorly, place the thumbs along the costal margin and the xiphoid process and make the same observations.

Unequal expansion of the thorax may be an indication of a collapsed lung or limited expansion due to pneumothorax, pneumonia, atelectasis, fluid, or a mass.

Fractured ribs from trauma as well as neurological impairment from various causes also cause asymmetrical chest wall movement. If unequal expansion of the chest is suspected, palpation is used to validate chest expansion.

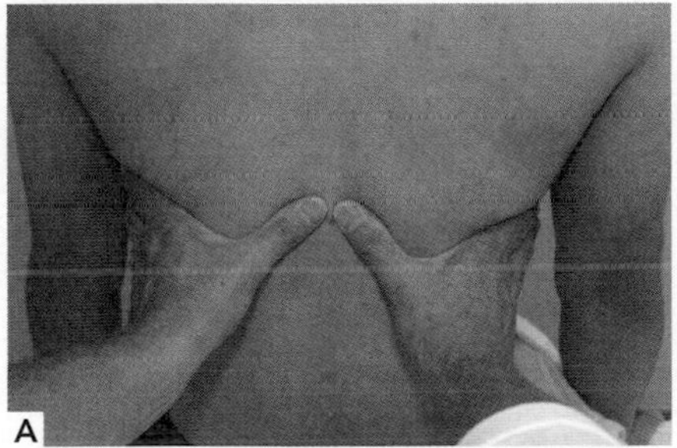

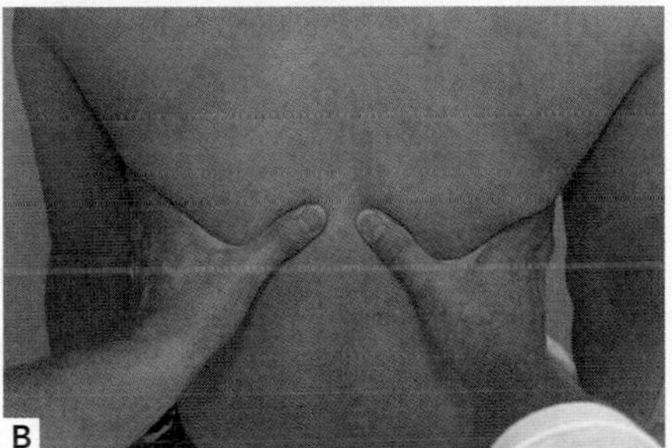

FIGURE 23-19A–B Hands placed on posterior thorax demonstrating proper hand placement for assessing thoracic expansion

Palpate the trachea for its position in the neck. Place the index finger on the superior point of the thyroid cartilage. From that point, lightly run the finger down the anterior aspect of the trachea (Figure 23-20). When the bottom of the trachea is reached, the finger should be just above or in the suprasternal notch. With the finger in this position the trachea should be midline.

Deviation of the trachea may be due to a number of conditions of the lungs. Atelectasis, thyroid enlargement, and pleural effusion may displace the trachea. A tension pneumothorax, tumor, or nodal enlargement may pull the trachea to one side.

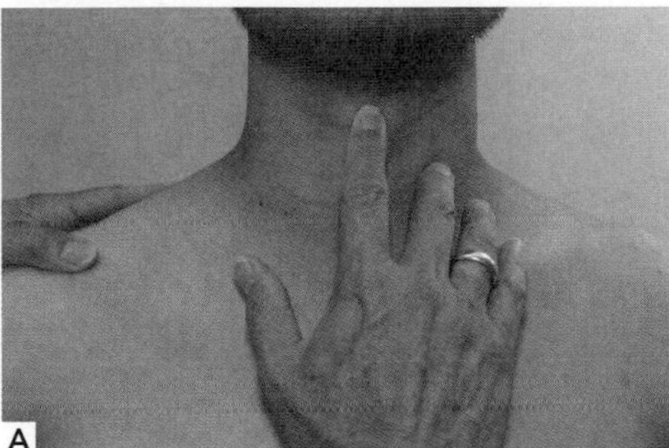

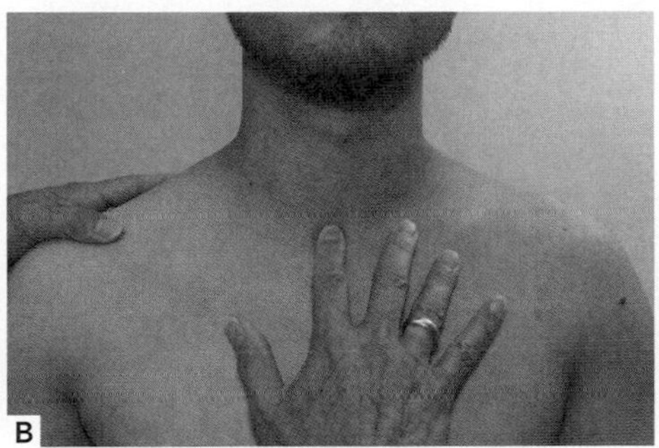

FIGURE 23-20A–B Palpation of the trachea: **a)** thyroid cartilage, **b)** suprasternal notch

Palpation Techniques and Expected Findings	Unexpected Findings

A patient who has had thoracic surgery or sustained any procedures is which collections of air (pneumothorax) or fluids (hemothorax) are removed, will most likely have a chest tube in place. A chest tube is inserted through the chest wall into the pleural space, allowing the air to escape and re-establishing the integrity of the pleural space (Figure 23-21).

In these patients, palpation is performed to assess for the presence of crepitus. With correct placement of the chest tube, palpation around the insertion site should demonstrate skin and underlying tissue that is free of any air.

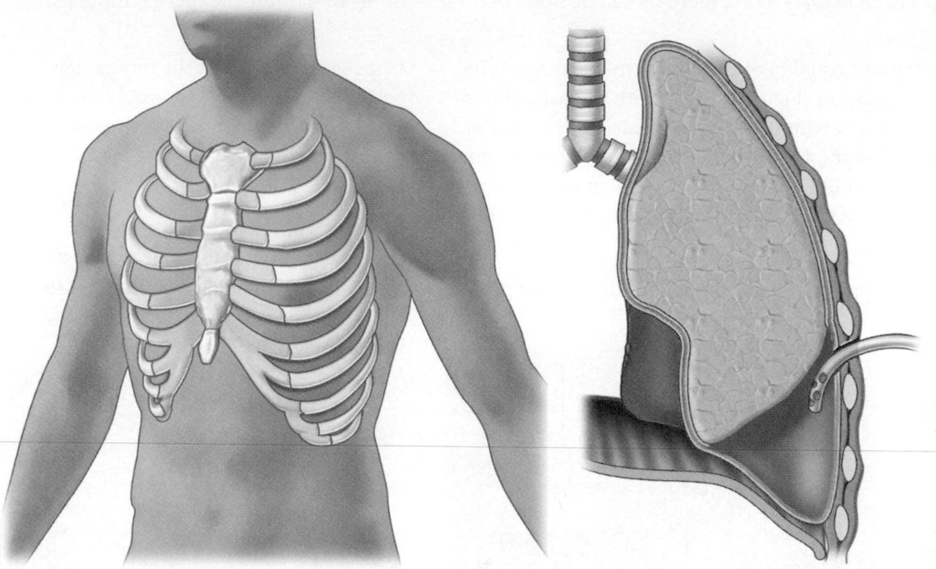

FIGURE 23-21 Chest tube placement

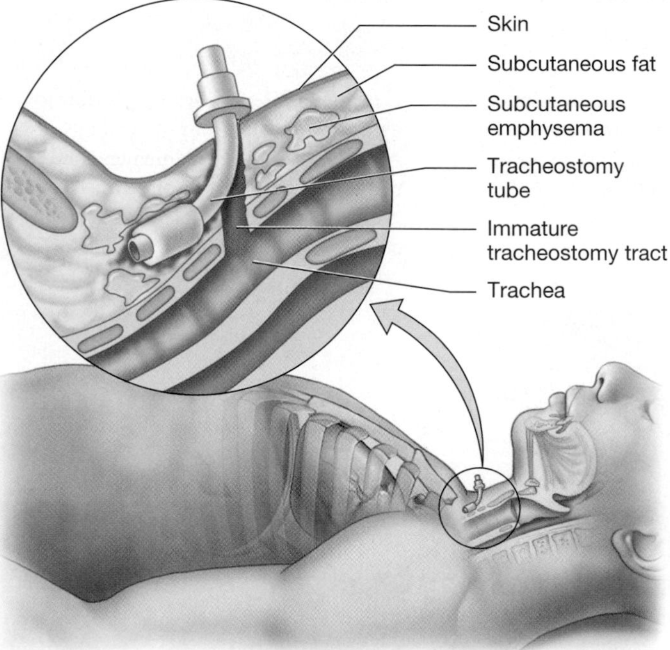

FIGURE 23-22 Crepitus

Unexpected Findings

In the presence of a chest tube, it is not unusual for the patient to develop and demonstrate crepitus, evidence of air within the subcutaneous tissues that is palpated as a bubbly sensation (Figure 23-22). Its presence is an indication that there is a leak somewhere within the pulmonary system that allows air to escape into the subcutaneous tissues. Crepitus is frequently palpated around the insertion site of a chest tube. When present, the surrounding area needs to be assessed frequently to monitor any progression or regression of the crepitus.

Palpation Techniques and Expected Findings	Unexpected Findings
During palpation of the chest wall, assess for the presence of any palpable vibrations, particularly if the patient complains of any pain on inspiration.	A sensation, palpated as a vibration, is evidence of a pleural friction rub. This may be felt more intensely on inspiration and is due to inflammation of the plural surfaces. As the pleura move over each other, the inflamed portions grate on each other creating vibrations. A vibratory sensation may also be felt in the presence of a cardiac murmur; therefore, the timing of the vibrations needs to be assessed in relation to the heart rate and ventilatory rate.

Palpation: Level III

Most significant chest wall injuries will be identified by physical examination. Bruising, grazes, or seat-belt signs are visible on inspection, and palpation may reveal the crepitus associated with broken ribs. Alert patients will complain of pain on palpation of the chest wall or on inspiration.

As noted previously, flail chest is identified as paradoxical movement of a segment of the chest wall, or indrawing on inspiration and moving outward on expiration. This is often better appreciated by palpation than by inspection. Use *gentle* palpation to locate the edges of the flail section.

Rib fractures are determined by palpation for bony abnormalities, localized tenderness, the feeling of "crepitus" or a grating feeling when the fracture sites move against one another.

Palpate the thorax to assess vocal or tactile fremitus, the vibratory sensations produced by vocalizations that can be felt with the palms or ulnar surface of the hands (Figure 23-23). Fremitus is assessed for the equality of the vibratory sensations, which should be equal. Instruct the patient to repeat words or phrases that are known to create vibrations, for example, "how now brown cow," "ninety-nine." As the patient repeats these words, the quality of the vibrations is compared bilaterally over the anterior and posterior chest. The provider may either use both hands to assess each lung simultaneously, or one hand may be moved for one area to the other, comparing symmetrical areas of the lungs.

Conditions that interfere with fremitus either increase or decrease vibrations. Solid material is a better conductor of sound than air, so any condition that causes consolidation of lung areas such as pneumonia, atelectasis, or a tumor will create more intense vibrations. Conversely, conditions that create air-filled areas such as pneumothorax, COPD, and emphysema will produce less intense vibrations.

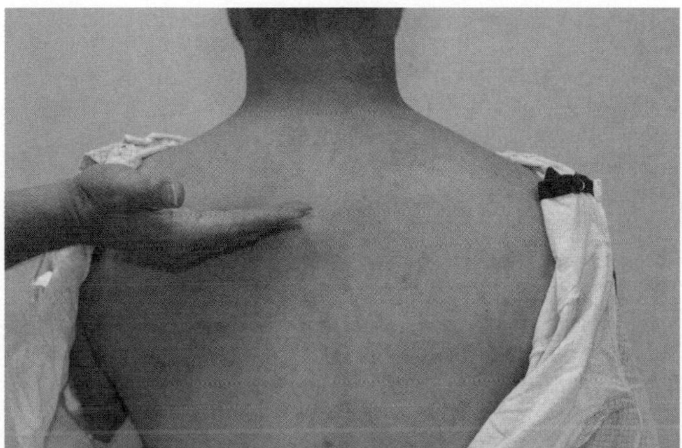

FIGURE 23-23 Palpation of posterior chest using ulnar side of hand to assess for fremitus

Percussion: Level II

Percussion is somewhat limited in its usefulness as far as the significance of data obtained, unless one is skilled in performing it. It requires a significant amount of practice to do it correctly and should not be used to validate or invalidate data unless one is skilled in its performance and is able to recognize subtle differences in the sounds obtained. Therefore, its use and usefulness is primarily determined by the provider and what data are needed so is most likely not appropriate to use until a Level II exam.

Percussion Techniques and Expected Findings	Unexpected Findings
Percussion of the thorax is done to determine the relative density of lung tissue (Figure 23-24). By itself, percussion is not that helpful, as the health care provider can only get a general idea of what is happening on the surface of the lung. Additionally, not all lung tissue is able to be percussed. The sound expected to be heard over lung tissue is resonance. 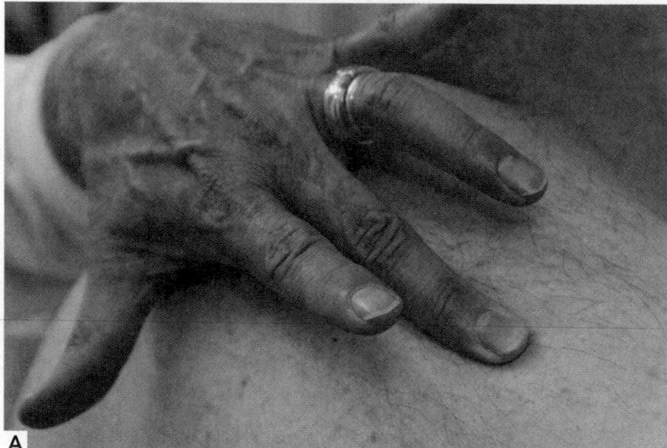 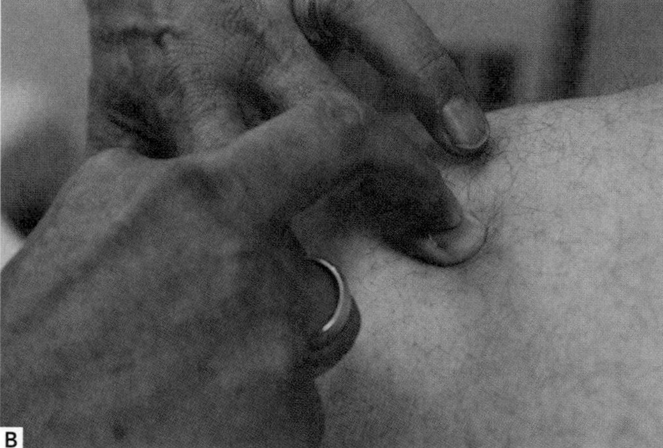 **FIGURE 23-24A–B** Proper placement of finger for percussion	Consolidation of tissue (pneumonia, atelactesis, or a tumor) or increasing the amount of air (COPD, emphysema, pneumothox) will cause changes in the sounds that are obtained through percussion. (Also refer to Chapter 7.) Dullness over lung tissue is associated with lung consolidation. Hyperresonance over lung tissue indicates an increase in air within the lungs.
Percussion follows a systematic approach, going from one side to the other, intercostal space by intercostal space (Figure 23-25). When percussing the lungs, compare symmetrical areas of the right and left lungs. This allows for comparison of sides related to the patient's condition and not to established parameters. Generally, start at the base of the neck and percuss laterally over the apices of the lungs, listening for resonance over lung tissue. Then proceed down the posterior thorax over the lung tissue between the spine and the scapula until the lower border of the scapula is reached. From that point on, the entire width of the lung may be percussed until the level of the diaphragm is reached. The position of the patient should be such that the arms are folded in front to move the scapula further apart and expose more lung tissue. Perform percussion of the lateral and anterior thorax in much the same way, moving across the chest and comparing symmetrical sites. When percussing, the anterior chest, the apices do not need to be percussed again. To expose the lateral areas, the patient may raise the arms. Again, the exact sequence may vary somewhat, but the need for a systematic approach that allows side-to-side comparison is essential.	Other causes of asymmetrical measurements may be due to either pulmonary (emphysema) or abdominal (tumors, ascites) conditions or pain due to trauma (fractured ribs).

Percussion Techniques and Expected Findings	Unexpected Findings

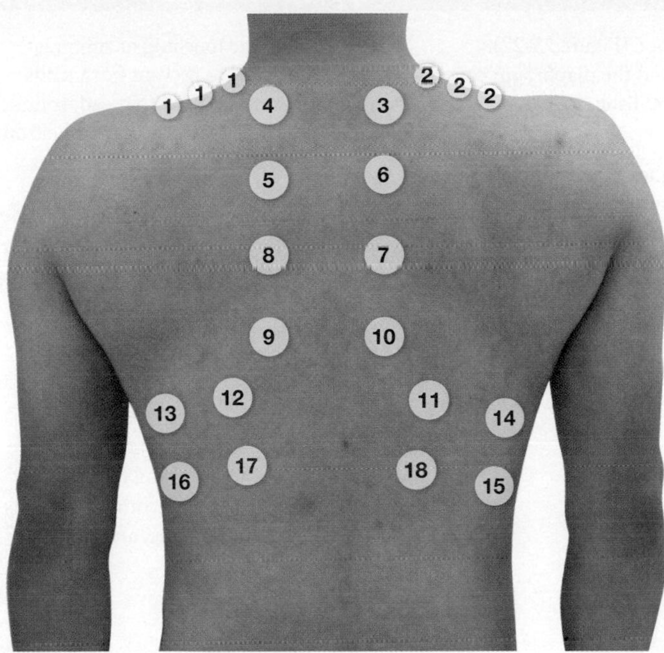

FIGURE 23-25 Percussion sequencing

Percussion is also used to assess diaphragmatic excursion. This measures the descent of the dome of the diaphragm during inspiration (Figure 23-26). The expected descent is approximately 3 to 5 cm and should be bilaterally equal; however, the right side of the diaphragm is displaced by the liver and its measurement may be higher than on the right.

The actual sequence for assessing diaphragmatic excursion may vary; however, assessment must be done at the end of both expiration and inspiration. A suggested sequence follows.

Stand behind the patient and instruct the patient to inhale deeply and exhale deeply and then hold the breath.

Begin percussing down the midscapular line midway down the back. The first sound should be resonance. Continue percussing until the sound changes to dullness.

Mark this point with a marker.

Ask the patient to take a couple of breaths and then take in a large breath and hold it.

Start percussing again either from the marked point or just above the point. The sound should be resonance again. Continue percussing down until resonance changes to dullness again.

Mark this point.

Measure the distance between the points to obtain the diaphragmatic excursion.

Repeat the procedure of the opposite side.

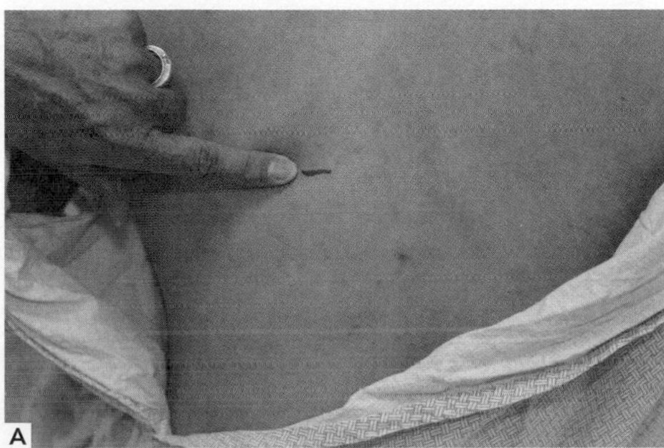

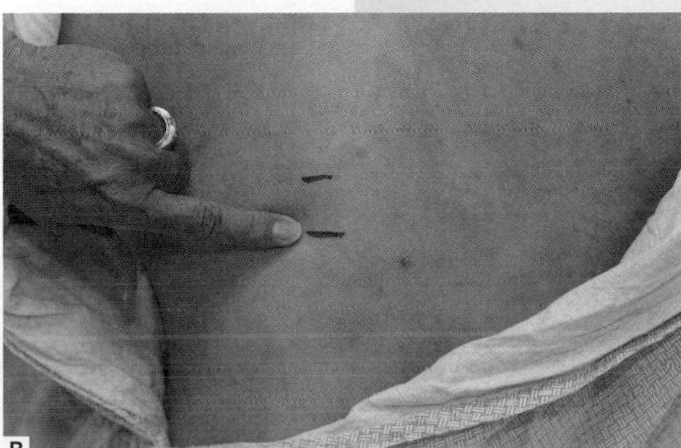

FIGURE 23-26A–B Assessing diaphragmatic excursion

Auscultation: Level I

Auscultation Techniques and Expected Findings	Unexpected Findings

Auscultation of the lungs is performed with the diaphragm of the stethoscope (Figure 23-27). The diaphragm is preferable over the bell as lung sounds are high pitched and the diaphragm covers more area to pick up the sounds. Place the diaphragm firmly on the skin and listen to sounds produced throughout one ventilatory cycle—inspiration and expiration.

Initial auscultation of the lungs provides information about air flow throughout the conducting airways and alveoli. The flow of air throughout the bronchial and alveolar systems creates characteristic sounds that can help to determine the patency of the airways and the presence of any unexpected conditions. In most instances, this can be confirmed with the identification of specific breath sounds; however, when in a critical situation, it is imperative to establish air moving in and out of the specific lobes of the lungs.

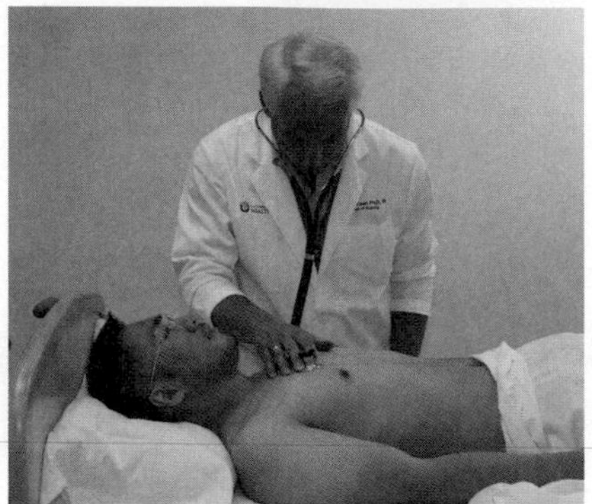

FIGURE 23-27 Proper placement of stethoscope on chest wall

Breath sounds produced by the flow of air into and through the lungs are characterized according to their intensity, pitch, quality, and duration. Audible sounds may not be produced well during normal breathing; thus to augment the intensity of breath sounds, instruct the patient to breathe through the mouth and take deeper than usual breaths. This increases the amount of air flow and facilitates hearing breath sounds.

PRACTICE POINT: Dizziness

Instruct the patient that breathing like this has the potential to cause dizziness and to inform you if this occurs. To minimize the possibility of causing this, auscultate the breath sounds as quickly as possible. If, however, more time is needed, stop and give the patient a break to breathe normally.

Auscultation generally starts on the posterior chest, but this is not mandatory. When auscultating the posterior chest, have the patient fold the arms in front with the head bent forward (Figure 23-28). This makes more lung area available for optimum assessment of breath sounds; the patient should also be as erect as possible. Have the patient raise the arms for auscultation of the lateral chest and sit erect when auscultating the anterior chest. If the patient's condition makes it difficult to assume these positions, the provider must adapt the techniques to the abilities of the patient.

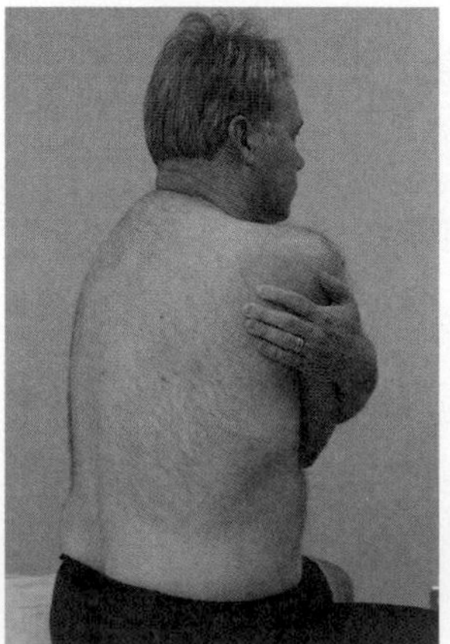

FIGURE 23-28 Proper position of patient when auscultating breath sounds

Unexpected Findings

Nothing should be touching or rubbing on the stethoscope to prevent extraneous sounds from interfering with breath sounds. Sources of extraneous noise may come from the following:

Bed clothing rubbing on the stethoscope

Stethoscope tubing rubbing on each other

Hairy chests in male patients

Ambient noise (TVs, radios, visitors)

Shivering of patient

If any of these sources of noise are interfering with auscultation, take appropriate measures to eliminate them: turn TVs and radios off, place bed clothes or gowns away from the stethoscope, and moisten chest hair.

Auscultation Techniques and Expected Findings

When auscultating the lungs, it is essential to compare symmetrical areas of the right and left lungs. This allows for comparison of sides related to the patient's condition and not to establish parameters (Figure 23-29). Generally, auscultation starts at the base of the neck and moves across the shoulder to assess the apices of the lungs. It then proceeds systematically, going from one side to the other, intercostal space by intercostal space, starting at the top of the spine, proceeding down the posterior thorax over the lung tissue between the spine and the scapula until the lower border of the scapula is reached. From that point on, the entire width of the lung may be auscultated until the level of the diaphragm is reached.

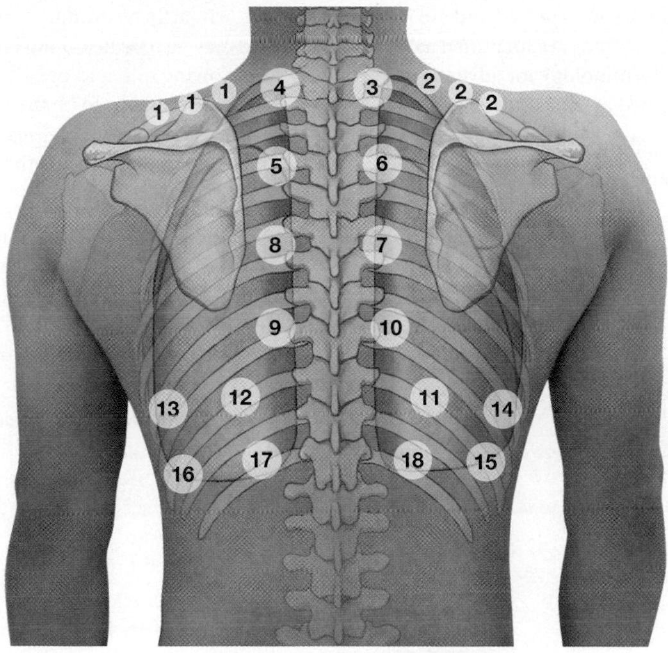

FIGURE 23-29 Auscultatory sites—proper progression from one to the other

The three prevalent breath sounds that are heard over lung tissue are bronchial, vesicular, and bronchovesicular. Each sound has its own unique characteristics that will help the provider determine what sound is being heard and where each sound should be heard (Figure 23-30).

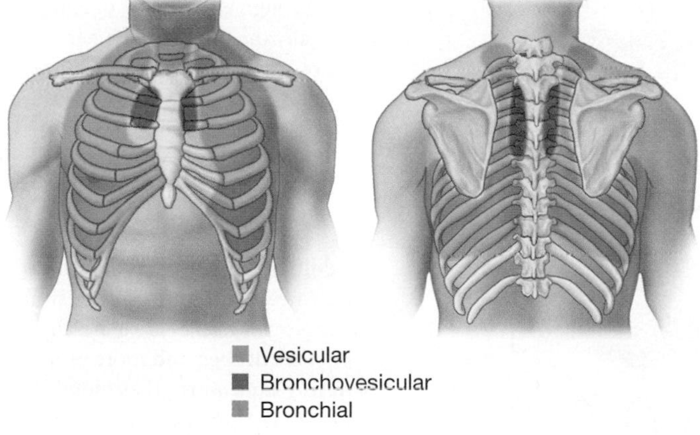

FIGURE 23-30 Three breath sounds in relationship to when and where heard anatomically

Bronchial breath sounds are produced by air flowing though the trachea and bronchi.

They are loud and harsh sounding with a high pitch. Sound is heard partially through inspiration and all of expiration.

Vesicular breath sounds are produced by air flowing through the terminal and respiratory bronchioles and alveoli. They are heard over the majority of lung tissue. They are low pitched and have a soft breezy quality. They are heard throughout all of inspiration and approximately one-third of expiration.

Unexpected Findings

Bronchial and bronchovesicular sounds should not be heard in any other anatomic location than their expected locations. When these sounds are heard away from their expected locations, it is an indicator of an underlying pulmonary condition, most likely causing pulmonary consolidation. Consolidated tissue is a better conductor of sound, therefore, bronchial and bronchovesicular sounds will be conducted through the consolidated lung tissue toward the periphery, where only vesicular sounds should be heard.

Auscultation Techniques and Expected Findings | **Unexpected Findings**

Bronchovesicular breath sounds are heard primarily over the R and L mainstem bronchi, where a combination of bronchial and vesicular sounds is heard. They are moderate in pitch and intensity and can be heard equally throughout inspiration and expiration.

Auscultation: Level II

Level II auscultation is essentially a continuation of Level I auscultation but involves some type of pulmonary alteration.

During auscultation, also listen for the presence of other sounds that may be superimposed over the three expected breath sounds (Figure 23-31). These sounds are unexpected and are indicators of underlying conditions of varying severity. These superimposed sounds are identified as adventitious sounds and are broadly categorized as crackles and wheezes. Terminology for adventitious sounds has been quite varied and consensus as to what they are identified as is nonexistent.

While adventitious sounds are generally considered to indicate pulmonary pathology and are not considered expected sounds, it is not unusual to hear crackles in patients without pulmonary pathology.

In the hospitalized patient, bedrest promotes the collecting of fluid in the bases of the lung causing crackles to be heard. This is particularly evident during the early morning assessment. In the absence of pathology, these sounds disappear after the patient does some deep breathing and coughing.

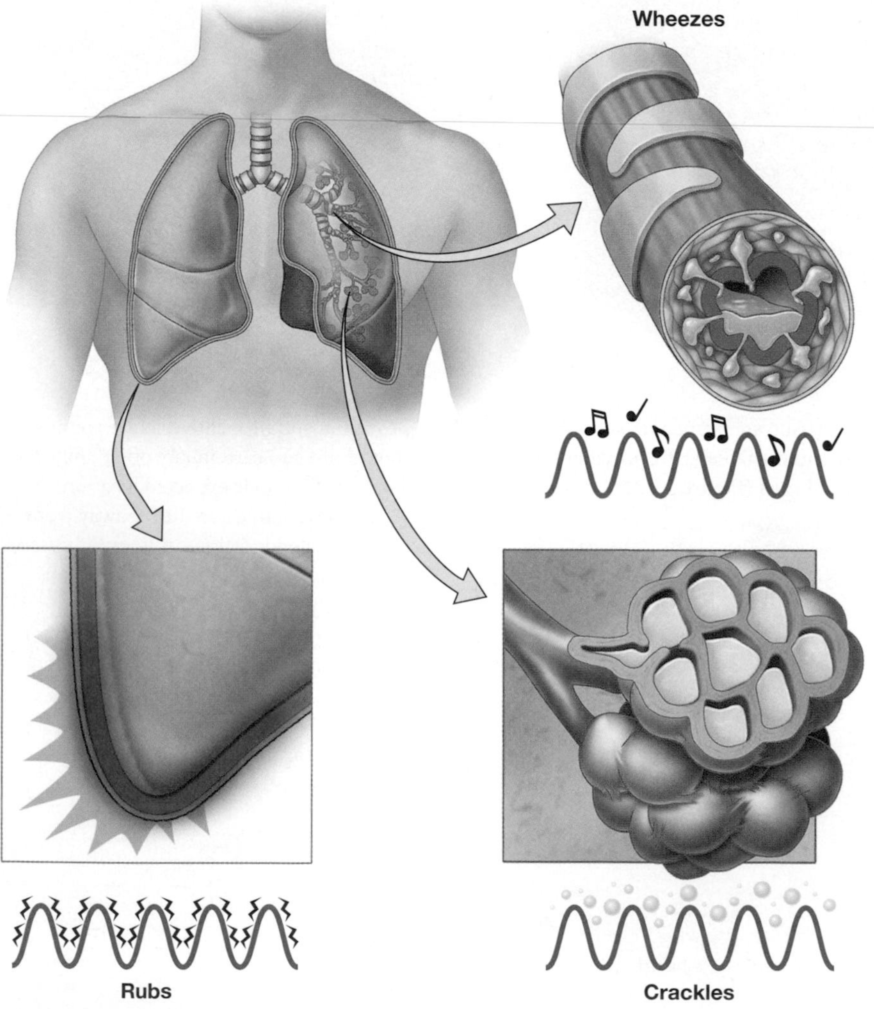

FIGURE 23-31 Adventitious sounds (wheezes, rubs, crackles)

PRACTICE POINT: Crackles (Discontinuous Sounds)

Discontinuous sounds that are heard as crackles can be compared to listening to popcorn popping. Each kernel pops at its own time so there is a constant popping sound. Another comparison could be rubbing bubble wrap. As the hand moves over the bubbles, each one makes a sound so there is continuous sound but comprised of multiple sounds of the bubbles being compressed.

Crackles are discontinuous sounds that are primarily heard during inspiration, but may also be heard during expiration. Air flowing into and opening collapsed alveoli is thought to be the cause of crackles. The asynchronous opening of the alveoli is responsible for the discontinuity of the sound.

- **Fine crackles** are heard toward the end of inspiration and are generally high pitched. End-inspiratory crackles most likely are caused by fluid collapsed alveoli at the periphery of the lung opening as air rushes in.
- **Medium crackles** are heard throughout the last half of inspiration, are lower in pitch, and more moist sounding. As the collapsed alveoli are located more toward the middle section of the lung, medium crackles are heard.
- **Coarse crackles** are low pitched and loud and are heard throughout most of inspiration. These represent collapsed alveoli that may be heard throughout the entire lung.
- **Wheezes**, in contrast to crackles, are continuous sounds with a musical quality. They are caused by air moving through a narrowed opening, specifically the bronchi. The narrowing or obstruction of the bronchi may be due to the presence of thick secretions (mucus plug), muscular spasm (asthma), or new growth (cancer). They may be heard on either inspiration or expiration or both.

Additional descriptors that characterize wheezes are **sonorous** or **sibilant**. Sonorous wheezes are generally lower pitched, deeper, and more pronounced during expiration. These sounds originate in the larger bronchi associated with tracheo-bronchitis.

Sibilant wheezes are more high pitched and originate in the smaller bronchi associated with asthma. These are also more musical in quality than sonorous with a whistle-like sound. They are also heard during inspiration or expiration.

Auscultation Techniques and Expected Findings

Unexpected Findings

Wheezes may be heard bilaterally or unilaterally. A foreign body or tumor may cause unilateral wheezes. Bilateral wheezes are associated with the bronchospasms of asthma or bronchitis. It is important to remember that adventitious sounds may occur together; causing a wide variety of sounds that can be heard. They may also come and go, so what one provider hears may not be the same as another provider. It is also important to initially establish the presence of expected breath sounds and then determine what adventitious sounds may also be present.

PRACTICE POINT: Wheezes vs. Stridor

In severe cases of bronchial narrowing, wheezing may be audible without the use of a stethoscope. These audible wheezes should not be confused with stridor. A wheeze will still have a musical quality associated with it whereas stridor is not musical. Wheezing results from narrowing of the bronchi and conducting bronchioles, commonly without an obstruction. Stridor is associated with some type of upper airway obstruction.

A **pleural friction rub** is a grating, leathery sound that is caused by inflamed, roughened visceral and parietal pleura rubbing over each other during inspiration and expiration. Its presence suggests pleurisy. It is a low-pitched sound and may be accompanied by pain. A friction rub may also be associated with pericarditis. To differentiate a plural rub from a cardiac rub, have the patient hold the breath—a plural rub will disappear, whereas a cardiac rub will be continuous.

Auscultation: Levels III and IV

Level III and IV auscultation represents additional auscultatory maneuvers that may be used to gather additional data related to pulmonary pathology.

Vocal resonance sounds are similar to fremitus; they are produced by vibrations within the lungs, which come from vocalizations by the patient (Figure 23-32). Vocal sounds are assessed by auscultation through the stethoscope. Resonant sounds are produced by greater vibrations. Vocalizations such as "how now, brown cow," and "ninety-nine" are commonly used phrases or words to cause vibrations. Vibrations are poorly conducted through air-filled tissue, but are augmented by solid tissue, so expected results will be muffled or indistinct vocal sounds. The expected finding is that the "eeee" would be heard as an "aaaa."

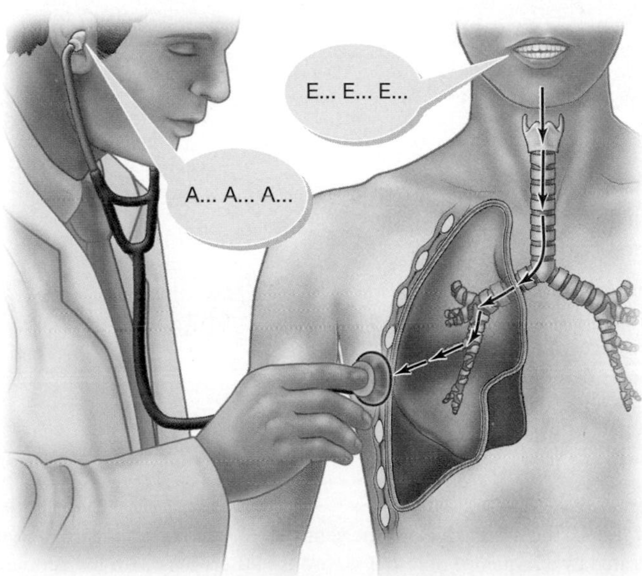

FIGURE 23-32 Characteristics of vocal resonance

Any condition that causes lung tissue to consolidate, such as pneumonia or atelectasis, will augment vocal sounds so that they become more distinct and pronounced.

Bronchophony is present if the vocalized words or phrases become more distinct or louder. In extreme conditions, even a whispered vocalization will be heard. This is called **whispered pectoriloquy**. Another assessment of vocal sounds is to have the patient say a continuous "eeeeee." If the "eee" can be clearly heard as an "eeee," **egophony** is present.

Developmental Applications

Techniques and Expected Findings	Unexpected Findings

Infants and Children

The infant is examined in much the same way as the adult. Inspection without disturbing the infant is important to obtain the necessary information. Palpation and auscultation are also performed, however, percussion is considered nonsignificant as the fingers of the health care provider are most likely too large for the infant's chest, particularly one that is premature.

The initial ventilatory effort of the infant is identified by the Apgar score (Table 23-7), taken at 1 and 5 minutes after birth. Ineffective ventilatory effort is frequently due to the maternal environment during labor.

Sedatives, analgesics, or a compromised blood supply all contribute to poor ventilations. Mechanical obstruction from mucus may also be a contributing factor.

Table 23-7 Apgar scoring system—infant evaluation at birth

	0	1	2
Heart rate	Absent	Slow (< 100 beats/min)	> 100 beats/min
Respiratory effort	Absent	Slow or irregular	Good crying
Muscle tone	Limp	Some flexion of extremities	Active motion
Response to catheter in nostril (tested after oropharynx is clear)	No response	Grimace	Cough or sneeze
Color	Blue or pale	Body pink, extremities blue	Completely pink

Add the scores of the five individual observations to get the full Apgar score. The lower the total, the more likely a problem.

Inspect the thoracic cage for size and shape, which should be round. Measure the chest circumference and compare it to the head circumference. The full term newborn's chest is approximately 30 to 36 cm, which is 2 to 3 cm smaller than the head circumference (Figure 23-33). This difference in circumference remains until approximately 2 years of age.

A premature infant as well as an infant with intrauterine growth retardation will demonstrate a greater difference between the two measures.

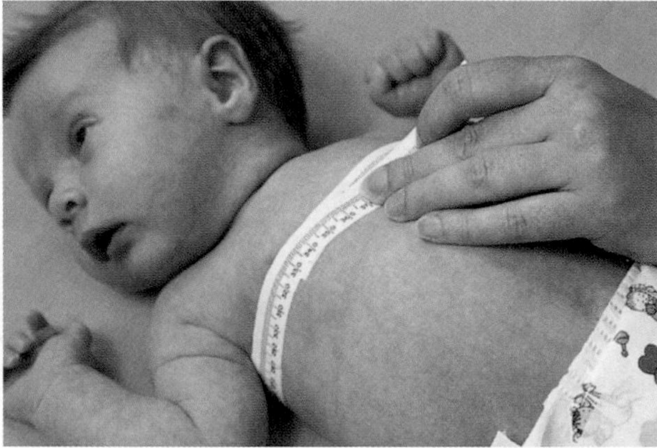

FIGURE 23-33 Measuring chest circumference

Cyanosis of the hands and feet (acrocyanosis) is a common manifestation in the newborn. (See Chapter 16.) In the presence of a cool environment, it is not uncommon for it to continue for a couple of days.

Count the ventilatory rate for 1 full minute. The most optimum time to count the infant's ventilations is during sleep. The range for a newborn is between 40 to 60 times a minute; however, a rate of 80 is not necessarily cause for concern. The ambient temperature influences the respiratory rate, most often by increasing it. Infants born by Cesarean section also demonstrate a more rapid rate than those delivered vaginally. The diaphragm is the primary respiratory muscle in the infant. The intercostal muscles are not fully developed, thus, when observing the infant's ventilations, more abdominal movement than thoracic movement is visible.

Infants are obligate nose breathers so it is not unusual to observe some slight nasal flaring. Ventilations are relatively regular, but the more premature the infant, the more irregular the ventilations may be. Periodic breathing is common. This is demonstrated by a sequence of rather vigorous ventilatory efforts followed by 10 to 15 seconds of apnea.

If the apneic periods become prolonged or are accompanied by central cyanosis, there is reason to become concerned. Periodic breathing is more common in preterm infants and should gradually decrease as term status is reached.

Techniques and Expected Findings	Unexpected Findings
Chest expansion should be symmetric.	If asymmetric expansion is observed, the infant's ability to fill both lungs is compromised and may be due to pneumothorax or a diaphragmatic hernia.
The infant's chest should be palpated for symmetry, any masses, and the presence of crepitus.	Crepitus may be present around a fractured clavicle, particularly after a difficult delivery and/or the use of forceps.
Auscultate the infant's chest for breath sounds. It is important for the infant to be quiet, which may require the health care provider to wait for a time until the infant stops crying or being restless. It is almost impossible to localize breath sounds due to the smallness of the chest and lungs.	Sounds are easily transmitted from one lung segment to the other; therefore, any absence of breath sounds may be overlooked.
Crackles and wheezes are frequently heard in the immediate newborn period. The opening of the airways along with the presence of amniotic fluid is responsible for these adventitious sounds.	Persistence of these sounds or asymmetric sounds is cause for concern.
Peristaltic sounds, movement, and mucus in the upper airway also contribute to adventitious sounds that may also be heard while auscultating the lungs.	Persistent intestinal gurgling sounds along with unilateral diminished breath sounds are suggestive of a diaphragmatic hernia.
Respiratory distress in the infant is accompanied by visible and auditory parameters. 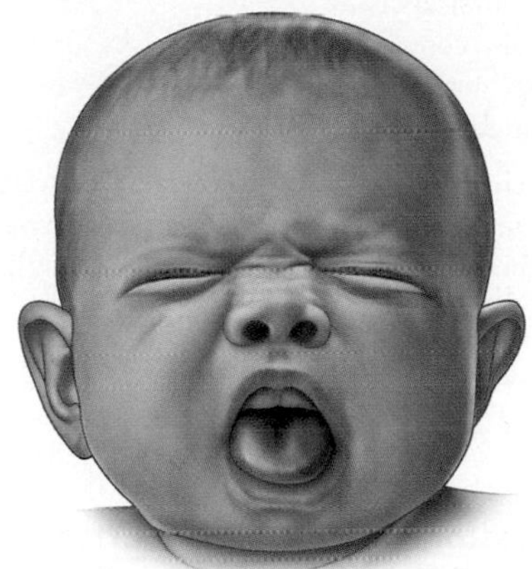 **FIGURE 23-34** Infant who demonstrates nasal flaring	Nasal flaring and retractions are easily observed. Nasal flaring is observed as a widening of the opening of the alae nasi with inspiration (Figure 23-34). Retractions are observed in the supraclavicular and sternal intercostal spaces. Frequently, retractions are accompanied by stridor, particularly in children. Its presence indicates severe difficulty in breathing and is caused by air being forced to move through a narrowed opening as occurs during obstruction, particularly laryngeal obstruction. Stridor may result in a prolonged inspiratory effort; inspiration may be three to four times longer than expiration. Respiratory grunting occurs when the infant is trying to force trapped air out of the lungs while still maintaining adequate air in the lungs. Respiratory distress may be demonstrated by a see-saw pattern of ventilation, which is visible as an alternating movement of the abdomen and chest. These parameters may also be observed in young children when experiencing respiratory distress.
By the age of 6 or 7, the breathing pattern changes from primarily nasal and abdominal to thoracic breathing in females, and abdominal breathing in males. The roundness of the chest also disappears and the chest configuration takes on the adult appearance of a 1:2 anteroposterior diameter to lateral diameter.	Persistent roundness of the chest is suggestive of a chronic obstructive disorder such as cystic fibrosis or asthma.
Ventilatory rates are faster than in adults for about the first 10 years; the rate gradually decreases as the child grows. By 10 to 12 years of age, the ventilatory rate should be that of an adult.	
The child's chest wall is thinner and more resonant than the adult's, resulting in hyperresonance being the dominant sound produced during percussion.	It may be easy to miss an underlying dullness due to consolidation, thus any change in sound should be further investigated. The size and thinness of the chest also allows for intrathoracic sounds to be more intense, thus bronchovesicular sounds predominate throughout the chest.

Techniques and Expected Findings	Unexpected Findings
The Pregnant Woman Pregnancy creates both structural and ventilatory changes. The uterus expands upward and forward, exerting pressure on the diaphragm, causing dyspnea. The expanding uterus also prevents complete expansion of the lungs resulting in a decrease of the functional reserve capacity, which is the volume of air within the lungs after a quiet exhalation. The tidal volume, the amount of air inhaled and exhaled during a usual breath, increases by about 40%, which also increases the minute volume. The ventilatory rate does not increase significantly, which indicates that ventilation is increased by deeper breathing and not by an increase in rate. The increased tidal volume is due mainly to high levels of progesterone, and to a lesser extent by estrogen. The increased tidal volume also causes hemoglobin to increase, which results in an increased oxygen-carrying capacity. The increased depth of ventilations produces a slight drop in the partial pressure of arterial carbon dioxide.	
The thoracic cage appears wider as well as the costal angle. This is more apparent during the third trimester when the enlarging uterus causes the diaphragm to rise, causing a widening of the rib cage at the base.	
The Older Adult It may be difficult for older individuals to breathe deeply and to hold their breath. This may be due to an inability to use respiratory muscles due to muscle weakness related to general physical disability or a sedentary lifestyle. There may be calcification of the rib articulations, which also contributes to a decreased chest expansion. This may also require the use of accessory muscles. When auscultating the older patient's lungs, pace the exam to accommodate the patient's breathing capabilities.	
Loss of subcutaneous tissue occurs with aging, which accentuates bony prominences. There is an increased thoracic curvature of the spine (kyphosis) accompanied by a flattening of the lumbar curve. (See Chapter 28.) This increases the AP diameter of the chest, giving it more of a barrel chest appearance. The kyphosis may be accompanied by a scoliosis, which further contributes to chest cage alterations.	Severe spinal curvatures may interfere with chest cage expansion and create difficulty with ventilations.

DOCUMENTATION

- **Inspection:** Spontaneous ventilatory effort at 16 breaths/min; ventilations smooth and effortless with equal anterior/posterior thoracic expansion. No need for aids or position to maintain ventilations. No bulges or ICS retractions. Thoracic configuration symmetrical with AP: lateral diameter of 2:1. Spine straight with lateral rib angle of 45°; costal angle <90°. Skin color without any evidence of cyanosis, no observable clubbing of fingers.
- **Palpation:** Trachea palpated at midline. No muscle tenderness or bulges of posterior thorax. Thoracic expansion equidistant from spine. No crepitus or vibrations palpated. Vocal fremitus equal bilaterally over posterior thorax.
- **Percussion:** Resonance percussed over posterior and anterior lung fields. No dullness. Diaphragmatic excursion 5 cm on R/L posterior chest. R side slightly higher than left.
- **Auscultation:** Vesicular sounds audible over anterior/posterior lung fields. Breath sounds clear without crackles/wheezes/rubs. Vocal resonance with muffled sounds obtained over posterior chest during bronchophony, egophony, and whispered pectoriloquy.

Electronic Charting

Pulmonary assessment information stored in the computer must include both current findings and relevant history. Findings from pulmonary function tests, lung scans, and other evaluations should be able to be correlated with physical symptoms. Electronic systems are being developed for automatic recording and analysis of lung sounds (Polat & Guler, 2004), but such systems are not yet in widespread use.

Expectations of Electronic Charting

Electronic charting systems typically include drug interaction checking. Drug checking should extend beyond drug–drug interactions. For example, beta-blockers are contraindicated in obstructive pulmonary diseases and the charting system should alert the user if medications are ordered that are contraindicated by the patient's diagnosis (Vinker, Kaiserman, Waitman, Blackman, & Kitai, 2006).

Electronic guidelines and protocols have been used for managing respiratory conditions. Clinical decision support systems integrate evidence-based protocols and guidelines with data from electronic records. For example, asthma and COPD guidelines have been implemented in electronic form (Kuilboer et al., 2006), as have protocols for management of ventilators (Gardiner, 2004).

Limitations of Electronic Charting

The quality of electronic data is important for making good decisions. Simple transformations that appear to be "common sense" to the clinician, such as recording FiO_2 as either a decimal (e.g., 0.90) or percent (e.g., 90), may not be understood by electronic systems unless intentionally programmed into the system.

Decision support systems can assist clinicians to navigate complex protocols, such as those used for ventilator management, but are only useful to the extent to which the "rules" apply to the specific patient. Patients can experience events not accommodated by protocol rules, so recommendations from decision support systems should always be evaluated for clinical appropriateness.

Summary

- The lungs and oxygenation status are assessed through the anterior and posterior thorax as well as integumentary findings through inspection, palpation, percussion, and auscultation.
- Internal anatomical structures of the pulmonary system are identified through external thoracic landmarks, which consist of visualized vertical and horizontal lines.
- Thoracic shape and structure is determined by the ribs and their attachment to the sternum and spinal column. Altered shape of any of these bones creates altered thoracic configurations ranging from cosmetic alterations to significant interference with adequate ventilations.
- The lungs participate in the processes of ventilation and respiration. Ventilation is the process of taking air into the lungs as well as expelling it through muscular contractions and relaxations. Respiration is the exchange of O_2 and CO_2 between the alveolar and capillary walls.
- Ventilations occur in various patterns that are related to oxygen needs of the body. Altered ventilation patterns are also associated with various lung alterations and pathologies. Awareness of another individual's ventilations in as indicator of some type of altered lung function.
- Air moving in and out of the lung during ventilations creates three types of breath sounds that are heard at specific locations on the posterior and anterior thorax. Lung alterations may also create certain types of sounds (adventitious) that are superimposed over the expected breath sounds.

Review Questions

1. When examining a patient's thorax, the landmark that the provider uses for the counting and identification of ribs and intercostal spaces is which of the following?
   1. suprasternal notch
   2. sternomanubrial angle
   3. mid-clavicular lines
   4. xiphoid process

2. The provider notes that a patient is able to breathe only when the head is elevated on two pillows. The provider documents this finding as which of the following?
   1. dyspnea
   2. hyperpnea
   3. hyperventilation
   4. orthopnea

3. A 16-year-old male patient is described as having pectus excavatum. The provider is aware that the manifestation of this condition would be which of the following?
   1. ribs that are positioned at a 90-degree angle
   2. an AP-lateral diameter that is 1:1
   3. a depression of the anterior chest wall
   4. a spinal column that is in the shape of an S

4. When caring for a 35-year-old patient who has just had thoracic surgery with placement of a chest tube, he should be assessed frequently by the provider for the presence of which of the following?
   1. crepitus
   2. sputum
   3. egophony
   4. friction rub

5. The provider notes breath sounds that are low pitched and breezy sounding when auscultating a patient's lungs. These sounds are described as which of the following?
   1. vesicular
   2. bronchial
   3. crackles
   4. adventitious

6. Percussion of the posterior lungs of a patient may be used by the provider to assess which of the following?
   1. fremitus
   2. diaphragmatic excursion
   3. thoracic expansion
   4. extrathoracic signs

7. The provider notes the presence of clubbing of the fingers when examining a patient. The provider is aware that frequent causes of this finding include which of the following: (Select all that apply.)
   1. cystic fibrosis
   2. chronic obstructive pulmonary disease
   3. congenital heart disease
   4. pneumonia
   5. pneumothorax

8. The provider is assessing a patient whose chief complaint is a cough that occurs on rising each morning. Which questions should the provider prioritize when interviewing this patient? (Select all that apply.)
   1. "Do you smoke cigars or cigarettes?"
   2. "Do you have frequent sinus problems?"
   3. "Have you been diagnosed with lung disease?"
   4. "Are you bringing up sputum with the cough?"
   5. "Is there a family history of respiratory problems?"

9. The provider notes the presence of stridor when performing a respiratory assessment of a pediatric patient. The provider is aware that this finding is due to which of the following?
   1. obstruction
   2. infection
   3. allergy
   4. reduced oxygen saturation

10. The provider is reviewing laboratory data as part of the assessment of a new patient. Arterial blood gas results reveal a pH of 7.32. The provider expects to find that the patient's pCO_2 is which of the following?
    1. 30
    2. 35
    3. 40
    4. 45

Conditions and Disorders

Atelectasis

Atelectasis is the collapse or closure of the lung resulting in the loss of lung volume leading to reduced or absent gas exchange. It may affect part or all of one lung. It is a condition where the alveoli are deflated, as distinct from pulmonary consolidation. Acute atelectasis may occur as a postoperative complication or a surfactant deficiency, which in premature neonates results in infant respiratory distress syndrome. In acute atelectasis, the lung has recently collapsed and is primarily notable only for airlessness; alveoli become deflated.

Pathophysiology

- Atelectasis may be obstructive or nonobstructive in etiology with different mechanisms responsible for tissue collapse.

Obstructive atelectasis may be caused by the following:

- Mucus plug (accumulation of mucus) in the airways, related to surgery, in cystic fibrosis, and severe asthma attacks.
- Inhalation of foreign body (toy, peanuts); — common in children Narrowing of major airways from disease or chronic infections, [fungal infections, TB, and other diseases that can scar and constrict major airways].
- Tumor in a major airway
- Blood clot that forms if significant bleeding into lungs can't be coughed out.

Nonobstructive atelectasis is associated with a loss of contact between the pleurae, compression, loss of surfactant or replacement of parenchyma tissue by scarring or infiltrates (Madeppa & Sharma, 2013). It may be caused by the following:

- Chest trauma
- Pleural effusion
- Pneumonia
- Pneumothorax
- Scarring of lung tissue
- Tumor

Subjective Data

- Most symptoms are determined by the rapidity with which the bronchial occlusion occurs, the size of the lung area affected, and the presence or absence of complicating infection.
- Cough, but not prominent
- Chest pain
- Breathing difficulty, rapid, shallow breathing

Objective Data

- Low oxygen saturation
- Pleural effusion (transudate type)
- Cyanosis (late sign)
- Increased heart rate
- Low-grade fever
- Faint or absent breath sounds
- Decreased chest wall expansion

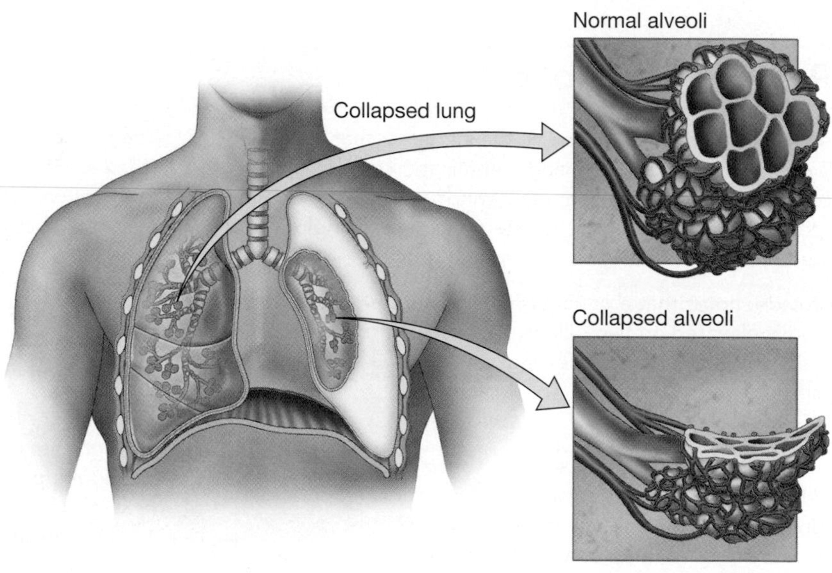

FIGURE 23-35 Collapsed lung

Pleurisy (Pleuritis)/Pleural Effusion

Pleurisy is an inflammation of the pleura in which the inflamed pleural layers rub against each other with every inhalation, causing severe sharp (pleuritic) chest pain. The pleural space can be invaded by fluid, air, and particles (effusion) from different parts of the body. In effusion of fluid, excess fluid accumulates in the pleural space, causing the two layers of the pleura to separate so they don't rub against each other when breathing, often relieving the pain. A large amount of extra fluid can push the pleura against the lung until the lung, or a part of it, collapses, making it hard to breathe. In some cases of pleural effusion, the fluid becomes infected resulting in an **empyema**.

Pathophysiology

The inflammation of the pleura can be caused by from numerous underlying conditions and include the following:

- An acute viral infection, such influenza
- Pneumonia if infected portion of lung involves surface of pleura
- TB and other infections
- Pulmonary embolism
- Trauma to the chest or after heart surgery
- Rib fractures

Subjective Data

- The defining symptom of pleurisy is a sudden sharp, stabbing, burning or dull pain in the right or left side of the chest during ventilations, increasing with deep breathing, coughing, sneezing, or laughing.
- The pain may stay in one place, or may spread to the shoulder or back. May become a fairly constant dull ache.

Objective Data

- Rapid, shallow breathing
- Ventricular tachycardia
- Pleural friction rub

- In some cases, the cause of pleurisy is idiopathic.

Depending on its cause, pleuritic chest pain may be accompanied by other symptoms:

- Dry cough
- Fever and chills
- Shortness of breath
- Sore throat followed by pain and swelling in the joints

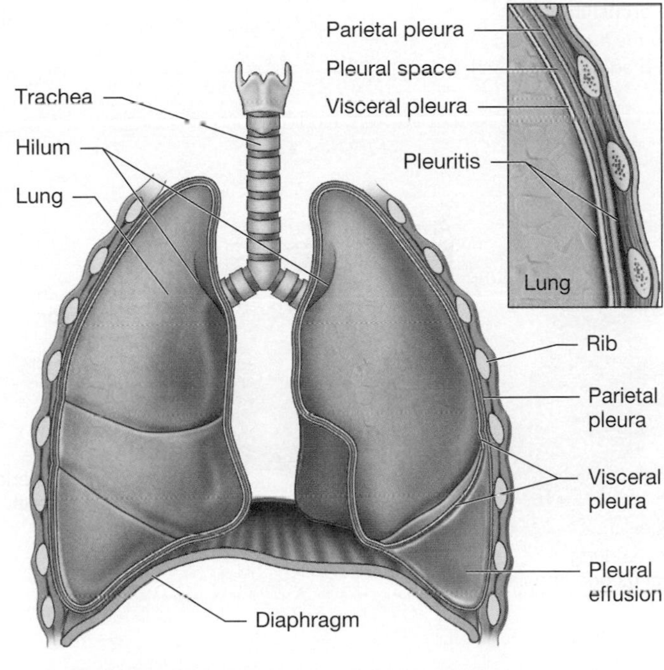

FIGURE 23-36 Pleural effusion

PRACTICE POINT: Pleural Effusion

A person can develop a pleural effusion in the absence of pleurisy. For example, pneumonia, heart failure, cancer, or a pulmonary embolism can lead to a pleural effusion.

Pneumonia

Pneumonia is an inflammatory condition of the lung, affecting primarily the alveoli. It is usually caused by a viral or bacterial infection, or less commonly by microorganisms, certain drugs and other conditions such as autoimmune diseases. It can range in seriousness from mild to life threatening, and is most serious for infants and young children, individuals older than age 65, and individuals with underlying health conditions or weakened immune systems. Lobar pneumonia affects a section of a lung, while bronchial pneumonia (bronchopneumonia) affects patches throughout both lungs. Pneumocystis carinii pneumonia (PCP) is caused by an organism believed to be a fungus; it may be the first sign of illness in many persons with AIDS.

Pathophysiology

- Pneumonia fills the lung's alveoli with fluid, hindering oxygenation.
- Viruses presented to the upper airway find their way to the lungs, where they invade cells lining the airways, alveoli, or lung parenchyma resulting in varying degrees of cell death.
- White blood (mononuclear) cells respond to the infection, initiating inflammation, often causing more lung damage
- Viruses also make the body more susceptible to bacterial infections; in this way bacterial pneumonia can arise as a co-morbid condition.
- Bacteria enter the lungs via small aspirations of organisms residing in the throat or nose.

Subjective Data

- Productive cough
- Fever accompanied by shaking chills (fever not very specific, as it occurs in many other common illnesses)
- Shortness of breath, sharp or stabbing chest pain during deep breaths, and an increased respiratory rate
- More severe signs and symptoms may include the following: blue-tinged skin, decreased thirst, convulsions, persistent vomiting, extremes of temperature, or a decreased level of consciousness.
- Bacterial and viral cases of pneumonia usually present with similar symptoms.
- Pneumonia caused by *Legionella* may occur with abdominal pain, diarrhea, or confusion

Objective Data

Physical findings often obtained include the following:

- Low blood pressure
- High heart rate
- Low oxygen saturation
- Ventilation rate faster than normal: occurring 1 to 2 days before other signs
- Decreased chest expansion on the affected side
- Harsh breath sounds (bronchial) from larger airways transmitted through the inflamed lung tissue
- Crackles heard over affected area during inspiration
- Percussion dulled over affected area; increased vocal resonance distinguishes pneumonia from a pleural effusion (decreased vocal resonance)

- While the throat always contains bacteria, potentially infectious ones reside there only at certain times and under certain conditions.
- A minority of types of bacteria such as *Mycobacterium tuberculosis* and *Legionella pneumophila* reach the lungs via contaminated airborne droplets.
- Bacteria can spread also via the blood.
- Once in the lungs, bacteria invade spaces between cells and between alveoli, where macrophages and neutrophils (white blood cells) try to inactivate the bacteria; also releasing cytokines, initiating immune system.
- This leads to the fever, chills, and fatigue common in bacterial pneumonia. The neutrophils, bacteria, and fluid from surrounding blood vessels fill alveoli resulting in consolidation seen on chest x-ray.

- Pneumonia caused by *Streptococcus pneumoniae* is associated with rusty colored sputum
- Pneumonia caused by *Klebsiella* may have bloody sputum often described as "currant jelly."
- Hemoptysis may also occur with TB, Gram-negative pneumonia, lung abscesses, and acute bronchitis.
- Viral pneumonia presents more commonly with wheezing than does bacterial pneumonia.

More severe signs and symptoms may include cyanosis.

- In older adults, confusion may be the most prominent sign
- In children under 5, fever, cough, and fast or difficult breathing may be the most-common signs

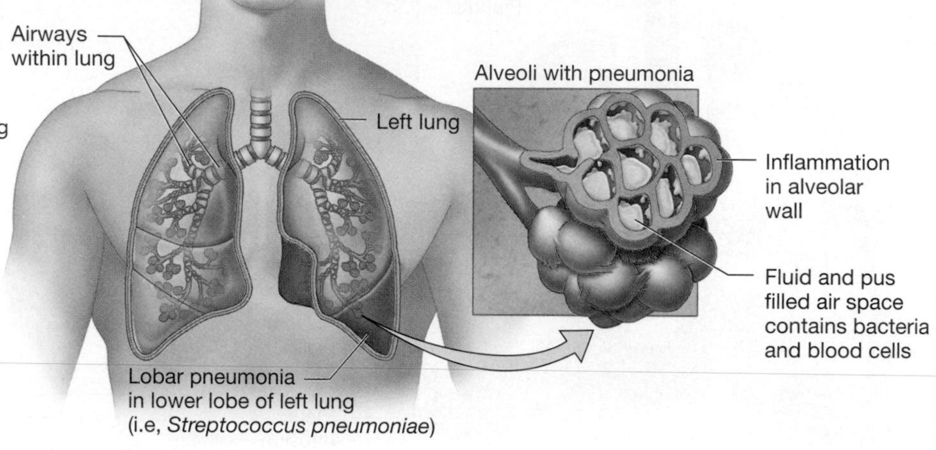

FIGURE 23-37 Pneumonia

Pneumothorax

Pneumothorax is an accumulation of air/gas within the pleural space that separates the lung from the chest. A **primary (spontaneous) pneumothorax (PSP)** occurs without an apparent cause and in the absence of significant lung disease. A **secondary (spontaneous) pneumothorax (SSP)** occurs in the presence of existing lung pathology, or blunt trauma or penetrating injury, which commonly occurs when chest wall is pierced (stab wound, gunshot wound, or surgery), allowing air to enter the pleural space; or some other mechanical injury compromises the integrity of the involved structures. The most common underlying abnormality cause of SSP is COPD. Cystic fibrosis has one of the most significant associations with SSP; greater than 20% reporting spontaneous pneumothorax. A **tension pneumothorax** is a life-threatening condition that develops when air is trapped in the pleural cavity under positive pressure, displacing mediastinal structures and compromising cardiopulmonary function.

Pathophysiology

- A pneumothorax can only develop if air is allowed to enter the pleural space, through damage to the chest wall or damage to the lung itself, or in some instances, microorganisms in the pleural space produce gas.

Subjective Data

- Acute onset of chest pain and SOB are predominant.
- Chest pain described as severe and/or stabbing, radiates to the ipsilateral shoulder, increasing with inspiration (pleuritic).
- PSP: Chest pain often improves over the first 24 hours, even without resolution of the underlying air accumulation.
- SSP: Chest pain is more likely to persist with more significant clinical symptoms.
- PSP: SOB/dyspnea is generally sudden onset
- SSP: Tends to be more severe with secondary because of decreased lung reserve.
- Anxiety, cough, and vague presenting symptoms (general malaise, fatigue) are not common manifestations.

Objective Data

Respiratory findings may include the following:

- Respiratory distress or respiratory arrest
- Tachypnea (or bradypnea as a preterminal event)
- Asymmetric lung expansion: mediastinal and tracheal shift to contralateral side (large tension pneumothorax)
- Unilateral distant or absent breath sounds
- Hyperresonance on percussion: rare finding; may be absent even in an advanced state
- Decreased tactile fremitus
- Adventitious lung sounds: ipsilateral crackles, wheezes
- Findings on lung auscultation vary depending on the extent of the pneumothorax.

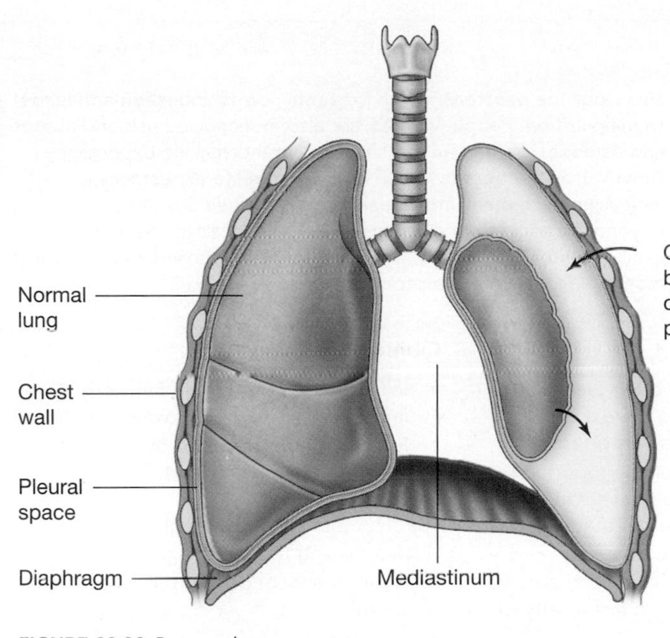

FIGURE 23-38 Pneumothorax

Cardiovascular findings may include the following:

- Tachycardia: Most common finding; if heart rate is faster than 135 beats/min, tension pneumothorax likely
- Pulsus paradoxus
- Hypotension: Inconsistently present finding; although typically considered a key sign of tension pneumothorax, hypotension can be delayed until its appearance immediately precedes cardiovascular collapse
- Jugular venous distention is generally seen in tension pneumothorax; may be absent if hypotension is severe
- Cardiac apical displacement is a rare finding

PRACTICE POINT: Degree of Pneumothorax

Importantly, the degree of pneumothorax often demonstrates limited correlation with the intensity of the symptoms; and physical signs may not be obvious if the pneumothorax is relatively small.

Hemothorax

Hemothorax is the accumulation of blood in the pleural space, which may come from the chest wall, lung parenchyma, heart, or great vessels. It is usually the result of blunt or penetrating trauma; significantly less common, it may be a complication of disease, iatrogenically induced, or develop spontaneously.

Pathophysiology

- Bleeding into the pleural space can happen with virtually any disruption of tissues of chest wall and pleura or the intrathoracic structures. Physiologic responses to a hemothorax demonstrated in two systems: hemodynamic and respiratory.
- Degree of hemodynamic changes related to amount of bleeding and rapidity of blood loss. Blood loss up to 750 mL causes no significant hemodynamic change. Loss of greater than 750 mL will cause the early symptoms of shock (i.e., tachycardia, tachypnea, and decreased pulse pressure).
- Significant signs of shock with signs of poor perfusion occur with blood volume loss of 30% or more (1500–2000 mL).

Subjective Data

- The space-occupying effect of blood within the pleural space may interfere with ventilations.
- A significant collection of blood results in dyspnea and chest pain.

Objective Data

- In trauma cases, abnormalities of ventilation and oxygenation may result, especially if associated with injuries to the chest wall.
- Tachypnea is common; shallow breaths may be noted. Findings include diminished ipsilateral breath sounds and a dull percussion note.
- If substantial systemic blood loss has occurred, hypotension and tachycardia are present. Respiratory distress reflects both pulmonary compromise and hemorrhagic shock.
- Children may have traumatic hemothorax without bony fractures of the chest wall.

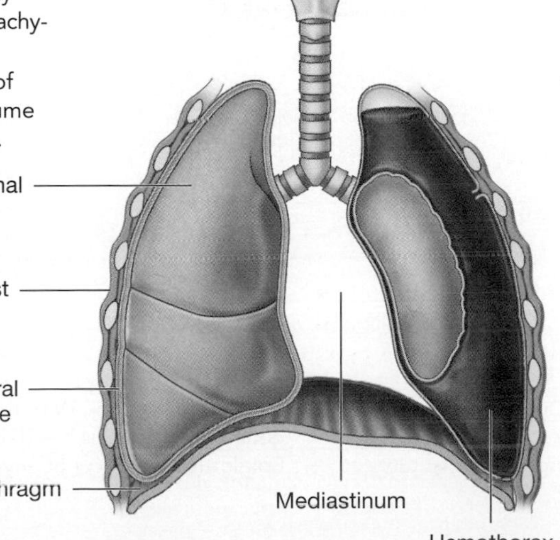

FIGURE 23-39 Hemothorax

Cystic Fibrosis (CF, Mucoviscidosis)

CF is an autosomal recessive genetic disorder that affects most critically the lungs, and also the pancreas, liver, and intestine. It is characterized by abnormal transport of chloride and sodium across epithelium, leading to thick, viscous secretions. Most of the damage in CF is due to blockage of the narrow passages of affected organs with thick, sticky mucus that blocks the airways in the lungs, making breathing difficult. Bacteria grow in this mucus, leading to life-threatening lung infections that can damage the lungs. The mucus also clogs the pancreas, which prevents normal digestion and leads to malnutrition. People with CF are also at increased risk of diabetes and osteoporosis and have a shorter-than-normal life expectancy. However, as treatments for CF improve, the life expectancy is increasing, with many individuals living into their 30s, 40s, and beyond. Screening of newborns for cystic fibrosis is now performed in all 50 states. As a result, the condition is diagnosed within the first month of life, before symptoms develop.

Pathophysiology

- An inherited disorder caused by a mutation in the gene for the protein cystic fibrosis transmembrane conductance regulator (CFTR).
- This protein regulates the components of sweat, digestive fluids, and mucus, and also regulates the movement of chloride and sodium ions across epithelial membranes.
- Most individuals without CF have two working copies of the CFTR gene.
- Requires inheritance of two defective CF genes, one from each parent. The parents most likely don't have the disease themselves.
- Individuals who inherit only one defective gene do not have CF but are carriers of the defective gene.

Subjective Data

- Most individuals are diagnosed with CF during infancy, so there are minimal symptoms that can be reported.
- Most symptoms would be reported by the parents and would reflect the manifestations of the disorder as indicated under objective data.
- Often the initial sign of CF that parents notice is the baby's skin tastes salty when kissed.

Objective Data

- Initial sign is often meconium ileus, or infant doesn't pass stool when first born.
- Rectal prolapsed caused by frequent straining to pass stool may be a sign of CF.

The thick and sticky mucus clogs the bronchioles causing the following:

- A persistent cough that produces thick sputum
- Wheezing
- Breathlessness
- Decreased ability to exercise
- Repeated lung infections
- Inflamed nasal passages or a stuffy nose
- The thick mucus affects nutrient absorption, leading to foul-smelling or greasy stools, poor weight gain and growth, intestinal blockage, particularly in newborns, and severe constipation.

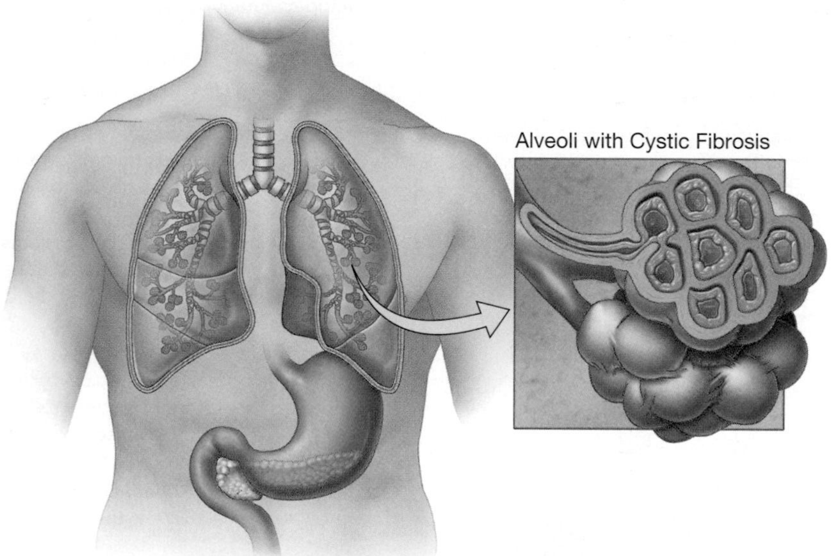

FIGURE 23-40 Cystic fibrosis

Epiglottitis

Epiglottitis is inflammation of the epiglottis. Due to its location in the airway, swelling of this structure can obstruct or completely close off the trachea, interfering with breathing, and constitutes a medical emergency. With the advent of the Hib vaccine, the incidence of epiglottitis has decreased, but has not been eliminated. Epiglottitis can occur at any age.

Pathophysiology

- Historically, the most common cause in children is Haemophilus influenzae type b (Hib) infection, the same bacterium that causes pneumonia, meningitis, and infections in the bloodstream.
- Hib spreads through infected droplets coughed or sneezed into the air. It's possible to harbor Hib in the nose and throat without becoming sick—though the potential to spread the bacteria to others exists.

Other possible causes may include the following:

- Swallowing a chemical or hot liquid that burns the throat or a foreign object
- Smoking drugs, such as crack cocaine
- Physical injury to the throat

Subjective Data

The early symptoms are insidious but rapidly progressive, and swelling of the throat may lead to cyanosis and asphyxiation.

In children, symptoms of epiglottitis may develop within a matter of hours, including:

- Severe sore throat
- Difficult and painful swallowing
- Anxious, restless behavior
- Greater comfort when sitting up or leaning forward

For adults, signs and symptoms may develop more slowly, over days rather than hours, and may include:

- Severe sore throat
- Difficulty breathing
- Difficulty swallowing

Objective Data

- Tripod position
- Fever
- Drooling/inability to handle secretions
- Stridor: A late finding indicating advanced airway obstruction
- Muffled voice
- Cervical adenopathy
- Hypoxia
- Respiratory distress
- Severe pain on gentle palpation over the larynx or hyoid bone
- Mild cough
- Irritability
- Tachycardia

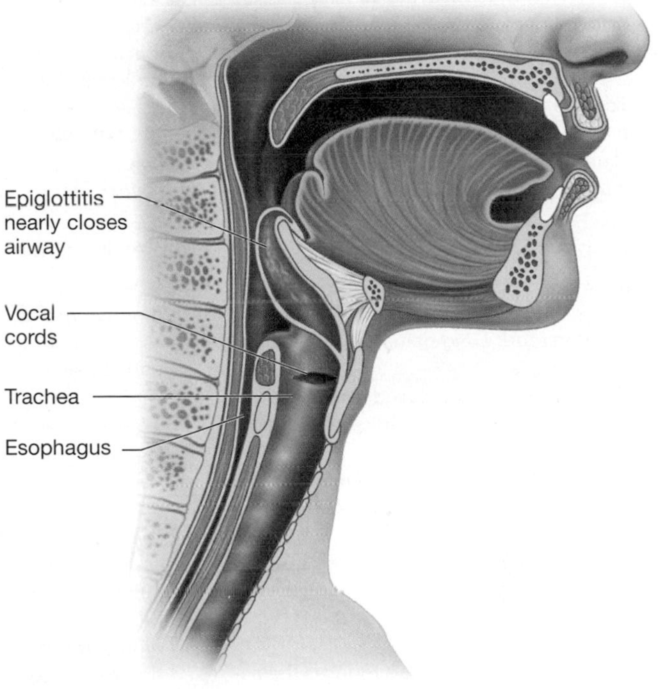

FIGURE 23-41 Epiglottitis

Croup (Laryngotracheobronchitis)

Croup is a respiratory condition usually triggered by an acute viral infection of the upper airway, which leads to swelling inside the throat, interfering with normal breathing and producing the classical symptoms of a "barking" cough, stridor, and hoarseness. It may produce mild, moderate, or severe symptoms, which often worsen at night. Children between the ages of 6 months and 3 years of age are at highest risk; it is estimated between 3%–5% of this age group are affected annually and is the most common cause of stridor. It is rarely seen in adults because their larger trachea and larynx can accommodate the inflammation without producing symptoms.

Pathophysiology

- Viral croup is caused by parainfluenza virus (types 1 and 2) in majority of cases. Infiltration of white blood cells (especially histiocytes, lymphocytes, plasma cells, and neutrophils) causes swelling of the larynx, trachea, and large bronchi leading to airway obstruction.

Subjective Data

- Usually begins with nonspecific respiratory symptoms, including rhinorrhea, sore throat, and cough.
- Fever and a hoarse voice are common
- Child's breathing may become noisy or labored.

Objective Data

- Within 1–2 days and enough inflammation, the characteristic signs of hoarseness, barking cough, and inspiratory stridor develop, often suddenly, along with a variable degree of respiratory distress often worse at night, and further aggravated by crying and coughing, as well as anxiety and agitation.

- Significant airway obstruction leads to dramatically increased work of breathing and stridor.
- The most common bacteria implicated are *Staphylococcus aureus, Streptococcus pneumoniae, Hemophilus influenzae,* and *Moraxella catarrhalis.*

Severity of the condition may occur if the child does the following:

- Demonstrates stridor both when inhaling and exhaling
- Begins drooling or has difficulty swallowing
- Patient seems anxious, agitated, or fatigued
- Breathes at a faster rate than usual
- Struggles to breathe
- Develops cyanosis

Chronic Obstructive Pulmonary Disease (COPD)

- This condition is also known as **chronic obstructive lung disease** (**COLD**), **chronic obstructive airway disease** (**COAD**), **chronic airflow limitation** (**CAL**) and **chronic obstructive respiratory disease** (**CORD**). It is the occurrence of chronic bronchitis and/or emphysema, a pair of commonly coexisting obstructive lung diseases in which the airways narrow over time. This limits airflow in and out of the lungs, causing shortness of breath (dyspnea).
- Clinically, chronic bronchitis is defined as a cough with sputum production on most days for 3 months of a year, for 2 consecutive years. The hallmark of chronic bronchitis is hyperplasia and hypertrophy of the goblet cells and mucous glands producing more mucus than usual in the airways, contributing to narrowing of the airways and a productive cough.
- In clinical practice, COPD is defined by its characteristically low airflow on lung function tests. In contrast to asthma, this limitation is poorly reversible and usually gets increasingly worse over time. COPD is the third leading cause of death in the United States.

Pathophysiology

Damage to lung tissue results from tobacco smoke; however, the exact mechanism is not well understood. Lung damage is caused by the following:

- Oxidative stress produced by the high concentrations of free radicals in tobacco smoke.
- Cytokine release due to inflammation as the body responds to irritant particles (tobacco smoke) in the airway.
- Tobacco smoke and free radicals impair the activity of antiprotease enzymes (alpha 1-antitrypsin), allowing protease enzymes to damage the lung.
- Narrowing of the airways reduces the airflow rate to and from the alveoli, limiting effectiveness of the lungs. The greatest reduction in airflow occurs during expiration because the pressure in the chest tends to compress rather than expand the airways.

Subjective Data

- SOB (dyspnea) one of the most common symptoms; commonly described as: "I feel out of breath," or "I can't get enough air in."
- Dyspnea generally first noted during vigorous exercise
- Dyspnea gradually worsens over the years, occurring during usual everyday activities.
- Dyspnea may occur during rest or be constantly present in advanced stages.
- Other symptoms of COPD include the following: persistent cough, sputum or mucus production, wheezing, chest tightness, and tiredness

Objective Data

- Few observable signs exist for COPD, although they can be present in other disorders. Some individuals have none of these signs.
- Common signs include the following: tachypnea, rapid breathing rate, wheezing or crackles, exhalation taking longer than inhalation, chest enlargement (particularly front-to-back distance, hyperaeration), active use of neck muscles to help with breathing, breathing through pursed lips, increased anteroposterior to lateral ratio of the chest (barrel chest)

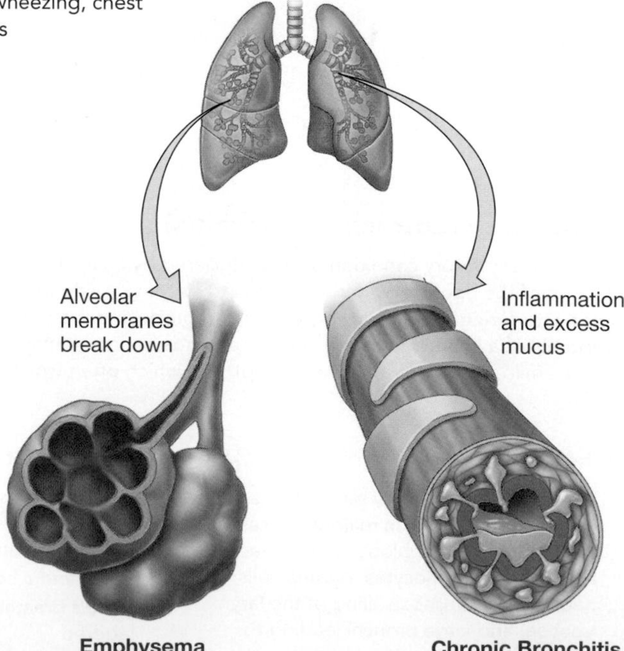

FIGURE 23-42 COPD

Emphysema

Emphysema is an enlargement of the air spaces distal to the terminal bronchioles, associated with destruction of their walls, reducing the surface area available for the exchange of oxygen and carbon dioxide. It is considered an obstructive lung disease because the destruction of alveoli makes them unable to maintain their functional shape during exhalation. It is most commonly related to long-term tobacco smoking and exposure to air pollution. In rare instances, it results from a genetic mutation, leading to alpha 1-antitrypsin deficiency. It can be identified as *primary* and *secondary* types; however, it is more commonly classified by location.

- *Panacinar* (*panlobular*) emphysema: Entire respiratory lobule (respiratory bronchiole to alveoli) has expanded. Occurs more commonly in the lower lobes (especially basal segments) and in the anterior margins of the lungs.
- *Centriacinar* (*centrilobular*) emphysema: Respiratory bronchiole (proximal and central part of the acinus) has enlarged. The distal alveoli are unchanged. More commonly found in the upper lobes and primarily associated with a history of cigarette smoking.

Pathophysiology

- Toxins (cigarette smoke) breathed into lungs, trapping harmful particles and causing localized inflammatory response.
- Chemicals released during inflammatory response eventually cause septal rupture, leading to a cavity larger than the sum of the two alveolar spaces.
- Due to the loss of mechanical support of the broken septa the new created space enlarges at the expense of the surrounding healthy parenchyma. The healthy parenchyma expansion is reduced in proportion to the amount of septal destruction.

Subjective Data

- SOB (dyspnea) on exertion, which usually begins gradually. The individual often starts avoiding activities that cause SOB, not becoming a problem until it starts interfering with daily tasks.
- Eventually causes SOB at rest.
- Productive cough that produces small amounts of colorless sputum from concomitant chronic bronchitis; usually worse in morning.

Objective Data

- The ventilation rate increases in proportion to condition severity.
- Use of accessory respiratory muscles and retractions of lower intercostal spaces are obvious.
- Cyanosis, elevated jugular venous pressure, and peripheral edema can be observed in advanced state.
- A forced expiratory time greater than 6 seconds is associated with severe expiratory obstruction.
- Thoracic examination reveals barrel chest, wheezing, diffusely decreased breath sounds, hyperresonance upon percussion, and prolonged expiration.

Asthma

Asthma is a common chronic inflammatory lung disorder that affects millions of individuals worldwide, characterized by variable and recurring symptoms, which are related bronchospasm that is partially or completely reversible. The airways are sensitive to a variety of stimuli, which may include viral illnesses, allergens, exercise, medicines, or environmental conditions. It is caused by a combination of complex and incompletely understood environmental and genetic interactions.

Pathophysiology

- Inflammation plays a critical role causing bronchospasms, but there is evidence indicating significant variability in the pattern of inflammation.
- Principal cells associated with airway inflammation include mast cells, eosinophils, epithelial cells, macrophages, and activated T lymphocytes. T lymphocytes release numerous cytokines, which are important for the regulation of airway inflammation.
- Acute bronchoconstriction is the consequence of immunoglobulin E-dependent mediator release when exposed to aeroallergens; the primary component of the early asthmatic response.
- Airway hyperresponsiveness/bronchial hyperreactivity is an exaggerated response to numerous exogenous and endogenous stimuli.

Subjective Data

- Symptoms include the following: wheezing, coughing, chest tightness, and shortness of breath
- Symptoms tend to come and go, and are related to the degree of airway narrowing in the lungs.

Objective Data

Mild episode:

- Individuals may be breathless after physical activity, but can talk in sentences and lie down flat
- May be agitated; the ventilatory rate is increased, and accessory muscles are not used.
- Heart rate is less than 100 bpm. Auscultation reveals moderate end expiratory wheezing.
- Rapid forced expiration may elicit wheezing that is otherwise inaudible. Oxyhemoglobin saturation on room air is 95% or greater.

Moderately severe episode:

- Ventilation rate increased.
- Accessory muscles of ventilation visible.
- Heart rate is 100–120 bpm and loud expiratory wheezing is heard.
- Oxyhemoglobin saturation on room air is 91%–95%.
- Breathlessness while talking; patient may assume a sitting position

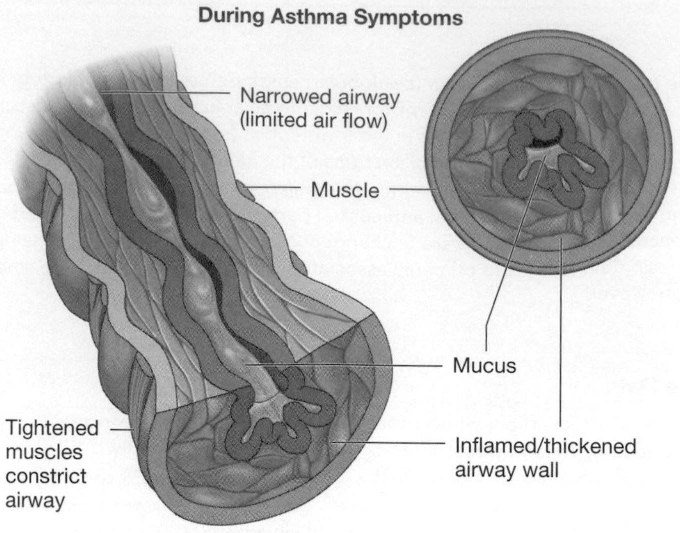

FIGURE 23-43 Asthma

Severe episode:

- Breathlessness during rest, uninterested in eating, sitting upright, talking in words rather than sentences, agitation
- Ventilatory rate is often greater than 30 bpm.
- Use of accessory muscles of ventilation, suprasternal retractions are commonly present.
- The heart rate is more than 120 bpm.
- Loud biphasic (expiratory and inspiratory) wheezing, and pulsus paradoxus is often present (20–40 mmHg).
- Oxyhemoglobin saturation on room air is less than 91%.
- Tripod position assumed as severity increases

PRACTICE POINT: Asthma Classification

Current guidelines for the classification of asthma are based on the severity of symptoms as follows:

- **Mild intermittent**: Attacks no more than twice a week and nighttime attacks no more than twice a month, lasting no more than hours to days. Attack severity varies, but no symptoms between attacks.
- **Mild persistent**: Attacks more than twice a week, but not every day; nighttime symptoms more than twice a month. Attacks sometimes severe enough to interrupt regular activities.
- **Moderate persistent:** Daily attacks and nighttime symptoms more than once a week. More severe attacks at least twice a week and may last for days. Attacks require daily use of quick-relief (rescue) medication and changes in daily activities.
- **Severe persistent:** Frequent severe attacks, continual daytime symptoms, and frequent nighttime symptoms. Symptoms require limits on daily activities.

Pulmonary Embolism (PE)

PE is a common and potentially lethal condition caused by obstruction of a main artery of the lung or one of its branches by an embolus. An embolus begins as a deep vein thrombosis that detaches and is carried in the blood to the lung, where it eventually reaches a point where it is larger than the lumen of the blood vessel, becomes lodged within the vessel, effectively cutting off blood supply to tissues distal to the embolus. Other material that can cause PE includes fat from marrow of a broken bone, part of a tumor, and air bubbles. PE is not a disease itself, but a complication of underlying venous thrombosis. As a cause of sudden death, massive PE is second only to sudden cardiac death.

Pathophysiology

- Thrombosis development is classically related to a collective group of causes known as Virchow's triad.
- Factors related to alterations in blood flow: refers to flow that has become slower, retrograde, or static due to surgery, prolonged immobility, surgery, pregnancy, obesity, and varicose veins.
- Factors in the vessel wall: refers to injury to the endothelium of the vessel wall. Damage of any sort (direct or indirect) releases cellular components that contribute to coagulation of blood and the formation of thrombi.

Subjective Data

Symptoms of PE are typically sudden in onset and consist of the following:

- dyspnea
- tachypnea
- chest pain of a "pleuritic" nature
- cough and hemoptysis

Objective Data

- Clinical signs include low blood oxygen saturation, tachypnea and tachycardia.
- More severe cases can include: cyanosis of lips and fingers, vascular collapse and circulatory instability due to decreased blood flow through the lungs and into the left side of the heart resulting in significantly lower blood pressure, and sudden death.

- Factors affecting the properties of the blood (procoagulant state) refers to microparticles in the blood that contribute to activation of the clotting cascade. The presence of these elements is related to certain diseases or conditions (cancer, pregnancy, hypertension, trauma, burns), or a congenital deficiency of protein C or S may exist.
- A primary element contributing to the procoagulant state is the presence of activated platelets. Activation occurs through various physiological processes.

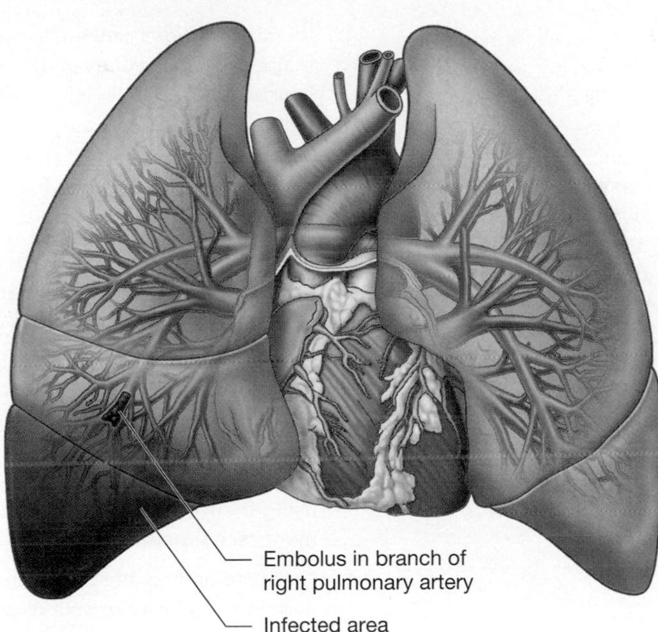

FIGURE 23-44 Pulmonary embolism

Other signs that can occur with pulmonary embolism include the following:

- Wheezing
- Unilateral swelling
- Diaphoresis
- Rapid or irregular heartbeat
- Weak pulse
- Lightheadedness or fainting
- Diagnosis is based primarily on validated clinical criteria combined with selective testing because the typical clinical manifestations are unable to be definitively differentiated from other causes of chest pain and SOB.
- Medical imaging is usually performed based on clinical data and an assessment of clinical probability.

24 Heart

The pain is excruciating. I suddenly find myself on the garage floor surrounded by trash and the barrels that fell with me. It hurts too much to call for help! I can hear hurried footsteps in the distance. I remember those hurried footsteps once belonged to me. *Dad? Dad! Are you OK? Dad!* Is it happening to me too? Is it going to end the same? Time is in slow motion. I glance over at the littered ashtray. I had quit cold turkey right before Emily was born, and then started smoking after dinner or during social events. Before I realized it, I was back to a pack a day. I reasoned that because the stress of raising three kids and work demands, I needed them to relax. How stupid my logic seems now. I catch a glimpse of Jake's football gear in the corner of the garage. He'd always begged me to practice with him, but I told him I didn't have time; I didn't want him to know I avoided anything that triggered shortness of breath and sweats. Lying on the floor of the garage, my chest feels as though a semi has parked on it. After the doctors told me I needed to change my eating habits, Cindy and the kids decided we would all eat healthier; they wanted to see me get better. And what did I do? I may as well have spat in their faces with all the sneaking around I did. How could I let my bad habits risk them losing their father? And Cindy—I can't leave her alone with the kids! They circle around me now as I hear the sirens in the distance. Their faces are tear-stained; I'm terrified, but I know I have to be strong.

LEARNING OUTCOMES

1. Identify the significant anatomic features and structures of the heart.
2. Describe the mechanical and electrical events of the cardiac muscle that occur within the cardiac cycle.
3. Describe a focused cardiac history based on the essential parameters associated with manifestations of cardiovascular conditions.
4. Explain the relationship between the anatomy and physiology of the cardiovascular system and the cardiac examination using the four physical assessment techniques.
5. Compare and contrast valvular and nonvalvular heart sounds and murmurs based on their unique characteristics.
6. Identify the relationship between lifestyle behaviors and cardiovascular diseases and appropriate prevention behaviors.

Cardiovascular disorders are common in both developed and developing nations. While the interplay of many factors contribute to the development of cardiovascular disorders, often the disorders result from lifestyle choices that interfere with optimal functioning of the heart and eventually other organs and systems. Manifestations of cardiovascular conditions (such as coronary artery disease and its sequel, cerebrovascular disease), peripheral artery diseases, aortic atherosclerosis and aneurysms, valvular heart disease, cardiomyopathy, stroke and arrhythmias may not be obvious until major damage has occurred. Careful assessment of individuals who present with signs and symptoms that characterize cardiovascular disorders is important to determine and differentiate causes of cardiovascular disease or other conditions.

The heart, one of the smaller organs in the body, works constantly to maintain delivery of oxygen and nutrients to all cells of the body. Its work begins within the first month of fetal development and continues until death. Over a person's lifetime, the heart contracts more than 4 billion times delivering more than 200 million liters of blood through the systemic circulation. The heart's work is supported by coronary arteries that supply more than 10 million liters of blood to the working muscle. The respiratory system provides the oxygen necessary for cellular function, and the nervous system regulates heart rate to meet changing requirements for oxygen.

Structure and Function

The heart, a four-chambered, muscular organ, functions as a side-by-side dual pump maintaining circulation of blood through the pulmonary and systemic circulation circuits (Figure 24-1). The heart is located in the midportion of the chest between the right and left lungs, superior to the diaphragm, known as the mediastinum (Figure 24-2). The sternum and the third to sixth ribs protect it. The external portion of the chest, overlying the heart is the precordium. The heart is shaped like an inverted cone with the broad section or base of the heart at the top, and the pointed section, or apex, at the bottom. Embryologically, these two parts start out in the opposite direction, but as the heart develops, it twists on itself to create a superior-positioned base and an inferior-positioned apex.

The four chambers of the heart comprise two upper chambers (atria) and two lower chambers (ventricles). The right-sided pump consists of the right atrium and right ventricle and pumps blood to the lungs for oxygenation. The left-sided pump consists of the left atrium and left ventricle and pumps blood to the rest of the body. The heart's pumping action is maintained by simultaneous contraction of the upper chambers and lower chambers.

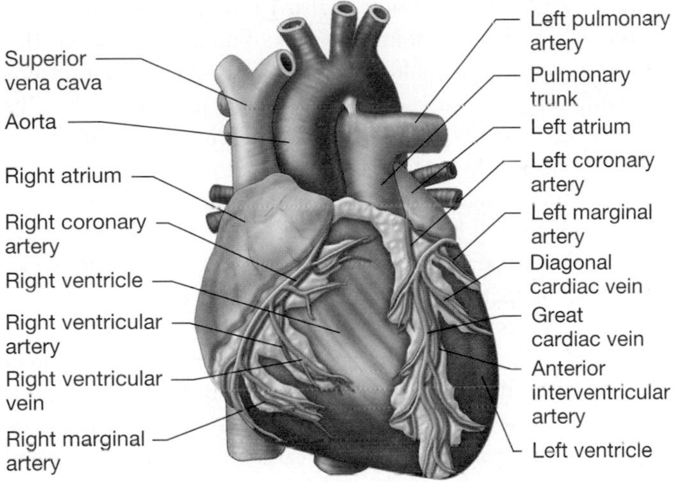

(a) Anterior view

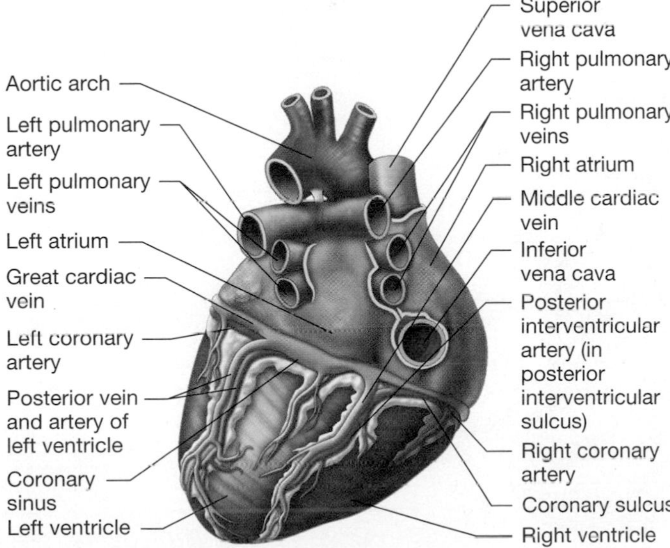

(b) Posterior view

FIGURE 24-1A–B a) Anterior and b) posterior view of heart

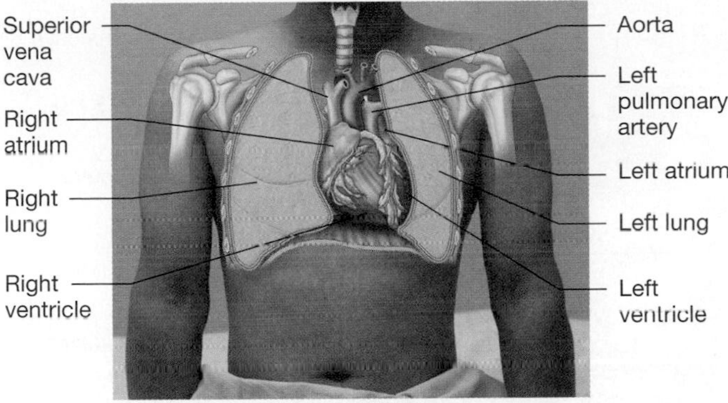

FIGURE 24-2 Position of heart in chest

The heart is positioned within the chest so that the right ventricle forms the anterior portion of the heart. The left ventricle is situated more posteriorly; however, due to its larger size, it extends anteriorly and becomes a part of the anterior portion of the heart at the apex. The right atrium lies superior and to the right of the right ventricle, forming the majority of the right border. The left atrium lies above and behind the left ventricle, forming the posterior aspect of the heart. The adult heart is approximately 12 cm long and 8 cm wide, with an antero-posterior diameter of 6 cm. The position of the heart varies greatly and is affected by individual body build, chest configuration, and diaphragmatic level. It is typically positioned more horizontally than vertically in the chest; however, with increased height, it may assume a more vertical position.

The four chambers are created by structures that separate the upper chambers from the lower chambers and the right side from the left side. The upper chambers of the heart are separated from the lower chambers by an **atrial-ventricular (AV) valve**, a tricuspid valve on the right, and a mitral valve on the left (Figure 24-3). The division of the heart into a right side and left side is achieved by the muscular cardiac septum. Another pair of valves, the **semilunar valves (pulmonic and aortic valves)**, separate the lower chambers of the heart from the two major blood vessels that carry blood away from the heart. These four valves are made of overlapping cusps or leaflets that open and close during ventricular contraction and relaxation, allowing blood to be ejected from a chamber, and also preventing blood from flowing backwards into a chamber. This configuration of the heart chambers and structural separations promotes and maintains blood flow within and through the heart in a unidirectional (forward) flow.

The heart muscle is composed of three layers—endocardium, myocardium, and pericardium (Figure 24-3). The **endocardium**, the innermost layer of the heart, lines the chambers of the heart, the valves, and the small muscles that control the opening and closing of the valves. The **myocardium** is the thick, middle layer of muscle that is primarily responsible for the heart's pumping action. The two lower chambers of the heart—the ventricles, which consist mostly of myocardial muscle—have the greatest role in maintaining circulation. The third layer, the **pericardium** is a tough, fibrous

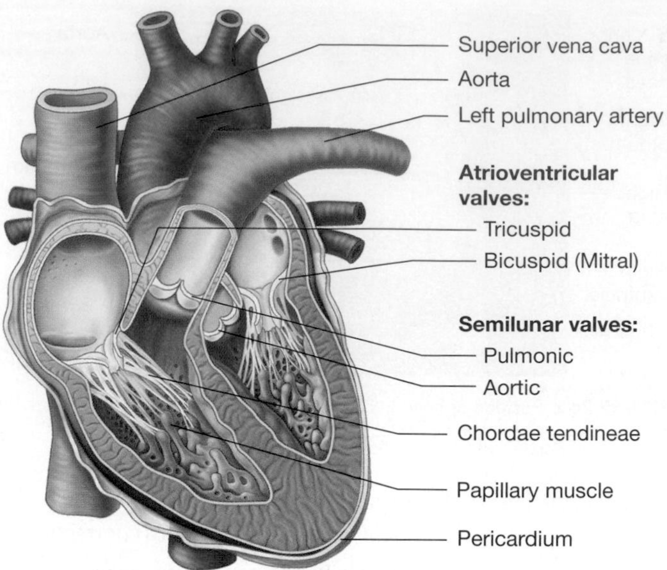

FIGURE 24-3 Cut away/cross section of heart

sac that surrounds and protects the heart. The pericardium actually consists of two layers: the pericardial layer and its inner layer, the **epicardium**. A small amount of lubricating fluid between these two layers allows the heart to pump with a minimum degree of friction. Epicardial tissue also extends to cover the **great vessels**, the major arteries and veins that enter and exit the heart.

The cardiovascular and peripheral vascular systems are closed systems, relying on pressure changes within the atria and ventricles to maintain the circulation of blood throughout the heart and body. Within a closed system, fluids (blood) flow from an area of greater pressure to an area of lower pressure. Additionally, pressures maintained within the system allow substances carried in the blood to enter or exit the blood stream. Changes in pressures within the chambers of the heart facilitate the opening and closing of the cardiac valves.

The opening and closing of the mitral and tricuspid valves is also aided by cartilaginous **chordae tendineae**, which are attached to the valve cusps and **papillary muscles**, which are attached to ventricular muscle. During atrial contraction and ventricular relaxation, ventricular expansion causes the chordae tendineae to pull the valve leaflets downward, separating the leaflets allowing blood flow through the valve into the ventricle. During ventricular contraction, the chordae tendineae are pushed upward so that the valve cusps join at their margins, creating a barrier so blood is unable to flow back into the atria (Figure 24-4).

The semilunar valves each have two cusps and separate the ventricles from the great vessels that exit from the heart. The aortic valve separates the left ventricle from the aorta, and the pulmonic valve separates the right ventricle from the pulmonary artery. There are no attachments to these valves that control their opening and closing; they open and close in response to changes in pressure that occur during systole and diastole.

As the ventricles fill with blood during ventricular relaxation, intraventricular pressure increases and eventually exceeds aortic pressure. Ventricular pressure is also increased just before contraction when myocardial muscles tense, but do not shorten. This isometric contraction rapidly increases intraventricular pressure, exceeding aortic pressure, causing opening of the aortic valve. The ventricles contract and blood is ejected into the aorta. After blood has been ejected, the ventricles relax and intraventricular pressure decreases, becoming lower than aortic pressure. This pressure gradient begins to pull blood back into the ventricles. As the blood begins to flow back, it catches the cusps of the aortic and pulmonic valves, causing them to shut, preventing further backflow of blood into the ventricles.

Blood is ejected from the heart into major arteries and flows into the heart through major veins, described as great vessels (Figure 24-5). These great vessels, located at the base of the heart, are the aorta, superior and inferior venae cavae, pulmonary arteries, and pulmonary veins. The aorta and pulmonary artery carry blood from the heart to the systemic and pulmonic circulation, respectively. The

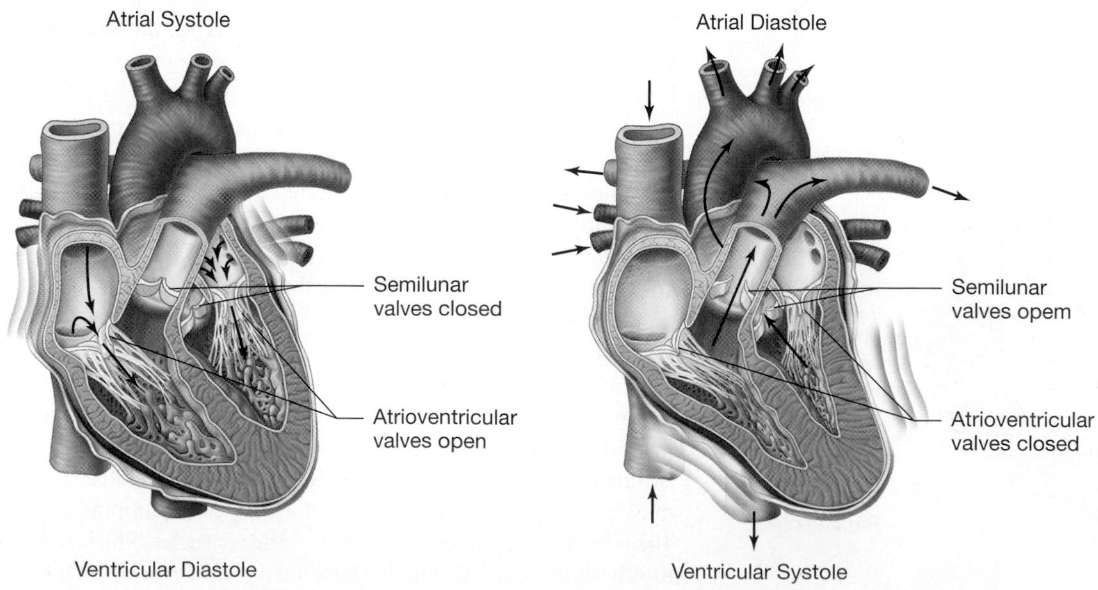

FIGURE 24-4 Position of chordae tendineae and mitral valve during ventricular systole/diastole

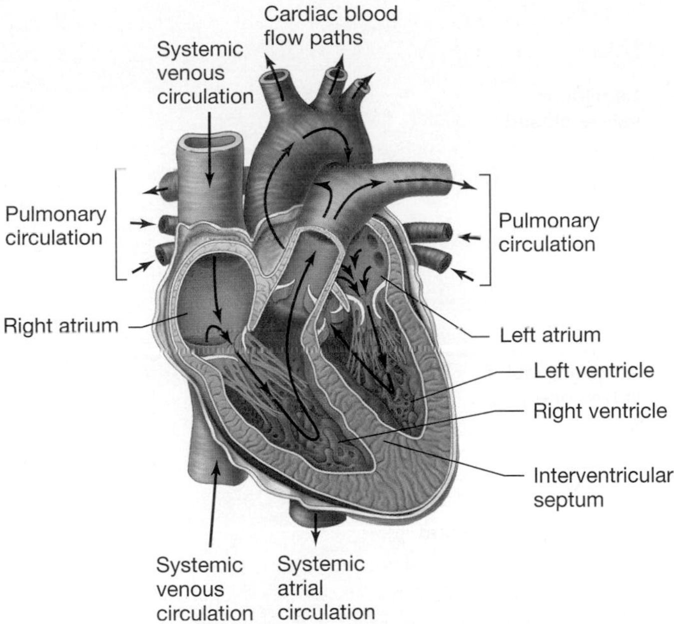

FIGURE 24-5 Blood flow through the heart

aorta branches into the subclavian and carotid arteries after exiting from the heart and the pulmonary artery splits into the right and left branches, bringing blood to the right and left lungs. The aorta carries oxygenated blood. In general, arteries carry oxygenated blood with the exception of the pulmonary artery that carries deoxygenated blood to the lungs and the uterine arteries in pregnancy, which then carry deoxygenated blood from the fetus to the placenta. The inferior and superior vena cavae deliver deoxygenated blood into the right atria and the four pulmonary veins carry oxygenated blood back to the left atrium.

The effectiveness of the pumping activity of the heart is related to its ability to adapt to the changing metabolic needs of the individual. The amount of blood circulated by the heart is dependent on the physiological need for oxygen. During regular, daily activity, the heart pumps approximately 4–6 liters of blood per minute, which represents its cardiac output (CO). Cardiac output is dependent on the heart rate (HR) and the stroke volume (SV) ($CO = SV \times HR$). The stroke volume is the amount of blood ejected with each ventricular contraction.

Stroke volume is determined by two components, preload and afterload. Preload is the volume of blood that is delivered to the ventricle during diastole. It also represents the length of ventricular muscle (amount of stretch) that occurs during diastole, just before ventricular contraction. During periods of increased metabolic demands, the heart increases CO by increasing SV and HR. During exercise, muscular contractions bring more blood to the right side of the heart, increasing the amount of blood ultimately delivered to the left side. To accommodate the increase in volume, the ventricular muscle fibers are stretched beyond their usual capacity. This increased stretch also increases the force of contraction (Starling's law).

Afterload is the amount of pressure the ventricles need to generate to exceed aortic pressure and open the aortic valve. Once the valve is opened, blood is rapidly ejected into the aorta.

Cardiac Cycle

Blood flows through the heart and through the circulation circuits as the result of regular contraction and relaxation of the heart. The contraction phase (or **systole**) and the relaxation phase (or **diastole**) form the cardiac cycle (Figure 24-6). The atria and ventricles have synchronized systolic and diastolic component and function so that when the atria are in systole, the ventricles are in diastole and vice versa. The two phases of the cardiac cycle, however, are primarily related to ventricular diastole and systole.

Diastole

During diastole, the ventricles are relaxed to allow blood to be ejected from the atria. The AV valves (tricuspid and mitral) are opened and because the blood-filled atria generate a higher pressure than the empty, relaxed ventricles, blood passively begins filling the ventricles. The mitral and tricuspid valves open as the chordae tendineae are pulled down as the ventricular muscle relaxes and lengthens.

This initial filling is identified as early diastolic filling or protodiastolic filling. As diastole progresses, the atria contract to push the last amount of blood into the ventricle during the late diastolic filling. This atrial contraction (systole) is frequently identified as the "**atrial kick**" and contributes approximately 24% of the blood volume ejected from the ventricle during contraction. Overall, diastole occupies approximately two-thirds of the cardiac cycle so that the heart is actually resting for a greater time period than it is working.

THINK LINK: Atrial Kick

The atrial kick adds momentum to the flow of blood into the ventricle, which helps to maintain the stroke volume and thus the cardiac output. Consider this to be like kicking a stationary football and measuring its distance. When a kicker simply stands behind the football and kicks it, the football has only the momentum of the kick and goes a certain distance. However, a kicker who is running before kicking the football passes the momentum of running to the football as it is being kicked. The momentum passed from the kicker to the football causes the football to go further.

The ejection of blood from the ventricles is not concerned with distance, but blood that is already in motion from the atrial kick will respond to ventricular contraction and increase the volume of blood ejected. Atrial kick is compromised in tachyarrhythmias like in rapid atrial fibrillation.

Systole

The blood in the ventricles plus the force of the atrial kick has now increased the pressure within the ventricles above the atrial pressure and aortic and pulmonic arterial pressure. The initial contraction of the ventricles increases ventricular pressure so that the AV valves close, preventing any blood from flowing backward into the atria. At the same time, the semilunar valves are forced open and blood is ejected into the aorta and the pulmonary artery. During ventricular systole, the atria are in diastole. They are receiving unoxygenated blood from the inferior and superior vena cavae and oxygenated blood from the pulmonary veins. At the completion of systole, the ventricular pressures are decreased and the cycle begins again. The decreased ventricular pressure also creates a vacuum that draws blood back into the ventricles. As blood begins to fill the ventricles, flowing

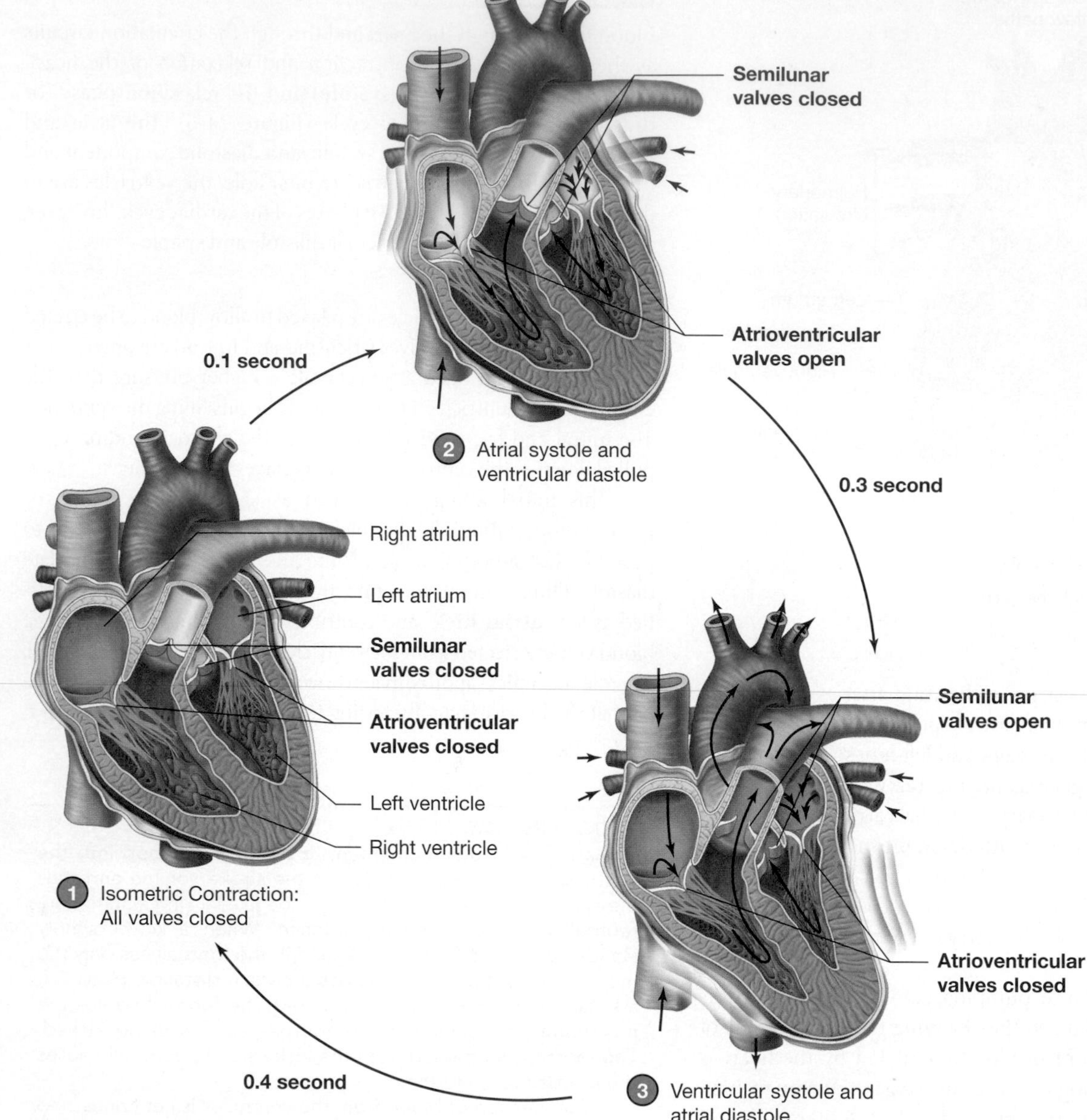

FIGURE 24-6 Cardiac cycle

into the ventricles, it catches the cusps of the valves and causes them to close, preventing the back flow of blood into the ventricle. Systole occupies the remaining one third of the cardiac cycle. As mentioned earlier, diastole occupies the initial two thirds.

Ventricular contractions occur almost simultaneously on the right and left sides of the heart with just a slight delay on the right. The pulmonary circulation functions at a lower pressure than the systemic circulation; however, even with the lower pressure, right ventricular contraction occurs slightly later than left ventricular contraction.

Heart Sounds

Ventricular contraction and relaxation also produce heart sounds, which are produced by the atrioventricular and semilunar valves. The cusps of the valve open to permit blood to flow through them during systole and close to prevent the backflow of blood during diastole. It is the closing of the valve cusps that produces the heart sounds.

Four heart sounds may be heard—S_1, S_2, S_3, and S_4. Heart sounds S_1 and S_2 are valvular sounds. They are consistent sounds that are closely associated with systole and diastole. Heart sounds S_3 and S_4 are not valvular sounds and may not always be present. When present, however, they are not always considered pathological findings and need to be evaluated within the context of the patient's condition and events within the cardiac cycle.

The two primary heart sounds are S_1 and S_2. S_1 is the heart sound produced by closing of the atrioventricular valves: tricuspid (T_1) and mitral (M_1) valves during ventricular systole. S_2 is produced by the closure of the semilunar valves: aortic (A_2) and the pulmonic (P_2) valves during ventricular diastole.

Electrical Conduction

The heart as a pump requires continuous and repetitive contractions to propel the blood through the circulatory system. The contractions of the cardiac cycle are regulated by the electrical conduction system, which is embedded within the muscle of the heart (Figure 24-7). This repetitive pumping cycle is maintained by autonomous stimulation of its electrical system, a property known as automaticity.

Each myocardial contraction begins with an electrical stimulus, initiated by autonomous depolarization of specific cells within the sinoatrial (SA) node, located in the right atrial wall. Prior to depolarization, cardiac cells are in a resting state, which is characterized as being polarized. Polarization of a cell is maintained at the cellular membrane by the accumulation of potassium and sodium ions. Potassium (K^{+2}) ions gather on the inside of the membrane and sodium (Na^{+2}) ions gather on the outside of the membrane. On the cellular level, the sarcolemma (plasma membrane) of an unstimulated cardiac muscle cell is polarized, that is, negatively charged inside with respect to the outside. The balance between K^{+2} inside the cell and Na^{+2} outside the cell contributes to the polarization or resting potential. In addition to potassium within the cell, there are also negatively charged ions, which cause the inside of the cell to be negatively charged.

In contrast to cardiac cells, noncardiac cells require some form of stimulation for depolarization to occur. Rapid depolarization occurs when fast opening Na^{+2} channels in the sarcolemma open and allow the influx of Na^{+2} ions into the cell, reversing the polarity of the cell membrane. This change in electrical charge causes the cell to contract, initiating an impulse that is transmitted throughout the cardiac conducting circuit. Before the SA node or any other cardiac cell can initiate another impulse, it must repolarize, returning Na^{+2} and K^{+2} to their original position along the cell membrane. This is carried out by Na^{+2} and K^{+2} pumps that carry them back to their original positions inside and outside the cell.

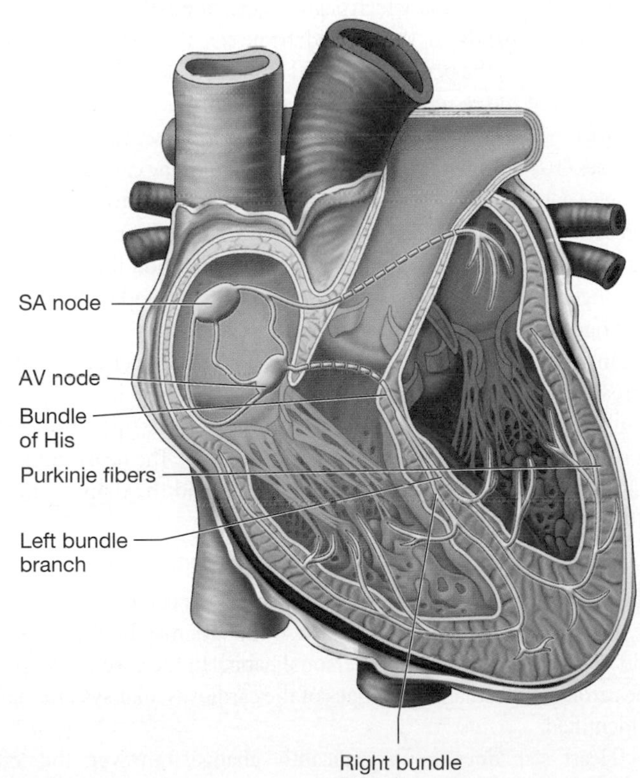

FIGURE 24-7 Electrical conduction through the heart muscle

From this impulse in the SA node, the electrical current travels through the right and left atria, causing atrial contraction. The current continues to the atrioventricular (AV) node, where it is slightly delayed. From the AV node, the current is conducted to the bundle of His, the right and left bundle branches, and then to the Purkinje fibers, which are distributed throughout the ventricular myocardium. Depolarization of the Purkinje fibers initiates ventricular contraction. Electrical events (conduction) occur slightly before the mechanical events (contraction).

The SA node is the primary initiator (pacemaker) of the electrical impulse and maintains this by depolarizing at a faster rate than the other parts of the heart. The SA node initiates an impulse approximately 80 times per minute; however, if for any reason the SA node fails, there is a back-up system. Any cell in the heart is capable of depolarizing to initiate an electrical impulse. This random electrical impulse may be generated elsewhere within the atria, the AV node, or ventricles. The AV node depolarizes itself approximately 60 times per minute and the ventricles are capable of depolarizing approximately 40 times per minute. These are called **intrinsic rates** (Table 24-1).

The Electrocardiogram

The electrical activity that occurs during depolarization and repolarization is reflected in an electrocardiogram (ECG) recording. The ECG shows a series of waves, intervals, and patterns that reflect electrical

Table 24-1 Intrinsic rates of depolarization

Supraventricular	
SA Node	60–100
AV Node	45–60
Bundle of His	40–45
Ventricular	
Right and Left Bundle	40–45
Purkinje fibers	20–40

(French, 2006)

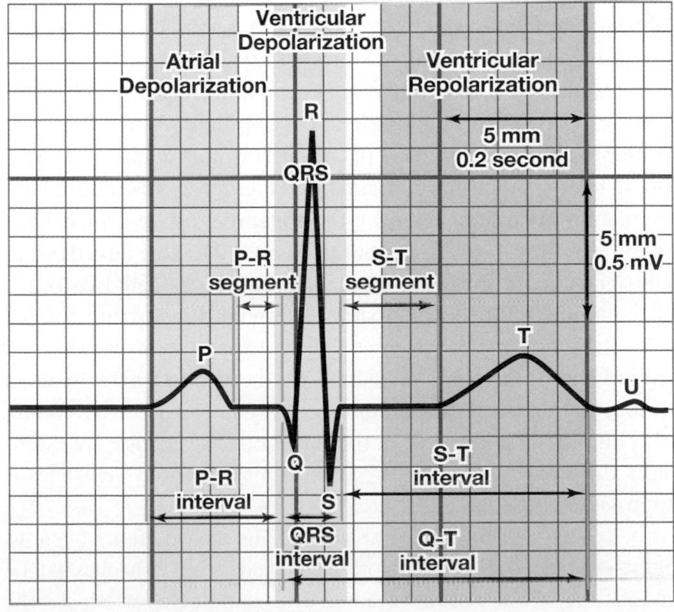

FIGURE 24-8 ECG waveform

conduction through the heart (Figure 24-8). Each complex represents one cardiac cycle. Each complex consists of the following components:

- P wave—positive deflection represents SA node impulse formation and atrial depolarization. A negative deflection may represent retrograde conduction.
- PR interval—the delayed conduction of the impulse through the AV node
- QRS complex—conduction through the ventricles causing ventricular depolarization
- ST segment—the beginning of ventricular repolarization
- T wave—ventricular repolarization

The deflection of the ECG waves is determined by the direction of electrical current, which starts from the SA node and progresses through the conduction pathway (Figure 24-8). The direction of sequential depolarization of the heart cells is described as a vector.

The transmission of electric current through the heart actually produces various vectors, but for purposes of the ECG tracing, there is one primary vector that is produced. The direction of flow is primarily related to increased electrical activity, and as the left side of the heart contains more muscle tissue, the overall trajectory of electrical activity flows towards the left (Figure 24-9). The position of the heart also directs the flow more horizontally than vertically as well as anteriorly. The overall trajectory of electrical current flow is also considered the heart's electrical axis. A deviation of the electrical axis indicates a shifting of the overall vector toward the right or left side of the heart.

The waves of the ECG complex are determined by whether the overall vector of the heart is directed toward or away from the positive electrode.

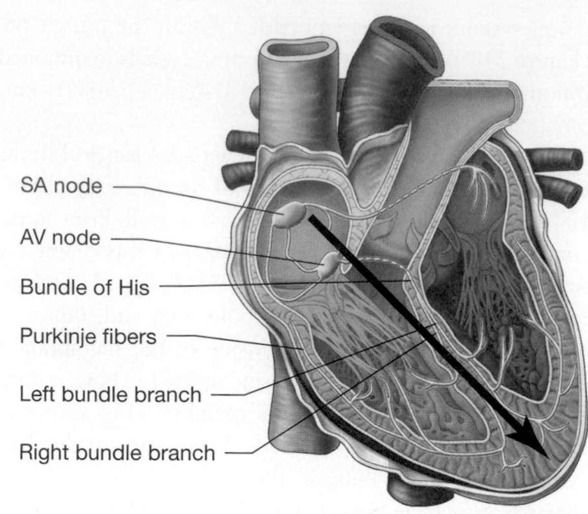

FIGURE 24-9 Electrical flow through heart conduction system [vector]

Developmental Variations

Developmental variations occur over the course of an individual's life span and events. Awareness of these variations is important to understand and recognize common age-related alterations or modifications of the cardiovascular system.

Infants and Children

During fetal development, the heart begins to function as a pump at approximately 28 days gestation. It assumes the shape of the adult heart very soon after that. Significant structural alterations are present throughout fetal development. As the lungs are nonfunctional, the right side of the heart is not required to pump blood to the pulmonary circulation (Figure 24-10). Pulmonary circulation is circumvented by the **foramen ovale**, which is an opening in the atrial septum that allows blood to flow directly from the right atrium into the left atrium. Approximately two-thirds of the blood from the right side is shunted directly into the left side. The blood that does enter the right ventricle is also shunted around the pulmonary circulation by the **ductus arteriosus**, a connection between the pulmonary artery and aorta. At this point, the pumping requirements of the right and left ventricle are essentially the same; therefore, the muscle mass of both ventricles is approximately equal.

At birth, the lungs become inflated and oxygenation of venous blood is required. These demands facilitate necessary changes in fetal circulation—closure of the foramen ovale and ductus arteriosis. The foramen ovale closes within 1 hour of birth due to pressure changes that now exist between the right and left sides. The ductus arteriosis closes somewhere between 10 and 15 hours after birth. The increased demand on the left side to maintain systemic circulation stimulates an increase in muscle mass. By about 1 year, the muscle mass of the left ventricle has increased to approximate the adult ratio of right ventricular mass to left ventricular mass of 1:2.

The position of the heart is more horizontal in the infant's chest than in the adult's. This results in an apex that is located higher on the chest at the fourth intercostal space (ICS). By about 7 years of age, the heart has achieved its adult position.

The Pregnant Woman

The blood volume of the pregnant woman increases approximately 40% over the nonpregnant volume. The increase is due mostly to an increase (>50%) in plasma, which begins to increase in the first trimester and rapidly expands in the second trimester. Because the plasma volume increases, the percentage of red blood cells decreases, lowering the hematocrit and resulting in physiologic anemia of pregnancy.

To accommodate the increase in blood volume, the heart rate also rises (10–15 bpm) with an overall increase in the cardiac output. The left ventricle grows in muscle mass and thickness to handle the increased load. During pregnancy, blood flow to the uterus, placenta, and breast increases, while hepatic and cerebral blood flow remains unchanged. Within 3–4 weeks after delivery, the blood volume and heart rate has returned to its prepregnancy parameters.

In spite of the increase in cardiac workload, arterial pressure decreases due to peripheral vasodilatation resulting in decreased peripheral resistance. Arterial pressure is at its lowest point during the second trimester and then gradually increases. The heart shifts to a more horizontal axis as the uterus enlarges and the diaphragm is shifted upward.

The Older Adult

It is difficult to isolate specific cardiovascular changes that occur in the older adult as many of these changes may be due to lifestyle, co-morbid diseases, and personal habits. In the absence of specific cardiac disease, aging changes of the cardiovascular system may be identified.

Heart size does not significantly change; however, the left ventricular wall thickens, and the valves are likely to calcify and become fibrotic. Systolic blood pressure increases gradually, which

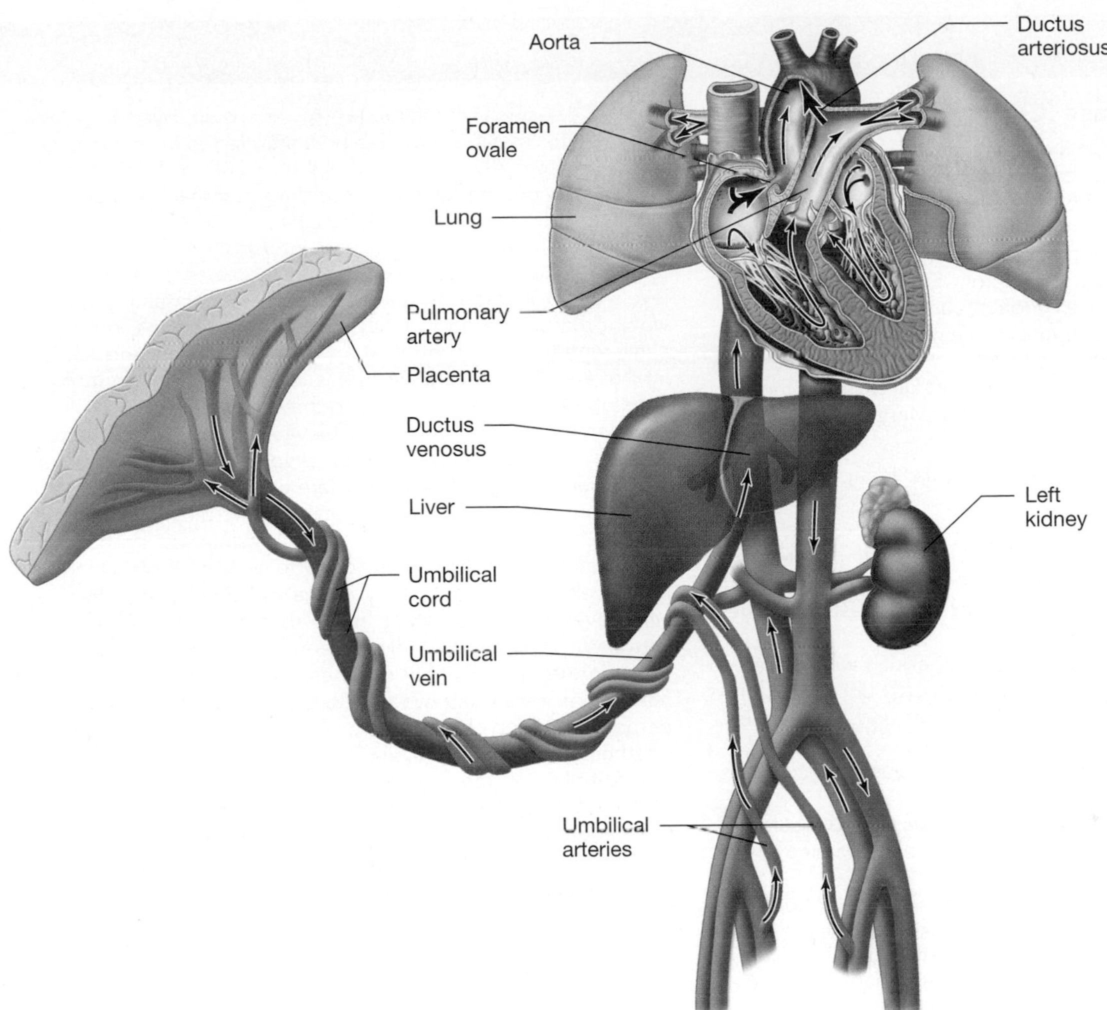

FIGURE 24-10 Fetal circulation

is due to stiffening of the arteries because of calcification of the vessel walls (**arteriosclerosis**). This stiffening also contributes to the increased workload of the heart and ventricular thickening. Diastolic pressure remains relatively constant; however, with the rising systolic pressure, there is a widening of the pulse pressure.

The heart rate slows down but the resting heart rate may not be significantly different. There is stiffening of the myocardium, which leads to impairment in filling and relaxation resulting in a lower stroke volume. There is also a decrease in diastolic compliance that contributes to a longer recovery period. The overall effect is a reduced capability to increase cardiac output and heart rate in instances where an increased myocardial demand exists. In spite of age-associated changes, the heart continues to maintain its contractility and pumping capacity so that it performs its function properly.

The electrical functioning of the heart may be compromised by fibrosis and sclerosis in the region of the SA node, which may allow for an increase in supraventricular and ventricular arrhythmias, or rhythm disturbances. **Ectopic beats**, heartbeats that originate in areas outside of the conduction pathways, are common in the elderly. They are usually asymptomatic; however, in the presence of co-morbid diseases, blood pressure and cardiac output may become compromised. Changes in electrical conduction like the slowing or blocking of conduction primarily occur within the AV node (AV blocks) or the bundle branches (bundle branch blocks). Repolarization may be delayed as well, resulting in ST-T wave abnormalities. Other manifestations result from multiple points of autonomous depolarization and accessory pathways, which include atrial fibrillation and flutter. Left ventricular hypertrophy, which may be due to hypertension and other remodeling processes, may also be evident.

THINK LINK: C-Reactive Protein/Homocysteine and Cardiac Disease

C-reactive protein (CRP) is produced by the liver and is a blood test marker for the presence of inflammation in the body. An increased CRP has been associated with atherosclerosis and heart disease. Atherosclerosis has been recognized to have an inflammatory aspect, which is thought to cause the increase in blood levels of CRP. The damage to the blood vessels caused by the atherosclerosis is seen as the cause of the inflammation. While increased blood levels of CRP are associated with cardiac disease, by themselves they are not diagnostic for the presence of disease. Homocysteine (HCY) is an amino acid in the blood that has also been linked to cardiovascular disease. Elevation of HCY in the blood has been weakly correlated as a risk factor for early development of cardiovascular disease but has yet to be established as a definitive cause (Clarke et al., 2012). Increased blood levels of HCY are also associated with lower levels of folate, and vitamins B6 and B12; however, it remains questionable as to whether administration of these substances significantly reduces any vascular events (Wierzbicki, 2007). There is evidence of any adverse effects associated with increased intake of them.

Health Promotion

Cardiovascular Disease (CVD)

Cardiovascular diseases (CVDs) are a group of heart disease conditions that are caused by narrowed, blocked, or stiffened blood vessels that supply blood to the heart, brain, and other parts of the body. These altered blood vessels prevent oxygen carrying blood from reaching these vital organs. Some of these conditions have modifiable risk factors and are not mutually exclusive. Other heart disease conditions are infectious, compensatory, or congenital in nature and create muscular, structural, or electrical alterations of the heart.

Healthy People 2020 topic area "Heart Disease and Stroke" has the following objectives (U.S. Department of Health and Human Services, 2009):

- HDS—1: Increase overall cardiovascular health in the U.S. population.
- HDS—2: Reduce coronary heart disease deaths.
- HDS—13: Increase the proportion of adults with elevated LDL cholesterol who have been advised by a health care provider on cholesterol lowering management including lifestyle changes and, if indicated, medication.
- HDS—14: Increase the proportion of adults with elevated LDL-cholesterol who adhere to prescribed LEL-cholesterol lowering management lifestyle changes and, if indicated, medication.
- HDS—15: Increase aspirin use as recommended among adults with no history of cardiovascular disease.
- HDS—16: Increase the proportion of adults aged 20 years and older who are aware of, and respond to, early warning symptoms and signs of a heart attack.
- HDS—20: Increase the proportion of adults with coronary heart disease or stroke whose low-density lipoprotein [LDL] cholesterol is at or below recommended levels.
- HDS—21: Increase the proportion of adults with a history of cardiovascular disease who use aspirin or antiplatelet therapy to prevent recurrent cardiovascular events.

In spite of declining mortality from heart disease because of improvements in diagnosis and interventions, cardiovascular disease remains a primary cause of death in the United States as well as worldwide. In 2008 in the United States, CVD accounted for 35%–40% (32.8%) of all deaths, which is more than all forms of cancer (National Heart, 2012). In 2008, there were 17.3 million deaths from CVD worldwide, representing 30% of all global deaths—with the majority of deaths occurring in low- and middle-income countries (World Health Organization, 2012). CVD is also a major contributor to disability as well as increasing health care costs.

The overall risk for developing CVD is quite high for individuals in the Unites States. Estimates are that 50% of males and 33% of females less than 40 years of age will develop CVD sometime in their life. Its prevalence is highest among individuals aged ≥65 years (19.8%) preceded by those aged 45–64 years (7.1%) and those aged 18–44 years (1.2%) (Morbidity and Mortality Weekly Report, 2012). The most significant pathology of heart disease is attributed to the buildup of atherosclerotic plaques in the arteries resulting in a narrowing of the interior lumen of the arteries and a decrease in the delivery of oxygenated blood to the heart muscle. The major causes of coronary heart diseases have been well defined. Most of them are considered modifiable, such as smoking, diets that are high in saturated fat, sedentary life, and obesity. Risk factors like hypertension, hyperlipidemia, and diabetes mellitus may also be controlled to improve cardiovascular outcomes.

Primary prevention is the most important factor in decreasing the incidence of cardiovascular disease, with lifestyle changes being the most significant intervention. These changes target the reduction in blood pressure, cholesterol, and glucose levels by an increase in aerobic activities; maintaining a body weight that is related to body size and proportions; moderate consumption of alcohol; limiting or reducing salt and sodium intake; and a dietary intake that is low in fat and high in fruits, vegetables, and low-fat dairy products.

For individuals who have elevated levels of cholesterol despite lifestyle changes, medications may be necessary. A number of drug classifications are used for this purpose; the most commonly used are the statins that block the production of the liver enzyme that is responsible for synthesizing cholesterol. While statins are used to reduce cholesterol and LDL levels in the blood, they may also be used in individuals who develop atherosclerosis in the absence of high cholesterol levels. Although cholesterol has been recognized as a significant factor in the development of atherosclerotic plaques, a certain number of individuals who experience a heart attack do not demonstrate high cholesterol levels, although there is evidence of atherosclerosis (Ogbru, 2009).

Antiplatelet medications, such as low dose aspirin and other antiplatelet therapy drugs, are also considered effective in prevention of heart attacks. Antiplatelet therapy prevents platelets from adhering to each other and thus prevents the formation of blood clots. Blood clots traveling in the blood stream through narrowed arteries may get stuck or trapped in the atherosclerotic plaque, further reducing or obstructing blood flow to the heart muscle.

Efforts to reduce blood levels of cholesterol by control of dietary intake of fats may also help in weight reduction. Over the past 20 years the prevalence of obesity has dramatically increased. Just over one-third (35.7%) of adults in the United States are obese and 12.5 million children (17%) aged 2–19 are obese (Ogden, Carroll, Kit, & Flegal, 2012).

While aerobic exercise is considered the most significant activity for weight reduction, any form of activity is preferred over none and helps in reducing cardiovascular problems. Giving up smoking is also considered a major step towards the reduction of CVD. Avoiding second-hand smoke is also an important consideration in prevention and reduction of risks for CVD. While smoking use has been declining in most developed, high-income countries, smoking and tobacco use are increasing in low-income and less-developed countries. If this pattern continues, it is estimated that globally, tobacco related deaths could reach 1 billion annually (Giovino et al., 2012). (Additional information on obesity and smoking is provided in Chapters 23 and 28.)

Evidence of the presence of risk factors for cardiovascular disease is seen as early as adolescence. The incidence of type 2 diabetes in children and adolescents in increasing, especially in minority ethnic groups (Vivian, 2006). While genetics does have a role in the development of type 2 diabetes, its increasing prevalence in younger individuals is most likely due to the increase in overweight and obese kids and teens (Dowshen, 2009).

Health Promotion *continued*

In the past 30 years, childhood obesity has tripled. Obesity in children aged 6–11 years of age increased from 7% (1980) to 20% (2008) and in the same time period, in adolescents aged 12–19 years the incidence increased from 5%–18% (Centers for Disease Control and Prevention, 2012).

Primary prevention for type 2 diabetes should begin in elementary and secondary schools as well as at colleges and universities. Screening efforts to detect high-risk individuals is essential as well as education regarding the promotion of heart healthy behaviors.

Clinical Context Exemplars

Situation A

Jim Payne is a 52-year-old male who presents to the ER with chest pain he describes as a "burning sensation" around the substernal and epigastric area that was brought on by exertion while taking out the trash. The chest pain was associated with nausea and relieved by rest. He attributed it the heartburn or gas as he had chili dog the evening prior. His wife and children accompanied him to the ER. His father died of a massive heart attack at age 52.

1. What elements of the history should be given top priority?
2. What should be the focus the physical examination?
3. What kind of symptom analysis information is needed to determine if chest pain is cardiac in origin?
4. What are the "not to miss diagnoses" that can hemodynamically compromise Mr. Payne?

Situation B

Mina Polanksi is a 54-year-old woman who comes into your office with epigastric pain radiating to her substernal area associated with lightheadedness, nausea, feeling warm, headaches, and just not feeling well. This pain occurs sometimes at rest and sometimes with exertion. Pain is described as sharp twinge, sometimes dull and sometimes as a heavy sensation on her chest. She had been having these episodes the last few months and presented to an urgent care where an electrocardiogram (ECG) was done and was told it was normal. They stated that it might just be hormone related.

1. Compare and contrast the presentations of Mr. Payne and Ms. Polanski.
2. How will either presentation affect your work-up?

Situation C

Mandy Der is 28 years old and 32-weeks' pregnant. She is being hospitalized for observation because of some vaginal bleeding. She is complaining of some shortness of breath, otherwise she feels reasonably well. During the examination a Grade II systolic murmur was heard. She also has a family history of diabetes and is concerned for her baby.

1. What is the significance of this murmur?
2. What will you tell Ms. Der?

Situation D

Kevin Barnes is 18 years old and is being worked up for open-heart surgery to replace his mitral valve. During your assessment when you are palpating his anterior chest, you feel some vibrations on his chest.

1. What would you expect to hear during auscultation of his heart sounds?
2. When listening to the heart sounds, where would you expect to hear what you suspect Mr. Barnes to have?

Situation E

Derek Carter is a 12-year-old boy who is receiving a sports physical for school. During auscultation of his heart, an extra sound is heard between S_2 and S_1. After listening for 30 seconds, the extra sound can be placed as occurring just after S_2.

1. What would you recommend to Derek and his mother regarding engaging in sports activity due to this particular finding?
2. Derek has a 15-year-old brother, and Derek is wondering if his brother would have the same finding? What would be an appropriate explanation?

SUBJECTIVE DATA

History of Present Illness (CC)

The patient may present to the provider with a variety of concerns that may be directly related to the cardiovascular system or other systems. Framing the questions will depend on the patient's age, gender, culture, race, emotional or mental status, health practices, and concurrent illnesses. All symptoms presented must be thoroughly assessed with a symptom analysis (COLDERRA).

Chest Pain (Angina Pectoris)

Chest pain comes from a variety of conditions; it is not always associated with cardiac disorders, so it must be carefully assessed to determine its origin.

Provider Inquiries	Clinical Reasoning/Logic
Characteristics: How would you describe the pain? (may be described as aching, sharp, tingling, chest twinges, burning, pressure, stabbing, crushing, tight band around the chest, viselike) (note use of clenched fist sign—Levine's sign) **O**nset: When did pain start (gradual or sudden)? Do you have pain now? What initiated the pain? Is pain related to other factors (eating, exertion, emotional situations, temperature, or sex)? Is this the first time it has occurred or have you experienced it previously?	Chest pain is the primary symptom that may indicate acute injury or damage to the heart muscle. Chest pain is also caused by other conditions, so it is important to determine if the pain is of cardiac origin or from other causes (see Differential Diagnosis).
Location: substernal, upper or lower chest, others: epigastric, neck, shoulder, jaw, back **D**uration: How long does the pain last? Is the pain cyclic or continuous in nature? Does it come and go? **E**xacerbation: What makes the pain worse (activity, exercise, eating, change in position of chest or thorax, breathing, or coughing)? How severe is the pain (1–10 scale)?	Patients may not know how long they have had the pain.
Radiation: Does the pain radiate to any other location (L arm, jaw, neck, back)? **R**elief: What makes the pain better or go away (rest, medications [what; how many], position change, complementary therapies)? **A**ssociated symptoms: Any other manifestations (nausea/vomiting, anxiety, dyspnea or SOB, diaphoresis, dizziness/syncope)?	You may need to explain the term radiation to some patients.

Differential diagnosis: chest pain

	Cardiac Angina/ Ischemic	Musculoskeletal	GI: Esophageal/ Peptic Ulcer	GI	Pleural
Characteristics	Pressure, crushing, stabbing, sharp	Tenderness	Burning; pressure-like, squeezing	Burning; gnawing	Sharp, intense
Onset	Early morning, after physical activity/effort, intense cold	Movement, twisting/ bending	Nonspecific, gradual onset; nocturnal lying flat	Nonspecific, gradual onset; nocturnal; empty stomach, spicy/ acidic meal, alcohol	After deep breathing/coughing, laughing, sneezing
Location	Substernal	Across chest	Substernal	Infradiaphragmatic, epigastric	Across chest
Duration	< 20 minutes	Hours	Variable		Hours to days
Exacerbation	Effort, activity, stress	Continued movement/ activity	Nonspecific, not related to activity	Nonspecific, not related to activity	Deep breathing, coughing, activity
Relief	Stopping activity/ effort NTG	Heat, NSAIDS, rest	Food	Food	Holding breath, shallow breathing, localized heat, analgesics
Radiation	Down L arm, to jaw, back	Localized	Occasionally to shoulder, neck, jaw, ear	Epigastric, radiating to lower bilateral chest	Variable
Associated S/S	Nausea, anxiety, diaphoresis, cyanosis	Nonspecific	Dysphagia	Nausea, abdominal tenderness	
Possible Causes	Angina: Prinzmetal's, unstable, CAD, mitral valve prolapse	Shoulder disorder (RA, bursitis, rotator cuff injury), costochondritis, herpes zoster	Hiatal hernia, cholecystitis, pancreatitis, dysmotility syndrome		Pulmonary HTN, pneumonia, pulmonary embolus

PRACTICE POINT: Levine's Sign

Levine's sign, clenched fist over the chest, is a classic manifestation of the individual experiencing chest pain of cardiac origin. While it is common for the patient to demonstrate this, it is not considered to be a reliable indicator. Specificity reported in the range of 78%.

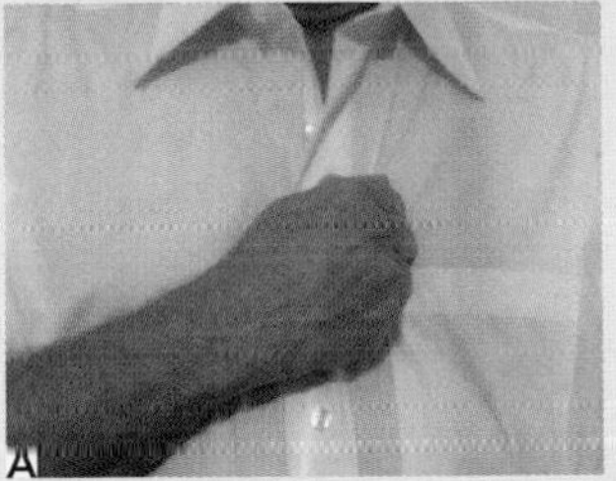

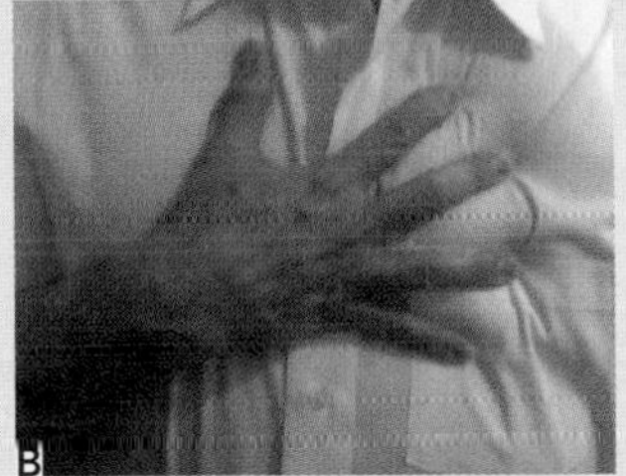

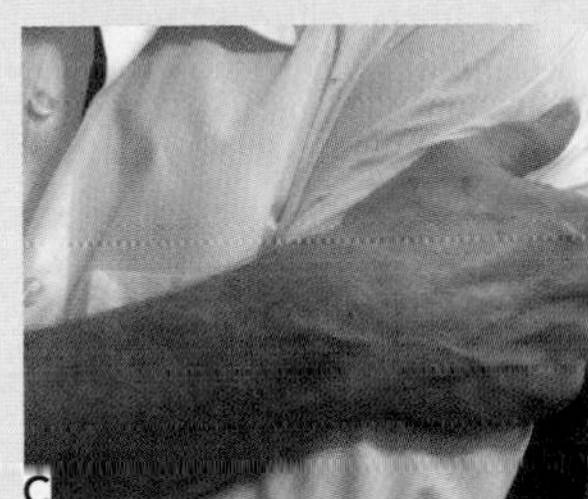

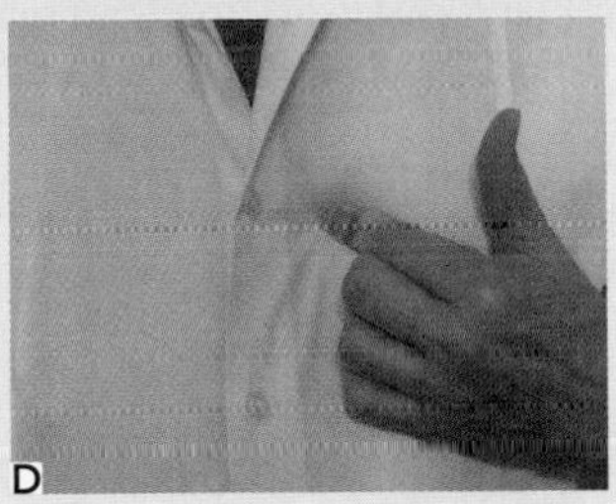

FIGURE 24-11A–D Characteristic gestures showing Levine's point

Prevalence of the Levine, palm, arm, and pointing signs were 11%, 35%, 16% and 4% respectively with sensitivities not exceeding 38% using troponins functional studies and coronary arteriogram. Specificities of Levine and arm signs ranged from 78% and 86% and positive predictive value did not exceed 55%. Pointing sign has specificity of 98% for evidence of nonischemic CP but with low prevalence. Diameter of chest discomfort seems to be associated with larger correlate with evidence of myocardial ischemia. Gestures articulate the size of discomfort with larger zone suggestive of ischemia.

Breathing Difficulties (Dyspnea, Orthopnea)

Respiratory manifestations often accompany cardiac conditions. The lungs are frequently affected with systolic or diastolic dysfunction of the heart. This is primarily due to accumulation of fluid within the alveoli in individuals with congestive heart failure.

Provider Inquiries	Clinical Reasoning/Logic
Characteristics: shortness of breath (SOB), increased rate/depth of breathing, air hunger, dyspnea on exertion (DOE), decline in activities due to shortness of breath?	Dyspnea can be an important sign of cardiac problems including cardiac ischemia and cardiomyopathy.
Onset: Acute or chronic? Intermittent or recurrent?	
Duration: How long do the episodes last?	Sleeping in an upright position causes fluid in the lungs to remain in the lower section of the lungs.
Exacerbation: Is there anything that makes it worse? Exercise, stress, or position? Time of day?	
Relief: What makes it go away? Activity reduction or discontinuance, position change like assuming upright position, increased number of pillows to sleep (pillow orthopnea)? Quantify number of pillows and compare with patient's baseline.	
Associated signs/symptoms: Are there other manifestations associated with episode? Paroxysmal nocturnal dyspnea [PND], chest pain, leg swelling, increase in weight?	

THINK LINK: Paroxysmal Nocturnal Dyspnea

Paroxysmal nocturnal dyspnea (PND) is characterized as an episode of shortness of breath or dyspnea that awakens an individual from sleep, often occurring about 1–2 hours after falling asleep and relieved by assuming an upright position. The individual may also experience coughing and wheezing and describe the feeling of suffocation. PND is an early sign of congestive heart failure and results from fluid reabsorption from peripheral interstitial spaces into blood. Additional theories include decreased adrenergic activity in the myocardium during sleep and reduced responsiveness of the respiratory center in the brain.

Cough

A cough, though frequently related to pulmonary function, is also often associated with cardiac conditions, primarily congestive heart failure, which causes an accumulation of fluid in the alveoli.

Provider Inquiries	Clinical Reasoning/Logic
Characteristics: Is the cough productive or dry?	A dry, persistent cough is a symptom of congestive heart failure.
Onset: Acute or chronic? Particular time of day that it occurs? (Worse at night?)	
Duration: Is the cough continuous or episodic? If episodic, how long do episodes last?	Unless CHF is acute in onset, a cough associated with CHF is chronic in nature.
Exacerbation: What makes it worse? (What position—lying down?)	Cough associated with CHF often gets worse at night.
Relief: What makes it go away? Any specific treatments used?	
Associated signs/symptoms: Coughing up blood, anxiety, SOB, leg swelling, chest pain weight gain?	In severe cases of CHF the sputum produced by coughing may be frothy and tinged with blood.

Provider Inquiries	Clinical Reasoning/Logic

Past Medical History

Information related to past medical history identifies any conditions that may affect or cause present cardiac condition or symptoms.

Childhood illnesses: Childhood diseases may have pathological manifestations in adult years. Rheumatic fever (unexplained fever, swollen joints, joint pain)?

Congenital heart disease?

Chronic illnesses: Hypertension, anemia, renal failure, bleeding disorders, diabetes, hyper/hypothyroidism, coronary artery disease, hyperlipidemia, congenital heart defects, congestive heart failure, stroke

Cardiovascular/peripheral vascular surgery?

Rhythm disorders, ECG abnormalities?

Provides information about previous cardiac conditions that may affect the present situation. Rheumatic fever is one of the most significant causes of structural alterations of the heart.

Hypertension, cardiovascular disease, hyperlipidemia, and diabetes are all associated with the development of significant heart disease.

Previous surgeries (coronary artery bypass grafts, femoral-popliteal bypass) are indicators of concurrent cardiovascular conditions. Any known cardiac conduction alterations may provide information related to present condition

Family History

Family History provides information regarding family member's illnesses or conditions as potential causes for chief complaint or presenting symptoms that may indicate a pattern of presentation associated with transmission of familial/genetic factors predisposing the individual to certain system related conditions/illnesses. Any of these may indicate a potential or actual cause of cardiac dysfunction.

Chronic illnesses: Diabetes, hypertension, heart disease (CAD), hyperlipidemia, CVA, arrhythmias

Congenital heart defects: Septal or valvular defects

Hypertrophic cardiomyopathy?

Sudden death syndrome (especially young or middle-aged individuals)?

Provides information as to any diseases or conditions that are familial or genetic and may provide information related to a patient's present condition/complaint.

Individuals with a family history of sudden death syndrome should be screened for evidence of cardiovascular disease as SDS may be the first and only manifestation of cardiovascular diseases.

THINK LINK: Sudden Death Syndrome

Sudden death syndrome is the unexpected death of an individual without any known diagnosis of a fatal condition. The individual may or may not have any cardiovascular disease. The primary mechanism of death is failure of the conduction system to produce electrical activity to sustain ventricular contraction. The most common cause is ventricular fibrillation, which may be caused by myocardial infarction, congestive heart failure, cardiomyopathy, myocarditis, and Wolff-Parkinson-White syndrome. For some individuals, sudden death may be the only manifestation of an underlying cardiac disease. Young individuals, especially teen athletes who experience sudden death are often found to have hypertrophic cardiomyopathy.

Personal and Social History

Personal and social history provides information related to habits, practices and/or environmental influences that may predispose the patient to the development of certain system related conditions/illnesses.

Employment: Physical/emotional demands, environmental hazards (chemicals, high temperatures)

Tobacco/smoking habits: Type (smoke, smokeless), how long (pack/years), age when started/stopped, tried to quit (successful), exposure to second-hand smoke?

Nutritional status: Usual daily intake (fats, sodium, preferences, dieting habits)?

Usual weight: Recent gain/loss (intentional/unintentional)?

Alcohol intake: Amount; frequency; increase in intake; ever told that he/she has a drinking problem; interference with job, social, or family relationships?

Personality characteristics: Anger, hostility, inability to relax, compulsive behavior, anxious, worrier?

Provides information as to any environmental conditions or personal behaviors that may predispose to cardiac involvement related to patient's present condition/complaint.

Provides information as to any environmental conditions or personal behaviors that may predispose to cardiac involvement related to patient's present condition/complaint.

Provider Inquiries	Clinical Reasoning/Logic
Activity: Hobbies, relaxation? Sports? Sedentary?	
Exercise: Type, amount, frequency, duration?	
Sex: Frequency of intercourse, practices, number of partners?	
Drugs/Toxins: Prescription/OTC: Antihypertensive, beta-blockers, calcium channel blockers, nitrates, diuretics, digoxin, aspirin/anti-coagulants, antihistamines, decongestants, herbs, anti-arrhythmics?	
Nonprescription: Cocaine, methamphetamine, club drugs, street drugs?	

THINK LINK: ***Women and Cardiovascular Disease***

Since 1999, when heart disease was recognized as a major health risk for women, many advances have been made by increasing awareness of risk factors and the implementation of CVD prevention strategies. As a result, deaths from CVD in women began to decline. However, that trend has been reversed, and the reversal is thought to be related to the obesity epidemic (Mosca et al., 2011). CVD rates are also higher in black women than in white women. This disparity also reflects the decreased awareness of heart disease and stroke among black women.

Much of what was known about CVD came from males, and it was assumed that the characteristics would be the same in women. It is now recognized that the "classic" signs and symptoms of heart disease are based on men's experiences and the signs and symptoms may be different for women. Chest pain in women, if present, often presents atypically; it may occur at rest, may come and go, and may not be relieved with rest. It may also be associated with symptoms like abdominal pain, SOB, inability to get breath in, numbness and weakness of arms, dizziness or lightheadedness, nausea, and just not feeling well. Weakness and unusual fatigue are also common. These symptom complexes may contribute to delay in the diagnosis as they may be attributed to something other than cardiac ischemia. They are commonly attributed to heart burn, indigestion, arthritis, stress, and being out of shape if shortness of breath is experienced with minimal exertion.

In spite of the better current understanding of angina and CAD in women, there is still the perception that women are at a lower risk for the development of CAD, and that angina in women has a more favorable prognosis (Vaccarino, 2006). However, while the symptoms of CVD may be manifest differently in men and women, the risk factors for causing CVD are not different.

Developmental Applications

Certain conditions or disorders may be related to certain age groups or situations. Inquiring to obtain age or condition specific information will provide further information for helping to determine causes of the chief concern as identified.

Infants and Children

Provider Inquiries	Clinical Reasoning/Logic
Ask the mother about her health during pregnancy, if possible	Did the mother experience any health related conditions during the pregnancy that may have affected development of the heart in the fetus (e.g., transposition of great arteries)? Rubella in first trimester, unexplained fevers, drug use (prescription, OTC, alcohol, illicit drugs, caffeine), hypertension?
Is your infant able to eat, nurse, finish bottle without tiring or with no cyanosis? Is there frequent crying or stopping during feeding. How long does it take to finish the bottle?	Generally, infants do not take more than 30 minutes to feed. If infant takes longer or needs to take frequent breaks, may be an indicator of a cyanotic heart defect.
Have there been any breathing changes (more heavily/rapid) during feeding?	If the infant is demonstrating difficulty with feeding, it may indicate that the increased work of feeding increases consumption of oxygen which then requires an increase in cardiac output. If enough oxygen cannot be inhaled during feeding, the infant needs to expend energy to breathe rather than eat.
Is the infant's weight gain as expected?	Failure to gain weight (failure to thrive) as expected is another indicator of feeding/eating difficulties and related to an increased consumption of calories and oxygen to maintain respiratory and cardiac function.

Provider Inquiries | **Clinical Reasoning/Logic**

Children

Are there any manifestations of failure to thrive? Is child at or near expected height/weight gain?

(Same reason as above)

Is your child able to play/keep up with siblings/friends without tiring (fatigue?)?

An indicator of increased fatigue related to increased efforts thus leading to increased oxygen consumption

Does your child ever assume a squatting position when at play/watching TV, or assumes a knee-chest position during sleep?

Squatting or knee chest position is observed in children with right to left ventricular shunts, most commonly associated with tetralogy of Fallot (see page 675). Squatting increases peripheral vascular resistance, which leads to decrease right to left shunting.

Does your child take naps longer than usual or more frequent than normal? Has your child ever complained of unexplained joint pains/fevers, nosebleeds, headaches?

The Pregnant Woman

Do you have any history of cardiac disease/surgery?

Do you ever experience dizziness/fainting upon standing?

Pregnant women with known cardiac disease need close monitoring for the development of cardiac decompensation due to the increased strain on her body and physiology. There is a higher incidence of maternal death as well as an increased risk for fetal demise and perinatal mortality (Ladewig, London, & Davidson, 2010).

Were there any indicators of cardiac disease during pregnancy—progressive/severe dyspnea, orthopnea, paroxysmal nocturnal dyspnea, hemoptysis, syncope with exertion, chest pain accompanying exertion?

Cardiac conditions that place the woman/fetus at high risk include pulmonary hypertension, complex cyanotic congenital heart defects, poor ventricular function, and Marfan's syndrome with marked aortic dilation.

How long, how treated?

An increase in blood pressure occurs with toxemia as well as proteinuria and the development of edema.

Did you have high blood pressure during this/other pregnancies? If high, when/how treated? Were there any accompanying signs/symptoms—edema, weight gain, proteinuria (protein in the urine)?

Drugs—Side effects, reactions (potassium excess—weakness, bradycardia, hypotension, confusion; potassium deficit—weakness, fatigue, muscle cramps, arrhythmias; digitalis toxicity—anorexia, N/V, diarrhea, HA, confusion, arrhythmias, halos, yellow vision)

The Older Adult

Are there any symptoms of cardiac disease—confusion, blackouts, dizziness, syncope, palpitations, coughing, sneezing, SOB, chest pain/tightness, fatigue, edema (location, pattern, time of day)?

The manifestations may result from a reduced blood supply to the brain due to vascular and circulation alterations.

Incontinence, constipation, impotence, heat intolerance (indicators of orthostatic hypotension)?

These manifestations are indicators of orthostatic hypotension.

Is there a history of known heart disease?

Coping capability: Family/individual?

Orthostatic hypotension?

The older adult has a decreased ability to adapt to stress, which may exacerbate existing cardiac diseases or indicate their presence.

OBJECTIVE DATA

The examination of the heart and cardiovascular system includes all four-examination techniques: inspection, palpation, percussion, and auscultation. The patient may be seated or in the supine position depending on patient's capability. The patient's position will determine the exact sequence of the examination, but you should develop a systematic approach that you use consistently for each examination. Maintain a comfortable ambient temperature as cold and chilling may cause the patient to be uncomfortable and may precipitate shivering, which may interfere with auscultation of heart sounds. A quiet environment is also important as heart sounds and other sounds are quite soft and may not be heard as well. Appropriate draping is necessary when examining an adult female patient. The left breast lies over a part of the heart that needs to be examined. During this part of the examination, gently displace the breast upward and ask the patient to hold it there.

The major focus of the cardiovascular exam is listening to the heart sounds; however, do not rush to this part of the exam or begin by listening to the heart. All information obtained is important so proceeding in a systematic manner beginning with inspection is necessary. In addition to the standard equipment, a light source that can provide tangential lighting is important.

When beginning the examination, the ideal location to stand is to the right of the patient. Throughout the exam, the patient may need to assume a variety of positions, which may require you to be flexible as well. The context of the exam will determine the need for position changes so provide an adequate time for position changes, especially if the patient is elderly.

The following is the suggested sequence for the complete examination of the heart according to the four techniques of data collection, followed by a break down into the taxonomy types of the exam.

Inspection

- General presentation/skin color,
- Capillary refill/clubbing
- Heaves or lifts
- Pulsations (apical)
- Jugular venous pulsation/distension
- ECG analysis: rhythm, 12-lead ECG

Palpation

- Peripheral pulses (rate, rhythm, quality)
- Heaves, lifts, thrills
- Apex beat (point of maximal impulse)
- Aortic pulsation

Percussion

- Estimate size of heart (if necessary)

Auscultation

- Blood pressure
- Carotid bruit
- Heart sounds in five auscultatory areas (rate, rhythm, S_1, S_2, splitting, S_3/S_4)
- Extra heart sounds (snaps, clicks, rubs, murmurs)
- Timing/duration
- Intensity
- Pattern
- Quality
- Location
- Radiation

Level I to IV Examination

The Level I to Level IV examinations are performed on a continuum, starting from a basic level and proceeding to a more comprehensive level based on provider's abilities and patient's presentation and location. It may start at the outpatient setting and may progress to the ED/ER, hospital unit bed, ICU, or specialty unit. Frequently all the elements from basic to comprehensive exam are done in one setting such as in a primary care setting or clinic.

The condition of the patient is the primary consideration in determining the type and amount of data needed to assess the patient's illness/disease/situation. The separation into levels is for general purposes and is meant to be descriptive rather than prescriptive. The purpose of leveling is to provide a framework to assist the learner in determining the appropriate data to collect.

Heart

	Level I	Level II	Level III	Level IV
Inspection	Skin color	Visible chest pulsations Rhythm analysis (Lead II, MCL_1) Jugular venous distension	12 lead ECG	Echocardiography Computer imaging Transesophageal echocardiography
Palpation	Radial/pedal pulse [presence, rate, rhythm, quality]* Capillary refill time	Brachial, femoral, popliteal, posterior tibial* Apex beat [PMI] Jugular venous pressure Thrill		Cardiac catheterization/PCTA Electrophysiology studies/mapping
Percussion		Borders of heart		
Auscultation	Blood pressure Heart sounds (S_1/S_2)	Identify extra heart sounds (S_3/S_4, splits, gallops) Carotid artery		Murmurs—Identify characteristics

Inspection: Level I

Inspection Techniques and Expected Findings	Unexpected Findings
Observe the patient's general presentation. Is the patient anxious, distressed, or neither? Skin color provides significant data about cardiovascular function. An optimally functioning heart is associated with skin that is warm to the touch, homogenous in coloring, and without significant moisture.	Skin pallor and cyanosis may suggest poor tissue perfusion. Skin diaphoresis may result from sympathetic stimulation as a result of diminished cardiac output.
Observe the hands and fingernails for any indicators of disease.	Cyanosis is best seen in the lips, nail beds, earlobes, mucous membranes or where skin is thin. It is due to arterial oxygen desaturation or increased oxygen extraction by the tissues.

Inspection Techniques and Expected Findings

Use the Schamroth's test to detect clubbing. When the distal phalanges of corresponding fingers of opposite hands are directly opposed, a small diamond-shaped "window" is typically apparent between the nail beds (Figure 24-12).

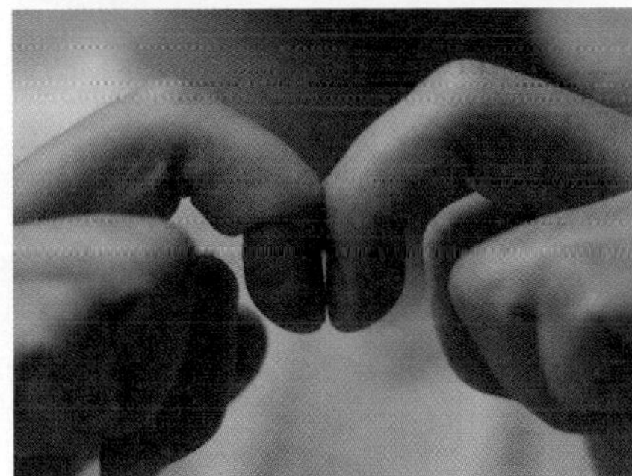

FIGURE 24-12 Schamroth's test

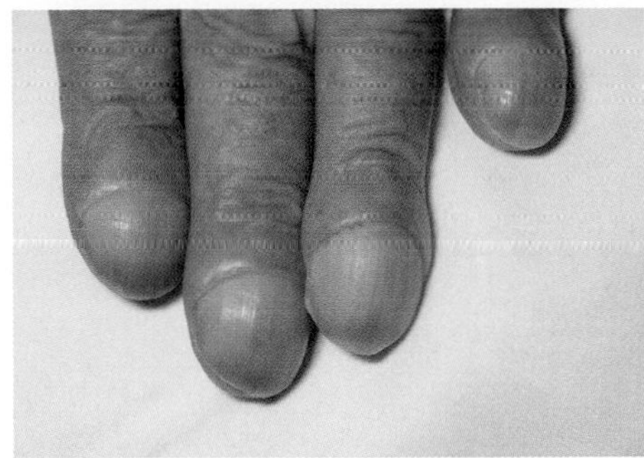

FIGURE 24-13 Nail clubbing is an unexpected finding
Source: Dr. M.A. Ansary/Science Source

Unexpected Findings

Splinter hemorrhages are tiny reddish brown vertical lines under the fingernail, thought to represent clot migration from infected heart valves in subacute bacterial endocarditis. They may be seen in other conditions such as trauma or vasculitis.

If this window is obliterated, the test is positive for nail clubbing, an increased convexity of the nail fold and loss of the normal, <165-degree angle between the nail bed and cuticle. It may indicate endocarditis and is a classic indicator of cyanotic congenital heart disease (Figure 24-13). It is not limited to cardiac conditions, and may be seen in pulmonary and GI conditions like malignancy, TB, chronic hypoxia, IBD, malabsorption, and liver cirrhosis.

Inspection: Level II

Observe the anterior chest for visible pulsations or movements. The apical impulse, also known as apex beat or point of maximal impulse, may be observed in the fifth left intercostal space along the midclavicular line in some individuals (Figure 24-14). It is generally not observed in healthy individuals unless the individual is quite thin and with very minimal developed chest musculature.

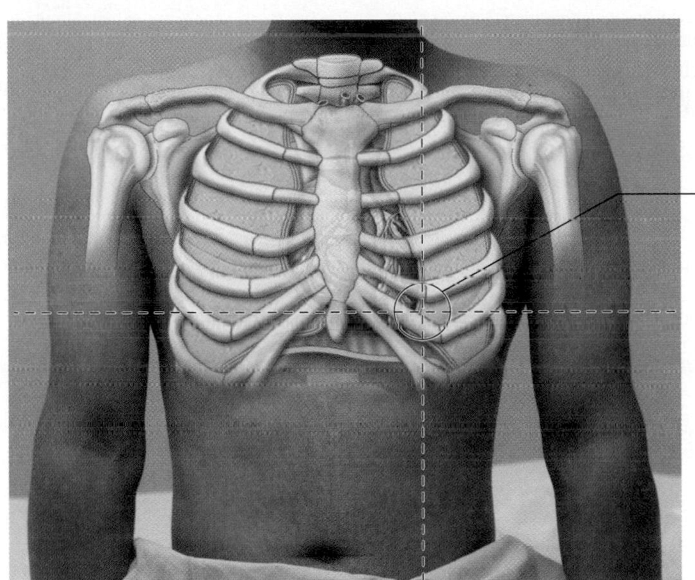

FIGURE 24-14 Location of apex beat on anterior chest

A visible apical beat may indicate left ventricular hypertrophy.

A lateral or inferior displacement of the apex impulse suggests cardiomegaly.

A dyskinetic (uncoordinated) impulse may be seen in ventricular dysfunction or aneurysm.

In emphysema or COPD, the impulse may be displayed inferiorly.

Forceful impulse may also be seen in hypertension.

In addition to a visible pulsation on the anterior chest, observe for **heaves** or **lifts**. If you suspect an increased force of contraction, place a pencil or any other straight object on the patient's precordium. The apex beat may also be found at other locations. Its presence is not necessarily pathologic, and often more visible when an individual sits up, bringing the heart closer to the chest wall.

In children, the apex beat may be seen in the fourth intercostal space medial to the nipple.

Next, observe the internal and external jugular veins of the neck (Figure 24-15). While the neck vessels are a part of the peripheral vascular system, pressure changes in the heart chamber are reflected in the jugular veins; changes are noted by measuring jugular venous pressure (JVP).

Jugular venous pressure is an indirect measurement of central venous pressure when there is no invasive central venous catheterization.

You will find the external jugular veins just above the clavicle, close to the insertion of the sternocleidomastoid muscle. JVP measurement relies on this visibility of the external jugular veins.

A heave or a lift is characteristic of a more forceful ventricular contraction suggesting hypertrophy. Excessive movement of the pencil or pen suggests the presence of a lift or heave.

In cases of dextrocardia, the apex beat may be seen on the right side.

Obesity, increased muscularity, large thorax, breast tissue, and diminished cardiac output interfere with its visualization. Tangential lighting of the precordium may help visualize the pulsations.

Inspection Techniques and Expected Findings	Unexpected Findings

The internal jugular veins, though more accurately representing the right atrial pressure, are buried within the sternocleidomastoid muscle and are therefore less visible.

The venous pulse is a visible ripple-like wave that is transmitted across the surface of the vein. (See Chapter 25 for further information.)

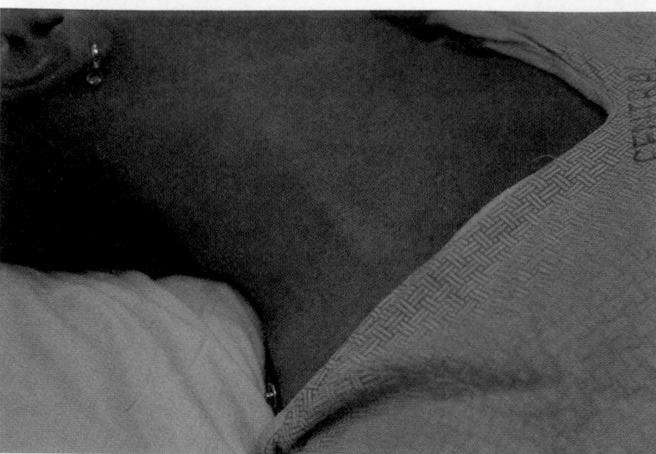

FIGURE 24-15 Observing external jugular veins

To measure JVP, begin with the patient in a supine position to aid visualization of the external jugular veins and locate the Angle of Louis (Figure 24-17). Position yourself to view the patient's neck from the right side. Tangential lighting on the neck with a penlight will be helpful.

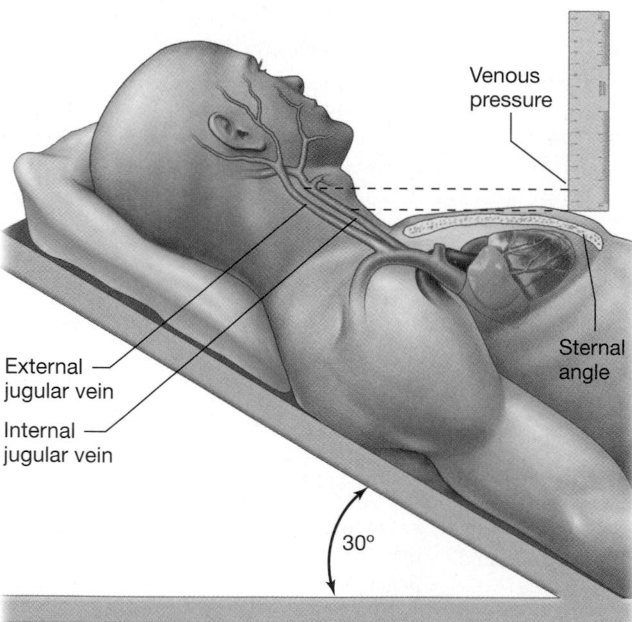

FIGURE 24-17 Patient positioned at 45-degree angle with provider looking across chest; lines drawn to measure JVP

In a supine position, gravity opposes the flow of blood into the right atrium causing distension of the neck veins, transmitting right atrial pressure changes up (retrograde) to the neck vessels (Figure 24-16) and making pulse pressure waves visible.

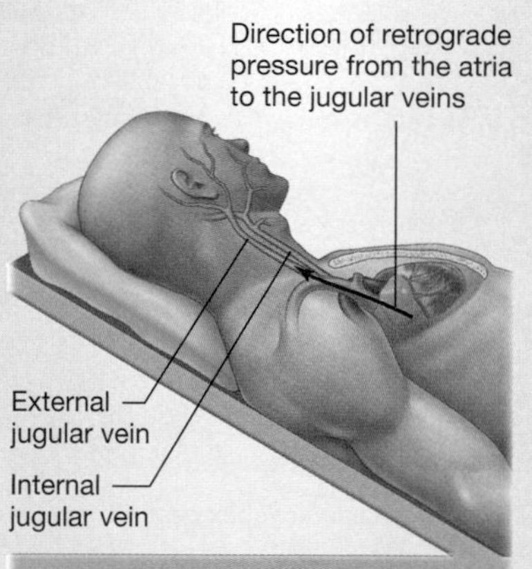

FIGURE 24-16 Retrograde reflection of right atrial pressure.

The jugular veins have direct communication with the superior vena cava, which directly connects to the right atrium allowing right atrial pressures to be reflected backward as pulse waves through the superior vena cava and to the jugular veins.

Inspection Techniques and Expected Findings

Next, use a pillow or raise the head of the bed to position the patient so that the neck is at a 45-degree angle. Now visualize a horizontal line (or use a ruler) that extends from the Angle of Louis through the neck. Visualize a second horizontal line that begins at the top of the distended jugular vein. The distance (in centimeters) between the horizontal lines as measured on a vertical line at 90 degrees to the horizontal lines is considered the right atrial pressure (see Figure 24-17).

Table 24-2 The JVP and carotid pulse differentiation

	JVP Pulsation	Carotid Pulsation
Wave/cardiac cycle	Two wave pulsation in one cardiac cycle	Only one beat
Palpability	Nonpalpable	palpable
Occludability	Occludable	Nonoccludable
Variability to position	Varies with position of the head	Does not vary with head up tilt
Variability with inspiration	Decreases with deep inspiration	Does not vary

ECG Analysis (Rhythm)

Perform a rhythm analysis to assess the competency of electrical conduction through the heart's conduction pathways. This measures the wave and interval parameters of the ECG complex to determine the presence of any rhythm disturbances or delays or blocking of electrical conduction, which may lead to lethal arrhythmias associated with any cardiac event.

Data for a rhythm analysis is obtained from an ECG tracing captured from electrodes with permanent polarity. Patients who require continuous monitoring of their heart activity generally have electrodes (chest leads) placed so that the ECG tracing is either Lead II or MCL1, meaning the ECG complex does not change unless the electrodes are actually moved and the heart's electrical activity is also constant, resulting in consistent ECG complexes.

The rhythm analysis begins with an understanding of the graph paper on which the ECG is printed (Figure 24-19). The graph paper is composed of large boxes that contain smaller boxes. Time is measured on the horizontal plane, so that one large box or the distance between two dark lines equals .20 seconds. Thus, each of the small boxes between the two dark lines is equal to .04 seconds. The amount of electrical activity (voltage) is measured on the vertical plane.

To perform an analysis, you will need calipers to facilitate accurate measurement of the waves and intervals (Figure 24-20). If one is not available, use a blank piece of paper and a pencil to mark the distance of each wave or interval.

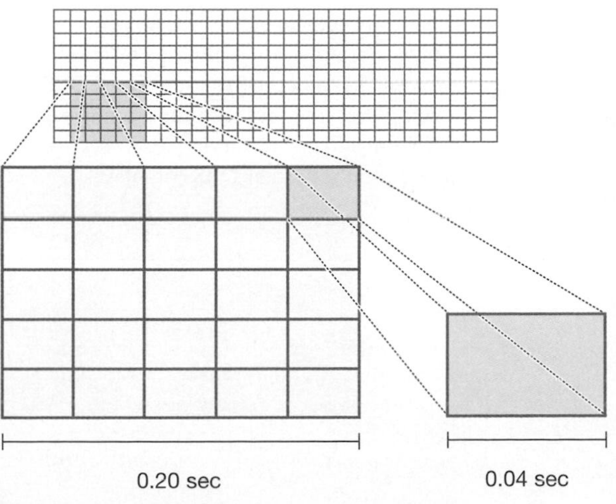

FIGURE 24-19 ECG graph paper

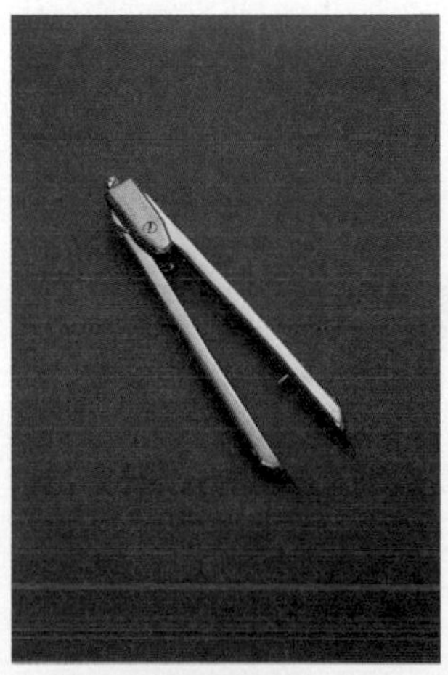

FIGURE 24-20 Calipers for rhythm analysis

Unexpected Findings

Any distension of the jugular veins above the clavicle with the patient positioned at 45 degrees is an unexpected finding and indicative of an increase in right atrial pressure, commonly resulting from right-sided heart failure (Figure 24-18). It should not be more than 3 cm above sternal angle. Also see Table 24-2 for the JVP and carotid pulse differentiation.

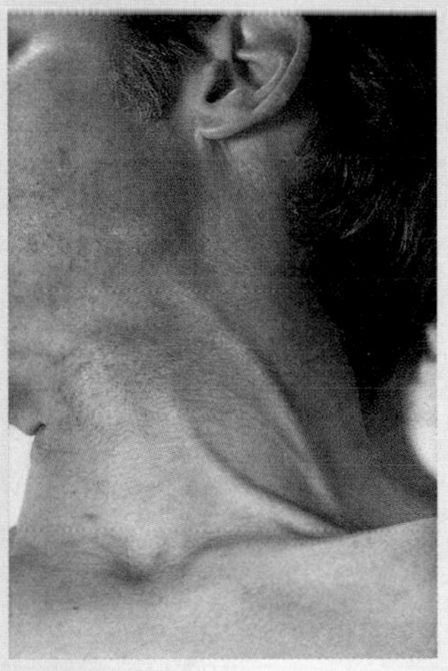

FIGURE 24-18 Jugular venous distension is an unexpected finding
Source: Wellcome Trust Library/Custom Medical Stock Photo

If there is previous damage to heart muscle, or there is evolving damage, the direction of electrical activity may result in characteristic alterations of the ECG complex, but the extent and location of damage cannot be determined from a rhythm strip.

Inspection Techniques and Expected Findings | **Unexpected Findings**

Using a systematic approach to rhythm analysis is essential to guide your analysis. The following is a suggested sequence, but this is not the only one that exists (Table 24-3). Each provider needs to find a sequence that is suitable for his or her own needs.

Table 24-3 Systematic approach to rhythm analysis

P wave	Establish presence/location of impulse generation
Ratio	P wave to QRS complex
Rhythm	equality of distance between QRS complexes
Rate	number of QRS complexes per established time unit
PR interval	conduction (depolarization) time from SA node through AV node
QRS complex	conduction (depolarization) time through bundle of His, Purkinje fibers of ventricles

Begin the rhythm analysis by identifying the presence of identical P waves (Figure 24-21a), which indicates that the S-A node in the atria is functioning as the pacemaker for the heart. Look at the configurations of each P wave to make sure that they are similar.

Absence of a P wave or altered wave configuration indicates that the pacemaker is somewhere else in the heart, most often in the atria or AV junction.

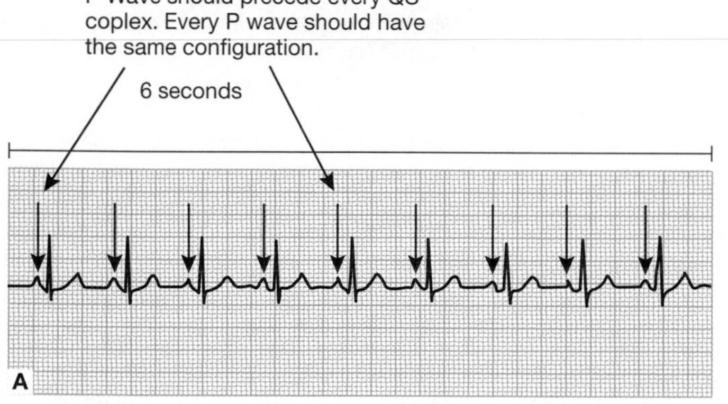

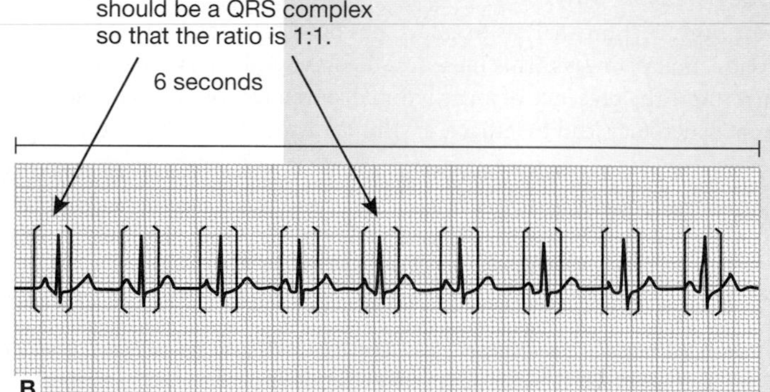

FIGURE 24-21A–B a. Assessment of P wave b. assessment of ratio [P wave to QRS]

Once you have established the presence of the P wave, determine that every P wave is followed by one QRS complex (Figure 24-21b). The ratio of P wave to QRS complex should be 1:1.

In certain rhythm alterations this ratio may be 2–3:1, which generally indicates some type of block within the conduction system.

Next, establish the rhythm by measuring the distance between QRS complexes (Figure 24-22). The QRS is generally used because it is large and comes to a point, making caliper placement easier.

Once you have identified the distance between two QRS complexes, place the calipers between the next two complexes, and then the next two. The distance between each QRS complex should measure out to be the same distance apart. A regular rhythm results from having only one pacemaker that is initiating each beat.

An irregular rhythm is present when there are ectopic beats, or QRS complexes (contractions) initiated by another pacemaker, not the SA node. These QRS complexes interfere with the established rhythm and create varying distances between the regular QRS complexes.

FIGURE 24-22 Assessment of rhythm [R to R distance]

Inspection Techniques and Expected Findings

Measure the rate by counting the number of QRS complexes in a 6-second strip and multiplying by 10. Six seconds on ECG paper is the time between two consecutive hash marks on the top of the graph paper (Table 24-4). To be more precise, you can measure the distance between two QRS complexes and count the number of small boxes between them. Table 24-4 gives the rate per number of small boxes. The expected adult rate is between 60 and 100 beats per minute.

Unexpected Findings

Above or below this range represents bradycardia and tachycardia, respectively.

Table 24-4 Calculation of heart rate according to number of small boxes

Boxes	Heart Rate	Boxes	Heart Rate	Boxes	Heart Rate
3	500	11	136	19	79
3.5	427	11.5	131	19.5	77
4	375	12	124	**20**	**75**
4.5	334	12.5	120	20.5	73
5	**300**	13	115	21	72
5.5	273	13.5	111	21.5	70
6	240	14	107	22	68
6.5	231	14.5	103	22.5	67
7	215	**15**	**100**	23	65
7.5	200	15.5	97	23.5	64
8	188	16	94	24	63
8.5	177	16.5	91	24.5	61
9	167	17	88	**24**	**60**
9.5	158	17.5	86	24.5	59
10	**150**	18	83	26	58
10.5	143	18.5	81	26.7	57

Note: numbers in bold represent one large box. A quicker calculation is to count the number of large boxes between R – R intervals. Refer to Figure 24-19 to see boxes.

The last two steps measure intervals of the ECG complex. First measure the PR interval by placing one point of the calipers on the beginning of the P wave and the other point on the beginning of the QRS complex (Figure 24-23). This is a measurement of the time it takes for an impulse to be conducted through the atria and through the AV node, and should be in the range of .12 to .20 seconds.

An interval greater than .20 seconds indicates some type of an AV block and a interval less than .12 seconds may indicate that the pacemaker of the heart is somewhere below the SA node.

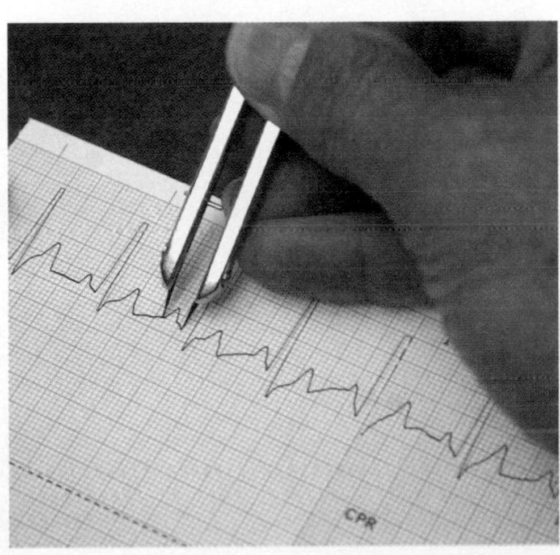

FIGURE 24-23 Assessment of PR interval

Inspection Techniques and Expected Findings

Measuring the QRS complex is the last step (Figure 24-24). It should be between .08 and .12 seconds, which measures the time it takes to conduct the impulse through the ventricles via the bundle of His, bundle branches, and Purkinje fibers.

A time interval greater than .12 seconds often represents some type of block within this ventricular conduction system.

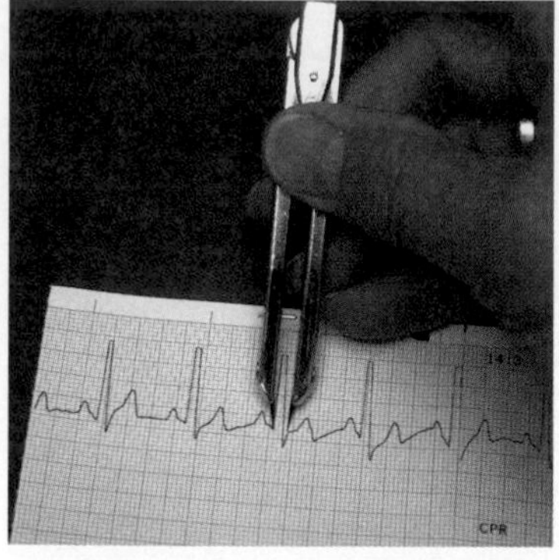

FIGURE 24-24 Assessment of QRS complex

Rhythm analyses when any of the six parameters are outside the expected criteria are identified as cardiac arrhythmias. Common arrhythmias are identified in Table 24-5 and further descriptions and characteristics of these arrhythmias are presented at the end of the chapter (Conditions and Disorders).

A rhythm analysis where all of the six parameters fall within the expected criteria is identified as Normal Sinus Rhythm [NSR].

Table 24-5 Common arrhythmias based on ECG wave form alterations

	NSR	Alteration	Arrhythmia
P wave	Present	Absent Altered configuration	Nodal rhythms Supraventricular tachycardias Wandering pacemaker
Ratio	1:1	Not 1:1	Atrial fibrillation Atrial flutter 2nd degree AV block (Mobitz II)
Rhythm	Regular	Not regular	Sinus arrhythmia Atrial fibrillation Atrial flutter Premature (ectopic) beats
Rate	60–100	Too fast > 100 Too slow < 60	Tachycardia Bradycardia
P-R Interval	.12–.20 seconds	> .20 seconds < .20 seconds Variable	1st degree AV block, 2nd degree AV block (Mobitz I) Nodal (junctional) rhythms 2nd degree AV block (Mobitz I)
QRS Interval	.06–.12 seconds	> .12 seconds	Bundle Branch Blocks

Inspection: Level III

Patients requiring a Level III inspection are experiencing some type of a cardiac event. In most situations, the patient is experiencing angina with the threat of developing into an acute coronary event, in the process of an acute coronary event or a completed coronary event. Individuals may also present with various types of arrhythmias or some type of cardiac trauma. In any of these situations, a 12-lead ECG would be obtained and analyzed for the presence of any damage to myocardial muscle.

Inspection Techniques and Expected Findings	Unexpected Findings
The 12-lead ECG analyses, in contrast to a rhythm analysis, are three dimensional methodical evaluations of the heart's electrical conduction. Interpretation of the 12-lead ECG identifies the location and extent of myocardial damage or death, and provides information related to any rhythm disturbances (arrhythmia). As previously described, the primary direction of conduction (vector) is downward, from the atria to the ventricles, toward the left side of the heart in an anterior orientation. To obtain a 12-lead ECG tracing, electrodes are placed at specific locations (see Figure 24-25) on the patient and then manipulated to be either positive or negative. Each lead of the ECG has a specific electrode designated as positive, which results in a distinct configuration of the ECG complex. The ECG leads are identified as bipolar or unipolar. Bipolar leads (I, II, III) have a negative and positive pole, whereas unipolar leads (aVR, aVL, aVF, V1-6) consist of only a positive pole (Figure 24-25). To correctly analyze the ECG, you must know what lead is positive or negative for each of the 12 leads and whether the electrical vector is directed towards or away from the positive pole.	Significant damage to the myocardium (infarction) alters the vector of the heart. The damaged or dead myocardial tissue is unable to conduct the electrical impulse, so the electrical conduction and the overall direction of the vector become redirected (Figure 24-26). The extent of redirection is dependent on the location and extent of the damage. Initial ECG alterations associated with an acute cardiac event will produce alterations in the ST segment and T wave. Alterations in the T wave and ST segment may be observed during the rhythm analysis, but are not necessarily involved in any rhythm disturbances. They are more related to changes in the amplitude and direction of electrical conduction. The two changes that are closely associated with myocardial ischemia, injury, and infarction are T wave inversion and ST segment elevation (Figure 24-27). While T wave inversion is primarily associated with myocardial ischemia, tall, flattened, and biphasic T waves may also be seen. Tall T waves occur very early in the ischemic process and may have disappeared before the patient is examined. Biphasic T waves may be present early but most likely will evolve into T wave inversion.

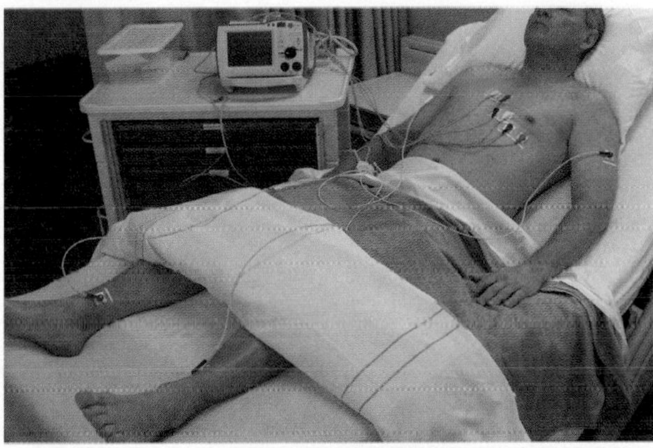

FIGURE 24-25 12-lead ECG poles [bipolar/unipolar]

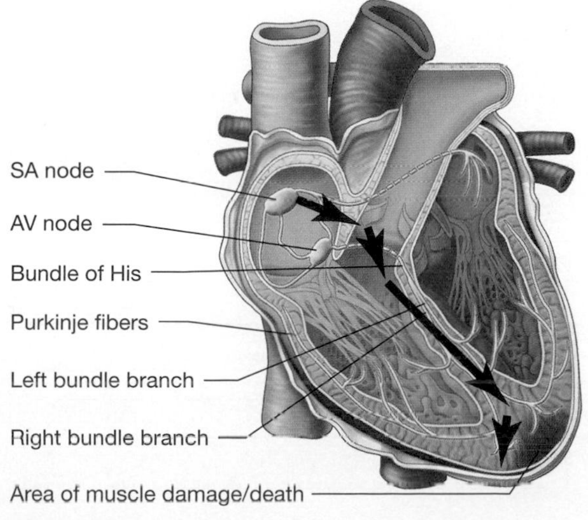

FIGURE 24-26 Altered vector

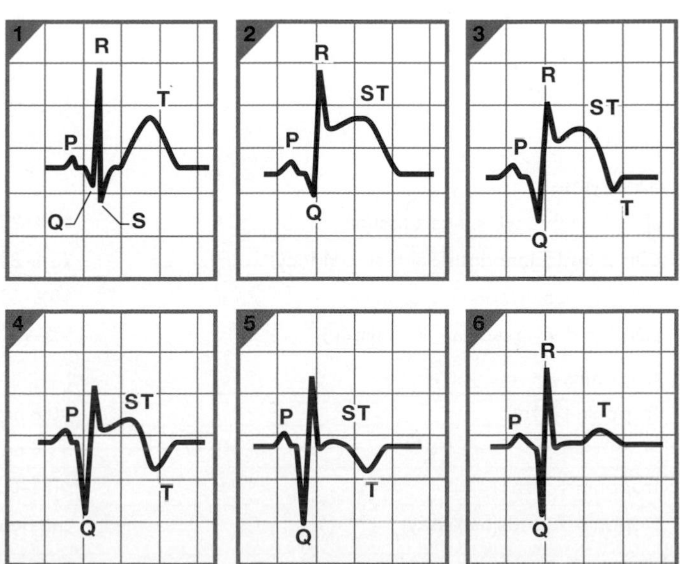

FIGURE 24-27 T wave, ST segment changes in Leads I, II, III, aVR, aVL, aVF

Inspection Techniques and Expected Findings	Unexpected Findings

PRACTICE POINT: ECG Changes

ECG changes by themselves are not considered diagnostic for myocardial infarction; they are a part of the overall diagnostic criteria that given their manifestations in the presence of other signs and symptoms determines whether a diagnosis of MI may be made.

ST segment elevation is considered another manifestation of acute myocardial ischemia, and is now used as a basis for classifying myocardial infarctions into two groups: STEMI (ST segment elevation) or NSTEMI (non-STEMI eleveation MI). NSTEMI is typically accompanied by an elevation of specific enzymes that provide evidence of actual muscle tissue necrosis (Earnest & Tadros, 2007). NSTEMI is limited in damage and not transmural.

Evaluation of an acute cardiac event or cardiac trauma also includes assessment for elevation of specific cardiac cell enzymes released into the blood (Table 24-6). When muscle cells and tissue are damaged or die, they release specific intracellular enzymes. Certain enzymes are released immediately and can be measured soon after the heart muscle is injured or dies, while others are released later and can be measured hours after the cardiac event.

Myocardial damage is suspected or confirmed if obtained blood enzyme levels exceed the expected parameters.

Table 24-6 Cardiac data: Enzymes and markers related to acute coronary event

Aspartate-Aminotransferase (AST)		**Reference Values**
	Adult	Male — 10–40 U/L
		Female — 9–25 U/L
	Newborn	2–3 times higher
	Aged	Slight increase
Creatine Kinase (CK)		
	Adult	Male — 40–150 U/L
		Female — 60–400 U/L
Isoenzymes		
CK - I Brain (BB)		0%–1%
CK - II Heart (MB)		<3% or 7.5 ng/mL
CK - III Muscle (MM)		95%–10%
Lactic Dehydrogenase (LDH)		
	Adult	45–90 U/L
	Pregnancy	Slight increase during labor/delivery, or other exercise
Newborn — 1st week of life		160–450 U/L
Children		60–170 U/L (decreases with age)
Elderly		55–102 U/L
Isoenzymes		
LDH 1(erythrocytes, heart tissue)		17%–27%
LDH 2 (reticuloendothelial tissue, kidney)		23%–28%
LDH3 (lungs, lymph nodes, spleen)		18%–28%
LDH4 (kidney, placenta, liver tissue)		5%–15%
Troponins		
Troponin I (cTnI)		<0.6 ng/mL
		>1.5 ng/mL (consistent with MI)
Troponin T (cTnT)		>0.1–0.2 ng/mL (consistent with MI)
Troponin T (Bedside Assay)		can detect values as low as 0.08 ng/mL

Inspection: Level IV

The level IV inspection would be advanced diagnostic tests and procedures that may provide further information as to what is the cause of the patient's complaints or manifestations.

Diagnostic tests and procedures

What	How	Why
Echocardiography (Echo)	Handheld device that emits high frequency sound waves that are received, read, and interpreted by a computer to produce images of the size, structure, and motion of heart	It provides information regarding the health of the heart and data regarding arrhythmias.
Computer Imaging (MRI, CAT, PET)	Magnetic field surrounding patient stimulates H+ atoms of body giving off radio signals that are received, read, and interpreted by a computer to produce images of heart	It provides detailed pictures of heart (chambers/valves) without an invasive catheterization.
MRA	Same as MRI but dye is used to image blood vessels	
Transesophageal Echocardiography (TEE) Same as Echocardiography	A transducer and a receiver are passed into the esophagus where ultrasonic sound waves are fed to a computer that produces images of heart.	It produces higher resolution images than echocardiogram because sound waves don't have to pass through skin, muscle, and bone before received by the computer.
Cardiac Catheterization (Cardiac Cath)	Small catheter inserted into femoral/radial artery and guided through artery to heart/ coronary arteries. Dye, fluoroscopy used to guide placement of catheter.	It visualizes coronary arteries for determining the extent of arterial occlusion by atherosclerosis.
PCTA (Percutaneous Transluminal Coronary Angioplasty)	Same procedure as for catheterization, but catheter tip contains stent that is placed at occlusion site of artery. When in place, a balloon inflates and expands the stent to reduce occlusion.	It opens up artery to restore blood flow to cardiac muscle.
Electrophysiology Studies	Electrode tipped catheter is placed in femoral vein and threaded and guided into heart with fluoroscopy. When in place, electrical impulses are sent through heart via cardiac conduction pathways to evaluate the conduction system.	It gives more detailed information than conventional ECG. It also helps to assess and diagnose various arrhythmias.
Mapping	An electrophysiology procedure, but uses more catheters/electrodes that are guided and placed at various points in the heart. Electrical impulses are sent to catheter electrodes.	It locates point of origin of an arrhythmia. If location identified, area is ablated (removal of point of origin by freezing/radiofrequency).

Palpation: Level I

Palpation Techniques and Expected Findings	Unexpected Findings
Your initial palpation of pulses may be limited to assessment of the most distal pulses, the radial and pedal. If the expected parameters of these pulses meet the criteria, you can assume that all prior pulses meet the expected criteria. Expected findings for all pulse locations are as follows: Rate: 60–100 Rhythm: Regular Amplitude: Quality +2 (Refer to Chapter 8, Vital Signs.)	Unexpected findings would be any patient assessment data that did not meet or fall within the expected criteria. A pulse rate of less than 60 is considered bradycardia, and is problematic if accompanied by any of the following symptoms: fainting, dizziness, weakness, fatigue, SOB, chest pain, confusion/memory problems, tiring easily during physical activity.

Palpation Techniques and Expected Findings	Unexpected Findings

PRACTICE POINT: Bradycardia

By itself, bradycardia doesn't indicate pathology. It is not unusual for an athlete in top condition or healthy young adults to have a heart rate in the 50s. Without an ECG, it is impossible to determine if there is a cause for it.

A heart rate greater than 100 is considered tachycardia. Increasing the heart rate is a physiological response to the need for more oxygen, which frequently occurs during strenuous activity or exercise. It also occurs from smoking, increased intake of caffeine, and frequently occurs with a fever.

The pulse should have a regular rhythm (evenly spaced palpable pulse waves)

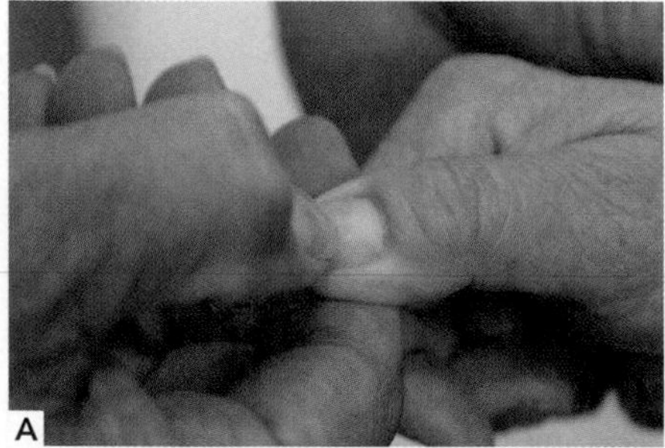
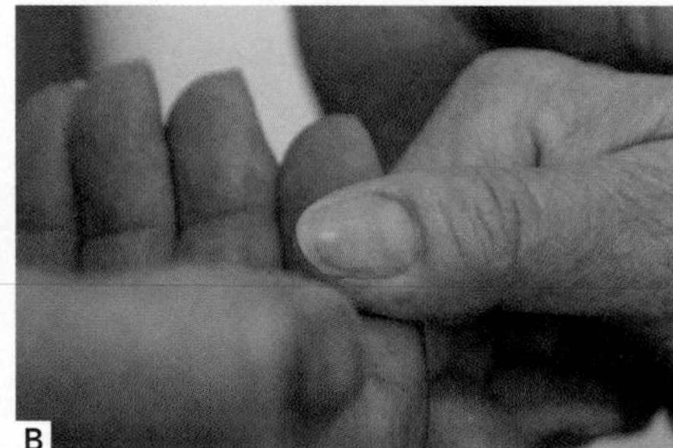

FIGURE 24-28A–B Capillary refill time (**a** & **b**)

Assess the quality and amplitude of the pulse. The pulse should feel palpable without exerting undue pressure over the site. Each pulse should also demonstrate the same quality.

THINK LINK: Absent Pedal Pulse

A palpable pedal pulse is absent in about 20% of the population. Before you decide that a patient lacks a pedal pulse, palpate over the foot's entire surface. The pulse may be located elsewhere than expected. If you still cannot locate it, check the posterior tibial pulse. If the pedal pulse is nonpalpable, assess other parameters (color, warmth, CRT) to assess for adequate perfusion of the foot.

CRT is a common indicator of peripheral tissue perfusion and state of hydration. It refers to the amount of time it takes for capillary circulation to return to the fingertips after capillary circulation is obliterated.

To assess CRT, hold the patient's fingernail above his or her heart level and exert pressure on the finger pad or nail bed by pinching it between your thumb and finger until it turns white (Figure 24-28a). Release the pressure while noting the time needed for color to return. Expected time is less than 3 seconds (Figure 24-28).

In neonates, pressure is exerted on the sternum for 5 seconds.

Unexpected Findings

Many individuals experience a periodic burst of tachycardia, which frequently produces palpitations (a conscious awareness of the heart beating).

It is unusual for an individual to have persistent tachycardia unless there is some underlying pathology. Many symptoms associated with bradycardia are also seen with tachycardia, and their occurrence indicates the need for further evaluation.

An irregular pulse rhythm has many causes.

A regular irregularity indicates that the irregular pulse rhythm occurs in a regular cycle.

An irregular irregular pulse rhythm indicates that there is no regular cycle to the irregular pattern. Its most common causeis atrial fibrillation, which is caused by multiple sites of the atria generating electrical impulses, all of which are conducted to the AV node. The AV node responds to only a certain number of atrial impulses, so that the impulses are conducted through the AV node vary, resulting in an irregular irregular ventricular rhythm.

A variation in pulse quality is related to variations in the stroke volume. Obstructed blood flow to the heart reduces the amount of blood delivered to the ventricles, thus reducing the stroke volume. A reduced amount of blood ejected from the ventricle causes a diminished expansion of the arterial wall, causing a decreased quality.

An arterial obstruction at a point in the artery before the pulse location may also cause a decreased pulse quality by effectively reducing the amount of blood that reaches the pulse location.

An increase in pulse quality indicates a greater stroke volume or a more forceful ventricular contraction, indicating a greater workload of the heart.

A prolonged CRT is suggestive of hypoperfusion and/or dehydration, frequently associated with hypovolemia.

In adults prolonged CRT is also suggestive of congestive heart failure and/or peripheral vascular disease; however, it is of questionable usefulness and value in providing clinical data (Mangione, 2008).

Palpation: Level II

Palpation Techniques and Expected Findings	Unexpected Findings

Palpate the other pulse locations for the brachial, femoral, popliteal, and posterior tibial. Use the same parameters for the remaining pulses (see Chapter 8).

If distal pulses (radial, pedal) are weak or variable, assess the proximal pulses to determine if the quality of the pulse is consistent in all areas or if the quality of the proximal pulses is different from that of the distal pulses.

Palpation of the precordium is done to assess for any palpable pulsations, heaves, or thrills The patient should be in the supine position with the total chest visible and the provider positioned to the right of the patient (see Figure 24-29).

A palpable lifting sensation under the sternum and anterior chest left sternal border suggests a central precordial heave, frequently associated with right ventricular hypertrophy (RVH). Severe RVH associated with congenital disorders may cause visible bulges at the left sternal border.

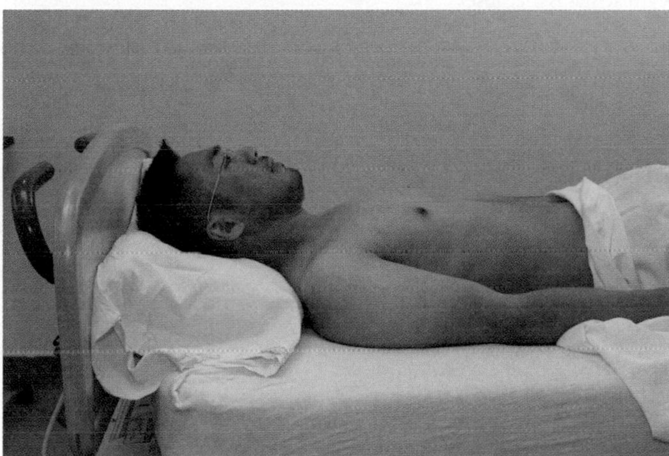

FIGURE 24-29 Patient position for palpation of precordium

Areas that are palpated are the left sternal border, left and right second interspace, and the epigastric area. Also palpate the chest for the presence of the apex pulse, or point of maximum impulse.

With warm hands, place your hand, or the proximal halves of the four fingers held together, on the patient's chest wall. Note the presence of any palpable pulsations). Do not use excessive pressure on the chest; let any movements rise up to the hand. Excessive pressure may hinder tactile input.

Also palpate for the presence of thrills.

Expected findings would be the absence of any pulsations or thrills.

Palpate the apex beat in the same location it was visible—fifth intercostal space, at or lateral to the midclavicular line. You may palpate the apex beat even if the pulsation is not visible.

After grossly locating the pulse, determine the exact location by moving one or two fingers to the spot (Figure 24-30). The pulse occupies a space that is no larger than a nickel (1–2 cm). It should feel like a gentle tapping against your fingers.

Displacement of the apex beat is often associated with ventricular enlargement. Displacement may be to the left or right, depending on the affected ventricle. In addition to displacement, the intensity may be increased or it may occupy a larger space.

Displacement to the left (laterally) and downward is suggestive of cardiomegaly or left ventricular hypertrophy.

A displacement to the right at the left sternal border accompanies R ventricular hypertrophy.

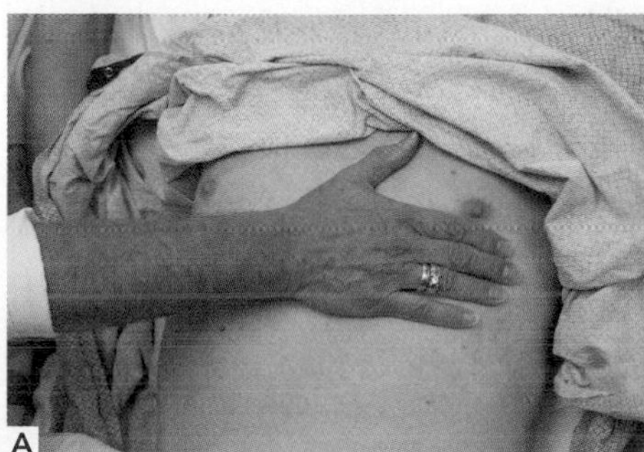

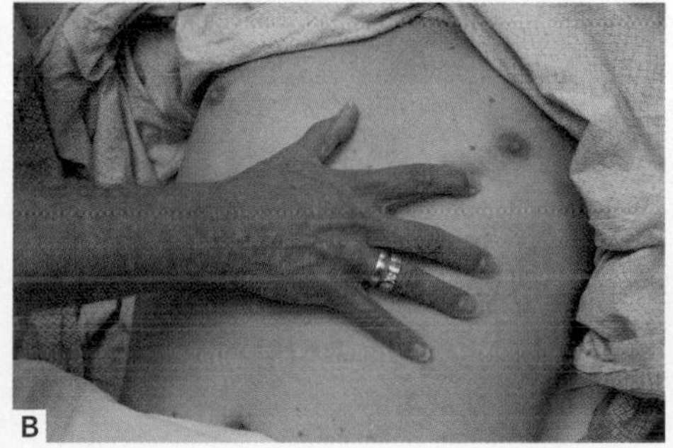

FIGURE 24-30A–B Location of the apical pulse

Palpation Techniques and Expected Findings	Unexpected Findings
If you are unable to locate the pulse in the supine position, turn the patient onto the left side to bring the heart closer to the chest wall. Still, the apex beat is palpable in only about one half of adults. The duration of the pulse is brief, occupying only the first part of systole. Once you locate the apex beat, place your other hand over the patient's carotid artery to relate the carotid pulse to the cardiac cycle. The two pulsations should be felt simultaneously.	

Percussion: Levels II–IV

Percussion is used to define the borders of the heart; however, its usefulness is limited because characteristics of the chest may hinder obtaining accurate data. For example, muscle mass, adipose tissue, and breast tissue may interfere with production of satisfactory percussion tones. Chest x-rays, scans, and echocardiography have become more reliable methods and have become the preferred means to determine cardiac size.

There is only one technique used in percussion and only one result that can be obtained, so the level at which it is used is based on the need for this information related to the patient's cardiac status. Because percussion is an advanced technique, a beginning provider would not use it in a Level I exam.

Percussion Techniques and Expected Findings	Unexpected Findings
In instances in which percussion is the only way to determine cardiac size, begin the procedure by starting percussion at the left anterior axillary line. Move the stationary hand medially toward the sternal border listening for the change from resonance to dullness. Proceed upward on the chest, interspace by interspace.	Unexpected findings would be borders of the heart that are percussed outside of the expected area, indicating an enlarged heart.
On the left side, cardiac dullness generally begins at the midclavicular line, fifth intercostal space. As you progress upward, the line slopes inward so that by the time you reach the second intercostal space, dullness coincides with the left sternal border. On the right side, the area of decreased resonance or relative dullness will be heard just at the right sternal border, indicating the right border of the heart. The absolute heart dullness extends approximately 3 to 4 cm to the left from the left sternal border. At each point where there is a change in percussion tone, make a mark with a pen so that the overall outline of the heart may be observed. Percussion in the left parasternal line estimates the superior heart border. The relative dullness starts at the third intercostal space, and the absolute dullness occurs at the fourth intercostal space. The inferior heart border is not amenable to precise percussion.	

Auscultation: Level I

Auscultation Techniques and Expected Findings	Unexpected Findings
Initial auscultation related to the cardiovascular system is obtaining the blood pressure and is data that has already been obtained during the vital sign assessment (see Chapter 8). Other parts of the exam related to auscultation are obtaining the apical pulse and heart sounds.	
Auscultate the carotid artery for the presence of a bruit by placing the diaphragm of the stethoscope over the location of the carotid pulse. The expected finding would be that no sound is heard. To obtain the apical pulse, place the diaphragm of the stethoscope over the precordium and listen for the sounds produced during the cardiac cycle (Figure 24-31). Each heartbeat consists of two sounds, frequently identified as "lub" and "dub." Most often one will be louder than the other. Counting the loudest sound is the easiest way to obtain the heart rate.	The presence of a bruit indicates atherosclerotic plaque build up on the interior lumen of the carotid artery. A carotid bruit is a risk factor for the development of a thrombus that breaks away, becoming an embolus and causing a stroke.

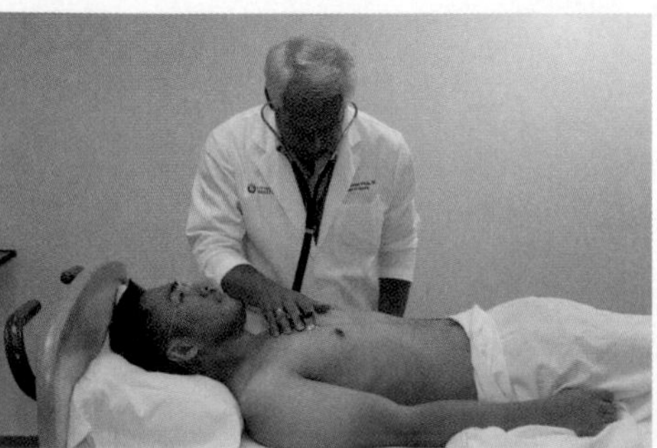

FIGURE 24-31 Auscultation of apical pulse

Auscultation Techniques and Expected Findings

The rhythm should be regular, but be aware of the presence of sinus arrhythmia in children and young adults. This occurs when the rhythm varies with the patient's ventilations, increasing at the end of inspiration and decreasing at the end of expiration.

The apical rate and rhythm are assessed in much the same way as the radial pulse rate and rhythm. The rate should range from 60 to 100, although age variations do exist.

PRACTICE POINT: Heart Sounds

Before auscultating heart sounds, inform the patient that it is common for this procedure to take more time than might be expected because the characteristics of the heart sounds need careful assessment. The amount of time does not indicate that there is something wrong with the heart.

It is essential that auscultation of heart sounds be done in as quiet an environment as possible. Heart sounds are low-frequency sounds that may be difficult to hear. It is also essential to maintain the patient's comfort, especially keeping the patient warm to prevent shivering and excessive movement—factors that interfere with hearing heart sounds. Avoid placing a cold stethoscope on exposed skin. If necessary, rub the stethoscope diaphragm on your clothing or hold the chest piece in your hands to warm it.

When listening to heart sounds, it is tempting to try to pay attention to all possible sounds at once. Avoid doing this. Learn to listen for and identify each sound before moving on to the next. It takes time to tune in to the various sounds, but it is an important to not rush and possibly miss something important.

Positioning the patient appropriately can help to identify heart sounds.

There are four positions for listening to heart sounds in which the patient may be placed; sitting and recumbent positions are the most common, but neither is better than the other (Figure 24-32). The patient's position is determined by where you are in the exam.

The other two positions are used to facilitate augmentation of the heart sounds. These are the left lateral decubitus position and sitting leaning forward. Either of these positions brings the heart closer to the chest wall, so the heart sounds may be easier to hear. These positions may also augment extra sounds and help to identify the presence of murmurs.

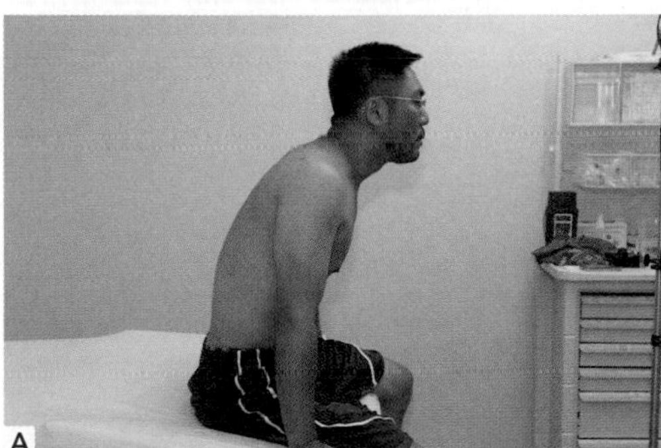

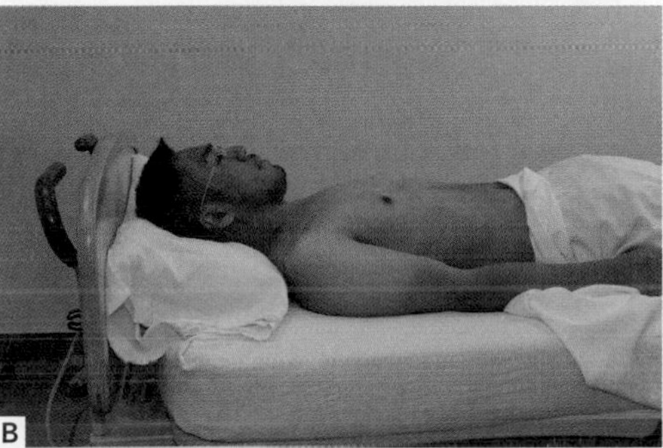

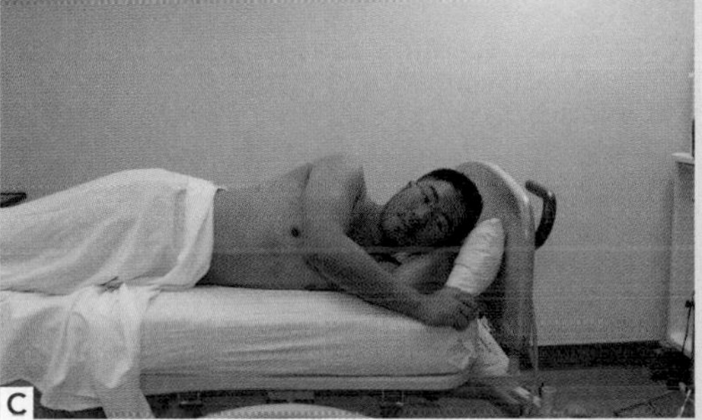

FIGURE 24-32A–C Positions for auscultation of the heart (a, b, c)

Unexpected Findings

If irregularities are heard, determine if there is a pattern to the rhythm or not. There may be regular irregularities or irregular irregularities (see earlier discussion). Count the pulse for one minute if the rhythm is irregular.

If you detect irregularities, assess for a pulse deficit, a discrepancy between the apical pulse and radial pulse. Generally, the apical rate will be greater than the radial rate. The pulse deficit is the difference between the peripheral rate and the apical rate.

THINK LINK: Pulse Deficit

A **pulse deficit** is most commonly associated with atrial fibrillation. Each impulse generated is capable of initiating ventricular systole. However, the AV node is unable to respond to each impulse, conducting it only when it has had time to repolarize and respond to another atrial impulse. AV node repolarization occurs irregularly, so its response to atrial impulses is sporadic.

In atrial fibrillation, each AV conducted impulse may not provide enough filling time for the ventricle, causing a reduced stroke volume, which may not be sufficient to create a palpable pulse wave. Thus, not every ventricular systole is included in the pulse count when only a radial pulse rate is taken.

Each ventricular systole, however, does create a heart sound. Thus, the apical pulse rate will be greater than the peripheral pulse rate. This difference is the pulse deficit.

Auscultation Techniques and Expected Findings | **Unexpected Findings**

Even though the heart sounds are produced by closure of specific valves, they are not heard directly over the anatomical location of the valves. Heart sounds follow the direction of blood flow and are transmitted to five auscultatory sites that coincide with the direction of the blood away from the heart valves (Figure 24-33). However, do not limit auscultation to those sites only, but establish a consistent routine, going from base to apex or apex to base. Begin auscultation by listening in each area with the diaphragm and then repeat the sequence with the bell.

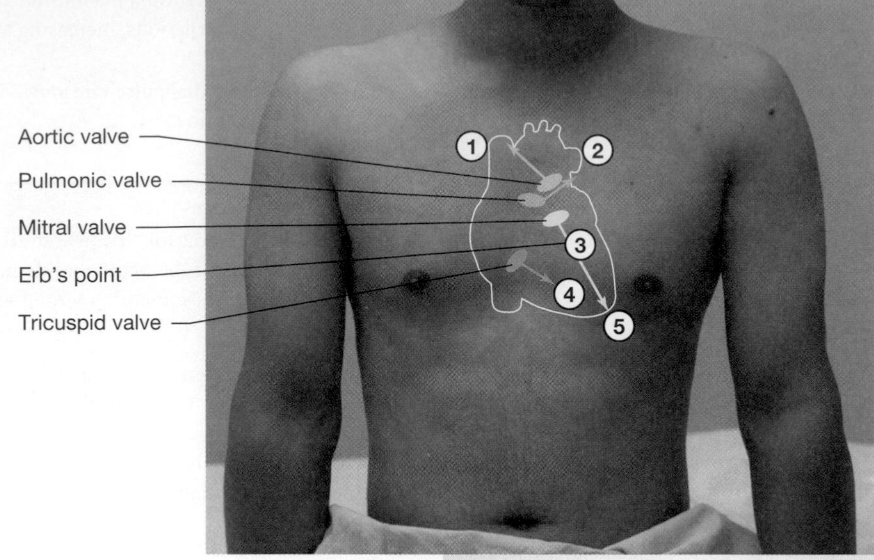

FIGURE 24-33 Locations of auscultatory sites on chest

The five auscultatory sites are identified and located in the following areas. Going from top to bottom and right to left they are as follows (Figure 24-33):

- Aortic area—second right intercostal space, R sternal border (Figure 24-34a)
- Pulmonic area—second left intercostal space, L sternal border (Figure 24-34b)
- Erb's point—third left intercostal space, L sternal border (Figure 24-34c)
- Tricuspid area—fourth left intercostal space, L sternal border (Figure 24-34d)
- Mitral area—fifth intercostal space, midclavicular line (Figure 24-34e)

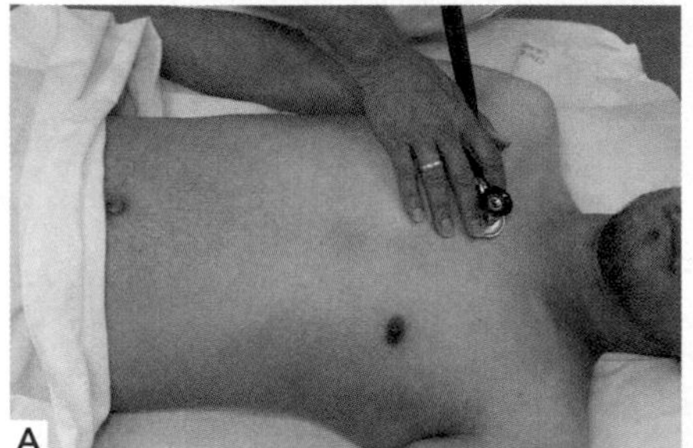

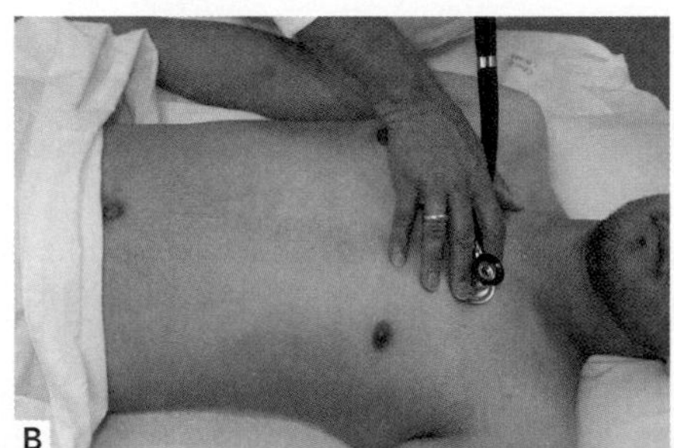

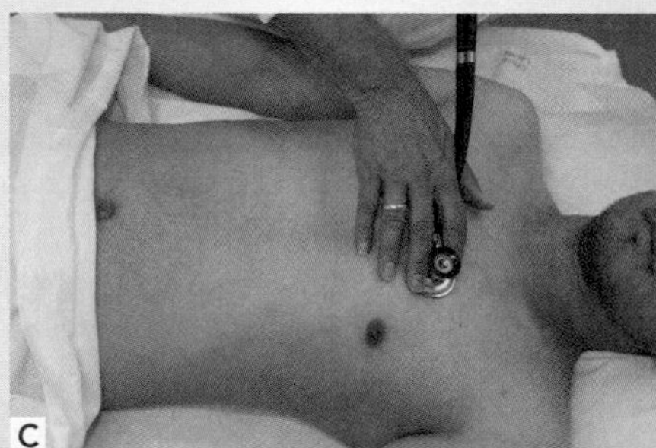

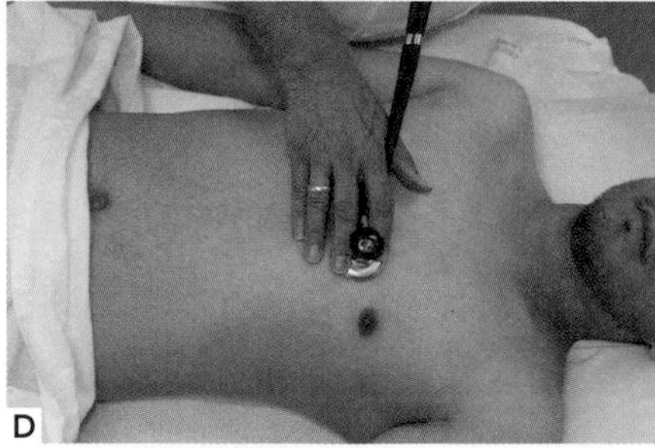

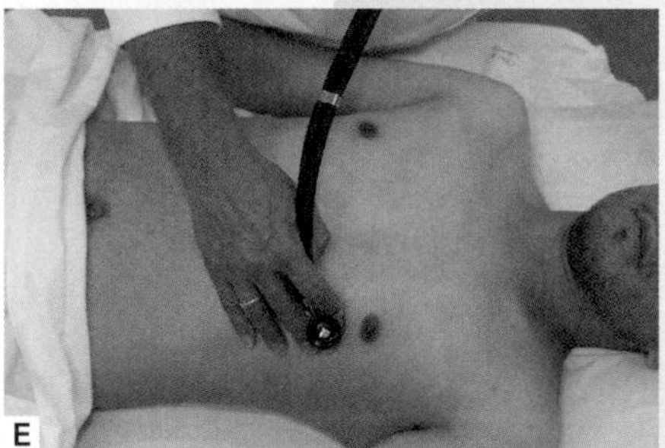

FIGURE 24-34A–E Five sites for heart auscultation: **a)** aortic area; **b)** pulmonic area; **c)** Erb's point; **d)** tricuspid area; **e)** mitral area

During auscultation, inch the stethoscope along, going from site to site. This allows you to appreciate the full spectrum of cardiac sounds. Pause long enough at each site to identify all the possible sounds. Initially this takes a minute or more per area. The following is a suggested routine for examining the heart sounds:

- Assess for rate and rhythm
- Identify and differentiate between valvular heart sounds (S_1/S_2)
- Identify the presence of extra (nonvalvular) heart sounds (S_3/S_4)/murmurs

PRACTICE POINT: Auscultation Tips

You may find it helpful to close your eyes while listening to heart sounds. This helps you to focus and concentrate fully on the heart sounds and not be distracted by other stimuli. Make sure that the earpieces of the stethoscope fit tightly into your ear canal. The tighter the fit, the greater the elimination of other extraneous sounds.

Do not listen through any clothing.

Do no let the tubing rub against clothing, side rails, or equipment to prevent hearing any extraneous noise.

Heart Sounds		Cardiac Cycle Timing	Ausculation Site	Position	Pitch
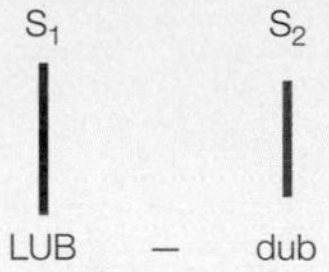 S_1 S_2 LUB — dub	S_1	Start of systole Closure of mitral (M1) and tricuspid (T1) valves	Best at apex with diaphragm	Position does not affect the sound	High Mitral closes (0.02 seconds) ahead of tricuspid, contributing the majority of S_1 sound
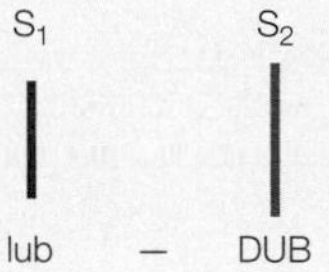 S_1 S_2 lub — DUB	S_2	End of systole Closure of aortic (A2) and pulmonic (P2) valves	Both at 2nd intercostal space (ICS); pulmonary component best at left sternal border (LSB); aortic component best at RBS with diaphragm	Sitting or supine	High Aortic closes before pulmonic valve, contributing the majority of S_2 sound
Splits					
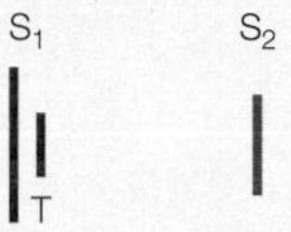 S_1 S_2 T	Split S_1	Beginning of systole	If normal, at 2nd ICS, LSB abnormal if heard at apex	Better heard in the supine position	High
S_1 S_2	Fixed Split S_2	End of systole	Both at 2nd ICS: pulmonary component best at LSB; aortic component best at right sternal border (RSB) with diaphragm	Better heard in the supine position	High
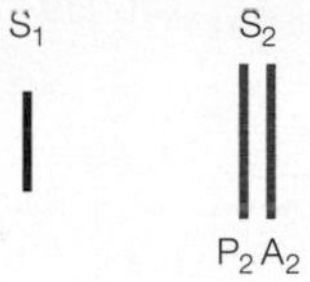 S_1 S_2 P_2 A_2	Paradoxial Split S_2	End of systole	Both at 2nd ICS; pulmonary component best at LSB; aortic component best at RSB with diaphragm	Better heard in the supine position	High
Expiration 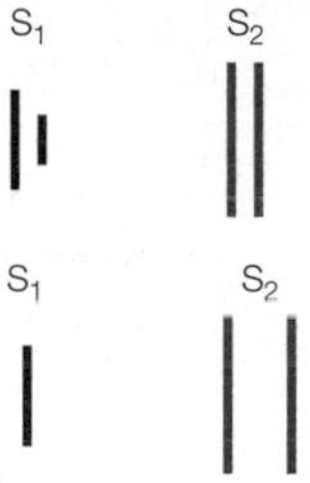 S_1 S_2 S_1 S_2	Wide Split S_2	End of systole	Both at 2nd ICS; pulmonary component best at LSB; aortic component best at RSB with diaphragm	Better heard in the supine position	High
Extra Heart Sounds					
Inspiration 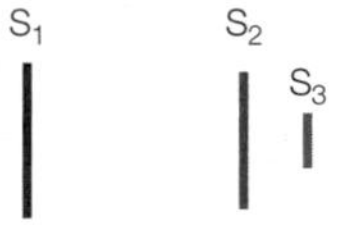 S_1 S_2 S_3	S_3	Early diastole right after S_2	Apex with the bell	Auscultated better in left lateral position or supine	Low
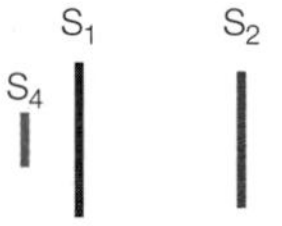 S_4 S_1 S_2	S_4	Late diastole right before S_1	Apex with the bell	Auscultated better in left lateral position or supine	Low

FIGURE 24-35 Schematic representations of heart sounds

Auscultation Techniques and Expected Findings

Heart sounds are characterized according pitch, intensity, duration, and timing in the cardiac cycle.

- Heart sounds are generally low pitched.
- The intensity or loudness of each sound varies with the auscultatory site.
- Heart sounds are of short duration and occur at specific times within the cardiac cycle.

To identify S_1 and S_2, you must determine and differentiate the characteristics of each sound (Figure 24-35).

In the context of the cardiac cycle, S_1 signals the beginning of systole and S_2 signals the end of systole and the beginning of diastole. When the heart rate is relatively slow, the distance between the two sounds may be used to help identify them. The distance between S_1 and S_2 (systole) is shorter than the distance between S_2 and the next S_1 (diastole).

As the heart rate increases, diastole shortens, so the distance between the sounds may be equal, thus not allowing differentiation based on timing.

A more reliable method of differentiation is based on the loudness (intensity) of S_1 and S_2 at each auscultatory site. At the base of the heart, S_2 is louder than S_1. The loudness of S_2 may vary, but it is still louder than S_1. The pitch of S_1 also is lower and slightly longer than S_2. Conversely, S_1 is loudest at the apex with a higher pitch and shorter duration than S_2 (Table 24-7).

Table 24-7 Differentiation of heart sounds

First Heart Sound (S_1)	Second Heart Sound (S_2)
Location:	**Location:**
Produced by mitral and tricuspid valve closures	Produced by aortic and pulmonic valve closure
$S_1 > S_2$ at apex	$S_2 > S_1$ at base
Two components: M_1/T_1	Two components: A_2/P_2
M_1 heard before T_1	A_2 before P_2
T_1 softer component	P_2 softer component
	A_2 most dominant of all heart sound components
Splitting:	**Splitting:**
Split heard best over tricuspid area	Split heard over pulmonic area or Erb's point (end of inspiration)
Overloading R side causes T_1 component to be heard	Paradoxical (reverse) splitting P_2 before A_2)
• RBBB	• S_2 split in expiration (single on inspiration)
"Wide splitting" more likely to be one of the following:	• LBBB. PDA, ASD
• $S_4 + S_1$ (apex)	• Mechanically caused LBBB (R ventricular pacemaker)
• S_1 + ejection click (apex or base)	Wide split—RBBB
• True wide, loud splitting before RBBB	Fixed split—unaffected by respiration
Loud S_1 à MS (closing snap), hyperkinetic states	• R ventricular output > L ventricular output
Diminished S_1 before 1st degree AV Block, MI, HRN (systemic/pulmonary)	• Large atrial septal defects, ventricular septal defect with R before L shunt, or R ventricular failure
	Split S_2 in expiration is always abnormal (Caution: Evaluate with patient in upright position before coming to this conclusion)
	Loud S_2 before systemic hypertension, MS, heart failure, AS/PS

Auscultation Techniques and Expected Findings	Unexpected Findings

Splitting of S_1 and S_2 occurs when the asynchronous closure of the valves is greater (0.03 seconds). It is more common for S_2 to be heard as a split sound than S_1. Closure of the aortic and pulmonic valves may be influenced by respirations. The usual cause of asynchrony is due to higher pressures and earlier depolarization on the L side of the heart.

Splitting of S_2 is most prominent at the end of inspiration when intrathoracic pressures are lowered and venous blood return to the R side of the heart is increased, increasing the blood volume and delaying closure of the pulmonic valve, called a physiologic split.

When pathology of the heart is the contributing factor to splitting (stenosis, septal defects, bundle branch block) it is considered a pathologic split. Splitting of S_1 is less common because closing of the tricuspid valve is too soft to hear. Occasionally, however, splitting may be heard at the tricuspid area, again during inspiration. (See Figure 24-35.)

Auscultation: Level II

Listen for the presence of extra heart sounds and/or murmurs.

Extra heart sounds, S_3 and S_4, are sounds heard in addition to S_1 and S_2 and are not created by valves closing (see Figure 24-35). Their presence is not always considered abnormal. When you hear them, place them in the context of the overall health and age of the patient. Both S_3 and S_4 occur during diastole and are thought to coincide with the two phases of ventricular filling. It is easier to differentiate between the sounds when they occur within the cardiac cycle. Differentiation of S_3 from S_4 is described in Table 24-8.

When present in adults, S_3 is considered pathological, indicating decreased ventricular compliance. It may be produced by either the R or L side of the heart and is often an initial sign of heart failure.

S_3 is a low-pitched, quiet sound that is difficult to hear.

S_3 occurs just after S_2 and is related to the first or early phase of ventricular filling. In this passive phase, blood flows from the atria to the ventricles, causing ventricular distension, which may initiate vibrations that are heard as S_3.

S_4 occurs just before S_1 and is related to the second phase of ventricular diastole. After blood has passively filled the ventricles, there is a vigorous atrial contraction that completes ventricular filling. This active phase causes vibrations of the valves, papillae, and ventricular walls, causing the S_4 sound. S_4 is a quiet, low-pitched sound that is difficult to hear.

S_4 can be a sign of decreased ventricular compliance, particularly coronary artery disease, cardiomyopathies, and hypertensive states (systemic and pulmonic).

Table 24-8 Differentiation of S_3 from S_4

Third Heart Sound (S_3)	Fourth Heart Sound (S_4)
Low-Frequency Sound	Low-Frequency Sound
1st phase of ventricular filling Ventricular distension à vibration	Second phase of ventricular filling (atrial contraction) Vibrations of valves, papillae, and ventricular walls
Heard just after S_2 (diastolic sound); later than OS	Heard just before S_1 with bell (late diastolic sound)
Heard best with bell—dull, soft sound; best in LL position	L ventricle—heard at apex; heard best in LL decubitus position during expiration
L ventricle—heard at apex; heard best in LL decubitus position; during expiration R ventricle—heard to R of apex; heard best at xiphoid of LLSB in supine position in inspiration (perhaps also over jugular)	R ventricle (less common)—heard at LLSB; during inspiration

Continued

Auscultation Techniques and Expected Findings | Unexpected Findings

Table 24-8 Differentiation of S_3 from S_4 *(continued)*

Third Heart Sound (S_3)	Fourth Heart Sound (S_4)
Incidence	**Incidence**
Common in children, young adults; one third of individuals < 30 years of age have S_3 (physiological).	May be common in late middle age or older without heart disease (physiologic)
Rarely persists after age 40; in women, may continue after age 40 Disappears when person sits up	
If heart condition present or suspected CHF implied by S_3 (pathological)	Heard at any age if decreased compliance of ventricles (CAD, cardiomyopathy), systolic overload (AS, HTN)
Accompanies conditions of volume overload (MR, AT TR), high cardiac output states (hyperthyroidism, anemia, pregnancy)	Loud S_4 suggests pathology
Accentuated	**Accentuated**
By left lateral decubitus position	Left lateral decubitus position
By hyperkinetic circulation	Draws near to S_1
Rhythm	**Rhythm**
S_3 gallop; protodiastolic gallop	S_4 gallop (presystolic) rhythm
"Ken-tu-cky"	"Ten-nes-see"

Both S_3 and S_4 are heard close enough to S_1 and S_2 that they may be mistaken for splitting of S_1 and S_2. The pitch and timing of the sounds helps to differentiate splitting from S_3 and S_4. S_2 is more commonly split than S_1; therefore, it more likely that you will encounter a split S_2, rather than S_3 (Table 24-9). It takes practice to identify all the heart sounds; however, knowing the difference between them will help you become more proficient in identifying the sounds. Table 24-10 will help to differentiate S_3 from and split S_2.

Table 24-9 Criteria for differentiating S_3 from split S_2

	S_3	Split S_2
Location	Heard best at apex or left lower sternal border (mitral site)	Heard best at base (pulmonic site)
Pitch	S_3 lower pitched than S_2	Pitch of both components remain the same
Timing	Timing not affected by ventilations	Heard best toward end of inspiration

The rhythmic pattern of the sound is also helpful in differentiating splits from S_3 or S_4. S_3 and S_4 have rhythmic cadences that are known as gallop rhythms. S_3 may be referred to as an S_3 gallop, ventricular gallop, or protosystolic gallop. The rhythm of S_3 resembles that of the word *Ken-tu-cky*. S_4 may be referred to as an S_4 gallop, atrial gallop, or presystolic gallop. The rhythm of S_4 resembles that of the word *Ten-ne-see*.

In some patients, both S_3 and S_4 may be heard. This produces a four-sound cadence that is identified as a quadruple rhythm. This is heard best at slow heart rates. When the heart rate speeds up, S_3 and S_4 may become fused and heard as one sound. When this occurs, the sound is identified as a summation gallop.

Classifications of Heart Murmurs				
Murmur	**Cardiac cycle timing**	**Auscultation site**	**Configuration of sound**	**Continuity**
Aortic stenosis	Midsystolic	RSB, 2nd ICS	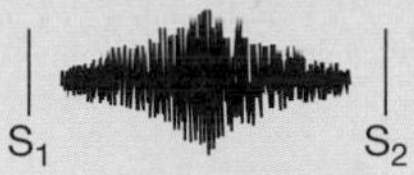 S_1 S_2	Crescendo-decrescendo, continuous
Pulmonary stenosis	Midsystolic	LBS, 2nd to 3rd ICS	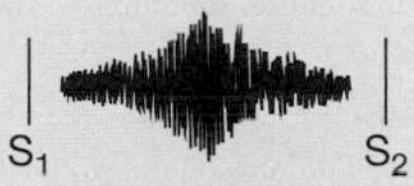 S_1 S_2	Crescendo-decrescendo, continuous
Mitral regurgitation	Systole	Apex	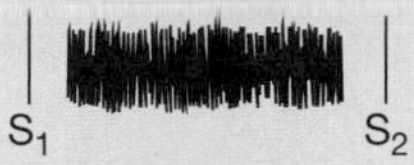 S_1 S_2	Holosystolic, continuous
Tricuspid regurgitation	Systole	4th ICS, LSB	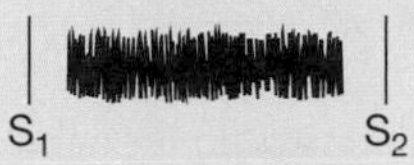 S_1 S_2	Holosystolic, continuous
Mitral stenosis	Diastole	Apical	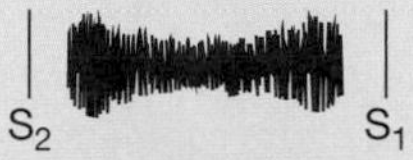 S_2 S_1	Rumble that increases in sound toward the end, continuous
Tricuspid stenosis	Diastole	Lower LSB	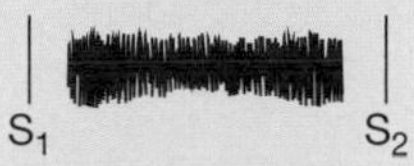 S_1 S_2	Rumble that increases in sound toward the end, continuous
Ventricular septal defect (left-to-right shunt)	Systole	3rd, 4th, 5th ICS, LSB	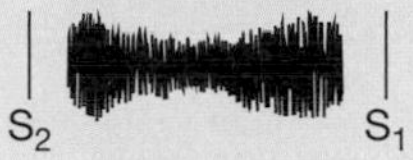 S_2 S_1	Holosystolic, continuous
Aortic regurgitation	Diastole (early)	3rd ICS, LSB	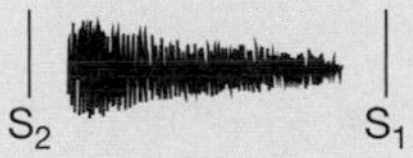 S_2 S_1	Decrescendo, continuous
Pulmonic regurgitation	Diastole (early)	3rd ICS, LSB	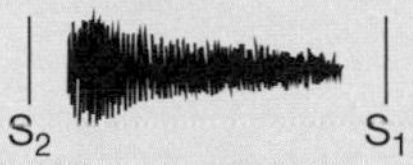 S_2 S_1	Decrescendo, continuous

Additional Heart Sounds					
Clicks	**Cardiac cycle timing**	**Auscultation site**	**Heart sound**	**Position**	**Pitch**
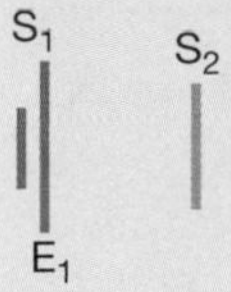 S_1 S_2 E_1	Early systole	2nd ICS, RSB for aortic click and apex with diaphragm	Aortic click	Sitting or supine position may increase the sound	High
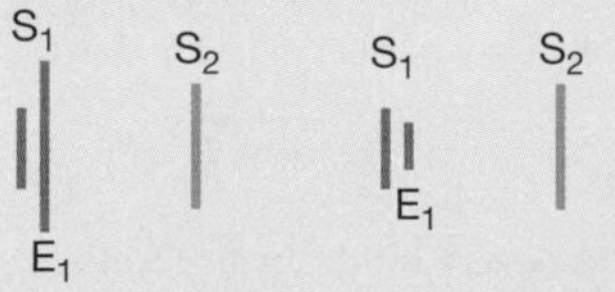 S_1 S_2 S_1 S_2 E_1 E_1	Early systole	2nd ICS, LSB for pulmonic click with diaphragm	Pulmonic	Sitting	High
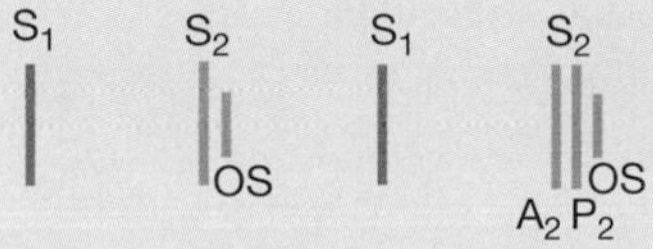 S_1 S_2 S_1 S_2 OS OS A_2 P_2	Early diastole	3rd to 4th ICS, LSB with diaphragm	Opening snap	Sitting or supine position may increase the sound	High
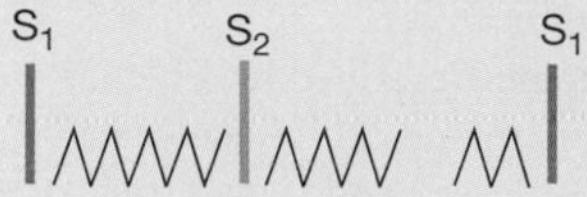 S_1 S_2 S_1	Can occur at any time	Best heard with the diaphragm, location variable	Friction rub	May be heard in any position, but best when the client sits forward	High, harsh in sound, grating

FIGURE 24-36 Schematic drawing of heart murmurs

Auscultation Techniques and Expected Findings	Unexpected Findings

Murmurs

Also listen for the presence of murmurs, which are not considered expected findings (Figure 24-36). Murmurs are characterized as prolonged or sustained sounds with a blowing, swooshing sound that is heard during or throughout systole or diastole.

Stenosis of the valves (obstruction of flow), regurgitation (backward flow of blood) through damaged valves, and septal defects (flow between chambers through opening in septum) are the major causes of murmurs.

Other causes include high output demands, altered blood flow in the great vessels, and aneurysms—dilation of the arteries, veins, or heart.

THINK LINK: Turbulent Blood Flow

Turbulent blood flow in the heart occurs as a result of impedance to forward flow. Blood flow through the heart is unidirectional, progressing from the upper chamber to the lower chamber and from the right side to the left side. Structural defects within the heart allow blood to flow backward between chambers or across from side to side. Murmurs are the sounds that are created by blood flowing through and across these defects and can be auscultated.

The initial identification of a murmur depends on whether it is diastolic or systolic.

First, you identify S_1 and S_2 and place the murmur within the appropriate location in the cardiac cycle.

Use additional descriptors to further clarify the murmur; these are early, mid, or late systole or diastole, or whether it was heard throughout the entire component of the cycle, pandiastolic/systolic or holodiastolic/systolic.

Systolic murmurs are heard as a continuous murmur that begins in systole (after S_1) and may persist throughout a part of diastole (after S_2).

Diastolic murmurs are heard beginning after S_2 and may persist into systole (after S_1).

Systolic murmurs may or may not be pathological; whereas, diastolic murmurs are always pathological.

Auscultation: Levels III/IV

Beyond identification as systolic or diastolic, additional characteristics help to determine a murmur's severity or intensity and need to be addressed (Table 24-10).

Table 24-10 Types of murmurs and where heard best: Possible etiologies

Aortic area (2nd ICS, R sternal border) Systole Aortic stenosis (radiation) Diastole Aortic insufficiency (radiation)	**Pulmonic Area** (2nd ICS L sternal border) Systole Pulmonic stenosis Atrial septal defect Diastole Pulmonic insufficiency Entire cycle Patent ductus arteriosis	
	Erb's Point (3rd ICS L sternal border) Systole Ventricular septal defect Aortic stenosis Diastole Aortic insufficiency	
	Right Ventricular Area (4th ICS L sternal border) Systole Tricuspid insufficiency Diastole Tricuspid stenosis	**Left ventricular area** (5th ICS MCL to PMI) Systole Mitral insufficiency Diastole Mitral stenosis

Timing: Murmur sounds are longer than heart sounds.

Pitch: May be high, medium, or low. Pitch of the murmur depends on quantity and rate of blood flow at the site of origin. Amount and characteristics of tissues between the site of origin and site of auscultation also determine pitch.

Loudness: Described according to six grades:

- Grade I—barely audible in a quiet room
- Grade II—clearly audible but faint
- Grade III—moderately loud, relatively easy to hear
- Grade IV—loud, associated with a thrill
- Grade V—very loud, thrill, easily palpable with patient in upright position leaning forward
- Grade VI—very loud, audible with stethoscope not in contact with chest; thrill palpable and visible

Pattern/shape: Described by whether the sound increases < (crescendo) or decreases > (decrescendo) over time, or does both <> (diamond pattern)

Quality: May be described as harsh, raspy, vibratory, musical, blowing, or rumbling

Auscultation Techniques and Expected Findings	Unexpected Findings
	Radiation: In addition to where the murmur is heard best, the sound may radiate to other areas on the precordium, back, neck, or axilla.
	Location: Identifies where murmur can be heard the loudest. As with S_1 and S_2, sound originates in a valve and travels in the direction of blood flow.
	Auscultation in all cardiac auscultatory sites allows the provider to determine where the murmur is heard best. Table 24-10 presents general guidelines for location.
Innocent and functional murmurs may both be considered nonpathological. Innocent murmurs, often heard in children and young adults, may be characterized as soft, short, and systolic. They generally disappear and are not indicators of potential cardiac problems.	Other sounds that may be heard during auscultation include opening snaps and ejection clicks (see Figure 24-36). These sounds are produced by valves that are thickened or roughened from pathological processes.
The functional murmur is due to increased blood flow in the heart that accompanies anemia, fever, pregnancy, and hyperthyroidism. Once the underlying condition is eliminated, the functional murmur disappears.	High-frequency ejection clicks occur very shortly after S_1, best heard at the base of the heart, and may originate from either the aortic or pulmonic valve. They are caused from blood being ejected through a stenotic valve or into a dilated chamber. Pulmonic ejection clicks are best heard at the left base and increase with expiration and decrease with inspiration.
	Aortic ejection clicks are best heard at the apex and are not influenced by respirations.
	A midsystolic click may be heard in the presence of mitral valve prolapse.
	Another extra heart sound is a pericardial friction rub, which indicates a pericardial inflammation that causes roughening of the pericardial surfaces so that they rub together throughout the cardiac cycle. It is a grating, leathery sound that overlies the other cardiac sounds and a high-pitched sound heard best with the diaphragm. It tends to be loudest during inspiration; however, in instances of a forced expiration the sound may become more audible. It tends to be a transitory sound that may come and go suddenly. It may be heard over the whole pericardium but frequently is heard best with the patient in an upright position, leaning forward.

Developmental Applications

Techniques and Expected Findings	Unexpected Findings

Infants

A significant change from fetal circulation to systemic and pulmonary circulation occurs within the first 24 hours after birth. Examination of the infant's cardiovascular system should thus occur within the first day of life, with a second examination done again within the next 48 to 72 hours.

Pay particular attention to the skin, lungs, and liver; dysfunction of the infant's cardiovascular system will be reflected in these organs.

The infant's skin and mucous membranes should be pink in color with variations of brown depending on the genetic makeup.

The heart rate is best obtained by auscultation rather than palpation of the radial artery. An infant's heart rate has a wide variability, ranging from 100–180/minute immediately after birth, then stabilizing to an average of 120–140/minute. The heart rate is responsive to activity and increases to 170/minute with vigorous crying and may decrease to 70–90/minute when sleeping.

The rhythm may be variable due to sinus arrhythmia.

Unexpected Findings: Of particular significance is the presence of central cyanosis—cyanosis of the skin, mucous membranes of the face, and upper body (Figure 24-37). Cyanosis that appears in the immediate neonatal period indicates the presence of congenital heart disease—that is, transposition of the great vessels, tetralogy of Fallot, severe septal defects, pulmonic stenosis, or tricuspid atresia.

Acrocyanosis, cyanosis of hands and feet in the absence of central cyanosis, is of minimal significance as it frequently disappears within a few hours to days after birth (see Chapter 16).

Other changes in skin color could be a purplish plethora due to polycythemia or an ashen-white color indicative of shock.

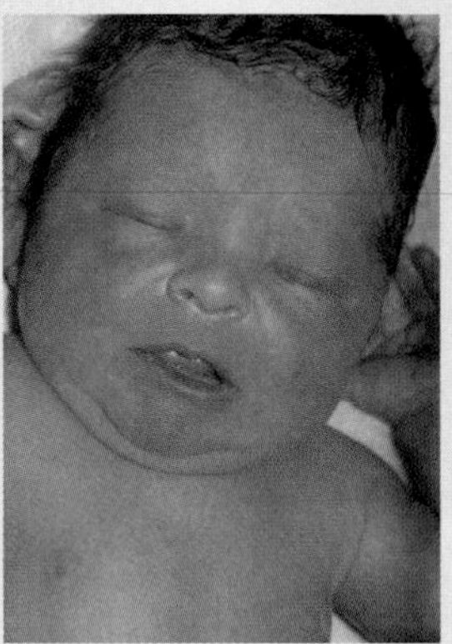

FIGURE 24-37 Central cyanosis of an infant
Source: St Bartholomew's Hospital, London/ Science Source

THINK LINK:* *Diaphragmatic Hernia
A diaphragmatic hernia is a condition in which the diaphragm fails to develop properly, allowing the abdominal organs to migrate through the hernia into the mediastinal cavity. These organs then compress the lungs and the heart, preventing them from developing properly. Depending on the severity of the diaphragmatic defect, the impact on the heart and lungs can vary. Surgery is necessary to correct the defect, but in severe cases the damage to the lungs and heart may be incompatible with life.

Children

Assess for signs of cardiac dysfunction.

The apex beat may be visible in children, particularly those with thin-walled chests.

Unexpected Findings: Indicators include poor weight gain, developmental delays, persistent tachycardia, and dyspnea on exertion, cyanosis, and clubbing. Clubbing is a late sign and may not be apparent until after the first birthday, even in the presence of severe congenital defects. Cyanosis is the most significant indicator of cardiac dysfunction.

Any obvious bulge on the chest is an indicator of cardiac enlargement. The elasticity of the child's chest wall, which is more cartilaginous, allows the enlarged heart to be more visible on the precordium.

The Pregnant Woman

Cardiac changes affected by pregnancy are a gradual increase in heart rate and an initial reduction in blood pressure. The blood pressure drops to its lowest point during the second trimester, then gradually rises during the third trimester.

The apex beat may be displaced 1–1.5 cm upward and laterally due to a change in heart position caused by the enlarging uterus. The overall degree of displacement depends on the position and size of the uterus.

Unexpected Findings: A sustained rise in blood pressure of 30 mmHg systolically or 15 mmHg diastolically should be evaluated for the presence of pregnancy-induced hypertension (PIH).

Techniques and Expected Findings	Unexpected Findings
The increase in blood volume has an effect on heart sounds. There is an increased intensity of S_1 as well as an increase in splitting of S_1 and S_2. A systolic ejection murmur is common, occurring in 90% of women and disappearing after delivery. Another murmur-type sound that may be heard is the mammary soufflé. This is often present just before delivery or during lactation. Increased blood flow through the internal mammary artery is responsible for creating this sound. It is best heard in the second, third, or fourth intercostal space as a continuous sound; however, it may be exaggerated during systole.	An S_3 may be present and is nonsignificant; however, an S_4 carries more significance and needs to be evaluated.
The ECG demonstrates no significant changes other than a left axis deviation that results from the change in the heart's position.	
The Older Adult A common finding in the elderly is gradual increase in systolic blood pressure. The diastolic pressure remains fairly constant, which results in a widened pulse pressure. Many elderly experience orthostatic hypotension, which results from a drop in blood pressure with rapid standing.	Heart sounds do not change to a great extent. Extra heart sounds indicate that S_3 and S_4 may be present. When present in the elderly, S_3 is most often an indicator of congestive heart failure (CHF). The presence of S_4 may or may not indicate cardiac pathology. If present, it is primarily the result of decreased left ventricular compliance. Murmurs, if present, are more likely to be caused by alterations associated with aging, such as calcification of the valvular apparatus or dilatation of the aorta and aortic annulus.
The apex beat may be more difficult to locate in the elderly due to an increase in the anteroposterior diameter of the chest. Obesity raises the diaphragm, further contributing to the difficulty in locating the apex beat.	
The heart rate varies widely and may be slower due to increased vagal tone. A frequent drop in heart rate may be an indicator of more serious cardiac pathology. The ECG may demonstrate occasional ectopic beats, which are common and nonsignificant.	

DOCUMENTATION

Once the examination is completed, the findings must be documented. Documentation data is determined by the type of exam performed. The following data represents a comprehensive examination. Data is described as related to expected findings. Unexpected findings would also be documented.

- **Inspection:** Skin warm and dry with uniform pigmentation. No clubbing of fingernails. No visible heaves or pulsations noted on anterior chest. Heart rhythm regular—normal sinus rhythm [NSR]/ECG. No ECG alterations noted.
- **Palpation:** No thrills or pulsations felt at aortic, pulmonic, tricuspid, mitral, and Erb's point. PMI located at fifth ICS lateral to MCL.
- **Auscultation:** Patient lying supine. Apical heart rate 74 with regular rhythm. S_1/S_2 heard clearly at aortic, pulmonic, tricuspid, mitral, and Erb's point. S_1 loudest at mitral and tricuspid points. S_2 loudest at aortic and pulmonic points. S_2 spilt at end of inspiration and heard best at pulmonic point. Without murmurs, gallops, S_3/S_4.

Electronic Charting

Expectations of Electronic Charting

Cardiovascular problems can be life threatening, and may require the patient to be treated in an intensive care unit. Cardiovascular information needs to be readily available, including information pertaining to cardiovascular medications and procedures, complications, electrocardiographic (ECG) rhythms and information regarding arrhythmias, and serum enzyme values. Images of various kinds (CT, MRI, echocardiograms, etc.) must be stored and made available to clinical users. This includes a range of imaging types, from simple drawings to complex videos. Special documentation may be needed to rapidly address the needs of patients with emergency conditions such as acute myocardial infarction.

Decision support modules can assist with or confirm decisions, such as the differential diagnosis of chest pain. Other decision support modules might identify unexpected values for vital signs or labs, based on age and gender-specific norms. Guidelines and protocols incorporated into electronic medical records provide an opportunity to improve the prevention of cardiovascular disease and stroke through preventive care reminders and risk calculators.

Many cardiovascular drugs interact with other medications, or have special precautions. Evaluation of possible drug–drug interactions is a common feature of electronic health records. Self care and home monitoring are prevention and treatment components for cardiovascular conditions. Many home ("personal") health records include data useful for the cardiovascular assessment, such as home blood pressure monitoring, weight and exercise logs, and medication sections.

Limitations of Electronic Charting

Interpretation of echocardiograms and radiographic studies requires complex, "fuzzy" logic and so can only be semi-automated. This type of decision making is intuitive for human users, but is difficult for computers. Automatic detection of certain arrhythmias such as ventricular fibrillation, and subsequent defibrillation with automatic devices (implanted or external) has become relatively common. Such devices have been found to be safe and effective in differentiating "shockable" rhythms from rhythms that should not be shocked. However, automatic interpretation of other arrhythmias is less well-established. You need to be able to interpret ECGs on your own, and not depend on computer-generated interpretations.

A study of nursing records for cardiac-surgery patients (Kim & Park, 2005) showed that while cardiovascular assessments were frequently documented, outcomes were less often documented. Outcomes related to disease management, insomnia, respiratory care, and pain control were more often documented than independent nursing activities such as education and emotional care. A survey of providers revealed that they do not document outcomes as often as they think they do; primarily related to insufficient time for documentation and lack of knowledge about what to document.

Summary

- The heart is a four-chambered dual pump that propels blood flow to and through the systemic and pulmonary vascular circuit. It is positioned in the mediastinum of the chest, protected by the sternum and rib cage.
- The cardiac cycle is composed of one ventricular contraction (systole) and one ventricular relaxation (systole). Ventricular contractions pump blood out of the heart into the vascular circuits. The regular cycle of contractions is regulated by the electrical conduction system that is imbedded within the heart's muscle. The ECG is a representation of electrical activity during 1 cardiac cycle. The ECG complex and is comprised of PQRST waves and intervals.
- The patient history of an individual with a cardiac condition presents with symptoms associated with chest pain, dyspnea, orthopnea, cough, and/or syncope. Other conditions are associated with chest pain and need to be ruled out. A thorough symptom analysis (COLDERRA) will help to determine the cause of chest pain.
- The cardiac assessment may use all four assessment techniques. The exam may be separated into four levels. Expected and unexpected findings will support the history data and relate to specific cardiac conditions.
- Heart sounds are composed of valvular and nonvalvular components. Expected heart sounds, identified as S_1/S_2 are synchronous valve closure sounds. Extra heart sounds, S_3/S_4 are nonvalvular sounds with a nonspecific origin. Split sounds are caused by asynchronous valve closure and are nonpathological unless heard in the presence of specific cardiac pathology. S_1/S_2 in combination with either S_3/S_4, or both, produce gallop rhythms.

Review Questions

1. During fetal development, blood is shunted around the pulmonary circulation through which of the following?
   1. Ductus venosis
   2. Foramen venosis
   3. Ductus arteriosis
   4. Foramen arteriosis

2. During the provider's examination of a female patient who is 7 months' pregnant you obtain the following data. Which would be considered an unexpected finding?
   1. A short, soft, and systolic flow murmur
   2. Increase in heart rate from a baseline of 74 bpm to 90 bpm
   3. An increase in systolic BP from a baseline of 115 to 158
   4. A displaced apex beat upward and laterally by 1 cm

3. While assessing a patient's cardiovascular system the patient asks the provider what causes the sounds that the provider listens to. The provider explains that heart sounds are produced by which of the following?
   1. Opening of the heart valves
   2. Closing of the heart valves
   3. A rapid drop in intraventricular pressure
   4. Rapid vibrations of the chordae tendinae

4. To augment heart sounds in a patient in the supine position, the provider should request that the patient to which of the following?
   1. Take a deep breath and hold it.
   2. Turn onto the left side.
   3. Breathe in rapidly through the mouth.
   4. Massage the carotid arteries.

5. During the examination of an adult male, the provider palpates the apex beat at the fifth ICS, just medial to the midclavicular line. The provider should interpret this finding as which of the following?
   1. An indicator of ventricular hypertrophy
   2. A symptom that accompanies aortic stenosis
   3. A warning sign of myocardial infarction
   4. An expected location for the apex beat

6. During auscultation of a patient's heart, the provider hears another sound between S_2 and S_1. The provider knows that a sound heard here could be which of the following?
   1. Systolic murmur
   2. S_3
   3. Venous hum
   4. Friction rub

7. The provider is assessing a patient's cardiac monitor. A change to which of the following arrhythmias will cause the provider to get emergency equipment and begin immediate cardiopulmonary resuscitation?
   1. Atrial fibrillation
   2. Left bundle branch block
   3. Ventricular fibrillation
   4. Second degree AV block

8. The provider is assessing a patient in the emergency room with a chief complaint of "chest pain." The provider recognizes that this pain is likely related to a noncardiac source if the patient does which of the following? (Select all that apply.)
   1. States that the pain was relieved by a dose of ibuprofen but has returned
   2. Indicates that the pain is mostly in the epigastric area
   3. Notes that the pain increases with a deep inhalation
   4. Reports that the pain is also in the arm and jaw
   5. Describes the pain as a pressure in the chest

9. The provider is reviewing cardiac assessment with a group of students. Which of the following statements should the provider include in this instruction regarding murmurs?
   1. Systolic murmurs are not considered pathologic.
   2. Diastolic murmurs are heard best with the diaphragm.
   3. Systolic murmurs only involve the semilunar valves.
   4. Diastolic murmurs are considered pathologic.

10. When assessing the electrocardiogram of a patient with atrial (Supra ventricular) tachycardia, the nurse expects that the ECG will reveal which of the following?
    1. Irregular rhythm
    2. Different P wave
    3. Increased QRS voltage
    4. Inverted T wave

Conditions and Disorders

Myocardial Infarction

Myocardial infarction (MI) is the irreversible death (necrosis) of myocardial muscle caused by a critical imbalance between oxygen supply and demand of myocardial tissue. The most common cause is a rupture of an atherosclerotic plaque with thrombus formation within a coronary artery, resulting in an immediate loss of blood supply to a section of the myocardium.

Pathophysiology

- Atherosclerosis is primary cause of MI (90% of the events) (Figure 24-38)
- After plaque ruptures, basement membrane exposed, activates aggregation of platelets
- Activation of coagulation cascade accumulation of fibrin, thrombus formation and vasospasm
- Degree of occlusion of the artery determines myocardial damage: cell ischemia, injury, or necrosis.
- Persistent ischemia or total occlusion of the artery results in acute coronary syndrome, which may progress to infarction.
- Myocardial cells can tolerate ischemia for approximately 20 minutes before they die. During ischemia their function is altered, but they remain viable and will recover if blood supply is restored in time.

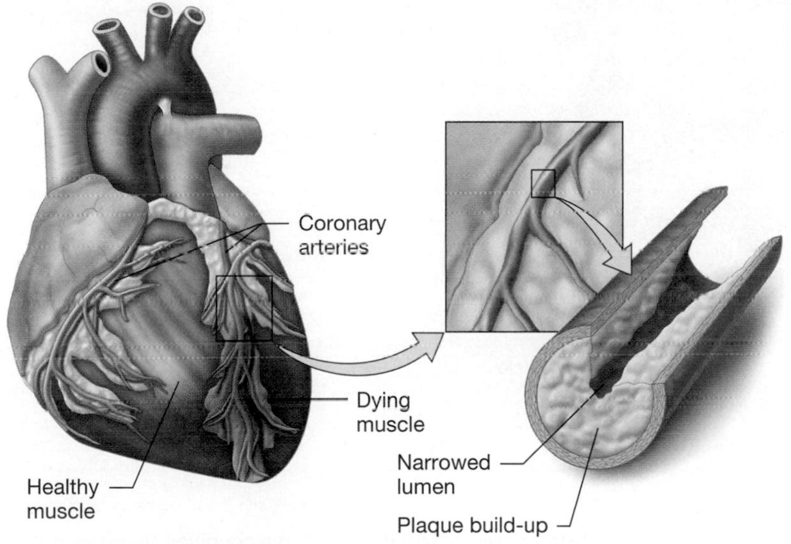

FIGURE 24-38 Myocardial infarction

- Total vessel occlusion; oxygen deprivation for > 4–6 hours ➔ irreversible myocardial necrosis Nonatherosclerotic causes of a MI are due to coronary artery vasospasm, which occurs in Printzmetal (variant) angina along with use of amphetamines and cocaine. Coronary emboli can also develop from an infected heart valve and occlusion can result from vasculitis. Severe, acute anemia can also result in oxygen deprivation and myocardial damage. Chest trauma from motor vehicle accidents or sports injuries have also been linked to MIs (Fenton, 2009).

Subjective Data

- Substernal chest pain, pressure-like sensation, radiate down left arm, up to jaw and/or neck
- Males—classic signs; but females—different presentation of symptoms

Objective Data

ECG changes reflective of cell damage and/or death; ST segment elevation, which is used to categorize myocardial infarctions into two groups: STEMI (ST segment elevation MI) or NSTEMI (non-STEMI elevation MI). STEMI is typically accompanied by an elevation of specific enzymes that provide evidence of actual muscle tissue necrosis (Earnest & Tadros, 2007).

Enzyme changes
Cardiac Data: Enzymes and markers related to acute coronary event
aspartate-aminotransferase (AST)
Adult male: >40 U/L
Female: >25 U/L
Creatine kinase (CK)
Adult Male: >150 U/L
Female: >400 U/L

Isoenzymes
CK - I Brain (BB) 0%–1%
CK - II Heart (MB): >3% or 7.5 ng/mL
CK - III Muscle (MM) 95%–100%
Lactic dehydrogenase (LDH)
Adult: > 90 U/L

Isoenzymes
LDH 1 (erythrocytes, heart tissue): > 27%
LDH 2 (Reticuloendothelial tissue, kidney) 23%–28%
LDH 3 (Lungs, lymph nodes, spleen) 18%– 28%
LDH 4 (kidney, placenta, liver tissue) 05%–15%
LDH 5 (liver tissue, skeletal tissue, kidney) 05%–15%

Troponins
Troponin I (cTnI) <0.6 ng/mL
>1.5 ng/mL (consistent with MI)
Troponin T (cTnT >0.1–0.2 ng/mL (consistent with MI)

Troponin T (Bedside assessment can detect values as low as 0.08 ng/mL.)

Congestive Heart Failure

Congestive Heart Failure (CHF) is a condition or syndrome where the heart fails as a pump and is unable to deliver adequate amounts of oxygenated blood to meet the body's demands. CHF occurs when the ventricular muscles have generally been damaged or overstretched for a long period of time, eventually losing their contractility so that the ejection force of the heart is diminished significantly.

Pathophysiology

- Damaged heart muscle due to coronary artery disease and myocardial infarctions, myocarditis, hypertension, chronic conditions (diabetes, hyper/hypothyroidism, emphysema)
- CHF caused by failure of one ventricle or both. If it originates in one ventricle, eventually it will affect the other one.
- Most commonly a chronic condition; signs and symptoms don't appear until an advanced state.
- Symptoms may appear suddenly; they usually develop over an extended period of time.

Subjective Data

- Symptoms of pulmonary involvement: fatigue progressing to dyspnea with exertion or when recumbent
- Additionally, shortness of breath, with persistent cough/wheezing
- May experience a sudden weight gain from fluid retention with the development of ascites (fluid in the abdomen), resulting in nausea, abdominal pain, and decreased appetite

Objective Data

Edema

- Pulmonary edema: crackles, SOB, dyspnea, productive cough (blood tinged, frothy sputum), jugular venous distension and increased JVP
- Bilateral peripheral pitting edema (lower extremities)
- Decreased BP, S_3, abdominojugular reflex

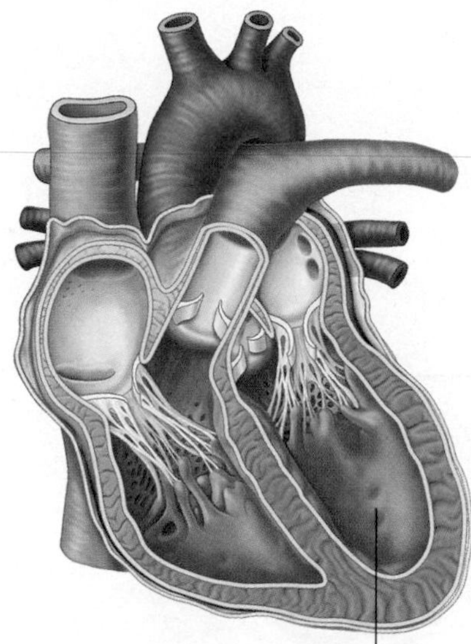

FIGURE 24-39 Congestive heart failure

Cardiomyopathy

Cardiomyopathy refers to heart diseases causing measurable deterioration of myocardial function resulting in loss of muscle contractility. Various causes include viral infections, chronic alcohol abuse, cocaine, or chemotherapeutic drugs. Lupus and congenital heart defects are also associated with heart muscle damage.

Acute stress myocardiopathy (ASM) is a condition that frequently follows intense emotional or physical stress, causing a rapid and severe weakness of heart muscle. Emotional stress may be caused by loss of a loved one (grief), fear, extreme anger, and surprise. Physical stressors include stroke, seizures, breathing difficulties (asthma, COPD), and severe hemorrhage.

Pathophysiology

- Functionally related to dilation (ventricular enlargement), hypertrophy (myocardial cell enlargement), or restriction (myocardial muscle stiffening)
- Dilation most common in males 20–60 years of age.

Subjective Data

- Presence of symptoms variable
- Chest pain
- SOB, dyspnea on exertion
- Fatigue
- Also symptoms of underlying disease/condition causing myopathy

Objective Data

- Edema (lower extremities), abdomen
- JVD
- ECG changes, arrhythmias

- It is hypothesized that during stress, the heart muscle is "stunned" by the massive amount of catacholamines that is released in response to the stress, resulting in acute left ventricular dysfunction (Lyon, Rees, Prasad, Poole-Wilson., & Harding, 2008). The myocardial cells in ASM undergo injury, but not death, which results in the possibility of a complete recovery from ASM if the condition is recognized and treated soon. However, in rare cases hypotension and CHF may develop and in even rarer cases, shock and life threatening arrythmias may occur.

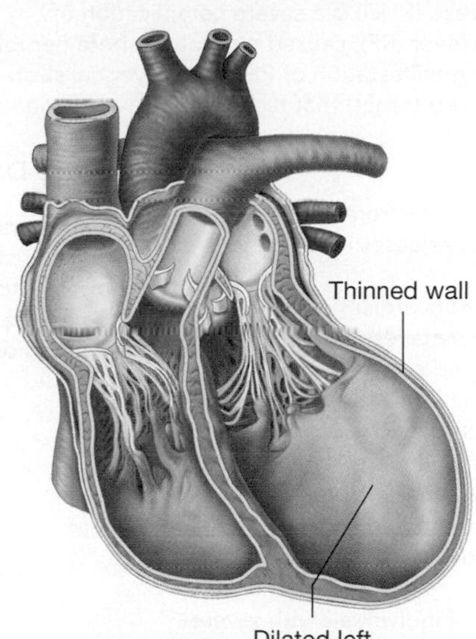

FIGURE 24-40 Cardiomyopathy

Infective Endocarditis

Infective endocarditis (IE), also known as bacterial endocarditis, is a bacterial infection and inflammation of the endocardium (Figure 24-41). Untreated, the bacteria damage the valves by promoting further bacterial growth, providing the groundwork for scarring of the valves. These scarred valves may cause stenosis or regurgitation. It is rare for individuals with normal hearts to develop IE. It is estimated that there are 29,000 new cases of IE per year (Petterson & Thomas, 2010).

Pathophysiology

- Bacteria causing IE normally exist on the body in the lungs, kidneys, mouth, and skin.
- Streptococcus viridans, a bacteria of oral cavity causes about 50% of IE infections (Levin, 2009).
- Bacteria enter the bloodstream, finding their way to the heart.
- Other bacteria include staphylococcus aureus and enterococcus.
- Bacteria may form infected clots that can become emboli and go to the brain, lungs, kidneys, or spleen.
- Individuals at risk for the IE often have preexisting conditions:
  - Artificial heart valve
  - Previous endocarditis
  - Damaged/scarred heart valves
  - Certain congenital heart defects
  - Hypertrophic cardiomyopathy
  - Individuals post transplant that develop heart valve abnormality
  - IV drug users are high risk

Subjective Data

- Chills with excessive sweating; particularly night sweats
- Muscle aches/pains as well as joint pain
- Fatigue, weakness, and shortness of breath with activity

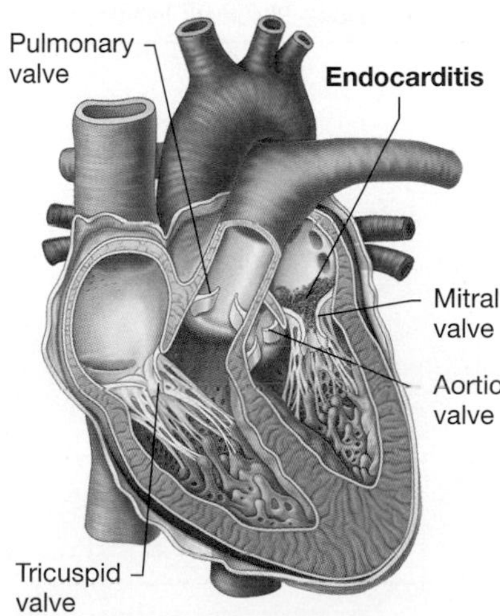

FIGURE 24-41 Infective endocarditis

Objective Data

- Fingernail alterations (splinter hemorrhages)
- Janeway lesions—red, painless skin spots on the palms and soles
- Osler's nodes—red, painful nodes on the pads of fingers /toes
- Pallor due to anemia
- Edema of lower extremities and abdomen

Rheumatic Heart Disease

Rheumatic heart disease (RHD) is a severe complication of untreated rheumatic fever (RF), caused by group A beta-hemolytic streptococcus. Initial manifestation of RF is a pharyngeal streptococcus infection (strep throat) that results in cytolysis toxin production capable of invading and damaging human tissue. Individuals most vulnerable to developing RF are between the ages of 5–15, but it may develop in adults.

Pathophysiology

- Damage to heart valves from autoimmune reaction that releases inflammatory cytokines
- Inflammation of endocardium causes edema of valve leaflets resulting in erosion along edges of leaflets.
- Persistent inflammation leads to deposition of small beadlike clusters of vegetation; contain fibrin and platelets
- These depositions cause progressive fusion causing scarring and hardening of valve leaflets, reducing their elasticity and the valve orifice
- 1% mortality rate of individuals with severe valve dysfunction in the acute phase (Chin, Chin, Siddiqui, & Sundell, 2012)

Subjective Data

- Joint inflammation causing tenderness/pain of wrists, elbows, knees, or ankles (polyarthritis)
- Stomach pains, anorexia, weight loss
- Shortness of breath and weakness

Objective Data

- Fever
- Joint inflammation leading to redness, swelling of the wrists, elbows, knees, or ankles (polyarthritis)
- Neuromuscular changes that may include jerky movements (sydenham chorea)
- Mitral valve regurgitation murmur frequently heard in acute RHD
- Congestive heart failure may result from acute RHD causing tachypnea, orthopnea, jugular venous distension, pulmonary crackles, hepatomegaly, a gallop rhythm, and peripheral edema

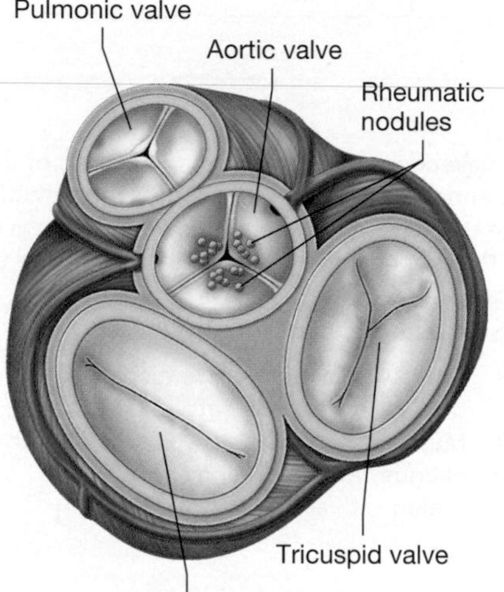

FIGURE 24-42 Rheumatic heart disease

Ventricular Hypertrophy

Ventricular hypertrophy is a condition in which the myocardium enlarges and results from an extra workload placed on the heart, generally due to the need for the ventricles to generate a greater force of contraction to maintain adequate cardiac output. It has a gradual onset and there are generally no symptoms until the heart muscle becomes worn out due to the extra work load placed upon it.

Pathophysiology

- Left ventricular hypertrophy (LVH) more common than right
- Most common cause of LVH is hypertension. Increased pressure within the arterial circulation makes it necessary for the left ventricle to generate a greater amount of pressure to open aortic valve and eject blood.
- Other causes of LVH include aortic stenosis, aortic regurgitation, and cardiomyopathy.

Subjective Data

- Shortness of breath
- Chest pain
- Awareness of a rapid heartbeat (palpitations)
- Dizziness
- Fainting
- Rapid exhaustion with increased activity

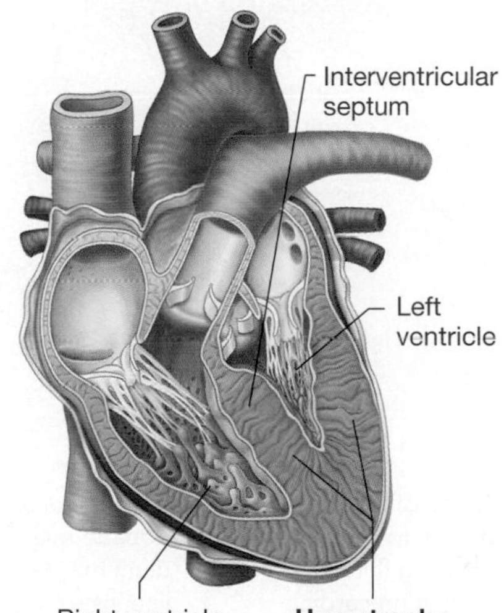

FIGURE 24-43 Ventricular hypertrophy

Objective Data

- Manifestations of RVH not evident until hypertrophy at an advanced stage.
- When they are evident, they are the same for LVH.
- Evidence of edema in lower extremities occur as ventricular muscle fails.

Pericarditis

Pericarditis is an inflammation of the pericardium, the outer layer of the heart. The two layers of the pericardium glide over each other during cardiac contractions due to approximately 20 mL of serous fluid between the layers. The space between the layers can accommodate approximately an additional 120 mL of fluid without compromising ventricular function. Additional fluid causes significant increase in pericardial pressure, which prevents the ventricles from completely relaxing during diastole, decreasing stroke volume and thus cardiac output, resulting in hypotension.

Pathophysiology

- Pericarditis has a multitude of causes, but these causes in most instances are unidentified or idiopathic; it may result from a minor viral illness or cold
- Other causes include myocardial infarction (Dressler's syndrome), cardiac surgery, infection (bacterial, viral, fungal), metastatic cancer, uremia, trauma, and rheumatic conditions (rheumatoid arthritis, systemic lupus erythematosus).
- Males affected more often than females; more common in adolescents and young adults

Subjective Data

- Most common symptom is chest pain, usually sharp and stabbing.
- If inflammation involves diaphragm, pain is generally worse with deep inspiration and may radiate to the shoulder blade. It frequently increases when lying flat and lessens if leaning forward.
- These symptoms may appear gradually or have an immediate onset. It may also radiate to the back, neck, or arm.
- Depending on the exact location of inflammation, other structures of mediastinum may be involved.
- Pain with deep inspiration and shortness of breath due to lung involvement; Painful swallowing may be due to inflammation close to the esophagus.

Objective Data

- Painful swallowing may be due to inflammation close to the esophagus.
- Predominant physical sign is a friction rub
- Rub is transient and may vary from hour to hour. Present in approximately half of the cases; best heard at lower left sternal border with patient leaning forward.
- Rub may be mistaken for a murmur, but unlike a murmur, its character changes from beat to beat and with positional changes.
- Heard as scratching or grating sound, very easy to hear.

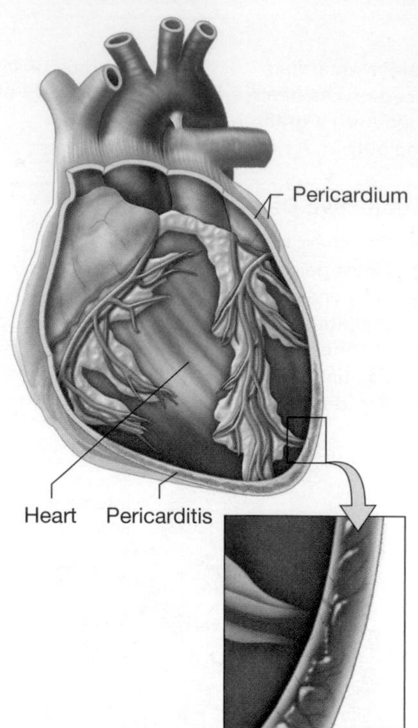

FIGURE 24-44 Pericarditis

Cardiac Tamponade

Cardiac tamponade is an accumulation of >120 mL of fluid in pericardial space due to pericarditis. It is often slow to develop, allowing time for the heart to adjust to the increasing fluid. Rapidly occurring tamponade often due to penetrating cardiac trauma and the pericardial fluid is blood (hemopericardium) rather than an effusion from pericarditis. A rapidly occurring tamponade may be life threatening. Other causes of hemopericardium may be due to penetration by pacemaker insertion, central line insertion, and cardiac catheterization. Tamponades have been known to develop hours to days after catheter penetration.

Pathophysiology

- With any inflammatory condition, fluid accumulates around the area. In pericarditis, the fluid accumulates within the space between the two pericardial layers.
- The rapidity with which fluid accumulates will determine the degree of cardiac compromise.

Subjective Data

- Anxiety, restlessness, chest pain, dyspnea, tachypnea, SOB—often when supine, relieved by sitting upright or leaning forward
- Syncope, light headedness
- Cyanosis
- Palpitations

Objective Data

- Jugular venous distension, hypotension, distant/muffled heart sounds
- Inflamed pericardium may become scarred and constricted, decreasing ventricular filling → hypotension, rapid/weak pulse, increasing paradoxical pulse.

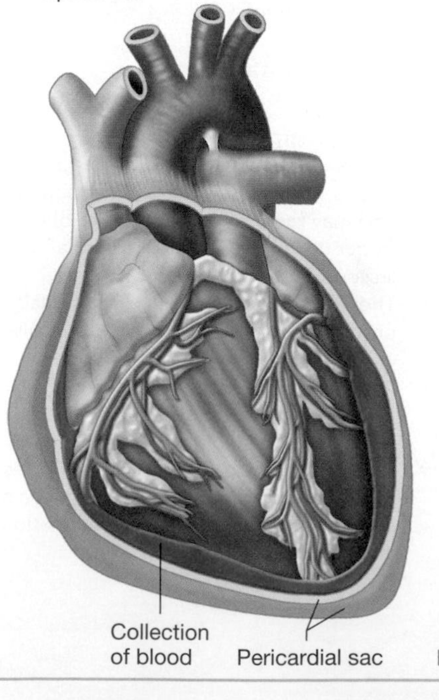

Collection of blood
Pericardial sac

FIGURE 24-45 Cardiac tamponade

Murmurs

Heart murmurs are heart sounds produced by turbulent blood flow through the heart chambers or an obstruction to the forward flow of blood through the heart. Most are caused by alterations of the heart valves or structural alterations of the septum that separates the sides of the heart. A ventricular aneurysm causes a murmur due to turbulent blood flow in and around the aneurysm.

Type	Where Heard Best (best heard with bell)	Characteristics
Diastolic Murmurs		
Mitral Stenosis		
• Smaller valve opening restricts forward flow of blood from left atrium to left ventricle. • Increased atrial contraction generated • Associated with rheumatic fever and infectious endocarditis	• Apex with patient in left lateral decubitus position	• Low, diastolic rumble, greater intensity in early/late diastole • Does not radiate • Quiet systole • Late diastolic thrill felt at apex • S_1 louder; palpable at left sterna border • S_2 split (accentuated P_2) • Opening snap after P_2 • Visible lift on right side of sternum if right ventricle hypertrophied • Decreased arterial pulse amplitude (quality)
Tricuspid Stenosis		
• Valves become calcified and restrict forward flow of blood from right atrium into right ventricle; occurs with mitral stenosis—uncommon to be single condition • Most common cause is rheumatic fever • Frequently associated with mitral stenosis; rarely a single event	• Over tricuspid area on chest (left sternal border)	• Mid-diastolic rumble, louder during inspiration (Carvallo's sign) • Diastolic thrill over right ventricle • Split S_2 during inspiration • Diminished arterial pulse amplitude • Visible jugular venous pulse

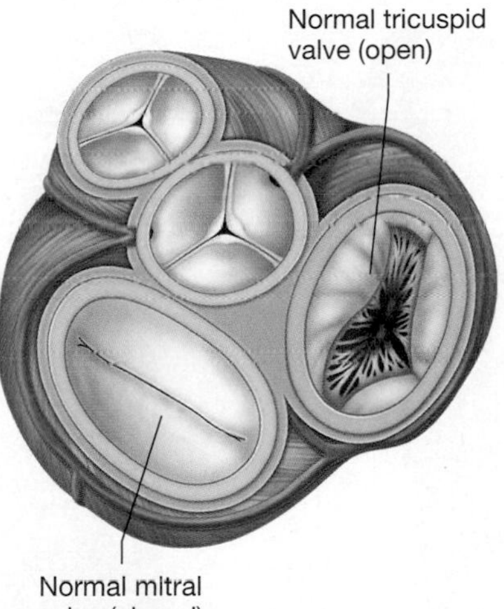

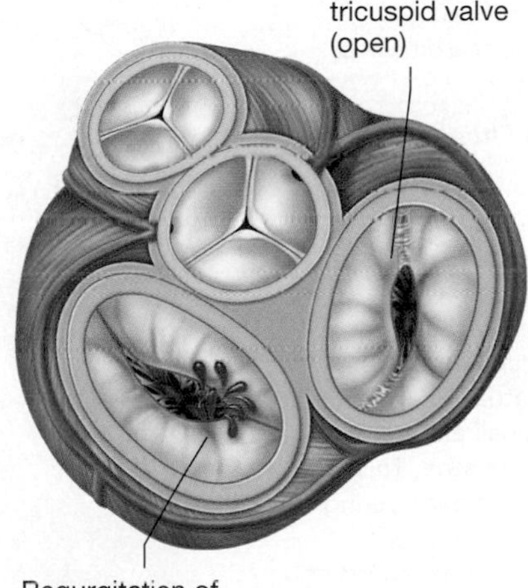

FIGURE 24-46 Stenotic/regurgitant valves

Type	Where Heard Best	Characteristics
Aortic Regurgitation		
• Valve leaflets fail to close completely, allowing back flow of blood from aorta to left ventricle. • Caused by rheumatic heart disease infectious endocarditis, syphilis, ankylosing spondylitis, aortic dissection, Marfan's syndrome	• Heard best with diaphragm at third left interspace at base with patient sitting, leaning forward; low pitched rumbling murmur at apex (Austin-Flint murmur)	• Early diastolic (onset of S_2), high pitched, blowing quality, S_1 soft, S_2 split • Bounding pulse (water hammer, Corrigan pulse) in brachial, carotid, and femoral arteries • Widened pulse pressure

Systolic Murmurs

Aortic Stenosis

- Calcification of valve cusps narrows valve orifice, restricting forward flow of blood from left ventricle into systemic circulation.
- Often related to congenital bicuspid valve (expected to be tricuspid)
- May cause sudden death in children/adolescents

- Heard best over aortic area (second ICS, RSB)

- Loud, harsh, ejection murmur, crescendo-decrescendo (diamond shaped)
- Radiates along left sternal border (to apex/carotid)
- Thrill over second/third intercostal spaces
- S_1 heard best at apex, may be ejection click
- Split S_2
- S_4 may also be present

Pulmonic Stenosis

- Narrowed valve orifice impedes forward flow of blood from right ventricle into pulmonary circulation.
- Almost always congenital defect

- Heard over pulmonic area, radiating to left and towards neck.

- Ejection murmur, loud/harsh/coarse
- Diamond shaped (<>)
- Thrill at second/third left intercostal spaces

Mitral Regurgitation

- Valve leaflets don't completely close, allowing backflow of blood from left ventricle into left atrium.
- Caused by rheumatic fever, myocardial infarctions, rupture of chordae tendineae

- Best heard at apex, radiates up to left axilla

- Holosystolic, with consistent level of sound, high pitched, harsh blowing quality
- May palpate thrill at apex
- S_1 diminished, S_2 increased intensity
- S_3 frequently present, S_3–S_4 gallop may appear late in disease

Tricuspid Regurgitation

- Valve leaflets don't close completely, allowing back flow of blood from right ventricle into right atrium.
- Frequently congenital in origin, also caused by infectious endocarditis, pulmonary hypertension

- Heard at left lower sternum, may radiate a few centimeters to the left
- Difficult to differentiate from aortic regurgitation during physical exam
- Heard at apex, left sternal border
- Best if patient upright (sitting/standing)

- Holosystolic murmur, soft, blowing in character, which increases on inspiration
- S_3 common, over tricuspid area, thrill at lame location
- Late systolic murmur with midsystolic clicks
- Intensity and timing highly variable

Pulmonic Regurgitation

- Valve leaflets don't close completely, allowing backflow of blood from pulmonary artery into right ventricle.
- Caused by infectious endocarditis and pulmonary hypertension

Murmurs Associated with Other Conditions

Mitral Valve Prolapse

- A condition in which the two flaps of the mitral valve do not open and close properly
- When the flaps are supposed to close during ventricular contraction, they may bulge upward into the atria.
- During this bulging, a small amount of blood may leak into the atria. This creates the clicking sound heard during auscultation.
- In severe cases, blood flows backward into the left atrium with the development of mitral regurgitation.
- MVP is the most common heart valve abnormality, being present in 5%–10% of the world's population.
- In MVP, there is altered formation of the structural protein collagen within the valves and chordae tendineae resulting in their thickening and enlargement (Figure 24-47).

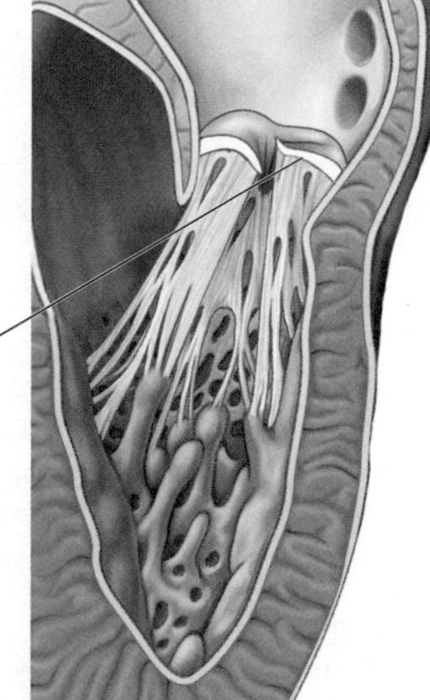

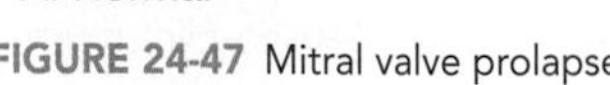
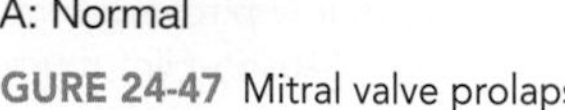

FIGURE 24-47 Mitral valve prolapse

Subaortic Stenosis

- A fibrous ring is present, usually 1–4 mm just below aortic valve.
- May be congenital, progressively becoming more severe

- Heard at apex, along the left sterna border
- Difficult to differentiate from aortic stenosis

- Holosystolic, diamond-shaped murmur, coarse sound.
- Palpable thrill at apex and right sterna border during systole
- S_2 usually split, S_3/S_4 often present

CONGENITAL HEART DEFECTS

Congenital heart defects (CHDs) are alterations of the heart's structures that occur during fetal development and are present at birth. Any part of the heart may be involved and the alterations range from simple to complex. Most CHDs either obstruct blood flow in the heart or vessels near it, or cause altered blood flow through the heart (American Heart Association, 2009).

CHDs are the most common type of birth defect. Annually, 35,000 babies are born with CHD, which correlates to 8 per 1,000 births. The majority of these defects are simple alterations that are easily repaired or may not require any intervention. Simple CHD refer to ventricular septal defect (VSD) and atrial septal defects (ASD), as well as patent ductus arteriosis (PDA), and coarctation of the aorta.

Ventricular Septal Defect

Ventricular septal defect (VSD) is one of the most common congenital heart defects. It may accompany other defects or occur by itself. A small VSD is usually asymptomatic and may spontaneously close. If the VSD does not close and the individual develops symptoms, surgery is then performed to close the septal opening.

Pathophysiology

- A VSD is an opening in the septum that separates the right and left ventricles, allowing blood to be shunted from the left ventricle back into the right ventricle.

Subjective Data

- Recurrent respiratory infections
- Larger VSDs associated with tachypnea, delayed growth, symptoms of CHF

Objective Data

- Arterial pulse diminished, JVP not affected
- Holosystolic, loud, coarse high-pitched murmur
- Best heard along left sternal border, third to fifth ICS

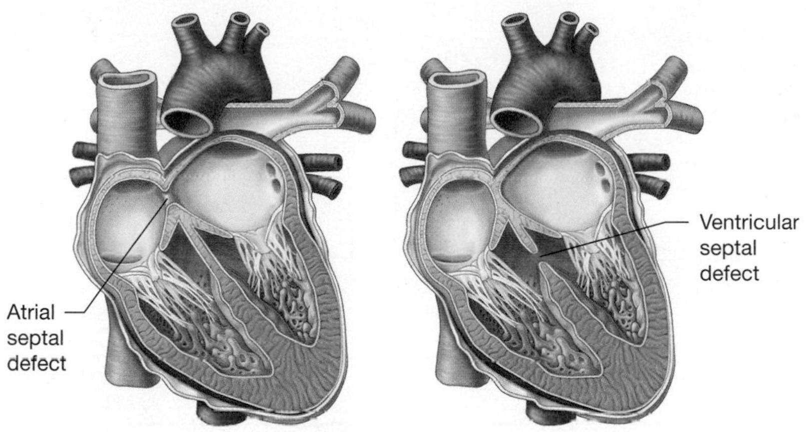

FIGURE 24-48A–B Septal defects **a)** ASD; **b)** VSD

Atrial Septal Defects

Atrial septal defects (ASDs) are less common in children, though more frequently diagnosed in adults due to late clinical manifestation. Small to moderate sized ASD may be asymptomatic until childhood or later into adulthood.

Pathophysiology

- An ASD is an opening in the septum that separates the right and left atria, allowing blood to be shunted from the left atria to the right atria.

Subjective Data

- Frequently asymptomatic
- Dyspnea
- Increased frequency of respiratory infections (children)

Objective Data

- Individuals with a larger ASD may become disabled by middle aged due to pulmonary alterations related to increased circulation due to the increased blood volume in the pulmonary circulation. These individuals have an increased risk for the development of the following:
  - Atrial fibrillation
  - Heart failure
  - Pulmonary overload/hypertension
  - Stroke
  - Palpitations (adult)
  - Conduction abnormalities

Patent Ductus Arteriosis

In fetal circulation a patent ductus arteriosus (PDA) shunts blood away from the pulmonary circulation in utero (Figure 24-49). Soon after birth, the ductus arteriosus closes so blood will enter the pulmonary circulation; however, a post birth failure to close results in maintaining a PDA. Failure of the PDA to close occurs in some premature infants and rarely occurs in full-term infants.

Pathophysiology

- A PDA will allow more blood to flow to the pulmonary circuit, overloading the pulmonary circulation, increasing work of the right ventricle.
- The larger the PDA, the greater the overload on the pulmonary circulation.
- When surgery is necessary, the PDA will be tied off, restoring effective pulmonary circulation.

Subjective Data

- Symptoms related to this include dyspnea, especially during or after activity, increased incidence of pneumonia, and delayed growth.

Objective Data

- Dilated, pulsatile neck vessels
- Widened pulse pressure
- Continuous, machine-like murmur (loud/harsh) at first to third ICS, lower sterna border
- Murmur not affected by postural changes

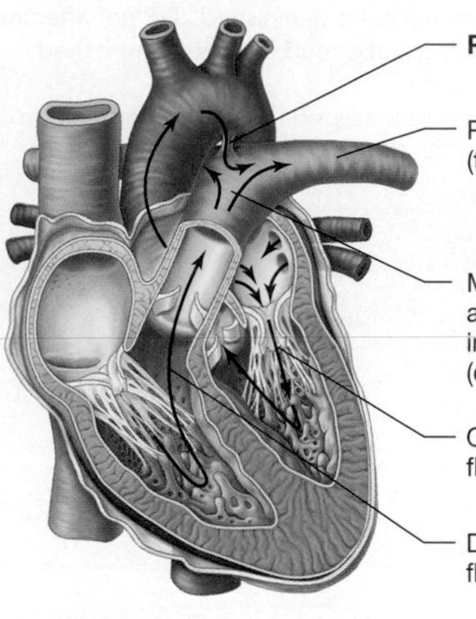

FIGURE 24-49 Patent ductus arteriosis

Coarctation of the Aorta

Coarctation of the aorta (COA) is a condition where there is a section of the aorta that is constricted or narrowed (Figure 24-50).

Pathophysiology

- Location of the constriction is commonly in the descending (thoracic) aortic arch, in the proximity of the origination of the left subclavian artery and ligamentum arteriossum (after the branches of the aorta that perfuse the upper body and before the aorta branches to perfuse the lower body).
- Cause of COA unknown but often accompanies other heart defects
- COA also associated with Turner syndrome
- Infants with severe COA need immediate corrective surgery to prevent heart failure and death.

Subjective Data

- Degree of constriction determines severity of symptoms.
- Those with less severe constriction may not exhibit symptoms until late childhood or adulthood.
- Infants with severe coarctation may demonstrate the following:
  - Pale skin
  - Irritability
  - Heavy sweating
  - Labored breathing
- When signs and symptoms develop in individuals with less severe narrowing they may include the following:
  - Hypertension
  - Shortness of breath (particularly after activity or exercise)
  - Headache
  - Muscle weakness
  - Leg cramps or cold feet
  - Nosebleeds

Objective Data

- Significant problem with coarctation is high blood pressure in upper part of the body.
- COA requires left ventricle to generate higher pressures to eject blood.
- COA frequently after subdivisions of aorta into major arteries for perfusing upper body; higher ventricular pressures result in hypertension of upper body.
- Pressure after coarctation greatly reduced; blood pressure not elevated in lower body
- Difference in the quality (amplitude) of pulse also evident. Higher ventricular pressures produce very forceful pulse wave.
- Palpation of the radial pulse demonstrates pulse that is characteristic of more forceful ventricular contraction; palpation of pedal or posterior tibial pulse demonstrates less forceful pulse.

- Untreated coarctation of the aorta may result in severe complications. Complications are primarily the result of sustained hypertension and may include the following:
  - Stroke
  - Rupture of the aorta
  - Premature coronary artery disease
  - Cerebral aneurysm
  - Liver/kidney failure

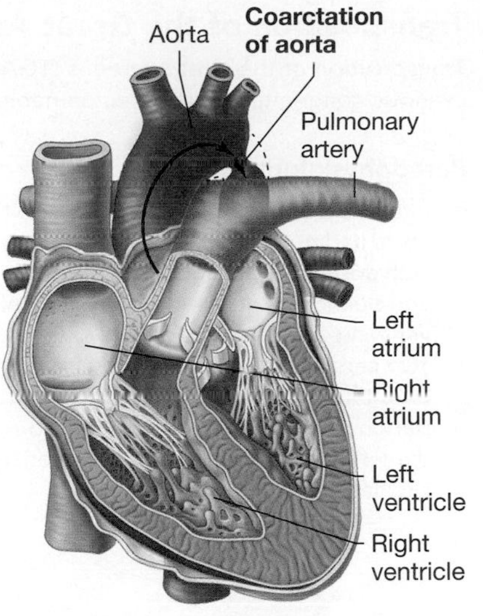

FIGURE 24-50 Coarctation of the aorta

COMPLEX CONGENITAL CARDIAC (CYANOTIC) DEFECTS

Complex CDDs result from significant alterations of heart's structures. Most instances require immediate surgery to save life of the infant. In utero, oxygenated blood from the mother maintains the viability of the fetus. At birth, when the infant's own heart and lungs take over circulation and oxygenation function, complex alterations restrict or prevent oxygenation of the blood, circulating unoxygenated blood and threatening viability of infant. For this reason, complex CHDs are also described as cyanotic defects.

Tetralogy of Fallot (TOF)

Pathophysiology

- TOF is characterized by four defects; the two significant alterations are a VSD and pulmonary valve stenosis. (Figure 24-51).
- Less significant alterations are hypertrophy of the right ventricle and an overriding aorta/aortic valve, where the aorta lies directly above the VSD.
- TOF bypasses pulmonary circulation so infant's blood fails to be oxygenated.

Subjective Data

- Dyspnea with feeding
- Slow/Delayed growth
- Exercise intolerance
- Paroxysmal dyspnea with loss of consciousness and central cyanosis (tetralogy spell)

Objective Data

- Parasternal heave with precordial prominence
- Systolic ejection murmur over third ICS; radiates to left side of neck
- S_2 heard without S_1
- Clubbing develops in older children.

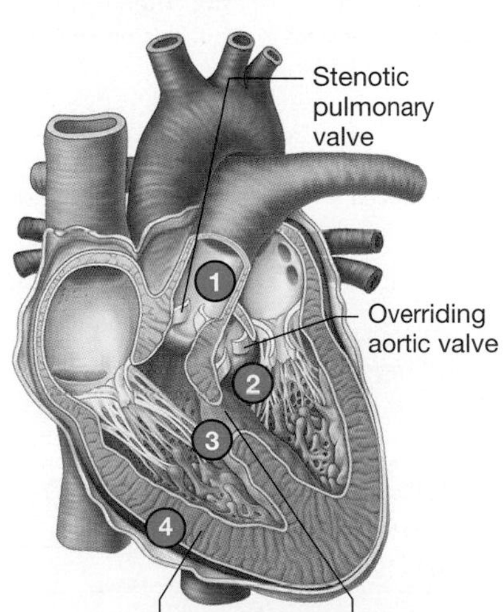

FIGURE 24-51 Tetralogy of fallot

Transposition of the Great Arteries

Transposition of the Great Arteries (TGA) is the most common cyanotic congenital heart defect in neonates. With appropriate and immediate intervention, the survival rate for neonates with TGA is >90%.

Pathophysiology

- Infants with TGV have a defect where the aorta and pulmonary artery are transposed with aorta connecting to right ventricle and pulmonary artery connecting to left ventricle.
- Two separate blood circulation circuits: blood from right ventricle returned to peripheral circulation, and blood from the left ventricle returned to pulmonary circulation.

Subjective Data

- No subjective data available; patient is a neonate.

Objective Data

- Cyanosis
- Shortness of breath
- Poor feeding
- Long-term manifestations
- Leaky heart valves
- Alterations of coronary arteries
- Arrhythmias
- Heart valve dysfunction
- Cardiomyopathy/CHF

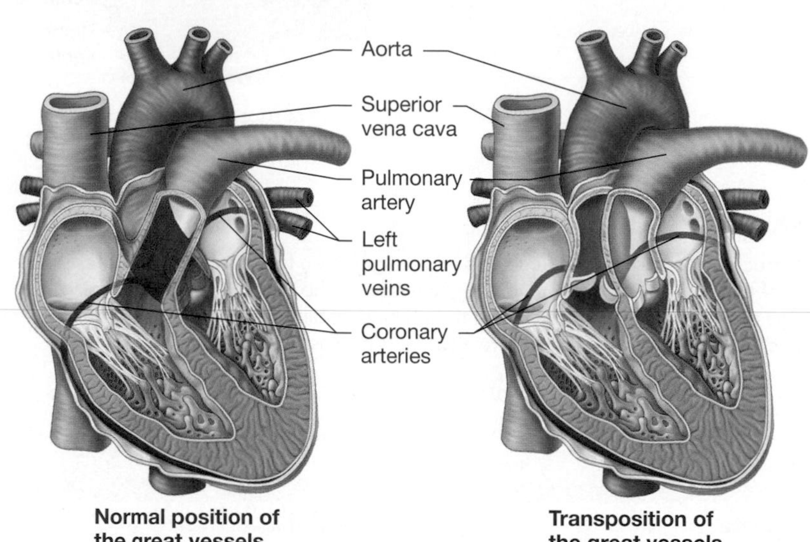

FIGURE 24-52 Transposition of the great vessels

CONDUCTION ALTERATIONS (CARDIAC ARRHYTHMIAS)

Cardiac arrhythmias occur when there is an alteration or interruption of the conduction system of the heart that are manifest through alterations of the ECG complex. Most arrhythmias are harmless, but not all of them. Most arrhythmias are treatable and allow the individual to experience a healthy lifestyle. Criteria for analysis of cardiac rhythms have been identified and described previously, and will be demonstrated throughout this section. Arrhythmias will also be categorized by alterations or variations related to each component of the criteria. There are other categorizing schemes that can be used, but this one will be presented here.

P Wave Alterations

The P wave may be absent due to failure of the SA node to depolarize or there is another site away from the atria that depolarizes and causes the atria to contract.

There are also P wave alterations that occur when there may be aberrant or multiple sites in the atria that depolarize independent of the SA node causing P waves with multiple configurations.

Nodal (Junctional) Rhythm

A nodal rhythm is characterized by an absent P wave or a PR interval < .08.

P wave: Absent, inverted	Rate: 60–100
Ratio: 1:1	PR interval: >.20 sec (If P wave is absent, there is no PR interval or it could be <.08 sec.)
Rhythm: Regular	QRS complex: .08–.12 sec.

- Nodal rhythms generally occur as an escape beat when the SA node has failed to generate an impulse or a tachycardia (Beinart, 2012). An escape beat (back up beat) results from depolarization occurring at another location initiated by failure of the SA node to depolarize. The impulse is most likely generated low in the atria, around the AV node, or within the AV node.
- Depending on where in the AV node the impulse is generated determines presence of P wave and PR interval (Figure 24-53).An inverted P wave results from the impulse being conducted upwards from the AV node, changing direction of vector.

- Presence and configuration of P wave are dependent on when atria contract. If impulse is generated high in the AV node, atria contract before the ventricles, but there is a shortened PR interval. If impulse is generated in the middle of AV node, atria may contract just before or during the first part of ventricular contraction, producing a P wave that is a part of the beginning of the QRS complex, and there is no measurable PR interval. If impulse is generated low in the AV node, the atria contract simultaneously with or possibly after the ventricles with the P wave buried in or after the QRS complex, so there is no visible/measurable P wave or PR interval.
- Regardless of where in the AV node the impulse in generated, it still travels the same pathway to and through the ventricles so the QRS complex retains its usual configuration.

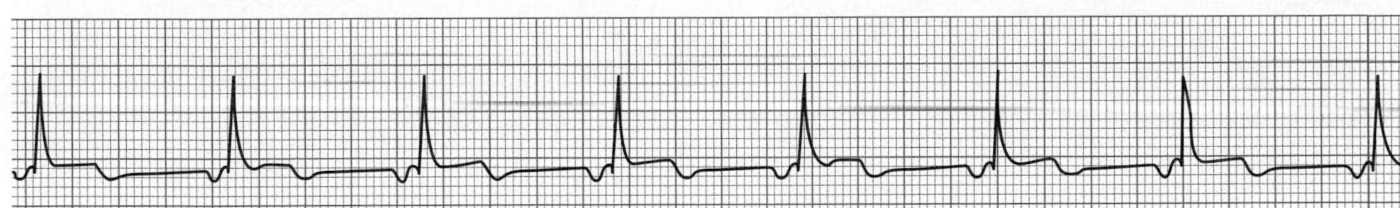

FIGURE 24-53 Nodal (junctional) rhythm

Supraventricular Tachycardias (SVT)

Supraventricular tachycardias are characterized by a ventricular rate that is greater than 100 with the impulse generated above the ventricles but not coming from the SA node. This impulse generating location can be either in the atria or AV node; however, these electrical impulses can reenter the atria and restimulate the atria before the SA node depolarizes.

P wave: Most likely absent or early	Rate: > 100
Ratio: 1:1	PR interval: Most likely absent or short
Rhythm: Regular	QRS complex: .08–.12 sec

- The presence and configuration of P wave depend on proximity of impulse generation site to the ventricles; the closer the site to the ventricles the greater the possibility that the P wave will be absent.
- QRS complex with usual configuration conduction through the ventricles is not altered.
- SVT often present in short runs rather than a consistent rhythm pattern. Short runs of SVT frequently are palpitations of the heart that are felt by patient and described as such.
- A variant type of SVT is Wolf-Parkinson-White syndrome. Individuals with this condition have an extra pathway for the impulse to travel from the atria to the ventricles. This pathway short circuits the functional pathway, disrupting the timing of SA impulse generation and causing a rapid heart rate. This variant rhythm may be life threatening.

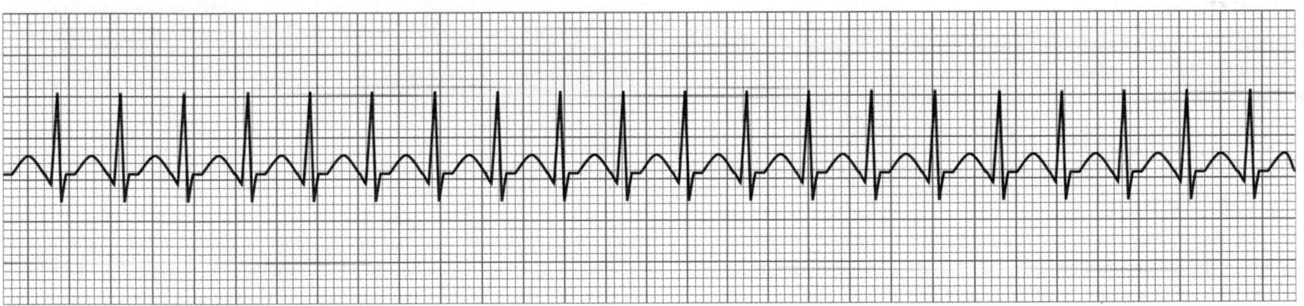

FIGURE 24-54 Supraventricular tachycardias.

Wandering Pacemaker

Wandering pacemaker occurs when there are multiple impulse generation sites.

P wave: present but with various configurations	Rate: 60–00
Ratio: 1:1	PR interval: somewhat variable (dependent on impulse generation site), but within .08–.20 sec
Rhythm: regular but there might be some slight irregularity	QRS complex: .08–.12 sec

- Multiple sites within the atria take turns (wander) depolarizing, accounting for the varied P wave configuration and slightly variable PR interval.
- The QRS complex is usual configuration.

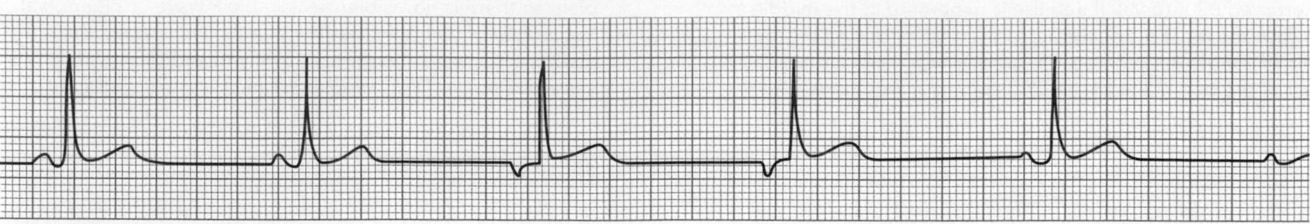

FIGURE 24-55 Wandering pacemaker

Sick Sinus Syndrome

Sick sinus syndrome occurs when the SA node remains the location for impulse formation but depolarization occurs irregularly so there is an irregular pattern to the rhythm usually associated with increased distances between R waves.

P wave: present	Rate: 60–100
Ratio: 1:1	PR interval: .08–.20 sec
Rhythm: irregular	QRS complex: .08–.12 sec

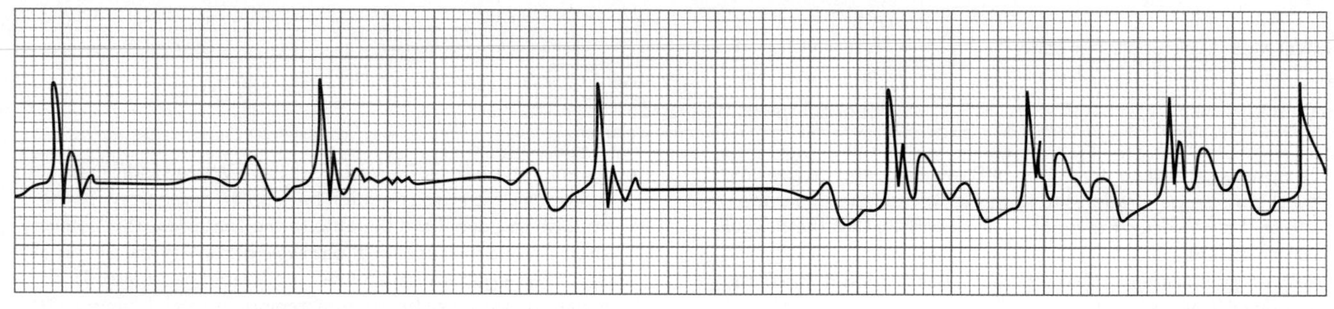

FIGURE 24-56 Sick sinus syndrome

Ratio Alterations

Ratio alterations are arrhythmias where there are a greater number of P waves to QRS complexes. The electrical impulses may be generated at other sites in the atria or there is some type of an AV node block so that only every third or fourth impulse is conducted through the AV node to the ventricles.

Atrial Fibrillation

Atrial fibrillation (AFib) is the most common serious arrhythmia and occurs when there are multiple sites in the atria that rapidly depolarize. Because of the rapidity of the depolarizations, atrial activity is represented by a baseline that is made up multiple P waves, known as fibrillatory waves. The AV node varies as to what impulse it will receive and conduct, so ventricular contraction is irregular. The QRS complexes remain consistent as conduction through the ventricular network is not affected.

P waves are not present but atrial fibrillatory waves are seen at rates of 600 bpm	Rate: ventricular rates are variable up to 240 bpm
Ratio: variable	PR interval: unable to measure
Rhythm: irregular	QRS complex; consistent configuration (.08–.12 sec)

- The onset of AFib generally occurs in the presence of conditions that damage heart muscle: hypertension, coronary artery disease, heart failure, and rheumatic heart disease.
- It also may occur for no apparent reason. Other conditions associated with AFib include hyperthyroidism and alcoholism. Idiopathic onset of AFib may be associated with aging.

- Initially, AFib may cause a serious reduction in cardiac output as the atria fails to contract, eliminating the "atrial kick." Eventually this loss may be adapted to with restoration of an adequate CO.
- Complications of AFib include clot (thrombus) formation within the fibrillating atria, which may break away and become an embolus resulting in pulmonary embolism, stroke, and heart failure.

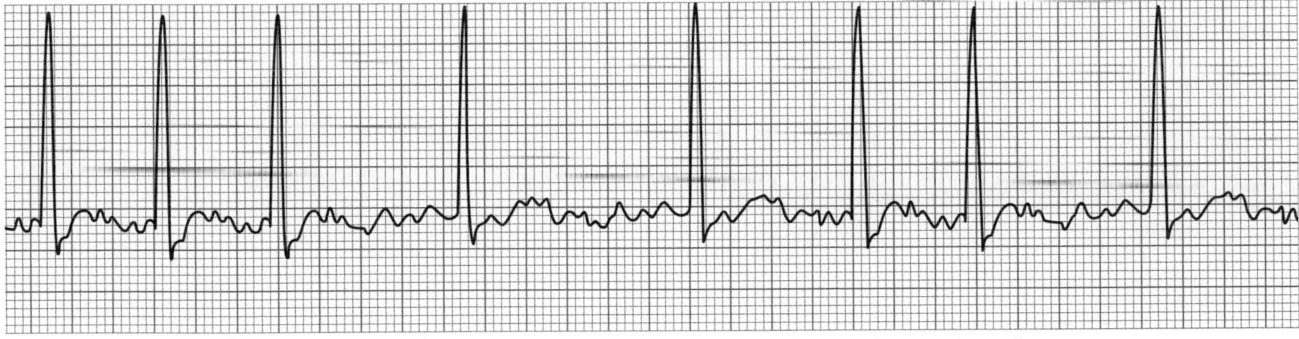

FIGURE 24-57 Atrial fibrillation

Atrial Flutter

Atrial flutter (AF) is similar to AFib with the exception of having a regular rhythm, providing a more consistent P wave pattern and P:QRS ratio. Instead of a baseline with an irregular pattern, the AF baseline demonstrates a saw-tooth pattern. Each flutter wave represents an atrial depolarization, generally from one site. The AV node conduction and ventricular response may be fixed 3–4:1 or it may vary. The QRS configuration remains consistent.

P wave: present (flutter waves)	Rate: 60–100 variable depending on conduction rate through AV node Flutter waves are usually 240–300 bpm
Ratio: fixed [3–4:1] or variable	PR interval: indeterminate
Rhythm: regular or irregular	QRS complex; .08–.12 (consistent configuration)

- Atrial Flutter is less common than AFib, but presents with similar symptoms and complications.

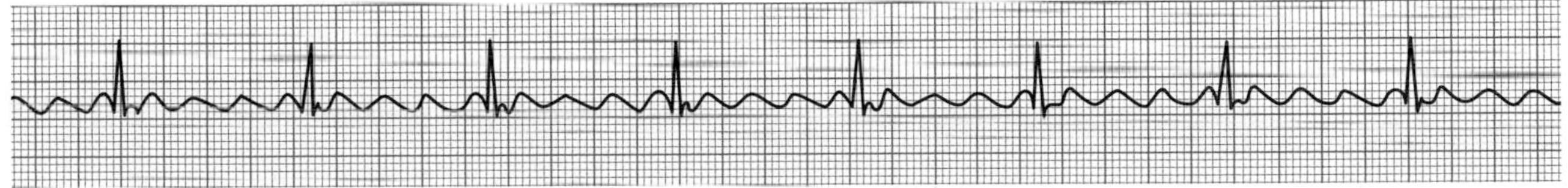

FIGURE 24-58 Atrial flutter

Third-Degree (Complete) Heart Block

Third-degree heart block (HB) occurs when the atria and ventricles depolarize and contract independently. There is a complete conduction block at the AV node, preventing any electrical impulses from reaching the bundle of His and bundle branches. As a result, the ventricles are stimulated by impulses arising in the AV node or lower in the conduction system (Budzikowski, Corsello, Daubert, & Shah, 2009).

P wave: present, consistent configuration	Rate: atrial rate (60–80) > ventricular rate (30–40)
Ratio: variable (inconsistent) atrial sites depolarize more rapidly than ventricular resulting in a greater number of P waves than QRS complexes	PR interval: inconsistent (as there is inconsistent rate of depolarization)
Rhythm: R to R interval consistent; P to P interval consistent	QRS complex: .08 to > .12 (depending on location of impulse generation; AV node [<.12], lower in conduction system [ventricles] [>.12])

- Third-degree heart block may result from a variety of conditions that cause infiltration, fibrosis, or a loss of connections within the conduction system at the AV node. It is a consequence of aging; however, there is a congenital form that is manifested in children. It is also associated with acute MI, drugs (calcium channel blockers, beta-blockers, quinidine, digitalis, lithium, tricyclic antidepressants), or cardiac procedures/surgeries.
- Initial onset of third degree block is potentially life threatening and has been linked to sudden death related to myocardial infarction. The individual may present with syncope (Stoke-Adams attack), lightheadedness, fatigue, dyspnea, and possibly angina.
- Unless third degree HB is caused by medication or some other known cause, treatment requires permanent pacemaker placement.

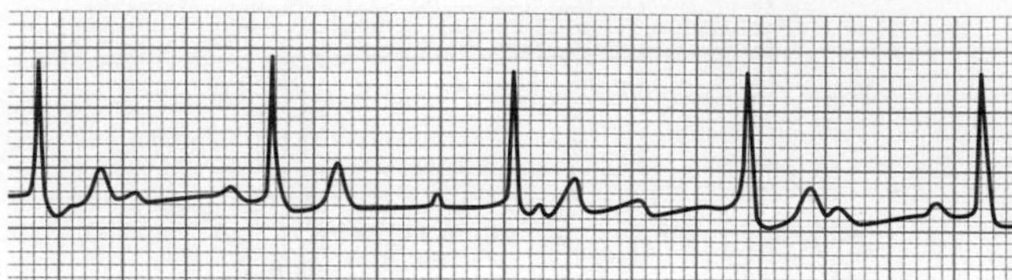

FIGURE 24-59 Third-degree (complete) heart block

Rhythm Alterations

Rhythm alterations are concerned with the regularity of cardiac contractions, which primarily measures the distance between two R waves (point of QRS complex). A regular rhythm has equally spaced QRS complexes; irregular rhythms have unequal distances between the QRS complexes. An irregular rhythm may be regularly irregular or irregularly irregular. A regular irregularity is when the irregular depolarization occurs in its own rhythm or pattern. Premature contraction or ectopic beats may occur on a regular cycle, such as between every fifth and sixth beat. Irregular irregularity has no identifiable pattern and heart contractions occur in an irregular pattern. Atrial fibrillation is the classic example of an irregular irregular pattern. Which atrial impulse will be conducted to the ventricles is a random occurrence so there is a random pattern to the heartbeat.

Sinus Arrhythmia

Sinus arrhythmia occurs when the SA node depolarizes on a slightly variable schedule so that the distance between QRS complexes is slightly irregular. The SA node remains the impulse generator, so time intervals and wave forms remain consistent. The irregular depolarizations are not significant in altering cardiac function, and the presence of sinus arrhythmia does not relate to any cardiac pathology.

P wave: present, consistent configuration	Rate: 60–100
Ratio: 1:1	PR interval: .12–.20
Rhythm: slightly irregular	QRS complex: .08–.12

- Sinus arrhythmia is associated with ventilations with the heart rate usually increasing during inspiration and decreasing during expiration.
- It is common in children and young adults and has no clinical significance except in elderly patients.

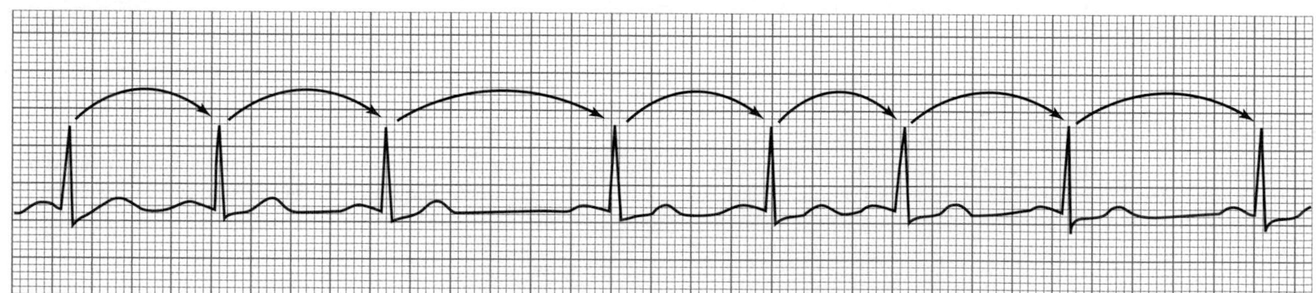

FIGURE 24-60 Sinus arrhythmia

Atrial fibrillation/flutter:
These arrhythmias have already been described.

Premature (Ectopic) Beats/Contractions

Premature beats are contractions that occur before their expected time within the cardiac cycle. Premature contractions may originate in the atria, AV node, or ventricles. Premature beats may be unifocal or multifocal. Unifocal beats come from the same impulse generation location so all ectopic complexes will be the same. Multifocal beats arise from various impulse generation sites, making these ECG complexes different from one another. Multifocal ventricular impulse generating locations may have severe or fatal consequences.

P wave: The presence of a P wave depends on where the early impulse was generated.

- If it occurs in the atria, there would be a P wave, but with a different configuration.
- If the impulse occurred in the AV node, there might or might not be a P wave. If one is present it could have an altered configuration or could be inverted.
- If the impulse was generated in the ventricles, there would be no P wave. There is atrial contraction, but it occurs at the same time as ventricular contraction, so the electrical activity of the atria, being much less than that of the ventricles, is not recorded on the ECG.

Rate: The rate would not be significantly altered unless the premature beats occurred in runs of premature contractions. The rate of the premature run of beats would be significantly different from the existing rate.

Ratio: If the P wave is present, the ratio would be 1:1

PR interval: Depending if there is a P wave, the PR interval may or may not be present. If there is a P wave, the PR interval may be within the identified parameters, but most likely different in time from the existing PR interval.

Rhythm: It is an irregular rhythm because the early beat is not a part of the existing pattern or occurrence within the cardiac cycle.

QRS complex; when the impulse is generated in the atria or AV node, the QRS complex will be consistent in its configuration. When the impulse is generated in the ventricles, the QRS complex will be significantly different from the existing complexes. It is often much wider and demonstrates different wave patterns.

- Premature ventricular contractions occurring after an MI is a serious development. An occasional unifocal PVC not of great concern, however other manifestations related to PVC determine its significance.
- Significant manifestations of PVCs include if they are multifocal, if they occur in couplets (two beats), or if they occur on or near the T wave (R on T phenomena).
- The T wave represents ventricular repolarization and is the time when the ventricles are most vulnerable to altered electrical activity. If PVC occurs during this time, it disrupts the repolarization and throws the electrical stability of the ventricles off so that multiple impulse generating sites emerge, inducing ventricular tachycardia or fibrillation.

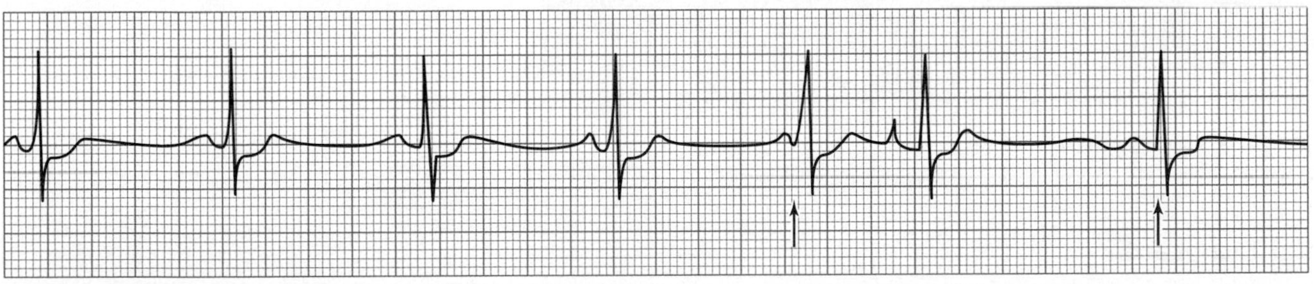

FIGURE 24-61 Premature beats (atrial, nodal [junctional], ventricular contractions)

Rate Alterations

Rate alterations are primarily slow (bradycardias) or fast (tachycardias). Age and physical condition are two major considerations when determining significance of fast or slow rates.

Sinus Bradycardia

Sinus bradycardia (SB) is generally not a lethal or significant arrhythmia unless it is present during exercise, a fever, or congestive heart failure. Persistent rates below 45 may be associated with certain medications such as digitalis, beta-blockers, and calcium channel blockers; however, in their absence, a rate below 45 is significant and may reflect dysfunction of the SA node.

P wave: present, consistent configuration	Rate: <60 (for adult)
Ratio: 1:1	PR interval: .12–.20
Rhythm: Regular	QRS complex: .08–.12

- SB is most often present in athletes who are well conditioned; it may also be present during sleep.
- Metabolic conditions such as hypothermia and hypothyroidism may also be the cause.

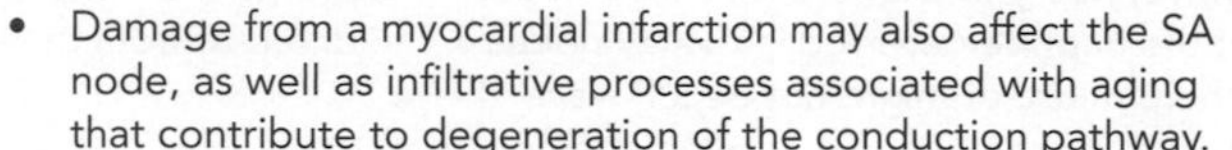

- Damage from a myocardial infarction may also affect the SA node, as well as infiltrative processes associated with aging that contribute to degeneration of the conduction pathway.

6 seconds

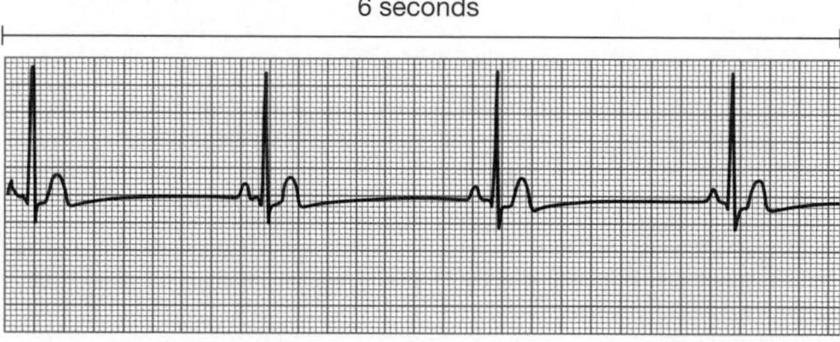

FIGURE 24-62 Sinus bradycardia

Sinus Tachycardia

P wave: present, consistent configuration	Rate: >100 [for adult]
Ratio: 1:1	PR interval: .12–.20
Rhythm: Regular	QRS complex: .08–.12

6 seconds

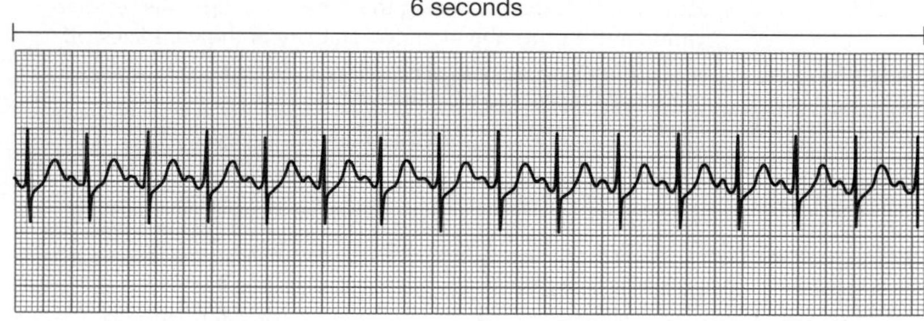

FIGURE 24-63 Sinus tachycardia

Atrial Tachycardia

Atrial tachycardia is when another location in the atria is depolarizing at a faster rate than the sinus node. It starts with a premature atrial contraction followed by a series, or runs of atrial generated beats. These runs may be short 6–10 beats, or they may go on for an extended period of time.

P wave: present, different configuration from sinus node generated P waves	Rate: >100
Ratio: 1:1	PR interval: .12–.20, different interval time from sinus node generated impulse
Rhythm: Regular	QRS complex: .08–.20, generally same configuration as sinus generated impulse

- Short runs may be associated with stress, high caffeine intake, or may not have any precipitating factor.
- Short runs are terminated when the SA node takes over as impulse generator.
- Generally, atrial tachycardia is not lethal, but it does represent some alteration of, or irritability of the atria. Often if a patient identifies the awareness of the heart beating (palpitations), it is atrial tachycardia. Although not always, atrial tachycardia may result in atrial fibrillation.

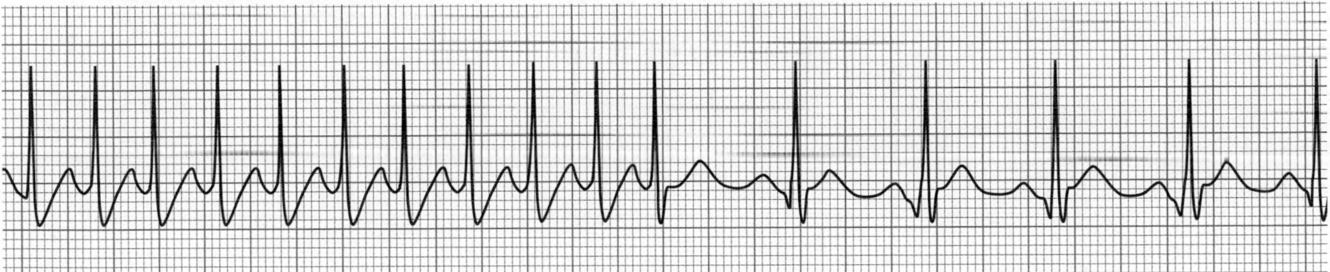

FIGURE 24-64 Atrial tachycardia

Nodal Tachycardia

Nodal tachycardia, like atrial tachycardia occurs when the AV node depolarizes at a faster rate than the SA node. It will also start with a premature nodal beat and be followed by a series of nodal generated beats. There may be only a short series of beats or an extended period of beats.

P wave: may or may not be present; if present will have an altered configuration	Rate: >100
Ratio: If P wave present, ratio of 1:1 will be present	PR interval: If P wave present, will have shorter interval than existing PR interval
Rhythm: Regular	QRS complex: .08–.12
Like atrial tachycardia, nodal techycardia is not significant for the development of severe manifestations.	

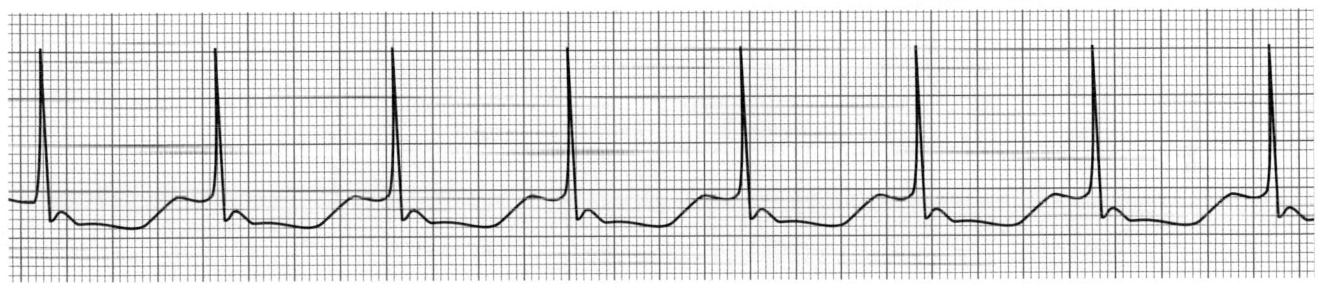

FIGURE 24-65 Nodal tachycardia

Ventricular Tachycardia

Ventricular tachycardia is frequently a significant and lethal arrhythmia. Some individuals tolerate a slow ventricular tachycardia, but most often it has more serious outcomes. It is precipitated by a premature ventricular beat with ensuing rapid ventricular contractions that are not synchronized with atrial contractions. Its lethal outcome is due to the rapid rate of the ventricles that does not allow for adequate ventricular filling, thus cardiac output is severely compromised and may result in death if not terminated quickly.

P wave: none	Rate: >100
Ratio: none	PR interval: none
Rhythm: generally regular, unless multifocal	QRS complex: >.12, much different in configuration from existing complexes

- Ventricular tachycardia is frequently preceded by premature ventricular contractions and are particularly lethal after an MI.
- Ventricular tachycardia often evolves into ventricular fibrillation, which is incompatible with life and frequently the cause of death from an MI. In ventricular fibrillation, the ventricles are not contracting but quivering so that there is no cardiac output.
- On the ECG there is only a wavy baseline and no evidence of ventricular contractions or QRS complexes.

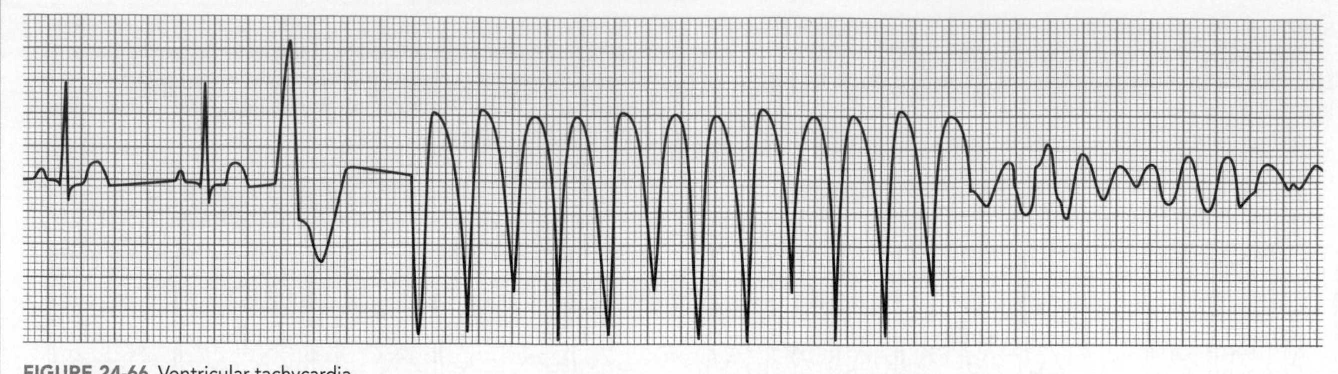

FIGURE 24-66 Ventricular tachycardia

PR Interval Alterations

PR interval alterations occur due to a delayed or blocked conduction of the impulse through the AV node. A delayed impulse goes through the usual conduction pathway so the P wave and QRS complex retain their expected configurations. If the impulse is blocked there is only a P wave without a subsequent QRS complex.

First-Degree AV Block

First-degree AV block occurs when the AV node takes a greater time to conduct the impulse to the ventricles. This is demonstrated by a PR interval that is greater than .20 sec.

P wave: present, consistent configuration	Rate: 60–100
Ratio: 1:1	PR interval: > .20
Rhythm: Regular	QRS complex: .08–.12

- By itself, first-degree block is not significant or lethal; however, it does represent an alteration of the AV node and may go on to produce second- or third-degree AV block.

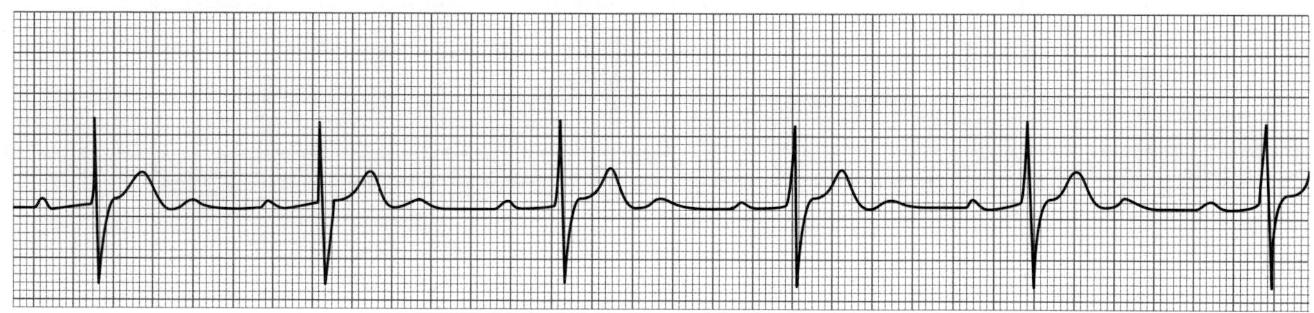

FIGURE 24-67 First-degree AV block

Second-Degree AV Block (Mobitz Type I)

Second-degree AV block has two types: Mobitz type I and Mobitz type II. Mobitz type I second-degree AV block is characterized by an incrementally increasing PR interval until an impulse is not conducted.

P wave: present, consistent configuration	Rate: 60–100
Ratio: 1:1, 2:1	PR interval: > .20
Rhythm: regular, irregular	QRS complex: .08–.12

The cycle then starts over and keeps on repeating itself. The ratio of P waves to QRS complexes is 1:1 until the impulse is completely blocked at the AV node; then there is a 2:1 ratio.

- Second-degree AV block represents an increasing conduction time through the AV node, which may eventually result in third-degree heart block or complete heart block. The PR interval may start out at .22 for the first beat, .26 for the second beat, .28 for the third beat, and then a fourth nonconducted P wave.

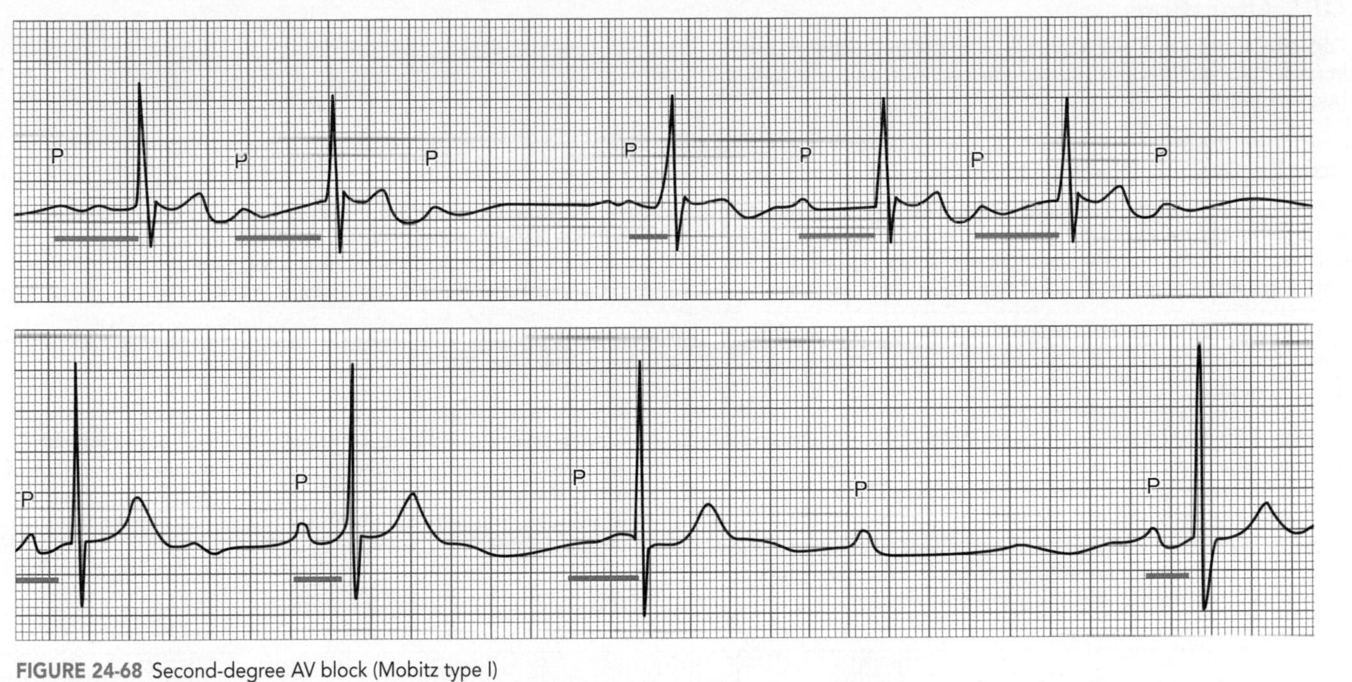

FIGURE 24-68 Second-degree AV block (Mobitz type I)

Second-Degree Heart Block (Mobitz Type II)

Arrhythmias identified as a block indicate that there is an alteration of the AV node or distal conduction system (bundle of His–Purkinje fibers), which delays or fails to conduct the electrical impulse.

Second-degree heart block (HB) II is characterized by every other SA impulse conducted to the ventricles. While a 2:1 ratio is most common, the number of P waves conducted may vary.

P wave: present	Rate: 60–100 (Variable depending on the conduction—The ventricular rate is usually a fraction of 300 bpm. Flutter waves are usually 240–300 bpm.)
Ratio: 2:1 (or greater); every other p wave not conducted	PR interval: <.20 sec
Rhythm: regular	QRS complex: .08–.12 sec

- The SA impulse that is conducted will also have an increase PR interval due to delayed conduction through the AV node.
- The QRS complex is within its time limits and has a consistent configuration.
- Second-degree HB type II is less common than type I (described next) and it is considered more severe, as it is concerned with the distal conduction system and may rapidly progress to third-degree HB or complete HB.

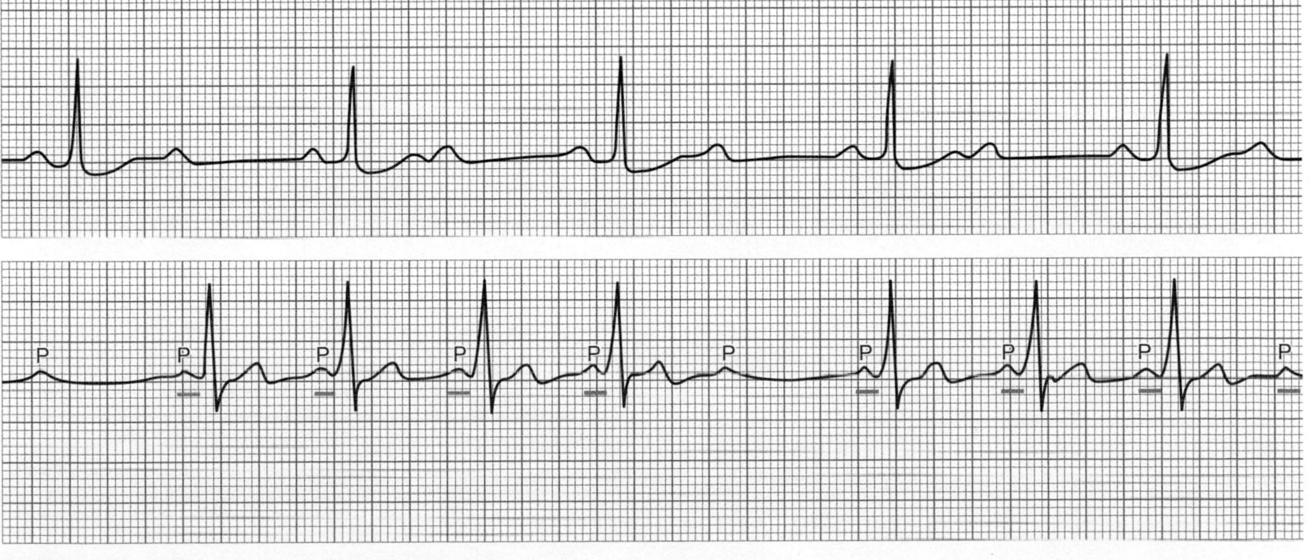

FIGURE 24-69 Second-degree heart block (Mobitz type II)

QRS Alterations

QRS alterations occur when there is aberrant conduction of the impulse through the ventricular conducting system, particularly the bundle branches.

Bundle Branch Blocks

A bundle branch block (BBB) occurs when the impulse conduction through the right and/or left bundle branches of the ventricle is delayed. Generally, impulse conduction is slower on one side, but both sides may be involved. Because of the slower conduction time, the width of the QRS complex is > .12. The slower conduction through the bundle branches may be due to coronary artery disease and myocardial damage from a MI, cardiomyopathy, myocarditis, hypertension, and scar tissue formation.

P wave: present, consistent configuration	Rate: 60–100
Ratio: 1:1	PR interval: .12–.20 (may be greater than .20)
Rhythm: regular	QRS complex. > .12 sec

- Right BBB may be present in healthy individuals with no underlying cardiac conditions, making RBBB the most common type. Left BBB is considered more significant than RBBB.
- Bundle branch blocks with no underlying cardiac conditions are generally asymptomatic and have no effect on cardiac function.
- When symptoms are present, they include syncope, lightheadedness (presyncope), dizziness, and bradycardia.
- Complications of BBB are similar whether the right or left side is affected, but LBBB are associated with an increased incidence of complications.
- Individuals who develop a BBB due to a MI are at a higher risk for developing complications and death.

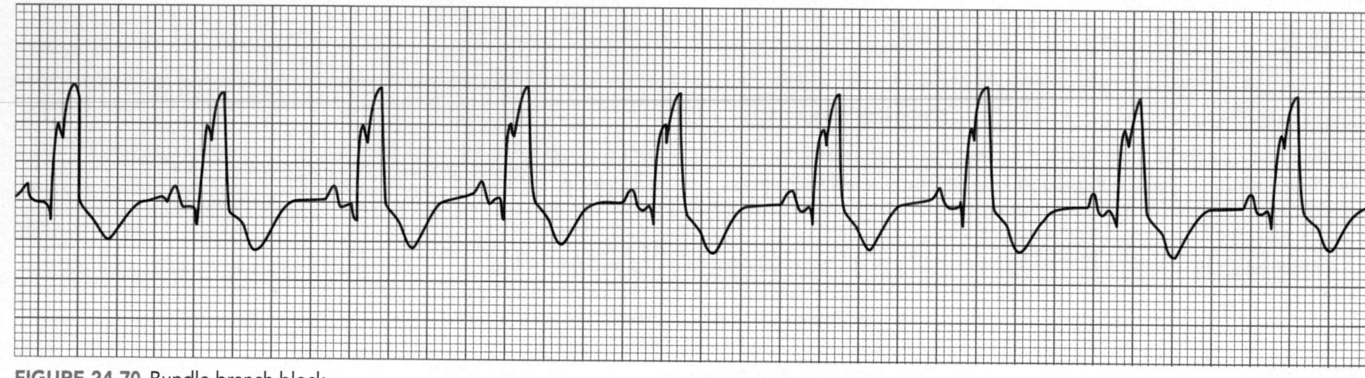

FIGURE 24-70 Bundle branch block

25

Blood Vessels

"All he needs is Tai Chi and our herbs!" Mr. Tender's wife has her arms crossed, already skeptical of my as-yet-unspoken recommendations. He is a 60-year-old Chinese immigrant with a 40 pack-a-year smoking history. He has hypertension and hyperlipidemia. He had a transient ischemic attack 2 years ago and bilateral claudication progressive over the past 6 months. Now his toes won't stop hurting. Mr. Tender was scheduled 2 weeks ago for amputation of his ischemic toes, which had gradually lost their pinkish hue in favor of a deep purple. Hours before his procedure, however, he developed cold feet (excuse the pun) and decided to get a second opinion. "He also needs relaxation and prayer!" Mrs. Tender leans forward and points a finger at me.

"See how she nags?" Mr. Tender begins. "This is why my pressure so high!"

"Your pressure high because you don't quit smoke!"

"Smoke not the problem!"

"Mr. Tender," I cut in, "I agree with your previous provider that your history of smoking has contributed to your health condition, and if you don't quit then your toes will only get worse." Mr. Tender frowns—he is obviously less than thrilled with the prospect of smoking cessation. "The good news is that the studies we performed did not demonstrate significant loss of blood flow. I think this can be reversed if you quit smoking and resume taking your medications to lower your blood pressure and cholesterol."

"What about the Tai Chi?" Mrs. Tender exclaims.

"Sure..." I say, slowly giving in, "Yes, you can certainly do Tai Chi, try herbs, and do relaxation exercises along with taking your medications will help."

Three months later, Mr. and Mrs. Tender are back for a follow-up appointment. I am surprised to see him enter my office in his normal work boots. As he takes them off to reveal nonswollen, pinkish toes, he reports that he has been able to return to his construction job.

"This is remarkable!" I blurt out.

"Tai Chi, relaxation, herbs." Mrs. Tender says with a satisfied grin. I open my mouth reflexively to rebut her claim and talk about the evidence behind behavior change and medical management, but I stop myself short. After all... *who can definitively say what worked?*

LEARNING OUTCOMES

1. Correlate knowledge of peripheral vascular system anatomy and physiology to physical assessment procedures.
2. Explain expected and unexpected characteristics and findings of a peripheral vascular assessment.
3. Summarize a patient history using the essential components of the peripheral vascular history and other related health history components.
4. Recognize differences related to the manifestations of venous alterations vs. arterial alterations.
5. Describe a peripheral vascular assessment using the appropriate assessment procedures with appropriate documentation of findings.
6. Summarize documentation findings related to expected and unexpected assessment findings of peripheral vascular system.

The peripheral vascular system is a component of the cardiovascular system and consists of muscular tubes that serve as the conduit for the delivery of blood to the body. The diameter of the tubes ranges from approximately 1.5 inches to the width of a single blood cell within the capillaries. The capillary bed is extensive in numbers and length. It is estimated that there are about 40 billion capillaries in the human body. Even though capillaries are short in length, the total number adds significantly to the overall length of the vascular system. It is estimated that the total length of the peripheral vascular system ranges from 60,000 miles in a child's body to 100,000 miles in an adult. The length in miles in an adult would circle the equator four times.

Structure and Function

Most tissues of the body have an extensive network of capillaries that supplies blood and necessary nutrients. Some areas or structures of the body are poorly vascularized or avascular. For example, tendons and ligaments are structures that are poorly vascularized, while the cornea, cartilage, and epithelia have no blood supply.

Systemic Blood Circulation

The peripheral vascular system circulation includes the systemic arterial and venous blood circuits. Circulation begins at the heart with the forceful ejection of blood through the aortic valve into the aorta (Figure 25-1). From the aorta, the major arteries **bifurcate** (branch) and continue to do so, subdividing into arterioles that end with the capillaries. After blood circulates through the capillaries, blood enters the venous portion of the capillaries, which begin and continue to **anastomose**, or join with each other, becoming major veins; the blood eventually is delivered to the heart by the superior and inferior vena cava. Where the arterial circuit ends and the venous circuit begins is not well demarcated; however, it occurs at some point within the capillary system.

The rhythmic contractions of the heart and forward motion of blood create a high-pressure system within the arteries, which influences their structure (Figure 25-2). The arteries consist of a thick, smooth muscle layer, which is divided into three layers, making them tougher, more tensile, and less distensible. The three distinct layers, called **tunics**, are the tunica interna, media, and externa. The innermost layer comprises the endothelium, which is simple squamous epithelium. It provides a smooth, friction-free surface for blood flow. The middle layer is made up of concentric circles of smooth muscle cells and is responsible for vasoconstriction and dilation. The outer layer is composed primarily of collagen fibers that are intersected with elastin fibers.

The venous system is a low-pressure system, which results in the veins being thinner and less sturdy than arteries. Their vessel walls are also composed of three muscular layers, but have very little smooth muscle. Pressure within the arterial system gradually falls so that by the time blood reaches the capillaries, there is hardly any pressure. Once blood has circulated through the capillary bed, there are no longer ventricular contractions to propel blood back to the heart. Instead, passive circulation through the veins depends on muscular movements that constrict the venous walls and move blood toward the heart. Without a propelling force to maintain blood circulation, blood is affected by gravity and tends to pool. To prevent pooling, veins are equipped with valves that open to let blood through and then close when blood is drawn backward by gravity.

Being thinner than the arteries, veins are more distensible so when there is an increase in volume of blood, the veins are able to expand and accommodate the extra volume. This compensation reduces the workload of the heart.

Arterial Pulse and Pressure

The peripheral vascular and the cardiovascular systems are closed systems due to the necessity of maintaining a certain level of pressure within them for optimum function. It is the various changes in the pressures along the vascular system that help to maintain blood flow. Any alteration that causes the system to open reduces the pressure within the system, compromising the delivery of blood throughout the body.

Each ejection of blood from the left ventricle creates a pressure wave that temporarily distends the arterial wall (Figure 25-3). Each distension produces a wave that is palpable at various points on the body and is referred to as the **arterial pulse**. A pulse wave consists of a steep rapid ascent wave that peaks and then begins a slower descent. The descent wave contains a **dicrotic notch**, which creates a mall secondary wave that is not palpable but is visible on an arterial pressure monitor.

Arterial pressure is a measurement of the force exerted against the arterial walls with each pulse wave. It consists of two measurements that reflect the components of the cardiac cycle. Systolic arterial pressure is the force exerted against the artery during ventricular contraction. Systolic arterial pressure is the highest pressure and is due to stroke volume, blood volume, and **vascular compliance** (distensibility) of the arterial wall. Compliance of the arterial wall can be thought of as the amount of stretch or distension an artery permits. As a person ages, the artery becomes stiffer due to arteriosclerosis, or a hardening of the arteries. As the stiffness of the artery increases, the compliance of the artery decreases.

Diastolic arterial pressure is the force exerted against the arterial wall when the ventricle is relaxed and filling with blood. Diastolic pressure is the lowest pressure that occurs during the cardiac cycle and is determined by the amount of **peripheral vascular resistance**, or the force that impedes the forward flow of blood. The peripheral vascular resistance is essentially regulated by the diameter of the blood vessel; the smaller the diameter, the greater the resistance. Arteriosclerosis also plays a role in peripheral vascular resistance. Atherosclerosis, or the buildup of plaques on the inside of the artery, is another determinant of distensibility and resistance.

The difference between the systolic and diastolic pressures is the **pulse pressure**. Determinants of the characteristics of the pulse and blood pressure are as follows:

- Stroke volume (amount ejected with each contraction)
- Viscosity (thickness) of the blood

PRACTICE POINT: Pulse Pressure

Pulse pressure has been largely ignored as having any significance relevance to cardiovascular disease. The systolic and diastolic pressures were perceived to be the parameters that related to the diagnosis of hypertension and these data were primarily assessed in determining the effectiveness of any interventions. Elevated diastolic pressures were emphasized as being more significant in determining the severity of hypertension. Recently, there has been a shift toward using the systolic pressure and the pulse pressure as significant indicators of cardiovascular risk. Elevated pulse pressures have now been positively correlated with an increased occurrence of cardiovascular events (Patel, Landers, Li, Mortimer, & Richard, 2011). Presently, studies have been conducted on males, which limit the ability to determine the effects of increased pulse pressure in females.

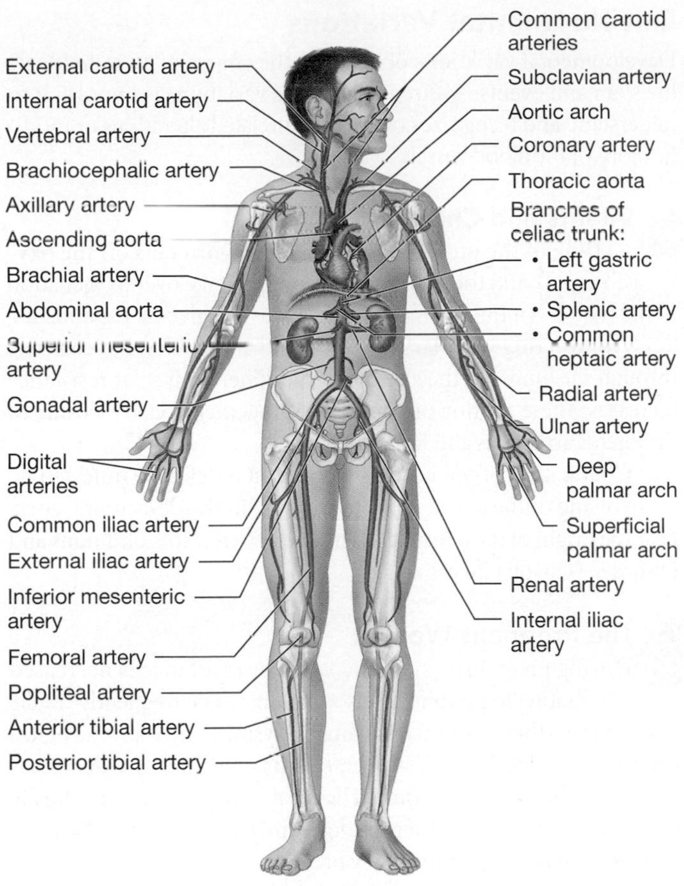

External carotid artery
Internal carotid artery
Vertebral artery
Brachiocephalic artery
Axillary artery
Ascending aorta
Brachial artery
Abdominal aorta
Superior mesenteric artery
Gonadal artery
Digital arteries
Common iliac artery
External iliac artery
Inferior mesenteric artery
Femoral artery
Popliteal artery
Anterior tibial artery
Posterior tibial artery
Common carotid arteries
Subclavian artery
Aortic arch
Coronary artery
Thoracic aorta
Branches of celiac trunk:
• Left gastric artery
• Splenic artery
• Common heptaic artery
Radial artery
Ulnar artery
Deep palmar arch
Superficial palmar arch
Renal artery
Internal iliac artery

FIGURE 25-1A Systemic arterial circulation

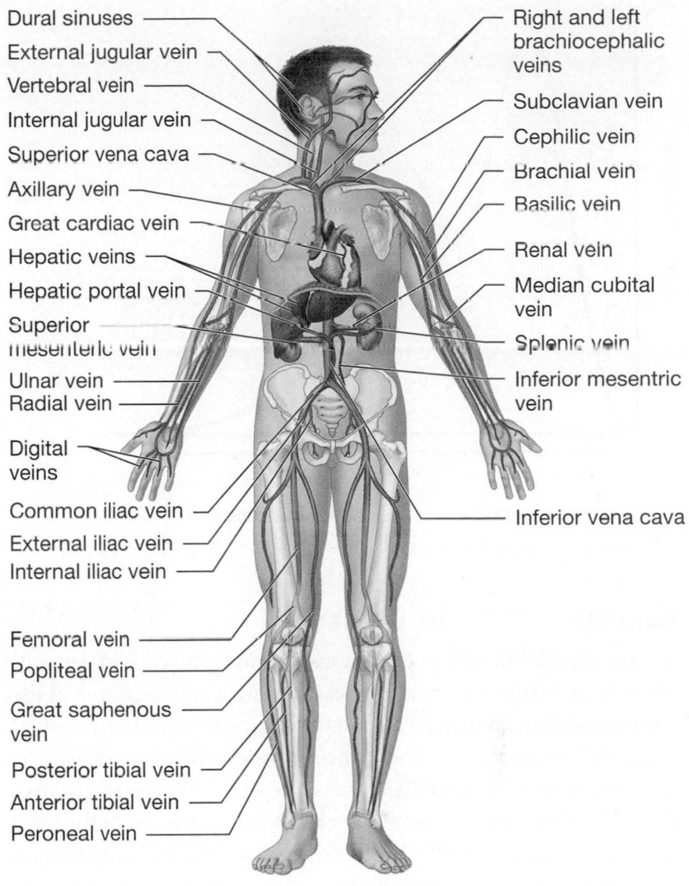

Dural sinuses
External jugular vein
Vertebral vein
Internal jugular vein
Superior vena cava
Axillary vein
Great cardiac vein
Hepatic veins
Hepatic portal vein
Superior mesenteric vein
Ulnar vein
Radial vein
Digital veins
Common iliac vein
External iliac vein
Internal iliac vein
Femoral vein
Popliteal vein
Great saphenous vein
Posterior tibial vein
Anterior tibial vein
Peroneal vein
Right and left brachiocephalic veins
Subclavian vein
Cephilic vein
Brachial vein
Basilic vein
Renal vein
Median cubital vein
Splenic vein
Inferior mesentric vein
Inferior vena cava

FIGURE 25–1B Systemic venous circulation

Valve
Tunica interna:
Endothelium
Basement membrane
Tunica media:
Smooth muscle
Tunica externa:
Adventitia
(a) Vein
Tunica interna:
Endothelium
Basement membrane
Internal elastic lamina
Tunica media:
Smooth muscle
External elastic lamina
Tunica externa:
Adventitia
(b) Artery
Endothelium
Basement membrane
(c) Capillary

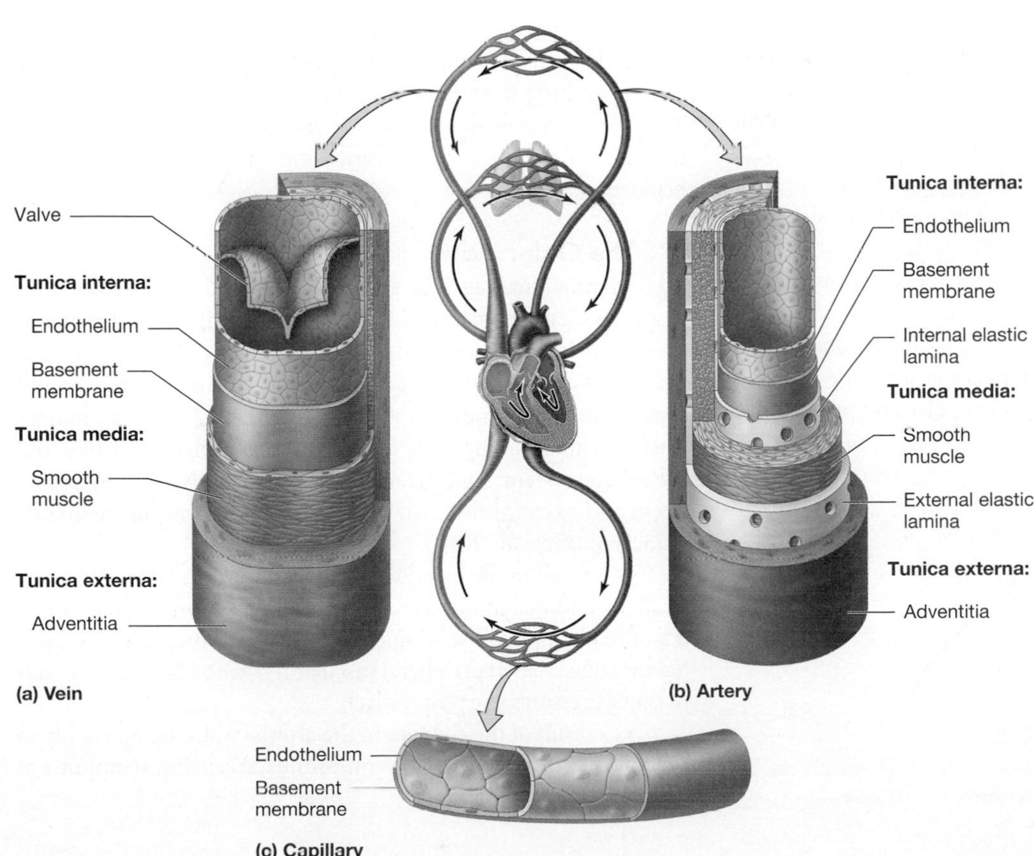

FIGURE 25-2 Anatomical structure of veins, arteries, and capillaries

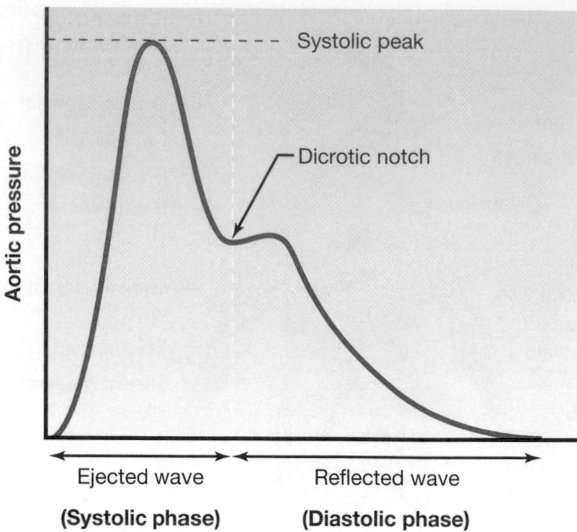

FIGURE 25-3 Arterial pulse wave

Venous Pulse and Pressure

Because blood flow within the venous system is passive and depends on muscular contraction to propel it to the heart, pressures in the venous system are much lower than the arterial system. The increased distensibility of the veins, due to their thinness and a lack of muscle, also contributes to the reduced pressures. Venous pressure corresponds to the pressure against which blood is delivered to the right side of the heart, rather than the pressures that expel and propel blood forward as it leaves the heart. Measurement of systemic venous pressure is generally not routinely done; however, venous pressure may be measured within the heart chambers and provides information related to overall pressures within the venous system. Measurement of **venous pressure** is not divided into systolic and diastolic as is the arterial pressure as there is no valve that opens and closes between the vena cavae and atrium. Increased pressures in the venous system are more of a reflection of **venous congestion**, or pooling of blood, which is an indication of inadequate delivery of blood to the right side of the heart. The most common site for measurement of venous pulse and pressure is at the jugular vein in the neck.

The **venous pulse** is created by changes in pressure within the right side of the heart caused by the filling of the chambers and opening and closing of the valves. There are five identifiable components of the venous pulse—three ascending peaks and two descending slopes (Figure 25-4). (Assessing the venous pulse and pressure are covered in Chapter 24.)

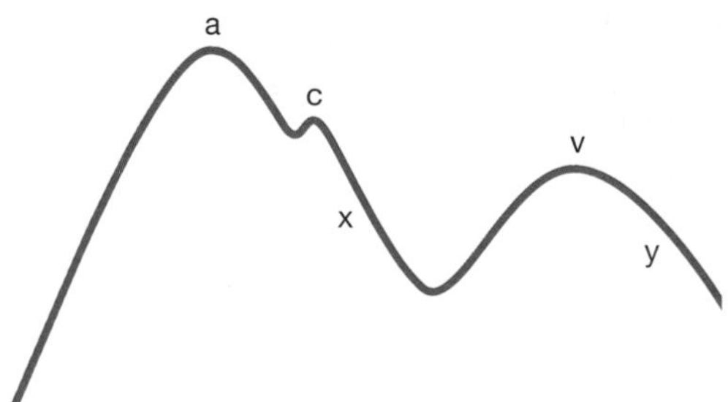

FIGURE 25-4 A venous pulse wave with C, V waves; X, Y descent

Developmental Variations

Developmental variations occur over the course of an individual's life span and events. Awareness of these variations is important to understand and recognize common age-related alterations or modifications of the blood vessels.

Infants and Children

Cutting of the umbilical cord in a newborn cuts off the oxygen supply and thus requires the lungs to take over oxygenation of the blood. An infant's first breath opens the alveoli, expands the lungs by lowering vascular resistance, and allows blood to circulate through the lungs. At the same time, peripheral vascular resistance increases. These shifting pressures work together to cause closure of the ductus arteriosus and foramen ovale.

Coarctation of the aorta is a congenital defect manifested by a narrowing of the aorta, most commonly in the descending aorta near the origin of the left subclavian artery. (Refer to Conditions and Disorders; Chapter 24 p. 674.)

The Pregnant Woman

During pregnancy, systemic vascular resistance is decreased contributing to peripheral vasodilation, which frequently results in palmar erythema and telangiectasis. Systolic and diastolic blood pressure also decreases; however, the diastolic pressure decreases more than the systolic pressure. The greatest decrease occurs during the second trimester and then gradually increases; however, the pressures remain below prepregnancy pressures.

Blood flow is frequently affected by the expanding uterus. Hypotension may occur in the third trimester, particularly when the woman is supine. Hypotension results from occlusion of the vena cavae, decreasing venous blood return to the heart. The enlarged uterus also causes occlusion of the pelvic veins and inferior vena cavae, resulting in stagnation of blood in the lower extremities. The increased pressures caused by venous occlusion results in an increase in dependent edema, varicosities of the legs and vulva, and hemorrhoids.

The Older Adult

As individuals age, the arteries become calcified (arteriosclerosis), causing narrowing of the lumen, diffuse intimal and medial thickening, increased stiffness, reduced compliance of central arteries, endothelial dysfunction, and impaired arterial wound repair and angiogenesis (Tau & Peterson, 2012). These changes start proximally at the aorta and then proceed distally throughout the arterial system. Superficial vessels, particularly of the forehead, neck, and extremities, also become tortuous and more visible (Rinckenbach et al., 2010).

As a result of the increasing stiffness, the arterial wall loses its elasticity and vasomotor tone; thus, the arteries lose their ability to adapt to changing physiological needs. Blood pressure also rises because of increased peripheral vascular resistance. Both systolic and diastolic pressures rise progressively.

As a result of the changes in the arterial walls, blood supply to the lower extremities may be compromised causing symptoms of **claudication**.

Health Promotion

Peripheral vascular health is essential to maintain the functioning of every organ system of the body; it is the conduit that connects organs and systems to each other. Diagnosis is critical, as peripheral vascular disease (PVD) can lead to catastrophic events that cause significant cellular, tissue and organ damage and may result in death. Individuals with PAD have four to five times higher risk of *heart attack* or *stroke*. The prevalence of peripheral vascular disease in the general population is 12%–14%, affecting up to 20% of those over 70 (10 million) (Shammas, 2007); however, 70%–80% of affected individuals are asymptomatic. Peripheral vascular disease also affects 1 in 3 diabetics over the age of 50. The incidence of symptomatic PVD increases with age and varies considerably depending on how PAD is defined and the age of the population being studied. Despite its prevalence and cardiovascular risk implications, only 25 percent of PAD patients seek treatment.

Hypertension

The objectives of *Healthy People 2020* within the Topic Area of Heart Disease and Stroke (HDS) are as follows:

- HDS—4 Increase the proportion of adults who have had their blood pressure measured with the preceding 2 years and can state whether their blood pressure was normal or high.
- HDS—5 Reduce the proportions of persons (adults, children and adolescents) with hypertension.
- HDS—11 Increase the proportion of adults with hypertension who are taking the prescribed medications to lower their blood pressure.
- HDS—12 Increase the proportion of adults with hypertension whose blood pressure is under control (U.S. Department of Health and Human Services, 2009).

Hypertension (high blood pressure) is a worldwide condition that remains an important public health challenge due to its morbidity and mortality costs to society. In the U.S., hypertension affects 75 million adults (Sakalihasan, Limet, & Defawe, 2005). Additionally, approximately 30% of American adults (59 million) over the age of 18 are considered pre-hypertensive, which increases an individual's chances of developing heart disease and stroke (Lizka, Mainous, King, Everett, & Egan, 2005). For these reasons, screening and early detection are paramount in its prevention and treatment.

Hypertension generally has an insidious onset with minimal to no manifestations of symptoms, which contributes to its significant morbidity and mortality and also leads to its description as the "silent killer." The prevalence of hypertension increases with age; the majority of individuals being aged 60 and older.

Certain ethnic populations are also at a greater risk for developing hypertension. It is more prevalent in non-Hispanic black populations, who also tend to develop it at an earlier age. Additionally, it is often more severe and this population experiences a higher incidence of early death from HTN related conditions (coronary artery disease, stroke, kidney failure). Non-Hispanic white populations are the next at risk populations with the Mexican American populations having the lowest risk. Other factors include the environment as well as genes that may interact in complex ways.

Due to the difficulty in defining HTN, it is classified according to specific parameters for individuals 18 years or older. The most recent recommendations come from the Seventh Report of the Joint National Committee on Prevention, Evaluation and Treatment of High Blood Pressure and places HTN in four classifications (expressed in mmHg):

- Normal—Systolic lower than 120, diastolic lower than 80
- Pre-hypertensive—Systolic 120—139, diastolic 80—89
- Stage 1—Systolic 140—159, diastolic 90—99
- Stage 2—Systolic equal to or greater than 160, diastolic equal to or greater than 100 (Sakalihasan et al., 2005)

These results are based on the average of two or more readings taken at each of two or more visits after initial screening. Prehypertension is a new category within the Joint National Committee report that describes individuals who are at risk for progression to HTN and require essential lifestyle modifications.

Pseudohypertension may be present in older adults who have thickened, calcified arteries. Significant higher cuff pressure may be needed to occlude a thickened brachial artery. This may result in an overestimated diastolic pressure. Pseudohypertension should be considered in instances when no organ damage occurs despite marked hypertension, when patients develop hypotensive symptoms on medications, and when calcification of the brachial artery is observed on radiologic examination. Direct measurement of intra-arterial pressure may be required if pseudohypertension is suspected.

Because of the unknown cause of HTN in most cases, specific screening and prevention strategies are not determined. However, lifestyle modifications are recommended for the prevention and control of HTN. These modifications include the following:

- Maintain healthy weight or lose weight if overweight.
- Be moderately physically active on most days of the week (aerobic activity—30–45 minutes).
- Follow a healthy eating plan (decrease sodium; maintain potassium, calcium, and magnesium for general health; reduce intake of saturated fat and cholesterol).
- Limit alcohol intake (no more than 1 oz (30 mL) of ethanol (e.g., 24 oz [720 mL] of beer, 10 oz [300 mL] of wine, 2 oz [60 mL] of 100-proof whiskey per day or 0.5 [15 mL] ethanol per day for women and people of lighter weight).
- Stop smoking.
- Manage stress and develop coping skills.

The DASH (Dietary Approaches to Stop Hypertension) eating plan is a strategy for reducing blood pressure by eating foods that are low in saturated fat, cholesterol, and sodium and that emphasizes fruits, vegetables, and fat-free or low-fat milk products. Studies of the DASH plan by the National Heart, Lung, and Blood Institutes demonstrated significant positive results. Participants who followed the plan and increased fruits and vegetables reduced their blood pressure (Cevallos, 2012; National Institues of Health, 2001).

Blood Disorders

Healthy People 2020 objectives within the Topic Area of Blood Disorders and Blood Safety (BDBS) are as follows:

- BDBS—12/13: Reduce the number of persons who develop venous thromboembolism (VTE); reduce the number of adults who develop venous thromboembolism (VTE) during hospitalization.

Bleeding and clotting disorders in regards to the peripheral vascular system focus on **hypercoagulopathies** and thrombophilia, both conditions in which individuals have an abnormality of blood coagulation that predisposes them to the development of thrombosis (blood clots). There are multiple causes of hypercoagulopathy syndromes, which have only been identified since 1993, and are primarily inherited. Five main categories of inherited hypercoagulable conditions have been identified:

- Qualitative/quantitative defects of coagulation factor inhibitors
- Increased levels/function of coagulation factors

Health Promotion *continued*

- Hyperhomocysteinemia
- Defects of the fibrinolytic system
- Altered platelet function (Palm, Trizna, & Goldman, 2011)

Although the exact incidence of VTE is unknown, each year, there are an estimated 900,000–1 million patients with evidence of VTE in the U.S., resulting in an estimated 300,000 deaths from pulmonary embolism (PE). Sudden death is the first symptom in about one-quarter (25%) of people who have a PE. The estimated 600,000 nonfatal cases of VTE result in several hundred thousand primary hospitalizations or extended hospital stays in patients who develop VTE while hospitalized (Raskob, Silverstein, Bratzler, Heit, & White, 2010). One-third (about 33%) of people with DVT/PE will have a recurrence within 10 years.

There are no specific manifestations of hypercoagulopathies making it difficult to determine individuals at risk. Often initial indicators are the formation of VTEs at a young age (<45 years) or recurrent formations. A strong family history of VTEs is a significant factor to consider in predicting one's predisposition to development of VTE. Presently, widespread testing for hypercoagulopathy is not recommended nor has it been determined that thrombophilia test results improve the ability to predict recurrence when compared with a clinical risk assessment (Saultz, Mathews, Saultz, & Judkins, 2010).

A major contributing factor to the development of VTE is immobility associated with any situation where it is difficult to move around. Postsurgical patients in hospitals have been widely recognized as high risk for developing VTE due to pain associated with movement and ambulation. More recently, individuals traveling on long flights have been identified as high risk for developing VTE (traveler's thrombosis).

While the condition is possible, the probability of developing VTE during air flight remains relatively low. In-flight conditions that contribute to developing VTE include lower than normal air pressure, dehydration, immobility; by themselves they do not appear to have a significant impact on VTE development. Their significance increases in individuals who are already at risk for developing VTE. The single most contributing factor in the development of VTE is a flight of 8 hours or more (Bartholomew, Schaffer, & McCormick, 2011).

Consensus on preventive measures for the development of VTE has yet to be reached. There is no specific test or screening tool that can be used to identify high-risk individuals within the general population.

Clinical Context Exemplars

Situation A

Mr. Tony Cooper is a 62-year-old male who is in the hospital for congestive heart failure. When the provider enters his room she observes that Mr. Cooper's veins in his neck are distended with some visible pulsations.

1. Why is it important for the provider to also observe the position of Mr. Cooper?
2. What is the significance of Mr. Cooper being in a 45-degree angle position in bed?

Situation B

Mr. Kent Thornton is a 52-year-old male who has been experiencing periods of forgetfulness and some periods of minimal black out. During the physical examination, a bruit is heard in the right carotid artery.

1. What is the significance of hearing a bruit in Mr. Thornton?
2. What is happening in the carotid artery to cause a bruit?

Situation C

Mrs. Grace Hawthorne is a 45-year-old female who is in for a routine physical. The following information is obtained from her history and physical: Occupation—hairdresser, BP—142/84, pulse—76, respirations—14; ht—5'6". Wt—260; smokes 1 ppd.

1. From the information given, why would Mrs. Hawthorne be at risk for the development of venous insufficiency?
2. What further information would you need to obtain to help assess her risk?
3. What visible manifestations would you need to look for during the exam?

SUBJECTIVE DATA

History of Present Illness (CC)

The individual may present to the provider with a variety of complaints that may be directly related to the peripheral vascular system or other systems. All symptoms presented must be thoroughly assessed with an appropriate symptom analysis.

Leg Pain/Cramps

Leg pain is a common complaint and symptoms often occur after an injury; however, pain can also occur due to medical conditions or nontraumatic reasons.

Provider Inquiries	Clinical Reasoning/Logic
Characteristics: Do you have limb pain?	Limb pain may be secondary to vascular or nonvascular causes. Non-vascular causes include deep venous thrombosis (DVT), musculoskeletal disorders, peripheral neuropathy and spinal stenosis.
Do you have spasms or leg pain at night?	Nocturnal leg cramps or restless leg syndrome must be differentiated from claudication. These are not associated with exercise.
	Claudication refers to a reproducible tight squeezing pain involving a defined group of muscles that is induced by exercise and relieved by rest. Many causes exist, with the most common one being arterial atherosclerosis or peripheral arterial disease involving aorto-iliac vessels to the popliteal vessels. Upper extremity claudication is less common. Leriche's syndrome has been used interchangeably with claudication.
Do you have "Charley horses" or cramping?	Charley horse is the colloquial term for muscle cramps associated with tightening or stiffness or sudden contraction of muscles, which may be the first signs of claudication. This can be due to poor circulation, fatigue, overexertion, mineral deficiency, medications or may be idiopathic (Aquarius, DeVries, & Van Berge Henegouwen, 2006).
Do you have a burning sensation?	People with neuropathy tend to describe their pain as a burning sensation, while those who have sciatica describe intense sharp pain. Sciatica may also cause changes in sensation along the path of the inflamed nerve root.
Onset: With activity/rest, what type of activity, how much activity, recent injury/immobilization?	
Location: Is the pain localized or generalized?	Pain in arterial occlusion is generally referred to the regional areas of flow. In venous insufficiency, pain is directly associated with the affected veins, skin changes and ulcerations. Pain is aggravated by movement of the joint in arthritis. Pain is intermittent in claudication based on demand for oxygen supply of the limb.
Duration: How long does pain last; intermittent/continuous?	
Exacerbation: Anything that makes the pain worse? Standing? Exercise?	Exacerbation by exertion and relief with rest suggest claudication, as in vascular ischemia. In venous insufficiency, pain is increased with standing and better with limb elevation and walking.
Relief: What makes pain go away; stopping activity?	Relief of pain with rest is characteristic of peripheral artery disease. Pain is increased with elevation of the limb in arterial occlusion and decreased in venous insufficiency.

Provider Inquiries	Clinical Reasoning/Logic
Radiation: Does pain go anywhere else?	Radiation of pain along the nerve distribution suggests spinal nerve compression.
Associated signs/symptoms: Increased tendency to bruise easily/bleed excessively?	In spinal neuropathy or degenerative disk disease, pain radiates following the involved dermatome.
Skin changes: Cold skin, pallor hair loss, redness or warmth over veins, visible veins, skin darkening (black), any odor? Ulcers, numbness or tingling of lower extremity and foot? Tired legs, swelling?	Cold skin or extremity, pallor, and loss of hair in that arterial distribution and sweat are seen in chronic arterial atherosclerosis. Darkening of skin with tissue breakdown and odor suggest gangrene.

THINK LINK: Leriche's Syndrome

This refers to occlusion of arterial blood flow from the aorta to the lower limb and manifest with leg weakness or numbness, claudication, erectile dysfunction, and weak lower extremity pulses. Conditions that resemble it include osteoarthritis, neurogenic claudication, or pseudoclaudication (pain due to neurospinal canal compression); pain here is relieved with sitting or lying down. Pain is induced by erect posture or lumbar lordosis exaggeration and relieved by leaning forward and straightening of the spine.

Swollen Ankles

Swollen ankles or leg swelling may be multifactorial in etiology. It may be from water retention, prolonged standing, lymphedema, renal causes, trauma, vascular occlusion or ischemia, venous insufficiency, blood clots, arthritis, or injured muscles ligaments and joints.

Provider Inquiries	Clinical Reasoning/Logic
Characteristics: Is the swelling noted in one leg (unilateral) or both (bilateral)? Vascular pathology affecting one or both lower extremities?	Swelling or enlargement of the ankles is commonly associated with venous disorders (venous insufficiency, varicose veins) due to incompetent valves that compromise venous return to the heart, resulting in venous congestion.
Onset: When does swelling occur? Does it progressively increase throughout the day? Do you remember when you first noticed the swelling?	Swelling initially starts in the ankles and as veins and valves become compromised swelling progresses upward.
Location: Ankles, progress upward, entire lower leg?	The most dependent part of the body is generally affected more. In chronic venous insufficiency swelling is directly related to degree of gravitational dependency.
Duration: Throughout day, only at night?	Venous insufficiency is worse by end of the day after prolonged standing or sitting and better after recumbency like in the morning.
Exacerbation: What makes worse (dependent position)?	Swelling decreases after elevation of limbs.
Relief: What makes better (elevation of legs)? What treatment used/tried? Effective?	
Associated signs/symptoms: Nocturia, polyuria, PND and orthopnea, shortness of breath, redness, ulcers, itching, pain or discomfort, discoloration, drainage, odor?	Redness and ulcers, pain and itching may occur in venous insufficiency, occlusive arterial disease and in neuropathy. Nocturia, PND, and orthopnea are commonly associated with congestive heart failure.

Past Medical History

Information related to past medical history helps identify any conditions that may affect or cause present peripheral vascular system condition or symptoms.

Provider Inquiries	Clinical Reasoning/Logic
Any cardiac surgeries/hospitalization for evaluation/treatment of vascular disorders? Rheumatic fever, joint swelling? **Chronic illnesses:** Hypertension, bleeding disorders, hyperipidemia, DM, thyroid dysfunction, thrombophlebitis, Raynaud's phenomena? History of DVT?	Cardiac risk factors such as smoking, hypertension, hyperlipidemia, family history, and age are similar risk factors in peripheral artery diseases and aneurysms are similar risk factors in atherosclerosis. Diabetes mellitus has also been found to be a significant factor in the progression of small vessel disease (Aboyans et al., 2006).

Family History

Family History provides information regarding family member's illnesses or conditions as potential causes for chief complaint or presenting symptoms that may indicate a pattern of presentation associated with transmission of familial/genetic factors predisposing the individual to certain system related conditions/illnesses. Any of these may indicate a potential or actual cause of peripheral vascular system dysfunction.

Provider Inquiries	Clinical Reasoning/Logic
Ask the patient about a family history for any of the following: Diabetes mellitus? Heart disease? Hypertension? CAD, hyperlipidemia? Hypercoaguability syndrome? Family history of venous disease?	Cardiovascular risk factors are similar for peripheral artery disease (PAD) as well. Also see risk factors under past medical history.

Personal and Social History

Information related to personal and social history identifies what personal habits, behaviors, or environmental factors might influence or cause present peripheral vascular system condition or symptoms.

Provider Inquiries	Clinical Reasoning/Logic
Employment: Physical demands (periods of standing), environmental hazards (heat, chemicals, dust)? **Tobacco Use:** Type (cigarettes, cigar, pipe, smokeless), age when started, how long, pack years; if stopped, how long ago? **Nutritional Status:** ht/wt (BMI), usual diet (fat intake), weight loss/gain, how much/over what time period, previous history of DVT hypercholesterolemia, hypertriglyceridemia? **Behavioral/Emotional Status:** Anger/hostility, unable to relax, compulsive behavior? **Lifestyle Activities:** Hobbies, exercise (type, frequency, duration, intensity), alcohol (amount, frequency, duration), drugs (prescription/nonprescription, street; frequency, mainline), alternative/complementary therapies?	Prolonged standing aggravates chronic venous insufficiency. Similarly, walking a lot on the job may trigger PAD symptoms. Smoking and the ratio of total to HDL cholesterol are significant factors in the progression of large vessel disease (Aboyans et al., 2006). Smoking also is a risk factor for chronic venous disease. Obesity is a risk for chronic venous insufficiency. Quality of life and interruption in activities of daily living may be affected by various vasculopathies. Prolonged standing, sedentary life, and smoking are risk factors for chronic venous diseases.

Developmental Applications

Certain conditions or disorders may be related to certain age groups or situations. Inquiring to obtain age or condition specific information will provide further information for helping to determine causes of the chief concern as identified.

Provider Inquiries	Clinical Reasoning/Logic
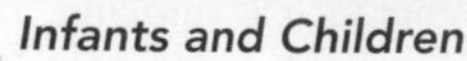 ***Infants and Children***	
Ask the parent or caregiver about a history of hemophilia, renal disease, coarctation of aorta?	Hemophilia can lead to hemarthrosis. Renal diseases like nephritic syndrome may cause edema on extremities, hypertension and may also lead to renal vein thrombosis and hypercoagulable state.
Leg pains during exercise?	
The Pregnant Woman	
Have you or are you experiencing headaches, visual changes, nausea/vomiting, epigastric pain, right upper quadrant pain, oliguria, rapid onset of edema (facial, abdominal, peripheral), hyperreflexia, proteinuria, or unusual bleeding/bruising?	There is increase plasma volume during pregnancy but BP generally lower due to decrease in peripheral resistance.
Have you or are you experiencing edema, varicosities, pain/discomfort?	Increased lower extremity edema during pregnancy due to pressure of the enlarging uterus on the iliac vessels. Varicosities are accentuated during pregnancy.
Are you taking any calcium supplements?	Calcium supplements (reduces risk of PIH).
The Older Adult	
Have you noticed any swelling of and/or sores developing on your legs and/or ankles? "If yes," can you tell me about it—location, pattern, frequency, time of day most evident? Interference due to condition? Does the swelling or the sores interfere with any of you routine or regular activities? Anything that you can't do that you could previously? What effect has this had on your physical and mental well being? Are you experiencing any pain in your legs during activities? Do you have to stop doing anything because of the pain? If yes, can you tell me: where, one side/both, walking distance before onset, duration, frequency? What medications are you taking? What specifically for pain?	A significant number of complications related to venous disease are more frequent in the elderly who often present late with advanced disease of active venous ulcerations (O'Hare & Earnshaw, 2008). Older adults often present with other conditions that affect the development and progression of venous disease as well as the possibility of concurrently having peripheral arterial disease.

THINK LINK: UNDER-DIAGNOSIS OF PAD

Approximately 12 million individuals in the United States are affected by peripheral arterial disease (PAD). In spite of this large number, it has been documented that many providers fail to obtain a relative history for PAD and also fail to recognize the subtle manifestations of this condition during the physical examination. This lack of recognition results in an under diagnosis of PAD and hinders the implementation of preventive strategies (Gey, Lesho, & Manngold, 2004).

OBJECTIVE DATA

The examination of the peripheral vascular system assesses parameters associated with blood circulation through the arterial and venous system—particularly the pulses, jugular veins, and measuring the blood pressure. Palpation of the arterial pulses is done at specific locations with comparisons made between contralateral pulses as well as comparison of the upper extremity pulses with those of the lower extremities. The veins are assessed for their ability to maintain blood flow within the extremities as the blood travels back toward the heart. Blood pressure is measured in both upper extremities with the patient lying supine or sitting. If clinically indicated, it may also be measured with the patient standing. Although not routinely done, the blood pressure may also be measured in both lower extremities.

Additionally, the extremities are assessed for the presence of excess fluid, color changes, skin appendages (hair/nails) as well as the overall condition of the veins. Specific provider procedures related to pathological conditions may also be performed when indicated.

Examination of the peripheral vascular system within the overall examination is performed when the provider is examining the upper and lower extremities. The exact point in the examination to do this depends on the systematic approach developed by the provider. The findings of the skin examination (Chapter 16) as well as the fundoscopic examination (Chapter 18) may give significant clues as to the integrity of the peripheral vascular system and possibly the presence of systemic alterations.

Inspection

- Extremities
  - Color, skin texture, and nail changes
  - Hair growth patterns
  - Atrophy
  - Edema
  - Varicose veins
- Jugular venous pulsation
- Jugular venous pressure
- Color change test
- Manual compression test
- Trendelenburg test
- Perthes test

Palpation

- Extremities
  - Temperature
  - Tenderness
  - Pitting edema
- Arterial pulses
  - Rate
  - Rhythm
  - Contour
  - Quality
- Radial arteries—Allen test
- Ankle-Brachial Index
- Abdominougular reflex

Homan's sign

Percussion*—not performed*

Auscultation

- Blood pressure
- Carotid arteries—bruits
- Doppler

Level I to IV Examination

The Level I to Level IV examinations are performed in a continuum, starting from a basic level and proceeding to a more comprehensive level based on provider's abilities and patient's presentation and location. The exam may start at the outpatient setting and may progress to the ED, hospital unit bed, ICU, or specialty unit. Frequently all the elements from basic to comprehensive exam are done in one setting such as in a primary care setting or clinic.

The condition of the patient is the primary consideration in determining the type and amount of data needed to assess the patient's illness/disease/situation. The separation into levels is for general purposes and is meant to be descriptive rather than prescriptive. The purpose of leveling is to provide a framework to assist the learner in determining the appropriate data to collect.

Blood Vessels (Peripheral Vascular System)

	Level I	Level II	Level III	Level IV
Inspection	Skin (color alterations) Extremities: Hair distribution (growth pattern), atrophy Edema (presence) Varicose veins	JV pulsation/distension Blood vessel dysfunction (arterial vs. venous alterations) Color change test	Blood vessel integrity (hemorrhage) Aortic Abdominal Aneurysm	
Palpation	Pulses (radial/pedal pulse) presence, rate, rhythm, quality Capillary refill Temperature changes	Pulses (carotid, brachial, femoral, popliteal posterior tibial) rate, rhythm, quality Edema (pitting) Homan's sign Allen test Abdominojugular reflex	Pulse (quality)	Trendelenburg test Manual compression test
Auscultation	Blood pressure Carotid artery (bruits)*	Blood pressure (Doppler) Ankle-Brachial Index	Lungs (pulmonary embolus)	

*technique may also be performed during assessment of the neck

Inspection: Level I

Inspection Techniques and Expected Findings	Unexpected Findings
Begin by inspecting the overall characteristics of the patient's skin, paying particular attention to the upper and lower extremities. Observe for any color alterations as well as any lesions that might be vascular (petechiae, ecchymosis, purpura) in origin. There should be no localized color changes, lesions or other alterations.	Localized areas of redness or pallor are generally indicative of alterations in circulation. Other physical findings may include a unilaterally cool extremity, a prolonged venous filling time, shiny atrophied skin, and nail changes. Physical signs can also help determine the extent and distribution of vascular disease. This includes the Buerger test (foot pallor with elevation of the leg and, in the dependent position, a dusky red flush spreading proximally from the toes). ***PRACTICE POINT: Color Changes*** An increased redness results from an increased blood flow or congestion of blood in a certain area. Paleness results from a lack of blood flow to the area.
Observe the overall hair distribution and growth patterns, particularly on the lower extremities. The presence of hair on the extremities varies from none at all to covering the whole body. If hair growth is evident, it should be equal in distribution bilaterally. The absence of hair is not a clinical predictor of the presence of PAD. Personal preference for body hair (shaving, waxing) will also determine whether any hair is visible. ***PRACTICE POINT: Tight Athletic Socks*** In some individuals, particularly males, it may appear that there is a well-defined line of demarcation related to hair growth. Before concluding that there is evidence of arterial insufficiency, ask the patient about the type of socks he usually wears. Tight athletic socks may wear the hair off. Other parameters, such as color and temperature, should be within expected range, contradicting the manifestation of hair loss.	Hair growth is dependent on adequate delivery of blood and nutrients to nourish the hair follicle; therefore, any areas where hair is absent should be considered suspicious and to be further assessed.
Skin should be mobile and elastic and able to be pinched. Extremities should also be bilaterally equal is size.	Skin that is tight and appears stretched may be an indication of the presence of edema, which is caused by fluid retained in the extra cellular and interstitial spaces. An indicator of compromised venous return to the heart, it is initially observed and palpated in the peripheral, dependent areas of the body. As the venous circulation becomes further impaired, edema moves toward the central portion of the body.
Check the nails for alterations.	Note any nail changes. (See Chapter 16.)

Inspection Techniques and Expected Findings	Unexpected Findings
Inspect the lower extremities for the presence of any manifestations of venous alterations that result from venous obstruction and venous insufficiency. Veins should not be visible on the surface of or through the skin. If any veins are visible, elevate the lower extremities; if veins and valves are not compromised, the distended veins will disappear.	Venous valves may appear as nodular bulges on the skin surface (Figure 25-5). The alterations vary according to the degree of obstruction and the speed at which the insufficiency develops. Pain is one of the first manifestations of venous alterations, but instead of being related to the degree of activity, it is more constant. The affected area is also warmer than expected due to venous congestion and also is erythematous and possibly cyanotic. The area is also swollen with visibly engorged superficial veins. Distended veins will not disappear if valves or veins are compromised. 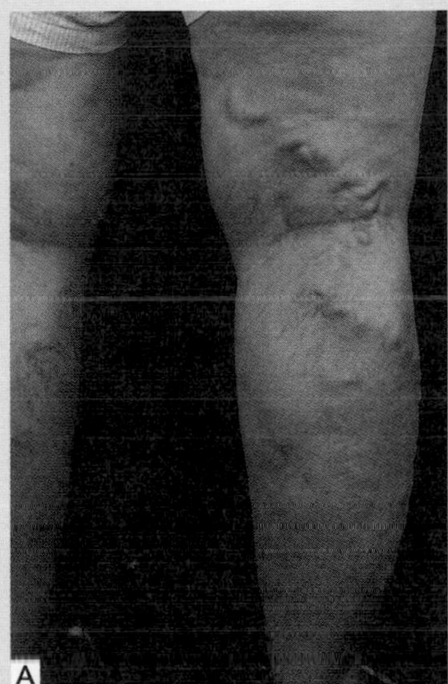 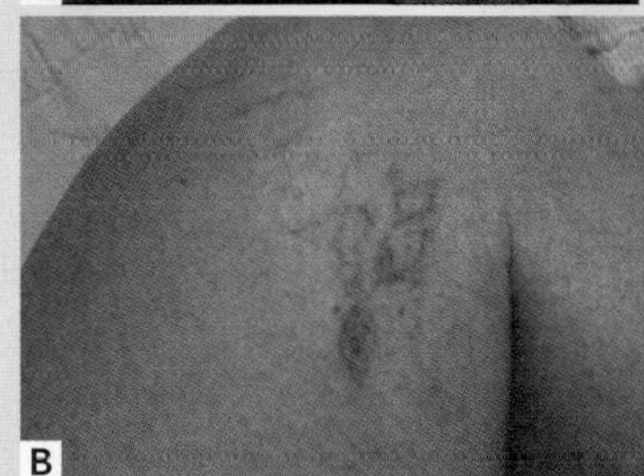 **FIGURE 25-5A–B** Venous alterations **a)** Varicose veins, **b)** Spider veins (telangectasias) *Source:* a. B. Slaven/Custom Medical Stock Photo
Observe the lower extremities for any manifestations of deep venous thrombosis (DVT).	Be aware of any redness, thickening, or tenderness that occurs along a superficial vein. DVT should be suspected if there is pain, swelling, and tenderness over a vein. Venous insufficiency creates an environment that is conducive to the development of a blood clot, or thrombus, in the vein. Blood that is not moving or stagnant allows the solid elements of the blood (platelets) to clump together, promoting thrombus formation.

Inspection: Level II

Inspection Techniques and Expected Findings	Unexpected Findings
Assess the jugular venous pulse and distention. Assessment of venous pressure is also a component of the peripheral vascular exam and has been covered in Chapter 24. The venous pulse is best observed when the patient is lying down with the head turned away from the side that is being assessed. When lying flat, blood will back up into the jugular veins causing them to be distended. [This is not true in all instances] If the veins are distended, it should be possible to observe ripples along the course of the vein, which is evidence of the venous pulse. It is not possible to identify all of the components of the venous pulse, but noting its presence is sufficient. In the absence of distension, it may still be possible to observe the venous pulse and noting its presence is aided by the use of tangential lighting.	Venous distension in this context is not an unexpected finding as it is intentionally caused for visualization of the venous pulse.
Assess lower extremities for the presence of skin breakdown or the presence of a venous **stasis ulcer** (Figure 25-6). The skin should be intact without any visible evidence of erosion, breakdown, or ulceration.	If evidence of ulceration is visible, it is generally located primarily on the inner part of the aspects of the lower limbs, just above the ankle, on one or both legs. 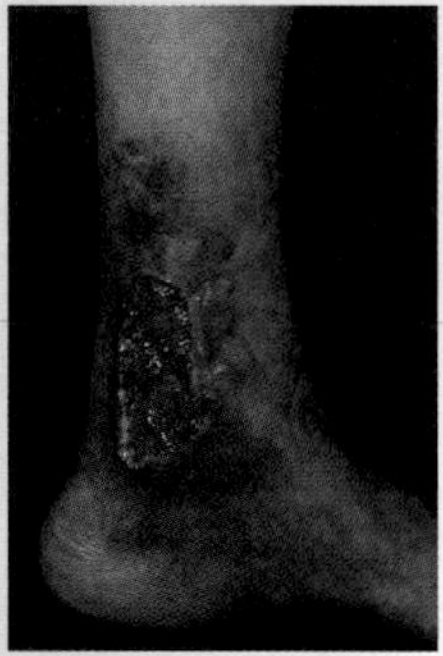 **FIGURE 25-6** Venous stasis ulcer *Source*: Biophoto Associates, Science Source Photos The base of the ulcer is usually red and covered with yellow fibrous tissue. The border of the ulcer is irregular in shape with surrounding skin that is often discolored and edematous. The surrounding skin also appears shiny and tight. Table 25-1 differentiates chronic leg ulcers.
Observe the lower extremities for any manifestations of arterial insufficiency and obstruction (peripheral arterial disease), which are due to a decreased supply of oxygen and nutrients to the affected area. Uncompromised blood flow to tissues results in skin that is warm, dry, and the same color as the patient's pigmentation.	Peripheral arterial disease (PAD) is most commonly due to a build-up of plaques on the interior wall of the arteries, which narrows the lumen of the artery. The manifestations of arterial insufficiency are the result of the tissue ischemia that develops because of lack of oxygen. The degree of the manifestations is determined by the degree of occlusion, how fast the occlusion develops, and the ability to develop collateral circulation. Initially, the patient will experience pain, characterized as a dull ache that frequently accompanies increased activity, such as exercise. Rest will alleviate the pain; however, it recurs again with activity. The pain will be distal to the occlusion.

Inspection Techniques and Expected Findings	Unexpected Findings
	The affected extremity distal to the obstruction will be cool to the touch as well as pale and possible cyanotic.
Also note signs of muscle atrophy and hair loss in the region.	If the occlusion it has been slow in developing, there will most likely be muscle atrophy as well as skin atrophy and a loss of hair growth.
If manifestations of arterial insufficiency and/or occlusion exist, perform the color changes test to evaluate the degree of occlusion. The legs should demonstrate pallor. With the patient lying supine, elevate the lower extremities about 12 inches off the table. Have the patient alternate dorsiflexion and plantar flexion to facilitate drainage of blood from the extremities. While still supporting the lower extremities, help the patient to turn on the table so that the lower extremities may be lowered. Note the time that it takes for color to return to the lower extremities (Figure 25-7). This should occur within 10 seconds or less. In addition to observing the return of color, observe the time that it takes for the superficial veins to fill, which should take place in about 15 seconds.	A delay in the return of color is an indicator of arterial occlusion. When the return of color takes 2 minutes or longer, the degree of occlusion is significant and the problem is severe (Figure 25-8).

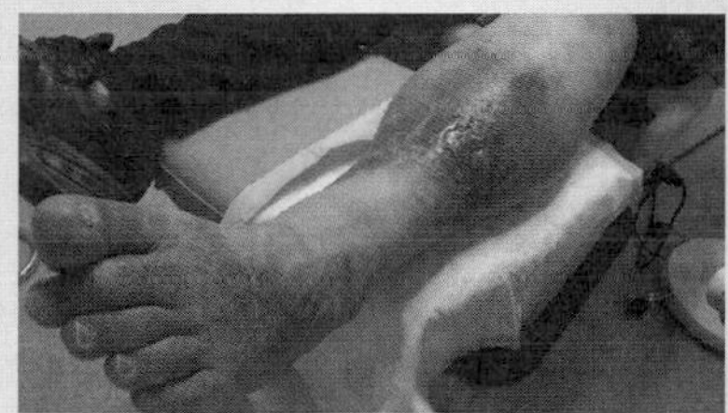

FIGURE 25-8 Color changes with venous occlusion/insufficiency
Source: B. Slaven/Custom Medical Stock Photo

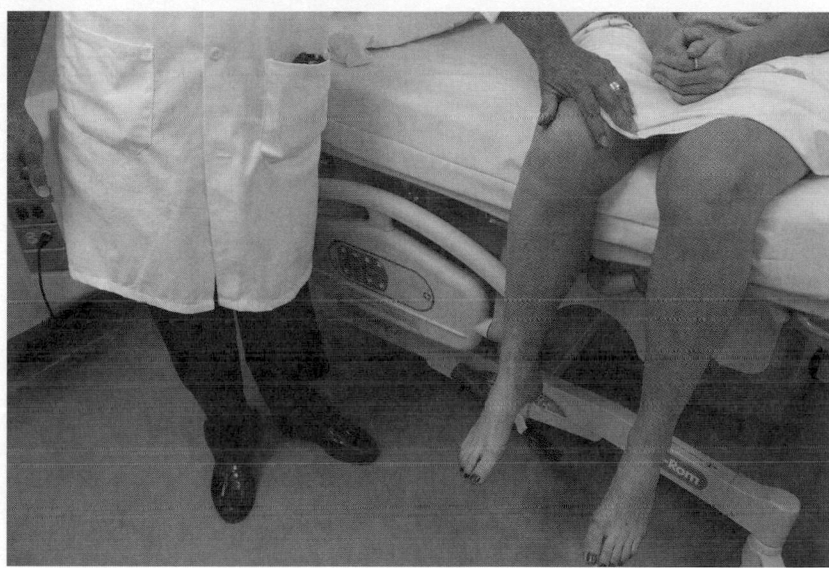

FIGURE 25-7 Postural color changes for arterial occlusion/insufficiency

Arterial ulcers are frequently observed on the feet, often over bony prominences like the heels and toes.

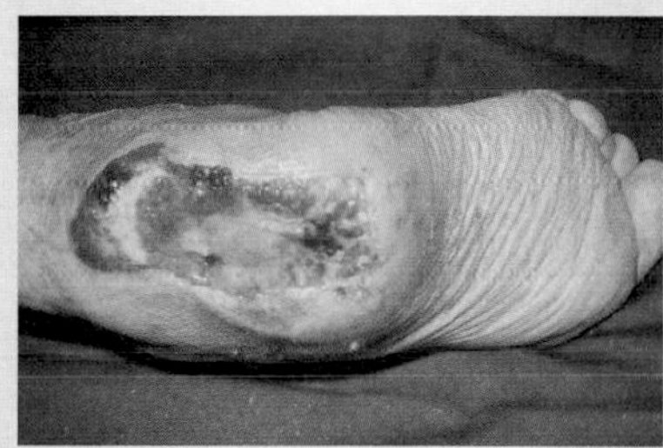

FIGURE 25-9 Ischemic ulcer
Source: Biophoto Associates/Science Source Images

Note the presence of any ulceration of tissue that is due to arterial insufficiency or occlusion. Arterial ulceration is identified or described as **ischemic ulcers** that develop as a result of decreased arterial blood flow to the area, usually after trauma, a break in the skin integrity that wasn't noticed, or physical pressure that is applied consistently over the area (Figure 25-9).

Table 25-1 Differentiation of chronic leg ulcers

Chronic leg ulcer refers to breaching of the integrity of the skin and subcutaneous tissues with longer duration (> 3 months). They are usually found below the knees except for the pressure ulcers which can be found on pressure points like sacrum and ischium due to immobility. Etiology ranges from venous insufficiency, arterial insufficiency, neuropathy like in diabetes, trauma or constant pressure, vasculitis, bacterial colonization or infection and/or combination of all these factors. They are costly to treat and frequently recur after healing.

	Venous Ulcers **(80% of all ulcers)** due to chronic venous insufficiency, DVT, and venous valve incompetence.	**Ischemic Ulcers** **(10%–15% of all ulcers)** due to inadequate arterial perfusion.	**Neuropathic Ulcers**–Seen in diabetics, due autonomic neuropathy and vascular insufficiency.

Continued

Table 25-1 Differentiation of chronic leg ulcers *(continued)*

Predisposing factors	Varicose veins, deep venous thrombosis, venous insufficiency/incompetence Usually associated with obesity, prolonged standing, immobility Multiple pregnancies\previous surgeries	Peripheral arterial disease (PAD), intermittent claudication, rest pain Usually with hypertension, diabetes, smoking, and atherosclerosis	Diabetics, those with impaired sensation of the feet or lower extremities
Location	Lateral and medial malleoli are the most common sites (ankle)	Over prominent osseous areas of feet, heels, and toes, and areas where there is pressure and skin shearing like between toes, tip of toes, over phalangeal heads, tend to be on the lateral aspect of leg like lateral malleolus	Location is where there is repeated trauma like metatarsal heads and DIP joints
Outer edges	Sloping Irregular, dry and scaly, dermatitis of surrounding area Granulation tissue healthy	Punched out Well demarcated, surrounded by fibrous tissue Granulation tissue minimal and pale	
Ulcer bed	Frequently covered with slough Hyperpigmentation Beefy red wound with granulation tissue	Wound bed may be pale, white, bluish, yellow or gray with little evidence of granulation tissue. There may be necrotic eschar, exposed tendons, and bone	Hyperkeratotic tissue overgrowth present like calluses and corns, with undermined borders
Exudate	Considerable Gelatinous and fibrinous exudate with weeping	Minimal	Low to moderate; infected ulcer may have purulent drainage
Pain	Not severe unless infected or significant edema Aching cramping, decreased with elevated extremity	Painful, even in absence of infection Acute, sharp, gnawing, decreases with rest and dependent position Pain may be localized to the ulcer or generalized and may be relieved by dependent position and increased with elevation of extremity (bothersome at night).	Painless unless an arterial component present Relieved by ambulation No sensation, or constant or intermittent numbness or burning; neuropathic ulcers are almost always accompanied by numbness and paresthesia
Edema	Extremity edema frequently associated with ulcer Usually present, foot to calf (unilateral, bilateral)	Uncommon. Affected limb may be atrophic. None or minimal, unilateral	
Accompanying characteristics	Eczema, hemosiderosis, pruritus	Gangrene may set in.	
Skin color	Brawny, brown, cyanotic when in dependent position	Pallor when elevated, redness in dependent position Skin around the lesion may be blanched, purpuric, with loss of hair on ankle and foot.	
Skin texture	Flaking, stasis, dermatitis, mottled Lipodermatosclerois—(hypertrophy or hardening of the overlying epidermis)	Thin, shiny, dry	Dry skin due to absence of sweating
Paresthesias	None	Possible	Yes
Pulses	+2, symmetrical	+1/0	Palapable
Skin temperature	Warm	Cool	Warm, unless there is arterial involvement
Hair loss	Not present	On ankle and foot	
Nails	No change	Thick, brittle	
Capillary refill	< 3 seconds	> 3 seconds	< 3 seconds if no associated arterial disease

Inspection: Level III

Inspection Techniques and Expected Findings	Unexpected Findings

A Level III inspection of the peripheral vascular system is observation for any evidence of vascular alterations that are caused by a tear in or a disruption to the integrity and continuity of the blood vessels. There should not be any evidence or manifestations of such an alteration.

The degree of bleeding is determined by the size of the vessel involved and the size of the disruption.

External Hemorrhage

External hemorrhaging is visible bleeding ranging from a minor loss of blood due to a superficial cut or abrasion to a major loss of blood (Figure 25-10). External bleeding is usually easy to recognize; a laceration of the skin bleeds, a person may cough or vomit blood, or a woman develops vaginal bleeding.

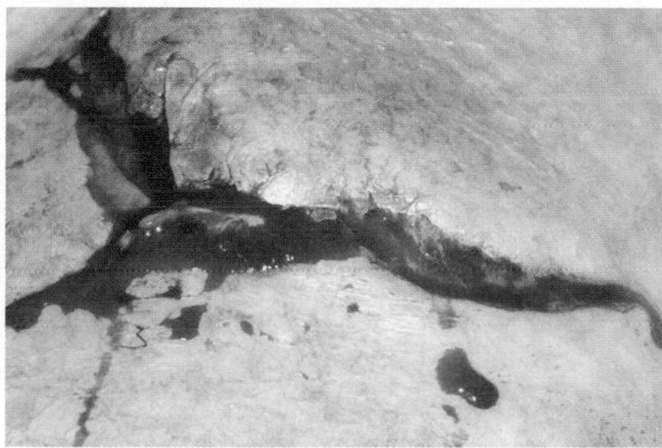

FIGURE 25-10 An externl hemorrhage is an unexpected finding.
Source: Dr P. Marazzi/Science Source

Active or uncontrolled bleeding (**hemorrhage**) may be caused by a myriad of actions or conditions and is either external or internal. A major loss of blood occurs with penetrating wounds or blunt trauma that goes deeper into tissues and may open larger vessels. The break in the vessel opens up to the environment, allowing the blood to escape out of the body.

The rapidity with which blood is lost is directly related to the size of the vessel affected as well as the number of vessels affected. Hemorrhaging from open veins is generally in a steady flow; whereas bleeding from opened arteries occurs in spurts due to the cardiac contractions that pump the blood through the arteries.

Internal Hemorrhage

Internal hemorrhaging may occur slowly enough so that manifestations of bleeding may not be readily apparent. The symptoms of internal bleeding vary depending upon what part of the body is involved or what organ system is damaged. Symptoms may be dramatic, arise gradually, or the patient may have no initial complaints. The amount of bleeding and the location are associated with the presentation and outcome.

The body can adapt and compensate for a slow hemorrhage for a significant amount of time. Alterations related to loss of blood may not be evident until the hemorrhaging and accumulation of blood interfere with physiological functions. Types of hemorrhages and their manifestations are identified and described in Table 25-2.

Hemorrhagic Shock

A rapid loss of blood has the potential to progress to hemorrhagic shock. Shock as a single condition has multiple causes. Patient's with hemorrhagic shock will present with or develop specific manifestations.

A dissecting or ruptured abdominal aortic aneurysm (AAA) causes massive hemorrhaging. The clinical manifestation of ruptured AAA usually includes excruciating pain of the lower back, flank, abdomen and groin. The bleeding usually leads to a hypovolemic shock with hypotension, tachycardia, cyanosis, and altered mental status. The mortality of AAA rupture is up to 90%; 65%–75% of patients die before they arrive at hospital, and up to 90% die before they reach the operating room. The bleeding can be retroperitoneal or intraperitoneal.

Hemorrhagic shock is caused by a rapid loss of blood volume leading to a reduction in tissue perfusion. Left untreated, shock will result in death.

The patient's skin will be pale with or without mottling and will also have increased ventilations that are characteristically rapid and shallow.

Table 25-2 Classification and characteristics of hemorrhage related to trauma

Category			Blood Volume Loss	Pulse rate	Blood pressure	Pulse pressure (mm Hg)	Capillary refill	Respiratory rate	Urine output
Grade	0	No bleeding							
Grade	I	Petechial bleeding	< 15% (750 mL)/ minimal	< 100	Normal	Normal or increased	Normal	14–20	> 30
Grade	II	Mild blood loss (clinically significant)	15%–30% (750–1500 mL)/ mild	> 100	Orthostatic	Decreased	Delayed	20–30	20–30
Grade	III	Gross blood loss, requires transfusion [severe]	30%–40% (2000 mL)/mod-erate blood loss	> 120	Hypotension	Decreased	Delayed	30–40	5–15
Grade	IV	Debilitating blood loss, retinal or cerebral associated with fatality	> 40% (2000 mL)/severe	≥ 140	Severe hypotension	Decreased	Delayed	> 35	Negligible

Inspection: Level IV

Level IV assessments may be used to obtain additional data regarding venous competency when other techniques or procedures are not available.

Inspection Techniques and Expected Findings	Unexpected Findings
The **Trendelenburg test** assesses valve competence. For this test, the patient is lying supine.	
With the lower extremity extended, have the patient flex the hip so that the lower extremity is at a 90-degree angle to the table. Note when the veins have emptied and then place a tourniquet about midway between the hip and the knee (Figure 25-11a).	
Once the tourniquet is in place, assist the patient to a standing position and observe the venous filling (Figure 25-11b). If the valves are competent, there will be a slow filling of the vein from the bottom.	
After about 20 to 30 seconds, remove the tourniquet and further assess venous filling.	
Competent valves will prevent blood from filling the vein from above.	Incompetent valves will allow rapid venous filling from above. Incompetent veins will allow the blood to pass through the valves and rapidly fill the vein from above.

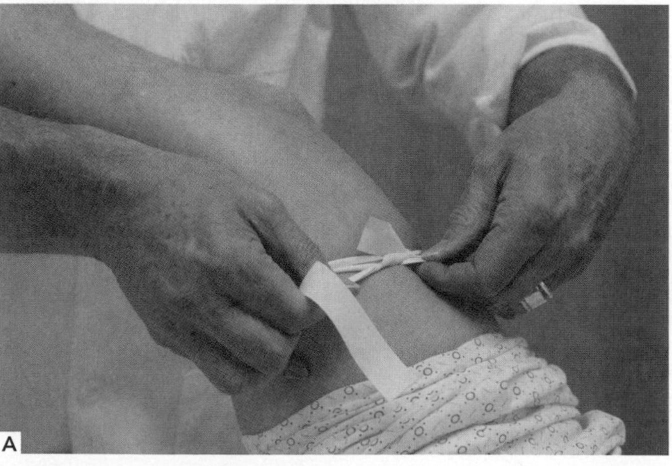

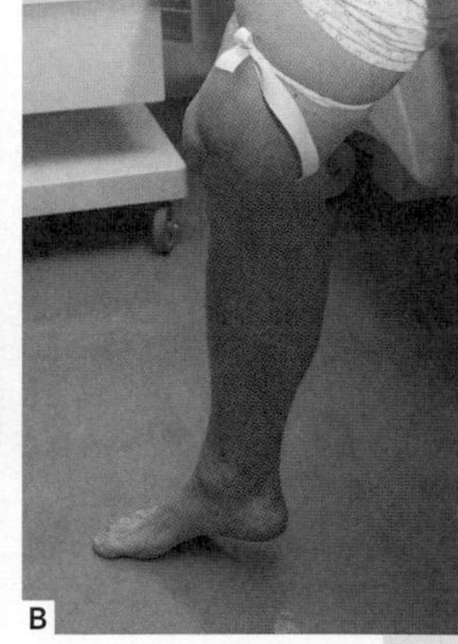

FIGURE 25-11A–B Trendelenburg test

Palpation: Level I

Palpation Techniques and Expected Findings	Unexpected Findings
Initial palpation of the skin is to determine if there are any areas of temperature changes. (See Chapter 16.) The temperature of the skin surface should be relatively consistent over the lower extremities and other parts of the body.	Areas of increased or decreased skin temperature are indicators of circulatory alterations. Skin temperature itself is not a reliable indicator as individuals may frequently complain about and demonstrate coldness in the distal areas of the upper and lower extremities that may or may not indicate a vascular alteration.
Capillary refill time of the lower extremities is done the same way as for fingernail capillary refill. (See Chapter 24.) Color should return in less than 3 seconds.	The color returns in greater than 3 seconds.
Palpate the radial and dorsalis pedis (DP) pulses for presence, rate, rhythm, and quality. In general, if these two most distal pulses are palpable and are within the expected parameters, it is safe to not palpate any of the other pulses.	
Pulses are best palpated at locations where they are close to the surface and located over bones or muscles. The locations of these pulses are identified in Figure 25-12a–g.	
The pulse is best palpated with the pads of the first and second finger. Exert pressure downward over the pulse location to establish the presence of the pulse. You may need to use varying degrees of pressure depending on the size of the patient's extremity and depth of the artery.	Absence of a pulse in an expected area may be an indicator of some type of arterial alteration. If difficulty is encountered in locating the specific pulse, it is helpful to palpate over a larger area with varying degrees of pressure to locate the specific point of impulse.

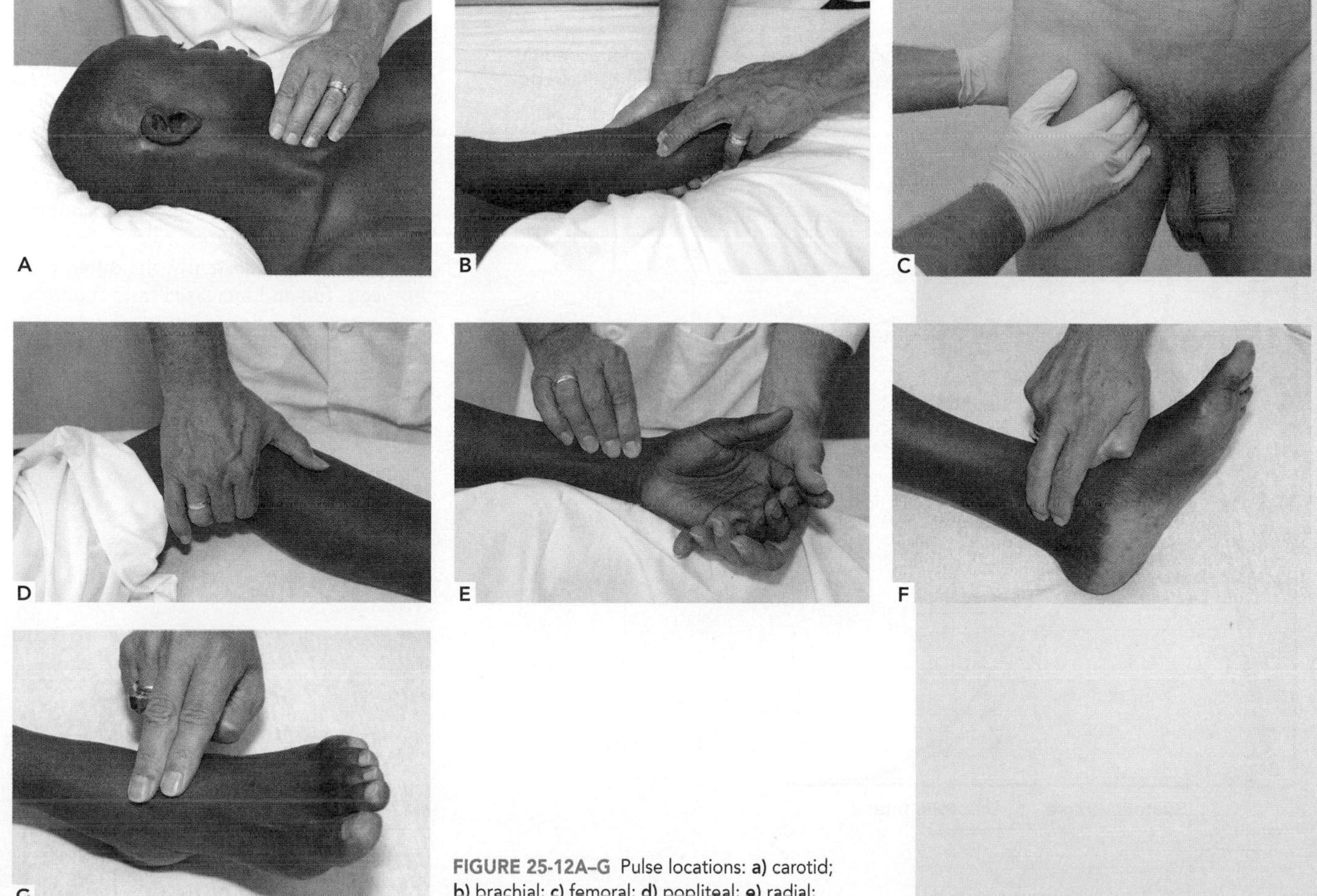

FIGURE 25-12A–G Pulse locations: **a)** carotid; **b)** brachial; **c)** femoral; **d)** popliteal; **e)** radial; **f)** posterior tibial; **g)** dorsalis pedis (pedal)

Palpation Techniques and Expected Findings	Unexpected Findings
The pulse is felt as a fluid wave underneath the skin. Each pulse wave results from the ejection of blood during one ventricular contraction. The carotid pulse is closest to the heart so it is often used to assess cardiac function and activity. The other pulses are located at varying distances from the heart and are obtained to assess the sufficiency of the total arterial circulation.	
Obtain the pulse rate by counting the number of pulse waves that are felt within one minute. The rate can also be obtained by counting the number of pulse waves in 30 seconds and multiplying by 2. This is recommended only if the pulse occurs in regular cycles. The resting pulse rate for an adult should be between 60 and 100 beats per minute; however, age, gender, and illness can affect the heart rate.	Heart rates over 100 or less than 60 are considered unexpected. By itself, the rate is not a reliable indicator of any alteration. Other parameters need to be obtained to determine if any alteration is present.
Determine the pulse rhythm. The expected finding is a regular rhythm that has an equal time period between pulse waves.	Irregular rhythms may be characterized as a regular irregularity or an irregular irregularity. A regular irregularity may be described as an alteration in the rhythm that occurs in a cyclical pattern. An irregular irregularity would be an alteration that has no particular type of pattern.
The quality of the pulse (**amplitude**) is the measurement of the force of ventricular contraction that produces the pulse wave. The integrity of the arterial wall will also have an effect on the quality of the pulse wave. The pulse quality is measured on a +3 scale. The descriptions associated with the +3 scale are as follows: +3 = full/bounding pulse +2 = expected +1 = diminished/barely palpable 0 = absent pulse The +2 or expected pulse quality is characterized as being palpable with a minimal amount of pressure and can only be obliterated with an increased amount of pressure applied over the pulse (Figure 25-13).	A +1 pulse is palpable only with an increased amount of pressure and can easily be suppressed with minimal pressure (Figure 25-13). A +3 pulse is easily palpated with a minimal amount of pressure and is difficult to suppress, even with increased pressure applied. A 0 (zero) pulse is the absence of any pulse wave.

PRACTICE POINT: Pulse Quality Measures

Another scale used to establish the quality of the pulses is a +4 scale. It differs from the +3 scale by including one more level above +2. +3 is described as "full, increased," and +4 is described as "bounding." There is no consistency as to when one scale should be used. Although the +4 scale is probably the scale most consistently, the difference between "full and increased" and "bounding" is not well defined.

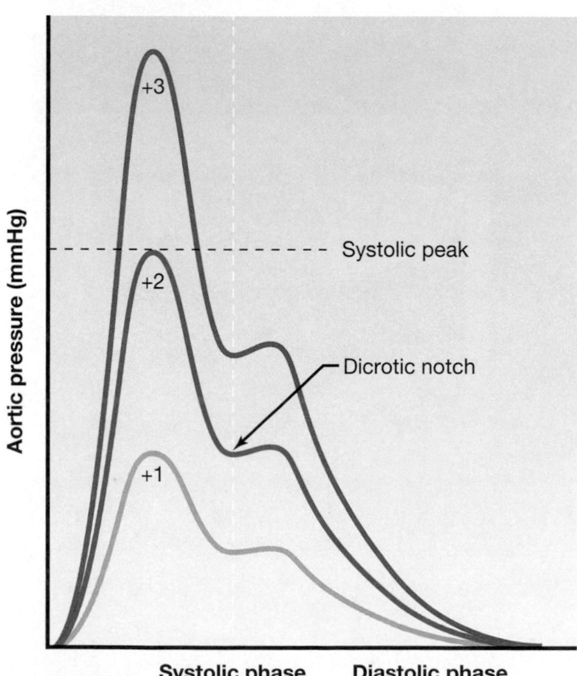

FIGURE 25-13 Diagram of pulse quality

Palpation Techniques and Expected Findings	Unexpected Findings
Assess the contour of the pulse waveform. The expected contour of the pulse waveform is a smooth upstroke that crests and then a smooth down stroke, with each component occupying 50% of the waveform. This may be visualized as having a rounded or dome-shaped appearance. The characteristics of the pulse wave should be symmetrical between both upper extremities and between the upper and lower extremities.	Any alteration present suggests an impaired circulation (Figure 25-14).

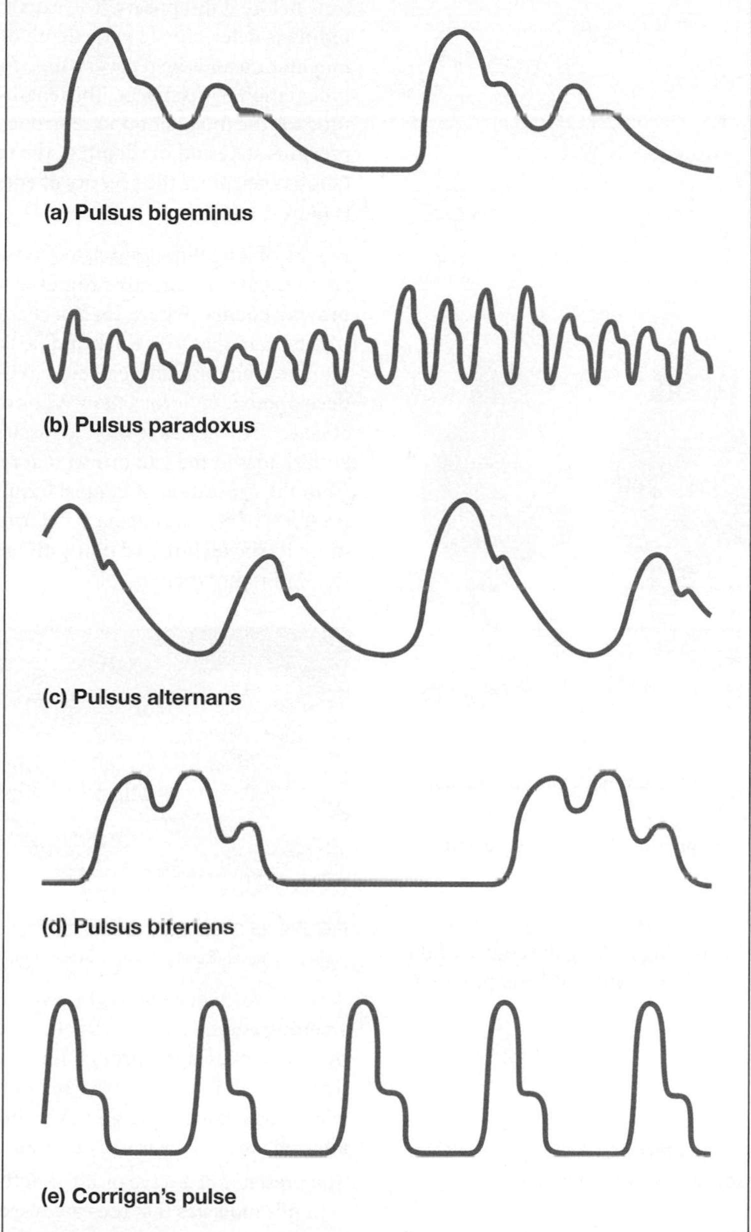

FIGURE 25-14A–E Changes in pulse wave contour

PRACTICE POINT: Patency of Distal Pulses/Absence of DP Pulse

The absence of a DP pulse is a finding in approximately 20% of individuals. While the absence of a pulse is of grave concern, when a DP pulse is not present, there may be adequate circulation and perfusion of the foot. This can be verified by other parameters related to circulation and perfusion. Often when the DP pulse is not palpable, the posterior tibial pulse is, which is an indicator of adequate circulation.

Additionally, if there are no color changes and if the foot is warm, this is evidence that circulation is adequate. It is not unusual for some individuals to also have cool feet.

Keep in mind that even though the provider may presume the patency of the other pulses, **confirming the presence of the distal pulses (radial, pedal), does not confirm the presence of any other pulse.**

Palpation: Level II

Palpation Techniques and Expected Findings	Unexpected Findings
Additional pulses (brachial, femoral, popliteal, and posterior tibial [PT]) are palpated when additional information is needed to determine integrity of the vascular system. The expected parameters associated with the pulse characteristics are the same as for the radial and DP pulses (60–100, +2, regular rhythm, with a consistent contour).	Findings that are outside the expected parameters would be unexpected.
Palpate the tissues of the lower extremities for the presence of edema. Palpate edematous areas of skin for the presence of pitting edema.	Edematous tissue has a spongy quality; you will feel some resistance when pressing into the tissue.

Palpation Techniques and Expected Findings

To palpate for edema, press your index finger into the skin, preferably over a bony prominence. Non-edematous tissues are easily palpated and offer minimal resistance to the finger pressure. If over a bony prominence, the finger tip will easily touch the bone (Figure 25-15).

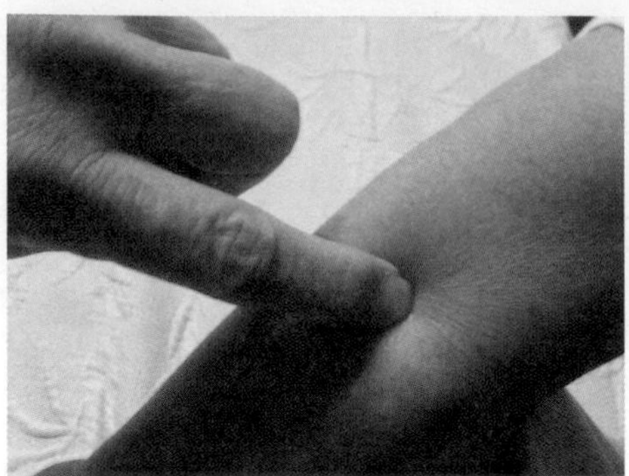

FIGURE 25-15 Provider indenting the skin of a patient

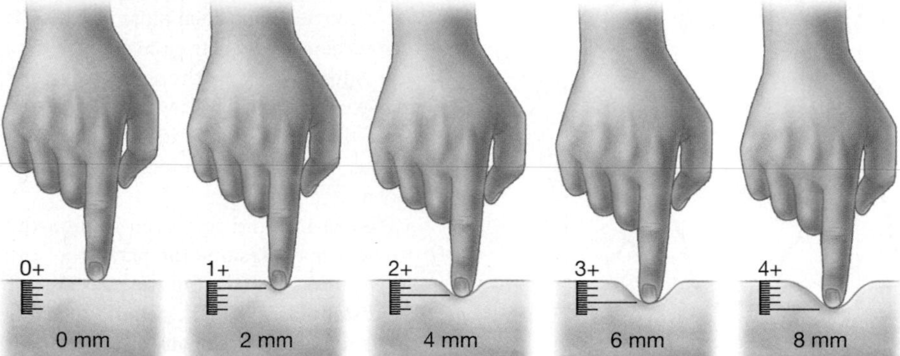

FIGURE 25-16 Edema evaluation by depth of indentation

Use the **manual compression test** to assess valve competency in a patient with varicose veins. It requires no additional equipment and is easy to perform.

With the patient standing or sitting, place one hand on the lower portion of the varicose vein (Figure 25-18).

Compress a vein with the thumb or finger of one hand.

With the finger of the second hand, empty the vein of blood by moving it along the course of the vein approximately 15 to 20 cm above the lower hand, toward the heart, while still compressing the vein with your other hand.

After you have moved your finger a short distance along the vein, remove it. A competent vein will allow filling only to the point of the first valve and will prevent a wave transmission.

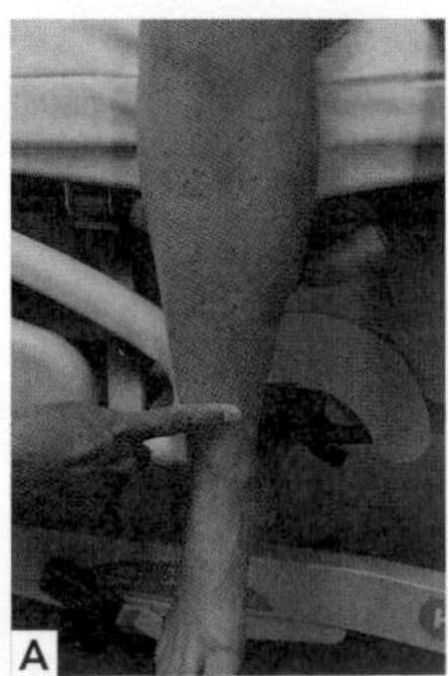

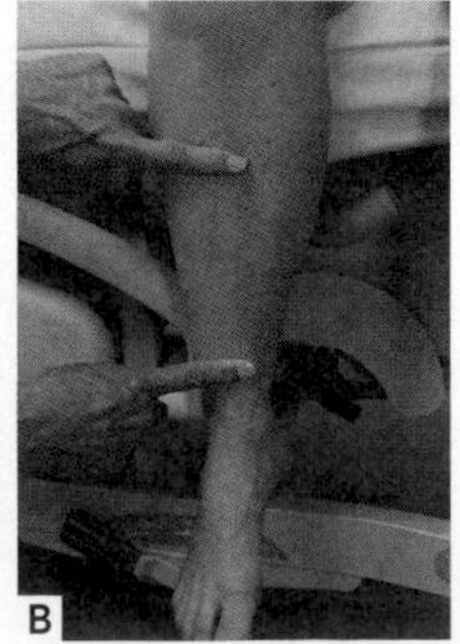

FIGURE 25-18A–B Manual compression test

Unexpected Findings

Non-pitting tissue edema will return to its previous state once the finger and pressure are removed.

Pitting edema is characterized by the indentation remaining for a period of time before it disappears. The extent of pitting is determined by the depth of the indentation and the recovery time for the indentation to disappear. The length of time for the indentation to return to its previous state and the depth of the indentation determines the severity of edema (Figure 25-16).

Edema of long duration related to vascular alterations frequently progresses into **brawny edema** (Figure 25-17), characterized by skin that feels thick and does not pit. These alterations are related to the development of fibrous tissue within the affected area. The skin is often discolored with shades of red and brown that result from the deposition of hemosiderin. The presence of brawny edema is determined more by the texture and non-pitting of the skin rather than its color.

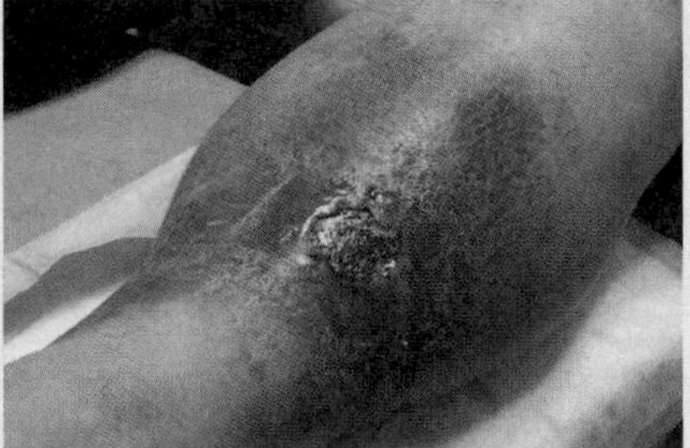

FIGURE 25-17 Brawny edema
Source: B. Slaven/Custom Medical Stock Photo

A severe form of edema is known as **weeping edema** and is characterized by fluid that escapes through the skin due the high interstitial pressure of the edematous tissues. The skin over the affected area will be warm and moist.

The presence of a wave or if the entire vein fills indicates that the valves are incompetent.

Palpation Techniques and Expected Findings	Unexpected Findings

Test for **Homan's sign**. For this procedure, the patient is lying supine with the lower extremities extended. The provider dorsiflexes the foot toward the tibia (Figure 25-19).

The expected result is that there is no discomfort or pain when the foot is dorsiflexed.

Unexpected Findings: Patient expression of pain with the dorsiflexion is a positive Homan's sign and may suggest DVT. This is however unreliable. This is not a specific indicator as pain in the calf may be present with other conditions—superficial phlebitis, Achilles tendonitis, gastrocnemius, plantar muscle injury, and lumbosacral disorders.

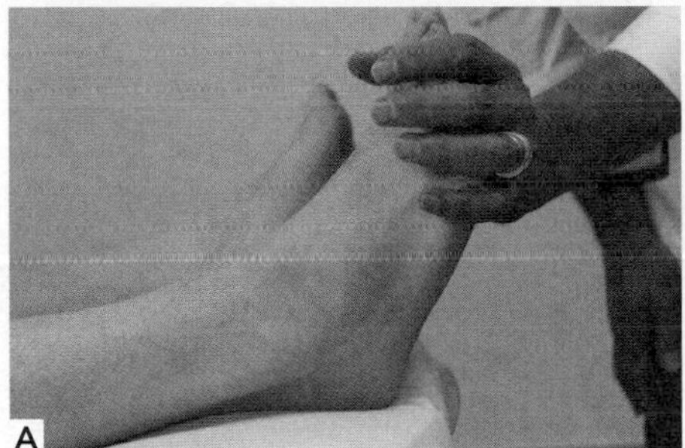
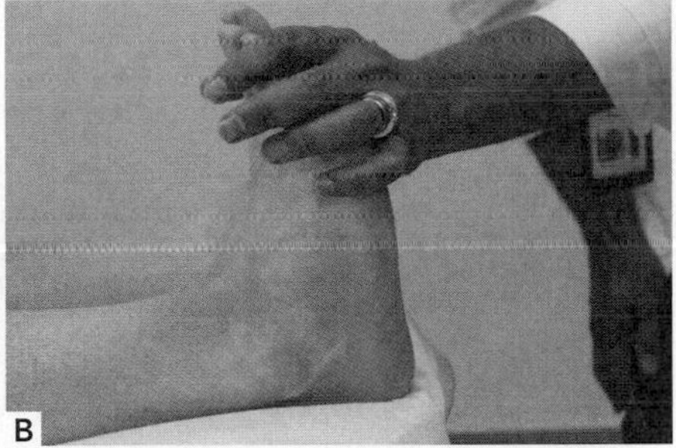

FIGURE 25-19A–B Health care provider performing Homan's sign test.

The Allen test is used to assess the competency and patency of the ulnar artery, which runs parallel to the radial artery on the ulnar side of the wrist.

The Allen test is primarily used to determine the presence of collateral circulation of the wrist when the radial artery is used for arterial pressure readings.

First, ask the patient to elevate the hand and make and release a fist several times and then to maintain the hand in a fist, which forces most of the blood from the area (Figure 25-20a). Next, with the patient still making fist, use both thumbs to put pressure on the patient's radial and ulnar arteries, occluding them both, which prevents blood from returning to the area.

After the arteries are occluded, have the patient release the fist and extend the fingers (Figure 25-20b). The palm and palmar aspects of the fingers should be pale.

Initially release pressure on the ulnar artery and observe for a color return to the palm and fingers as blood from the ulnar artery perfuses the area (Figure 25-20c). A return of color to the palm and fingers indicates that the ulnar artery is patent and the patient has an adequate collateral circulation.

Unexpected Findings: If color fails to return to the palm and fingers, release the radial artery and observe the return of color. If there color returns only when the radial artery is released, the patient does not have adequate collateral circulation.

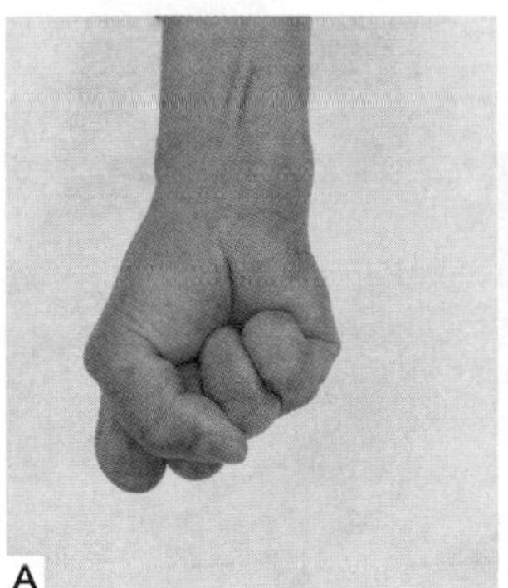
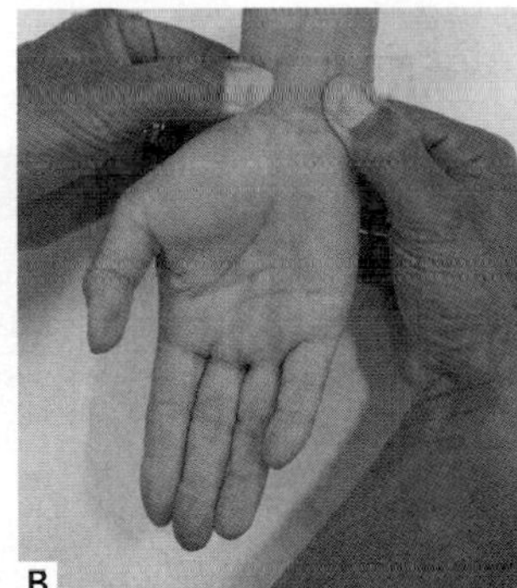
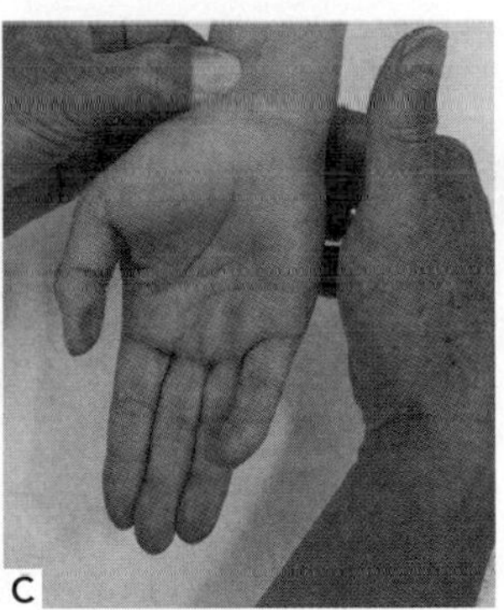

FIGURE 25-20A–C Allen test

If the venous pressure is elevated or if there is a possibility of heart failure, the provider may perform the **abdominojugular reflux** (Figure 25-21):

Place the patient in the supine position. The head may be resting on a pillow or folded towel.

Instruct the patient to breathe regularly through an open mouth (this prevents doing the Valsalva maneuver which could produce a false positive) (Cook & Simel, 2009).

Place one hand in the right-upper quadrant and exert continuous pressure over the area.

Observe the jugular vein for an increase in venous pressure and simultaneous distension.

Unexpected Findings: The abdominojugular reflux is not diagnostic for heart failure, as all patients will demonstrate an elevated venous pressure with this maneuver; however, it is exaggerated in the presence of heart failure and useful in evaluating this condition.

If heart failure is present, the veins will distend and remain distended.

Palpation Techniques and Expected Findings	Unexpected Findings
Maintain pressure for about 30 seconds. This forces blood out of the liver sinusoids and adds it to the volume of venous blood. If the heart can handle this increased volume, the venous pressure will increase momentarily and then return to its prior level.	A positive abdominojugular reflux is present if there is an increase in jugular venous pressure of 3 cm or greater and is sustained for greater than 15 seconds. A positive abdominojugular reflux is not necessarily indicative of heart failure; it is an indication that the right ventricle is unable to accommodate an increased venous return (Mangione, 2008).

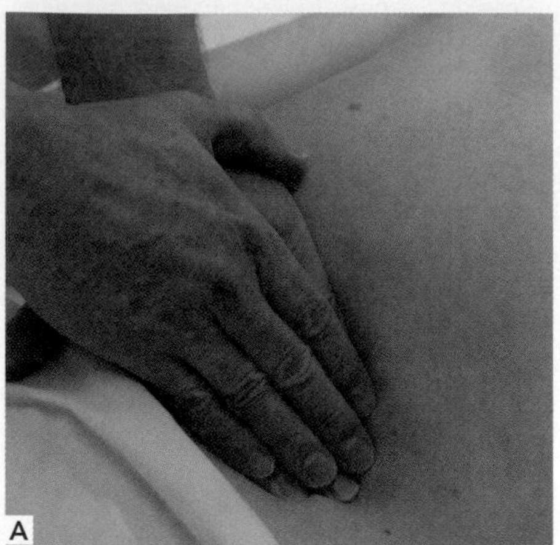
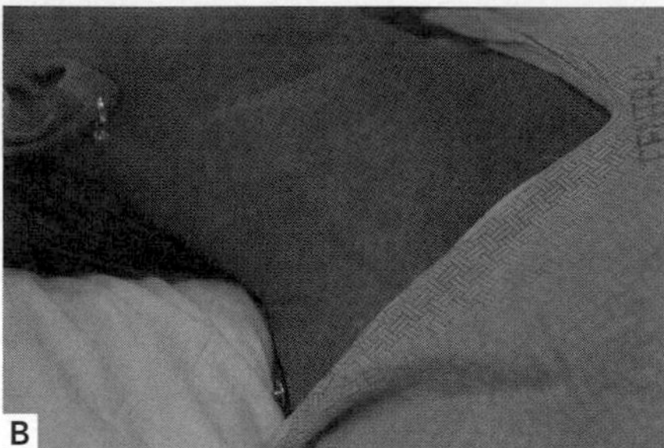

FIGURE 25-21A–B Abdominojugular reflux

Palpation: Level III

The patient with hemorrhagic shock will present with classic manifestations that are easily obtained with light palpation. Palpation of the skin and radial pulse are the primary focus for assessing a patient in shock.	Initial palpation of the skin will find it cool and clammy. Palpation of the radial pulse will find it weak and thready (1+) as well as rapid.

Palpation: Level IV

Classic tourniquet tests for saphenous or perforator incompetence or deep venous occlusion (Trendelenburg test, Ochsner-Mahorner test, Perthes test) are rarely used today; they are mostly of historic interest and should be used in rare instances, when duplex scanning or Doppler studies are not available.

Auscultation: Level I

Auscultation Techniques and Expected Findings	Unexpected Findings
Initial auscultation of the peripheral vascular system is accomplished by taking the blood pressure. (See Chapter 8.) Occasionally, it may be difficult to hear the Korotkoff sounds and to obtain the blood pressure with a stethoscope. Patients who are in shock or have a significant amount of fatty tissue of the antecubital fossa over the brachial artery are instances where distinct Korotkoff are difficult to hear. In these instances a **Doppler,** which is an ultrasonic stethoscope may be used. It amplifies the vascular sounds of the pulses and circulation.	Obtaining the blood pressure with a Doppler will provide only a systolic reading as it doesn't pick up differences in sounds, only the sound of flowing blood, In addition to obtaining the blood pressure, the Doppler may be used to validate the presence of the pulse via sound when it is difficult to palpate the pulse.

PRACTICE POINT: Doppler

A Doppler is an ultrasonic stethoscope that detects blood flow velocity rather than augments sounds. It detects changes of the transmitted ultrasound wave that occurs when it bounces off the moving blood cells in the vessel. Obtaining a Doppler signal indicates blood flow, but not the sufficiency of perfusion. When using a Doppler, first apply transmission gel to the skin area. The gel creates a seal that blocks air as ultrasound waves do not transmit through air. Next place the tip of the stethoscope directly over the area, manipulating the tip as needed to pick up sounds. Arterial blood flow is heard as a pumping, intermittent sound that reflects the pulse wave.

Also use auscultation to listen to arteries for the presence of bruits (Figure 25-22). The bell of the stethoscope is used because vascular sounds are low pitched. When auscultating arteries, the expected finding is the absence of any sounds.	A rhythmic, low-pitched, "buzzing," motorlike sound heard over an artery is most likely caused by a bruit.

Auscultation Techniques and Expected Findings	Unexpected Findings

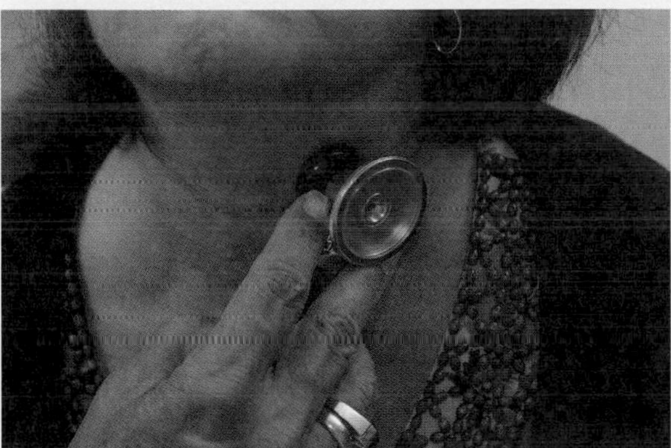

FIGURE 25-22 Auscultating the carotid artery

The presence of a **bruit** is an indication of turbulent blood flow. These sounds are generally produced at the site of auscultation; however, they may be referred sounds from a cardiac murmur. The carotid artery is most commonly the artery auscultated and is frequently the only artery auscultated; however, bruits may be present in any artery, so the temporal, abdominal aorta, renal, iliac, and femoral pulse locations also should be auscultated for bruits

THINK LINK: Bruits and CVA/TIAs

The presence of bruits in the carotid artery is a significant warning for the development of transient ischemic attacks (TIAs) and/or cerebral vascular accidents (CVAs). TIAs occur when small amounts of the plaque on the arterial wall break off and travel to the brain, interfering with blood supply to various parts of the brain. These are usually nonpathological and the manifestations disappear. However, if a large portion of the plaque breaks off and travels to the brain, much of the blood supply to a section of the brain is cut off and there is destruction of brain cells (CVA), which may cause death or leave the individual severely impaired. Identifying the presence of bruits allows for appropriate interventions to be implemented and prevent TIAs and CVAs from occurring. The significance of TIAs and stroke is addressed in Chapter 27.

When auscultating the carotid artery for bruits, occasionally the provider will also pick up a **venous hum**, a continuous, soft, hollow sound that is louder during diastole.

This is relatively rare in adults and is more common in pediatric patients. It is heard just below the right clavicle. The sound may be eliminated by maneuvers that affect venous return—lying supine, changing head position, and jugular venous compression. In adults it may be mistaken for a carotid bruit and in children it may be mistaken for the murmur of PDA. In adults, it may be present with anemia, thyrotoxicosis (hyperthyroidism), and pregnancy.

THINK LINK: Bruits—Vascular Whitewater

Bruits are audible sounds arising from turbulent blood flow. They are better indicator of atherosclerosis than stroke risk. It is unlikely to hear a bruit if artery is less than 40% occluded. If stenosis is more than 90%. Bruit may be absent. Imagine a bruit as "whitewater" of the blood. Blood flows through the arterial system unobstructed, much like the flow of water in a river or stream. Without obstacles, the flow of water is relatively quiet and inaudible. Yet as soon as the water encounters an obstacle, it must change course and makes a more noticeable sound. Many obstacles, such as rocks, logs and so on, create whitewater, which can be very loud and audible. The same thing happens in the vascular system. Plaques that form on the arterial wall are the obstacles that interfere with the smooth flow of blood, creating vascular whitewater that is audible through the stethoscope.

Auscultation: Level II

Auscultation is also used to assess the degree of peripheral arterial disease (PAD) by obtaining the **ankle-brachial index** (ABI). This is the ratio of the blood pressure of the lower extremity to the blood pressure in the upper extremity. The ABI is determined by the following (Figure 25-23).

Obtain the systolic blood pressure in either the posterior tibial or dorsalis pedis artery with a Doppler stethoscope.

Obtain the systolic blood pressure over the brachial artery. This may be obtained with a regular BP cuff.

Divide the ankle systolic BP by the arm systolic pressure to determine the ABI. The expected result of the ABI is an index value of >0.9 to 1.4. A reading of <0.9 with symptoms of PAD is diagnostic with sensitivity of 95% and 100% specificity (Khan, Farooqui, & Niazi, 2008).

The ankle-brachial index is a reliable, noninvasive procedure that will aid in the diagnosis of PAD.

Auscultation Techniques and Expected Findings	Unexpected Findings

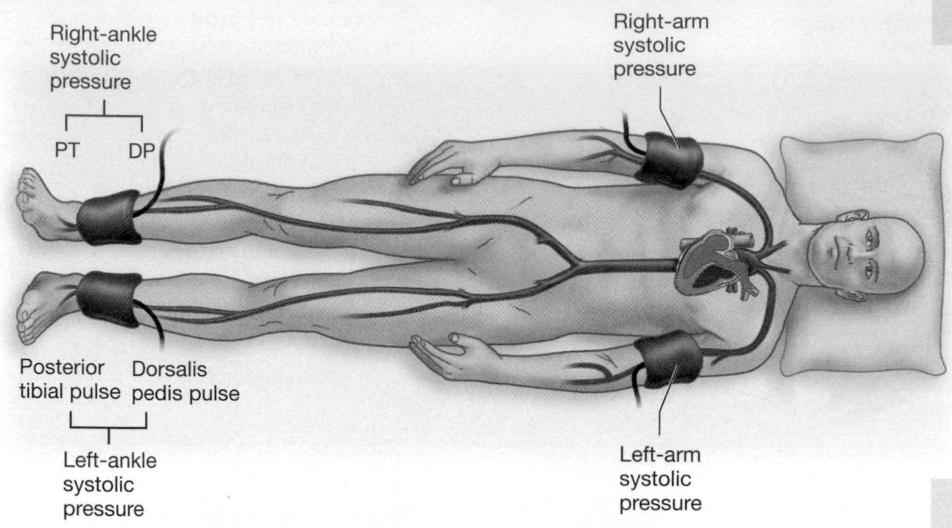

Right ABI	Average right ankle pressure / Average brachial artery pressure
Left ABI	Average left ankle pressure / Average brachial artery pressure

Interpretation of ABI	
>1.30	Noncompressible
0.91–1.30	Normal
0.41–0.90	Mild-to-moderate peripheral arterial disease
0.00–0.40	Severe peripheral arterial disease

FIGURE 25-23 Ankle-brachial index

Auscultation: Levels III and IV

Evidence for determining the presence of a pulmonary embolus is obtained through auscultation of the lungs. There are no specific peripheral vascular parameters associated with pulmonary embolism other than there may be a history of or other evidence indicating that the patient is high risk for hypercoagulopathies.

Auscultation in pulmonary embolism may reveal expected lung findings. In acute pulmonary embolism, signs may appear after obstruction compared to chronic pulmonary embolism.

Auscultation findings of the lungs of patients with a possible PE may reveal the presence of crackles, wheezes, or a plural rub, accentuated pulmonic component of the second heart sound. Massive PE may reveal right ventricular failure manifested by increase JVP, right sided S_3 and a right parasternal lift.

Loud P_2 in acute severe pulmonary embolism may be heard.

Developmental Applications

Techniques and Expected Findings	Unexpected Findings

Infants and Children

Pulses that are palpable in the newborn are the brachial, radial, and femoral. As with adults, changes in the quality of the pulse are indicative of alterations.

A weaker pulse may be associated with peripheral vasoconstriction, possibly associated with a decreased cardiac output.

Blood pressure in an infant is difficult to obtain with the usual procedures. If obtaining blood pressure is necessary, use the Doppler to provide the best results.

Techniques and Expected Findings	Unexpected Findings
Blood pressure is usually not regularly obtained until the infant is three years old. Blood pressure in children aged 3 and older should be taken annually. Cuff size is very important to obtain accurate readings. Ranges of blood pressure vary throughout childhood. Blood pressure results vary throughout childhood and expected readings can be determined using the following formula: *Systolic range* 1–7 years of age = age in years + 90 8–18 years of age = [2 × age in years] + 83 *Diastolic range* 1–5 years of age = 56 6–18 years of age = age in years + 52 (Muscari, 2005) The blood pressure in the infant ranges from 60 to 96 mmHg systolic and from 30 to 62 mmHg diastolic.	A bounding pulse is present with a patent ductus arteriosis that produces a large left-to-right shunt. Pulses that vary in quality between the upper and lower extremities and/or absent femoral pulses are consistent with coarctation of the aorta. A sustained elevated blood pressure in the infant is generally considered to be significant. Hypertension in the infant can be the result of multiple conditions—thrombosis due to use of an umbilical catheter, renal artery stenosis, coarctation of the aorta, renal cystic disease, neuroblastoma, Wilm's tumor, hydronephrosis, adrenal hyperplasia, or central nervous system disease. Hypertension in children is rare but becoming more common due to the increase in obesity in children. Most causes of hypertension in children are related to renal disease, renal arterial disease, pheochromocytoma, or coarctation of the aorta.
Capillary refill time for infants and children under 2 years of age is generally rapid: less than 1 second. A prolonged refill time, greater than 2 seconds, is consistent with dehydration or hypovolemic shock.	
In the first 24 to 48 hours, an infant may demonstrate cyanosis of the hands and feet (acrocyanosis).	This is not associated with any circulatory alterations and is more a reflection of ambient temperature, which is often cooler than the uterine environment. It should disappear within a couple of days.
As discussed previously, when auscultating the neck of the child, a venous hum may be heard.	Venous thrombosis is rare in children and most often caused by placement of venous access devices or congenital hypercoagulation syndromes.
The Pregnant Woman During the first trimester, the blood pressure falls and reaches its lowest point around weeks 16 to 20. After this point, the blood pressure gradually rises until it reaches prepregnancy levels at term. During the third trimester the parameters increase to 130 mmHg systolic and 85≈mmHg diastolic. An increase of 30 or more mmHg systolic or 15 mmHg diastolic over the first trimester baseline blood pressure requires close scrutiny.	Blood pressures that would be considered nonsignificant in the nonpregnant woman may be indicators of potential problems for the pregnant female. During the second trimester, a systolic blood pressure of 125 or greater or a diastolic pressure of 75 mmHg or greater suggests a problem. A continuously elevated systolic pressure of 140 mmHg or higher or a diastolic pressure of 90 mmHg or higher is cause for concern for a blood pressure disorder in pregnancy.
The pregnant woman will also demonstrate diffuse bilateral pitting edema in the lower extremities, particularly in the evening. The development of varicose veins is also common as well as hemorrhoids.	
The Older Adult The dorsalis pedis and posterior tibial pulses become more difficult to locate in the elderly adult. Superficial blood vessels also appear distended and tortuous.	Arteriosclerosis results in an elevation of blood pressure, particularly the systolic pressure. Hypertension in the elderly is associated with consistent pressures greater than 140 mmHg systolic and 90 mmHg diastolic. Systolic BP rises more than the diastolic, therefore, there is an increase in pulse pressure.

DOCUMENTATION

Once the examination is completed, the findings must be documented. Documentation data are determined by the type of exam performed. The following data represent a comprehensive examination. Data are described as related to expected findings. Unexpected findings would also be documented.

- **Inspection:** Extremities are uniform in color without any areas of increased redness, pallor, or cyanosis. Skin smooth and supple without any edema. Hair growth patterns equal without any evidence of hair loss. Extremities equal in size and no evidence of varicose veins. Jugular venous pulsations visible bilaterally when patient in supine position. Visible jugular venous distension disappears when patient in 45-degree-angle position.
- **Palpation:** Upper/lower extremities with consistent temperatures, no areas of increased/decreased temperatures. Nontender to palpation and without pitting edema. Capillary refill bilaterally instantaneous in fingers and toes.
- **Peripheral pulses:** 72 bpm, regular rhythm, smooth contour

	Right	Left
Carotid	+2/3	+2/3
Brachial	+2/3	+2/3
Radial	+2/3	+2/3
Femoral	+2/3	+2/3
Popliteal	+1/3	+1/3
Posterior Tibial	+2/3	+2/3
Dorsalis Pedis	+2/3	+2/3

- **Auscultation:** Carotid arteries without bruits, no venous hum. Ankle-Brachial Index .98. No bruits or vascular sounds in abdomen.

Electronic Charting

Expectations of Electronic Charting

Peripheral vascular information stored in the computer must include both current findings and relevant history. Findings from extremity Doppler exams must be stored and made available in a timely manner. Data regarding peripheral vascular system examination should include how a parameter was measured (e.g., standing versus sitting) in addition to storing the value of the parameter.

An electronic record should be able to automatically assist with calculations such as computing body mass index (BMI) from height and weight, or determining pulse pressure from systolic and diastolic blood pressure. Decision support modules, such as alerts for extreme values, need to take into account patient characteristics. For example, reference ranges that define hypertension need to be both age and gender sensitive.

Limitations of Electronic Charting

National consensus has determined that peripheral artery disease is an appropriate proxy when screening for coronary artery disease. Despite national guidelines, patients who have peripheral artery disease have been significantly under-treated with respect to overall cardiovascular risk management (Rehring, Stolpart, Sandhoff, J.A., & Hollis Jr., 2006). For example, compliance with national cholesterol guidelines is significantly worse for patients who have peripheral vascular disease but who do not have documented coronary disease (Maviglia, Teich, Fiskio, & Bates, 2001).

Electronic records, by integrating full examination, laboratory, and pharmacy data, can help to identify patients with peripheral artery disease and improve risk management. However, data must be well documented to be useful. An evaluation of computerized charting in a surgical database found a large portion of data for cardiovascular and peripheral vascular conditions (Bezanson, Strickland, Kinney, & Weintraub, 2002). The quality of electronic data is also important for making good decisions. Significant variability can be found when administrative (billing) data are compared to clinical data, for example.

PRACTICE POINT: Documentation

Correct documentation of pulse quality should be in the form of a fraction with the denominator indicating the scale (+3 or +4) used and the numerator the palpated quality.

Summary

- The peripheral vascular system is a series of branching arteries that end at the capillaries that then begin to join together to form the veins that eventually deliver blood to the heart.
- Pressures within the peripheral vascular system maintain its blood flow and are the result of ventricular contractions and its property as a closed system.
- Assessment of the peripheral vascular system is concerned with the integrity of the blood vessels and the adequacy of blood flow to all the tissues of the body as well as measuring various pressures within the system.
- Significant alterations associated with the peripheral vascular system include hypertension, reduced blood flow and supply to parts of the body, and the development of blood clots that may break away and be transported within the arteries and veins.
- Life-threatening conditions are associated with structural changes to the vascular wall, which could be the creation of an opening of the vascular wall resulting in bleeding, or a weakening of the vascular wall that enlarges and may eventually rupture, also resulting in bleeding. Any break or opening in the system results in a reduction in pressure that may be life threatening if the break or opening is large enough to cause rapid and/or massive loss of blood.

Review Questions

1. To determine the presence of decreased arterial circulation to the lower extremity, the provider would ask the patient about the presence of which of the following?
   1. pain with walking
   2. redness with elevation
   3. muscle twitching with activity
   4. edema in the morning

2. When assessing the vascular system of an older adult the provider should keep in mind that as arteriosclerosis increases, there will also be an increase in which of the following?
   1. heart rate
   2. vascular resistance
   3. numbness and tingling
   4. edema

3. During the history, the patient indicates that there has been an increase in redness of the lower extremities and that there appears to be an increase in size of the ankles. During the examination, the provider may also expect to do which of the following?
   1. Observe visible pulsations in the veins of the lower extremities.
   2. Palpate an increase in temperature of the lower extremities.
   3. Auscultate the presence of bruits in the iliac veins.
   4. Palpate a +3 pulse in the posterior tibial artery.

4. The provider is examining a 27-year-old pregnant female who is in her second trimester and in for her routine check-up. During the examination, the provider could expect to find which of the following?
   1. widened pulse pressure
   2. +1 pedal pulses
   3. decreased systolic pressure
   4. bigeminal pulse

5. During the initial assessment of a newborn infant, the examiner would be concerned about possible pathology associated with which of the following?
   1. varying heart rate between 120–140
   2. absent popliteal pulse
   3. capillary refill of < 2 seconds
   4. +2 pulses of upper extremities, +1 pulses of lower extremities

6. When assisting with the examination of a patient with a suspected abdominal aortic aneurism, the provider should expect to find that the patient (Select all that apply.)
   1. is a young female.
   2. has a history of hypertension.
   3. is a smoker.
   4. has a cardiac arrhythmia.
   5. presents with primarily GI symptoms.

7. The provider is called to see a patient with a complaint of sudden onset of chest pain. The provider can assist in determining whether the patient's symptoms may be due to a pulmonary emboli by asking the patient about which of the following?
   1. a prior history of chest pain
   2. medication and diet history
   3. presence of cough
   4. anxiety associated with the symptoms

8. The provider is about to perform a routine assessment of an adult patient's peripheral pulses. The provider is aware that in most cases, the assessment can include which of the following?
   1. just the pulses of the upper extremities
   2. only the pulses that have had past abnormal assessments
   3. only the dorsalis pedis and radial pulses
   4. the femoral and carotid pulses only

9. A patient tells the provider that he has been told that he has prehypertension. When assessing this patient the provider would expect to find that the patient's blood pressure is which of the following?
   1. 110/70
   2. 132/84
   3. 140/92
   4. 160/100

10. The provider is preparing to conduct discharge teaching with a patient admitted for control of new onset hypertension and his family. The provider would plan to include which of the following measures that may assist in control of this patient's blood pressure? (Select all that apply.)
    1. Exercise aerobically 1–2 times per week for at least 20 minutes.
    2. Omit all alcohol intake from the diet.
    3. Maintain a weight that is in the healthy range for height.
    4. Identify healthy coping behaviors.
    5. Increase red meats and other sources of iron in the diet.

Conditions and Disorders

Raynaud's Phenomenon/Disease

Raynaud's phenomenon is a vasospastic disorder causing discoloration of fingers, toes, and occasionally other areas. It may also cause nails to become brittle with longitudinal ridges. It is believed to be the result of vasospasms that decrease blood supply to the respective regions. Stress and cold are classic triggers of the phenomenon. Raynaud's phenomenon includes **Raynaud's disease** ("Primary Raynaud's phenomenon"), which is idiopathic, and **Raynaud's syndrome** (*secondary Raynaud's*), caused by some other instigating factor, most commonly connective tissue disorders such as systemic lupus erythematosus. It often develops in young women in their teens and early adulthood.

Pathophysiology

- Primary Raynaud's is thought to be at least partly hereditary, although specific genes have not yet been identified. Smoking and caffeine worsens frequency and intensity of attacks, and there is a hormonal component. An exaggeration of vasomotor responses (hyperactivation) of the sympathetic nervous system to cold or emotional stress, causing extreme vasoconstriction of peripheral blood vessels, leading to tissue hypoxia.
- The specific pathophysiology of Raynaud's is still not known.

Subjective Data

- May cause pain, discoloration (paleness), and sensations of cold and/or numbness within affected extremities.
- Feeling of tightness or fullness of the affected area.
- When blood flow returns to the affected area, it is often accompanied by swelling, tingling, and a painful "pins and needles" sensation.
- Primary Raynaud's disease is often considered "being allergic to coldness."
- Patients are also more likely to have migraine and angina.

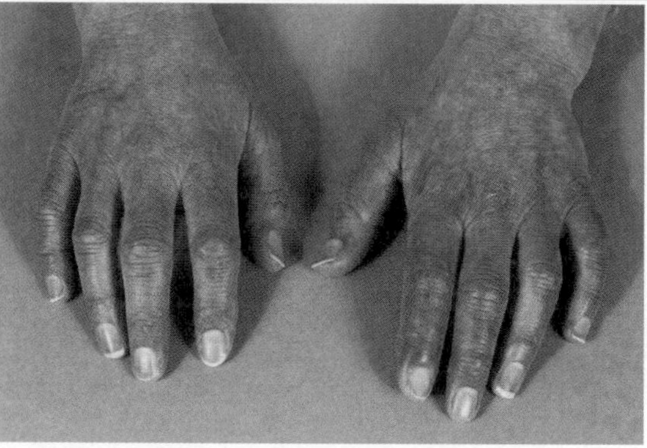

FIGURE 25-24 Raynaud's phenomenon
Source: SPL/Custom Medical Stock Photo

Objective Data

- When exposed to cold temperatures, the blood supply to the fingers or toes, and in some cases the nose or earlobes, is markedly reduced; the skin demonstrates pallor, and becomes cold and numb.
- Cyanosis in affected area when oxygen supply is depleted.
- Events are episodic; when episode subsides or the area is warmed, the blood flow returns and the skin color demonstrates rubor, and then returns to normal.
- Chronic, recurrent cases of Raynaud's phenomenon can result in atrophy of the skin, subcutaneous tissues, and muscle.
- In extreme cases, the secondary form can progress to necrosis or gangrene of the fingertips.

Hypertension (HTN)

HTN refers to chronic elevated BP >140/90 and in the U.S. is the most common reason for clinic visits of non pregnant patients. The most common type of hypertension (90%–95%) is considered essential or without an identified cause; in approximately 5%–10% of cases, HTN is secondary to an identified cause. Secondary causes include primary renal disease, oral contraceptives, primary hyperaldosteronism, pheochromocytoma (a rare, catecholamine-secreting tumor that may precipitate life-threatening hypertension), renovascular disease, Cushing's, and other endocrine conditions (thyroid disorders, hyperparathyroidism diabetes), coarctation of the aorta, and obstructive sleep apnea (OSA). Hypertension is a risk factor for stroke, MI, heart failure, aneurysms, PAD, cognitive dysfunction, dementia, hypertensive retinopathy and nephropathy. Obstructive sleep apnea (OSA) is a sleep-disordered breathing condition that results from recurrent inspiratory collapse of the upper airway, and has been determined to be a risk factor for developing hypertension (Das & Khayat, 2009).

Pathophysiology

- Caused by increased sympathetic neural activity, which enhances beta adrenergic responsiveness, and increased angiotensin II activity.
- Other contributing factors include mineralocorticoid excess, genetics, and reduced nephron mass.

Subjective Data

- Generally asymptomatic.
- Individuals may complain of occipital headaches, dizziness, vertigo, altered vision, tinnitus, and near fainting.

Objective Data

- Physical findings are related to involvement of end organ such as eyes and heart.
- Fundoscopic exam may reveal arteriolar narrowing or nicking, hemorrhages, cotton wool spots and infarcts.

- Endothelial dysfunction and vascular inflammation also contribute to the increased peripheral resistance; initially with a normal cardiac output.
- HTN progression results in hypertrophy of the myocardium, eventually leading to heart failure.

- Palpitations, sweats, pallor, and anxiety may be presenting complaints in pheochromocytoma.

- Physical findings associated with secondary hypertension, such as moon face, acne, truncal obesity, buffalo hump, and purplish striae may be seen in Cushing's, and renal artery bruits may be heard in renal artery stenosis.

Abdominal Aortic Aneurysm (AAA)

An aortic aneurysm, a focal dilatation of the abdominal aorta, is a common and potentially life-threatening condition. The abdomen is the most common site of dilatation resulting in an **abdominal aorta aneurysm (AAA)** usually at the infrarenal region. Aneurysms are not symptomatic unless dissection or ruptures occur. Risk factors for AAA include older age, male, Caucasian, positive family history, smoking, presence of large vessel aneurysm, and atherosclerosis. The major risk for expansion and rupture is a large diameter of aneurysm, increased velocity of diameter expansion and female gender. Abdominal aortic diameter of 3 cm or more is considered aneurysmal. Large aneurysms (> 5.5 cm) are a high risk.

Pathophysiology

- A localized, weakened, enlargement of the aorta, increasing the diameter of the aorta by 50% (Pearce, 2011)
- Its cause is multifactorial and linked to transmural inflammatory changes, abnormal collagen remodeling and cross linking, loss of elastin and smooth muscle cells, and expansion.
- AAA rupture is secondary to progressive weakening, expansion of aneurysm, ulcerations, and dissection.

Subjective Data

- AAA is commonly asymptomatic unless dissection or rupture occurs, in which case pain is most common manifestation.
- Pain increases risk for rupture. Pain is constant and not dependent on change in positions.
- Pain from limb ischemia may occur in distal embolization of the thrombus or debris. These emboli may be multiple.
- Fever, fatigue, malaise and weight loss may be seen in infected aneurysms.
- GI symptoms: fullness, nausea, vomiting

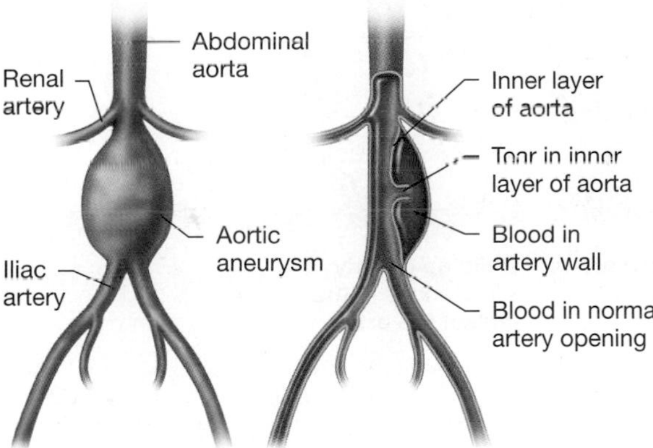

FIGURE 25-25 **A)** AAA **B)** Dissecting AAA

Objective Data

- Pulsatile abdominal mass, limb ischemia, light fever, weight changes related to inflammation, or infection of the aneurysm
- The classic triad of symptoms with a ruptured AAA are as follows: 1) back pain, with or without abdominal pain, 2) hypotension, and 3) pulsatile abdominal mass; however, only about 25%–50% of individuals present with these and often demonstrate signs and symptoms of other diagnoses (Assar & Zarins, 2009).
- Ecchymosis such as:
    - Grey Turner sign—flank ecchymosis in rupture of AAA into the retroperitoneal region
    - Cullen sign (perumbilical ecchymosis)
    - Fox's sign (proximal thigh ecchymosis)
    - Bryant's sign (scrotal ecchymosis); may be seen with other pathologies (pancreatitis, ruptured ectopic hepatocellular hematoma)
- Carotid and radial pulse asymmetry suggest aortic dissection.

Chronic Venous Insufficiency (CVI)

Also called *impaired musculovenous pump*, this is a chronic disorder that commonly affects women. Risk factors include advancing age, family history of venous disease, increased body mass index, smoking, a history of lower extremity trauma, prior venous thrombosis, and, in women, pregnancy.

Pathophysiology

- CVI is a result of venous valvular incompetence, obstruction to the venous flow, and failure of the venous pump.

Subjective Data

- Common symptoms are leg pain or discomfort, itching, aching, heaviness, dragging sensation on legs, fatigue of legs, numbness, and tingling.

Objective Data

- Stasis dermatitis may be the first manifestation with chronic leg swelling, hyperpigmentation, discoloration, eczematous changes and lichenification, thickening of

- Venous insufficiency creates an environment that facilitates the pooling of blood, resulting in stagnant blood flow that allows platelets to clump together, promoting thrombus formation.
- Legs are usually affected, although upper arms may be involved in conditions like malignancy, procedure-related sequelae and trauma.

the skin and underlying tissue (lipodermatosclerosis), varicosities, telangiectasias, reticular veins, cellulitis, and ulcers.

Peripheral Artery Disease (PAD)

PAD refers to the systemic luminal narrowing of the non-coronary arteries generally caused by atherosclerotic plaques. Narrowing of the arteries may also be caused by inflammation and thrombosis but PAD is the most common etiology.

Risk factors are advancing age, male gender, ethnicity (African American), family history, genetic factors, smoking hypertension, DM, hyperlipidemia, metabolic syndrome, and homocystinuria.

Pathophysiology

- The luminal narrowing is due to accumulation of lipid and fibrous material between the intimal and medial layers of the arteries.
- The imbalance of oxygen supply and demand leads to the ischemic manifestations characteristic of this condition.

Subjective Data

- Painful cramping of legs with exertion, changes in color of legs, changes in toenail, cold legs, hair loss, leg numbness and weakness, nonhealing sores.
- In severe cases, ischemic pain at rest may occur.
- Symptoms depend on the severity and location of occlusion.
- Claudication, which is reproducible pain on lower extremities (from buttocks to calves depending on location of occlusion), exertion relieved by rest.

Objective Data

- Frank ischemia-like tissue loss, necrosis, and gangrene.
- See Table 25-1.

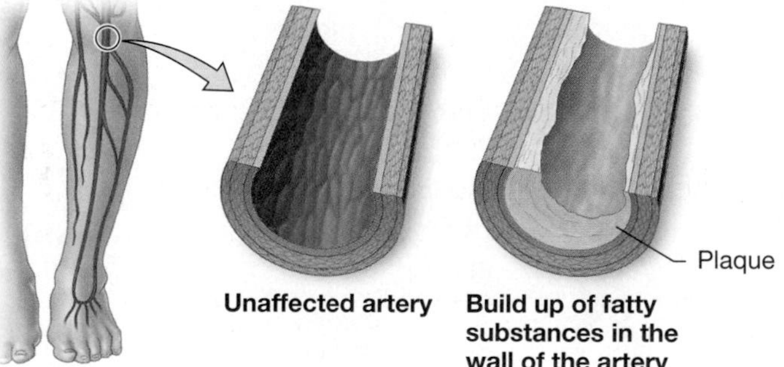

FIGURE 25-26 Peripheral arterial disease (PAD)

Arteriovenous Malformation (AVM)

AVM is a connection between arteries and veins that bypasses the capillaries. It is usually asymptomatic but can cause pain and bleeding. It can develop anywhere there are blood vessels but is most common in the brain and spinal cord. Most AVMs are congenital malformations, which can cause hemorrhage, headaches, and seizures when they are in the brain. They are generally incidental findings for diagnosis of unrelated disorders.

Pathophysiology

- An AVM is an anomalous connection between arteries and veins. They are often associated with the brain and spinal cord. It is a congenital condition in which there is a failure of the embryonic tissues to fully develop and differentiate into a capillary bed in the location of the lesion.

Subjective Data

- There are no specific manifestations of AVM that would alert one to its presence.
- Approximately 50% of individuals with an AVM will experience the first symptoms when the malformation has ruptured, causing bleeding into the brain.

Objective Data

- Bruit maybe heard over the site of the AVM.

- In essence, blood is shunted from the artery to the vein without going through capillaries, depriving the organ of oxygenated blood. AVM lacks the dampening effect of capillaries and therefore subjected to the high pressure arterial flow leading to fragility and bleeding.
- The other 50% may experience seizures, headaches, and progressive weakness or numbness.
- An occasional patient may hear a noise in the head, which can compromise hearing and sleep.
- Sudden rupture of the AVM causes signs and symptoms that accompany a stroke. These manifestations include a sudden, severe headache with focal neurologic deficits (weakness, numbness, or paralysis); loss of vision; difficulty with speech; and an extreme unsteady gait.

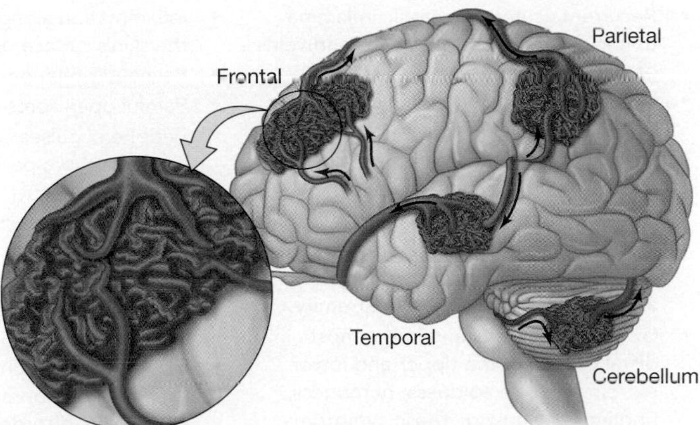

FIGURE 25-27 Examples of AV malformation locations, enlarged to show their structure

Giant Cell Arteritis

Giant cell arteritis refers to chronic vasculitis involving large and medium sized vessels. It occurs usually between the ages of 50 to 75 with mean age of 72. Although the inflammation may be widespread, it frequently involves the cranial nerve vessels with loss of vision as the most feared complication if not treated. Vessels like the thoracic aorta, cervical arteries, and external carotid arteries are frequently involved. The intracranial vessels are rarely involved.

Pathophysiology

- Inflammation of the arteries involving the cranial branches from the aortic arch is the proposed pathogenesis.
- Both the humoral and cellular arm of the immune system have been implicated in its pathogenesis.
- Age, genetic factors, and infection may play a role in its pathogenesis.

Subjective Data

- Localized new headache
- Jaw claudication or tonic contraction of muscles with chewing
- Systemic symptoms may include fatigue, low-grade fever, weight loss
- Joint pains or polymyalgia rheumatica symptoms (aching and stiffness of shoulders, hips, torso and neck in the morning)
- Visual symptoms amaurosis fugax (transient monocular visual loss), due to ischemia of retina, choroid or optic nerve or retinal arterial occlusion, diplopia, bitemporal hemiaopia, and homonymous hemiaopia
- Associated symptoms may include cough, arm claudication
- Other unusual symptoms: tongue pain, sore throat, dysarthria, hearing impairment

Objective Data

- Tenderness along the temporal artery
- Thickening of temporal artery
- May have diminished pulses—temporal artery, radial, carotid, brachial, femoral, and pedal
- Synovitis of joints
- Fundi exam may reveal cotton wool spots, optic disc pallor or blurred margins or may have Marcus Gunn pupil (afferent papillary defect) on the swinging flashlight test
- Visual findings range from pale, blurred disk, to bitemporal hemianopsia and homonymous hemianopsia depending on involved vessel
- Bruit may be heard on the large and medium vessels (temporal artery, carotids, supraclavicular vessels, femoral, brachial vessels)
- In presence of associated aoritc aneurysm—a murmur of aortic regurgitation may be heard.

Thromboangiitis Obliterans (TO) (also known as Buerger's Disease)

This is a recurring, segmental, progressive, inflammatory, nonatherosclerotic, occlusive vascular disease resulting in a highly cellular, inflammatory intraluminal thrombosis of small and medium arteries and veins of the hands and feet, with relative sparing of the internal elastic lamina. TO primarily affects men between the ages of 20 and 40 and is strongly associated with use of tobacco products, mostly from smoking, but also from smokeless tobacco. Cessation of smoking promotes an excellent prognosis; however, continuation of smoking results in progression of the disorder, frequently requiring amputation.

Pathophysiology

- Although the condition was recognized and the pathology described over 100 years ago, its pathogenesis is poorly understood.
- It has been hypothesized that tobacco may initiate an immune response or it may expose a clotting defect. Either of these processes could initiate inflammation of the vessel wall, resulting in vasculitis and ischemic changes in distal parts of limbs.
- In the acute phase, inflammatory thrombi develop in the arteries and veins primarily in the distal extremities.
- In the subacute phase, the thrombus becomes progressively more organized and stable within the small to medium-sized arteries and veins
- In the chronic phase, inflammation is no longer present and only organized thrombus and vascular fibrosis remain (Mohler III & Olin, 2013).

Subjective Data

- Recurrent acute and chronic inflammation and thrombosis of arteries and veins of the hands and feet.
- Increased sensitivity to cold caused by the impaired circulation.
- Color changes in extremity, ranging from cyanotic blue to reddish blue.
- Skin becomes thin and shiny.
- Reduced hair growth in the affected area, often resulting in the need for amputation of the involved extremity
- Gradual onset, starting in the most distal vessels of the upper and lower extremities with coldness, numbness, tingling, or burning. These symptoms may develop before objective evidence of disease.
- Raynaud's syndrome is common.
- Intermittent claudication (pain) in affected extremity (usually arch of foot or in the leg; rarely in the hand, arm, or thigh) during activity and use that eases with rest, but may progress to rest pain.
- Persistent or severe pain may cause affected area to feel cold, sweat excessively, and become cyanotic
- Ischemic ulcers eventually develop in most patients and may progress to gangrene, often resulting in the need for amputation of the involved extremity.

Objective Data

- Inflammation along a vein just below the skin's surface due to a blood clot.
- Raynaud's phenomenon
- Painful open sores on fingers and toes
- Peripheral pulses are impaired or absent in one or more pedal arteries and often at the wrist.
- Positive Allen's test in young men who smoke and have extremity ulcers
- Pallor with elevation and rubor with dependency frequently occur in affected hands, feet, or digits.
- Ischemic ulceration and gangrene, usually of one or more digits, may occur early in the disorder but not acutely.
- Noninvasive tests show greatly decreased blood flow and pressure in the affected toes, feet, and fingers.

The Brain and Nerves

26

I have learned that 3:30 a.m. phone calls are never good news. "Hello?" My voice is groggy and distant. The crackling over the line tells me that this call is indeed from the Philippines, and I brace myself for the worst. "Dad has been missing for three days." I tell my sister that I will be on the next flight out of San Francisco.

One week later, he is still nowhere to be found. The 10 of us are all gathered at the family house, reminiscing about our father, who always seemed to have a joke and a smile ready. As a momentary silence falls over us, the phone rings. My brother picks up, exchanges a few quiet words, and puts the receiver down slowly. "They found him under a bridge!"

Not just any bridge, as it turns out; the bridge on the block where we used to live, more than 20 kilometers away. He was found emaciated, dehydrated, with shrunken temples, but in good spirits, sitting alone with a can filled with coins and pesos. How did he get there? Alas, in a man of 95 years, with severe dementia, that is a question that will forever remain unanswered. He had begun wandering years ago, but he always seemed to return home. This time was no different, but for the home that he chose to return to.

Before heading back to the states, I take my father for a walk through the neighborhood. I am surprised that he recognizes me as his daughter and knows that I am a nurse, although he cannot recall my name. As a retired civil engineer, he points to nearly every building that we pass—homes, shopping centers, restaurants—and informs me that he built and owns them all. His voice swells with pride as he promises me everything as inheritance, and I burst into laughter. "What will I do with all of these buildings? I work in a hospital, you know." I say to him. "Then I shall build you one here so you can help everyone!" Tears roll down my eyes as I continue laughing. My father, demented though he is, is still entertaining me after all these years, and whether he remembers it later or not, I am proud to share this moment with him.

LEARNING OUTCOMES

1. Correlate knowledge of the neurological anatomy and physiology to physical assessment techniques.
2. Explain the significant anatomic features and structures of the neurological system.
3. Compare and contrast the divisions and the major functions of the neurological system.
4. Describe the patient history using the essential components of the neurological history.
5. Explain the components of the physical examination of the neurological system and specific assessment techniques used on patients within specified levels.
6. Correctly describe expected and unexpected results of the physical examination.
7. Explain the relationship between expected and unexpected examination findings and the patient's physiological status.

The neurological system coordinates all the physiological functions of the body. Its various components maintain and control both voluntary and involuntary actions. With the exception of the brain and spinal cord, the neurological system is not confined to a specific space or location within the body, but is spread throughout it. This means it is impossible to assess the neurological system without involving some other system. Even though the neurological system is very complex in its structure and function, most of the techniques used in the assessment process as well as the results are very simple to perform and interpret.

Structure and Function

The neurological system consists of two main divisions—the central and peripheral nervous systems (Figure 26-1). Within these divisions, multiple pathways connect the various components of the nervous system are responsible for the mental function and processing of the brain. These pathways are referred to as the wiring of the nervous system, and are not necessarily the same within each individual. It is the organization and development of the wiring of the nervous system that makes it so complex.

Central Nervous System

The **central nervous system** consists of the brain and spinal cord and is responsible for processing the information needed to maintain control and coordination of the various responses for physiological functions.

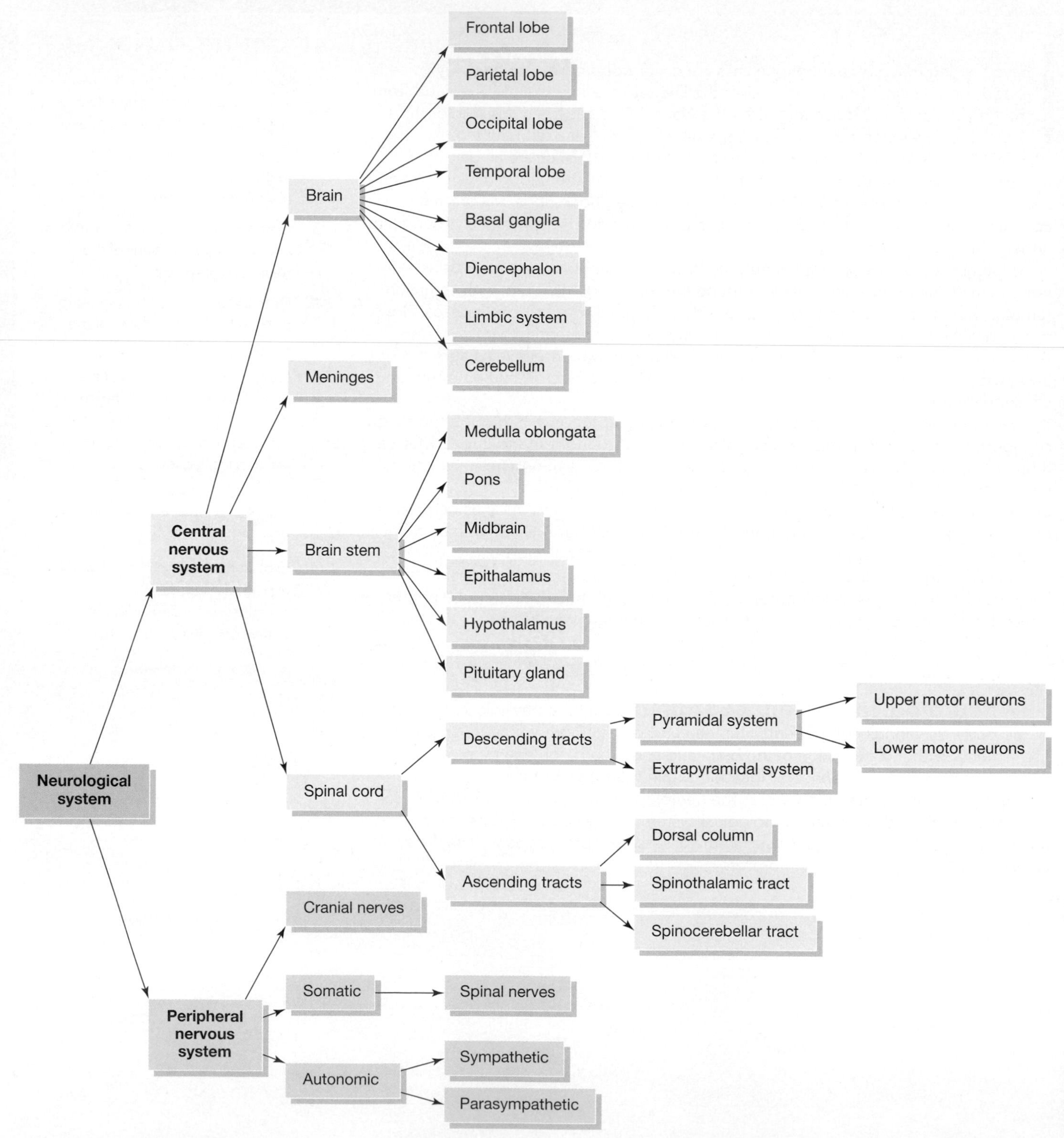

FIGURE 26-1 Organization of the nervous system
Source: Courtesy of Dr. Peter Rudd, Stanford University

Brain

The brain is an organized aggregate of functional nerve cells (neurons) that is encased in and protected by the cranium. Neurons belong to three categories: sensory, motor, and interneurons (Figure 26-2). An interneuron (internuncial neuron) is any neuron that connects afferent and efferent neurons in a reflex arc. The billions of neurons within the brain are assembled into multiple, sophisticated circuits in which neurons process and respond to sensory stimuli to produce a specific functional action, be it decision making or specific behaviors (Chiu & Cline, 2010).

The connections and transmissions of impulses through these pathways are facilitated by neurotransmitters (dopamine, norepinephrine, acetylcholine, and serotonin) that are secreted by cells within the brain. Synapsis between specific neurons establishes the formation of the multiple neural circuits. It is estimated that each neuron can connect with more than 1,000 other neurons making the number of neuronal connections in the trillions (Stiles & Jernigan, 2010).

The brain also contains structural non-neuronal components identified as **glial cells** of which there are three types: (1) ogliodendrocytes, (2) astrocytes, and (3) microglia (Figure 26-3). The **ogliodendrocytes** are responsible for the formation of myelin sheaths that surround the nerve fiber. The functions of the **astrocytes**

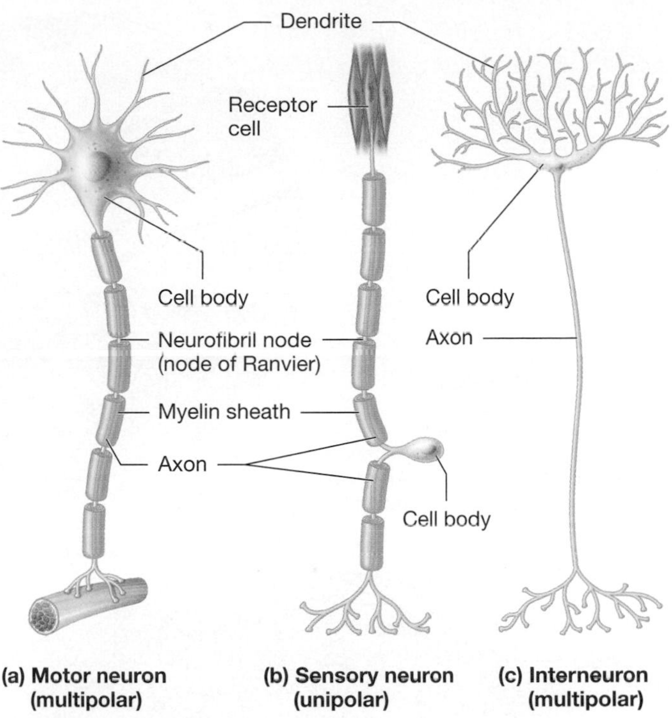

FIGURE 26-2 Types of neurons

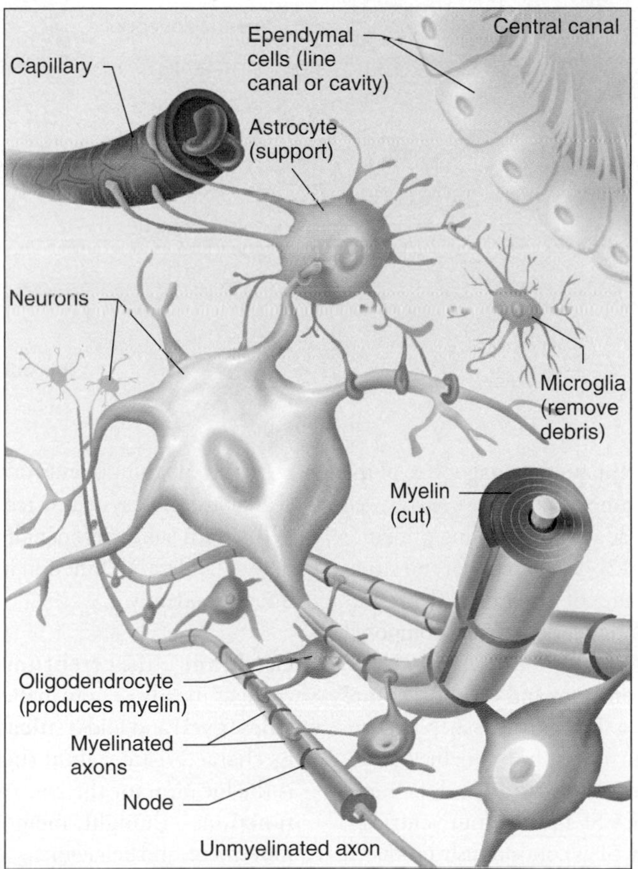

FIGURE 26-3 Glial cells

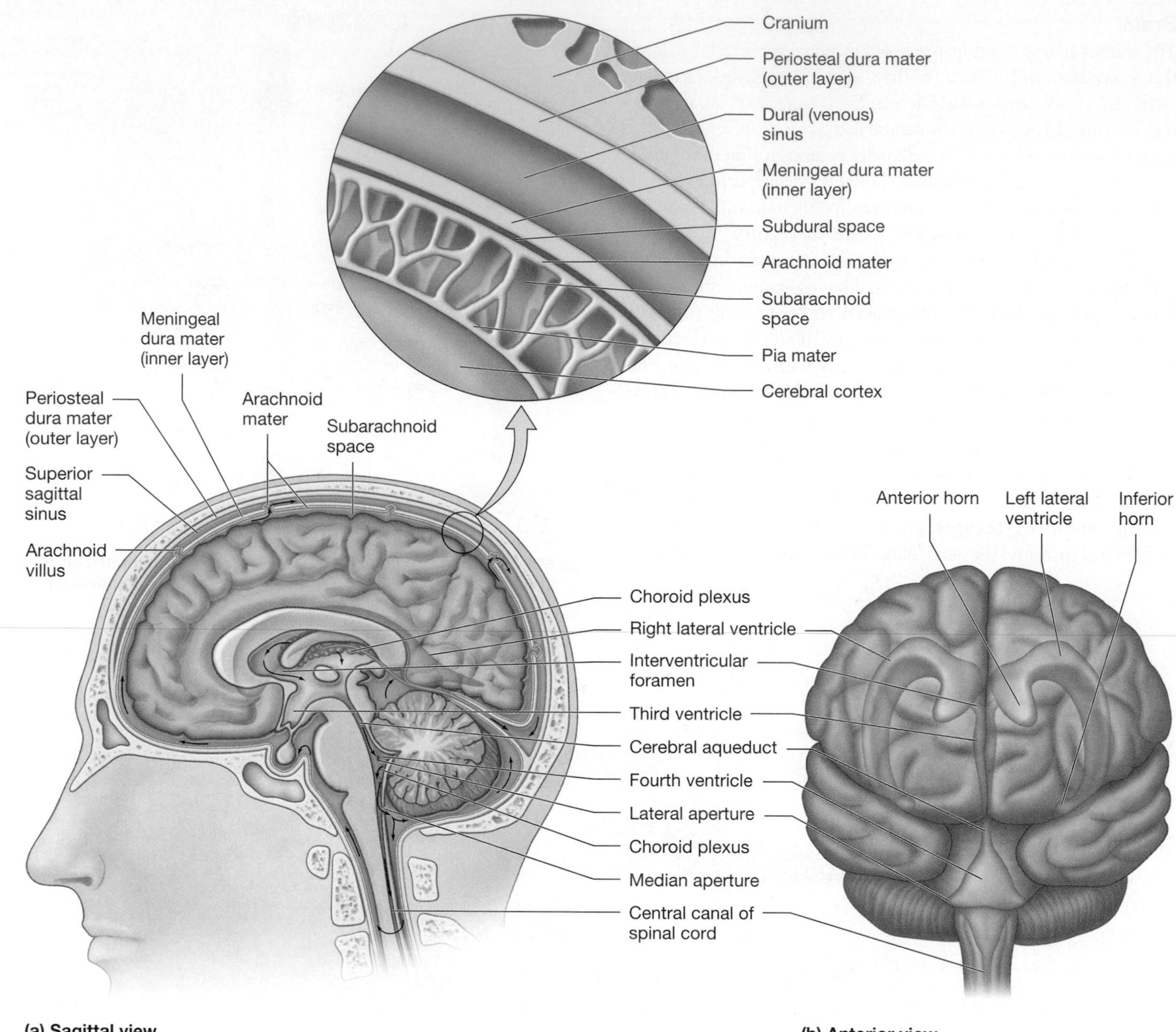

FIGURE 26-4 Meninges and ventricles

are not clearly identified. The **microglia** are the phagocytes of the nervous system that contribute to immune defense processes as well as the trimming process that takes place in the refining of neural circuits (Stephan, Barres, & Stevens, 2012). The functional and structural cells of the brain constitute the matter of the brain with the gray matter composed of functional units, and the white matter composed of structural units.

In addition to the cranium, the **meninges** and **cerebral spinal fluid (CSF)** are also a part of protecting the brain. The meninges are three layers of connective tissue that surround the brain: the outside layer (**dura mater**), the middle layer (**arachnoid**), and the inner layer or **pia mater** (Figure 26-4). The CSF fills the four ventricles, providing a cushion for the brain. The CSF is continuously produced by the **choroid plexus** within the ventricles of the brain flowing through them and the arachnoid spaces that extend down the spinal cord. Excess CSF is removed from circulation through the arachnoid villi in the spinal cord and absorbed into the venous circulation.

The subcomponents of the brain include the cerebrum, diencephalon, limbic system, cerebellum, and the brain stem (Figure 26-5). While each subcomponent has a unique and specific function, they do not necessarily function independently of each other, but rather interdependently.

Cerebrum The **cerebrum** is the largest portion of the brain and consists mostly of gray matter. Its outside surface consists of many loops (**gyri**) and folds (**sulcus**) of nervous tissue that gives the brain its characteristic walnut shell appearance. The **cerebral cortex** is the location for the control and integration of humans' highest functions—thought, memory, reasoning, sensation, voluntary movement, and behaviors.

The cerebrum is subdivided into two hemispheres, connected to each other by the **corpus callosum** that also connects the counterpart areas of each hemisphere (see Figure 26-5). The hemispheres are also divided into anterior and posterior sections by the central

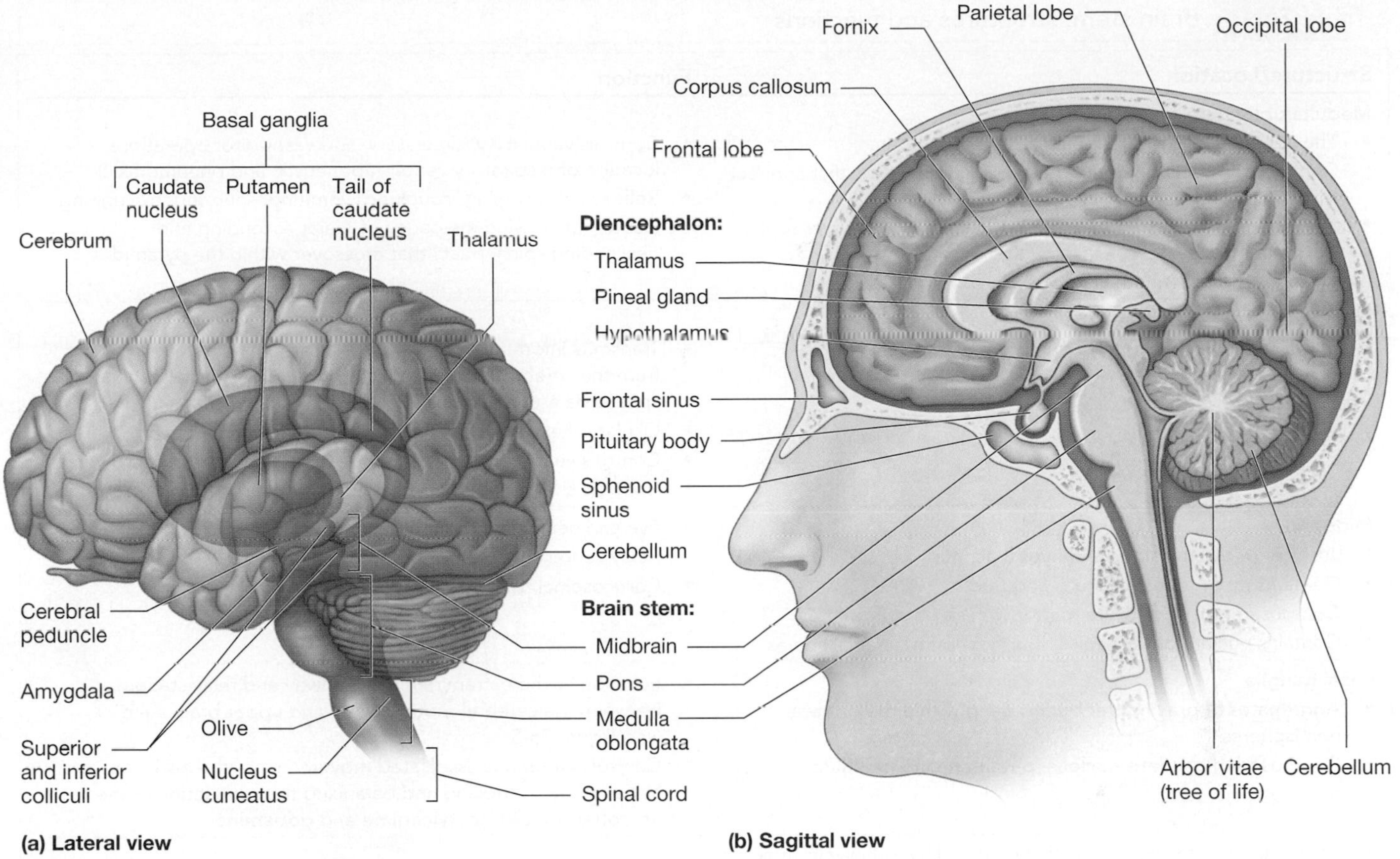

(a) Lateral view (b) Sagittal view

FIGURE 26-5 The brain and its subcomponents

sulcus. On each side of the central sulcus are the precentral gyrus and the postcentral gyrus.

Each hemisphere is composed of four lobes—frontal, parietal, occipital and temporal (Figure 26-6). Although described as lobes, they are not well defined and refer more to specific areas of the cerebrum rather than a specific section. Each lobe is responsible for mediating certain functions. The **basal ganglia** are also contained within the cerebral hemispheres.

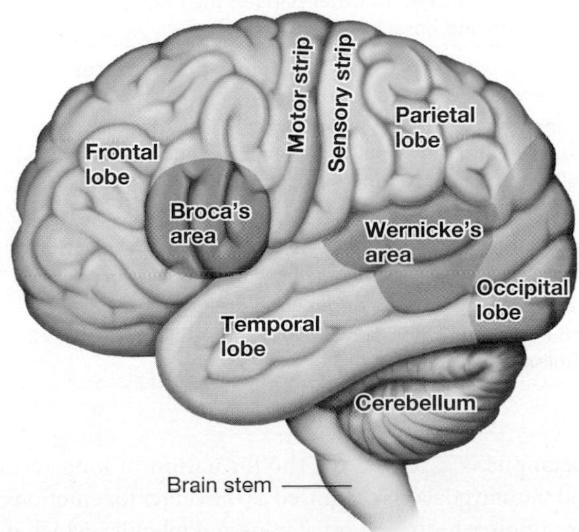

FIGURE 26-6 Lobes of brain, surface anatomy of lobes

The **frontal lobe** is primarily responsible for an individual's personality, behavior, emotions, and intellectual function. The **precentral gyrus** (motor cortex) of the frontal lobe is the primary motor area that initiates voluntary activity and also controls fine motor movement. The frontal lobe is also the origination of the corticospinal tracts that are located and travel through the spinal cord. **Broca's area** in the frontal lobe is responsible for mediating motor speech expression.

The **parietal lobe** is primarily responsible for receiving, processing, and interpreting sensory data. It facilitates the interpretation of tactile stimuli (pain, pressure, temperature, size, shape), as well as sight, sound, taste, and hearing stimuli. The **postcentral gyrus** is part of the parietal lobe and is the primary sensory area.

The **occipital lobe** is primarily responsible for the reception and interpretation of visual stimuli.

The **temporal lobe** is primarily responsible for auditory perception and interpretation and location or source of sound. It is also involved with the integration of taste smell and balance. **Wernicke's area** in the temporal lobe is responsible for speech and language interpretation and comprehension.

The **brain stem** is located between the cerebrum and the spinal cord, connecting the cerebral cortex and the spinal cord. The brain stem regulates many involuntary functions (Table 26-1).

Limbic System The **limbic system** is a wishbone-shaped grouping of gray matter that includes parts of the diencephalon and cerebrum. Some of its gray portions include the anterior

Table 26-1 Brain stem: structures and functions

Structure/Location	Function
Medulla oblongata • The continuation of the spinal cord into the brain. • Contains the ascending and descending fiber tracts that connect the spinal cord to the brain. • Site where the descending corticospinal tracts cross over to the opposite side. • Contains nuclei for cranial nerves VIII–XII.	• Controls ventilatory, circulatory, and vasomotor operations; location of respiratory center (apeneustic and pneumotaxic) • Reflexes: Swallowing, coughing, vomiting, sneezing, hiccupping • Center for relaying messages of major ascending and descending spinal tracts that crossover within the pyramid
Pons • Middle section of the midbrain	• Transmits information between brain stem and cerebellum, and from the cerebral cortex to the contralateral cerebellar hemisphere via ascending and descending fiber tracts. • Ocular reflexes: Pupillary action and eye movements • Controls ventilations (portion of respiratory center located here) • Controls skeletal muscle movement with corticospinal tract
Midbrain • Just below the thalamus and hypothalamus • Contains many motor neurons and tracts • Composed mostly of white matter with some gray matter • Contains nuclei from the third, fourth, and fifth cranial nerves	• Eye and head movement reflexes • Relay center for auditory pathway • Corticospinal tract pathway
Basal ganglia • Aggregates of gray matter buried deep within the cerebral hemispheres • Composed of **caudate nucleus**, **putamen**, and **pallidum**	• Function as the extrapyramidal pathway and relay station between the cerebral motor cortex and upper brain stem (see Figure 26-5) • Controls automatic associated movements of the body; this is achieved by controlling and balancing the production of the neurotransmitters **acetylcholine** and **dopamine**.
The **diencephalon** consists of the thalamus and hypothalamus. It also contains the lateral geniculate nucleus and the posterior lobe of the pituitary gland.	
Thalamus • The channel to the cerebral cortex.	• Relay center for impulses between cerebrum, cerebellum, pons, and medulla • Transmits sensory impulses (not olfactory) to and from cerebrum prior to delivery to their appropriate sensory areas. • Integrates impulses between motor cortex and cerebrum, mediating skeletal muscle movements and motor response.
Epithalamus • Dorsal posterior segment of the diencephalon • Includes the habenula and their interconnecting fibers (habenular commissure, the stria medullaris and the pineal body).	• Location of pineal body • Regulates sexual development and behavior • Some functions of its components include the secretion of melatonin by the pineal gland, and regulation of motor pathways and emotions. • Connects the limbic system to other parts of the brain (wired with limbic system and basal ganglia).
Hypothalamus	• Center for major processing of internal stimuli that regulates autonomic nervous system activities • Regulates temperature control, water metabolism, osmolarity of body fluids, eating behaviors, sleep, anterior and posterior pituitary gland, and neuroendocrine function
Lateral geniculate nucleus **Posterior lobe of the pituitary gland**	• Receives all signals from the optic nerve where they are processed and sent to the appropriate visual regions of the cerebral cortex • Releases antidiuretic hormone and oxytocin. • Controls hormonal regulation of growth, lactation, vasoconstriction, and metabolism

nucleus of the **thalamus**, **limbic lobe**, **mammillary bodies**, **amygdala**, and **hippocampus**. The limbic system is responsible for mediating primitive behaviors, visceral responses to emotional stimuli, and biologic rhythms, all of which are necessary for survival. The hippocampus is essential for the formation of long-term memory and the amygdala is recognized as the center for emotions. It transmits impulses to the hypothalamus and medulla, which in turn activate the sympathetic nervous system (fight response).

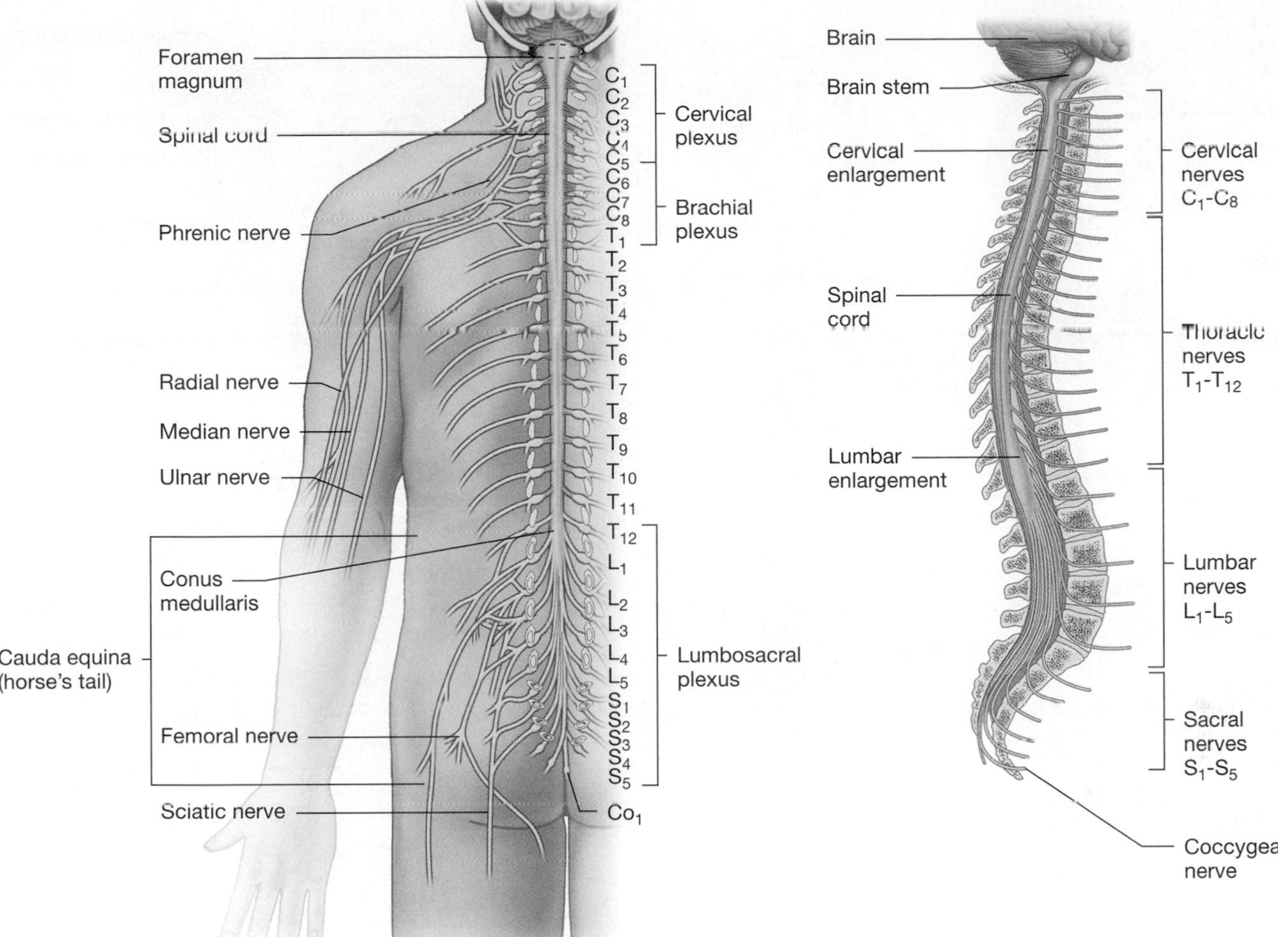

FIGURE 26-7 Spinal cord and spinal nerves

Spinal Cord

The spinal cord is a long cylindrical-shaped, ropelike structure that is a continuation of the medulla and passes through the vertebral canal of the spinal column (Figure 26-7). It begins at the foramen magnum of the skull and terminates at L1 or L2 of the vertebral column. It is composed of sensory (ascending), motor (descending), and autonomic fiber tracts that transmit nerve impulses between the brain and the body. The ascending and descending tracts are contained within the myelinated, white matter. The gray matter, which contains the nerve cell bodies, is shaped like an H in the central portion of the cord. The wing extensions of the gray matter are identified as the posterior and anterior horns. In addition to functioning as the conducting pathway for nerve impulses, the spinal cord functions as the connection center for reflexes.

Descending Spinal Tracts The descending spinal tracts originate in the brain and transmit motor commands impulses to various muscle groups to regulate muscle tone and voluntary actions. The spinal tracts are classified according to their point of origination and termination; thus, descending tracts begin in the brain and terminate in the spinal column. The descending spinal tracts are composed of two systems, the **pyramidal** (direct) and the **extrapyramidal** (indirect). The direct pathways in the pyramidal system are the lateral and anterior **corticospinal** tracts and the lateral and anterior **corticobulbar** tracts (Figure 26-8).

The pyramidal system pathway originates in the pre-motor cortex of the cerebrum. The impulse travels from the cortex to the brain stem or spinal cord via the pyramids located in the medulla. The fibers that transmit these impulses constitute the corticospinal tract. At the pyramids, approximately 90% of the fibers **decussate** (cross over) to the opposite side of the brain. The remaining fibers continue to travel down on the same side as their origin. The fibers that cross over are referred to as the lateral corticospinal tract; the fibers that remain on their original side form the anterior corticospinal tract. Pyramidal fibers that synapse with cranial nerves in the brain stem make up the corticobulbar tract.

The pyramidal system consists of and functions as a two-neuron system, the upper motor and lower motor neurons. **Upper motor neurons** are unable to exit the central nervous system. The pyramidal tract is a significant upper motor neuron tract. Upper motor neurons must synapse with lower motor neurons to transmit impulses and deliver messages to the muscles.

Lower motor neurons consist of the spinal and cranial nerves. All spinal nerves have a lower motor neuron component because they are both motor and sensory. Not every cranial nerve has a lower motor neuron component as there are some that are only sensory. The cell bodies of these neurons are located in the brain stem, however, their axons can exit from the central nervous system and synapse with the muscles they innervate.

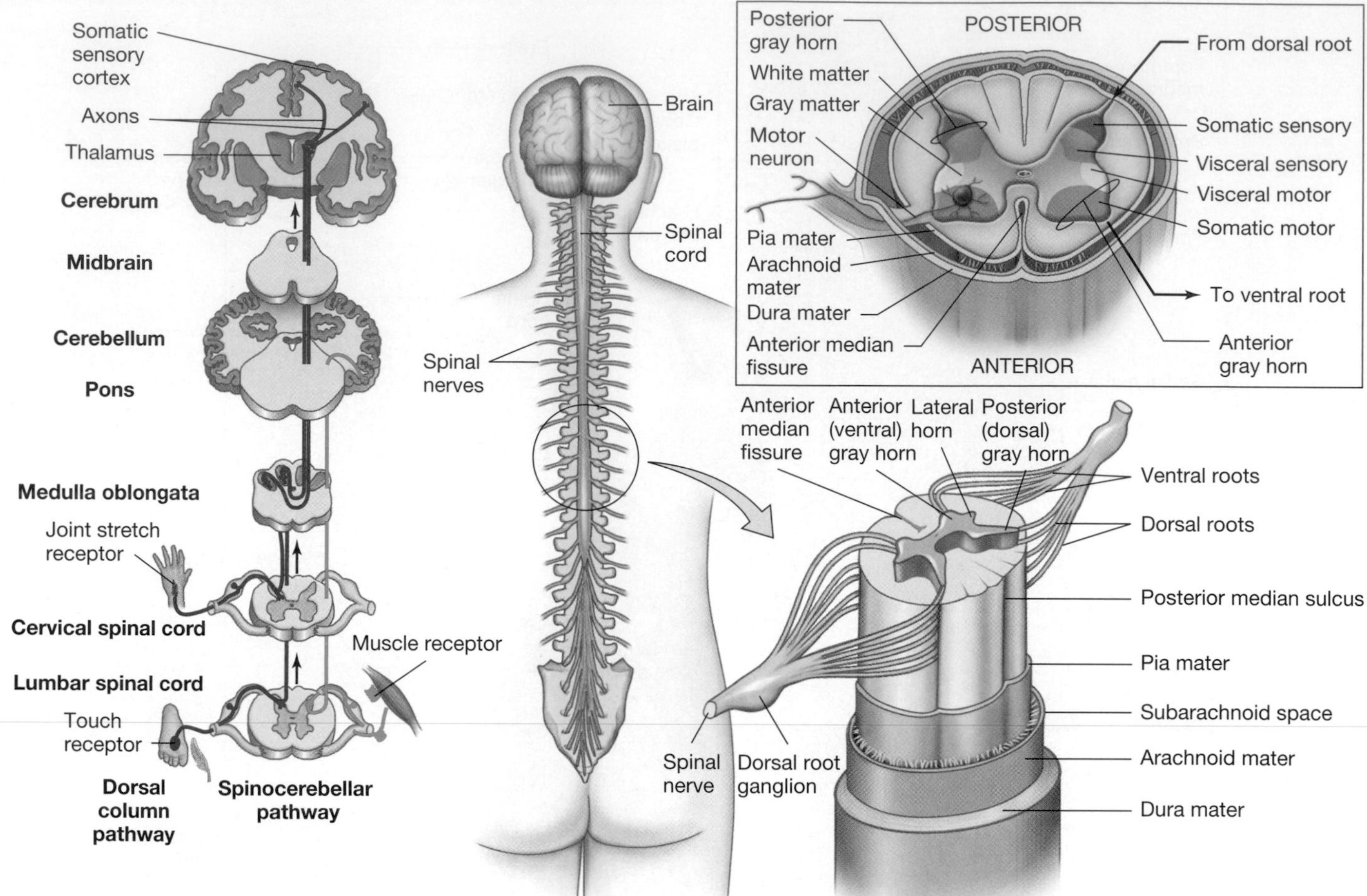

FIGURE 26-8 Spinal cord/cross section with tracts

The extrapyramidal system is primarily concerned with involuntary muscle movement to maintain posture, balance, and reflexes. Impulses that travel in the extrapyramidal pathway originate in the cerebellum as well as the red nucleus, the substantia nigra, and the reticular formation. There are four tracts that comprise the extrapyramidal system—**rubrospinal**, **reticulospinal**, **tectospinal**, and **vestibulospinal**. All four tracts terminate in the spinal nerves. The extrapryamidal system is only a lower motor neuron system.

Ascending Spinal Tracts The ascending tracts originate in the spinal column and transmit sensory impulses to the brain where they terminate in various areas of the brain (see Figure 26-8). Sensory impulses travel from sensory receptors in the skin or other areas through afferent fibers in peripheral nerves. The impulse enters the spinal cord through the dorsal root and ascends to the brain. The ascending tracts consist of three pathways—the **dorsal column**, the **spinothalamic tract**, and the **spinocerebellar tract**.

The dorsal column system consists of the **fasciculus gracilis** and **fasciculus cuneatus**, and transmit highly critical sensory impulses to the brain. The speed and accuracy of their impulse transmission are faster and better than transmission of impulses in the spinothalamic tract. The dorsal columns are responsible for transmitting sensations related to **proprioception**, fine touch and vibration to the medulla oblongata.

Sensations associated with proprioception allow an individual to locate each segment of the body in space. This ability for spatial perception of the body is a highly refined process that makes possible the detection of very minute movement positions, or changes in position. Fine touch is associated with the ability to identify forms and objects by simple touch. Two-point discrimination sensations are also conveyed by the dorsal columns. Vibratory sensations up to 700 cycles per second are also transmitted through the dorsal columns.

The spinothalamic pathway consists of two tracts—the **lateral spinothalamic** and **ventral spinothalamic tract**. These tracts transmit crude sensations that are slower and less accurate than the dorsal columns. The lateral spinothalamic tract conducts pain and temperature sensations and the ventral spinothalamic tract conducts sensations for pressure and simple touch.

The spinocerebellar tract relays information pertaining to unconscious proprioceptive sensation. Receptors in joints, tendons, and muscles transmit impulses concerning muscle tone, position of the body, and movement of muscles through the spinocerebellar tracts to the anterior lobe of the cerebellum. The spinocerebellar pathway consists of two tracts—the **posterior** and **anterior spinocerebellar tracts**.

Peripheral Nervous System

The major responsibility of the **peripheral nervous system** is sending and receiving sensory and motor impulses to and from the central nervous system. It consists of the spinal nerves and **ganglia** (groups of nerve cell bodies) outside the central nervous system that are the conduits for the afferent and efferent impulses that travel

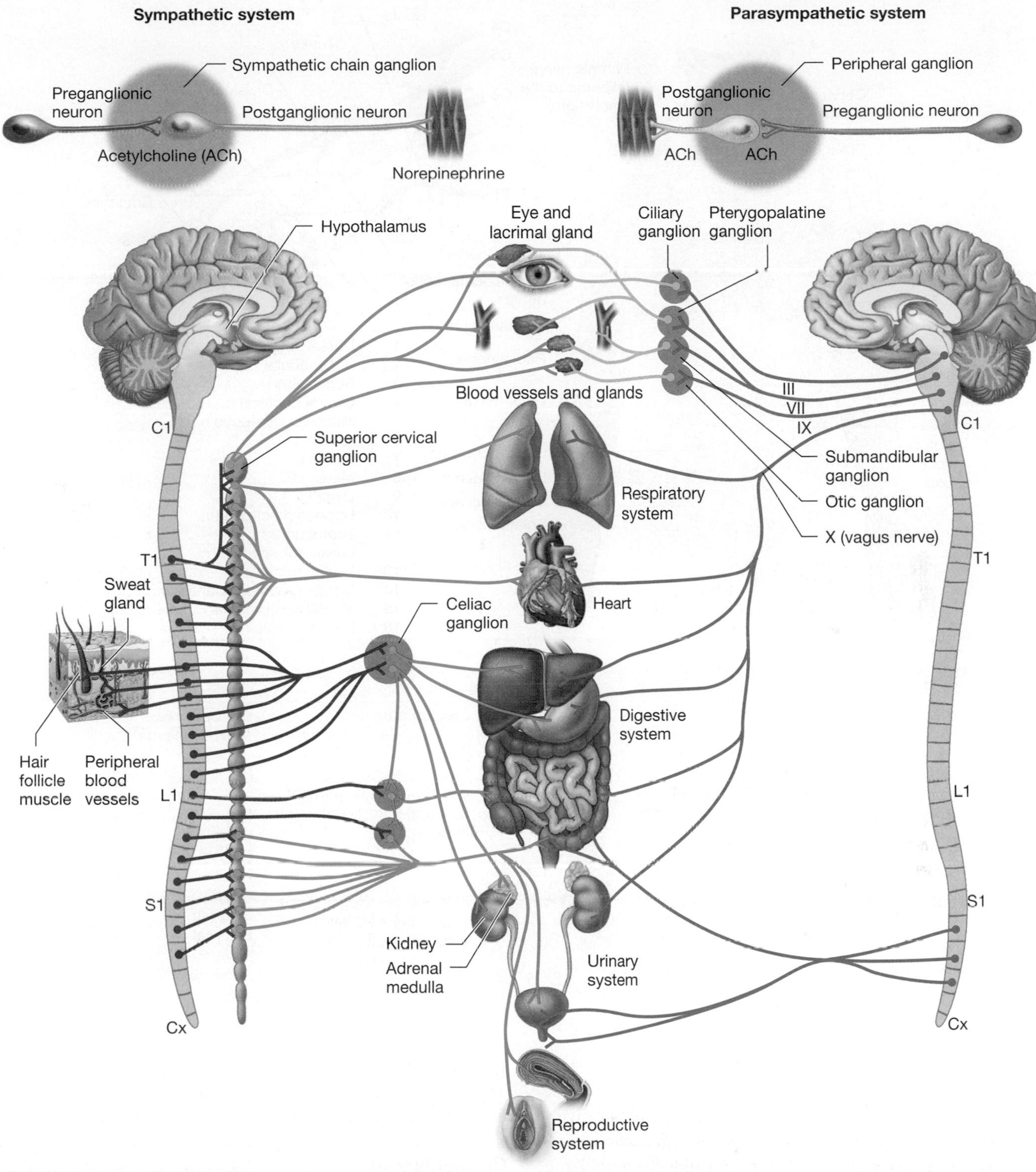

FIGURE 26-9 Location of PNS ganglia

between the sensory receptors throughout the body and the spinal cord. Nerve fibers do not contain cell bodies. Cell bodies are contained within and comprise the ganglia that are distributed throughout the body (Figure 26-9).

The peripheral nervous system is divided into two subsystems—the **somatic** and **autonomic systems**. The somatic nervous system primarily innervates skeletal muscle and is responsible for coordinating voluntary movements. The autonomic nervous system is composed of two divisions: the

PRACTICE POINT: Remembering Cranial Nerves

A traditional mnemonic frequently used to remember the names of the cranial nerves is "**O**n **O**ld **O**lympus **T**owering **T**op **A** **F**inn **A**nd **G**erman **V**iewed **S**ome **H**ops." The capital letter of each word indicates the initial letter of the 12 cranial nerves. More difficult is to remember the function of the cranial nerve, whether a cranial nerve is sensory, motor, or both. Another mnemonic can be memorized to help identify the specific functions of the nerve. In this case, **S** = sensory, **M** = motor, and **B** = both. "**S**ome **S**ay **M**arry **M**oney **B**ut **M**y **B**rother **S**ays **B**ad **B**usinesses **M**arry **M**oney."

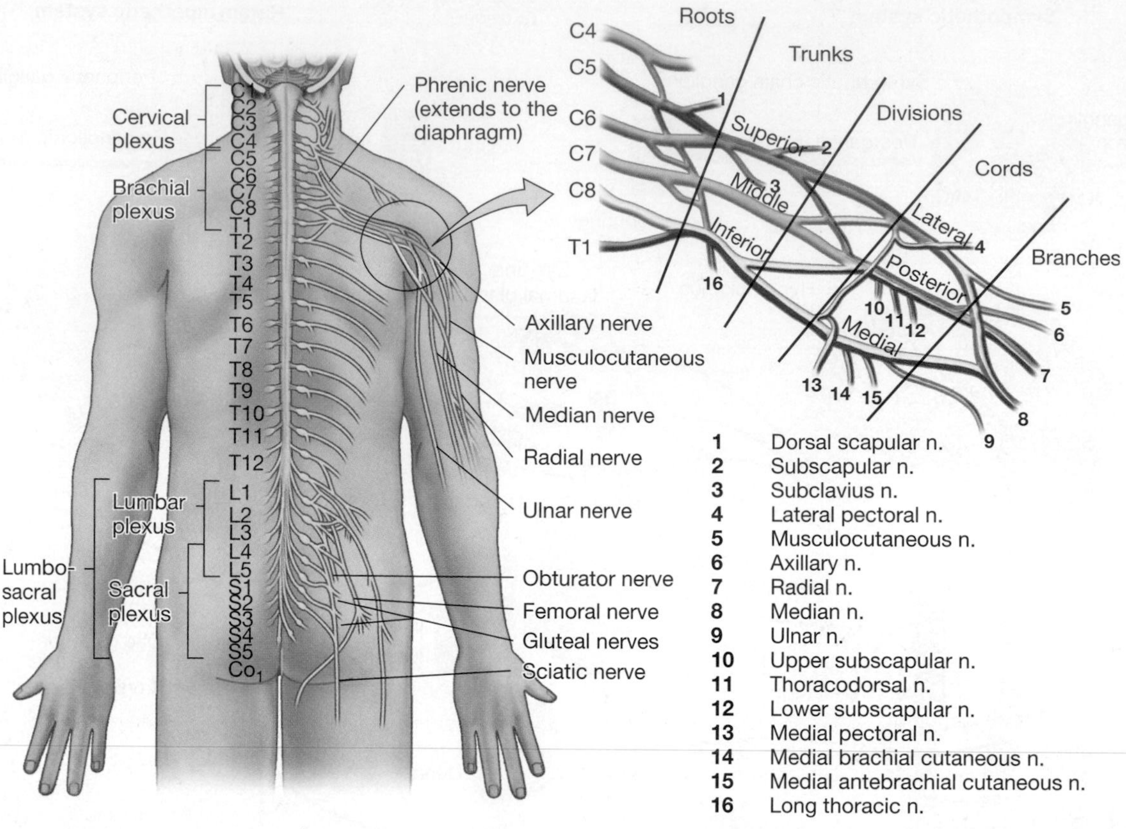

Spinal nerve plexuses

Plexus	Location	Spinal nerves involved	Region supplied	Major nerves leaving plexus
Cervical	Deep in the neck, under the sternocleidomastoid muscle	C1–C4	Skin and muscles of neck and shoulder; diaphragm	Phrenic (Diaphragm)
Brachial	Deep to the clavicle, between the neck and the axilla	C5–C8, T1	Skin and muscles of upper extremity	Musculocutaneous Ulnar Median Radial Axillary
Lumbosacral	Lumbar region of the back	T12, L1–L5, S1–S4	Skin and muscles of lower abdominal wall, lower extremity, buttocks, external genitalia	Obturator Femoral Sciatic Pudendal

FIGURE 26-10 Peripheral nerves that form brachial plexus

sympathetic and **parasympathetic systems**. Together, these two divisions function to coordinate and maintain multiple involuntary activities that contribute to physiological homeostasis. Essentially the sympathetic system is responsible for mobilizing energy during times of emergency, the "fight or flight" activities; and the parasympathetic system is responsible for conservation and restoration of energy for routine maintenance functions. The overall functioning of the body is maintained by a balance between the "rest and relaxation" or "rest and digest" activities of the parasympathetic system and the "fight or flight" activities of the sympathetic system.

In some organs, there is dual innervation so that there are opposite effects that occur when either system is activated. In other instances, there is only sympathetic innervation so that the opposite response is brought about by deactivation of the sympathetic system.

The nerves that comprise the peripheral nervous system consist of cranial nerves and spinal nerves.

Cranial Nerves

The 12 paired **cranial nerves** originate from the brain or brain stem (see Figure 26-10). These are peripheral nerves that innervate structures of the head and neck. One exception is the vagus nerve that also innervates the heart, respiratory muscles, stomach, and gall bladder. Cranial nerves are identified either by their function or their relationship to adjacent structures, appearance, distribution, composition, or location (Oommen, 2013; Table 26-2). Cranial nerves are also classified as sensory nerves, motor nerves, or both. Additionally, some cranial nerves also have parasympathetic properties. Knowledge of the cranial nerves makes it easier for the provider to remember their function, making their assessment self-evident.

Table 26-2 Cranial nerves and their functions

Cranial Nerve Name		Function
CN I	Olfactory	Sensory—smell
CNII	Optic	Sensory—vision
CN III	Occulomotor	Motor—eye muscle movement Parasympathetic—pupil constriction lens accommodation
CN IV	Trochlear	Motor—eye muscle movement
CN V	Trigeminal	Motor—muscles for chewing Sensory—sensation of face and scalp, cornea, mucous membranes of mouth and nose
CN VI	Abducens	Motor—lateral movement of eye
CN VII	Facial	Motor—facial muscles, eye lid (closure) labial speech Sensory—taste on anterior two-thirds of tongue (sweet and salt) Parasympathetic—saliva and tear secretion
CN VIII	Auditory (Acoustic)	Sensory—hearing and balance
CN IX	Glossopharyngeal	Motor—vocal sounds and swallowing (pharynx) Sensory—taste on posterior one-third of tongue (bitter and sour); gag reflex (pharynx)
CN X	Vagus	Motor—talking and swallowing (larynx and pharynx) Sensory—generalized sensations from carotid body, carotid sinus, pharynx, and viscera Parasympathetic—carotid reflex
CN XI	Accessory (Spinal)	Motor—trapezius and sternocleidomastoid muscles (contraction)
CN XII	Hypoglossal	Motor—movement of tongue for speech articulation and swallowing

Spinal Nerves

The 31 pairs of **spinal nerves** exit from the spinal cord and are aligned alongside the vertebral column (see Figure 26-10). Each pair exits the spinal cord as **dorsal** and **ventral roots** and then merge to form the spinal nerve. The dorsal root is an afferent sensory nerve that transmits sensory impulses into the spinal cord, whereas the ventral root is an efferent motor nerve that transmits motor impulses to effector muscles and glands. The dorsal root also contains the **dorsal root ganglion**. Each ganglion is comprised of the cell bodies and axons of these sensory neurons. The spinal nerve exits the spinal cord through the intervertebral foramen. The bone structure and width of each vertebra creates a vertebral canal, which is where each ganglion is located so it is protected from injury.

Spinal nerves are identified by their respective vertebrae so that there are 8 paired cervical nerves, 12 paired thoracic nerves, 5 paired lumbar nerves, 5 paired sacral nerves, and 1 pair of coccygeal nerves. Spinal nerves consist of both sensory and motor fibers. Each pair of spinal nerves innervates a specific area of the body known as a **dermatome**. Knowledge of dermatomes allows for the identification of extent and location of damage to the spinal cord after trauma.

Certain spinal nerves, as they exit the spinal cord through the ventral root, do not go directly to their specific structure of origin. Instead of direct innervation, they form a plexus, which is an interconnection of nerve fibers that form new combinations of fibers to become peripheral nerves (see Figure 26-8). The four plexuses of spinal nerves are (1) cervical, (2) brachial, (3) lumbar, and (4) sacral. The spinal nerves involved in creating the brachial plexus and peripheral nerves that emerge from the plexus are listed in Table 26-3. The interconnection of these nerves allows for compensation by other nerves to occur if nerves within the plexus are damaged. The second through eleventh thoracic nerves do not form a plexus and are identified as the intercostal or thoracic nerves.

Reflexes

Reflexes are subconscious actions and reactions that are vital defense mechanisms for the nervous system. They initiate an immediate response to alert and protect an individual from potentially painful or harmful stimuli or situations. They also function to maintain proper muscle tone and balance.

A **reflex arc** is a neural pathway that controls an action reflex. Most sensory neurons do not pass directly into the brain but synapse in the spinal cord. This rudimentary transmission of impulses allows reflex actions to occur rapidly by activating spinal motor neurons without signal routing to the brain (Figure 26-11).

Monosynaptic refers to the presence of a single synapse with immediate transmission of the impulse from the afferent nerve to the efferent nerve at the level of the spinal cord. An example of this is the patellar knee jerk. By contrast, in polysynaptic reflex pathways, one or more interneurons connect afferent (sensory) and efferent (motor signals) allowing processing or inhibition of polysynaptic reflexes within the spinal cord.

Deep tendon reflexes (DTRs) are monosynaptic spinal segmental reflexes that assess the competency of cutaneous innervation, motor supply, and cortical input to the matching spinal segment. DTRs are easily assessed by tapping the tendon that is connected to the muscle spindles of the muscle. Tapping initiates a sensory impulse that travels in an afferent nerve to the dorsal root where it enters the spinal cord. It synapses with a motor neuron in the anterior horn where it then exits via an efferent nerve at the ventral horn and travels back to the muscle where it initiates a response.

Superficial reflexes are segmental motor reflex responses to scratching of the skin. They indicate the competency of cutaneous innervation and corresponding motor flow. Superficial reflexes are more complex than DTRs as they are polysynaptic and ascend and descend through the spinal cord.

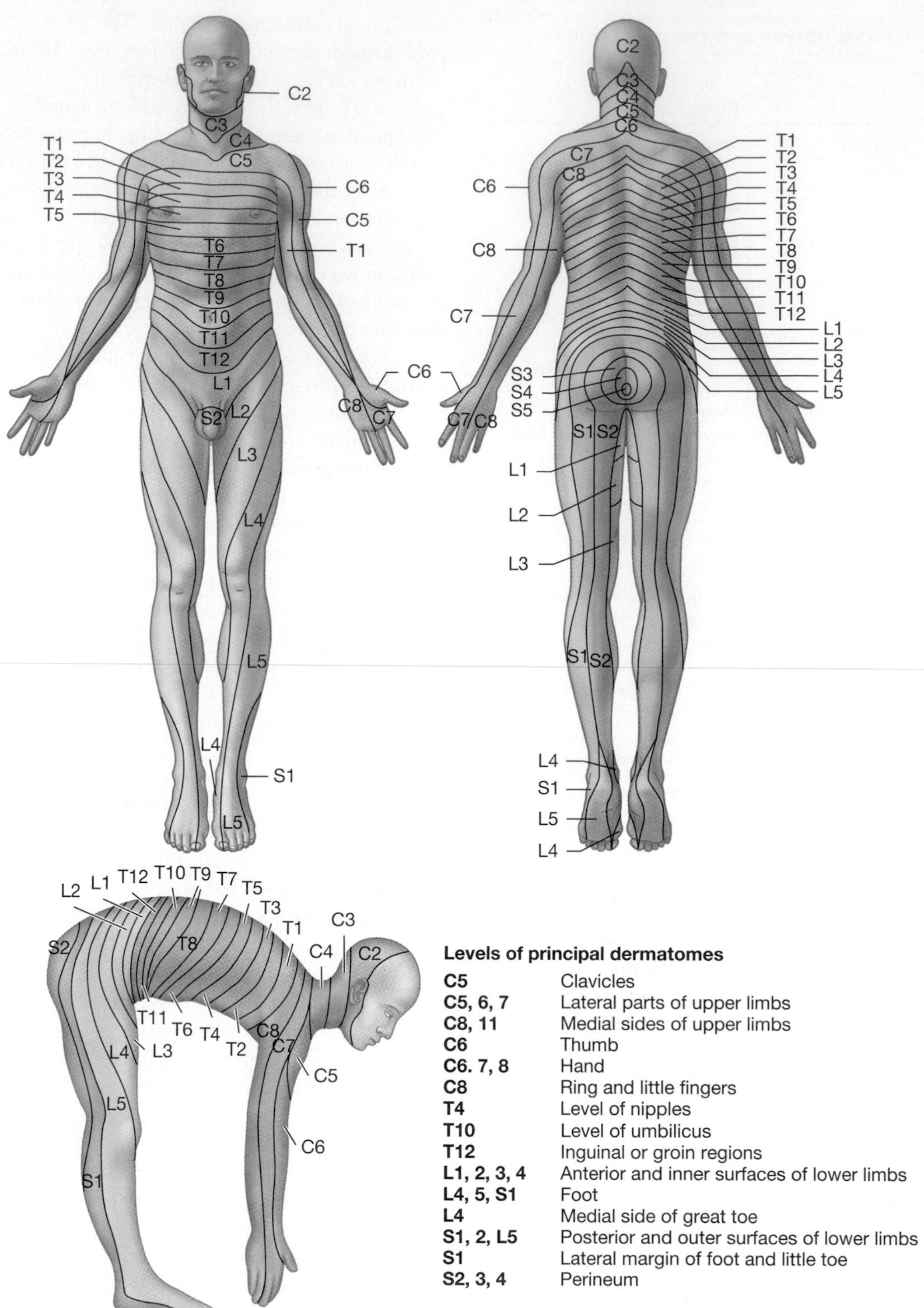

Levels of principal dermatomes

C5	Clavicles
C5, 6, 7	Lateral parts of upper limbs
C8, 11	Medial sides of upper limbs
C6	Thumb
C6. 7, 8	Hand
C8	Ring and little fingers
T4	Level of nipples
T10	Level of umbilicus
T12	Inguinal or groin regions
L1, 2, 3, 4	Anterior and inner surfaces of lower limbs
L4, 5, S1	Foot
L4	Medial side of great toe
S1, 2, L5	Posterior and outer surfaces of lower limbs
S1	Lateral margin of foot and little toe
S2, 3, 4	Perineum

Dermatome mapping

THINK LINK: Dermatome Mapping

The systematic distribution of dermatomes is determined during embryological development. Initially, the embryo becomes segmented into somites that are innervated by the adjacent spinal cord segment or cranial nerve. The section of the somite that is predetermined to develop into skin is identified as a dermatome. These dermatomes have been identified and mapped. The dermatome map may look somewhat confusing, particularly in the extremities because the relationship of the dermatome to the spinal nerve doesn't appear to be logical. This is because the dermatomes become somewhat distorted during development and the distribution map is most often depicted on a human that is in the upright position. The relationship between the spinal nerve and its corresponding dermatome is easier to understand if the dermatomes are viewed on a body that is in a quadrapedal (four-legged animal) position. Each dermatome receives its densest innervation from its corresponding spinal nerve; however, the dermatome may also be innervated by other adjacent spinal nerves (Berne & Levy, 2002).

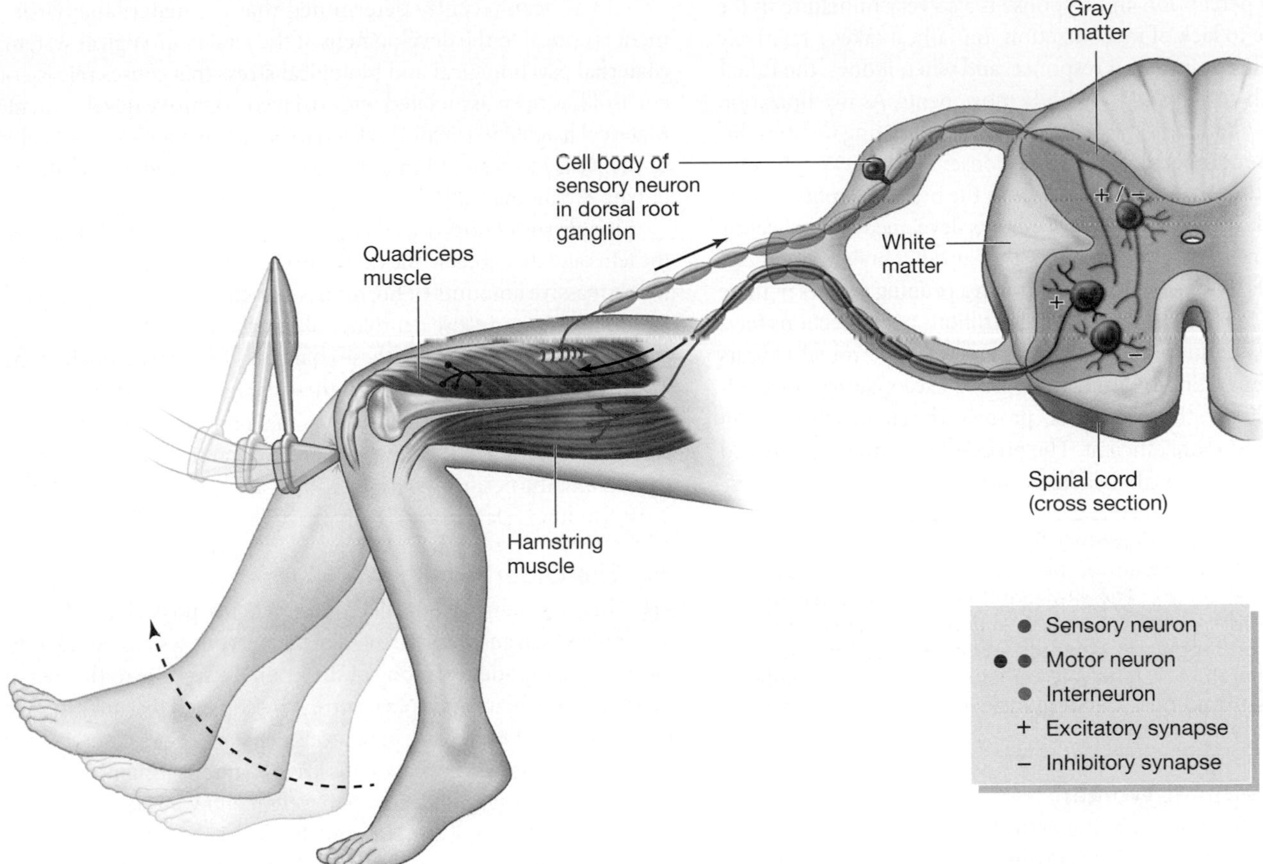

FIGURE 26-11 Reflex arc

Developmental Variations

Developmental variations occur over the course of an individual's life span and events. Awareness of these variations is important to understand and recognize common age-related alterations or modifications of the brain and nerves.

Infants and Children

The nervous system begins to form within the first 3 weeks of fetal development. The three sections of the brain, forebrain, middle brain, and hind brain, are identified by week 4. It has long been thought that an infant was born with all the neurons that one was ever going to have. More recently, however, there has been a change in thought and there is growing consensus that neurons continue to develop throughout a lifetime.

Brain growth and development is extremely complex and appears to occur in spurts of activity. At birth, most of the brain's cells are already present; however, the connections between the cells that form the circuits or pathways are not formed. The experiences and sensations that the infant encounters significantly impact the formation of these connections. The development of the brain continues throughout childhood and is thought to continue on through early adulthood. Even though by this time the wiring of the brain is well established, new circuits related to learning and acquisition of motor skills develop throughout the remainder of an individual's lifetime.

At birth, the nervous system is quite immature. There is minimal cortical activity so that the spinal cord and medulla are primarily responsible for motor activity. Responses by the newborn are primarily primitive reflexes that are present. As the brain grows and develops and cortical activity increases and voluntary activity emerges, these primitive reflexes are inhibited causing them to disappear at expected times. The disappearance of these reflexes is a measurement of nervous system maturation. Persistence of these reflexes beyond their expected disappearance is an indication of CNS dysfunction. Any intrusive event during this first year of development can interfere with maturation of the CNS system and have significant effects on future brain function.

The major growth in the brain and nervous system as well as myelinization occurs during the first year. Nervous system development in the infant proceeds in a systematic manner, progressing in a **cephalocaudal** (head, neck, trunk) and **proximodistal** (inner to outer) order, following the pattern of myelinization of the peripheral nervous system. As the nervous system develops, the infant achieves mastery and control of the motor system, achieving milestones along the way. The initial milestone is the lifting of the head, and the final milestone is walking. Each succeeding milestone is more complex and requires more coordination. Although the progression and development of the nervous system occurs sequentially, the age at which the milestones are achieved may vary considerably from infant to infant.

Sensory perception and response is also very immature in the newborn due to lack of myelinization. Initially, it takes a relatively strong stimulus to initiate a response, and when it does, the infant responds with crying and total body movements. As myelinization proceeds, the infant becomes more precise in localizing the stimulus and making a more accurate motor response.

During this process, circuits within the brain are continuously being formed. The total number of circuits developed is significantly greater than the number of circuits within an adult brain. Recent evidence suggests that the brain goes through a pruning process of these connections. During the first 10 years, trillions of connections have been formed so at this point, the brain is super dense. Around 11 years of age, the brain begins to eliminate, or prune, excess connections, primarily according to the "use or lose" process. The circuits that remain are stronger and more efficient. The process of forming circuits and pruning continues throughout adolescence and into early adulthood.

THINK LINK: The Teenager's Brain

Pruning begins in the back of the brain, moving forward toward the prefrontal cortex. The prefrontal cortex is the center of control that is responsible for evaluating consequences, forms judgments, and regulates impulses and emotions. The teenager's brain, therefore, is relatively immature and helps to explain the impulsivity and poor decision making that characterize this developmental stage.

The Pregnant Woman

No specific changes of the neurological system during pregnancy are identified. Hypothalmic-pituitary neurohormonal changes are well established to maintain the pregnancy. Physiological changes may occur and include contraction or tension type of headaches and acroparesia. Headaches may become worse with postural changes and new situational or environmental conditions that precipitate stress and anxiety. **Acroparesia,** numbness and tingling of the hands, may be experienced and is caused by postural kinking of the blood vessels at the thoracic outlet. These symptoms may be mistaken for carpal tunnel syndrome. Carpal tunnel syndrome may also occur during pregnancy and resolves generally after delivery of the fetus. Both may be aggravated in a recumbent position thus interfering with sleep.

DTRs should be +2 when assessed. Increased (+3/+4) or brisk reflexes are an indication of the possibility of preeclampsia or other conditions like hyperthyroidism.

It has been recently determined that the maternal environment is critical to the development of the fetal neurological system. Maternal psychological and biological stress that causes release of cortisol has been associated with delayed cognitive development. Maternal heightened anxiety related to her pregnancy and the health of the fetus has resulted in a reduction in gray matter in children (Glynn & Sandman, 2011).

It is also recognized that there is a reciprocal relationship between the fetus and the mother. The exposure of the pregnant woman's brain to the massive amounts of hormones secreted during the perinatal period is known to cause neurological changes within the brain; however, the extent and effect of these changes is unknown. Much of the evidence supports the notion that these changes are mediated by the placenta as well as maternal behaviors that promote bonding and the care and nurturing of the newborn are programmed and developed throughout the perinatal period (Kim et al., 2010; Kinsley & Meyer, 2010; Sandman, Davis, Buss, & Glynn, 2011).

The Older Adult

The older adult is more likely to experience physiologic changes rather than anatomic changes of the nervous system. As an individual ages, a gradual atrophy of the brain occurs due to the loss of neurons in the brain and spinal cord. It is estimated that after the age of 50, there is a 1% decrease in neurons per year. The vast numbers of brain neurons, however, makes this loss of neurons insignificant. The loss of neurons causes a decrease in weight and volume of the brain such that by 80 years of age, the brain has lost 15% of its weight.

The speed of nerve conduction decreases causing the reaction time of the elderly to also decrease. There is also an increased delay at the synapse resulting in a slower traveling time for an impulse. This may result in a diminished sense of smell and taste as well as decreased sensation of pain and touch.

In spite of the loss of neurons, the elderly experience minimal changes in the function of memory storage. There is a decrease in the speed of learning and processing information, and also their reaction to simple and complex stimuli is slower. Thus, they may need more time when asked to perform certain activities.

The loss of neurons also affects the muscular system. There is an overall loss of muscle bulk that reduces muscle strength. There may also be a decrease in muscle tone, particularly around the face and neck. There is also a decreased agility that results in impaired fine motor coordination.

Health Promotion

The central nervous system is constantly sending, receiving, and processing information that is necessary for maintenance of vital functions, mobility and motor coordination, and sensory interpretation, Optimal function and performance of the nervous system requires uninterrupted transmission of all this information. Unlike other tissues and organ of the body, damage or injury to the nervous system is unable to be repaired and restored. Keeping the nervous system intact and preventing injury to the nervous system are dependent on awareness of potential threats, internal and external, and by avoiding behaviors and activities that are considered risky with a high probability for accidents and injuries. Internal threats to nervous system damage are alterations within the vascular structures that diminish or obstruct blood flow, particularly to the brain.

Stroke, Brain Attack

To achieve the goals within the topic area Heart Disease and Stroke (HDS), one of the objectives of Healthy People 2020 is:

- HDS—3 Reduce stroke deaths. (U.S. Department of Health and Human Services, 2009)

Health Promotion *continued*

A **stroke** (previously identified as cerebral vascular accident or CVA) occurs when the source of blood to an area of the brain is disrupted causing injury to (ischemia) and death of (infarction) brain tissue. Individuals who are more likely to sustain a stroke are those that demonstrate the characteristics or risk factors shown in Table 26-3.

Strokes are the primary cause of neurological problems in the U.S. making it the third overall cause of death. Facts regarding stroke include the following:

- Stroke kills almost 130,000 Americans each year—that's 1 in every 19 deaths.
- On average, one American dies from stroke every 4 minutes.
- Every year, more than 795,000 people in the United States have a stroke. About 610,000 of these are first or new strokes. One in four are recurrent strokes.
- Stroke costs the United States an estimated $38.6 billion each year. This total includes the cost of health care services, medications, and missed days of work.
- Stroke is a leading cause of serious long-term disability (Members et al., 2012).

The risk of having a stroke varies with race and ethnicity. African Americans' risk of having a first stroke is **nearly twice** that of whites. Hispanic Americans' risk falls between that of whites and African Americans. American Indians/Alaska Natives and African Americans are more likely to have had a stroke than are other groups. Moreover, African Americans are more likely to die following a stroke than are whites. (Cruz-Flores et al., 2011). Unless intervention is started early in the course of the event, individuals who survive a stroke are often left with multiple disabilities that may leave them dependent on others for daily care.

Strokes are often preceded by **transient ischemic attacks** (TIA), transient neurologic dysfunction caused by focal brain, retinal or spinal cord ischemia without infarction. This is defined by the absence of end organ injury using imaging techniques. These are essentially minor strokes that often cause no permanent disability, but are a warning sign that a stroke may be imminent. Symptoms are not dissimilar from stoke, but are transient, lasting minutes in low flow TIA and hours in embolic TIAs. Recognition of TIA is important as these patients may benefit from preventive therapy or revascularization of the large vessel like the carotid artery.

Stroke Warning Signs The inability of one-third of Americans to identify symptoms of a stroke means that a stroke is often not treated as an emergency, which presents a major problem for those experiencing a stroke. This leads to critical delays in receiving appropriate early interventions. These delays may be decreased by asking the individual specific questions using the FAST action plan.

- *Face*—Ask the person to smile. A stroke can cause one side of the face to droop. Abrupt dimming of vision or a sudden severe headache with no known cause is also a warning sign.
- *Arms*—Ask the person to raise both arms. If one arm drifts downward, that could signal a stroke, which can trigger weakness, numbness, and paralysis of an arm of leg, particularly on one side of the body. Unexplained loss of balance or a sudden fall are clues to support focal neurological dysfunction.
- *Speech*—Ask the person to repeat a simple sentence. Stroke victims may slur their words, have trouble speaking or understanding speech, or not be able to talk at all.
- *Time*—If the person has any of these symptoms, call 911. Stroke is a life-or-death emergency in which every minute counts. To have any hope of reversing the effects, a patient must receive thrombolytics within 3 hours if they are eligible or get the clot-dissolving agent, tissue plasminogen activator (tPA) within 3 hours, or the Merci Retriever procedure within 8 hours (Nor, A. M. et al., 2004; Nor, S. M. et al., 2004; Sacco et al., 2006).

Prevention Recognizing stroke risk factors and adopting a healthy lifestyle are the best steps to prevent a stroke or avoid having another stroke. Many stroke prevention strategies are the same strategies to prevent heart disease. In general, healthy lifestyle recommendations are identified in Table 26-4.

Spinal Cord Injuries

For the topic area of Injury and Violence Prevention (IVP), there is the following objective:

- IVP—3 Reduce fatal and nonfatal spinal cord injuries.

Spinal cord injury (SCI) is an insult or damage to the spinal cord that results in a significant alteration that may be temporary or permanent of its motor, sensory, or autonomic functions. Damage to the spinal cord results in the inability to transmit sensory and motor information to the brain for interpretation and response.

The majority of individuals who sustain SCI are Caucasian males (80%) between the ages of 16–30 (50%–70%) who engage in risky behaviors without wearing appropriate protective safety gear (12%) or combine alcohol/drugs with driving (46%). Individuals who survive the initial impact are faced with an extended period of rehabilitation as well as a lifetime of adapting and coping with the significant physiological alterations caused by SCI. The financial cost for SCI patients and their families is also significant ($15,000–$30,000/year) and impacts the health care system in terms of cost and resources.

Prevention of SCI could be drastically reduced by avoiding or creating situations that are high risk for sustaining traumatic injuries. The thrill of "taking risks" and living on the edge are major deterrents to implementing preventive actions. While these internal motivators will always be there, knowledge of the risks involved and planning for them will help to reduce the incidences of head and spinal cord injuries. Recognition of the need for safety measures with regard to sports and recreational activities and taking personal responsibility for safety measures are other means for preventing SCIs.

In spite of statistics that indicate prevention is the most compelling factor, there are still many individuals who fail to employ safety and preventive measures. Using seatbelts and head protection when riding a bicycle or motorcycle is the best way to prevent the head from receiving direct force impacts related to encounters with another vehicle or the ground. "Fall proofing" a house is also essential to prevention of head injuries. Awareness of water depth and not diving into unknown water are necessary precautions to take to prevent spinal cord injuries.

PRACTICE POINT: *Onset of Symptoms*

It is sometimes difficult for the patient to determine the time of onset of symptoms. A practical question is "when was the last time you felt normal?" Use simple commands like can they walk, talk, use a phone, or lift their arms.

Table 26-3 Risk factors for strokes

Older adult; after 55 risk doubles every decade	High serum levels of fibrinogen, beta lipoproteins, cholesterol, hematocrit
Male (slightly higher risk)	Diabetes mellitus
History of stroke or TIAs	Drug abuse (cocaine)
Hypertension	High dose contraceptives
Smoking	High estrogen levels
Chronic alcohol intake (> 3 drinks per day)	Post menopausal females
History of cardiovascular disease (CAD, CHF, rhythm abnormalities (atrial fibrillation), mitral valve prolapse	Overweight
Sleep apnea	African American

Table 26-4 Risk reduction for strokes/brain attacks

Monitor blood pressure regularly; regular exercise	Regular blood tests to measure cholesterol, hematocrit
Stop smoking	If diabetic, follow treatment plan
Limit alcohol intake to < 3 drinks per day	Monitor blood sugar regularly if diabetic
Schedule regular health care checkups	Avoid drugs (cocaine)
Diet low in fat and cholesterol	

Clinical Context Exemplars

Situation A

An 18-year-old male is brought into the ED with a suspected spinal cord injury from a motor vehicle accident. He wasn't ejected from the car, but was bounced around the inside two to three times. He has a cervical collar on and is complaining of inability to move his legs and feet. After stabilizing the patient, the location of the spinal cord lesion needs to be identified. The exam is started by assessing the patient's ability to feel superficial pain. The patient indicates that he senses the touch over his face, upper extremities, and upper chest. The sensations disappear approximately below the nipple line.

1. Where would you expect the location of the spinal cord lesion to be? What is your rationale for placing it in this location?
2. Would this be an upper motor neuron disorder or a lower motor neuron disorder?

Situation B

A 24-year-old female is admitted to the ICU with a diagnosis of traumatic (closed) head injury. On your initial assessment of her level of consciousness, she requires a very loud voice to get her to open her eyes and when her eyes are open; she stares blankly and does not seem to focus on any object. She rapidly returns to her previous state. What level of consciousness would you put her in? The only motor response that can be obtained is a withdrawal of her hand when her fingernail is pinched.

1. What score would she be given on the Glasgow Coma Scale?
2. On the next day she is unresponsive, and when a painful stimulus is applied she draws her hands up to her chest and internally rotates her hips.
3. What does her response to painful stimuli indicate? What other optic finding would you expect to obtain? Why?

Situation C

When testing the sensory component of the neurological system, the 45-year-old male patient indicates that he cannot feel light touch sensation but is able to feel vibratory sensations in his lower extremities.

1. What sensation would you next use to assess his sensory function and why?

Situation D

The following data regarding cranial nerve functioning for a 58-year-old male has been recorded. PERRLA, able to sense touch and superficial pain in all three divisions, facial symmetry noted, sound lateralizes to R ear, bone conduction greater than air conduction, swallows without difficulty, shoulder shrug equal. (*Note:* This is not necessarily correct documentation.)

1. What data is unexpected?
2. What CN is involved?
3. What might the patient be experiencing? What other tests might be used to validate your thinking?

SUBJECTIVE DATA

History of Present Illness (CC)

The patient may present to the provider with a variety of concerns that may be directly related to the neurological system or other systems. Framing the questions will depend on the patient's age, gender, culture, race, emotional or mental status, health practices, and concurrent illnesses. All symptoms presented must be thoroughly assessed with a symptom analysis (COLDERRA).

Pain

Refer to Chapter 8 regarding general assessment of pain. Assessment of "neurologic-specific" type pain refers to pain associated with neurological structures, such as headaches elated to meningitis or encephalitis, neck pain, trigeminal neuralgia, sciatica, or shingles. (See Conditions and Disorders.)

Headache/Facial Pain (HA)

Symptom analysis for headaches is covered in Chapter 20.

Peripheral Neuropathy/Radiculopathy

Radiculopathy (peripheral neuropathy) is nerve root compression most commonly the lumbosacral and the cervical spinal nerves, caused by disc herniation or spondylosis (spinal stenosis, resulting from degenerative disc disease or arthritis). Compression of spinal nerve root leads to local edema, ischemia, and inflammation (Table 26-5). Osteophytes or disc herniation may directly impinge on the nerve roots or the spinal cord or may lead to instability and misalignment of the spine (degenerative spondylolisthesis) causing pain and neurologic deficits. The lumbosacral spine is vulnerable to disc herniation due to its mobility (L_4–S_1) disc. Radiculopathic symptoms follow the level lower than the exit of the nerve root.

Peripheral neuropathy, polyneuropathy, and neuropathy are used interchangeably although are distinct entities. Peripheral neuropathy is less specific but refers to conditions affecting the peripheral nervous system including radiculopathies and mononeuroplathies. Polyneuropathy refers to a generalized, homogeneous process affecting several peripheral nerves with distal ones mainly affected. Neuropathy is even a more general term used in disorders of the central and peripheral nervous system. It is often difficult to distinguish symptoms from disorders of the central nervous system like in strokes, spinal cord lesions, and brain tumors from polyneuropathy. In polyneuropathy, sensory precedes the motor symptoms. Longer axons are affected first, thus symptoms begin in the lower limbs.

PRACTICE POINT: Red Flags for Headaches

- Acute, new or severe headaches that changed from previous patterns
- New onset of headaches in adults above 50 years of age
- Headaches with high fever and other systemic signs
- Headaches on exertion, valsalva, early morning or at night
- Headaches with meningismus
- Headaches with seizures or new focal neurological signs
- Progressive and worsening headaches that is changed from baseline
- Headaches with worsening

Provider Inquiries	Clinical Reasoning/Logic
Characteristics: Describe the pain (deep/superficial, aching, boring, throbbing, sharp/dull, stabbing, burning, freezing, electric-like pain, pressing, stinging cramping, gnawing, shooting, pins and needles, crawling sensation?).	Description of pain is less important here. Sensory symptoms like numbness, tingling and burning, freezing, electric-like pain are usually the typical initial sensory symptoms of peripheral neuropathy.
Onset: When did pain start? Gradual or sudden? Associated with fever or injury?	Acute neuropathies require urgent assessment. Motor nerves (control muscles), sensory nerves, or autonomic nerves (control automatic like heart rate, body temperature and breathing) may be affected. In acute neuropathies, such as Guillain-Barré syndrome, symptoms appear suddenly, progress rapidly, and resolve slowly as damaged nerves heal. In chronic forms, symptoms begin subtly and progress slowly. Some people may have periods of relief followed by relapse. Others may reach a plateau stage where symptoms stay the same for many months or years. Some chronic neuropathies worsen over time, but very few forms prove fatal unless complicated by other diseases.
Location: Where is pain felt? Unilateral or bilateral, multiple nerve involvement?	In multiple mononeuropathies, nerves that are not contiguous may be involved like median nerve and sciatic nerve.
Stocking glove distributions?	"Stocking glove "distribution in chronic axonal polyneuropathy seen in diabetes or uremia.

Provider Inquiries	Clinical Reasoning/Logic
Duration: How long have you had pain? How long do episodes last? Constant or intermittent, progressive?	Axonal neuropathies progresses over years.
Exacerbation: Anything that increases the pain (intensity)?	
Radiation: Does the pain travel along a specific path?	Radiculopathy follows the nerve root distribution.
Relief: What measures have been taken to relieve pain (heat, cold)? Medications (opioids, anti-inflammatories, ASA, NSAIDS)?	
Associated signs/symptoms: Motor symptoms like weakness, gait abnormality, twitching, fasciculations, autonomic symptoms, cramps, spasms, imbalance and loss of coordination	In Gullian-Barré motor precedes sensory symptoms.
Atypical BP and HR, decreased sweating, bladder incontinence, gastroparesis, malabsorption, diarrhea, constipation, nausea and vomiting, impotence	Motor symptoms are commonly seen in damage to the motor nerve.
	Atypical BP, HR and other involuntary symptoms may accompany autonomic nerve dysfunction.

Table 26-5 Nerve root compression syndromes

Nerve Root	Pain Pattern	Weakness	Reflex Loss
C_2	Occipital, eyes		
C_3	Neck, trapezius		
C_4	Neck, trapezius		
C_5	Neck, shoulder, lateral UE	Deltoid	Biceps, brachioradialis
C_6	Lateral forearm, first two digits	Biceps	Biceps, brachioradialis
C_7	Posterior forearm, 3rd digit	Triceps	Triceps
C_8	Medial forearm, 4th/5th digit	Finger abduction, grip	
T_1	Neck, medial arm, and forearm	Thumb abduction, distal thumb flexion, finger abduction and adduction	
L_1	Inguinal region	Hip flexors (rarely)	
$L_{2, 3, 4}$	Anterior thigh to knee to the medial aspect of the lower leg and to the arch of the foot	Hip flexors, knee extension and hip adduction	Patellar
L_4	Lateral aspect of leg to dorsum of the foot and first two toes	Weakness of foot dorsiflexion, toe extension, foot inversion and eversion	
L_5	Back, radiating into buttock, lateral thigh, lateral calf and dorsum foot, great toe	Hip abduction, knee flexion, foot dorsiflexion, toe extension and flexion, foot inversion and eversion	
S_1	Back, radiating into buttock, lateral or posterior thigh, posterior calf and lateral or plantar foot	Hip extension, knee flexion, plantar flexion or the foot	Achilles
$S_{2, 3, 4}$	Sacral or buttock pain radiating into the posterior aspect of the leg or perineum	Weakness may be minimal, with urinary and fecal incontinence as well as sexual dysfunction	

Dizziness (Lightheadedness/Vertigo)

Symptom analysis for dizziness (lightheadedness/vertigo) is covered in Chapter 19. Vertigo is associated with peripheral (Chapter 19) or central causes. Central causes include tumors (acoustic neuroma), TIAs/strokes, migraine headaches, multiple sclerosis, as well as brain stem ischemia and cerebellar infarction or hemorrhage.

Seizures

Seizures represent the physical manifestation of abnormal, excessive, disorganized firing of neurons in the cerebral cortex. They are paroxysmal, generally lasting seconds to minutes followed by a postictal (after the seizure) component of fatigue, confusion, somnolence, and headaches. They are classified as epilepsy when seizures recur over a period of time after resolution of the acute events or triggers or with no obvious provocation or precipitant. Epilepsy may be due to brain tumors, congenital malformations, and inborn errors of metabolism, trauma (shaken baby syndrome, child abuse), intracranial infections (meningitis, encephalitis, sepsis), cerebral degeneration, strokes, and vasculopathy. Most clinical information related to description of seizure activities is obtained from family members or witnesses to the activities.

Provider Inquiries	Clinical Reasoning/Logic
Characteristics: Petit mal (absence) or grand mal? Partial or generalized? Loss of consciousness? Or interruption of seizures by calling the child's name or touch? Interruption of activities?	Petit mal or absence, involves a brief, sudden lapse of consciousness. In true absence, there is usually interruption of activities like talking, eating, or playing in children; while daydreaming is usually during sedentary activities like sitting at a school desk. Absence seizures are not interrupted by calling the person's name or tactile stimulation. Grand mal is characterized by generalized tonic-clonic movements. Generalized tonic-clonic seizures typically start with a scream/shriek and abrupt loss of consciousness followed by jerking within few seconds to a minute—associated with tongue biting, frothing in the mouth, and urinary incontinence. Complex partial seizures are also associated with loss of consciousness.
Stereotypic?	Stereotyped seizures have similar clinical presentations with every seizure.
Onset: At what age did seizures begin? Are seizures preceded by an aura, such as: irritability, tension, confusion, blurred vision, mood changes, smells/odors, or focal motor seizure activity, black outs, buccal lingual activities, déjà vu, psychic experiences, memory impairment, inability to move, eyes rolling up. drooling, confusion, talking difficulty, shaking, rhythmic movement like shaking, bicycling, hand waving, out of body experiences? How much time is there between the onset of the aura and seizure? Do automatisms, such as eyelid fluttering, chewing lips, smacking, or swallowing occur?	Petit mal seizures occur most commonly in individuals under age 20 (children ages 6 to 12), it is rare to experience onset after 20. In children a higher proportion of seizures are due to congenital brain malformations. Seizure in children presents differently than adults. Etiologies of seizures include electrolyte abnormalities (hyponatremia, hypocalcemia), fever, toxins, drugs, intracranial bleed or neoplasms, trauma, ischemia, perinatal asphyxia, neurometabolic/neurodegenerative disorders. They may also be idiopathic. Patients with history of stable, controlled epilepsy often experience seizures during acute insult like hypoxia brain injury, hypoglycemia, electrolyte imbalance, hypocalcemia or hypomagnesemia, infections, and head trauma. In older adults, strokes, neoplastic and degenerative disorders are frequently causes. An **aura** is a perceptual disturbance experienced by some migraine sufferers before a migraine headache, and the telltale sensation experienced by some people with epilepsy before or after a seizure. Auras refer to the site of the cortex where seizures originate, often associated with temporal lobe seizures. They may generally look like simple partial seizures—flashing lights when it originates in the occipital cortex or jerking of face, arm and leg opposite the side of the motor cortex involved. The characteristics of an aura may help in locating the focus of the seizure.

Provider Inquiries	Clinical Reasoning/Logic
	An aura is often the first sign that a person is going to have a seizure. It may last from several seconds up to 60 minutes before a seizure. Most people who have auras have the same type of aura every time they have a seizure.
	Occasionally a generalized/grand mal seizure may present with focal clinical signs (automatisms) at the onset which then proceeds to generalization. These focal signs at times are mistaken as auras. Careful questioning of the family members is crucial.
Location: Is there a specific area of the body where the seizure starts?	Partial seizures begin in a specific area or location of the brain. The most common types of partial seizures are as follows:
Location can also refer to where in the brain the seizure may originate, particularly partial (localized) seizures.	
Does the patient remain conscious during the seizure or lose consciousness?	Simple partial seizures—do not affect consciousness or awareness.
	Complex partial seizures—do affect level of consciousness; patient may become unresponsive or lose consciousness completely.
	Partial seizures with secondary generalization—begin as simple or complex partial seizures, but then spread (generalize) to the rest of the brain and look like generalized tonic-clonic seizures. These two types can easily be confused, but are treated differently. Most tonic-clonic seizures in adults begin as partial seizures and are caused by partial epilepsy. Generalized tonic-clonic seizures are more common in children.
Duration: How long do the seizures last? Is this consistent or do they vary?	Absence seizures recur frequently during the day and last for few seconds, rarely more than 10–30 seconds.
Frequency?	
Exacerbation: Are there any known triggers for the seizures?	Catamenial seizures occur during menstruation.
	Intense physical exertion, or psychological stress, menstruation, stress, flashing lights, fever in children, loud music, lack of sleep, and medications that lower seizure threshold are known triggers for seizures.
Intense crying prior to seizure?	Intense crying prior to seizure activity suggests a breath-holding spell.
Relief: How do you (or does the individual) feel after the seizure (weakness, paralysis, confusion, drowsiness, headaches, muscle aching)? What medications are you taking?	Postictal state—confusion, tiredness, headache, somnolence
Associated signs/symptoms: Skin color change (face/lips)?	Automatisms are auras and simple partial seizures.
Cyanosis? Pallor?	In fainting or syncope, patient is generally pale not cyanotic.
Todd's paralysis—transient neurologic paralysis that may last for hours or rarely few days after an epileptic seizure?	Seen in seizures and not with other causes of loss of consciousness like syncope. These helps strengthen the diagnosis of seizures.

Provider Inquiries	Clinical Reasoning/Logic
Loss of consciousness or no LOC?	Seen in generalized seizures.
	Seen in tonic/myoclonic seizures.
Loss of control of muscles?	Seen in atonic seizures where muscle tone is lost and person collapses to the ground.
Weakness, confusion fatigue, headache, and somnolence after a vigorous muscle contractions and LOC?	These are postictal signs and symptoms that suggest seizure, not syncope as the cause of loss of consciousness.
	These help strengthen the diagnosis of seizures.
Stiffening/sudden muscle contractions of groups of muscles?	Muscle activities seen in seizures but are not specific. Seen in tonic/myoclonic seizures.
Scream or shriek, tongue biting, frothing in the mouth and urinary incontinence?	

Weakness

Muscle weakness (**myasthenia**) may be an indicator of peripheral nerve damage, disorder of the neuromuscular junction, the muscle itself, or it can be from a central lesion like stroke or mass lesion in the brain. It may also be an accompanying symptom of systemic disorders like malignancy, cachexia, infection, prolonged bedrest, malnutrition, depression, and inflammatory disorders. Symptoms of weakness must be objectively assessed to differentiate primary weakness from fatigue or from asthenia.

Provider Inquiries	Clinical Reasoning/Logic
Characteristics: Weakness associated with pain in the muscle or joint?	Weakness associated with muscle tenderness localizes the condition to the muscle.
Focal or Generalized? Is it weakness or paralysis (inability to move a part)?	
Is it an inability to perform specific task like combing hair or climbing stairs? Fatiguing weakness, or—weakness with continuous activity or effort, for example combing of hair or reaching for an object or putting up curtains or painting?	Joint pains may contribute to weakness as the person may not be able to move the limb. Focal weakness/paralysis of the face or left side of body suggests central nervous system lesions (ischemic stroke, vascular or mass lesions in the brain), peripheral nervous system or neuromascular disorder, neuropahty.
	Generalized weakness is seen as a constitutional symptom associated with deconditioning, malnutrition, or other systemic inflammatory or infectious disease.
	Fatiguing weakness as an activity progresses is characteristics of a neuromuscular junction condition like myasthenia gravis.
Onset: Acute or chronic? Did it occur suddenly? Is it progressive?	Acute onset of weakness or paralysis is seen in TIA or stroke.
	Neuromuscular disorders are generally chronic except in inflammatory conditions like Guillane-Barré or infectious like viral, parasitic, bacterial (Campylobacter).
	Progressive weakness is seen in ALS or MS (Multiple sclerosis).

Provider Inquiries	Clinical Reasoning/Logic
Location: Asymmetric or symmetric?	Asymmetric weakness is likely secondary to CNS and peripheral nervous system disorders.
Unilateral or bilateral?	
If symmetric, is it proximal (neck [axial], deltoids, hips and, proximal thighs)? An example is inability to get up from a chair or raise arms above shoulders.	Bilateral proximal muscle weakness is seen in myopathy.
Is the weakness distal (forearm, wrist, hand, feet)? Example: weakness in dorsiflexion or plantar flexion, foot drop, plantar	Bilateral distal weakness is characteristic of early motor neuron disorder or peripheral neuropathy.
	Proximal muscle weakness is seen in myopathies, muscular dystrophy, inflammatory muscle disorders like polymyositis, dermatomyositis, Cushing's, thyroid disease, electrolyte abnormalities, drugs (steroids, alcohol, cocaine) or systemic infections (viral, bacterial (Lyme, fungal, parasitic), or rhabdomyolysis.
Duration: Persistent?	
Exacerbation: Anything that increases manifestations of symptoms? Have they been getting increasingly worse? Sleep or activities like painting, needle point, computer work?	These activities may aggravate carpal tunnel syndrome. Myasthenia gravis gets worse with continuous effort and better with rest.
Radiation: Sensation travel to any other part of body?	In Guillain-Barré, paralysis is ascending.
Relief: Anything that provides relief from pain? Control of glucose? Rest? Wrist splint? Cessation of triggering activities?	Drugs help improve neuromuscular disorders.
	Control of glucose may improve diabetic neuropathic symptoms.
	Wrist splints may improve carpal tunnel syndrome by decreasing the impingement along the carpal retinaculum.
Associated signs/symptoms: Confusion, trouble speaking, or understanding speech, headache, impaired vision (one or both eyes), pain, shortness of breath, joint stiffness, stiff neck, fever, sensory deficits, incontinence?	Paralysis, speech difficulty, and severe headache may accompany stroke.
	Paralysis and meningitis may present with confusions, change in mental status plus fever or stiff neck.
	Shortness of breath and joint pains suggest non-neuromuscular disorders as cause of weakness.
	Incontinence and other gastrointestinal problems like gastroparesis, and urologic abnormality like incontinence and impotence suggest autonomic dysfunction associated with peripheral neuropathy.
Muscle pain?	Myopathies like Polymyositis can be associated with muscle tenderness.

Paresthesias (Numbness)

Paresthesia is a condition in which a distorted sensation of burning, numbness, tingling, itching or prickling is felt somewhere on the body despite the absence of external stimuli. It can also be described as a feeling of pins-and-needles or skin-crawling sensation. Paresthesia is commonly felt in the extremities, such as the hands, feet, fingers, and toes, but it can occur in other parts of the body. It can be caused by a wide range of conditions affecting the nervous system at any level.

Provider Inquiries	Clinical Reasoning/Logic
Characteristics: How do you experience this sensation? Some patients may describe loss of or diminished sensitivity/numbness (**anesthesia** or **hypesthesia**) Have you lost sensation in any areas? If yes, is the loss in the same area as the numbness (paresthesia)?	The patient should be encouraged to describe his symptoms in detail in his own words. Common descriptions include burning, stabbing, pins and needles, prickling, stinging, and sharp shooting pains. Painful paresthesias suggest an inflammatory or ischemic process such as vasculitis. Shooting pains are characteristic of nerve entrapment. Burning pains are characteristic of paresthesias affecting small unmyelinated fibers. Paresthesias may occur as part of a migraine aura or have an onset at the same time as the headache, and they typically last <1 hour from the onset of the headache.
Onset (acute, sub-acute, chronic): When did you first start experiencing numbness? Was it sudden, or did it occur over a period of time (seconds, minutes, hours, days, weeks)?	A sudden onset suggests ischemia (stroke or trauma). Symptoms that evolve over several seconds suggest epilepsy. Symptoms that evolve over • Minutes suggest migraine, panic attack, or fish poisoning (if the patient has ingested fish within the previous 8 hours). • Hours to days suggest infectious or toxic-metabolic. • Days to weeks suggest infectious, toxic-metabolic, or immune-mediated. An insidious onset is characteristic of inherited neuropathies, neoplastic or degenerative disorders.
Can you identify a particular stimulus that causes sensation?	*Dysesthesia* refers to unpleasant sensations perceived in response to normally nonnoxious stimuli; when normal stimuli are perceived as painful, *allodynia* is the descriptor use.
Location: Can you determine the location of the sensations? Is there a consistent pattern associated with feeling? One side or both? Symmetrical?	The location/distribution/pattern of the symptoms provides clues to level of lesion. Numbness of part of one limb: peripheral nervous system lesion. Unilateral numbness of both limbs (with or without the trunk): brain lesion. Bilateral numbness below a specific dermatomal level: a spinal cord lesion. Bilateral numbness not corresponding to a specific dermatomal level: polyneuropathy, multiple mononeuropathy, or a patchy spinal cord or brain disorder.

Provider Inquiries	Clinical Reasoning/Logic
Duration: Is the sensation constant, or intermittent (relapsing)?	Paresthesias that do not persist are most likely related to a neurologic lesion. Pressure on a nerve frequently causes transient paresthesias: individuals who cross their legs, sit too long on a toilet seat, drape an arm over back of chair, or lean on one elbow while holding a newspaper in that hand. Many individuals have fleeting paresthesias of unknown cause and no significance. Persistent paresthesias reliably imply an alteration of sensory pathways.
Associated signs/symptoms: Any changes in mood? Trouble sleeping or concentrating? Increased urination? Rapid breathing? Tingling in the extremities? Light-headedness?	Nervousness, shakiness, tremor, restlessness, irritability, insomnia, poor concentration, heart palpitations, racing heart, sweating, dizziness, diarrhea, lump in throat and frequency of urination may accompany paresthesias. Patients may also experience hyperventilation, which can cause paresthesia around the lips, lightheadedness and tingling in the extremities. If incontinence is present with leg paresthesia, this may suggest poliomyelitis, cauda equina tumor or metastatic tumor of the lumbar spine.

Tremors

Tremors are involuntary rhythmic oscillations or shaking of muscles in the body with variable amplitude but reasonably constant frequency. They are different from the shaking seen in seizures. They are often symmetric. Parkinson's disease is a chronic progressive neurodegenerative disorder characterized by rest tremor. There are tremors that mimic Parkinson's, for example Lewy body dementia, Huntington's disease, progressive supranuclear palsy, drug induced like in use of neuroleptics and other dopamine antagonist (tardive dyskinesia) and essential tremors.

Provider Inquiries	Clinical Reasoning/Logic
Characteristics: Is it resting or action tremor? Shaky voice, head shaking, shaky penmanship, shaking of hands or feet, lips or face, limb shakes? Does it get worse when reaching for a target?	Resting tremors occur when a person is in a recumbent or sitting position when the body is supported; they are disabling as the individual has to be constantly active to dampen the tremors. Action tremors occur during voluntary activities. This type includes intention tremors, which are aggravated as the target activity is almost reached. Essential tremors are the most common resting tremors, having about a 50% chance of genetic inheritance. Hands are mostly affected but may involve the head, tongue, voice, legs, and trunk. Parkinson's tremor is a resting tremor, therefore worse while resting and improves with voluntary activity. It can also get worse when a person is being observed.
Onset: Acute or chronic? Did it occur suddenly? If chronic, is it progressive? Does it follow certain activities, taking or stopping drugs? Did it appear after certain conditions/illnesses?	Cerebellar tremors are intention tremors that are worse when reaching a target. They can be due to masses in the cerebellum, multiple sclerosis, or stroke. It may be also from chronic alcoholism.

Provider Inquiries	Clinical Reasoning/Logic
	Tremors may be secondary to non-neurologic causes: drugs like stimulants (caffeine), antidepressants, alcohol excess or withdrawal, benzodiazepine withdrawals, stress, hyperthyroidism, and liver failure, and neurologic causes (Multiple sclerosis, stroke, TBI, brain stem and cerebellar conditions, neurodegenerative process like Parkinson's)
	Tremors from alcohol withdrawal or thyroid disorders or hepatic encephalopathy may be acute. Essential tremors are often chronic.
Location: Asymmetric or symmetric? Unilateral or bilateral? Upper body or lower body?	Essential and Parkinson's tremors may start on one side but may affect both sides as they progress.
Duration: Intermittent or persistent?	Acute tremors may only persist for the duration of the etiologic event. Essential tremors, resting tremors are usually persistent.
Exacerbation: Does is get worse with stress with voluntary actions, when body is recumbent, fever, caffeine, rest, or movement or at rest, medicines?	Essential tremors may be aggravated by adrenergic stimuli like stress, caffeine, and certain drugs. Fever, exhaustion, stress and heightened emotion increase these tremors.
Radiation: Does the tremor move from one part of the body to other parts?	They may start in one side of the body and progresses to involve both sides.
Relief: Is it better with activity or with rest, with decrease caffeine or stressors?	
Associated signs/symptoms: Voice changes, other neurological changes?	Voice changes may also be seen in dystonia.
Bradykinesia, gait abnormalities like shuffling gait, rigidity, and postural instability?	Bradykinesia and gait abnormalities are seen in Parkinson's disease.
Ataxia, dysarthria, titubation, nystagmus?	These changes may accompany the cerebellar tremors and make cerebellar lesions more likely when present.
Mental status changes, falls, Babinski, supranuclear gaze palsy, dementia prior to diagnosis of tremor, dysautonomia?	Mental status changes are symptoms and signs that suggest other conditions other than Parkinson's tremors or essential tremors.

Past Medical History

Past medical history provides knowledge related to previous conditions that may have effect on present neurological system.

Provider Inquiries	Clinical Reasoning/Logic
Childhood Illnesses: Meningitis, encephalitis, history of febrile seizures or epilepsy, congenital malformation, deformities, poliomyelitis?	Changes later in the child's neurological status may be explained by the past medical history.
Chronic Illnesses: Cardiac (CAD), peripheral vascular, DM, hypertension, epilepsy? Stroke, aneurysms?	CAD, HTN, DM and hyperlipidemia are risks for strokes.
Neurosurgery: Surgery to brain, spinal cord (what, when, outcomes)? Any residual effects of surgery?	Surgery and instrumentation may put patients at risk for infection and change in neurological status.
Trauma: Head trauma, spinal cord trauma, birth trauma, accidents (what, when, outcomes)? Catastrophic/life-threatening situations (experience/observe), PTSD?	A past history traumatic brain injuries may have an impact on present neurological condition/symptoms. (Refer to Chapter 17 for further discussion of TBI.)

Family History

Family history provides information regarding family member's illnesses or conditions as potential causes for chief complaint or presenting symptoms that may indicate a pattern of presentation associated with transmission of familial/genetic factors predisposing the individual to certain system related conditions/illnesses. Any of these may indicate a potential or actual cause of neurological dysfunction.

Provider Inquiries	Clinical Reasoning/Logic
Illnesses/Disorders: Epilepsy, headaches, alcoholism, mental retardation, anxiety, depression, bipolar, suicide, learning difficulties (dyslexia, attention deficit disorder [ADD]), Alzheimer's, multiple sclerosis (MS), amyotrophic lateral sclerosis (ALS), brain tumors, strokes/brain attacks, myasthenia gravis?	Family history of certain conditions like migraine, brain cancer, aneurysms contribute to the risk of having such disorders when the appropriate clinical history is suggestive.
Hereditary Disorders: Huntington disease, muscular dystrophy, neurofibromatosis, Tay-Sachs disease?	
Medical Conditions: Thyroid disease, hypertension, DM?	

Personal and Social History

Information related to personal and social history identifies what personal habits/behaviors or environmental factors might influence or cause present neurological condition or symptoms.

Environmental/Occupational Conditions: Exposure to toxins (lead, arsenic, organic solvents, other); operate dangerous equipment, work at heights?	These are known agents that may have negative effects on the neurological system.
Wear head protection? **Ability to care for self:** Hygiene, ADLs communication, shopping, work requirements? **Sleeping patterns:** Consistency?	Wearing protective gear during work, sports activities, recreation, etc. Important to prevent head and/or spinal cord injuries. Ability to care for self and engage in daily activities are dependent on an intact and functional neurological system.
Drug use: Alcohol, mind-altering street drugs, medications; use of alcohol and/or mind altering drugs when driving, or using dangerous equipment? **Coordination:** Maintain balance, hand eye coordination?	Substances that impair neurological function should not be taken when engaging in work or recreational activities that require an intact and functional neurological system.

Developmental Applications

Certain conditions or disorders may be related to certain age groups or situations. Inquiring to obtain age or condition specific information will provide further information for helping to determine causes of the chief concern as identified.

Infants and Children

How was mother's health during pregnancy? Medications (prescription, street drugs), alcohol use? Infections/exposure to infections (TORCH—toxoplasmosis; other [syphilis, TB], rubella, CMV, herpes)? Toxemia, bleeding, trauma/stress, persistent vomiting, HTN?	Prenatal and delivery history have impact on infants' neurological development and maturation.
Birth history: APGAR score, gestational age, birth weight, presentation, instruments, length of labor, fetal distress (vaginal/cesarean delivery)?	Apgar scores determine necessity of further intervention at the neonatal stage. Antepartum events like fetal distress and hypoxia may lead to some neurological impairments in infants. Hypoxia or perinatal asphyxia may lead to cerebral palsy and other neurologic complications.
Respiratory status: Immediate breathing, need O_2, apnea/cyanosis? Need resuscitation/ventilator?	
How was neonatal health? Jaundice (appearance/cause), infections, seizures, irritability, sucking/swallowing coordination?	There are risks for vertical transmission of bacteria from colonized mothers like Group B strep, which can lead to sepsis, bacteremia, and meningitis in the neonates.

Provider Inquiries	Clinical Reasoning/Logic
Congenital anomalies?	Malformations and anomalies often are a result of defect in embryonic developments. These may be evident and screened at birth.
Hypotonia/hypertonia in infancy?	Tone and posture vary according to gestational age.
Achievement of developmental milestones (age attained)? Smiling, head control in prone position, grasping, transferring objects between hands, rolling over, sitting crawling, independent walking, toilet trained? Loss of previously achieved skill: Change in progress of development (always been slow, or slowed down after expected progression)?	Checklists of developmental milestones, which include motor, language, behavioral, socio-emotional and mental health domains help detect developmental delay and disabilities in children.
Self-care abilities: dressing, feeding, toileting? **Impulsive behavior:** Difficulty with change, poor organizational skills, uncontrolled anger, poor social skills, problems at school (especially with peers)?	To obtain information regarding any delays in child's development and maturation related to chronological age.
Impairment in gaze-to-gaze behavior, lack of ability to share enjoyment, or lack of social reciprocity, stereotyped and repetitive use of language, patterns of behavior or activities? Health conditions?	Screening for autism. This is indicated in children with delayed language and communication milestones.
Headaches, vomiting, lethargy, personality changes?	These may be indicators or causes of neurological dysfunction.
Seizure activity: Associated with fever, frequency, duration, characteristics of movement?	Febrile seizures are common cause of convulsions in infants. Neurologic sequelae are rare following febrile seizures in infancy.
Uncoordination/clumsiness: Unsteady gait, progressive muscle weakness, falling, problems negotiating stairs, difficulty getting up after lying down?	Motor and postural dysfunction are common in cerebral palsy. In infants CP may be manifested by neurobehavioral signs like irritability, poor feeding, difficult to handle and cuddle, and poor visual attentions.
Environment: Exposure to toxic elements in environment such as toxic chemicals, lead, radioactive tailings, air quality?	There are biologic effects of toxins and radiation exposure and they include growth retardation, malformations, neonatal death, and poor functioning and cancer.
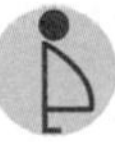 ***The Pregnant Woman*** Gestational weeks (EDC)? Health Status?	The mother's health during past pregnancies and any problems that may affect present pregnancy are important know to prevent birth defects of the nervous system.
Seizure activity: Convulsions, past history, pregnancy induced hypertension; frequency, duration character of movement? **Headache:** Onset, frequency, duration, associated with hypertension, visual changes?	Mismatch between placental supply and fetal demands can result in impaired fetal growth or fetal growth restrictions. Maternal factors include substance abuse, infections, vasculopathy like preeclampsia, hypoxemia, starvation, other toxic exposures like drugs. Fetal growth restrictions or small for gestational age appear to be at increased risk for neurodevelopmental abnormalities and decreased cognitive performance.
Nutritional status: Dietary supplements (folic acid), prenatal vitamins, calcium?	Elements necessary to promote fetal neurological development.

Provider Inquiries	Clinical Reasoning/Logic
The Older Adult **Mobility difficulties:** Increased stumbling, falls, unsteadiness, decreased agility? More difficult in dark? Home safety modifications? **ADLs:** Anything interfering with? What social activities? Toileting (fecal/urinary incontinence)? **Sensory deficits:** Visual, hearing, anosomia? Constant or intermittent? Getting worse? What is patient doing about it? Transient neurological symptoms (paresthesias, visual disturbances, one sided weakness, loss of speech)? **Environment:** Exposure to toxic agents or environmental elements (what and how long exposed?)	Any deficits in mobility, functional abilities, self care may be due to neurological causes.

OBJECTIVE DATA

The neurological examination is very easily incorporated into the overall examination. Additionally, a majority of data regarding the neurological system can be obtained without actually asking the patient to perform specific maneuvers. Many involuntary and common actions that the patient demonstrates will provide this information. For example, facial expressions used during conversation and the history demonstrates CN VII activity, swallowing, talking, and responding appropriately to questions are all observations that can be made through focused observation and provide data regarding neurological function. The motor system is frequently assessed when doing musculoskeletal maneuvers. The two systems are interdependent and data obtained are used for both systems.

The primary assessment technique for the neurological system is observation. While palpation and percussion may be used to elicit responses, it is still the activity associated with each response that is observed. The procedures will be organized according to levels, but it is not as easy to differentiate when and what observations are used as there are multiple tests that can be used that essentially give the same data. The extent of the exam is also guided by the nature of the patient's condition and degree of dysfunction. Regardless of what level of exam is done, the sequence for the neurological exam follows the same sequence.

- LOC (mental status)
- Cranial nerves
- Motor function (descending motor tracts)
- Sensory function (sensory ascending tracts)
- Reflexes

Level I to IV Examination

The Level I to Level IV examinations are performed in a continuum, starting from a basic level and proceeding to a more comprehensive level based on provider's abilities and patient's presentation and location. It may start at the outpatient setting and may progress to the ED/ER, hospital unit bed, ICU, or specialty unit. Frequently all the elements from basic to comprehensive exam are done in one setting such as in a primary care setting or clinic.

The condition of the patient is the primary consideration in determining the type and amount of data needed to assess the patient's illness/disease/situation. The separation into levels is for general purposes and is meant to be descriptive rather than prescriptive. The purpose of leveling is to provide a framework to assist the learner in determining the appropriate data to collect.

Brain and Nerves

	Level I	Level II	Level III	Level IV
Inspection	**LOC**	**LOC**	**LOC**	**LOC**
	State of Awareness/ Arousal Orientation (X 3/4) Mini Mental Status Exam Follows commands	State of Awareness/ Arousal Glascow Coma Scale	Glascow Coma Scale: Identify degree of brain injury due to internal or external trauma Clinical severity	State of Awareness/ Arousal Orientation Mental Status Exam

Continued

Brain and Nerves (*continued*)

	Level I	Level II	Level III	Level IV
Inspection	**Cranial Nerves**	**Cranial Nerves**	**Cranial Nerves**	**Cranial Nerves**
	CN III (tested) Gross observation of CN Function	CN II – XII (not smell and taste)–determined by patient's condition/LOC Fundoscopy	CN II – XII (not smell and taste)–determined by patient's condition/LOC Fundoscopy	CN I – XII [Inclusive of all tests]
	Motor Activity	**Motor Activity**	**Motor Activity**	**Motor Activity**
	Purposeful/voluntary movements Balance/coordination (gait) Symmetry	Response to tactile stimuli Coordination/proprioception Cerebellar function (one of each) Rapid alternating movements Hand flips Leg cross/uncross Finger to thumb Accuracy of movement Finger to nose Finger to finger Heel to shin Response to tactile stimulation (posturing)	Response to tactile stimulation (posturing)	Balance/equilibrium Romberg Gait (heel to toe) Tandem walking
	Sensory Perception	**Sensory Perception**	**Sensory Perception**	**Sensory Perception**
	Response to verbal stimuli Pain (perception/physical manifestations)	Sensory: Superficial pain/touch (distal) Temperature Position sense	Sensory: Superficial pain/touch (dermatomes)	Vibration (additional joints) Position of joints (Cortical Sensory Function) Stereognosis Graphesthesia Two-point discrimination Extinction phenomena Point location
	Additional Tests	**Additional Tests**	**Additional Tests**	**Additional Tests**
				x-ray CT Scan MRI
Palpation	**Reflexes**	**Reflexes**	**Reflexes**	**Reflexes**
	DTRs: Biceps, patellar, achilles	DTRs: Triceps, brachioradialis	Pathological reflexes	DTRs: Superficial plantar, Abdominal
			Superficial reflexes–plantar	

Inspection: Level I

Inspection of neurological function in Level I is related to patients who do not have any significant neurological impairments that would produce unexpected results of any consequence.

Inspection Techniques and Expected Findings | **Unexpected Findings**

Begin the initial patient encounter with the assessment of the patient's level of consciousness (LOC), the initial component of the mental status. Consciousness is dependent on two interdependent functions: awareness and arousal. Both states are assessed in determining the LOC. In the Level I exam it is essential to establish the patient's LOC as a baseline for future comparisons.

Awareness is determined by the patient's orientation to person, place, and time.

It is expected that the patient is oriented to time (day, month, year), place (where located at this time), and person (who the patient is and recognition of other individuals).

Unexpected Findings: Unexpected findings would be that the patients is unable to determine what date it is, what the location is, and unable to recognize self or other familiar faces.

> ***PRACTICE POINT: Time Orientation***
>
> It is important to keep in mind that patient's in hospitals experience a disruption to their regular daily activities, thus it is very easy to lose track of time, which may result in the inability to determine what date it is. The provider must determine whether the patient has simply lost track of time or is truly unable to determine the date. Some coaching to help the patient determine the date may be needed.

Arousal is evaluated by the degree of stimuli that is needed to elicit wakefulness. The LOC also provides an assessment of brain function. The validity and reliability of the rest of the neurological exam is dependent on an optimum functioning brain.

Expected findings for the patient's LOC and brain functioning is of an individual who is awake, alert, and responds appropriately to verbal and environmental stimuli and is grounded in reality.

Unexpected Findings: Unexpected findings indicate that the patient's LOC is characteristic of one of the five states of altered consciousness represented by variations in awareness and arousal: (1) confused, (2) lethargic, (3) obtunded, (4) stuporous, or (5) comatose. Characteristics of these states have been described in Chapter 7.

> ***PRACTICE POINT: Sequence of Loss of Orientation***
>
> Disorientation frequently occurs with organic brain dysfunction, particularly delirium and dementia. Orientation is generally lost in a sequential order—first to time, then to place, and infrequently to person. Various conditions and disorders may be associated with specific orientation losses. Time disorientation is associated with anxiety, depression, and organic brain syndrome. Disorientation to place is found with psychiatric disorders and organic brain syndromes, disorientation to person results from cerebral trauma, seizures, or amnesia.

An additional assessment of LOC can be made by observing the patient's ability to follow commands. The patient that provides appropriate responses to history questions and demonstrates what is requested does not have an impaired LOC.

Another opportunity to test the patient's ability to follow commands is to ask the patient to squeeze the provider's two fingers. This request is frequently done for assessment of motor activity so it can be deferred until that portion of the exam.

The patient should be able to follow a simple command and grasp the providers extended fingers and squeeze them.

Unexpected Findings: Unexpected findings would be that the patient is unable to understand and follow a simple command.

Mini Mental Status Exam (MMSE)

If there is any question as to the cognitive abilities of the patient, or cognitive changes (forgetfulness, difficulty understanding spoken/written communication, and trouble finding words) it is appropriate to administer the MMSE (see Chapter 7).

In addition to assessing the patient's orientation, the MMSE also assesses registration, attention and calculation, recall, and language (Santacruz & Swagerty, 2001).

The range of scores for the MMSE is 0–30. A patient that scores within the range of 25–30 is considered to be without any cognitive impairment.

Unexpected Findings: Scores within the range of 20–24 indicate mild cognitive impairment, 10–19 is considered moderate cognitive impairment, and >10 is considered severe impairment.

> ***PRACTICE POINT: MMSE Cutoff Points***
>
> The exact number for differentiating between levels of cognitive impairment is not standardized. Patients who score around cutoff scores will need further assessment. The MMSE is only a screening tool, so its value is to be able to document any change in scores over time, not necessarily to diagnose a specific level of impairment. Scores on the MMSE are also affected by educational level and age so the patient's obtained score needs to be evaluated in light of these variables.

Inspection Techniques and Expected Findings	Unexpected Findings

Cranial Nerves

Cranial nerve assessment is an essential component of the neurological exam. When conducting a neurological exam by itself, cranial nerve assessment is the first component of the exam. When an integrated physical assessment is conducted, cranial nerve assessment is often done with the assessment of the head and motor and sensory innervations of various structures.

For the Level I exam, testing cranial nerve (CN) III (oculomotor) is most important because it is an indicator of brain function. Although the oculomotor nerve itself innervates the majority of the eye muscles, parasympathetic fibers from the Edinger Westphal nucleus travel in the third CN, which regulate the pupil and lens and control pupil constriction and lens accommodation.

To test CN III, shine a direct light (penlight, ophthalmoscope light) on to the pupil and observe for pupillary constriction.

An intact third CN will cause the pupil to constrict when a beam of light is directed on it, indicating that there is no damage to the oculomotor nerve.

The remaining 11 CNs are not generally tested unless there is a specific reason to do so. Even if not specifically tested, observation of the patient's activities and behaviors provides adequate information as to the overall motor functioning of the CNs (Table 26-6).

Unexpected findings would be related to anything that might cause inequality of the pupil's reaction to light. (Pupil alterations are further described in Chapter 18.)

Motor Activity

Motor activity is dependent on appropriate innervation of muscles so that this component of the neurological exam is also assessing the integrity of the muscular system; often referred to as a neuromuscular assessment. A significant amount of the muscular assessment will be covered here and the remaining components will be discussed in Chapter 27.

Observations related to motor activity in Level I are concerned with the patient's ability to initiate purposeful and voluntary movements of the extremities. Expected findings would be that the patient is able to control movements in response to one's needs for a specific activity.

The need for a certain action or function may be observable or not. The need for the patient to scratch an itch is an individual sensation that prompts the patient to initiate scratching of the skin surface. Reaching for an object such as a glass of water is observable and allows the provider to determine the need for such an action.

Unexpected findings would be that the patient is unable to initiate controlled voluntary and purposeful movements either due to weakness, paralysis, or the presence of involuntary movements (tremors).

Voluntary and purposeful movements should also be executed with a smooth and coordinated effort.

Movements may also be controlled and voluntary but not purposeful in a meaningful way. Patients who experience hallucination may visualize ants crawling on the bed and or bed clothes with the patient picking at the ants—which are invisible to the provider.

Table 26-6 Cranial nerve testing of motor activity by observation

CN II	Optic	Observe patient's ability to move around freely without bumping into objects. Eyes observed to focus on specific objects.
CN III, IV, VI	Oculomotor, Trochlear, Abducens	Observe parallel eye movements. Location of corneal light reflex
CN V	Trigeminal	Observe jaw movements when talking.
CN VII	Facial	Observe facial movements and expressions.
CN VIII	Auditory	Assess patient's ability to hear questions and provide appropriate responses to inquiries, and converse appropriately.
CN IX	Glossopharyngeal	Observe patient's ability to swallow, articulate words.
CN XII	Hypoglossal	Observe ability to swallow, observe tongue movement during conversation.

Balance and Coordination

The patient's gait is commonly your first observation during the initial patient encounter. Observe patients who are ambulatory while they are walking around the room or unit. Assess the characteristics of the gait, noting the coordination, rhythm (cadence), and sequence of movements (Figure 26-12).

Inspection Techniques and Expected Findings	Unexpected Findings

The patient's gait should have a smooth, rhythmic cadence with equal amount of time in the swing and stance phase with opposite arm movements. There should also be symmetry in the length of the leg swing. The lower extremities should also swing in a straight line without any circular or rotating movements.

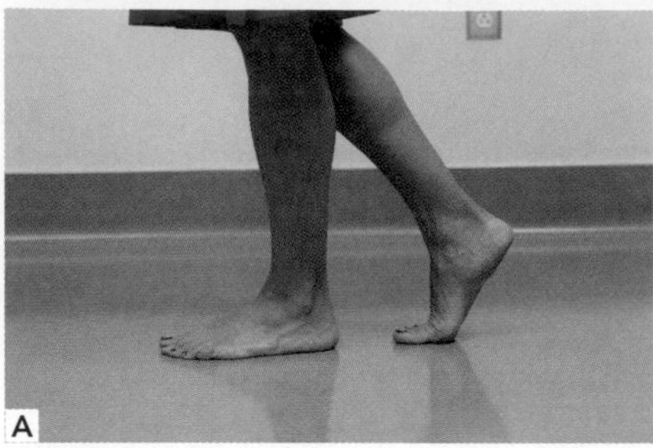

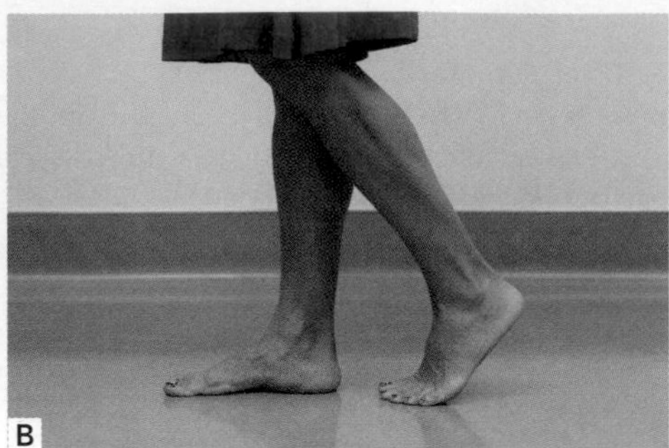

FIGURE 26-12A–B Sequence of steps that constitute the gait

The gait sequence occurs in a number of steps. In general, each lower extremity goes through a swing and stance phase, with specific motions related to each phase. These movements can be described as follows:

- Heel Strike: The first heel strikes the floor and then comes into full contact with the ground.
- Foot Flat: The second heel pushes off, leaving contact with the ground. The first foot flattens on the ground.
- Mid-stance: Body weight is distributed evenly over all aspects of the foot because the second foot is off the ground.
- Acceleration: The leg swing is accelerated as weight is removed from the second foot.
- Mid-swing: The second foot is lifted and moves ahead of the weight-bearing foot, swinging through.
- Deceleration: The second foot slows in preparation for the heel strike.

Unexpected findings would include shuffling, widely placed feel, toe walking, foot flop, leg lag, scissoring, and loss of arm swing, staggering, or reeling.

Any unexpected findings related to the gait will be exaggerated by having the patient walk heel to toe (tandem walking). Instruct the patient to walk in a straight line by touching the heel of one foot with the toe of the opposite foot (Figure 26-13). The patient should be able to maintain continuous contact between the heel and toe. Slight swaying may be observed and is an expected finding. Unexpected finding would be extending the arms for maintaining balance, instability, a tendency to fall, and any lateral swaggering or reeling.

Unexpected findings may be the result of ethanol intoxication, weakness, faulty position sense, vertigo, and leg weakness. These causes should be ruled out before they may be attributed to a cerebellar lesion. See Chapter 27 for more information on unexpected gaits.

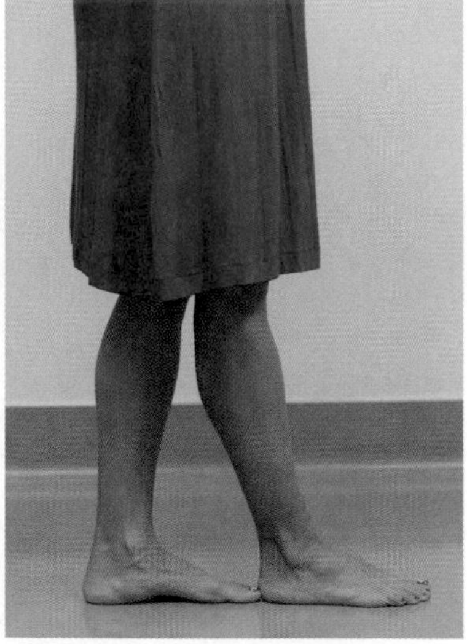

FIGURE 26-13 Tandem walking

Sensory Function

Specific sensory responses at this level are not generally assessed unless there is an indication that the patient is experiencing a sensory deficit. Sensory awareness may decline to a certain extent, but should not be extinct in individuals without neurological impairment.

Unexpected findings would be that the patient is unable to respond appropriately to verbal stimuli. This may be due to neurological alterations such as deafness or an altered level of consciousness. If there is no response to verbal stimuli, stronger stimuli may be needed to elicit a response from the patient.

Inspection Techniques and Expected Findings	Unexpected Findings

The initial response of the patient should be in response to the verbal stimuli from the provider such as an introduction or a question as to the patient's condition or need to be seen. The expected findings would be that the patient responds appropriately to a question or request from the provider and be able to engage in conversation throughout the examination.

General responses to touch or other stimuli will provide adequate information in regards to the patient's overall sensory functioning.

Pain is always a concern and frequently present in hospitalized patients. Pain control is a significant part of the management of the patient's condition. (Pain assessment is covered in Chapter 8.)

Painful stimuli may need to be used to elicit a motor response in patients who are stuporous or comatose.

The expected responses would be that the patient is able to perceive touch and that pain if present is adequately controlled.

Inspection: Level II

The Level II exam is performed on individuals who are experiencing or recovering from some form and degree of neurological impairment. Individuals may also be recovering from surgical intervention to reduce or prevent negative outcomes associated with the type of trauma experienced. The most frequent types of neurological impairments in patients in this level are head trauma, strokes, infections (encephalitis/meningitis), and spinal cord injuries.

LOC

Assessment of the patient's level of consciousness may be done with the **Glascow Coma Scale (GCS)**. The GCS is used clinically to quantify an individual's LOC and overall neurological impairment. It may be used for any type of patient and is primarily used when an individual demonstrates an altered LOC due to head trauma or other hypoxic events. The GCS assesses the function of the cerebral cortex and brain stem by scoring the individual's behavior in three functional categories: eye opening, verbal response, and motor response. There are adult, infant, and young child versions. Table 26-7 outlines the categories used for the GCS and the scoring of the responses from the patient.

The GCS allows the provider to assess the patient's LOC at specific intervals to determine whether the patient is improving or deteriorating. Each category has specific criteria that correlate with an assigned score. The patient's best response in each category is matched to the scoring criteria. The highest possible score is 15 and the lowest score is 3; the lower the score, the greater the degree of neurological damage.

Table 26-7 Glasgow coma scale

Category	Patient Response	Scoring
Best eye opening response (record "c" if eyes closed by swelling)	Spontaneously	4
	To speech	3
	To pain	2
	No response	1
Best motor response to painful stimuli—press at fingernail bed Record best upper limb response	Obeys verbal commands	6
	Localizes pain	5
	Flexion—withdrawal	4
	Flexion—abnormal	3
	Extension—abnormal	2
	No response	1
Best verbal response record "e" if endotracheal tube in place, "t" if tracheostomy in place	Oriented X 3	5
	Conversation—confused	4
	Speech—inappropriate	3
	Sounds—incomprehensible	2
	No response	1
Add the numbers from each category. Maximum score = 15, minimum score = 3		

Unexpected findings would be a GCS <15. The lowest score possible is 3; the lower the score, the greater the degree of neurological damage. A lower score indicates a deeper coma and poor prognosis. Individuals with a GCS of 3–8 are considered comatose. Individuals with an initial score of 3–4 have a >95% incidence of death or persistent vegetative state.

Inspection Techniques and Expected Findings	Unexpected Findings

Cranial Nerves

For the Level II exam, all cranial nerves may be tested or just selected ones, depending on the patient's condition. Testing of each CN has already been described in previous chapters. For review purposes, Table 26-8 briefly describes testing of each CN. For a more detailed description, refer back to specific chapters.

Unexpected results would be an incorrect or absent action/response controlled by the CN.

Expected results would be a correct demonstration of the action/response controlled by each CN.

The appearance of CN II on examination of the retina is related to the degree of ICP.

Pupillary response to light (CN III) is a primary concern for individuals with brain injuries.

Direct damage or trauma to the oculomotor nerve occurs because intracranial pressure is increasing, compressing CN III due to brain stem herniation, resulting in unilateral or bilaterally fixed pupil dilation.

The margins of the optic CN on the retinal background, when visualized through an ophthalmoscope, are well defined.

Increasing ICP increases the pressure on CN II causing it to swell. As the swelling increases, the margins of the optic disc become less distinct resulting in **papilledema** (Figure 26-14).

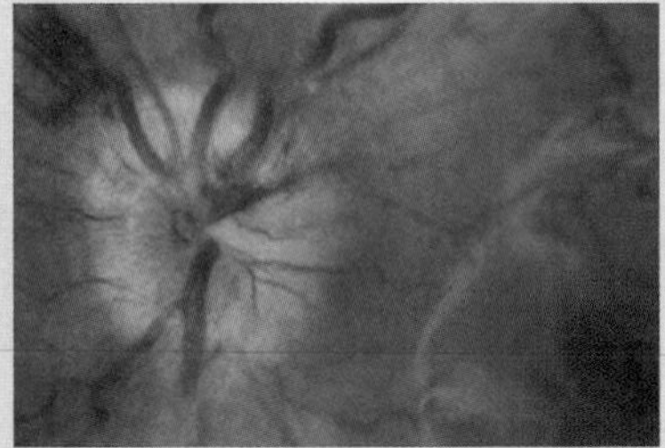

FIGURE 26-14 Papilledema
Source: Custom Medical Stock Photo

Table 26-8 Testing cranial nerves and their functions

Cranial Nerve	Name	Chapter	Function	
CN I	Olfactory	20	Sensory—smell	Differentiate specific odors
CNII	Optic	18	Sensory—vision	Snellen Visual Chart, Jaegar card, newsprint at arm's length
CN III	Occulomotor	18	Motor—eye muscle movement Parasympathetic—pupil constriction, lens accommodation	Extraocular movements Direct light on pupils
CN IV	Trochlear	18	Motor—eye muscle movement (downward/inward)	Extraocular movements
CN V	Trigeminal	17	Motor—muscles for chewing Sensory—sensation of face and scalp, cornea, mucous membranes of mouth and nose	Palpate TMJ Apply sharp/dull end to 3 divisions of nerve; light touch (cotton swab) to same areas
CN VI	Abducens	18	Motor—lateral movement of eye	Extraocular movements
CN VII	Facial	17	Motor—facial muscles, eye lid (closure), labial speech	Observe facial symmetry when making requested facial movements (faces).
		20	Sensory—taste on anterior two-thirds of tongue (sweet and salt) Parasympathetic—saliva and tear secretion	Apply sugar/salt to anterior portion of tongue.
CN VIII	Auditory (Acoustic)	19	Sensory—hearing and balance	Whisper test, rubbing finger test; Weber, Rinne tests
CN IX	Glossopharyngeal	20	Motor—vocal sounds and swallowing (pharynx) Sensory—taste on posterior one-third of tongue (bitter and sour); gag reflex (pharynx)	Observe speaking ability (word formation) and for ability to swallow. Apply lemon juice, vinegar (sour), tonic water (bitter) to posterior section of tongue.

Continued

Inspection Techniques and Expected Findings				Unexpected Findings

Table 26-8 Testing cranial nerves and their functions *(continued)*

Cranial Nerve	Name	Chapter	Function	
CN X	Vagus	20	Motor—talking and swallowing (larynx and pharynx) Sensory—generalized sensations from carotid body, carotid sinus, pharynx, and viscera Parasympathetic—carotid reflex	Observe for midline elevation of uvula during phonation (aahhhhh).
CN XI	Accessory (Spinal)		Motor—trapezius and sternocleidomastoid muscles (contraction)	Feel for symmetrical and equal shoulder elevation by placing hands on shoulders while patient shrugs them.
CN XII	Hypoglossal	20	Motor—movement of tongue for speech articulation and swallowing	Observe for midline protrusion of tongue.

THINK LINK: Herniation

Herniation occurs when increasing intracranial pressure leads to a descent of the brain through openings in the base of the skull. The most common cause of increased brain mass is a space-occupying tumor and cerebral edema. Two locations for herniation are the tentorial notch and the foramen magnum. Tentorial herniation occurs when the temporal lobe shifts across the edge of the tentorium cerebelli. Tonsillar herniation occurs when the cerebellar tonsils are forced through the foramen magnum. Both types of herniation are life threatening due to compression of the midbrain and brain stem. A significant finding related to herniation occurs when the third CN is compressed, causing unilateral or bilateral fixed and dilated pupils. Herniation can also occur without an increase in intracranial pressure where a mass lesion like hematoma occurs at the border of brain compartments.

Motor, Proprioception, and Cerebellar Function (Rapid rhythmic alternating movements)

Assessment of motor, proprioception, and cerebellar function tests the patient's coordination, fine motor skills, and balance. These motor responses can only be performed by patients who are awake and alert who can respond to verbal stimuli.

Descending Tracts	Motor Activity Assessed
Direct (pyramidal) **Corticospinal** (lateral and ventral)	Rapid, rhythmic alternating movements Voluntary movement Deep tendon reflexes Plantar reflex
Indirect (extrapyramidal) Reticulospinal (medial, ventral and lateral) Tectospinal Vestibulospinal Rubrospinal	Posture and Romberg Gait Instinctual motor reactions

Assess motor activity by the patient's ability for muscle movement and coordination by demonstrating the ability to perform rapid alternating movements (RAM). Proprioception and cerebellar functions primarily assess the functioning of the medial and lateral reticulospinal motor tracts of the spinal cord. The ability of the patient to respond appropriately and perform the requested motor action is also assessing the patient's ability to comprehend and follow directions.

An alert and oriented individual will respond appropriately to verbal stimuli and obey a command for movement.

Assess coordination by directing the patient to perform activities that may require simultaneous movements, fine motor control, accuracy and repeating actions. A straightforward activity to assess these characteristic movements is to have the patient demonstrate the finger-to-nose test.

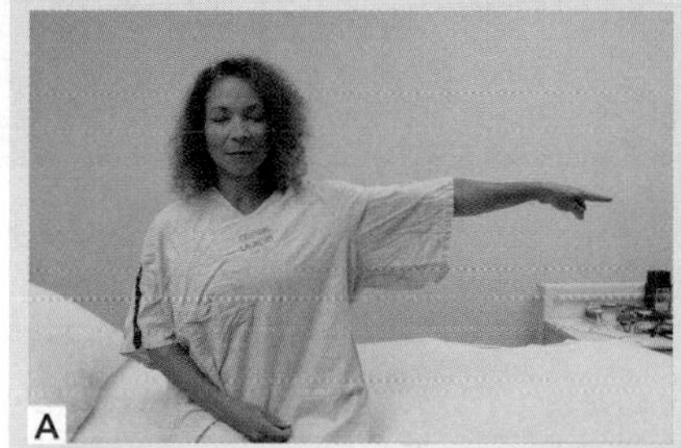

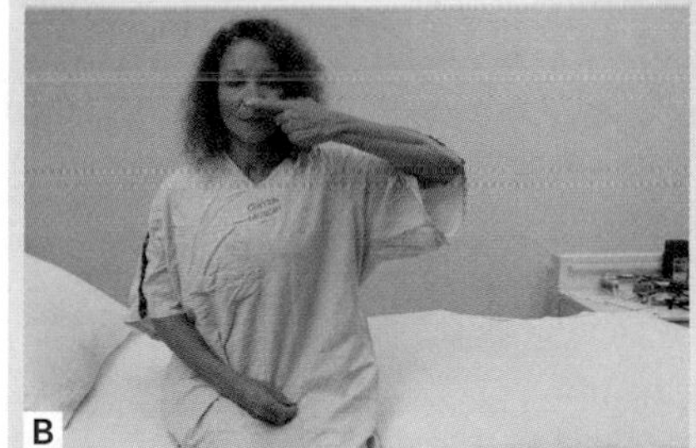

FIGURE 26-15A–B Testing coordination—finger to nose

Finger-to-Nose Test

Instruct the patient to close the eyes and extend both arms out toward the sides. Ask the patient to alternately touch the nose with the index finger of either hand (Figure 26-15).

Have the patient increase the speed at which the fingers touch the nose.

A patient with an intact neurological system will be able to move the upper extremities in a purposeful and controlled manner to accurately bring the finger toward the nose.

Unexpected findings would be uncoordinated actions, misses touching the nose several times, or downward drift of the arms (unable to maintain testing position).

Inspection Techniques and Expected Findings | **Unexpected Findings**

Accuracy in touching the nose depends on **proprioception**, the ability of the patient to perceive oneself in space without the aid of visual stimuli. Essentially, the patient has to be internally aware of the location and position of the nose to be able to touch it with both left and right fingers. The patient also demonstrates coordination in alternating movement of the extremities when touching the nose.

Hand Flip

The patient should be seated for this test with the forearms resting on the upper part of the lower extremities. Instruct the patient to rapidly, with both hands, pat the upper legs, alternating between the palm and back of the hand (Figure 26-16). Ask the patient to perform this maneuver as fast as possible.

Cross/Uncross Legs

To test the lower extremities, instruct the patient to cross and uncross the legs as rapidly as possible.

Thumb to Finger

An additional test is to have the patient touch each finger with the thumb of the same hand, starting with the index finger to the little finger and back (Figure 26-17). Instruct the patient to demonstrate this action simultaneously and as rapidly as possible.

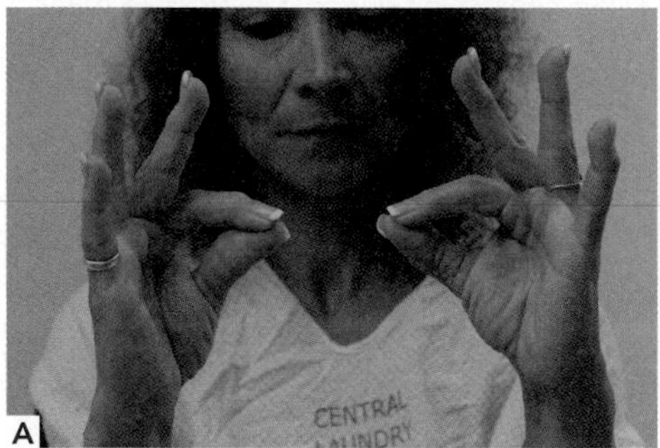

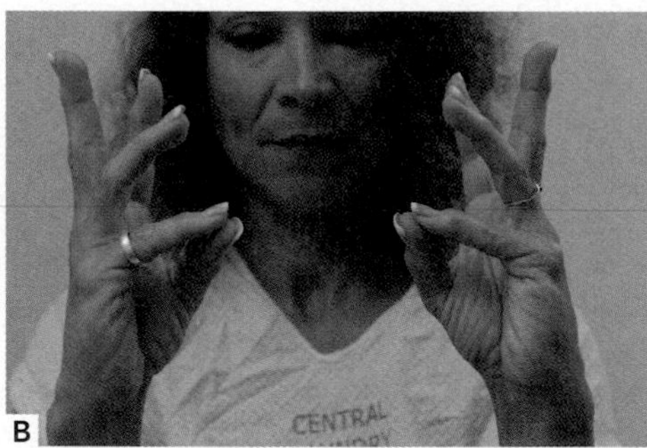

FIGURE 26-17A–B Patient demonstrating touching each finger to thumb

The patient should be able to perform these tests with smooth coordinated movements.

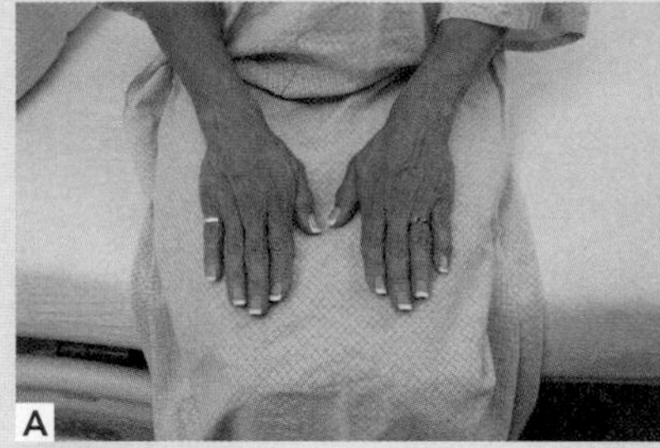

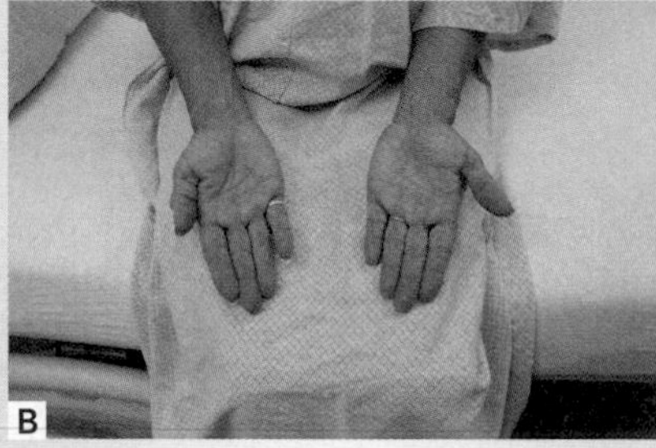

FIGURE 26-16A–B Testing coordination: RAM demonstrating turning of hands on thighs

Unexpected results would be stiff, slowed, nonrhythmic, or jerky movements.

Dysdiadochokinesis is the term used to describe the inability to perform rapidly alternating movements as may be seen in patients with multiple sclerosis.

Accuracy of Movements: Point-to-Point Movements

Finger-to-Finger Test

Standing in front of the patient, position your index finger approximately 18” from the patient. Instruct the patient to use her index finger to alternately touch her nose and then your finger while keeping her eyes open.

After the patient touches your finger, move it so the patient will have to relocate your finger and direct her finger to the new location (Figure 26-18). Change location several times. Repeat the procedure with the other hand.

The patient’s movements should be smooth, rapid, and accurate. (The Finger-to-Finger test, described previously, also tests point-to-point movements).

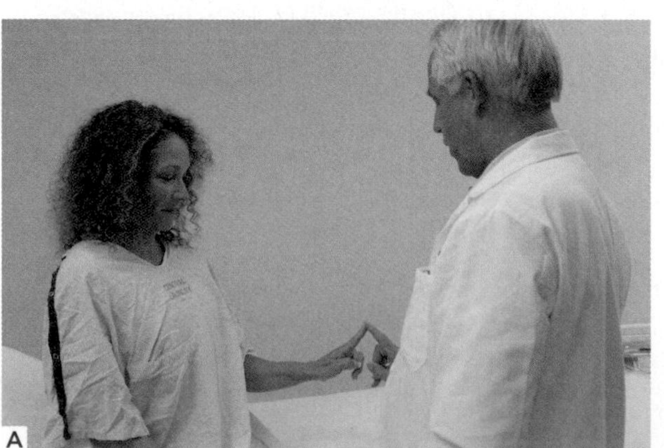

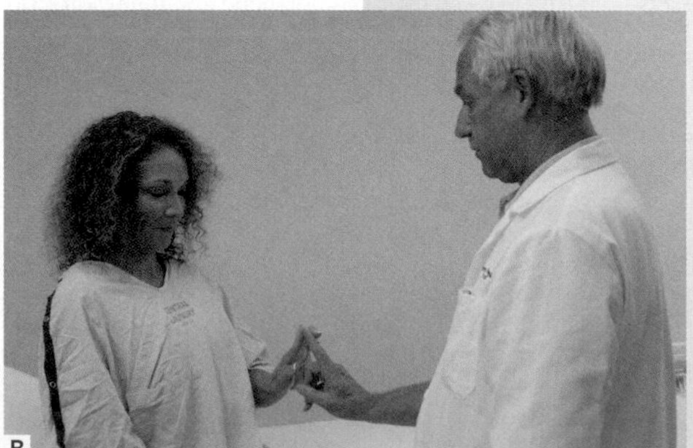

FIGURE 26-18A–B Patient demonstrating touching provider’s finger in two different locations

Inspection Techniques and Expected Findings

Heel-to-Shin Test

This test is performed with the patient in either the sitting or supine position. Instruct the patient to place the heel of one foot on the knee of the opposite leg and run the heel down the shin from the knee to the ankle (Figure 26-19). Repeat the procedure on the opposite leg. The patient should run the heel down in a smooth, straight line and coordinated movement.

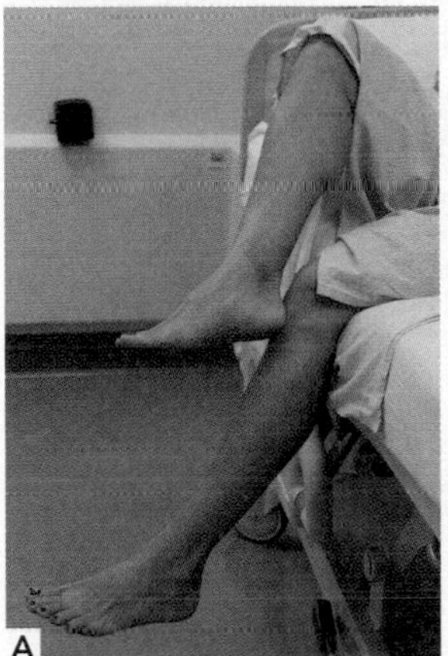
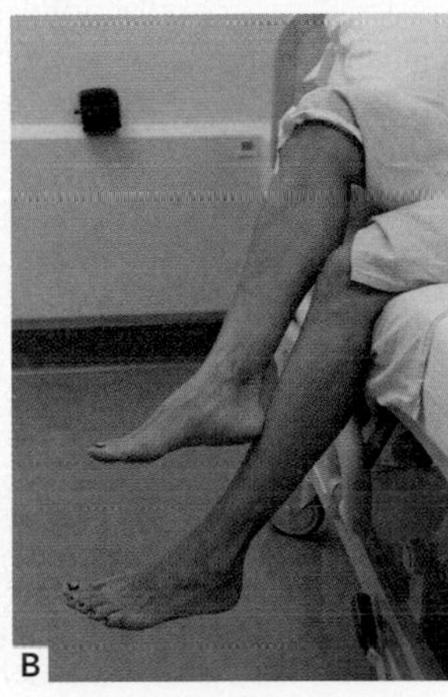
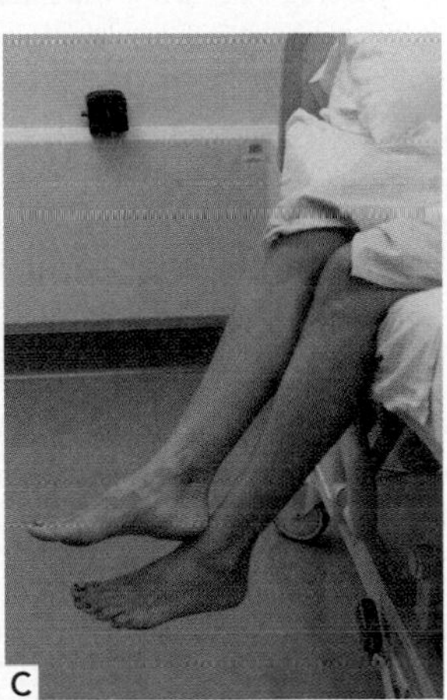

FIGURE 26-19A–C Heel to shin test: Patient demonstrates placing heel of one foot on kneecap of other leg and moving it down the shin

Altered Motor Response

Patients who have sustained any type of brain trauma may not be able to demonstrate any motor activity. As the patient transitions into altered levels of consciousness an increased intensity of stimuli is required to obtain a motor response. Louder verbal stimuli may be needed. When the individual does not respond to louder verbal stimuli increased tactile stimulation, such as vigorous shaking may be added.

When there is no response to verbal stimuli with increased tactile stimulation, the patient's response to painful tactile stimuli is assessed.

Apply a painful stimulus by pinching the individual's fingertip or pinching the shoulder section of the trapezius muscle (Figure 26-20). The initial response to painful stimuli is withdrawal from the source of the pain. The patient may attempt to pull the pinched finger hand away or may move the pinched shoulder away.

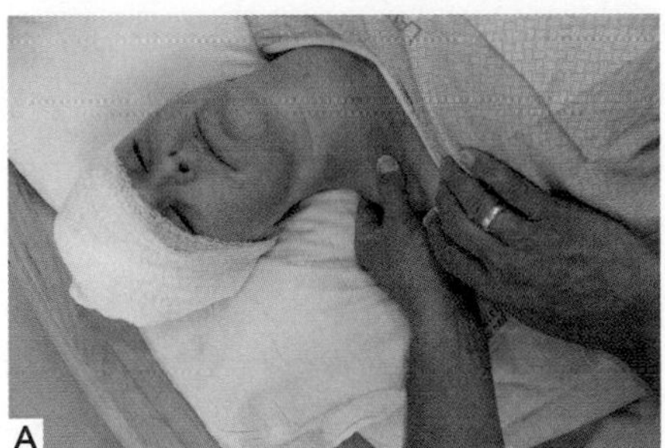
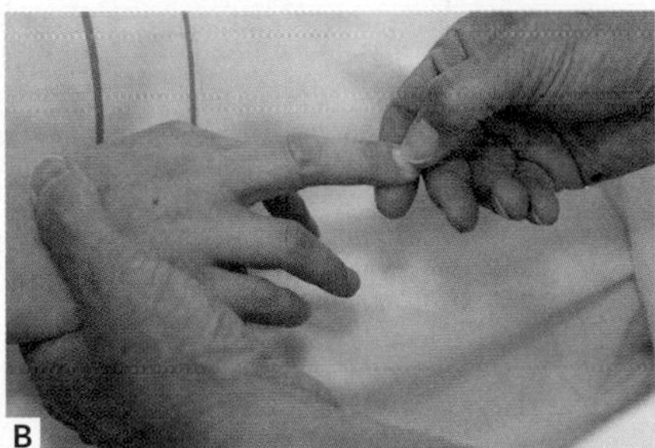

FIGURE 26-20A–B Provider pinching shoulder section and fingertip

Deepening levels of coma result in the absence of attempts to withdraw from painful stimuli; instead the patient demonstrates decerebrate and decorticate posturing.

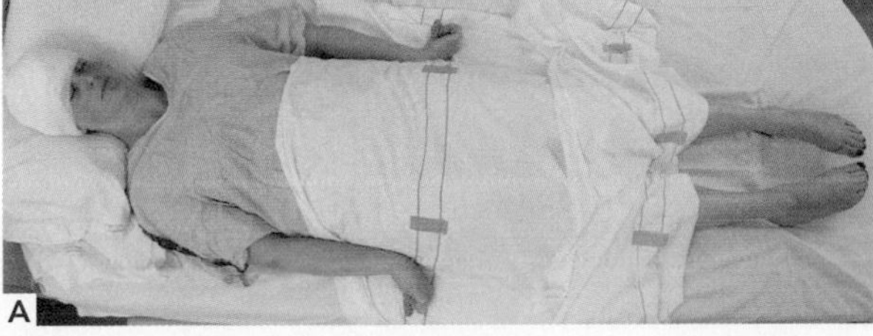
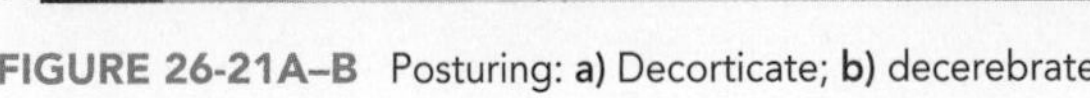
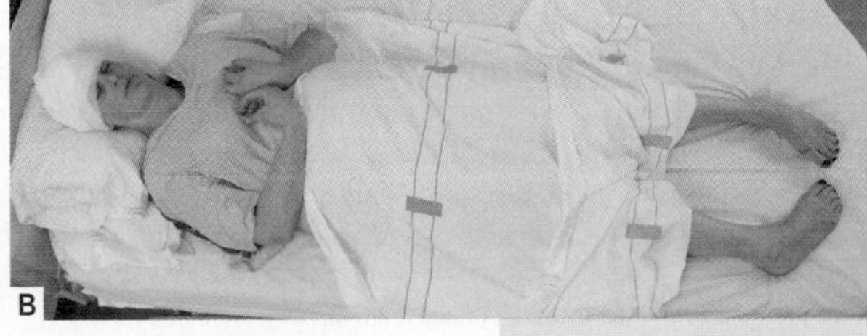

FIGURE 26-21A–B Posturing: **a)** Decorticate; **b)** decerebrate

Unexpected Findings

Unexpected findings would be consistently missing the provider's finger, which may be indicative of cerebellar dysfunction. **Dysmetria** is the term used to describe the inability to perform point-to-point movements by over- or under projection of the fingers.

Inability to coordinate these movements may be due to a loss of motor strength, proprioception, or a cerebellar lesion.

Posturing is a primitive motor reflex to painful stimuli. Its presence always accompanies coma and is an indication of severe brain damage (Figure 26-21).

Decorticate posturing is characterized by rigid flexion of the upper extremities (elbows, wrists and fingers with arms held tightly to the sides of body, lower extremity extension with internal rotation, and plantar flexion of the feet). It is demonstrated when there is a lesion of the corticospinal tracts with preservation of the brain stem.

Inspection Techniques and Expected Findings

PRACTICE POINT: Painful Stimuli

The description "painful stimuli" most likely creates anxiety in the novice health care provider and appears antithetical to therapeutic interventions in the provision of medical and nursing care. A fundamental tenet of medical and nursing practice is to first "do no harm" or "inflict no pain." The term "painful stimuli" is somewhat of a misnomer. Obviously, it is not the intent to inflict pain on an individual. A better meaning of the term is that it represents a sensation that is strong enough to elicit a response in an individual. In a conscious individual, the degree of "painful" is minimal—just enough so that the stimuli is felt or located. As the level of consciousness deteriorates, the strength of the stimulus is increased so that the patient experiences a sensation of discomfort or distress rather than actual pain. A reasonable analogy to discomfort is the sensation felt when a blood pressure cuff is inflated to the point where an uncomfortable sensation of pressure is felt. It is a dull type of pain and an endurable sensation for a brief period of time without any serious consequences. One does not necessarily interpret taking a blood pressure as inflicting pain, but relative to the sensation felt at the height of inflation, it fits into the description of "painful stimuli."

Sensory Function

Evaluate the primary sensory function status of patients with conditions that affect the neurological system. Primary sensory responses are mediated by the spinothalamic sensory tracts of the spinal cord.

Ascending Tracts	Sensation Assessed
Dorsal columns	Vibration Deep pressure Position sense Stereognosis Point location Two-point discrimination
Spinothalamic Lateral Ventral	Superficial pain Temperature Superficial touch Deep pressure
(ventral and dorsal)	Proprioception

A comprehensive neurological examination would test sensory function for each dermatome corresponding to each major peripheral nerve. For the Level II examination, perform distal testing on the hands, lower arms, abdomen, feet, and lower legs. If the distal portions of the periphery produce expected results, it is relatively safe to assume that no alterations exist within the proximal areas. Ask the patient to close their eyes.

Begin each test by using minimal intensity of the stimuli and gradually increasing the intensity until the patient is aware of the stimulus. In specific areas, such as back, buttocks, or thickened areas, a stronger intensity of stimulation may be needed initially as these are areas of decreased level of sensitivity.

Perform contralateral testing to make comparisons between sides. For every kind of stimulus, the expected findings should demonstrate the following:

- Minimal differences between the sides
- Correct perception of each sensation
- Identification of side of body being tested
- Location of sensation and where located relative to previous stimuli, that is distal or proximal.

Assess primary sensory function with superficial light touch and superficial light pain.

Superficial (Light) Pain

With the patient's eyes closed, touch the patient's skin lightly with the sharp and dull points of a bent paper clip, broken tongue blade, pen, or any other object that has a distinct sharp and dull point (Figures 26-22 and 26-23). Before testing, it is helpful to touch the patient's skin with both the ends and inform the patient when the dull and sharp points are being used. This provides the opportunity for the patient to establish and differentiate what each one feels like before being asked to identify each point.

Unexpected Findings

Decerebrate posturing is demonstrated when there is damage to the upper brain stem and indicates a deteriorating motor response.

Lack of any motor response with muscle flaccidity is the worst possible motor response and is characteristic of severe damage to the brain and most likely a terminal situation (Merck Manual, 2005).

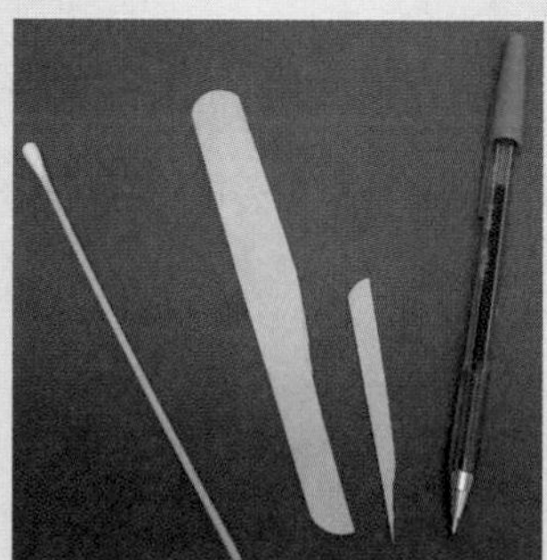

FIGURE 26-22 Objects that may be used for testing superficial pain

Inspection Techniques and Expected Findings	Unexpected Findings

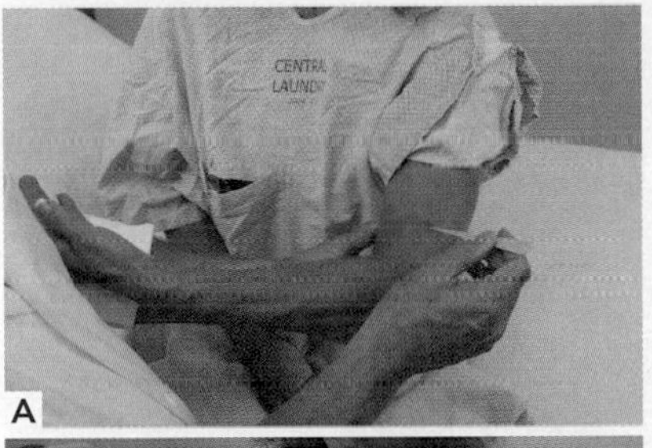
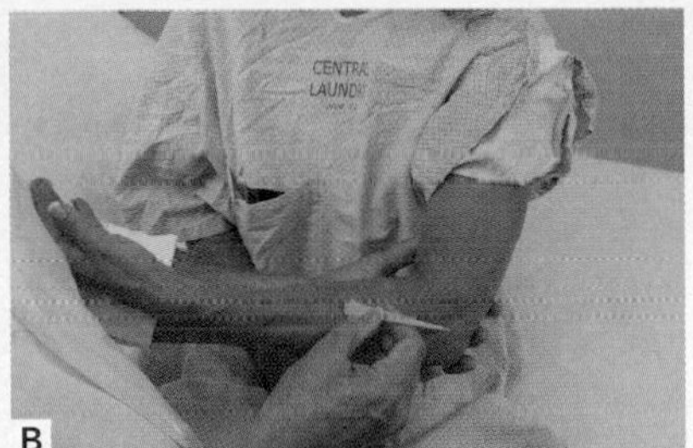
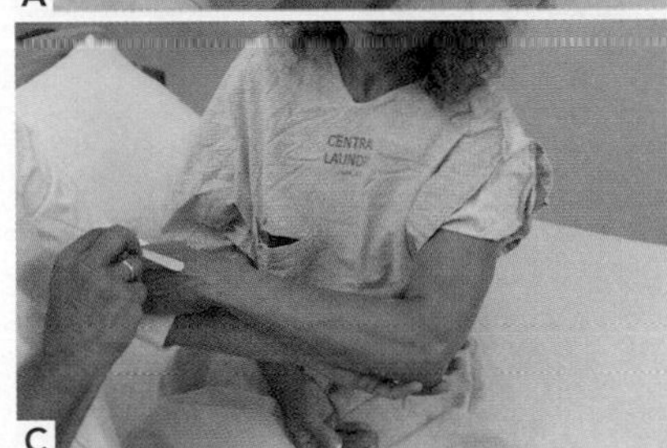

FIGURE 26-23A–C Testing superficial pain by placing sharp/dull instrument on surface of skin at different locations on body

Light Touch

For light touch, use a cotton ball, cotton tipped swab or other soft material to produce the sensation of touch. Follow the same procedure as for light pain, however, wait two seconds between each touch to avoid a summative effect. Instruct the patient to indicate when the sensation is felt by identifying whether it was perceived as sharp or dull (Figure 26-24).

Expected results would demonstrate the patient's ability to correctly identify when the skin was touched and differentiate between sharp and dull sensations.

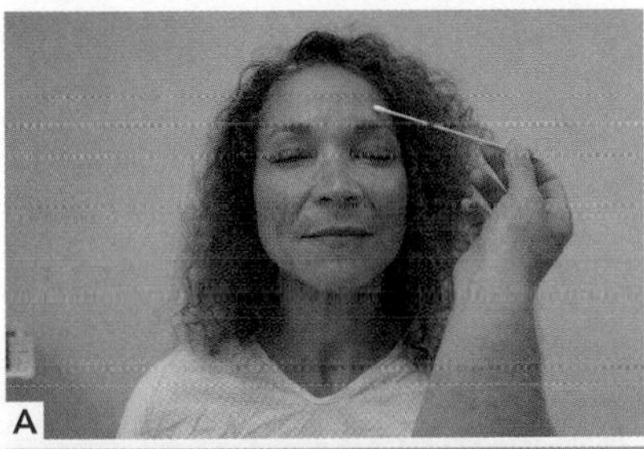
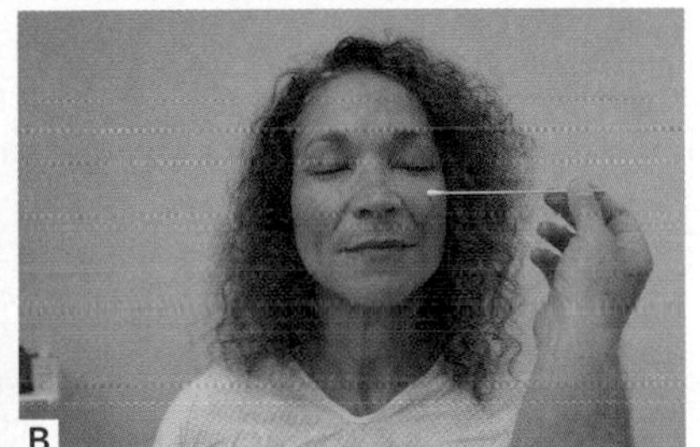
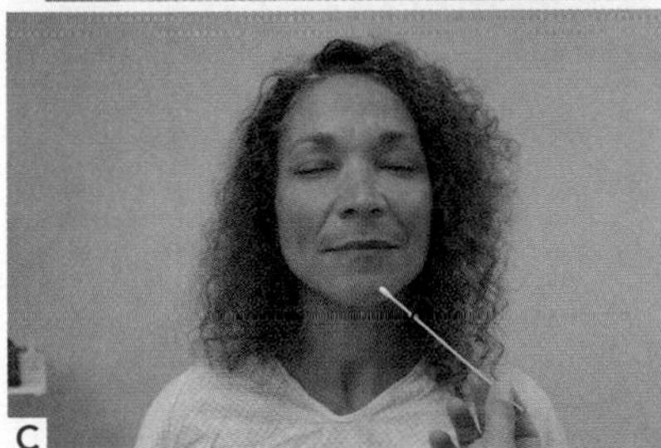

FIGURE 26-24A–C Testing light touch by placing cotton swab on surface of skin at different locations on body

Temperature

To test temperature sensation recognition, use test tubes that have been filled with hot and cold water. Touch the patient's skin with either the hot or cold test tube and have the patient indicate where the touch is located and if it was hot or cold (Figure 29-25). Temperature sensations are transmitted through the lateral spinothalamic tract of the spinal cord.

Expected findings would be the patient correctly identifying the hot and cold sensations when applied to the skin surface.

PRACTICE POINT: How Hot Is Hot?

When filling the test tubes with water, the water used for hot should not be hot enough to cause damage to the patient's skin. To determine if it is too hot, hold it in your hand for 10–15 seconds. You should be able to hold the test tube comfortably for that length of time. If you feel the test tube getting hotter to the point where you can't hold on to it, the temperature of the water is too hot.

Unexpected findings would be the inability to perceive touch/pain sensation and incorrect identification of touch locations. Asymmetrical responses would also be unexpected.

Unexpected findings would be the inability of the patient to correctly identify the hot and cold sensations when applied to the skin surface.

Inspection Techniques and Expected Findings	Unexpected Findings

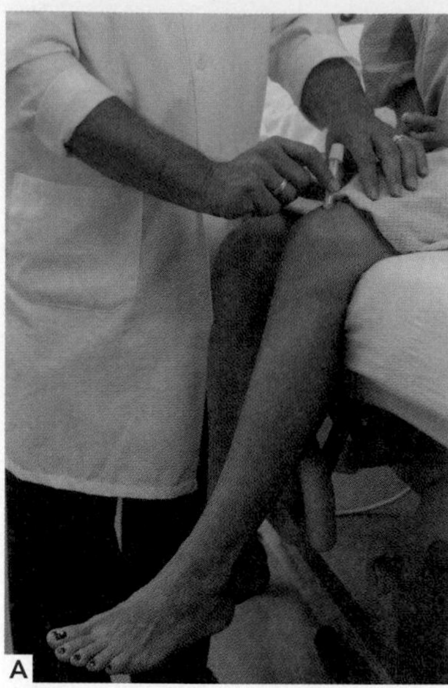
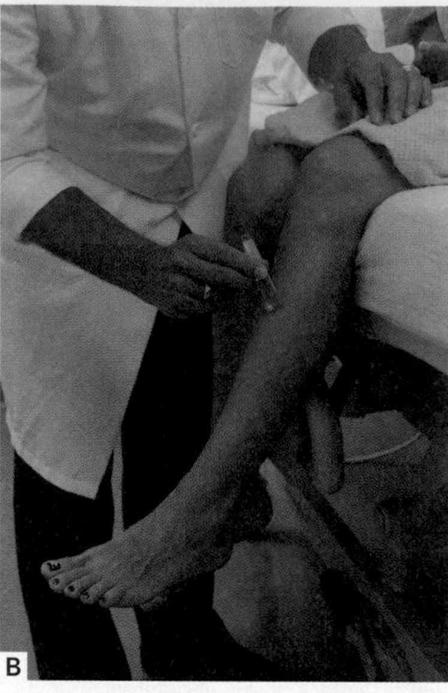
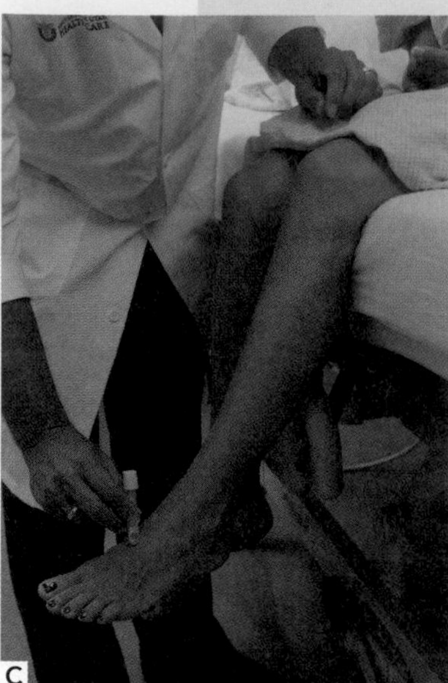

FIGURE 26-25A–C Testing temperature sensation—provider holding test tube of water to surface of patient's skin

Ask the patient to close their eyes and place the stem of a vibrating tuning fork on various bony prominences (Figure 26-26). Use a tuning fork with a lower frequency (128 or 256 Hz) because it has a slower reduction of vibration. The sensation of vibration is transmitted through the posterior column sensory tract.

Place the vibrating tuning fork on a specific joint, such as the sternum, shoulder, elbow, wrist, finger joints, knee, ankle, or toes. Begin at the most distal location and if the patient is able to identify the sensation, it is not necessary to proceed further. Assess both sides and compare the patient's perceptions.

The patient should feel a buzzing or tingling sensation; have the patient indicate when and where the vibrations are felt. You may also extinguish the vibrations and have the patient indicate when the sensation stops. You may also place a nonvibrating tuning fork on a site to determine if the patient is able to discriminate between sensations.

Unexpected results would be the inability to identify the sensation either in a localized area or over the entire extremity.

Expected results would be that the patient is able to identify the sensation and indicate when and where the sensation is perceived.

There may also be differences between the upper and lower extremities. Loss of sensation in the lower extremities is often due to peripheral neuropathy that accompanies diabetes and alcoholism.

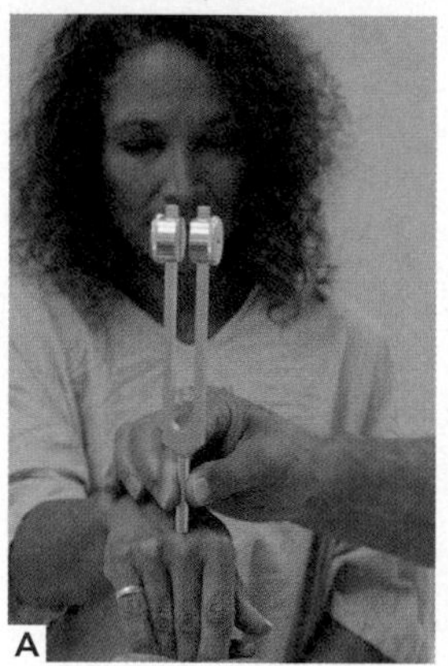
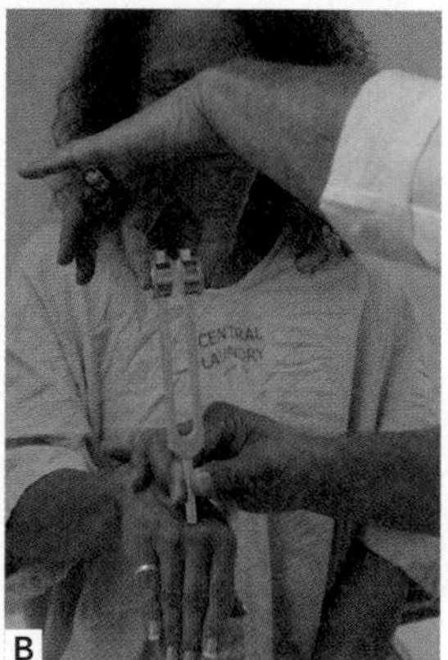

FIGURE 26-26A–B Testing the posterior column sensory tract placing a tuning fork over bony prominence

Position Sense

Sensory function is also assessed by position sense or **kinesthesia**, the patient's ability to identify passive movements of the digits of the upper and lower extremities. Usual digits are the big toe and either the index or middle finger.

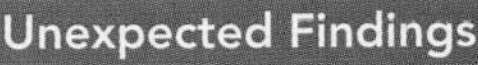

Inspection Techniques and Expected Findings

Hold the digit by the sides to avoid giving the patient pressure cues as to the movement of the digit (Figure 26-27). The movement is either up or down from a neutral position. Have the patient identify in what direction the digit was moved. Move each digit about 4–5 times and vary the pattern, returning to the neutral position before each up or down movement. Repeat the procedure so that the great toe of each foot and a finger of each hand are tested. Expected findings would be that the patient is able to correctly identify how the digit position has moved.

Unexpected Findings

Unexpected findings would be that the patient is unable to distinguish the digit position changes.

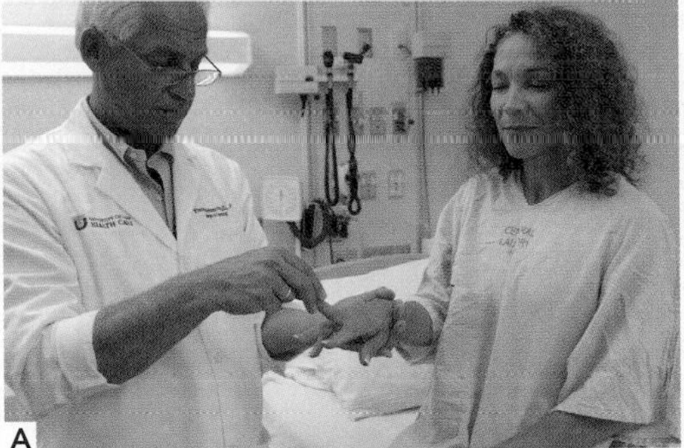

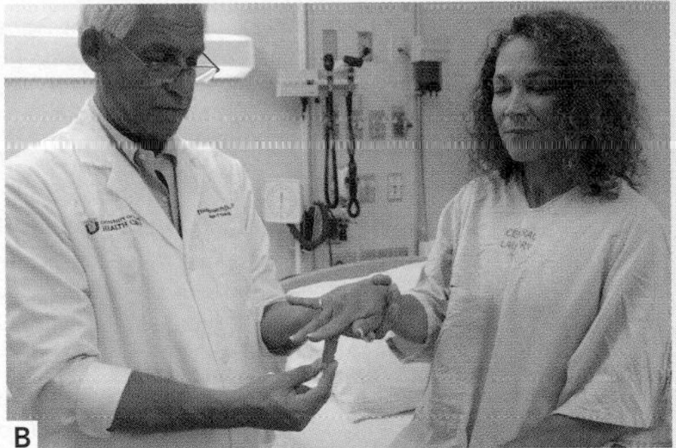

FIGURE 26-27A–B Assessing position sense (kinesthesia)

Inspection: Level III

A Level III exam is primarily performed on an individual who is experiencing some type of acute head injury in which the patient's skull/brain has been damaged from encountering a hard surface. These injuries could range from a minor concussion to massive brain injury from accidental trauma (gunshot wound, motor vehicle accident). Severe brain damage may also result from an acute stroke caused by a blood clot or hemorrhage from a ruptured blood vessel. Additionally, individuals may present with spinal cord injury.

Individuals who present with head trauma are likely to demonstrate some degree of amnesia. External signs of head injury or basilar skull fracture, focal neurologic deficits, associated alcohol intoxication or drug abuse, or a history of loss of consciousness mandates a thorough evaluation for intracranial injury.

See Box 26-1 for warnings signs of head injury and Table 26-9 for physical evidence of head trauma.

Box 26-1 Head Injury

Warning Signs
Increasing headache
Change in level of consciousness
Projectile vomiting
Bleeding from nose or ears/CSF
Raccoon's eyes or Battle's sign
Dilated pupils
Seizure
Cushing's Triad–increasing blood pressure, lowering pulse, change in breathing pattern

Table 26-9 Physical evidence of head trauma

Battle's Sign	Ecchymosis (bruising) observed behind the ear over the mastoid May not appear until 2 days post-injury
Raccoon eyes	Periorbital ecchymosis
CSF otorrhea	Cerebrospinal fluid leaking through the ears
CSF rhinorrhea	Cerebrospinal fluid leaking through the nose
Halo sign	Blood stain surrounded by a yellowish stain (CSF), usually observed on bed linins/pillows
Hemotympanum	The presence of blood in the tympanic cavity of the middle ear

LOC/Mental Status

The Glascow Coma Scale is used to establish awareness and arousal as well as motor activity.

Clinical severity is graded by GCS:

- Mild, GCS 13–15
  - Normal to lethargic
  - Mildly disoriented
- Moderate, GCS 9–12
  - Lethargic to obtunded
  - Follows commands with arousal
  - Confused
- Severe, GCS 3–8
  - Comatose, no eye opening or verbalization
  - Does not follow commands
  - Motor exam: ranges from localizing to posturing

Table 26-10 American Spinal Injury Association (ASIA) method for classifying spinal cord injury (SCI) by neurologic level.

ASIA Impairment Scale (AIS)	Steps in Classification
A = Complete. No sensory or motor function is preserved in the sacral segments S4-5. **B = Sensory Incomplete.** Sensory but not motor function is preserved below the neurological level and includes the sacral segments S4-5 (light touch or pin prick at S4-5 or deep anal pressure) AND no motor function is preserved more than three levels below the motor level on either side of the body. **C = Motor Incomplete.** Motor function is preserved below the neurological level**, and more than half of key muscle functions below the neurological level of injury (NLI) have a muscle grade less than 3 (Grades 0–2). **D = Motor Incomplete.** Motor function is preserved below the neurological level**, and *at least half* (half or more) of key muscle functions below the NLI have a muscle grade ≥ 3. **E = Normal.** If sensation and motor function as tested with the ISNCSCI are graded as normal in all segments, and the patient had prior deficits, then the AIS grade is E. Someone without an initial SCI does not receive an AIS grade. ** For an individual to receive a grade of C or D, i.e. motor incomplete status, they must have either (1) voluntary anal sphincter contraction or (2) sacral sensory sparing *with* sparing of motor function more than three levels below the motor level for that side of the body. The International Standards at this time allows even non-key muscle function more than 3 levels below the motor level to be used in determining motor incomplete status (AIS B versus C). NOTE: When assessing the extent of motor sparing below the level for distinguishing between AIS B and C, the ***motor level*** on each side is used; whereas to differentiate between AIS C and D (based on proportion of key muscle functions with strength grade 3 or greater) the ***neurological level of injury*** is used.	The following order is recommended for determining the classification of individuals with SCI. **1. Determine sensory levels for right and left sides.** *The sensory level is the most caudal, intact dermatome for both pin prick and light touch sensation.* **2. Determine motor levels for right and left sides.** *Defined by the lowest key muscle function that has a grade of at least 3 (on supine testing), providing the key muscle functions represented by segments above that level are judged to be intact (graded as a 5).* *Note: in regions where there is no myotome to test, the motor level is presumed to be the same as the sensory level, if testable motor function above that level is also normal.* **3. Determine the neurological level of injury (NLI)** *This refers to the most caudal segment of the cord with intact sensation and antigravity (3 or more) muscle function strength, provided that there is normal (intact) sensory and motor function rostrally respectively.* *The NLI is the most cephalad of the sensory and motor levels determined in steps 1 and 2.* **4. Determine whether the injury is Complete or Incomplete.** *(i.e. absence or presence of sacral sparing)* *If voluntary anal contraction =* ***No*** *AND all S4-5 sensory scores =* ***0*** *AND deep anal pressure =* ***No****, then injury is* ***Complete****.* *Otherwise, injury is* ***Incomplete****.* **5. Determine ASIA Impairment Scale (AIS) Grade:** **Is injury Complete?** **If YES, AIS=A** and can record ZPP (lowest dermatome or myotome on each side with some preservation) NO ↓ **Is injury Motor Complete? If YES, AIS=B** (No=voluntary anal contraction OR motor function more than three levels below the motor level on a given side, if the patient has sensory incomplete classification) NO 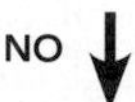 **Are at least half (half or more) of the key muscles below the *neurological* level of injury graded 3 or better?** NO 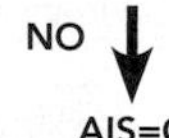 AIS=C YES ↓ AIS=D **If sensation and motor function is normal in all segments, AIS=E** *Note: AIS E is used in follow-up testing when an individual with a documented SCI has recovered normal function. If at initial testing no deficits are found, the individual is neurologically intact; the ASIA Impairment Scale does not apply.*

Source: American Spinal Injury Association: International Standards for Neurological Classification of Spinal Cord Injury," revised 2013. Reproduced by permission of the American Spinal Injury Association, Atlanta, GA.

Inspection Techniques and Expected Findings	Unexpected Findings

Cranial Nerves

Primarily CN assessment is generally limited to CN II and CN III, as previously described. However, when the patient's condition may necessitate CN testing, other ones may be included in the assessment.

Motor Activity

Assessment of the patient's motor activity is essentially the same as the Level II examination.

Sensory Examination: Primary Sensory Responses

The primary sensations of light touch and light pain have already been described in Level II. In situations where the patient may have a spinal cord injury primary sensations may be assessed within each dermatome. Knowing where or up to what dermatome sensation is felt can help in determining where the spinal cord has been injured or severed.

In addition to light touch and pain, primary sensation can also be assessed by recognition of temperature changes.

Inspection: Level IV

The Level IV exam is commonly done on individuals who are not hospitalized or seeking emergency care. The comprehensive exam includes any or all the other tests identified and described in each level. Placement of tests or techniques within this level does not preclude their use in other levels.

Inspection Techniques and Expected Findings	Unexpected Findings
LOC/Mental Status	
The provider may want to do a complete Mental Status Exam as previously described (Chapter 7), or may opt to use the Mini Mental Status Exam (MMSE).	MMSE scoring is used to determine the patient's cognitive function. The complete mental status exam is not scored so determining the degree of unexpected results is somewhat subjective. Age, education, and cultural variables need to be taken into account when evaluating the results of the mental status exam.
X-ray, MRI (magnetic resonance imaging), and CT (computerized tomography) can sometimes diagnose head and brain injuries by showing areas of fracture, hemorrhage, or other kinds of tissue injury.	These techniques are usually employed initially in the case of any head trauma to check for life-threatening bleeding or swelling in brain tissue.
However, traumatic brain injury (especially if mild) often involves scattered disconnection among neurons and supportive tissue, stretched and damaged axon membranes (known as diffuse axonal injury), chemical injury due to neurotransmitter toxicity, and cellular dysfunction due to changes in brain chemistry.	These kinds of changes to brain cells often do not result in sufficient change in the tissue density to be detected by conventional imaging techniques.
Often, more elaborate imaging techniques such as SPECT (single-photon emission computed tomography) or PET (positron emission tomography) can detect changes due to brain injury because these techniques measure brain cell metabolism, not tissue density.	

Cranial Nerves

CN I (Olfactory)

The olfactory nerve is sensory and tested by having the patient smell and correctly identify common odors, such as coffee, vanilla, tobacco, peppermint, or oranges (Figure 26-28).

Begin by having the patient breathe through each naris to establish their patency. Have the patient close her eyes and occlude one naris.

Next, hold the odor under the naris and have the patient inspire deeply to distribute to odor to the olfactory mucosa (Figure 26-29). Repeat the procedure on the other naris but using a different odor.

The patient should identify each odor correctly and discriminate between different odors. Therefore, repeat the procedure two or three times using different odors.

Any other CNs (II–XII) are tested in the same manner as previously identified and described.

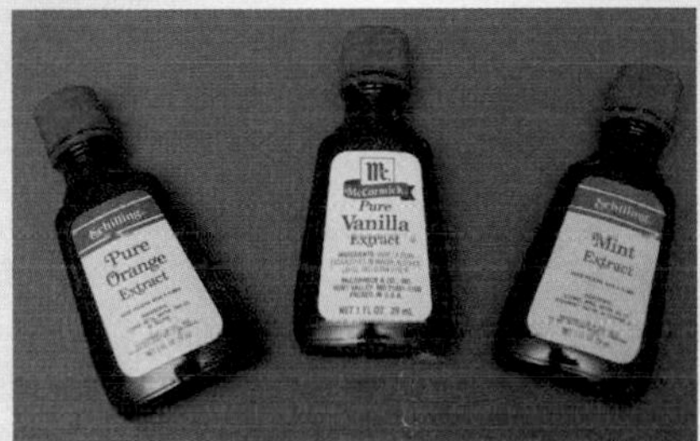

FIGURE 26-28 Examples of substances used for CN I (olfactory) testing

Unexpected Findings: Dysfunction of the olfactory nerve may result in **parosomia** (altered sense of smell) or **anosomia** (loss of smell).

The common cold is frequently the cause of dysfunction. Dysfunction may also result from trauma or fractures of the cribriform plate of the ethmoid bone.

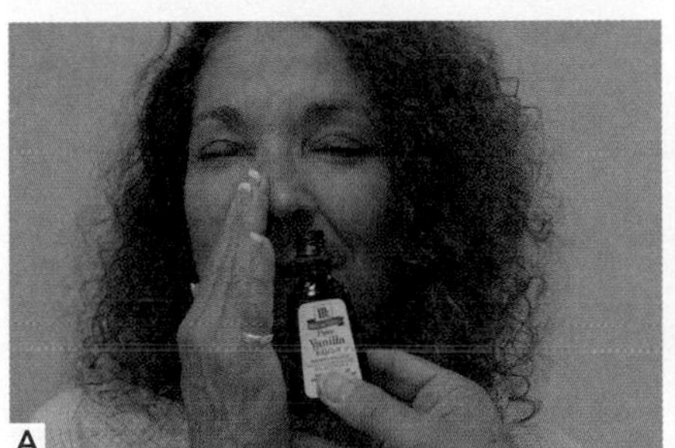

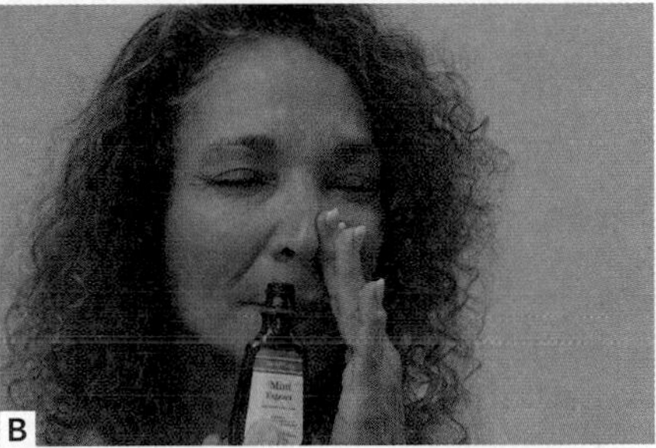

FIGURE 26-29A–B Assessing CN I by placing aromatic substance under patient's nose

Motor, Proprioception, and Cerebellar Function

Balance and Equilibrium

Testing for the patient's ability to maintain balance and equilibrium is done by using the Romberg test and assessing gait. These activities are coordinated by the lateral and anterior corticospinal motor tracts of the spinal cord.

Inspection Techniques and Expected Findings	Unexpected Findings

Romberg Test

For the Romberg test, the patient stands with her feet together and arms at the side. Instruct the patient to close the eyes for approximately 30 seconds (Figure 26-30).

Observe the patient's ability to maintain an upright position. The provider should be positioned in close proximity to the patient in order to catch the patient if she begins to fall. The patient may demonstrate slight swaying back and forth, but there should be no danger of falling.

To achieve balance, an individual requires two out of the following three transmissions to the cortex: (1) visual confirmation of position, (2) nonvisual confirmation of position (including proprioception and vestibular input), and (3) a properly functioning cerebellum (Padma Srivastava, 2012).

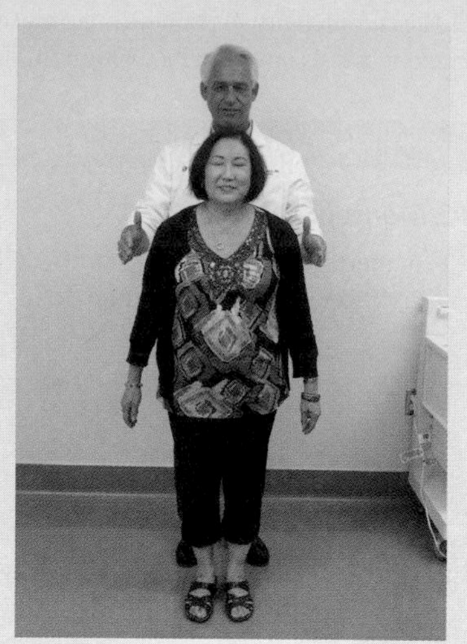

FIGURE 26-30 Testing balance—Romberg test

A positive Romberg indicates the possibility of cerebellar ataxia, vestibular dysfunction, or sensory loss. In some instances, the patient will lose balance with the eyes closed but be able regain balance when the eyes are opened. This is also a positive Romberg and is generally associated with a lesion of the cerebellum.

Expected findings would be that the patient is able to maintain equilibrium and balance for a period of 30 seconds. If the patient loses balance, it is considered a positive Romberg.

If the patient demonstrates a positive Romberg, then any further tests of cerebellar function should not be attempted. A patient's age should also be considered when determining further testing.

Additional information regarding distal muscular weakness may be elicited by the patient walking on toes and heels. Toe walking is sensitive to plantar flexion and heel walking is sensitive for dorsiflexion of the ankles.

Further assessment of balance may be done with the following maneuvers.

You may also have the patient stand with feet slightly apart. Push the patient's shoulders with enough force to cause a loss of balance. Be close enough to break the patient's fall if necessary. Expected results would be that the patient would be able to recover balance quickly to avoid falling.

Another test is to have the patient stand on one foot for approximately 5 seconds with their eyes closed and their arms out (Figure 26-31). Repeat the procedure with the opposite leg.

The patient should be able to maintain balance on one foot for 5 seconds. However, slight swaying is expected.

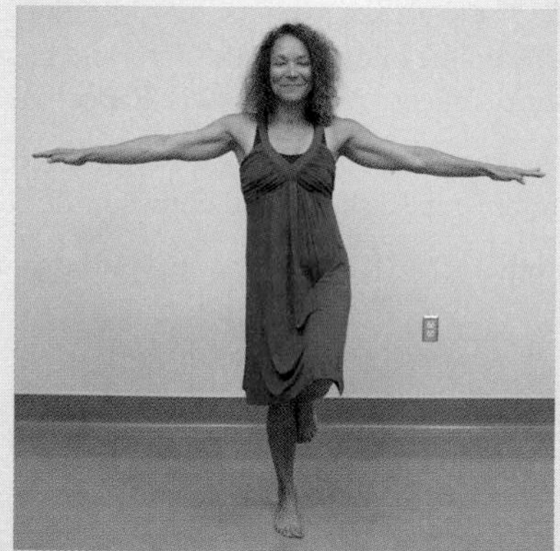

FIGURE 26-31 Assessing balance by having patient stand on one foot with eyes closed

Next, ask the patient to hop in place on one foot, with eyes open. Repeat the procedure with the opposite leg. The patient should be able to hop on one foot while maintaining balance for approximately 5 seconds. Assess the patient for loss of coordination, instability, and the need to continuously put the opposite foot on the floor to maintain balance.

Assess the patient for loss of coordination, instability, and the need to continuously put the opposite foot on the floor to maintain balance.

Inspection Techniques and Expected Findings	Unexpected Findings
Additional tests include asking the patient to do a shallow knee bend—first with one leg and then with the other (Figure 26-32). Depending on the age of the patient, the provider may need to offer some support to the patient, such as allowing the patient to hold on to the provider's hand or supporting the patients elbow. For elderly patients, it is more appropriate to ask them to rise from a sitting position or step up and down on a sturdy stool instead of hopping and knee bends.	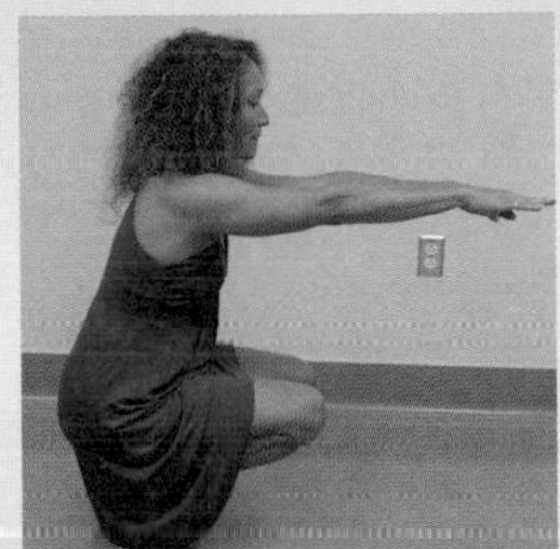 **FIGURE 26-32** Patient in "knee bending" position

Palpation: Level I

Palpation Techniques and Expected Findings	Unexpected Findings
Motor Activity If there is no evidence of neurological impairment, the patient's natural motor activity can be observed to determine ability, purposefulness, if voluntary, and equality. Motor activity in an individual with no neurological impairment should demonstrate the ability to voluntarily move all extremities for some reason or purpose. Extremity movement of both sides should be equal. Motor activity is also assessed by asking the patient to squeeze your fingers. Extend your index and middle finger and place them in the palm of the patient's hands. Instructs the patient to "squeeze" your fingers (Figure 26-33). This assesses the patient's ability to follow commands and the symmetry of the motor activity as well as muscle strength. The patient should follow the provider's instructions and demonstrate equal and symmetrical strength with the squeeze.	Unexpected results would be an inability to follow the instructions or unequal or unsymmetrical grip strength. 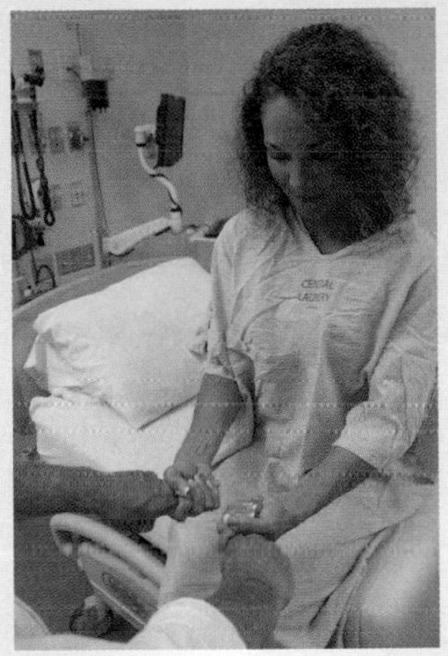 **FIGURE 26-33** Patient squeezes provider's fingers to assess motor activity
The same assessment may be done with the lower extremities. Place your hands on the dorsal aspect of the patient's feet and slightly dorsiflex them, providing minimal resistance. Ask the patient to push with both feet against your hands, again demonstrating equal and symmetrical strength. Expected results would be that the patient is able to dorsiflex the foot against resistance exerted by the provider.	Unexpected results would be that the patient is unable to dorsiflex the foot against resistance, or there is weak or unequal strength with dorsiflexion.
Deep Tendon Reflexes Assessment of the reflexes is generally not a part of an overall general assessment of the patient, unless there is a reason to do so. When necessary to test deep tendon reflexes (DTRs), the biceps and patellar reflexes could easily be tested. These are described in the next level.	
Palpation: Level II	
Deep Tendon Reflexes Deep tendon reflexes (DTRs) are obtained by striking certain tendons that are attached to a muscle. Striking the tendon causes it to contract the muscle it is attached to. A visible movement of the extremity controlled by the muscle is evidence of an intact reflex arc.	Absent reflexes or hyperactive reflexes suggest a motor neuron disorder. Absent reflexes are associated with lower motor neuron disorders and hyperactive reflexes are associated with upper motor neuron disorders.

Palpation Techniques and Expected Findings

Obtaining a visible reflex action is dependent on having the attached muscle relaxed. If the reflexes are difficult to elicit due to tense muscles, have the patient focus on another object or contract an alternate muscle group. You may also use distraction by maintaining a conversation with the patient. This is using **reinforcement** to obtain the DTRs (Figure 26-34).

When obtaining reflexes in the upper extremities, have the patient clench the jaw and teeth as hard as possible.

When testing the lower extremities, have the patient hook the fingers of one hand around the fingers of the other hand and pull.

Palpate for the tendon that is being tested rather than randomly tapping the area. Once the tendon has been located, hold the reflex hammer securely between the thumb and forefinger and tap the tendon using a quick flick of the wrist. If the reflex response is not obtained on the first tap, gradually increase the force of the tap.

The reflexes are assessed by comparing the responses on both sides of the body. Expected results would be symmetrical visible or palpable responses.

DTRs are scored on a +4 scale (Table 26-11).

Table 26-11 Deep tendon reflex grades

Grade	Description
0	Absent response (no evidence of contraction)
+1	Weak response (decreased, but still present, hyporeflexive)
+2	Expected (normal) response
+3	Hyperactive response
+4	Hyperactive response with clonus (repetitive shortening of the muscle after a single contraction)

Biceps Reflex (Spinal Nerves C_5/6; Musculocutaneous Nerve)

The biceps tendon passes through the antecubital fossa. To best locate the tendon, instruct the patient to flex the elbow. Palpate the antecubital fossa; the biceps tendon will feel like a hard cord.

Once it is located, support the patient's upper arm with the thumb placed over the tendon and the hand and rest of the fingers placed just above the elbow. Support the patient's forearm with your forearm.

To elicit the reflex, take the reflex hammer and strike your thumb tendon directly with the reflex hammer (Figure 26-35). Tapping the tendon causes contraction of the biceps muscle with visible or palpable contraction of the biceps tendon and elbow.

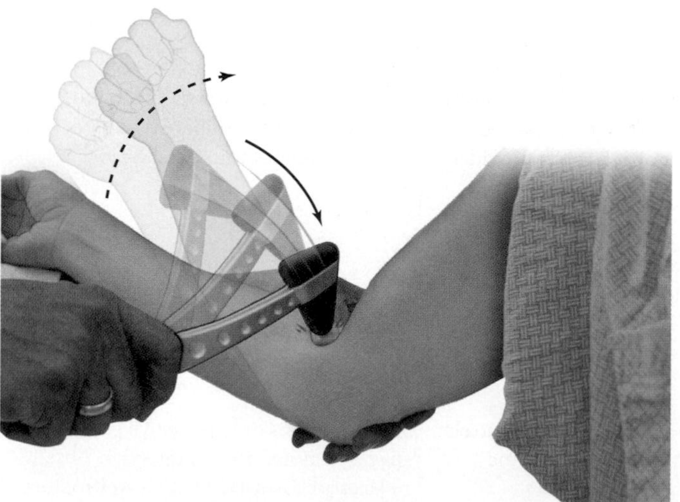

FIGURE 26-35 Testing the biceps reflex

Unexpected Findings

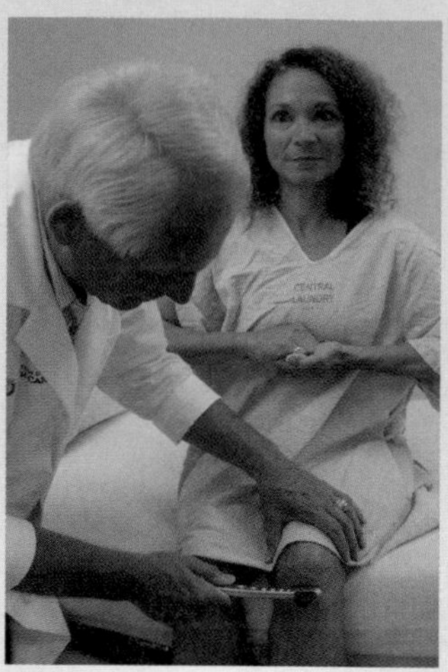

FIGURE 26-34 Reinforcement

An unexpected finding would be the absence of a reflex action. Lack of a reflex may indicate neuropathy of a lower motor neuron disorder.

Palpation Techniques and Expected Findings	Unexpected Findings

Patellar Reflex (Spinal Nerves L2–4; Femoral Nerve)

The patellar tendon is located just below the kneecap. Have the patient sit on the edge of the examining table, far enough over the edge so the lower legs can hang freely (Figure 26-36).

Strike the patellar tendon directly with the reflex hammer. Striking the patellar tendon causes contraction of the quadriceps muscle, resulting in extension of the lower leg.

Unexpected Findings: An unexpected finding would be the absence of a reflex action. Lack of a reflex may indicate neuropathy of a lower motor neuron disorder.

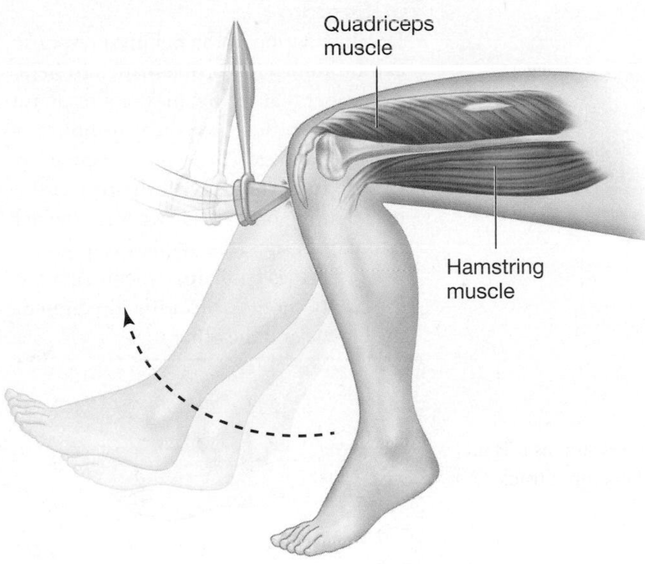

FIGURE 26-36 Testing the patellar reflex

Achilles Reflex (Spinal Nerves L_5—S_2; Sciatic Nerve)

The Achilles tendon is located directly behind the ankle. Have the patient in a sitting position on the edge of the examining table with the legs hanging freely. In this position, the feet are plantar flexed (Figure 26-37). To obtain optimum results, slightly dorsiflex the foot so that it is in a neutral position. Strike the Achilles tendon directly with the reflex hammer. Striking the Achilles tendon causes contraction of the gastrocnemius muscle resulting in plantar flexion of the foot.

Unexpected Findings: An unexpected finding would be the absence of a reflex action. Lack of a reflex may indicate neuropathy of a lower motor neuron disorder.

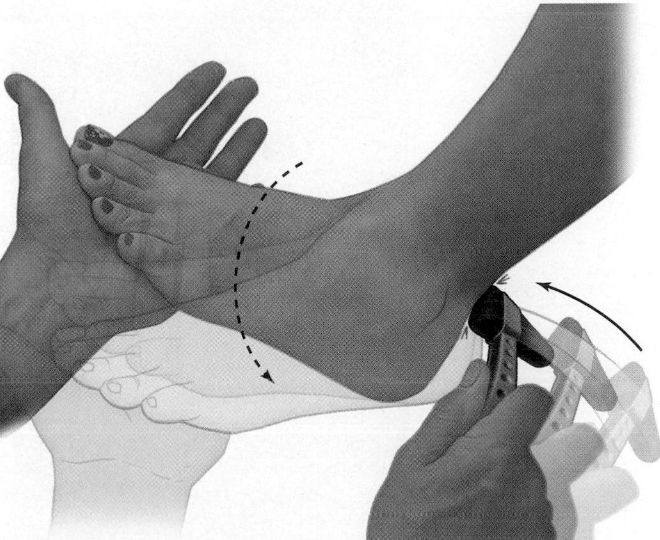

FIGURE 26-37 Testing Achilles reflex

Palpation Techniques and Expected Findings

Clonus is predominantly tested in the ankle. Begin by placing one hand under the patient's knee and the other hand around the ball of the foot. Briskly dorsiflex the foot and observe for the presence of clonus.

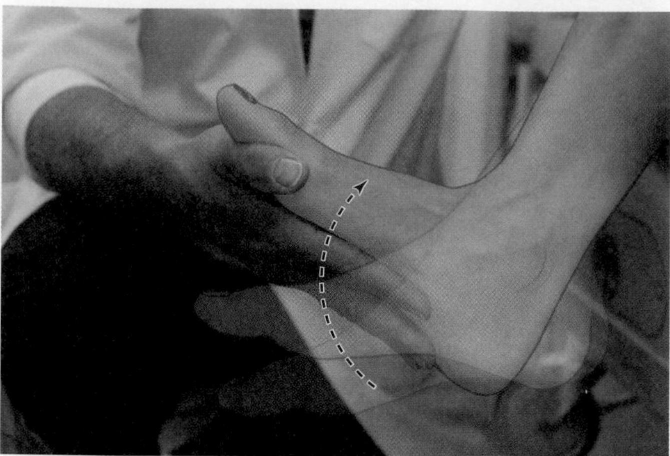

FIGURE 26-38 Testing for the presence of clonus

Superficial Reflexes

These are not routinely assessed with the exception of the plantar reflex, which is tested as it is an indicator of motor development related to the upper motor neurons of the corticospinal track.

Plantar Reflex (L_4 and 5, S_1 and 2)

The plantar reflex assesses spinal nerves T_{12}, L_1 and 2. It is elicited by stroking the lateral side of the foot, from heel to ball, moving across the ball to the medial side of the foot (Figure 26-39). The foot is stroked with a blunt instrument that may be the provider's finger, a tongue blade, or the tip of the reflex hammer. The plantar reflex may be difficult to obtain in conscious, ticklish patients and they may have some degree of an extensor response. Using a firm touch when stroking the foot may help to avoid this; unconscious patients will not present this problem. The plantar reflex is characterized by plantar flexion of the toes.

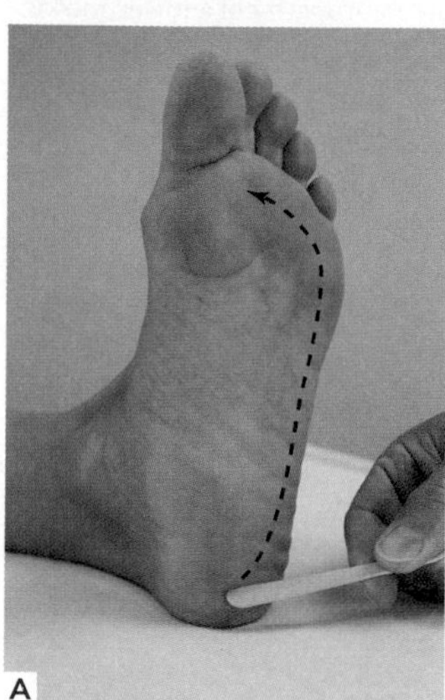

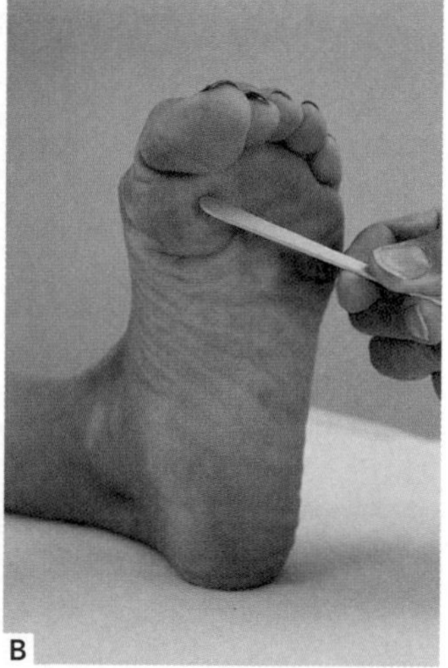

FIGURE 26-39A–B Assessing the plantar reflex

Unexpected Findings

An expected response for reflexes is a single muscle contraction with response. If hyperactive reflexes are obtained, assess for the presence of **clonus,** a repeated contraction of the reflex (Figure 26-38).

PRACTICE POINT: Babinski Response

Documentation of the Babinski response can be somewhat problematic. To help, remember that the Babinski is a response and not a reflex. A typical response is that toes all flex. An atypical response is the big toe extends with the rest of the toes fanning out. This is what is referred as Babinski sign (the atypical response is where the toes point up). Documentation for clarity should reflect the direction of the big toe and the other toes.

The unexpected response is dorsiflexion of the great toe with or without fanning of the other toes, identified as the **Babinski response** and may be described as a positive Babinski (Figure 26-40). Its presence is considered an expected response in children under the age of two. When present in older individuals, it may represent lesions of the pyramidal tract.

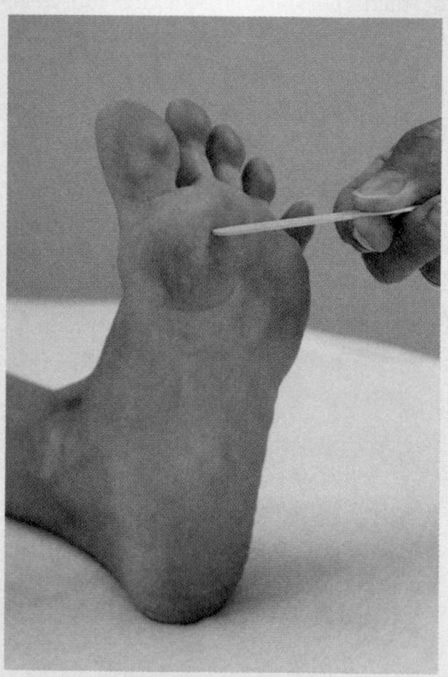

FIGURE 26-40 The Babinski response is an unexpected response

Palpation: Level III

Pathological reflexes are only obtained when some pathological condition exists; therefore they are not routinely assessed. They may be used to rule out or confirm the presence of certain conditions.

Palpation Techniques and Expected Findings	Unexpected Findings

Meningeal Signs (Meningismus)

These signs are assessed when there is a high index of suspicion for meningeal inflammation from infection (meningitis, encephalitis) or subarachnoid hemorrhage. These signs are neck mobility, Brudzinski's sign, and Kernig's sign. Additional tests may be performed to determine the level of brain function.

Neck Mobility (Nuchal Rigidity)

Before the neck is tested for mobility, the possibility of injury to the cervical vertebrae or cervical cord must be ruled out. To test for neck mobility, have the patient in a supine position. Place your hands behind the patient's head and flex the neck forward as far as possible (Figure 26-41).

The neck should be supple and easily flexed without any pain or resistance to flexion.

Unexpected results would be pain on flexion and resistance to flexion.

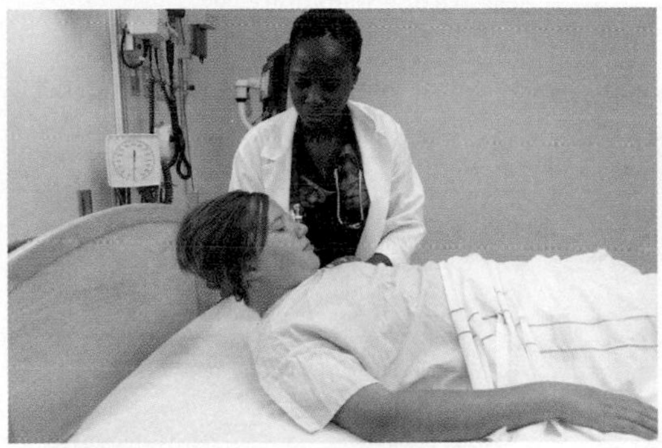

FIGURE 26-41 Testing nuchal rigidity

Brudzinski's Sign

The presence of Brudzinski's sign is assessed during the test for neck mobility. As the patient's neck is flexed, observe the response of the hips and knees to this maneuver (Figure 26-42).

Expected findings would be that the hips and knees remain relaxed and motionless.

Unexpected results would be pain and flexion of the hips and knees to neck flexion.

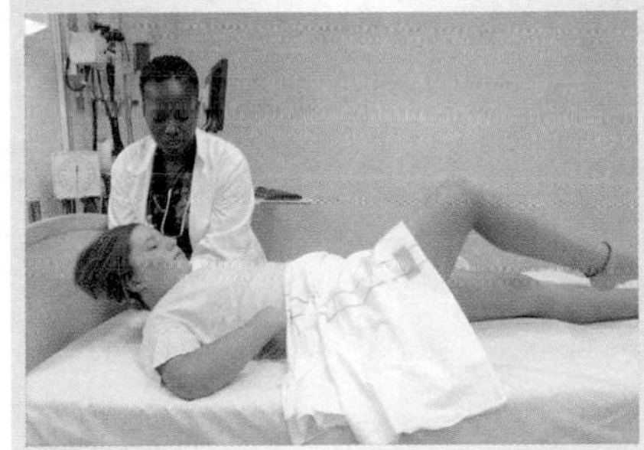

FIGURE 26-42 Testing Brudzinski's sign

Kernig's Sign

To test for Kernig's sign, flex the patient's leg at both the hip and knee, and then straightening the knee. Expected results are the absence of pain during the maneuver (Figure 26-43).

Unexpected results are pain and an increased resistance to knee extension.

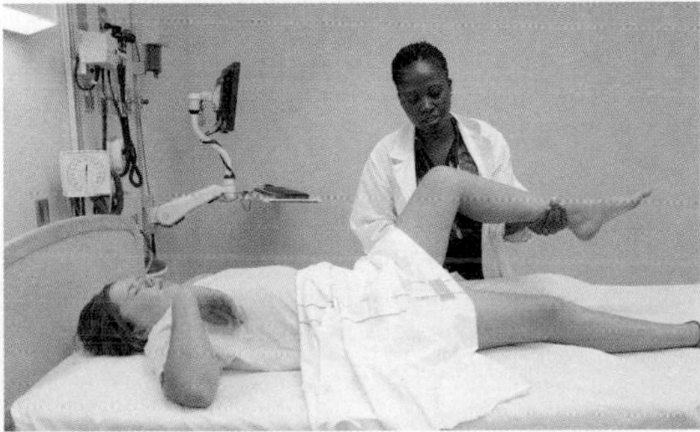

FIGURE 26-43 Testing Kernig's sign

Palpation Techniques and Expected Findings	Unexpected Findings

Reflexes

Oculocephalic Reflex

The **oculocephalic reflex** or "doll's eye movements" is performed on comatose patients to assess brain stem function. It is not possible to observe this reflex in an awake and alert patient as conscious control over eye movements is difficult to eliminate. The **oculocephalic reflex** maintains stable images on the retina during eye movements. This reflex is demonstrated by eye movements that go in the opposite direction of the head so that a right head turn will cause the eyes to move to the left.

To perform this test, lift the eyelids so the eyes will remain open. Turn the patient's head to one side and observe the movement of the eyes.

If the brain stem is intact, the eyes will move to the opposite side so that the iris is observed in the medial and lateral corners of the palpebral fissures.

Unexpected Findings: Unexpected results occur in the presence of a brain stem lesion, either in the pons or midbrain. When the patient's head is moved to one side, the eyes remained fixed, positioned in the center of the eye, and continuously look forward (Figure 26-44). This is considered a negative or absent doll's eyes.

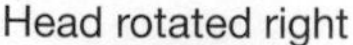
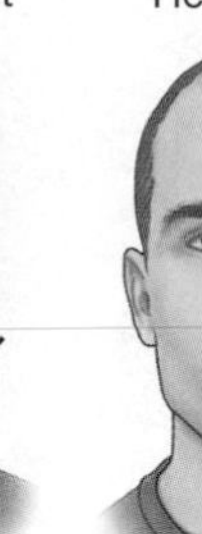
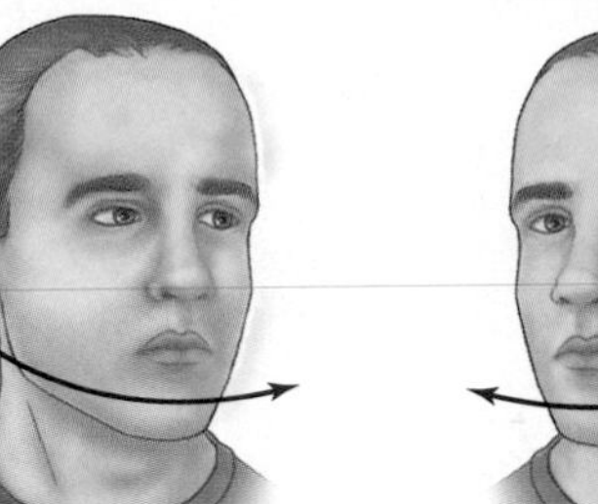
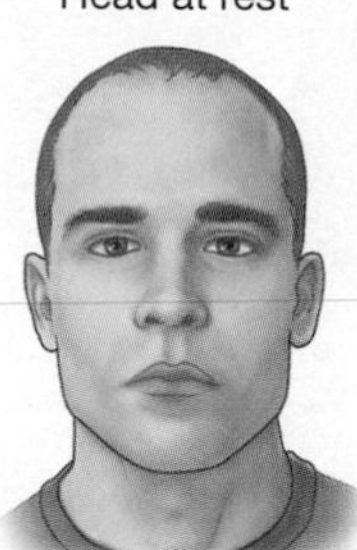
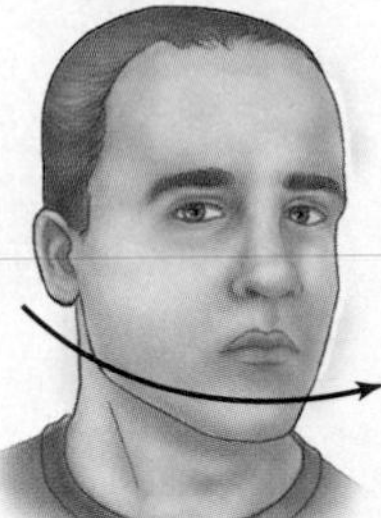

FIGURE 26-44 Testing oculocephalic reflex or "doll's eye movements" on an unconscious patient

Oculovestibular Reflex (Cold Caloric Test)

To perform this test, irrigate the patient's ear canal with 50-100 cc of cold water.

Unexpected Findings: In the comatose patient, when cold water is used, the eyes will move towards the opposite side, whereas warm water will cause the eyes to move toward the same side. The caloric reflex test is used to determine brain stem function which may result in the diagnosis of brain death.

Frontal Release Signs (Reflexes)

Frontal release signs are assessed when there is a concern regarding frontal lobe function. Frontal release signs are actually primitive reflexes that can be demonstrated in adults.

The return of primitive reflexes indicates that the reflexes are no longer suppressed, but released from frontal lobe suppression.

Deep tendon reflexes that may be assessed on the patient with an altered level of consciousness are the biceps, patellar, and Achilles reflex.

Unexpected Findings:

Palmomental reflex—manifests as a twitch of the chin muscle when the eminence of the palm is stroked. The twitch should be observed to occur on the same side as the stroked palm. This reflex may be present in the elderly, so should not necessarily be considered an indicator of any brain alteration.

Snout reflex—is observed as a pouting or pursing of the lips when the closed lips are tapped near the midline. Its presence is another indicator of brain damage that may be caused by dementias, metabolic encephalopathies, closed-head injuries, and hydrocephalus.

Palpation Techniques and Expected Findings

Unexpected Findings

Globellar reflex—manifests as blinking in response to repetitive tapping on the forehead. The blinking is observed only in response to the first few taps.

Palpation: Level IV

Palpations for Level IV are additional tests that may be used if more data is needed.

Sensory Function

Sensory: Cortical Sensory Responses

Cortical sensory functions are assessed by fine touch; they provide information about the patient's cognitive ability to interpret and discriminate tactile stimuli. Cortical sensory responses are transmitted by the posterior columns of the spinal cord. The patient's eyes need to be closed for each of these tests.

Stereognosis

Test stereognosis by placing a familiar object (e.g., key, paper clip, coin) in the palm of the patient's hand and ask him or her to identify the object by touch and manipulating the object (Figure 26-45). Repeat the procedure with the other hand, only use a different object. The patient should be able to correctly identify the object in each hand.

The inability to identify the object (**astereognosis**) may be due to a parietal lobe lesion or sensory cortical lesions.

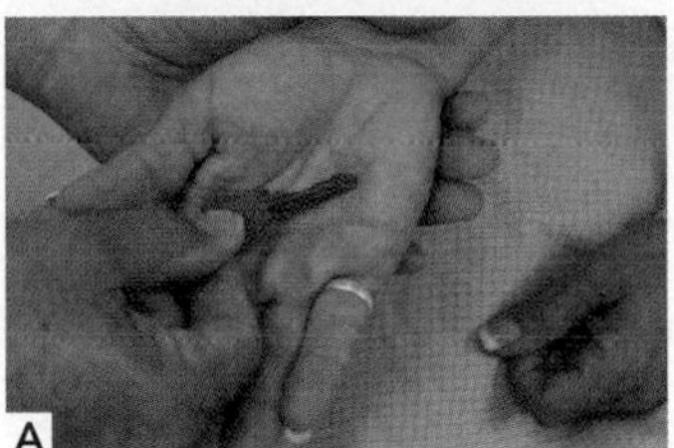

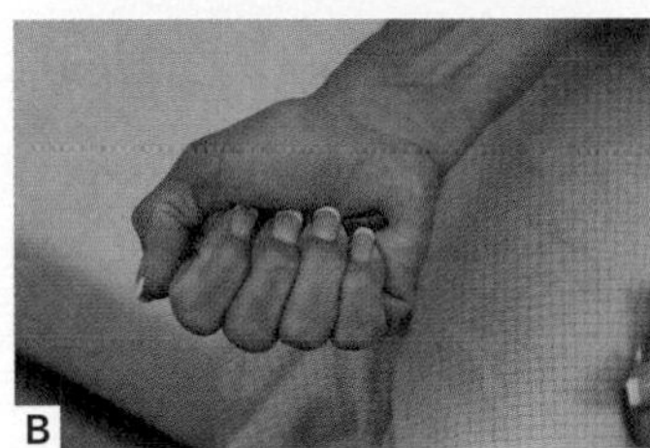

FIGURE 26-45A–B Provider places familiar object onto patient's palm

Graphesthesia

Test graphesthesia by writing a letter or number on the patient's palm (Figure 26-46). It is permissible to tell the patient whether you are going to write a letter or a number so that the patient would know whether it was the number 7 or the letter L. Repeat the procedure with the other hand only use different numbers or letters. Other locations on the body may be used, but the palms are most commonly used. Graphesthesia may be substituted for stereognosis when the patient is unable to move the hand or fingers well enough to identify an object.

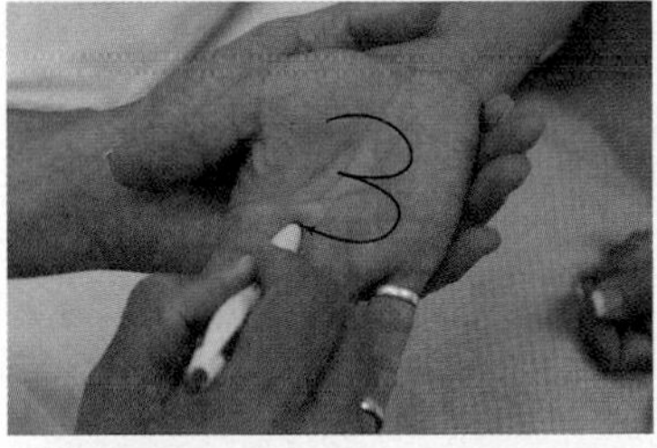

FIGURE 26-46 Provider traces the number 3 on the patient's palm to test graphesthesia

Extinction

Extinction assesses whether the patient is able to feel touch at simultaneous locations on the skin. Touch the patient with a sharp point at the same location on both sides of the body. The patient should feel touch at both locations.

Point Location

Point location assesses the ability of the patient to locate the point of touch after the stimulus has been removed. With the patient's eyes closed, touch an area of the patient's skin and withdraw the stimulus. Instruct the patient to identify where on the body the touch was felt (Figure 26-47). The patient should be able to identify where the touch occurred. Table 26-12 shows the minimal distance between points for two point discrimination.

Table 26-12 Minimal distance between points for two point discrimination

Body Part	Minimal Distance (mm)
Tongue	1 mm
Fingertips	2 mm
Toes	3–8 mm
Palms of hands	8–12 mm
Chest/forearms	40 mm
Back	40–60 mm
Upper arms/thighs	75 mm

Palpation Techniques and Expected Findings

Unexpected Findings

Two-point discrimination is the ability to discern whether the skin is being touched by two distinct points or one and is assumed to reflect how finely innervated an area of skin is. The smallest distance between two points that still results in the perception of two distinct stimuli is documented as the patient's two-point threshold. Performance on the two extremities can be compared for discrepancies.

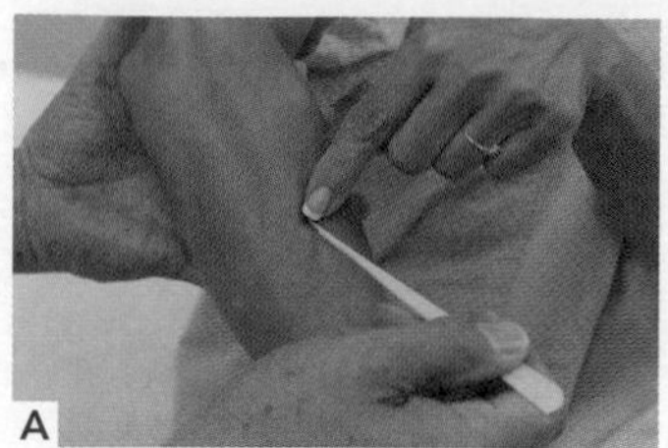

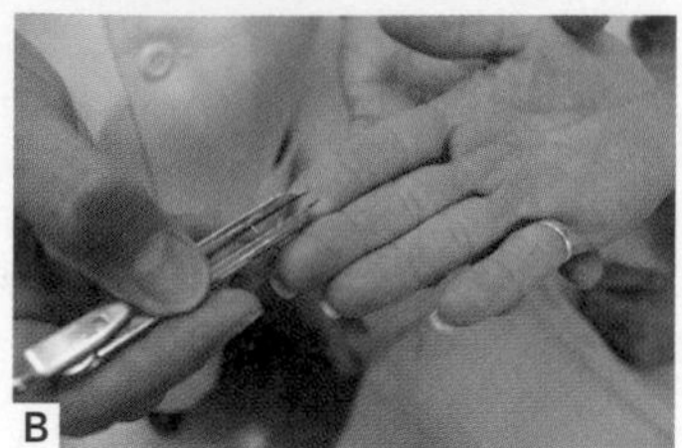

FIGURE 26-47A–B Testing cortical sensory point location: A is testing point location; B is testing 2 point discrimination

Reflexes

Additional DTRs that may be assessed are the triceps and brachioradialis. It is a bit more difficult to obtain these reflexes as the tendons connecting to the muscle are not as well defined or palpated.

Triceps Reflex (C_7/8; Radial Nerve)

The triceps tendon is located posterior to the olecranon process. Support the patient's upper arm and let the forearm hang freely (Figure 26-48).

Locate the triceps tendon with the thumb of the other hand.

Once it is located, take the reflex hammer and strike the tendon directly with the reflex hammer. Tapping the tendon causes contraction of the triceps muscle with visible or palpable extension of the elbow.

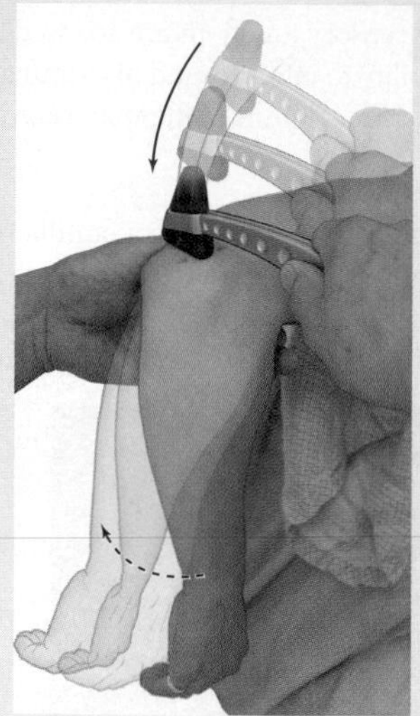

FIGURE 26-48 Testing triceps reflex

Brachioradialis Reflex (C_5/6; Radial Nerve)

The brachioradialias reflex is easiest to elicit with the patient sitting and the forearm resting loosely on the upper leg or supported by the provider's hand (Figure 26-49). The brachioradialis muscle tendon is unable to be seen or palpated. The tendon crosses the radius at the base of the wrist into the radial styloid process (radial side of wrist around 4 inches proximal to base of thumb).

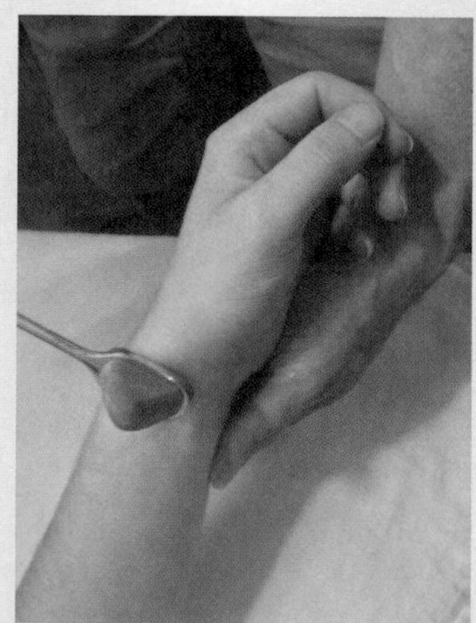

FIGURE 26-49 Brachioradialis reflex

Palpation Techniques and Expected Findings	Unexpected Findings

The reflex should cause slight wrist extension and/or radial deviation, supination, and slight elbow flexion.

Superficial Reflexes

Additional superficial reflexes include the corneal/conjunctival, abdominal, and cremasteric. The level of control in the spinal cord is identified after the specific reflex.

Corneal/Conjunctival Reflex

If CN V and VII have been completely examined, the conjunctival and corneal reflexes have been tested. The expected response for both reflexes is bilateral blinking.

Abdominal Reflexes

Abdominal reflexes may be assessed during the abdominal exam and are assessed in each of the four quadrants of the abdomen. The upper two quadrants are innervated by spinal nerves T_7, 8, and 9, and the lower two quadrants are innervated by spinal nerves T_{10} and 11.

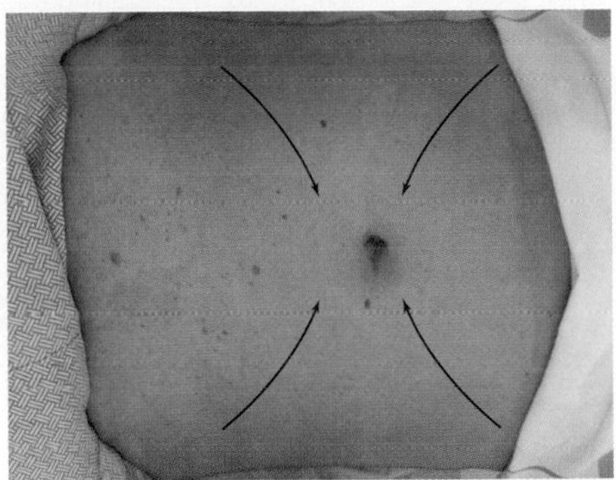

FIGURE 26-50 Testing superficial abdominal reflexes

With the patient in the supine position, stroke each quadrant of the abdomen with the end of the reflex hammer or tongue blade.

For upper quadrant reflexes, stroke downward and towards from the umbilicus.

For lower quadrant reflexes, stroke upward and towards from the umbilicus (Figure 26-50). For each stroke, there should be contraction of the rectus abdominus muscle that pulls the umbilicus toward the stroked side.

Unexpected Findings: A diminished response may be the result of obesity or stretched muscles from pregnancy. Lack of any response suggests a lower motor neuron disorder or destruction of sensory pathways from the skin area that was stimulated.

Cremasteric Reflex

The cremasteric reflex, which assesses spinal nerves T_{12}, L_1 and 2, is present and tested only in males. The patient may either be standing or supine for this procedure with the genitalia fully exposed. Stroke the inner thigh from proximal to distal and observe the testicle and scrotum on the stroked side (Figure 26-51). The testicle and scrotum should move upward. Repeat the procedure on the opposite side.

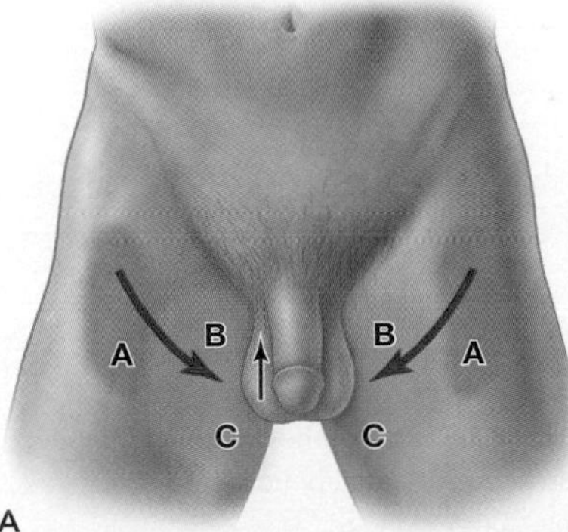

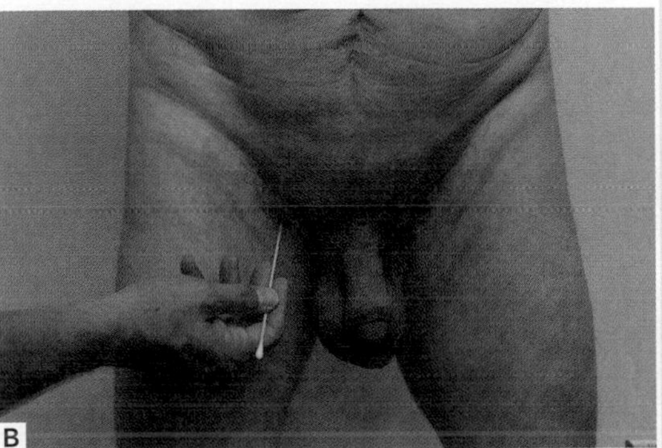

FIGURE 26-51 Testing cremasteric reflex. Area A represents the area of sensory fibers controlled by the genitofemoral nerve; area B represents that controlled by the ilioinguinal nerve; arrow C shows the direction and location where the skin must be stroked to elicit this reflex.

Developmental Applications

Techniques and Expected Findings	Unexpected Findings

Infants

The neurological exam in infants is adapted to the infant's age and ability to cooperate with the provider. Much of the neurological exam is based on the patient following directions or responding to a particular stimulus and providing a verbal or nonverbal reaction. In the newborn neither can be obtained, therefore critical observations of the infant's behavior and movement provide the information needed. Adaptations to the exam are also necessary to accommodate for the lack of patient cooperation. The gestational age of the infant also needs to be considered when evaluating infant responses and activity. Neurological development in the infant is also monitored and assessed by the presence and disappearance of specific primitive reflexes.

Mental Status

The optimum time for evaluation of the infant's mental status is between feedings. Interruption during feeding causes excessive crying and if just fed, the infant is more interested in sleep than being examined. Essential observations for the mental status include spontaneous eye opening, facial and extremity movement, and responses to stimuli. Alertness is determined by the length of eye opening and spontaneous movement of the face and extremities. These states of alertness are greatly influenced by prior activities and time of feeding.

A lethargic infant is unable to maintain an alert state.

An irritable infant is agitated and cries with minimal stimulation and does not respond to comfort or soothing actions.

Cranial Nerves

The cranial nerves are not tested directly, but astute observations made during the examination or modifications will provide adequate data regarding cranial nerve function. These observations are described in Table 26-13.

Table 26-13 CN examination adaptations for infants and children

Cranial Nerve	Observations/Modification of CN Examination
CN I	Infant—pass strong smelling substance (peppermint, cloves) under nose, assess for startle response, grimace or sniffing (not tested in newborns)
CN II	If child is old enough to cooperate, use Snellen E chart, HOTV or picture chart for vision testing Fields of vision may be tested, but may need to immobilize child's head.
CN III, IV, VI	Infant—size, shape, equality of pupils; optical blink reflex (when eyes open, shine light and note rapid closure); eyes follow movement Child—use light source to assess direct and consensual pupil response to light; move object through cardinal fields of vision (EOMs), may need to immobilize head "Doll's eye movement"—rotate infants head side to side, note eyes moving in the opposite direction (head right—eyes left)
CN V	Infant—rooting; sucking reflex Child—observe eating cookie/cracker (equality/strength of jaw movements); touch areas of trigeminal nerve distribution with cotton, observe child bat it away.
CN VII	Infant—symmetry of facial expressions, when crying/smiling Child—observe facial symmetry when smiling, talking, frowning, crying; have child show teeth, demonstrate puffed cheeks and have child imitate faces
CN VIII	Response to loud noise
CN IX, X	Infant—swallowing, gag reflex; coordinated sucking and swallowing Child elicit gag reflex
CN XI, XII	Infant—pinch nose, observe infant's mouth open and tongue elevate in midline Child—have child stick out tongue and shrug shoulders

Motor Activity

Assess motor activity by observing the infant's spontaneous activity coordination and smoothness of movement. The coordination of sucking and swallowing is also controlled by the cerebellum. Observing the resting posture of the infant provides information regarding muscle tone. Preterm infants have minimal tone with extremities in extension. In contrast, the term infant will demonstrate flexion of all the extremities.

Jerky movements are unexpected and require that the infant be evaluated for structural or metabolic disorders (Yang, 2004).

Techniques and Expected Findings

The fists are flexed tightly for about the first 3 months, but occasionally they will be opened, gradually opening up for longer periods of time. Reaching for and grasping objects appears around 2 months. By 6 months, the infant takes objects with one hand and 1 month later transfers objects from hand to hand. By 10 months, there is purposeful releasing of objects. These movements should be smooth and coordinated with no tremors or constant overshooting of movements.

Muscle tone for head control is an important milestone in infant motor development. Two maneuvers assess head control. First, have the infant in a supine position and then hold on to the wrists, pulling the infant up to a sitting position. The term infants head will be held in almost the same plane as the body. When the infant is in the sitting position, the head will be balanced briefly and then flop forward.

The second maneuver is to lift up the infant in a prone position with one hand supporting the chest. The term infant maintains the head at a 45-degree angle or less from the horizontal. Additionally, the back is straight or slightly arched with the elbows and knees slightly flexed. At 3 months of age, the infant will raise the head and arch the back (Figure 26-53).

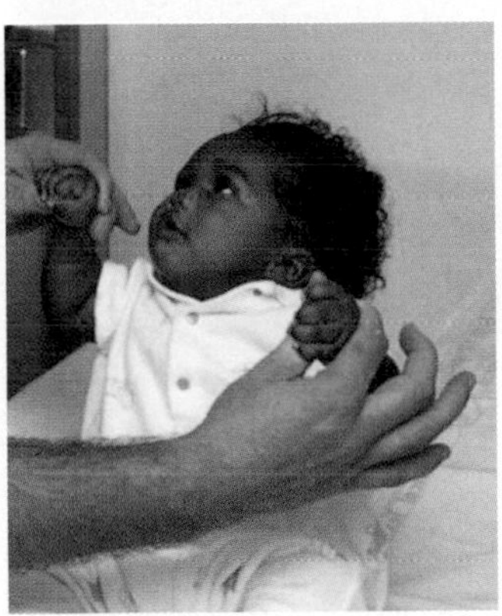

FIGURE 26-53 Infant in prone position in provider's hands

Sensory

In the infant, very few of the sensory procedures will be used. Infants generally have hypoesthesia, therefore requiring a stronger than normal stimulus to elicit any responses. The infant's response to pain is crying and withdraws all extremities. Around 7 to 9 months of age, the infant is able to localize the stimulus and demonstrates a more specific withdrawal.

Reflexes

Deep tendon reflexes that are present in the infant are the biceps, brachioradialis, patellar, and Achilles. When testing reflexes in the infant, use your finger, not a reflex hammer. The results should be the same as for the adult; however, it is not unusual to observe clonus. The Plantar reflex is not of help as a Babinski response is present in infants until 16 to 24 months of age.

Primitive Reflexes

The appearance and disappearance of **primitive reflexes** is of great importance in determining neurological development (Figure 26-54). These reflexes appear in a predictable sequence in relation to the infant's chronological age. When performing these maneuvers, observe the infants movement, which should be smooth and symmetrical. The primitive reflexes are identified and described in Table 26-14.

Unexpected Findings

By 4 months of age the infant should hold the head up and not flop forward.

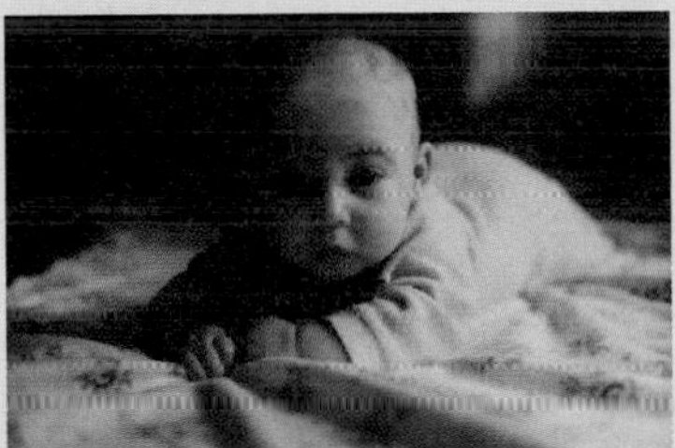

FIGURE 26-52 Infant demonstrating head control

Failure to disappear or to return is an indicator of neurological damage. If the Primitive Reflexes are retained past the first year of life (at the very latest), they can interfere with social, academic, and motor learning. Basically, the perception of our inner and outer environments and our responses to them may be disturbed.

Techniques and Expected Findings

Even more important than their presence is their disappearance because it indicates that the neurological system is maturing and suppressing their actions.

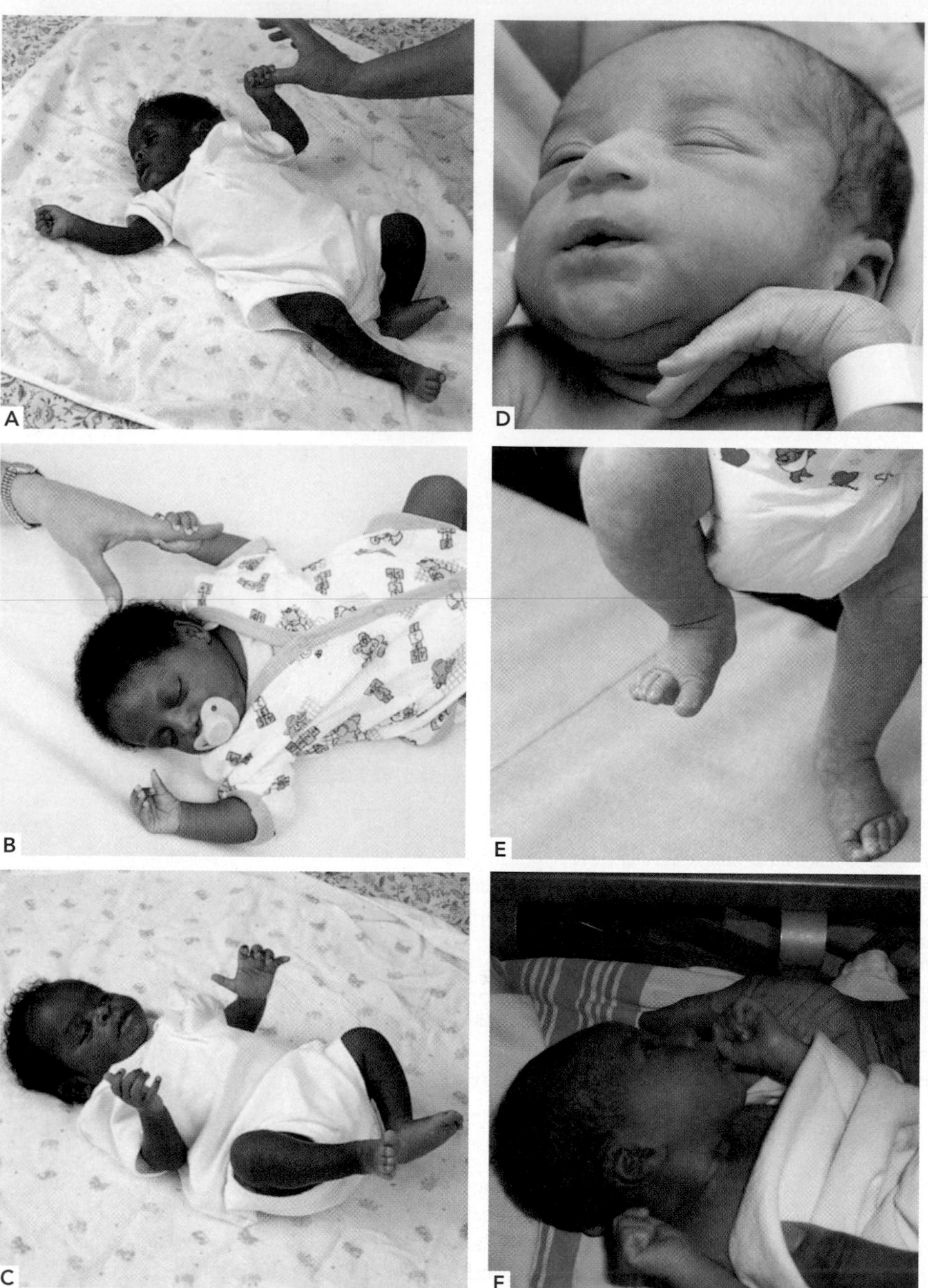

FIGURE 26-54A–F Primitive reflexes. **a)** tonic neck reflex; **b)** palmar grasping reflex; **c)** moro reflex; **d)** rooting reflex; **e)** stepping reflex; **f)** sucking reflex

Source: a, c, d: George Dodson/Lightworks Studio/Pearson Education

Unexpected Findings

Table 26-14 Primitive reflexes

Reflex	Procedure	Expected Results	Appears	Disappears
Rooting	Lightly stroke infant's cheek near mouth	Infant turns head toward stroked side and opens mouth	Birth	3–4 months
Sucking	Touch lips with gloved finger	Infants begins to suck	Birth	10–12 months
Palmar grasp	Place your finger in infants hand, approaching from ulnar side.	Infant grasps fingers (may be able to pull infant to sitting position)	Birth	3–4 months
Plantar grasp	Gently push your thumb into the ball of the infants foot	Toes curl down tightly	Birth	8–10 months
Babinski response	Stroke up the lateral side and across the ball of the infant's foot.	Toes fan out	Birth	18–24 months
Tonic neck reflex (fencing position)	With the infant supine, turn the head to one side with the chin over the shoulder.	Ipsilateral arm and leg extends; opposite side arm and leg flex	2–3 months	4–6 months
Moro	Startle the infant (loud noise, lowering body position rapidly).	Symmetrical abduction and extension of arms and legs, fanning of the fingers, and curling the index finger and thumb to form a C; then brings both arms and legs	Birth	1–4 months
Placing reflex	Position yourself and infant near a table. Hold infant in an upright position with hands under the arms. Let the dorsal (upper) part of the foot touch the underside of the table.	Infant flexes hip and knee followed by extension at the hip to position foot on the top of the table.	After 4 days	Varies
Stepping reflex	Hold infant upright with feet positioned on a flat surface.	Infant takes regular alternating steps.	Birth to 8 weeks	Before voluntary walking
Galant's (truncal incurvation)	Suspend infant in prone position resting on your arm or on a flat surface. Stroke down one side of the infant's back about 4–5 cm from the spine.	Infant curves trunk toward stoked side.	Birth	4–6 months
Landau	Suspend infant in supine position with one hand support upper chest and other hand supporting the abdomen and hips, infants legs should extend from hand supporting hips.	Infant lifts head and extends spine on a horizontal plane.	3 months	12–24 months
Parachute	Firmly support infant while holding prone; lower infant slowly toward a flat surface.	Infant should extend arms/legs in an attempt to protect self.	9 months	Persists

Techniques and Expected Findings	Unexpected Findings

Child

Assessment of the child's neurological system is sequenced in the same manner as for an adult with certain modifications.

Mental Status

Observe the child's behavior during play activities, the reactions to the parent(s), and cooperation with the parent(s) and provider. The Denver II instrument is a valuable tool to evaluate the child's progressive development related to gross and fine motor skills, language, and personal–social skills.

Cranial Nerves

Examination of the cranial nerves requires some modifications to elicit the child's response. Many of the procedures used to test the neurological system may be turned into games to be played with the child. This helps to gain the child's cooperation and makes the examination less threatening. Modifications for the CN exam are identified and described in Table 26-13.

Strabismus

Strabismus is characterized by misalignment of the eyes. When demonstrated, the cover-uncover test may be used. See Chapter 18.

Unexpected Findings: Strabismus is suspected when there is an asymmetric corneal light reflex. It may be described as an esotropia (eye turned inward) or an exotropia (eye turned outward). Strabismus results in amblyopia or double vision.

Motor

The motor assessment can be made by watching the child during play, while on the lap of their parents and performing any activity, and during dressing and undressing. Manipulation of objects is also a way to observe the child's gross and fine motor skills, posture and movement. The Denver II also provides information related to fine and gross motor skills. The child's skills and abilities, as determined by the Denver II, are compared to the developmental milestones that are appropriate for the age of the child.

Unexpected Findings: Developmental reflexes often are not appropriately integrated or inhibited in children with CP. Thus, delay in the disappearance or exaggeration of a developmental reflex may be an early indication of motor disability. An obligatory developmental reflex (a response that persists for as long as the stimulus is applied) is abnormal at any age.

Also observe the child's gait. The child just beginning to walk will have a wide-based gait, whereas the older child will walk with the feet closer together. The older child also has a better sense of balance and is able to recover quicker when unbalanced. Heel-to-toe walking, jumping, and hopping are all skills that develop in the early years. By 4 years of age the child should be able to balance on one foot for about 5 seconds and by age 5 should be able to balance for 8 to 10 seconds.

Observe the child's actions and movements when moving from a supine position to a sitting position and then to a stand. Pay particular attention to the neck, abdominal, arm, and leg muscles. The child should curl up in the midline to sit up and then push off the floor with both hands to stand.

Fine motor coordination may be assessed by the finger-to-nose test. Make sure that the child is capable of understanding the directions for the test. Demonstrate the procedure to the child, and then have the child do it with the eyes open and then with the eyes closed. A child of 4 to 6 will not have fully developed fine motor coordination so if the child comes within 2 to 5 cm (1 to 2 inches) of the nose, it is an acceptable result.

Sensory

Sensation testing is frequently not done in toddlers and preschoolers; their responses are generally not reliable and findings imprecise. Depending on the age and cooperation of the child, light touch may be assessed by having the child point to where the touch or tickling was. Discrimination between rough and smooth surfaces is an alternate method. Test of vibration, position, stereognosis, graphesthesia, or two-point discrimination is routinely not done in children under the age of 6. Superficial pain is generally not tested until the child is older than 6 and then is done in the same manner as with the adult, using a broken tongue blade or bent paper clip. Make sure that the child can differentiate between sharp and dull. When testing graphesthesia, use geometric figures rather than numbers and letters.

Reflexes

DTRs are not tested in children under the age of 5 due to their lack of cooperation and inability to relax. If they are tested, use a finger or edge of the diaphragm on the stethoscope rather than a reflex hammer to strike the tendon. Distraction of the child may be the only way to get the child to relax enough to obtain the reflexes.

Techniques and Expected Findings	Unexpected Findings

Neurological Soft Signs

In some older children, **neurological soft signs** may be present.

Soft signs are developmental, neurological findings that may indicate a possible neurological deficit or maturational delay. They are behaviors and activities that exist past their expected disappearance time and still present in a child.

Soft signs can be apparent in fine and gross motor, sensory, and reflex functions. When multiple soft signs are present in a child, the probability the child will have learning disabilities increases. Soft signs are identified and described in Table 26-15.

Table 26-15 Neurological: developmental soft signs

Activity	Soft Sign Indicators	Age for Concern If Indicators Still Present
Walking, running gait	Stiff legged with a foot slapping quality, unusual posturing of the arms	3 years
Heel walking	Difficulty remaining on heels for a distance of 10 feet	7 years
Tiptoe walking	Difficulty remaining on toes for a distance of 10 feet	7 years
Tandem gait	Difficulty walking heel-to-toe, unusual posturing of arms	7 years
One foot standing	Unable to remain standing on one foot longer than 5–10 seconds	5 years
Hopping in place	Unable to rhythmically hop on each foot	6 years
Motor stance	Difficulty maintaining stance (arms extended in front, feet together, and eyes closed), drifting of arms, mild writhing movements of hands or fingers	3 years
Visual tracking	Difficulty following object with eyes when keeping the head still; nystagmus	5 years
Rapid thumb to finger test	Rapid touching thumb to fingers in sequence is uncoordinated; unable to suppress mirror movements in contra lateral hand	8 years
Rapid alternating movements of hands	Irregular speed and rhythm with pronation and supination of hands patting the knees	10 years
Finger to nose test	Unable to alternately touch provider's finger and own nose	7 years
Right-left discrimination	Unable to identify right and left sides of own body	5 years
Two-point discrimination	Difficulty in localizing and discriminating when touched in one or two places	6 years
Graphesthesia	Unable to identify geometric shapes drawn in child's open hand	8 years
Stereognosis	Unable to identify common objects placed in own hand	5 years

The Pregnant Woman

The neurological examination of the pregnant female is the same as that for a nopregnant female of the identical age. Deep tendon reflexes should be obtained on the initial visit to serve as baseline responses.

Hyperreactive reflexes are a concern for the development of pre-eclampsia.

The Older Adult

The neurological exam for the older adult is the same as for the adult. These patients may have a slower response time to instructions, especially those that require coordination of movements. Knowledge of the patient's medications is important to determine if their actions on the nervous system are responsible for slowness of response time and tremors or anxiety.

Techniques and Expected Findings	Unexpected Findings
Cranial Nerves	
Although smell and taste are frequently not done, the elderly often demonstrate a decreased sensation for both.	The sweet and salt tastes are impaired first. Other changes in the cranial nerves include a reduced upward gaze and convergence, sluggish papillary response to light changes, decreased corneal reflex, middle to high frequency loss, and a diminished gag reflex.
Motor	
A decreased bulk of muscles is often observed and is most apparent in the hands, which is manifest by guttering between the metacarpals. The muscles of the dorsal hand often appear wasted even when there is no joint dysfunction. Grip strength remains quite strong despite the thin, atrophic appearance of the hands.	
The gait of an elderly individual may be slower and more deliberate with slight anteroflexion of the upper body and slight flexion of the arms and knees. The gait is characterized by short, uncertain steps due to a diminished sense of proprioception. Shuffling may be observed as speed and balance diminish with age.	
Other observations related to motor activity include **senile tremors** and **dyskinesias**. Senile tremors (also known as *essential, familial tremors*) are common, benign tremors that include intention tremors of the hand, head nodding up and down, and tongue protrusions. Dyskinesias are the repetitive movements in the jaw, lips, or tongue that may accompany senile tremors.	These are distinguished from Parkinson's tremors in that they are not associated with rigidity, which is characteristic of Parkinsonism tremors.
Sensory	
Sensory changes in the elderly adult include impaired vibration and tactile sensation, as well as impaired position sense. A stronger stimulus may be needed for the patient to feel these sensations.	
Reflexes	
The older adult commonly demonstrates a diminished response or even absent deep tendon reflexes. The lower extremities are often affected before the upper extremities. The Achilles and plantar reflex may be difficult to obtain and may even be absent in some older adults. Superficial reflexes may also be absent.	

DOCUMENTATION

Documentation will represent a comprehensive examination. Whatever procedures and techniques used for a neurological exam should be documented as such.

Mental Status Documentation for mental status is provided in Chapter 7 (LOC/orientation is a component of the Mental Status Documentation).

Cranial nerves

CN I -Correctly identifies and discriminates odors bilaterally

CN II—Vision 20/20 OS, 20/30 OD uncorrected, 20/20 -2 both eyes uncorrected. Visual fields without and field deficits.

CN III, IV, and VI—No ptosis demonstrated, EOMs intact with smooth, conjugate movement through 6 cardinal fields of vision.

CN V—Equal muscle contraction palpated bilaterally. Correctly identifies touch in 3 divisions of CN V, correctly differentiates between sharp and dull touch in 3 divisions. Corneal reflex with bilateral blink.

CN VII—Symmetrical and equal facial movements demonstrated in all expressions. Able to maintain closure of eyelids against resistance. Able to sense and differentiate sweet a salt tastes on tongue.

CN VIII—Able to repeat whispered words correctly. Able to hear finger rub equally bilaterally. Weber test without lateralization, Rinne test with AC 2X BC bilaterally.

CN IX, X—Swallows effortlessly. Uvula and soft palate rise midline upon phonation. Gag reflex present bilaterally. Able to sense and differentiate between bitter and sour tastes on tongue.

CN XI—Shoulder shrug equal bilaterally. Able to turn head in both directions and maintain position against resistance.

CN XII—Tongue protrudes midline. Pushes against tongue blade equally bilaterally.

Motor: Proprioception and Cerebellar Systems

Coordination and Fine Motor Skills

Rapid arm movements and leg crossing and uncrossing movements smooth and coordinated; finger to thumb movements smooth and coordinated at rapid pace. Able to touch nose with finger and correctly locates provider's finger at different spatial positions. Able to run heel straight down opposite leg with smooth and coordinated movements.

Balance and equilibrium

Able to maintain self in upright position with eyes closed for 30 seconds. Able to recover balance when pushed. Able to maintain balance on one foot for 5 seconds, and able to hop in place on each foot without losing balance.

Gait with smooth and coordinated movements, equal time in swing and stance phase with opposite arm swing. Able to walk heel to toe forward and backward without difficulty. Maintains consistent contact between heels and toes.

Sensory

Primary Sensations

Correctly identifies superficial touch and pain sensations over extremities, abdomen, and chest, differentiating between sharp and dull correctly. Differentiates warm and cold correctly over same areas. Squeezing the trapezius muscle produced discomfort bilaterally.

Vibration sensations felt bilaterally equal over thumb joints, knees, and toes. Correctly identifies position of great toes when moved up or down.

Cortical Sensory Functions

Correctly identifies a key and paper clip in R and L hand respectively. Correctly identifies the letters D and M, and the numbers 8 and 4 in the R and L hand respectively. Able to feel two points at 4 mm on the fingertips, and 70 mm on upper arms. Able to feel touch simultaneously on contralateral areas of the body. Able to correctly locate point of touch after stimulus withdrawn.

Reflexes

Superficial Reflexes

Abdominal reflexes present in all 4 quadrants. (Male) Testicle rises on same side as stimulus. Toes with plantar flexion bilaterally after sole of foot stroked.

Deep Tendon Reflexes

DTR	R	L
Biceps	+2	+2
Triceps	+2	+2
Brachioradialis	+2	+2
Patellar	+2	+2
Achilles	+2	+2

Electronic Charting

Expectations of Electronic Charting

Electronic charting for the neurological system should be tailored to the specific needs of the specialty. Charting templates can help clinicians to organize and document detailed neurological examinations. Other templates can remind clinicians to ask pertinent questions of patients with specific disorders such as multiple sclerosis or Parkinson's disease. Almost any form of electronic charting should include calculators for scores such as the Glasgow Coma Scale, function independence measures, and other scoring algorithms. Calculators for common scales are even available for personal digital assistants (PDAs). Ideally, calculators and templates should be "smart" forms that are "aware" of other patient data, for example, by presenting the clinician with age-appropriate versions of templates and scales.

Continuous monitoring of the central nervous system is common in the intensive care unit. Intracranial pressure is a common form of continuous monitoring, but many other techniques exist for continuous CNS monitoring. All such devices should, ideally, record their findings directly into electronic charting systems.

Computers are integrated into most neurological evaluation equipment, such as EEGs and EMGs. Decision support algorithms integrated within the equipment can aid in detecting specific waveforms, and can combine multiple measurements to create reports that assist with easier recognition of abnormal findings. Picture archiving and communications systems (PACS) store images electronically, and give clinicians rapid access to diagnostic images and reports.

Limitations of Electronic Charting

Use of electronic charting in general is growing rapidly, but electronic charting for specialties such as neurology lags behind general usage. The reason, in part, is because medical records must be tailored for the specific needs of the specialty; a detailed neurological examination requires a much different level of detail than routine assessments.

Decision support algorithms integrated into neurological evaluation equipment can assist with interpretation of the signals. Many of these systems, however, have a high rate of false positive results; for example, it is common to have the automated system indicate that an EEG shows epileptic waveform patterns that are not relevant to the clinical situation. As with any automated system, preliminary reports generated by the equipment should be interpreted with caution until the test result is analyzed by an expert.

There is a lack of universal standards for how to document the unique needs of neurological examinations. However, progress is being made and such standards may exist within the next few years.

Summary

- The neurological system is distributed throughout the body and controls multiple physiological and mental activities. Because of this, observation is the primary assessment technique necessary to assess the neurological system.
- The largest components of the neurological system are the brain and spinal cord that are connected to each other at the foramen magnum at the base of the cranial vault. The brain and spinal cord receive and interpret stimuli that are delivered to them by afferent and efferent nerves throughout the body.
- There are two divisions of the neurological system, the central (CNS) and peripheral (PNS) systems. The CNS consists of the brain and spinal cord while the PNS consists of the spinal and cranial nerves. The PNS is also further divided into the autonomic nervous system, which consists of the sympathetic and parasympathetic divisions.
- The patient history is focused on the presence of pain (headaches), neuropathy, dizziness, paresthesias, tremors, seizures, weakness as indicators of nervous system conditions or alterations.
- The neurological examination consists of five specific areas for assessment: level of consciousness, cranial nerves, motor function, sensory function, and reflexes. Each level of examination assesses part of each area.
- While the neurological system is complex, many of the assessment techniques are quite simple to perform and observe; however, documentation is not as simple and should describe the patient's ability to perform each test.
- Unexpected results of the neurological system are not necessarily life threatening or altering and even significant alterations may result in devastating consequences, but may still allow individuals to live a meaningful and productive life.

Review Questions

1. To assess a patient's cerebral functioning, the provider would ask the patient which of the following?
   1. "Have you experienced and dizziness in the past month?"
   2. "Have you noticed any change in your muscle strength?"
   3. "Have you experienced any loss of memory in the past 6 months?"
   4. "Have you noticed any heart rhythm disturbances recently?"
2. To assess patient's level of consciousness, the provider should initially use which of the following?
   1. verbal stimuli
   2. painful stimuli
   3. olfactory stimuli
   4. tactile stimuli
3. When assessing a patient's cerebellar function, the provider would want to observe the patient doing which of the following?
   1. changing position in a chair
   2. walking into the exam room
   3. eating a meal
   4. rolling over in bed
4. When assessing the patient with head trauma, the provider should pay particular attention to which of the following?
   1. pupil reaction
   2. corneal reflex
   3. nystagmus
   4. extraocular movements
5. When assessing the patient's reflexes, to obtain the Achilles reflex, the provider would hit the tendon located
   1. in the patient's antecubital fossa.
   2. just below the knee.
   3. behind the ankle.
   4. just above the wrist.
6. During the assessment of a 1-year-old, after stroking the bottom of the infant's foot, the provider observes dorsiflexion of the great toe with fanning of the toes. This finding is generally associated with which of the following?
   1. developmental delay
   2. expected findings
   3. hyperreflexia
   4. clonus
7. During the health history, the provider asks the patient if she has experienced any paresthesias. The patient indicates that she doesn't understand what the provider is asking. To clarify, the provider should ask the patient if she ever experienced sensations related to which of the following?
   1. shooting pain
   2. double vision
   3. dizziness and vertigo
   4. numbness and tingling
8. The patient is able to touch his nose with his finger for both upper extremities. Based on this finding, the provider is able to conclude that the patient's
   1. CNs III, IV, and VI are functioning normally.
   2. reflex arcs are intact.
   3. cerebellum is intact.
   4. brain stem is functioning.
9. The provider is performing a neurological assessment on a 5-year-old child. The provider would be concerned if which neurological soft signs are noted in the assessment? (Select all that apply.)
   1. running with a stiff-legged gait and foot slapping quality
   2. maintaining toe walking for only 5 feet
   3. inability to remain standing on one foot for 5 seconds
   4. inability to identify common objects when placed in the hand
   5. inability to identify right and left side on their own body
10. To assess the motor function of a CN X the provider should ask the patient to do which of the following? (Select all that apply.)
    1. Identify a common object placed in the hand.
    2. Read aloud from a newspaper.
    3. Differentiate sharp from blunt stimuli.
    4. Drink water from a cup.
    5. Smile.

Conditions and Disorders

Stroke

Sometimes referred to by the older term **cerebrovascular accident (CVA)**, stroke is the rapid loss of brain function due to an interrupted or severely reduced blood supply to a part of the brain. Strokes are often preceded by **transient ischemic attacks** (TIA), transient neurologic dysfunction caused by focal brain, retinal or spinal cord ischemia without infarction, which is defined by the absence of end organ injury. These are essentially mini strokes that often cause no permanent disability, but are a warning sign that a stroke may be eminent. Symptoms are not dissimilar from stoke (see below), but they are transient, lasting minutes in low flow TIA and hours in embolic TIAs. Their recognition is important as these patients may benefit from preventive therapy or revascularization of the large vessel like the carotid artery.

Pathophysiology

- Brain tissue ceases to function if deprived of O_2 for more than 60–90 seconds; after approximately 3 hours brain tissue suffers irreversible injury possibly leading to death, (infarction.)
- Atherosclerosis disrupts the blood supply by narrowing the lumen of blood vessels causing a reduction of blood supply by the formation of blood clots within the vessels.
- Embolic infarction occurs when emboli formed elsewhere in the circulatory system, typically the heart, as a consequence of atrial fibrillation, or in the carotid arteries, break off, enter the cerebral circulation, then lodge in and occlude brain blood vessels.
- Hemorrhagic strokes result in tissue injury by causing compression of tissue from an expanding hematoma or hematomas. This can distort and injure tissue. In addition, the pressure may lead to a loss of blood supply to affected tissue with resulting infarction, and the blood released by brain hemorrhage appears to have direct toxic effects on brain tissue and vasculature Inflammation contributes to the secondary brain injury after hemorrhage.

Subjective Data

- Symptoms typically start suddenly, over seconds to minutes, and most commonly do not progress further.

Symptoms depend on the area of the brain affected; the more extensive the area of brain involved, the more functions most likely to be lost. They may include:

- Stumbling, sudden dizziness, loss of balance/coordination, or trouble walking.
- Trouble with speaking and understanding, confusion, word slurring, difficulty understanding speech.
- Facial, arm, or leg paralysis or numbness that may develop suddenly, especially on one side of the body.
- One side of the mouth may droop when trying to smile.
- Trouble with seeing in one or both eyes, such as suddenly blurred or blackened vision, or seeing double.
- A sudden, severe headache, which may be accompanied by vomiting, dizziness, or altered consciousness.

Objective Data

- Various findings are able to predict the presence or absence of stroke to different degrees.
- Sudden-onset face weakness, arm drift (a person, when asked to raise both arms, involuntarily lets one arm drift downward), and abnormal speech are the findings most likely to lead to the identification of a case of stroke.
- Similarly, when all three of these are absent, the likelihood of stroke is significantly decreased.

Meningitis/Meningoencephalitis

Refers to the inflammations of the leptomeninges surrounding the brain and spinal cord and may be caused by bacteria, virus, mycobacteria, fungaus, spirochetes, or parasites. **Bacterial meningitis** can be community or hospital acquired. Most common pathogens for community acquired meningitis are streptococcus pneumonia, neisseria mengitidis, and listeria monocytogenes. Staphylococcus and gram negative bacilli are the most common offending organisms in hospital acquired. **Viral meningitis** is caused by common viruses, such as enteroviruses, HSV, HIV, West Nile, herpes, mumps and LCM (lymphocytis choriomeningitis virus). Encephalitis is distinguished from meningitis by the presence of cerebral dysfunction like altered mental status, motor and sensory deficits, altered behavior and personality changes, speech or movement disorders. **Aseptic meningitis** refers to meningitis with negative culture.

The differentiation may be difficult as some patients will present with both clinical features, thus the term meningoencephalitis.

Pathophysiology

- Caused by invasion of the meninges by bacteria, either through the blood stream or direct extension from the sinuses, skull fractures, indwelling catheters.

Subjective Data

- Fever
- Stiff neck
- Headache increased with a jolt (induced by rapidly rotating head to sides)
- Change in mental status like lethargy and confusion

Objective Data

- High fever, in small number of cases may have hypothermia
- Nuchal rigidity
- +Kernig's
- +Brudzinski
- Lethargy

- Microorganism penetrates the blood–brain barrier leading to more inflammation and release of cytokines that stimulate other tissues to participate in an immune response.
- The blood–brain barrier becomes more permeable, leading to edema. that leads to increased intracranial pressure, making it difficult for blood to enter the brain, depriving brain cells of oxygen resulting in brain, cell death.

- Arthralgias
- Rash
- Photophobia
- Nausea
- Vomiting
- Diarrhea may be present in viral meningitis
- Blurred vision
- Phonophobia
- Irritability, drowsiness, and poor feeding in infants

- Obtundation
- Altered sensorium
- Seizures
- Papilledema
- Focal neurological deficits
- Ataxia, nystagmus, and cranial nerve palsies have been associated with *Listeria monocytogenes* caused meningitis. Petechia and purpura are caused by *Nisseria meningitidis* meningitis.
- Arthritis
- Hearing loss may be a late manifestation.
- Bulging fontanel in infants
- Hypotension, sepsis, and circulatory collapse in extreme cases with bleeding from DIC (disseminated intravascular coagulation)
- Decreased LOC, posturing, cranial nerve abnormalities and loss of papillary reflex as brain swells and herniation occurs.

Multiple Sclerosis (MS)

MS is the most common autoimmune and inflammatory demyelinating disease of the central nervous system. The disorder is characterized by relapses and remissions and affects younger women more than men with 1.4–2.3: 1 ratio. Higher frequencies are in geographic areas like Northern Europe, Southern Canada, Northern U.S., New Zealand, and Australia. Asians, African and American Indians seem to be less affected. There is some genetic susceptibility and vitamin D seems protective. Progression of disability is variable but it is usually slow. Progressive rather than relapsing disease is a poor prognosticator.

Pathophysiology

- Main characteristics are the formation of lesions (plaques), inflammation, and myelin destruction. These features interact in complex, not yet fully understood ways to produce the characteristic neurodegeneration and in turn the clinical symptoms of the disease.
- Damage is believed to be caused by the person's own immune system attacking the nervous system.
- Proposed pathogenesis include inflammatory and autoimmune activation followed by neurodegeneration leading to activation of lymphocytes and macrophages leading to blood brain–barrier disruption, myelin, oligodendrocytes and axonal loss.

Subjective Data

Multiple symptoms at the onset such as the following:

- Visual symptoms—scotomas, central vision loss, double vision (diplopia)
- Sensory symptoms (dysesthesias) in limbs or face manifested by pain, numbness, tingling, tightness, cold sensation, radicular pain, and intense itching
- Problems with gait and balance, pain, ataxia, vertigo, bladder incontinence, neurogenic bladder
- Lhermitte's sign (electric shocklike sensation through back and limb when the neck is flexed)
- Fatigue
- Trigeminal neuralgia
- Painful tonic spasms
- Bowel dysfunction (constipation and incontinence)
- Sexual dysfunction
- Heat sensitivity
- Depression

Objective Data

- Acute transverse myelopathy
- Optic neuritis—acute or subacute
- Marcus Gunn pupil
- Disc edema and optic cup pallor
- Atypical vibration and position sense
- Decreased pain and light touch—patchy in distribution in the face, limbs, and trunk (nondermatomal)
- Uhthoff phenomenon—increase in body heat
- Cognitive dysfunction like diminished speed in processing information, mild memory impairment, not frank dementia
- Motor: Paraparesis, paraplegia
- DTRs may be hyperreflexic with clonus or may be diminished
- Spasticity
- Gait and coordination disorder, intention tremors in the limbs and head, nystagmus
- Slurred speech, scanning speech

Amyotrophic Lateral Sclerosis (ALS), Lou Gehrig's Disease, or Motor Neuron Disease (MND)

ALS is a relentless, mixed motor neuron neurodegenerative disorder that leads to a linear pattern of progressive weakness, disability, and eventually death. There are no relapses or remission. The symptoms and signs progress in a linear function. It is now known that it shares similar etiology and pathophysiology with primary lateral sclerosis, primary muscular atrophy, and progressive bulbar palsy. ALS affects both upper and lower motor neurons. Its cause is unknown.

Pathophysiology

- Alteration in RNA processing, superoxide dismutase I mediated toxicity, cytologic and mitochondrial derangement, inflammatory activation and growth factor abnormalities have been proposed to contribute to the pathogenesis of ALS.

Subjective Data

- Asymmetric limb weakness is one of the most common initial symptoms. It may begin as hand or shoulder weakness or foot drop.
- Weakness, incoordination, and stiffness, poor hand dexterity, spastic gait, imbalance
- Bulbar symptoms like dysarthria with slow speech and strained voice
- Dysphagia—swallowing difficulty leading to choking and coughing with swallowing
- Cramps
- Heavy legs
- Tripping, falls
- Paresthesias
- Respiratory muscle weakness
- Weight loss (less common)
- Autonomic symptoms like excessive sweating and constipation are later complaints.

Objective Data

- Progressive unilateral weakness that starts in the limb and progresses to involve the contralateral side is the common initial presentation. It also affects the bulbar and axial regions.
- The presence of upper and lower motor neuron signs in one limb is suggestive of ALS.
- Lower motor neuron signs like weakness and atrophy of muscles fasciculations.
- Upper motor neuron signs like increased tone, spasticity, clonus, increased reflexes, and Babinski.
- Pathologic reflexes like crossed adductors, jaw jerk, and Hoffman's sign
- Slowness of movement
- Gait abnormalities like spastic gait
- Imbalance
- Foot drop
- Extrapyramidal signs (tremor, bradykinesia, postural instability, as in Parkinson's) and supranuclear palsy.
- Subtle frontotemporal cognitive dysfunction may precede or follow the motor neuron presentation.
- Pseudobulbar affect (crying and uncontrolled laughter)
- Dysarthria
- Diaphragmatic and respiratory muscle weakness leads to respiratory depression.

Myasthenia Gravis (MG)

MG is a common neuromuscular condition in which weakness is caused by circulating antibodies that block acetylcholine receptors at the post-synaptic neuromuscular junction. The hallmark of the condition is a fluctuating degree of weakness in the ocular, bulbar, limb, and respiratory muscles. MG is associated with various autoimmune diseases like Hashimoto's and Graves, DM Type I, SLE, rheumatoid arthritis and demyelinating CNS diseases.

Pathophysiology

- MG is autoimmune disorder with antibodies directed against the nicotinic acetylcholine receptor and the motor end plate receptor that stimulates muscular contractions.

Subjective Data

- Muscle weakness worsens with sustained effort and improves with rest.

Common symptoms are as follows:

- Weakness and fatigue of a specific muscle group
- Muscles of eye and eyelid movement, facial expressions, chewing, talking, and swallowing are especially susceptible. The muscles that control breathing and neck and limb movements can also be affected.
- Diplopia
- Dysphagia
- Dysarthria

Objective Data

- Signs are worse with continuous effort or activity
- Ptosis
- Weakness of facial muscles
- Respiratory muscle paralysis
- Proximal muscle weakness
- Dropped head syndrome due to neck extensors weakness

Guillain-Barré Syndrome (GBS)

GBS is an acute immune-mediated polyneuropathy, affecting the peripheral nervous system that is usually triggered by an infection. It can result in life-threatening complications, particularly if the respiratory muscles are affected or there is autonomic nervous system involvement. Symptom progression is usually 2 to 4 weeks. Symptoms lasting more than 8 weeks are suggestive of chronic inflammatory demyelinating polyradiculopathy. Recovery is expected starting 2–4 weeks, after disease progression halts.

Guillain-Barré syndrome is rare, at 1–2 cases per 100,000 people annually; but is the most common cause of acute nontrauma-related paralysis. If nerve cell body is not destroyed, peripheral nerve regeneration may take place; if nerve cell body dies, unable to regenerate.

Recovery usually starts after the fourth week from the onset of the disorder. Approximately 80% of patients have a complete recovery within a few months to a year, although minor findings may persist, such as areflexia. About 5%–10% recover with severe disability, with most of such cases involving severe proximal motor and sensory axonal damage with inability of axonal regeneration.

Pathophysiology

- It is postulated that an acute infection like respiratory or gastrointestinal infections trigger an immune response directed toward the myelin and axons of the peripheral nerves.
- Campylobacter infection is the most common infection causing GBS, but it has also been caused by, flu, and meningococcal vaccinations, viral infections (cytomegalo hepatitis, Herpes simplex/ zoster, HIV), bacterial infections (H–influenza, E-coli) after surgery, trauma, or bone marrow transplantation.

Subjective Data

- Paresthesias, in fingers, toes, or both that may spread to upper body
- Muscle weakness that results in unsteady gait and can evolve into paralysis.
- Difficulty with eye movement, facial movement, speaking, chewing or swallowing
- Severe pain in lower back
- Difficulty with bladder control or intestinal functions
- Difficulty breathing
- Lack of sweating
- Palpitations

Objective Data

- Symmetric muscle weakness to paralysis with absent or diminishes deep tendon reflexes. The signs progresses over a period of 2 weeks.
- Severe respiratory depression in about 10%–30% of cases; oculomotor weakness may be present.
- Autonomic dysfunction like tachycardia, urinary retention, orthostasis, bradycardia in some cases, ileus, lack of sweating and arrhythmias occur about 60%–70% of cases.
- Diagnosis is usually made by nerve conduction studies and studies of the cerebrospinal fluid.
- Rapid heart rate
- Low or high blood pressure

Trigeminal Neuralgia or Tic Douloureux

This refers to the paroxysmal intense, incapacitating, sharp or stabbing facial pain along the trigeminal nerve distribution. It is one of the most common causes of facial neuralgia especially in the elderly. The attacks tend to wax and wane, with each attack typically lasting for few seconds to minutes. Remission sometimes last few months to a few years.

TN affects lifestyle choices as common activities (triggers) such as eating, talking, shaving, and brushing teeth can initiate an attack. Wind, high-pitched sounds, loud noises such as concerts or crowds, chewing, and talking aggravates the condition in many patients.

Pathophysiology

- Usually caused (80%–90%) by compression of the trigeminal nerve root by an aberrant loop of veins or arteries as it enters the pons.
- Other causes may be from schwannomas (acoustic neuroma), meningioma, epidermoid cysts, AVM or aneurysms.
- Chronic compression causes injury to the myelin sheath of the nerve.

Subjective Data

- Intense, severe unilateral pain in any of distribution of the trigeminal nerve (CN V). It may be bilateral. It commonly involves the V_2 (maxillary) and V_3 (mandibular) branches of the trigeminal nerve.
- Pain described as stabbing electric shocks, burning, pressing, crushing, exploding, or shooting pain that becomes intractable.
- Dull pain in between attacks
- Facial spasms
- Trigger areas along the distribution of the nerve, primarily near the midline, when touched during an examination may initiate the onset of an attack.

Objective Data

- There are no classical manifestations of TN as it is primarily related to pain.
- Facial expressions would characterize pain, but nothing that is specific to TN.

Cerebral Palsy (CP)

CP is a term that describes a group of disorders of movement, muscle tone, or posture that is caused by injury or abnormal development in the immature brain, most often before birth. The diagnosis of cerebral palsy (CP) depends upon a combination of findings, including motor delay, neurologic signs, persistence of primitive reflexes, and atypical postural reflexes. Infants with expected functional development and behavior who have mild hypertonia or hyperreflexia should be observed. If these manifestations remain isolated, in most cases will resolve progressively after the child reaches 9 months of age.

Pathophysiology

- Etiology is unknown but thought to be injury to the developing brain from hypoxia, infection, asphyxia, or trauma during pregnancy, delivery, or a few years after birth. CP more commonly seen in multiple births and prematurity.

Subjective Data

- Data for the history will most likely come from parents.
- Typical history includes poor feeding in the neonatal period. The baby often is irritable, sleeps poorly, vomits frequently, is difficult to handle and cuddle, and has poor visual attention
- Neurobehavioral indicators suspicious for CP are excessive docility or irritability.
- Babies may be stiff or floppy with spinal curvature, small head
- Delays in reaching motor skills milestones, such as pushing up on arms, sitting up alone, or crawling
- Favoring one side of the body, such as reaching with only one hand or dragging a leg while crawling

Objective Data

- Contractures
- Stiff muscles with normal reflexes (rigidity) or exaggerated reflexes (spasticity)
- Balance and muscle coordination difficulty (ataxia). Difficulty with precise motions, such as picking up a crayon or spoon.
- Tremors or involuntary movements (athetosis)
- Abnormal oral motor patterns include tongue retraction and thrust, tonic bite, oral hypersensitivity, and grimacing. Excessive drooling or difficulty with swallowing. Difficulty with sucking or eating
- Delays in speech development or difficulty speaking due to large range of jaw movement and inappropriate placement of the tongue during articulation
- Poor head control may be an early motor sign. However, increased neck extensor and axial tone may make head control appear better than it actually is.

Spinal Cord Injury (SCI)

SCI is damage to the spinal cord resulting in either temporary or permanent neurologic deficits or disability in the cord's motor, sensory, or autonomic functions. Accidental injury is the most frequent cause of SCI, which may be due to motor vehicle accidents, falls, sports injuries, recreational activities (diving into shallow water), industrial accidents, gunshot wounds, and assault (Zieve & Hoch, 2012). Other causes may be related to conditions that can affect the tissue and bones that surround and protect the spinal cord. Conditions that weaken bone structure such as osteoporosis and rheumatoid arthritis may cause collapse or fractures of the vertebrae from trauma that ordinarily would not cause SCI. Narrowing of the vertebral foramen (spinal stenosis) may impinge on the spinal cord. Events that cause swelling of the spinal cord due to inflammation or hemorrhage also result in damage to the spinal cord.

Pathophysiology

- The primary pathology associated with SCI is a transection of the cord, resulting in its inability to transmit nerve impulses to and from the brain below the level of injury.
- Determining the extent of damage and classification of the injury is generally not possible until approximately 72 hours after the initial incident due to the inflammatory response that causes swelling in and around the spinal cord that may cause some temporary symptoms that will resolve once the swelling is reduced.

Subjective Data

Immediate symptoms of spinal cord injury after an accident may include the following:

- Significant back pain or pressure in the neck, head or back. Pain/intense stinging sensation caused by damage to the nerve fibers in spinal cord.
- Weakness, lack of coordination or paralysis in any part of the body
- Numbness, tingling or loss of sensation in hands, fingers, feet or toes
- Loss of sensation, including the ability to feel heat, cold and touch
- Loss of bladder or bowel control
- Difficulty with balance and walking

Objective Data

- The degree and severity of damage to physiological systems is determined by the level of the spinal cord that is damaged as well as the extent of damage to the cord.

Classification of SCI is determined by whether the injury causes any of the following:

- **paraplegia** (loss of muscle strength in lower extremities) or
- **tetraplegia** (loss of muscle strength in all 4 extremities) and if the damage is incomplete or complete.

Combining these terms results in four classifications:

- Incomplete tetraplegia

- Incomplete cord lesions may evolve into more complete lesions.
- More commonly, the injury level rises 1 or 2 spinal levels during the hours to days after the initial event. A complex cascade of pathophysiologic events involving free radicals, vasogenic edema, and altered blood flow accounts for this clinical deterioration.
- Adequate oxygenation, perfusion, and acid–base balance are necessary to prevent extension of the spinal cord injury.

- Impaired breathing after injury
- An oddly positioned or twisted neck or back

- Complete tetraplegia
- Incomplete paraplegia
- Complete paraplegia
- Spinal cord damage within the cervical vertebrae results in tetraplegia; damage to the other sections of vertebrae produce paraplegia.
- A complete classification indicates that there is a complete loss of motor and sensory function below the level of cord injury.
- An incomplete classification is associated with variable sensory and motor losses.

27

Bones and Muscles

From what I read about patients with myotonic dystrophy, Mrs. Styler will be lucky if she's ever discharged. Only 49, she's been in and out of hospitals over the past few years for respiratory problems. Most recently, on a trip to Europe, she developed pneumonia and after 3 months, has not bounced back, and is unable to breathe on her own. Her muscular weakness is profound. She can hardly hold her eyelids closed, nor plantar flex her ankles against minimal resistance. Mr. Styler told me that the clues to his wife's disease had been present for a long time, recalling that when they were dating in their 20s, she "had a funny gait." Pulling out old photos, he pointed out the temporal wasting characteristic of the condition, even when Mrs. Styler was a teenager. Despite these signs, the diagnosis was not made until she was 46.

Now, Mrs. Styler has been hospitalized for more than a month, making steady progress toward extubation. Every day I repeated her neuro and strength examination. She was moderately sedated to help her tolerate the mechanical ventilator. I noted the settings—tidal volume, respiratory rate, peak inspiratory pressure. On the third week, we began weaning her from the ventilator. She tolerated this well, maintaining her oxygen saturation levels.

On the fifth week, we gather around her bedside to remove her breathing tube. My eyes are glued to her vital sign monitor, and it is only when I hear her husband sobbing that I take in what is happening around me. Mr. Styler has not heard his wife speak in more than 120 days. For all practical purposes, I have known her only as a series of parameters and lab results. She is not a machine, but a real person. The resident pulls the breathing tube back through her trachea and out her mouth. Mrs. Styler coughs heavily, catches her breath, and we all witness her first words: "Thank you."

LEARNING OUTCOMES

1. Explain the composition, structure, and function of the musculoskeletal system.
2. Describe the expected findings associated with examination of the musculoskeletal system.
3. Compare and contrast the manifestation of altered conditions of the musculoskeletal system.
4. Describe age-related changes that affect the composition, structure, and function of the musculoskeletal system.
5. Describe appropriate techniques and procedures used to assess the musculoskeletal system.
6. Document history and characteristics of the musculoskeletal system related to assessment findings.

The bones and muscles provide the framework, stability, and mobility for the body. Bones have the unique characteristics of being hard, strong, and inflexible, accounting for their weight-bearing capability. In addition to weight bearing, bones protect various sections of the body as well as provide areas for blood cell production.

Muscles are attached to bones at various points and function as pulleys to move the joints and engage in the work of the body. Work and movement are carried out by flexion and extension of various muscle groups. Muscles also provide strength for work. Muscles comprise the bulk of the composition of the body and also give the body its characteristic form and shape. Injuries to bones and muscles are common as they are often subjected to trauma in their role of protecting the body from external forces.

Structure and Function

Bone

Bone consists of osteocytes (bone cells) that are embedded within a matrix of collagen, calcium carbonate and calcium phosphate (Figure 27-1). These elements, when combined, form hydroxyapatite, the substance that provides bones with strength and density. The four different types of bones are based on their shape and structure, which also determines their function (Table 27-1). The major function of bones is to form the skeleton, an interconnection of joints and levers that provide for various types and degrees of movement. The point where two bones come together and articulate is the joint. Joints with the greatest degree of movement are those that are formed by connections between or with long bones. The degree of joint movement is the most common way of classifying the joints (Table 27-2).

Diarthrotic joints are also described as synovial joints. These joints provide the greatest amount of freedom, but also experience the most wear and tear. To reduce the risk of damage from constant use, synovial joints have extra components. The ends of bones creating the joint are covered with cartilage—a tough, smooth, and flexible protective tissue that reduces friction and allows the bone ends to glide over each other. These joints are also surrounded by synovial tissue that creates the joint capsule. The synovial tissue contains cells that secrete synovial fluid that provides lubrication for the joints as well as nourishment for the cartilage.

Diarthrotic joints are held together by ligaments, which are strong, dense, flexible cords of collagen and elastic connective tissue fibers and provide support by attaching bones in various ways. They may encircle a joint, by gripping it obliquely, or by lying parallel to the

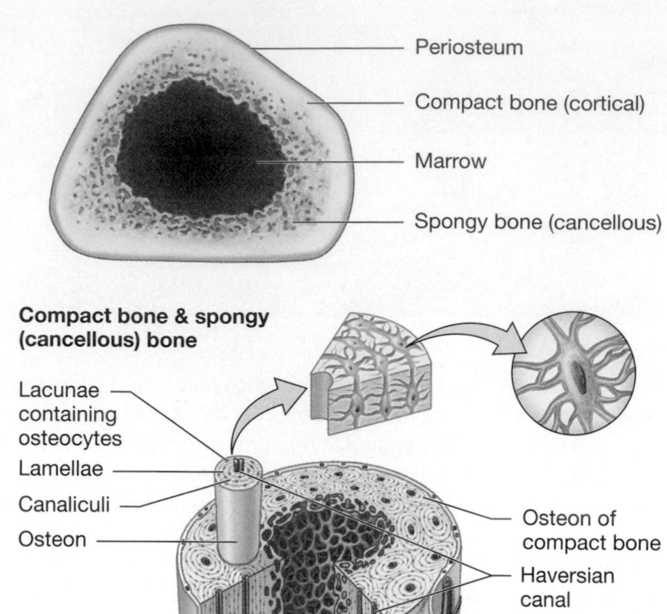

FIGURE 27-1 Bone cells (osteocytes) and types of bone

Table 27-1 Classification of bones by shape

Long bones	Bones of arm, legs, fingers, and toes (movement)	
Short bones	Bones of wrists and ankles (movement)	
Flat bones	Ribs, shoulder blades, hip, and cranial bones (support and protection)	
Irregular bones	Vertebrae, facial bones (support and protection)	

Table 27-2 Classification of joints by degree of movement

Classification	Movement	Type	Location	Characteristics	Example
Synarthrotic	Immovable	Suture	Cranial sutures	Joined by thin layer of fibrous tissue	
Amphiarthrotic	Partial movement	Symphysis	Vertebrae Symphysis pubis	Bones connected by fibrocartilage disk	
		Syndesmosis	Radius–ulna articulation	Bones connected by ligament	
Diarthrotic	Full movement (synovial membrane surrounds joint capsule, cartilage covers the ends of bones, ligaments hold bones together)	Ball and socket	Hip	Movement in all planes; widest degree of motion	
		Hinge	Elbow	Flexion and extension	
		Pivot	Atlantoaxial	Rotation	
		Condyloid	Wrist, between radius and carpals	Motion in two planes at right angles to each other (no radial motion)	
		Saddle	Thumb at carpal–metacarpal joint	Motion in two planes at right angles to each other (no axial motion)	
		Gliding	Intervertebral	One surface moves over another surface	

bone's end. Ligaments strengthen and stabilize joints by permitting movement only in certain directions and restricting certain types of movement.

Bone Maintenance

Bone is in a constant state of dynamic equilibrium, of creating and destroying for the purpose of bone remodeling. Remodeling involves changing the composition of collagen and matrix to adapt and accommodate various stresses placed on the bone. Remodeling is regulated by osteocytes, of which there are two types—osteoblasts and osteoclasts. Osteoblasts are responsible for calcium deposition and osteoclasts are responsible for calcium removal. Blood levels of calcium are also regulated by osteocytes; when blood calcium is high, osteoblasts deposit calcium in the bone, and when blood levels of calcium are low, osteoclasts remove calcium from the bone.

Blood Cell Production

A non-movement or support function of bone is the formation of blood cells (hematopoiesis) within the bone marrow, the flexible tissue in the interior of bones. In humans, red blood cells are produced in the heads of long bones at a rate of approximately 500 billion blood cells per day. Marrow is also a key component of the lymphatic system, producing the lymphocytes that support the body's immune system.

The two types of bone marrow are red marrow, which produces red cells, platelets, and most white cells; and yellow marrow, which is mainly made up of fat cells. At birth, all bone marrow is red; with age, more and more of it is converted to the yellow type so that an adult's bone marrow is approximately 50% red. Red marrow is found mainly in the flat bones, such as the pelvis, sternum, cranium, ribs, vertebrae and scapulae, and in the cancellous ("spongy") material at the epiphyseal ends of long bones such as the femur and humerus. Yellow marrow is found in the medullary cavity, the hollow interior of the middle portion of long bones. In cases of severe blood loss, the body can convert yellow marrow back to red marrow to increase blood cell production.

Muscle

The muscles are attached to the bones and joints to help move them in a coordinated way, enabling voluntary activity. Muscles consist of (1) skeletal, (2) smooth, and (3) cardiac muscle tissue. Most abundant, skeletal muscle is attached to the bones of the skeleton and functions to facilitate mobility and movement for work or other activities. Movement and mobility is carried out through contraction and relaxation of the muscles. Joint movement is dependent on intact innervation of the muscles so that the neuromuscular junction functions to transmit neurological messages from the brain along the appropriate nerve pathways indicating what action is needed and for how long (Figure 27-2). Because skeletal muscle movement is dependent upon specific brain messages for its activity, it is considered to be under voluntary control. Any damage or trauma to the nervous system that interferes with or prevents the delivery of these neurological messages inhibits muscular contractions and may have serious consequences for the affected individuals.

Muscles are arranged within the body to allow variety of movements. Muscle arrangement facilitates antagonistic or synergistic movements. Antagonistic movement occurs when there is the need

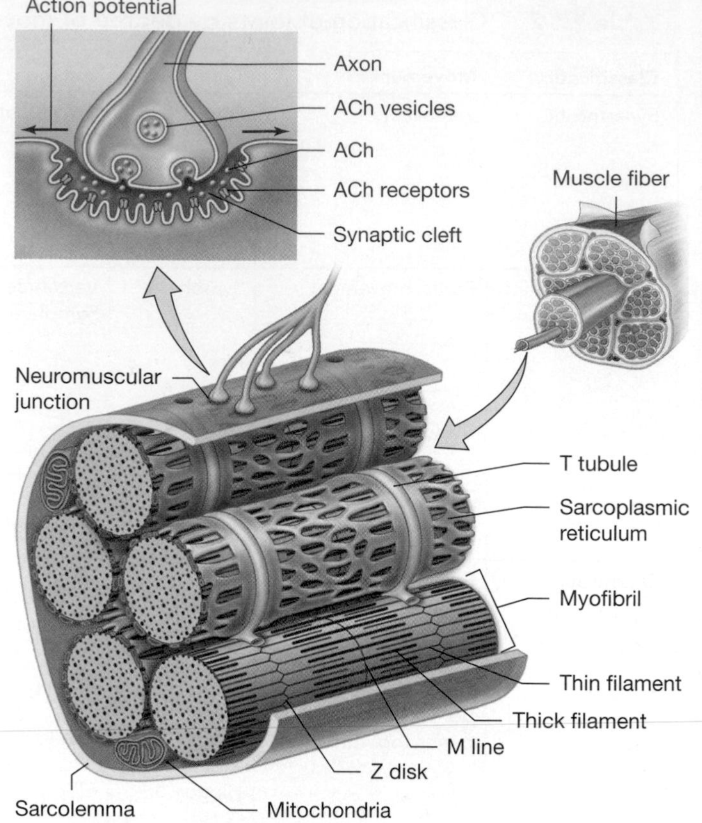

FIGURE 27-2 Neuromuscular junction and structure of muscle cells

for an opposing or opposite function. This is primarily needed with diarthrodial joints that are capable of a wide range of movement. The most common types of opposing movement are flexion and extension. Muscle contraction results in shortening of the muscle fibers causing flexion of a joint. To return to a neutral position, flexion must be overcome, which is facilitated by muscles that cause extension. Synergistic movement is the result of muscle groups working together to enhance muscle strength or to reduce the stress placed on muscle groups. Specific actions of muscles are identified in Table 27-3.

Muscle tone results from antagonistic forces and is necessary for stability and support during weight bearing, to maintain an upright and other positions, and for coordinated movements. It is the opposing action of flexion and extension that creates muscle tone. Flexion is slightly stronger than extension so that, for the most part, muscles are in a resting state of slight contraction. Contraction requires only a few muscle fibers so alternating among the fibers prevents muscle fatigue. Muscle tone is also demonstrated as a slight resistance to passive movement.

Muscles are attached to bones by tendons, which are strong, fibrous connective tissue. Tendons unite with the fascia that covers the muscle and with the periosteum that covers the bone. Each muscle has two tendons that are attached to different bones. The origin is the more immobile or stationary attachment; the insertion is the attachment that is more mobile or moveable. Muscles generally span over a joint made up of the two bones to which they are attached. Contraction of the muscle applies pull on its insertion, moving the bone in a particular direction.

Table 27-3 Functional actions of muscles

Action	Definition	Description
Flexion	Decrease in the angle of the joint	Bending elbow toward the shoulder 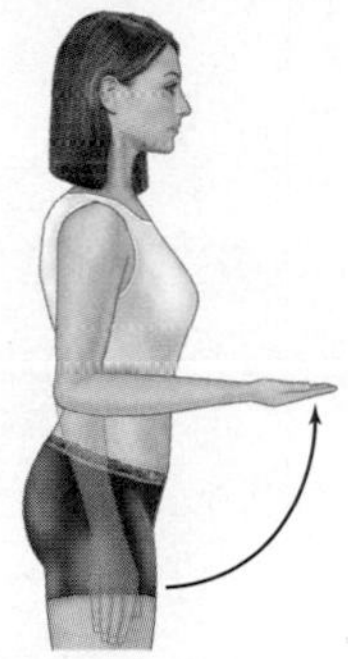
Extension	Increase in the angle of the joint	Bending elbow away from the shoulder 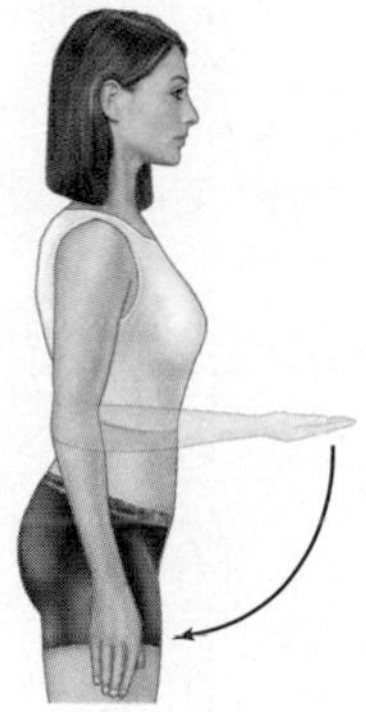
Adduction	Move close to the midline	Swinging arm (at shoulder) or leg (at hip) toward middle of body 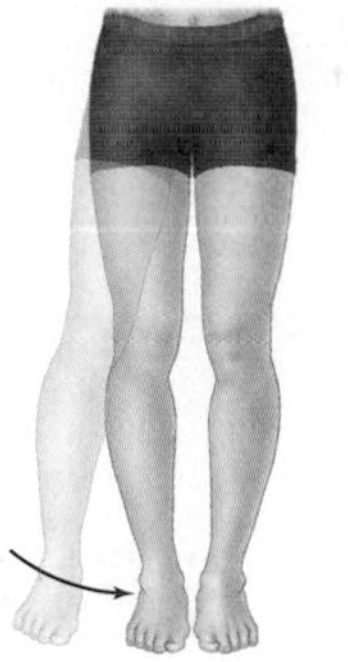
Abduction	Move away from the midline	Swinging arm (at shoulder) or leg (at hip) away from middle of body 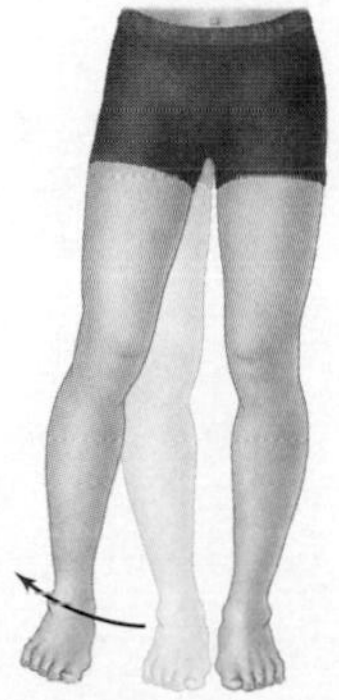

Continued

Table 27-3 Functional actions of muscles *(continued)*

Action	Definition	Description
Rotation	Moving a bone around its longitudinal axis	Holding the arm straight and moving the shoulder to create a circle 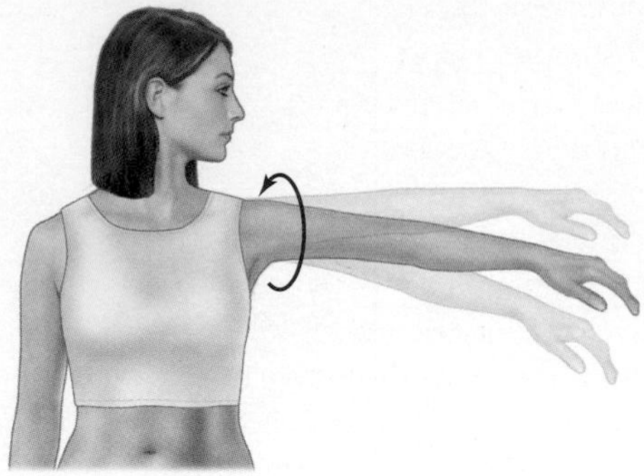
Pronation	Turn the palm down	Turning the palm down so that the palm is directed toward the floor 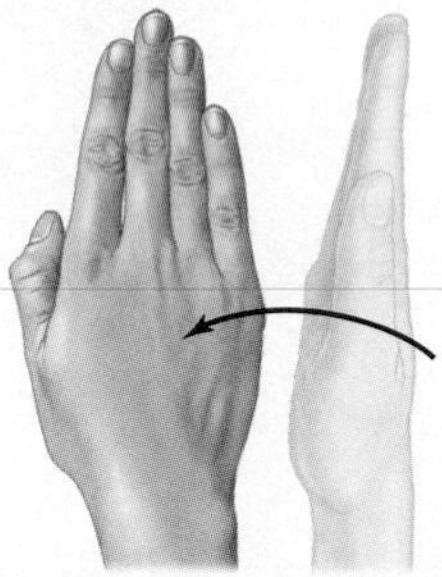
Supination	Turn the palm up	Turning the palm so that the palm is directed toward the ceiling 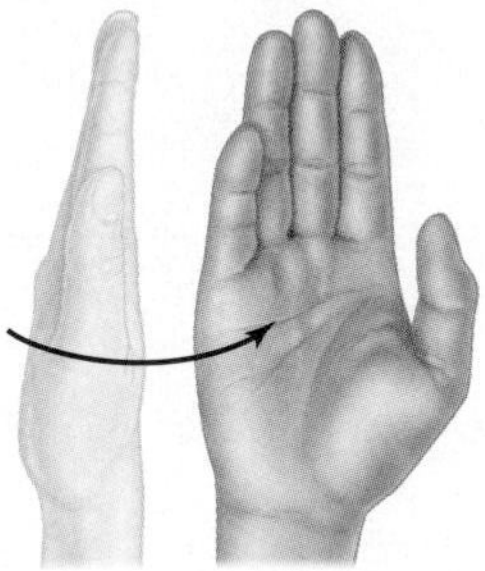
Dorsiflexion	Elevation of the foot	Pointing the toes so that they are pointed toward the knee 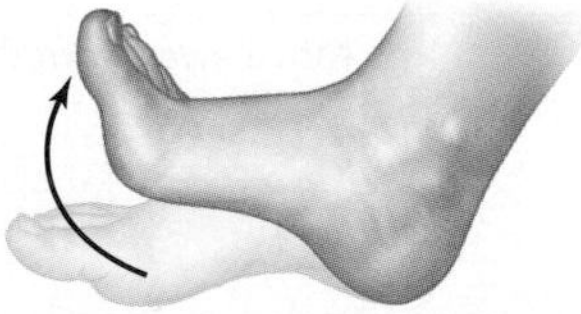
Plantarflexion	Lowering of the foot	Pointing the toes so that they are pointed away from the knee 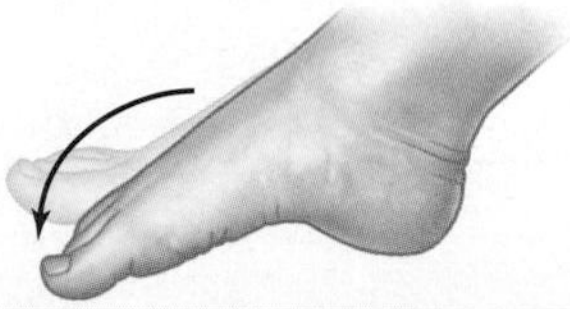

Groups of muscles function together to provide and coordinate the necessary movements of joints to perform specific actions. These groups of muscles can be divided into six areas of the body: head and neck, trunk, upper extremities, shoulder, lower extremities, and hip.

The two other muscle types, smooth and cardiac, are not directly a part of the musculoskeletal system. These muscle types are involuntary and controlled by the autonomic nervous system; they are primarily associated with tissues and organs that are responsible for carrying out the vital functions that maintain life.

Cardiac muscle is found only in the heart and is a combination of smooth and skeletal muscle. Contraction of heart muscle is responsible for maintaining blood circulation (see Chapter 24). Smooth muscle is found in the walls of the digestive tract, bladder, some ducts, blood vessels, and other internal organs. Smooth muscle fibers are elongated and thin, forming sheets rather than bundles.

The Skeleton

The human skeleton consists of two divisions: the axial skeleton and the appendicular skeleton (Figure 27-3).

Axial Skeleton

The axial skeleton is composed of the central bones of the trunk, which include the facial bones of the skull, hyoid bone, vertebrae, ribs, and the sternum.

Skull and Facial Bones

The skull is made up of 8 cranial bones and 14 facial bones. Additionally, there are the 3 ossicles of the middle ear and the hyoid bone. The bones of the skull and face are identified and described in Figure 27-4.

The joints of the skull bones are essentially fused, which makes them immobile. The edges of the skull bones where they attach to each other are described as sutures. The facial bones are also immobile with the exception of the mandible. The joints of the facial bones are also sutures. The condyles of the mandible and the mandibular fossae of the temporal bone create a condyloid joint that allows articulation of the bones with each other. This joint functions as a hinge to allow the jaw to open and close the mouth and also permits gliding action, allowing lateral movement as well as protrusion and retraction.

The Spine

The spine is composed of individual bones designated as vertebrae (Figure 27-5). They are further classified according to their location relative to the specific region of the back: cervical, thoracic, lumbar, sacral, coccygeal.

The 12 thoracic vertebrae connect with the posterior section of the ribs. The lumbar vertebrae are located in the small of the back and are considered the strongest of the vertebrae. The sacral vertebrae are fused into one sacral bone that articulates with

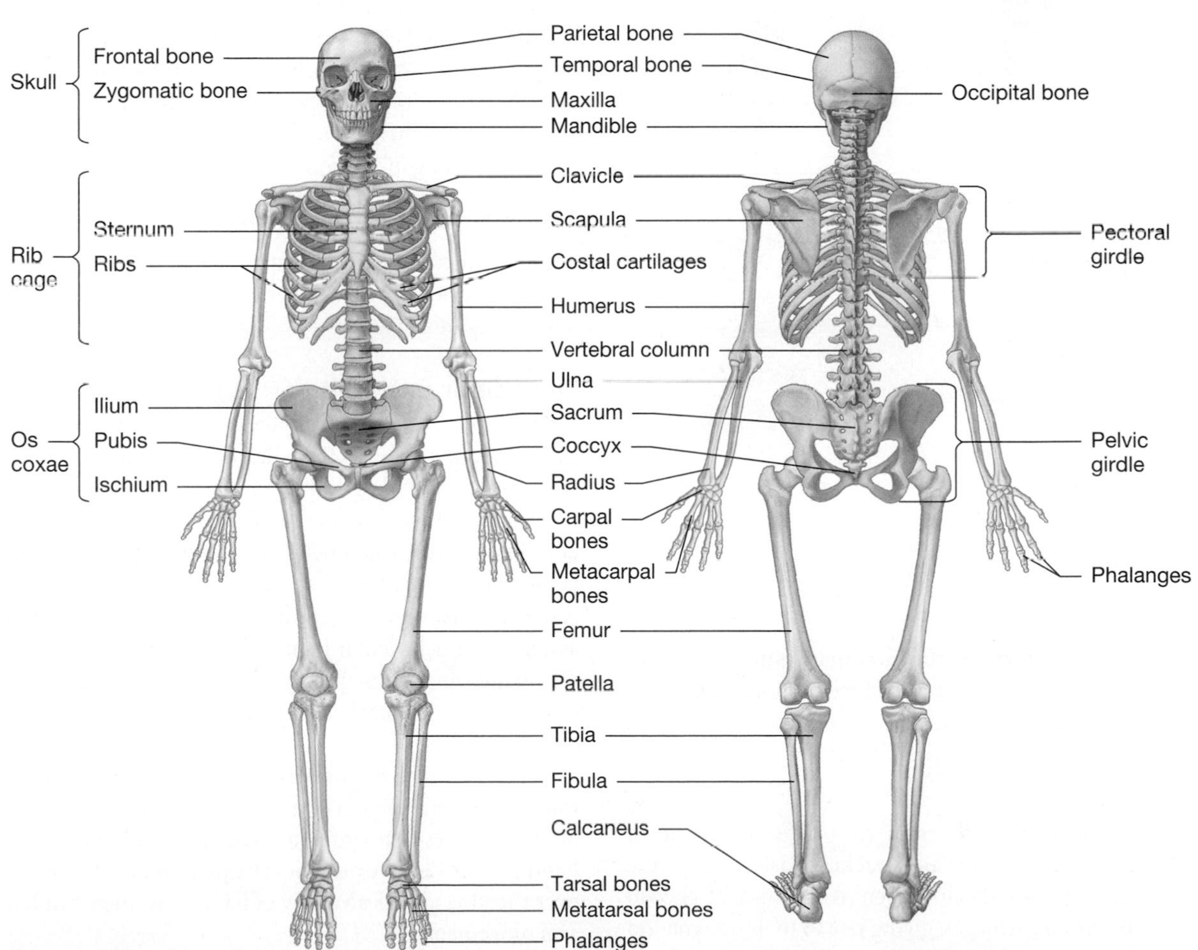

FIGURE 27-3 Axial skeleton and appendicular skeleton: Blue = axial; Tan = appendicular

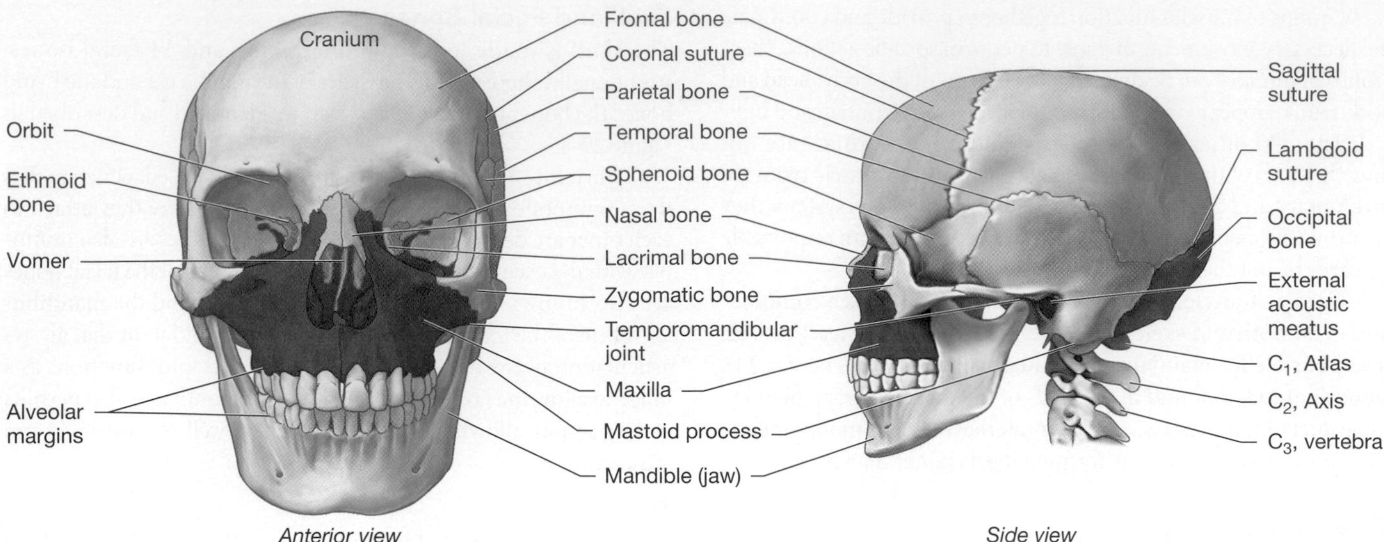

FIGURE 27-4 Bones of the skull and face

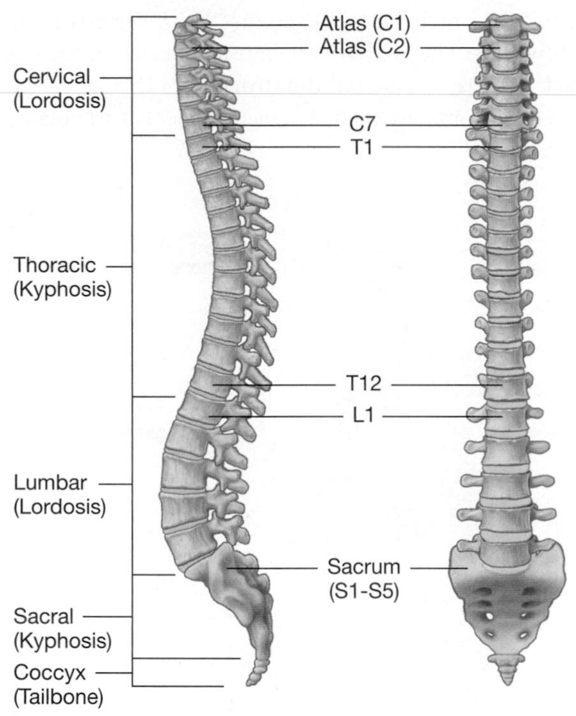

FIGURE 27-5 Bones of spine

the two bones of the hip, forming the sacroiliac joint. The four to five coccygeal vertebrae (coccyx) are also fused to form one bone. These vertebrae are remnants of tail vertebrae and attach to some perineal muscles.

Rib Cage

The rib cage consists of 12 pairs of ribs plus the sternum (Figure 27-6). All 12 pairs of ribs are attached posteriorly to the thoracic vertebrae. Anteriorly, the first seven ribs are also attached to the manubrium by costal cartilages, giving rise to their designation as true ribs. The next three pairs of ribs are referred to as false ribs as their costal cartilages merge with the cartilage of the seventh rib. The last two pairs of ribs are referred to as floating ribs as they have no attachment to the manubrium.

The sternum is made up of three parts: the manubrium, the body, and the xiphoid process. The overall function of the rib cage is to protect the heart and lungs, as well as some upper abdominal organs: the liver and spleen. Its other important function is to enlarge the thoracic cavity during ventilations. The ribs are pulled upward and outward by the external intercostal muscles, which expands the lungs, facilitating inhalation.

The Appendicular Skeleton

The appendicular skeleton is made up of the peripheral bones and includes the bones of the upper extremities, hip, and lower extremities (see Figure 27-3).

The Upper Extremities

The shoulder girdle consists of the scapula (shoulder bone) and clavicle (collar bone), which attach the upper extremities to the axial skeleton (Figure 27-7). A group of four muscles reinforce and maintain the position of the shoulder joint. These muscles along with the tendons make up the rotator cuff. Two additional joints also contribute to the articulation of the shoulder girdle. The acromioclavicular joint is the articulation between the acromion process and the clavicle, and the sternoclavicular joint is the articulation of the clavicle with the manubrium. These points of attachment and articulation of the clavicle serve to brace the scapulae and prevent too forward a motion of the shoulders.

The bones of the upper extremity include the humerus, the radius, and the ulna. The radius and ulna articulate with each other at the wrist forming a pivot joint that permits turning the hand palm side up or down. The position of the radius crossing over the ulna allows a variety of hand movements independent of arm movements.

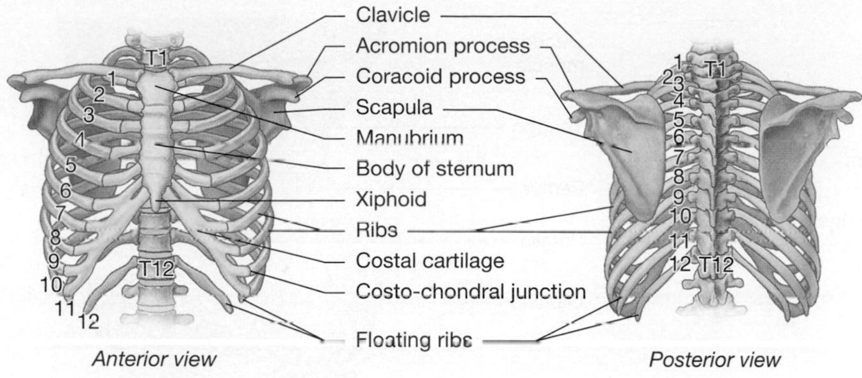

FIGURE 27-6 Rib cage

Wrist and Fingers The radius and ulna also articulate with the carpal bones of the wrist, creating condyloid joints (Figure 27-8). The eight carpal bones also articulate with each other, resulting in gliding joints, as well as articulating with the five metacarpal bones of the hand. The metacarpals articulate with the phalanges, or bones of the fingers. The joint between the metacarpal and phalanges is identified as the metacarpophalangeal (MCP) joint. Each thumb has two phalanges and each finger has three phalanges. The joints of the phalanges are hinge joints while the carpometacarpal joint of the thumb is a saddle joint, permitting the thumb to cross over the palm and engage in gripping. The joints between the phalanges are identified as the proximal interphalangeal (PIP) joints and the distal interphalangeal (DIP) joints.

The Hip and Lower Extremities

The hip, or pelvic girdle, is made up of two hip bones, the coxae or innominate bones (Figure 27-9). Each hip bone consists of three sections: the ilium, the ischium, and the pubis. The two pubic bones are separated from each other with a fibrous cartilaginous disk at the symphysis pubis. This disk allows the two pubic bones to articulate with each other.

The cup-shaped depression in the iliac bone just above the ischium is the acetabulum, where the hip bone articulates with the head of the femur. The acetabulum is a deep socket, which is necessary as the hip is a weight-bearing joint. The depth of the acetabulum also prevents the hip from being easily dislocated.

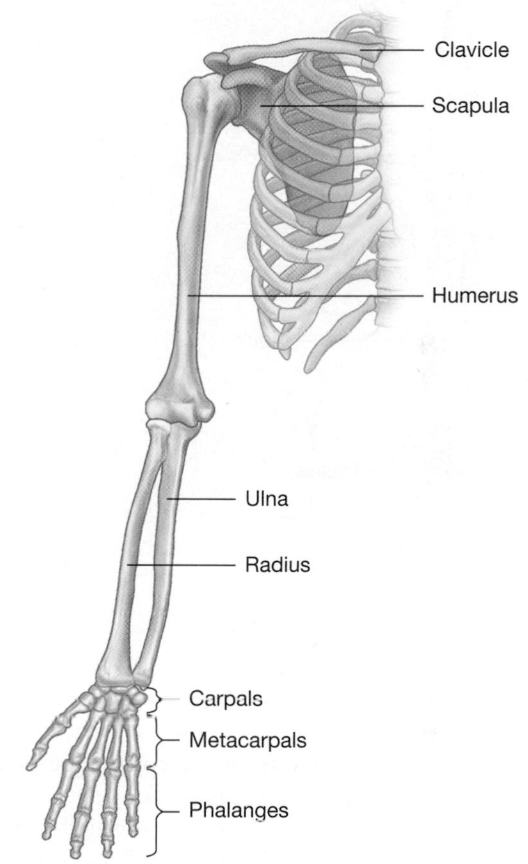

FIGURE 27-7 Shoulder and arm bones

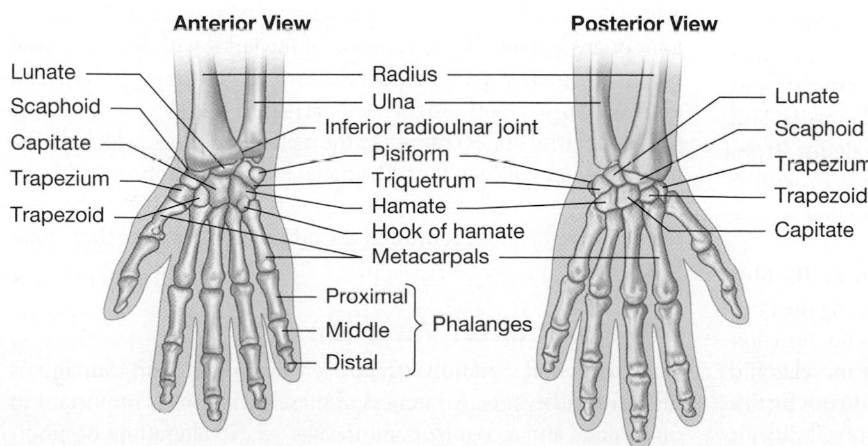

FIGURE 27-8 Bones of the wrist and fingers

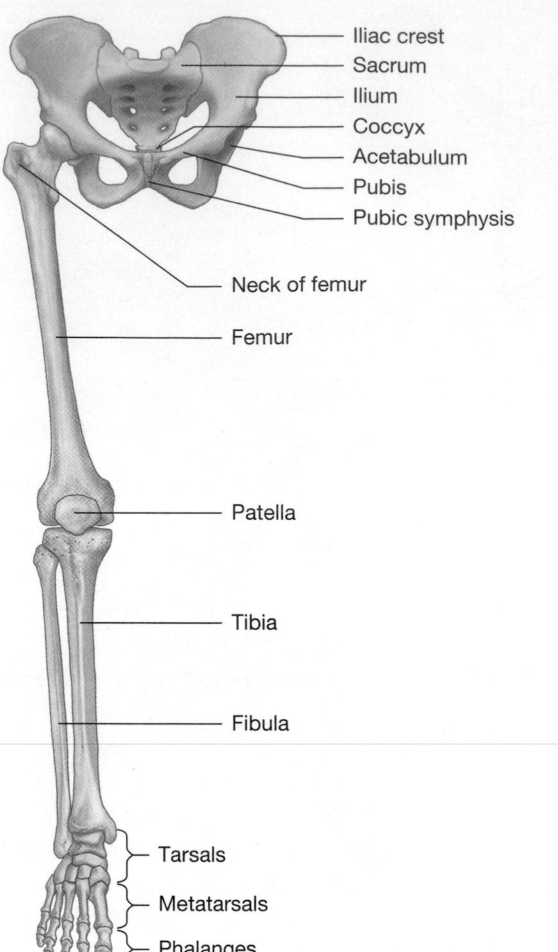

FIGURE 27-9 Bones of hip and leg

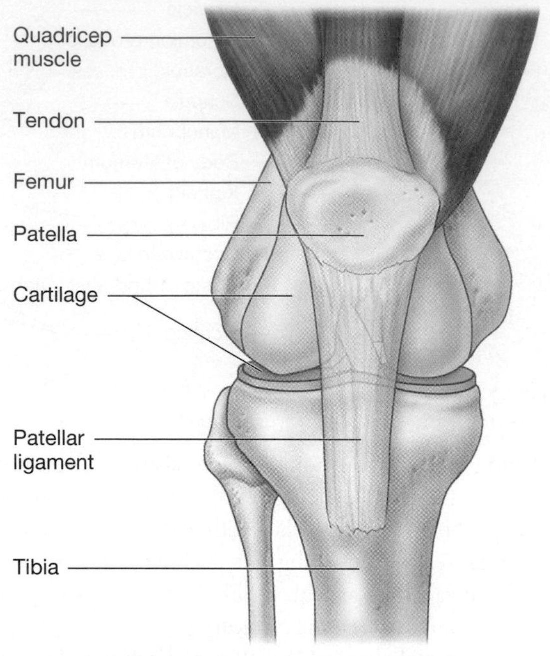

FIGURE 27-10 The knee joint

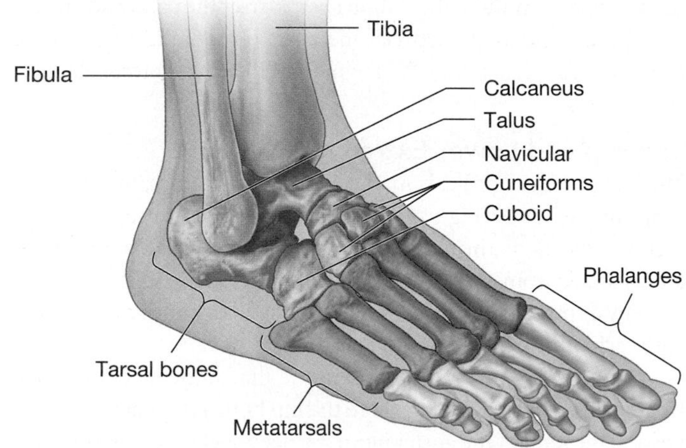

FIGURE 27-11 Bones of the ankle and foot

Leg The upper portion of the leg (thigh) consists of a single, long bone known as the femur. The head of the femur that fits into the acetabulum of the hip is connected to the body of the femur by a section of bone that can be referred to as a neck.

At the distal end of the femur, it articulates with the tibia forming the knee joint (Figure 27-10). The knee, like the elbow, is a hinge joint. The knee joint also consists of the patella, or knee cap, that is situated anterior to the knee. The knee joint and patella are also comprised of fibrocartilaginous disks and multiple ligaments that support and provide stability for the knee. The fibrocartilaginous disks are the medial and lateral meniscus and cushion the tibia and femur. There are also two sets of ligaments, the cruciate and collateral ligaments. The collateral ligaments provide medial and lateral stability to the knee and prevent varus and valgum stress. The cruciate ligaments cross obliquely within the knee, providing anterior and posterior stability. There are also bursae that reduce friction between the articulating bones.

The bones of the lower leg include the tibia and fibula. The tibia is the weight-bearing bone with its upper section forming the knee joint. The fibula is not a part of the knee joint and does not function in weight bearing. It does provide an attachment for muscles and helps to stabilize the ankle joint. The tibia and fibula do not form a pivot joint like the radius and ulna. This provides more stability for the lower leg and foot, aiding in providing support for the body.

Ankle and Foot The ankle consists of seven tarsal bones. The largest of these is the calcaneus, which is the bone of the heel. The talus bone articulates with the tibia forming a hinge joint known as the tibiotalar joint or ankle joint. The articulation of the tarsal with the metatarsal bones form gliding joints that facilitate inversion (turning inward) and eversion (turning outward) of the foot (Figure 27-11).

Four tarsal bones connect to the metatarsal bones, which are the five long bones of each foot. The metatarsal bones connect with the phalanges, which are the bones of the toes. Like the fingers, the great toe has two phalange bones and the other four toes have three phalange bones.

Developmental Variations

Developmental variations occur over the course of an individual's life span and events. Awareness of these variations is important to understand and recognize common age-related alterations or modifications of the bones and muscles.

Infants and Children

The initial skeletal system of the fetus is composed of connective tissue that eventually develops into cartilage that eventually calcifies, or ossifies, into bone. Bone growth continues throughout infancy and childhood. There is a rapid growth during infancy, which slows down but continues during childhood. There is a second rapid growth spurt during adolescence.

Bone growth is influenced by a variety of internal and external factors. Genetic factors are the primary regulators of bone growth. An individual's height is determined by the length to which bones are genetically programmed to grow. Genes responsible for bone growth are inherited from both parents.

Nutritional factors also play an important role in promoting bone growth. Minerals—primarily calcium and phosphorous—protein, are essential building blocks for the development of the matrix that comprises bone structure. Vitamin D is also necessary for the absorption of calcium and phosphorus from the small intestine. Vitamins A and C are also necessary for adequate ossification (hardening) of the bone matrix. Children who are nutritionally deficient fail to grow appropriately and may not achieve their genetic potential for height.

Physical factors, primarily exercise, are essential for bone maintenance and growth. Bones respond to stress, which refers to weight bearing, their primary function. Without this stress, calcium is removed from the bone at a faster rate than it is replaced. Extensive periods of non–weight bearing result in weaker and more fragile bones.

Endocrine factors, through hormones, also are responsible for appropriate growth and maintenance of bone integrity (Table 27-4, Figure 27-12).

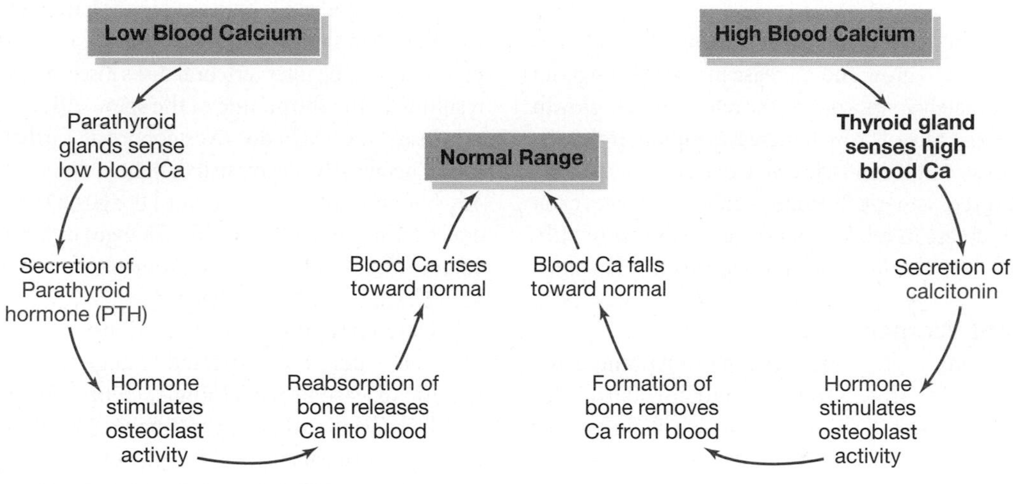

FIGURE 27-12 Hormones related to bone growth

Table 27-4 Hormones regulating bone growth and maintenance

Hormone	Produced by	Action(s)
Regulators of Bone Mass and Distribution		
Growth Regulators		
Growth hormone	Anterior pituitary gland	Increases rate of mitosis of chondrocytes and osteoblasts
		Increases rate of protein synthesis (collagen, collagen matrix)
		Main regulator of height
Estrogen	Ovaries/testes	Promotes closure of the epiphyses of long bones
Testosterone		Helps retain calcium in bones to maintain strong bone matrix
		In adults, maintains bone mass by suppressing spongy bone remodeling
		Inhibit resorption by stimulating osteoplastic apoptosis and preventing osteoblast/osteocyte apoptosis (loss of hormones accelerates osteoclast activity, favoring resorption)
Thyroxine (T_4)	Thyroid	Increases rate of protein synthesis
		Increases energy production from all food types
Calcium (Ca^{++}) Regulators		
Calcitonin	Thyroid	Inhibits osteoclast activity allowing osteoblasts to form bone tissue
Parathyroid hormone	Parathyroid	Increases the reabsorption of calcium from bones to blood (increases blood calcium)
		Increases the absorption of calcium by small intestines and kidneys
Vitamin D (Calcitriol)		Hormone-like effects; often considered a calcium regulatory hormone
		Necessary for Ca^{++} absorption from intestines

During adolescence bone growth occurs primarily in length as well as diameter. Bone growth in diameter is the result of the accumulation of new bone tissue around the shaft of the bone. Growth in length occurs at the **epiphysis** or growth plate. Epiphysis is a transverse disk growth center located at the ends of long bones. The epiphysis continues longitudinal bone growth until there is closure of the epiphyseal plate around 20 years of age. A major concern related to bone growth is any trauma or infection at the epiphyseal plate, which places the bone at risk for delaying bone growth or developing a deformity.

Skeletal changes are also observed in the contour of the spinal column. At birth, the spinal column has a C shape, which will eventually become S shaped, that is formed by the cervical and lumbar curve. The anterior curve begins to develop at around 3 to 4 months of age, when the infant begins to raise its head. Later, around 1 year to 18 months, as the infant begins to walk, the lumbar curve begins to appear.

Muscle fibers of the fetus are in place around the fourth to fifth month and continue to grow and increase in mass throughout childhood. At approximately 2 years of age, the rate of muscle growth increases. At puberty, the rate of growth increases rapidly, primarily due to the increase in size of the muscle cell. Up until puberty, girls' muscle cell size increases at a greater rate than boys'; however, at puberty the rate of increase in cell size of boys exceeds that of girls. The length of muscle fibers also increases as bone growth takes place.

The Pregnant Woman

Skeletal adaptations to pregnancy are the result of increased levels of hormones. Estrogen, relaxin, and corticosteroids cause an increased elasticity of the ligaments and a softening of the cartilage in the sacroiliac, sacrococcygeal, and symphysis pubis joints of the pelvis. These changes begin to occur around the twelfth to the twentieth week of gestation.

The initial change in the posture of the pregnant female is a gradually developing lordosis of the lumbar spine. This change compensates for the increasing size of the uterus by shifting the center of gravity back to the lower extremities. Mechanical factors shift the pregnant woman's balance, increasing the strain on the lower back muscles, which is frequently felt as lower back (lumbar) pain. Rarely is herniation of a disk a cause of back pain.

The shift in balance as well as the loosening of the symphysis pubis may also cause pelvic pain. Loosening of the pelvic joints allows for increased mobility and possible joint separation that may cause asymmetry and pelvic joint pain.

An additional compensation for lordosis is an anterior flexion of the neck and shoulder girdle, which frequently places increased pressure on the ulnar and radial nerves and is felt as numbness, aching, and weakness of the upper extremities. These manifestations are often present during the third trimester of pregnancy.

Cramps of the gastrocnemius, thigh, or gluteal muscles may occur during the second trimester. The cause is unknown and they may be quite painful. They occur most often during the night or after initiating muscle activity after waking from sleep.

The Older Adult

The most significant skeletal change in the elderly is the development of osteoporosis, which occurs because of a shift in the balance between bone growth and bone destruction, with bone destruction outpacing bone growth. This condition occurs in all the elderly, but predominates in post-menopausal females and is more frequent in whites than blacks. The lack of estrogen is the primary cause in females and results in a decrease in bone density and calcium deposition.

The loss of bone density is distributed throughout the skeleton but most commonly affects the vertebrae and the long bones. This affinity for the long bones increases the potential for fractures in the elderly.

A loss of height is another manifestation of skeletal aging. This is not due to a shortening of the bones but a shortening of the vertebral column. The intervertebral disks lose water and become thinner resulting in the shortening of the spine. Additionally, the vertebrae may lose some height due to osteoporosis, further contributing to the loss of height. The decrease in height (1 cm per decade) starts in the 40s, but may not be evident until the 60s. Decreasing stature accelerates during and after the 70s. Changes in the vertebrae and spinal column also result in the development of a kyphosis and a compensatory backward tilt of the head.

Osteoarthritis is so prevalent in the elderly that is it often considered an expected change with aging rather than a specific disease process (Hugle, Geurts, Nuesch, Muller-Gerbe, & Valderrabano, 2012). Approximately 75% of the elderly population experience osteoarthritis, although only about 30% demonstrate any symptoms and only 10% experience a significant disability.

Another significant change of the joints is the development of osteophytes (bone spurs) on the ends of long bones as well as on the spine.

Fat and subcutaneous tissue distribution changes during the adult years and later with a loss of fat in the face and an increase in fat in the abdomen and hips. There is a loss of fat and subcutaneous tissue and a deterioration of cartilage around the joints. This results in marked bony prominences as well as joint pain. With aging, there is also loss of fat and subcutaneous tissue from the periphery, which is most noticeable in the upper extremities.

The muscles are also affected by aging with an absolute loss of muscle mass resulting in a decrease in size that may be accompanied by atrophy and weakness. Collagen also collects in the muscles and is followed by fibrosis of connective tissue and the loss of stretch in the tendons. In addition to the loss of mass, there is a decrease in strength and muscle tone, as well as decreased agility, speed of movement, and endurance.

Health Promotion

Musculoskeletal conditions are the primary cause of disabilities in the U.S. MS disorders that have the greatest impact on the overall health and quality of life issues are arthritis and its associated rheumatic disorders, osteoporosis, and chronic back pain. The potential for living longer and working longer increase the need for reducing the impact that inactivity and disability related to these disorders has on individuals with these MS conditions.

Goals of *Healthy People 2020* related to the topic area of Arthritis, Osteoporosis, and Chronic Back Conditions (AOCBC) follow.

Health Promotion *continued*

Arthritis

- AOCBC—1: Reduce the mean level of joint pain among adults with doctor-diagnosed arthritis.
- AOCBC—2–5: Reduce the proportion of adults with doctor-diagnosed arthritis who experience a limitation in activity due to arthritis or joint symptoms; find it "very difficult" to perform specific joint-related activities; have difficulty in performing two or more personal care activities, thereby preserving independence; report serious psychological distress.
- AOCBC—6: Reduce the impact of doctor-diagnosed arthritis on employment in the working-aged population.
- AOCBC—7/8: Increase the proportion of adults with doctor-diagnosed arthritis who receive health care provider counseling; have had effective, evidence-based arthritis education as an integral part of the management of their condition.
- AOCBC—9: Increase the proportion of adults with chronic joint symptoms who have seen a health care provider for their symptoms.

More than 15% of the population of the U.S. (43 million) and 20% of adults have one type of arthritis—**osteoarthritis (OA)**, also known as degenerative joint disease (DJD), or **rheumatoid arthritis (RA)**. These percentages make arthritis one of the most common conditions in the U.S. as well as having a significant impact on each individual's life.

Arthritis is characterized by inflammation of the joints, resulting in joint pain (arthralgia). In OA, the cartilage on the ends of the bones becomes inflamed. This type is often the result of everyday wear and tear on the joints and primarily affects weight-bearing joints. As such, it is primarily seen in older adults. In RA, the lining of the joint becomes inflamed. It can have multiple causes, and affects any joints. RA can be seen in individuals of all ages; however, it is still predominately a condition of older individuals. Differentiation between OA and RA is identified in Table 27-5.

Limitations on activities of daily living is one of the most severe consequence of arthritis, affecting approximately 7 million individuals, making it the major cause of disability. Arthritis is second to heart disease as the cause of work-related disability. The loss of independence related to arthritis disability affects not only the individual, but other family members and/or care givers.

A limitation on activity and/or disability also impacts the overall quality of life for these individuals, particularly in relation to their health. Individuals with arthritis are consistently worse off in health-related issues or activities. Various measures to improve health-related quality of life may be used, but they most commonly relate to "healthy days," pain free days, or ability days (days without limitations or restrictions on activities).

The economic impact of arthritis is also substantial related to health care costs as well as loss of productivity due to lost work days. In 2004, OA resulted in over 11 million physician and outpatient visits, 662,000 hospitalizations, and more than 632,000 total joint replacements, with accompanying hospital costs of $22.6 billion. Additionally, an estimated $3.4–13.2 billion is spent per year on job-related OA costs (Lubar et al., 2010).

As with other conditions related to pain, arthritis has significant negative effects on individual's mental health status as well as overall health status. Although not a specific cause of death, death rates for individuals with certain types of arthritis are higher than those for the general population.

The overall outlook for the impact of arthritis is that it will only increase. In 2010, it was estimated that 50 million adults in the U.S. indicated that they were diagnosed with some form of arthritis (OA/RA), gout, lupus, or fibromyalgia (Centers for Disease Control, 2010). By 2030, it is estimated that 67 million Americans older than 17 years of age will have some form of physician diagnosed arthritis (Hootman & Helmick, 2006).

Table 27-5 Differential characteristics of rheumatoid arthritis and osteoarthritis

Manifestations	Rheumatoid Arthritis	Osteoarthritis
Average of onset	3rd and 4th decade (gradual or sudden [24–48 hours], sometimes weeks to months)	5th and 6th decade (insidious, develops over years)
Weight	Normal or underweight	Generally overweight
Condition of bones	Osteoporosis	Condensation of articular margins
Joints involved	Any joint in body	Primarily knees, spine, and fingers
Joint involvement progression	Migratory, symmetrical	Not migratory
Appearance of joints	Periarticular swelling; synovial proliferation and thickening Fusiform soft tissue enlargement of finger joints	Without swelling, effusion common with minimal synovial involvement Heberden's/Bouchard's nodes
Subcutaneous (rheumatoid) nodules	Appear in 10%–20% of cases	Not seen
Stiffness (duration)	At least 1 hour; frequently longer; more remarkable after rest	Few minutes
Pain	May occur at rest; sleep disturbance possible	With motion and prolonged activity; relieved by rest
Heat (erythema)	Sometimes present	Unusual; very slight if present
Tenderness localized over involved joint	Almost always, most sensitive symptom of inflammation	Common
Crepitus	Medium to fine	Coarse to medium with movement
Course of disease	Usually progressive with spontaneous exacerbations and remissions	Stationary or slightly progressive
Termination	Ankylosis and deformity	No ankylosis, usually no deformity

Health Promotion *continued*

There will also be a proportional increase in direct and indirect costs.

Reduction in the incidence of arthritis begins with identification of risk factors associated with its development. Joint injury from recreational or occupational accidents is related to developing osteoarthritis at a later age. Obesity is recognized as contributing to osteoarthritis of the knee, possibly contributing to hip and hand involvement. Obesity is also related to the progression and severity of osteoarthritis.

Potential identification of at-risk individuals may be possible with genetic research with the anticipation that interventions may prevent or reduce the severity of arthritis. Present interventions and treatment are focused on pain and symptomatic relief; however, many sufferers fail to use approved interventions because of the prevailing belief that arthritis is an expected aspect of aging and that nothing can be done.

Education and land or water exercise programs have also been successful in reducing pain by up to 20% above what was attained with usual health care practices. Education to dispel myths as well as promoting effective interventions and treatment is also expected to reduce the overall impact arthritis has on affected individuals.

Osteoporosis/Chronic Back Conditions

- AOCBC—10–12: Reduce the proportion of adults with osteoporosis, hip fractures among older adults, and activity limitation due to chronic back conditions.

Osteoporosis is characterized by a significant reduction in bone mass or density and deterioration of bony architecture (Hobar, 2005; National Osteoporosis Foundation, 2008). It occurs when there is a shift in the balance of bone remodeling, with bone destruction occurring at a greater rate than construction, resulting in a loss of calcium and other minerals. Its exact cause is not identified, but a combination of genetic and environmental factors affect peak bone mass and the rate of bone loss (Hobar, 2005). A decreased bone density is initially described as **osteopenia** (American Association of Clinical Chemistry, 2006); however, a significant decrease in density that results in weakness and the possibility of fracture is described as osteoporosis.

Osteoporosis is more common in females with approximately 13%–18% of females older than 50 affected. Males are less commonly affected, with approximately 3%–6% of males over 50 affected. These percentages translate into 4–6 million females and 1–2 million males over 50 with osteoporosis. The incidence of osteopenia is greater in both genders, but the distribution is less dramatic related to gender. Approximately 37%–50% of females and 27%–47% of males over 50 have osteopenia.

The most significant health-related consequence of osteoporosis is an increased risk for fractures. Osteoporosis-related fractures are approximately 1.5 million annually. More females (33%) experience a fracture due to osteoporosis than males (12%). Health care costs for osteoporosis-caused fractures are estimated to be $13.8 billion annually.

Although any bone fracture can be osteoporosis related, hip fractures are the most common type and have the most significant impact on health care costs and individual consequences. The risk for osteoporosis-related fracture increases with age so that by the age of 90, 17% of females and 6% of males will experience a hip fracture. The incidence rate for females has remained relatively constant, but the incidence rate for males is increasing. Most hip fractures are related to falls or minor trauma and present with inability to bear weight and shortening with external rotation of the affected limb. In some instances, the hip may be fractured without a history of trauma. This type of fracture may allow for weight bearing and walking. In these instances, the fracture is most likely a stress fracture related to severe osteoporosis. The individual may complain of pain, but it is less intense and often in the anterior groin or thigh (Bhatti & Ertl, 2005).

There is significant morbidity and mortality associated with hip fractures. On average, 1-year mortality rates after injury range from 15%–20% (Brunner & Kuo, 2003), with males having a higher death rate than females. Functional impairments are also more likely to be present in individuals with hip fractures than in those with other serious medical conditions including heart attack, stroke, and cancer. For example, approximately 40% of individuals with hip fractures are able to engage in all activities of daily living, and 54% are able to walk without some type of assistance (Rao & Cherukuri, 2006).

Prevention of development of osteoporosis, decreasing bone loss after it develops, and reducing the risk for fractures are identified interventions to reduce the overall consequences that result from its occurrence. Prevention of osteoporosis is primarily aimed at lifestyle changes related to nutrition, smoking and alcohol, and exercise. Nutrition is focused on increasing the amount of calcium and vitamin D in the diet. The goal is to increase the bone mass, particularly during adolescence, so that bone loss during aging will be more gradual, thus delaying its onset. If the patient is also overweight, weight reduction is important. Giving up smoking as well as reducing alcohol intake is also recommended. Activities that increase stress on the bone, such as exercise and walking, will also serve to increase bone calcium contributing to a delayed onset. Screening for osteoporosis is also recommended to initiate early treatment and prevent fractures. Bone mineral density (BMD) is the primary test for predicting fractures. Individuals who should have bone density testing include the following:

- Post-menopausal females below 65 who have risk factors for osteoporosis
- All females over 65
- Post-menopausal females with fragility fractures
- Females considering treatment that will be determined by BMD results
- Females on long-term hormone replacement therapy
- Males who demonstrate fractures after minimal trauma. Recent guidelines from the National Osteoporosis Foundation recommend a BMD test for males 70 and older (Preidt, 2008).

Individuals with evidence of osteopenia on x-rays or have a condition known to be high risk for osteoporosis.

Chronic back pain may be defined as pain that persists for longer than 12 weeks. It is often referred to as low back pain (LBP) with approximately 97% being mechanical (non-specific) in origin (Kinkade, 2007). Regional back pain results from overuse of a mechanical structure causing muscle strain, irritation, inflammation. Other types of back pain result from trauma, deformity, or degeneration of an anatomical structure (rupture/herniation of nucleus pulposus, fracture, and spondyloarthropathy) (Bhangle, Sapru, & Panush, 2009). Acute LBP is generally responsive to therapy and has a favorable prognosis; however, chronic LBP has a less favorable prognosis and often results in limitations on activity and disability. The impact of LBP, like that of arthritis, is demonstrated in increased health care costs and decreased productivity.

Back pain develops in 15%–45% of individuals annually with approximately 2%–8% progressing to chronic LBP. Annually, 3%–4% of the U.S. population become temporarily disabled with 1%–2% becoming totally or permanently disabled due to LBP.

Health Promotion *continued*

It is second to the common cold as the most frequent cause of work time loss and primary care office visits, costing the U.S. more than $100 billion/year in health care costs and productivity losses (Wheeler, Wopf, Staiger, & Deyo, 2013).

The most frequently cited causes of LBP are work-related factors, accounting for 27%–50% of LBP problems in adults. Work-related factors include heavy lifting, forceful movements, awkward positions, and whole-body vibrations. Personal factors also play a significant role in the development of LBP. Non-modifiable factors relate to age, gender, and certain anthropomorphic (height and body type) measurements, history of LBP, and spinal abnormalities. Modifiable factors include weight, physical fitness, smoking, trunk muscle strength, and flexibility and elasticity of lumbar and hamstring muscles.

Prevention of LBP is best carried out by identifying activities at work or home that have the potential for causing back problems, and developing new ways of managing the physical requirements of work or other activities. A greater understanding and utilization of ergonomic principles are a significant component of exploring alternative work methods and activities. Exercises that increase muscle strength and endurance are also recommended. Weight reduction may also be necessary as are exercise and nutritional changes.

Clinical Context Exemplars

Situation A

During the assessment of a newborn, the mother is present and observes you palpating the clavicle, moving the hips in and out, and looking at all the creases in the infant's posterior thighs. The mother wants to know what you are doing and why you are doing it.

1. How would you explain to the mother what you are doing?

Situation B

During the taking of a history for a 15-year-old female, she indicates that she has noticed that her clothes don't seem to fit right. If she wears a skirt of a dress, it appears crooked and the hemline is not straight. She also has noticed that her shoulders appear to be uneven.

1. During your assessment, what would you expect to observe when observing the patient's back?
2. What procedures would you want to perform to validate your observations?
3. What information would you want to give to the patient?

Situation C

A 45-year-old female is getting her yearly physical. She is complaining of some joint pain in her hands. Her family history is positive for arthritis, but she can't remember which type family members had.

1. What information—history and physical exam—would you need to obtain to determine what type of arthritis this patient has?

Situation D

An 80-year-old male states that he thinks he is getting shorter. He used to be 5′ 11″ and when he was recently measured he was about 5′ 9.5″. He can't seem to figure out why this is happening.

1. How would you explain this to him?
2. What other information would you provide him with?
3. As a part of his examination, what other information would you want to obtain and what would you ask?

SUBJECTIVE DATA

History of Present Illness (CC)

The patient may present to the provider with a variety of concerns that may be directly related to the musculoskeletal system or other systems. Framing the questions will depend on the patient's age, gender, culture, race, emotional or mental status, health practices, and concurrent illnesses. All symptoms presented must be thoroughly assessed with a symptom analysis (COLDERRA). A major focus to the history component is the degree to which functional capabilities (activities of daily living) are affected.

Joint Pain

The most common subjective complaints related to the musculoskeletal system are joint pain and loss of function/movement. Joint dysfunction refers to abnormal function or movement of a joint in a particular area of the body and is present whenever joints, muscles, and nerves are not functioning at optimum efficiency. It is common in the regions of the low back and neck, but is often also present in the mid-back, shoulders, knees, ankles, or wrists. The most common locations for joint dysfunction are the temporomandibular joint (TMJ) and the sacroiliac (SI) joint. Joint pain and swelling may be secondary to any of these different conditions: rheumatoid arthritis (RA), osteoarthritis (OA), systemic lupus erythematosus (SLE), gout, septic arthritis, psoriasis, inflammatory bowel disease, Mixed Connective-Tissue Disease (MCTD), viral causes (hepatitis B/C, parvovirus, HIV), and calcium pyrophosphate deposition (pseudogout).

Provider Inquiries	Clinical Reasoning/Logic
Characteristics: Any pain? How is pain felt? Is it aching, sharp/dull, or shooting? Do you have joint stiffness or limitation of movement? Gradual or immediate onset? Constant or intermittent? Grating present? Severity of pain (1–10)? Disabling?	Type and severity of pain may help in determining type of arthritis and effects on daily life. Acute, disabling pain occurs in gout. Acute joint pain is usually seen in septic arthritis, and gout or pseudogout, although RA may also present acutely. The patient's response will validate your understanding of the patient's verbal description. A response of "sore or aching" pain usually relates to muscle pain, "throbbing" as a descriptor usually relates to bone pain. Pain in SI can range from dull aching to sharp and stabbing, as well as transient numbness, prickling, or tingling. With TMJ, limited movement or locking of the jaw, making it difficult to open or close the mouth.
Onset: When does pain start? Any particular time of day? Any known recent injuries?	Acute arthritis of less than 6 weeks suggests processes like viral, septic arthritis, or traumatic arthritis. RA pain—worse in the morning; usually symptoms are chronic for more than 6 weeks. OA pain—worse in evening/night, also increases with weight bearing or with activities. Tendinitis—worse in the morning and gets better through the day. Sudden onset of pain in great toe, ankle, or knees suggests gout. Trauma is also a risk for OA.
Location: Where does pain start? Where is pain located? Unilateral or bilateral? Which joints affected? Does it affect multiple joints or one joint? Does it affect small joints or large joints?	RA—symmetrical/bilateral joints and multiple small joints of the wrist and hands, MTP. OA— generally asymmetric, affects DIP. Lupus may affect any joint. Gout is usually asymmetric. (Oligoarthritis or symmetric polyarthritis usually has distal involvement, usually DIP. OA and psoriatic arthritis usually affect DIP joints, although there can be DIP involvement in RA.)
Duration: How long does pain last? How often does it occur?	Duration of pain helps in determining type of arthritis. Duration of pain in RA is usually longer (an hour), and shorter in OA, while gout pain is longer. Pain comes and goes with TMJ.
Exacerbation: What makes pain worse (movement, position, time of day, change in weather, temperature changes)? Does your job require repetitive motion/movement?	Movement increases most joint pain, movement in RA decreases pain. RA pain increases with changes in barometric pressure. Bone pain—no increase with movement; SI pain increases with physical activity or with prolonged or sustained positions (e.g., sitting, standing, lying). Bending forward, stair climbing, hill climbing, and rising from a seated position can also provoke pain. Pain is reported to increase during sexual intercourse and menstruation in women.

Provider Inquiries	Clinical Reasoning/Logic
Relief: What makes pain better (heat/cold, rest, position, movement, medications)? What remedies have you used? Effective?	Resting and elevating the affected body part usually decreases the pain.
Radiation: Does pain travel or move anywhere? If so, where?	Some conditions/disorders (acute rheumatic fever, leukemia, juvenile rheumatoid arthritis) are associated with migratory arthritis. Pain that travels through the face, jaw, or neck is associated with TMJ dysfunction.
Associated signs/symptoms: Anything that accompanies pain? Stiffness, swelling, heat, redness? Joint locking or giving way? Nodules or deformity? Bony enlargement of joint? Fever, fatigue, dry eyes, myalgias, weight loss, pleuritis, pericarditis, neuropathy, or carpal tunnel syndrome? Rashes or plaques? Nail pitting, tenosynovitis, dactylitis (swelling of entire finger or toe)? Ocular involvement (uveitis)? SI joint involvement or spondylitis?	Bony enlargement of joint is associated with OA. Deformity of hands is common in RA and in psoriatic arthritis. Morning stiffness in RA lasts usually 30 minutes to an hour. RA and gout are usually inflammatory, so there may be redness, warmth, and swelling. Crepitation occurs during active ROM in OA. Swelling, warmth, and redness (inflammation) are associated with RA, septic arthritis, and gout. Fever may be seen in RA and septic arthritis. Constitutional symptoms and other extra-articular signs are common in RA. Psoriatic arthritis is highly likely in the presence of psoriatic plaques or history of psoriasis, although they can have other forms of arthritis as well. Nail pitting is also seen in psoriatic arthritis. Uveitis is seen in ankylosing spondylitis and psoriatic arthritis. Sacroiliitis and spondylitis are associated with ankylosing spondylitis and psoriatic arthritis. Patients with severe and disabling sacroiliac joint dysfunction can suffer from insomnia and depression. Sometimes earaches, dizziness, and hearing problems occur with TMJ.
Muscle/Pain or Myalgia **Myalgia**, or muscle pain, is a symptom of many diseases and disorders. Unusually excessive exertion (overuse or over-stretching of a muscle or group of muscles), trauma, and viral infections are among the most common causes. Myalgia without a traumatic history is often due to viral infections. Longer-term myalgias may be indicative of a metabolic myopathy, some nutritional deficiencies, or chronic fatigue syndrome.	
Characteristics: Soreness or pain? How is it felt (aching, cramping)? Weakness/fatigue? Muscle spasms, muscle tightness?	Cramping/aching pain associated with myalgia. Weakness associated with involvement of musculoskeletal/neurological disorders. Proximal weakness—**myopathy**, distal weakness—neuropathy Pain with weakness suggests primary muscular disorders. Soreness may be perceived as a dull, aching pain in the affected muscle, often combined with tenderness and stiffness associated with delayed onset muscle soreness.

Provider Inquiries	Clinical Reasoning/Logic
Onset: When first noted? Anything that initiates condition? Acute or gradual in onset? Does it occur in the morning? Subacute myalgias? Chronic? Recent start/discontinuation of drugs? Any recent accidents/injuries/strenuous activity?	Sudden pain may occur after trauma or strenuous exertion. Acute myalgia with constitutional symptoms suggests bacterial infection, viral influenza, acute hepatitis, or sepsis. Acute pain on neck, shoulder or upper arms/shoulder girdle, or hip suggests polymyalgia rheumatica (PMR). Morning acute myalgia is suggestive of PMR or inflammatory arthritis like RA or SLE and inflammatory myalgias. Subacute onset is associated with medications like statins seen weeks after initiating therapy. Chronic myalgia is seen in chronic hepatitis, vitamin D deficiency, hypothyroidism, fibromyalgia, myofascial syndrome, somatization disorder, and depression.
Location: Where located? Localized/generalized, diffuse?	Diffuse or generalized myalgias are characteristics of systemic infections like viral, bacterial, and spirochetal diseases, rheumatological diseases, fibromyalgia, medications, mitochondrial diseases, autoimmune diseases and endocrine diseases like adrenal and thyroid diseases.
Localized myalgias—occur in a specific region?	Localized myalgias are seen in trauma, overuse, overexertion, bursitis, tendinitis, myofascial pain syndrome or compartment syndrome. Acute pain on neck, shoulder, upper arms, and hip girdle is characteristic of PMR. With medications like statins, myalgias can also start
Proximal myalgias (upper arms, shoulder and hip girdle, and neck)?	proximally and symmetrically. Proximal muscle pain is seen in dermatomyositis and steroid myopathy. Acute, severe focal pain is seen in compartment syndrome.
Duration: How long does it last? How long has it been experienced?	Chronic multiple sites of muscle pain is seen in myofascial pain syndrome and fibromyalgia.
Exacerbation: What makes it worse (position, activity, temperature changes, sudden movement, stress)? Exertion? Medications? Trauma?	Acute trauma with severe, focal muscle pain and swelling suggest compartment syndrome. Statins may exacerbate myalgia.
Relief: What makes it better (rest, massage, position (elevation), heat/cold applications, splints, medications)?	Muscle pain that occurs during/after strenuous activity generally indicates a "pulled" or strained muscle. These types of injuries usually respond well to R.I.C.E. therapy: **Rest.** Reduce/stop normal activities. **Ice.** Place an ice pack or bag of frozen peas on the sore area for 15 to 20 minutes three times a day. **Compression.** Use a compression bandage to reduce swelling. **Elevation.** Elevate foot to help reduce swelling.

Provider Inquiries	Clinical Reasoning/Logic
Radiation: Does it travel or move anywhere? If so, where?	
Associated signs/symptoms: Malaise, weakness? Fever, swelling, warmth? Constipation, fatigue, hoarse voice?	Malaise or weakness is seen in pyomyositis, abscess, muscle infarct and compartment syndrome.
Do you have fever, or swelling/warm in the affected area? Do you have constipation, fatigue, or voice hoarseness? Do you have areas of hyperpigmentation? Myalgias with red/violaceous scaly papules on extensor surface of MCP and IP joints, upper eyelids, or malar region? Medications? Bursitis or joint pains? Trauma? Any cramps with myalgias?	Presence of fever suggests infections (viral, bacterial, sepsis) or pyomyositis. Myalgia with fever, malaise, and joint pain may be seen in inflammatory arthritis. Fatigue, weight gain, hoarse voice, and constipation with myalgias suggest hypothyroidism. Muscle pain, weakness, and hyper-pigmentation may be seen in adrenal insufficiency. Myalgias with weakness may be seen in statin or fibrates (anti-lipidemic) drugs users and may be seen weeks after starting the medications. Weakness is also seen in PMR, fibromyalgia, and myofascial pain syndrome. Joint pain, swelling, and myalgias are seen in psoriatic and other inflammatory joint diseases like SLE and RA. Compartment syndrome may be a result of trauma. Cramps are seen in electrolyte abnormalities, neurologic diseases, dehydration, medication use, unusual positioning, or are exercise induced.

Back Pain

Back pain is one of the most common medical problems and is one of the most common reasons people go to a health provider or miss work. Back pain often develops without a specific cause that can be identified with a test or imaging study. In about 85% of people, the physiologic cause of back pain is unidentifiable. Red flags for potentially serious causes of back pain include trauma, unintentional weight loss, unexplained fever, history of infections, immunosuppression, diabetes, history of cancer, IV drug use, prolonged steroid use, osteoporosis, age above 50 in women or men with compression fractures or osteoporosis, age above 70, focal neurological deficits, cauda equina syndrome, duration longer than 6 weeks, and prior surgery.

Provider Inquiries	Clinical Reasoning/Logic
Characteristics: How is pain felt (aching, tearing, burning, shooting, tingling/numbness)?	Back pain is experienced as a dull, constant ache to a sudden sharp pain. Acute, sharp, localized pain in the neck, upper/lower back—especially after lifting heavy objects or other strenuous activities indicates muscle strain and spasm and generally gets better.
Onset: Is it acute after lifting, trauma, sports activities, weight lifting, heavy lifting? Gradual or sudden? Prolonged and felt even when supine or during sleep? Under age 40?	Acute pain may occur after certain sports and injury. Subacute persistent pain, especially in a person with diagnosis of cancer, is suspicious for cancer involvement of the bone. In men under 40, persistent back pain, especially involving the sacroiliac joint, suggests ankylosing spondylitis.
Location: Is the pain unilateral/bilateral? Does it occur in one area on back (upper, middle, lower)?	Location may vary depending on cause or areas of spine involvement. Persistent aching/stiffness anywhere along the spine
Duration: How long does pain last? Constant/intermittent?	In most instances it lasts only days to weeks; 40%, however, will experience a recurrence and may go on to develop chronic back pain.

Provider Inquiries	Clinical Reasoning/Logic
	Acute back pain—1 month or less
	Chronic back pain > 3 months. Persistent pain after 6 weeks is worrisome and deserves a work up, especially with attended risk factors (see red flags).
Exacerbation: What makes pain worse (coughing, sneezing, position, posture, activity)?	Pain that increases when coughing/sneezing or Valsalva are seen in disc herniation. Most back pain is better when one assumes lying positions. Degenerative disc disease is worse with standing or walking, and relieved by sitting or lying positions and leaning forward. Low back pain is worse with lying down and may indicate infectious or malignant cause of pain. Peripheral neuropathy is usually not affected by change in position or activity.
Relief: What makes pain better (position/posture, hot/cold applications, medications, therapy/other providers/treatment)? Is it relieved by lying down?	Persistent pain unrelieved by rest, such as sitting or supine position, is worrisome.
Radiation: Does pain travel anywhere? If so, where?	Nerve root irritation like in sciatica will manifest with back pain radiating to posterior-lateral leg to the ankle and foot.
Associated signs/symptoms: Any neurologic symptom, such as numbness, tingling, and weakness following a nerve distribution? Bladder and bowel incontinence with numbness or loss of sensation around the rectal region and groin?	Numbness, tingling, sensory loss, and weakness are usually associated with nerve root involvement. Saddle anesthesia is seen with bowel and bladder incontinence, and weakness on the lower extremity suggests cauda equina syndrome, which can be due to tumor or midline disc herniation.
Weight loss, fatigue?	Weight loss is a constitutional symptom, and when seen in a person with persistent back pain suggests infection, inflammatory or neoplastic involvement of the spine.
Fever? Urinary symptoms?	Fever, dysuria, and burning during urination may indicate bacterial urinary tract infection. Fever and persistent, nagging back pain may also be seen in vertebral osteomyelitis.

Past Medical History

Past medical history provides information as to previous illnesses or conditions that may have an effect on the musculoskeletal system.

Experienced any trauma: Incident, what bones/muscles affected (fracture, sprains, strains, dislocations); complications (failure to heal, infection); outcomes; residual effects?	It is important to determine if there may be a previous incident that may have predisposed the patient to musculoskeletal disorder.
Surgery: For what; procedure (arthroscopy, open incision); complications; outcomes?	Complications may arise after surgery, like infection or inflammation.
Chronic conditions: Cancer, renal/neurological disorder, arthritis (DJD, RA)?	Unrelenting back pain in a patient with malignancy suggests neoplastic involvement with a tumor.
Skeletal: Disorders, deformities (describe)?	

Provider Inquiries	Clinical Reasoning/Logic
Weight conditions: Have there ever been any issues/concerns related to your weight? If obesity, how long? If recent weight gain, over what time period?	Increased weight places increased stress on joints, which may cause or hasten onset of osteoarthritis.

Family History

Family history provides information regarding family members' illnesses or conditions as potential causes for chief complaint or presenting symptoms that may indicate a pattern of presentation associated with transmission of familial/genetic factors predisposing the individual to certain system-related conditions/illnesses. Any of these may indicate a potential or actual cause of musculoskeletal dysfunction.

Provider Inquiries	Clinical Reasoning/Logic
Congenital conditions of hip/foot?	
Spinal conditions: Scoliosis/back problems, spinal stenosis?	
Rheumatic disorders: Arthritis (DJD, RA), ankylosing spondylitis, gout?	
Genetic conditions: Osteogenesis imperfecta, rickets, muscular dystrophy, calcium/phosphate disorders?	
Weight problems?	Excessive weight puts added stress on the skeleton, creating joint difficulties and weight-bearing alterations.

Personal and Social History

Personal and social history provides information related to habits, practices and/or environmental influences that may predispose the patient to the development of certain system-related conditions/illnesses.

Provider Inquiries	Clinical Reasoning/Logic
Working conditions: Heavy lifting (use of back support), repetitive motions, potential for injury/trauma (use protective gear/wear)? Job stress, satisfaction with job, prolonged standing?	Repetitive joint movements predispose to carpal tunnel syndrome. Heavy lifting predisposes to lower back pain. Job stress and dissatisfaction are risk factors for lower back pain.
	Participation in sports activities increases risk for trauma, particularly if no protective gear used.
Exercise patterns: Frequency, type (weight bearing/stress on joints), precautions (shoes, warm up/cool down)? Any injury/trauma from exercise?	Sedentary lifestyle precipitates muscle weakness and contributes to poor coordination and skills.
Sun exposure?	Daily UV exposure (20 minutes) needed for vitamin D synthesis.
Nutrition: Calcium, vitamin D, calorie, protein intake?	Decreased protein intake interferes with proper bone growth and muscle tone.
	Low Ca++ intake decreases bone density, increasing risk for osteoporosis.
	Decreased vitamin C interferes with proper bone and tissue healing.
	Milk (lactose) intolerance reduces Ca++ intake leading to osteoporosis.
Habits: Smoking, alcohol, substance abuse (frequency, amount)?	Smoking, caffeine, and alcohol increase the risk for developing osteoporosis. Substance abuse is a risk factor for lower back pain.
Functional abilities: Mobility (walking, stair climbing, housework; [any restrictions]), personal care (washing, bathing, grooming, elimination)?	

Developmental Applications

Certain conditions or disorders may be related to certain age groups or situations. Inquiring to obtain age- or condition-specific information will provide further information for helping to determine causes of the chief concern as identified.

Provider Inquiries	Clinical Reasoning/Logic
Infants and Children	
Birth history: Delivery problems (trauma, use of forceps, shoulder injury); presentation (head first)?	Traumatic births increase risk for fractures, especially of the clavicle.
Low birth weight/premature; need resuscitation, ventilator support (how long)?	Periods of anoxia associated with decreased muscle tone.
Hip dislocation, club foot: How treated, any problems? Any difficulty with walking?	Early intervention necessary for some deformities to prevent long lasting complications. Some deformities may self-correct; others may require surgery.
Broken bones/dislocations: Which ones, how treated, outcomes? Any noticeable deformities?	
Developmental progress: Fine motor and gross motor development appropriate for age? **Coordination:** Mobility (muscle flaccidity/spasticity)?	Fine and gross motor developmental tasks require neuromuscular coordination.
Activity: Sports involvement—type, protection, injuries? Adult supervision?	Involvement with sports increases risk for musculo/skeletal injuries. Adult supervision to prevent major injuries.
The Pregnant Woman	
Are you experiencing muscle cramping?	If not presenting complaint, do symptom analysis with COLDERRA.
Back pain: Weeks of pregnancy? If this is not first pregnancy, determine if this is a new symptom or has occurred with previous pregnancies. Type of shoes worn?	Lordosis develops during last trimester.
Going to breastfeed?	Breastfeeding increases requirements for vitamin D.
The Older Adult	
Activities of daily living: Are you able to participate in/perform daily routine activities related to your care needs (preparing meals, eating, toileting, shopping)? Do you have mobility/safety issues (climbing stairs, risk for falling)?	Helps to determine capabilities of individual to care for self and prevent injuries.
Weakness: Have you experienced/do you experience any muscle weakness?	Muscle weakness is common as individual ages.
Balance and coordination: Increase in falls/stumbling? Any injuries? Changes in mobility? Do you use or think you need aids (cane, walker)?	Older adults have an increased incidence of falls often due to a change in posture that affects balance. The loss of balance may be due to sensory/motor disorders (inner ear infection, side effects of medications). Use of walking aids may help with ambulation but may also be a cause of falls if they are not used correctly.
Pain/stiffness in joints: Limitation of movement?	
Muscle cramps?	
Medications?	

OBJECTIVE DATA

Objective data are obtained through inspection and palpation. The overall focus for the MS exam is to examine for symmetry and alignment. The examination of the muscles and bones is easily incorporated throughout the whole exam. Observation of the patient throughout the exam will provide clues as to whether the patient is experiencing any musculoskeletal deficits or not.

Inspection

- Skeleton
  - Alignment—linear arrangement of bones
    - Spine
    - Upper/lower extremities
    - Joints—swelling, redness, deformity
  - Movement/coordination
    - Gait ROM
    - Tests
- Muscles—symmetry of right and left sides [atrophy/hypertrophy]
  - Size (mass)

Palpation

- Skeleton
  - Joints
  - Warmth
  - Pain
- Muscles
  - Mass
  - Bulk
  - Strength

Percussion*—not performed*

Auscultation*—not performed*

Level I to IV Examination

The Level I to Level IV examinations are performed on a continuum, which starts from a basic level to a more comprehensive level based on the provider's abilities and knowledge as well as the patient's presentation and location. It may start at the outpatient setting progressing to the ED, hospital unit bed, critical care unit, or specialty unit. Frequently all the elements from basic to comprehensive exam are done in one setting, like in a primary care setting or clinic.

The condition/illness of the patient is the primary consideration related to the type and amount of data needed to assess the patient's condition/illness/situation. The arrangement of skills into levels is for general purposes and is meant to be descriptive rather than prescriptive. The purpose of arranging into levels is to provide a framework to assist the learner in determining the appropriate data to collect.

Bones and Muscles

	Level I	Level II	Level III	Level IV
Bones and Muscles				
Inspection	General movement, coordination Skeletal alignment (symmetry, position, posture) Skeletal alignment (anterior, posterior, lateral) Joints (shape, size/symmetry) Extremity length measurement	Mobility (movement/coordination [gait])	Skeletal alignment (linear continuity of bone): fractures, dislocations	Straight leg raising test Femoral stretch test Thomas test Trendelenburg test
	Muscle Mass: Size/shape, symmetry Muscle tone		Pain: knee, back, joint (strains, sprains)	

Bones and Muscles *continued*

			Dislocation Hawkins Kennedy test	
		Phalen's test		
	GALS (ROM)	ROM active/(passive)		
Palpation	GALS Joints (temperature, pain, effusion, crepitus)	Bulge test Ballottment	Neer test Drop arm test	Specific joints (TMJ, wrist, hips, knee)
		Muscle strength		Bragard stretch test Tinel's sign Snuffbox tenderness Drawer test McMurray test Lachman test
		Examine knee/ shoulder		

Inspection: Level I

The Level I examination is primarily concerned with general observation of overall mobility, movement, and coordination. The axial/appendicular skeletal structures are observed for alignment, symmetry, and the presence of any gross alterations as well as muscles for mass, symmetry, and tone. Much of the information for Level I may be obtained during the General Assessment (Chapter 7).

Inspection Techniques and Expected Findings	Unexpected Findings
Mobility and Coordination Smooth, coordinated, and effortless movement is dependent on appropriate innervation of muscles so that motor impulses can be transmitted from the brain to the muscles resulting in muscle contraction and relaxation. The quality of muscle movement is also considered as the motor exam component for the neurological exam (Chapter 26). Observe overall muscle movement for smoothness, coordination, and effort. Observe for any limitations of movement that may be related to pain or deformities. Muscle dysfunction as well as nerve damage may also be noted to limit movement. The patient is expected to be able to voluntarily move the extremities freely without excessive effort and pain. Movements should also be coordinated and purposeful and without any limitations due to pain or deformities.	Muscle movements that are uncoordinated or ROM that is limited, and muscle size and shape that is asymmetrical would be significant for some type of dysfunction. Unexpected observations would be movements that are involuntary, uncoordinated, and do not appear to be purposeful. (More specific alterations are described in Chapter 7.)
General movement/coordination General movement and coordination can be easily observed when patient walks into room as well as when changing positions during the exam. These movements should be smooth, voluntary, and coordinated.	
Skeletal Alignment Initially, observe the overall skeletal alignment from behind (posterior view) (Figure 27-13). With the patient's back exposed, observe the straightness of the spinal column as well as the lower extremities.	Alterations in alignment are described as deviations toward or away from the midline of the body.
The head should also be in alignment with the three sections of the spinal cord as well as the gluteal cleft.	A lateral curvature of the spine is an indicator of **scoliosis**.

Inspection Techniques and Expected Findings

The spine should be in a straight line (midline) from the neck to the hips.

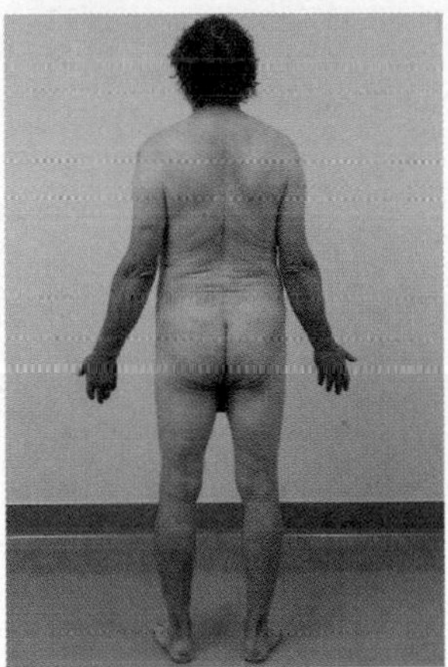

FIGURE 27-13 Posterior view of patient; note alignment of head with gluteal cleft

Observe for symmetry of skinfolds and muscles.

The lower extremities should be in a straight line between the hips and the ankles with the heel of the foot firmly placed on the floor. The arms should be hanging freely on the sides of the body, also in a straight line. The head should be held upright and positioned on the midline of the body. The shoulder blades should be symmetrically positioned on the sides of the upper trunk.

Inspection of the anterior trunk and lower extremities should demonstrate the same characteristics (Figure 27-15). From the anterior view, the knees should be in a straight line between the hips and ankles and the feet should be flat on the floor, pointing directly forward in a symmetrical manner or slightly toward the outside.

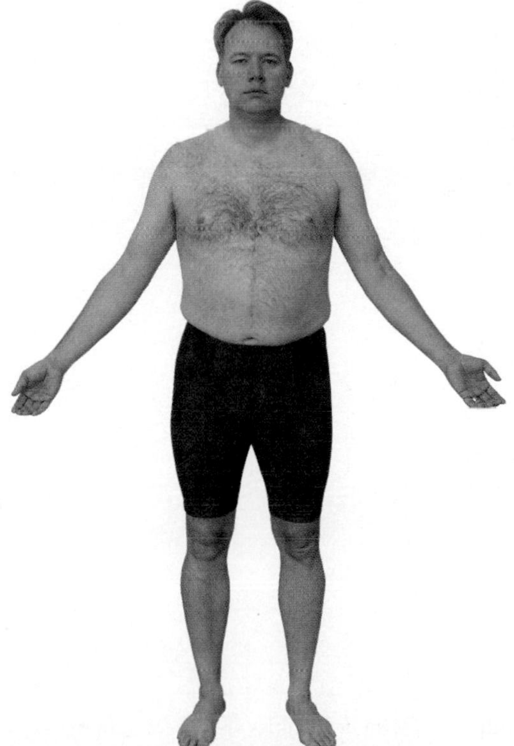

FIGURE 27-15 Anterior view of patient

Unexpected Findings

Bones that deviate toward the midline are described as **varus** deformities; bones that deviate away from the midline are described as **valgum**. The most common deviations observed related to alignment of the lower extremities are bowleg (genu varum) and knock-knee (genu valgum) (Figure 27-14).

THINK LINK: Genu Varum/Valgum

At first glance genu varum and genu valgum appear to be switched. In genu varum the knees looked bowed, and in genu valgum; the knees look closer together. The reason for the appearance of the knees is actually the misalignment of the tibia. In bowlegged people, the tibia is angled inward, giving the knees the outward appearance; in knock-kneed people, the tibia is angled outward, giving the knees the inward appearance. Therefore, it is the direction of the tibia that is used to evaluate the appearance, not the knees, even though the common description of these conditions is related to the knees.

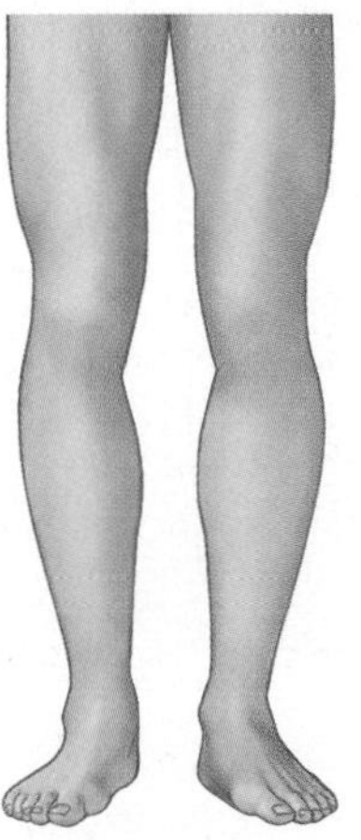

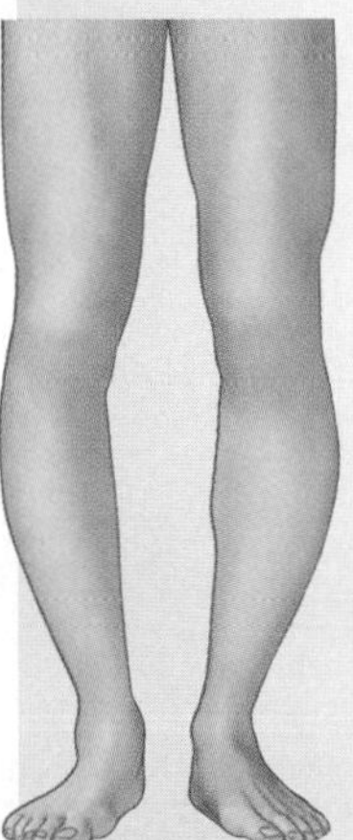

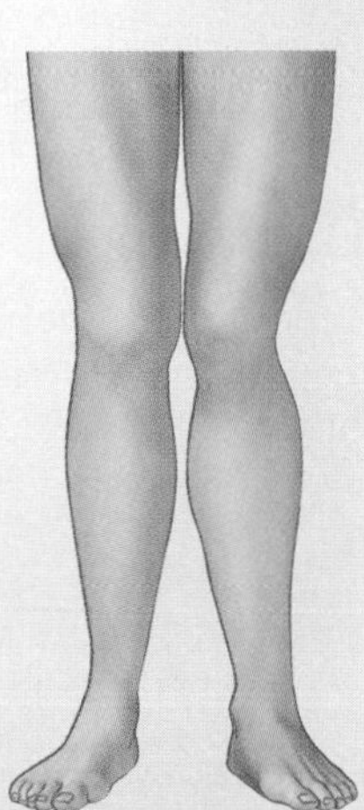

FIGURE 27-14 Alterations of tibia alignment

Inspection Techniques and Expected Findings	Unexpected Findings
Also observe skeletal alignment from the side with the patient standing upright without any forward or backward leaning (Figure 27-16). From the side, the spinal column should demonstrate three distinct curves—cervical, thoracic, and lumbar. The cervical and lumbar curves are concave and located at their anatomical locations. The thoracic curve is convex and positioned between the cervical and lumbar curves.	Unexpected findings would be an exaggerated thoracic curve (kyphosis) or lumbar curve (lordosis) of the spine (Figure 27-17). **Lordosis** is common in obese patients as well as those who are pregnant. If lordosis is the result of pregnancy, it should disappear after the birth of the infant. **Kyphosis** is commonly seen in elderly patients. A **gibbus**, a sharp, angular deformity, is associated with a collapsed vertebra or osteoporosis.

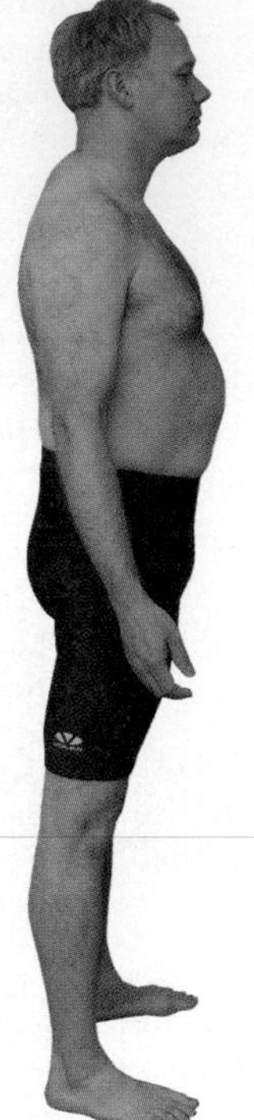

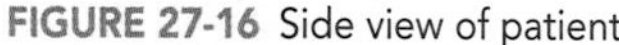

FIGURE 27-16 Side view of patient

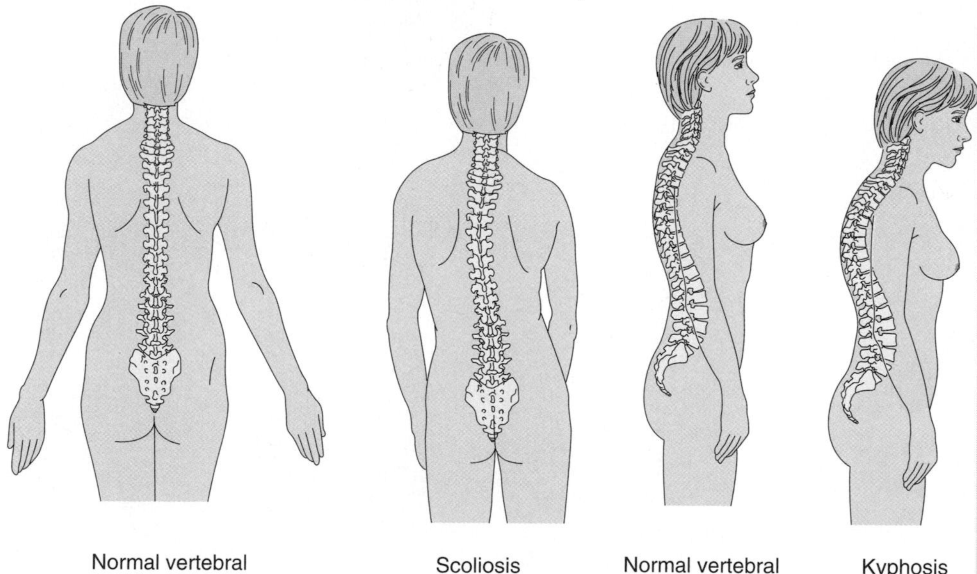

FIGURE 27-17 Curvature alterations of spine

Joints

Inspection Techniques and Expected Findings	Unexpected Findings
Observe finger joints/knuckles (PIP, DIP) for size, shape, and symmetry. PIP/DIP joints of both hands should be equal in size, shape, and symmetry.	Joint deformities are observed in the presence of rheumatoid arthritis (RA) or osteoarthritis (degenerative joint disease, DJD). Common manifestations of both conditions are joint enlargement

Inspection Techniques and Expected Findings

Unexpected Findings

(Figure 27-18). Joint involvement in RA is bilaterally symmetrical and affects multiple joints, with the hands and fingers being the most common locations. As the condition progresses, the following later deformities may develop:

Ulnar deviation: Flexion of the fingers toward the ulnar side of the hand

Swan-neck: Hyperflexion of the DIP joints and hyperextension of the PIP joints

Boutonnières: Hyperextension of the DIP joints and hyperflexion of the PIP joints.

Joint involvement in DJD is asymmetrical and may involve one or two joints. Joints will be swollen due to soft tissue damage and effusion (fluid) into the joints. Joints commonly have hard, nontender nodules bony overgrowths (**osteophytes**) on them. DIP joint nodules are known as **Heberden's nodes**; PIP joint nodules are **Bouchard's nodes.**

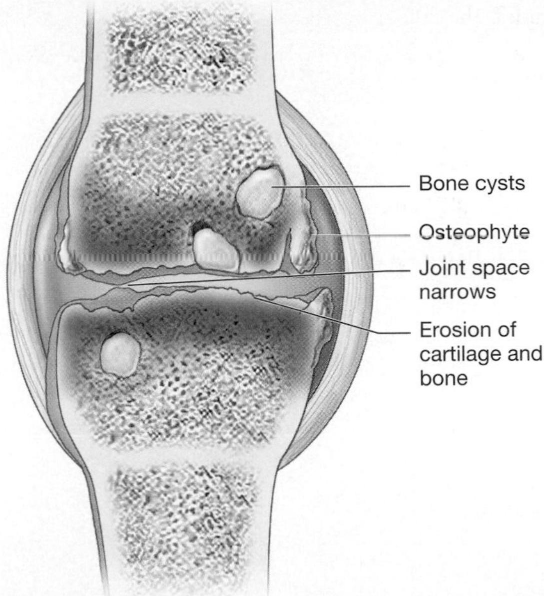

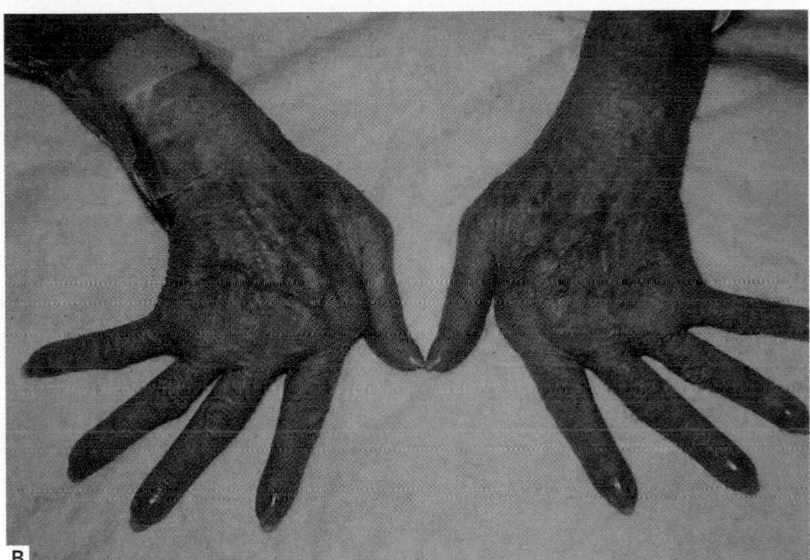

FIGURE 27-18A–B Unexpected findings: **a)** Osteoarthritis; **b)** Joint alterations in arthritis

Extremity Length

When a difference in length is suspected or observed between the paired extremities, measurement of extremity length is done (Figure 27-19).

Measure the leg length from the anterior superior iliac crest to the medial malleolus. The measuring tape will cross over to the medial side in proximity to the knee.

Measure the arm length from the acromion process to the tip of the middle finger. Expected findings would be a measured limb length that is identical or a difference that is not greater than 1 cm.

Lower extremities with a difference of >1 cm

Inspection Techniques and Expected Findings	Unexpected Findings

When measuring the circumference of the extremities, no specific landmarks are used as reference points, so it is necessary to obtain measurements using identical locations on both extremities. The expected and unexpected findings would be the same as for limb length.

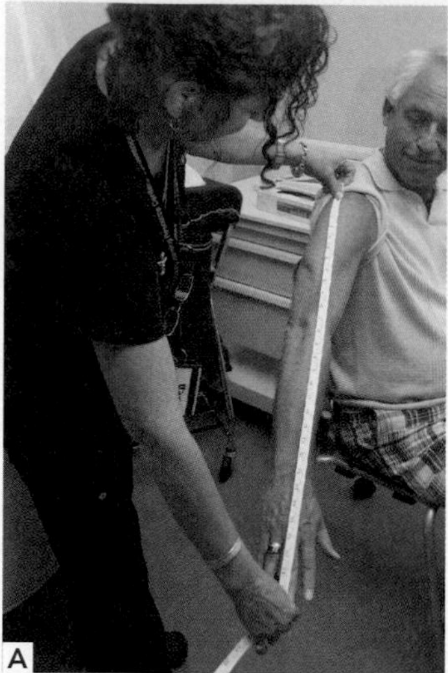

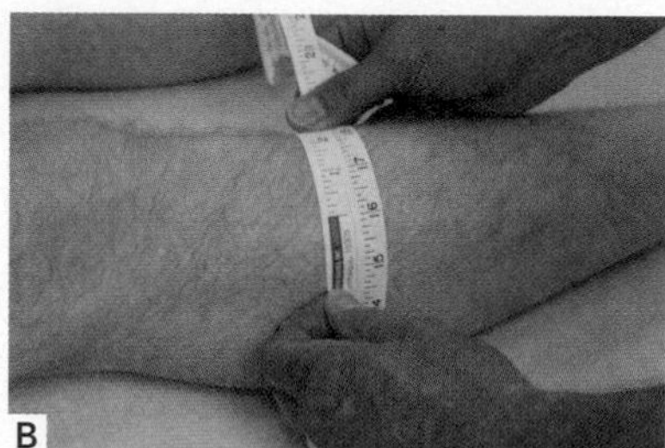

FIGURE 27-19A–B Limb measurement: length and circumference

Muscle Mass

Observe muscles for shape and symmetry of size. Muscles should demonstrate a symmetrical appearance as well as equality in muscle mass (bulk) or size.

Muscles are expected to be bilaterally equal in size and shape and demonstrate coordinated movement.

From behind the patient, observe the shoulder girdle and paraspinal muscles, gluteal muscles, and calf muscles.

From the front, observe the quadriceps muscle group. All muscle groups should be symmetrically equal in bulk and size.

Observe for the presence of atrophy or hypertrophy and whether it occurs bilaterally or unilaterally. Confirmation of atrophy or hypertrophy can be obtained by measuring the circumference of an extremity.

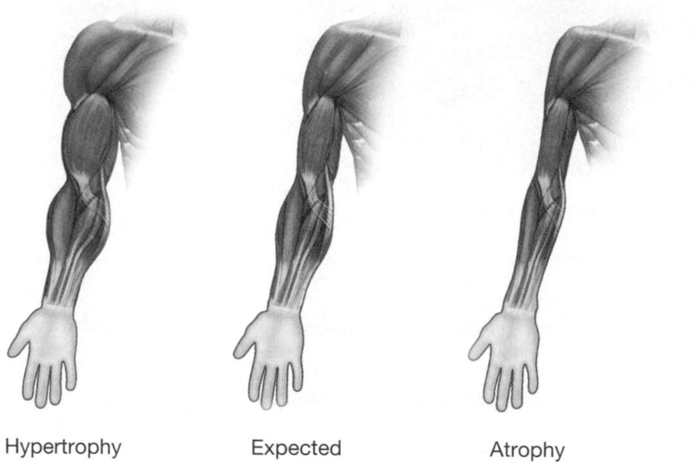

FIGURE 27-20 Muscle hypertrophy and atrophy

Unexpected Findings:

Symmetry is not absolute, as there may be a slight variation in size and bulk. Generally, the predominant side of the individual may be slightly larger than the non-dominant side, particularly in individuals engaged in manual labor in which the dominant side is often used for various work-related actions.

If there is a systemic condition that affects the individual, there most likely will be bilateral involvement. A localized condition would most likely be responsible for unilateral involvement.

Muscle atrophy and hypertrophy are characterized as a loss or gain of muscle mass (circumference; Figure 27-20).

Muscle atrophy occurs as a result of non-use or non-weight bearing of an extremity. Extremities that have been in a cast for a bone fracture are often smaller in size when the cast is removed.

Hypertrophy is the result of an increase in size of the muscle cells producing an overall increase in the muscle itself. It occurs most commonly as a result of weight lifting.

Muscle Tone

Observe the patient's muscle movement tone. Movements should be coordinated and smooth and the patient should be able to flex and extend muscle groups at will.

Unexpected Findings:

Loss of muscle tone is demonstrated in two forms—spastic or flaccid. Both extremes of muscle tone make it impossible to support body weight; thus the individual is unable to assume an upright position.

Inspection Techniques and Expected Findings	Unexpected Findings
	Spastic muscle tone is stiff and rigid, thus making it extremely resistant to passive movement. The muscles are in a state of hyperflexion and hyperextension. Spasticity is frequently associated with upper motor neuron disorders.
	Flaccid muscle tone is characterized by extremities that are floppy and offer no resistance to passive movement. Muscles are in a state of hypoflexion and hypoextension.

GALS

Historically, examination of the MS system has been perceived to be less important than other systems (Walker & Kay, 2002).

To increase the frequency of MS examinations, a screening tool was developed to assist the provider in detecting significant MS alterations. This screening tool is known as **GALS**, which stands for **g**ait, **a**rms, **l**egs, and **s**pine.

Although the following sequence does not specifically follow the same order as the GALS Screening Tool, all elements of the GALS examination are included.

Observe ROM in certain joints (Figure 27-21). While observing the patient from the front, note the elbow in full extension. Instruct the patient to tilt the head from side to side so that the ear touches the shoulder to observe lateral extension of the neck.

Next instruct the patient to move the head backward as far as possible and then touch the chin to the chest to observe for neck extension and flexion.

Next have the patient touch the side of one knee, then the other without bending the legs to observe lateral flexion of the spine.

While still in front, have the patient place the hands behind the head and push the elbows back to observe shoulder adduction and external rotation as well as elbow flexion.

Next have the patient bring the arms down and place them behind the small of the back, observing internal rotation and extension. Return the arms to anatomical position and observe anterior shoulder bulk and note elbow extension if not done previously.

Unexpected findings would be inability to move the joints through the expected ROM. The significance of the joint limitation needs to be determined by the patient's age and the presence of any joint-limiting condition.

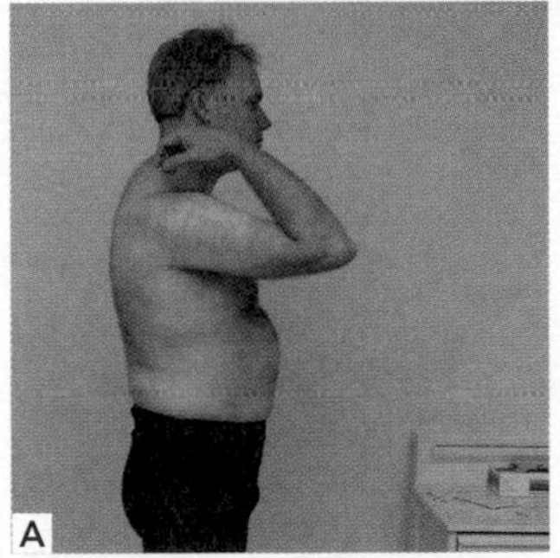

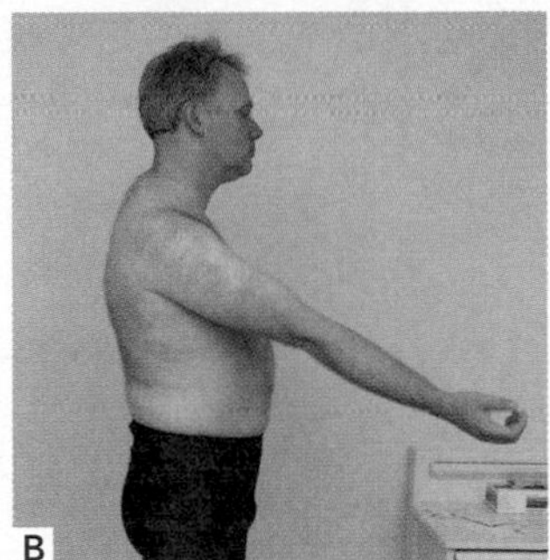

FIGURE 27-21A–B Example of ROM for GALS screening exam

Inspection: Level II

Mobility

The most common observation of coordinated movement is to observe the patient's gait; however, in a critical situation it is unlikely that this observation would be possible. Any movement that the patient attempts should be voluntary, with smooth and coordinated efforts to facilitate movement (Figure 27-22).

Alterations in gait are a reflection of conditions that affect the musculoskeletal or neurological system. Specific conditions often have unique gait characteristics

Inspection Techniques and Expected Findings	Unexpected Findings
Observe the patient when walking into the exam room or have the patient walk toward the wall and back. The patient's head should be held erect. Observe for symmetry and smoothness of movement as well as the elements and sequence of the two phases of gait—**swing** and **stance phase**. The stance phase is characterized as weight bearing with the foot in contact with the ground. The swing phase is characterized as no weight bearing with no contact with the ground. Each phase can be broken down into steps (Table 27-6). Each phase should occupy 50% of each cycle. Also note the motion of the arms, which should swing in the same direction as the opposite leg so that when the left leg is in the swing phase, the right arm should also be swinging in the same direction.	that help to identify what condition the patient may have. Altered gait patterns, usual causes, and unique characteristics are identified and described in Table 27-7 and Figure 27-23.

Table 27-6 Phases of a gait and their descriptions

Stance	Heel strike	Heel comes in contact with floor. Quiet, controlled, smooth and coordinated. Knee in extension.
	Foot flat	Foot flattens, entire foot in contact with ground.
	Mid-stance	Weight is distributed evenly over entire foot.
	Push-off	Hyperextension of MTP joints, heel of foot lifted off the ground, weight transferred to ball of foot.
Swing	Acceleration	Quadriceps contract, initiating the forward swing of the foot. Knee flexed, shortening the leg allowing for ground clearance. Ankle dorsiflexes also allowing ground clearance.
	Midswing	Ankle in dorsiflexion while leg is moving forward
	Deceleration	Contraction of hamstring muscles, decelerating the forward swing in preparation for heel strike

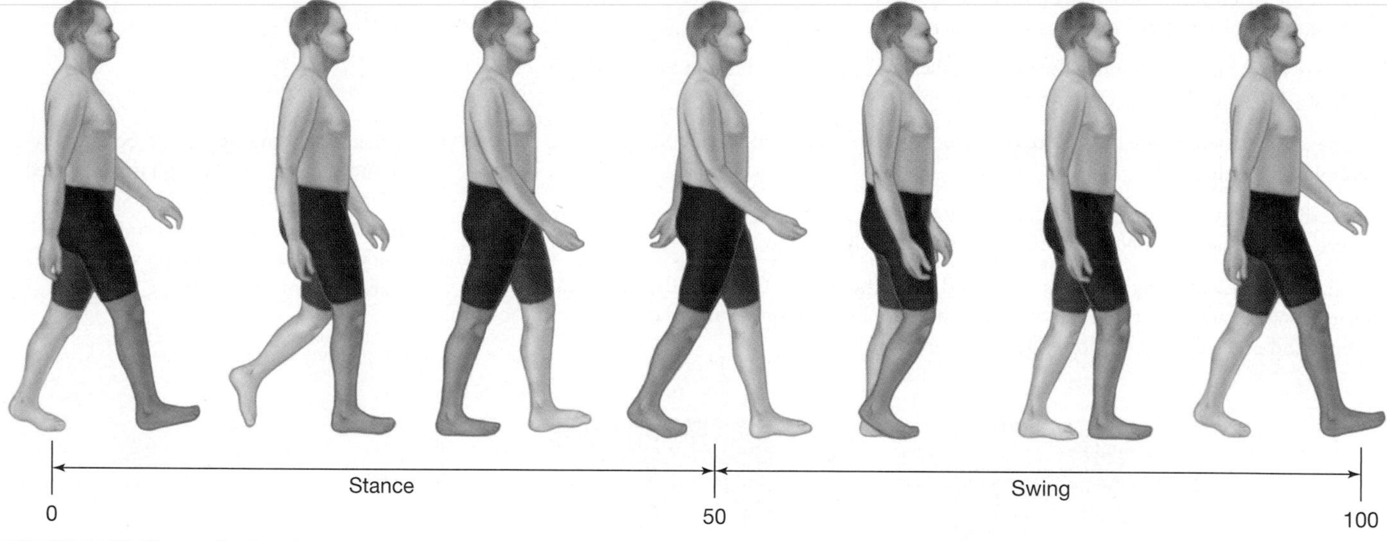

FIGURE 27-22 Phases of gait cycle

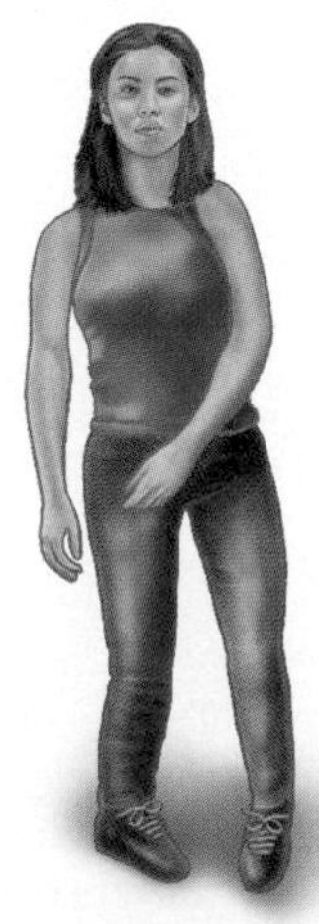
Spastic gait

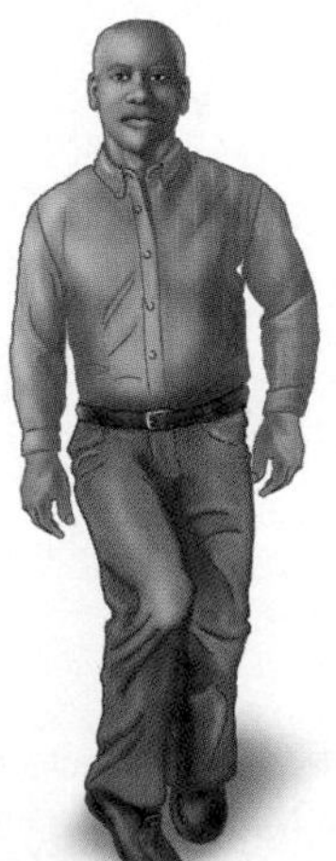
Scissors gait

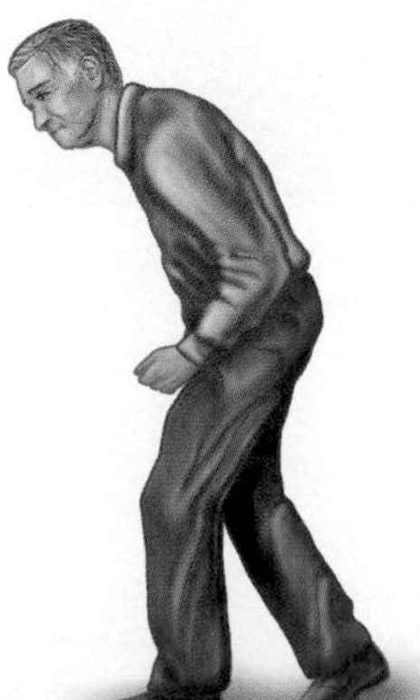
Propulsive gait

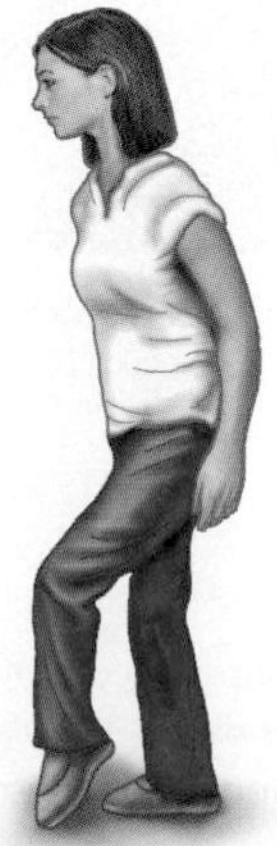
Steppage gait

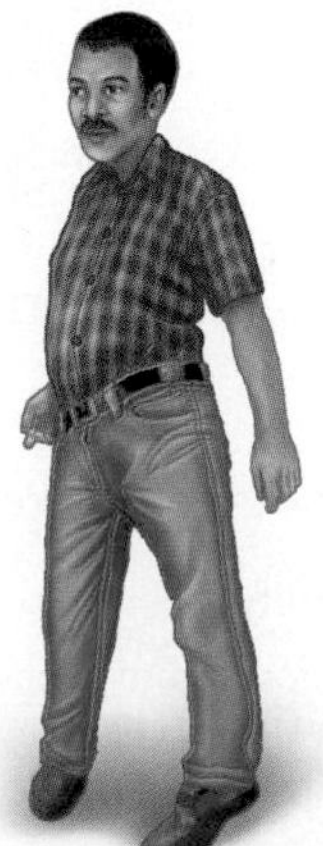
Waddling gait

FIGURE 27-23 Gait alterations

Inspection Techniques and Expected Findings | **Unexpected Findings**

Table 27-7 Altered gaits

Gait Pattern	Common Cause	Characteristics
Spastic hemiparesis	Stroke (CVA)—lesion of corticospinal tract	Affected arm in abduction with internal rotation of the shoulder, pronation of the forearm and flexion of wrists and fingers. Affected leg is stiff and extended with foot in plantar flexion. Tilting the affected side of the pelvis upward and dragging or swinging of the foot in a circular motion results in forward movement. When dragging the foot, the toe is often scraped.
Spastic diplegia	Cerebral palsy (lesion/injury of pyramidal system)	Stiff legs (spastic) are extended and the thighs cross forward on each other with each step. The steps tend to be short and the ball of the foot is dragged across the floor/ground.
Steppage	Foot drop (lower motor neuron disease)	Foot is plantarflexed necessitating excessive elevation of hip and knee to get foot off of ground. Foot is brought down to the floor with a slap.
Dystrophic (waddling)	Muscular dystrophy	Legs positioned far apart to maintain wide base of support; weak hip abductor muscles result in weight shifting from side to side, exaggerated pelvic tilt with waddling gait. Lordosis also a common manifestation.
Cerebellar ataxia	Lesion of cerebellum or cerebellar pathways	Feet are wide based with steps that are variable in length with an irregular rhythm resulting in a staggering gait (feet thrown outward) with a lurching quality, and trunk swaying side to side.
Sensory ataxia	Loss of position sense of legs (polyneuropathy or damage to posterior column)	Feet wide based and unsteady gait; slow and deliberate steps, watching ground for visual navigation. Feet thrown forward and outward, bringing them down on the heels first and then toes, creating a slapping sound (slapping gait)
Parkinsonian gait	Basal ganglia defects caused by Parkinson's disease	Stooped posture with rigid body held; head and neck forward, hips and knees slightly flexed. Elbow and wrist flexed—decreased arm swing. Hesitation on initiating walking, although when going has difficulty stopping. Steps short with shuffling.
Tabetic gait	Tabes: gradual, progressive wasting of the body associated with any chronic disease	High stepping gait; legs wide apart and brought down forcefully, stamping the heel on the ground.
Dystonia	Chorea (Huntington's, Syndham's)	Involuntary, jerky, dancing movements, irregular in pattern, sometimes bizarre.
Antalgic gait (limp)	Sprain, strain (painful limb or joint)	Gait pattern that is asymmetric, stance phase reduced to limit weight bearing on affected leg.

ROM

Measure joint ROM by how easily specific types of joints (diarthrodial) can move through their expected degrees of movement.

Active ROM is observed when the patient is able to move the joints independently without any support or help from the provider.

Any time there appears to be any limitation of movement, use passive ROM, which occurs when the patient needs help to move a joint. This may be confined to one or a few joints, or the patient may require help to move all the joints.

To observe ROM, have the patient place the joint in its neutral position. Ask the patient to then move the joint through its direction and extent of movement.

Joint movement should be smooth and effortless and the expected degrees of movement should be easily attained.

If pain and tenderness result in limitation of movement, measure the degree of movement with a goniometer (Figure 27-24). The same can be used if there is an increase in ROM.

Pain and tenderness are common causes of limitation of movement. The significance of the joint limitation needs to be determined by the patient's age and the presence of any joint-limiting condition.

Crepitus may be heard as a grating sound from bone moving over bone, as occurs in osteoarthritis or rheumatoid arthritis. Occasionally a "crack" may be heard when the joint is moved. This occurs when a ligament or tendon slips over the bone during motion and is commonly heard in the knee when doing a knee bend.

Inspection Techniques and Expected Findings	Unexpected Findings

First place the goniometer with the 0 point centered over a joint that is in its neutral position. Have the patient then extend or flex the joint and measure the angle of movement with the goniometer.

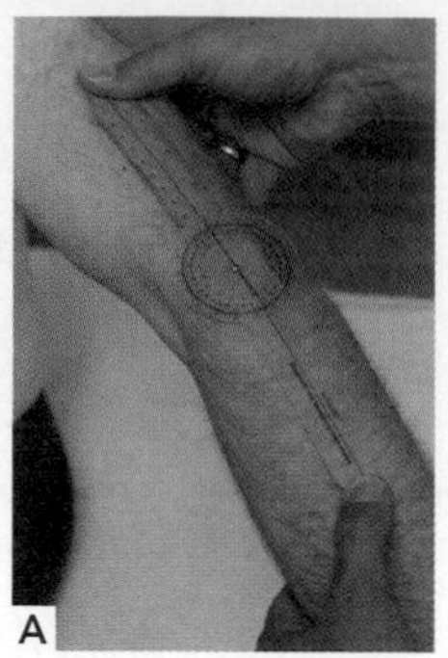

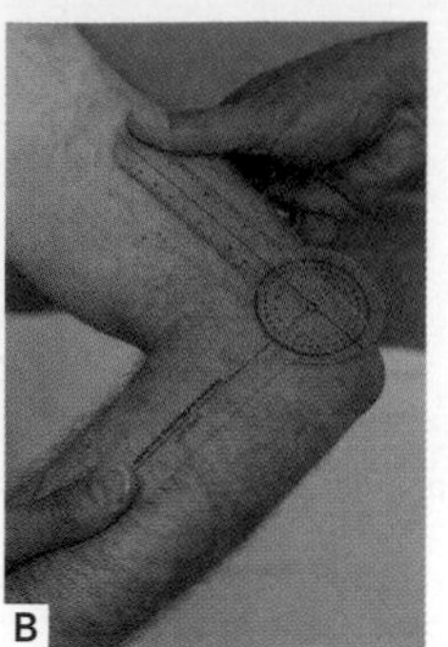

FIGURE 27-24A–B Goniometer placed over joint in neutral position and then after joint movement

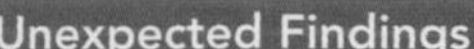

PRACTICE POINT: Movement Demonstration

You may need to demonstrate movement for the patient. To make sure that the patient understands the directions for ROM movements, it is helpful for the provider to request the patient to copy the movements as they are demonstrated to the patient.

Head and Neck

To assess ROM, request that the patient (Figure 27-25):

Bend the head forward touching the chin to the chest. Observe for 45 degrees of flexion.

Bend the head backward pointing the chin to the ceiling. Observe for 45 degrees of extension.

Bend the head to each side, touching each ear to the shoulder for lateral flexion. Observe for lateral bending of 40 degrees.

Turn the head side to side, with the chin pointing toward each shoulder for lateral rotation. Observe for 70 degrees of rotation.

Unexpected results would be the inability to move the neck through the expected degrees of movement, or the presence of pain or stiffness.

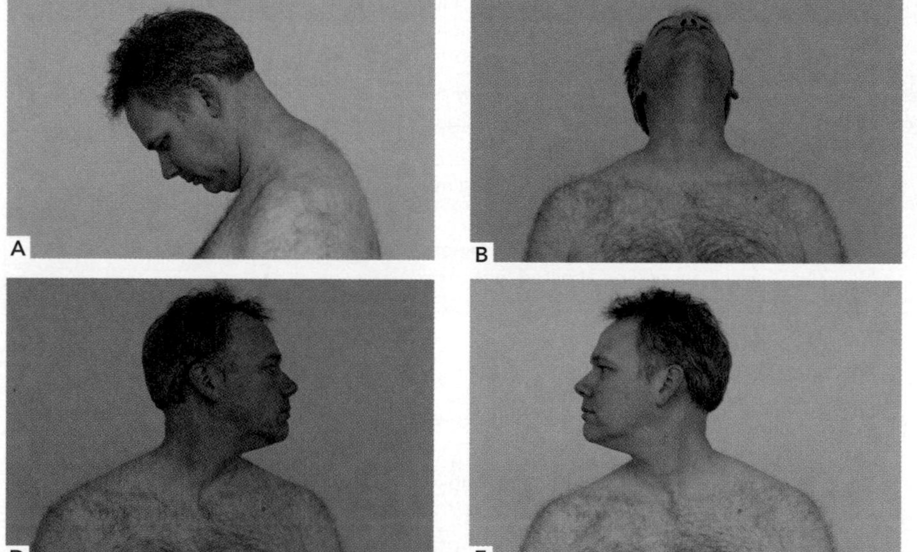

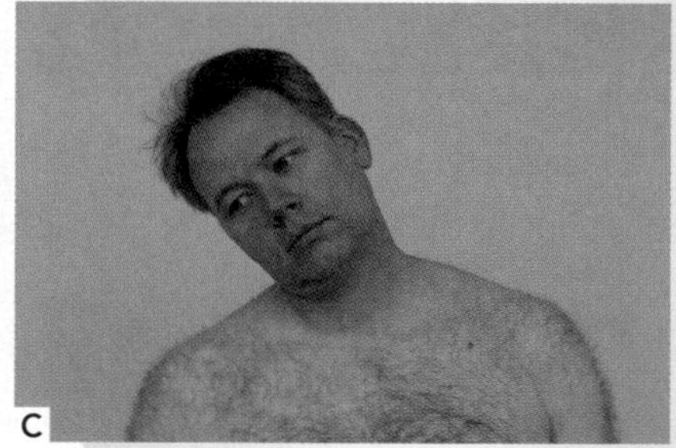

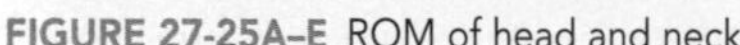

FIGURE 27-25A–E ROM of head and neck

The temporomandibular joint (TMJ) is the articulation of the mandible with the temporal bone of the cranium. The joint should move smoothly and should be without tenderness, crepitus, and locking. There may be an audible or palpable pop or clicking when the joint moves, but this is not significant. (This also tests for CN V motor aspect for the neurological exam.)

Unexpected findings would be the inability to move the TMJ through the expected maneuvers. Pain is also unexpected.

To assess ROM, request that the patient (Figure 27-26):

- Open and close the mouth. Observe for a 3–6 cm space between the upper and lower jaw when it is open.
- Move the lower jaw from side. Observe for a 1–2 cm movement in each direction.
- Move the jaw (chin) in and out. Observe for movement in both directions.

Inspection Techniques and Expected Findings	Unexpected Findings

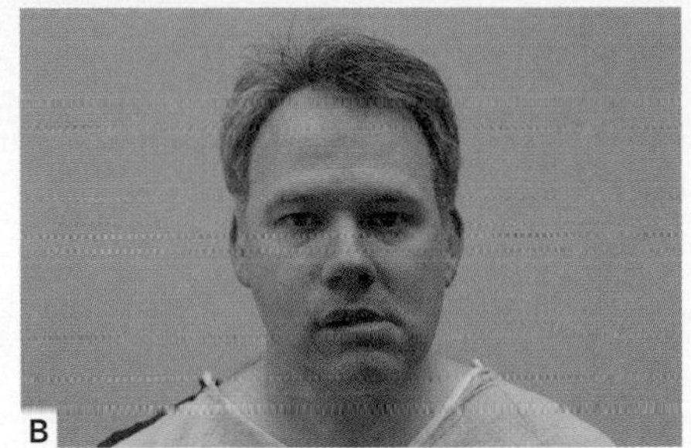

FIGURE 27-26A–B TMJ assessment

Back/Spine (Cervical, Thoracic, Lumbar)

Observe the three sections of the spine for alignment with the head and each other and the head with the shoulders. The three sections of the spine should be in alignment with each other at the midline.

Observe for landmarks on the posterior chest. Not all spinous processes may be visible; however, C_7 and T_1 should be visible as they are the most prominent. Other landmarks include the scapula, iliac crests and paravertebral muscles.

Unexpected findings would be an exaggerated thoracic (kyphosis) or lumbar curve (lordosis) of the spine. A gibbus, a sharp angular deformity, is associated with a collapsed vertebra or osteoporosis.

Observe for bilateral symmetry of the shoulder, scapular, and iliac crest heights (Figure 27-27).

Shoulder, scapular, and iliac crest heights should be equal.

- Bend forward, trying to touch the toes. Observe for 75–90 degrees of flexion.
- Bend backward at the waist as far as possible. Observe for 30 degrees hyperextension.

Pain suggests impingement or tendonitis.

- Bend sideways at the waist as far as possible. Observe for 35 degrees of lateral bending.
- Twist the upper trunk from side to side at the waist as far as possible, keeping the pelvis and lower extremities stable. Observe for 30 degrees of rotation.

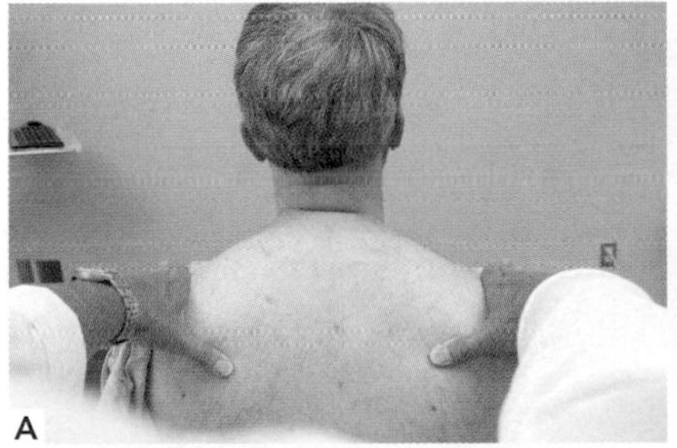
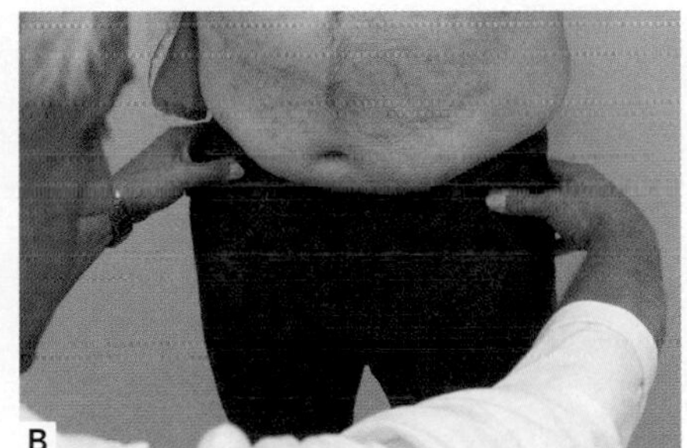
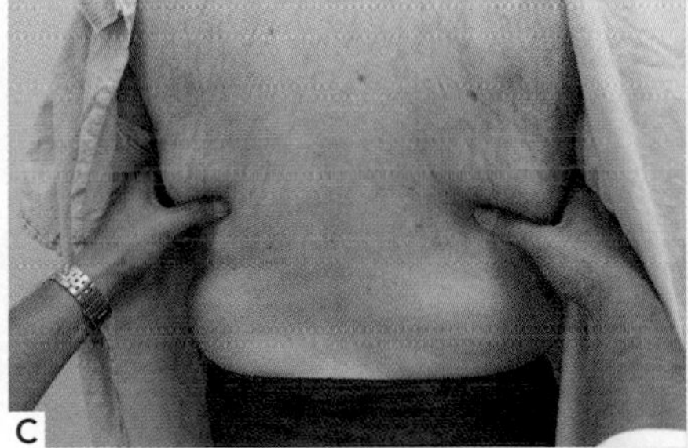
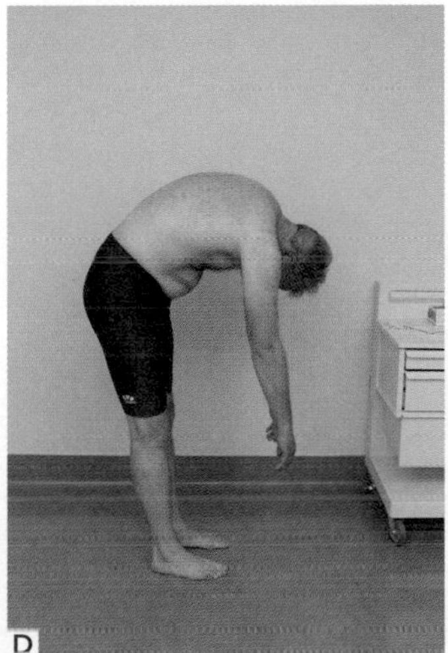
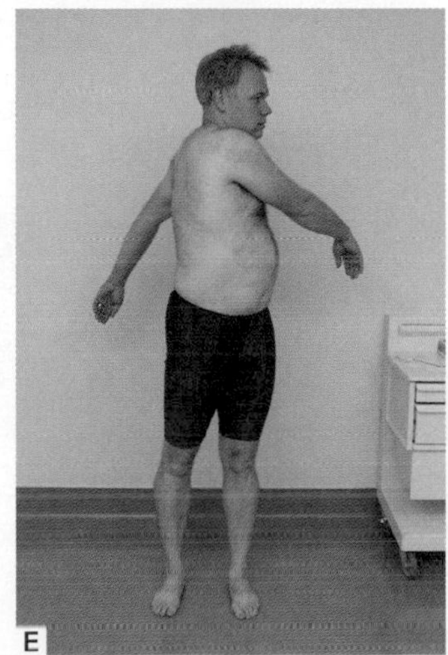
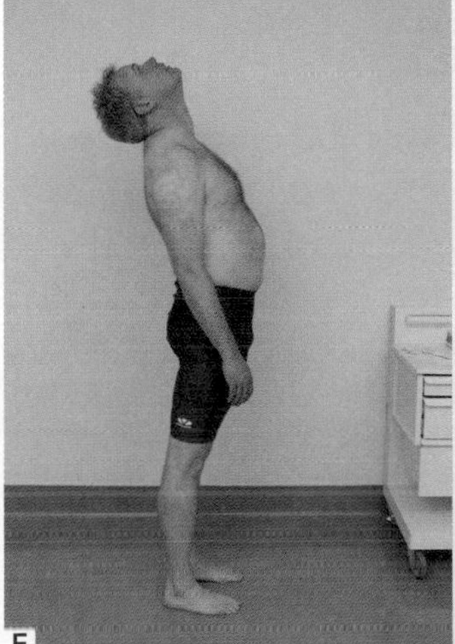

FIGURE 27-27A–F Assessing back/spine for alignment and ROM

Inspection Techniques and Expected Findings	Unexpected Findings

Upper Extremities (Shoulders)

Observe the shoulders for symmetry of the bones (shoulder girdle, scapulae, and clavicle) and muscles. The size and contour of all shoulder structures should be symmetrical. Additionally, the patient may be asked to place both hands against a wall and push against it. Observe for any asymmetry of the scapulae. To assess ROM, ask the patient to (Figure 27-28):

- Shrug the shoulders. Observe for symmetrical elevation of the shoulders.
- Raise both arms forward and straight up over the head. Observe for forward flexion of 180 degrees.
- Extend both arms behind the back. Observe for hyperextension or 50 degrees.
- Lift both arms laterally, moving them to straight up over the head. Observe for shoulder abduction of 180 degrees.
- Swing each arm across the front of the body. Observe for adduction of 50 degrees.
- Place both arms behind the hips with the elbows directed outward. Observe for internal rotation of 90 degrees.
- Place both arms behind the head with the elbows directed outward. Observe for external rotation of 90 degrees.

Unexpected findings would be inability to demonstrate the standard degrees of movement for the shoulder. Pain with movement is also an unexpected result.

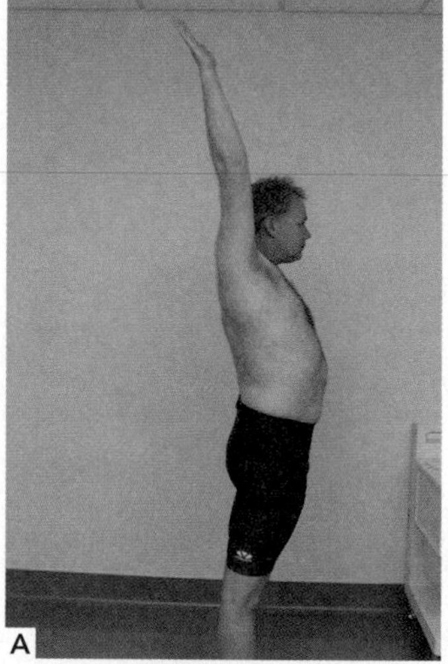
A

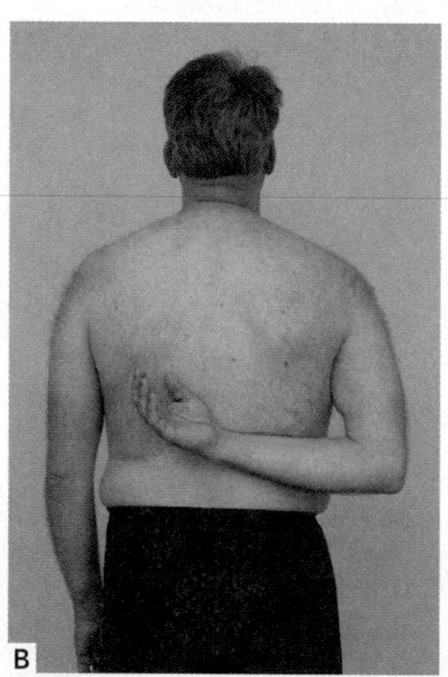
B

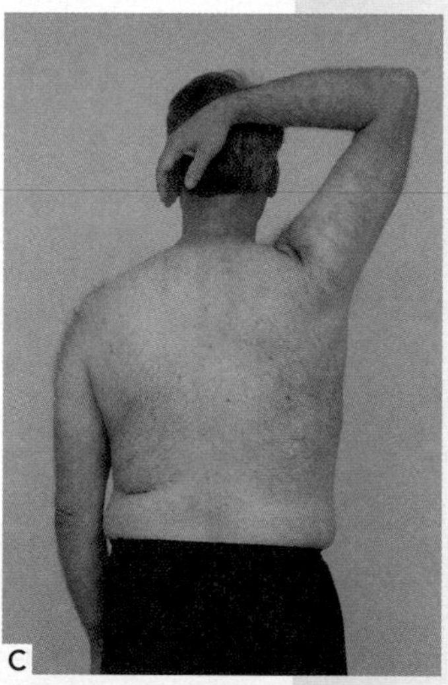
C

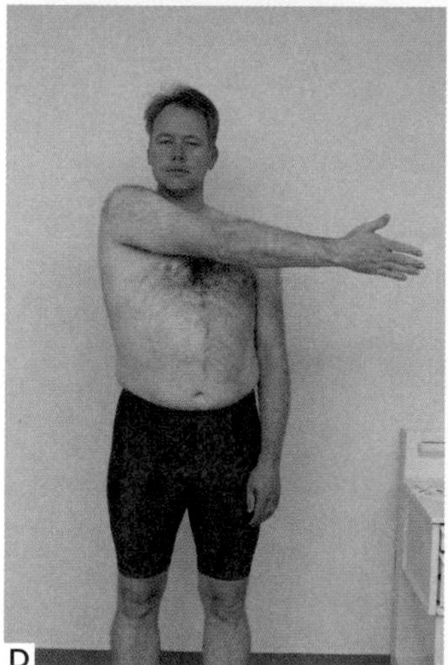
D

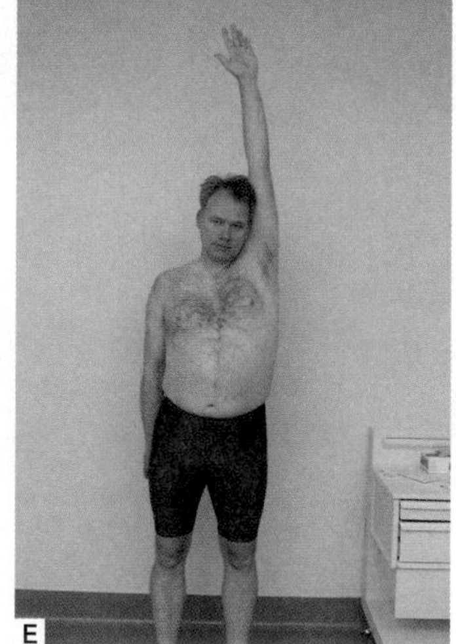
E

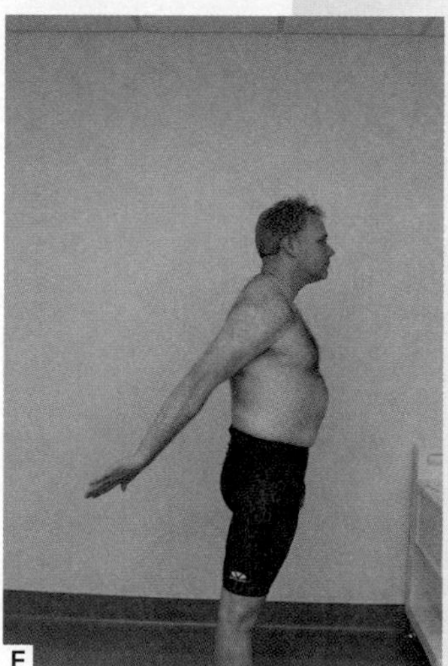
F

FIGURE 27-28A–F ROM/muscle strength of upper extremities: shoulders

Inspection Techniques and Expected Findings	Unexpected Findings

Upper Extremities (Elbows)

Observe the elbows' contour and size in the flexed and extended positions. They should appear symmetrical and should be free of any nodules, redness, or swelling. To assess ROM, request the patient to do the following (Figure 27-29):

- Fully extend the elbow (0 degrees) and then bend the elbow up toward the shoulder as far as it will go and then straighten it. Observe for flexion of 180 degrees and 180 degrees at full extension.
- Flex the elbow to a right angle (90 degrees) and place the ulnar side of the hand on a solid surface. Rotate the hand, alternating between palm side up (supination) and palm side down (pronation). Observe for 90 degrees of movement in both positions.

Unexpected findings would be inability to demonstrate the standard degrees of movement for the upper extremity. Pain with movement is also an unexpected result.

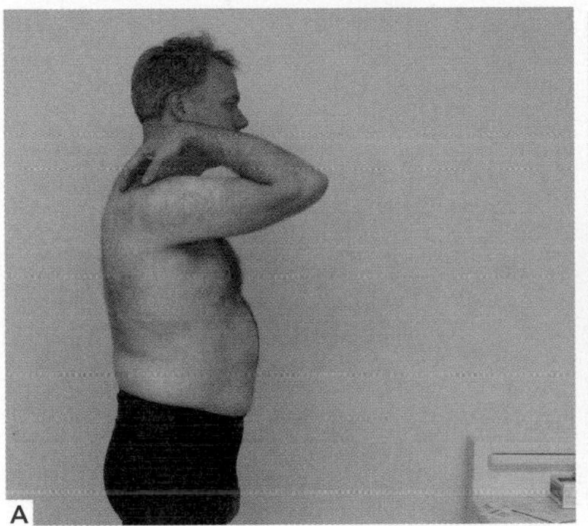

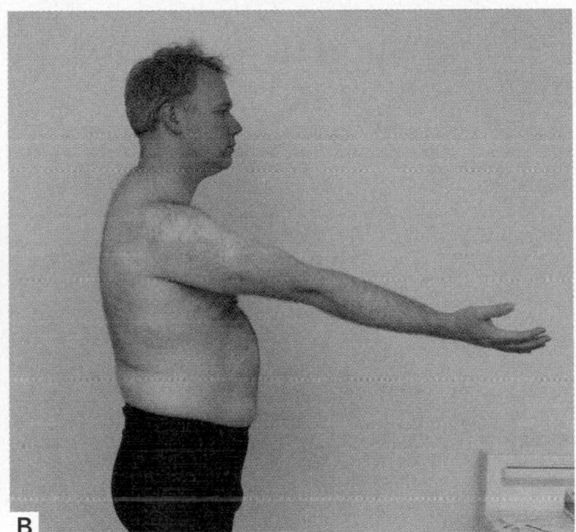

FIGURE 27-29A–B ROM upper extremities: elbow

Upper Extremities (Wrist and Hand)

Observe the joints of the hand and wrist for expected characteristics, alignment, swelling, redness, and any bumps or deformities. Also make note of the number of digits present and their integrity. Observe for phalangeal and palmar creases. The palmar aspect of the hand has a concave appearance characterized by a central depression. Surrounding the depression are two rounded elevations known as eminences. Just below the thumb is the thenar eminence and on the little finger side is the hypothenar eminence.

The dorsal aspect of the hand has no specific landmarks or characteristics. Tendons may be visible as they cross vertically from the metacarpal joint to the wrist. Also note horizontal creases across the dorsal aspect of the fingers. When the fingers are extended, note the bunching of the skin over the PIP and DIP joints (knuckles), creating oval creases over the joints. When the fingers are extended, they should be in alignment with each other and point forward without any lateral or medial deviation. The fingers should gently taper from the MCP joints to the tip and terminate with a translucent fingernail (fingernail description is in Chapter 16). To assess ROM, request the patient to (Figure 27-30):

- With the fingers extended in the neutral position (0 degrees) bend the fingers forward (flexion) at the MCP joints. Return to the neutral position and bend the fingers backward and upward (hyperextension). Observe for flexion of 90 degrees and hyperextension of 30 degrees.
- Touch the thumb to each fingertip and to the base of the little finger and then make a fist. Observe that the patient can perform all these actions. The patient can perform these separately or simultaneously.
- Spread the fingers apart and then bring them back together. Observe that the patient is able to perform these actions.

Unexpected findings would be the presence of Heberden's nodes, Bouchard's nodes, swan neck and boutonnière deformities, and ulnar deviation of the fingers. Other unexpected findings would be the absence of digits or parts of digits, most commonly caused by trauma.

Inspection Techniques and Expected Findings | **Unexpected Findings**

- Bend the wrist so that the hand points toward the ceiling (extension) and then toward the floor (flexion). Observe for 90 degrees of flexion and 70 degrees of extension.
- With the wrists supinated (palm down) and in the neutral position, move the hand to the right and left. Observe for radial movement of 20 degrees and ulnar movement of 55 degrees.

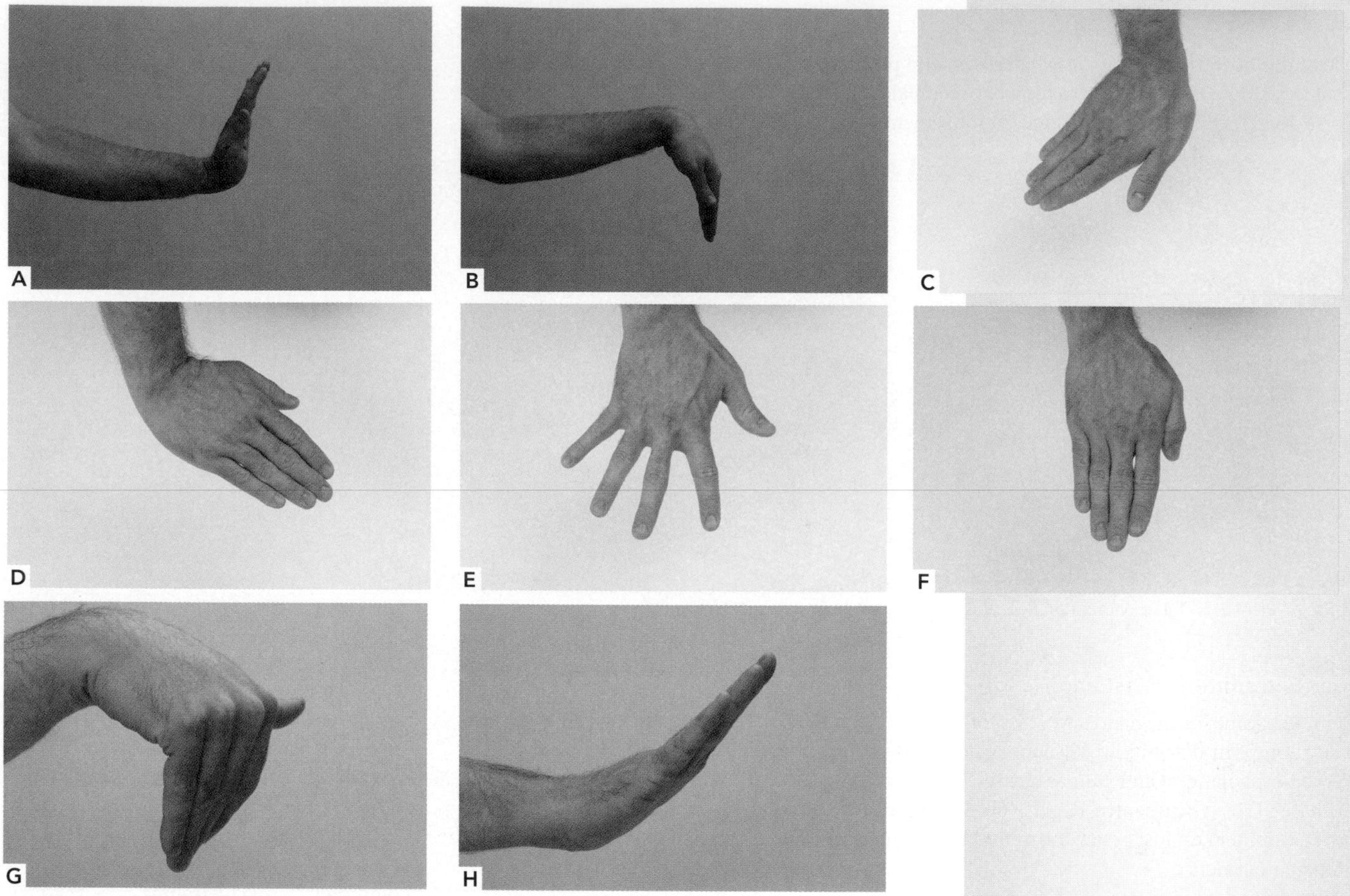

FIGURE 27-30A–H ROM upper extremities: wrist and fingers

Median Nerve

Diagnostic procedures are used primarily to assess the integrity of the median nerve that innervates the palm of the hand and the radial side of the hand (palmar aspect of the thumb, index and middle finger, and one-half of the ring finger).

A maneuver that is used to assess for CTS is the Phalen's sign.

Perform Phalen's sign by having the patient fully flex the wrists and place the backs of the hands together, holding this position for 60 seconds (Figure 27-31).

Unexpected Findings:

Carpal tunnel syndrome (CTS) is caused by compression of the median nerve as it passes through the carpal tunnel in the wrist.

Numbness and tingling along the distribution of the median nerve from the wrist to the hand is suggestive of CTS.

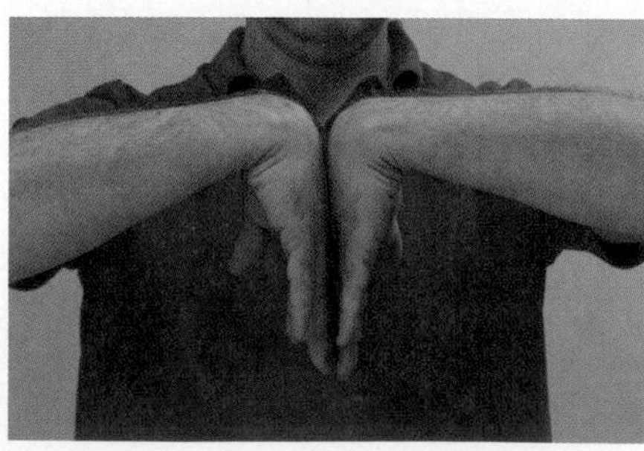

FIGURE 27-31 Phalen's sign

Inspection Techniques and Expected Findings

Lower Extremities (Hip)

Observe the hip for symmetry by noting equality in height of the iliac crests and the greater trochanter.

Posteriorly, note the symmetry of the gluteal folds, both in number and level. Also note the size of the buttocks and assess for symmetry. The patient's gait should be even and smooth, indicating that the lower extremities are of equal length. To assess ROM, request the patient to do the following (Figure 27-32):

- Maintain the leg in a straight position (neutral position with knee extended) and lift the leg off of the table to a vertical position. Observe for 90 degrees of hip flexion.
- Swing the leg in a straight line backward from its neutral position. Observe for 30 degrees or less of hyperextension of the hip.
- Flex the knee and raise the knee up toward the chest while keeping the opposite leg straight and on the table. Observe for hip flexion of 120 degrees.
- While still supine, maintain the leg in neutral position and swing the leg from one side to the other (adduction and abduction). The provider may lift up the opposite leg to allow for full movement of the extremity being tested. Observe for 30 degrees adduction and up to 45 degrees of abduction.
- While supine, flex one knee. Keeping the foot flat on the table, move the knee toward the knee of the opposite leg, causing internal rotation of the hip.
- After this maneuver, move the leg toward the side placing the lateral ankle on the knee of the opposite leg, causing external rotation of the hip. Place a hand on the patient's flexed knee and gently move the knee down toward the table. Observe for 40 degrees of internal rotation and 45 degrees of external rotation.

Unexpected Findings

Unexpected findings would be inability to demonstrate the standard degrees of movement for the lower extremity and hip. Pain with movement is also an unexpected result.

PRACTICE POINT: Back Arching

Note if there is any arching of the back. This maneuver needs to be done with the patient standing or in a prone position on the exam table or bed.

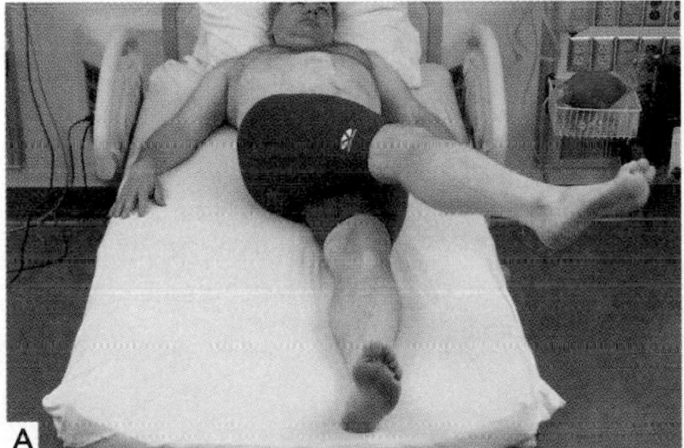

A

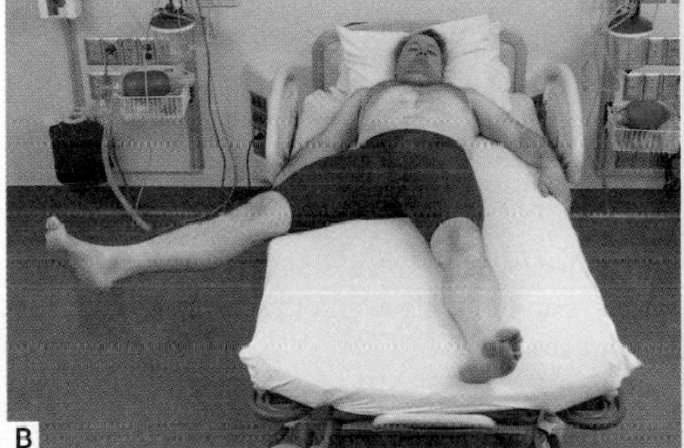

B

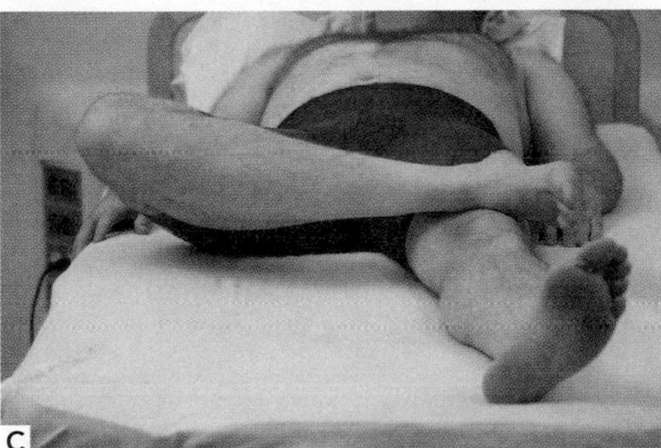

C

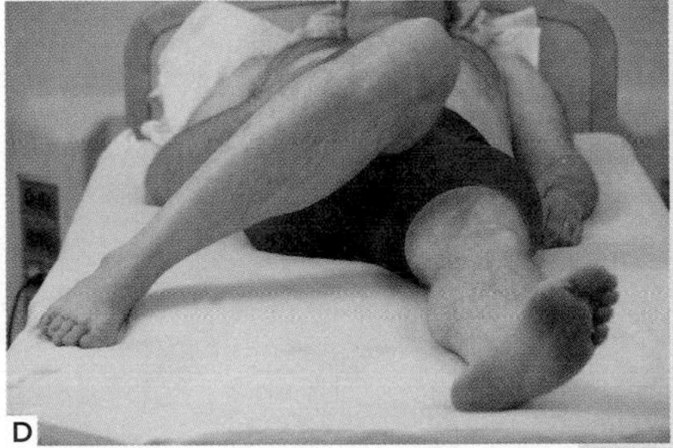

D

FIGURE 27-32A–G ROM lower extremities: hip

Inspection Techniques and Expected Findings	Unexpected Findings

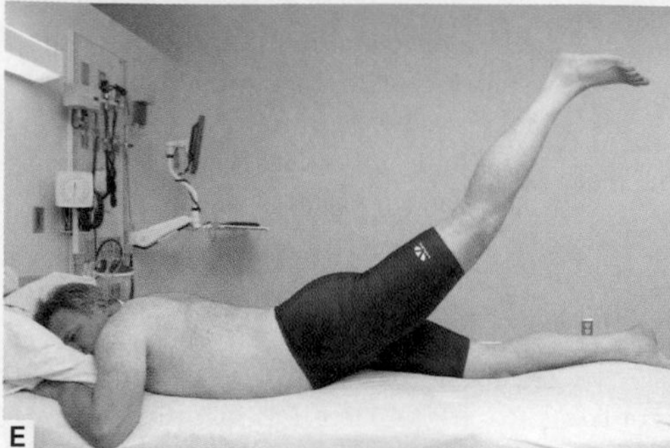

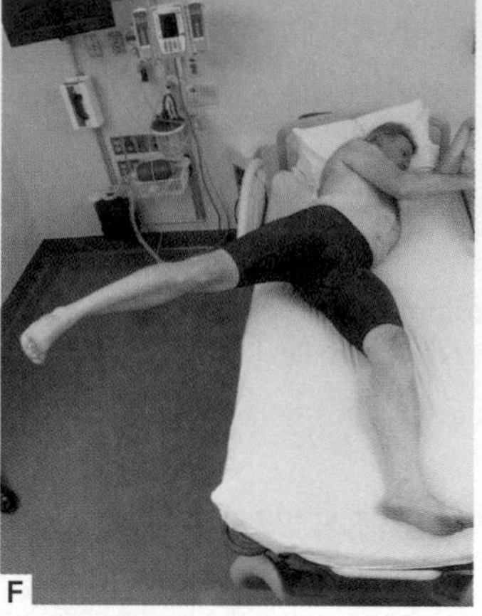

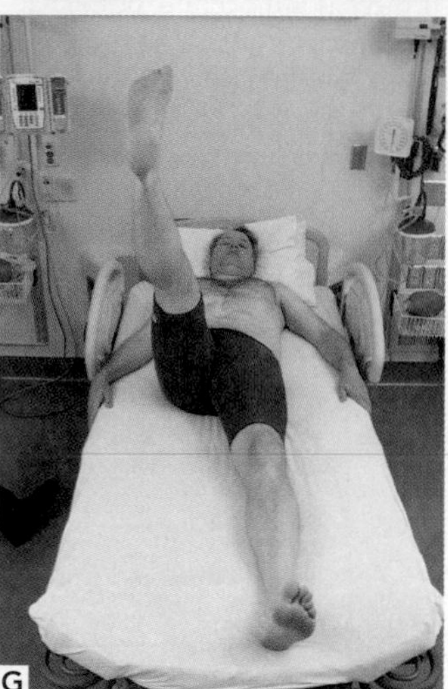

FIGURE 27-32A–G ROM lower extremities: hip *continued*

Lower Extremities (Leg and Knee)

Inspect the knee and popliteal space in both the flexed and extended position.

Unexpected findings would be an effusion of fluid in the suprapatellar pouch. This is manifested as a convex bulging of the suprapatellar pouch.

When the knee is flexed, observe the patella for its depressions along the side of the knee and above the patella. The knee should have no swelling or fluid bulges, and the skin over the knee should be smooth, the same color of skin, and without any lesions.

Observe the leg for alignment. The bones of the upper part and lower part of the leg should be in a straight line; however, an angular deviation of the femur and tibia of up to 15 degrees is acceptable. To assess ROM, request the patient to do the following (Figure 27-33):

- Bend each knee. Observe for 130 degrees of flexion,
- Straighten each knee (return to neutral position). Observe for full extension, with some individuals demonstrating 15 degrees of hyperextension.

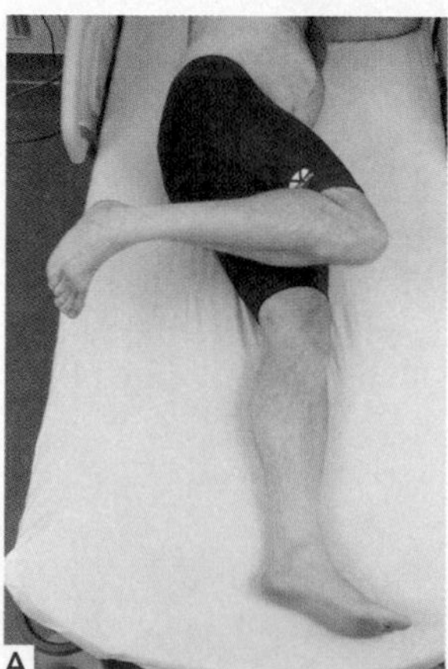

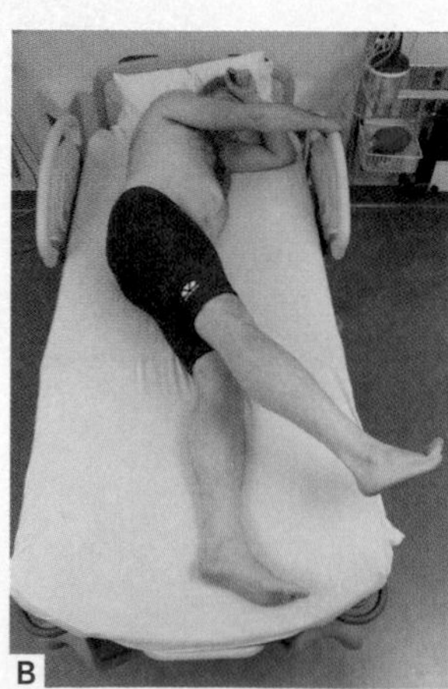

FIGURE 27-33A–B ROM/muscle strength: legs/knees

Inspection Techniques and Expected Findings	Unexpected Findings

Lower Extremities (Ankle and Foot)

Inspect the ankles and feet with the patient sitting and when weight bearing (standing). Landmarks for the ankle are the medial and lateral malleolus and the Achilles tendon. Expect the skin to be smooth over the rounded prominences of the malleoli as well as over the entire foot, without any lesions, and a color that is consistent with the rest of the body.

Unexpected findings would be the presence of thickened, hardened skin, which may be corns or calluses. These lesions may also be yellow in color. See Chapter 16.

Assess the contour of the foot as well as the presence of the toes, their position and size. The dorsal aspect of the foot is slightly rounded, particularly over the arch. Note that the alignment of the foot should be in a straight line with the tibia. Weight bearing should fall on the middle of the foot. This may be visualized as an imaginary line that starts at the heel and extends through the midfoot to between the second and third toes. The foot should also present with a longitudinal arch along the medial aspect of the foot. Expect to observe a portion of the medial section of the foot that is slightly curved and does not touch the floor.

Unexpected findings would be a minor misalignment of the feet with the tibia. Observe that the feet and toes either point inward (pes varus) or outward (pes valgus) (Figure 27-34). A shift in weight bearing may result from a misalignment of the forefoot, pronation of the heel, and pain and injury. Unexpected results would be a higher or lower arch. A flat foot (pes planus) is observed when the foot remains flat on the floor, even when not weight bearing. Opposite of a flat foot is a higher arch (pes cavus), which is frequently described as a high instep.

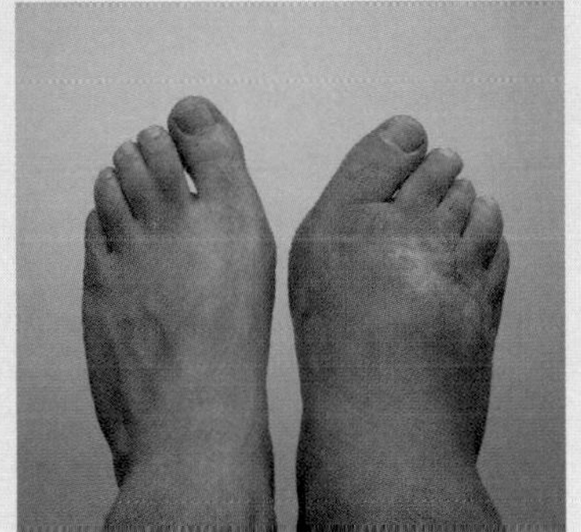

FIGURE 27-34 Pes varus/valgus
Source: A. Bartel/CMSP

The toes should be straight and pointing forward, and flat against the floor. To assess ROM, request the patient to do the following (Figure 27-35):

- Lift the foot up (dorsiflexion) so the toes point toward the ceiling. Observe for dorsiflexion of 20 degrees.
- Lower the foot (plantarflexion) so the toes point toward the floor. Observe for 45 degrees of plantarflexion.
- Bend the foot at the ankle so that the sole of the foot is directed inward (inversion) and then outward (eversion). Observe for inversion of 30 degrees and eversion of 20 degrees.
- Rotate the ankle by having the patient point the great toe toward the other foot (adduction) and then away from the other foot (abduction). The provider may have to stabilize the leg if the patient turns the leg rather than the ankle. Observe for 20 degrees of adduction and 10 degrees of abduction. Overall rotation of the ankle can be observed by having the patient draw an imaginary circle with the great toe.
- Bend and straighten the toes. Observe each toe for the ability to flex and extend.

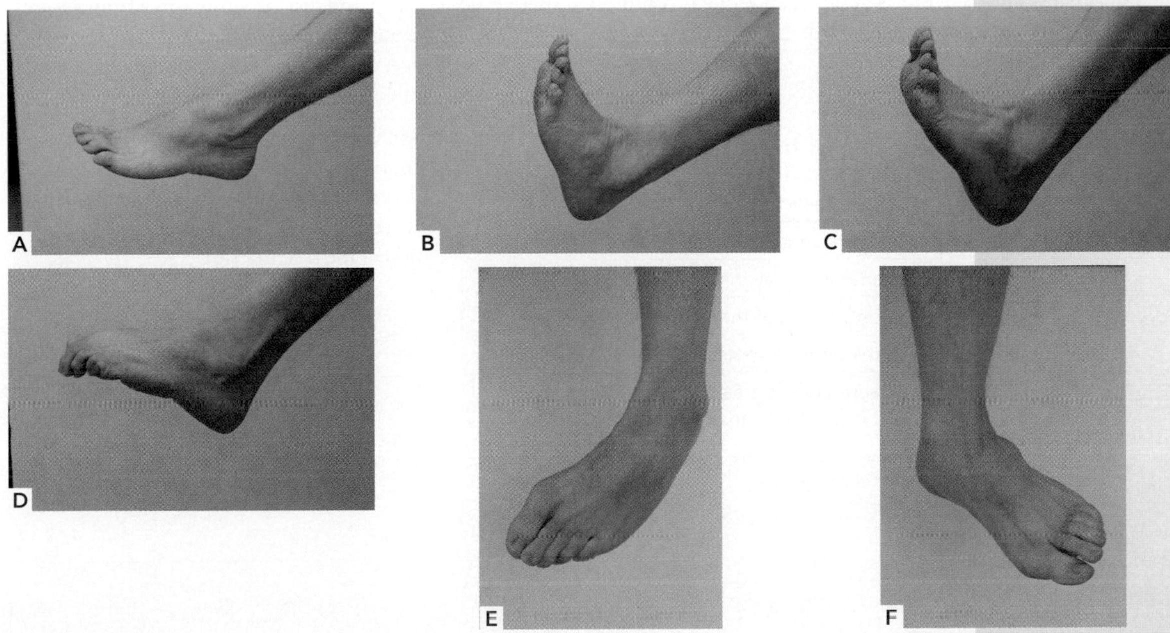

FIGURE 27-35A–F ROM of lower extremity: ankle and foot

Inspection Techniques and Expected Findings	Unexpected Findings

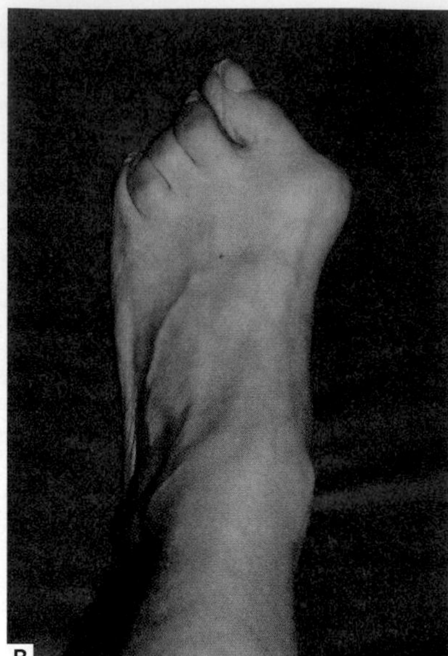

FIGURE 27-36 Toe alterations
Source: a. Biophoto Associates/Science Source

Unexpected findings of the toes are commonly due to ROM alterations (Figure 27-36). Unlike alterations of the fingers, toe alterations are not necessarily caused by arthritic conditions. A hammer toe results from hyperextension of the metatarsalphalangeal (MTP) joint with flexion of the PIP joints. This is similar to boutonnière deformity of the fingers.

A claw toe is hyperextension of the MTP joint with flexion of the toes PIP and DIP joints.

A mallet toe is due to a flexion deformity at the DIP joint of the toe. Hallux valgus is a lateral deviation of the great toe and may overlap onto the second toe. The enlarged joint at the base of the great toe becomes a pressure point and may become inflamed.

Inspection: Level III

Skeletal Alignment

A fracture is a disruption to the liner continuity of a bone. Fractures occur when there is a greater stress placed upon bone and soft tissue than they can tolerate. Direct stress, most commonly caused by a direct blow or crushing force related to trauma, is a major cause of a fracture. Other types of forces that cause fractures are related to indirect stress that is caused by torsion (twisting), extreme muscle contraction. Diseased bone, such as that found in osteoporosis or malignancies, is responsible for pathological fractures.

Depending on the amount of trauma associated with the fracture, observation of the surrounding tissue also provides important data. In simple fractures in which the bone is not displaced and does not protrude through the skin, edema and ecchymosis at the fracture site is common. If there is no disruption to the vascular system, ecchymosis is not observed.

Table 27-8 Classification and description of fractures

Classification of Fractures	Characteristic manifestations
Non-displaced	Bone remains in anatomical position/alignment
Displaced	Bone is out of anatomical alignment
Incomplete (greenstick)	Break through only a part of the bone thickness
Complete	Break through the entire thickness of bone
Closed (simple)	Soft tissue and surrounding area not severely disrupted; bone does not protrude through skin.
Open (compound)	Soft tissue and surrounding area disrupted and bone protrudes through skin

Classification and descriptions of bone fractures are identified in Table 27-8 and Figure 27-37.

Displacement of the bone may cause deformity, which may be observed as a change in length, shape, or alignment. Muscle spasms may also be observed in the muscles surrounding the fracture. Open and displaced fractures from severe trauma result in more severe tissue damage, with exposed tissue and bleeding often present.

Along with a disruption to the linear continuity of the bone, there may be some degree of deformity to the extremity that is caused by muscle spasms and contraction at the fracture site.

Inspection Techniques and Expected Findings | Unexpected Findings

Proximal
Midshaft
Distal
Transverse
Oblique
Spiral
Comminuted
Segmental
Butterfly
Impacted

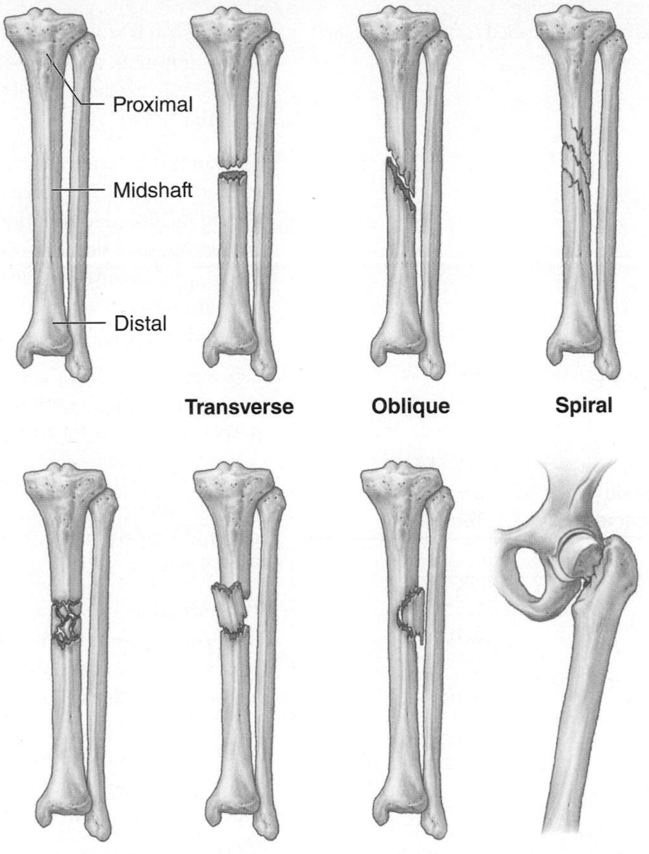

FIGURE 27-37 Types of fractures

Dislocation and Subluxation

Dislocations and subluxations are conditions associated with joints. Observations related to dislocations and subluxations include joint deformity as well as loss of movement of the related joint and extremity Pain is also present and severe. In severe situations, neurovascular function may be impaired.

Normal anatomy
Subluxation
Dislocation

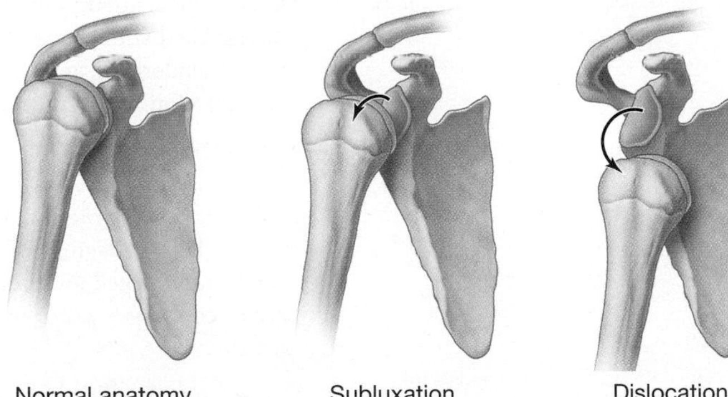

FIGURE 27-38 Dislocation and subluxation

A dislocation is a disruption in the continuity of a joint so that the articulating surfaces are not in contact with each other.

A subluxation is an incomplete dislocation (Figure 27-38). Both conditions result from injury or trauma and commonly occur in active adults. The involved ligaments and surrounding soft tissue may also sustain damage.

Inspection Techniques and Expected Findings

Contusions, Strains, and Sprains

Observe for contusions, strains, and sprains. Both strains and sprains can be described as first, second, or third degree.

The characteristic manifestations of types of musculoskeletal injuries are described in Table 27-9.

Table 27-9 Musculoskeletal injuries

Musculoskeletal component	Fracture Bone	Dislocation Joint	Sprain Ligament	Strain Tendon
Characteristics				
Pain	0-3	4-7–8-10	0-3–4-7	0-3–4-7
Swelling (edema)	0-3–4-7	0-3	0-10	0-10
Bruising (contusions)	0-10	0-10	0-10	0-10
Disfigurement (deformity)	Likely	Significant	Minimal to none	Minimal to none
Function/ mobility	Loss of function/ movement	Loss of function/ movement	Restricted	Restricted
Tenderness/ sensitivity	8-10	4-7-8-10	4-7	4-7
Crepitus/grating	Yes	No	No	No
Muscle spasms	Yes	No	No	Yes

0 - 3 mild 4 - 7 moderate 8 - 10 severe

Unexpected Findings

A **contusion** is soft tissue damage that is usually minimal, causing hemorrhaging into the subcutaneous, adipose, or muscular tissue.

A **strain** is due to overusing a muscle, ligament, or joint structure or using it beyond its intended functional ability. A strain may be a one-time injury or it may be a consequence related to continuous or constant overuse resulting in a gradual rather than a sudden onset.

A **sprain** is a partial or complete tear or rupture of the ligament fibers that surround a joint capsule.

Manifestations include bruising of the area with evidence of ecchymosis, pain, and limited movement of the affected area.

Strain Degrees

First degree: results from mild stretching of a muscle or tendon accompanied by pain and tenderness on palpation and possible muscle spasms. Generally no loss of movement, edema, or ecchymosis occurs. Pain suggests impingement or tendonitis.

Second degree: results from moderate stretching or tearing of a muscle or tendon. It is accompanied by severe muscle spasms and pain with passive movement. Additionally, edema and ecchymosis are present following the injury.

Third degree: caused by severe stretching with complete disruption of the tendon and muscle that produces intense muscle spasms, tenderness, and edema with a loss of motion.

Sprain Grades

A sprain is most commonly the result of a sudden, twisting motion, producing minimal hemorrhaging accompanied by edema and reduced joint functioning. Sprains commonly occur in the ankle and knee joints.

Grade 1 sprain: mild, with possible tearing of the ligament fibers with minimal, localized bleeding, tenderness, and swelling. The joint remains stable.

Grades 2-3: more tearing of the ligament, with up to one-half of the fibers torn in grade 2 (moderate) and a complete tearing of the ligament in grade 3 (severe). In both grades, there is swelling, ecchymosis, tenderness, pain with movement or palpation, and loss of joint function.

Inspection Techniques and Expected Findings	Unexpected Findings
A common cause of shoulder pain and disability related to strains is a rotator cuff tear. A torn rotator cuff occurs when one or more of the tendons of the muscles of the rotator cuff are partially or completely torn, so that it is no longer attached to the head of the humerus. Individuals who present with shoulder pain should be evaluated for a torn rotator cuff.	
The **Hawkins Kennedy test** assesses rotator cuff injury and impingement (Figure 27-39).	
For this test, forward flex the patient's arm to 90 degrees in front of him or her, and then flex the elbow to 90 degrees. When in this position, ask the patient to internally rotate the shoulder while applying resistance with external rotation. There should be not pain in the shoulder.	Pain with this maneuver indicates rotator cuff injury.

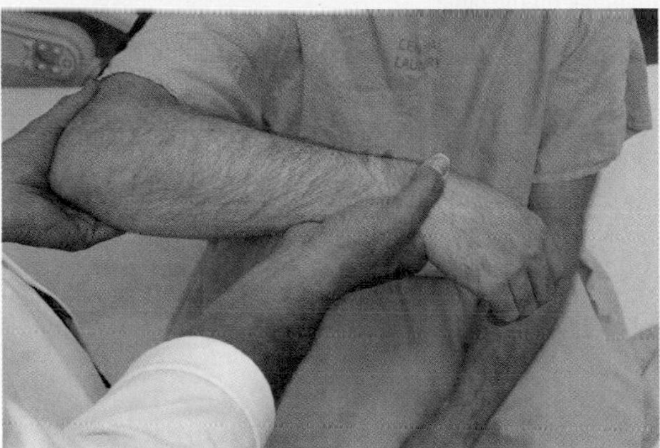

FIGURE 27-39 Hawkins Kennedy test

Inspection: Level IV

Patients who present with low back or hip pain may be evaluated with diagnostic procedures that assess for herniated disks or nerve root inflammation as well as hip dysfunction.

Straight Leg Raising Test

Inspection Techniques and Expected Findings	Unexpected Findings
Begin with the patient in the supine position with the legs extended and neck slightly flexed (Figure 27-40). Instruct the patient to raise one leg, keeping the knee extended. There should be no pain.	Pain below the knee that follows a $L_{4/5}$ or S_1 dermatome distribution indicates nerve root compression or tension. The inability to raise the leg greater than 30 degrees without pain is identified as Lasègue's sign. The pain is frequently relieved with flexion of the knee. Pain below the knee that follows a dermatome pattern may be associated with disk herniation.

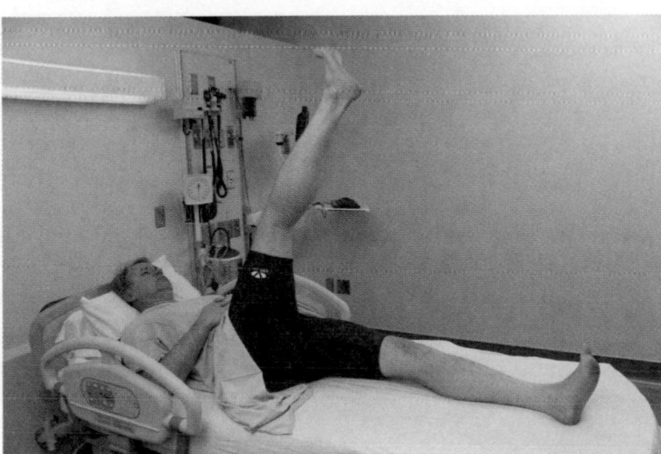

FIGURE 27-40 Straight leg raising test

Femoral Stretch Test

Inspection Techniques and Expected Findings	Unexpected Findings
Perform to assess for nerve root inflammation at the level of $L_{1/2/3}$ and sometimes L_4. Instruct the patient to assume a prone position and extend the hip. There should be no pain.	Pain associated with leg extension indicates nerve root involvement.

Inspection Techniques and Expected Findings	Unexpected Findings
Diagnostic Procedures used for assessing hip dysfunction include the Thomas test and the Trendelenburg test. These tests are used primarily to assess for muscular alterations.	
Thomas Test	
Perform to assess for flexion contractures of the hip muscles (Figure 27-41). Begin with the patient lying supine with both lower extremities extended.	If the extended leg does not remain flat, a flexion contracture is most likely the cause.
Instruct the patient to flex one hip by bringing the knee up toward the chest. As the hip becomes flexed, the lumbar spine should flatten.	Weakness of these muscles is most commonly due to osteoarthritis of the hip.
Once the spine is flat, observe the opposite leg, which should remain flat on the table.	
Trendelenburg Test	
Perform to detect weakness of the gluteus medius hip adductors (Figure 27-42). Begin with the patient standing. Instruct the patient to stand on one leg and then the other and observe the pelvis for any tilting. Individuals without any muscle weakness will demonstrate an elevation of the pelvis on the side of the lifted leg.	Those with muscle weakness will demonstrate an elevation of the opposite pelvis.

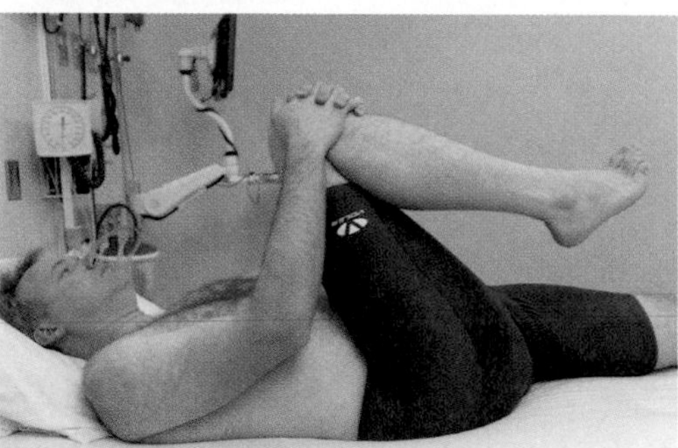

FIGURE 27-41 Thomas test

FIGURE 27-42 Trendelenburg test

Palpation: Level I

Palpation Techniques and Expected Findings	Unexpected Findings
Joints	
If there is any indication of swelling or redness of any joints, they may be palpated for temperature and tenderness. Perform palpation on each joint and its overlying skin. The joints should be aligned and be the same temperature as the surrounding skin. They should also be firm, and without any nodules, swelling, or redness.	Unexpected findings would include tenderness and pain with movement as well as manifestations of inflammation (increased temperature, redness, and swelling). If the synovial membrane is thickened, it will give a joint a "doughy" or "boggy" feel.
GALS Examination	
Palpation in the GALS examination is primarily concerned with any pain in the joints of the hands and feet. Gently squeeze across the MCP and MCT joints, assessing for tenderness or other evidence of joint disease from inflammatory or degenerative processes (Figure 27-43).	Swelling is often due to accumulation of fluid within the synovial sac. If this is present, the free fluid will be localized and freely moveable around the joint. While squeezing, observe the patient's face for any evidence of pain. Facial expressions seldom conceal pain even if the patient verbally indicates no pain.

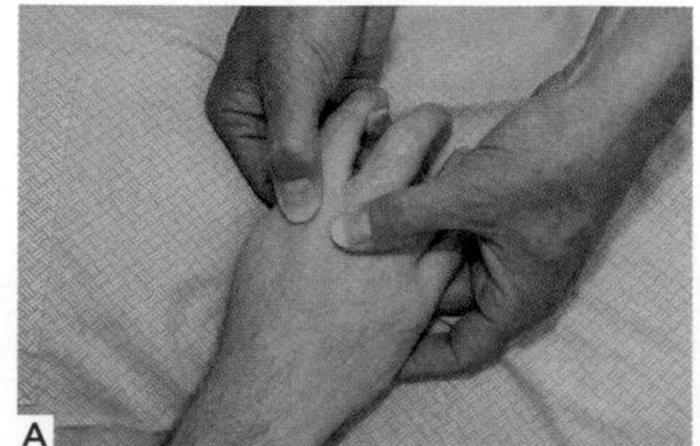

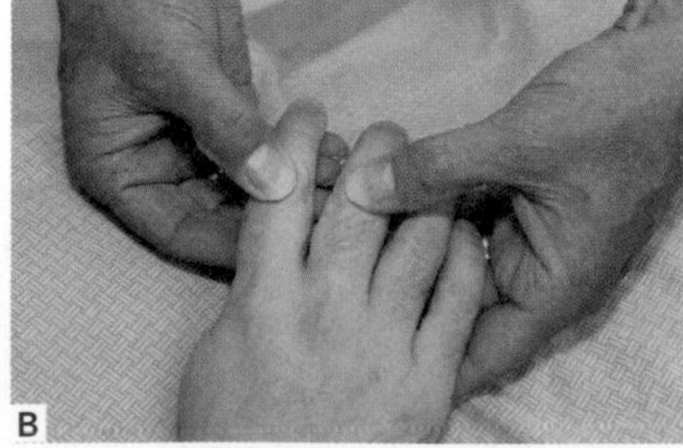

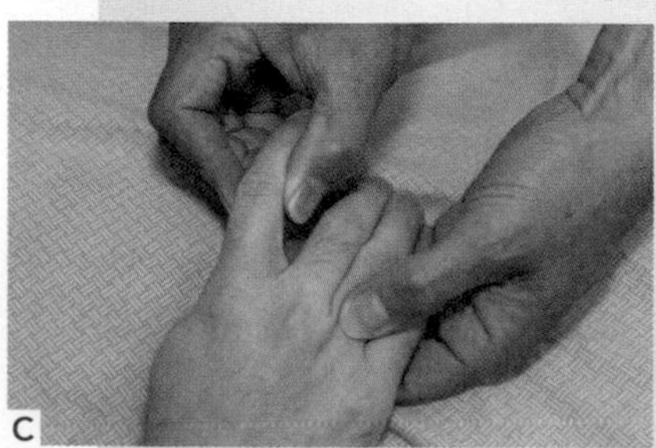

FIGURE 27-43A–C Palpation of joints

Palpation: Level II

Palpation Techniques and Expected Findings | **Unexpected Findings**

Muscle Strength

The major focus of Level II palpation is testing for muscle strength. Muscle strength is graded on a 0–5 scale (Table 27-10).

Test muscle strength by having the patient flex or extend a certain group of muscles while applying a counter force, attempting to extend or contract the muscle. The expected response is that the patient is able to overcome the counterforce and maintain the position of the muscle group. A score or grade is then assigned, depending on how much the patient was able to resist the counter force. Strength is measured on a five-point scale.

Unexpected findings would be a grade of +4 or lower.

Table 27-10 Muscle strength

Grade	Description
0	No muscle activity or movement A 0/5 score means the patient is unable to create any visible or noticeable contraction in a specific muscle. This occurs when a muscle is paralyzed, such as after a stroke, spinal cord injury, or cervical or lumbar radiculopathy. Sometimes pain can prevent a muscle from contracting at all.
+1	Minimal evidence of movement; trace of contraction A 1/5 score occurs when muscle contraction is noted but no movement occurs. The muscle is not strong enough to lift the particular body part against gravity or move it when in a gravity-reduced position.
+2	Complete ROM with gravity removed This muscle-strength grade is assigned when muscle can contract but cannot move the body part fully against gravity. When gravity is reduced or eliminated during a change in body position, the muscle is able to move the body part through its full range of motion.
+3	Complete ROM against gravity A 3/5 grade means that the patient is able to fully contract the muscle and move the body part through its full range of motion against the force of gravity. But when resistance is applied, the muscle is unable to maintain the contraction.
+4	Complete ROM with some resistance A 4/5 grade indicates that the muscle yields to maximum resistance. The muscle is able to contract and provide some resistance, but when the physical therapist presses on the body part, the muscle is unable to maintain the contraction.
+5	Complete ROM with full resistance This means the muscle is functioning normally and is able to maintain its position even when maximum resistance is applied.

Head/Neck

To assess neck strength, request the patient to do the following:

- Touch the chin to the chest while you apply resistance under the chin.
- Move the back of the head toward the spine while you apply resistance to the back of the head.
- Turn the head toward the right/left while you apply resistance to the same side of the head that is turning (Figure 27-44).
- Tilt the head towards the right or left while again applying resistance to the same side of the head that is tilting

Expected results would be that the patient would be able to overcome the applied resistance and achieve a grade of 5/5.

Unexpected results would be that the patient was unable to overcome the applied resistance and achieve a grade of 0–4/5.

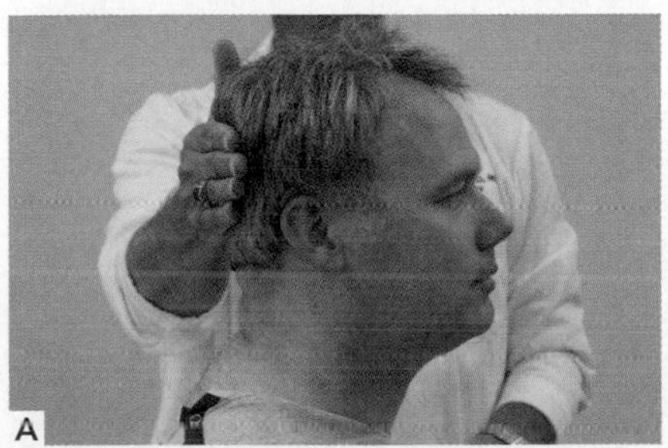

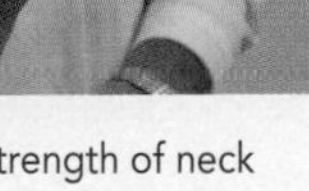

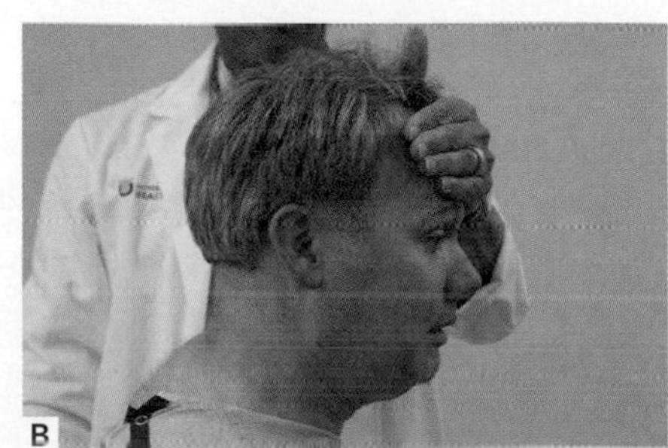

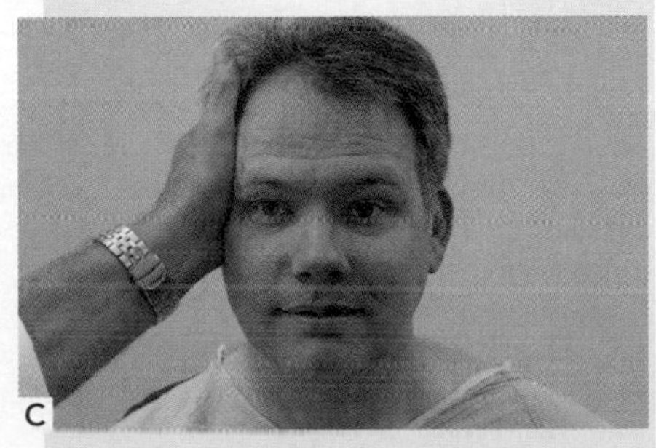

FIGURE 27-44A–C Muscle strength of neck

Palpation Techniques and Expected Findings	Unexpected Findings

Temporomandibular Joint

To assess the temporalis and masseter muscles, request that the patient do the following (Figure 27-45):

- Clench the teeth while you palpate for equal muscle strength and contraction.
- Open the mouth while you place a hand underneath the patient's chin. As the patient opens the mouth, apply an opposing force (upward pressure) against the bottom on the jaw; palpate the patients muscle strength as the jaw opens against resistance.

Unexpected results would be that the patient was unable to overcome the applied resistance and achieve a grade of 0–4/5.

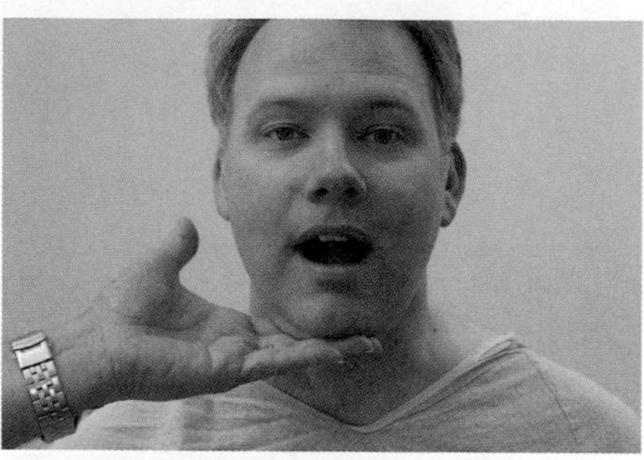

FIGURE 27-45 Muscle strength of TMJ

Spine

Palpation of the spine is done along the spinal processes and includes palpation of the paravertebral muscles. The paravertebral, sternocleidomastoid, and trapezius muscles should be firm, equal in size, without any tenderness or spasms.

With the patient standing, palpate the spine and paravertebral muscles by moving the fingers of one hand down the middle of the spine to assess for subtle changes in the alignment of the spine.

Also run your index and middle fingers down the sides of the spine, noting any subtle changes in alignment or any muscle tenderness or spasms (Figure 27-46). The spine should be straight without any muscle tenderness or spasms.

Perform these same procedures with the patient bending over and touching the toes. The spine should remain straight with the lumbar curve becoming convex as the patient bends forward.

Unexpected results would be that the patient was unable to overcome the applied resistance and achieve a grade of 0–4/5.

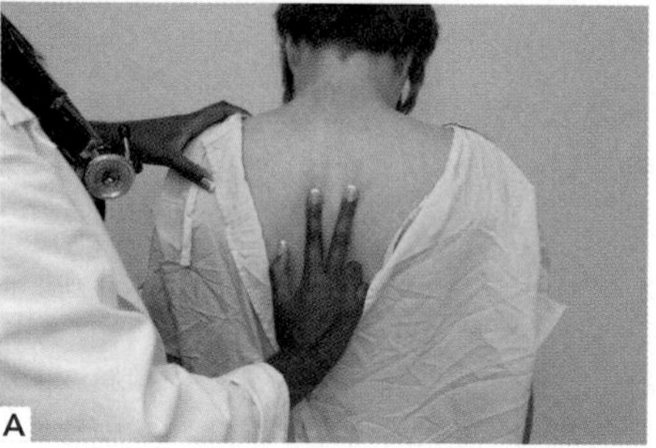

FIGURE 27-46A–B Assessment of the spine

Upper Extremities (Shoulder)

Palpate the shoulder area (clavicle, acromioclavicular joint, scapula, coracoid process, greater tubercle of the humerus, subacromial bursa, biceps groove, and area muscles.) All structures and muscles should be symmetrical without any tenderness, swelling, or muscle spasms.

Instruct the patient to do the following:

- Shrug the shoulders with your hands placed on the tops of both shoulders (Figure 27-47). As the patient attempts to shrug the shoulders, apply opposing downward pressure.
- Attempt to overcome resistance and maintain shrugged shoulders as you palpate for symmetrical muscle strength.

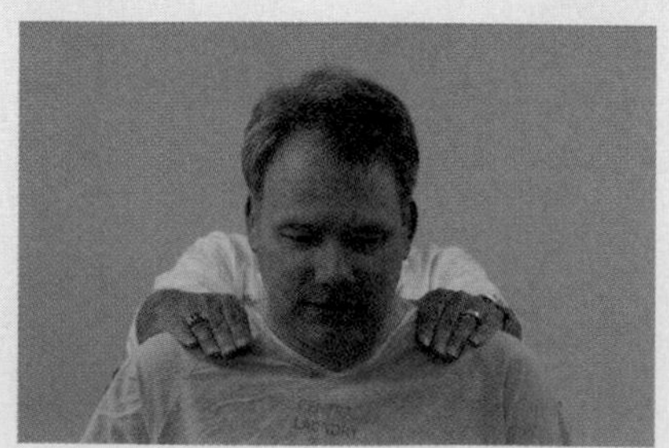

FIGURE 27-47 ROM/muscle strength: shoulder

Palpation Techniques and Expected Findings	Unexpected Findings

Upper Extremities (Elbow)

Palpate the elbows with the elbow flexed about 70 degrees and supported with the provider's hand and arm.

Palpate the extensor surface of the elbow, the olecranon process, and the medial and lateral epicondyles.

Palpate the grooves on either side of the olecranon process, noting any swelling, tenderness, or thickening of the synovial membrane.

Place the elbow on a solid surface or support/stabilize the patient's elbow with one hand.

Place the other hand around the patient's wrist and instruct the patient to flex the elbow against a pulling resistance applied at the patient's wrist (Figure 27-48a).

Next instruct the patient to extend the elbow against a pushing resistance at the patient's wrist (Figure 27-48b). The patient should be able to overcome the resistance and maintain the elbow in flexion or extension.

A boggy, soft, or fluctuant swelling as well as point tenderness of the lateral epicondyle or along the grooves of the olecranon process and epicondyles with pain with supination and pronation of the elbow are unexpected findings. These manifestations may be indicative of a tendonitis or epicondylitis.

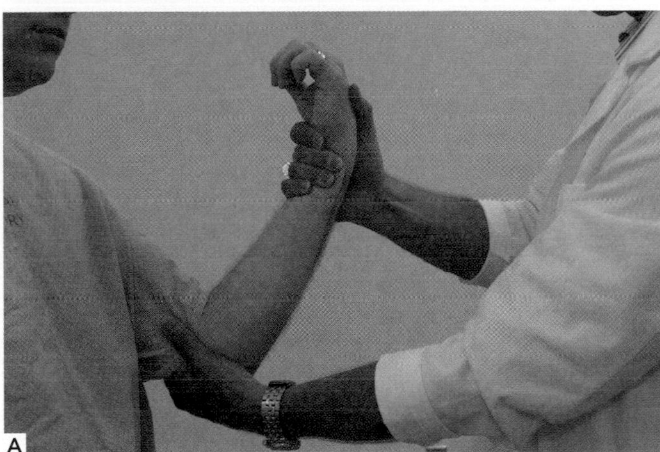

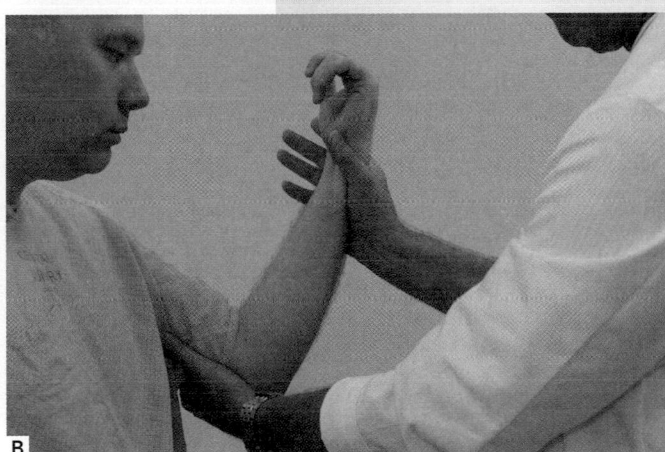

FIGURE 27-48A–B ROM/muscle strength: elbow

Upper Extremities (Wrist/Fingers)

Palpate the joints of each finger and wrist, noting any unusual characteristics. The wrist and MCP joints are palpated with the thumb and the DIP and PIP joints with the thumb and index finger. The joints should feel smooth and there should not be any increased temperature.

Unexpected findings would include rough surfaces, swelling, bogginess, nodules, and tenderness. A solid mass palpated over the dorsal aspect of the wrist is commonly a ganglionic cyst.

To assess muscle strength, have the patient flex and hyperextend the wrist and maintain its position while an opposing force is applied by the provider (Figure 27-49). The patient should be able to overcome resistance and maintain the wrists position.

Unexpected results would be that the patient was unable to overcome the applied resistance and achieve a grade of 0–4/5.

Squeeze two fingers of the hand (index and middle finger) to assess for finger strength.

Strength of the fingers can also be assessed by having the patient abduct (spread the fingers) and adduct (bring them back together while applying an opposing force) (Figure 27-49c–d). The patient should be able to overcome resistance and maintain the position of the fingers.

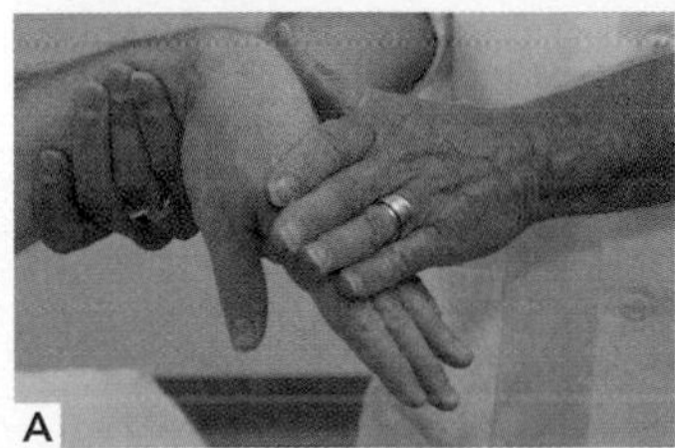

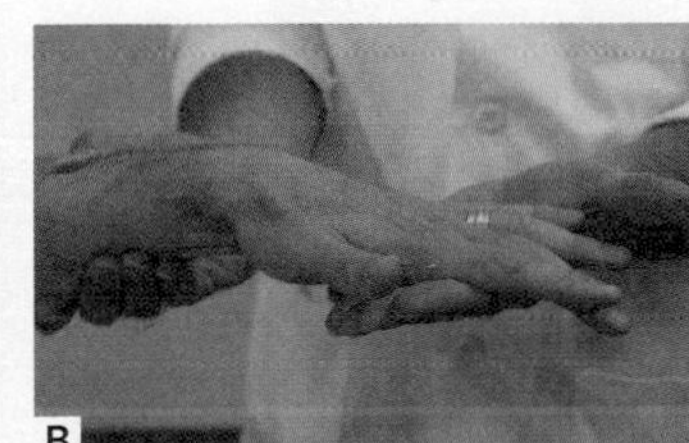

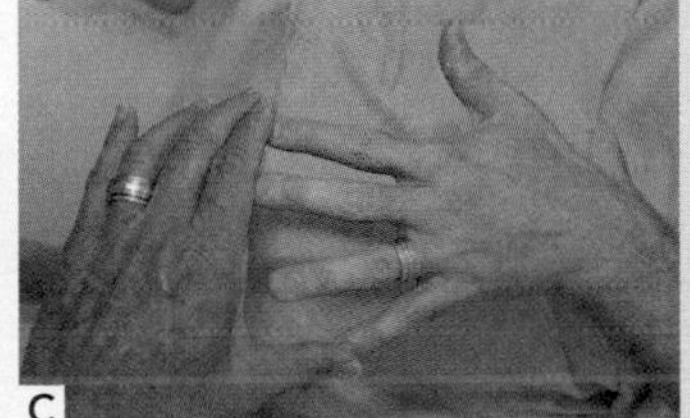

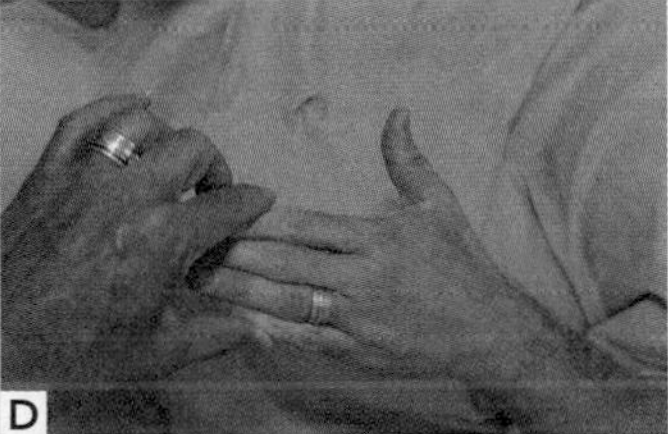

FIGURE 27-49A–D ROM/muscle strength: wrist and fingers

Palpation Techniques and Expected Findings	Unexpected Findings

Median Nerve (Carpal Tunnel Syndrome)

Perform **Tinel's sign** by percussing the patient's wrist with the index or middle finger at the location where the median nerve passes through the carpal tunnel, which is formed by the carpal bones and the flexor retinaculum muscle (Figure 27-50).

Tapping the median nerve should not elicit any tingling along the path of the median nerve.

Unexpected Findings: Tingling along the path of the median nerve from the wrist to the hand is a positive indicator for carpal tunnel syndrome.

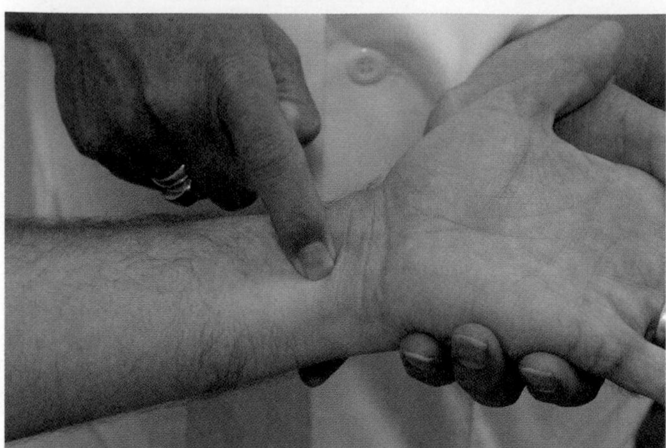

FIGURE 27-50 Assessing for Tinel's sign

Lower Extremities (Hip)

Palpate the hip joints when the patient has resumed a supine position. Position your hands over the iliac crest, applying pressure to determine if the hips are stable and without tenderness. Expect the hips to be stable with smooth joints.

Unexpected Findings: Unexpected findings would be the presence of crepitus as well as pain or tenderness.

Request the patient to flex the knee and hip, and apply an opposing force. Follow the same procedure except with the knee extended.

Request the patient to place the leg in its neutral position with the knee extended and try to elevate the leg against an opposing force (Figure 27-51). In all situations, the patient should be able to overcome the resistance and maintain the leg in its original position.

Hip strength may also be tested by having the patient abduct and adduct the leg while you apply the opposing force. The patient should be able to overcome resistance and maintain the position of the leg (Figure 27-51).

Another variation is to have the patient cross and uncross the legs while in a sitting position. Apply a counter force in an attempt to prevent the crossing and uncrossing.

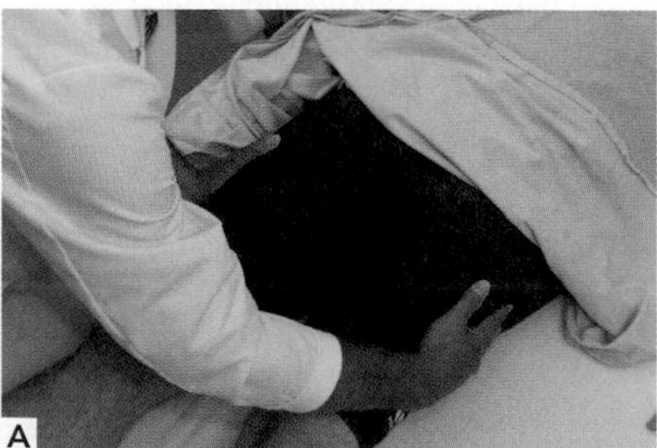

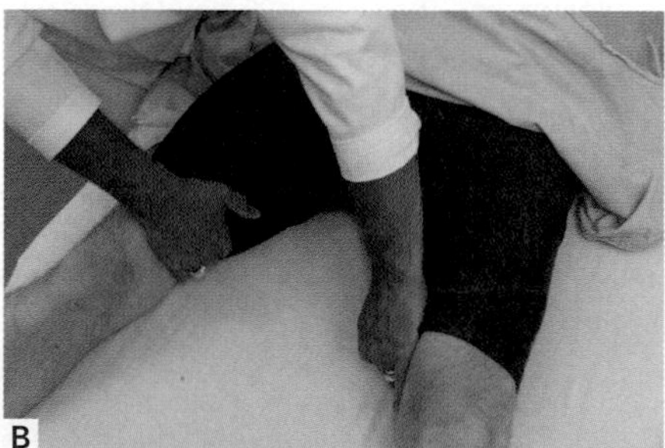

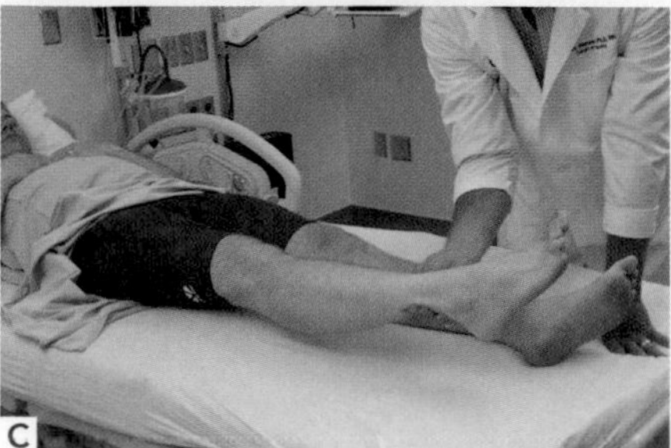

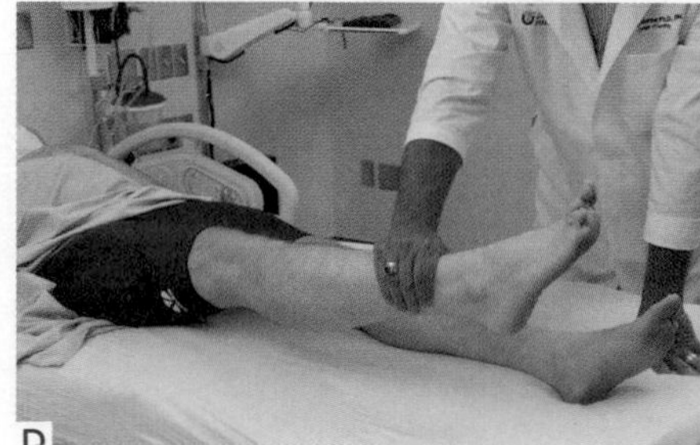

FIGURE 27-51A–D ROM/muscle strength: hip

Palpation Techniques and Expected Findings	Unexpected Findings

Lower Extremities (Knee)

Palpate the popliteal space, assessing for any swelling and tenderness (Figure 27-52). (This may be done simultaneously when palpating for the popliteal artery.)

Begin by placing a hand on the quadriceps muscle about 10 cm above the knee. Move down toward the knee in a grasping motion until the suprapatellar pouch is reached. Palpate the tibiofemoral joint noting the patella, suprapatellar pouch, and infrapatellar fat pad.

Any swelling that is noted around the knee joint needs to be further evaluated to determine whether it is from soft tissue damage or "opens up," excess fluid within the joint. One can be differentiated from the other by the bulge sign and patellar ballottement.

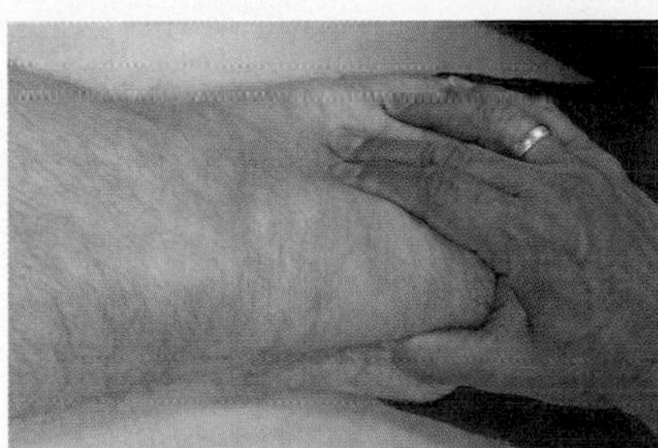

FIGURE 27-52 Knee palpation

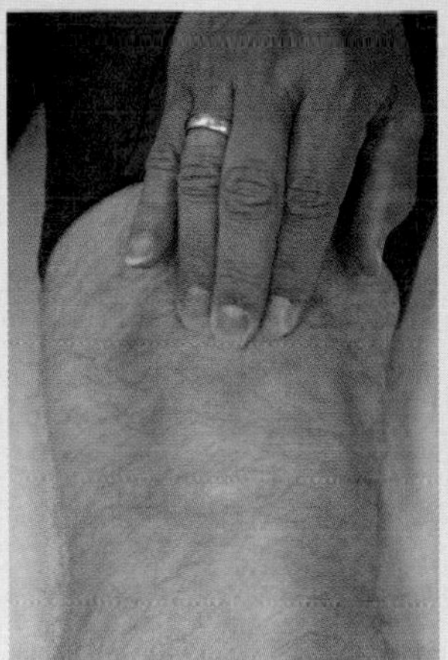

FIGURE 27-53 Ballottement

The tissues and muscle should feel firm and solid and the joint should be smooth, with no tenderness, warmth, bogginess, thickening, or nodules.

Ballottement of the patella is performed when there is a larger amount of fluid present (effusion).

Place a hand above the patella, with the thumb and index finger on the lateral and medial aspect of the joint (Figure 27-53).

Apply pressure with the thumb and finger, compressing the suprapatellar pouch and moving fluid into the knee joint.

With the opposite hand, push the patella sharply toward the femur.

If there is no fluid, the patella is already firmly set against the femur.

The bulge sign helps to determine if there is fluid in the suprapatellar pouch. The bulge sign is done with the knee extended and flat on the table or bed.

Begin by firmly stroking upward on the medial collateral ligament aspect of the patella. Use two to three firm strokes to displace any fluid that may be present. Next externally rotate the ankle and apply outward (valgus) pressure. If the knee joint "opens up," gently tap the lateral aspect of the patella and observe for any fluid that returns to the medial side. As the fluid returns, it will create a bulge, confirming the presence of fluid.

Joints

Palpate the MTP, PIP, and DIP joints and note for temperature, swelling, and tenderness or pain.

Use the thumb and fingers of both hands for palpation of the joints.

Palpate the Achilles tendon as well as the anterior surface of the ankle and the lateral and medial malleoli, noting any alterations on the skin surface or joint tenderness and pain. The skin and joints should feel smooth without any visible lesions or any tenderness and pain. The Achilles tendon should feel like a firm cord and without any tenderness or pain.

Inflamed joints of the toes present with increased temperature, tenderness, swelling, and redness and are commonly due to rheumatoid arthritis, septic joints, fractures, or tendonitis.

If the patient experiences episodes of gout, the MTP joint of the great toe presents with symptoms of inflammation as well as a nodule (tophus) on the joint. Occasionally the tophus will present with draining.

Palpation Techniques and Expected Findings	Unexpected Findings
Request the patient to plantar flex and dorsiflex the ankle with the provider applying an opposing force (Figure 27-54). The patient should be able to overcome the opposing force and maintain the ankle in plantar flexion and dorsiflexion.	Unexpected findings would be manifestations of inflammation with pain and tenderness, the presence of nodules or other lesions, and joints that feel rough. Individuals with hyperlipidemia may have a thickened Achilles tendon.

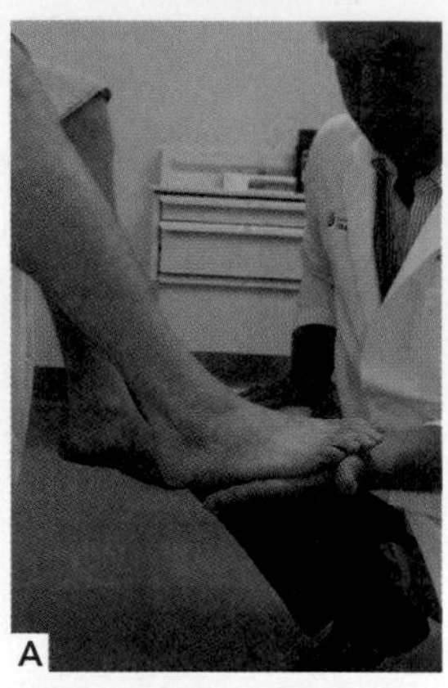
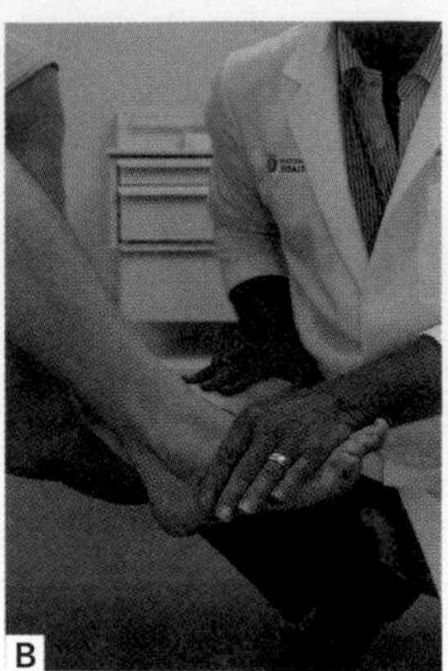

FIGURE 27-54A–B ROM/muscle strength: ankle and foot

Palpation: Level III

Fracture site

Palpation of the fracture site, as well as internal trauma, causes pain and tenderness at the fracture site and surrounding tissue.

Muscle spasms may also be palpated in the surrounding area. Pain impulses from the periosteum are sent to the muscle, causing powerful tonic contractions of the surrounding muscles. The muscle spasms are also an attempt to reduce the fracture and pull the bones back into position. Additionally, there may be evidence of crepitus, which is a grating sound or sensation caused by bone rubbing on bone.

Individuals may present in the emergency department or clinic for shoulder pain that may be caused by a rotator cuff tear. Three assessment maneuvers are suggested to use to determine whether or not a tear exists.

The active **painful arc test** requires the patient to actively abduct the arm from a neutral position. The patient should be able to do this without experiencing pain.

Unexpected Findings: Pain with active abduction is considered a positive test. This test will be positive if the patient cannot control the arm adduction movement, and the arm drops to the patient's side Severe pain with the adduction movement is also a positive test.

Drop-Arm test

The **drop-arm test** is used to assess for rotator cuff tear (Figure 27-55).

Have patient actively abduct the shoulder to 90 degrees. If the patient cannot do this, you should do so passively, and then ask the patient to slowly lower the arm. Patients without a rotator cuff tear should be able to do this smoothly and in a coordinated manner.

Unexpected Findings: If there is a rotator cuff tear (supraspinatus), the arm will drop to the side.

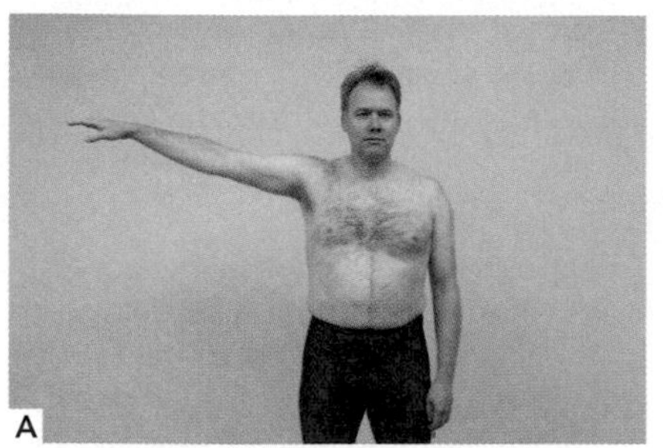
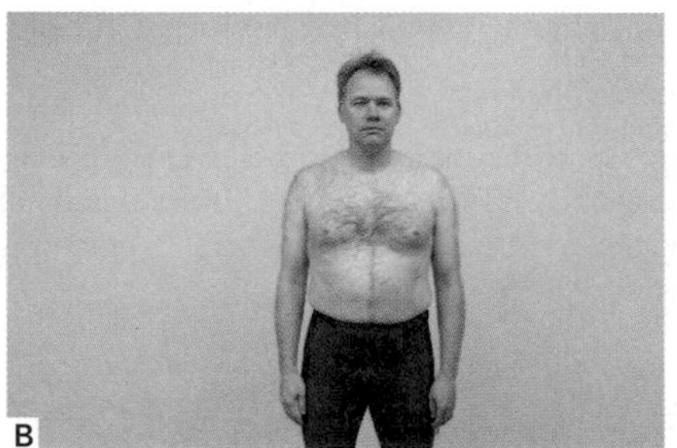

FIGURE 27-55A–B Drop arm test

Testing for **weakness in external rotation** (infraspinatus muscle): To test for this, have the patient adduct the arm (shoulder) with the elbow at 90 degrees and attempt to externally rotate the arm. The provider attempts to resist this movement with the hand. Patients without a rotator cuff tear should be able to overcome the resistance.

Palpation Techniques and Expected Findings	Unexpected Findings
Another cause of shoulder pain can be shoulder impingement syndrome (SIS), which is a combination of shoulder symptoms, examination findings, and radiologic signs related to the compression of structures around the glenohumeral joint when the shoulder is elevated (Simons, Kruse, & Dixon, 2013). Examination techniques for presence of SIS are the Neer's test and Hawkins-Kennedy tests.	Patients with a rotator cuff tear will not be able to overcome resistance. Pain is a positive sign of impingement.
Neer's test **Neer's test** (impingement sign) occurs when the rotator cuff tendons are compressed by the greater tuberosity against the anterior acromion under the coracoacromial arch (Galatz, 2010). To perform the Neer's test, have the patient pronate the arm and then bring up the arm so that the shoulder is fully flexed (150 degrees). Place one hand on the patient's scapula, and grasp the forearm with your other. Rotate the arm internally (thumb pointed downward). Forward flex arm, positioning hand over the head. (Figure 27-56). Patients without SIS will not experience pain. 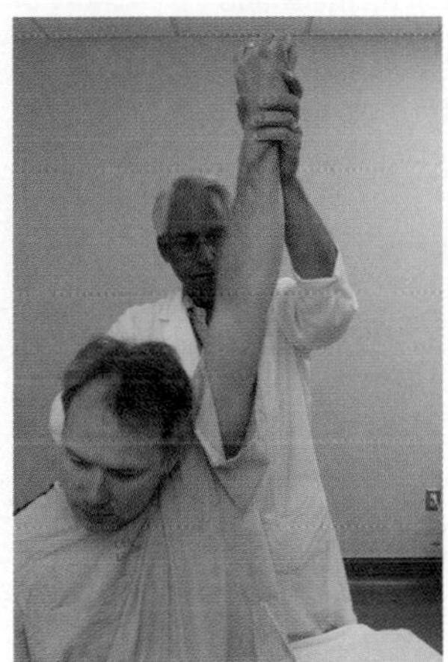 **FIGURE 27-56** Neer's test	Pain elicited with this maneuver is positive for rotator cuff pathology.
Palpation: Level IV	
Bragard stretch test The **Bragard stretch test** is used for the same purpose as the straight leg raising test. Start with the patient in the same position. Place one hand under the heel of one leg and slowly raise the leg until pain is experienced. Lower the leg slightly and dorsiflex the foot quickly and internally rotate the leg. Have the patient identify the most distal point where the pain is felt. After this maneuver, have the patient sit on the edge of the table leaning slightly forward. The provider then instructs the patient to extend the knee while applying resistance.	Pain below the knee with the leg elevated to less than 70 degrees that is augmented by dorsiflexion and internal rotation is highly suggestive of a herniated disk at $L_{4/5}$ or S_1. Pain with extension of resistance accompanied by attempts to lean backward to lessen the pain is an indicator for sciatic nerve tenderness.
Snuffbox tenderness test The **Snuffbox tenderness test** is performed by identifying the anatomic snuffbox that is located between the extensor pollicis longus and brevis muscles (Figure 27-57). A triangular depression is formed when the wrist is ulnar deviated and the thumb abducted and extended. Press down firmly with the thumb or index finger. 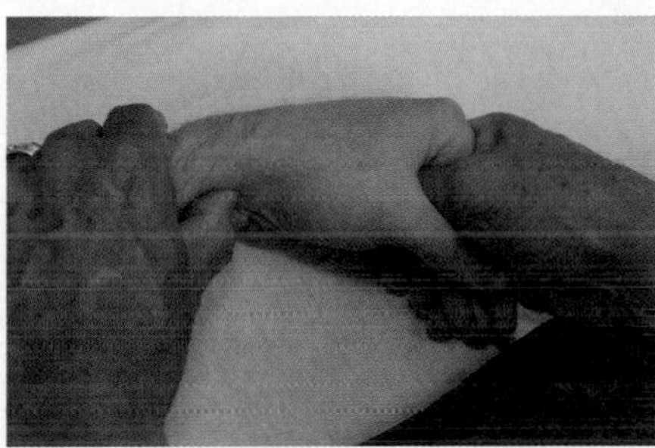 **FIGURE 27-57** Snuffbox tenderness	Any tenderness or pain with compression of the site highly suggests a scaphoid fracture.

Palpation Techniques and Expected Findings	Unexpected Findings

Diagnostic Procedures

Diagnostic procedures used for assessing knee dysfunction include the **McMurray, Lachman,** and **drawer tests**. All four are used primarily to assess for knee injuries related to ligaments and the menisci. These entire procedures are done with the patient in the supine position with the legs fully extended.

PRACTICE POINT: McMurray Test

When doing the McMurray test, flex the knee to the maximal pain-free position. With the leg supported, externally rotate the foot and then gradually extend the knee, keeping the tibia externally rotated. To test the lateral meniscus, perform the same maneuver, only with the foot internally rotated.

Varus/Valgus tests

Use the McMurry test to determine if a tear exists in the lateral or medial meniscus (Figure 27-58). Begin by flexing one knee and position the hand over the top of the knee with the thumb over one joint line and index and middle finger over the opposite joint line.

A palpable or audible click with extension is significant for a tear of the lateral meniscus.

With the other hand, support the heel to maintain knee flexion and rotate the tibia medially and laterally, paying attention for an audible click.

If the patient experiences pain, it confirms an injury.

Next, laterally rotate the tibia and extend the knee beyond 90 degrees. To examine the lateral meniscus, return the knee to full flexion and apply a medial rotation to the tibia, then extending the knee once again.

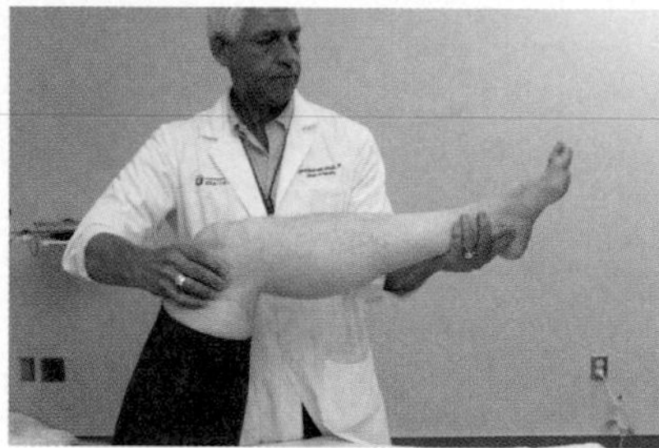

FIGURE 27-58 McMurray test

Perform the Lachman test to assess the integrity of the anterior and posterior cruciate ligaments (ACL/PCL) (Figure 27-59). Start by flexing one leg 15–20 degrees while keeping the heel on the table.

With one hand, grasp the thigh above the knee, stabilizing the femur, and place the other hand around the proximal tibia. For the best results, have the patient relax the hamstring muscles. Instruct the patient to move the tibia with a forward or anterior motion.

If the tibia moves out from under the femur, the possibility of an injured or torn ACL is high. Repeat the procedure using posterior stress. If the tibia moves back under the femur, the possibility of an injured or torn PCL is high.

The absence of a definite end point is suggestive of a tear of the anterior cruciate ligament.

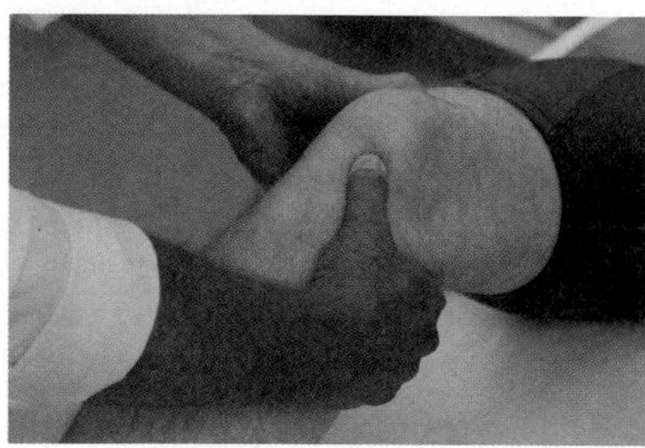

FIGURE 27-59 Lachman test

PRACTICE POINT: Lachman Test

For the Lachman test, the thigh muscles should be relaxed and supported. Flex the knee 30 degrees and grasp the distal femur from the lateral side and the proximal tibia from the medial side. Maintaining the knee in a neutral position, lift or pull anteriorly on the tibia while stabilizing the femur. Observe for the extent of bony translation of the tibia relative to the femur and the presence or absence of a definite end point when full translation is reached.

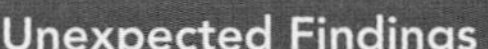

Palpation Techniques and Expected Findings	Unexpected Findings
Perform the Anterior/Posterior Drawer test to assess the stability of the anterior and posterior cruciate ligaments (Figure 27-60). Instruct the patient to flex one knee to 90 degrees, keeping the foot flat on the table. Grasp the lower leg with the thumbs on the ridge of the anterior tibia and pull forward.	If the tibia moves out from under the femur, there is a high probability that the ACL is torn or injured. In the same position, push backward on the leg. If the tibia moves back under the femur, there is a high probability that the PCL is torn or injured.

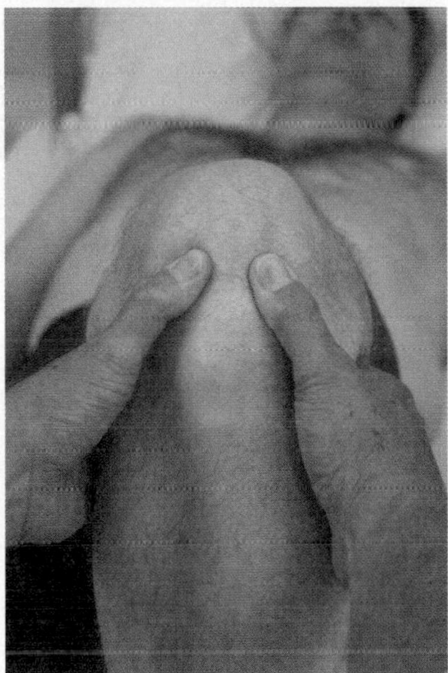

FIGURE 27-60 Drawer test

Palpation Techniques and Expected Findings	Unexpected Findings
The **varus**, or **adduction**, **stress test** evaluates the lateral collateral ligament. To perform this test, place the patient's knee in 30 degrees of flexion. While stabilizing the knee, adduct the ankle. The valgus, or abduction, stress test evaluates the medial collateral ligament. To perform this test, place the patient's knee in 30 degrees of flexion. While stabilizing the knee, abduct the ankle. (Figure 27-61).	If the knee joint *adducts* greater than normal (compare with the uninjured leg), the test is positive. This is indicative of a lateral collateral ligament tear. If the knee joint *abducts* greater than normal (compare with the uninjured leg), the test is positive. This is indicative of a medial collateral ligament tear.

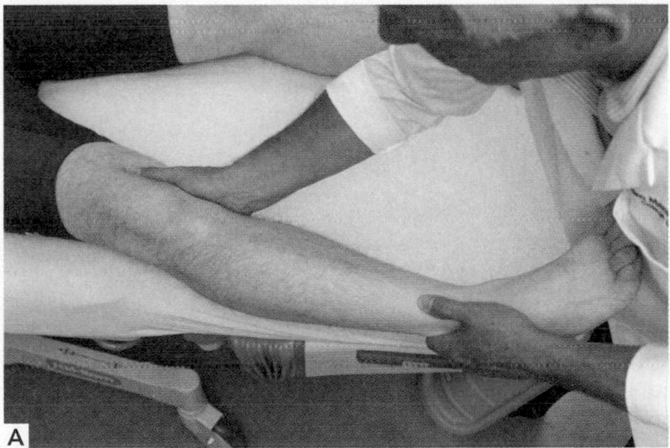

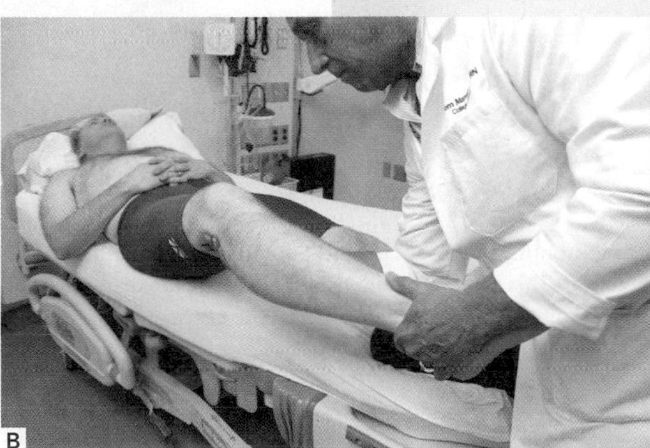

FIGURE 27-61A–B Varus/valgus stress test

Developmental Applications

Techniques and Expected Findings	Unexpected Findings

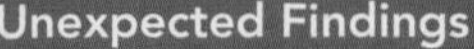

Infants

Examination of the infant is important to identify any alterations of the MS system so that early intervention may reduce or eliminate any adverse conditions.

Most skeletal alterations or malformations are genetic in origin; however, various environmental influences may also contribute to their development. Fetal position in the uterus may also predispose to certain conditions. Traumatic births or use of instruments during birth may also contribute to skeletal alterations.

The infant should be completely undressed and lying on a table. A warming table is necessary for examination of the newborn. Overall, observe the infant for symmetry relative to size and position. The lower and upper extremities should demonstrate bilaterally equal size, length, and joint flexion and extension. The axillary, gluteal, popliteal, and femoral creases should also be symmetrical (Figure 27-62).

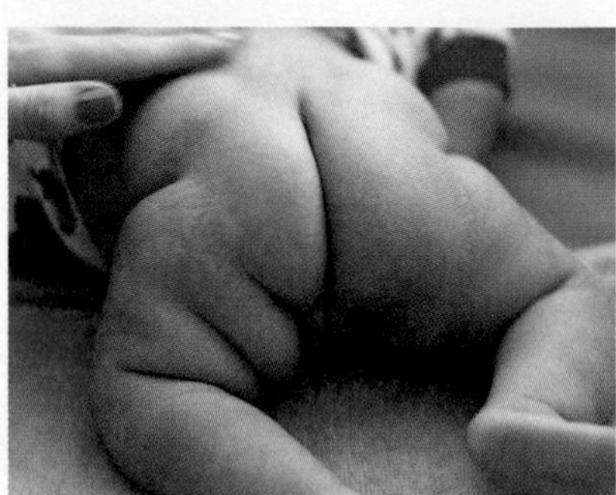

FIGURE 27-62 Examination of infant: posterior skin folds

Examine the infant's back by picking up the infant, supporting the neck and head with the fingers and the rest of the body on the forearm or supporting the infant's buttocks with the other hand. The expected curves of the spine are not yet apparent, so the infant's spine assumes a C shape (Figure 27-63). This shape remains until the infant can sit without support. Inspect the length of the spine and observe for any tufts of hair, dimples, cysts, or masses.

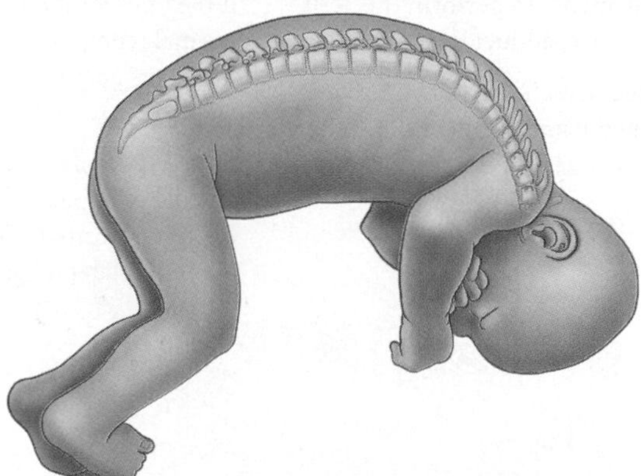

FIGURE 27-63 Infant back exam: C spine

At approximately 2 months, the infant should demonstrate the ability to lift the head and trunk from a prone position. This provides evidence of adequate forearm muscle development and strength, as well as promoting the development of the cervical spinal curve.

In utero positioning may cause some minor alterations in skeletal alignment. Often the infant's feet are positioned in a varus or valgus position. Metatarsus adductus (MTA) (pigeon toe) is commonly observed as adduction and inversion of the forefoot, occurring in approximately one out of 1000–2000 live births, with first-born infants more likely to be affected (Figure 27-64). There is no gender difference and infants with MTA may be at increased risk for a hip dysfunction known as developmental dysplasia of the hip.

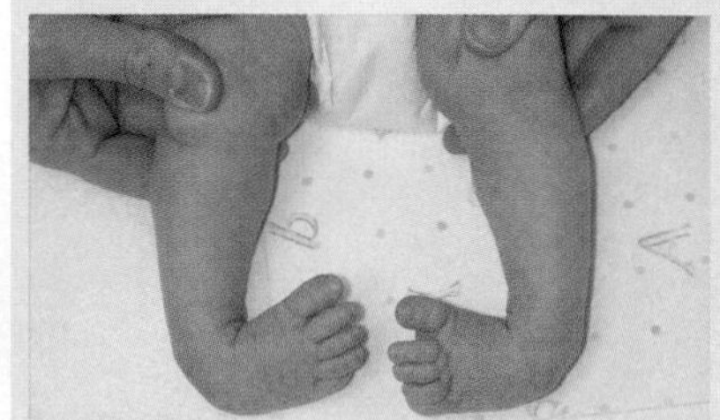

FIGURE 27-64 Metatarsus adductus in infant
Source: K.Shea, M.D./CMSP

Techniques and Expected Findings

Unexpected Findings

Tibial torsion, a twisting of the tibia that manifests as bowleggedness with adduction and inversion of the foot, is another common positional alteration in alignment. It is most common in children between the ages of 18 months and 3 years of age (Duderstadt, 2006). It frequently resolves with growth and weight bearing without any complications, but yearly evaluations should be performed.

If the thumbs are not parallel, tibial torsion is present.

Any of these may indicate the possibility of a spinal cord alteration such as spina bifida, meningocele, or myelomeningocele.

In MTA the midline of the foot is shifted so that it passes through the third and fourth toes rather than the second and third toes. The foot also demonstrates a high arch with a wide gap between the second toe and the great toe that deviates inward. MTA is frequently correctable and is described as flexible MTA. This type requires frequent, gentle manipulation of the foot to achieve correct alignment. A correctable, faulty alignment demonstrates flexibility by straightening out with gentle abduction of the forefoot. Approximately 85% of these cases correct themselves as the infant begins to stand and start walking and require no further treatment. The other 15% do not improve and may become less flexible and require further treatment.

Examination for tibial torsion begins with the infant/child prone on the exam table. Flex one knee to 90 degrees and align the midline of the foot parallel to the femur. Grasp the medial and lateral malleoli with the thumb and index finger of one hand and the patella with the same fingers on the same side of the leg. The expected finding would be the thumbs parallel to each other.

Examine the hips for the presence of hip dislocation or subluxation using the Barlow and Ortolani tests, which should be performed at every newborn exam during the first year (Figure 27-65).

If the femoral head is dislocated, a clunk or feeling of movement may be felt as the head dislocates. This is considered a positive Barlow's and indicates hip dislocation.

Begin the Barlow test with the infant supine on the examination table with hip and knees flexed to 90 degrees. Grasp the infant's leg with the thumb on the inside of the thigh with the base on the knee and the fingers on the outside of the leg positioned on the greater trochanter. Next adduct the thigh while gently applying downward pressure on the femur. This maneuver attempts to dislocate the head of the femur from the acetabulum. Expected results would be that the femoral head remains in the acetabulum and any movement is smooth without any sounds. High-pitched clicks are not unusual and commonly are heard.

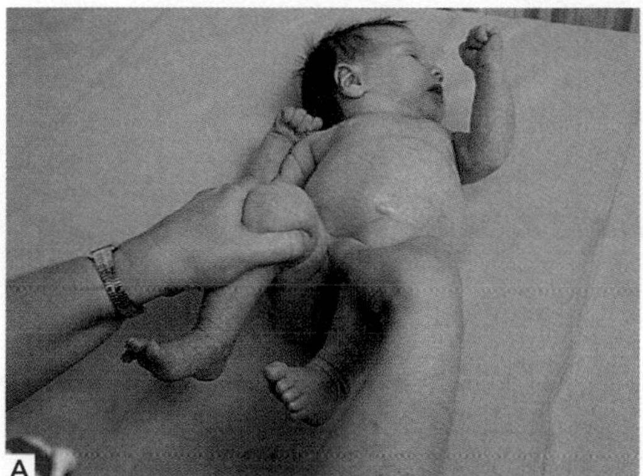

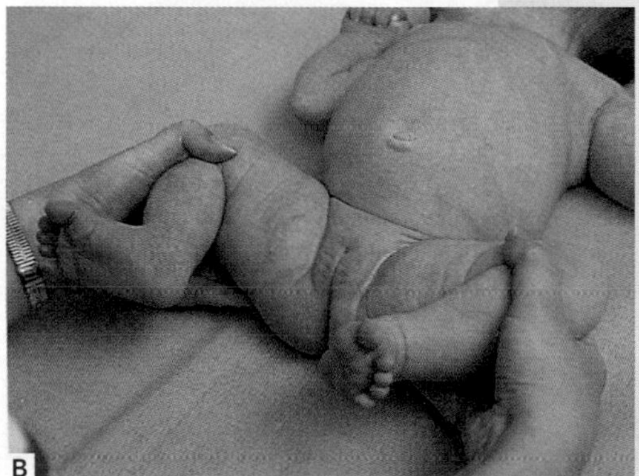

FIGURE 27-65A–B a) the Barlow maneuver; b) the Ortolani maneuver

Techniques and Expected Findings

The **Ortolani test** is then done, which relocates the dislocation caused by the Barlow test. With the fingers in the same position, gently abduct the hips while maintaining the downward pressure. With the fingers on the trochanter, apply an upward pressure on the trochanter. This movement is also expected to be smooth without any sounds.

The **Allis test** is another test for hip dislocation that compares leg length (Figure 27-66). With the infant still supine, keep the infant's feet flat on the table while flexing the knees to 90 degrees. With the knees at eye level, observe the height of the knees. It is expected that the knees are equal in height.

Palpate the clavicles to assess for any fractures that may be the result of a traumatic delivery.

In addition to palpation for evidence of injury during birth, the upper extremities should be assessed for full range of motion. The arm is adducted with inward rotation but with an appropriate hand grip (Duderstadt, 2006).

The infant's hands are most often fisted with opening occurring periodically. When the hand is fisted, the thumb is placed within the fingers. To examine the hand, pry the fingers open and inspect the dermatoglyphic characteristics observing the palmar and phalangeal creases of each hand. Also inspect the infant's feet (Figure 27-67).

Palpate the infant's muscles to assess muscle tone. Grasp the muscles to determine firmness. Also observe for the presence of spasticity or flaccidness, noting whether it is localized or generalized if present. Passive range of motion is used to assess joint mobility.

Assess muscle strength by holding the infant under the axilla in an upright position. Expected muscle strength is demonstrated by the infant being securely wedged between the hands and maintaining the upright position.

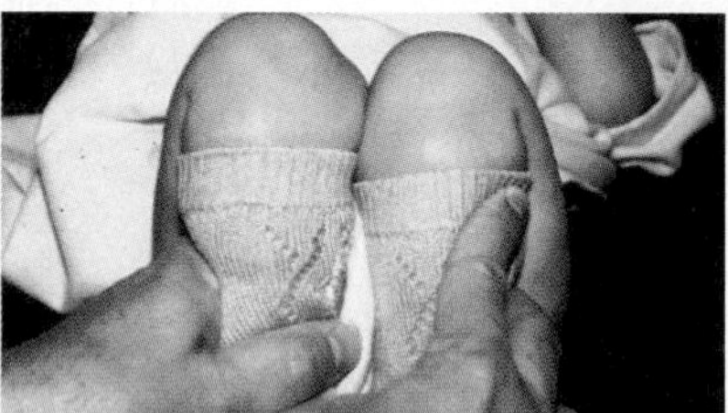

FIGURE 27-66 Allis test
Source: Used with permission International Hip Dysplasia Institute

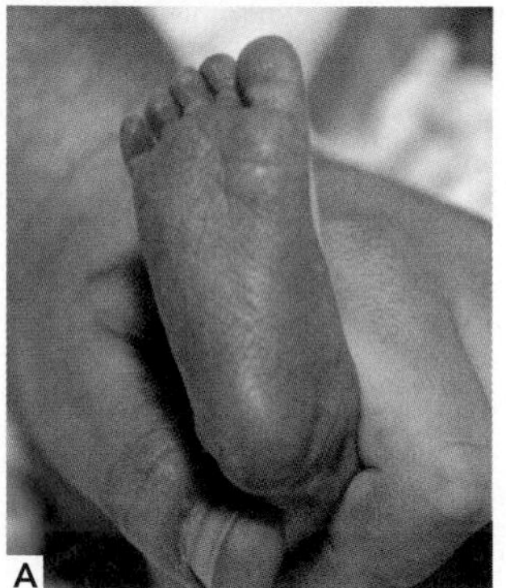

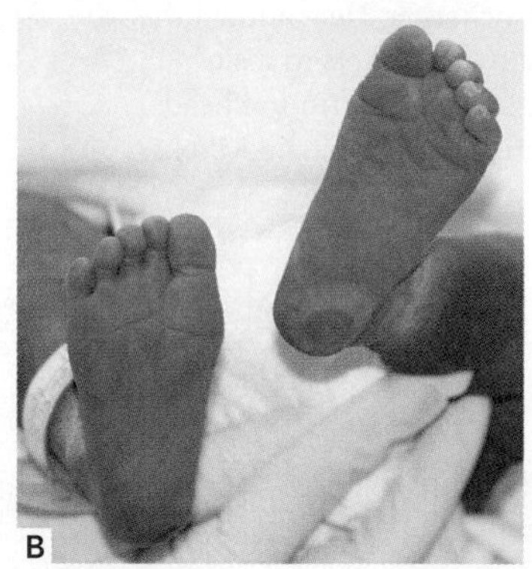

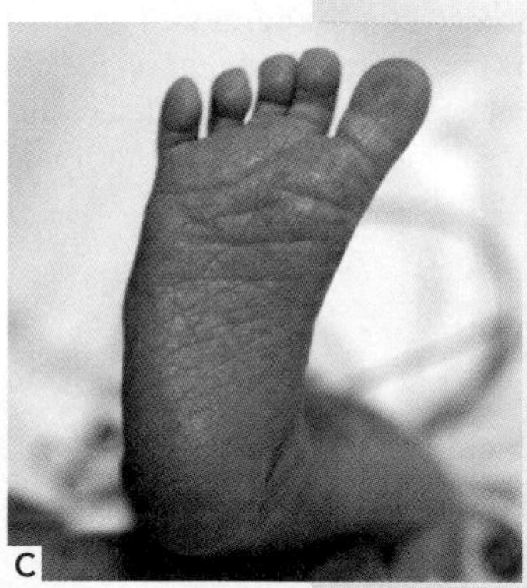

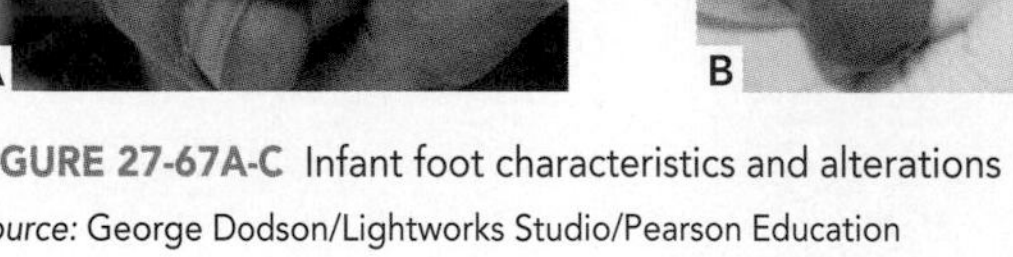

FIGURE 27-67A-C Infant foot characteristics and alterations
Source: George Dodson/Lightworks Studio/Pearson Education

Children

Development of the musculoskeletal system in children can be easily observed by watching the activities of the child during play or when interacting with parents or others. Picking up toys and playing with them; balanced, coordinated and smooth movements during play; and getting around by oneself are all indicators of appropriate musculoskeletal development. Additional activities that allow evaluation of joint ROM, bone stability, and muscle strength include hopping, climbing, jumping, and rising from a sitting position. Assessment of appropriate activities related to age is related to knowledge of the expected sequence of motor development.

Unexpected Findings

If the fingers relocate the femoral head in the acetabulum, a clunk or movement felt when the head is relocated is a positive Ortolani's sign for dislocation of the hip.

If one knee is lower than the other, hip dislocation is the probable cause.

Bony irregularities, crepitus, and tenderness are common indicators of fractures. If a clavicular fracture is not identified early, a palpable bony prominence is frequently present later on. This is the callus that forms as the bone shapes and remolds itself during healing.

Erb's palsy may result from injury to the fifth and sixth cranial nerves that demonstrates no spontaneous abduction of the shoulder muscles of flexion of the elbow.

Also note the presence of a palmar crease, **syndactyly** (webbed fingers) or **polydactyly** (more than five fingers/toes).

Weakness of the shoulder muscles is demonstrated by the infant slipping between the hands.

Genu varum is present when there is greater than 2.5 cm (1 inch) between the knees. Persistent genu varum may be an indication of rickets. Persistent genu valgum is also associated with rickets as well as syphilis and poliomyelitis.

Techniques and Expected Findings	Unexpected Findings

With the child in a standing position, observe the contour of the spine and abdomen. Lordosis is commonly present in children as is a protuberant abdomen.

Observe alignment of the lower extremities to note any changes present in the legs and feet (Figure 27-68). Genu varum and valgum may be present and best observed with the child standing with the medial malleoli together and facing the examiner.

True flat feet in children is uncommon. Physiological flat feet present in children, pre-school and up, is most likely caused by weak ligaments (Duderstadt, 2006).

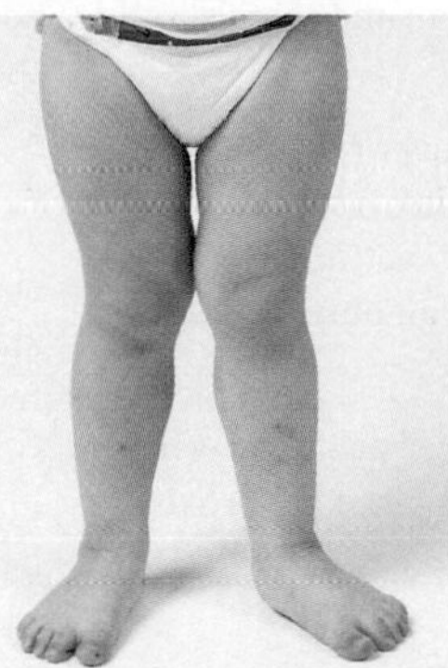

FIGURE 27-68 Child standing: anterior view

Genu varum is common in the first year after the child begins to walk and may be manifested with a waddling type gait. Genu varum generally resolves spontaneously without intervention.

Genu valgum (knock-knee) is present when there is greater than 2.5 cm between the medial malleoli with the knees placed together. Genu valgum is common in children between 2 and 4 years of age.

Inspect the child's feet also for any evidence is misalignment. Observe the longitudinal arch of the foot and foot position when bearing weight. Until the age of 3, the arch is obscured by a fat pad, giving the appearance of flat feet (pes planus). In an older child that appears to have flat feet, have the child stand on tip toes and observe for the appearance of the arch.

Metarsus adductus that has been diagnosed at birth should have resolved but may persist until 3 years of age. Further follow-up and treatment may be required.

Observe the position in which the child sits, or ask parents about it. Also observe the child getting up from a sitting position.

The W position or reverse tailor position is often observed in children with intoeing that accompanies femoral anteversion. This position places stress on the hip, knee, and ankle joints.

Overall generalized muscle weakness, common to muscular dystrophies, is demonstrated by the child placing the hands on the thighs and pushing the upper body up; this is known as the Gower sign (Figure 27-69).

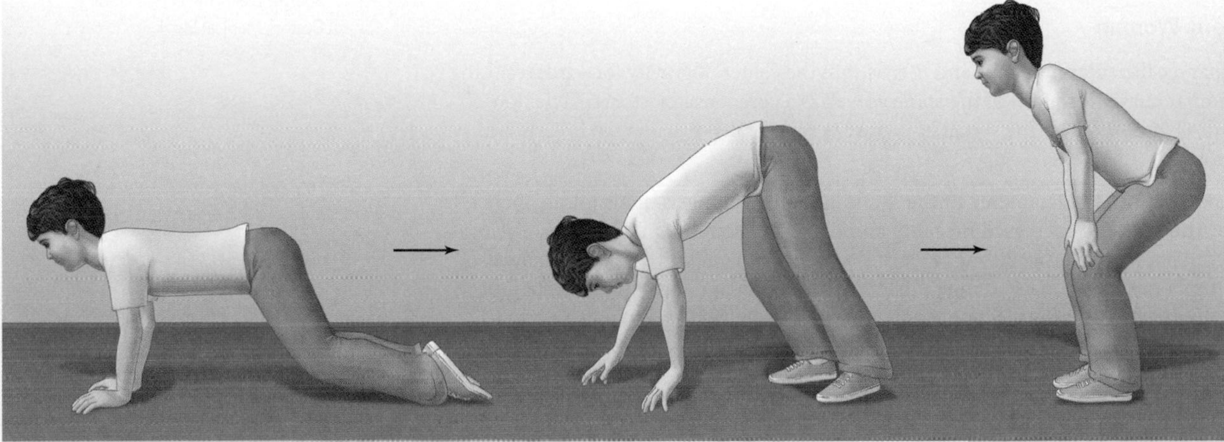

FIGURE 27-69 Gower's sign

Techniques and Expected Findings	Unexpected Findings

Adolescents

Examination of adolescents' MS system proceeds in the same manner as for the adult.

The spine needs particular attention to detect any postural or spinal deformities. Adolescents who participate in sports activities will frequently present for a sports physical, which requires special attention to bones and joints for sports safety and prevention of injuries.

The shoulders and scapulae should be symmetrically equal in height and position, and there should be no lateral curvature or rib hump apparent with forward flexion of the spine.

Routine screening of preadolescent and adolescent females for scoliosis is no longer recommended. However, any subjective or objective information that may suggest scoliosis should be followed up. Subjectively, the patient or parent may note that there is difficulty in getting some clothes to fit— hem lines and waist lines may appear uneven. There may also be an observation of unevenness of the shoulders as well as a curvature of the spine.

To assess for scoliosis, observe the posterior chest for evidence of curvature as well as the forward bend test. In the forward bend test, ask the patient to stand straight with the feet placed approximately 12 inches apart and to then slowly bend over and touch the toes (Figure 27-70).

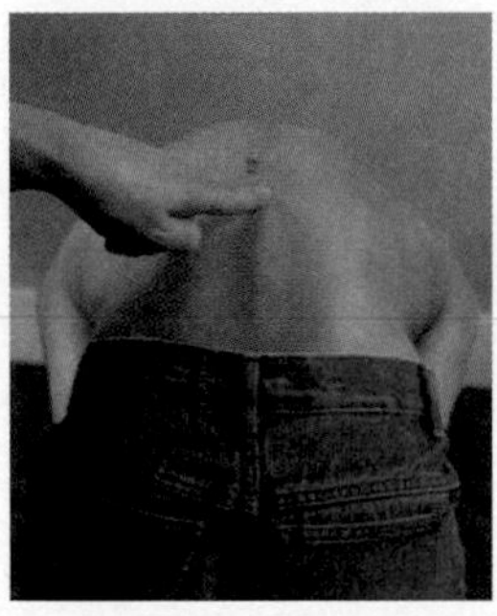

FIGURE 27-70 Inspection of the spine for scoliosis.
Source: George Dodson/Pearson Education

Poor posture in adolescents may result in a slight kyphosis with rounded shoulders.

Scoliosis is a spinal deformity that usually presents during the preadolescent/ adolescent growth spurt. In scoliosis, there is a lateral curvature of the thoracic spine (Figure 27-71). Scoliosis presents as two types—idiopathic (structural) and functional. Idiopathic scoliosis most commonly occurs in females age 10 and above. The cause is unknown and requires intervention (neck brace and/or surgery) to prevent the curvature from increasing. Functional scoliosis does not have spinal rotation, does not progress, and often presents with no additional problems.

If the patient has structural scoliosis, the curvature of the spine will be apparent in the standing position and as the spine curves forward.

The shoulders and scapula may also be observed to be unequal in height. In the forward position, it may appear as if the ribs hump together. If the scoliosis is the functional type, the spine will straighten out during forward bending and the curvature will disappear.

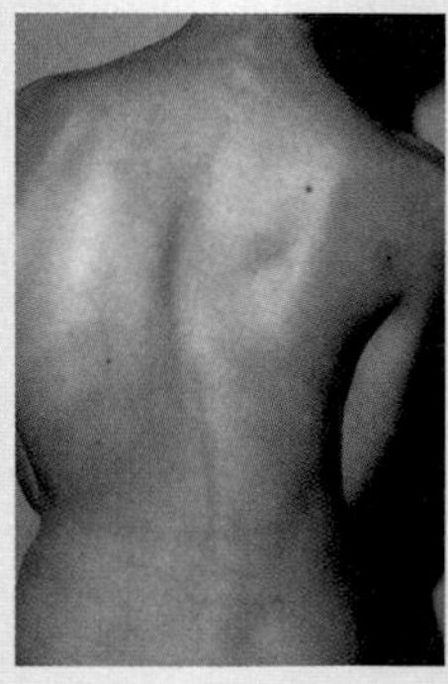

FIGURE 27-71 Scoliosis
Source: Wellcome Image Library/ Custom Medical Stock

The Pregnant Woman

During pregnancy, the enlarging fetus and uterus shift the center of gravity forward, resulting in an increased lumbar curve (lordosis) of the spine as well as a compensatory forward flexion of the cervical spine (Figure 27-72). The spinal curvature is exaggerated by enlarged breasts and stooped shoulders.

The hormone relaxin acts on the ligaments of the sacroiliac and symphysis pubis joints, increasing their elasticity, thus causing increased mobility and decreased stability of the joints. These skeletal changes contribute to the "waddling" gait of the pregnant female. The patient may also indicate that the hip bones feel "loose" or may move when walking and may also complain of pain in the inner thigh when standing. Some women may also experience carpal tunnel syndrome in the last trimester. Increased fluid is the probable cause and the symptoms disappear after delivery.

Techniques and Expected Findings | Unexpected Findings

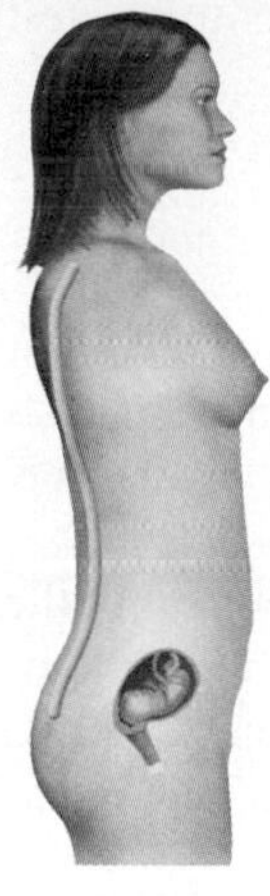
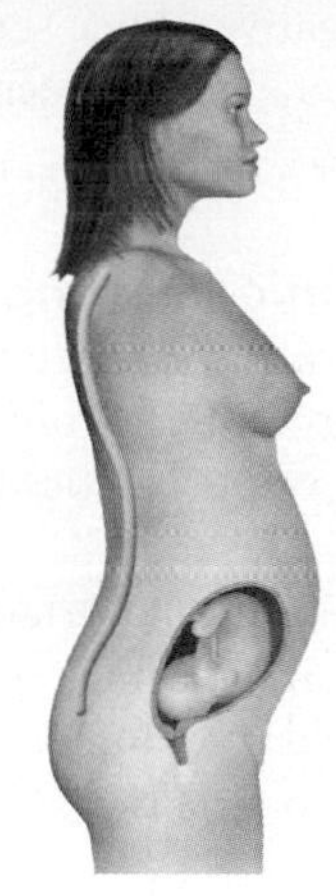
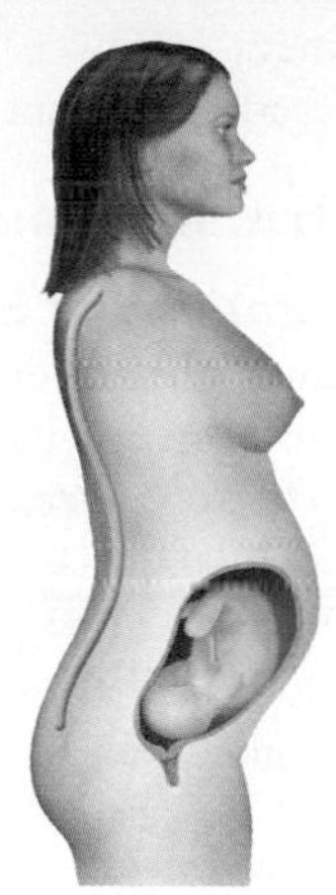
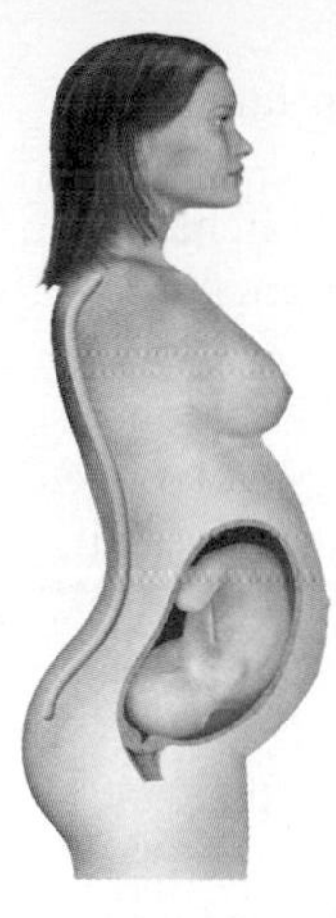
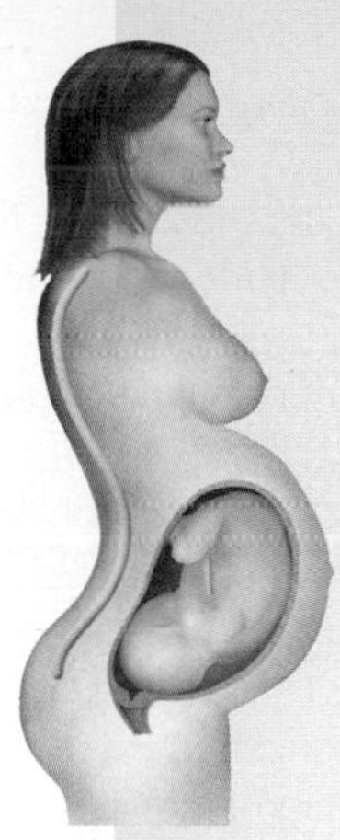

FIGURE 27-72 Pregnant female posture

The Older Adult

The examination of the MS system of the elderly patient proceeds in the same manner as for the adult with the need to allow for more time for the patient to participate in certain maneuvers. There is a wide variety of ability and muscle agility within the elderly population, so it is necessary to individualize the examination.

Almost every adult experiences postural changes associated with aging. There is a decrease in height, due to shortening of the spine, which creates the appearance of elongated upper extremities. The vertebrae may also collapse, due to osteoporosis, also causing the spine to become shorter. A kyphosis frequently is present and may be accompanied by a scoliosis (**kyphoscoliosis**). This is frequently described as the "dowager's hump" as it is mostly seen in females (Figure 27-73). To compensate for the kyphosis, the head and neck may demonstrate a backward tilt. The feet may be positioned further apart to increase the base of support, and the upper extremities may be held away from the body to aid in maintaining balance. The hips and knees may also be positioned in slight flexion.

Bone density decreases and the development of osteoporosis is a primary concern in the elderly. Bone destruction occurs at a greater rate than bone construction, which is the reason for the development of osteoporosis.

Joint alterations, primarily rheumatoid and osteoarthritis are present in varying degrees of severity. As a result, ROM in certain joints may be decreased. Muscle strength may also be decreased, but should still demonstrate the ability to perform actions and move in opposition to gravity. Overall muscle mass decreases, contributing to muscle weakness, and is most often the result of atrophy related to disuse or loss of nerve function related to medications or diabetes.

A significant assessment of the elderly is a functional assessment that determines the patient's ability to adequately engage in and safely perform activities of daily living. The functional assessment may easily be done during the health history.

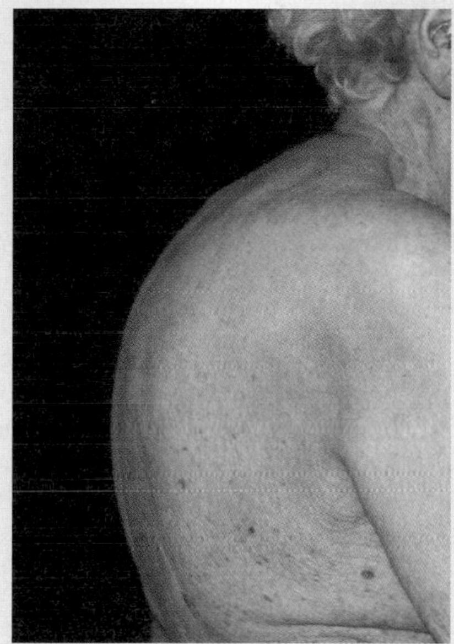

FIGURE 27-73 Dowager's hump/kyphosis

Source: Dr. P. Marazzi/Science Source

DOCUMENTATION

- **Inspection:** Gait smooth, rhythmic, and coordinated; walks with ease without limping. Arms at side and swing in opposition to legs. Posture erect with spine midline and expected cervical, thoracic, and lumbar curves. Spine straight without any lateral/medial curvatures or accentuated spinal curves. Knees in straight line between hips and ankles. Feet point forward. Upper extremities/lower extremities equal in length without any observable deformities. Muscle mass bilaterally equal in UE/LE's.

No redness, swelling noted in joints. Without varus/valgus deformities.

Range of Motion:

Neck—Able to flex, extend, hyperextend, rotate, and laterally flex.

Shoulder—Active ROM demonstrating flexion, extension, hyperextension, adduction, abduction, internal/external rotation, and circumduction.

Elbows—Full ROM evident through flexion, extension, pronation, and supination.

Wrist—Able to perform flexion, extension, hyperextension, and radial/ulnar flexion.

Fingers—No loss of flexion, extension, hyperextension, abduction, or adduction.

Thumb—Performs active flexion, extension, abduction, and opposition with no noted loss of mobility.

Trunk—Flexes and extends with difficulty. Lateral flexion intact. Patient refuses to perform rotation or hyperextension; states she wishes to protect her lower back from further injury.

Hip—No loss of movement noted.

Knee—Flexes and extends with difficulty.

Ankle—Patient able to perform eversion/inversion, plantar flexion, and dorsiflexion.

Toes—Able to actively flex, extend, abduct, and adduct with difficulty.

Muscle mass equal bilaterally in all major muscle groups. All muscle groups demonstrate tone that allows individual to support own weight; demonstrates flexibility and ability to freely move and control movement and activities. Muscle strength +5 for neck, shoulder, elbow, wrist, finger, hip, knee, and ankle muscles.

- **Palpation:** Joints nontender without evidence of effusion, masses, or crepitation. Muscle strength equal bilaterally in all areas—able to overcome resistance to flexion and extension in all major muscle groups (ocular, facial, neck, deltoids, biceps, triceps, wrists, fingers, hamstrings, gluteal, abductor and adductor muscles, as well as quads, ankles, and feet).

Specific Joints:

TMJ—Smooth mandibular action without clicking or pain upon opening of jaw.

Wrist—Phalen's test without numbness.

Hips—Thomas test negative—extended leg flat on table.

Knees—Drawer test negative—knee stable; McMurray test negative—no pain upon rotation and extension.

Electronic Charting

Expectations of Electronic Charting

A study by the American College of Rheumatology noted that use of information technology and electronic charting systems is rapidly becoming crucial for viable practice (Mosley-Williams & Williams, 2005).

Diagnostic imaging can be an important component of the musculoskeletal assessment, and imaging reports should be readily accessible. The system should accommodate assessments such as tests for balance and stability, bone density assessments, and similar evaluations.

Musculoskeletal system problems can be acute or chronic. Electronic systems should allow review of previous history. For example, growth charting should be able to span multiple encounters, and documentation regarding birth defects or chronic conditions should be able to carry forward between encounters.

Self-care and home treatment can be an important part of the care of chronic problems. Use of an electronic charting system has been associated with a higher number of self-care topics discussed with a patient (Arar & Pugh, 2006). Nutrition, exercise, and weight gain/loss can be tracked at home and may be ideal components of an electronic personal health record (PHR). PHRs are becoming increasingly common, and data from those records can be a useful part of the musculoskeletal assessment when looking for changes over time.

Limitations of Electronic Charting

Although electronic health records are becoming widespread, it is still difficult to share data between different systems. Tracking change over time becomes more difficult when records need to be shared across multiple electronic systems.

Use of electronic charting, like other computer use, can be associated with repetitive motion injury and similar musculoskeletal problems.

Summary

- The musculoskeletal system is composed of the bony skeleton and muscles that are attached to them. The bones and muscles work together as a system of levers that provide the support and movement of the joints that allows for mobility. Functional muscle activity also depends on appropriate innervation with the ability to transmit and receive impulses. Bone metabolism is also responsible for maintaining calcium balance.
- The bony skeleton is assessed for structure and alignment, and the joints are assessed for movement by range of motion. Synovial joints should allow smooth movement throughout the expected degrees of motion. The muscles are assessed for strength and tone, which allows the muscles to move the joints and maintain an upright position.
- Alterations of the musculoskeletal system prevent performance of expected function by altering the alignment of the skeleton, preventing joint movement, and altering muscle tone. Damage to nerves also alters muscular function.
- Growth of the bony skeleton occurs through the elongation of the long bones. During puberty growth hormone stimulates the epiphyseal plate, causing it to increase osteoblastic activity and promote linear growth. When an individual reaches adult height, the epiphyseal plate becomes inactive; however, bone

metabolism remains active throughout life through osteoblastic and osteoclastic activity.

- Bone mass or density is lost as people age, especially in women after *menopause*. The bones lose calcium and other minerals and may develop osteoporosis, increasing the risk for fractures in older adults. The joints become stiffer and less flexible. Fluid in the joints may decrease, and the cartilage may begin to rub together and erode, causing the symptoms associated with osteoarthritis. Minerals may deposit in and around some joints (calcification).
- Changes in the muscle tissue, combined with normal *aging changes in the nervous system*, causes muscles to have less tone and ability to contract. Muscles may become rigid with age and may lose tone, even with regular exercise.

Review Questions

1. The provider is working with a patient who has sustained an injury to the brachioradialis muscle. The provider would expect that this patient may have limitations in movement of which of the following?
   1. extension of the forearm
   2. flexion of the forearm
   3. adduction of the upper arm
   4. abduction of the upper arm
2. The provider is caring for a patient with a degenerative disorder affecting the skeletal muscles. The provider plans care for the patient with the knowledge that skeletal muscle is (Select all that apply.)
   1. voluntary in its activity.
   2. required for body movement.
   3. required for maintenance of circulation.
   4. necessary for peristalsis.
   5. responsive to autonomic control.
3. While assessing range of motion during a physical assessment, the provider asks the patient to adduct the right arm. The provider directs the patient correctly by asking the patient to do which of the following?
   1. Move the arm away from the body.
   2. Move the arm toward the midline of the body.
   3. Turn the arm so the palm is downward.
   4. Turn the arm so that the palm is facing upward.
4. A pregnant female patient presents to the provider with complaints of low back pain. The provider may identify a cause of this pain by inspecting for which of the following?
   1. ataxia
   2. lordosis
   3. scoliosis
   4. kyphosis
5. A 45-year-old female tells the provider that she is concerned that she has osteoporosis. The best response for the provider to give to the patient is which of the following?
   1. "If your mother doesn't have the disease, it is unlikely that you will develop it."
   2. "As long as you drink milk and exercise, you really have nothing to worry about."
   3. "Screening for the disease is really the only way to know if you have it."
   4. "You have no risk factors for osteoporosis, so there is no cause for concern."
6. When caring for a patient with rheumatoid arthritis, the provider should expect that the affected joints will (Select all that apply.)
   1. be stiff for a few minutes after arising.
   2. be painful at night.
   3. be symmetrical.
   4. feel warm to the touch.
   5. have no deformity.
7. When assessing an elderly patient with osteoarthritis, the provider notes crepitation with joint movement. The provider is aware that crepitus is produced by which of the following?
   1. roughened articular surfaces moving over each other
   2. tendons or ligaments that slip over bones during motion
   3. joints that are stretched when placed in hyperflexion or hyperextension
   4. an inflamed bursa
8. The provider is testing the muscle strength of a patient by
   1. asking the patient to lift a heavy object and observing muscles for the degree of contraction.
   2. appling an opposing force when the individual puts a joint in flexion or extension.
   3. measuring the degree of force that it takes to overcome joint flexion or extension.
   4. measuring the degree of flexion and extension of a joint with a goniometer.
9. The provider completes an assessment of a patient with carpal tunnel syndrome and documents which of the following as supportive of that diagnosis?
   1. "Thomas test is negative bilaterally."
   2. "The snuffbox tenderness test is bilaterally negative."
   3. "The patient displays a positive Phalen's sign."
   4. "Pain rated by the patient as 4/10 noted with Trendelenburg test."
10. The provider is aware that when assessing an individual for scoliosis the following manifestations will be noted in functional scoliosis:
    1. A lateral spinal curvature that remains visible in the standing and bending position.
    2. A lateral curvature of the spine that remains at less than 20 degrees.
    3. A lateral spinal curvature that is visible in the standing position, but disappears when the individual bends over.
    4. A lateral curvature of the spine that affects only the thoracic area or the lumbar area, but not both.

Conditions and Disorders

Carpal Tunnel Syndrome (CTS)

CTS is an entrapment neuropathy that causes paresthesia, pain, numbness, and other symptoms along the distribution of the median nerve resulting from its compression at the wrist in the carpal tunnel. Its cause is thought to be a combination of genetic and environmental factors. Certain conditions, which include: diabetes, obesity, pregnancy, hypothyroidism, heavy manual work, or work with vibrating tools, are also considered predisposing factors.

Most people relieved of their carpal tunnel symptoms with conservative or surgical management find minimal residual or "nerve damage." Long-term chronic carpal tunnel syndrome (typically seen in the elderly) can result in permanent nerve damage, (i.e., irreversible numbness, muscle wasting, and weakness). As of 2010, 8% of U.S. workers reported ever having carpal tunnel syndrome and 4% reported CTS in the past 12 months, with the prevalence higher among females and workers aged 45–64.

Pathophysiology

- The pathophysiology is not well understood but can be considered compression of the median nerve traveling through the carpal tunnel.
- Cause of compression may include a decrease in the size of the canal, an increase in the size of the contents, or both. Simply flexing the wrist to 90 degrees will decrease the size of the canal.
- The superficial sensory branch of the median nerve, which provides sensation to the base of the palm, branches proximal to the TCL and travels superficial to it. Thus, this branch is spared in carpal tunnel syndrome, and there is no loss of palmar sensation.

Subjective Data

- Symptoms typically start gradually with a vague aching in the wrist that can extend to the hand or forearm.
- Tingling or numbness in fingers or hand, especially thumb and index, middle or ring fingers, but not little finger. As the disorder progresses, the numb feeling may become constant.
- Pain radiating from the wrist up the arm to shoulder or down into palm or fingers, especially after forceful or repetitive use. Usually occurs on the palm side of forearm.
- A sense of weakness in hands and tendency to drop objects.

Objective Data

- Compression of the median nerve as it runs deep to the transverse carpal ligament (TCL) causes atrophy of the thenar eminence and weakness of the flexor pollicis brevis, opponens pollicis, and abductor pollicis brevis.
- Sensory loss in the digits supplied by the median nerve.

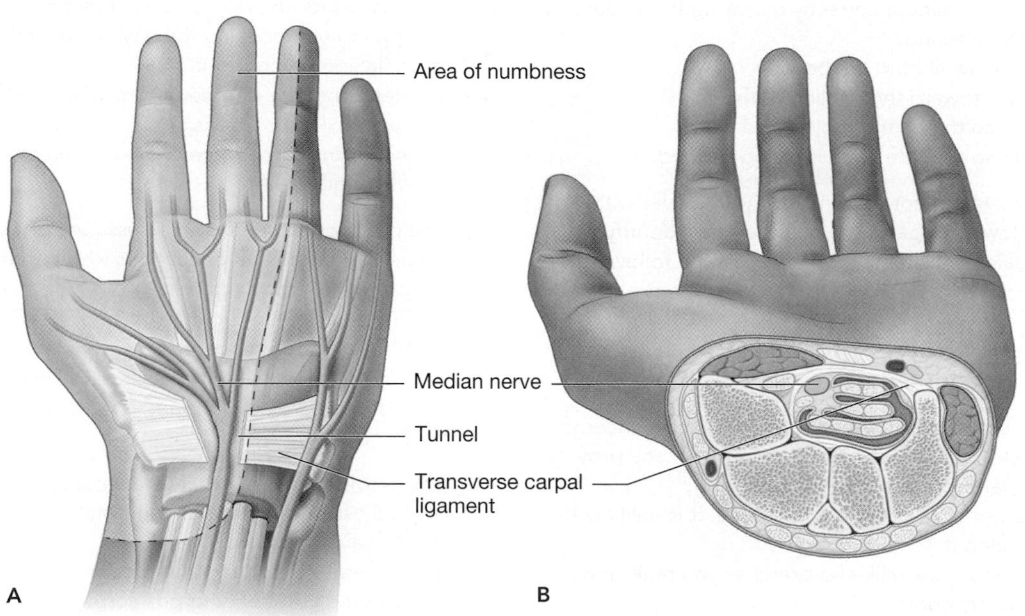

FIGURE 27-74 A–B Carpal tunnel syndrome

Muscular Dystrophy (MD)

MD is a diverse group of inherited muscular disorders that have common characteristics that cause progressive fiber degeneration. MD affects individuals of all ages, but is more prevalent in children. Symptoms may begin to appear in infancy or later in childhood. The pattern of inheritance occurs through X-linked recessive, autosomomal dominant, or recessive mechanisms, as well as spontaneous mutation. Duchenne/Becker MD are the most common types in children, predominately affecting males and occurring in approximately 1 per 3500 male births (Cleveland Clinic, 2008). MD is incurable and most individuals die within their 20s, usually of cardiopulmonary failure.

Pathophysiology

- Muscle damage is due to the absence of certain proteins that are required for muscular strength and stability (Do, 2007).
- Damaged muscle fibers are eventually replaced with fibrous and fatty tissue that cause pseudohypertrophy. The muscles become weak and eventually lose the ability to support body weight.
- The disease progression generally occurs in a proximal to distal direction.

Subjective Data

- Clumsy movement
- Difficulty climbing stairs
- Unable to jump/hop as expected
- Tip toe walking
- Leg pain
- Facial weakness

Objective Data

- The progressive degeneration of the muscles leads to muscle weakness that eventually affects ambulation and may interfere with cardiopulmonary function.
- Severe contractures and a rapidly progressive scoliosis.
- It is estimated that for every 10 degrees of thoracic scoliosis curvature, there is a 4% decrease in the forced vital capacity (Do, 2007).
- May also include ptosis, atrophy, scoliosis, calf deformation, contractures, cardiomyopathy, and arrhythmias

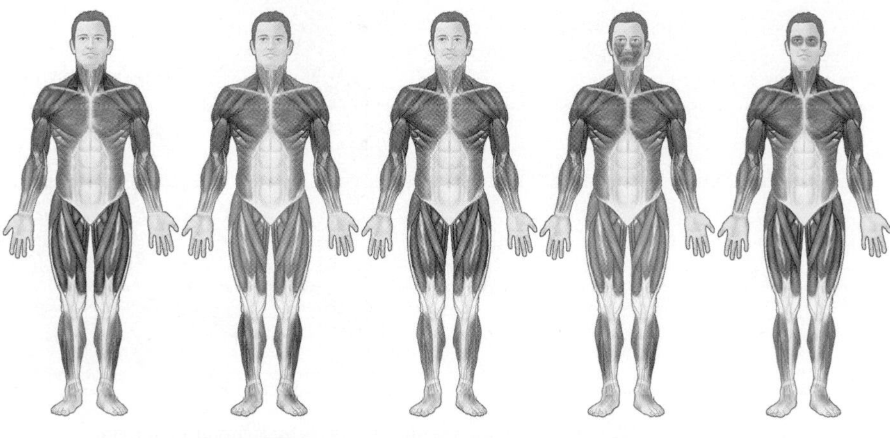

FIGURE 27-75 Muscles affected by MD

Ankylosing Spondylitis (AS)

AS is a chronic inflammation of the spine (vertebrae) and the sacroiliac joints causing pain and stiffness in and around the spine. Spinal mobility is eventually lost as the vertebrae and intervertebral disks fuse and become ossified with new bone. The areas most commonly affected are the joint between the base of the spine and pelvis, vertebrae in the lower back, places where the tendons and ligaments attach to bones, cartilage between breastbone and ribs, and hip and shoulder joints. Males are 2–3 times more likely to have AS than females. Although it can be seen in all ages, symptoms frequently begin to appear in the teens and 20s.

Pathophysiology

- Evidence suggests that AS it is genetically inherited.

Subjective Data

- Low back pain located over the sacrum with radiation to the groin, buttocks, and down the leg.

Objective Data

- Cervical vertebrae become fused late in the disease progression, severely restricting neck mobility and rotation.

- May develop chronic inflammatory cauda equina syndrome (CES), a rare neurological manifestation in patients with long-standing AS caused by compression of the low back nerve roots that causes paralysis and cuts off sensation to the legs, and radiculopathy (shooting pain caused by pressure on the nerves) secondary to fracture or compression of the nerve roots (Liu, Lin, Lo, & Chang, 2011).
- Nearly all diagnosed individuals (90%–95%) have the human leukocyte antigen (HLA) B27 (Peh, 2005), however, only 1% develop the condition.
- Two other associated genes are ARTS1 and IL23R, which appear to participate in the immune function (Sheil, 2008).
- Tumor necrosis factor-alpha (TNF α) and IL-1 are also implicated in AS.
- Pain and stiffness in lower back and hips, especially in the morning and after periods of inactivity
- Pain that improves during the day, is better with activity, and worse with inactivity. (This helps distinguish AS from mechanical low back pain.)
- Gradual ascending pattern from the lumbar region to the thoracic spine and then the cervical spine
- Improvement in response to anti-inflammatory medications
- Approximately 25% of people experience proximal joint (hips, knees) involvement.
- Breathlessness on exertion. In long-standing disease, a small percentage of patients may develop fibrosis in the upper lobes of the lungs.
- As the spine becomes rigid and fused, the expected curves of the spine are lost, resulting in a stooped appearance. Additionally, there is C_1–C_2 subluxation (partial displacement), a tendency for spinal fractures with minor trauma, and spinal stenosis in the cervical or lumbar regions.
- In addition to spinal involvement, other manifestations of AS include peripheral arthritis, iritis, pulmonary involvement, along with renal and cardiac alterations.
- Peripheral (hip) joint involvement. Eventually, the joints of the shoulder, wrist, hand, and foot are affected.

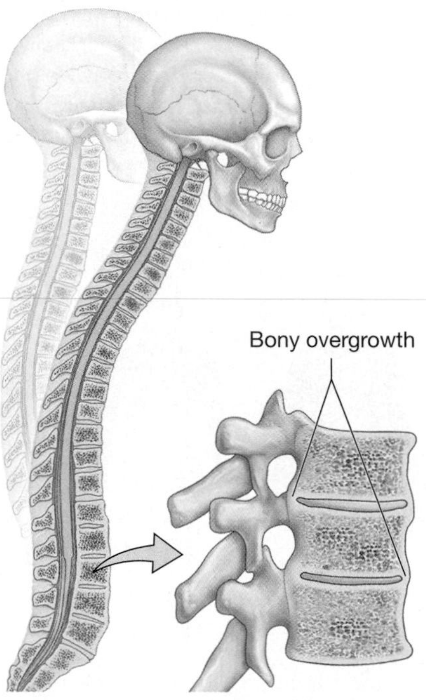

FIGURE 27-76 Ankylosing spondylitis

Osteogenesis Imperfecta (OI)

OI is another genetic disorder that is caused by gene mutations that code for type I procollagen (Plotkin & Pattekar, 2008). As a result, bones fail to grow and develop properly, leading to weak bones that are brittle and break easily. OI is also described as "brittle bone disease." The actual number of individuals with OI in the U.S. is not known; however, estimates place the number between 20,000 and 50,000.

Pathophysiology

- The severity and characteristics of OI vary dramatically among patients, including family members.
- The majority of cases are classified into four types (I, II, III, IV), ranging from mild to severe, and are caused by a dominant mutation for coding type I collagen.

PRACTICE POINT: OI and Child Abuse

The parents of a child with OI are often suspected of child abuse due to the frequency of bone fractures. OI is not that common of a condition that is seen in the emergency department. It is important for the examiner to keep in mind this possibility and not pre-judge the parents as abusers. It is a difficult condition to have to deal with, and to be suspected of child abuse only makes the situation harder for everyone.

Subjective Data

- Manifestations of Type I include "loose" joints (hyperlaxity), muscle weakness, continuous bone pain that does not go away, and skull deformities resulting from frail bones as an infant.

Objective Data

- There may also be bone fractures at birth from in utero fractures or from the birth itself.
- Limb deformities and shortening are common and affect the individual's function and mobility.
- Kyphoscoliosis frequently creates adverse effects on respiratory function.
- The individual's face has a triangular shape and the sclera may demonstrate a blue, purple, or gray hue.

Fibromyalgia

This is a chronic condition that is characterized by pain in the muscles, joints, ligaments, and tendons. It is accompanied by fatigue and multiple "tender spots" that are painful to the touch and commonly located in front of the knees, the elbows, hip joints, and around the neck (Figure 27-77).

Females are 9 times more likely to develop fibromyalgia than males, but the severity is greater in males (Winfield, 2007). Many people who have fibromyalgia also have tension headaches, temporomandibular joint (TMJ) disorders, irritable bowel syndrome, anxiety, and depression.

Pathophysiology

- The cause is unknown, but current thought focuses on "central sensitization," a theory that proposes that individuals with fibromyalgia have a lower threshold for pain due to an increased sensitivity in the brain to pain signals (Mayo Clinic Staff, 2007).
- It is thought that repeated nerve stimulation causes changes in the individual's brain, specifically an increase in the levels of neurotransmitters that signal pain.
- Neurons that receive pain signals seem to develop a memory of the pain, overreacting to pain signals. Therefore, pressure that is not perceived as pain in an individual who doesn't have fibromyalgia is perceived as pain in the individual with fibromyalgia (Winfield, 2007).

Subjective Data

- The severity of the pain is variable and is responsive to activity, stress, and changes in the weather.
- Characterized by additional pain when firm pressure is applied to specific tender points.
- Pain is frequently characterized as a deep ache or burning, with possible muscle spasms.
- Other symptoms include sleep disturbances, fatigue, irritable bowel syndrome, numbness and tingling, headaches and jaw pain, and an increased sensitivity to odors, noise, and bright lights.
- Depression due to the chronic pain and frustration.

Objective Data

- In patients with fibromyalgia, the only reproducible finding on physical examination is tenderness in soft-tissue anatomic locations.
- The tender point examination requires that the provider know where to palpate and how much pressure to apply (Goldenberg, 2013).

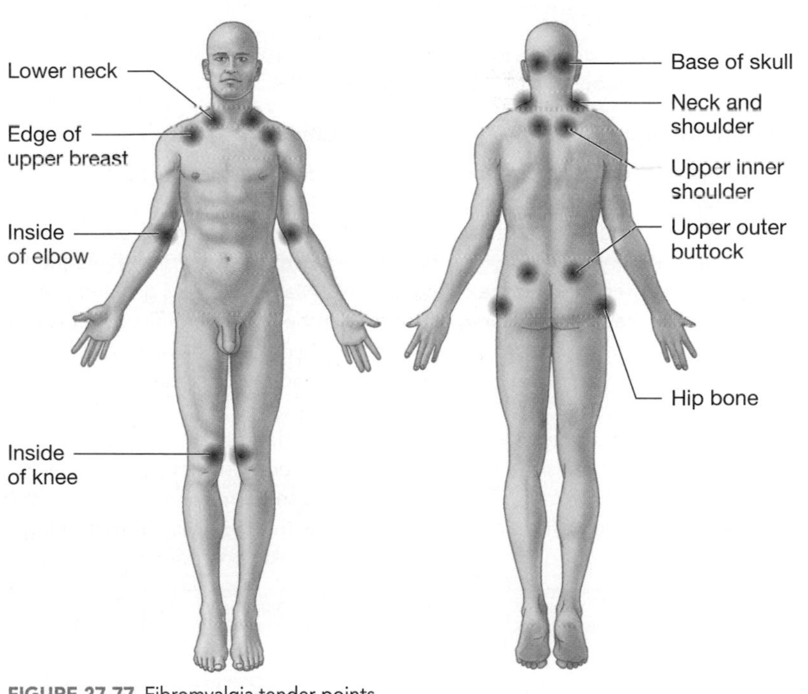

FIGURE 27-77 Fibromyalgia tender points

Gout Podagra

Gout is a metabolic, medical condition usually characterized by recurrent attacks of acute inflammatory arthritis—a red, tender, hot, swollen joint. The metatarsal-phalangeal joint at the base of the big toe is the most commonly affected (approximately 50% of cases). However, it may also present as tophi, kidney stones, or urate nephropathy. Men are more likely to get gout, but women become increasingly susceptible to gout after menopause.

Pathophysiology

- A disorder of purine metabolism; occurs when uric acid crystallizes in the form of monosodium urate, precipitating in joints, on tendons, and in the surrounding tissues, triggering a local immune-mediated inflammatory reaction.
- It is caused by elevated levels of uric acid in the blood. The uric acid crystallizes, and the crystals deposit in joints, tendons, and surrounding tissues.
- High levels of uric acid in the blood (hyperuricemia) is the underlying cause.

Subjective Data

- Presents in many ways
- Usually a recurrent attack of acute inflammatory arthritis—metatarsal-phalangeal joint affected most often
- Also affects heels, knees, wrists, and fingers
- The affected joint or joints are swollen, tender, and red.
- Joint pain usually begins over 2–4 hours at night.
- Pain likely to be most severe within the first 12 to 24 hours after it begins.
- Lingering discomfort lasts from a few days to a few weeks—later attacks are likely to last longer and affect more joints.
- Fatigue and high fever are less common symptoms.

Objective Data

- Long-standing elevated uric acid levels (hyperuricemia) may result in other symptomatology, including hard, painless deposits of uric acid crystals known as tophi.
- Extensive tophi may lead to chronic arthritis due to bone erosion.
- Elevated levels of uric acid may also lead to crystals precipitating in the kidneys, resulting in stone formation and subsequent urate nephropathy.

Osteomyelitis (OM)

OM is an infection localized to bone. Infections can reach a bone by traveling through the bloodstream or spreading from nearby tissue. It can also begin in the bone itself if an injury exposes the bone to infectious microorganisms.

Pathophysiology

- Microorganisms may infect bone through the bloodstream, local infection, or penetrating trauma (including surgery).
- Leukocytes enter infected area, releasing enzymes that destroy bone, causing necrosis.
- The body may try to make new bone around the necrosis.
- Encompasses all of the bone (osseous) components, including the bone marrow. When it is chronic, it can lead to bone sclerosis and deformity.

Subjective Data

- Symptoms vary greatly.
- Fever or chills
- Swelling, warmth, pain, and redness over the area of the infection
- May cause no signs and symptoms, or they may be difficult to distinguish
- Symptoms develop quickly in children and may include irritability and lethargy.
- Patients with diabetes, peripheral neuropathy, or peripheral vascular disease may not have pain or fever, with the only symptom being an area of skin breakdown that does not heal.

Objective Data

- Local signs of inflammation (tenderness, erythema, swelling, and warmth) are often only objective manifestations.

The Abdomen

28

I find myself staring at the empty chair at the head of the table as I lay out the serving dishes of rice and adobo chicken. My eyes are red from crying, but the tears are thankfully absent for the moment. "Dinner time!" I call from the foyer. Our two beautiful kids—Stefan and Michele—scurry down the stairs and climb into their seats, grinning. I need to maintain my composure for their sake. My husband, still looking fit and healthy despite his diagnosis, walks in and takes his spot at the head of the table. He's wearing a sweater vest over a shirt and tie as if he had just come from work. "So what's for dinner?" he smiles at me.

We eat mostly in silence, the kids fidgeting in their chairs from time to time. They know that their father has pancreatic cancer—we told them only a few days after we found out ourselves—but they cannot possibly understand the complexities of the disease or how it's going to shake this family. "I'm worried about you, Julie," my husband had said a few days ago. "The kids are going to be teenagers soon, and you're so busy at the hospital. How are you going to manage?" I'm lost in thought over the inevitable loss of my husband but struggling not to let him go. Tears well in my eyes. Just then, Stefan looks up from his plate, directly into his father's eyes: "How much time did they give you, Daddy?" A solitary tear streams down my right cheek as I muffle a short gasp with my napkin. My husband sets his fork down and places Stefan in his lap. "I can't tell you that, son, but what I can tell you is that I'm going to fight this with everything I can." Michele tugs at my dress, "Mommy, you make people better. Why don't you make Daddy better?" All I can do is smile down at her, tears pouring down my face. My memory of my husband is from the next moment, looking back across the table to see him holding Stefan. He is rocking him back and forth slowly, the light from the chandelier outlining them both like a silhouette. But everything, even his face, is blurred by tears.

LEARNING OUTCOMES

1. Describe the composition, structure, and function of the gastrointestinal organs as well as the organs of elimination.
2. Explain the expected findings associated with examination of the gastrointestinal and renal systems.
3. Compare and contrast the manifestations of altered conditions of the gastrointestinal and the renal systems.
4. Recognize age-related changes that affect the composition, structure, and function of the gastrointestinal and renal systems.
5. Explain appropriate techniques and procedures used to assess the gastrointestinal and renal systems.
6. Explain appropriate documentation of the patient's history and characteristics of the gastrointestinal and renal systems examination to correctly reflect assessment findings.

The abdomen is a large cavity that contains the organs of the gastrointestinal (GI), reproductive, and elimination systems. While all the abdominal organs are necessary for maintaining life, the functions of the liver and kidneys are essential for sustaining life. Loss of hepatic and renal function results in death. Life may be maintained in the absence of kidney function, but with liver failure, death is inevitable.

Structure and Function

The majority of abdominal organs belong to the GI system, which are separate but are connected and coordinate with each other to facilitate all the processes related to the breakdown of foods into nutrients required to sustain vital cellular functions. The functions of the GI organs include ingestion, digestion, absorption, and elimination of food substances. Alterations of GI organs significantly impact the effectiveness and efficiency of these processes and often require interventions to maintain their functionality.

The spleen and the reproductive and elimination organs do not participate in digestion. The spleen is primarily a lymphatic organ, and the kidneys participate in maintaining fluid and electrolyte balance. The kidneys, like the liver, play a role in the elimination of fluid and other metabolic waste from the body, but they have no direct function related to digestion.

External Borders

The abdominal organs are secured in place and bordered by other anatomic structures. The posterior aspect is bordered by the spine and the paravertebral muscles. The superior border is the diaphragm, and the inferior border is composed of pelvic organs that have peritoneal lining. The sides and anterior aspect include the lower rib cage and the abdominal muscles. The anterior muscles are large and flat, and are composed of four layers: the rectus abdominis, external and internal obliques, and the transversus abdominis (Figure 28-1). The midline of the rectus abdominis muscles consists of a tendinous seam (linea alba) that unites the muscles and extends from the xiphoid process to the symphysis pubis. The umbilicus is also aligned within the linea alba. The peritoneum is the inner lining of the abdominal cavity that forms a protective cover for many abdominal organs. Folds of the peritoneum form additional structures that are the greater and lesser omentum, a double fold around the stomach, and the mesentery, a fanlike fold that covers the small intestine and attaches it to the posterior abdominal wall.

Internal Viscera

The multiple organs of the abdomen are often referred to as viscera, which are further differentiated into solid viscera, or organs that maintain a specific, characteristic shape, and hollow viscera, tubular organs that contain air and assume various shapes that are consistent with their contents. When these organs are empty, they collapse, losing any characteristic or unique shape. The hollow organs consist of the alimentary tract (Figure 28-2).

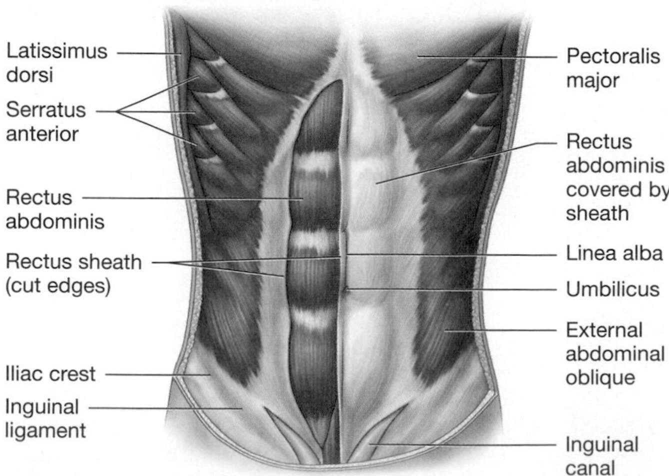

FIGURE 28-1 Abdominal muscles

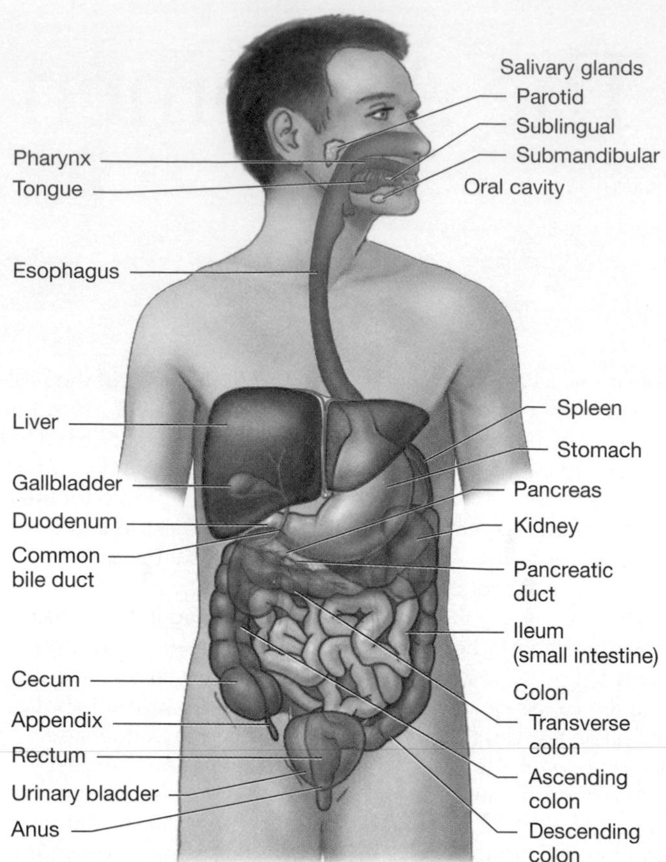

FIGURE 28-2 Anatomic structures of abdominal cavity and alimentary tract

Alimentary Tract

The alimentary tract occupies the greatest amount of space in the abdomen. It consists of a long (30 feet), hollow tube that originates at the mouth and terminates at the anus. Along the course of the alimentary tract, it is subdivided into specific sections with specified functions. These sections are the mouth, esophagus, stomach, small intestine, and large intestine.

Mouth Although the mouth is generally assessed during the head and neck exam, it functions as part of the alimentary tract. The tongue and teeth begin the process of digestion by chewing the food, tearing it apart so saliva can act on it. Enzymes secreted in the saliva begin to act on food to break it down into nutrients that can be absorbed. Food passes into the throat through the voluntary act of swallowing, which begins when the tongue pushes the food back into the throat. Swallowing initiates an involuntary series of complicated and coordinated events that moves the food into the esophagus.

Esophagus A continuation of the throat, the esophagus is a hollow tube that connects the pharynx to the stomach and transports the swallowed food into the stomach by peristalsis, successive waves of muscle contractions controlled by the autonomic nervous system. About 10 to 13 inches long, the esophagus is located posterior to the trachea, descending through the mediastinum and diaphragm, and opening into the stomach. No actual digestion occurs in the

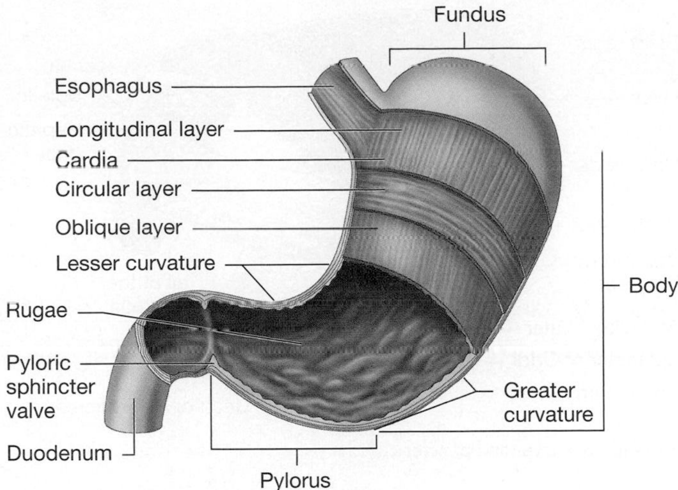

FIGURE 28-3 Stomach with identified sections

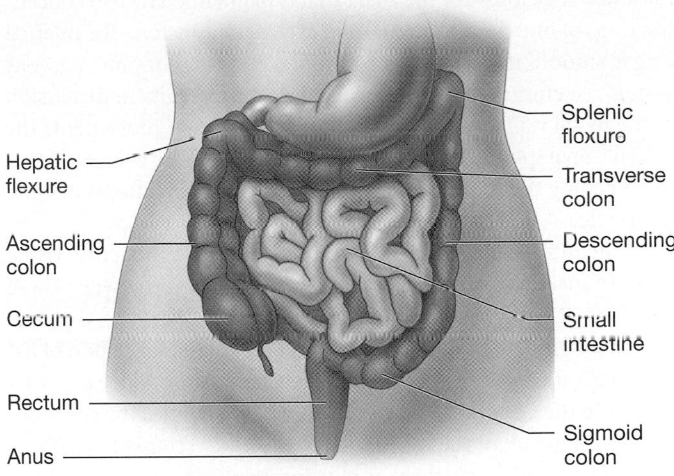

FIGURE 28-4 Large intestine with identified sections

esophagus. The passage of food into the stomach is controlled by two sphincters located where the esophagus merges with the stomach. The upper esophageal sphincter opens to allow food to exit the esophagus and closes after food enters the stomach. The lower esophageal sphincter prevents food from re-entering the esophagus.

Stomach The stomach is a flask-like, hollow organ that is transversely positioned just below the diaphragm in the upper abdominal cavity. It is divided into three portions: the fundus, body, and pylorus. The fundus is the upper portion and lies above and to the left of the esophageal sphincters; the body is the largest portion, comprising the middle two-thirds of the stomach; and the pylorus is the most distal portion, which connects to the small intestine at the pyloric sphincter (Figure 28-3).

Small Intestine The digested food passes from the stomach to the small intestine through the pyloric sphincter, which separates the stomach and small intestine. The small intestine is approximately 21 feet in length and coiled within the abdominal cavity; like the stomach, it is divided into three sections. The first section, the duodenum, accounts for the first foot and appears as a C curve around the head of the pancreas. Bile from the gallbladder and pancreatic enzymes enter the duodenum through the duodenal papilla, which is approximately 3 inches below the pyloric sphincter. Certain minerals such as calcium and iron are absorbed in the duodenum. The next section, the jejunum, accounts for the next 8 feet of the intestine, where fats, starches, and proteins are further broken down. The remaining 12 feet accounts for the last section, the ileum, where water, vitamin B_{12}, and bile salts are absorbed.

> ***THINK LINK: Transit Time through the GI System***
> Once food enters the digestive system, it travels a winding route through which it will be broken down by various enzymes to extract the vital nutrients. The composition of the meal determines how long it will take for the food to travel the distance through the length of the stomach and intestine. A typical meal will be in the stomach about 2 hours as the stomach muscles reduce solids to a liquid. A meal high in protein may require and extra hour or two; a meal high in fat may require up to 6 hours. From the stomach, the food passes into the small intestine, where it may take 3–5 hours to move through it. From the small intestine it passes into the large intestine, where water is extracted and the leftover residue is transported to the rectum for elimination. Approximately 80%–90% of the water that is passed into the large intestine is reabsorbed in the transit through the large intestine. Passage of food through the entire length of the intestines may be as little as 4 hours but may take up to 72 hours.

Large Intestine, Rectum, and Anus The remaining products of digestion are passed into the large intestine through the ileocecal valve. This initial section of the large intestine is the cecum, which is a blind pouch approximately 2–3 inches long. Attached to the cecum is the appendix. The remaining length of the large intestine, which is about 4–5 feet long, is identified according to the direction of food movement through it. The content of the large intestine is propelled through it by contractions of the colon wall.

The ascending colon starts at the cecum and goes up the right posterior abdominal wall to the inferior surface of the liver (Figure 28-4). At the liver, it turns and becomes the transverse colon. This turning point is known as the hepatic flexure. The transverse colon proceeds across the midline towards the spleen. At the spleen it turns downward at the splenic flexure and becomes the descending colon. The descending colon progresses down the left abdominal wall to the edge of the pelvis. At this point, it turns medially and inferiorly to become the sigmoid colon. From the sigmoid colon it becomes the rectum and terminates at the anus, the end point of the alimentary tract.

The main function of the large intestine is to absorb the water that remains as part of the undigested food. Approximately 1 quart of liquid is delivered to the large colon each day with 80%–90% of water absorbed. The final 6 inches of the large intestine is the rectum, which is where waste material accumulates. Within the walls of the rectum, there are three semilunar folds, which are known as Houston's valves. The large intestine terminates at the anal canal, which is about 2.5–4 cm long and exits the abdomen into the perineum, which is the anus. The closure of the anal canal is maintained by two concentric rings of muscle, the internal and external sphincters. The internal ring is smooth muscle that is controlled by the autonomic nervous system. Accumulation of feces in the rectum results in distension of the rectal wall that initiates the urge for a bowel movement. The external anal sphincter is striated muscle and is under voluntary control, keeping the rectal contents in place until the appropriate time for its release.

The internal anal canal is lined by columns of mucosal tissue that are fused, forming the anorectal junction. In between these columns of tissue are spaces, known as crypts, where anal glands empty. Inflammation of these glands may cause the formation of fissures and/or fistulas. A ring of veins that anastomose with each other comprise the *zona hemorrhoidalis,* which encircles the columns. Another network of veins is located in the lower segment of the rectal canal. Dilation of either set of veins results in the formation of internal or external hemorrhoids.

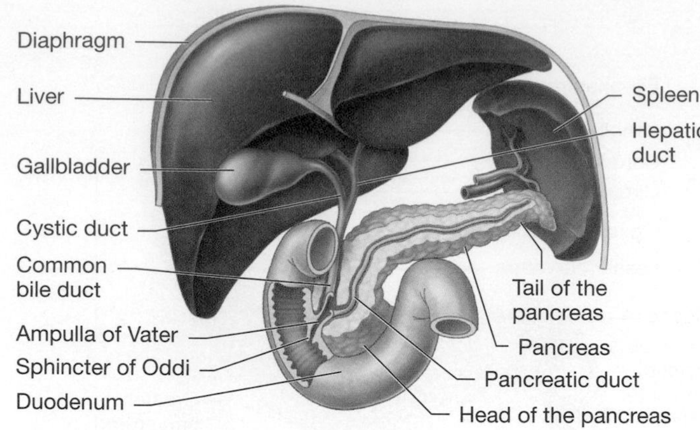

FIGURE 28-5 Liver and pancreas

Solid Visceral Organs

The other abdominal organs are the solid visceral organs. These organs—the liver, gall bladder, pancreas, spleen, kidneys, ureters, and bladder—vary in function, some of which are unrelated to digestive processes. Gender-specific reproductive organs are the uterus and ovaries in females, and the prostate gland in males.

Liver The liver is a large organ positioned in the right upper section of the abdomen and composed of four lobes. Its superior border is the diaphragm, and its inferior border encompasses the gall bladder, stomach, duodenum, and the hepatic flexure of the colon. It is triangular in shape with the widest surface along the right abdominal wall and the narrowest surface at the sternal border (Figure 28-5). The lobule is the functional unit comprised of liver cells (hepatocytes), which secrete bile that drains from the small bile ducts on the hepatocytes (canaliculi). These merge to create larger ducts that eventually form the hepatic duct. The hepatic duct merges with the cystic duct from the gallbladder, forming the common bile duct, which drains into the duodenum.

A unique feature of the liver is its vascular structure, receiving both arterial and venous blood (Figure 28-6). Arterial blood is delivered from the aorta by the hepatic artery and venous blood is delivered by the portal vein. Venous blood comes from the digestive tract and spleen. Both vessels branch extensively throughout the liver, making it a highly vascularized organ. Blood is transported out of the liver by three hepatic veins that then empty into the inferior vena cava. Additionally, branches of the hepatic artery and portal vein, as well as bile ducts, surround the periphery of the liver.

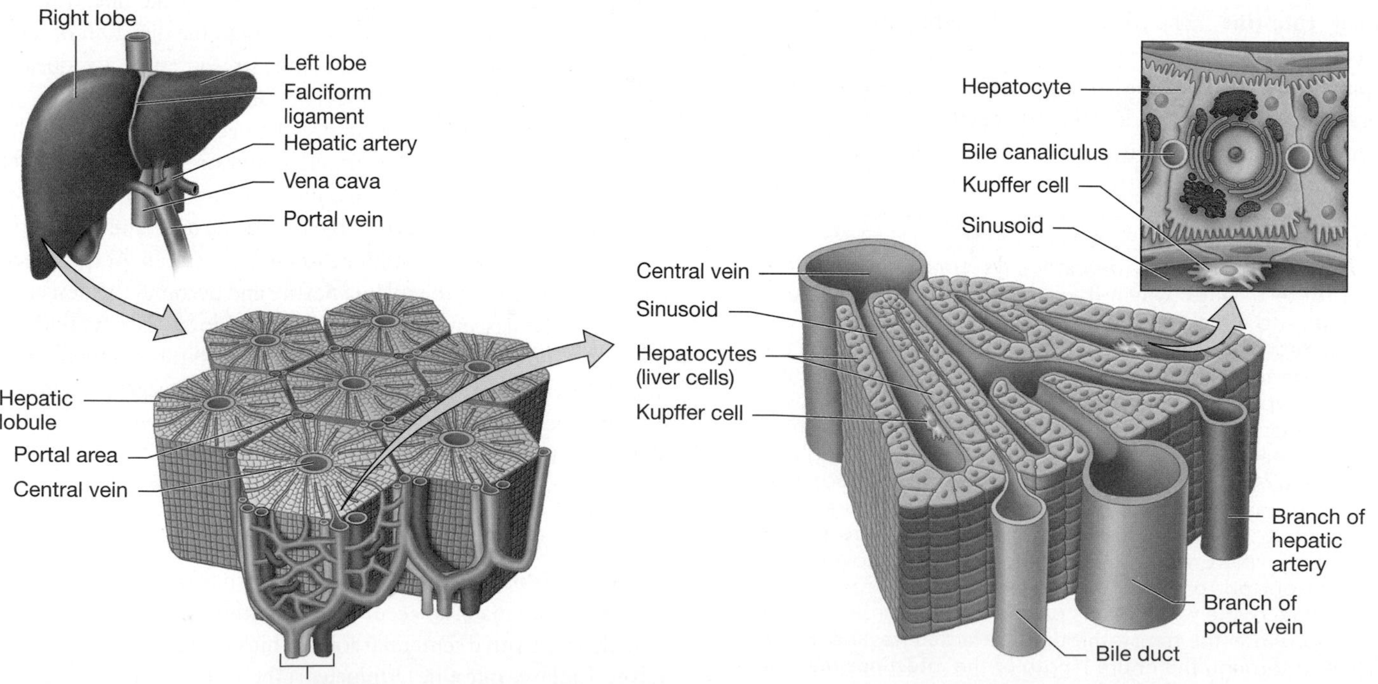

FIGURE 28-6 Liver hepatocytes and lobule

In addition to the secretion of bile for the breakdown of fats, the liver also performs a significant role in the metabolism of fats, carbohydrates, and proteins. Fats that have been broken down by digestion return to the liver as fatty acids that are then converted into two carbon components that then enter the tricarboxilic acid cycle. The liver also uses cholesterol for the formation of bile salts. Fat is also synthesized in the liver from carbohydrates and proteins.

The liver is also responsible for producing the majority of circulating proteins in plasma that are essential for coagulation and immunoglobulins.

Participation or initiation of non-metabolic/digestive processes are also a part of the liver's function. It serves as a reservoir for vitamins and iron. It also detoxifies harmful substances and plays a role in the metabolism of certain drugs. Blood coagulation is dependent on the liver's ability to synthesize prothrombin and fibrinogen. Finally, it also converts fat soluble substances, most notably bilirubin, to water soluble substances, which can be excreted through the kidneys.

Gallbladder The gallbladder is a small, pear shaped sac that is positioned on the inferior surface of the liver (see Figure 28-5). It is approximately 4 inches in length and primarily responsible for concentrating and storing the bile produced by the hepatocytes. Bile is composed of bile salts, cholesterol, and pigments, making it greenish-yellow in color. Its function is to maintain an alkaline pH of the small intestine so that fats can be emulsified and absorbed.

Pancreas The pancreas is positioned behind and below the stomach, with its head located in the curve of the duodenum and the body stretched across the abdominal cavity with the tip almost reaching the spleen. The pancreas is a gland with both exocrine and endocrine functions. The exocrine function facilitates digestion, with the acinar cells secreting inactive digestive enzymes that empty into the pancreatic duct. The pancreatic duct runs the length of the organ, releasing its contents into the duodenum, just adjacent to the common bile duct.

The islet cells are responsible for its endocrine function by secreting the hormones glucagon and insulin. Insulin and glucagon are secreted directly into the blood, regulating the blood glucose level. Every organ, except the brain, requires insulin for transporting glucose into the cells.

Spleen The spleen is located in the upper left section, just above the left kidney and under the diaphragm. The spleen is found exclusively in vertebrates (Brendolan, Rosado, Ccarsetti, Selleri, & Dear, 2007). Specific functions of white and red pulp are described in Chapter 21.

Kidneys, Ureters, and Bladder The two kidneys are considered abdominal organs; however, they are retroperitoneal, meaning they are located outside the abdominal peritoneum. The kidneys are positioned at the level of T_{12} to L_3 in the area described as the costovertebral angle (Figure 28-7). The left kidney is positioned slightly higher than the right, most likely because the liver is positioned directly over the right kidney.

Each kidney is composed of approximately 1 million nephrons, which are its functional units. Each nephron is a filtering unit that receives blood for removal of waste, excess electrolytes, and other organic acids. The blood supply to the kidneys is through the renal artery that delivers approximately one-eighth of the cardiac output. The blood is filtered at a rate of approximately 125 mL per minute in the adult male and 110 mL per minute in the adult female.

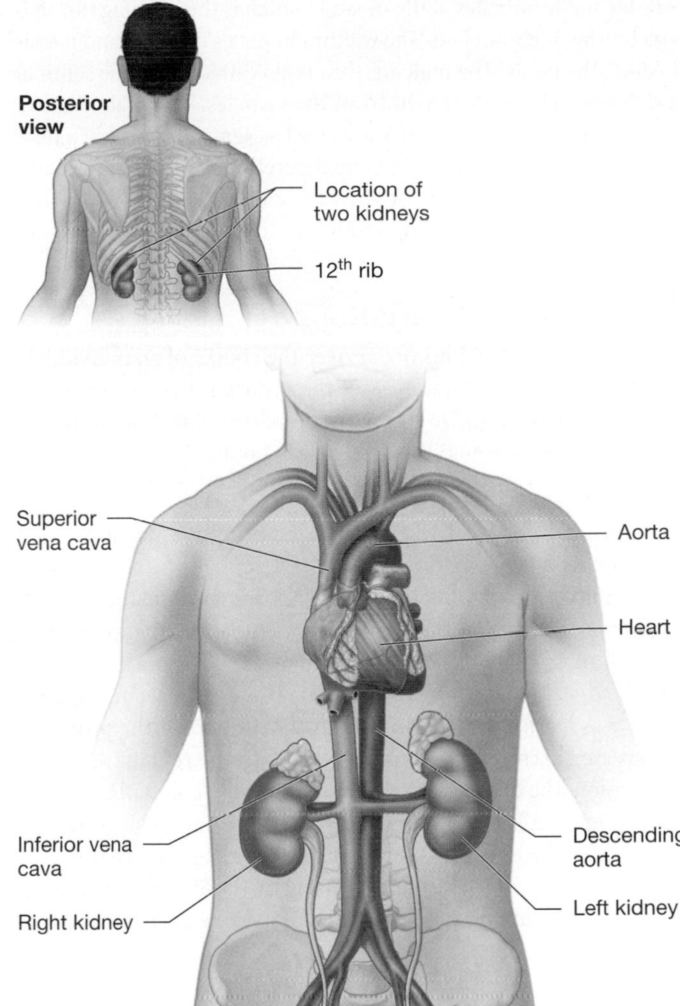

FIGURE 28-7 Renal position

Excess water, electrolytes, and other waster products that are secreted in the nephrons are excreted as urine. Urine passes into a collecting tubule that empties into the renal pelvis and leaves the kidney via the ureters. Urine is transported through each ureter by peristaltic waves. The ureters connect to the bladder, which is the reservoir for urine until it is excreted out of the body.

The bladder is a hollow, muscular organ that is located just above the symphysis pubis in the lower part of the abdominal cavity. It has a capacity of approximately 400–500 mL in the adult. Urine is retained in the bladder by constriction of the urinary sphincter. Relaxation of the sphincter allows the urine to be excreted via the urethra. The urethra is a single tube that is attached to the lower surface of the bladder and terminates at the meatus, which is the opening through which urine is eliminated. The urethra in males is longer and passes through the penis. The male urethra is also attached to the seminal vesicles, which stores semen from the testicles. The male urethra serves as a passage way for urine as well as semen that is ejaculated during sexual intercourse. The female urethra is much shorter and terminates at the meatus in the vulva; its sole purpose is the excretion of urine. The structure and function of the reproductive organs are covered in Chapters 29 and 30.

Developmental Variations

Developmental variations occur over the course of an individual's life span and events. Awareness of these variations is important to understand and recognize common age-related alterations or modifications of the gastrointestinal and urinary systems.

Infants and Children

During the 4th week of gestation, the primitive gut has formed from the dorsal section of the yolk sac. Initially a hollow tube, it divides into three sections: the foregut, the midgut, and the hindgut. The foregut evolves into the esophagus, stomach, upper portion of duodenum, liver, biliary system, and pancreas. The midgut evolves into the distal duodenum and the small intestine, cecum, appendix, the ascending colon, and a significant part of the proximal transverse colon. The hindgut evolves into the remaining transverse colon, the descending colon, the sigmoid colon, the rectum, and the upper part of the anal canal. By the 7th week of gestation, a portion of the hindgut is separated into a rectum and a urogenital sinus that becomes the anal opening by the 8th week. Anorectal malformations are frequently due to alterations during this partitioning process.

The motility of the GI system progresses in a cephalocaudal direction so that by the 17th week, the fetus is able to ingest and swallow amniotic fluid. The presence of amniotic fluid in the fetus' GI system produces meconium, the end result of fetal metabolism. By the 36th to 38th week, the GI system is capable of supporting extrauterine life, although the adult characteristics related to elasticity, musculature, and control are not fully developed until the child is 2–3 years old.

Liver development begins as a bud that evolves from the distal section of the foregut. The fetal liver is responsible for the production and development of red blood cells, which begins during the 6th week of gestation. This function also accounts for the large size of the liver. Additionally, bile is produced in the liver at the 16th week of gestation, giving the meconium a dark green color. Glycogen production and storage begins during the 9th week.

The spleen begins development in the 5th week, arising from the dorsal aspect of the midgut. Red cell production begins and evolves from cells within the yolk sac. As the fetus develops, red cell production stops and lymphoid precursors begin to migrate into it.

The pancreas begins as dorsal and ventral buds that develop from mesodermal cells of the foregut (Brendolan et al., 2007). Pancreatic islet cells begin producing insulin at 12 weeks' gestation. Eventually the ventral and dorsal buds fuse to form the main pancreatic duct.

The kidneys begin to develop during the 5th to 8th week of gestation, beginning urine production by the 8th week. At the same time, the bladder begins functioning as the reservoir for the urine. Nephron development continues until week 36, at which time it stops. Each kidney contains about 1 million nephrons.

The Pregnant Woman

The abdomen of the pregnant woman is significantly affected by the enlarging uterus. The lack of anterior bones surrounding the abdomen allows it to expand and accommodate the uterus without significantly compromising other abdominal organs and function. Nausea and vomiting are the earliest manifestations of pregnancy that are related to the GI system, and may be present even before the woman realizes she is pregnant.

Visible changes occur with the stretching of the abdominal skin and muscles, causing changes in the contour of the abdomen. Contour changes may also occur with changes in fetal position, particularly when the fetus descends into the pelvis prior to birth. An early change is the appearance of the linea nigra on the midline of the abdomen, beginning at the symphysis, up to the umbilicus or higher. Stretching of the skin may also cause the development of striae, or stretch marks (see Chapter 16). As the abdominal muscles become stretched, the rectus abdominis muscles may separate (diastasis recti), allowing the abdominal contents to protrude. Another visible change is the flattening of the umbilicus; however, protrusion of the umbilicus is also possible.

The enlarging uterus also has effects on the internal organs. During the second trimester, pressure of the lower esophageal sphincter is reduced and accompanied by a decrease in velocity of peristaltic waves. Gastric emptying time is not affected; however, movement through the intestines is increased during the 2nd and 3rd trimester. The pyloric sphincter is also relaxed, which may allow for a reflux of alkaline duodenal contents back into the stomach. This leads to heartburn, which frequently is associated with pregnancy.

Distension of the gallbladder is common, causing a loss in tone as well as a decreased emptying time. Retention and secretion of bile increases the formation of cholesterol crystals, increasing the potential for the formation of gall stones. Gallstones are more prone to develop during the 2nd and 3rd trimester.

The kidneys demonstrate a slight enlargement (1 cm) in length. Hormones and pressure from the enlarging uterus cause the renal pelvis and ureters to dilate. The ureters also elongate, forming single and double curves of varying sizes and angulation. Retention and stasis of urine may result in pyelonephritis with bacteriuria, which may or may not be associated with any symptoms. Renal changes may persist as long as 3 to 4 months after the pregnancy has ended.

The bladder is compressed during pregnancy as well as demonstrating increased sensitivity, which causes frequency and urgency of urination during the first and third trimester. During the third trimester, bladder compression may also be due to fetal descent into the pelvis. When this occurs, incontinence may also become a problem, even if there is a minimal amount of urine in the bladder.

The intestines are displaced upward, laterally, and to the back, which results in decreased peristalsis and increased water absorption. Bowel sounds are decreased and constipation and increased flatus are commonly experienced. Blood circulation is increased to the pelvis causing an increase in venous pressure and the development of hemorrhoids.

After delivery, the uterus rapidly begins to return to its prepregnancy size. In the immediate postpartum period, the uterus size decreases to approximately its size at 20 weeks' gestation. By the end of the first week, its size is further decreased to about its size at 12 weeks' gestation. Muscle tone is gradually restored over a 6–7 week period to the pelvic floor muscles and pelvic supports.

The Older Adult

Aging has some significant effects on the function of the GI system of the elderly; however, healthy individuals appear to have no critical alterations. Overall changes in fat and muscle composition may change the overall body appearance. Beginning around the age of 40–50, an individual begins to experience a loss of fat-free mass, primarily from muscles and bone, and an increase in fat. The increase in fat is an absolute increase as well as a relative increase due to a declining muscle mass (Chang, Beason, Hunleth, & Colditz, 2012; Ritz, 2000).

A major alteration is the slowing of intestinal motility related to a slower and weaker peristalsis, which contributes to a lower resting pressure of the lower esophageal sphincter, as well as a delay in the emptying of gastric contents. As a result, an increased possibility for reflux of gastric contents into the esophagus exists.

The reduction in motility is most likely the result of changes in the neurons of the central nervous system as well as changes in collagen that increase resistance to stretching of the intestinal wall. Functional alterations of the GI system may be a reflection of adverse changes elsewhere in the body. There may also be a reduction in blood supply to the intestines related to changes associated with reduced blood volume or reduced oxygenation of blood.

Secretion and absorption are also affected, but not as significantly. Epithelial atrophy of the GI tract results in decreased secretion of digestive enzymes and mucus, creating a loss of the gastric mucosal barrier. The mucosal cells become less differentiated, which causes a decreased secretory ability, making them more susceptible to damage from physical and chemical agents. These agents include drugs, alcohol, and caffeine as well as ingested carcinogens. Long-term infection with bacteria (*H. pylori*) may also be a cause of mucosal cell damage. There is also the potential for drug solubility and absorption to be adversely affected.

The liver decreases in size and mass due to the loss of hepatocytes in size and number (Ritz, 2000). Blood flow to the liver is also decreased due to a reduction in cardiac output that goes along with aging. Consequences of these changes result in a reduction in hepatic enzymes and its ability to regenerate. These changes also affect drug metabolism and clearance. Liver function studies are rarely affected and there is no substantial evidence that there are significant alterations in protein and energy metabolism.

The gallbladder does not demonstrate any significant changes in its structure or function. The bile ducts widen to some extent and there may be a decrease in bile storage. Biliary lipids, phospholipids, and cholesterol may increase, predisposing to the development and formation of gall stones.

The pancreas is largely unaffected by aging. There is no significant change in the organ's size; however, there is a widening of the pancreatic duct and its branches. There is some increase in fibrous tissue and fat deposition that contributes to atrophy of the acinar cells, but this does not seem to have any physiologic implications. In high-risk adults, this may increase the possibility of adult onset diabetes.

Health Promotion

Health promotion for the abdomen and renal system includes preventing or reducing the incidence of alterations related to multiple organs. Goals of *Healthy People 2020* related to the abdomen and GI system are found under the topic areas of Cancer (C), Immunization and Infectious Diseases (IID), Nutrition and Weight Status (NWS), and Chronic Kidney Disease (CKD).

Colorectal Cancer

Goals for the topic area of Cancer are as follows:

- C–5/9: Reduce the colorectal cancer death rate and invasive colorectal cancer.
- C–16: Increase the proportion of adults who receive a colorectal cancer screening based on the most recent guidelines in 2008 (U.S. Department of Health and Human Services, 2009).

Colorectal cancer (CRC) is the second overall leading cause of cancer-related deaths in the U.S. Gender- based statistics indicate that for females, CRC is third leading cause of cancer deaths behind lung and breast cancers; for males it is third behind lung and prostate cancers. In females who are of Hispanic, American Indian/Alaska Native, or Asian/Pacific Islander descent, CRC becomes the second leading cause of death (Fingerote, 2009).

Risk factors for CRC are related to age, personal or family history of polyps or CRC, inflammatory bowel disease, lack of physical activity, and a high-fat/low-fiber diet. Increasing fiber in the diet, however, has not been definitively related to reducing one's risk for CRC (Gund & Zleve, 2009). A diet that is high in red meat, smoking, and obesity have also been linked to CRC. In 2002, 3.2% of new cancers were attributed to obesity (National Cancer Institute, 2009).

In the majority of instances, CRC begins as a benign polyp that slowly evolves into cancer. Colon cancer does not have any specific early symptoms so that by the time CRC is diagnosed the cancer may be in a more advanced stage. There are early indicators of cancer, but they are not definitive. The early indicators include the following:

- Abdominal pain and tenderness of the lower abdomen
- Blood in the stools
- Changes in bowel habits (diarrhea, constipation)
- Intestinal obstruction
- Narrow stools
- Anemia that cannot be explained
- Unexpected weight loss
- Nausea and vomiting, although this indicator does not appear until later in the course of the CRC

Screening remains the optimal way for preventing CRC. Initially a mass may be palpated in the abdomen or rectum during a physical, which necessitates further investigation with imaging tests. Imaging tests are a significant aid in the diagnosis of

Health Promotion *continued*

CRC as are the colonoscopy and sigmoidoscopy. Both procedures require the insertion of a thin, flexible plastic tube with an attached camera into the rectum and colon through the anus. Advancing the tube allows the camera to send images of the colon to a video monitor. If any polyps are observed, they may be removed to prevent their transformation to cancer. The colonoscopy is a more comprehensive procedure as it is advanced through the entire colon. The sigmoidoscopy is advanced only through the rectum, sigmoid colon, and most of the descending colon.

An early screening test is looking for the presence of occult (unobservable) blood in the stool. False negatives are relatively common with this test as well as false positives, so testing for occult blood should not be done without an imaging test.

Another test that is used is the barium enema. This is a radiological test that produces images via x-rays of the colon. Barium is introduced into the colon and rectum, producing a contrast that highlights tumors, if present. Tumors that are small may not be picked up with the use of barium. If a tumor is detected, a CAT (computerized axial tomography) scan is usually done for a more definitive picture of the tumor and whether it is localized or has spread.

Hepatitis

Goals for the topic area of Immunization and Infectious Diseases are as follows:

- IID—1: Reduce, eliminate, or maintain elimination of cases of vaccine-preventable diseases (new hepatitis B cases).
- IID—7/10: Achieve and maintain effective vaccination coverage levels for universally recommended vaccines among young children (3 doses hepatitis B [hep B], 2 doses hepatitis A vaccine by age 19–35 months) and maintain vaccination coverage levels for children in kindergarten (3 or more doses of hepatitis B vaccine).
- IID—15: Increase hepatitis B vaccine coverage among high-risk populations.
- IID—23: Reduce hepatitis A.
- IID—24/25: Reduce chronic hepatitis B virus infections in infants and young children (perinatal infections); reduce hepatitis B.
- IID—26/27: Reduce new hepatitis C infections; increase the proportion of persons aware they have a hepatitis C infection.

Hepatitis is an inflammation of the liver that may be caused by infection, alcohol, medications, chemicals, toxins, or immune disorders that result in diffuse hepatocellular necrosis. There are five identified types of hepatitis that have certain characteristics. These five types are identified and described in Table 28-12.

Hepatitis also manifests as acute or chronic. Acute viral hepatitis may cause serious illness and may progress to fulminant acute hepatic failure, which may be fatal, accounting for 4000–5000 deaths per year (Buggs & Lim, 2009). Individuals with acute viral hepatitis may recover and not have any major residual effects. Recovery from acute hepatitis produces life-long immunity and does not progress to a chronic condition. These characteristics are mostly associated with hepatitis A.

Chronic hepatitis carries an even higher rate of morbidity and mortality, resulting in 16,000 deaths per year. The majority of deaths (70%) are due to hepatitis C and 20% are due to hepatitis B; the remaining 10% result from a combination of hepatitis B and C.

Overweight and Obesity

Goals for the topic area of Nutrition and Weight Status are as follows:

- NWS—8: Increase the proportion of adults who are at a healthy weight.
- NWS—9/10: Reduce the proportion of adults who are obese; reduce the proportion of children and adolescents who are considered obese.
- NWS—11: Prevent inappropriate weight gain in youth and adults.

Overweight and obesity are significant health concerns with their incidence increasing substantially. Obesity is no longer a concern for individuals in the early and middle adult stages, it is becoming more and more prevalent in children and adolescents. Recent statistics indicate that in the years 2003–2006, one-third of adult males were obese and a little over one-third of females were obese. For the same years, 16.3% of children and adolescents between 2 and 19 years were considered obese (Centers for Disease Control and Prevention, 2009).

No accepted standard for the definition of obesity exists. The body mass index (BMI) is the most frequently used parameter; it is calculated based on an individual's height and weight (refer to Table 13-7, p. 236). Although the BMI is an indicator of the amount of body fat, it is not a direct measure of body fat, which makes it possible for an individual with well-developed muscles to have a BMI that indicates being overweight, when in reality there is minimal body fat. The BMI also does not give information regarding the distribution of body fat. For adults, having a BMI between 25 and 28.9 is overweight and a BMI of 30 or greater is obese. Various other parameters may also be used to estimate body fat and its distribution. These include skinfold thickness measurement, hip-to-waist circumference ratio, and waist circumference.

Fat is now recognized as a complex endocrine organ (Gosnell, 2008). Obesity is associated with **visceral** and **subcutaneous fat**. Visceral (yellow) fat is deposited within the abdomen, surrounding vital organs and hanging off of the stomach. While seemingly inert, it produces over 100 hormones and chemicals that perpetuate fat storage (Whittington, 2005). Visceral fat is primarily associated with males and is significantly linked to the development of cardiovascular and other diseases. Subcutaneous (brown) fat, in contrast, contains energy generating mitochondria and is considered beneficial. It is deposited in the hip, buttocks, and thigh areas and found predominately in females.

Females are also at risk of increasing the deposits of visceral fat and incurring the same risk for the development of certain diseases and conditions. Visceral fat appears to produce estrogen in postmenopausal females, increasing their risk for estrogen-dependent breast cancers (Whittington, 2005).

Obesity in the United States is the second leading cause, after tobacco, of preventable deaths. Overweight and obesity are not simply a problem of an increase in fat. Obesity increases the risk of developing many other serious conditions, significantly compromising one's health status and include coronary heart disease, type 2 diabetes, cancer, hypertension, dyslipidemia, stroke, liver and gallbladder disease, sleep apnea and respiratory problems, osteoarthritis, abnormal menses, and infertility (Centers for Disease Control, 2009).

Health Promotion *continued*

While obesity is primarily caused by an increased intake of calories, it is also recognized that other factors contribute to its development, such as genetic, metabolic, behavioral, environmental, cultural, and socioeconomic elements. The availability and abundance of food as well as decreasing physical activity also contribute significantly to obesity.

The prevalence of obesity and attempts to lose weight also have a significant impact on economics. Billions of dollars are spent annually on attempts to lose weight through dieting that consists of diet programs, diet foods, diet books, and diet pills. The cost of treating obesity-related conditions is estimated at $45 billion dollars. Businesses also lose an estimated $20 billion dollars annually due to absences caused by obesity-related conditions or illnesses.

A significant and disturbing concern is the increasing prevalence of obesity in children and adolescents. Overweight and obesity acquired as a child or adolescent persists into adulthood, greatly increasing the risk for other health problems and conditions in adulthood.

The safest and most effective way to lose weight is to eat less and exercise more. Although it sounds very simple, it often includes making significant lifestyle and environmental changes, which are not always easy to do. A change in mindset is often also needed, which may require some professional intervention.

Chronic Kidney Disease (CKD)

Chronic kidney disease is the most significant cause of chronic kidney failure. The course of the disease begins with renal damage of some sort, going through various stages of renal insufficiency, and ultimately results in end-stage renal disease, at which point the individual must go on dialysis or receive a kidney transplant in order to survive.

- CKD-1: Reduce the proportion of the U.S. population with chronic kidney disease.

Symptoms of CKD are not immediately recognized, so it is difficult to estimate how many individuals are affected, making it also difficult to estimate how many of these will ultimately develop end-stage renal disease (ESRD). This also makes it difficult to initiate early intervention to prevent the progression of the disease.

Often the damage to the kidney takes place over many years. The most common causes of kidney damage are diabetes and hypertension. Other significant causes leading to kidney damage include glomerulonephritis, interstitial nephritis, genetic and congenital conditions, and polycystic kidney disease. The incidence of CKD has been increasing over the past decades, which has been attributed to the increase in cases of type 2 diabetes. In the decade between 1987 and 1997, the incidence of diabetes-related renal failure went from 45 per million to 124 per million.

The potential for developing CKD is higher in individuals who are African American, Native Americans, or Alaska Natives. These individuals are more prone to develop diabetes, hypertension, proteinuria, as well as exposure to environmental agents. There is also a significant family history for these conditions. It seems logical that strategies for prevention should focus on these groups.

Individuals within these groups should be screened and treated for any of these predisposing conditions. Control of blood sugar as well as hypertension with appropriate medications has been demonstrated to slow or halt the progression of CKD. These interventions should be initiated early in the course of the disease; however, in the early stages of CKD symptoms are insidious and often unrecognized.

THINK LINK: Nonalcoholic Fatty Liver Disease

Although not a specific condition that is targeted by *Healthy People 2020* related to liver disease, nonalcoholic fatty liver disease (NAFLD) is a growing concern as a nonalcoholic cause of liver damage. NAFLD is a broad spectrum liver disease that results in the deposition and accumulation of fat in the liver. The development of NAFLD is highly correlated with obesity, causing concern that as the incidence of obesity increases, so will the incidence of NAFLD. Presently, NAFLD is the most common liver disease in the U.S., accounting for 24% of all liver diseases (Lee, 2009). Even though NAFLD is not associated with excessive alcohol consumption, the altered substrate metabolism of NAFLD has obesity as a critical pathogenic element. This results in microscopic characteristics that closely resemble liver damage associated alcoholic cirrhosis (Croke & Sampson, 2012).

Deposition of fat in the liver (steatosis) is of two types: isolated, or with necroinflammation and fibrosis that progresses to nonalcoholic steatohepatitis (NASH), advanced fibrosis, and cirrhosis, and may result in hepatocellular cancer (Heidelbaugh & Bruderly, 2006). Along with obesity, NAFLD is associated with type 2, which appears to be related to insulin resistance, which occurs in both conditions (Tendler, 2013).

Clinical Context Exemplars

Situation A

An individual with hepatitis A is on the medical unit of the local hospital. Before you go into the room to assess the patient, what skin manifestations of hepatitis might you expect to observe and why?

1. What questions would you want to ask the patient regarding what symptoms are present and why would you ask them?
2. The patient expresses concern about the long-term consequences of having hepatitis. What information would you provide to alleviate some anxiety?
3. Specifically the patient wants to know if it can be contracted again and what effect this should have on the liver.

Situation B

Your next-door neighbor has just been diagnosed with GERD and a hiatal hernia. You are being sought out by the neighbor to help in understanding this condition.

1. What information should be given to your neighbor regarding the cause and manifestations of the condition?
2. The neighbor also wants to know more about the hiatal hernia, such as if it will get worse, and how it happened. What should you tell him?
3. Another concern expressed was whether the condition could eventually become cancerous. How would you address this concern?

Situation C

A patient on your hospital unit has been admitted with the diagnosis of possible bowel obstruction. When you go in to assess the individual, you observe that the abdomen is rather distended. The patient didn't appear to be obese, so you initially reason that it is probably not due to fat.

1. What do think is most likely the cause of the distension and why?
2. How would you determine what might be causing the distension?
3. When you listen to the abdomen, you are surprised to hear hyperactive bowel sounds. Why would these be present and what is their significance?

Situation D

An elderly patient is being seen for a yearly checkup. The major concern this patient expresses is fatigue and lack of energy. During the history, you also find out that there is a history of heavy drinking as well as chronic ulcers.

1. What possible cause might there be for the fatigue and lack of energy? What is your reasoning for this?
2. How would you validate your suspicions regarding the cause?
3. What long-term problems would you be concerned about?

SUBJECTIVE DATA

History of Present Illness (CC)

The patient may present to the provider with a variety of concerns that may be directly related to the abdomen (GI system) or other systems. Framing the questions will depend on the patient's age, gender, culture, race, emotional or mental status, health practices, and concurrent illnesses. All symptoms presented must be thoroughly assessed with a symptom analysis (COLDERRA).

Abdominal Pain

Due to the number of organs located in the abdomen, identifying a source and cause presents quite a challenge. Acute abdominal pain accounts for 5%–10% of all emergency department visits (White & Counselman, 2009). Abdominal pain is a common manifestation in the primary outpatient care setting and in the emergency department. Etiology varies from benign conditions like gastroenteritis and irritable bowel syndrome to more life-threatening conditions like perforated ulcer, ruptured abdominal aneurysm, or peritonitis. Differential diagnosis and treatment are based on clustering of symptoms, appropriate history, risk factors, and physical findings.

Provider Inquiries	Clinical Reasoning/Logic
Characteristics: What does the pain feel like—dull, sharp, burning, gnawing, stabbing, cramping, achy, or colicky?	Characteristics of the pain help in identifying its cause. Deep pain or visceral pain is associated with organs and is relatively dull and difficult to localize. Superficial pain or parietal pain frequently is associated with inflammation of the peritoneum and is sharp and in a specific location.
Onset: Did the pain have a gradual or an immediate onset? Gradual onset of pain is more common with chronic disorders or slow developing conditions whereas immediate onset indicates a more acute situation. Were you engaging in any activity when it first occurred?	See Table 28-1. Knowledge of onset of pain helps with the differential diagnoses of abdominal pain.
Location: Where is the pain located? Identifying the location helps to determine what organ may be involved.	See Table 28-2. Localizing the pain often helps with determining visceral organs involved.

Provider Inquiries	Clinical Reasoning/Logic
Duration: Is the pain constant or intermittent? When does it occur? Does there seem to be a pattern or cycle of the pain?	Some types of pain are associated with other physiological functions (menstrual cycle, gallbladder contraction, eating certain foods). Identification of a cycle or pattern helps to associate the pain with other functions.
Exacerbation: What, if anything, makes the pain worse? Position, food, medications, alcohol, activity, stress/anxiety?	Appendicitis/peritonitis pain is aggravated by motion or coughing; gastritis pain is increased by ingestion of foods/alcohol. Peptic ulcer pain is made worse by empty stomach.
Relief: What, if anything, relieves the pain? Position, food, medications, activity, rest? Use of any complementary therapies?	
Radiation: Is the pain felt elsewhere or has it moved from its original location? Certain abdominal pain radiates to other sources.	In some instances abdominal pain may be a referred from a source outside the abdominal cavity.
Associated signs/symptoms: Is the pain associated with any other manifestations? Nausea/vomiting, diarrhea, distention, constipation, gas, fatigue, stress, rectal bleeding or other discharge? Weight loss? Other manifestations associated with the pain will help in identifying its source or cause. Any known food allergies or food intolerances? Rash in dermatomal distribution? Morbilliform rash?	Presence of fever suggests infection or inflammation. Distension and constipation or no bowel movement suggests obstruction. Weight loss, blood in the stools, and other constitutional signs are alarm symptoms and help in determining causes of abdominal pain. Dermatomal rash suggest herpes zoster and morbilliform rash may be seen in viral gastroenteritis or hepatitis.

Table 28-3 lists the numerous possible causes of gastrointestinal pain.

Table 28-1 Onset of pain, sensation, and temporal characteristics

Sudden onset (full pain in seconds)	Rapid onset (initial sensation to full pain over minutes to hours)	Gradual onset (hours)
Perforated ulcer	Strangulated hernia	Appendicitis
Mesenteric infarction	Volvulus	Strangulated hernia
Ruptured abdominal aortic aneurysm	Intussusception	Chronic pancreatitis
Ruptured ectopic pregnancy	Acute pancreatitis	Peptic ulcer disease
Ovarian torsion or ruptured cyst	Biliary colic	Inflammatory bowel disease
Pulmonary embolism	Diverticulitis	Mesenteric lymphadenitis
Acute myocardial infarction	Ureteral and renal colic	Cystitis and urinary retention
		Salpingitis and prostatitis

Table 28-2 Potential causes of pain by location

Location of Pain	Organs Involved	Associated Conditions
Right Upper Quadrant	Stomach, liver, kidney, gallbladder/biliary tract, hepatic flexure	Acute cholecystitis, biliary colic, acute hepatitis (hepatomegaly), NAFLD, cancer, cirrhosis, duodenal ulcer, right lower lobe pneumonia
Right Lower Quadrant	Ascending colon, appendix, ovary, fallopian tube	Appendicitis, cecal diverticulitis, ectopic pregnancy, tubo-ovarian abscess, ruptured ovarian cyst, ovarian torsion
Left Upper Quadrant	Pancreas, spleen, colon, kidney	Gastritis, acute pancreatitis, splenic pathology (splenomegaly), bowel obstruction or intussusception, colon cancer, gas, left lower lobe pneumonia
Left Lower Quadrant	Sigmoid and descending colon, ovary, fallopian tube	Diverticulitis, ectopic pregnancy, tubo-ovarian abscess, ruptured ovarian cyst, ovarian torsion
Midline (epigastric, perumbilical, suprapubic)	Stomach, pancreas, small intestine, bladder, uterus, cecum/appendix, rectum	Appendicitis (early), gastroenteritis, pancreatitis, ectopic pregnancy, Mittelschmerz, ruptured ovarian cyst, pelvic inflammatory disease, endometriosis, urinary tract infection
Right Flank	Liver, kidney	Renal colic, pyelonephritis, hepatomegaly
Left Flank	Spleen, kidney	Renal colic, pyelonephritis, splenomegaly

Table 28-3 Causes of abdominal pain

Condition	Demographics/Risk	Etiology	Pain Characteristics	Location	Associated Signs/Symptoms	Relieved by	Made worse by	Exam findings
Abdominal Aortic Aneurysm (AAA)—may lead to rupture or dissection	Ages 40–70, peak 65–75 History of hypertension, alcoholism, smoking, FH of aneurysm, genetic factors, connective tissue disorders (Marfan's, Ehlers-Danlos), relapsing polychondritis, and pseudoxanthoma elasticum	Exact cause is unknown; may be caused by atherosclerosis, infection, trauma, arteritis, or cystic medial necrosis.	Usually asymptomatic unless it expands to exert pressure to surrounding organs, or in leakage, rupture or dissection. Sudden, steady, throbbing (unbearable), ripping, excruciating back pain, flank pain, abdominal or groin pain in dissection. In rupture-shock symptoms	Midline, over aneurysm, may radiate to back, flank.	Nausea, vomiting Signs and symptoms of shock–sweating, dizziness (in rupture or dissection)			Palpable mass, abdominal mass (pulsating), bruits, difference/decrease in femoral pulses shock-hypotension, tachycardia, cyanosis, and altered mental status in rupture (signs of hypovolemic shock) Grey Turner sign (flank echymosis-retroperitoneal bleed)
Appendicitis	Any age (peak age is 10–20 years) M > F	Acute inflammation of appendix secondary to obstruction of the appendiceal lumen leading to vascular obstruction from swelling, then necrosis and suppuration	Colicky to progressive, then constant	Periumbilical or epigastric; localizes at McBurney's point [RLQ].	Nausea/vomiting, anorexia after onset of pain Low grade fever	Staying still in recumbent position	Moving, coughing	Guarding, tenderness, rebound tenderness fever Positive obdurator (flexing and internal rotation of the hip) and iliopsoas signs (passive extension of knee and hip or active flexion of hip by pt) RLQ hyperesthesia Increased tenderness to palpation on the right iliac fossa when patient lies on left side
Cholelithiasis (biliary gall stones)/ cholecystitis	Adults; females > males 5 Fs (forties, female, fat, flatulence, fertile)	Obstruction of the cystic duct (CBD) by gallstones leads to inflammation and secondary infection by intestinal microorganisms. Stones may obstruct distally the CBD, or Ampulla of Vater, obstructing the pancreatic duct causing CBD obstruction and pancreatitis, respectively. Gallstones may form due to bile high cholesterol/ bile salts ratio and stasis in the gall bladder from infrequent or incomplete emptying,	May be asymptomatic for years. Episodic, colicky to constant pain, or severe 15 min to hours (after fatty meal)	RUQ/epigastric area; may radiate to R scapular region or right shoulder.	Anorexia, nausea, vomiting, jaundice, temp < 98.6, dark urine Fever in cholecystitis		Fatty foods	Tenderness palpation/ percussion. Positive Murphy's RUQ (tenderness/rigidity) + Murphy's sign, palpable gallbladder Jaundice and clay-colored stools in CBD obstruction or gallstone pancreatitis Fever Pancreatitis if the pancreatic duct is obstructed at the ampulla.
Small or large bowel obstruction	Older adults, history of abdominal surgeries, adhesions, hernias, Crohn's, volvulus neoplasms, intussusception or intestinal atresia in children In large bowel obstruction—neoplasm, constipation, inflammatory bowel diseases, adhesions, narcotics, endometriosis may cause the obstruction.	Mechanical obstruction to the normal forward passage of intestinal contents due to barriers (adhesions, tumor, strictures), or slowing of peristalsis from drugs.	Colicky, abrupt onset, severe, intermittent	Diffuse or localized to central mid-abdomen	Nausea, bilious or feculent vomiting, less frequent stools or no stool Diarrhea/constipation No passage of gas or stools	Relief of obstruction	Antidepressants, anti-cholinergics, pain medications, or any drugs that decrease motility	Hyperactive bowel sounds or no bowel sounds Abdominal distention Tenderness to palpation—(localized or diffuse)

Continued

Table 28-3 Causes of abdominal pain *(continued)*

Condition	Demographics/Risk	Etiology	Pain Characteristics	Location	Associated Signs/Symptoms	Relieved by	Made worse by	Exam findings
Diverticulosis/ diverticulitis	Older adults Males >40 Advancing age, constipation, diet low in fiber, connective tissue disorders (Ehlers-Danlos, Marfan's), and genetic predisposition	Weakness of the muscle layers in the colon lead to saclike outpouching of the colonic wall. This is thought to be due to increased intra-colonic pressure; associated with low fiber intake.	Intermittent, dull, cramping (often gradual onset), May be localized	Epigastric, radiating down L side (LLQ) of abdomen (after eating), may radiate to back	Flatulence, diarrhea, constipation Fever in diverticulitis	Passing gas, bowel movement	Eating	Palpable LLQ mass Fever in diverticulitis Tenderness to palpation usually at the LLQ, borborygmi, mild distension
Ectopic pregnancy	Women of child-bearing age; menstrual irregularity History of salpingitis/ PID History of ectopic pregnancy, tubal surgery, tubal ligation and tubal pathology, chronic IUD use	Fertilized egg implants outside the uterine cavity (usually Fallopian tube). Growing embryo outgrows tube, creates pressure, release of prostaglandins, and bleeding; eventually ruptures.	Sudden onset Persistent, if ruptured, agonizing	Lower quadrant or pelvis–side depends on which Fallopian tube; radiating to left shoulder due to irritation of the diaphragm from blood leakage	Early pregnancy vaginal bleeding Abdominal pain Symptoms of pregnancy, and amenorrhea Pain with urination or bowel movement or urge to defecate due to blood in the posterior cul de sac		Pain sometimes increased with urination or bowel movement	There may be no physical findings in unruptured ectopic pregnancy. Tenderness on lower abdomen, or adnexa; palpable adnexal mass on affected side, Blood in vaginal vault, cervical motion tenderness If ruptured, signs of shock, orthostatic change in vital signs, rigid abdominal wall, + Kehr sign (pain in the tip of the shoulder due to blood in the peritoneal cavity), + Cullen test (periumbilical ecchymosis)
Peptic ulcer disease (PUD), gastric ulcers (GU), duodenal ulcers (DU)	Ages 30–50, males > females Alcoholism, NSAID/ Salicylates/steroids/ bisphosphonate use *H pylori*	Inflammation to breakdown of gastric mucosa or duodenum may be due to NSAID or *H. pylori.* Other factors contribute, (ZE syndrome).	Gnawing, burning (sudden onset) GU—during meals or (1–2 hours after meal), DU—2–5 hours after meals, mid-morning, mid-afternoon, middle of night. DU may disappear for a while and then reappear weeks to months later.	Epigastric pain, may radiate to the back 2–5 hours after a meal (DU), or at night, and during meals (GU), Location may be in the LUQ or RUQ. Sudden, diffuse or localized intense pain in penetration or perforation	Hemorrhage, nausea, vomiting, fever, diarrhea, constipation, or other IBS symptoms Epigastric fullness, early satiety, belching nausea or vomiting after a meal Reflux like dyspepsia Weight loss.	Antacids Food intake in DU	Alcohol Empty stomach in DU and food intake in GU, NSAID, aspirin, and steroids	Epigastric tenderness or in RUQ, LUQ in other cases In perforation, there may be signs of peritonitis.
GERD/ esophagitis	Older adult 35% in children (newborn) Obesity, hiatal hernia, Zollinger-Ellison syndrome. Medicines (prednisone, NSAID), hypercalcemia, scleroderma	Failure of GES to prevent regurgitation of stomach contents into LE; may be caused by hiatal hernia.	Burning pain	Epigastric; may radiate to jaw.	Weight loss Aspiration Dysphagia Nausea Chest pain In children, spitting, coughing, vomiting, crying for food and then removing bottle or breast to cry, wheezing, failure to gain weight	Lying recumbent	Sitting in upright position	No specific exam findings
Abdominal wall pain	Postoperative incisions, shingles, hernia, trauma, hematomas, vigorous exercise Neuropathies (zoster) Myofascial pain syndromes	Stimulation of cutaneous innervations from pressure, inflammation or trauma. Pain is outside the abdominal cavity	Localized, sharp, pinching pain tends to be chronic, unless related to trauma Superficial pain with trigger points and increased pain when the abdomen is tensed (sitting up)	Localized to a region or muscle group or cutaneous innervation		Relief may be obtained from splinting, sitting or reposed position.	Aggravated by tensing of the abdominal wall, movement, coughing, stretching, or walking.	Trigger point tenderness— + Carnett's test (palpation of tender spot during resting recumbent position with increasing pain as the patient sits up or tenses abdomen).
Irritable bowel syndrome (IBS)	Young women, female to male ratio of 2:1	Alteration in GI motility with visceral hypersensitivity with impaired transit of gas and colonic contents	Chronic, recurrent crampy, abdominal pain with variable intensity	LLQ hypogastric area, may be nonspecific.	Mucus in stools Pain with gas, bloating, distension Alternating constipation or diarrhea Belching Anxiety, chest pain, dyspepsia, reflux Intense pain associated with nausea and/or vomiting, followed by explosive diarrhea	Food Emotional stress	Passage of stool or gas	Nonspecific tenderness to palpation and abdominal distension during acute attacks No specific physical findings in between attacks.

Continued

Table 28-3 Causes of abdominal pain *(continued)*

Condition	Demographics/Risk	Etiology	Pain Characteristics	Location	Associated Signs/Symptoms	Relieved by	Made worse by	Exam findings
Mesenteric ischemia (MI) (occlusive [OMI] or nonocclusive [NOMI])	Older adult All risk factors for atherosclerosis—hypertension, diabetes, coronary heart disease, MI, valvular heart disease, heart failure. peripheraly vascular disease Hypercoagulable states Drugs (cocaine, vasodilators) that reduce perfusion Intra-abdominal malignancy Cardiac arrhythmias (atrial fibrillation) Smoking Following procedures like CABG with long aortic cross-clamp time, dialysis, which may decrease perfusion Other processes that reduce perfusion (sepsis, aortic insufficiency) Vasculitis	Reduction in arterial blood flow to the mesentery due to occlusion from an embolus or thrombosis, vasospasm or hypoperfusion from low cardiac output states	Depends on whether it is OMI or NOMI OMI: Severe, rapid onset periumbilical pain that is out of proportion with physical findings NOMI: Variable/subacute or absent abdominal pain in Small bowel ischemia tends to have more severe pain than in colonic ischemia which presents with lower abdominal pain with anorexia Pain is sudden in embolism compared to the insidious pain in thrombotic processes.	Initially periumbilical, then generalized	Nausea and vomiting Early satiety Weight loss Postprandial pain Forceful bowel evacuation Anorexia Diarrhea (may be bloody), constipation, shock (hypotension), tachycardia	Eating may increase symptoms		Normal abdominal examination initially Abdominal distension As it progresses, abdominal wall rigidity, and other peritoneal signs with guarding, rebound tenderness and absent bowel sounds may be present. Hypotension Shock Tachycardia Signs of acidosis + occult blood in the stools
Pancreatitis	Older adult Alcoholism, cholelithiasis Pneumonic Medications (corticosteroids, diuretics, anticonvulsants, chemotherapy, estrogens, diabetic drugs, atypical antipsychotics) Inherited traits Cystic fibrosis Procedures (ERCP) Congenital conditions (pancreas divisum) DM, autoimmune, pregnancy, pancreatic cancer, stones, or sludge, hyperlipidemia, hypothermia, hyperparathyroidism, mumps	Acute inflammation of pancreas due to alcohol or cholelithiasis Drugs (valproic acid, tetracycline, hydrochlorothiazide, Lasix), CA, trauma, surgery, ulcer with pancreatic involvement	With gallstones: Sudden onset, excruciating, knife like pain; with steady and progressive localized pain with maximum intensity within 20 minutes When due to alcohol, drugs, metabolic and hereditary causes, pain is less abrupt and poorly localized and persists for several hours to days.	Epigastric periumbilical or RUQ and rarely LUQ may be felt in one or both flanks, may radiate to back (in alcohol pancreatitis or from hereditary or metabolic causes). In gallstones pancreatitis, pain is abrupt onset that is localized and progressed to maximum intensity within 20 min.	Nausea and vomiting, fever, shock, diaphoresis Dyspnea due to diaphragmatic irritation from pancreatitis, pleural effusion, or ARDS	Lying supine	Leaning forward or bending forward	Dependent on severity Epigastric tenderness + grey Turner sign + Cullen sign Abdominal distension and hypoactive bowel sounds from ileus, jaundice, icterus if common bile duct is obstructed by gallstones or edema at head of the pancreas Fever, tachypnea, tachycardia, or hypotension in severe pancreatitis In chronic condition, symptoms of decreased pancreatic function—steatorrhea DM
Peritonitis—also called an acute abdomen	No age preponderance Ruptured or perforated PUD, cholecystitis, diverticulitis, bowel strangulation, acute salpingitis, abdominal trauma, peritoneal dialysis, inflammatory bowel disease, perforation from tumor, spontaneous bacterial peritonitis in alcoholic liver disease with cirrhosis and ascites. Noninfectious peritonitis may be due to surgical causes, blunt abdominal trauma, endometriosis, familial Mediterranean fever.	Inflammation of the peritoneum due to perforation or disruption of any part of the GI tract, trauma, infection, or other noninfectious causes.	Gradual onset; dull aches; severe, sharp, unrelenting pain; Acute severe, sharp	Localized related to organ inflammation Pain with deep inspiration	Loss of appetite, thirst, nausea and vomiting, bloating/distension, fever, chills	Lying still, deep breathing, assuming flexed position (reduces tension on abdomen)	Coughing, moving	Diffuse abdominal rigidity Rebound tenderness to light palpation Guarding Increased pain when bumped Fever tachycardia In later stages, hypotension, hypovolemia, Sepsis Reduced urine output, unable to pass gas or stool. Rebound tenderness. Hypoactive or absent bowel sounds Shallow, rapid ventilations. Guarding; hypotension, rapid heart rate

Continued

Table 28-3 Causes of abdominal pain *(continued)*

Condition	Demographics/Risk	Etiology	Pain Characteristics	Location	Associated Signs/Symptoms	Relieved by	Made worse by	Exam findings
Volvulus	Children—in first year of life is associated with malrotation of intestines during fetal development. May occur later in life (middle-age and elderly men who are institutionalized and debilitated like in Parkinson's disease and schizophrenia) Patients with constipation, redundant colon, Duchenne's muscular dystrophy Sigmoid volvulus may occur in Crohn's disease, pregnancy, Chagas disease.	Twisting of the bowel leads to obstruction and ischemia of the bowel. Common sites are the cecum and sigmoid colon.	Severe, acute pain Continuous and severe in sigmoid volvulus	Referred to umbilicus and hypogastric area	Nausea Vomiting Lack of stools or constipation Abdominal distension Anorexia			Bilious vomiting, bloody stools, abdominal distension, dehydration with weight loss, visible peristaltic waves

THINK LINK: Hepatic Tenderness

Individuals who have hepatitis often experience pain and/or tenderness in the right upper quadrant (RUQ). Pain of this nature is primarily the result of hepatocyte swelling leading to hepatic enlargement resulting in stretching of the hepatic capsule. It is the stretching of the hepatic capsule that causes the pain, not anything related to damage per se to the hepatocytes or structural components of the liver.

Nausea and Vomiting

Nausea and vomiting may be due to central nervous system (CNS); gastrointestinal causes; food poisoning; medication side effects; infections like viral infections, hepatitis, and meningitis; systemic causes like diabetic ketoacidosis (DKA), gastroparesis, renal failure, and hepatic failure; advanced malignancy, especially with liver involvement; psychogenic causes; or in severe abdominal pain like pyelonephritis and pancreatitis, pregnancy, migraine; or in labyrinthitis or inner ear conditions.

Provider Inquiries	Clinical Reasoning/Logic
Characteristics: How would you describe the vomit (emesis)? Color, presence of blood, coffee grounds, undigested food, particular odor, number of times stomach contracts? Ever experienced dry heaves? Does nausea occur without vomiting? Do you feel better after vomiting?	Bright red blood emesis is seen in esophageal varices, Mallory-Weiss tear, Boerhaave's syndrome, or in vigorous upper GI bleed from peptic ulcer disease (PUD). Feculent emesis is seen in mechanical or non-mechanical intestinal obstruction. Emesis with undigested food may be seen in gastroenteritis. Bilious emesis is seen in obstructions, like in volvulus, small bowel obstruction, biliary obstruction, or gallstones pancreatitis.
Onset: When did the nausea/vomiting start? Is there a pattern or cycle associated with other activities (pain, meals, eating certain foods)? Is there any identifiable stimulus for vomiting? Any type of pattern or relationship to other functions or time of day? Any recent infections/head trauma?	Timing of vomiting may help in defining its etiology. Vomiting right after a meal may be an indication of food poisoning as the cause, but also may indicate gastritis or an ulcer or bulimia.

Provider Inquiries	Clinical Reasoning/Logic
	Vomiting 1 to 8 hours after a meal may also be associated with food poisoning due to salmonella or staphylococcus, which takes longer to cause symptoms.
	Pregnant women, individuals with uremia, and chronic alcoholics often experience early morning nausea and vomiting (Seller, 2007).
Duration: How long does vomiting last? Is there a single or multiple times during the episode?	Continuous vomiting places the patient at risk for dehydration and electrolyte imbalance. Vomiting that lasts longer than 24 hours needs medical evaluation.
Exacerbation: What, if anything, makes the vomiting worse? Odors, foods, activities?	Vomiting may be caused by noxious odors or certain type smells like during pregnancy or in migraine. Activity may worsen nausea and may lead to vomiting.
Relief: Anything that relieves or prevents nausea/vomiting? Medications (antacids), position, complementary therapies, foods, hydration?	Nausea and vomiting may be better if patient stops eating like in gastroenteritis. Medications may be needed to prevent continuous vomiting for specific causes (chemotherapy).
	Vomiting can be prevented by consuming small amounts of clear, sweetened liquids such as soda pop, fruit juices (except orange and grapefruit because these are too acidic), and popsicles. Drinks containing sugar calm the stomach better than other liquids. Rest either in a sitting position or in a propped lying position.
	Often vomiting makes the migraine pain go away.
Associated signs/symptoms: What other manifestations, if any, accompany the nausea/vomiting? Changes in bowel functions (diarrhea, constipation), pain, fever, or chills?	Vomiting bright red blood associated with hypotension calls for emergent treatment and procedures.
	Red flags include vomiting with any of the following: fever, stiff neck, and mental status changes; hypertension; peritoneal signs; no bowel sounds and progressive bowel distention
Headaches accompany vomiting?	Individuals with migraines often complain of nausea or discomfort in the stomach. It is estimated that almost three-quarters of those with migraines have nausea.

Indigestion (Dyspepsia)

Dyspepsia is commonly described by patients as indigestion. It refers to symptoms like postprandial fullness, early satiety or inability to finish a common, usual meal, or epigastric pain or fullness or discomfort. It may be caused by a wide variety of gastrointestinal disorders like PUD, gastric malignancy, gallbladder disease, gastroparesis, GERD to metabolic, systemic, drug-induced, and functional causes.

Provider Inquiries	Clinical Reasoning/Logic
Characteristics: How do you experience indigestion? Feeling full/loss of appetite, bloating, nausea, excessive gas (frequent burping or passing gas), heartburn/pain?	Description per patient may vary.
Onset: When did indigestion start, or is there anything specifically that initiates indigestion? Any particular time of day that it starts? How frequently do you experience indigestion? Sudden or gradual onset?	Commonly a sensation of fullness during or after a meal. After a meal, there may be a feeling of being overly full.
Location: Localized or general?	Generally the pain is in the epigastric area.
Duration: How long does episode last? Constant or variable in length?	
Exacerbation: Anything, if any, that makes it worse? Position, food? NSAID, steroid, or salicylate use? Smoking?	Alcohol increases risk, mediations (ASA, steroids, NSAIDs), raises NSAID, induces dyspepsia like gastritis or PUD.
Relief: Anything, if any, that makes it better? Position, food, antacids, rest, activity?	Small, low-fat meals several times through the day, and abstaining from alcohol, coffee, smoking may provide relief. Rest periods.
Radiation: Does the epigastric pain or discomfort radiate to the back or shoulders or arms?	Radiation to jaw and arms is suspicious for cardiac ischemic pain. Radiation to the back suggests PUD or early pancreatitis.
Associated signs/symptoms: Cough, heartburn, retrosternal chest pain and regurgitation?	Cough, heartburn, and regurgitation suggest GERD.
Anything associated with indigestion? Specific foods, timing of food intake, nausea/vomiting? Association with epigastric pain or LUQ or RUQ pain?	Epigastric pain, LUQ, or RUQ pain are suspicious for PUD.
Weight loss, anorexia, early satiety, dysphagia, vomiting? Joint pains?	Weight loss, anorexia, dysphagia, and vomiting are suspicious for malignancy. Abdominal pain, diarrhea, weight loss, and joint pains are seen in Whipple's disease.
Association with fatty food intake, RUQ pain and nausea or vomiting?	These suggest gallbladder disease like gallstones.

Change in Bowel Pattern/Characteristics

Any changes in patterns of bowel movements or characteristics must be assessed in relation to what is considered normal for the patient. While it is generally thought that normal is having one bowel movement per day, that is not necessarily considered to be a universal standard.

Diarrhea and constipation are common gastrointestinal complaints. Diarrhea may be due to infections, GI conditions like malabsorption and pancreatic insufficiency drug, other systemic conditions, psychiatric causes may be present in obstructions., food intolerance. It may be self-limited as in viral infections or persistent as in IBD or colitis.

Constipation may be due to IBS, lack of fiber or fluids in the diet, rectal pain from hemorrhoids, side effects of drugs like narcotics and antidepressants, endocrine disorders (hypothyroidism), neurodegenerative disorders (Parkinson's, MS), motility dysfunction, or malignancies.

Provider Inquiries	Clinical Reasoning/Logic
Characteristics: What is the character of change? What is usual pattern for bowel movements (daily, every other day, more than once per day, time of day)? What is usual color? Diarrhea or constipation?	Individuals vary as to their usual patterns. Some individuals will have bowel movements once a day. Some may have two or three per day and others may have two or three bowel movement a week. See Table 28-4 for stool color changes. Distinct odor of stools is characteristic of *C. difficile* colitis ("neuro smell")—difficult to describe. Fatty stools floating in the toilet and stuck to sides of the toilet bowl are seen in malabsorption. Mucus in the stools may be seen in IBS or infectious causes of diarrhea.

Provider Inquiries

Table 28-4 Stool color changes

Color of Stools	Cause/Condition
Black melena	Blood from upper GI tract/stomach (ulcers, esophageal varices) Iron (supplements, iron-rich foods) Medications with bismuth (Pepto-Bismol) Black licorice Blueberries Large amounts of spinach/other greens
Red (hematochezia)	Blood from lower intestines (inflammatory bowel disease, hemorrhoids) Red dye (gelatin, popsicles, Kool-aid) Tomatoes (juice/soup)/beets
Pale/clay colored	Lack of bile salts (hepatitis, cirrhosis, liver cancer) Common bile duct obstruction from stones or malignancy
Green	Antacids containing aluminum hydroxide Green, leafy vegetables (large amounts) Green dye (gelatin, popsicles, Kool-aid) Iron supplements (very dark—> black) Salmonella, Giardia (diarrhea), or *C. difficile*
Orange	High intake of beta-carotene (orange-colored fruits and vegetables) Rifampin (drug)
Bloody diarrhea	Gastroenteritis Regional enteritis Rectal/anal bleeding Food poisoning (Salmonella, *E. coli*) Chemical/plant poisoning Hemolytic uremic syndrome Ulcerative colitis Shigellosis Campylobacter Yersinia
Blood in stools	Amebiasis Colitis Dysentery Enterohemorrhagic *E. coli* infection Food poisoning Cancer Gastritis Cirrhosis Intussusception Thrombocytopenia Diverticular disease
Rectal bleeding/BRBPR—Bright Red Blood Per Rectum	Anal fissure Anal/rectal cancer Polyps/polyposis Crohn's disease Diverticular disease Hemorrhoids Pancytopenia Proctitis

Clinical Reasoning/Logic

Alternating constipation and diarrhea is seen in IBS (irritable bowel syndrome).

Pellet-sized stools (goat's stools) are characteristics of constipation.

Blood may also be in the feces without causing any color change. This is blood that is occult, or hidden. Routine testing for occult blood should be done to determine if this is in fact the case. See Table 28-4.

Provider Inquiries	Clinical Reasoning/Logic
Diarrhea: Watery, amount, explosive, color, does it contain blood, food, oil, or fat, or have a particular odor?	Acute diarrhea, especially with travel history, suggests infections causes from viral, bacterial, or parasitic causes.
Constipation: Any blood noted? Is it black/tarry in appearance or mucoid?	Chronic diarrhea is seen in malabsorption or psychiatric causes.
Onset: When was change first noticed? Anything noted that initiates change? Frequency of changes? Gradual or sudden? Any noted pattern associated with particular foods, other changes (diet, work, sleep patterns, medications)? Recent travel?	Chronic constipation may be due to drugs.
Acute? Chronic?	Acute and progressive constipation may be seen in mechanical intestinal obstruction.
Duration: How long does episode last? How many episodes per day? Does it end spontaneously or do you need to use medications or diet modifications?	Duration of diarrhea or constipation helps in determining etiology and treatment planning. Self-limiting diarrhea with no signs of dehydration may simply need conservative oral hydration.
Exacerbation: What, if any, makes change worse or prolongs the episode?	Antidepressants and narcotics aggravate constipation. Milk may aggravate acute infectious diarrhea or chronic diarrhea like in malabsorption.
Relief: What, if any, makes change better or shortens the episode? Medications, food, activity, fluid intake? Complementary therapies?	Patients may use OTC or herbal remedies to relieve constipation of diarrhea.
Associated signs/symptoms: Fever with diarrhea and blood in the stools?	These suggest infectious like bacterial colitis or inflammatory bowel disease (IBD).
Non-gastrointestinal symptoms like sexual dysfunction, headaches, dysmenorrhea, depression, anxiety, fibromyalgia symptoms?	Non-gastrointestinal symptoms suggest IBS.
Associated with gas, distension and belching, and sensation of incomplete emptying?	IBS may be associated with fatigue, generalized pain and headaches, and anxiety disorder.
Persistent constipation with distension and pain?	Gas, distension, and alternating constipation and diarrhea, along with intermittent cramping, are seen in IBS.
Pain with bowel movement? Do you have an urge to evacuate without success (tenesmus)?	If there is no bowel movement, especially with abdominal distention, a work up for small bowel obstruction is warranted.
Resolution of pain with bowel movement?	Pain with bowel movement with sensation of need to empty the bowels despite an empty bowel is seen in infectious colitis, IBD, anorectal abscess.
	Pain with bowel movement is seen in IBS.
	Weight loss and bloody diarrhea may be seen in inflammatory bowel disease and malignancy.
	Fever and acute bloody diarrhea suggest colitis from infectious causes like *C. difficile* colitis or diverticulitis.
	Nocturnal pain and change in bowel habits argue against IBS.
	Signs of dehydration suggest severe diarrhea.

THINK LINK:* *Change in Bowel Habits 1 of 7 Signs of Cancer

A significant change in bowel elimination pattern is recognized as one of the seven signs for cancer. A significant change in the characteristics (color, consistency, composition) of the feces is also important to recognize as this may also be associated with the presence of cancer. Weight loss and other constitutional signs like fatigue, anorexia, family history of cancer, and advancing age point to malignancy as a legitimate concern.

Red flags: Change in bowel movement associated with the following are alarming and considered as red flags:

1. Bloody stools
2. Weight loss
3. Progressive pain, especially nocturnal pain
4. Rectal bleeding
5. Small bowel obstruction
6. Persistent nausea and vomiting
7. Fever
8. Dehydration

Loss/Changes of Appetite

Loss of appetite (anorexia) may result from stress, changes in diet, indigestion, decrease in gastric emptying, changes in taste and smell, acute diseases like appendicitis or colitis, or chronic diseases (liver and renal diseases), chronic heart disease (heart failure), pulmonary disease (COPD, chronic inflammation) or infection (HIV, TB, hepatitis), autoimmune diseases, malignancy, neurodegenerative disorders, endocrine causes (adrenal insufficiency), stroke, swallowing difficulties, dental pain or conditions, drugs, toxins or psychiatric causes like depression and anorexia nervosa. It is also frequently reported in the elderly.

Provider Inquiries	Clinical Reasoning/Logic
Characteristics: Can you taste the food? Does food taste good? Have you noticed any change in your sense of smell? Have you noticed any changes in your mood? Any recent major stresses? Any new or changes in medications? Any pain? Any unusual tastes in your mouth? Has eating been enjoyable in the past? Previous eating habits?	There are multiple causes of anorexia that can be physical or psychological.
Onset: Is there a specific time that you can identify when you lost your appetite? Anything happen around the time you lost your appetite? Acute or chronic?	Onset of stress or depression may coincide with loss of appetite. Acuity helps in determining causes of anorexia and its management.
Duration: Has this happened previously?	If anorexia has been experienced previously, is there an association between this time and previous incidences?
Exacerbation: Anything that seems to make loss of appetite worse? Odors, types of food?	Certain odors, smells, presentation of foods may increase how one experiences anorexia.
Relief: Anything that seems to increase desire for food/eating?	Certain odors, smells, foods may decrease the sensation of anorexia.
Associated signs/symptoms: Frequently experience indigestion, heart burn? Food intolerances/allergies? Other constitutional findings like weight loss?	Other types of GI disturbances may cause anorexia. Anorexia accompanied by weight loss and other constitutional findings suggests neoplasm and anorexia nervosa.

Urinary Elimination Alterations

Urinary alterations may present in various ways and may be related to changes in volume, color frequency, clarity, content, and concentration. They may also occur separately or together in various combinations. They could also represent a primary problem or secondary ones related to other disease processes. There are also differences in presentation related to age and gender. Individuals may also be hesitant to bring up or admit to having problems associated with urinary elimination.

Provider Inquiries	Clinical Reasoning/Logic
Characteristics: Describe what you're experiencing. Pain/burning with urination (**dysuria**), frequency (increased number of times per day), urgency (need to immediately urinate), hesitancy (difficulty in starting urination), and nocturia (having to urinate during sleep)?	Burning, pain, frequency may indicate bladder infection. Loss of muscle tone may cause incontinence (females). Dysuria, voiding that is either painful or difficult, may result from stricture of the urethra, urinary infections, injury to the bladder and/or the urethra. Burning during micturition is often due to an irritated urethra. Burning following urination may be a result of bladder infection. Frequency may result from increased fluid intake, cystitis, stress, or pressure on the bladder. Men with enlarged prostate gland experience urgency, frequency, and hesitation (delay and difficulty in initiating voiding).
What color is your urine? Is it Blood/red or dark?	Dark amber urine associated with kidney, liver disorders, dehydration.

Provider Inquiries	Clinical Reasoning/Logic
	Red or orange urine may come from blood (trauma, menstruation, instrumentation, kidney stones, glomerulonephritis, bladder infection, neoplasms), pigments (rhabdomyolysis, myoglobinuria, porphyria), medications (pyridium, rifampin, cyclophosamide, warfarin, senna), and food (beets, rhubarb, blackberries).
Other color of urine? Green urine? Black urine?	Green urine in administration of methylene blue, propofol, and amitriptyline. Black urine is seen in hemoglobinuria, myoglobinuria or ochronosis (alkaptonuria).
Are you experiencing incontinence?	Incontinence may be seen in infection, stress incontinence, overactive bladder, and other neurological conditions like cognitive decline, dementia, seizure activity, neurogenic bladder in MS (multiple sclerosis), medications, obesity, prostate conditions, excess caffeine or alcohol, pregnancy, estrogen deficiency, or functional causes.
Onset: When were symptoms first noted? Associated with any trauma, accidents, and illnesses? Gradual or rapid onset?	Acute symptoms are seen in stones and infections. Chronic symptoms are seen in psychiatric causes and chronic infection like prostatitis, interstitial cystitis. A sudden onset of symptoms related to urge or stress incontinence associated with infection; gradual onset of stress incontinence symptoms primarily after menopause of oophorectomy associated with estrogen deficiency (Seller, 2007).
Location: If pain, where located? (Suprapubic (lower, mid abdomen), flank (back), urethral (pain when urinating)?)	Flank pain suggests kidney processes like stones or pyelonephritis. Cystitis, bladder infection, interstitial cystitis present with suprapubic or pelvic pain or discomfort.
Duration: Constant or intermittent manifestations? Length of time manifestations experienced?	Acute onset is associated with stones and infection.
Is there blood in urine (hematuria)? If so, is it transient (intermittent)?	Transient hematuria may be seen after intercourse or after vigorous exercise and may also be seen in malignancy, prostatitis, and cystitis.
Do you experience persistent (constant) hematuria?	Persistent hematuria is seen in kidney stones, malignancy, and glomerulonephritis.
Do you experience painful urination (dysuria) or the immediate need to urinate (urgency)? Are your symptoms intermittent or persistant (chronic)?	Interstitial cystitis can present with intermittent or recurrent symptoms of urgency and dysuria.
Do you have a burning sensation with urination?	Chronic presentation of dysuria, bladder pressure, and burning with urination and hematuria may be seen in interstitial cystitis.
For males, do you experience hesitation, frequency, urgency, or nocturia? If so, it it transient or constant (persistent)?	Symptoms of benign prostatic hypertrophy/hyperplasia (BPH) fluctuate most likely due to changes associated with bladder tone, bladder neck obstruction, and tone of the prostate and capsule (Seller, 2007).

Provider Inquiries	Clinical Reasoning/Logic
Exacerbation: What, if anything, makes it worse? Position? Fluid intake? Instrumentation?	Females: Incontinence (leaking) may occur with sneezing, laughing, coughing, or running. Catheterization, prostate biopsy, stents placement, and urethral dilation are associated with changes in urination. Hematuria or rhabdomyolysis may be seen after vigorous exertion.
Relief: What, if anything, makes it better? Position, heat, medications, fluid intake?	Individuals may decrease fluid intake of caffeine or alcohol to decrease incidences of incontinence or need to urinate. Decreased fluid intake may result in dehydration and stasis increases possibility for urinary tract infections and development of kidney stones (urolithiasis).
Radiation: If pain is present, is it felt in another part of the body? Where?	Blood in the urine associated with flank pain radiating to the groin, testicles, and inner thigh suggests kidney stones.
Associated signs/symptoms: Fever, chills? Known exposure to bacterial, viral, parasitic infections? Pain with intercourse? Nausea and vomiting?	Fever, chills, back pain are associated with pyelonephritis, prostatitis, and kidney stones. Pain with intercourse may be seen with interstitial cystitis. Nausea and vomiting are seen in renal colic from stones.

Past Medical History

Past medical history provides information as to previous illnesses or conditions that may have an effect on the abdominal organs.

Any known GI or renal disorders: ulcers (peptic of duodenal), inflammatory bowel disease, intestinal obstruction, pancreatitis, cirrhosis, kidney stones?	Knowledge of past medical illnesses helps in determining cause for current symptoms.
Any known infectious disorders? Hepatitis, urinary tract infections (cyctitis, pyelonephritis)? If so, how many? How treated? Any long-term effects? Scarlet fever? Exposure to tuberculosis?	
Any abdominal or renal surgeries? If so, for what? Any postoperative complications/alterations?	Procedures like endoscopic retrograde chonalgiopancreatography (ERCP) may place a person at risk for pancreatitis. Abdominal surgeries are risk factors for adhesions and later complications like small bowel obstruction.
Any blood transfusions? For what? How long ago?	Blood transfusion is a known risk factor for hepatitis B and C.
Any other major illnesses? Cancer (rectal—both genders), (breast, ovarian, endometrial—females), (prostate—males)? Arthritis, renal disease, cardiac disease?	History of cancers, autoimmune disease, or atherosclerosis helps in narrowing differential diagnoses.

Family History

Family history provides information regarding family members' illnesses or conditions as potential causes for chief complaint or presenting symptoms that may indicate a pattern of presentation associated with transmission of familial/genetic factors predisposing the individual to certain system-related conditions/illnesses. Any of these may indicate a potential or actual cause of GI or renal dysfunction.

Provider Inquiries	Clinical Reasoning/Logic
Any known GI or renal disorders—gallbladder disease, ulcers, inflammatory bowel disease, renal stones, polycystic disease, renal tubular acidosis, and renal cancer?	Family history is important as there are conditions that predispose an individual to conditions like polycystic kidney disease, inflammatory bowel discasc, malignancy, aortic aneurysm, diabetes, cystic fibrosis, and other malabsorptive diseases.
Malabsorption syndromes: cystic fibrosis, celiac disease?	Genetic factors play a role in celiac sprue and cystic fibrosis.
Hirschsprung's disease, aganglionic megacolon	Genetic basis for Hirschsprung's have been shown.
Colorectal cancers or predisposing conditions—familial adenomatous polyposis, hereditary non-polyposis colorectal cancer?	Familial adenomatous polyposis is inherited where individuals are at risk to develop colon cancer at earlier age like late thirties.

Personal and Social History

Personal and social history provides information related to habits, practices, and/or environmental influences that may predispose the patient to the development of certain system related conditions/illnesses.

Provider Inquiries	Clinical Reasoning/Logic
Any changes noted to occur in any of the following areas: bowel habits, change in caliber or stools urination, menstruation, weight, appetite?	Changes in any of these symptoms help to determine the cause of presenting concern.
Medications—past and present. Steroids, aspirin, antibiotics, antihypertensives, nonsteroidal?	Medications are commonly associated with almost any presenting complaint and also help in management. Antibiotic use is a risk factor for *C. difficile* colitis or antibiotic-related diarrhea. NSAIDs, steroids, and salicylates are common causes of dyspepsia and PUD.
Alcohol intake—past and present? Frequency, amount, type?	Alcohol has been implicated in gastritis, PUD, alcohol liver disease, pancreatitis, cholelithiasis, and malignancy—(esophageal cancer, colorectal, pancreatic, hepatocellular cancers), and renal dysfunction.
Coffee/tea intake—frequency, amount?	Coffee and tea may be a source of irritant and may cause dysuria and frequency *or* urination cancers.
Tobacco use?	Tobacco has been associated with risks for cancers of the esophagus, pancreas, liver, bowel, and bladder as well as atherosclerosis, abdominal aortic aneurysm, mesenteric ischemia, impotence, preterm delivery, taste disruption.
Drug vaccinations—up to date, hepatitis A/B vaccinations?	Hepatitis and zoster vaccine
Diet/exercise?	Weight gain/obesity of major concern due to its association with other major threats to health (NAFLD—obesity, atherosclerosis). Exercise helps intestinal motility and improve transit time.
Weight gain/loss not planned?	Weight loss is a worrisome finding in patients with abdominal complaints.
Bowel and renal?	Baseline bowel and bladder habits are necessary information to determine departure from baseline.
Exposure to any toxic agents around home, at work?	Toxins may present with abdominal pain.
Physical/psychological changes?	Stress may increase symptoms of IBS and inflammatory bowel disease, interstitial cystitis.

Provider Inquiries	Clinical Reasoning/Logic
Trauma at work, physical activity, abuse?	Trauma to abdomen may present with acute abdomen, gross hematuria, pancreatitis as after ERCP.
Any recent travel?	Travel puts individuals at risk for food-associated infections, infectious diarrhea, caused by salmonella, shigella, viral, *E. coli*, cholera; parasitic diseases caused by *Entamoeba histolytica*, giardia, cryptosporidium, listeria; food-borne diseases like hepatitis A; and contaminated water.

Developmental Applications

Certain conditions or disorders may be related to certain age groups or situations. Inquiring to obtain age or condition specific information will provide further information for helping to determine causes of the chief concern as identified.

Infants/Children

Provider Inquiries	Clinical Reasoning/Logic
What was the infant's gestational age and birth weight?	Preterm infants and those weighing less than 1500 grams are at high risk for necrotizing enterocolitis.
Did the infant pass first meconium stool within 24 hours?	Validates the patency of the anus.
Is the infant breastfed or bottle fed? If bottle fed, how is formula tolerated?	Most newborns need 8–12 feedings per day (every 2–3 hours).
If breastfed, does infant appear satisfied after feeding? How frequent does the infant feed?	If poor technique, or infant is not sucking well, the infant may not be getting an adequate amount of milk. Indicators of getting enough to eat are steady weight gain, content between feedings, six wet diapers and three bowel movements per day by 5th day.
Has the infant been introduced to new foods? How tolerated?	New foods should be introduced one at a time to determine tolerance and possibility of allergens.
How often does toddler/child eat? Regular or irregular feeding patterns?	It is not unusual for toddlers/children to have their own feeding pattern. If child appears satisfied, is gaining weight appropriately, and primarily eating nutritious foods, there is no cause to worry or be concerned.
Does child eat non-foods (grass, ice, clay, chalk, dirt, or sand)?	It is not unusual for children to attempt to eat nonfood items, but they should be able to distinguish food from nonfood by 2 years. If child ingests paint chips, this may result in lead poisoning if older paint has been used that contains lead.
Pattern of bowel movements? Ever experience constipation? Amount of fluids ingested? Toilet trained/ready for toilet training?	By age 2 the child has two formed bowel movements per day. If child has fewer bowel movements than usual or complains of pain during a bowel movement, he or she may be constipated. A child who usually has a bowel movement every two days is not constipated, if the bowel movement is reasonably soft and not difficult or painful to pass. Maintaining adequate hydration is essential to prevent constipation. Children are at risk for constipation during toilet training. If a child is not ready/interested in using the toilet, may avoid going to the bathroom (called withholding),

Provider Inquiries	Clinical Reasoning/Logic
	which can lead to constipation. Children who have experienced a hard/painful bowel movement are more likely to withhold, which worsens the problem.
If child is overweight: How long has weight been a problem? Any significant changes—diet, family, school? Weight problems in family? How active is child?	Reduced physical activity and increased intake of soft drinks, carbohydrates, etc. contribute to weight gain. Significant changes in child's life may cause eating to become a coping mechanism. Weight problems often run in families.
Extreme weight loss, particularly in adolescents (male and female)? How did weight loss occur, over what period of time? How often do you feel tired, fatigued, and hungry? What do you usually eat, how often? How do you perceive your body?	Extremely thin adolescents (male and female) with recent of continuing weight loss may have anorexia nervosa.
 ***The Pregnant Woman*** History related to possible pregnancy-alterations of GI and renal system covered in Chapter 30.	
 ***The Older Adult*** Are you experiencing any problems with urinary elimination (dribbling, incontinence, initiating urine flow, polyuria, and nocturia) or bowel patterns (constipation, diarrhea)? Urinary tract infections? Fluid intake adequate?	Older females may have weakened pelvic floor muscles, which don't provide adequate support for bladder, resulting in loss of bladder control causing leaking. Males may experience enlarged prostate glands, which may result in hesitancy and frequency nocturia. If urinary problems are present, individuals may decrease their fluid intake to reduce urine output; however, adequate fluid intake is necessary for regular bowel movements and prevention of urinary tract infections (UTIs). A reduction in gastric motility may cause constipation. UTI is the most common infectious problem among older adults, both in the community and institutional settings. UTIs may be the cause of mental changes in older adults.
Any changes in dietary habits and/or intake? Any changes in teeth?	Changes in smell and taste, decreased saliva secretion may cause a reduction in food intake (food may not taste good, etc.). Decreased gastric motility results in delayed emptying of stomach and reduced feelings of hunger. Alterations in teeth (missing teeth, poorly fitting dentures, periodontal disease) may contribute to difficulty in chewing food.

OBJECTIVE DATA

Objective data for the abdominal exam is obtained through inspection, auscultation, palpation, and percussion. When doing the abdominal exam, the sequence of techniques is altered so that auscultation precedes palpation and percussion. This is so that activity of the intestines (bowel sounds) will not be influenced by the maneuvers of palpation and percussion.

For purposes of identification of underlying organs and documenting findings, the abdomen is divided into four quadrants or nine regions (Figure 28-8). The four quadrant approach is most commonly used; however, for organs that are midline and cross the upper or lower quadrants, the nine region approach is frequently used. To divide the abdomen into four quadrants, perpendicular lines are drawn through the umbilicus. The vertical line extends from the xiphoid process to the symphysis pubis, and the horizontal line bisects the vertical line at the umbilicus. These quadrants are identified as the upper and lower right and left quadrants.

The nine region approach requires two horizontal and two vertical lines. The two vertical lines are extensions of the midclavicular lines into the groin. The two horizontal lines are created by drawing one line across the chest at the lower edge of the costal margin and drawing the second line across the lower abdomen at the edge of the iliac crests. The nine regions are the right and left hypochondriac, lumbar, and inguinal regions that make up the outer six regions. The three inner regions are the epigastric, umbilical, and hypogastric (suprapubic) areas. The anatomical location of the abdominal organs in the four quadrants or nine regions is laid out in Table 28-5. In addition to the division of the abdomen, there are other landmarks that are useful in describing locations on the abdomen (see Figure 28-8).

When examining the abdomen, it is important for the abdomen to be as relaxed as possible. This is achieved by placing a pillow under the patient's knees or having the patient flex the knees. A pillow under the head or slight elevation of the bed or table is also recommended. The patient's arms should also be extended alongside the body. Having the patient's hands placed under the head stretches the abdominal muscles, making it more difficult to examine the abdomen, particularly doing palpation (Figure 28-9). Also instruct the patient to breathe slowly and through the mouth. Patients may often hold their breath and tense up when anticipating something uncomfortable or that may cause pain, or if they are ticklish. Concentrating on their breathing will help to eliminate this possibility.

Drape the lower abdomen so that the pubic area is accessible, with another drape or the patient's gown placed across the upper chest. Male patients may not object to having the entire upper abdomen and chest exposed; however, female patients should expect that their breasts are not exposed. If the breasts are large, they may have to be displaced for adequate exposure of the upper chest. The provider may do this or may ask the patient to lift her breasts up during the examination. Having the patient do this should not interfere with maintaining relaxation of the abdomen as the arms are still in position along the side of the body.

Table 28-5 Abdominal organs in each quadrant (4/9)

Right Hypochondriac	**Right Upper Quadrant**	**Epigastric**	**Left Upper Quadrant**	**Left Hypochondriac**
Right lobe of liver	Liver and gallbladder	Pyloric end of stomach	Left lobe of liver	Stomach
Portion of gallbladder	Pylorus	Duodenum	Spleen	Spleen
Portion of duodenum	Duodenum	Pancreas	Stomach	Tail of pancreas
Portion of right kidney	Head of pancreas	Portion of liver	Body of pancreas	Upper pole of left kidney
Right adrenal gland	Right adrenal gland	Portion of gallbladder	Left adrenal gland	Left adrenal gland
	Portion of right kidney		Portion of left kidney	
Right lumbar	Portions of ascending and transverse colon		Portions of transverse and descending colon	**Left lumbar**
Ascending colon				Descending colon
Lower half of right kidney		**Umbilical**		Lower half of left kidney
Portion of duodenum and jejunum		Lower duodenum		Portions of jejunum and ileum
	Right Lower Quadrant	Jejunum and ileum	**Left Lower Quadrant**	
	Lower pole of right kidney		Lower post of left kidney	
Right Inguinal	Cecum and appendix		Sigmoid colon	
Cecum			Portion of descending colon	
Appendix	Bladder (if distended)		Bladder (if distended)	**Left inguinal**
Ilium (lower end)	Right ovary and salpinx	**Hypogastric**	Left ovary and salpinx	Sigmoid colon
Right ureter	Uterus (if enlarged)	Ilium	Uterus (if enlarged)	Left ureter
Right spermatic cord	Right spermatic cord	Bladder	Left spermatic cord	Left spermatic cord
Right ovary	Right ureter	Uterus (pregnant)	Left ureter	Left ovary

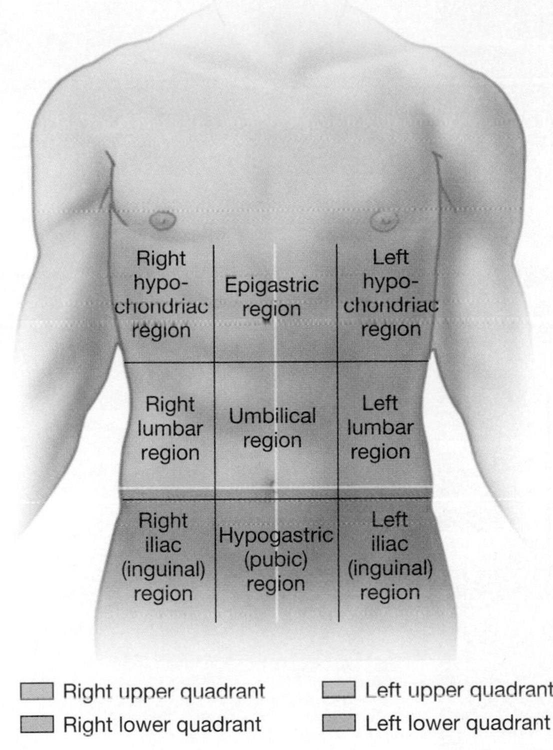

FIGURE 28-8 Abdomen divided into four quadrants and nine regions

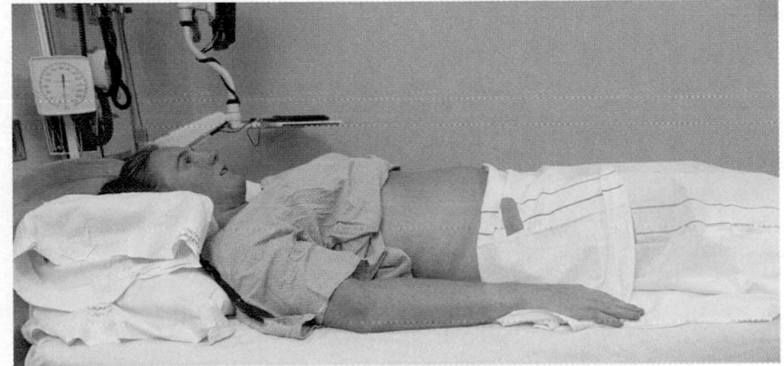

FIGURE 28-9 Position of patient for abdominal exam

It is also important for the patient to have an empty bladder. This is for the patient's comfort and preventing any interference with palpation. Palpation of a full bladder may be uncomfortable for the patient. If the patient may have difficulty with urinary incontinence, palpation of the bladder may initiate leaking and cause embarrassment for the patient. A full bladder may also give the impression that there is an abdominal mass when there is none.

Inspection

Contour
Skin—surface condition/characteristics (symmetry)
Umbilicus
Rectum

Palpation

Light/deep—Turgor
Organomegaly
Contents
Rectum/prostate
Abdominal reflexes

Auscultation

Bowel sounds
Vascular sounds

Percussion

Tympany vs. dullness
Liver/spleen—location/size
CVA tenderness

Level I to IV Examination

The Level I to Level IV examinations are performed on a continuum, which starts from a basic level to a more comprehensive level based on provider's abilities and knowledge as well as the patient's presentation and location. It may start at the outpatient setting progressing to the ED, hospital unit bed, critical care unit, or specialty unit. Frequently all the elements from basic to comprehensive exam are done in one setting like in a primary care setting or clinic.

The condition/illness of the patient is the primary consideration related to the type and amount of data needed to assess the patient's condition/illness/situation. The arrangement of skills into levels is for general purposes and is meant to be descriptive rather than prescriptive. The purpose of arranging into levels is to provide a framework to assist the learner in determining the appropriate data to collect.

Abdomen

	Level I	Level II	Level III	Level IV
Inspection	Skin (landmarks, scars, bruising, color) Contour (shape) Symmetry (upper to lower/right to left quadrants); visible bulges	Contour (visible movements) Skin (surgical incisions/ dressings) Umbilicus (position, contour, color, herniation) Visible hernias Rectum (skin surrounding anus)	Contour (traumatic disruption) Skin	Contour Skin
Auscultation	Bowel sounds (presence, timing, loudness)	Bowel sounds/ vascular sounds	Bowel sounds/ vascular sounds	Bowel sounds/ vascular sounds
Palpation	Turgor Light: pain/ tenderness Contents (fluid, air)	Fluid/air Deep: Organ position/size/ tumors Rectum Prostate Gland*	Deep: Guarding aortic pulsations	
Percussion	Fluid/air	Ascites (fluid wave, shifting dullness)		CVA tenderness
	Bladder distension			

*Considered an abdominal organ but has reproductive functions so is covered in Chap 29

Inspection: Level I

Inspection Techniques and Expected Findings

Inspection of the abdomen focuses on the surface characteristics of the skin and the contour of the abdomen. The skin should be intact without any evidence of a break in continuity or significant changes in color; color should be uniform and consistent with the skin color of the rest of the body. Depending on sun exposure, the abdomen color may be slightly paler than other sun exposed areas.

Inspect and assess any scars for their origin and the length of time they have been there.

The surface of the skin over the abdomen should be smooth and symmetrical without any evidence of localized bulges or protrusions.

Unexpected Findings

Surgical scars are generally linear in direction, contiguous, and smooth to the touch.

Traumatic scars may be larger and not necessarily contiguous or linear and may also contain a greater amount of scar tissue, making them feel rougher than the other skin. Traumatic scars may also appear somewhat patchy.

Old scars are lighter in color and may be somewhat recessed in the skin, while newer scars are pink to purple in color and may be slightly elevated.

Note and describe any other skin lesions. Common lesions include macules and papules in association with rashes, nodules, tumors, and possible areas of loss of pigmentation (patches).

Any localized bulges or protrusions may indicate the presence of a hernia, nodules, or tumors.

Inspection Techniques and Expected Findings

The contour of the abdomen is shaped by the contents within it and spans the area from the rib margins to the pubis. Assess the abdominal contour by looking horizontally, across the patient at the level of the abdomen. This may require sitting in a chair or flexing the knees to view across the abdomen's surface. Abdomens are commonly described as flat, scaphoid, rounded, or distended (Figure 28-10). The expected finding is a flat abdomen that demonstrates a surface that is level on the horizontal plane and is the standard for comparison.

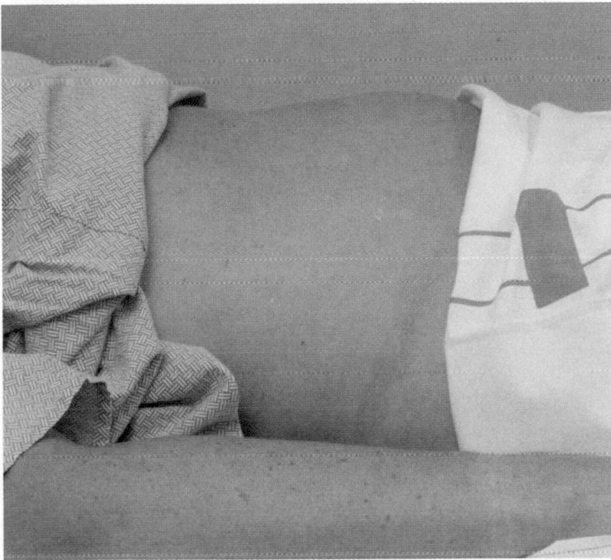

FIGURE 28-10 Abdominal contour

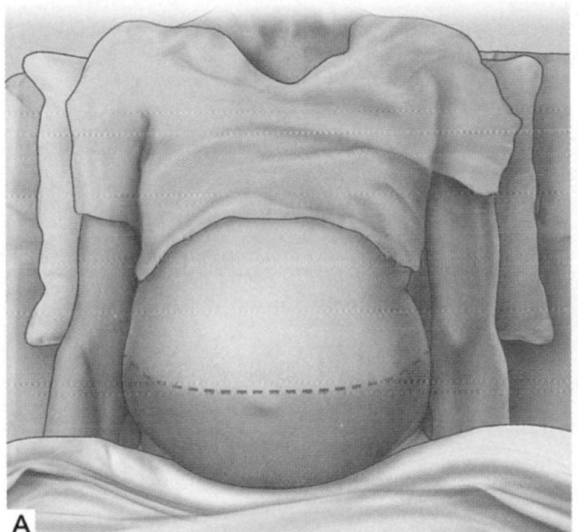

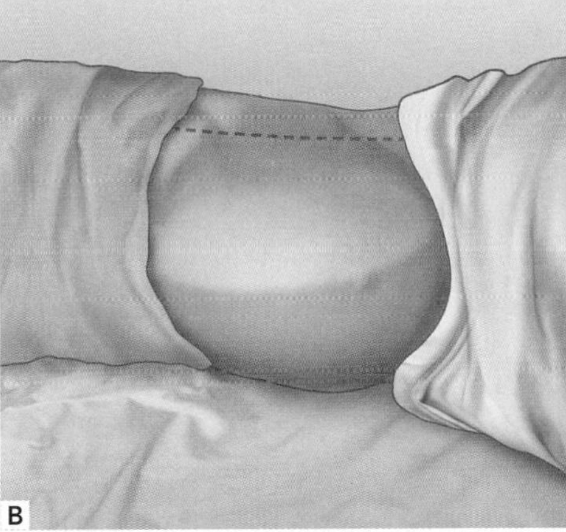

FIGURE 28-12A–B **a)** Bulging flank from fluid in the abdomen when patient is lying down; **b)** Reduced bulging when patient lies on side

Unexpected Findings

A scaphoid abdomen demonstrates a surface that is concave, giving the abdomen a sunken appearance.

A rounded abdomen demonstrates a surface that is convex, with the abdomen increasing in vertical width and then decreasing, reaching its highest level at the umbilicus.

A distended abdomen demonstrates a surface that is excessively rounded with the vertical width greatly increased (Figure 28-11). The point where a rounded abdomen becomes a distended abdomen is not well differentiated, so absolute criteria are not possible.

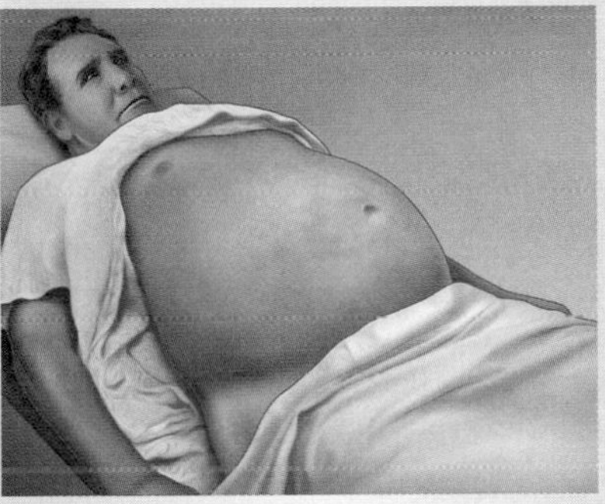

FIGURE 28-11 Distended abdomen

A distended abdomen may be filled with fluid or air. Differentiating between the two may be accomplished with various techniques.

The effects of gravity on the abdominal contents as well as knowledge of the properties of air and fluid help to differentiate the contents.

Fluid is free within the abdomen, so it will be drawn downward. When the patient is lying on the back, fluid is drawn downward into the flank area. Bulging flanks will thus be observed in a fluid-filled abdomen. When the patient is turned onto the side, the fluid will drain from the flank, reducing any bulging (Figure 28-12).

Fat, on the other hand, is attached to abdominal structures and not free floating. It may be present in the flank area when the patient is on the back, but when turned to the side, it will remain stationary and not be removed from the area.

Air, even though it is free within the abdomen, does not move around that much. An air-filled abdomen may appear as fluid; however, there is no noticeable accumulation in the flank area. When the patient is turned to the side, air may be drawn into the flank area, but its presence will not make a significant change in the flank's appearance (Figure 28-12).

Inspection Techniques and Expected Findings	Unexpected Findings
Observe symmetry by comparing the upper and lower sections, and right and left sections of the abdomen. The upper quadrants should be symmetrical with the lower quadrants and the right and left quadrants the same. Observe the abdomen for any bulges, which may indicate the presence of a hernia. There should not be any noticeable bulges.	The contour of the abdomen may appear asymmetrical in the presence of a hernia, a weakening of the muscles of the abdominal wall that allows abdominal contents to protrude to the surface. It is visible as a small lump or bump on the surface of the abdomen. Hernias have various causes and may or may not present as an emergency. They are generally described by their location on the abdomen and whether they are reducible or non-reducible. Most common, a reducible hernia means that its contents can be easily reduced or pushed back into its original location when pressure is applied. The contents of a nonreducible hernia cannot be pushed back, or the contents remain permanently until the hernia is repaired. It may become critical if the blood supply is cut off and the possibility of severe damage or death of the tissue of the hernia exists. Also called a *strangulated hernia*, it requires immediate attention and intervention. (Further information on hernias is in the Level II exam section.)

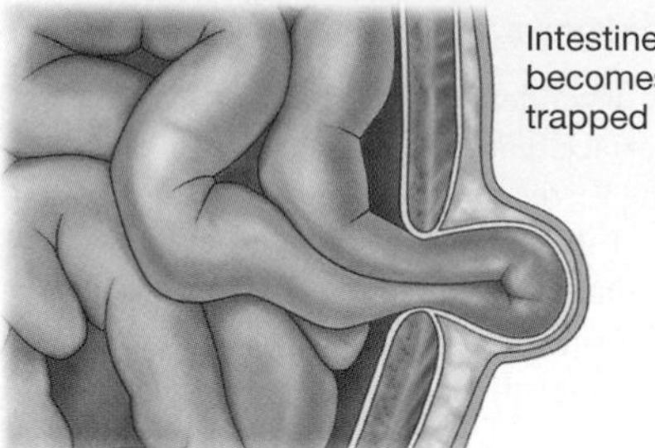

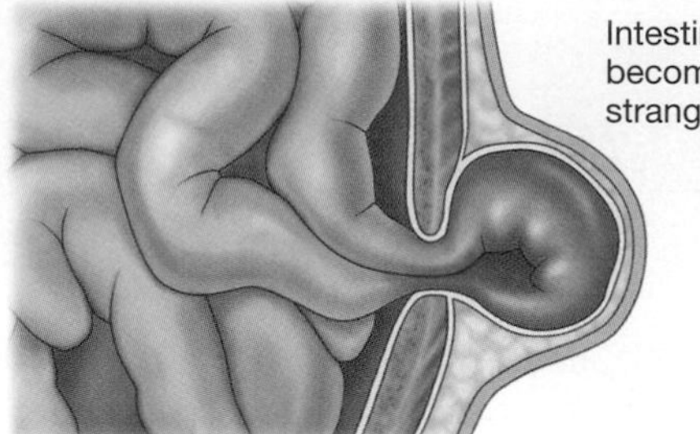

FIGURE 28-13 Nonreducible (strangulated) hernia

PRACTICE POINT: Distended Abdomens and Breathing Difficulties

It is important to remember that distended abdomens, whether they are filled with air or fluid, push up on the diaphragm, limiting its ability to contract and allow full expansion of the lungs. This may cause breathing difficulties for these individuals, particularly when supine. In the supine position, gravity pulls the fluid upward against the diaphragm. If the patient is able to have the head elevated, gravity will pull the fluid downward, away from the diaphragm, facilitating lung expansion. In obese individuals, the excessive weight of the fat may make it difficult for the intercostal muscles to contract and raise the rib cage. For these reasons, assess individuals with enlarged abdomens for any breathing difficulties.

Inspection: Level II

Inspection Techniques and Expected Findings	Unexpected Findings
Observe the contour of the abdomen for any movement. Movement associated with ventilations should demonstrate a smooth and even pattern. Males tend to be abdominal breathers, so abdominal movement is more observable in males.	Shallow breathing or limited movement of the abdomen in males suggests peritonitis or some other type of inflammation.
Peristalsis is generally not directly observed on the surface of the abdomen. Aortic pulsations are also generally not observed; however, they may be present in thin individuals.	Any ripple-like movement across a portion of the abdomen is unexpected and considered a possible indication of a bowel obstruction. Significant pulsations that are observable may indicate in increased pulse pressure or the presence of an abdominal aortic aneurysm.
Observe the characteristics of the umbilicus related to its location and contour. It should be centrally positioned on the midline of the abdomen (Figure 28-14). It is characteristically inverted or may protrude slightly.	Unexpected findings would be a displaced umbilicus laterally, downward or upward. Inflammation, swelling, or bulging around the umbilicus may indicate the presence of a hernia.
Postoperative patients will most likely have some type of dressing the covers the surgical site. In some instances, drainage equipment may be present to remove expected fluids from the site.	Note and describe any bleeding or other drainage from the site.

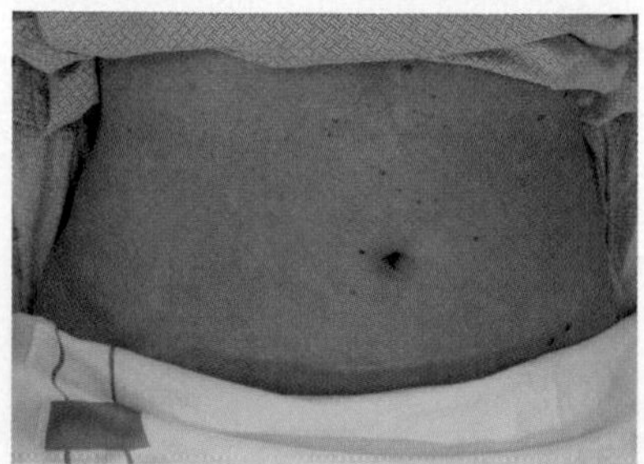

FIGURE 28-14 Umbilicus

Inspection Techniques and Expected Findings	Unexpected Findings

Hernias may not be directly observed on the abdomen and appear only when intra-abdominal pressure is increased. To observe for their presence, ask the patient to take a deep breath and hold it. This maneuver contracts the diaphragm, lowering it into the abdomen and compressing the abdominal organs. Any muscular weaknesses or hernias will protrude creating a visible bulge or mass.

Hernias may occur elsewhere on the body, but the majority are located on the lower torso, the abdominal wall hernias (see Figure 28-15). Hernias are commonly described according to their location on the abdomen or what specific structure may be involved.

An incisional hernia results from a weakness in the muscle that develops after a surgical incision (Figure 28-15). This occurs in approximately 2%–10% of abdominal surgeries.

Inguinal hernias, although they involve the protrusion of abdominal contents, are not located directly on the abdomen. Inguinal hernias present as bulges in the groin area. (These hernias are covered more extensively in Chapter 29.)

Another hernia located in the groin area is a femoral hernia.

Other less common types of hernias are identified and described in Table 28-6.

Begin the rectal examination with inspection of the sacrococcygeal and perianal areas. The skin of the perianal area in the adult is somewhat more pigmented in color and coarser than the skin over the buttocks. The skin should be smooth and without any evidence of dimpling or skin lesions.

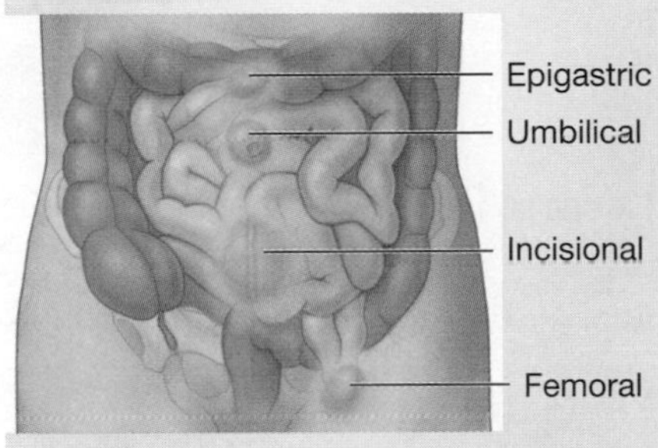

FIGURE 28-15 Examples of hernias

Table 28-6 Examples of hernias

Type	Location	Characteristics
Common Hernias		
Incisional	Site of abdominal surgery	Protrudes from the area around the surgical scar, and may return even after repair
Femoral	Appears just below the inguinal crease, about mid-thigh	Results from passage of abdominal contents through the femoral canal, the opening through which the femoral artery, vein, and nerve leave the abdomen to enter the thigh. This is generally a tight space, but may enlarge to permit passage of abdominal contents. Women are more likely to develop. Carry a high risk of becoming non-reducible and strangulated.
Umbilical	Protrusions of abdominal contents around the umbilicus. Mostly seen in infants at birth, but may appear later in adult life.	Relatively common, represent 10%–30% of all hernias. Those occurring in later years are due to increased intra-abdominal pressure caused by obesity, heavy lifting, coughing, straining at bowel movements, chronic lung disease, ascites, or pregnancy (females).
Less Common Hernias		
Epigastric hernias	Between navel and lower border of rib cage, along midline (linea alba)	Contain fatty tissue, not intestine; painless and non-reducible
Obturator hernias	Protrudes through obturator of pelvic bone.	Very rare; develop in females. Do not appear as bulge, and may cause nausea and vomiting.
Spigelian hernias	Diastasis recti—appear several inches from midline along edge of rectus abdominis muscle	Quite rare

Inspection Techniques and Expected Findings	Unexpected Findings

Inspect the anus by spreading the buttocks apart. If lighting is poor, a penlight or lamp may be necessary. Inspect the anus and surrounding skin, noting the presence of any skin tags, skin lesions, external hemorrhoids, fissures, or fistulas.

During inspection, ask the patient to bear down, which will make any of these alterations more apparent.

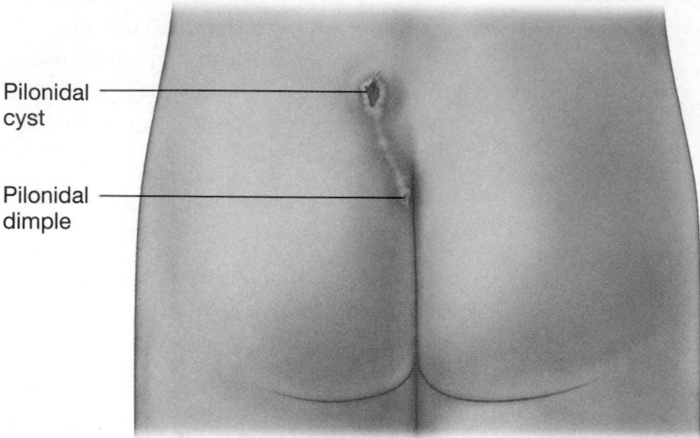

FIGURE 28-16 Pilonidal dimple and cyst

Unexpected findings would include pilonidal dimpling with or without tufts of hair (Figure 28-16). These are manifestations of a pilonidal cyst or sinus. These were previously considered congenital anomalies; however, these theories are questionable at present (Doerr, 2009).

Present thinking is that they are caused by penetration of loose hairs into the skin, causing an inflammatory reaction. They appear to be related to excessive and repetitive trauma or pressure. They are more common in males, particularly between the ages of 15–24, and rarely occur after 40. Pilonidal cysts are generally not problematic, but they may be complicated by formation of an abscess, infection, or fistula.

Other unexpected findings include anal (venereal) warts and hemorrhoids (external). Reddened, irritated perianal skin may be caused by fungal infections in adults and pinworms in children.

Inspection: Level III

Observe individuals who present with nontraumatic acute abdominal pain for skin color changes. Inspection of the abdomen from traumatic causes focuses on alterations of the skin surface. Abdominal trauma may be identified as either blunt or penetrating. Blunt trauma occurs from a forceful impact of the abdomen with another object causing abdominal injury. The injuries may be caused by compression, crushing, shearing, or deceleration of the abdominal organs.

Individuals who may have had intra-abdominal bleeding will most likely manifest with pale skin. Individuals who may have a liver disorder will present with skin that is jaundiced.

Penetrating abdominal trauma is caused by some object or weapon that directly enters the abdominal cavity, causing direct damage and injury to the organs and structures of the abdomen. The force behind the object is strong enough to penetrate through the skin and muscles before entering the abdomen; therefore there is damage to the skin as well as the underlying organs. Hemorrhaging of varying severity is most likely present and related to the severity of the injury as well as what organ(s) is/are involved. Blood is lost directly to the outside and does not accumulate within the abdominal cavity.

The most common actions associated with blunt trauma are motor vehicle collisions, assaults, recreational accidents, or falls (Udeani & Reinberg, 2009). There may be evidence of bruising on the skin surface, but force behind it or its size prevents it from breaking through skin surface. Hemorrhaging is a frequent complication of blunt trauma, with blood accumulating in the abdominal cavity. Bleeding may be from the traumatized liver, spleen, or blood vessels.

Ecchymosis that is visible in the skin of the abdomen suggests the presence of an active intra-abdominal or retroperitoneal hemorrhage. Periumbilical ecchymosis (Cullen's sign) or flank ecchymosis (Grey Turner sign) may be present in as many as 3% of individuals with acute pancreatitis, but not until a few days after onset. Rarely, it may accompany ectopic/ruptured pregnancy, but is not considered to be diagnostically significant. In the absence of significant manifestations of abdominal conditions, ecchymosis may indicate a bleeding disorder.

Inspection: Level IV

There are no specific observations that need to be made in Level IV that are not part of the Level I and Level II observations.

Auscultation: Levels I–IV

Auscultation for the abdominal exam is done prior to palpation and percussion. While different from the usual sequence of examination techniques, it is done this way because palpation and percussion performed prior to auscultation could alter the characteristics of the bowel sounds.

The purpose for auscultation of the abdomen is to document the presence of bowel sounds and any other sounds. There is no gradation of bowel sounds; thus there is no need for leveling auscultation for the abdominal exam. With practice and expertise, the provider will refine they technique for auscultation and be able to identify and differentiate various sounds.

Auscultation Techniques and Expected Findings	Unexpected Findings
Listening for bowel sounds begins with lightly placing the stethoscope on the abdomen. The stethoscope must be warm because a cold stethoscope may cause the abdominal muscles to contract. Initially place the stethoscope in the right lower quadrant and then move up, across, and down to listen in the other three quadrants (Figure 28-17). Their presence or absence in each quadrant is an important parameter to assess in postoperative and posttraumatic patients. 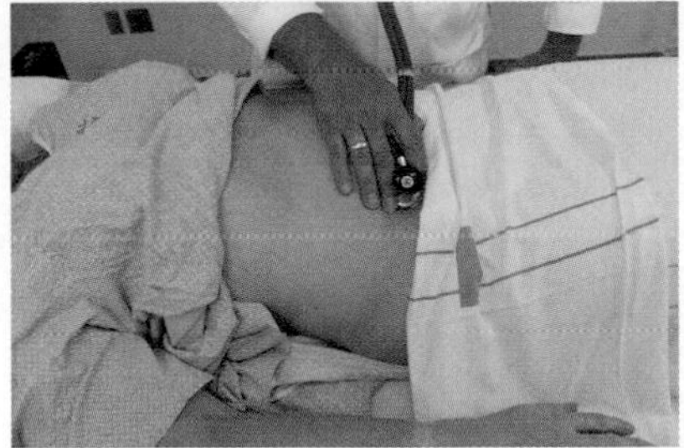 FIGURE 28-17 Auscultation of the abdomen	***PRACTICE POINT: Bowel Sounds*** Bowel sounds are not specifically associated with a particular location and are widely distributed through the abdomen, and because they echo throughout the abdomen, listening for and documenting their presence in one location is sufficient unless more specificity is needed. If so, then listening for bowel sounds in all four quadrants is done.
Bowel sounds are produced by peristalsis through the alimentary tract, primarily the intestines, occur in irregular cycles, and are heard from 5–35 times per minute. The hollow intestines allow bowel sounds to echo throughout the abdomen. Bowel sounds are commonly referred to as high-pitched clicks and gurgles. Gurgles are more descriptive of the sounds than clicks. There is also a rumbling characteristic to the sound, somewhat like thunder. The sound may be likened to the sound of air moving through a fluid, as heard when air is blown through a straw that is immersed in a glass of water. The actual sound is not significant as it may vary, but their presence is of great importance. Bowel sounds are low pitched, but are adequately heard with the diaphragm. The bell component may be used, but in most instances pressing the bell tightly against the skin in essence creates a diaphragm.	Alterations in timing and pitch are most commonly associated with alterations of the abdomen or abdominal organs. Altered bowel sounds are described as either hypoactive or hyperactive. Hypoactive bowel sounds are heard less than 3–4 times per minute. Hypoactive or absent bowel sounds are commonly associated with peritonitis and paralytic ileus. Paralytic ileus is common after abdominal surgery or trauma. Disruption to the intestines by handling during surgery or from significant trauma can cause them to stop functioning for a period of time. The return of bowel sounds is then important to identify.
Borborygmi are hyperactive bowel sounds that are loud and prolonged; heard without a stethoscope and described frequently as stomach growling. They occur frequently when one is hungry. Auscultation of the abdomen for the presence of bowel sounds may give evidence as to the severity and duration of the obstruction.	Hyperactive bowel sounds are not necessarily associated with an increase in occurrence; however, this might be the case in some instances. They are frequently higher in pitch and result from air and fluid under increased pressure, thus are frequently an early indicator of bowel obstruction.

Auscultation Techniques and Expected Findings	Unexpected Findings
PRACTICE POINT: Establishing Absent Bowel Sounds The absence of bowel sounds is a significant finding and indicates a potential problem. The length of time that the provider needs to listen over the abdomen in order to establish the absence of bowel sounds has not been clearly identified. Previous requirements indicate that only after listening for 5 minutes in each quadrant can it be documented that bowel sounds are absent. Practically speaking, listening to the abdomen for 20 minutes seems rather inefficient and ineffective. Current recommendations vary from listening for at least 1 minute over various parts of the abdomen (White & Counselman, 2009) to listening for 2–3 minutes with no indication as to where.	Borborygmi may also be an indicator of a bowel obstruction, a partial or complete blockage of the small or large intestine that prevents transportation of food, fluid, or gas through the intestines. As with hernias, the blood supply to the tissues distal to the obstruction may end abruptly, causing death of the affected tissues. This is also referred to as ischemic bowel or strangulated bowel. In the early stage of the obstruction, the bowel sounds will be hyperactive as there is an attempt by the intestines to eliminate the obstruction. In the late stages, the bowel sounds are hypoactive or may be absent.
Auscultate for vascular sounds after auscultating for bowel sounds, using the bell of the stethoscope. Auscultate over the aorta, renal, iliac, and femoral arteries for the presence of bruits (Figure 28-18). Vascular sounds, unlike bowel sounds, are not well transmitted throughout the abdomen; therefore the stethoscope should be directly over the site corresponding with the specific artery. Expected findings would be the absence of any vascular sounds.	Unexpected findings would be the presence of bruits heard over a particular artery. If present, a thorough exam of the peripheral vascular system in the lower extremities is essential.
Other sounds that may be heard during auscultation are vascular sounds, typically bruits due to atherosclerosis of the major abdominal arteries. Unless it is specifically known that these may be heard during auscultation, vascular sounds may not be identified while listening for bowel sounds. This is especially true if bowel sounds are assessed by listening in one location. Don't try to listen for bowel sounds and vascular sounds at the same time. If vascular sounds are heard during auscultation, first pay attention to the characteristics of the bowel sounds and then give your attention to the vascular sounds. 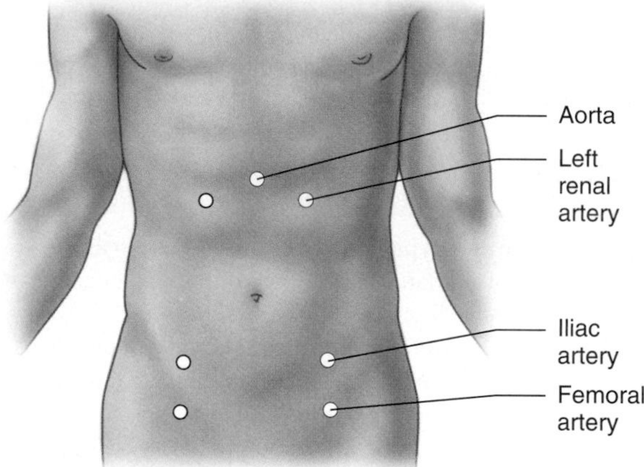 FIGURE 28-18 Sites for auscultating vascular sounds	Another unexpected sound is a friction rub, a grating, leathery sound caused by inflamed tissues rubbing over each other. In the abdomen, it is associated with inflammation of the peritoneum surrounding an organ resulting from a tumor, infection, or an infarct. They are best heard with the diaphragm and correlate with ventilations. A venous hum may be heard in the epigastric region and around the umbilicus. This is heard with the bell and as a soft, low-pitched, continuous sound. It is present when collateral circulation between the portal and systemic systems is increased.

Palpation: Level I

Palpation Techniques and Expected Findings	Unexpected Findings
The skin of the abdomen should also be smooth, mobile, and reflect adequate hydration by returning immediately to its original location after it has been pinched together.	The skin of dehydrated patients will demonstrate tenting.
Palpate the organs of the abdomen for the presence of masses, fluid, and tenderness as well as for size, mobility, and consistency. Not all organs are palpable. Before initiating palpation, determine if the patient has an empty bladder; a full bladder may cause discomfort or give the impression of an abdominal mass or tumor.	

Palpation Techniques and Expected Findings

Palpation is usually performed with the provider on the right side of the patient, or vice versa if the provider is left-handed (Figure 28-19).

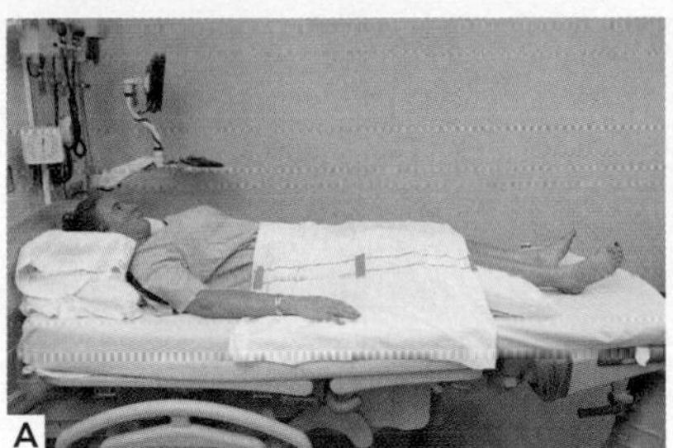
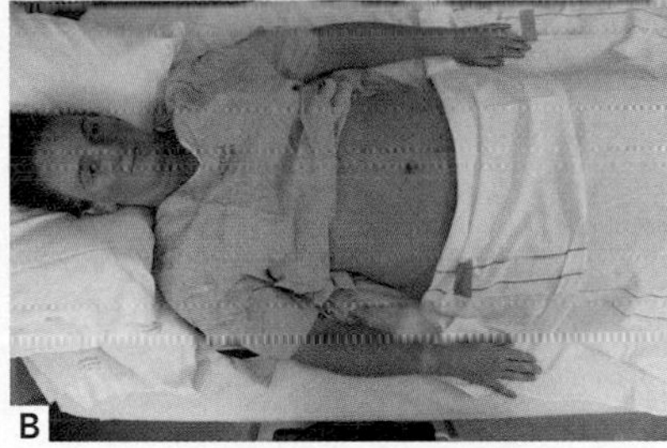

FIGURE 28-19A–B Position for palpation

The patient's abdominal muscles must be relaxed, which is accomplished through patient positioning as described previously.

Make sure your hands are warm to prevent involuntary muscle contraction in response to applying cold hands. Perform palpation in two stages: light and deep. Palpation of patients who are overweight or obese is ineffective.

Light palpation is done initially to determine the presence of any tenderness or pain. It is performed using the palmar surface of the hand and fingers, with the fingers approximated with each other (Figure 28-20). Lightly depress the abdomen no more than 1 cm, using a gentle, circular motion as the hand is moved over the surface of the abdomen in all four quadrants. When moving from one location to the other, lift the hand off the skin surface. Sliding or dragging the hand between areas may initiate a tickling response from the patient. Palpation is usually begun in the RLQ; however, if the patient has indicated the presence of pain or tenderness in that area, start in a different location and end in the affected area. The abdomen should feel smooth, with a consistent degree of softness.

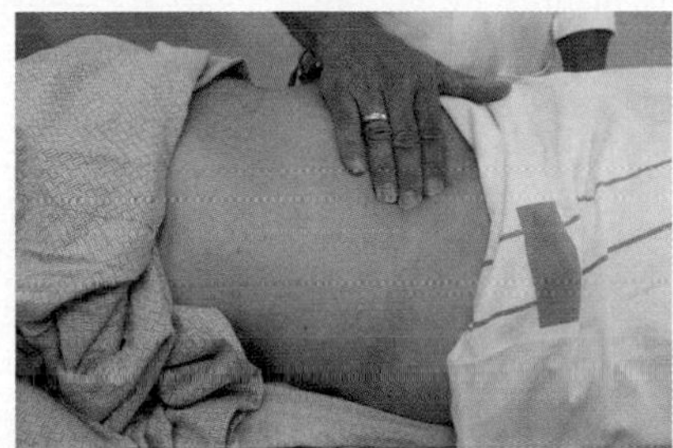

FIGURE 28-20 Light palpation

An area of tenderness may also be determined with cutaneous hypersensitivity. This is done by pinching the skin together between the thumb and index finger and gently lifting the fold of skin up, away from the underlying muscle. Another way to assess is to gently stimulate the skin with a tapered point. In both instances, have the patient describe the sensation. If the area is hypersensitive, the patient will indicate pain or an increased sensation in the area.

This should be performed prior to beginning palpation and can be accomplished by assessing skin turgor on the abdomen.

PRACTICE POINT: The Ticklish Patient

Palpation of a ticklish patient presents a challenge, but may be done using certain techniques. First, use slow, firm strokes. When moving from one location to another, pick the hand up off the abdomen; moving it lightly across the skin may initiate a tickling response. Another technique is to initiate palpation by using the patient's own hand. It is generally impossible to tickle oneself, so using the patient's hand helps to reduce tickling stimuli. Place the patient's hand on the abdomen where you plan to begin, and then place your hand over the patient's hand. This is basically the bimanual technique, using the patient's hand as the bottom one. Begin palpation with your fingers slightly beyond the patient's. As palpation proceeds, gradually move your hand off the patient's hand until you are doing the palpation. It also helps to have the patient not look at the abdomen during the procedure so that when your hand slides off the patient's, the patient doesn't see it.

Unexpected Findings

Depending on the degree of surgery or trauma to the abdomen, palpation may cause more pain to the patient than is necessary. If determining recovery from peritoneal irritation or inflammation, light palpation may be used to determine whether pain is resolving or not.

Pay close attention to the patient's facial expressions as he or she may indicate pain when it is denied or minimized verbally.

Muscle rigidity may occur if pressing too deeply or too quickly. Rigidity will also occur when approaching an area of tenderness. Proceed cautiously when around the tender area.

Palpation: Level II

Palpation Techniques and Expected Findings	Unexpected Findings

Before beginning deep palpation, it may be appropriate to do moderate palpation, which is performed in the same manner as light, only with a greater amount of pressure, palpating deeper into the abdomen.

Deep palpation follows moderate or light palpation, depending on the condition of the patient. Deep palpation reaches deeper into the abdomen and more thoroughly identifies abdominal organs, any enlarged organs (organomegaly), and any elusive masses.

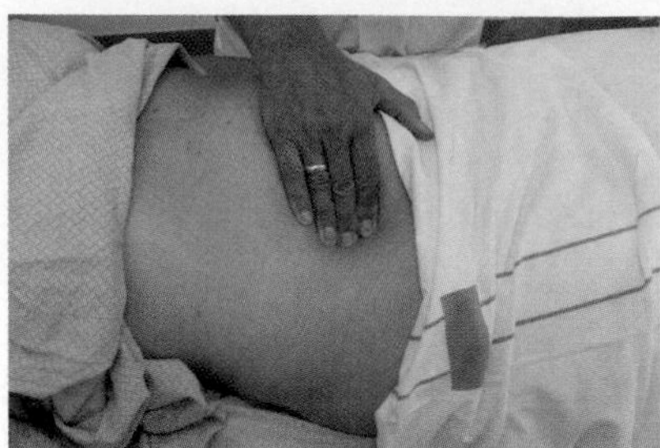

FIGURE 28-21 Deep palpation

For deep palpation, use the same technique with the exception that the hand approaches the abdomen in a more vertical position than previously (Figure 28-21). Use a slow, circular motion, lifting the fingers off the skin surface in between each palpation. Deep palpation may be more uncomfortable for the patient, but in the absence of any inflammatory conditions, it should not elicit true tenderness. Deep palpation may elicit tenderness not obtained on light or moderate palpation, but should be differentiated from the uncomfortable sensation experienced.

Deep palpation may also be performed directly or indirectly. Direct palpation is performed with one hand doing the pressing and feeling.

Indirect palpation is performed with one hand placed over the other. In this manner, the bottom hand is doing the feeling and the top hand is doing the pressing. Using two hands is also referred to as the bimanual technique (Figure 28-22).

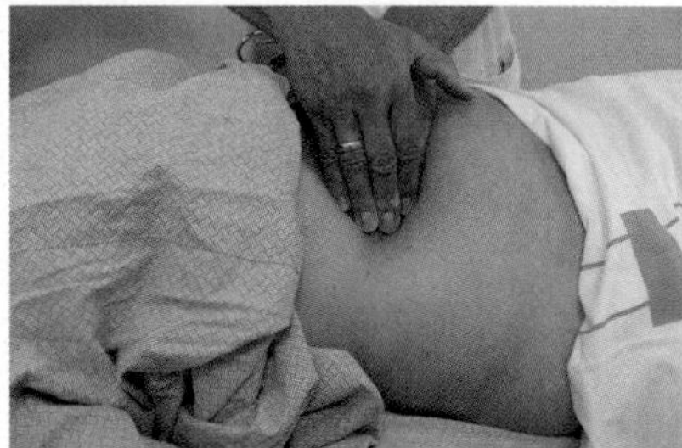

FIGURE 28-22 Bimanual (indirect) palpation technique

Deep palpation is also used to palpate the liver and spleen. Palpation of the spleen is described in Chapter 21.

Because the liver lies in the upper right quadrant and is protected by the lower right rib cage, it is only possible to palpate its lower edge. Inform the patient about possible discomfort if it takes extra downward pressure to palpate for the liver edge, but it should not be painful.

To begin palpation, place the left hand, palm side up, under the right lumbar region parallel to the costal arch. (If needed, use the left hand to elevate the right side of the thorax in a slightly higher position, facilitating palpation.)

Place the fingers of the right hand flat on the upper right abdomen, parallel to the costal arch and with the index finger below the lower border of the liver. Generally use the radial side of the right index finger to palpate.

Request the patient to breathe in calmly and deeply through the mouth. (*During inspiration, the liver is displaced caudally by the contracting diaphragm.*) While the patient is inhaling, make a careful, gliding motion with the right hand in the cranial direction. It may also help to have the patient hold inspiration a bit longer so that the lower edge of the liver is at its lowest position.

If the border of the liver is not felt, repeat this process after repositioning the palpating hand slightly in the cranial direction (Figure 28-23). Repeat this process until you reach the right costal arch.

Unexpected Findings

Tenderness not evident on light palpation may be elicited during moderate palpation.

Any masses that are palpated should be assessed for location, size, shape, consistency, mobility, pulsatility, and tenderness.

A pulse that is directed laterally indicates the possibility of an aortic aneurysm.

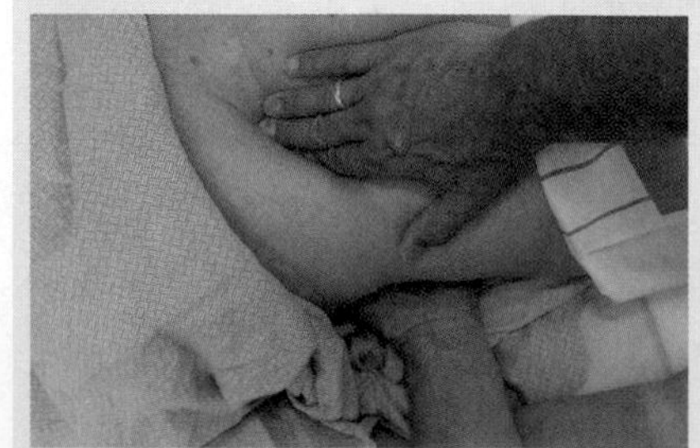

FIGURE 28-23 Palpation of the liver

Palpation Techniques and Expected Findings	Unexpected Findings
This procedure can also be performed by placing the right hand on the upper right abdomen so that the fingertips point in the direction of the costal arch. The liver edge may be difficult to palpate. Less abdominal tissue makes it easier to palpate and possibly feel the lower edge of the border. The costal margin is generally considered the lower edge of the liver, so it should not be easily palpated below this margin. If the liver edge is palpated, it should feel smooth, firm, and without any nodules or bumps. The patient may experience some discomfort while you apply pressure during inspiration, but there should not be any tenderness or pain.	
The hooking method is another technique to palpate the lower edge of the liver. To perform, stand to the right of the patient's chest at a slight angle, somewhat parallel to the right costal margin. Place the fingertips on the lower edge of the costal margin, curling them over the edge of the right costal margin (Figure 28-24). Ask the patient to take a deep breath, and gently, but firmly, pull inward and upward with your fingers. 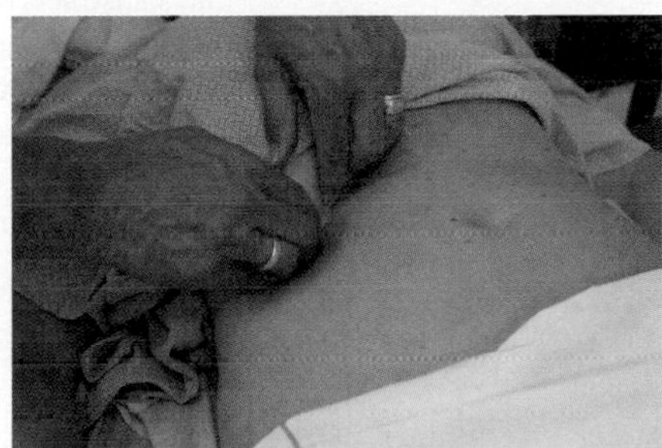 **FIGURE 28-24** Hooking technique	A hard, firm liver suggests cancer. Palpable hard nodules frequently occur with tumors, metastatic cancer, late cirrhosis, or syphilis. Tenderness may result from vascular engorgement associated with congestive heart failure, acute hepatitis, or abscess. A liver more than 1-3 cm below the costal margin is considered enlarged (unless pressed down by the diaphragm). Enlargement may be due to hepatitis, liver tumors, cirrhosis, and vascular engorgement.
Other organs that may be palpated but not necessarily routinely are the gallbladder, kidneys, and bladder. Evaluation for cholecystitis may be done by having the patient take a deep breath during deep palpation. The kidneys are considered non-palpable; however, in certain individuals the lower pole of the right kidney may be palpable. Palpating the kidneys is performed from the patient's right side with the provider's left hand reaching over the patient and placing in on the left flank. Place the right hand along the patient's left costal margin. Have the patient take in a deep breath and as this occurs, lift the left flank up with the left hand and palpate deeply with the right hand. Reverse sides but have the same position and location of the hands as for the left. Another technique that may be used is to capture the kidney. This maneuver requires that you move to the left side when trying to capture the left kidney, and move back to the right side for the right kidney. Place your hands in the same location as before, and instruct the patient to take in a deep breath. At the peak of inspiration, press the fingers of both hands together, attempting to capture the kidney in between them. Have the patient exhale and simultaneously release the fingers. A captured kidney may be felt between the fingers as it returns to its original place.	The gallbladder is not palpable unless it becomes inflamed. When the inflamed gallbladder makes contact with the provider's fingers, pain will result and the patient will abruptly stop inhaling. This response is known as Murphy's sign.
The bladder may be palpated to determine whether it is distended with urine or not. This is not routinely performed unless there is a question as to whether the patient is unable to empty the bladder, or the patient may complain of the urge to urinate but is unable to do so. Generally, the bladder is not palpable unless it is distended with urine. If it is necessary to determine if the bladder is distended, percussion may be used. The borders of the bladder can be identified by where the percussion tone changes from tympany to dullness when percussing in the suprapubic area. Palpation is also used to perform the rectal examination, which consists of palpation of the anal sphincter, anal ring, and anterior, posterior, and lateral rectal walls. To perform the rectal exam, the patient needs to be positioned appropriately. Depending on the age and mobility, the patient may assume one of three positions. Appropriate draping is also necessary for patient comfort and modesty.	A distended bladder is palpated as a smooth, round, nontender mass in the symphysis pubis area. Palpating a full bladder may be uncomfortable for the patient.

Palpation Techniques and Expected Findings	Unexpected Findings
Begin the exam by putting a glove on the examining hand and lubricating the index finger. Place the lubricated finger on the anal opening and exert a gentle pressure (Figure 28-25). While doing this, ask the patient to bear down to relax the external sphincter.	
As the sphincter relaxes, slip the finger into the anal canal. Inform the patient that he or she will feel the need to have a bowel movement, but that this will not occur.	
With your finger at the external sphincter, test its tone by asking the patient to tighten the external sphincter around your finger. There should be an even contraction of the sphincter around your finger and no discomfort.	A loose or weak contraction may indicate a neurological alteration.
At this point, rotate your finger to palpate the muscular anal ring. This should feel smooth with even pressure felt on the finger. Note the presence of any nodules or other lesions.	An extremely tight contraction may indicate scarring or spasticity from a fissure or other lesion, inflammation, or anxiety related to the exam.
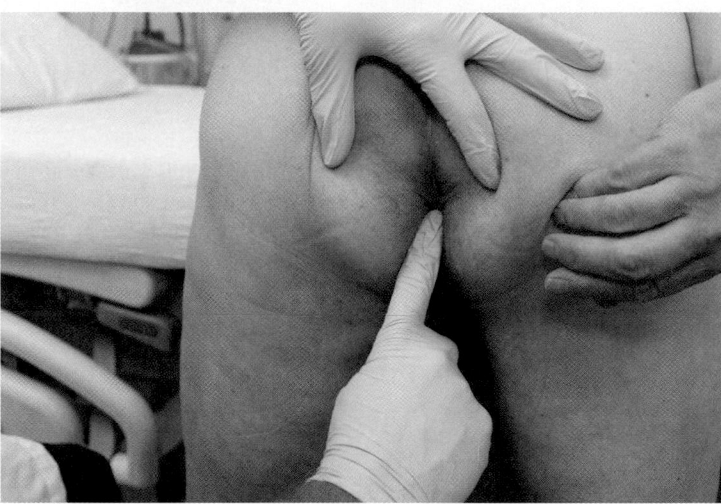 FIGURE 28-25 Palpation of rectum	The presence of an anal fissure of fistula may cause severe tenderness and pain that local anesthesia may be necessary to complete the exam. Rectal pain frequently accompanies a local alteration such as irritation, hardened feces (constipation), fissures, or thrombosed hemorrhoids. Note the presence of any nodules, masses, polyps, or tenderness. The presence of any of these requires a more thorough follow up examination by colonoscopy or sigmoidoscopy. In females, a uterus that is retroverted or retroflexed may be palpated through the rectal wall. It may also be possible to palpate the cervix through the anterior rectal wall. This is covered in Chapter 30.
Next, insert your finger all the way into the rectum, approximately 6–10 cm, and then rotate your finger as you palpate the posterior and lateral rectal walls (Figure 28-26). The rectal walls should feel smooth, even, without interruption.	Note also any blood or pus that may be present. Color changes of the stool may provide information as to what conditions may be present.
Next, rotate the finger to palpate the anterior rectal wall. The anterior rectal wall should feel the same as the posterior rectal wall. In males, this position is used to palpate the prostate gland. This portion of the exam is covered in Chapter 29.	Light-colored stools, tan or gray, are associated with liver conditions that alter bilirubin metabolism and lead to jaundice.
After palpation of the anterior wall, ask the patient to bear down again. This allows your finger to reach a few more centimeters into the rectum. When this is completed, slowly withdraw your finger and examine it for any fecal material. If any is present, it should be soft and brown.	Black, tarry stools are associated with upper intestinal bleeding. Lower intestinal bleeding may not create any color change, but blood may be observed in or on the stools. Occult blood, blood that is not directly visible, that may be present can be tested for by a guaiac test.
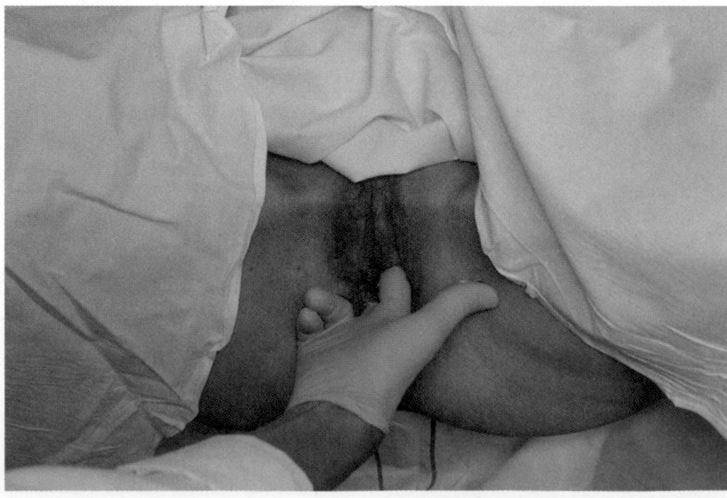 FIGURE 28-26 Palpation of rectal walls	

Palpation: Level III

Level III palpation is performed on patients who present to emergency facilities for treatment. The most common causes or conditions that initiate the need for emergency care are acute abdominal pain and abdominal trauma.

Palpation Techniques and Expected Findings	Unexpected Findings

Acute abdominal pain is caused by an intra-abdominal process resulting in severe pain. There are myriad causes of acute abdominal pain, which may be related to six broad categories: [1] inflammatory, [2] mechanical, [3] neoplastic, [4] vascular, [5] congenital defects, and [6] traumatic.

Three types of pain associated with abdominal alterations are visceral, parietal, and referred.

Visceral pain originates in the abdominal organs; it is characterized as a dull sensation and is poorly localized. **Parietal pain** originates from the peritoneum, commonly due to an underlying irritation or inflammation; it is characterized as sharp and intense and is localized to a specific area.

Referred pain is felt at a site or area that is away from the pathological organ (Figure 28-27).

Examples of each include the following:

Inflammatory—appendicitis, PID

Mechanical/neoplastic—obstruction disorders

Vascular—thrombosis/embolism, hemorrhage

Congenital—duodenal atresia, diaphragmatic hernia

Trauma—stab/gunshot wounds, blunt abdominal injuries

PRACTICE POINT: Carnett's Test: Differentiating Visceral from Peritoneal Pain

First, identify the location of maximal tenderness. Next, instruct the patient to lift the head off the table during palpation. This maneuver contracts the abdominal muscles and produces "induced guarding." If the patient indicates an increase in pain, or increased tenderness, this is a positive result and suggests abdominal wall tenderness/peritonitis. If the patient reports feeling better, the test is negative and is more likely to be organ tenderness.

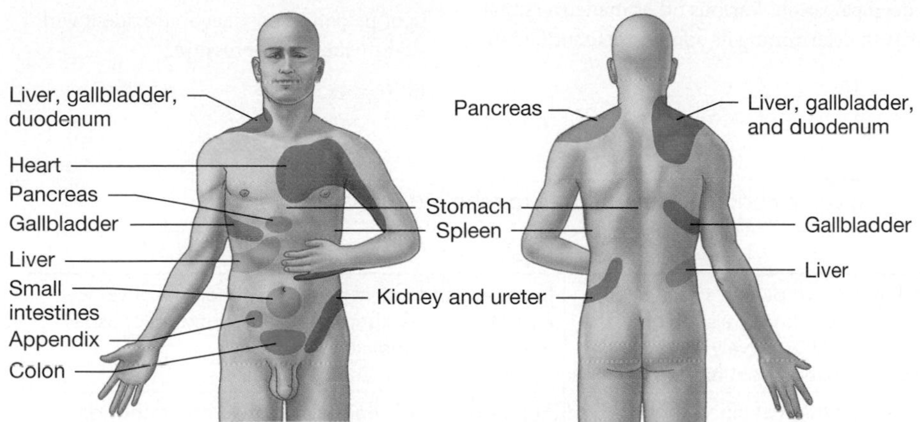

FIGURE 28-27 Sites of referred pain

PRACTICE POINT: Rebound Tenderness

Rebound tenderness is described as tenderness elicited indirectly by the sudden release of a deeply palpating hand and has been considered the clinical benchmark for the presence of peritonitis. Its use as a diagnostic maneuver, however, has been identified as unnecessary, and cruel and unusual punishment. Gentle percussion of the abdomen is more precise and localizing (Whang, Ashley, & Zinner, 2008). In instances in which the patient has not complained of pain and pain is elicited with rebound tenderness, it is an appropriate maneuver and should be documented as such.

Palpation Techniques and Expected Findings	Unexpected Findings
Abdominal trauma may be nonpenetrating or penetrating. Palpation of patients with penetrating abdominal trauma in the Level III examination is contraindicated. Light palpation of the patient with blunt abdominal trauma is primarily used to identify and locate areas of tenderness. It may also be used to determine if a hernia is reducible or not. Before initiating palpation, have the patient point to the location with the greatest pain so this location may be assessed last and with less pressure. In addition, the provider may ask the patient to cough. It is helpful to the provider if the patient can differentiate tenderness, which is localized, from pain, which tends to be more diffuse. Ask the patient to indicate if it hurts more when pressing on the abdomen. Follow up by placing the palm side of the hand over the rectus abdominis muscle and gently pressing down. Ask the patient to take a slow and deep breath in. Continue by palpating the abdomen lightly with one finger. Start as far away as possible from the identified area of tenderness. Gradually move toward this location. If there is an area of significant tenderness, repeat the examination several times. The presence of guarding is an indicator that caution should be exercised during the remainder of the exam. Deep palpation is used to identify enlarged organs and/or the presence of any masses, which can be solid or pulsatile. Before doing deep palpation, perform intermediate or moderate palpation. Use clinical judgment to determine progression to deep palpation. Various other maneuvers that may be used to assess peritoneal tenderness and assist in determining its source are identified in Table 28-7.	If inflammation is suspected, the patient will be able to indicate the location of the pain. Guarding or rigidity of the muscle is an indication for the presence of peritonitis. Voluntary guarding is the conscious contraction of the abdominal muscles due to anticipation of pain or an attempt to reduce ticklishness. Involuntary guarding is a protective reflex that causes flexion of the abdominal muscles to protect the internal organs. Localized tenderness should provide consistent results upon reexamination. If the tenderness is diffuse and without muscle rigidity, inflammation of the peritoneum is unlikely. Tenderness that is not apparent with light palpation may become evident with slightly increased pressure.

Table 28-7 Indicators of peritoneal irritation in acute abdomen (alternatives to rebound tenderness)

Maneuver	Procedure	Findings
Psoas sign	Place right hand above patient's right knee; have patient flex right knee (raise thigh) against resistance. Alternatively, have patient turn side to side, extend right hip/leg.	Increased abdominal pain with either maneuver is a positive psoas sign, suggesting irritation of psoas muscle by appendicitis.
Obturator sign	Flex patient's right thigh at hip; with knee bent, rotate the leg internally at hip.	Right hypogastric pain is a positive obturator sign, suggesting irritation of obturator muscle by an inflamed appendix.
Cutaneous hyperesthesia	At a series of points down the abdominal wall, gently pick up a fold of skin between thumb and index finger without pinching the skin. Should not be painful at any area.	Localized pain in all or part of RLQ may accompany appendicitis.
Rovsing's sign	Apply pressure in LLQ.	Pain in RLQ is a positive Rovsing's sign, suggesting appendicitis.
Other Signs That Are Significant in Acute Abdomen		
Murphy's sign	Occurs during moderate to deep palpation.	Abrupt interruption of inspiration during palpation of RUQ suggests acute cholecystitis.
Kehr's sign	Severe pain in left shoulder	Splenic rupture Ectopic pregnancy rupture
McBurney's sign	Tenderness localized at point 2/3 distance for anterior iliac spine to umbilicus in RLQ	Appendicitis
Cullen's sign	Bluish discoloration around umbilicus	Retroperitoneal hemorrhage (hemorrhagic pancreatitis) Rupture of abdominal aortic aneurysm
Grey-Turner's sign	Discoloration of flank area	Retroperitoneal hemorrhage (hemorrhagic pancreatitis) Rupture of abdominal aortic aneurysm

Palpation: Level IV

No specific palpation maneuvers are needed for a Level IV examination. Instead, specific palpation techniques at this level are based on the patient's condition and presenting manifestations. In some instances the provider may want to assess abdominal reflexes (Chapter 26).

Percussion: Level I

Percussion Techniques and Expected Findings

Percussion is performed to assess size and density of abdominal organs and for the presence of air, fluid, and masses. Abdominal percussion is generally performed indirectly, with the provider hitting a finger that is placed on the abdomen with a finger of the opposite hand (Figure 28-28).

Percussion follows the same order as palpation. Avoid or assess last identified areas of tenderness. Percussion of the abdomen should produce tympany over areas that are primarily filled with air or are hollow (stomach, small and large intestines).

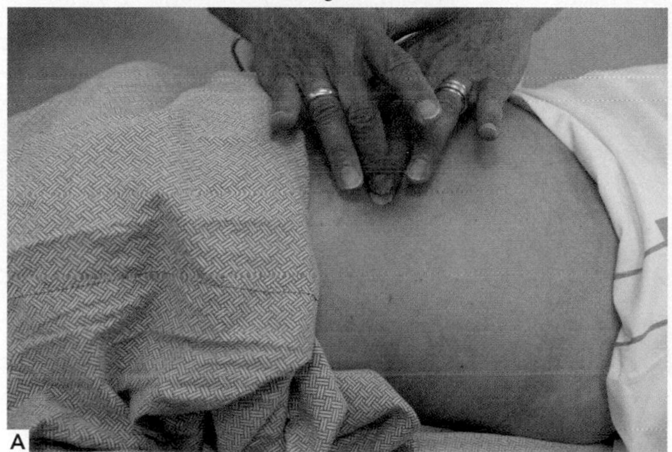

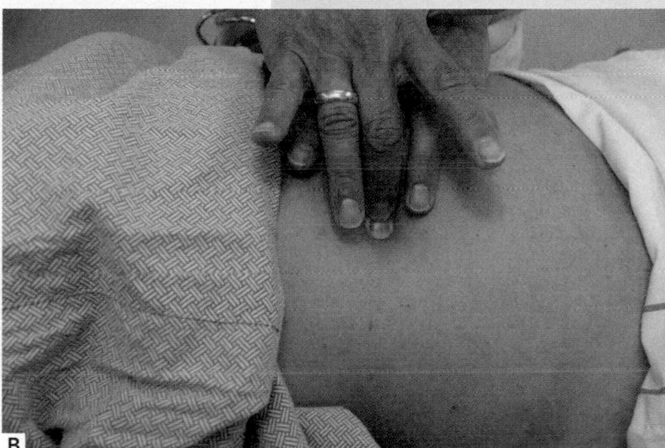

FIGURE 28-28A–B Percussion of the abdomen

Percussion is typically used to differentiate air from fluid in a distended abdomen. Initial percussion of the abdomen will either result in a tympanic sound (air) or a fluid wave (fluid). An increased amount of air in the abdomen will intensify the tympany associated with abdominal percussion.

A palpable fluid wave may also be assessed with the use of a third hand, which may be the patient's or another provider's. Begin by placing the ulnar side of the third hand on the patient's abdomen at the midline, pressing down firmly. The third hand prevents a false positive by inhibiting the transmission of the wave through mesenteric adipose tissue. The fluid wave maneuver is the most specific for detecting abdominal fluid.

Another technique to determine the presence of fluid in the abdomen is "shifting dullness." The outcome of this maneuver is dependent again on the physical properties of fluid and air and relies on the fact that air will float on top of water. Any air present in the abdomen will rise to the top and create an air bubble.

With the patient supine, begin percussing the sides of the abdomen, beginning at the umbilicus and moving downward.

Next, have the patient turn over and lie on one side. Percuss the abdomen again, starting at the top of the patient's side and moving toward the umbilicus. Any air should rise above the fluid and be at the top portion of the patient's side. There should be a point again where the sound shifts from tympany to dullness. Mark this point and compare it to the other shift point. The second point should be above the first point. The shift in the level of tympany with position change will measure at least 3 cm when ascites is present.

THINK LINK: *Fluid Wave*

Fluid in the abdomen (ascites) responds to percussion in much the same way as free water does. A pebble dropped in still water initiates a series of waves that travel in enlarging concentric circles away from the initial impact. Fluid in the abdomen will produce the same effects. Waves will be visible in the skin overlying the abdomen, away from the point of percussion.

Unexpected Findings

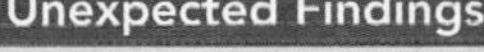

Dullness is produced when percussing over solid organs or other masses.

If percussion is performed above the diaphragm, resonance (lung tissue) will be heard.

The initial sound obtained should be tympany due to air at the top of the abdomen.

At some point below the umbilicus, when the level of the fluid is reached, the sound should shift to dullness. This point should be marked and should also be equidistant for the umbilicus on both sides of the abdomen.

Percussion: Level II

Percussion Techniques and Expected Findings	Unexpected Findings

After general abdominal percussion, use percussion to measure the size of various organs, with the most common being the width of the liver.

Liver Width

Percussing for liver width involves determining where percussion tones change, specifically from resonance to dullness and tympany to dullness.

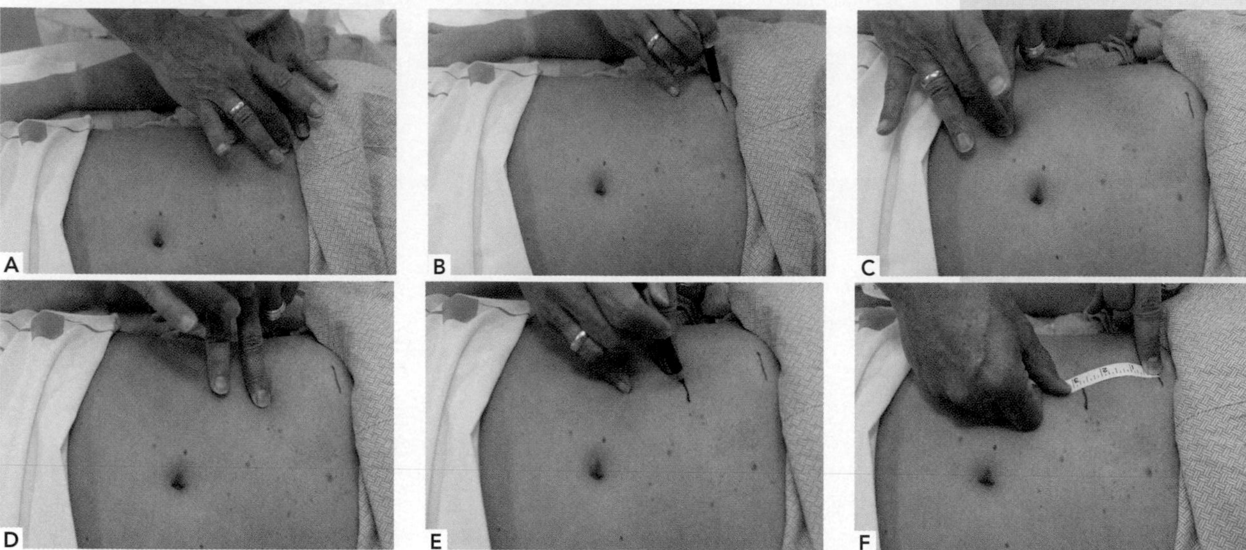

FIGURE 28-29A–F Percussion for liver width

Begin the procedure at the right midclavicular line, below the costal margin where the percussion tone is resonance (Figure 28-29). The lower border of the liver generally is aligned with the costal border. Continue percussing up the midclavicular line until the percussion tone changes to dullness. Note this point with a marking pencil.

Move up the midclavicular line to a point where resonance is heard. The nipple may be used as a starting point. The upper border of the liver generally begins at the level of the fifth to seventh intercostal space. Begin percussing down the midclavicular line until the resonance turns to dullness. Note this point also with a marking pencil. Measure the distance between these two points to estimate the width of the liver. This should be about 6 to 12 cm or 2 ½ to 4 ½ inches.

A distance greater than this indicates an enlarged liver, and a smaller distance suggests liver atrophy.

Scratch Test

This is another method to determine liver width. While it does not necessarily use percussion, because it involves determining liver size, it will be described here. It does use auscultation, but one is not listening to actual physiological sounds, which are artificially produced.

Begin the scratch test by placing the diaphragm of the stethoscope over the liver, slightly above the costal border (Figure 28-30). With the ear pieces in place, begin lightly scratching the patient's skin in the mid-clavicular line. The scratching may be started either above or below the liver. Listen to the scratching sound and note when there is a change in the sound. There is not a specific change as there was when percussing for the liver borders, but there will be a noticeable sound change. Note the point of change from above and below the liver.

Again, the distance between these two points indicates the width of the liver.

The scratch test may be more useful in certain individuals who present with difficulties for eliciting audible percussion sounds.

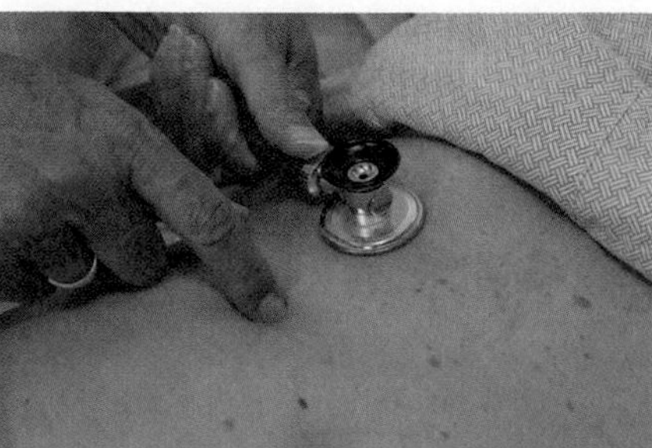

FIGURE 28-30 Scratch test

Percussion: Level III

Percussion Techniques and Expected Findings	Unexpected Findings
Percussion of the abdomen in a patient with abdominal pain or trauma is generally not indicated and does not necessarily contribute any additional information to assist with diagnosis.	Fluid (blood or ascites) in the abdomen will give an overall dull sound, thus not allowing for any comparison of sounds obtained.
Assess retroperitoneal pain, which may indicate renal involvement, by percussion of the back at the costovertebral angle (CVA) (Figure 28-31). This is accomplished by giving a substantial blow with a fist right over the CVA. This can be accomplished by direct or indirect percussion.	Pain associated with this maneuver is suggestive of kidney pathology.

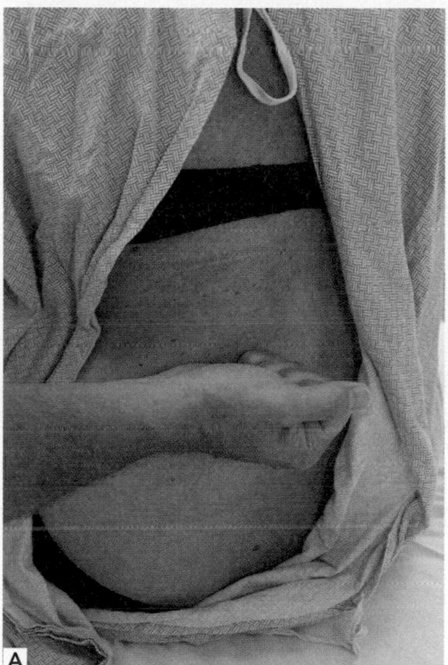

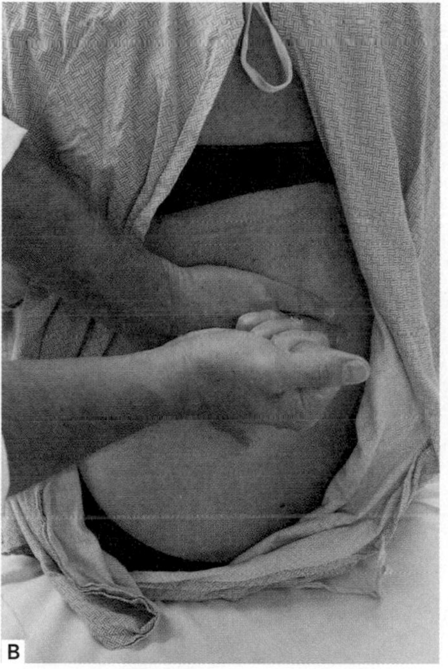

FIGURE 28-31A–B CVA percussion: **a)** direct; **b)** indirect

Developmental Applications

Techniques and Expected Findings	Unexpected Findings
Infants and Children The optimal time for inspecting the infant's abdomen is when the infant is relaxed and relatively quiet. Sucking on a pacifier or on a bottle may help the infant relax. The infant's abdomen appears protuberant due to the underdeveloped abdominal musculature, but should not protrude above the level of the chest.	An abdomen that is scaphoid in contour accompanies dehydration. A scaphoid abdomen also suggests the presence of a diaphragmatic hernia.
A portion of the umbilical cord (stump) remains attached to the abdomen and should be dry and odorless, without any redness, induration, or increased warmth around it. Within a week it becomes hard, turns black, and falls off within 10 to 14 days. Once the cord has detached, there should be no apparent discharge.	The presence of only one artery is suggestive of other congenital anomalies. A serous or serosanguineous discharge indicates infection.
The abdomen should be symmetrical with the possibility of a fine, superficial, venous pattern on the surface of the skin. Respiratory and abdominal movements should be synchronous with a slight bulging of the abdomen noted at the start of inspiration. Pulsations are commonly observed in the epigastric area. Peristaltic movements may occasionally be observed, but they are not considered an expected finding. Peristaltic activity is best observed when looking across the abdomen.	If movements are observed more frequently or become more visible, an intestinal obstruction is a possibility.

Techniques and Expected Findings	Unexpected Findings

The abdominal contour through toddlerhood remains convex, appearing as a potbelly (Figure 28-33). This appearance gradually disappears; however, in some children that are past 5, the abdomen will assume a convex shape when supine. When this is apparent, the abdomen should not protrude above an imaginary line that extends from the xiphoid process to the symphysis pubis. Children remain abdominal breathers until 6 or 7 years of age; but if it continues past this age, it suggests a thoracic problem. Abdominal breathing that appears restrained may be due to peritoneal inflammation or an acute abdomen.

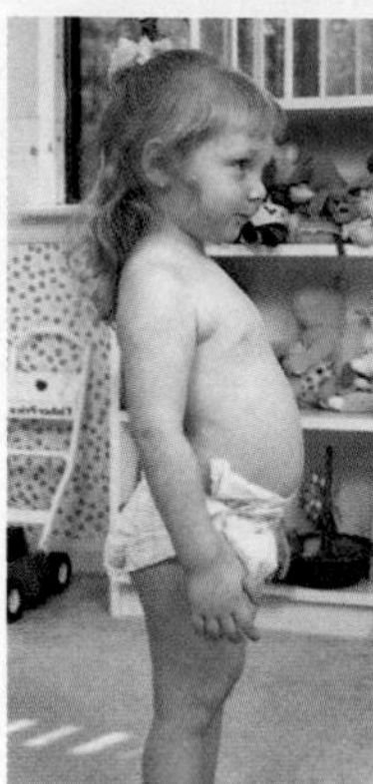

FIGURE 28-33 Toddler with pot belly

Two alterations may be observed in the early neonatal period and infancy. The first is an umbilical hernia, which is a bulge around the umbilical cord (Figure 28-32). It commonly appears within the first 2–3 weeks and becomes noticeably prominent when the infant is crying. It is easily reduced, but it usually returns. Umbilical hernias may appear quite large; however, the size does not determine significance. The size of the opening is a more appropriate measure of its size. Its maximum size is reached by 4 weeks and is usually gone by 1 year.

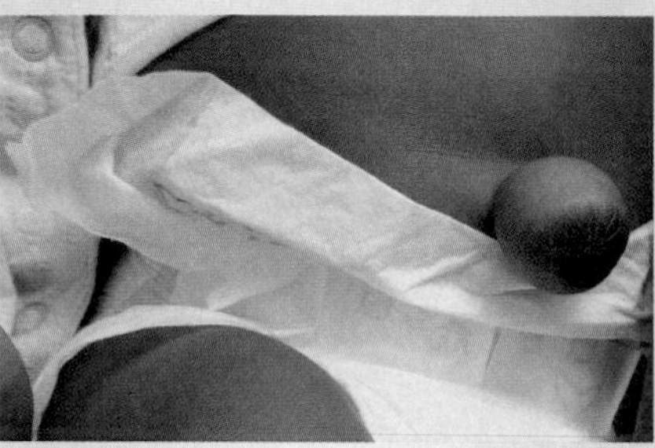

FIGURE 28-32 Umbilical hernia
Source: George Dodson/Lightworks Studio/Pearson Education

The second alteration is a separation of the rectus abdominis muscle, also known as *diastasis recti*. The separation may be 1–4 cm wide at the midline, extending from the xiphoid process to the umbilicus. This occurs when the rectus abdominis muscles do not approximate at the midline. Generally, there is no need to close the opening and it is expected to resolve within the first few years. Herniation through the diastasis recti is cause for concern and indicates a need for repair. Diastasis recti that persist up to the age of 6 requires further evaluation.

Auscultation of the newborn's and infant's abdomen follows the same procedure as for adults. The presence of bowel sounds should be apparent 1 to 2 hours after delivery. Bowel sounds should be heard every 10 to 30 seconds. Assess infants with a scaphoid abdomen for the presence of bowel sounds in the chest.

A scaphoid abdomen suggests an absence of abdominal organs; thus bowel sounds heard in the chest would indicate that organs have entered the chest through a diaphragmatic hernia.

During auscultation, listen for the presence of any vascular sounds. There should not be any bruits or venous hums present.

THINK LINK:* *Congenital Diaphragmatic Hernia

A diaphragmatic hernia develops in utero when the abdominal organs are developing on the outside of the abdomen. During that time, the diaphragm closes and fuses. In some fetuses the diaphragm fails to develop properly. As a result, when the abdominal organs migrate back to the abdominal cavity, they also herniate into the thoracic cage. With abdominal organs in the thoracic cage, the lungs and their vascular supply fail to develop properly. There are degrees of severity with the most severe resulting in respiratory difficulty at birth leading to respiratory failure along with persistent pulmonary hypertension. On the other end, the diaphragmatic hernia may be so small that there are minimal respiratory problems evident at birth and may not show up for years. Mortality associated with CDH is approximately 60%, which translates into approximately 750 infant deaths annually.

Techniques and Expected Findings

Palpation of the infant's and child's abdomen is done primarily for the same purposes as palpation of the adult abdomen; to identify areas of tenderness, organ enlargement, masses, ascites, and indicators of peritonitis. An infant or young child is most likely to be uncooperative during palpation. Giving the infant a pacifier or bottle and distracting the child with a toy or stuffed animal may help in getting cooperation. Examining the child on the parent's lap may also provide a greater sense of security and help toward getting cooperation (Figure 28-34).

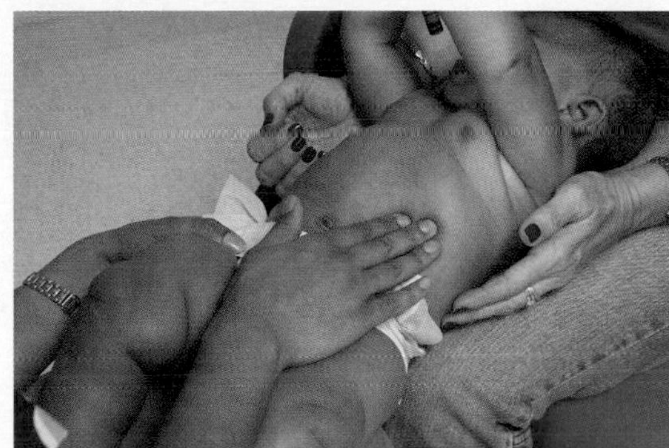

FIGURE 28-34 Palpation of the abdomen

Like in adults, the abdomen needs to be relaxed. Flexing the knees and hips promotes relaxation of the abdomen. Infants often have their knees flexed; however, grasping the infant's feet in one hand and flexing the knees is a technique used to relax the abdomen.

Perform light palpation first to determine the borders of the liver and spleen and the presence of any superficial masses. It is not uncommon for the liver to be palpated 1–2 cm below the right costal margin. The liver may be palpated by placing the right hand's fingertips on the midclavicular line just below the costal margin. Gently press upward, noting a firm tap with inspiration. Continue pressing upward until the liver edge may be felt again. The distance between the liver edge and the costal margin should not exceed 3 cm.

In the same manner, palpate the spleen by placing the fingertips just below the costal margin in the left midclavicular line, feeling for a firm tap on inspiration. It is not unusual to palpate a spleen in 5%–10% of children (Duderstadt, 2006).

During palpation, observe the infant's facial expressions for any indication of tenderness. The infant and young child will have difficulty localizing the tenderness or describing its characteristics. Distracting the infant or child with a toy or talking to the child during palpation, allows the provider to watch for changes in facial expressions.

Deep palpation is done next, feeling for the presence of any masses. Transillumination will differentiate fluid filled (cystic) masses from solid masses. A sausage-shaped mass in the left lower quadrant is commonly associated with stool in the sigmoid colon. If present, it is a common indication of constipation.

Percussion of the abdomen produces greater tympany than in adults due to an increase of abdominal air caused by swallowing air during feeding and crying. It can also be used to determine organ size and borders. Percussion of the liver borders is done the same way as for adults. The upper border of the liver should be located approximately at the fifth intercostal space at the mid clavicular line. Up until 3 years of age, female infants have a larger liver span than males; but after age 3 the male's liver enlarges at a greater rate than females. Liver span of infants is detailed in Table 28-8.

Unexpected Findings

A renal bruit may be an indication of renal artery stenosis or the possibility of a renal arteriovenous fistula. Both sounds are difficult to hear. Renal artery stenosis produces a high-frequency, soft sound whereas the arteriovenous fistula sound is continuous. Listening over the flank of the infant may help in assessing their presence.

Constriction of the pupils is also a visible indication when a tender area is being palpated. Palpating for rebound tenderness may be done, but extreme caution should be taken to prevent causing severe pain.

Light will pass through a fluid mass but will cast a shadow with a solid mass. If pulsations are observed, palpate for aortic enlargement. Any palpable mass should be manipulated very cautiously until a malignancy has been ruled out.

Any dullness that is heard will be due to more solid tissue related to masses of fluid.

Techniques and Expected Findings | **Unexpected Findings**

Table 28-8 Liver span in infants, children, and adolescents

Age	Male (cm)	Female (cm)
6 months	2.4	2.8
12 months	2.8	3.1
2 years	3.5	3.6
3 years	4	4
4 years	4.4	4.3
5 years	4.8	4.5
6 years	5.1	4.8
8 years	5.6	5.1
10 years	6.1	5.4
12 years	6.5	5.6
14 years	6.8	5.8
16 years	7.1	6

The Pregnant Woman

Assessment of abdominal changes during pregnancy is covered in Chapter 11.

The Older Adult

The techniques of performing an abdominal exam on an older adult do not differ from those used on younger adults. Anatomic and physiological changes may require some adjustment and may affect the findings. Caution is needed in requesting the elderly to change or assume various positions. Musculoskeletal alterations may make movement and position changes very difficult if not impossible.

A significant change of the abdomen in the elderly is a loss of connective tissue and muscle mass resulting in a thinner and less firm abdominal wall. This may, however, make palpation easier and may allow for more accurate findings. In spite of the loss of adipose tissue in the extremities, fat continues to be deposited in the abdomen. Fat deposition and the loss of muscle tone give the elderly abdomen a rounded contour.

Changes in the pulmonary system can produce changes in the abdomen also. As the upper and lower borders are both lower, the liver span is not significantly altered and should remain between 6 to 12 cm. The liver, however, does decrease in size after 50, which may also decrease the liver span at the midclavicular line.

Decreased motility of the intestines in the older adult commonly results in complaints of intestinal problems. Regular bowel movements seem to be a great concern to the elderly and will often have personal remedies or interventions to maintain regularity. Constipation is a common occurrence, particularly in older adult females, and stool in the sigmoid colon is more likely to be palpated. Lack of exercise and dietary fiber are also factors that contribute to constipation. Decreased intestinal motility also affects absorption of nutrients. Changes in the structural features of the intestine or barriers to diffusion by mucosal cells are the leading factors interfering with absorption.

Enlargement of the lungs due to emphysema and/or COPD depresses the diaphragm, pushing the liver down so that the upper and lower borders may be 1 to 2 cm lower than the usual locations.

If constipation is chronic or severe in character, a fecal impaction may occur.

Common disorders of the elderly (rheumatoid arthritis, infections, diverticula, mental disorders) contribute to absorption problems.

THINK LINK: ***Pernicious Anemia***

Pernicious anemia (PA) is an anemia that results from vitamin B_{12} deficiency. Vitamin B_{12} is absorbed in the stomach and is necessary for red cell growth and maturation. It is also dependent upon the presence of intrinsic factor (IF) within the stomach. Older adults that suffer from chronic gastritis or who have immune destruction of the mucosal gastric cells experience a deficiency of IF. Lack of vitamin B_{12} leads to altered and uncharacteristic development of red cells. The development of PA occurs gradually and is easily treated. Failure to treat it though will ultimately result in the individual's death.

Older adults may develop an intestinal obstruction. Common causes are hypokalemia, myocardial infarction, and infections, particularly pneumonia, sepsis, peritonitis, and pancreatitis. Indicators of an obstruction include vomiting, distention, diarrhea, and constipation. Severe obstructions may reduce or block blood flow to the area, which may result in infarction that turns to gangrene. Mesenteric artery ischemia is a complication that has a high morbidity and mortality rate.

Techniques and Expected Findings	Unexpected Findings
	Cancers of the GI system carry a higher incidence rate as age increases. The GI organs may be the primary sites for cancers, or they may be secondary to metastasis from other primary sites. In many GI organ cancers, the onset of symptoms occurs relatively late, making the mortality rate very high. Even when symptoms do appear, they are nonspecific and can be related to multiple GI conditions.
Recent studies have also identified that depressive symptoms in the elderly result in an increase in abdominal obesity, particularly visceral fat, that is independent of overall obesity (Vogelzangs et al., 2008).	These results suggest that there may be an underlying pathophysiological pathway linking depression to obesity. It also may provide and explanation as to why diabetes and cardiovascular disease often occur with depression.

DOCUMENTATION

- **Inspection:** Abdomen contour predominately flat and symmetrical with only slight rounding. No signs of inflammation or evidence of hernia around umbilicus. Without scars, rashes, lesions, pulses, or masses. White striae on upper lumbar region with an inverted umbilicus.
- **Auscultation:** Bowel sounds present in all four quadrants, loudest in RLQ. No bruits heard over epigastrium (aorta) or iliac and renal arteries.
- **Percussion:** Tympany percussed in all four quadrants. Liver dullness of 8 cm heard at R MCL, lower edge of costal margin.
- **Palpation:** Light—no masses/tenderness in all four quadrants. Deep—No masses/tenderness noted. Liver border barely palpable at costal margin, smooth and firm, without tenderness or nodules. No CVA tenderness bilaterally.

Electronic Charting

Expectations of Electronic Charting

Electronic charting should accommodate not only the abdominal assessment, but also related information such as medications, social habits (alcohol, tobacco, drugs, caffeine, etc.), and preventive health care such as vaccinations, diet, and exercise. The family history, social history, and environmental history should be included, as well.

Electronic charting should automatically compute measures such as body mass index (BMI) based on the entered height and weight. Electronic systems that include medication alerts should accommodate age-related changes to abdominal systems that can affect drug metabolism and clearance.

Electronic records can support complex information over time, facilitating management of chronic conditions such as diabetes (Orzano et al., 2007). There is an increasing need to manage genomic information such as genetic tests for conditions such as colon cancer (Atreja, Achker, Jain, Harris, & Lasher, 2008). In addition, electronic charting can promote efficient outcomes research and clinical trials (Atreja et al., 2008). For example, electronic charting was shown to improve documentation of quality assurance measures in bariatric surgery patients (Parikh, Yermilov, McGory, Ko, & Maggard, 2007).

Limitations of Electronic Charting

Information relevant to the abdominal examination may be organized as separate systems in electronic charting. While it should be easy to navigate between the different parts of the assessment, the information may not be directly linked.

Technology alone is not sufficient for achieving optimal clinical outcomes. While technology can support information management, clinicians must interpret and decide how to act on the information. For example, interpretation of BMI based on standard threshold values of BMI does not give information regarding the distribution of body fat, and BMI thresholds may be misleading in certain ethnic groups, in elderly patients, or in patients who are athletic or muscular.

Summary

- The abdomen contains the primary organs of digestion as well as the spleen and kidneys. The kidneys are primarily organs of elimination and the spleen functions as a part of the immune activities of the lymphatic system.
- The organs within the abdomen perform multiple functions so that expected findings reflect optimal functioning of each organ in maintaining the processes of digestion, elimination, and lymph/immune activities.
- The multiple organs within the abdomen may also undergo changes that interfere with digestion and elimination resulting in a multitude of conditions and disorders that range from minor dysfunction to significant life-threatening situations.
- The organs within the abdomen are functional at birth and do not go through any significant changes as one ages. The major age-related change is the slowing down of intestinal

motility, but there are no significant consequences due to this change. The expanding uterus of a pregnant woman crowds and displaces abdominal organs, but these changes are temporary and of no significant consequence.

- Assessment of the abdominal organs uses all four assessment techniques. For assessment of the abdomen, auscultation is performed after observation, prior to palpation and percussion so that abdominal sounds have not been affected by manual stimulation.

Review Questions

1. The provider is performing an assessment of the alimentary canal on a patient with a gastrointestinal complain. To fully assess this area, the provider will include which of the following? (Select all that apply.)
   1. inspection of the oral cavity
   2. auscultation of bowel sounds
   3. palpation of the liver
   4. percussion of the spleen
   5. palpation of the rectal walls
2. The provider is examining a patient with a diagnosis of hepatitis B and has anticipated that
   1. the patient may have rebound tenderness upon deep palpation of the right lower quadrant.
   2. dullness will be noted in the epigastric area upon percussion.
   3. pain will result when the right upper quadrant is palpated.
   4. peri-umbilical pain will be the patient's primary complaint.
3. The provider notes that documentation of a prior physical examination revealed that the patient reported pain when the examiner tested for CVA tenderness on the right side. The provider is aware that this finding is
   1. significant of possible kidney pathology.
   2. considered normal in adult patients.
   3. probably the result of a spinal injury.
   4. related to a recent stroke.
4. The provider is performing auscultation of the abdomen to note the presence of the patient's bowel sounds. The provider is aware that normally bowel sounds
   1. occur only after a meal.
   2. can be heard at about 5–35 times per minute.
   3. should be assessed only in the symptomatic patient.
   4. are loud and high-pitched in nature.
5. The provider is teaching a student the technique of auscultating the abdomen for vascular sounds. What information should the provider include in this instruction? (Select all that apply.)
   1. The presence of bruits and hums should be the expected finding.
   2. Vascular sounds are not well transmitted through the abdominal wall.
   3. The vessels included in the assessment are the aorta, renal, iliac, and femoral arteries.
   4. The stethoscopes should be positioned directly over the arteries.
   5. This assessment can be combined with the auscultation of bowel sounds for efficient use of time.
6. The provider is examining the abdomen of a 4-month-old child and is having difficulty gaining the cooperation of the child to complete palpation. The best strategy for the provider to use is to
   1. ask the parent to leave the room until the assessment is complete.
   2. restrain the child while the examination is performed.
   3. omit palpation of the abdomen from the examination until the child is able to cooperate.
   4. grasp the infant's feet in one hand and flex the knees while the examination is performed.
7. When assessing the abdomen of the older adult, the provider should anticipate that the assessment will reveal
   1. an increase in peristaltic activity noted by more frequent bowel sounds.
   2. tympanic sounds noted on percussion of the liver.
   3. a decrease in liver size noted on percussion.
   4. chronic tenderness over the right upper quadrant.
8. When performing an abdominal examination of a patient, the order in which the provider performs the techniques of examination is which of the following?
   1. inspection, palpation, percussion, auscultation
   2. inspection, percussion, auscultation, palpation
   3. inspection, auscultation, palpation, percussion
   4. auscultation, inspection, percussion, palpation
9. The provider documents that a patient's abdomen has a scaphoid contour. This indicates that the patient's abdomen is
   1. rounded.
   2. convex.
   3. concave.
   4. distended.
10. The provider uses the technique of shifting dullness when assessing a patient's abdomen to test for which of the following?
    1. abdominal bleeding
    2. peritoneal irritation
    3. ascites
    4. borborygmi

Conditions and Disorders

Diarrhea

Diarrhea is an increase in the frequency of bowel movements, an increase in the looseness of stool, or both. **Absolute diarrhea** is more than five bowel movements a day or liquid stools. **Relative diarrhea** is an increase in the number of bowel movements per day or an increase in the looseness of stools compared with an individual's usual bowel habit. Increased amounts of water in stool can occur if the stomach and/or small intestine secrete too much fluid, the distal small intestine and colon do not absorb enough water, or the undigested, liquid food passes too quickly through the small intestine and colon for enough water to be removed. An adult with diarrhea may pass more than one quart of stool per day.

Pathophysiology

- Stools are looser whether or not the frequency of bowel movements is increased, which is caused by increased water in the stool.
- Acute diarrhea: most common, generally lasts a few days to a week, often results from a bacterial, viral, or parasitic infection, and resolves spontaneously.
- Chronic diarrhea: defined in several ways, but almost always lasts more than 3 weeks. Prolonged diarrhea (>2 days) indicates possible more serious condition, places person at risk for dehydration.

Can be categorized into five major types:

- Secretory diarrhea occurs when too much fluid is secreted into the intestine.
- Osmotic diarrhea occurs when undigested or nonabsorbed food molecules pass into the colon, raising osmotic concentration, drawing fluid and electrolytes into the large intestine.
- Motility-related diarrhea: hypermobility of intestinal muscles causes rapid movement of food through the intestines, preventing absorption of nutrients and water. May be due to a vagotomy or diabetic neuropathy, or occur in those individuals who have had portions of their bowel removed.
- Exudative diarrhea: presence of blood and pus in the stool, as in inflammatory bowel diseases (Crohn's disease, ulcerative colitis) or severe infections (*E. coli*, other forms of food poisoning).
- Inflammatory diarrhea: damage to mucosal lining or brush border, leading to a passive loss of protein-rich fluids and a decreased ability to absorb these lost fluids.

Subjective Data

- Patients with mild dehydration may experience thirst and dry mouth.
- Secretory: bowel movements are frequent and watery. Pain is not common, no signs of inflammation.
- May be watery, but stop once ingestion of food or offending dietary substance stops
- Intestinal hypermotility may cause cramping abdominal pain.
- Travel outside the U.S., particularly to underdeveloped countries, is a frequent cause of "traveler's diarrhea."
- Suspect bacterial food poisoning if more than two individuals develop diarrhea after ingesting the same food
- Bacterial infections may also be caused by drinking contaminated water, such as when camping.

Objective Data

- Moderate to severe dehydration may cause orthostatic hypotension with syncope, diminished urine output, severe weakness, shock, kidney failure, confusion, acidosis, and coma.
- Electrolytes are lost when diarrhea is prolonged/severe, causing mineral or electrolyte deficiencies, especially sodium and potassium. Abnormalities of chloride and bicarbonate also may develop.
- Irritation of anus due to frequent passage of watery stool containing irritating substances.

Gastroesophageal Reflux Disorder (GERD)

GERD is a chronic symptom of mucosal damage that is caused by liquid contents from the stomach, which usually contains acid, pepsin, and possibly bile entering the lower portion of the esophagus. GERD is a chronic condition requiring some type of continuous therapy. Medications as well as some alterations to diet, posture and position, and eating habits will generally control the reflux and prevent further complications.

Pathophysiology

- Caused by alterations in the lower esophageal sphincter, such as relaxation, impaired expulsion of gastric reflux from the esophagus, hiatal hernia.
- Lack of mucous secreting cells place acids in contact with the esophageal lining.
- These changes may be permanent or temporary.

Subjective Data

Common symptoms:

- Heartburn: burning sensation in chest, sometimes spreading to throat, and sour taste in mouth
- Regurgitation of food or acid reflux
- Dysphagia
- Sensation of a lump in the throat

Less-common symptoms:

- Hoarseness or sore throat/dry cough
- Pain with swallowing (odynophagia)
- Increased salivation

Objective Data

- There are a few obvious signs related to GERD:
  - Narrowing of the esophageal stricture causes damage to LES cells from acid exposure, causing formation of scar tissue/narrowing, causing difficulty swallowing.
  - Esophageal ulcer caused by stomach acid, which may bleed, cause pain, and make swallowing difficult.
  - Precancerous changes to the esophagus (Barrett's esophagus) cause color and composition alterations of the tissue lining of LES. Associated with increased risk of esophageal cancer and occurs in approximately 10% of individuals with GERD (Marks, D., 2009).

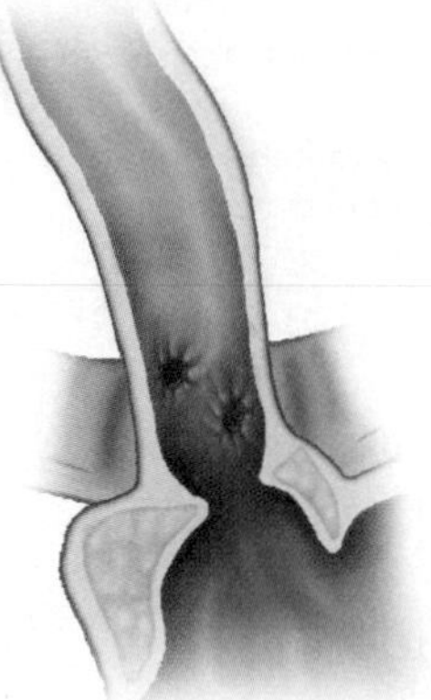

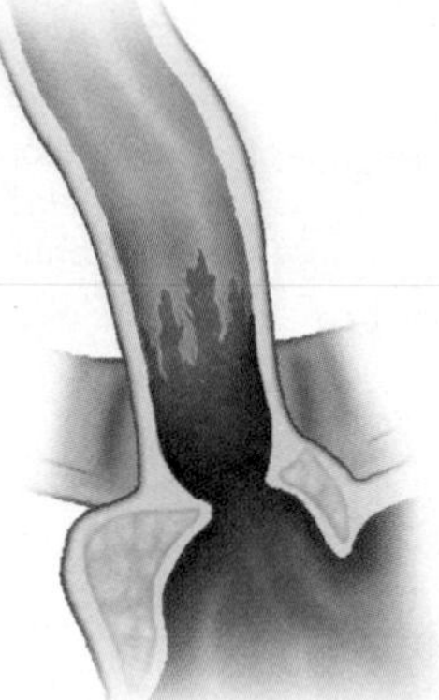

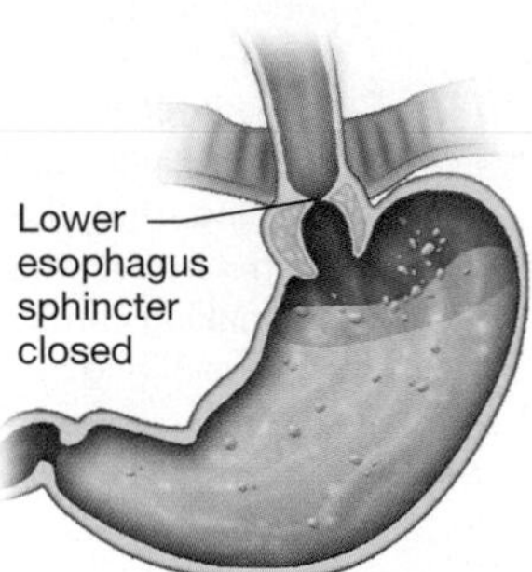

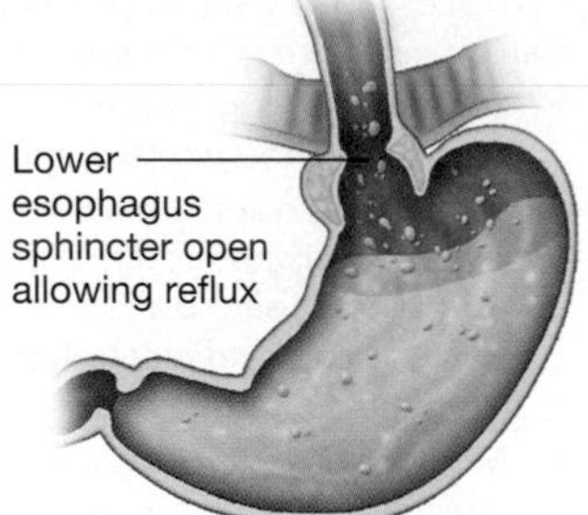

FIGURE 28-35 Causes of gastroesophageal reflux disease (GERD)

PRACTICE POINT: GERD

It is estimated that one-third of adults in the U.S. experience symptoms of GERD at least monthly, and approximately one-tenth experience it weekly or daily. It may also be present in infants and children. Risk factors that increase its likelihood of developing include the following:

- Hiatal hernia, due to mechanical and motility factors
- Obesity: increasing body mass index is associated with more severe GERD (Hajar, Castell, Ghomrawi, Rackett, & Hila, 2012)
- Zollinger-Ellison syndrome (increased gastric acidity due to gastrin production)
- Hypercalcemia: can increase gastrin production, leading to increased acidity
- Scleroderma and systemic sclerosis, which feature esophageal dysmotility
- The use of medicines such as prednisolone

Hiatal Hernia (HH)

A hiatal hernia is characterized by an upper section of the stomach that has been pushed upward into the mediastinal cavity through the esophageal opening of the diaphragm. It is a common condition, being present in approximately 15% of the population, but only a minority actually demonstrates any symptoms (Marks, J. W., 2009). It occurs most frequently in females and older adults, occurring in 70% of individuals over 70 (Qureshi, 2009).

Pathophysiology

- Sliding hiatus hernia is most common (95%); gastroesophageal junction moves above the diaphragm together with some of the stomach. May be pulled up and down (slides) through the diaphragm during eating and swallowing.
- Rolling (paraesophageal) hiatus hernia: part of the stomach herniates through esophageal hiatus, lying beside esophagus, without movement of the gastroesophageal junction (5% of hiatal hernias).

Subjective Data

- Asymptomatic in most cases
- Symptoms and manifestations are basically the same as for GERD, as well as the potential for the same complications.
- Acid reflux
- Severity of symptoms unrelated to hernia size

Objective Data

- Physical examination usually unhelpful.
- Certain conditions may predispose to the development of hiatal hernia, such as muscle weakening and loss of elasticity with age, pregnancy, obesity, and abdominal ascites.
- Diagnosis typically made through an upper GI series, endoscopy, or high-resolution manometry.
- Complications include gas bloat syndrome, dysphagia, dumping syndrome, excessive scarring, and achalasia (rare).
- Strangulated hernia or obstruction symptoms include early satiety, pain with eating, nausea or vomiting, inability to have a bowel movement or pass gas.

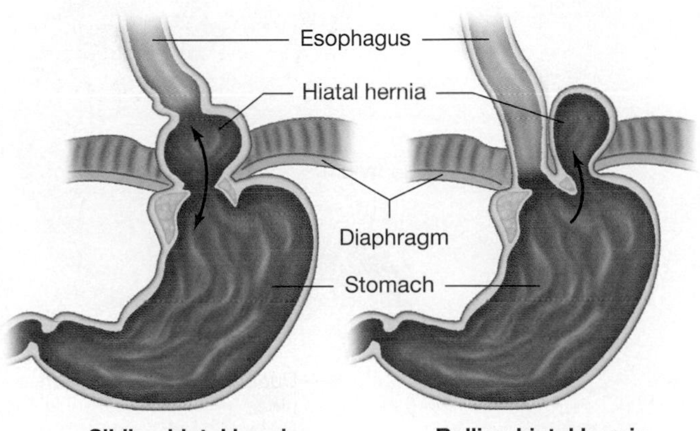

FIGURE 28-36 Hiatal hernia

Peptic Ulcer Disease (PUD)

PUD results from an imbalance between factors promoting mucosal damage (gastric acid, pepsin, *H. pylori* infection, NSAID use) and those influencing gastroduodenal defense (mucus, bicarbonate, prostaglandin, and mucosal blood flow). Individuals at an increased risk of peptic ulcers are those who

- are infected with *H. pylori* (80% of all ulcers believed to be associated with this bacterium).
- use NSAIDs (70% of Americans older than 65 years use NSAIDs at least once weekly, and about 34% take these drugs on a daily basis).
- smoke (may increase the risk of peptic ulcers in people who are infected with *H. pylori*).
- drink alcohol (alcohol can irritate and erode stomach mucous lining and increase amount of stomach acid that's produced).

Pathophysiology

- An ulcer occurs when there is a break in the protective mucosal barrier, allowing acid to come into contact with the inner lining of the stomach, precipitating autodigestion.

Two types of ulcers—

- Duodenal: most common, results from break in the duodenal mucosa.
- Gastric: generally located in the antral portion of the stomach.

Subjective Data

- May demonstrate wide variety of symptoms or be asymptomatic; in rare cases, potentially life threatening complications (bleeding) may occur.

Symptoms may include the following:

- Pain or discomfort (usually in the upper abdomen)
- Bloating
- Early sense of fullness with eating
- Lack of appetite
- Nausea

Objective Data

- Diagnosis confirmed with tests (endoscopy, barium contrast x-rays, esophagogastroduodenoscopy (EGD), which are typically ordered if symptoms do not resolve after a few weeks of treatment, or when they first appear in a person over age 45 or with other symptoms, such as weight loss. This is because stomach cancer can cause similar symptoms.

- May heal spontaneously, but frequently return. Without known cause, removal will usually prevent return. In the case of *H. pylori*, treatment with antibiotics is often successful to eliminate the bacteria.
- May bleed (minimal or severe). Those that perforate through the stomach wall may cause massive bleeding and considered an emergency situation. These individuals may present with manifestations of an acute abdomen.

- Vomiting
- Blood in the stools
- Symptoms of each ulcer may be different.
- Duodenal ulcer symptoms—burning, gnawing, aching, or hunger-like pain, primarily in epigastric region. Pain may occur or worsen when the stomach is empty, usually 2–5 hours after a meal or between 11 p.m. and 2 a.m., when acid secretion tends to be greatest. Sequence known as "pain—food—relief."
- Pain localized in epigastric area is common with both types of ulcers, particularly within the first 2 hours after eating a meal.

- Severe ulcers that resist treatment may indicate an underlying condition.

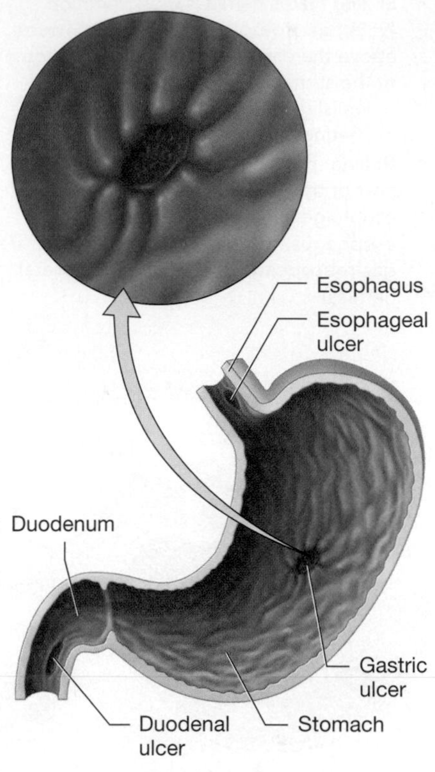

FIGURE 28-37 Peptic ulcer disease (PUD)

INFLAMMATORY BOWEL DISORDERS

Inflammatory bowel disease (IBD) consists of two conditions known as ulcerative colitis and Crohn's disease (Table 28-9). The exact causes of either condition are unknown but are related to genetic factors, immune alterations, and environmental factors. They are both characterized by a dysregulated immune response to host intestinal microflora. In the process, white blood cells enter the lining of the intestines, producing chronic inflammation. Both conditions are chronic in nature and are associated with inflammatory alterations of the small and large intestines.

Ulcerative Colitis (UC)

UC is characterized by ulceration of the colon mucosa that progresses proximally from the rectum to the colon (Figure 28-38). The severity ranges from mild to severe, depending on the degree of colon involvement. It may be in remission for some years after an initial acute phase or may become chronic with periodic recurrences of symptoms. Chronic, recurring UC may be a precursor to colon cancer.

Pathophysiology

- Inflammation originates in mucosal cells with infiltration of white cells and mast cells.
- Destruction of the mucosa results in the loss of surface area for absorption as well as increased transit time through the colon, producing large volumes of watery diarrhea.
- Products of inflammation and inflammatory debris primary causes of tissue damage. In severe inflammation, bleeding may occur and small areas of erosion coalesce into larger ulcers.
- Abscesses may form that end in necrosis and ragged ulceration of the mucosa.

Subjective Data

- LLQ cramps that are relieved with defecation
- Fecal urgency with tenesmus (ineffective straining at stool)
- In moderate states, bleeding increases and abdominal pain and tenderness may exist, but are not severe.
- Characterized by intermittent periods of exacerbations and remissions

Objective Data

- Bloody diarrhea is hallmark manifestation.
- Large volumes of watery diarrhea that may also contain purulent mucus.
- In mild to moderate states there are fewer than 5 movements/day, intermittently with rectal bleeding. Stools may be formed or loose in consistency.
- In a severe state, individuals may have 6–10 bloody stools/day that results in anemia, hypovolemia, and hypoalbuminemia.

Crohn's Disease

CD is a type of inflammatory bowel disease that results in ulcerations of the intestinal lining of any part of the gastrointestinal tract from mouth to anus. Unlike UC, which is confined to the large intestine, CD is frequently found in the small intestine, particularly the ileum.

Pathophysiology

- Associated ulcerations extend into the deeper layers of the intestinal lining.
- Skip lesions, or areas of CD that are separated by healthy tissue
- Cause unknown, though some strains of bacteria have been hypothesized to cause the condition, no substantial evidence exists to support this theory.
- Activation of the immune system is a prevailing belief; however, it is not known if the activation results in the condition or the condition results from the activation (NIH, 2006).
- Like UC, CD goes through periods of relapse and remission.

Subjective Data

- Symptoms of CD include abdominal pain (RLQ), diarrhea, and weight loss.
- Patients may also experience rectal pain and rectal bleeding.
- Other, less frequently occurring symptoms are poor appetite, fever, night sweats.

Objective Data

- Specific alterations of the anal area occur in approximately one-third of individuals with CD, including anal sphincter tissue swelling, ulcer/fissure formation within anal sphincter, anal fistulae formation between anus or rectum and surrounding skin of the anus. Fistulae may drain mucous and pus.
- There may also be formation of abscesses in the anal and rectal area.
- Individuals with severe Crohn's disease may also experience arthritis, eye inflammation, skin disorders, inflammation of the liver or bile ducts, delayed growth or sexual development (in children).

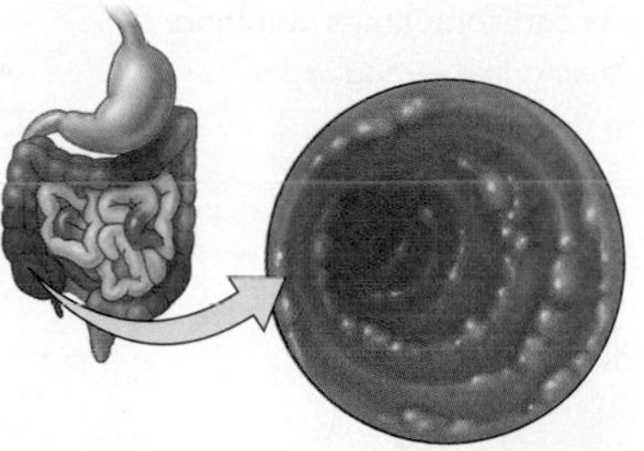

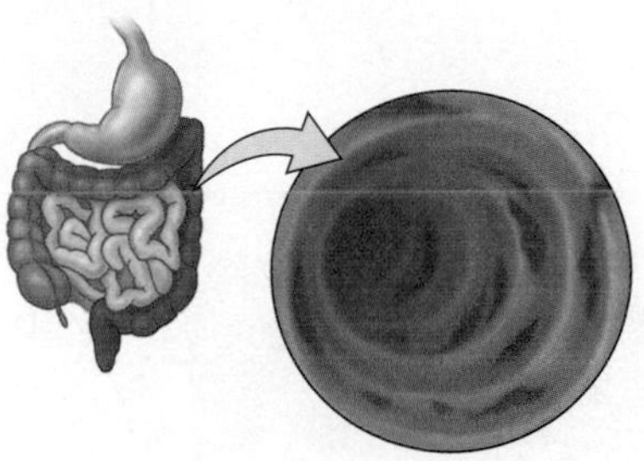

FIGURE 28-38 Ulcerative colitis and Crohn's disease

Table 28-9 Comparison of Ulcerative colitis and Crohn's disease

Characteristics	Ulcerative Colitis	Crohn's Disease
Age of onset	Nonspecific (adolescence/early adulthood)	Nonspecific (adolescence/early adulthood)
Family history	Less common	More common
Gender distribution	Males and females equal	Males and females equal
Risk for cancer	High	High
Pathology		
Lesions located	Colon and rectum; lesions continuous	GI tract (mouth to anus); skip lesions
Tissues affected (ulcers/inflammation)	Mucosal layer	Entire intestinal wall
Frail mucosa	Common	Common
Fistulas/abscesses	Rare	Common
Strictures/obstruction	Rare	Common
Signs/Symptoms		
Abdominal pain	Occasionally	Common
Diarrhea	Common	Common
Bloody stools	Common	Less common
Abdominal mass	Rare	Common
Fat in stools	Rare	Common
Treatment		
Medications	Anti-inflammatory, immunomodulators	Anti-inflammatory, immunomodulators
Surgery	Yes—will cure condition.	No—will not cure; condition often returns after surgical removal of affected area.

Diverticulosis

This is the most common structural alteration of the large intestine or colon and can occasionally occur in the small intestine. It is characterized by the formation of small pouches (diverticula) or herniations through the lining of the colon. The exact incidence of diverticulosis remains unknown but it is known to increase in numbers as the population ages increasing in prevalence to 50%–66% in patients older than 80 years (Matrana & Margolin, 2009).

Pathophysiology

- The most likely cause for diverticula formation is either a weakness of the wall of the colon or an increase in intracolonic pressure, or a combination of these factors; however, evidence is increasing that implicates a low-fiber diet that is a significant contributing factor.
- Diverticulitis (infection/inflammation) occurs as a result of small pieces of stool becoming trapped in these pouches.

Subjective Data

- Most individuals do not experience any discomfort or symptoms.

Symptoms may last from a few hours to a week or more and include the following:

- Tenderness in the LLQ, with severe pain that may come on suddenly that sometimes worsens with movement. Pain may also initially be mild with gradual intensity that develops over days (most common symptom).
- Fever and chills
- Bloating and gas
- Diarrhea or constipation
- Nausea and sometimes vomiting
- Not feeling like eating

Objective Data

- Simple diverticulitis: localized abdominal tenderness affected area, fever
- LLQ tenderness most common (most diverticula occur in sigmoid colon)
- RLQ, mimicking acute appendicitis, can occur in right-sided diverticulitis
- Complicated diverticulitis: formation of tender, palpable mass
- Older adults and some patients taking corticosteroids may have unremarkable findings, even in the presence of severe diverticulitis
- Diagnostic tests may include abdominal CT scan, ultrasound, x-ray.
- Complications include the development of bleeding, formation of abscesses, perforation of the bowel with resultant peritonitis, formation of fistula, and bowel obstruction. All complications require immediate intervention to prevent them from progressing to more serious consequences.

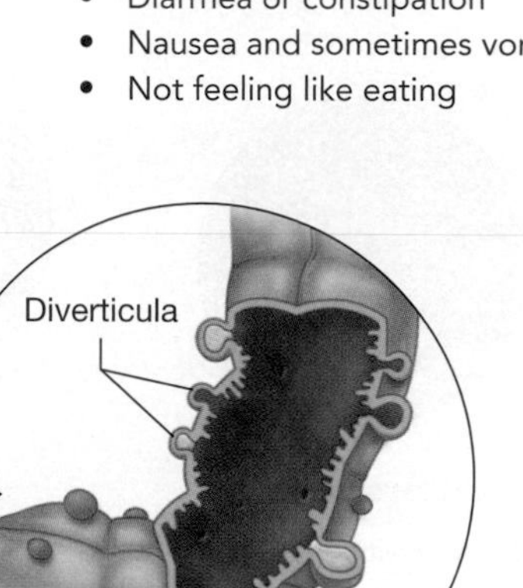

FIGURE 28-39 Diverticulosis

Gastric Cancer

This is the second most common cause of cancer-related death in the world, and it remains difficult to cure in Western countries, primarily because most patients present with advanced disease. In the United States, stomach malignancy is currently the 14th most common cancer (Cacebe, Mehta, & Fisher, 2013). Treatment may also be affected by its location. Approximately 40% of GC originates in the lower section, 40% in the middle section, 15% in the upper section, with about 10% of cancers involving more than one section.

Pathophysiology

- A slow, progressive cancer that may develop over years.
- Median age of onset in U.S.: 70 for males, 74 for females (Cacebe et al., 2013). Slightly higher incidence in males than females.
- The majority (90%–95%) are adenocarcinomas, arising from mucosal tissue lining inside of the stomach.

Subjective Data

- Early symptoms are vague and nonspecific, resulting in delays in diagnosing its presence. Often, by the time the diagnosis is made, the cancer is in an advanced stage.

As the cancer grows, the most common symptoms are as follows:

- Discomfort or pain in the stomach area
- Dysphagia
- Nausea and vomiting

Objective Data

- All physical signs are late events; by the time they are evident, the cancer is invariably too far advanced for curative procedures.

Signs may include the following:

- Palpable enlarged stomach with succussion splash
- Hepatomegaly
- Periumbilical metastasis (Sister Mary Joseph nodule)

- Spread by various means, the tumor can grow through stomach wall and invade adjacent organs or spread to close lymph nodes where it spreads through the blood stream; gastric cancer metastasizes to other organs.
- Table 28-11 identifies the four types of gastric cancers.
- Unexplained weight loss
- Feeling full or bloated after a small meal
- Vomiting blood or blood in stool
- Most often, these symptoms are not due to cancer. Other health problems, such as an ulcer or infection, can cause the same symptoms.
- Enlarged lymph nodes such as Virchow nodes (left supraclavicular) and Irish node (anterior axillary)
- Blumer shelf (shelflike tumor of the anterior rectal wall) may also be present.
- Weight loss
- Melena or pallor from anemia
- Paraneoplastic syndromes such as dermatomyositis, acanthosis nigricans, and circinate erythemas are poor prognostic features.

PRACTICE POINT: Succussion Splash

A succussion splash is a sound obtained when a patient has free fluid and air/gas in a hollow organ or body cavity. It can be elicited to confirm intestinal or pyloric obstruction due to pyloric stenosis or gastric carcinoma, and may also be heard with hydropneumothorax, a large hiatal hernia, or over a normal stomach. To obtain this sign, gently shake the abdomen by holding either side of the patient's pelvis. If a splashing noise is heard, either with the naked ear or with the aid of a stethoscope, the test is considered to be positive. The test is not valid if the patient has consumed food or fluid within the last 3 hours.

Table 28-10 Risk factors for developing gastric cancer

Risk Factor	Characteristics	Supporting Data
Gender	Males have 2× more incidences of cancer than females.	
Age	Most individuals > 50	Median age—70 (males); 74 (females). Gastric cancers in younger individuals a more aggressive type.
H. pylori infection	*H. pylori* infection worldwide; person-to-person transmission	Long-term infection causes atrophic gastritis—precancerous condition
Diet	Foods preserved by smoking, salting, or pickling Foods that contain nitrites and nitrates (bacon, ham, processed meat) Large amounts of red meat—well done or barbecued	Nitrates and nitrites combine with other nitrogen-containing substances forming N-nitroso compounds that are known carcinogenic agents.
Tobacco use	Smokers have twice the rate of cancer than non-smokers.	Tobacco use irritates lining of stomach.
Previous stomach surgery	Surgery to remove part of stomach and pyloric valve	Bile, pancreatic juices can back up, causing irritation and inflammation of stomach lining.
Stomach polyps	Small growth in lining of stomach	Most noncancerous, adenomatous polyps may be precancerous.
Familial cancer syndromes	Hereditary nonpolyposis colon cancer and familial adenomatous polyposis Mutations of BRCA1/BRCA2	Increased risk for development of gastric cancer
Family history	Parent or sibling with incidence	Increased risk for development of gastric cancer
Pernicious anemia	Associated with atrophic gastritis	Lack of intrinsic factor for B_{12} absorption. PA treated, still slightly at risk for gastric cancer
Blood type	Type A blood	Reasons unclear, individuals with type A higher risk than other blood types
Country of origin	Japan, Korea, Eastern Europe, Latin America	Increased ingestion of foods that are smoked, heavily salted, or pickled Increased incidence of infection with *H. pylori*
Body build/weight	Obesity	Extra weight associated with some cancers, including gastric cancer.

Table 28-11 Types of gastric cancers

Type of Cancer	Origination	Characteristics
Adenocarcinomas	Start in glandular cells of stomach's innermost lining.	Majority of stomach cancers (90%–95%)
Lymphomas	Cancers of immune system in stomach wall	Some aggressive Others slow growing (MALT) lymphomas 4% of stomach cancers
Carcinoid tumors	Originate in the stomach's hormone producing cells	Slow growing, with less frequent metastasis 3% of stomach cancers
Gastrointestinal stromal tumors (GISTs)	Develop from cells called interstitial cells of Cajal (part of autonomic nervous system) in the wall of the GI tract.	May occur from esophagus—most in stomach (60%–70%). Specific gene mutation allows treatment with new molecular target drugs aimed at inhibiting such mutations (Tarn & Goodwin, 2005).

Hepatitis

Described as inflammation of the liver, hepatitis is characterized by the presence of inflammatory cells in the liver tissue. The condition may be self-limiting or may progress to fibrosis and cirrhosis. Acute hepatitis lasts less than 6 months, while chronic persists longer. It can also be caused by toxic substances (alcohol, some medications, industrial organic solvents, and plants), other infections and autoimmune diseases. A small proportion of people with acute hepatitis progress to acute liver failure, in which the liver is unable to clear harmful substances from the circulation. This may lead to confusion and coma due to hepatic encephalopathy and the production of blood proteins that cause peripheral edema and bleeding. This may become life-threatening and occasionally requires a liver transplant (Table 28-12).

Pathophysiology

- Hepatitis viruses (HVA, HVB, HVC, HVD, and HVE) cause most cases worldwide. Viruses A, C, D, and E are RNA viruses, whereas HVB virus is a DNA virus (Dienstag, 2013).
- After inoculation, HV is transported across the intestinal epithelium traveling through the mesenteric veins to the liver.
- Virus enters hepatocytes and replicates exclusively within the cytoplasm via RNA-dependent polymerase. The exact mechanism of injury is not clearly understood, but evidence indicates the role of a cell-mediated immune response.
- HV is then shed from the hepatocyte to the sinusoids and bile canaliculi, and then to the intestines through bile, whereby fecal excretion occurs.
- The course of the disease varies by individual and etiologic agent, although typically progresses through four stages (Table 28-13).

Subjective Data

- Initial, nonspecific flulike symptoms, common to almost all acute viral infections. May include malaise, muscle/joint aches, fever, nausea/vomiting, diarrhea, headache.
- Acute hepatitis: profound jaundice, anorexia, malaise, loss of appetite, aversion to smoking among smokers, dark urine, abdominal discomfort
- Acute viral hepatitis is more likely to be asymptomatic in younger people.
- Chronic hepatitis: nonspecific symptoms (malaise, tiredness, weakness) or no symptoms.
- Occurrence of jaundice indicates advanced liver damage.

Objective Data

- Physical findings usually minimal, apart from jaundice in a third and tender hepatomegaly in about 10%.
- Some exhibit lymphadenopathy (5% of patients) or splenomegaly (5%).
- Extensive damage to liver and cirrhosis lead to weight loss, easy bruising and bleeding tendencies, peripheral edema, accumulation of ascites in peritoneal cavity.
- Cirrhosis may lead to complications: esophageal varices, hepatic encephalopathy, hepatorenal syndrome
- Commonly identified on blood tests performed either for screening or to evaluate nonspecific symptoms.

THINK LINK:* *The Silent Killer

Hepatitis C has earned the title of "silent killer," with an estimated number of 4.9 million individuals infected with the virus. It is transmitted by blood-to-blood contact and is recognized as the most common chronic blood-borne infection. The highest risk factor for infection with HCV is a history of intravenous drug use, causing two-thirds of new cases (Moore, Hawley, & Bradley, 2009).

Table 28-12 Characteristics and features of viral hepatitis

	Hepatitis A (HAV)	Hepatitis B (HBV)	Hepatitis C (HVC)	Hepatitis D (HVD)	Hepatitis E (HVE)
Transmission	Fecal–oral, parenteral, food/water	Blood/body fluids, sexual	Blood/body fluid, sexual, needle sticks	Blood/body fluids, sexual, fecal–oral (needs HVB to replicate)	Fecal–oral
Incubation period	2–7 weeks (30 days)	30–180 days (28 days)	15–150 days	30–180 days (35 days)	15–60 days (45 days)
Onset	Acute with fever	Insidious	Insidious	Insidious	Acute
Perinatal transmission	Not established	Yes	Yes	Rare/not documented in U.S.	Not established
Immunity	Yes	No	No	No	No
Signs/Symptoms	Fatigue, nausea, vomiting, high fever, hepatomegaly, jaundice, dark urine, anorexia, and rash	Gradual onset of fatigue, malaise, anorexia; RUQ pain, liver tenderness, jaundice; dark urine, light stools, nausea, vomiting, pruritis	Similar to HBV. 80% may not have symptoms.	Co-infection with HVB; co-infection leads to more severe disease course (one-third go to develop fulminant hepatitis)	Self-limiting condition similar to HVA infection. 10% progress to fulminant condition

Table 28-13 Four stages of hepatitis

Stage	Description	Characteristics/Manifestations
Stage 1	Viral replication	Individual asymptomatic
		Serologic and enzyme markers on laboratory panels
Stage 2	Prodromal	Onset of anorexia, nausea, vomiting, taste alterations, arthralgias, malaise, fatigue, urticaria, and pruritis. May develop aversion to cigarette smoke.
Stage 3	Icteric	Urine becomes darker and stools become lighter clay colored.
		Jaundice begins, RUQ pain with hepatomegaly
Stage 4	Convalescent	Resolution of symptoms and jaundice.
		Liver enzymes become WNL

Cirrhosis

This is a consequence of chronic liver disease; chronic alcoholism is the most common cause (40% of cirrhosis-related deaths). Other major causes include nonalcoholic fatty liver disease (NAFLD) and chronic hepatitis. Chronic viral hepatitis B or C can infect the liver for years, causing progressive liver damage that results in cirrhosis. Hepatitis C is more likely to cause cirrhosis than Hepatitis B. Other causes of cirrhosis include genetic disorders and altered biliary duct conditions. Genetic disorders result in hemochromatosis or Wilson's disease in the liver and other organs. Biliary duct conditions cause damage to or destruction of the bile ducts that allows bile to accumulate in the liver (see biliary atresia under Infants and Children).

Pathophysiology

- The pathological hallmark of cirrhosis is distortion of hepatic architecture by scar tissue that replaces parenchyma and formation of regenerative nodules, blocking the portal flow of blood through the organ and altering normal function.
- Damage to hepatic parenchyma activates the stellate cell, which becomes contractile and obstructs blood flow. It also leads to a fibrotic response and proliferation of connective tissue.
- The fibrous tissue bands (septa) separate hepatocyte nodules, which eventually replace the entire liver architecture, leading to decreased blood flow throughout.

Subjective Data

- Patients often have no signs or symptoms until liver damage is extensive.
- In the early stage of cirrhosis, symptoms are vague and nonspecific.
- The individual may experience fatigue and weakness, along with a loss of appetite, nausea and vomiting, and weight loss.
- As the liver damage increases, jaundice and itching develop due to decreased processing of bilirubin and accumulation of bile pigments in skin.

Objective Data

The following signs may occur in the presence of cirrhosis or as a result of the complications of cirrhosis. Many are nonspecific and may occur in other diseases and do not necessarily point to cirrhosis. Likewise, the absence of any does not rule out the possibility of cirrhosis.

- Spider angiomata or spider nevi caused by an increase in estradiol
- Palmar erythema caused by altered sex hormone metabolism
- Nail changes:
  - Muehrcke's lines from inadequate production of albumin
  - Terry's nails also due to hypoalbuminemia
  - Clubbing

- The spleen becomes congested, leading to hypersplenism and increased sequestration of platelets.
- Portal hypertension is responsible for most severe complications of cirrhosis.

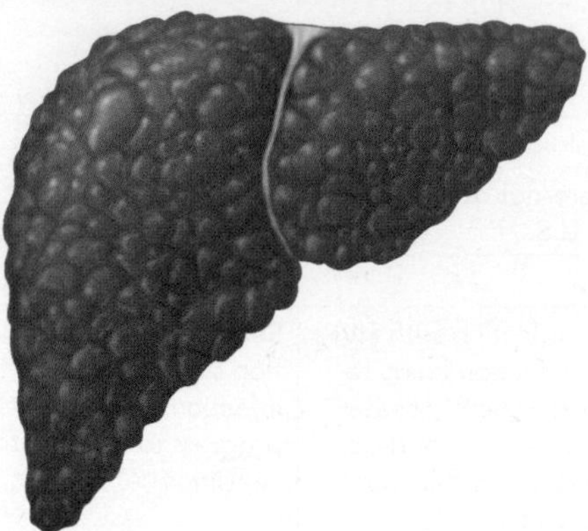

FIGURE 28-40 Cirrhosis of liver

- Easy bruising of the skin becomes apparent due to the decreased production of blood clotting factors.
- Sensitivity to medication caused by decreased metabolism of the active compounds.
- Gynecomastia caused by increased estradiol (occurs in up to 66% of patients)
- Hypogonadism: impotence, infertility, loss of sexual drive, testicular atrophy because of primary gonadal injury or suppression of hypothalamic or pituitary function
- Ascites
- Caput medusae. In portal hypertension, periumbilical collateral veins may dilate.
- Urine may also appear dark.

Disease progression results in development of serious, life-threatening complications:

- Hepatic encephalopathy
- Asterixis
- Fetor hepaticus (musty odor in breath)
- Portal hypertension
- Spontaneous bacterial peritonitis
- Esophageal varices
- Portacaval anastomosis
- Hepatocellular carcinoma

PRACTICE POINT: Cirrhosis

Once a patient develops complications of cirrhosis, he or she is considered to have decompensated disease. The high morbidity and mortality of cirrhosis is secondary to these devastating complications. The quality of life and survival of patients with cirrhosis can be improved by the prevention and treatment of these complications. If the cause of the cirrhosis is removed or treated, the formation of scar tissue is arrested, and further damage is arrested. However, if the cause is not removed or treated, eventually scar tissue formation exceeds cellular regeneration and liver functions fail. Cirrhosis is generally irreversible, and treatment usually focuses on preventing progression and complications. In advanced stages of cirrhosis, the only option is a liver transplant.

Liver Cancer (HCC)

Primary liver cancer, identified as hepatocellular carcinoma (HCC), is relatively rare in the U.S. with only about 18,000 cases diagnosed in 2006 (Gangloff, 2007). Secondary liver cancer results from metastasis of cancer cells to the liver from another cancer site.

Hepatocellular carcinoma is the most common form; it begins in the hepatocytes. Other types of cells in the liver can develop cancer, but these are much less common. In most cases, the cause of liver cancer is cirrhosis. Patients with hepatitis B or C are at risk for liver cancer, even if they have not developed cirrhosis. The incidence of liver cancer has increased somewhat over the past two decades and is expected to continue increasing over the next 20 years. This increase is most likely due to the increased incidence of hepatic B and C infections, which along with cirrhosis are the primary risk factors for developing HCC (Stuart & Stadler, 2013).

There is no conventional chemotherapy for HCC as evidenced by the absence of any significant benefits to its use. One contributing factor to its ineffectiveness is that the cirrhosis-related cancer impairs the liver's ability to metabolize drugs, making them ineffective.

The rates of hepatitis B and C have been declining over the past two decades; however, two other conditions have been identified as significant risk factors for HCC: diabetes and obesity. How they contribute to HCC is still being investigated; however, both are known causes of NAFLD and/or cirrhosis.

Pathophysiology

- Chronic infection with hepatitis C may predispose liver to injury and inflammation with an increased cell turnover, contributing to cellular transformations that may result in malignancies.
- Hepatitis B virus genetic material can inset itself into healthy liver cells, which initiates cellular mutations and excessive cell growth that may lead to cancer.

Subjective Data

- Symptoms of HCC are not evident until the later stages of the disease, making early diagnosis difficult, particularly in those that have no risk factors.

When signs and symptoms do appear, they may include the following:

- Unexplained weight loss
- Loss of appetite
- Upper abdominal pain

Objective Data

- Later manifestations may include the following:
  - Jaundice
  - Ascites
  - Hepatomegaly
  - Alcoholic stigmata (Dupuytren contracture, spider angiomata)
  - Asterixis
  - Pedal edema

- Liver cells are known to undergo multiple genetic defects or mutations as they multiply, making liver cancer difficult to treat—there is a continuous shift in the target, so that what may work for one doesn't always work for another.

- Nausea and vomiting
- General weakness and fatigue
- Abdominal swelling
- Jaundice
- White, chalky stools
- Additional evident symptoms consist of URQ pain that may extend to the shoulder and back and full feeling after small meals.

- Periumbilical collateral veins
- Enlarged hemorrhoidal veins

Cholecystitis/Cholelithiasis

Cholecystitis is inflammation of the gallbladder, most commonly due to obstruction of cystic duct with gall stones (90% of cases). Acalculous cholecystitis is an acute necroinflammatory disease of gallbladder and accounts for the other10% of cases of acute cholecystitis.

Cholelithiasis is the presence of gall stones in the gall bladder; it may exist by itself or progress to cholecystitis. Uncomplicated cholecystitis has an excellent prognosis; however, more than 25% of patients require surgery or develop complications. Delayed diagnosis of acute cholecystitis increases morbidity and mortality.

- Not everyone who has gallstones will go on to develop cholecystitis.
- Cholelithiasis and cholecystitis may present as a single episode or may recur on multiple occasions.

Pathophysiology

- Risk factors are increasing age, female gender, obesity, rapid weight loss, certain drugs, and pregnancy.
- Individuals of Native American (Pima), Hispanic, Mexican American, and Scandinavian heritage have higher incidence of cholelithiasis (Vorvick, 2009).
- Obstruction of the cystic duct results in the accumulation of bile within the gallbladder, causing it to distend. Distension of the gallbladder compromises blood flow and lymphatic drainage causing swelling and inflammation, predisposing to the development of mucosal ischemia and necrosis. Further complications, infection, and perforation may also develop.

Subjective Data

- Predominant symptom of cholecystitis is severe, sharp RUQ abdominal pain that may also be felt in the right shoulder or back.
- Other characteristics associated with the pain include nausea and vomiting, increasing pain during a deep breath, pain that lasts longer than 6 hours, and often occurs after eating, especially a meal that contains a fair amount of fat.
- Other symptoms may include fever, heartburn/indigestion, and excessive gas.
- Tenderness over the abdomen when it's touched
- Sweating
- Chills
- Abdominal bloating
- Patient may notice clay-colored stools and jaundice.

Objective Data

- Cholecystitis is usually diagnosed by a history of subjective data, as well as examination findings:
  - Low grade fever
  - Tender RUQ with or without Murphy's sign
- Subsequent laboratory and imaging tests are used to confirm the diagnosis and exclude other possible causes.
  - Visible gallstones on ultrasound helps confirm diagnosis of cholecystitis.
  - CT scan and MRI are also useful in the detection of cholecystitis.
  - Endoscopic Retrograde Cholangiopancreatography (ERCP) may be useful to visualize the anatomy.

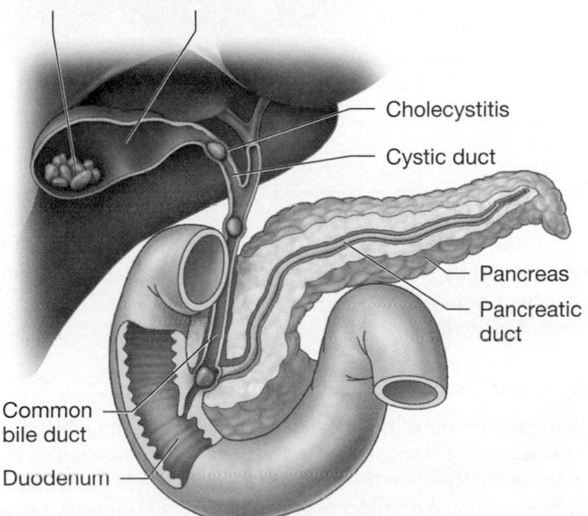

FIGURE 28-41 Cholelithiasis (gallstones) and cholecystitis (blockage and inflammation)

Pancreatitis

This is an inflammation of the pancreas that occurs when pancreatic enzymes (especially trypsin) that digest food are activated in the pancreas instead of the small intestine resulting in autodigestion. It may be acute—beginning suddenly and lasting a few days, or chronic—occurring over many years. The two major causes of pancreatitis are alcohol abuse and cholelithiasis. Gallstones are the single most common etiology of acute pancreatitis. Alcohol is the single most common etiology of chronic pancreatitis. Chronic pancreatitis can lead to diabetes or pancreatic cancer.

Pathophysiology

- Alcohol acts at the cellular level by causing intracellular accumulation of digestive enzymes that are activated and released prematurely. It also increases the permeability of ductules, allowing enzymes to reach pancreatic cells (Khoury & Deeba, 2009). The protein content of enzymes is increased and the bicarbonate levels and trypsin inhibitor concentrations are decreased, leading to the formation of protein plugs that obstruct outflow from the pancreas. The end result is damage and destruction to the pancreas.
- Cholelithiasis is the second most common cause of pancreatitis. A gallstone may obstruct the pancreatic duct, preventing the pancreatic enzymes from entering the duodenum, thus accumulating in the pancreas. Pancreatitis of this nature is more common in females over 50 years of age.
- Chronic pancreatitis begins with an acute episode. If scarring of the pancreas occurs during the acute episode, it is unable to return to its previous healthy state. The acute episode then turns into a chronic condition in which there is continuous damage to the pancreas that worsens over time.

Subjective Data

- Acute pain, characterized as a severe, burning pain in upper middle or upper left abdomen, which may radiate to the back.
- Pain with a gradual onset, which may have been present for a few days and may increase in intensity after eating or when lying on the back
- Nausea that may be associated with vomiting that worsens with eating.
- Fever
- Jaundice
- Tender, swollen abdomen
- Unexplained weight loss due inadequate breakdown of food
- Fatigue, lethargy, irritability, confusion, and headache.

Objective Data

- The physical examination will vary depending on severity and presence of internal bleeding.
- Blood pressure may be elevated by pain or decreased by dehydration or bleeding.
- Heart and respiratory rates are often elevated. Increased heart rate may be due to the pain and/or fever, or an indicator of internal bleeding.
- The abdomen is usually tender but to a lesser degree than the pain itself. Bowel sounds may be reduced from reflex bowel paralysis.
- If the acute episode becomes severe and progresses to infection or bleeding, the individual is at risk for becoming dehydrated and having low blood pressure.
- If the blood pressure becomes extremely low, the situation may progress to shock.

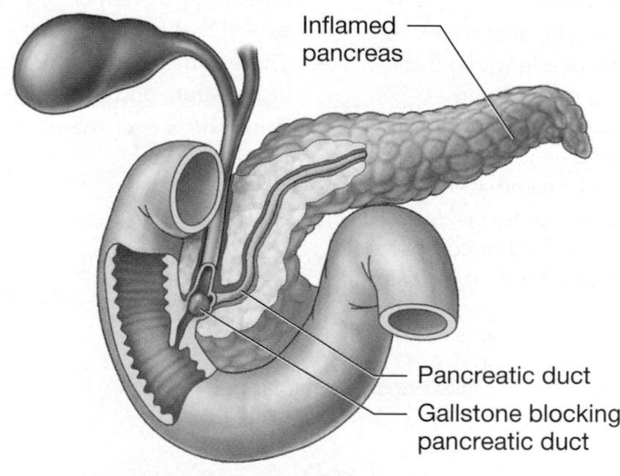

FIGURE 28-42 Pancreatitis

Pancreatic Cancer

This is a highly aggressive cancer that has often metastasized by the time of diagnosis. Like liver cancer, pancreatic cancer is highly resistant to treatment and carries a high mortality rate. Pancreatic cancer is considered curable only when it is discovered in its earliest stages.

Pathophysiology

- Pancreatic cancer may originate as one of three types of cancer. The most common type, pancreatic adenocarcinoma, arises from the exocrine glands.
- The other two types are intraductal papillary mucinous neoplasia and neuroendocrine carcinoma (islet cell tumor) (Kuo & Fisher, 2009).

Subjective Data

- Early symptoms of pancreatic cancer are vague and nonspecific and become apparent only when the cancer is well advanced. As the cancer progresses, symptoms begin to appear and often begin with the onset of pain.

Objective Data

- The initial presentation varies according to location of the cancer.
- Malignancies of the head of the gland typically present with jaundice, possibly in combination with darkened urine.

- The development of pancreatic cancer may involve the over-expression of oncogenes, inactivation of tumor suppressor genes or the deregulation of various signaling proteins (Sarkar, Banerjee, & Li, 2007).
- No well-established risk factors exist for the development of pancreatic cancer.
- Smokers have been found to develop pancreatic cancer two to three times the rate for nonsmokers.
- Age and gender—older males are more likely to develop pancreatic cancer. Most cases occur after age 60, while cases before age 40 are uncommon.
- Blacks have a higher incidence than whites.
- 5%–10% of pancreatic cancer patients have a family history of pancreatitis as well as some other genetic syndromes (BRCA2 gene mutation, Lynch syndrome, and familial atypical mole-malignant melanoma [FAMMM])
- Typically, pancreatic cancer first metastasizes to regional lymph nodes, and later to the liver or to the peritoneal cavity and, rarely, to the lungs; it rarely metastasizes to bone or brain.

- Pain in the upper abdomen that typically radiates to the back
- Heartburn—acid stomach
- Poor appetite or nausea and vomiting
- Diarrhea, loose stools
- Significant weight loss (cachexia)
- Itching as the salt from excess bile can cause skin irritation.
- Tiredness, irritability, and difficulty eating because of pain also exist.
- Pulmonary embolisms due to pancreatic cancers producing blood-clotting chemicals
- Development of diabetes mellitus or elevated blood sugar levels may occur months or even years before diagnosis with pancreatic cancer, suggesting new onset diabetes in an elderly individual may be an early warning sign of pancreatic cancer.
- Clinical depression has been reported in association with pancreatic cancer, sometimes presenting before the cancer is diagnosed (Mayr & Schmid, 2010).

- Cancer of the head of the pancreas (75% of cases) obstructs the common bile duct as it runs through the pancreas (may also cause pale-colored stool and steatorrhea).
- The recent onset of atypical diabetes mellitus
- Recent but unexplained thrombophlebitis (Trousseau syndrome) when blood clots form spontaneously in the portal blood vessels, the deep veins of the extremities, or the superficial veins.
- Previous attack(s) of pancreatitis are sometimes noted.

Urinary Tract Infections (UTIs)

UTIs (acute cystitis, bladder infection) are common occurrences and result from bacteria that ascend up the urethra into the bladder. When it affects the lower urinary tract it is known as a simple cystitis (bladder infection), and when it affects the upper urinary tract it is known as pyelonephritis, a kidney infection. Pyelonephritis, if it occurs, usually follows a bladder infection but may also result from a blood-borne infection.

Pathophysiology

- The main causal agent of both types is *Escherichia coli*; however, other bacteria, viruses, or fungi may rarely be the cause.
- The downward flow of urine is a primary means of preventing bacteria from ascending up the urethra into the bladder. Dehydration or infrequent urination interferes with this protective function.
- Women are more prone to develop a UTI because of the short urethra and the proximity of the urethra to the rectal area, allowing rectal bacteria to colonize the perineum.
- Sexual intercourse and family history have also been identified as contributing factors.

Subjective Data

- Patients with UTIs may be asymptomatic.
- Symptoms may include the following:
- Strong, persistent urge to urinate
- Dysuria
- Passing frequent, small amounts of urine
- Pelvic pain, in women
- Rectal pain, in men
- In older adults and in the very young, symptoms may be vague or nonspecific.

Objective Data

- Signs of a UTI may include all or any of the following:
  - Pyuria (pus in urine)
  - Urine that appears red, bright pink or cola-colored— a sign of hematuria
  - Strong-smelling urine
  - Present costovertebral angle (CVA) tenderness

PRACTICE POINT: UTIs in the Older Adult

Older adults with serious UTIs rarely have a fever or other common symptoms, resulting in over diagnosing and over treating on the basis of nonspecific clinical signs and symptoms (Beveridge, Davey, Phillips, & McMurdo, 2011). Often there is confusion or a delirium-like state, agitation, hallucinations, and change in behaviors, which are seen as early stages of dementia. These patients may also exhibit signs of poor motor skills, dizziness, and falling, while some present to a health care provider with sepsis as the first symptom. Diagnosis can be complicated by the fact that many elderly people have preexisting incontinence or dementia.

THINK LINK: Cranberry Juice and UTIs

Cranberry juice has often been identified with prevention of UTIs. It was thought to interfere with the pH of the urine, making it more acidic so that bacteria would not survive. The change in pH was due to the presence of large amounts of vitamin C. The amount of juice that needed to be ingested to achieve this was quite large. More recently, cranberry juice has been found to prevent the adhesion of bacteria to the transitional wall epithelium in the bladder. This property was particularly successful against certain types of *E. coli*, the most common bacterium that causes a UTI. The volume of cranberry juice needed to achieve protection is not as large as that needed for altering urinary pH.

Glomerulonephritis (GN)

GN refers to several renal diseases that usually affect both kidneys and cause injury and destruction of the renal glomeruli. It may be acute or chronic. Not strictly a single disease, its presentation depends on the specific disease entity. Acute GN may be caused by infections such as strep throat. It may also be caused by other illnesses, including systemic lupus erythematosis, Goodpasture's syndrome, Wegener's disease, and polyarteritis nodosa.

Pathophysiology

- Acute post-streptococcal glomerulonephritis (PSGN) is the model of acute GN, caused by a group A beta-hemolytic streptococcus infection, which usually starts at a distant location, most commonly the throat, and then migrates to the kidneys. Acute GN is defined as the sudden onset of hematuria, proteinuria, and red blood cell (RBC) casts.
- The damage begins with an inflammatory response in the glomeruli, causing cellular proliferation, sclerosis, and fibrosis, decreasing glomerular blood flow and filtration rate.
- A decreased glomerular blood flow leads to renal failure. In most instances, recovery occurs without any significant loss of renal function or a reoccurrence of the disease.
- In certain situations, the course of the disease continues to become a chronic condition that ultimately terminates in the development of renal failure.
- Except in PSGN, the exact triggers for the formation of the immune complexes are unclear.

Subjective Data

- The first indication that something is wrong may come from symptoms or from the results of a routine urinalysis.

The early symptoms of the acute disease are as follows:

- General ill feeling, and loss of appetite
- Fatigue from anemia or kidney failure
- Abdominal pain
- Swelling of face, hands, feet, and abdomen
- Pink or cola-colored urine from hematuria
- Urinating less than usual (oliguria)
- Cough and shortness of breath, dyspnea on exertion
- Diarrhea
- Fever
- Joint or muscle aches
- Foamy urine due to excess urine protein
- Headache

Objective Data

The physical manifestations of acute GN include the following:

- Anemia
- Fluid retention and edema (periorbital and/or pedal)
- Hypertension due to fluid overload (in 75% of patients)
- Crackles (i.e., if pulmonary edema)
- Elevated jugular venous pressure
- Ascites and pleural effusion (possible)
- Early diagnosis and prompt treatment are important to prevent kidney failure.
- Two conditions often associated with chronic GN are diabetes mellitus and systemic lupus erythematosus.

ACUTE RENAL FAILURE

Acute renal failure is a sudden and severe cessation of renal function. Causes of acute renal failure include nephrotoxic agents, infectious agents, reduced blood flow, or obstruction of the urinary tract. Initial treatment is to remove or treat the underlying cause. If treatment is initiated quickly, there may be recovery of renal function without any significant impairment. During the recovery phase of acute renal failure, dialysis may be needed on a temporary basis to replace renal function until the kidneys are able to function.

Nephrolithiasis (Kidney [renal] stones)

Kidney stones are composed of calcium salts, uric acid, cystine, and struvite and tend to form in alkaline urine. Other factors affecting stone formation include urine temperature, concentration of the urine, and ionic strength. Renal stone formation is more prevalent in males than females. Pain generated by renal colic is primarily caused by dilation, stretching, and spasm because of the acute ureteral obstruction.

Pathophysiology

Likely the result of two basic actions:

- Supersaturation of the urine by stone-forming constituents. A low fluid intake, with a subsequent low volume of urine production, produces high concentrations of stone-forming solutes in the urine The resulting calculi cause symptoms when they become impacted within the ureter as they flow with the urine into the bladder.
- Deposition of stone material on a renal papillary calcium phosphate nidus. This is most likely responsible for calcium oxalate stones.

Subjective Data

- Stones that grow to sufficient size (usually at least 3 millimeters [0.12 in.]) can cause obstruction of the ureter when passing into the ureter resulting in proximal urinary tract dilation, and spasms associated with classic renal colic.
- Acute onset of severe flank pain radiating to the groin and genital areas, gross or microscopic hematuria, nausea, and vomiting not associated with an acute abdomen are symptoms that most likely indicate renal colic.
- Fever may also be present and hematuria is common.

Objective Data

- Significant CVA tenderness/pain that can radiate to the upper or lower abdominal quadrant as a ureteral stone migrates distally is common.
- Abdominal examination usually is nonsignificant. Bowel sounds may be hypoactive, related to a mild ileus, which is often the case in patients with severe, acute pain.
- Small kidney stones may be spontaneously passed out of the kidneys into the urine and eliminated. Larger stones may need to be surgically removed or treated with high frequency sound waves that cause the stone to break up into smaller pieces that can then be eliminated.

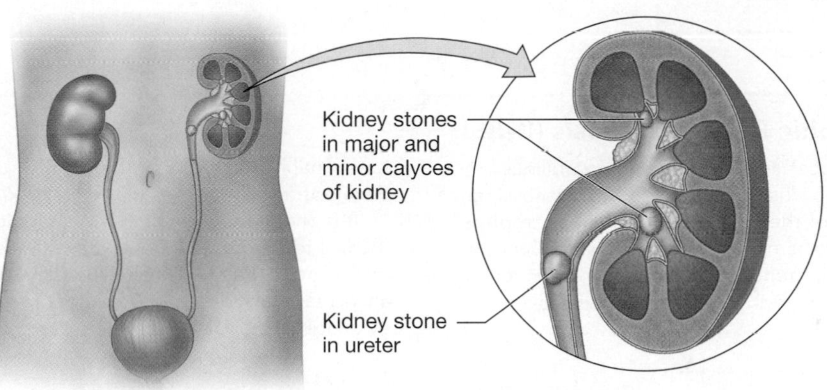

FIGURE 28-43 Nephrolithiasis

Conditions and Disorders: Infants and Children

Intussusception

This is intestinal obstruction in children caused by the prolapsing, or telescoping of one portion of the intestine into another. This "telescoping" often blocks food or fluid from passing through and also cuts off the blood supply to the part of the intestine that's affected. It can lead to a bowel perforation, infection and death of bowel tissue.

Pathophysiology

- Approximately 75% of cases of intussusception in children are considered idiopathic due to no clear disease trigger or pathological lead point.
- Believed to be secondary to an imbalance in the longitudinal forces along the intestinal wall, which can be caused by a mass acting as a lead point or by a disorganized pattern of peristalsis (e.g., ileus in the postoperative period).

Subjective Data

- Early symptoms can include lethargy, nausea, vomiting (sometimes bile stained [green color]), and intermittent moderate to severe cramping abdominal pain, causing pulling of the legs to the chest area.
- Dyspnea with paroxysms of pain
- Fever is not a symptom; however intussusception can cause a loop of bowel to become necrotic, secondary to ischemia due to compression of arterial blood supply. This leads to perforation and sepsis, which causes fever.

Objective Data

- Hallmark physical findings are a right hypochondrium sausage-shaped mass and emptiness in the right lower quadrant (Dance sign). This mass is hard to detect and is best palpated between spasms of colic.
- Abdominal distention is frequently found if obstruction is complete.
- Early on occult blood in the stools is the first sign of impaired mucosal blood supply. Later on, frank hematochezia and the classic currant jelly stools appear.
- Fever and leukocytosis appear with development of transmural ischemia and infarction.

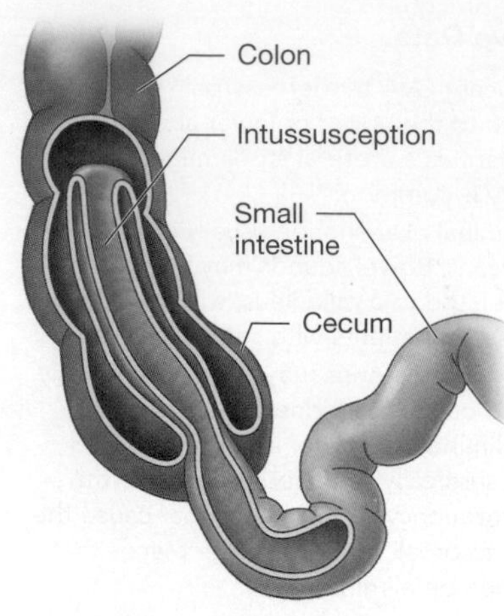

FIGURE 28-44 Intussusception

PRACTICE POINT: Intussusception

This condition is diagnosed most often in infancy and early childhood (ages of 3 and 36 months), striking about 2000 infants (1 in every 1900) in the U.S. in the first year of life and occurs three times more frequently in boys than in girls. Its incidence begins to rise at about 2 to 3 months of life, peaks at 4 to 9 months of age, and then gradually declines at around 18 months. In adults, intussusception represents the cause of approximately 1% of bowel obstructions and is frequently associated with neoplasm, malignant or otherwise. Intussusception occurs most frequently in the fall and winter months during viral season, but may occur at any time of the year. Approximately 30% of patients have a recent history of a viral illness.

Infantile Hypertrophic Pyloric Stenosis (IHPS)

This is a condition that causes severe projectile non-bilious vomiting in the first few months of life caused by a stenosis, or narrowing, of the pylorus of the stomach, due to hypertrophy of the muscle surrounding the pylorus, which spasms when the stomach empties. In pyloric stenosis, it is uncertain whether there is a real congenital narrowing or whether there is a functional hypertrophy of the pyloric sphincter muscle. Typically develops in male babies in the first 2–6 weeks of life.

It is one of the most common alterations that occur within the first few months of life, and five times more common in white males and full-term infants (Mayo Clinic Staff, 2009). There is also an increased incidence in Down syndrome infants and there is also evidence to support a familial tendency (Evers, 2006).

Pathophysiology

- Marked hypertrophy and hyperplasia of the two muscular layers of the pylorus results in obstruction of the pyloric sphincter and blocking food from entering the infant's small intestine.
- The pyloric canal becomes lengthened, and the whole pylorus becomes thickened. The mucosa becomes edematous and thickened. In advanced cases, the stomach becomes markedly dilated in response to near-complete obstruction.
- The causes of infantile hypertrophic pyloric stenosis are multifactorial. Both environmental factors and hereditary factors are believed to be contributory.
- Possible etiologic factors include deficiency of nitric oxide synthase containing neurons, abnormal myenteric plexus innervation, infantile hypergastrinemia, and exposure to macrolide antibiotics.

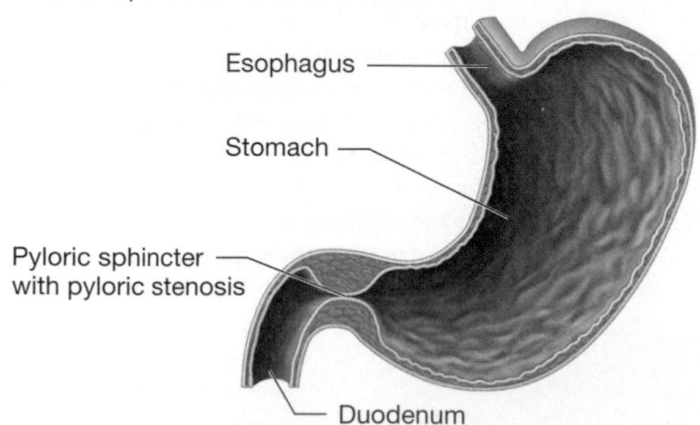

FIGURE 28-45 Pyloric stenosis

Subjective Data

- Some infants present with poor feeding and weight loss, but others demonstrate normal weight gain.
- Constant hunger, belching, and colic are other possible signs that the baby is unable to eat properly.
- Changes in bowel movements or constipation
- Problems gaining weight
- General signs of dehydration and malnutrition: baby cries without tears, fewer wet diapers, poor weight gain, weight loss, marasmus, decreased urinary output, lethargy, and shock
- Jaundice

Objective Data

- In as many as 60%–80% of the infants with IHPS, a firm, nontender, and mobile hard pylorus that is 1–2 cm in diameter, described as an "olive," may be present in the right upper quadrant at the lateral edge of the rectus abdominis muscle. This is best palpated after the infant has vomited and when calm, or when the gastric contents have been removed via nasogastric tube.
- Infants with IHPS begin vomiting for no apparent reason, gradually increasing in force until it becomes projectile vomiting. Vomiting usually occurs right after eating and consists of food that has just been ingested plus retained food from previous feedings. It is uncommon for any blood to be present in the vomit (Mayo Clinic Staff, 2009). The infant frequently demonstrates hunger after vomiting.
- Left untreated, the infant will develop severe fluid and electrolyte imbalance, malnutrition, and weight loss that may be fatal in a period of 4–6 weeks. Signs of dehydration include depressed fontanelles, dry mucous membranes, decreased tearing, poor skin turgor, and lethargy.
- Gastric peristalsis may be visible just prior to vomiting as the peristaltic waves try to overcome the obstruction.

Meconium Ileus (MI)

This is a lower or distal intestinal obstruction due to impaction of thick, tenacious meconium, a substance that consists of intestinal gland secretions, bile acids and bile salts, and amniotic fluid. Meconium fills the entire intestine prior to birth and is passed from the rectum within the first 24–72 hours after birth. In addition, complications such as ileal atresia or stenosis, ileal perforation, meconium peritonitis, and volvulus with or without pseudocyst formation can occur in association with meconium ileus.

Failure to pass a meconium stool may also be an indication of imperforate anus (IA), in which the infant has an anal canal that ends blindly and has no anal opening. It is frequently associated with alterations and malformations of the muscles and nerves that are involved in anal functioning (Rosen & Beals, 2009). IA is often accompanied by fistula formation that connects to the perineum and may be an indication of other congenital malformations. While not a fatal condition, there may be long-term consequences related to fecal and urinary incontinence.

Pathophysiology

- Meconium ileus results from the lack of digestive enzymes in utero. It is frequently associated with cystic fibrosis and is often its first manifestation.
- Meconium of this nature also contains albumin, which is not an expected substance of meconium (Evers, 2006). Detection of albumin is used as a screening for diagnosis of cystic fibrosis.

Subjective Data

- As this condition is noted shortly after birth, there is no specific subjective data.

Objective Data

- The infant with MI usually presents with abdominal distension that develops over the first few days after birth. There is failure to pass the meconium and the infant may begin to vomit within the first few hours to days of life.
- If the infant also has CF, pulmonary problems may also be present.
- Hyperactive bowel sounds will also be present.

Biliary Atresia (BA)

This is an uncommon progressive, idiopathic, fibro-obliterative congenital alteration characterized by the absence or obstruction of hepatic bile ducts throughout the liver and/or the common bile duct between the liver and the small intestine. BA is the most frequent cause of neonatal jaundice for which surgery is indicated and the most common reason for a liver transplant in children. As a birth defect in newborn infants, it occurs in 1/10,000 to 1/15,000 cases in live births in the U.S. Anomalies associated with BA include cardiac lesions, polysplenia, situs inversus, absent vena cava, and a preduodenal portal vein.

Pathophysiology

- Pathogenesis of this disorder remains poorly understood and varies widely. BA is categorized into three types based on the predominant site of atresia:
  - Type I: atresia restricted to the common bile duct
  - Type II: atresia of the common hepatic duct
  - Type III: atresia of the right and left hepatic duct
- The cause is an intrauterine injury, which may be related to chromosomal alterations, drugs, toxins, viral infections, or immune reactions.
- The destruction of the biliary tracts is related to the developmental stage of the fetus in utero.
- Progressive destruction of the bile ducts leads to biliary cirrhosis, portal hypertension, or liver failure. Fibrosis and cirrhosis may develop within the first 3–6 months after birth. Biliary atresia is fatal within 2 years if not treated.

Subjective Data

- As BA presents in early infancy, there are few, if any, specific symptoms noted as the majority of infants with biliary atresia (BA) are born at full term, have a normal birth weight, and initially thrive and seem healthy.

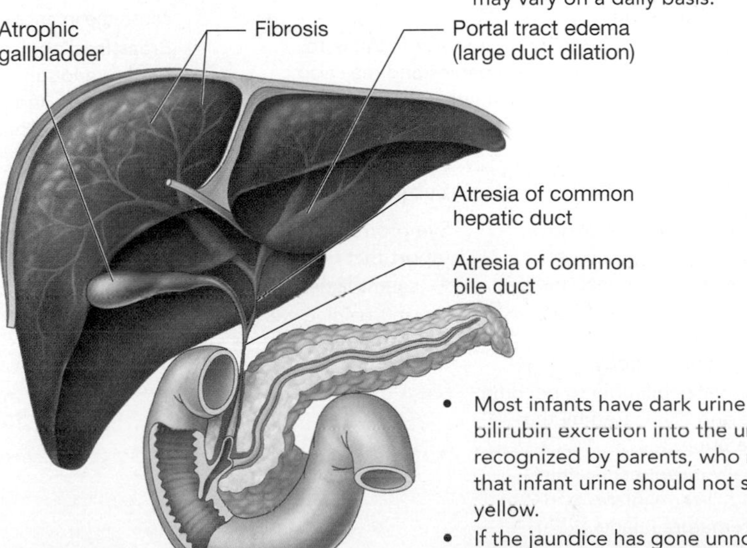

FIGURE 28-46 Biliary Atresia

Objective Data

- Jaundice is the initial sign of BA, which may only be seen in the sclerae. The onset of jaundice occurs between birth to 8 weeks, and is highly unlikely to appear later.
- Some infants have acholic stools, which often go unrecognized because the stools are pale but not white and the stool color may vary on a daily basis.
- Most infants have dark urine because of bilirubin excretion into the urine; often not recognized by parents, who may not realize that infant urine should not stain a diaper yellow.
- If the jaundice has gone unnoticed and the child's disease has progressed, there may be a firm, enlarged liver and spleen.

Necrotizing Enterocolitis (NEC)

This is a devastating condition primarily seen in premature infants, where portions of the bowel undergo necrosis. It is the second most common cause of morbidity in premature infants; however, it also presents in full-term infants. Annually, 1500 to 2000 infants die from NEC (20%–30% mortality rate), with those requiring surgery having the highest rate (Neu & Walker, 2011). The mean gestational age for affected infants is 31 weeks (Evers, 2006). The more mature the GI tract, the less the risk of developing NEC.

Although early recognition and aggressive treatment of this disorder has improved clinical outcomes, NEC accounts for substantial long-term morbidity in survivors of neonatal intensive care, particularly in premature very low birth weight infants (birth weight below 1500 g). Complications of NEC include the development of intestinal strictures and short bowel syndrome. Infants with short bowel syndrome will most likely require continuous total parenteral nutrition.

Pathophysiology

- The overall mechanism of injury is the reduction of blood flow to the mucosa resulting in hypoxic injury, with mucosal edema, hemorrhage, and necrosis.
- The exact cause is unknown, but is presumed to be related to immaturity of the GI immune system. Specific etiologic causes include infections (gram-positive and gram-negative bacteria, fungi, and viruses have been isolated), colonization of endotoxins, and the effects of medications and oral feedings, which initiate the release of proinflammatory cytokines by the mucosa.
- Left untreated, it results in bowel necrosis, perforation, and death.

Subjective Data

The clinical presentation of NEC includes nonspecific aspects of the history, such as the following:

- Apnea
- Lethargy
- Poor tolerance to feedings

Objective Data

- Manifestations of NEC appear in premature infants within the first 14 days after birth; full-term infants will present earlier.
- Primarily affects the GI tract, but in severe cases, can cause profound impairment of multiple organ systems.

Initial symptoms may be subtle and can include any of the following:

- Delayed gastric emptying with retained gastric contents
- Abdominal distention/tenderness, or both
- Ileus/decreased bowel sounds
- Redness or abnormal color of abdomen (advanced stages)
- Hematochezia
- Bloating or swelling of abdomen
- Frequent vomiting (possibly green in color)
- Bloody stool
- Systemic signs, such as apnea, bradycardia, decreased peripheral perfusion, labile body temperature, and hypoglycemia, are indicators of physiologic instability and disease progression.

Physiologic Jaundice

This is a short-term, nonthreatening situation that occurs within the first week in healthy infants. It is not considered to be critical; however, treatment with fluorescent (ultra violet) lighting is used to hasten the conjugation of bilirubin. Risk factors for physiologic jaundice include the following:

- Premature birth. A premature baby is generally not able to process bilirubin as quickly as full-term babies and may also feed less and have fewer bowel movements less bilirubin eliminated in the baby's stool.
- Bruising during birth. Bruising results in a higher level of bilirubin from the breakdown of more red blood cells.
- Blood type. A mother's blood type that is different from the infant's may have received maternal antibodies through the placenta that cause the infant's blood cells to break down more quickly.
- Breastfeeding. Infants who are having difficulty nursing or not getting enough nutrition from breastfeeding may develop dehydration and low intake of calories, contributing to the onset of jaundice.

Pathophysiology

- The cause is related to a breakdown of excess red cells, which release bilirubin, at a greater rate than the liver can handle. Bilirubin released from red cells is unconjugated, a state that cannot be eliminated from the body.
- The liver conjugates bilirubin to become water soluble and eliminated by the kidneys in the urine.
- Jaundice usually disappears within 1 to 2 weeks in full-term infants and 2 to 4 weeks in premature infants.
- If the jaundice does not disappear, then other causes of liver dysfunction must be considered.

Subjective Data

Symptoms would relate to the parent's report that the infant

- seems listless, sick or difficult to wake.
- isn't gaining weight or is feeding poorly.
- makes high-pitched cries.

Objective Data

- Primary objective data are skin that appears yellow and/or whites of the infant's eyes that look yellow.
- Long-term hyperbilirubinemia may cause kernicterus (bilirubin encephalopathy), which may result in brain damage.
- Unconjugated bilirubin is fat soluble, so in the presence of excess bilirubin, it is deposited in the brain, which is toxic to brain cells and may result in cerebral palsy and hearing and speech disorders.

BLASTOMAS

A **blastoma** is a type of cancer or neoplasm, more common in children, that is caused by malignancies in immature, undifferentiated (blast) cells that contain minimal to no structural cells. The most common blastomas in childhood are **neuroblastoma** and **nephroblastoma.**

Neuroblastoma

Neuroblastoma is the most common extracranial solid cancer in infants and account for approximately 7% of cancers in children. It is a neuro-endocrine malignant tumor of primitive nerve cells arising from any neural crest element anywhere along sympathetic nervous system (SNS).

Children under 5 have the highest incidence; rarely does it occur in children older than 10 years. Children with a family history of neuroblastoma are at higher risk for developing the disease; however, familial neuroblastoma accounts for a very small percentage of neuroblastomas. More commonly, a cause is never identified. The group of scientists at the Smurfit Institute of Genetics at Trinity College in Dublin identified that the CHD5 gene is "deleted" in children with the worst form of neuroblastoma., resulting in neuroblasts that are incapable of growing into mature nerve cells (Heffernan, 2013).

Pathophysiology

During fetal development, neuroblastic cells migrate from the neural crest to peripheral organs in the neck, chest, and abdomen, during which neuroblasts differentiate into adult neuronal tissue that forms the sympathetic chain and adrenal medulla.

- Neuroblastoma is neuronal tissue derived from the neural crest that remains or becomes undifferentiated after reaching its peripheral location, adopting the appearance of small, round blue cells with neuritic processes (Davenport, Blanco, & Sandler, 2012).
- Approximately one-third of neuroblastomas originate in the adrenal gland; another third originate in the sympathetic ganglia of the abdomen; and the rest originate in the ganglia of the chest or pelvis. Often by the time of diagnosis, the tumor has metastasized.
- Neuroblastoma behavior is unlike those of other malignancies. In some instances, the cells die for no reason and the tumor disappears. Or, the cells may spontaneously mature into ganglion cells that no longer divide, becoming a ganglioneuroma.

Subjective Data

- Early, nonspecific, vague symptoms include fatigue, loss of appetite, fever, joint pain, weight loss, and irritability.
- Neuroblastomas may secrete certain chemicals that irritate other normal tissues, causing signs and symptoms called paraneoplastic syndromes.

Objective Data

Signs of NB depend on primary tumor locations and metastases if present. Metastatic disease is manifested by hepatomegaly, subcutaneous nodules, blue or purple lesions (blueberry muffin baby), and bone pain, which is caused by bone marrow infiltration (Davenport et al., 2012).

- Adrenal gland tumors can cause high blood pressure and an increased heart rate.
- An abdominal tumor may cause pain, distension, hepatomegaly, a nontender mass, and diarrhea/constipation.
- A chest tumor may cause breathing problems (wheezing, chest pain, cough).
- A tumor pressing on the spinal cord may cause back pain, weakness, and paralysis.
- Bone lesions in the legs and hips may cause pain and limping.
- Metastasis may also involve the orbits of the eyes, creating an ecchymotic discoloration of the upper and lower lids, creating a raccoon-like eye appearance.

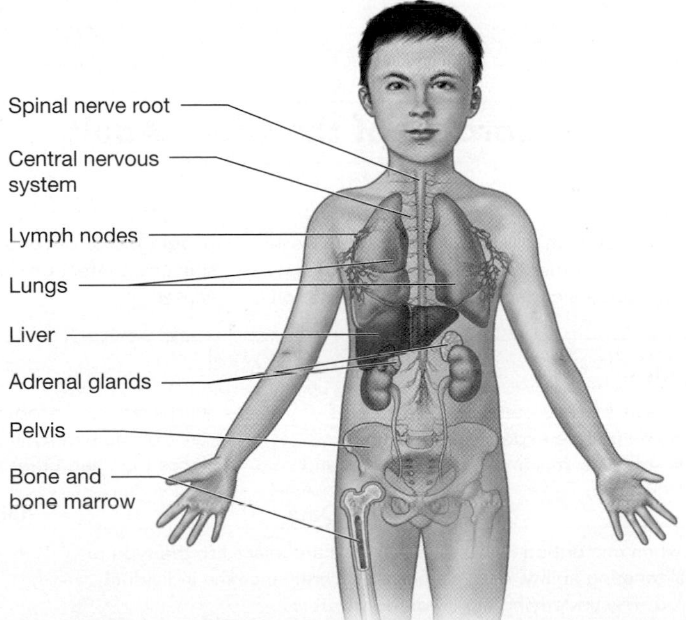

FIGURE 28-47 Common sites for neuroblastoma

Nephroblastoma (Wilms' Tumor, WT)

This is a malignant tumor of the kidney. Like neuroblastomas, nephroblastomas arise from immature kidney cells and begins in utero. It is one of the most common childhood cancers of the abdomen and the most common type of kidney cancer in children; however, the overall survival for most patients with WT is 90% (Ko & Ritchey, 2009). The highest incidence of Wilms' tumor is at 3 years of age and rarely occurs after age 8. There are a number of recognized syndromes associated with an increased predisposition toward developing WT.

Pathophysiology

- One or both kidneys may be involved. The size of the tumor may be quite large; however, it usually remains encapsulated, so metastasis is rare. If it does metastasize, the lungs are most commonly affected.
- The exact cause of Wilms' tumor is unknown but is attributed to multiple genetic alterations. There is a familial genetic link, but it only represents 1%–2% of newly diagnosed cases (Ko & Ritchey, 2009).
- Risk factors include being female, being black, family history.

Subjective Data

- Unlike most cancers, Wilms' tumor does not generally interfere with a child's health—even though it may become very large, there are usually no symptoms that are obvious to the child or parent.
- Parents might also find a lump in the belly.
- Only rarely will the child complain of abdominal pain.

Objective Data

- The tumor is most often palpated during a routine exam of the abdomen.

Other manifestations may include the following:

- Hematuria
- Nausea and vomiting accompanied by loss of appetite and weight loss
- Fever
- Constipation
- General malaise
- High blood pressure in some instances.

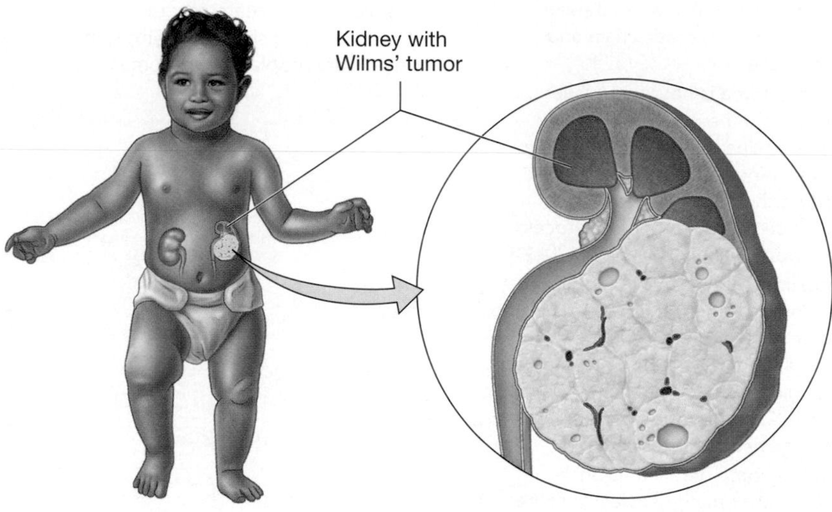

FIGURE 28-48 Nephroblastoma (Wilms' Tumor)

Conditions and Disorders of the Older Adult

INCONTINENCE

Incontinence is generally associated with loss of voluntary control over urinary and bowel functions. As with other alterations that become manifest in the elderly, incontinence is not an expected manifestation of aging. Loss of control over bladder and bowel elimination has a significant effect on one's quality of life and may have one of many causes.

Urinary Incontinence

Urinary incontinence is the inability to control the release of urine from the bladder. Some people experience occasional, minor leaks—or dribbles—of urine. It is an underdiagnosed and underreported problem that increases with age—affecting 50%–84% of the elderly in long-term care facilities—and at any age is more than two times more common in females than in males.

Pathophysiology

- Incontinence occurs when micturition physiology, functional toileting ability, or both have been altered. The underlying pathology varies among the different types of incontinence.

Subjective Data

- Symptoms are related to the type of urinary incontinence the individual demonstrates.
- Also see Table 28-14.

Objective Data

- The primary objective data would be evidence of urinary leakage on underclothes, protective pads, or bed sheets, etc.
- Also see Table 28-15.

- Urinary incontinence in elderly females is often related to a reduction in estrogen, which weakens the tissues around the pelvic floor and bladder outlet, decreases the muscle tone of urethral smooth muscle (urethral hypermobility secondary to poor anatomic pelvic support).
- Urinary incontinence in elderly males is most commonly related to prostatic hypertrophy, which may result in a radical prostatectomy for prostate cancer or transurethral resection of the prostate for benign prostatic hyperplasia. This results in a decline in the rate of urinary outflow, urinary retention, and a decreased stability of the detrusor muscle.
- Causes other than gender-related aging changes may also contribute to urinary incontinence. These include delirium, drugs (anticholinergics and diuretics), infections, and diabetes. Other causes of incontinence may be remembered by using the mnemonic DRIP (see Table 28-14).
- Acute incontinence that is not reversed with treatment is considered persistent and causes continuing problems in management is classified into the following four categories and managed accordingly: (1) stress, (2) urge, (3) overflow, and (4) functional. Characteristics of these categories are described in Table 28-15.

Table 28-14 Reversible causes of urinary incontinence

D	Delirium (confusion), dehydration
R	Retention, restricted mobility (unable not enough time to get to toilet)
I	Impaction (stool), infection, increased urine output (excess fluid intake, alcoholic or caffeinated beverages, diuretics, [peripheral edema, congestive heart failure], or metabolic disorders [hyperglycemia or hypercalcemia])
P	Polyuria, pharmaceuticals, psychological disorders (depression, behavioral disorders)

Table 28-15 Urinary incontinence

Type of Incontinence	Characteristics	Manifestations
Stress (urine leakage associated with increased abdominal pressure)	Small volume incontinence with cough, sneezing, laughing, running; history of prior pelvic surgery	Pelvic floor relaxation; cystocele, rectocele; lax urethral sphincter; loss of urine with provocative testing, atrophic vaginitis; post-void residual < 100 mL
Urge (involuntary leakage accompanied by or immediately preceded by urgency)	Uncontrolled urge to void; large-volume incontinence; history of CNS disorders such as stroke, multiple sclerosis, parkinsonism	Unexpected findings only as related to CNS disorder; post-void residual < 100 mL
Overflow (incomplete bladder emptying secondary to impaired detrusor contractility or bladder outlet obstruction)	Small volume incontinence, dribbling, hesitancy; in men, symptoms of enlarged prostate, nocturia, dribbling, hesitance, decreased force and caliber of stream	Distended bladder; prostate hypertrophy; stool in rectum, fecal impaction; post-void residual > 100 mL
	In neurogenic bladder; history of bowel problems, spinal cord injury, or multiple sclerosis	Evidence of spinal cord disease or diabetic neuropathy; lax sphincter; gait disturbance
Mixed (combination of stress and urge incontinence; it is a more common type of incontinence in older women)	Shares symptoms of both stress and urge incontinence.	
Functional (the inability to hold urine due to reasons other than neuro-urologic and lower urinary tract dysfunction)	Change in mental status, impaired mobility, new environment Medications: hypnotics, diuretics, anticholinergic agents, alpha-adrenergic agents, calcium-channel blockers	Impaired mental status, mobility Impaired mental status or unexpected findings only as related to other physical conditions.

Bowel (Fecal) Incontinence

Bowel incontinence is also considered a major problem of the elderly. Any alterations in the neuromuscular functions that control bowel elimination contribute to the development of incontinence. Control of bowel function becomes more of a problem in the presence of diarrhea.

Bowel incontinence is the recurrent inability to voluntarily control the passage of bowel contents through the anal canal and expel it at a socially acceptable location and time, causing stool to leak unexpectedly from the rectum.

It ranges from an occasional leakage of stool while passing gas to a complete loss of bowel control.

Pathophysiology

- Aging results in a decreased muscle mass of the rectum and a weakening of the external sphincter. This, along with any other neurogenic problems or alterations in intestinal motility, contributes to bowel incontinence.
- Bowel incontinence may be related to four categories of causes: (1) neurogenic, (2) muscle atrophy, (3) constipation, and (4) diarrhea. These categories are further described in Table 28-16.

Subjective Data

- The direct (primary) symptom is the inability to control or manage the passage of gas or stools, which may be liquid or solid, from the rectum, which becomes worse without treatment.
- Symptoms of fecal leakage (FL), such as loss of small amounts of brown fluid and staining of the underwear may occur after defecation. Indirect (secondary) symptoms are the result of leakage causing pruritus ani (intense itching sensation from the anus), perianal dermatitis, and UTIs.
- Due to embarrassment, people may only mention secondary symptoms rather than acknowledge incontinence.
- Additionally, patients may not be able to make it to the toilet in time and experience diarrhea, constipation, and gas and bloating.

Objective Data

- Any major underlying cause will produce additional signs, such as protrusion of mucosa in external rectal prolapse.

Table 28-16 Categories of bowel incontinence

Type	Cause	Mechanisms	Conditions
Neurogenic	Damage to nerves that sense stool in rectum and urge to defecate	Nerve impulses interrupted, so messages regarding need to have bowel movement not transmitted	Childbirth Constant straining Spinal cord damage Stroke Diabetes mellitus Multiple sclerosis
Muscle dysfunction	Injury to muscles of rectum and anal sphincters, causing them to weaken and to be unable to hold stool properly	External sphincter damage—urgency: Need to rush to bathroom as soon as need felt. If not reached in time, loss of stool on the way. Internal sphincter damage—soft stool or small portions of stool leak out without person realizing it is occurring. May occur after having a BM or with activity (walking, bending, sports). Scarring and stiffening of rectum from surgery, radiation, inflammatory bowel disease reduces holding capacity of rectum.	Childbirth (episiotomy, use of forceps) Surgical operations Injuries Rectal cancer/treatment Aging
Constipation	Stool becomes impacted causing formation of large mass that becomes dry and hard; unable to be evacuated.	The muscles of the rectum and intestines stretch and weaken allowing watery stools further up the colon to leak around mass.	Immobility Medications Some nerve diseases (Parkinson's)
Constipation	Stool becomes impacted causing formation of large mass that becomes dry and hard; unable to be evacuated.	The muscles of the rectum and intestines stretch and weaken allowing watery stools further up the colon to leak around mass.	Immobility Medications Some nerve diseases (Parkinson's)
Diarrhea	Loose, watery stools are more difficult to control. Causes or worsens incontinence.	Individuals with diarrhea often have high pressure waves in colon, which may be so intense that create extreme urgency and need to find bathroom immediately.	Infection Inflammatory bowel disease/irritable bowel syndrome

Male Genitalia

29

Up two sets to one and late into the fourth set, Marcus lines up a crosscourt forehand and cocks his racket high behind his shoulder. He's on the run, and the shot stretches him to the limits of his famed arm-span. The ball catches the face of the racket squarely and curls over the net and out of reach of his opponent. Marcus's leading foot strikes the clay hard, and he slides into a full split. Bringing his left leg around to the front to pivot up to a stand, Marcus cries out as a searing pain in his groin forces him back to the ground. A pulled muscle? This feels different; this pain is deep, constant, intolerable. Marcus slides a hand over his lower abdomen, gently probing in an attempt to discover the source of his discomfort. It's emanating from his right testicle. *I've been through worse*, he thinks, rising to his feet.

At first the pain seems to improve as he limbers up. However, his groin screams between points, but he wills this to the back of his mind. Nevertheless, the next three games slip away, and he finds himself embroiled in a long fifth set. Two hours later, he emerges from the locker room in tears and hardly able to stand.

Three hours pass before he goes to the emergency department, his testicle swollen like a melon and turning blue. The doctors are unimpressed with his stubbornness on the court, and Marcus grits his teeth in response to their grim expressions. Defeat might not have been in his vocabulary, but the next word from the doctors would linger there for the rest of his life: *orchiectomy*.

LEARNING OUTCOMES

1. Explain the composition, structure, and function of the male reproductive organs.
2. Summarizes the expected findings associated with examination of the male reproductive system.
3. Compare and contrasts the manifestations of altered conditions of the male reproductive system.
4. Explain age-related changes that affect the composition, structure, and function of the male reproductive system.
5. Explain appropriate techniques and procedures used to assess the male reproductive system.
6. Recognize appropriate data from the patient's history and characteristics of the male reproductive system and correctly document them in accordance with assessment findings.

The organs of the male reproductive system are specialized to produce, maintain, and transport sperm (male reproductive cells) and protective fluid (semen); to discharge sperm within the female reproductive tract; and to produce and secrete male sex hormones. Male reproductive organs are primarily external with some being internal. Their function is not fully mature until a male reaches puberty. Mature male reproductive and sexual function is associated with libido, erection, ejaculation, and orgasm.

Structure and Function

The male reproductive organs consist of the external structures: the penis and scrotum, which contain the testicles and epididymides, and the internal seminal vesicles, Cowper's gland, and prostate gland.

External Structures

The penis consists of a tube, the urethra, which is encased in sponge-like tissue that is capable of enlarging and becoming more firm (Figure 29-1). The urethra begins at the bladder extends the length of the penis, terminating at the end of the penis as a slitlike opening. The urethra, a part of the renal system, is the conduit for the passage of urine from the bladder through the meatus. The urethra also has a male reproductive function as the conduit for deposition of semen in the female vagina.

The spongy tissue that occupies the majority of space in the penis, giving it its shape and structure, consists of corpus spongiosum and two corpora cavernosum. Each cavernosum consists of smooth muscle surrounded by a tough, fibrous connective tissue framework, the **tunica albuginea**. The cavernosum and spongiosum extend internally into the pelvic area and are attached to the pelvic bone. Each cavernosa contains blood sinuses that fill with blood, causing the tissues to expand and become firm, producing an erection. The filling of the sinuses is brought about by arterial dilation that is a response to the release of nitric oxide and parasympathetic impulses.

The two corpora cavernosum form the lateral and dorsal sides of the penis. The corpus spongiosum, which contains the urethra, enlarges distally to form the glans penis. The shaft of the penis extends from the base to the glans. The penis is covered by a thin layer of relatively loose skin that is darker in color and does not contain any subcutaneous tissue. The skin folds on itself at the distal end, forming the foreskin, or prepuce, that covers the glans. Circumcised males have had the foreskin removed.

At the base of the penis, the skin becomes the scrotum a sac of skin that contains two testicles (see Figure 29-1). The internal scrotum is divided by a septum, with a testicle on each side. The scrotal skin also consists of thin cremasteric muscle, which contracts or relaxes the scrotum relative to temperature fluctuations. Spermatogenesis (sperm production) requires a temperature lower than body temperature, thus the cremasteric muscle controls the temperature by increasing or decreasing the distance between the testes and the body. The scrotal skin is also coarse in appearance and covered with wrinkles that are called **rugae**. These manifestations are more apparent when the scrotum is contracted. Like the penis, the scrotum is often darker in appearance that the rest of the skin, but unlike the penis, contains hair. Additionally, there is a dark, vertical, linear line in the middle of the scrotum identified as the **raphe** that is formed when the non-differentiated genital folds fuse at the midline.

The testicles are ovoid-shaped structures that produce sperm and testosterone. They do not begin their primary function until an individual has started puberty. Each testicle is approximately 4 × 3 × 2 cm and is suspended within the scrotum by a spermatic cord (see Figure 29-1). Each testis is subdivided internally into lobes that each contains several seminiferous tubules. Within the seminiferous tubules are **spermatogonia**, stem cells that generate sperm; they become efferent tubules that connect within the epididymis.

Attached to each testicle is a comma-shaped **epididymis**, which curves over the posterior portion of each testis, and consists of a tightly coiled duct that collects the immature sperm from the seminiferous tubules. During the travel through the tubules, which may be 12 or more days, the sperm mature and receive testosterone and other nutrients to enhance their fertilization properties. The tubules then become a single tube, the **vas deferens**, which is encased within the spermatic cord. The spermatic cord is a connective tissue sheath attached to the testicle that contains the vas deferens as well as testicular blood vessels and nerves. Once the vas deferens passes through the inguinal canal it passes over the bladder and connects with the **seminal vesicle**.

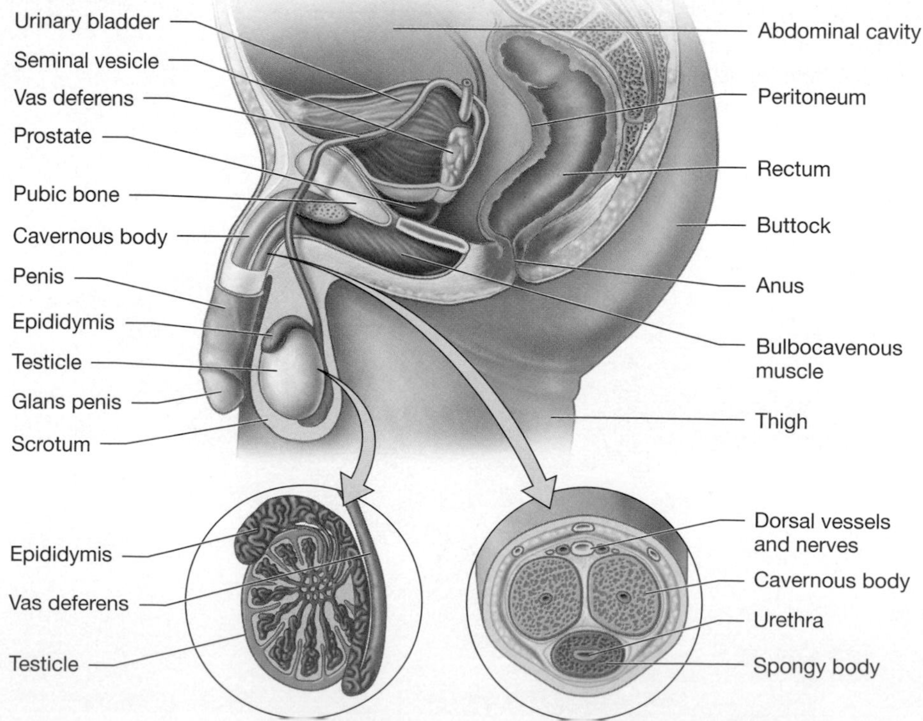

FIGURE 29-1 Anatomy of male genitalia

Internal Structures

The seminal vesicle is a paired glandular pouch that is located above the prostate gland on each side of the bladder and collects and stores semen, the fluid that contains sperm and other components that are ejected during orgasm. Each seminal vesicle contains a series of tubes that are lined with secretory epithelium that contribute the majority of the fluid in each ejaculate. These secretions are rich in fructose, an energy source for the sperm, and prostaglandins. The specific role of the prostaglandins is not known. The seminal vesicles merge with the vas deferens as it passes through to form the ejaculatory duct. Each ejaculatory duct merges with the urethra through which semen is discharged.

THINK LINK: Composition of Semen

Semen is a combination of various substances. While sperm is thought to be the main composition of semen, various other substances are included to nourish and maintain viability of the sperm. Semen contains the following:

- 3–7 mL/ejaculation
- 60,000,000 sperm/mL
- Mucus (Cowper's gland)
- Fructose (seminiferous tubules)
- Initially thick → thin

The Cowper's gland (bulbourethral gland) is another paired, pea-sized exocrine gland that is located at the base of the penis. Each gland is composed of several lobules held together by a fibrous covering. Each lobule consists of a number of secretory cells that connect to a single duct that connects with the ducts of other lobules to form a single excretory duct. This duct is approximately 2.5 cm long and opens into the urethra at the base of the penis.

Cowper's gland produces a clear, viscous secretion known as pre-ejaculate. This fluid helps to lubricate the urethra for the passage of sperm, as well as neutralizing and removing any residual acidic urine and any foreign matter. It also acts as an external lubricant for the penis making it analogous to the female Bartholin's glands.

The prostate gland is positioned at the base of the bladder, surrounding its neck and urethra as it exits the bladder (Figure 29-2). The prostate gland consists of smooth muscle as well as a complex of 30 to 50 tubular or saclike glands that secrete fluids into the urethra and ejaculatory ducts. It is about the size of a walnut and made of a center lobe and a lobe on each side. During ejaculation, the muscular glands of the prostate contract to propel the prostate fluid and semen forward through the urethra.

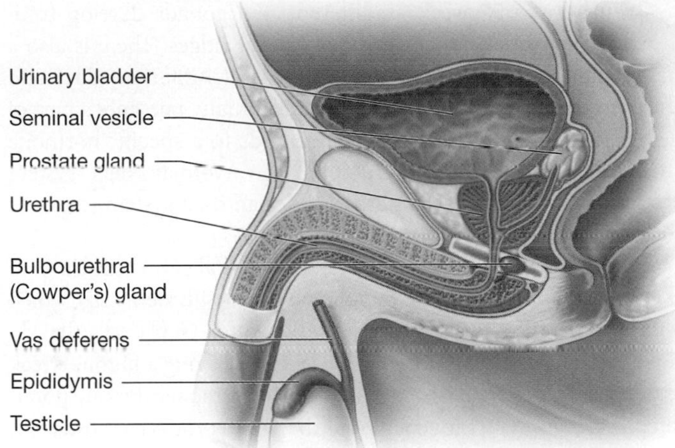

FIGURE 29-2 Internal structures

The prostate glands primary function is to secrete a milky, white, slightly alkaline fluid that is part of the seminal fluid. Fluid from the prostate also contains fibrinolysin, which liquefies the coagulated semen to most likely facilitate sperm motility. In humans, the prostate contributes 15%–30% of the semen.

Developmental Variations

Developmental variations occur over the course of an individual's lifespan and events. Awareness of these variations is important to understand and recognize common age-related alterations or modifications of the male reproductive system.

Infants and Children

During the initial 8 weeks of gestation the fetus is sexually undifferentiated. Sexual differentiation is determined by genes found on the X and Y chromosomes. In males, the Y chromosome contains the male-specific area that encompasses almost all the active genes essential for testicular formation. The development of male genitalia is dependent on the presence of androgens, particularly **Dihydrotestosterone (DHT)**, a biologically active metabolite of the hormone testosterone that is responsible for the formation of male sex-specific characteristics (facial/body hair growth and deepening of the voice). In the absence of testosterone, female genitalia will develop (Figure 29-3).

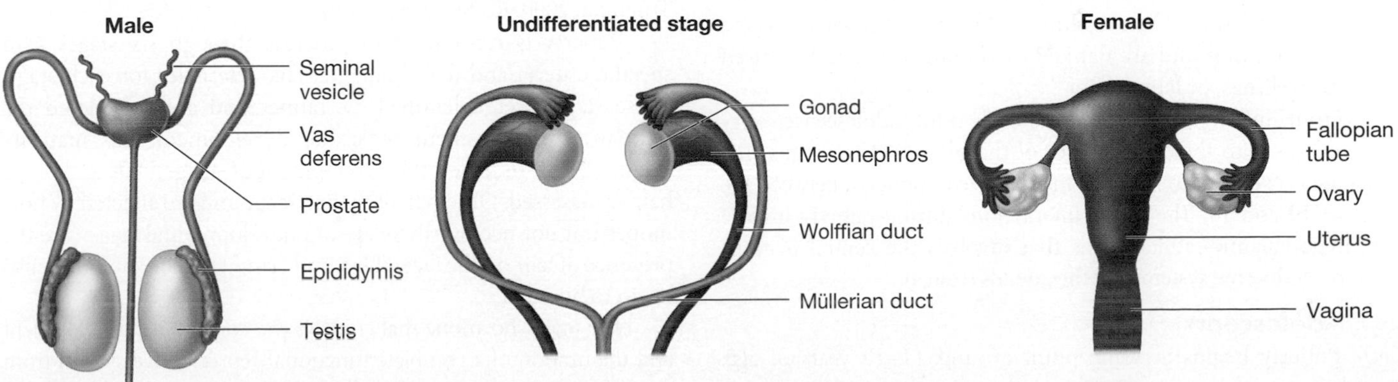

FIGURE 29-3 Duct system and eventual structures formed

During the 5th week, undifferentiated gonads develop from a mass of mesoderm identified as gonadal ridges. There is also a paired duct system, the paramesonephric (Müllerian) duct and the mesonephric (Wolffian) duct that eventually becomes a part of genital differentiation. Each duct responds to a specific hormone that determines its final structure. The Wolffian duct system responds to testosterone, and the Mullerian duct system responds to estrogen (Figure 29-3).

Once the gonadal ridges appear, primordial germ cells travel to them from another location populating them with stem cells, which will become either spermatogonia or oogonia. Germ cells that do not arrive at the genital ridge fail to develop, leaving a fibrous streak characteristic of gonadal agenesis. Once the gonadal ridges are populated with stem cells, the genetic male begins to produce testosterone, causing the gonadal ridges to develop into testes.

The testes organize by developing testis cords, which are primitive seminiferous tubules that mature into semen-producing tubules at the onset of puberty. The seminiferous tubules contain two primitive cell types–**Leydig and Sertoli cells**, which remain dormant until puberty.

Under the influence of testosterone, a few testis tubules link up with neighboring mesonephric tubules on each side of the mesonephric duct system. The combined mesonephric tubules along with their mesonephric ducts eventually become the vas (ductus) deferens and ureters. The testes also produce another hormone (Müllarian inhibitory factor) that causes the paramesonephric duct system to degenerate. Eventually, the testes descend from their abdominal location into the scrotum. Around the 4th fetal month the testes have descended next to the internal inguinal ring, where it remains until around the 7th fetal month. At this point the testicle passes through the internal ring, inguinal canal, and external ring to its position in the scrotum. In some instances, the testicles will not have totally descended into the scrotum (**cryptorchidism**); however, descent should occur within the postnatal period.

Like the internal structures, the external genitalia is undifferentiated, consisting of a **genital tubercle** (i.e., a knob) and a pair of **urogenital folds** flanked by a pair of **genital swellings**.

At 3 months the external rudimentary structures begin to assume male or female characteristics. In the male, the tubercle and the united urogenital folds combine as the penis, thereby continuing the urethra to its end; the genital swellings shift toward the anus, fuse, and become the scrotum. In the female, the tubercle remains small, and becomes the clitoris; it does not contain the urethra. The urogenital folds remain unclosed as the lesser labia minor and are flanked by the unshifted and unfused genital swellings, or labia major.

From infancy through childhood until adolescence, very little occurs with the development of the reproductive organs. The prostate is expected to reach its mature size at puberty, between the ages of 10 and 14. The major interactions during puberty involve the hypothalamic-pituitary axis that involves the central nervous system, endocrine system, and the gonads (testes).

> ***THINK LINK:* *Sexual Differentiation/Gender Identity***
>
> Sexual differentiation occurs as a result of a specific chain of events that determine what pathway will be followed that determines what sexual organs will develop. The first determination is the genetic gender based on the chromosomes present—XX or XY. The genetic gender then controls the differentiation of the gonads, what hormones will be produced, what duct system will predominate, and what external genitalia will develop.
>
> Gender identity is based on individual identification as male or female, which results from genetic and hormonal activity as well as the structure and appearance of the reproductive organs. Gender identity thus determines expression and behaviors associated with each gender. These are also determined by pre- and postnatal environmental factors. Societal expectations regarding gender expression also determine gender identity, and are referred to as gender roles.
>
> In most instances, sexual differentiation is closely associated with gender identification; however in a small number of instances, gender identity is not associated with one's genetic gender and differentiation. Such individuals may have gender identity disorder (GID). Individuals with GID identify with the opposite gender rather their genetic gender. Characteristics of GID range from wearing some intimate undergarments to actual cross dressing, externally wearing articles of clothing that are associated with the opposite gender. Individuals with severe GID may eventually undergo gender reassignment surgery to remove the external characteristics of one's genetic sex and create external characteristics of one's gender identity.

Adolescents

Puberty begins at some point around 11–12 years of age; however, the onset varies by gender and ethnicity. The specific trigger for initiating puberty has yet to be established. Puberty is a time of complex interrelated physiological and chemical processes that facilitate sexual and reproductive development and maturation. Sex hormones are produced and released in greater amounts, causing specific changes. Early-onset puberty as well as late-onset puberty can be somewhat distressing to adolescents when it is realized that there are significant differences in their appearance when compared to their peers.

Growth and maturation of reproductive structures and processes during puberty expend a significant amount of energy, so at the onset of puberty, it is imperative that the central nervous system receives information that energy resources are sufficient and available, with the primary energy reserves provided by fat (Mann & Plant, 2002). The messenger for this information is presently thought to be the hormone **leptin**; however, its exact role is yet to be determined. It is not clear whether leptin serves as the triggering agent or has a more permissive action for the onset of puberty (Clayton & Trueman, 2000; Rutters et al., 2009).

Puberty is recognized to progress through six stages with specific criteria and developmental characteristics for each stage. These stages were identified by Tanner and are considered the standard for assessment of sexual development and maturity (Figure 29-4). In males, the development of the genitals and pubic hair are assessed. Other changes that occur and are affected by hormones but not necessarily related to developmental stages are the presence of hair on the face, chest, and armpits. Male shoulders also begin to broaden.

The major hormone that controls the continuous development and maturation of a complete functional reproductive system from fetal life to puberty is gonadotropin releasing hormone (GnRH) that is released through the hypothalamic-pituitary-gonadal axis. GnRH acts on luteinizing hormone (LH), which in the male acts on the testicular Leydig cells to produce testosterone. Evidence suggests that high level of gonadotropin is required for fetal gonad maturation. Leydig cells also respond to follicle stimulating hormone (FSH), which increases the response of Leydig cells to LH. FSH is, in turn, regulated by two other protein complexes identified as activin and inhibin. Activin enhances FSH biosynthesis and secretion, whereas inhibin reduces FSH synthesis and secretion as well as GnRH release from the hypothalamus.

The release of GnRH is regulated by the GnRH pulse regulator, a group of neurons in the hypothalamus that secrete GnRH in a synchronized manner (Kim, 2007; Pinon, 2002; Figure 29-5). The pulsatile release of GnRH is required for gonadotropin release (Lee, Lee, & Chow, 2008). Sustained levels of GnRH result in reduced levels of gonadotropins in the blood.

In males, sperm production (spermatogenesis) may begin around 9–10 years of age; however, they do not produce mature sperm until they are 14–15 years of age. At birth, the seminiferous tubules contain Sertoli cells, which contain primordial sperm cells and testosterone producing Leydig cells. Leydig cells disappear by 6 months but then reappear at 9–10 years and begin spermatogenesis.

Older Adults

As males age, serum levels of testosterone decrease to the point where 25% of males over 70 have testosterone levels in hypogonadal range. Age-related changes are due to deficits in all levels of hormones related to the hypothalamic-pituitary-gonadal axis.

> **THINK LINK: DHT and Hair Loss**
>
> Male pattern baldness or androgenetic alopecia (AA) is a progressive hair loss condition where the hair line recedes from the top and front of the head. The agent responsible for this condition is dihydrotestosterone (DHT).
>
> When DHT reaches the scalp, it initially binds with the androgen receptor on the hair follicle. When this occurs, hair growth is interrupted and delivery of essential nutrients and oxygen are blocked. The growth cycle of each hair is also interrupted causing hair to become finer and finer through each cycle. The growing phase of the hair is also reduced so eventually the ability to grow terminal hair is lost. The hair follicles will gradually shut down and stop producing hair.

After adolescence, males remain fertile throughout the remainder of their lifespan. Unlike females, changes in the male reproductive system occur gradually. Aging changes in the male may be referred to as **andropause**; however, a specific time or process does not indicate its onset.

Aging changes primarily affect the testes. A reduction in testicular mass occurs, but levels of testosterone do not significantly decrease. Sperm production is continuous with a slight decline in production time of mature sperm. The quality of the sperm is questionable as the rate of conception declines with age; however males in their late 80s and 90s have been able to father children. The time it

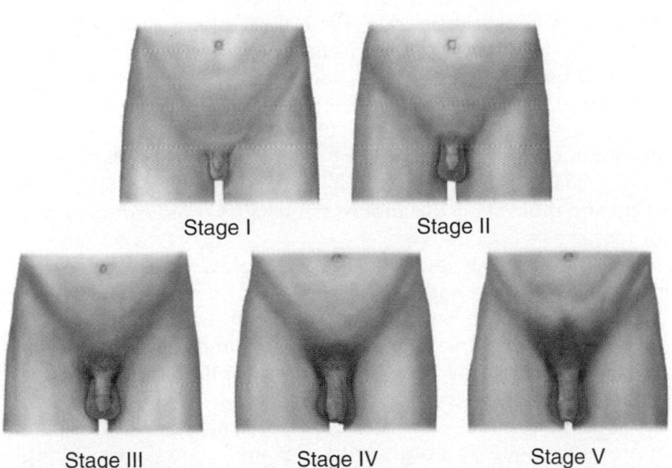

FIGURE 29-4 The Tanner stages of male pubic hair and external genital development with sexual maturation. Stage I, Preadolescent, hair present is no different than that on the abdomen. Testes, scrotum, and penis are the same size and shape as in a young child. Stage II, pubic hair is slightly pigmented, longer, straight hair, often still downy, usually at base of penis, sometimes on scrotum; enlargement of scrotum and testes. Stage III, pubic hair is dark, definitely pigmented, curly pubic hair around base of penis; enlargement of penis, especially in length, further enlargement of testes, descent of scrotum. Stage IV, pubic hair is definitely adult in type but not in extent, spread no further than inguinal fold. Continued enlargement of penis and sculpturing of glans, increased pigmentation of scrotum. Stage V, hair spreads to medial surface of thighs in adult distribution. Adult stage, scrotum ample, penis reaching nearly to bottom of scrotum.

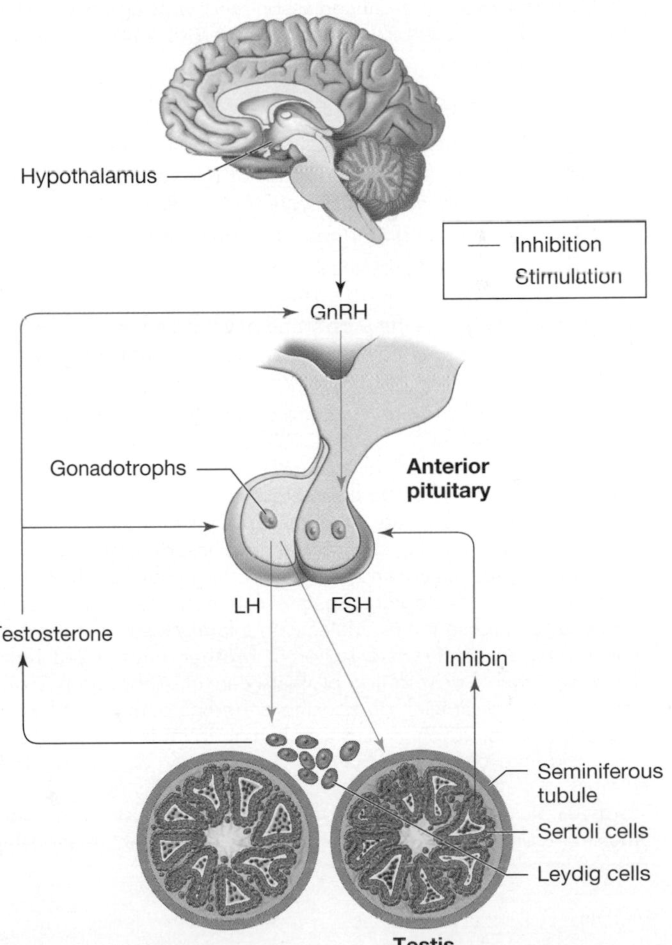

FIGURE 29-5 GnRH regulator

takes to attain an erection increases while the time it takes to maintain an erection decreases. The volume of ejaculate generally remains constant; however there may be an increase, but this is most likely caused by a decrease in sexual activity.

The accessory structures related to fertility go through changes also, but not enough to significantly impair their function. The epididymis, seminal vesicles, and prostate gland lose some of their surface cells, but maintain their production of fluid that accompanies the sperm (Table 29-1). Around the age of 50, the size of the prostate and the amount of its secretions commonly decrease. In contrast, the size of the prostate often increases after midlife and often contributes to difficulties in urination. Prostate enlargement may result from inflammation or malignancy.

Table 29-1 Aging characteristics of prostate gland after age 40

Outer Region	Inner Region
Atrophy of smooth muscle and proliferation of connective tissue	Increase in the number of cells present (hyperplasia)
Flattening of secretory epithelium	

The muscles of the scrotum lose their tone resulting in the scrotum becoming more pendulous. Pubic hair decreases in volume and also may become finer in texture. Some males may also experience a total loss of pubic hair.

Health Promotion

Health promotion related to the male reproductive system does not have its own objective, but is addressed in other topic areas: cancer and sexually transmitted infections (U.S. Department of Health and Human Services, 2009). Prostate cancer is the second most common type of cancer in males, second only to lung cancer (Oneill, 2009). Annually, there are about 20,000 new cases accompanied by a death rate of 30,000 (Soni & Hardin, 2009). It is primarily a cancer associated with aging with less than 1/100,000 cases in 40-year-old men to 1146/100,000 in 85-year-old males.

Prostate Cancer

- C—7 Reduce the prostate cancer death rate.
- STD—1 Reduce the proportion of adolescents and young adults with Chlamydia trachomatis.
- STD—6 Reduce gonorrhea rates (males aged 15–44 years).
- STD—7 Reduce sustained domestic transmission of primary and secondary syphilis (among males).
- STD—10 Reduce the proportion of young adults with genital herpes infection due to herpes simplex type 2.

It is generally thought that if a male lives long enough, eventually he will develop prostate cancer. It has been projected that in males over 80, between 50%–80% of them have prostate cancer in some state of development. In males over 90, 90% of them will have some stage of prostate cancer.

The cause of prostate cancer is not known but it is related to certain known factors such as race, genetics, diet, and chemical exposure. Males of African American heritage have a 1.5–2 times greater risk of developing prostate cancer. It also occurs at an earlier age in these males. Males with a family history of prostate cancer, especially if it is a father or brother, have a 2–3 times increased risk of developing prostate cancer. Although prostate cancer may be familial, no specific gene has been identified as a cause (Oneill, 2009). A diet that is high in fat is also related to the incidence of prostate cancer. Accordingly, obesity doubles the risk of developing prostate cancer, particularly an aggressive form (Hitti, 2007). Obesity also increases the risk in younger males (Medical College of Georgia, 2005). The exact relationship between obesity and prostate cancer is yet to be determined. One theory proposes that obesity increases production of testosterone which may promote the development of cancer cells (Mayo Clinic Staff, 2009).

Exposure to certain chemicals like cadmium has been recognized as a potential cause of prostate cancer. Recent studies have also examined the relationship between Bisphenol-A (BSA), an estrogen mimicking chemical and prostate cancer. There is no known relationship between the frequency of sexual activity and development of prostate cancer (Soni & Hardin, 2009).

Early detection is quite difficult as early signs/symptoms frequently are not evident. Most prostate cancers are detected incidentally during a rectal examination. When symptoms occur, it is most likely due to urinary bladder obstruction caused by constriction of the urethra by the enlarging prostate gland. Other symptoms may include blood in the urine, painful ejaculation, and erectile dysfunction, but these are relatively uncommon and nonspecific. Often by the time medical attention is sought for treatment of late occurring symptoms—fatigue, malaise, and weight loss—the cancer is in an advanced stage and most likely has metastasized. The most common site for metastasis is bone.

Prostate cancer is a relatively slow growing cancer so the individual may have had prostate cancer for an extended period of time. Depending on the rate of growth and the individual's age at diagnosis, treatment may be minimal to none. Some prostate cancers may grow aggressively, which requires more conventional cancer therapy.

The most effective method for determining the presence of prostate cancer is a digital rectal examination (DRE). During the rectal examination, the prostate gland is palpated by the examiners gloved finger to detect any changes in the consistency and surface characteristics of the prostate gland. Additionally, a blood test for **prostate specific antigen (PSA)** may be done. Increased levels of PSA do occur in prostate cancer; however, increased levels are also evident in other prostate gland alterations, so its usefulness as a screening tool is questionable.

Health Promotion *continued*

Use of DRE and PSA data for early detection of prostate cancer has not significantly reduced the incidence of prostate cancer. Although PSA was expected to increase early detection, no clear relationship between PSA levels and prostate cancer could be determined. It was clear the significantly increased levels of PSA were associated with prostate cancer, there were also incidences where PSA level was not increased in the presence of prostate cancer. Even though DRE has been considered essential for detecting prostate cancer, its use has not significantly reduced morbidity and mortality from prostate cancer. Since it has been determined that the benefits of screening for prostate cancer do not significantly outweigh the risks, routine screening beginning at a certain age is not recommended. Clearly, if an individual is at high risk for developing prostate cancer, routine screening should be considered; however, the most recent guidelines stress the importance of the decision to begin screening as a shared, informed decision between the patient and provider based on consideration and analysis of the risks and benefits.

Objectives for sexually transmitted infections are identified and discussed in Chapter 14.

Clinical Context Exemplars

Situation A

During the taking of the history of a 25-year-old male, he indicates that when he was about 5 years old he had surgery to get one of his "balls" down into his scrotum. He also states that "no one told me what that was about. What happened and why did I have to have that done?"

1. How would you respond to his question?
2. He also is curious if there might be any problems related to his condition or if there is anything that he needs to be aware of.
3. He also wants to know if there is anything that could have been/can be done to prevent this from happening and that if he gets married and has children, if his sons will also have this.

Situation B

A 16-year-old male is being seen because of delayed puberty. Genetic testing was done and it was confirmed that he had Klinefelter's syndrome. He and his parents are quite upset that he was not diagnosed earlier so something could have been done about it. How would you respond to the teenager's and parents' concerns?

1. While delayed puberty may have been the initial reason for having him evaluated, knowing that there are other manifestations of KS, what further information would you want to obtain to help determine a course of treatment?
2. As this is their only child, the parents are concerned about their son's future related to marriage and fathering children. What response would you give them regarding their concerns?

Situation C

A 70-year-old widowed male is being seen because he "wants to get back in the saddle" with some of his female friends. He says that it's been 4 years since his wife died and he needs more than just companionship. You consider it important to provide some education to him so you inquire as to what type of protection he intends to use. He responds "I don't need to use protection, I probably won't be able to father a child and all my lady friends are too old to get pregnant." How would you respond to his reasoning?

1. You also recommend that he be screened for prostate cancer. When this is recommended to him he states, "No one is sticking their finger up my butt. Isn't there an easier way to find out about this?" How would you respond?
2. He also responds by saying, "It's probably unlikely that I would have any prostate problems." What additional information would you want to obtain to help determine his risk status for prostate cancer?

SUBJECTIVE DATA

History of Present Illness (CC)

The patient may present to the provider with a variety of concerns that may be directly related to the male genitalia system or other systems. Framing the questions will depend on the patient's age, gender, culture, race, emotional or mental status, health practices, and concurrent illnesses. All symptoms presented must be thoroughly assessed with a symptom analysis (COLDERRA).

Pain

Primary pain of the penis/genitals is a rare occurrence and most commonly occurs as secondary to a local external or internal condition, or referred pain (Nishihara, 2000). Males who experience genital pain without any obvious manifestations or alterations may be experiencing **male genital pain syndrome (MGPS)** (Harris, 1998). Further examination may identify a source of the pain. Referred pain from sensory nerves innervating organs associated with the genitalia must also be considered.

Provider Inquiries	Clinical Reasoning/Logic
Characteristics: How do you experience the pain? How to best describe it (burning, tenderness, numbness, tingling, spasmodic, colicky, sharp, dull, ache)? Does it increase/decrease? Generalized or localized? Any change in the contour/shape of penis?	Generalized pain associated with urinary tract infections. Dull, aching pain associated with epididymitis. Acute pain in testicular area associated with testicular torsion. Inguinal hernias not painful unless strangulated.
Onset: When did the pain begin? What initiates pain (ejaculation, urination, erection)? Acute or chronic in nature? Any specific activity/trauma? Vasectomy?	Pain with erection associate with priaprism, Peyronie's disease, and phimosis. Pain with urination associated with urinary tract infections. Chronic pain occurs after vasectomy in 1%–15% of males (Keoghane & Sullivan, 2010). Gradual, increasing scrotal/testicular over days characteristic of epididymitis.
Location: Where is pain felt (penis, scrotum, testicles, groin, and suprapubic area)? In lower back?	Pain may be experienced on surface associated with contact dermatitis, allergies. Pain in groin or scrotum associated with inguinal hernias. Testicular pain primarily from condition of testicle—epididymitis, orchitis, hydrocele, or tumor. Pain of the glans associated with balanitis.
Duration: How long does pain last (constant, intermittent)?	Priaprism pain with erection > 4 hours, need to seek treatment. Prolonged priaprism may scar penis. Scrotal pain longer than 3 months is considered chronic and often no contributing cause is determined.
Exacerbation: What makes pain worse (intercourse, erection, urination, prolonged erections)?	Pain exacerbated with priaprism. Urination may increase pain in non-gonococcal urethritis or STIs.
Relief: What brings relief? Heat, cold, loss of erection?	Pain from priaprism relieved when erection reduced.
Radiation: Is pain felt elsewhere, away from genitals; if so, where? Constant or intermittent?	Abdominal pain with decreased appetite, nausea and vomiting may be referred pain from testicular torsion. Or other conditions that affect the scrotum.
Associated signs/symptoms: Any discharge (if so character of it)?	A discharge is frequently associated with STIs or urethritis.

Swelling, Masses, or Enlargement of Scrotum/Testicles

Scrotal masses are associated with several disorders that cover a wide range of conditions including benign, congenital alterations to life-threatening malignancies and acute surgical emergencies. Some may be associated with pain, but many are not and may only be found incidentally during a physical examination. Scrotal edema may also occur without any precipitating causes.

Provider Inquiries	Clinical Reasoning/Logic
	Enlargement of the scrotum may be caused by extra contents within scrotum from inguinal hernias. It is also felt as dull ache. Bumps/lumps on surface of testicle are associated with testicular cancer. Varicoceles and hydroceles often cause scrotal enlargement that can be felt.
Characteristics: What does enlargement feel like—surface characteristics (smooth, bumps, firm, soft, fluid)? Any pain—if so where, characteristics? Noticeably enlarging—if so, how fast? Feeling of fullness/dragging in scrotum? Symmetry of scrotum?	Asymmetrical scrotum is associated with inguinal hernia that has passed into the scrotum.

Provider Inquiries	Clinical Reasoning/Logic
Onset: When swelling/enlargement first noticed? Immediate/gradual? Any recent trauma?	Pain after trauma may indicate injury to scrotal contents, causing swelling. Standing up may cause transient pain or discomfort from transmission of abdominal pressure into the scrotum.
Location: Specific location—testicle, scrotum, groin?	Varicoceles, hydroceles are commonly noted on the left side.
Duration: How long has it been present? Constant or intermittent?	Intermittent, painless groin swelling associated with inguinal hernia. Scrotal swelling that increases over days associated with epididymitis.
Exacerbation: What makes it worse (erection, urination, temperature changes, lack of support)?	Standing may increase pain/discomfort.
Relief: What provides relief (heat, support)?	
Radiation: Is feeling or pain felt/perceived elsewhere?	
Associated signs/symptoms: Any redness or warmth?	Redness and warmth of the scrotum often related to inflammatory/infectious causes within the scrotum.
Penile Lesions/Discharge Penile lesions and/or discharge are frequently associated with STIs and related to specific bacteria or viruses.	
Characteristics: Appearance of lesion (size, color, raised/flat, crust)? Appearance of discharge (color, consistency, spontaneous discharge, volume, odor)? Vesicles? Warts?	Syphilis and gonorrhea have characteristic lesions that are frequently external and easily identifiable. A urethral discharge is more commonly associated with gonorrhea than syphilis. Viral lesions are caused by the herpes simplex variety and human papilloma virus (HPV). Herpes infections cause the development of vesicles within the genital area and are intermittent in their appearance. HPV is manifested as genital warts. Cancer (squamous cell) of the penis is quite rare and may be associated with either of the above sexually transmitted infections. Males who are uncircumcised are at a higher risk for developing penile cancer than those who are circumcised.
Onset: When first noticed? Gradual or rapid? Constant or intermittent? Exposure to STIs?	
Location: Where on penis/groin?	
Duration: How long outbreak lasts?	
Exacerbation: Anything that makes it worse?	
Relief: Anything that makes it better (medications, lotions)?	
Associated signs/symptoms: Redness, itching, increasing size, painful/difficulty with urination or ejaculation? Is patient circumcised or not?	Dermatologic lesions of the penis may be caused by many other conditions, so it is important to remember that not all penile lesions are either infectious or cancerous.

PRACTICE POINT: Testicular Self-Exam (TSE)

It is necessary to determine the patient's awareness and knowledge regarding what, how, and when to perform **testicular self-exam (TSE)**. Formulate questions to obtain this information from the patient.

Awareness of TSE?	Has been previously informed about TSE or has been made aware of it through magazines, brochures, advertising, etc.?
What knowledge of TSE?	Regular TSEs are the best way to identify alterations on surface of testicle that may be indicators of testicular cancer.
What knowledge related to how to perform?	Gently palpate the surface of the testicle through the scrotum with the testicle between the thumb and the index/middle finger. Surface of testicle should be smooth.
What knowledge of when to perform?	Should perform monthly. Best when in shower as the heat causes the scrotum to relax and allows the testicles to hang lower, making them easier to palpate. Identify a specific date of the month to perform. No male monthly cycle to indicate a best time to perform the exam. Pick a date and stick to it.

Erectile Dysfunction

Erectile dysfunction (ED) is a common problem and has become of greater interest in the past few years. Most commonly it is associated with inability to attain or maintain an erection; however, erections may also last too long, leaving the patient with a prolonged erection. Curvature of the penis in any direction may also occur with erections.

Provider Inquiries	Clinical Reasoning/Logic
Characteristics: Describe problem: difficulty in achieving/maintaining erection, erection lasting too long, curvature of penis—if so, in what direction?	Peyronie's disease may cause curvature of the penis, painful erections, general pain, and affect a man's desire to engage in a function during sex.
Onset: When difficulty first noted? Immediate or gradual in onset? Any idea about what may be the cause (known conditions/situations—medical or marital)?	There may be psychological/emotional causes of ED as well as physical.
Duration: If problem in maintaining an erection, how long does erection last? Do you have erections at all, i.e., wake up in the morning with an erection?	If able to have erections intermittently, or notes erections at other times, there is probably a psychological cause rather than physical.
Exacerbation: Anything that makes it worse? What medications taking?	Many medications are known to cause difficulty in attaining/maintaining erections.
Relief: Anything that relieves situation? Medications? Devices?	Viagra and other medications may be helpful in achieving an erection.
Associated signs/symptoms: Anything else noted when experiencing difficulty?	

Fertility Difficulties (Infertility)

Infertility is not just a female's problem. Females are more likely to seek evaluation and treatment for it than males; however, approximately 40% of fertility difficulties are related to male causes. Answers to previous questions as well as family, personal and social history will also provide needed information relating to fertility problems.

Provider Inquiries	Clinical Reasoning/Logic
Characteristics: Any difficulties with intercourse (pain, difficulty penetrating)?	Penile disorders (Peyronie's disease, priaprism, phimosis, erectile dysfunction) may affect a male's ability to engage in sexual intercourse.
Any gels/lubricants used to assist in intercourse? Use of alcohol/tobacco? Frequency of intercourse?	Some gels/lubricants may have anti-sperm properties. Alcohol/tobacco also associated with infertility problems.
Knowledge of reproductive physiology (timing of intercourse with ovulation)? Libido (intensity of sex drive)?	Understanding of timing intercourse with ovulation may help patient to determine optimum timing for intercourse.
	Heat is an antagonist to sperm production. Saunas, hot tubs, etc, possible cause of fertility problems. Boxers recommended as they allow scrotum to descend as needed. Briefs keep scrotum confined next to body. Biking can also cause problems due to tight fitting biking shorts and some seat designs.
Onset: Last time had intercourse? How long trying to create pregnancy (unprotected intercourse)? When stopped using birth control methods? Type of birth control methods used?	Infertility is generally diagnosed after one year of unprotected intercourse.
Duration: Same information as onset	
Exacerbation: Lifestyle factors: factors that may increase temperature in scrotum (tight clothing/underwear, frequent hot baths/saunas, employment in high temperature environment/radiation)?	Heat is detrimental to sperm production and motility. Other environmental hazards include pesticides, lead, paint, mercury, benzene, boron, and heavy metals.
Medications/Drugs? History of sexually transmitted infections, childhood diseases—mumps?	Multiple drugs may interfere with libido or cause erectile dysfunction. Recreational use of drugs also known cause of infertility.
	Prior STIs may have caused scarring that interferes with transporting sperm. Mumps as a child may cause testicular damage.
Associated signs/symptoms: History of cryptorchidism, decrease in volume of ejaculate? Varicocele? Diagnostic tests performed?	Varicocele is often a primary cause of infertility, which can often be reversed with surgical intervention.

THINK LINK:* *Cycling and Fertility Problems

While exercise is recommended for producing healthy sperm, the type of exercise may have detrimental effects (Leibovitch & Mor, 2005). Cycling has been associated with low sperm counts and total motile sperm, contributing to fertility problems (Wise, Cramer, Hornstein, Ashby, & Missmer, 2011). While there is a causal relationship, a specific cause/effect connection has yet to be established. Cycling for more than 5 hours per week appears to be an important factor; however, more studies need to be done to establish a direct relationship. It is thought that the tight fitting Lycra biking shorts increase the temperature of the scrotum creating a warmer environment for the testicles, decreasing sperm production. There is also some thought that there may be some trauma within the pelvic area related to the type of bike seat that is used. Seats that allow the body weight to be supported by the perineum rather than the ischial tuberosities are the cause of injury, primarily to the pudendal nerve resulting in neuropathy, which may be a cause of fertility problems.

Past Medical History

Information from the past medical history is important to determine if any previous medical condition or situation is a possible cause of present complaint of condition. Depending on how much of a history has been done to determine the patient's present condition (chief concern), some of the information related to past medical history may have already been obtained.

Provider Inquiries	Clinical Reasoning/Logic
Any surgical procedures for alterations associated with genitalia: undescended testicle, hypospadias, epispadias, varicocele, prostate gland, hernia repair, sterilization?	Previous surgeries may cause **retrograde ejaculation** (semen goes into bladder instead of out the urethra). History of cryptorchidism associated with increased risk for testicular cancer. Epispadias/hypospadias may interfere with urination and ejaculation.
Any history of sexually transmitted infections: If so—type, one or more infectious incidences, treatment, effectiveness, any subsequent problems?	STIs may have caused scarring, blocking passage of sperm.
Any chronic illnesses: cancer (testicular/prostatic), diabetes (type 1 or 2), arthritis, peptic ulcer disease/GERDS, high blood pressure, neurological or vascular alterations? If so, what medications taking for condition?	Multiple medications are often a cause of fertility problems. Interference with blood flow to genital area may lead to ED. Blood pressure medication also associated with ED.

Family History

Family history provides information regarding family member's illnesses or conditions as potential causes for chief complaint or presenting symptoms that may indicate a pattern of presentation associated with transmission of familial/genetic factors predisposing the individual to certain system related conditions/illnesses. Any of these may indicate a potential or actual cause of male reproductive system dysfunction.

Provider Inquiries	Clinical Reasoning/Logic
Fertility alterations in any siblings?	Siblings with fertility difficulties may indicate some familial tendencies.
History of cancer (prostate, testicular, or penile) or hernias?	Cancers may have a familial predisposition.

Personal and Social History

Information regarding personal and social activities may provide clues as to cause of present condition or the potential for future alterations or conditions.

Provider Inquiries	Clinical Reasoning/Logic
Employment type? Potential for trauma or alterations of suprapubic/genital areas, or exposure to environmental toxins and/or radiation? What protection measures taken?	Exposure to toxins, chemicals, radiation may be basis for fertility problems.
What protection measures for sports or exercise activities—protective device (cup) for contact sports, bike riding (exercises or sport)?	Appropriate protection to prevent trauma to genitals.
Any children? If so, how many?	An indicator of fertility, if infertility is a problem.
Sexually active? If so, how many partners? Partner male/female/or both? Satisfaction with sexual activity? What concerns?	Multiple partners increase possibility of contracting STIs.
Protection against STIs—what, frequency of use? Knowledge/familiarity of STIs—transmission, cause, treatment, signs/symptoms?	It is important for the patient to describe extent and depth of knowledge. Simply asking the patient if he knows about STIs does not provide any data whether there is comprehension and application of that knowledge, particularly related to prevention.

Provider Inquiries	Clinical Reasoning/Logic
Use of street (recreational) drugs, alcohol?	Smoking may cause misshapen and sluggish sperm. Smoking may also damage sperm's DNA increasing risk for growth/development problems as well as risk of cancer. Marijuana decreases sperm motility. Heavy drinking decreases quantity/quality of sperm.
What knowledge of TSE? What knowledge related to how to perform? What knowledge of when to perform?	Regular TSE increases chances of finding early testicular cancer.

Developmental Applications

Certain conditions or disorders may be related to certain age groups or situations. Inquiring to obtain age or condition specific information will provide further information for helping to determine causes of the chief concern as identified.

Infants and Children

Provider Inquiries	Clinical Reasoning/Logic
Mother's use of hormones during pregnancy (DES)?	Hormones may be administered to prevent miscarriage. Use of DES associated with development of testicular cancer.
Circumcision: If done, by whom? Any complications? If not done; hygiene measures, any interference with urination?	During the neonatal period, the foreskin is firmly attached to the glans and may not be retractable. Forcible retraction should not be done until the foreskin has separated from the glans. It is not uncommon for it to exist into childhood and adolescence. It is important to determine parent's knowledge related to this and the importance of appropriate hygiene measures to be taken.
Any congenital alterations? Hypospadius, epispadias (displaced meatus), undescended testicle, ambiguous genitalia?	Early treatment has better outcomes.
Swelling of scrotum during crying or bowel movement?	If present, possible indicator of inguinal hernia.
Parental concerns with early sexual development—masturbation, sexual exploration, questions of child?	Precocious puberty may be an indicator of hormonal dysfunction.
Any discolorations, bruises, sores, c/o pain on or around genitalia?	Bruising of genital area may be an indicator of abuse.

Adolescents

Information from adolescents is best obtained without parents present.

Provider Inquiries	Clinical Reasoning/Logic
Knowledge of reproductive function and sexual activity? How information obtained and from whom?	Knowledge of sexuality/reproductive functioning increases recognition of need for protection if sexually active.
Development of secondary sex characteristics—nocturnal emissions, enlargement of penis/testicles, pubic hair? When started? Pain in breast area? Any breast enlargement? Any concerns related to sexual development? Masturbation, genital size? Gynecomastia?	Concern for appropriate, age related development. Gynecomastia development is not unusual, but should disappear; however, in a small percentage of males it remains into adulthood. Provides opportunity for adolescent to ask questions and express concerns.
Sexually active? When began, contraception used? Frequency of use? How many partners?	Provides opportunity to discuss issues related to protection options and prevention of STIs.
Knowledge and performance of TSE?	Provides opportunity to inform adolescent about performing TSE on a regular basis.

Older Adult

Sexuality and sexual activity are often overlooked or denied, but there is no specific age after which an individual should not engage in sexual activity.

Provider Inquiries	Clinical Reasoning/Logic
Changes in sexual activity—frequency, partner?	
Restrictions related to sexual activity: partner available, environment, opportunity/availability for sex, loss of libido, physical limitations, pain, medical conditions (diabetes, arthritis, high blood pressure, prostate surgery) medications takes, and depression?	Recognizes that the elderly male may still be interested in sexual activity and provides him with the opportunity to address any issues. More than likely, there is hesitation on the part of the patient to bring up the topic and asking questions related to sexuality indicates it is not a taboo subject.
Changes in sexual response experienced—longer time to achieve/maintain erection, less forceful ejaculation, rapid loss of erection, longer intervals between erections?	Provides the opportunity to present these topics/issues for the older male to discuss without having to overcome the possibility of fear and anxiety to bring them up.

OBJECTIVE DATA

Assessment of the male genitalia involves inspection and palpation. For this assessment, the patient may be either standing or lying down, depending on where the exam it is being performed. If the patient is standing, then the provider should be seated and facing the patient.

Assessment of the genitalia involves exposing, observation, and touching parts of the body that are considered private and not to be exposed, particularly to an individual of the opposite gender. This may cause apprehension in individuals, as well as invading or an invasion of personal space.

It is most important for the provider (male and female) to act in a professional, direct, matter-of-fact way, with or without a chaperone. By managing the genitalia assessment as just another aspect of the physical exam, the provider projects confidence and assures the patient that there is nothing to be embarrassed about. It is also important to not apologize for having to perform this exam. This communicates embarrassment on the part of the provider, making the patient question the importance of this component of the exam.

A major fear of the male patient is the possibility of developing an erection during the examination. If this does occur, assure the patient that this is a physiological reaction to touch and that it is not perceived to be sexual in context. The possibility of this occurring during the exam should be told to the patient before the exam. Also indicate that it will not necessarily interfere with the exam and there is no need to stop the exam until the erection is gone. If this has not been mentioned prior to the exam and it occurs during the exam, it makes it more difficult to explain to the patient and more than likely may cause embarrassment.

To reduce the chances of developing an erection, use a firm and deliberate touch during the exam. Hesitancy in touching or manipulation of the penis and scrotum, or a light touch most likely communicates discomfort to the patient. Also, involve the patient as much as possible, making him feel he has some control in this situation.

It is also important for the provider to be aware of behaviors that have been demonstrated throughout the rest of the exam. For instance, if procedures have been explained to the patient throughout the exam, keep on explaining procedures, et cetera during the genitalia exam. By treating this portion of the exam no different than any other communicates that this is simply examining another part of the body that is no different than examining any other part.

***THINK LINK:** Use of Chaperones*

The use of chaperones during a genitalia examination of either gender is relatively inconsistent. The primary purpose of having a third party present during this part of the exam is to legally protect both the provider and patient. In most instances, the setting implied a male physician examining a female patient and most often the chaperone was another female. However, in today's society and health care environment, it is not unusual for a female physician to examine a male patient, which begs the question as to whether a chaperone should be present during the male genitalia exam. Research has reported that far fewer female providers use chaperones than their male counterparts when performing a genital exam on a patient of the opposite gender. Surprisingly, studies also found that patients often were uncomfortable with a third party in the room. Thus, what appears to be a relatively easy solution to a problem, becomes more complicated than expected. The general consensus on handling this issue is to offer the presence of a chaperone to all patients, whether it is patients of the same gender or opposite gender. If the patient refuses to have a chaperone present, documentation of such is an absolute necessity.

Inspection

Pubic hair—distribution and general characteristics, infestations

Penis—Characteristics, configuration, color, lesions, discharge, erectile state, foreskin, jewelry/piercing, appliances

Scrotum—surface characteristics, color, asymmetry

Groin (Inguinal and femoral area)—bulges

Semen analysis

Palpation

Pubic hair—texture

Penis—consistency, tenderness, foreskin retraction

Scrotum/contents (testes, epididymides, vas deferens)—configuration, surface characteristics, tenderness, fluid, consistency, nodules

Groin—inguinal/femoral bulges

Percussion*—not performed*

Auscultation*—not performed*

Level I to IV Examination

The Level I to Level IV examinations are performed on a continuum, which starts from a basic level to a more comprehensive level based on the provider's abilities and knowledge as well as the patient's presentation and location. It may start at the outpatient setting progressing to the ED, hospital unit bed, critical care unit, or specialty unit. Frequently all the elements from basic to comprehensive exam are done in one setting like in a primary care setting or clinic.

The condition/illness of the patient is the primary consideration related to the type and amount of data needed to assess the patient's condition/illness/situation. The arrangement of skills into levels is for general purposes and is meant to be descriptive rather than prescriptive. The purpose of arranging into levels is to provide a framework to assist the learner in determining the appropriate data to collect.

Male Genitalia

	Level I	Level II	Level III	Level IV
Inspection	Hair pattern/distribution	Presence of bulges with bearing down	Alignment of erect penis	Physical characteristics r/t gender/ genetic composition
	Configuration r/t age, development	Lesions (description)	Scrotum (inflammation)	Infertility work-up
	Lesions (presence)		Evidence of trauma	
	Meatus location			
	Presence of foreskin			
	Scrotum (presence of testes, skin characteristics)			
	Presence of parasites			
	Characteristics of urine (color, amount, clarity, odor, SP. Gr.)			
Palpation		Shaft of penis (consistency, nodules, tenderness, induration)	Scrotum (tenderness)	Cremasteric reflexes
		Retractable foreskin		
		Scrotum [testes surface characteristics, mobility, vas deferens)		
		Inguinal/femoral hernias		
		Prostate gland		

Inspection: Level I

Inspection Techniques and Expected Findings	Unexpected Findings
Begin initial inspection with observation of pubic hair and its distribution. Pubic hair is coarser than scalp hair and ranges from relatively straight to curly. The pattern of hair growth is generally in the shape of a diamond with the lower triangle surrounding the genitalia and the upper triangle extending up to the umbilicus. The amount of hair in the upper triangle varies, but a diamond pattern is often visible (Figure 29-6). Hair is also present on the scrotum and around the anus.	

Inspection Techniques and Expected Findings

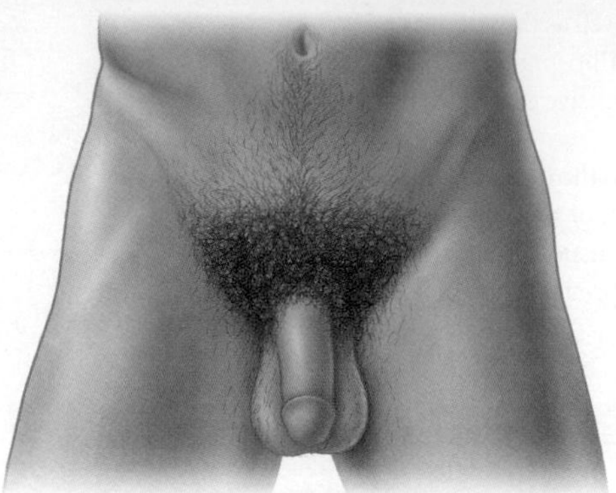

FIGURE 29-6 Male pubic hair distribution

Inspect the genital hair and surrounding skin is for the presence of parasitic infestations (Figure 29-7).

> ***PRACTICE POINT: Manscaping/Male Grooming***
>
> It is becoming more popular and acceptable for males to groom or shave their pubic area, which may range from total removal of pubic hair to trimming and pruning to reduce its length and coverage. It may also include shaping the distribution of the hair.
>
> Certain medical conditions (adrenal gland underactivity/Addison's disease) or infections (fungal/ringworm) are also known to cause a loss of pubic hair.

Simultaneously while inspecting the pubic hair, observe the configuration and position of the penis and scrotum in relationship to age and developmental stage, and any external conditions that might be visible on the surface of the skin.

The skin covering the shaft of the penis should be smooth, elastic, and hairless without any evidence of lesions or growths. The skin is often darker in appearance than the rest of the skin.

The configuration of the penis should demonstrate a straight, cylindrical tube that extends from the midsection of the groin (symphysis pubis). In general the dimension of the erect adult penis is 5.5–6.2 in. in length and 4.7–5.1 in. around.

The position of the penis is described as flaccid or erect. The flaccid penis hangs loosely from the body with the dorsal surface of the penis exposed (see Figure 29-8). In the flaccid state, the dorsal vein should be visible; it generally hangs in the midline; however, in the erect state there may be some deviation to one side or the other.

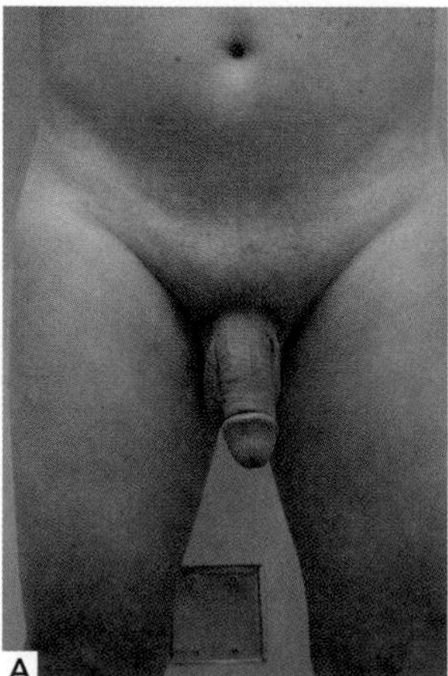

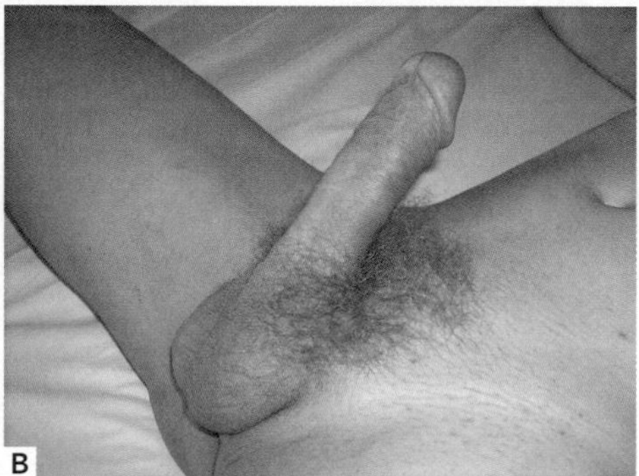

FIGURE 29-8A–B Penis: a) flaccid; b) erect

Unexpected Findings

In the postoperative patient, pubic hair may be absent due to prostate or bladder surgery.

There should be no hair present on the penis.

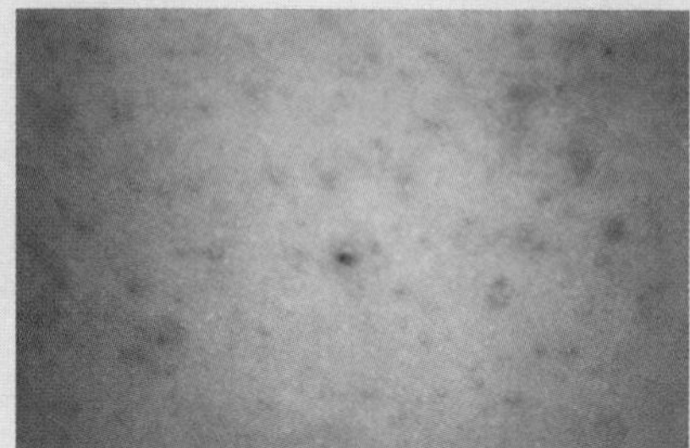

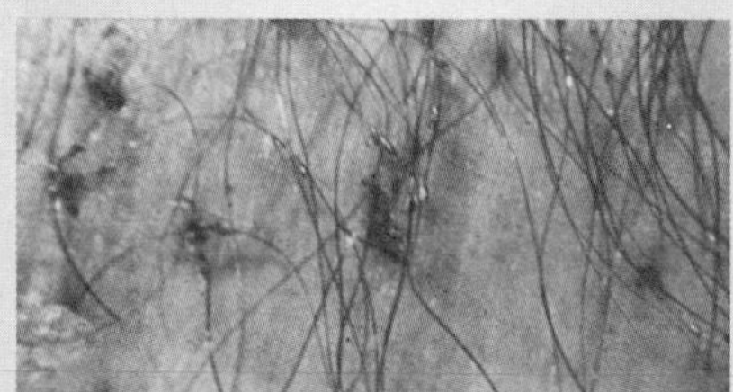

FIGURE 29-7 a) Rash caused by scabies infestation; **b)** pubic lice
Source: CDC/Joe Miller

The adult erect penis that measures < 2" (7 cm) but demonstrates the expected configuration is referred to as a **micropenis**.

Inspection Techniques and Expected Findings

The erect penis is engorged with blood that causes it to extend horizontally from the body or directed upward, exposing the ventral surface of the penis. In some individuals, the erect penis may demonstrate a curvature either to the right or left.

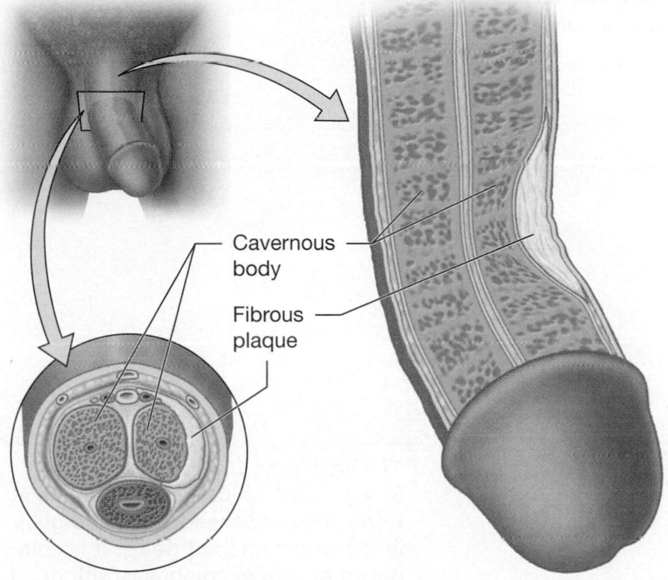

FIGURE 29-9 Peyronie's disease (bottleneck deformity)

THINK LINK: Dorsal/Ventral Sides of the Penis

When referring to the dorsal and ventral surface of the penis, at first glance it seems to be backwards. The reference to the surface of the penis relates to its position in a quadruped. In most male animals, the penis is encased in a sheath that suspends the penis in a stationary position. In this way, the dorsal aspect of the penis is facing the ventral side of the abdomen. Whether the penis is flaccid or erect, its position does not vary.

In the human male, the direction and position of the penis is different in the flaccid or erect position. In the flaccid state, the dorsal aspect of the penis is foremost and in the erect state, the ventral aspect is foremost. Therefore, when referring to the dorsal or ventral aspect of the penis, the reference to the side does not change, only the position of the penis.

Inspect the glans at the end of the penis, which resembles a rounded cap placed on the end. It is separated from the penile shaft by a ridge that slightly flares at its lower edge (corona). The glans may be pinker in color than the shaft but without evidence of redness or other color changes (Figure 29-10). The amount of blood in the penis helps to determine the overall color.

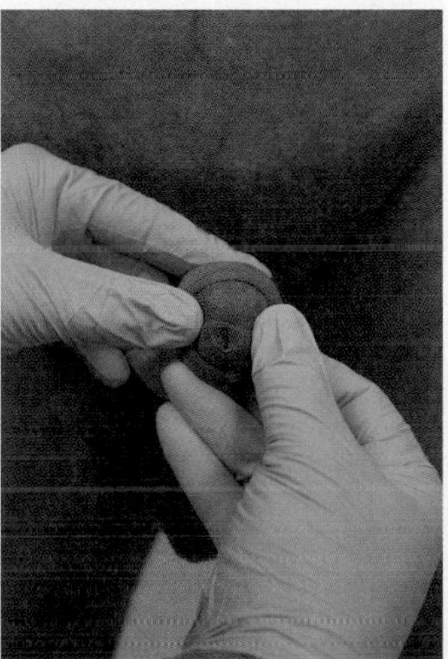

FIGURE 29-10 Glans—urethral meatus

Unexpected Findings

A condition in which there is a bend or curvature of the penis during erection is known as **Peyronie's disease** (Figure 29-9). This is caused by the formation of a hard fibrous layer of scar tissue (plaques) in the tunica albuginea surrounding the corpus cavernosum (Pourbagher, Turunc, Pourbagher, Guvel, & Koc, 2005). The erection may also be accompanied by pain.

The bend in the penis is determined by where the fibrous scar tissue develops. If it is on the ventral portion, the penis will bend upward and if on the dorsal aspect will cause a downward bend. This generally is not considered a significant alteration unless there is a problem with penetration during intercourse. This may be due to an injury or it may be due to failure of the corpus cavernosa to develop equally on both sides of the penis.

In some instances, the fibrous tissue will develop on both sides, causing an indentation of the penis known as "bottleneck" (Mayo Clinic, 2009). When present, the fibrous tissue may be palpated in the penile shaft in the flaccid state.

The cause of Peyronie's disease is not known, but possibilities that have been identified include penile trauma, autoimmune disorder, inherited collagen abnormality, and medications. Effective treatment may be achieved through medical intervention with drugs or surgical removal of the lesion.

Inspection Techniques and Expected Findings	Unexpected Findings

The foreskin may or may not cover the glans depending on whether the patient is circumcised or uncircumcised.

If the patient is uncircumcised, the glans may be covered with the foreskin (prepuce). Even in circumcised males, a small portion of the foreskin may remain. The foreskin may also vary in size. It may just encircle the glans or it may cover it completely and taper to a point that extends beyond the tip of the penis (Figure 29-11).

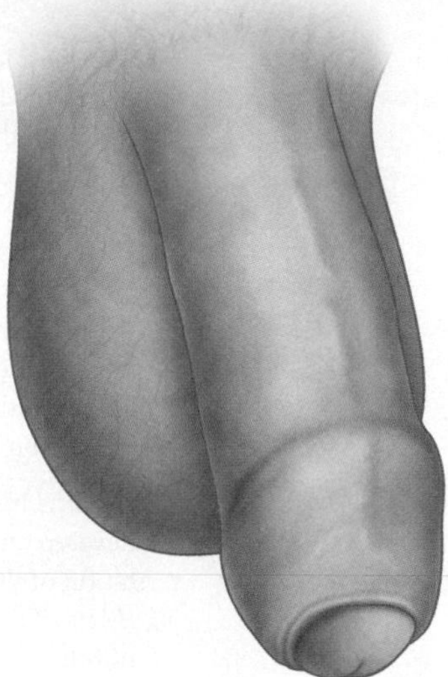

FIGURE 29-11 Foreskin on uncircumcised penis

THINK LINK: SMEGMA

Smegma is a whitish, oily material that forms between the foreskin and glans in the uncircumcised penis. It is composed of sebum combined with dead skin cells. Its function is to keep the glans moist and act as a lubricant to facilitate sexual intercourse. Very little smegma is produced during childhood, but increases during adolescence until sexual maturity.

In the erect position, the foreskin may be drawn back so as to expose the glans, or there may be enough slack in the skin to still cover the glans. When the foreskin is retracted, the glans may be covered with a whitish substance known as **smegma**. If present, it should be odorless.

Inspect glans for position of urethral meatus, a small, vertical slitlike opening that is located at the tip of the glans. Also observe for any evidence of a discharge from the meatus.

Unexpected: The urethral meatus may be located anywhere along the ventral/dorsal surface of the penis. In **hypospadias** it is located on the ventral surface. In **epispadias** it is located on the dorsal surface. (See Conditions and Disorders)

A clear, viscous substance is considered an expected finding. If meatus not present, inspect shaft of penis for other locations.

Unexpected: Purulent drainage associated with infections/inflammation.

The presence of any metal piercing should also be noted.

PRACTICE POINT: Genital Piercing

Genital piercing is a practice that is becoming more popular with both genders (Griffin, 2003). Piercing of body parts is common in many cultures; however, genital piercing is largely a recent Western practice. While personal feelings towards genital piercings range widely, health care providers must be careful regarding their expression. A common reaction is to "pathologize" the practice and the individual with piercings; however, studies have found that many individuals with genital piercings are not that different from mainstream society (Armstrong, Caliendo, & Roberts, 2006). The most common problems that genital piercings cause are infections, bleedings, nerve damage, or allergic reactions (Meyer, 2000), and may present relatively soon after the procedure. Infections left untreated may be life threatening or cause sterility (Griffin, 2003). Long-term complications may include priaprism, urethral stricture, and paraphimosis (Meltzer, 2005). A major need for health care providers is to know how to remove genital piercing hardware. Improper removal may cause or exacerbate complications related to piercing.

Inspection Techniques and Expected Findings

Inspect the genital area for the presence of any lesions. The penis should be free of any lesions.

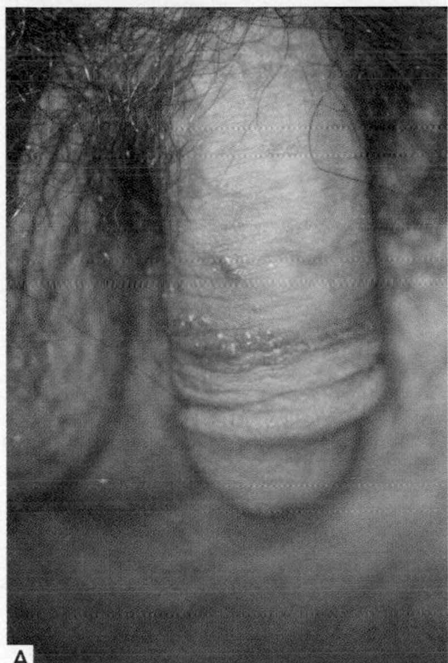

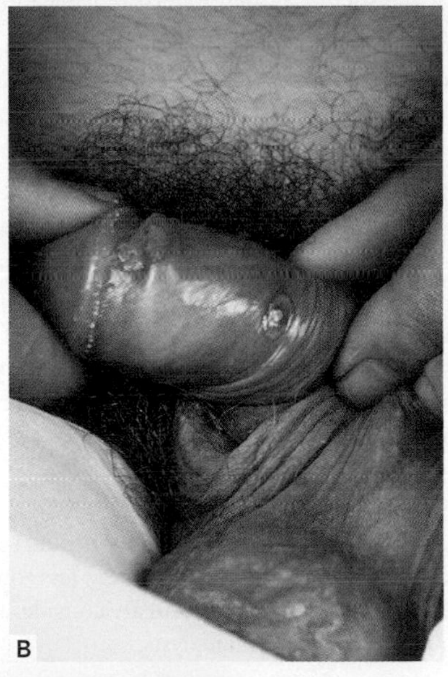

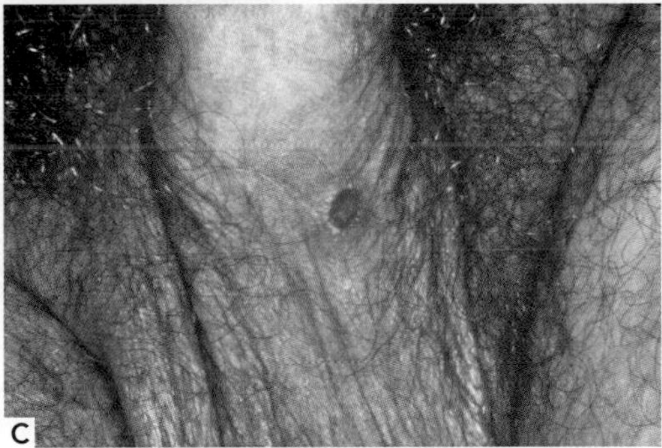

FIGURE 29-12A–C Examples of genital lesions: **a)** Wart caused by HPV (*Source:* CDC/Susan Lindsley); **b)** Chancre caused by Haemophilus ducreyi infection (*Source:* CDC/Dr. Pirozzi); **c)** Syphilitic chancre (*Source:* CDC/Dr. N. J. Fiumara; Dr. Gavin Hart)

Table 29-2 Penile lesions

	Ulcerating	Non-ulcerating
Infectious		
Viral	Genital herpes HSV type 2	Genital warts (HPV/viral)
Bacterial	Chancre/syphilis	2° syphilis
	Chancroid/soft chancre	
	Granuloma inguinale	
	Lymphogranuloma venerum	
Cutaneous conditions		Psoriasis
		Lichen planus/sclerosis
		Dermatitis
		Drug eruptions
Inflammation	Balanitis/balanoposthitis	
Infestations		Scabies
		Pediculosis

Unexpected Findings

The presence of any lesions on the genital organs should be noted along with their characteristics. Commonly, genital lesions are associated with STIs; however, not all lesions necessarily indicate the presence of a STI (Figure 29-12).

Lesions that are associated with STIs are often easily identified by their characteristics. Specific STIs related to specific lesions are syphilis, genital herpes, and chlamydia. The absence of lesions does not necessarily rule out their presence as some lesions are present only at certain times.

Lesions on the genital area are unexpected findings and may be related to a benign skin condition, STI, parasitic infestation, or non-infectious cutaneous conditions (Table 29-2).

Inspection Techniques and Expected Findings	Unexpected Findings
Assess the scrotum for symmetry, skin condition, and color. The ambient room temperature will most likely affect its position and thus the symmetry of testicular suspension. Also inspect for the presence of visible lumps or additional contents. Inspect the scrotum for configuration, uniformity and condition of skin. To inspect, move the penis to the side to expose the anterior scrotal sac. This may be done by the provider or requesting the patient to hold his penis. When the scrotum is hanging loosely, the left testicle hangs lower than the right one. This is due to a longer spermatic cord on the left testicle. In some individuals this may be reversed with the right side lower than the left.	Asymmetry of the scrotum is most likely due to swelling or edema of the scrotal contents.
The external appearance of the scrotum should demonstrate a deeper, redder pigmentation than the rest of the body with skin that is wrinkled (**rugae**) or rough with visible sebaceous glands. The roughened appearance is more apparent when the scrotum is retracted and closer to the body. The midline **raphe** should also be visible, which again is more easily observed in the retracted scrotum (Figure 29-13). In contrast to the hairless characteristic of the penis, the scrotum will have sparse hairs visible on the surface.	In certain conditions, not related to the genitalia, the scrotum may appear thickened due to edema. Frequently the edema is also characterized by pitting. Conditions related to this manifestation are related to fluid retention caused by hepatic, renal, or cardiac diseases.
When contracted, the scrotum has a more uniform appearance; when relaxed, the unequal suspension of the testes provides a more asymmetric appearance and the skin is thinner and less rough in appearance. Small lumps that may be apparent on the surface of the scrotum are considered an expected finding and are small sebaceous cysts, also known as epidermoid cysts.	Under certain circumstances, these cysts may enlarge and secrete and discharge an oily substance.

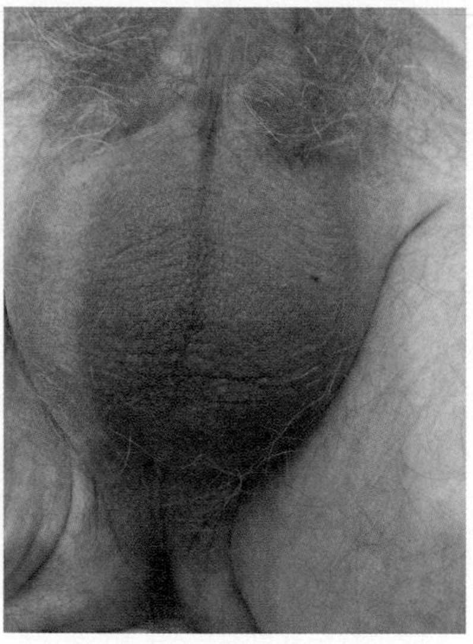

FIGURE 29-13 Inspection of the scrotum (rugae/raphe)

PRACTICE POINT: Temperature Changes and Scrotum Size

The scrotum demonstrates and elastic quality allowing it to expand and contract in response to temperature changes. Optimum sperm production occurs at just slightly below body temperature; therefore the scrotum serves as the regulator of temperature. In cool temperatures, the scrotum contracts, bringing the testicles closer to the body. Conversely, in warm temperatures it expands, allowing the testicles to hang lower and be removed from body heat.

Inspection: Level II

The Level II assessment is performed on patients with unstable conditions and who have significant pathological alterations. Data gathered is associated with more depth and/or detail requiring more time, skill, and effort. More than one system is generally involved and changes in the patient's conditions and assessment parameters have the potential to shift drastically and quickly.

Inspection Techniques and Expected Findings	Unexpected Findings
If the patient has experienced any type of surgery of the genital area, an indwelling urinary catheter is frequently inserted through the penis into the bladder which allows for continuous drainage of urine. Urine is yellow in color, ranging from very light to very dark depending on its concentration.	The patient who has had renal, bladder, or prostate gland surgery may have urine that contains blood, turning it to various shades of orange. It may also contain visible clots. Certain medications and other conditions may also cause the urine to demonstrate other color changes.

Inspection Techniques and Expected Findings	Unexpected Findings

Inspect the glans for evidence of inflammation. The glans is covered with smooth skin that is without lesions or redness. The skin covering the glans may be slightly darker in color than the skin of the shaft and may also appear purple in color.

Inflammation of the glans and the mucous membrane beneath it is known as **balanitis**. It can present as acute or chronic and caused by irritation or infectious agents (Figure 29-14).

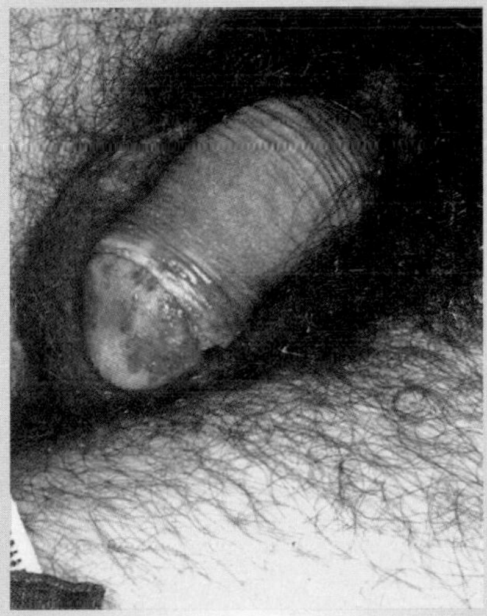

FIGURE 29-14 Balanitis
Source: CDC/Dr. N.J. Fiumara

Lastly, inspect the inguinal and femoral area for any evidence of bulging. This is ideally done with the patient standing; however, it is permissible to inspect for this with the patient lying supine in bed.

Any bulging that is visible is most likely due to a hernia.

Instruct the patient to "bear down" as if having a bowel movement. While the patient is doing so, again observe the area for any evidence of bulging. There should be no evidence of bulging in the area.

During inspection of the inguinal and femoral area, also observe for any evidence of lymph node enlargement.

Any inflammatory or infectious process may cause enlargement of the horizontal and vertical lymph nodes.

Inspection: Level III

An alteration in the integrity or continuity of the penis may be caused by traumatic injury. Traumatic injury may consist of penile fracture, penile amputation, penetrating penile injuries, and penile soft tissue injuries, which are considered urologic emergencies, commonly requiring surgical intervention (Santucci & Broghammer, 2009). Traumatic injury may be occur in common actions (zipping up a pants' fly) to devastating injury caused by penetrating trauma, experienced by military personnel due to improvised explosive devices (IED) used in the Middle East conflicts over the past years.

Inspect for any evidence of a break in the continuity or alignment of the penis or any break in skin integrity of the genitals or within the genital area.

Penile fracture results from the traumatic rupture of the corpus cavernosum due to sudden blunt trauma or an abrupt lateral bending of the erect penis, breaking the markedly thinned and stiff tunica albuginea. The fracture of the tunica albuginea causes hemorrhaging into one or both of the corpora cavernosum. When both corpora are involved, there is often urethral damage also.

Inspection Techniques and Expected Findings	Unexpected Findings
Penile fracture is relatively rare; however, it is also thought to be under reported due to embarrassment (Santucci & Broghammer, 2009).	In most instances, penile fracture occurs during sexual intercourse, with the penis accidentally falling out or disengaging from the vagina and hitting the partner's perineum or pubis, or some other hard object. There may be a popping or cracking sound with the immediate loss of erection. Pain is also associated with the fracture, but ranges from minimal to severe, depending on the amount of damage. Classic presentation of a fractured penis is deformity, swelling, and ecchymosis, commonly identified as the **"eggplant" deformity**. The shape of the penis often assumes an "S" shape, with the penis deviated away from the tear. If the urethra is also involved, there will be blood present at the meatus.
Penile amputation consists of complete or incomplete severing of the penis.	Amputation of the penis is rare with 65%–87% the result of self-mutilation due to acute psychosis or gender dysphoria. (Thomas, Santucci, & Morey, 2007). Other instances are frequently related to traumatic assaults. Physical evidence of amputation is obvious. Historical data is vital to determine the mental state of the individual as a possible cause related to self-mutilation. Reattachment of the penis depends on preservation of the severed part, the integrity and condition of the graft site, and whether the individual's mental state will be a risk for reamputation. If reattachment is not possible, penile reconstruction is done with the primary focus of maintaining the ability to void in the standing position. Participation in sexual intercourse is primarily dependent upon the remaining length of the penis. Penetrating and soft tissue injuries are generally due to trauma from shrapnel, gunshot, stabbing, infection, burns, human and animal bites and degloving injuries related to machinery involvement. Injuries can involve either or both corpora, the urethra, or be confined to just soft tissue. Penetrating injuries are most commonly seen during military combat. Gunshot wounds are the most common cause of non-combat injuries. Stab wounds are quite rare. Trauma to the penis is rarely a single reason for seeking medical attention. In most instances, other injuries are also present and if life threatening, should take precedence over genital injury. Presentation of penile injury is often self-evident and depends on the specific cause. As with other injuries, blood in the meatus is evidence of urethral involvement.

Inspection Techniques and Expected Findings	Unexpected Findings
	In the absence of other life-threatening injuries, surgical reconstruction is indicated and should begin as soon as possible to prevent infection. Minor, superficial injuries may be treated nonsurgically.
A nontraumatic emergency condition that relates to a Level III exam is **priaprism**.	Priaprism is the presence of a persistent erection that is not related to sexual stimulation or desire. It may occur in both circumcised and uncircumcised males and frequently accompanied by pain. As with paraphimosis, the earlier treatment is sought, the greater the chances are of maintaining the function and structure of the penis. Low-flow priaprism is most common, with continuous accumulation of blood in the cavernous tissue as well as venous stasis. Prolonged venous accumulation and stasis results in ischemia and cavernosal artery thrombosis (Al-Qudah, Al-Omer, Parraga-Marquez, Santucci, & Wanlheim, 2009) that leads to fibrotic changes and a loss of the ability to achieve an erection.

THINK LINK: *Priaprism and Sickle Cell Disease*

Priaprism is a serious complication associated with sickle cell disease (SCD), which is a blood disorder that affects African Americans. The incidence of priaprism in males with SCD is estimated to be between 30%–45 % (Nolan, Wyszynski, Farrer, & Steinberg, 2005). The exact mechanism is unknown; however recent studies suggest that it results from an increase in hemolysis of the red cells that decreases the availability of nitric oxide, which is necessary for venous dilatation to allow for blood to drain from the erect penis. This type of priaprism is characteristic of a low-flow priaprism.

Inspection: Level IV

A Level IV exam would include the cremasteric reflex. This is also a component of the neurological exam (Chapter 26) when doing a comprehensive neurological assessment. When indicated, assess the cremasteric reflex in the presence of scrotal pain.

An intact cremasteric reflex is the elevation of the testis and scrotum due to stimulation and contraction of the cremasteric muscle (see Chapter 26).

Inspection Techniques and Expected Findings	Unexpected Findings
Inspection may also include transillumination of the scrotum, which is done by shining a bright light through the scrotum (Figure 29-15). It is commonly performed after palpation when additional scrotal contents are palpated. Transillumination helps to determine if the palpated mass is filled with fluid or a solid material.	A fluid-filled mass (**hydrocele**) will allow the light to pass through it whereas a solid mass (**spermatocele,** hernia) will cast a shadow, outlining the mass. A hernia will become smaller when reduction is performed, unless it is incarcerated, which requires immediate surgery.

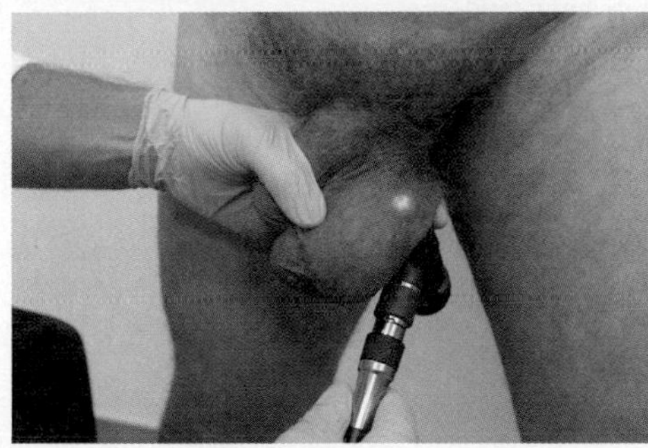

FIGURE 29-15 Transillumination

Transillumination is best performed with the patient standing. This allows for better positioning and manipulation of the light along the side or behind the scrotum for optimum observation.

Palpation: Level I

Palpation Techniques and Expected Findings	Unexpected Findings
Palpation of the penis and scrotum for a Level I exam is often unnecessary. Instances where palpation may be appropriate would be to assess the mobility of the foreskin and retraction of the foreskin to observe the glans. If the foreskin is present, it should be easily moved over the glans and be positioned behind it; a small amount of smegma may be covering the glans. If present, it should be odorless. Lesions may also be obscured by the foreskin, so retraction will allow for observation of the glans and other areas for the presence of any lesions. Palpation of the penis should always be done with the use of gloves.	If the foreskin is not able to be retracted over the glans, it should not be forced. **Phimosis** is the term used to describe this condition. Physiologic phimosis may be present through childhood and into adolescence (Figure 29-16).

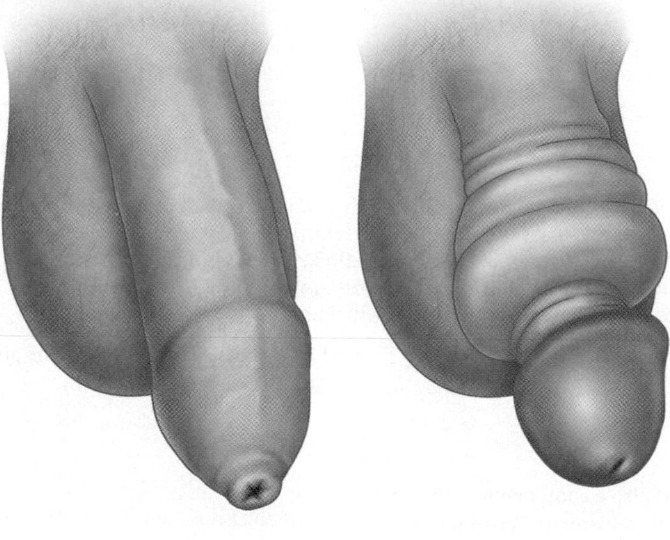

FIGURE 29-16 **a)** Phimosis; **b)** paraphimosis

Palpation: Level II

Palpation Techniques and Expected Findings	Unexpected Findings
Palpation of the penis is done to assess consistency of the internal structures and for the presence of internal alterations. To palpate the penis, grasp its shaft between the index finger and thumb at the base of the penis and compressing the penile tissue between them down the shaft (Figure 29-17). The flaccid penis tissue should be soft, but firm and easily compressed, without any tenderness, or areas of hardness. The urethra may be palpable in the midline of the penis. Palpation of the penile shaft is performed to assess for any tenderness or induration. The flaccid penis should be easily compressed with a spongelike softness and free from any nodules or hardened areas. When the glans is reached, gently squeeze the top and bottom to open the urethral meatus. Assess the meatus for color and any discharge. The opening should be moist and pink without any evidence of discharge.	As already identified, fibrous scar tissue causing Peyronie's disease may be palpated.

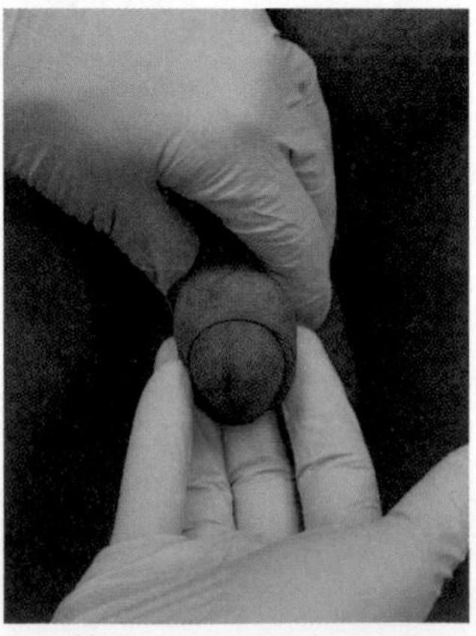

FIGURE 29-17 Palpation of penis

Palpation Techniques and Expected Findings	Unexpected Findings
When the possibility of a urethral inflammation exists, due to gonorrhea or another infection, determine the presence of a discharge. The decision to determine this is also based on the patient's history for the presence of a discharge.	If a discharge is present, it will be brought forward to exit through the meatus. The discharge is then collected for culturing and sent to the laboratory.
Assess for discharge by "milking" the urethra. Hold the penis with one hand and place the index finger of the other hand at its base of the penis (Figure 29-18). Move the index finger down the shaft, compressing the urethra from the base to the tip.	

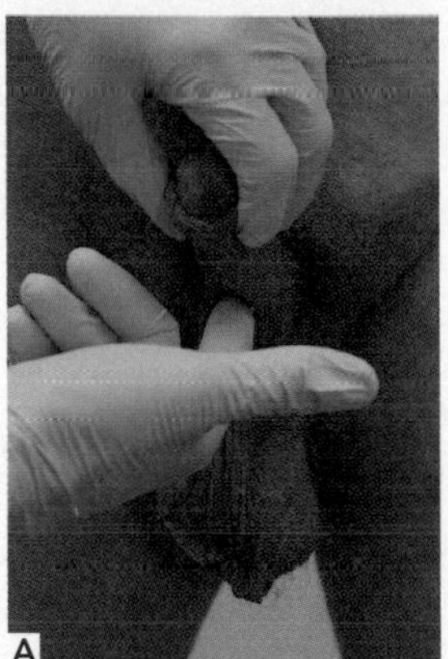

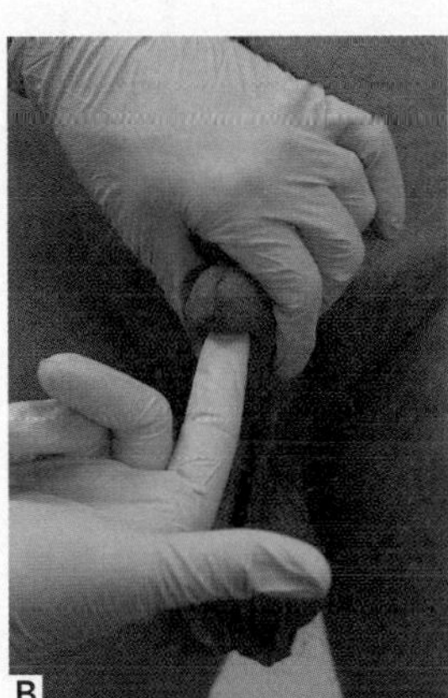

FIGURE 29-18A–B Milking the urethra

Palpation of the scrotum is primarily performed to assess the contents of the scrotum—testes, epididymis, and vas deferens. Gently palpate the testes between the thumb and first two fingers. The testes are extremely sensitive to pressure, so gentle compression is necessary. The testes should feel smooth, without any evidence of nodules or growths, and have a rubbery texture. The testes should also be equal in size, ovoid in shape and freely moveable (Figure 29-19).

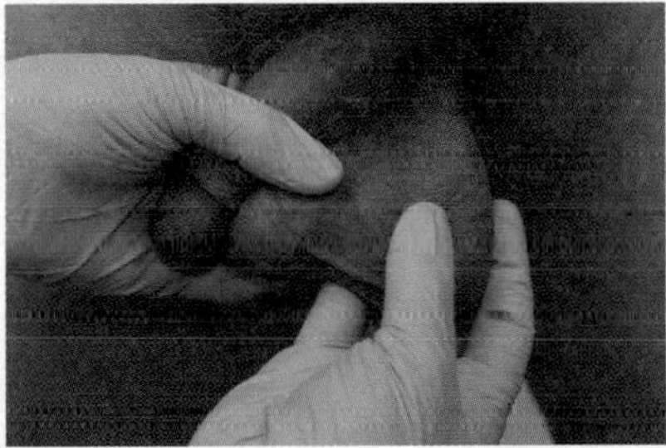

FIGURE 29-19 Palpating the testicles

Palpation Techniques and Expected Findings	Unexpected Findings
Palpate the epididymis on the posterolateral surface of the testes; it should feel smooth, discrete, and be nontender. The epididymis moves with the testes, but can also move independently. The texture of the epididymis can be described as a cluster of soft noodles.	A spermatocele may be felt when palpating the epididymis. It is a benign cystic accumulation of sperm that develops from the head of the epididymis.
Palpate the vas deferens along the side of the scrotum as it leaves the testes and ascends upwards to the inguinal canal. Because the vas deferens, along with arteries and veins, are contained in the spermatic cord, it is nearly impossible to specifically identify each structure. The vas deferens may be felt as a smooth, soft, pliable cordlike structure.	During palpation of the vas deferens, the presence of additional cord like structures may be evidence of a **varicocele**, which is due to dilatation and tortuosity of the veins accompanying the spermatic cord. It most often occurs on the left side and may be painful. The patient may also identify a "tugging" of "pulling" sensation in the scrotum accompanied by a dull ache.

Palpation Techniques and Expected Findings

Palpating for the presence of an inguinal hernia and palpation of the prostate gland are the last components of the male genitalia exam.

Perform palpation for a hernia with the patient standing. Begin the assessment by placing the index finger alongside the scrotum and pressing upward until the inguinal canal is reached (Figure 29-20). Allow for enough loose skin from the scrotum to permit comfortable insertion of the finger. It is also helpful if the patient can flex the leg of the side that is being examined. Inform the patient that some pressure may be experienced as the finger passes through the scrotum but that it should not be painful.

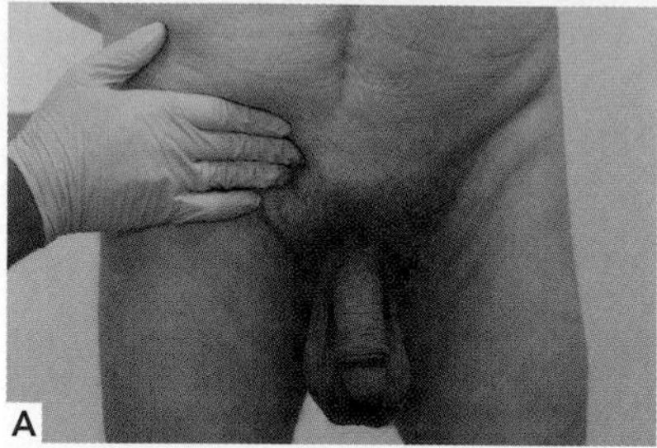

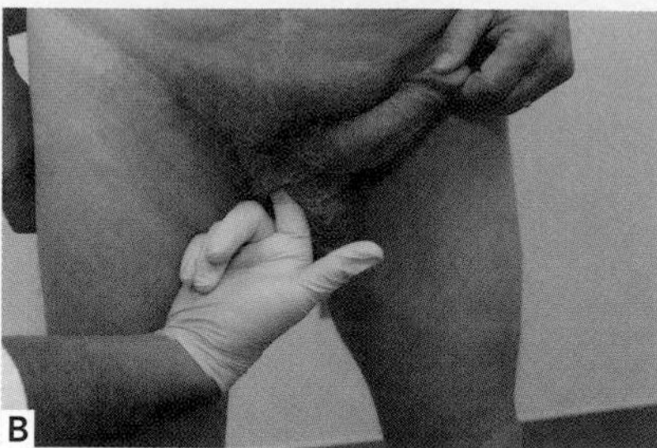

FIGURE 29-20A–B Palpation for inguinal hernia

When the finger reaches the inguinal canal, palpate around the canal opening for any evidence of muscle mass that protrudes through the canal.

If the finger encounters any mass or resistance, do not progress any further.

If no mass or resistance is felt, request that the patient to "bear down" while you feel for the sudden presence of a "mass" touching your finger. The expected result is that there is nothing that comes in contact with your finger.

Unexpected Findings

A varicocele may not be visible and most likely observed only when the patient is standing. It may be described as small, moderate, or large. A small varicocele is palpable only during the Valsalva maneuver, a moderate varicocele is palpable without the Valsalva, and a large varicocele is visible as a bulging of the side of the scrotum. The classic description of a varicocele is like a "bag of worms."

The sudden presence of a mass touching the fingertip is evidence of an inguinal hernia.

An inguinal hernia is caused by a weakness in or around the inguinal canal, allowing a loop of intestine to pass through or around the canal. Inguinal hernias may be indirect and direct.

A hernia, if present, will be palpable just below the inguinal ligament.

An **indirect inguinal hernia** is when the intestine passes through the inguinal canal, beginning at the internal ring and passing through the external ring (Figure 29-21). It may also pass into the scrotum where it may be palpated as a mass. If it has not entered the scrotum, it may be palpated or it touches the finger when the patient bears down as requested. Indirect hernias are often bilateral, so palpation of both inguinal canals is important. Indirect hernias are more common in children and young males.

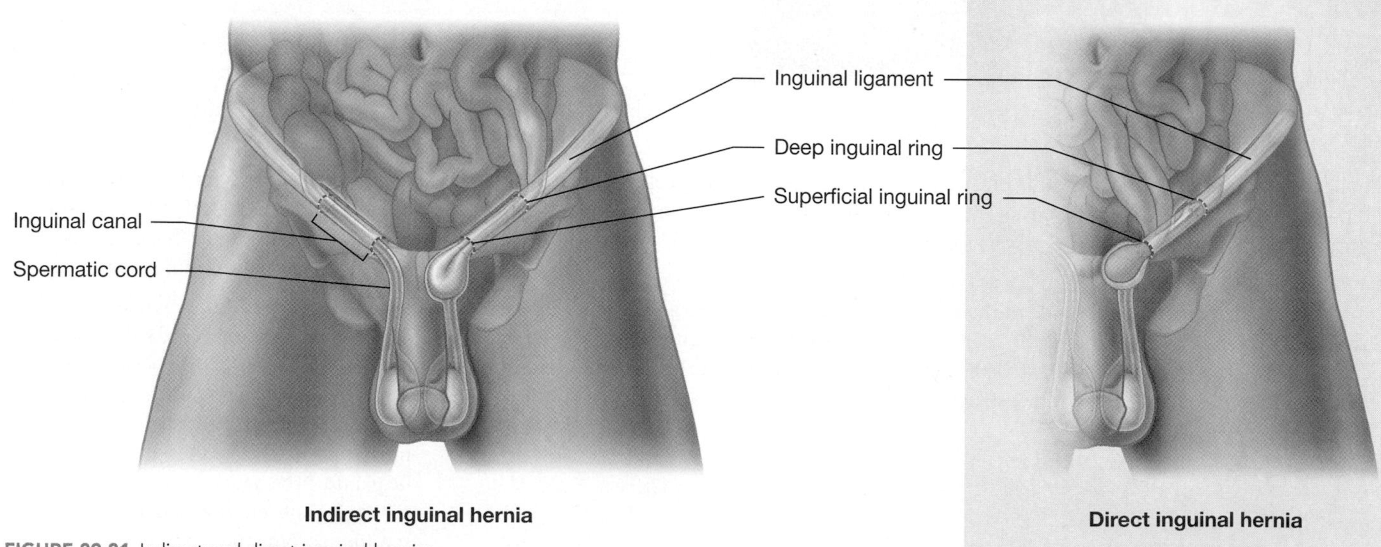

FIGURE 29-21 Indirect and direct inguinal hernias

Palpation Techniques and Expected Findings	Unexpected Findings
	A **direct inguinal hernia** occurs when the loop of intestine passes through the external ring directly, not first passing through the internal inguinal ring. It is caused by degeneration of connective tissue and abdominal muscle, causing them to weaken. It seldom enters the scrotum, but may be felt hitting the finger when the patient bears down. While both types of hernia touch the finger, the direct hernia will be felt more on the side of the finger and the indirect will be felt as touching the tip of the finger. While it may be possible to distinguish between the two types by palpation, it is not clinically significant as both types will need to be repaired. Direct hernias are more common in males over the age of 40.
The presence of a femoral hernia is determined by placing the hand over the inguinal area while the patient is "bearing down." There should not be any bulging palpated.	A **femoral hernia** involves the passing of the intestine through an expanded femoral ring, which is near the inguinal canal, but there is no direct connection between them. The femoral hernia also has no connection to the scrotum. The femoral ring is where the femoral blood vessels exit the abdominal cavity, and when it becomes weakened, also allows the intestine to exit. It is characterized by a bulging in the femoral area of the groin as well as palpating a mass that is felt in the same manner as inguinal hernias. Pain may accompany a femoral hernia and may become severe. They are less common than inguinal hernias and occur more frequently in females.

PRACTICE POINT: Turn Your Head and Cough

A common directive to males when examining them for inguinal hernias is "turn your head and cough." While it was generally understood the reason for coughing, turning the head didn't seem to have anything to do with a hernia. Turning the head while coughing was done to protect the examiner from having the person cough directly over him, avoiding the possibility of the transmission of viruses and bacteria during the cough. It is now more likely that the examiner will request the patient to simply bear down during the exam, rather than direct the patient to turn and cough. Bearing down also provides a more even buildup of intra-abdominal pressure rather than the quick, explosive build up and release from a cough.

Palpation Techniques and Expected Findings	Unexpected Findings
Palpation of the prostate is performed with the rectal exam of the male. The rectal exam is described is Chapter 28.	
The prostate gland is considered a component of the male reproductive system but is located internally. After the walls of the rectum have been palpated, palpate the posterior surface of the prostate, the only palpable portion. Assess the size, contour, consistency, and mobility of the prostate gland. The expected characteristics of the prostate gland are a diameter of about 4 cm that should not protrude more than 1 cm into the rectal wall.	Greater than 1 cm is an indication of enlargement. Enlargement of the gland may be due to hypertrophy or cancer. Hypertrophy of the prostate causes the gland to feel rubbery or boggy whereas cancer causes it to feel hard and nodular. A hard and nodular prostate may also be due to calculi or chronic fibrosis, so one should not jump to conclusions when palpating a hard and nodular prostate gland.
The consistency should be firm and smooth with slight mobility. The median sulcus, which divides the gland into right and left lobes, should be palpable, and overall there should be no tenderness associated with palpation	

Palpation: Level III

Palpation Techniques and Expected Findings	Unexpected Findings
Palpation of the penis in the presence of trauma is generally not performed. Additional data from palpation is not particularly necessary to determine a specific condition.	
Palpation of the scrotum in the presence of pain or inflammation is tenuous. It is questionable as to whether additional information obtained from palpation will facilitate an appropriate examination and/or diagnosis.	Inflammation is associated with **epididymitis** and/or **orchitis**.
	Orchitis that is secondary to epididymitis is known as epididymo-orchitis. In both conditions, the majority of incidences only involve one testicle.
	Acute scrotal pain may also indicate a **testicular torsion (TT)**, which must be differentiated from epididymitis, as a delay in treating TT may result in the loss of the testicle (Table 29-3). It most frequently occurs in adolescent males aged 12–18 years (Rupp & Zwanger, 2009).

Table 29-3 Differential diagnosis: testicular torsion and epididymitis

Torsion	Epididymitis
Twisting of testis on spermatic cord	Bacterial infection (STD or UTI)
Babies to teens	Teens to adults
Acute pain	Gradual onset of pain
Vomiting, nausea	Fever
Scrotal discoloration	Dysuria, pyuria
Lack of cremasteric muscle	Redness of scrotum
Surgical emergency	Uretheral discharge
	Nodular epididymis

PRACTICE POINT: Urinary Catheter Inspection

Individuals who have had surgery on either the external or internal reproductive organs will most likely have an indwelling urinary catheter in place. This is a tube that is inserted through the urethra into the bladder to provide for continuous drainage of urine from the bladder.

Proper assessment of the catheter is to determine that it is placed properly by noting the presence of urine in the drainage tubing. The catheter should be positioned so that there is no pulling on the catheter. In some instances there may be traction applied to the catheter as a method to prevent bleeding from the surgical site, particularly on the prostate gland.

The drainage system/collection bag should be placed in a position that is lower than the patient. This facilitates drainage of the bladder by the effect of gravity. The drainage tubing should also be positioned in such a way that there are no loops of the tubing hanging down, preventing the free flow of urine into the collection bag.

Developmental Applications

Techniques and Expected Findings	Unexpected Findings
Infants and Children The genitalia of the male infant are inspected for the presence of any anomalies or deformities, incomplete development, and sexual ambiguity.	
Inspect the penis for size and placement of the meatus. The non-erect infant's penis is 2–3 cm. It is not uncommon for the penis to become erect, and when so, it should project straight. For the first 3 months the foreskin is frequently tight and may be retracted some to visualize placement of the meatus. The foreskin should not be retracted forcefully as this may cause tearing and result in the	When the urethra exits on the ventral side of the penis the condition is identified as hypospadias and when it exits of the dorsal side it is hypospadias.

Techniques and Expected Findings

formation of adhesions between the prepuce and glans. The meatus should be visible on the tip of the glans. When possible, observe the force of the urinary stream which should be strong and emerge from the meatus in a straight line.

In some infants, the meatus does not exit at the tip of the glans, but is located on either the dorsal or ventral side of the penis.

Inspect the scrotum for size, shape, characteristics, and the presence of testes. The scrotum of the full term infant should be loose with the presence of rugae and a midline raphe. The scrotum of the newborn frequently appears to be larger in proportion to the penis, frequently due to edema of the scrotum.

Palpation of the infant's penis is generally not performed. Palpation of the scrotum is done to determine the presence of two testes. Before palpating the scrotum, position the thumb and index finger of one hand over the inguinal canal to prevent the testicle from retracting back into the inguinal canal. While positioning the thumb and index finger, gently palpate the area for any soft masses in the inguinal canal. If a mass is palpated, gently push it downward to determine if it can be pushed into the scrotum.

Palpate both halves of the scrotum between the index finger and thumb of the opposite hand to determine the presence of the testes. In the full-term infant, both testicles should have descended into the scrotum and be palpable. The size of the infant's testicle is approximately 1 cm in diameter. If a testicle is pushed into the scrotum with pressure, it is considered to be descended.

While palpating the scrotum, try to prevent eliciting the cremasteric reflex, a response to cold and sudden touching that may pull the testicle up into the inguinal canal. To prevent the cremasteric reflex, have warm hands and palpate gently. Also palpating down from the inguinal canal is recommended.

Palpating the scrotum may also reveal the presence of other masses. Differentiating between solid or fluid-filled masses can be done with transillumination.

Inspection and palpation of the genitalia of a toddler, child, and adolescent are no different than as already described. The penis and testicles size will begin to enlarge during puberty as well as the development of secondary sexual characteristics.

The Older Adult

The assessment of the genitalia for the older adult male proceeds in the same way as described for the adult. Visible changes in the genitalia may be evident.

Secondary sex characteristics that are dependent on testosterone begin to diminish; there is an overall reduction in muscle mass as well as facial and body hair. The reduction in production of testosterone allows for an increase is follicle stimulating hormone (FSH) and luteinizing hormone (LH). This is not an absolute increase but a relative increase due to the reduction in testosterone.

The testes become less firm with age and lose a significant number of seminiferous tubules, resulting in a decreased production of sperm. The reduction in sperm production does not necessarily affect the fertility of the patient as males in their 80s and 90s have been known to father children.

The scrotum of the older adult male loses some of its tone and becomes elongated and pendulous (Figure 29-22). A major problem with this is that the elderly patient may sit on the scrotum, resulting in trauma or excoriation of the surface.

Penis size may become somewhat smaller, although no well-documented evidence supports that this is a common experience. Blood circulation may be somewhat reduced and cause the penis to look smaller. Also, in obese individuals, fat deposition in the groin and pubic area makes the penis appear smaller. Other changes the patient may identify are that it takes longer to achieve and maintain an erection as well as a decreased firmness with a decreased force of ejaculation.

Unexpected Findings

Failure to palpate one or both testicles in the scrotum is evidence that the testicles have not descended (cryptorchidism), occurring frequently in premature infants. It also is present in approximately 3%–5% of term infants (Docimo, Silver, & Cromie, 2000). While the initial finding of cryptorchidism is not significant, failure of the testicle to descend by 6 months is a concern and treatment should be considered to prevent the development of potential long term consequences. Possible consequences of cryptorchidism include testicular cancer, subfertility, testicular torsion, and inguinal hernia.

Shining a light through the scrotum will create a shadow is the mass is solid and light will pass through a fluid-filled mass (most likely a hydrocele); a solid mass is most likely a hernia. A hernia will also get smaller when reduction is attempted whereas a hydrocele will not change in size. Hydroceles are common in children under 2 years of age.

While each child's development will progress at its own pace, any apparent delays in development need to be addressed with the child and parents.

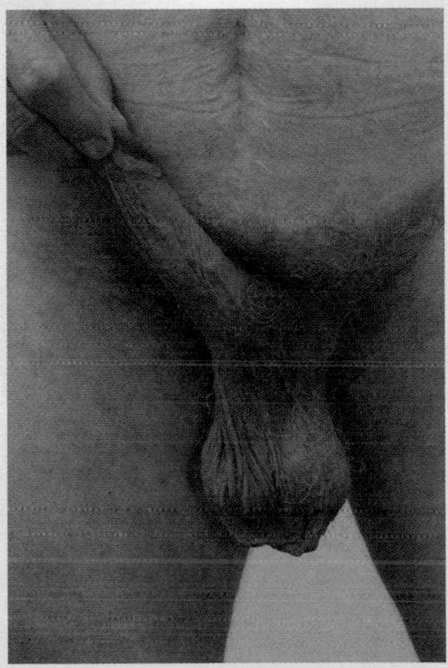

FIGURE 29-22 Loss of muscle tone in the scrotum of the older male

DOCUMENTATION

History

Patient presenting for yearly physical. No complaints of pain in groin and adjacent structures. Denies any swelling or enlargement of testicles or scrotum. Is able to achieve and maintain an erection with no noticeable curving or deviation of penis. Able to engage in intercourse with partner without any problems related to pain or ability to penetrate partner. Does use condoms during sexual activity. Has not fathered any children but does not perceive that he would have any fertility problems. Has not noted any lesions on penis or scrotum and has not noted any urethral discharge. Past medical history not significant. Denies any history of surgical procedures related to any alterations of genitalia. No history of STIs and no chronic conditions that have affected sexual functioning. No family history of prostate, testicular, or penile cancers. Employment of a nature that does not pose a threat to potential damage to genitalia. Does ride bike and is aware of potential fertility problems associated with particular bike seats.

Is sexually active with female partners and uses condoms for protection of STIs. Does have multiple partners but states is "monogamous" with one partner at a time. Satisfied with amount of sexual activity and ability to engage in intercourse. Is able to identify major STIs and manifestations associated with them. Does have knowledge of TSE but not sure if he performs it correctly.

Physical Exam

Pubic hair in diamond shape extending up to umbilicus. Texture coarse and curly. No evidence of parasite infestation. External genitalia with typical male characteristics and configuration. Penis in flaccid state with meatus exiting at tip of glans. No redness of meatus observed. Skin color consistent with overlying body skin, is smooth without any obvious lesions. Circumcised with a small remnant of foreskin the covers one half of the glans. Scrotum hanging freely with left testicle slightly lower than right. Testicles appear symmetrical in size and shape. No bulging or redness observed. Skin of scrotum slightly darker than penis and rest of skin. No bulges noted in inguinal and femoral regions.

Shaft of penis soft to palpation with spongy/rubbery consistency. No areas of hardness or tenderness. Scrotum contains two testicles that are symmetrical in size and shape and with a firm, rubbery texture. Slight tenderness to minimal palpation. Surface smooth without nodules or other surface alterations. Spermatic cord palpated without evidence of pain tenderness or additional structures. No evidence of inguinal or femoral hernia when inguinal canal and femoral canal palpated.

Electronic Charting

Expectations of Electronic Charting

Electronic charting should accommodate the entire reproductive assessment, including related information such as sexual activity, protection measures for sports or exercise activities, and protection measures for STIs. Charting should accommodate age-appropriate developmental assessments. Ideally, the system should accommodate modifiable graphics of the internal and external reproductive system to facilitate documentation.

Patients may be embarrassed about aspects of the reproductive assessment. Electronic charting should provide appropriate measures to protect patient privacy and confidentiality.

Electronic charting systems are increasingly accommodating genomic information. Reproductive counseling may soon include counseling patients on the basis of genome-wide data.

Limitations of Electronic Charting

While electronic charting is increasingly integrated into health care, the technology is not equally well developed in all areas. The particular charting system in use may or may not have structured documentation in place for reproductive assessments, or the male reproductive system documents may not be as well developed as documentation of the female reproductive system. Documentation may need to be developed within your charting system, or you may need to document on unstructured forms such as free-text clinical notes. Unstructured documentation limits the ability to access data for longitudinal care, and to re-use data for research or quality improvement (Roth, Lim, Pevnick, Asch, & McGlynn, 2009).

Summary

- Male reproductive organs are primarily external with some being internal. Their reproductive function is not fully mature until a male reaches puberty. The penis also contains the urethra, which is the conduit for the elimination of urine from the bladder.
- The male reproductive organs are assessed by observation and palpation. The external organs (penis and scrotum) demonstrate a specific male configuration, and in the adult are accompanied by secondary sexual characteristics (diamond shaped pubic hair presentation).
- Altered conditions of the male reproductive organs and system are caused by infections, inflammation, congenital anomalies, anatomic alterations and genetic (chromosomal) dysfunction.
- The full development and maturation of reproductive function begins at puberty (adolescence) that causes growth of the penis and testicles as well as the initiation of sperm production. During childhood, there are no reproductive functions and the penis primarily functions in the elimination of urine. Reproductive functions do slow down as the male ages, however fertility remains and sperm production continues through a male's life.
- Subjective and objective data obtained from the history and physical is documented in a way that correctly and appropriately describes the individual and unique characteristics of the male patient and are in agreement with each other.

Review Questions

1. When teaching a patient about the structure and function of male genitalia, the provider should include which of the following statements? (Select all that apply.)
   1. Male sexual function is associated with libido, erection, ejaculation, and orgasm.
   2. The urethra is a structure of the urinary and reproductive systems.
   3. Penile erection occurs in response to a central nervous system signal.
   4. The prostate gland is primarily responsible for testosterone production.
   5. The prostate gland is important in ejaculation.
2. When conducting an examination of the male reproductive system the provider includes which of the following structures in inspection? (Select all that apply.)
   1. Cowper's gland
   2. corpora cavernosum
   3. glans penis
   4. vas deferens
   5. scrotum
3. The provider is assessing a young man who reports that his female partner has been diagnosed with Chlamydia. The provider should expect that the patient will
   1. have a red raised rash on his penis.
   2. have no symptoms of the infection.
   3. report drainage from the penis.
   4. exhibit flulike symptoms.
4. When assessing a male patient the provider notes that the patient has several vesicles in the genital area. The patient reports that this has occurred in the past, but he did not seek treatment because the problem resolved. The provider expects that the patient has contracted which of the following?
   1. syphilis
   2. chlamydia
   3. epididymitis
   4. herpes
5. The provider is conducting an education program for men at a senior center. When addressing concerns about cancer the provider should include that a major risk factor for the development of prostate cancer is which of the following?
   1. ethnicity
   2. onset of puberty
   3. age
   4. history of STIs
6. When assessing a male patient, he develops an erection during the genitalia examination. The most appropriate action for the provider is to do which of the following?
   1. Quietly leave the room until the erection resolves.
   2. Continue with the exam as if nothing has happened.
   3. Cover the erection and go to another area to continue the exam.
   4. Engage the patient in conversation to draw attention away from the erection.
7. The provider documents that a patient admitted to the emergency room has an "eggplant deformity." This term is commonly used to describe the assessment findings associated with which of the following?
   1. penile fracture
   2. testicular torsion
   3. priaprism
   4. hypospadias
8. When examining a male toddler's genitourinary system, the provider notes the presence of a collection of fluid in the scrotum. The provider is aware that this finding is likely which of the following?
   1. a femoral hernia
   2. epispadias
   3. the result of an STI
   4. a hydrocele
9. To assess the cremasteric reflex, the provider should do which of the following?
   1. Stroke the shaft of the penis on the dorsal side.
   2. Stroke the inner aspect of the thigh.
   3. Pinch the underside of the scrotum.
   4. Pinch the spermatic cord.
10. The provider is performing a rectal examination on a healthy male patient and expects that upon palpation the prostate gland will be
    1. rubbery.
    2. tender.
    3. firm and slightly mobile.
    4. hard and nodular.

Conditions and Disorders

CANCER

Penile Cancer

Penile cancer is quite rare in most developed countries. In the U.S. the incidence rate is 1/100,000 per year (National Cancer Institute, 2009). In other areas of the world, particularly Asia, Africa, and South America, they represent 20%–30% of all cancers in males (Brosman, 2013). Squamous cell carcinoma is the most prevalent type of penile cancer (Hakenberg & Protzel, 2012). Although rare (<2%), melanoma cancers of the penis have been confirmed. While the exact cause is unknown, a relationship to human papillomavirus infection has been identified (American Cancer Society, 2013; Gross & Pfister, 2004). Other risk factors include age > 60, phimosis, poor personal hygiene, early age at first intercourse and multiple sexual partners (Pizzocaro et al., 2010). The long-held belief that that penile cancer may be caused by exposure to carcinogens contained in smegma has not been confirmed (Van Howe & Hodgest, 2006). As with other cancers, use of tobacco products also increases the risk for developing cancer.

Early diagnosis and treatment is essential to preventing metastasis, which may be lethal. Initial metastasis is to the femoral and inguinal lymph nodes. Untreated penile cancer is often fatal within 2 years. Superficial carcinoma can be easily resected while more invasive cancers may result in partial or complete penectomy. Radiation may be an effective substitute for surgery in certain individuals but there are very few candidates for this therapy. Chemotherapy is used when there is evidence of metastasis.

Pathophysiology

- Majority originates on glans or prepuce, presenting as a sore/lesion that doesn't heal, a papule or pustule, wartlike growth, or reddened area.
- These symptoms are not necessarily specific to penile cancer so diagnosis may be delayed.
- Delay in a diagnosis is also due to embarrassment, guilt, fear, ignorance, and personal neglect (Brosman, 2013).

Subjective Data

- Few symptoms are associated with the development of penile cancer. Even with significant local tissue destruction, pain is rare.
- Patients with advanced metastatic cancer may report weakness, weight loss, and fatigue; the penile lesion may bleed.

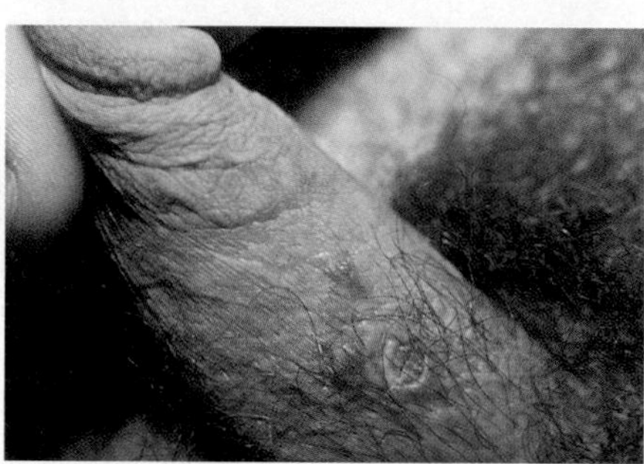

FIGURE 29-23 Penile cancer
Source: CMSP

Objective Data

- Lesion that fails to heal within 4 weeks
- Subtle induration in the skin, a small, a papule, a pustule, a warty growth, or a reddened area on the glans, or a rash
- Shallow erosion or deep ulceration with rolled edges
- Because majority of patients with penile cancer are uncircumcised, phimosis is often present and obscures the tumor, allowing it to grow undetected.
- Frequently, men do not seek medical attention until the tumor has eroded through the prepuce, causing it to become malodorous due to infection and necrosis.
- Change in color of the penis (redness)
- Bleeding from penis or under the foreskin

Testicular Cancer

This is the most common solid malignancy affecting males between the ages of 15 and 35, although it accounts for about 1% of all cancers in men (Steele, Richie, Oh, & Michaelson, 2013). Incidence remains highest in developed nations with primarily Caucasian populations (Rosen, Jayram, Drazer, & Eggener, 2011).

Patients with cryptorchidism have a four to eight times higher risk of developing germ cell tumor. It is generally believed that the presence of a tumor contributes to cryptorchidism; when cryptorchidism occurs in conjunction with a tumor then the tumor tends to be large. Removal of one testicle does not cause infertility or relate to other possible sexual problems. For cosmetic reasons, a prosthetic testicle may be placed in the scrotum. Testicular cancer is highly treatable and frequently cured when caught in its early stages. Even caught in advanced stages, it is considered curable. Complications occur and it becomes lethal when it has advanced to the point of metastasis. Initial treatment is surgical removal of the testicle. Radiation and chemotherapy may be implemented if it has metastasized.

Pathophysiology

- Testicular germ cell tumors have too many chromosomes, and most often they are triploid to tetraploid.
- Classified as seminomas or nonseminomas, depending on which types of cells are present.
- Risk factors include inguinal hernias, Klinefelter syndrome, mumps, orchitis, sedentary lifestyle, and early onset of male characteristics.

Subjective Data

- Sharp pain or dull ache in the lower abdomen or scrotum
- Feeling of "heaviness" in the scrotum
- Low back pain if tumor spreads to lymph nodes

While uncommon, if spreads to other organs, symptoms may include dyspnea, cough, hemoptysis, and lump in neck due to lymph node metastases

Objective Data

- Lump in one testis, which may or may not be painful
- Gynecomastia from hormonal effects of ß-hCG

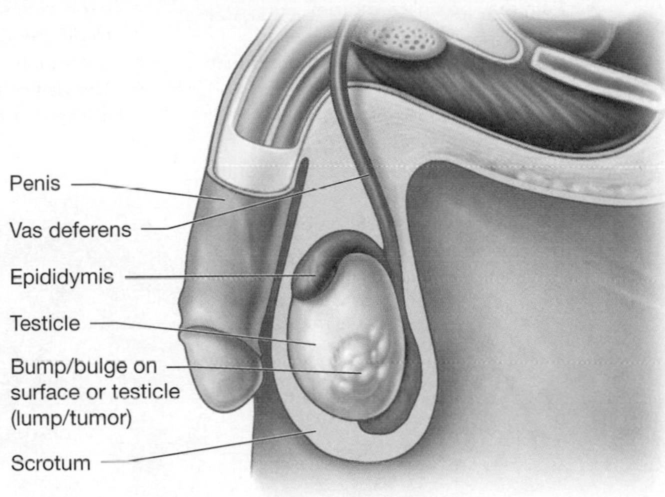

FIGURE 29-24 Testicular cancer

Paraphimosis

This occurs when the foreskin in the uncircumcised or partially circumcised male is retracted behind the glans penis and cannot be returned to its normal position, impeding blood flow to the glans penis with potential for permanent damage and gangrene.

Pain may or may not be present. The goal of treatment is to return the foreskin to its appropriate location. Manual reduction is initially tried and if unsuccessful, surgical reduction is required.

Pathophysiology

- Cause is often not known, but frequently occurs after penile manipulation and a failure to replace the foreskin to its original position.
- Most frequently occurs after retraction of the foreskin during detailed penile examination, cleaning, urethral catheterization, or cystoscopy.
- Being prudent with foreskin manipulation is the most important key in preventing paraphimosis.

Subjective Data

- Swelling of the penis
- Penile pain

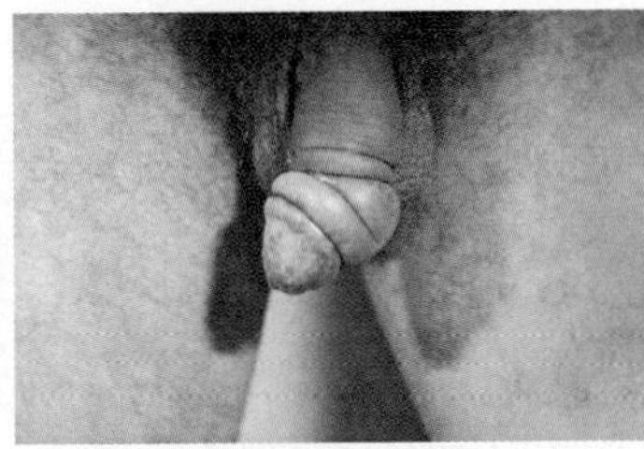

FIGURE 29-25 Paraphimosis
Source: CDC/Susan Lindsley

Objective Data

- Edema and tenderness of the glans penis
- Painful swelling of the distal retracted foreskin
- A constricting band of tissue proximal to the head of the penis at the coronal sulcus
- The penile shaft appears flaccid and unaffected
- With ischemia of the glans penis, the skin color will change from the normal pink color to blue or black. In addition, the ischemic glans penis will be firm to palpation rather than soft.

Epididymitis

Inflammation of the epididymis characterized by discomfort or pain in of the epididymis. Must be differentiated from testicular torsion, which is a true urologic emergency. In some instances, the testicle also may become inflamed (epididymo-orchitis). Males of any age can get epididymitis, and is the fifth most common urologic diagnosis in males aged 18–50 years.

Pathophysiology

- Most often caused by a bacterial infection or by a STI (gonorrhea, chlamydia).
- Manifestations of orchitis are the same as those for epididymitis.
- Abscess formation of either the epididymis or testicle is a potential complication.
- Sepsis is also a possible complication. Either may affect the fertility of the involved testicle. Bilateral involvement, although rare (10%), may result in infertility or sterility (Tubridy & Sinert, 2009).

Subjective Data

Acute:

- Gradual onset (days) of unilateral, tender, swollen, indurated epididymis
- Redness/warmth of scrotum

Chronic:

- Pain may be only symptom
- Testicle pain (mild to severe) and tenderness, which may get worse with a bowel movement
- Painful intercourse or ejaculation
- Dysuria, frequency, or urgency
- Fever and chills (in only 25% of adults with acute epididymitis but in up to 7 of children with the condition)
- Usually, no nausea or vomiting (in contrast to testicular torsion)

Objective Data

- A lump on the testicle
- Enlarged inguinal lymph nodes
- Discharge from the penis
- Blood in the semen
- Cremasteric reflex if prior responses as expected, no change with epididymitis (helps to differentiate from testicular torsion)
- Scrotum may fill with fluid (hydrocele).
- The gait of the patient may also demonstrate a limp due to pain.

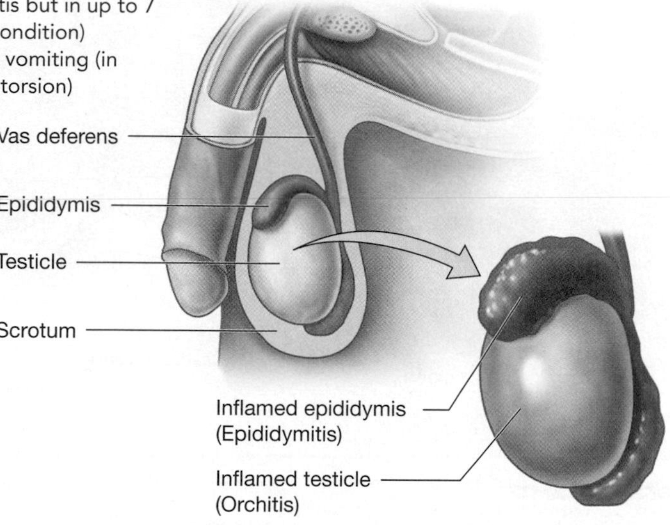

FIGURE 29-26 Epididymitis and orchitis

Testicular Torsion (TT)

TT is the result of a twisting of the spermatic cord, which accounts for as many as 26% of cases of acute scrotum. TT is a urologic emergency that must be differentiated from other manifestations of testicular pain; blood flow to the testicle is cut off, and if surgery is not immediately performed, the affected testicle may be lost. Although it can occur at any age, including prenatal and perinatal periods, most commonly occurs in adolescent males; it is the most frequent cause of testicle loss in that population. The majority of TT develop spontaneously but in 4%–8% of cases is related to sports/physical activity and/or trauma.

Pathophysiology

- Caused by twisting of the spermatic cord and the blood supply to the testicle.
- In mature attachments, the tunica vaginalis is firmly attached to the posterior lateral aspect of the testicle, so that the spermatic cord is relatively immobile.
- If the attachment of the tunica vaginalis to the testicle is higher than it should be, the spermatic cord can rotate within it, which can result in intravaginal torsion (bell clapper deformity); occurs in about 12%–17% of males and is bilateral in 40% (Spanierman, 2009).

Subjective Data

- Intravaginal testicular torsion produces a sudden onset of severe unilateral scrotal pain (duration of pain of less than 6 hours) followed by inguinal and/or scrotal swelling. Pain may lessen as the necrosis becomes more complete.
- Approximately one-third of patients also have gastrointestinal upset with nausea and vomiting. In the pediatric population, nausea and vomiting has more significance.
- Fever, vomiting, history of trauma or activities

Objective Data

- The physical examination is helpful, but imperfect, in diagnosing acute testicular torsion. Absence of cremasteric reflex and abnormal testicle direction have been significantly associated with a diagnosis of testicular torsion.
- The physical examination, moreover, may be difficult to perform, as the testicle is typically very tender and patients are often in significant discomfort. Patients may also have a reactive hydrocele or massive scrotal edema, making testicular examination even more difficult.

- Patients rarely report voiding difficulties or painful urination.
- Although a negative Prehn's sign (relief of pain with elevation of the testicle) is classically thought to be a predictor of torsion, this is unreliable for diagnosis.

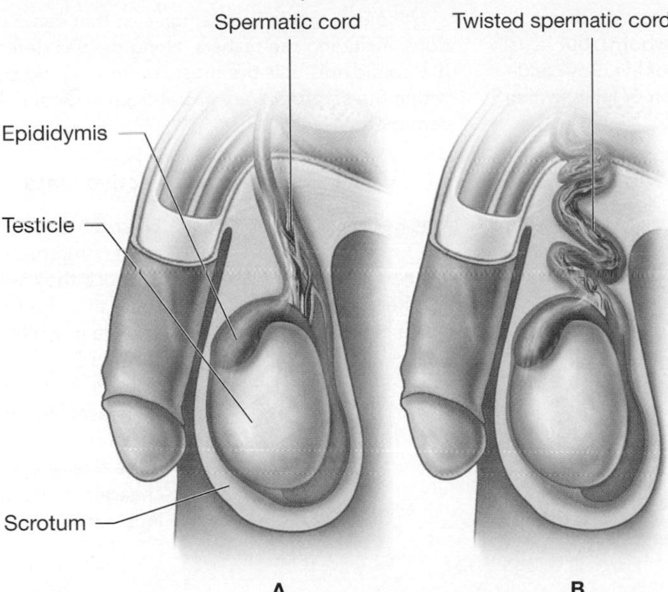

FIGURE 29-27 a) Testicle with expected structures; b) Testicular torsion

Urethral Displacement (Hypospadias/Epispadias)

Hypospadias is a birth anomaly of the urethra in the male in which urinary meatus is displaced anywhere along a line (the *urethral groove*) running from the tip along the underside (ventral aspect) of the shaft to the junction of the penis and scrotum or perineum, occurring in approximately 1 per 250 male births (Gatti, Kirsch, & Snyder, 2009).

First degree: Urethral meatus opens on the underside of the glans penis (50%–75% of cases); frequently an isolated birth anomaly without detectable alterations of the remainder of the reproductive or endocrine system.

Second degree: Urethra opens on the shaft; minority of infants, primarily those with more second or third degrees of hypospadias, have additional structural anomalies of the genitourinary tract.

Third degree: Urethra opens on the perineum (20%–30% of cases).

Epispadias is a rarer, unrelated type of urethral malformation, which is a failure of midline penile fusion earlier in embryogenesis. The cause is unknown but does not involve androgens. It is less common than hypospadias, occurring in 1 per 117,000 newborn boys. Frequently associated with bladder exstrophy, a rare birth defect in which the bladder develops outside the abdomen and is exposed inside out.

Pathophysiology

- Exact cause unknown, and in some instances it is inherited.
- As the penis develops in a male fetus, androgenic hormones stimulate the formation of the urethra and foreskin. Hypospadias results when a malfunction occurs in the action of these hormones, causing the urethra to develop abnormally.

Subjective Data

- Hypospadias is present at birth with diagnosis based on appearance rather than subjective data.

Objective Data

- Opening of the urethra at a location other than the tip of the penis
- Downward curve of the penis (chordee); most often with third-degree placement
- Hooded appearance of the penis because only top half is covered by foreskin
- Abnormal spraying during urination
- Up to 10% of boys with hypospadias have at least one undescended testis, and a similar number have an inguinal hernia.
- Treatment involves surgery to reposition the urethral opening and, if necessary, straighten the shaft of the penis.

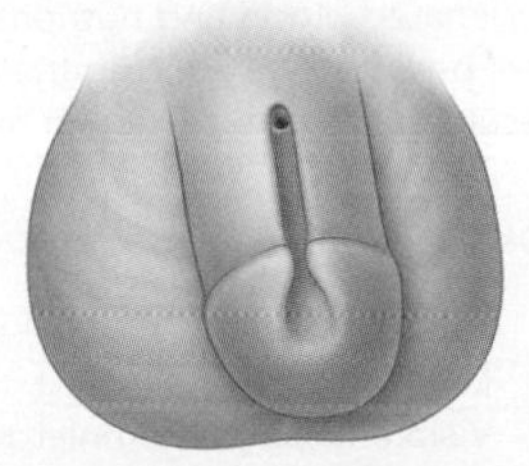

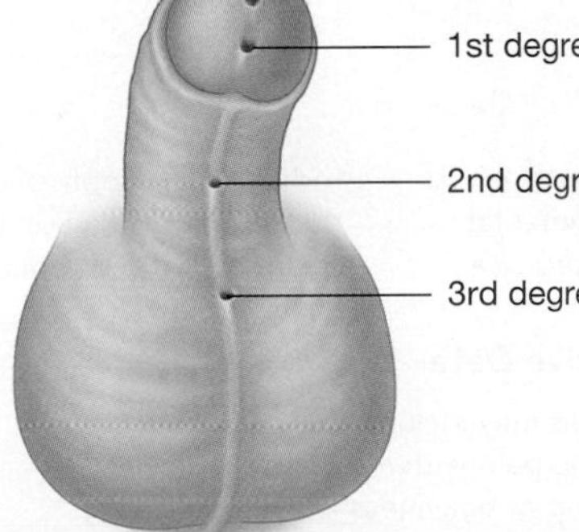

FIGURE 29-28 a) Urethral meatus on dorsal surface (epispadius); b) Urethral meatus on possible sites along ventral surface (hypospadius)

Hydrocele Testis and Spermatocele

A hydrocele is an accumulation of fluids around a testicle that results in swelling of the scrotum. Common in newborns, but usually disappear without treatment within the first year of life. Boys and men may develop a hydrocele due to inflammation or injury within the scrotum.

A spermatocele is a benign cyst that can develop in varying locations, including the testicle, along the vas deferens, and the head of the epididymis. It is the most common cystic condition encountered within the scrotum. Vary in size from several millimeters to many centimeters.

Pathophysiology	Subjective Data	Objective Data
Hydrocele • Requires an imbalance of scrotal fluid production and absorption. • Can develop as a result of inflammation within the scrotum. Inflammation may be the result of infection of the epididymitis or testicle, or orchitis. • May also develop due to a scrotal or groin injury or surgery. • May occur with cancer of the testicle or left kidney (rare). This type can occur at any age but is most common in men older than 40. • May occur in infants undergoing peritoneal dialysis.	• Often a hydrocele does not cause symptoms. • Symptoms, when present, can include pain, swelling, or redness of the scrotum or a feeling of pressure at the base of the penis.	• Enlargement/swelling of scrotum most common. • Because they are fluid-filled, light will shine through them. • Testicle may not be palpable due to surrounding fluid. • Size can sometimes be increased or decreased by applying pressure to abdomen or scrotum. • If the size of the fluid collection changes, more likely to be due to an inguinal hernia.
Spermatocele • Specific cause unknown	• Generally painless • Larger spermatoceles may cause discomfort.	• Vary in size from several millimeters to many centimeters. • Often discovered as incidental scrotal masses found on physical examination or via self-inspection of the scrotum and testicles.

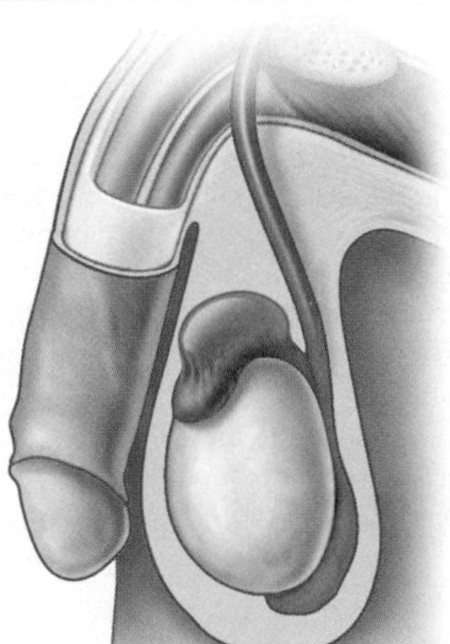

FIGURE 29-29 a) Hydrocele; **b)** spermatocele

Varicocele

This is dilation and tortuosity of the veins of the pampiniform plexus in the scrotum which drains the testicles. They have a detrimental effect on sperm production, which is progressive and related to a reduction in supply of oxygenated blood and nutrient material to the sperm production sites, persistently reducing the quality and the quantity of the sperms, resulting in the reduction in fertility over time.

Pathophysiology	Subjective Data	Objective Data
• Idiopathic: develops when valves within veins of spermatic cord do not function properly; similar process as varicose veins. Resulting backflow of blood into the pampiniform plexus causes increased pressures and vein dilation. • Develop slowly	Symptoms may include the following: • Aching pain within scrotum • Feeling of heaviness in the testicle(s) • In most instances, the individual is asymptomatic and frequently seeks treatment for infertility at which time the varicocele may be discovered.	• Atrophy of the testicle(s) • Low testosterone • Visible or palpable enlarged vein

- Most common in males between 15–30 years of age; and rarely develop after the age of 40. They occur in 15%–20% of all males.
- The majority (98%) of idiopathic varicoceles occur on the left side.
- The cause for the dysfunction of the venous valves remains unknown.

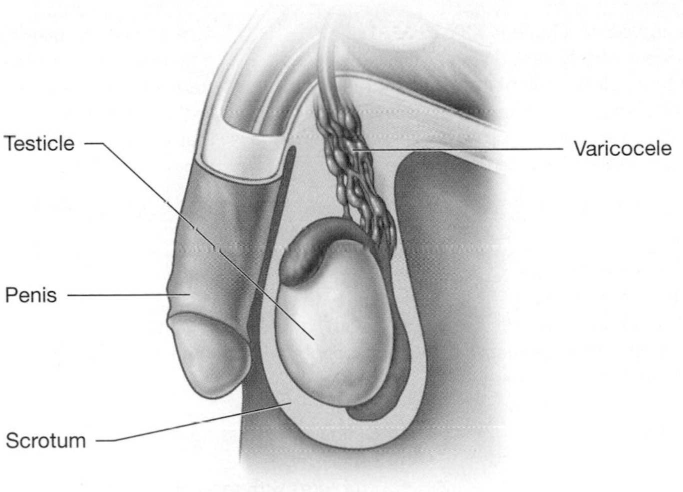

FIGURE 29-30 Varicocele

Prostatic Enlargement

The enlarged prostate gland in elderly males is a significant alteration that affects bladder function in males. The two causes of prostate gland enlargement are benign prostatic hyperplasia (BPH) and prostatic cancer.

- **Benign prostatic hyperplasia (hypertrophy)** (BPH) is a common manifestation in aging males. Growth of prostate cells begins by the age of 40 and continues throughout the remainder of life. By age 50, 50% of males are affected; and by age 70, 95% of males are affected. While histologic indicators may be present in affected males, clinical manifestations are only found in 25% and require treatment. Other contributing factors thought to contribute to BPH include use of anabolic steroids, diet, genetic predisposition, and environmental toxins.
- **Prostate cancer** is the most common cancer in males and usually appears after the age of 50. The risk of developing prostate cancer increases with age so that 75% of cases of prostate cancer are identified in males over 75.

Pathophysiology

- Prostatic enlargement depends on dihydrotestosterone (DHT) that binds to androgen receptors in the cell nuclei, potentially resulting in BPH.
- Both the glandular epithelial cells and the stromal cells undergo hyperplasia, with stromal hyperplasia being the most common.
- Hyperplasia causes prostate to encircle the urethra and impedes bladder emptying; this results in the clinical BPH manifestations.
- Initial treatment is monitoring symptoms when there are minimal manifestations.
- Medications may be given that inhibit the growth of the prostate.
- Surgery to remove part of or total gland when other options unsuccessful.

Subjective Data

- Major BPH manifestations relate to urinary elimination difficulties, including the following:
  - increased frequency of urination
  - difficulty starting/stopping urination
  - weak urine stream
  - feeling that bladder has not completely emptied
  - urinary retention/ painful urination
  - loss of small amounts of urine due to a poor urinary stream
  - In severe cases, total obstruction of the bladder may lead to bladder retention and hypertrophy and bladder and kidney infections.

Objective Data

- Palpation of the prostate through the rectum may reveal a markedly enlarged prostate.
- Usually affects the middle lobe.
- Also feels smooth and rubbery.

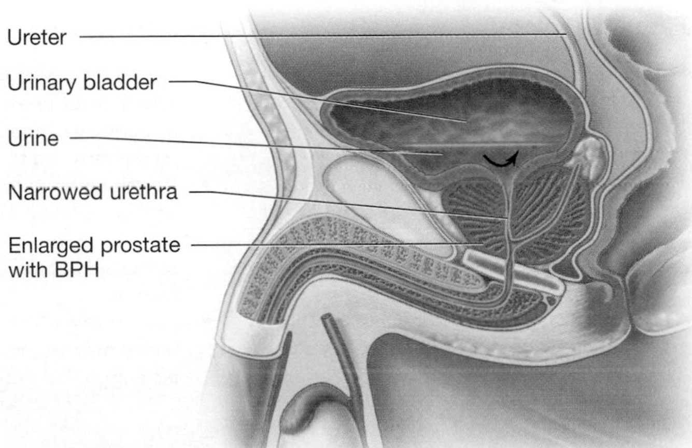

FIGURE 29-31 Benign prostatic hypertrophy (BPH)

CHROMOSOMAL ALTERATIONS

XXY (Klinefelter's Syndrome, KS)

In this condition, the genotype of a male is XXY instead of XY. The manifestations of KS are widely varied with some individuals demonstrating minimal to no signs. It is believed to be the most common chromosome alterations in humans with an incidence of 1 per 500–1000 male births resulting in approximately 3000 affected males born annually (Chen, 2009). This represents approximately 40% of male fetuses that are carried to term. Most variants of KS are much rarer, occurring in 1 in 50,000 or fewer newborns. Researchers suspect that it is under-diagnosed because it may not be identified in people with mild signs and symptoms. Additionally, the features of the condition vary and overlap significantly with those of other conditions.

Pathophysiology

- Related to the X and Y chromosomes.
- Most often, KS results from one extra copy of the X chromosome in each cell (47, XXY) that interfere with male sexual development, often preventing the testes from functioning normally and reducing the levels of testosterone.

Subjective Data

- Infants:
  - Delay in speaking
  - Quiet, docile personality
- Adolescents:
  - Low energy levels
  - Shyness
  - Difficulty expressing feelings or socializing
  - Problems with reading, writing, spelling or math
  - Attention problems
- Adults:
  - Infertility
  - Decreased sex drive

Objective Data

In infants, may include the following:

- Weak muscles, slow motor development, undescended testicles at birth.

In adolescents and adults, may include the following:

- Taller than average
- Longer legs, shorter torso and broader hips
- Absent, delayed or incomplete puberty
- After puberty, less muscular bodies and less facial and body hair
- Enlarged breast tissue
- Small, firm testicles
- Small penis
- Gynecomastia
- Weak bones

PRACTICE POINT: KS

Previously, KS was thought to be a risk factor for developing testicular cancer, however recent evidence does not support that presumption. It has been found to be associated with breast cancer in men and prostate cancer; furthermore, men with Klinefelter's syndrome may be at substantially elevated risks for non-Hodgkin lymphoma, and, perhaps, lung cancer (Swerdlow, Scheomaker, Higgins, Wright, & Jacobs, 2005).

DISORDERS OF SEXUAL DEVELOPMENT (DSD)

Ambiguous Genitalia

Ambiguous genitalia (AG) broadly identifies DSD as a condition where there is failure of the infant's external genitalia to differentiate and therefore are not well defined or there are characteristics that resemble both genders. Gender assignment or reassignment is not addressed immediately, but when a team of specialists is put together that can assist with the physiological, psychological, and sociological aspects of AG.

Pathophysiology

- Congenital adrenal hyperplasia (CAH) is the most common cause of ambiguous genitalia and represents a medical emergency due to the salt wasting nephropathy that develops in 75% of infants with AG (Hutcheson & Snyder III, 2012). If not recognized immediately, the resulting hypotension may result in vascular collapse and death.
- CAH affects males and females.
- In females, there is an overproduction of androgens causing male appearing genitalia.

Subjective Data

- Family history of genital ambiguity, infertility, or unexpected changes at puberty suggests a genetically transmitted trait.
- Recessive traits frequently occur in siblings, while X-linked abnormalities are more likely to appear in males who are scattered sporadically across the family history.
- History of early death of infants in a family may suggest previously missed adrenogenital deficiency.

Objective Data

Male infant may demonstrate the following characteristics:

- Small penis (micro penis) that is less than 2–3 cm or 0.8–1.2 inches that appears to be an enlarged clitoris (enlarged clitoris is common in female infants at birth).
- Urethral meatus may be located along, above, or below the penis; may also be located on the peritoneum, further contributing to a female appearance.
- Small, slightly separated scrotum giving the appearance of labia.

- In males, there may be a reduction in production of androgens causing female appearing genitalia.
- A disruption of the steps that determine sex can result in a mismatch between the external genitals and the internal sex organs or the chromosomal sex (XX or XY).
- Lack or deficiency of male hormones in a genetic male fetus can cause ambiguous genitalia, while exposure to male hormones during development results in ambiguous genitalia in a genetic female.
- Mutations in certain genes can influence fetal sex development. Chromosomal abnormalities (missing or extra sex chromosome) may be the cause.
- Alteration or absence of short arm of the Y-chromosome (contains Testis-determining factor) may cause gonads to develop into ovaries (Hutcheson & Snyder III, 2012).
- Other causes in females are prenatal exposure to male hormones or tumors that may produce male hormones.
- Maternal drug ingestion, particularly during first trimester, when virilization may be produced exogenously in a gonadal female.
- History of maternal virilization may suggest an androgen producing maternal tumor (arrhenoblastoma); this is rare.
- Undescended testicles are frequently a manifestation (Lewis, 2007).

Genetically female infants may demonstrate the following:

- Enlarged clitoris (resembling a penis)
- Fused labia or folded labia (resembling a scrotum)
- Lumps that may be palpated within the fused labia

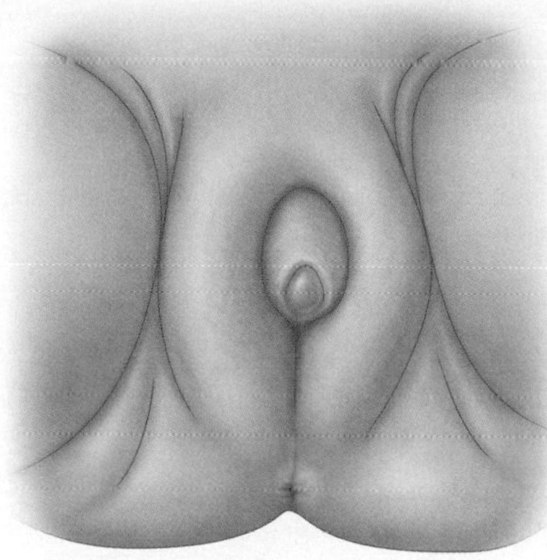

FIGURE 29-32 Ambiguous genitalia

30 Female Genitalia

Linda Bergstrom, RN, CNM, PhD, FACNM
Marianne F. Moore PhD(c), CNM

"There's no way, Anna, and that's the end of the discussion!" Her mother takes the insurance approval form and holds it over the paper shredder. "An HPV vaccination? I might as well be buying her condoms!"

As it turns out, Anna has been sexually active for the past year, and on birth control for the past two. The reason for her current predicament? A legal complication. Under California law, Anna is allowed to begin oral contraceptives without parental consent (with coverage through the state), but needs to go through her mother's insurance for an HPV vaccination because she is a minor.

Mrs. Ludgate, in period seven health class, had made it abundantly clear that cervical cancer is the third most common gynecological malignancy, and that the mortality rate is greater than 50%. Human papillomavirus is the cause, and you get it from sexual activity. Women who start having sex earlier are at greater risk, as are those with multiple and high-risk partners. Anna perked up and took meticulous notes because this all seemed to apply to her. How might she protect herself from infection? The HPV vaccine, Mrs. Ludgate had said.

Statistics had spoken to Anna, so perhaps the same approach would work on her mother.

"Mom, times have changed. Did you know that 40% of 16-year-olds have already had sex? I'm not saying that I am, but if something happens then I don't want to get an HPV infection."

"I know what you're really after, Anna, and you can forget about it. Times haven't changed so much that a girl should give up her chastity just because her friends do. You're better than that, and I won't have you thinking otherwise!" Anna feels a deep pit of anxiety well up in her stomach; dozens of paper strips curl through the shredder and wilt at the base of the trash can.

LEARNING OUTCOMES

1. Apply concepts of growth and development in the care of women.
2. Explain anatomical and physiological genital system in women and any pathophysiological alterations that may be experienced.
3. Describe the elements of an assessment of the female reproductive system.
4. Recognize expected and unexpected findings of an assessment of the female reproductive system.
5. Explain the elements on an appropriate patient history in preparation for examination of the female reproductive system.
6. Explain the elements of examination of the female reproductive system using appropriate techniques and document findings.

Outside of care during pregnancy, most care given to women for their genital system is either screening for a few serious problems such as cancer or sexually transmitted infections (STIs) or assistance with contraception. Most gynecologic care occurs during early and middle adulthood, and most women who receive gynecologic care do not have major diseases or problems with other systems primarily because of their age. Unless gynecologic symptoms or issues are present, children do not need to receive gynecologic care until just before the initiation of sexual activity, and older women can cease routine screening care at certain ages depending upon their individual situations.

Structure and Function

The female reproductive system is designed for conception, growth and development, and giving birth to a new human being. Additionally it is associated with and the location for sexual pleasure. Over the course of a lifetime, most women experience no major alterations in the function of this system. Developmental milestones, such as puberty and menopause, generally happen at the expected times in a lifespan and are unproblematic. There may be secondary effects on the physiology of this system from other systems, especially the endocrine system, but this system itself generally does not produce secondary problems in other systems.

The female reproductive system is divided into three components, (1) the external genitals, (2) the internal genitalia, and (3) the bony pelvis. The organs of this system are located in close proximity to organs of the digestive and urinary systems, which may become a problem for the provider when dealing with a symptom like pain in the abdomen, since it can be difficult to determine the exact system that is causing the pain. The whole system is an open one so that it is possible for microorganisms or other foreign substances to gain entry into the abdominal cavity by ascending through this system. The key physiological function for this system is the menstrual cycle.

External Genitalia

Vulva or **pudendum** is the general term for the external female genitalia. The vulva is comprised of the mons pubis, labia majora, labia minora, prepuce, clitoris, vaginal vestibule, vestibular glands, vaginal orifice, perineum, frenulum, fourchette, urethral opening, and anus (Figure 30-1).

The mons pubis is a layer of adipose tissue, covered with hair after puberty, which sits atop the symphysis pubis (bone). The labia majora consists of folds of adipose tissue that arise from the mons and extend down to the perineal area. Inside the labia major are the labia minora. In many women these are not visible unless the labia majora are separated. The labia majora join anteriorly to form a hood or prepuce that covers the clitoris. The clitoris is a small, round erectile organ that produces sexual pleasure and is very sensitive to touch. The clitoris is the erectile homologue of the penis, and is composed of two small corpora cavernosa and surrounded superiorly by the prepuce and inferiorly by folds of the labia minora, which are called the frenulum. Posteriorly, the labia minor join to form the **fourchette** or area just below the vaginal opening.

The generally flat area inside the folds of the labia minora is the vestibule or vestibular area. There are six openings: the urethral opening, the vaginal orifice, and two sets of paired glands, Bartholin's and Skene's. The glandular openings are not easily visible. Skene's glands are found on each side of the urethra and drain fluid from urethral glands. Bartholin's glands are found just inside the vaginal orifice and secrete the mucous used for vaginal lubrication especially during sexual activity.

The vaginal **vestibule** (orifice) is the largest opening; it may or may not be covered by a thin layer of tissue called the hymen. The vaginal opening can have a large variety of shapes and sizes. Once a woman has given birth vaginally, the vaginal opening is more enlarged and more irregularly shaped.

The fourchette is the flat place below the vaginal opening that is still encircled by the labia. The perineum is the flat area outside the fourchette that is located in between the vagina and the anus. This area is also known as the pelvic floor and consists of layers of muscles. These muscles form the sphincters, which cause the anus, vagina and urethra to open and close.

Internal Genitalia

The organs of the internal female genitalia are the vagina, the uterus that is divided into different parts, the fallopian tubes and the ovaries (see Figure 30-2).

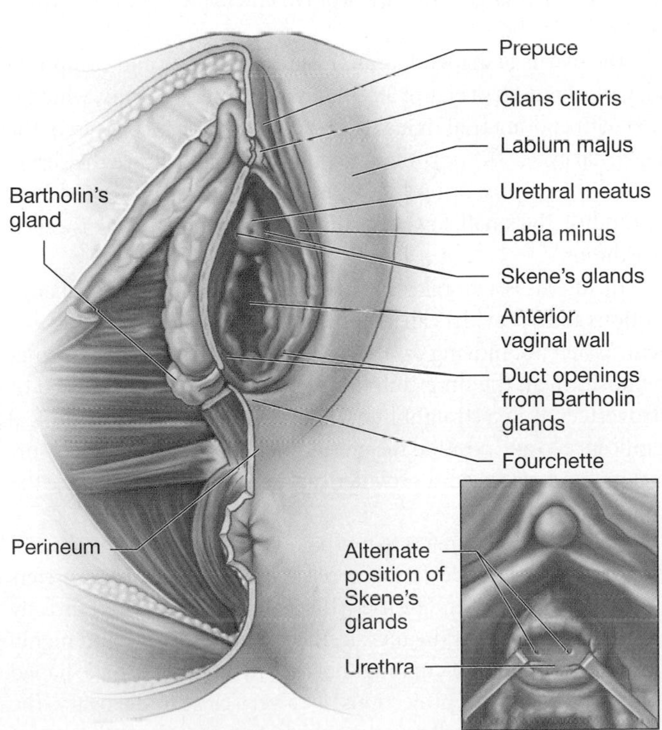

FIGURE 30-1 External female genitalia

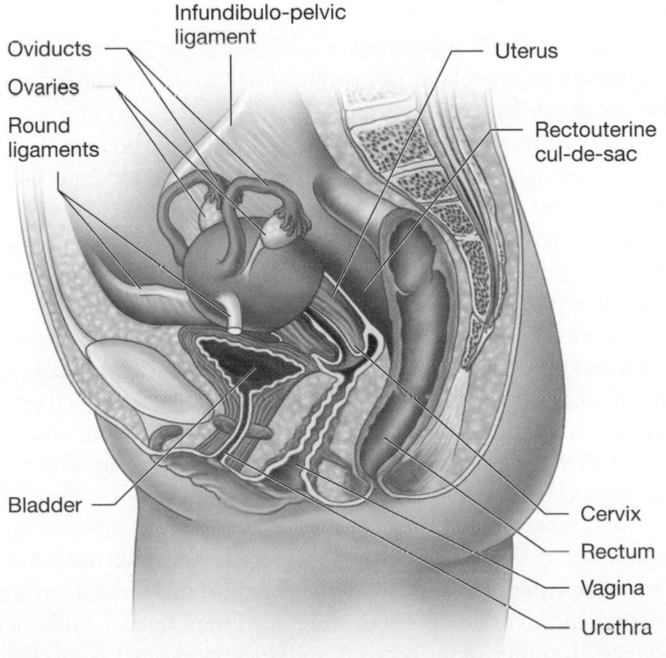

FIGURE 30-2 Internal female genitalia

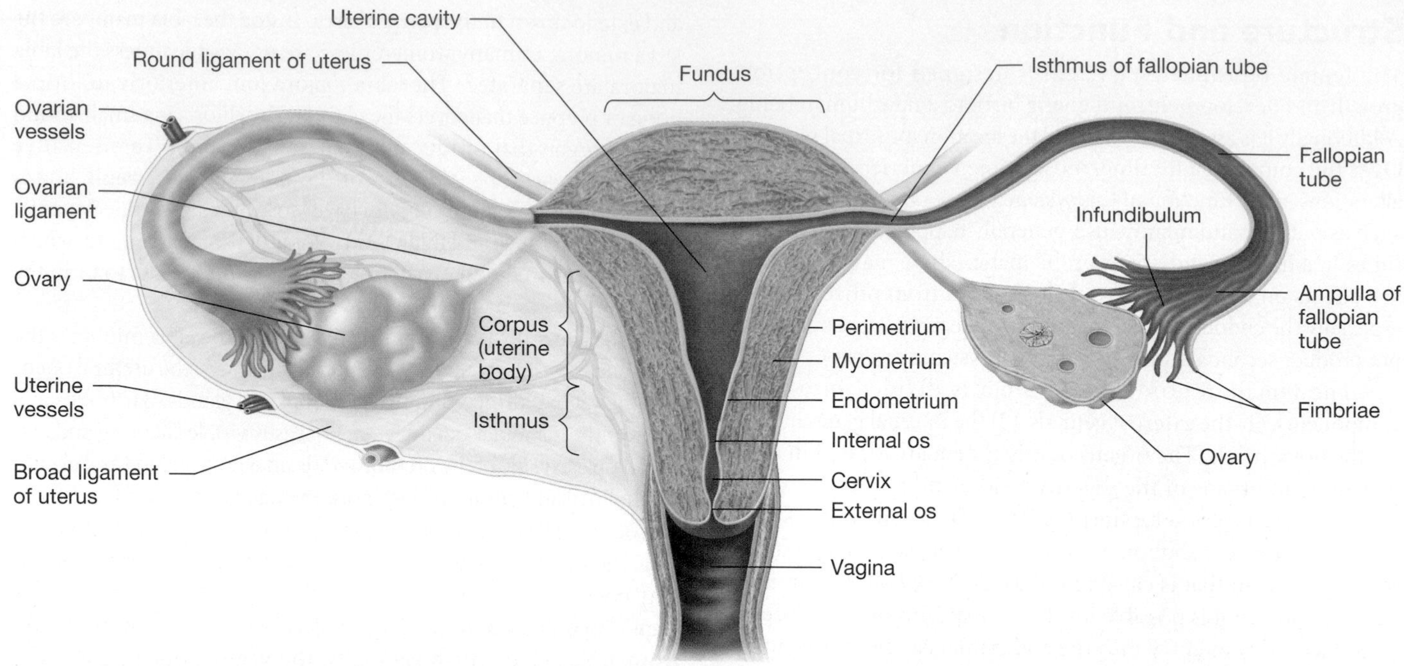

FIGURE 30-3 Structures of the uterus

The vagina begins at the vestibule on the external genital area and extends upwards and backwards. It normally is a collapsed tube, but is easily opened by the insertion of some foreign body such as fingers, a penis, or a speculum. If a fetus' head is able to pass through the bony pelvis, the vagina will stretch sufficiently to allow passage of the infant's whole body. Women have given birth vaginally to babies over 13 pounds, which is an indication about how much ability this organ has to stretch. The vagina is lined with stratified epithelial tissue. In the premenopausal woman, the vagina is generally covered with multiple folds of tissue known as rugae. No matter what the woman's race, the vagina is pink-colored, similar to the inside of the mouth.

The normal pH of vaginal tissue is 3.8–4.5. The vagina provides a habitat for bacterial flora, primarily kinds of lactobacillus (bacteria that can secrete lactose).

Connective tissue, called septum, on the top and bottom, separate the vagina from the urethra and the anus. The posterior portion of the vagina contains a blind pouch called the pouch of Douglas. The small pockets at the terminus of the vagina around the sides of the cervix are called **fornices** (anterior, posterior, and lateral). These areas are very thin and pelvic organs can be palpated through them.

The lower portion of the uterus, called the cervix, extends down into the vagina and is observed by a provider with the use of a speculum. Similar to the vagina, it is also covered with stratified epithelial tissue on the outside, which makes the tissue of both organs look similar. In a woman who has never experienced a vaginal birth the opening of the cervix is small and round, about the size of a cotton applicator. After a woman has had a vaginal birth, the opening assumes an irregular shape, often appearing as a small slit instead of a round opening. The cervix is actually a short tube, which has an internal, and an external os (opening) that can be open in differing degrees. The lining of the cervix, the endocervical canal, is covered with columnar epithelium, which looks redder and rougher than the external cervix. Sometimes the movement of the speculum as it pushes into the fornices causes the epithelial tissue on the outside to be stretched backwards, which then allows for visualization of the tissue of the internal os. This happens commonly during pregnancy. The junction between the two kinds of tissue on the cervix is called the squamocolumnar junction.

The uterus is the organ of gestation for a developing fetus. The uterus of a woman who has never been pregnant (nullipara) is about 5.5 to 8 cm long, 3.5 to 4.0 cm wide, and 2.0 to 2.5 cm thick. Once a woman has had a pregnancy, the uterus, in the nonpregnant state, becomes a bit enlarged until the woman enters menopause at which point it diminishes.

The uterus is shaped like an upside down pear and composed of layers of muscles (Figure 30-3). It has an interior cavity, which is lined with endometrial tissue that responds to the hormones of the menstrual cycle. The portion of the uterus located above the cervix is called the *corpus,* or body. The top of the corpus is referred to as the fundus. The small, lower portion just above the cervix is called the isthmus.

The uterus is a mobile organ. Sexual arousal causes it to change positions and a provider can temporarily manipulate it during assessment. When not moving or being manipulated, the uterus assumes one position all the time: anteflexed or anteverted, retroflexed or retroverted, or in a straight line (Figure 30-4). There is no clinical significance to any position the uterus might assume, and unless surgical methods are used, a provider cannot permanently change the position of the uterus.

The term **adnexa** refers to two paired sets of organs, one set each on the right and left side. In this application, the *adnexa uteri* refers to the fallopian tubes and ovaries. The fallopian tubes insert directly into the upper sides of the uterus. They are soft, pliable and highly mobile tubes about 10 cm long that end in a trumpet-bell shaped fimbriated (finger-like projections) area very close to the ovary. The tubes are lined with small muscles, which contract in a rhythmic way to facilitate transportation of an ovum down into the uterine cavity.

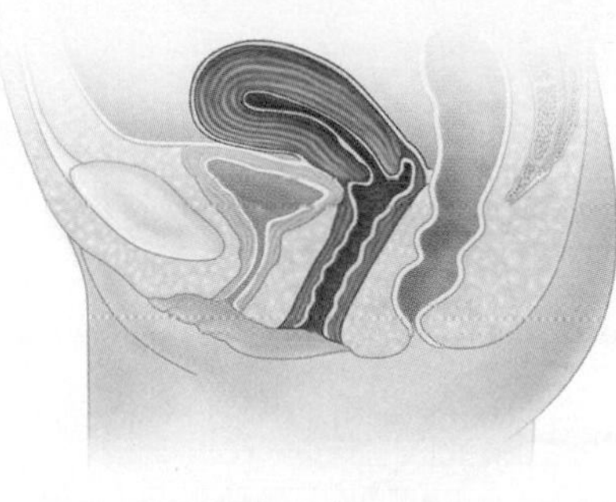

(a)

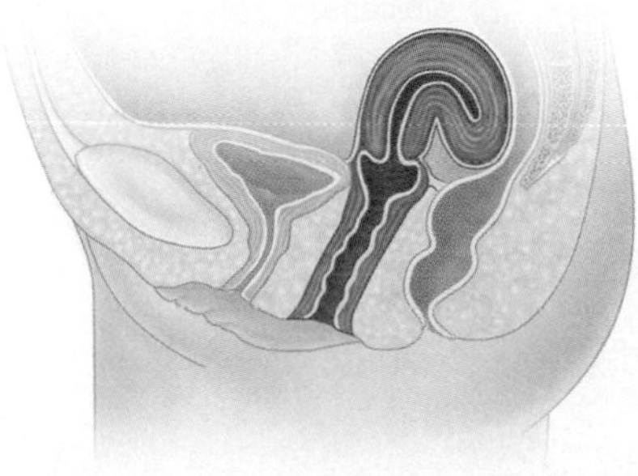

(b)

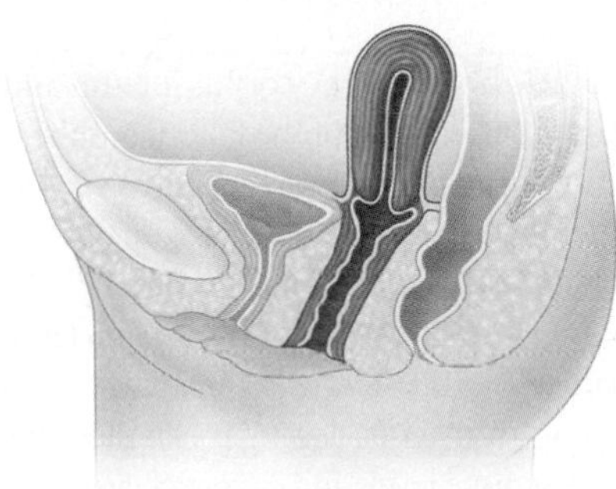

(c)

FIGURE 30-4A–C Positions of the uterus: **a)** Anteflexed (anteverted); **b)** retroflexed (retroverted); **c)** in a straight line

The ovaries are oval-shaped organs about 3 cm long, 2 cm wide, and 1 cm thick (see Figure 30-3). At birth, the ovaries contain all the immature eggs a woman will have for her lifetime. They are endocrine organs, which secrete the hormones estradiol, progesterone, and androstenedione and testosterone. These hormones initiate sexual development, maintain secondary sexual characteristics, regulate the menstrual cycle, cause the development and release of ova, and maintain pregnancies.

Four pairs of ligaments (cardinal, uterosacral, round and broad) support all the internal organs of the female reproductive system (Figure 30-5).

Bony Pelvis

The pelvis is part of the musculoskeletal system and has no function for sexuality or reproduction, but it does provide support for all the organs of the abdominal cavity. It can also be a barrier to the birth of a fetus. Occasionally fetuses are too large to fit through their mother's pelvic opening, a condition called fetal-pelvic or **cephalo-pelvic disproportion**. This condition is always unique to the particular fetus. A fetus that is smaller may very well be born successfully through the same-sized pelvic opening.

The pelvis appears as a single bone, but is actually four bones (see Figure 30-5). These are the paired innominate bones on each side, which consist of the ilium, ischium, and pubis (2); the sacrum (1), and the coccyx (1). The pelvis also has four joints that have very little movement. During pregnancy these joints relax a bit under the influence of two hormones, estrogen and relaxin, which soften up the cartilage, in anticipation of the birth process. In late pregnancy the symphysis can actually separate a bit, which causes pain especially when walking.

Menstrual Cycle

The menstrual cycle is characterized as a sequence of repeating changes in the endometrial lining of the uterus in preparation for implantation of a fertilized ovum. The menstrual cycle commences with the onset of puberty (menarche) and continues until menopause. While the menstrual cycle consists of a period of 21–35 days, it is the 4–5 days of menses or bleeding that is generally referred to as "the period" (Figure 30-6).

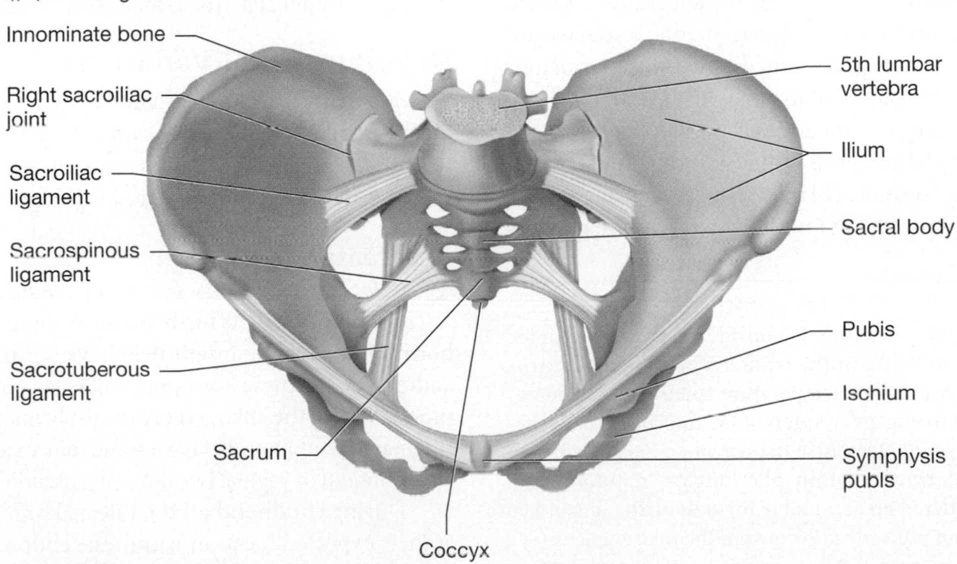

FIGURE 30-5 Pelvic bones with supporting ligaments

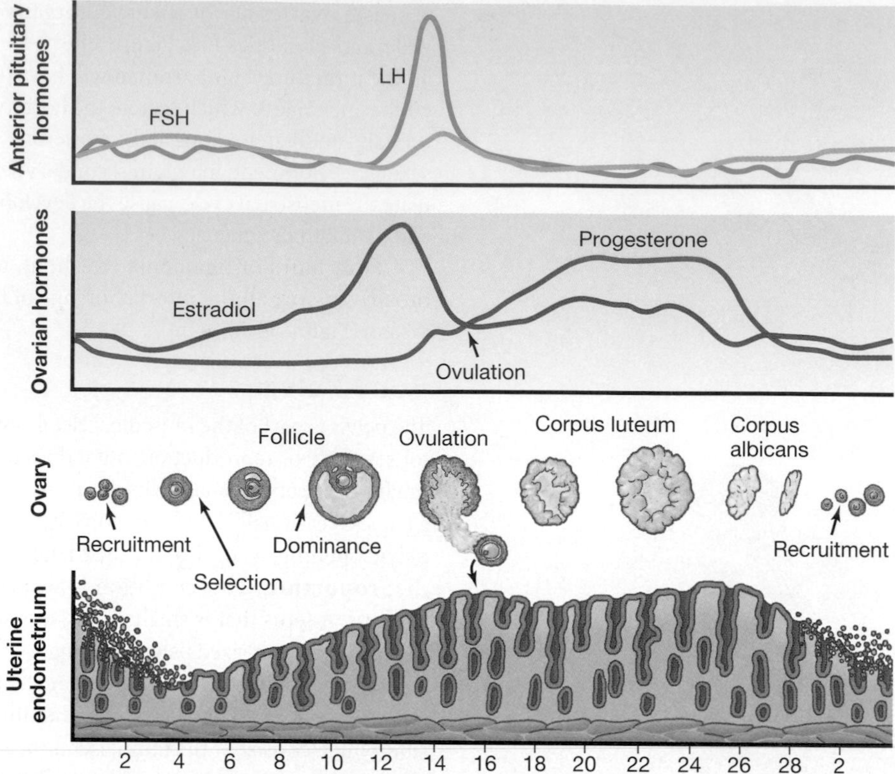

FIGURE 30-6 The menstrual cycle. Note the relationship between the levels of FSH, LH, and progesterone and events like ovulation, development of the lining and menses.

For purposes of calculation, the first day of the menses (bleeding) is the beginning of the menstrual cycle, when hormone levels are relatively low and which lasts for the first 5–6 days. Bleeding is actually caused by the suppression of hormones that facilitated the increase in endometrial tissue in preparation for implantation. Suppression of hormones causes a sloughing of the endometrial lining, and creates the menstrual flow, which consists of blood and tissue. Also during this time, approximately six follicles in the ovaries are developing into mature ova that are capable of being fertilized by sperm, usually on one ovary or the other.

Between day 6 and 7, estradiol levels rise and (usually) one follicle becomes dominant, taking up more estradiol to increase its growth and nourish the ovum (egg) inside the follicle. As ovulation (release of the ovum) nears (day 11–12) progesterone is secreted and begins to rise. Estradiol levels peak immediately prior to ovulation and the follicle is like a bubble about to burst. Rising estradiol levels also cause the uterine lining to grow and become blood filled.

On the day of ovulation, both follicle stimulating hormone (FSH) and luteinizing hormone (LH) levels peak, causing the follicle to rupture, expelling the ovum into the abdominal cavity. The ruptured follicle becomes the corpus luteum and begins secreting progesterone. The fimbriae of the fallopian tube capture the egg, drawing it in for transportation into the uterus via the fallopian tube.

> ***PRACTICE POINT: Rise in Temperature***
>
> The period of time after ovulation is considered the fertile time and is accompanied by a rise in the woman's body temperature (basal temperature). Noting this temperature spike can be used as a marker for couples to engage in intercourse to produce a pregnancy; or to not engage in intercourse to prevent a pregnancy from occurring. This is considered family planning or "natural birth control" and is considered an acceptable form of birth control by some religions. It is not precisely known what the time frame is for a woman's fertile period, so there is the possibility that a pregnancy may result if intercourse occurs too close to ovulation.

Following ovulation, estradiol level drops slightly and is maintained; however, progesterone continues to peak. If the ovum is fertilized and implantation in the uterus occurs, rising hCG levels tell the corpus luteum to remain and progesterone remains so that there is no menses. Without signals from a developing pregnancy, the corpus luteum deteriorates, progesterone levels and estrogen levels drop off, and menstruation occurs by day 21 to day 35 (depending on the woman). Many women maintain a regular cycle of menstruation throughout their lifetime; however, there are some women who have an irregular pattern, making it very difficult to determine when ovulation actually occurs.

Developmental Variations

Developmental variations occur over the course of an individual's lifespan and events. Awareness of these variations is important to understand and recognize common age-related alterations or modifications of the female reproductive system.

Infants and Children

Refer to Chapter 29 for the discussion on in utero gender differentiation. At birth, because of the influence of maternal hormones, a female infant may have a prominent labia minora and/or clitoris. These hormones will recede on their own in a short time, allowing the enlarged organs to shrink to their expected size. A female infant may also have some milky vaginal discharge, and a small amount of vaginal bleeding, or a pseudo period.

During childhood all the internal organs remain very small at their expected location within the abdominal cavity. The labia minora are tiny and difficult to see. The labia majora and mons are hairless and smooth.

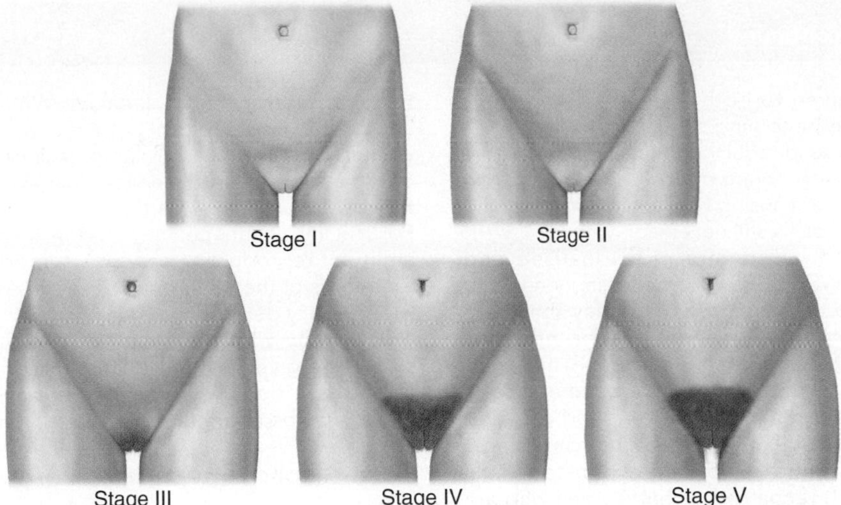

FIGURE 30-7 The Tanner stages of female pubic hair development with sexual maturation. Stage I: Preadolescent—no growth of pubic hair. Stage II: Soft downy straight hair along the labia majora is an indication that sexual maturation is beginning. Stage III: Sparse, dark, visibly pigmented curly pubic hair on labia. Stage IV: Hair coarse and curly, abundant but less than adults. Stage V: Lateral spreading in triangle shape to medial surface of thighs. Stage VI: Further extension laterally and upward.

Adolescents

With the onset of puberty, the ovaries secrete more estrogen, which stimulates the growth and development of the reproductive tract and causes the development of secondary sexual characteristics (Figure 30-7). The first signs are usually breast and pubic hair development. The menstrual cycle begins (menarche) towards the end of puberty. The whole process takes about 3 years to complete. The age of **menarche** in the population has been gradually decreasing over time. It now usually happens between the ages of 11 and 13 in the United States. The various organs develop somewhat independently of each other and at unknown rates. For example, an adolescent girl could become pregnant before actual menarche if sexual intercourse occurs after the ovaries are fully functional.

The Older Adult Woman

Ovarian function begins to diminish gradually, becoming irregular at around age 40. As the cessation of menstrual periods approaches (perimenopause), the periods become irregular in frequency, duration, and amount. Pregnancy is still possible, although less probable, until menopause is assured.

Menstrual periods generally cease totally sometime in a woman's 50s, a period called *menopause*. Once menstrual cycles have not occurred for 12 consecutive months, the woman is considered postmenopausal. Secondary symptoms of menopause may manifest, such as hot flashes. Androgens and testosterone also decrease, which may cause a slight, generalized loss of muscle mass and strength, and decreased libido. Most women have no difficulty with this life transition time; it is simply another transition they experience.

After menopause, all external pelvic structures become smaller, secondary to a general loss of subcutaneous fat. Skin is drier and shinier. Pubic hair is sparse, gray or white colored, or absent. The urinary meatus may be more prominent secondary to relaxed musculature or prolapse. The vaginal introitus may have a smaller opening making either digital or speculum exam very difficult, or it may be gaping, especially in a multiparous woman. The vagina will have fewer or absent rugae, be paler in color, shorter and smaller in size, and drier. Vaginal dryness may make sexual activity and pelvic examination more painful. There may no longer be surrounding fornices, and the recto-vaginal septum should be thinner. The cervix may also have a smaller opening, making adequate sampling for a Pap test difficult. The uterus is smaller and may not be palpable at all. The ovaries should not be palpable secondary to their small size. (Palpable ovaries in an older woman would be a sign that a provider should follow up on.) Obvious prolapse of various organs may be present (see Conditions and Disorders).

Health Promotion

Cervical Cancer

Healthy People 2020 topic areas Cancer (C), Family Planning (FP), and Maternal, Infant and Child Health (MICH) have the following objectives (U.S. Department of Health and Human Services, 2009).

- C—04/10: Reduce the death rate from cancer of the uterine cervix; reduce invasive uterine cervical cancer.
- C—15: Increase the proportion of women who receive a cervical cancer screening based on the most recent guidelines in 2008 (age adjusted to the year 2000 standard population). Increase the proportion of women who were counseled by their providers about Papanicolaou (Pap) tests.

All women are at risk for the development of cervical cancer. Approximately 12,000 women over the age of 30 develop cervical cancer. Cervical cancer is known to be caused by various strains of the human papillomavirus (HPV), which is quite a common virus in women. Not every woman with HPV will develop cervical cancer, so other factors contribute to its development. These other factors include having multiple sex partners (both the woman and her partner), becoming sexually active at an early age, a history of other sexually transmitted infections, smoking, and a weakened immune system (often associated with AIDS). When found early, cervical cancer can be successfully treated resulting in long survival and a satisfactory quality of life.

Health Promotion *continued*

New HPV vaccines given to both young women (11–12 years old) and men before becoming sexual active, or by the early 20s, show great promise in reducing the incidence of cervical cancer, causing it to be a very rare disease. The vaccines do not cover all potentially cancer causing HPV strains, so screening for cervical cancer via Pap tests is still necessary.

Screening recommendations are individualized and change every few years. Women do not necessarily need to have Pap tests during gynecological visits, but they should be counseled about screening recommendations for them and their life circumstances. Most guidelines for screening recommend starting at age 21. The frequency of screening is generally mutually decided on by the patient and provider based on the presence of risk factors. The American Cancer Society (ACS) and the American College of Obstetricians and Gynecologists (ACOG) recommend that women who are 21–29 years of age, sexually active and have a cervix should have a Pap smear every 3 years with HPV testing if any abnormal tissue is found. After age 30, until age 65, women should have a Pap smear and HPV testing every 5 years, or can have the Pap smear with HPV testing for any abnormals every 3 years. In addition to the Pap test, the HPV DNA test may also be performed. which is done to determine if the woman is infected with any of the cancer causing HPV viruses.

Reproductive Health

- FP—07: Increase the proportion of sexually active persons who receive reproductive health services.
- FP—07: Increase the proportion of sexually active persons aged 15 to 19 years who use condoms to both effectively prevent pregnancy and provide barrier protection against disease.

Additional preventive measures include the use of condoms with every sexual encounter. It is not known whether condom use directly prevents HPV infections, but condom use is associated with a lower rate of cervical cancer.

Access to reproductive health services is regulated by local, state, and national public health policy issues as well as the beliefs, mores, and values of any local, state, or national society. Additionally, beliefs related to gender, age, rights, and purpose are also significant influences on the availability of and access to reproductive health services. While reproductive health and related issues affects both men and women, it is primarily women who bear the burden of lack of access and availability of reproductive health services. Family planning programs are the most crucial services that need to be available to women. Political involvement on any level related to access to and availability of reproductive services is important both to increase awareness of the need for such services and to influence public health policy decision making.

Women who are vulnerable to unintended pregnancy should be given patient education about possible effects of alcohol use during very early pregnancy, before the woman might even be aware that she is pregnant.

Fetal Alcohol Spectrum Disorders (FASD)

- MICH—25: Reduce the occurrence of fetal alcohol syndrome (FAS).

Fetal alcohol spectrum disorders (FASD) is a group of congenital conditions caused by maternal consumption of alcohol with subsequent fetal exposure. There is a wide variety of manifestations of FASD and a diagnosis of fetal alcohol syndrome (FASD) is based on characteristics related to three areas: (1) characteristic facial anomalies, (2) growth retardation, and (3) CNS involvement (Cannon, Dominique, O'Leary, Sniezek, & Floyd, 2012).

Alcohol is a known **teratogen**, crossing the placenta immediately and entering the fetal circulation. Alcohol is known to reduce neural cell progenation and increase cellular death by apoptosis (Burd, Cotsonas-Hassler, Martsolf, & Kerbashian, 2003). Additionally, amniotic fluid acts as a reservoir for alcohol, extending fetal exposure to alcohol.

It has been determined that two or more drinks per day places the fetus at risk for FAS. Most infants with FAS were born to women who consumed at least 8–10 drinks per day. The greater the number of drinks per day the greater the risk for and infant born with FAS. Even though one drink per day may be considered "safe," to completely prevent the incidence of FAS women should abstain from alcohol during pregnancy (Kesmodel et al., 2012).

PRACTICE POINT: Papanicolaou Tests

Cells from the exo- and endocervix are physically scraped off with a number of different devices. These cells may be mounted immediately onto dry slides and fixed in place with a spray chemical (a special fixative for this purpose or ordinary hairspray). In the laboratory these slides are stained and then examined microscopically by specially trained technicians (cytotechnicians) supervised by pathologists.

A modern proprietary collection system using liquid media (Thin-Prep) is in common use; this system has better reliability compared to the dry slide method. In this case, the cells are shaken off of the collection implements into the liquid media, and the small jar with the liquid is sent directly to the laboratory where the slide for examination is prepared under specific product directions.

Computerized systems for examining the Pap test slides (e.g. Auto-Pap made by Tri-Path Imaging Inc.) are also now in common use. These systems, when accompanied by visual confirmation by humans for certain slides, also have increased reliability compared to older methods.

Pap test specimens collected via liquid media can also be analyzed for evidence of some strains of the HPV virus. Use of information from HPV testing plus results of Pap tests themselves help providers to make individualized recommendations for cervical cancer screening in the future.

Clinical Context Exemplars

Situation A

Shawna is 17 years old and presents at your family planning clinic. She tells you that she won't need much time—she just needs a prescription of the pill that her girlfriend takes. Upon asking, you find that she takes no medications, has had no other surgeries except for a myringotomy and tubes at age 2, and has been having intercourse for the last 6 months.

1. What do you think about the level of Shawna's understanding concerning contraception?
2. What is positive here? What is challenging?
3. What should you ask her about to help you decide which exams to set up for or consider?

Shawna says her boyfriend doesn't like condoms so she hasn't used them much. She is worried because "he still talks to his ex-girlfriend." She hopes that the pill will prevent STIs.

4. What should be done at this exam? Per ACOG guidelines, does Shawna need a Pap at this time?
5. What needs to be further assessed and discussed in these comments Shawna has made?

Situation B

Maryanne, a 38-year-old, arrives complaining of increasingly heavy menses. Says she wants the Copper-T IUD that was placed 8 years ago removed, but is unsure of what she would do for contraception at that point. She is G4P4, with her last delivery 8 years ago.

1. What is a common cause of heavier bleeding in IUD patients?
2. What should you assess in this woman?

Upon questioning, Maryanne states that she has no new sexual partners, and her menses has been getting heavier for about 3 months now, and cramping has been increasing. She denies pain with intercourse. She denies nausea, breast changes, or other s/s of pregnancy, but a pregnancy test is done (concern for possible ectopic) and is negative. A GC and Chlamydia test was done in the last 4 months, but is repeated due to pain and bleeding.

3. What else needs to be considered?
4. How can she be tested for this?

The wet mount shows yeast. On bimanual, the uterus is slightly enlarged on one side.

5. In light of the bleeding, what should be done?

SUBJECTIVE DATA

History of Present Illness (CC)

Women who are experiencing a problem with their reproductive system may present with problems that are caused by or related to disorders of the gastro-intestinal, urinary, or the endocrine system. Sorting out which system is causing the symptom or difficulty can present a diagnostic reasoning challenge. The patient may present to the provider with a variety of concerns that may be directly related to the reproductive system or other systems. Framing the questions will depend on the patient's age, gender, culture, race, emotional or mental status, health practices, and concurrent illnesses. All symptoms presented must be thoroughly assessed with a symptom analysis (COLDERRA).

Pelvic Pain

Pelvic pain is the primary problem that causes women to seek care for their reproductive system. The provider needs to carefully differentiate pain from this system versus pain from either the digestive or urinary systems. (Appendicitis is the most common surgical emergency in pregnancy.) Pain may be a late but solitary symptom of ovarian cancer.

Provider Inquiries	Clinical Reasoning/Logic
Characteristics: Are you experiencing pressure or burning? Is the pain stabbing, constant, or wave-like? Does it feel like what you think labor is like?	**Vulvodynia** is pain in the vulvar area with no known cause and may be characterized as burning, stinging, or rawness. A burning pain is single most common symptom of vulvodynia. Endometriosis is another cause of pelvic or abdominal pain and is caused by endometrial tissue that is distributed throughout the abdomen and responds to hormonal stimulation just as uterine endometrial tissue does.
Onset: Does the pain occur especially in relationship to the menstrual cycle (before, during, after)?	Endometriosis pain often occurs with menses. Pain of ectopic pregnancy may be acute in onset and unilateral. **Mittelschmertz** is abdominal pain that occurs during the middle of the menstrual cycle when the egg is released from the ovary. Symptoms of vulvodynia usually begin suddenly.

Provider Inquiries	Clinical Reasoning/Logic
Location: Localized or more generalized across the abdomen/pelvic area?	Endometriosis pain may be generalized abdominal pain or low back pain. Vulvodynia may be generalized and felt in the entire vulvar area or may be localized to the vaginal orifice area.
Duration: How long does the pain last? Does it come and go within a short amount of time (a few minutes)?	Vulvodynia may go on for months to years.
Exacerbation: Any particular activities that make it worse? Especially activities relating to urination, having a bowel movement or sexual activity? Wear tight fitting/nylon underwear? Contact with hot water? Biking, horseback riding?	Pain with vulvodynia may occur with activities or at rest. These activities are thought to increase symptoms of vulvodynia.
Relief: Anything that has been tried that gives relief? Cold compresses, Sitz baths?	No known interventions/activities that relieve pain of vulvodynia.
Radiation: Does the pain go anywhere else?	
Associated signs/symptoms: Especially related to the urinary or digestive systems; bleeding or vaginal discharge of any kind?	Pain in the lower abdomen can arise from the digestive or urinary system. Most STIs do not cause pain, but if pain is present along with positive tests for gonorrhea or chlamydia, this can be a serious complication known as pelvic inflammatory disease (PID).
Previous yeast infection or vaginitis?	Women with vulvodynia may have a history of yeast infections or vaginitis.
Anxiety, depression, sleep disturbances, sexual dysfunction?	Frequently accompany vulvodynia.

Vaginal Bleeding (Dysfunctional Uterine Bleeding)

Dysfunctional uterine bleeding (DUB) is the most common cause of unexpected vaginal bleeding during a woman's reproductive years. Changes in the amount and characteristics of menstrual bleeding may be typical changes that occur during a lifetime. For example, as menopause approaches one period may be quite heavy and the next one very light. Intracycle bleeding may be a benign occurrence after coitus or a symptom of cervicitis caused by a STI. Heavy bleeding, even if caused by "benign" changes such as the growth of uterine fibroids, can be so severe as to cause incapacitation and anemia severe enough to require transfusions. Light or absent bleeding not caused by prescribed hormones may not be a gynecological problem, but instead may signify an endocrine problem such as diabetes or thyroid disorders. This may also be one of the irregularities associated with approaching menopause. Bleeding that happens in a postmenopausal woman always needs investigation. This is the classic symptom associated with endometrial cancer.

PRACTICE POINT: Estimating Quantity of Bleeding

Asking a woman how many pads/tampons she has used may give misleading information because many women change a pad/tampon long before it is thoroughly soaked. Instead of asking for the number of pads/tampons used, ask the patient to compare the number of pads/tampons used during a typical menstrual period and the number of pads used since bleeding started.

Provider Inquiries	Clinical Reasoning/Logic
Characteristics: Quantity (how much)? Spotting, or does it soak through pads/tampons in a short amount of time? Is it bright red (fresh) or brownish (older)? Clots? How big? How many pads are soaked in 24 hours?	There are many possible variations on what constitutes irregular bleeding; the provider needs to obtain a clear description of what is happening with this woman at this time.
Prolonged (>7 days) or excessive (>80 mL/day) or occurring at regular intervals?	Heavy bleeding commonly comes from the uterus, while staining, spotting or light bleeding may be from any part of the genital tract.
Occurring at irregular and more frequent than expected intervals?	**Menorrhagia**—Prolonged (>7 days) or excessive (>80 mL/day) uterine bleeding occurring at regular intervals
Prolonged/excessive bleeding at irregular and more frequent intervals that expected?	**Metrorrhagia**—Uterine bleeding occurring at irregular and more frequent than normal intervals
Variable amounts occurring between regular menstrual intervals?	**Menometrorrhagia**—Prolonged or excessive uterine bleeding occurring at irregular and more frequent than normal intervals
Spotting occurring just before ovulation, typically from decreasing estrogen levels?	
Recurrence of bleeding in a menopausal woman at least 6 months to 1 year after cessation of cycles?	
No uterine bleeding for 6 months or longer?	

Provider Inquiries	Clinical Reasoning/Logic
	Intermenstrual bleeding—Uterine bleeding of variable amounts occurring between regular menstrual periods
	Midcycle spotting—Spotting occurring just before ovulation, typically from declining estrogen levels
	Postmenopausal bleeding—Recurrence of bleeding in a menopausal woman at least 6 months to 1 year after cessation of cycles
Onset: In relation to the menstrual cycle or how long ago until coming in for care?	Information that may provide clues as to cause for the bleeding.
Recent intercourse?	Bleeding that occurs consistently after intercourse suggests cervical pathology
Recent onset of menarche?	
Symptoms of menopause?	
Location: Certain it is coming from the vagina and not the rectum?	Patients may confuse urethral, vulval, or anal bleeding with vaginal bleeding. Bleeding with urination suggests a urinary tract infection. Bleeding with bowel movements suggests hemorrhoids.
Duration: How long have you been experiencing bleeding alterations? Intermittent or constant?	Information related to whether this is an acute onset or has been chronic.
Exacerbation: Does anything you do make it worse?	
Relief: Does it stop on its own?	
Associated signs/symptoms: Labor pains? Pelvic/abdominal pain? Vaginal discharge other than bleeding?	DUB associated with abdominal pain should be considered a high suspect for miscarriage, ectopic pregnancy.
	Lower abdominal pain, fever and/or vaginal discharge cause for concern related to infection (pelvic inflammatory disease, endometritis)
	Dysmenorrhea, dyspareunia or infertility suggest endometriosis
	Changes in bowel/bladder habits/function may be due to extrauterine bleeding or mass effect from neoplastic tumor
	Galactorrhea, heat/cold intolerance, hot flashes may indicate an endocrine cause
Vaginal Discharge Vaginal discharge can be physiologic and therefore benign; it can be symptomatic of a mild vaginal infection, such as yeast or bacterial vaginosis (BV), or a severe infection, such as gonorrhea or chlamydia (G/C) or trichomoniasis.	
Characteristics: Color, odor, amount? Itching (where, intensity, frequency)?	Benign discharge is usually colorless and odorless.
	Vaginal itching frequently associated with infectious conditions.
Onset: In relationship to the menstrual cycle?	Bacterial vaginosis (BV) tends to wane and wax in conjunction with the menstrual cycle.
Duration: How long ago before seeking care?	
Relief: Anything you have done to make it better or does it get better on its own?	

Provider Inquiries	Clinical Reasoning/Logic
Associated signs/symptoms: Itching or skin irritation, bleeding, does your partner have anything similar?	STIs may cause discharge that causes skin irritation. Partners can have the same symptoms as the woman when they share the same STI. Males may have more pronounced discharge in the case of gonorrhea compared to the woman who may notice little to none.

Additional Concerns

There may be instances when a female patient requires an assessment for significant concerns and not necessarily for treatment of specific symptoms or complaints. While a complete symptom analysis may not be appropriate, adapting components of COLDERRA may be appropriate and helpful.

Infertility (Inability to Achieve a Desired Pregnancy)

Technically the diagnosis of infertility cannot be made until a couple has been trying unsuccessfully to achieve a pregnancy for 12 months, but for women over 35 years, some providers shorten the time interval to 6 months. Many women who are anxious about conceiving seek care after only a few months of trying. Infertility may be a problem exclusive to the woman, exclusive to the male partner, or result from a combination of male and female factors. When a woman with a male partner seeks care for infertility, the partner should also see his provider at the same time. Women without a male partner may also present for care in order to achieve a pregnancy with technological help.

Provider Inquiries	Clinical Reasoning/Logic
Characteristics: Ever achieved a pregnancy at all or achieved a pregnancy but had a miscarriage (especially if more than once) or achieved a pregnancy in the past with a different partner?	Inability to sustain a pregnancy is caused by factors different from the inability to ever achieve a pregnancy. If the woman had successful pregnancies with a different partner, she will still need evaluation for herself, but the provider may want to wait for evaluation of the present partner before doing expensive, difficult or invasive procedures on the woman.
Onset: Any past or present conditions/illnesses/practices that may have caused fertility issues with self or partner?	Thyroid conditions, kidney disorders, diabetes, Cushing's disease, or history of STIs are known causes of infertility in females. Exposure to chemicals and pesticides, as well as heat may impair sperm production in males. Poor nutrition, obesity, and use of alcohol, tobacco, or drugs are also factors related to infertility. A varicocele in males may also impair fertility. Men over 40 years of age are also less fertile than younger men.
Duration: How long have you been trying to get pregnant? When was the last time you used contraception? What kind?	Long-acting hormonal contraception may take several months to be totally cleared from a woman's system.
Associated signs/symptoms: Characteristics of the menstrual cycle? (Ask woman to keep accurate track of cycle and all its characteristics on a calendar or chart for a few months, including frequency and timing of intercourse with a male partner if applicable.) Have you ever had a successful pregnancy? Has your partner ever had a successful pregnancy? Is this a new partner for you? Any history or symptoms that might suggest diabetes, thyroid or other endocrine problems? Any history of STIs? What medications do you take?	The woman will need careful general assessment to rule out endocrine system problems like thyroid or diabetes at the beginning. If known to be preexisting, the provider will look closely at how well these problems are managed. STIs like gonorrhea or Chlamydia can have cause permanent scarring of fallopian tubes with resulting infertility. Various medications, especially in combinations, may have effects on endocrine or immune systems. Some medications are known teratogens and will need to be changed as measures are taken to try to achieve a pregnancy.

Desire to Prevent a Pregnancy

Women commonly seek care in order to receive a prescription for hormonal contraception or for insertion of intrauterine devices. Diaphragms and cervical caps can only be provided by prescription. Some women just want advice about this topic and may prefer to use over the counter products like condoms and spermicides or may intend to use planned abstinence in relationship to the menstrual cycle.

Provider Inquiries	Clinical Reasoning/Logic
Duration: Desire for temporary, long-term but reversible or nonreversible methods. How long does she intend to use her planned method? How important is it to her that she not become pregnant?	It is important to try to match the kind of contraception to be used in relationship to a woman's long and short-term goals about pregnancy. The woman's attitude toward the importance of preventing a pregnancy also helps when looking at the effectiveness of different methods.
Relief: What methods has she used in the past? How successful or not successful was she in using these methods? Did she like them? Does she want to use them again? Why or why not?	If a woman has used something successfully in the past, the method she used may be a good one to use again. Conversely, a bad experience may make a woman reluctant to even try it again.
Associated signs/symptoms: Does she have any health problems that contraindicate one method or another? If she used hormonal methods in the past, did she ever have any danger signs of high blood pressure, stroke or blood clots? Does she have true migraines?	Hormonal contraceptive methods may be contraindicated in light of preexisting health conditions or past medical/surgical history especially blood clots and stoke. Hormonal contraception may exacerbate pre-existing migraines.
Concern with Sexual Activity Women may seek care for counseling about their sexual practices. They may want reassurance that something they do, have done, or are thinking about doing is normal or usual.	
Characteristics: What exactly are you concerned about? If pain is the issue, then characteristics of the pain. What is your goal about this issue (make it go away or improve, be reassured, learn something)? Concern about STIs?	Pain (dysparcunia) during sexual activity is not uncommon. Women's concerns may actually be about their partners, especially for an issue like lack of desire or ability of the partner. Women who experience desire, especially if this causes her lifestyle problems, may also seek care.
Onset: Recent or long standing issue? If pain is the issue, relationship to menstrual cycle	
Location: If pain is the issue, exact location?	
Duration: If pain or another physical symptom, how long does it last?	
Exacerbation: Anything make it worse?	
Relief: Anything make it better?	
Associated signs/symptoms: What other health problems do you have? What medications do you take? Does this issue interfere with your lifestyle in any way? Is your partner concerned or affected? What does your partner do, say, think or believe?	Women may seek care for their own lack of sexual desire; this is a very common side effect of many medications that may be prescribed for other health problems and may accompany many chronic health problems such as diabetes and depression, or be related to hormonal contraception and sex hormone-binding globulin (SHBG) effects.

Past Medical History

Past medical history identifies the information needed to determine whether there is any prior incidences/events that may have contributed to the present situation.

Provider Inquiries	Clinical Reasoning/Logic
Do you have diabetes of any kind? Did you have any kind of diabetes while you were pregnant?	Diabetes is often the cause of secondary gynecological problems, especially in polycystic ovary syndrome (PCOS), infertility or unusual menstrual patterns.
Is there anything wrong with your thyroid gland?	Abnormal thyroid hormone levels can also cause secondary gynecological problems.
Do you have any kind of bleeding or clotting disorders?	Systemic clotting problems may result in abnormal gynecological bleeding, especially excessive bleeding.
Have you ever had a stroke?	In the presence of history of stroke, use of various hormones may be contraindicated.
Do you have migraine headaches?	Various hormones used therapeutically may exacerbate migraines.
What medications do you take now or regularly? What do you take them for?	Therapeutic hormones may interact with a variety of medications, e.g., birth control pills may make some antibiotics less effective.
Menstrual History	
How old were you when you began to have periods? How old were you when you stopped having them? How many days in between the first day of one period and the first day of the next one? How many days does a cycle usually last? Any bleeding or spotting in the middle of a cycle? How heavy/light is the bleeding on the various days? How does it change, if it changes?	Understanding what happened or is happening typically or usually for a woman is crucial to help understand any problems related to the menstrual cycle. This history can be taken once upon first encounter in a gynecological setting. Unless the woman is complaining of a menstrual cycle problem, it does not need to be repeated or even updated. It is unnecessary information for most encounters in urgent care, non-gynecological settings or during a pregnancy.
Do you have any other problems or issues associated with your periods? Pain at any time? How severe? Over time, have your periods changed? If so, how? Any concerns related to changes? Have changes required you to make any lifestyle changes?	Pain associated with menstruation (dysmenorrheal) occurs in approximately 50% of menstruating women. Causes are thought to be related to psychogenic factors, hormone imbalances, and increased prostaglandin secretion. Pain by itself is not considered pathological; however, in some women, changes in the hormone level at various stages of the month generate accompanying systemic symptoms associated with **premenstrual syndrome** (PMS). These may include headaches, fatigue, cravings, fluid retention/bloating, irritability, mood fluctuations, anxiety/depression, and sleep dysfunction. Women during the menopausal years may seek care for symptoms associated with menopause including hot flashes, sleep disorders, and vaginal dryness.
When did you first experience symptoms?	There's no specific time of onset associated with PMS but it is helpful to know how long the woman has been experiencing manifestations.

Provider Inquiries	Clinical Reasoning/Logic
How long do manifestations last?	PMS symptoms occur right after ovulation and typically end with the onset of menses. PMS manifestations present during the last half of menstrual cycle.
Does anything that makes it worse?	Underlying medical/psychological conditions may mimic or worsen manifestations.
Has anything you have tried make it better, such as medications (OTC), reducing caffeine, avoiding salt, quit smoking, reduce alcohol intake, reducing intake of refined sugars?	These are general management actions that may help reduce symptoms.
Family History	
Family history provides information regarding family members' illnesses or conditions as potential causes for chief concern or presenting symptoms that may indicate a pattern of presentation associated with transmission of familial/genetic factors predisposing the patient to certain system-related conditions/illnesses. Any of these may indicate a potential or actual cause of female reproductive system dysfunction.	
Ovarian cancer in your mother or a sister?	Ovarian cancer in a first-degree female relative may be a risk factor for the same cancer.
Any family members with diabetes, thyroid, or other endocrine system diseases?	Family history of endocrine problems, especially diabetes or thyroid diseases may confer risk of these problems for the patient.
Any family history of bleeding or clotting diseases?	Some clotting or bleeding disorders may run in families.
Any family history of multiple, naturally achieved pregnancies?	Multiple pregnancies may run in families.
Was or is there any problem with violence in your present or past family or your partner's family of origin?	Sexual abuse of women or children may be passed through generations by example.
Personal and Social History	
Information about personal and social activities may help to explain certain problems, may identify potential lifestyle modifications to improve general health, and may help the provider to give culturally appropriate care.	
Tobacco: Use at all? Secondary exposure? If exposure, how much? Ever tried to stop; ever successfully stopped, even for a short time? (Many women are able to quit or cut back their intake considerably during a pregnancy.)	Tobacco exposure is related to many problems, and counseling to stop or cut back is an appropriate health teaching topic, no matter what the purpose of the visit.
Alcohol: Use at all? How much? How often? Any binge drinking? Ever tried to quit? Want to quit?	Excessive alcohol intake or Illegal drug use may put the patient at increased risk for contacting STIs or for experiencing abuse.
Drugs: All drugs taken including prescription, illegal, OTC, counter, nutritional supplements, and herbal preparations?	If the woman is being seen for infertility, modifications in prescription drugs may be needed.
Nutrition: What is your usual diet?	If there are other red flags in other systems, be alert to the possibility of anorexia nervosa or bulimia.
Employment/hobbies: Sports, dancing, other strenuous physical activities? Chemical exposures? Other physical demands? Excessive heat exposure? At risk for occupational exposure to violence (e.g. law enforcement or military occupations)?	Menstrual periods can disappear when a woman has a problem with anorexia or bulimia or with excessive exercise, especially in some activities such as gymnastics or ballet dancing. Menstrual or fertility problems may result from environmental chemical exposure.

Provider Inquiries	Clinical Reasoning/Logic
Home neighborhood: Any known exposures to environmental pollutants including agricultural chemicals?	Large varieties of chemical compounds are known teratogens or can be endocrine disrupters.

Developmental Applications

Certain conditions or disorders may be related to certain age groups or situations. Inquiring to obtain age or condition specific information will provide further information for helping to determine causes of the chief concern as identified.

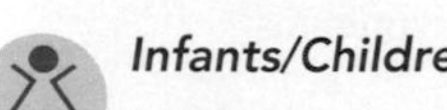

Infants/Children

Problems urinating?

Problem with itching, rash, vaginal discharge of genitals?

Any signs of trauma to the genital area? Bruising? Pain?

Been touched between your legs when not wanted to?

If any issue involving the female reproductive system is the presenting problem or is brought up unasked by a caregiver, the provider should immediately suspect abuse as a problem. A child who needs evaluation for sexual abuse needs to be seen in a specialty setting by providers specifically trained to do an appropriate evaluation. If sexual abuse is suspected, the general provider should make sure the child is safe, take care of an immediate or urgent problems within his/her scope of practice and refer the patient immediately to specialized care. A forensic exam will be needed, and the primary provider should do nothing that might interfere with obtaining biologic specimens that could be used as evidence. Also see Chapter 14.

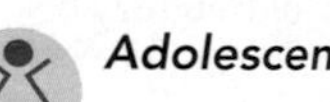

Adolescents

Have you begun to engage in sexual activities yet?

What kind of activities are you engaged in?

Have you used any kind of birth control or protection?

What are you worried or concerned about? What do you need from this visit?

PRACTICE POINT: Speaking the Same Language

The provider should know up-to-date, local street slang for the various medical terms and be prepared to substitute language in order to communicate clearly.

Changes associated with menarche may bring adolescents in for care. The young woman may only need teaching and reassurance about what is normal development. Young women who are having problems, especially if they have become sexually active, need extra care, time, and sensitivity to get a thorough and accurate assessment of subjective issues. The provider needs to be willing and able to adapt his or her language to casual or slang terms. For many young people, the performance of oral sex only is sometimes not considered to be true sexual activity. If a young woman is sexually active, then ask her the same questions as would be asked of a more mature woman. Providers should arrange some amount of time to see the adolescent alone if the young woman is accompanied by an adult.

Provider Inquiries	Clinical Reasoning/Logic
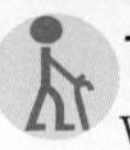 ***The Older Woman*** What are you concerned about today? Have you ever had this problem before? Once you went through menopause, did you ever have any bleeding after that? Have you ever had a pelvic exam? What was your experience with pelvic exams in the past? Do you have any problems with joint pain or hip difficulties?	Older women may have health issues that have resulted in a variety of communication difficulties. They may also have various musculoskeletal problems that will require modification of examination procedures. Most older women do not seek routine gynecologic care; they may only seek care if they are having problems.
Do you have regular gynecologic care?	Many older women are especially embarrassed to have to seek gynecological care and may ignore symptoms for quite some time because they don't want to undergo gynecological examinations. Some women may never have had gynecologic care in the past especially if they never had problematic symptoms or never used prescription contraception. Providers need not ask questions about past pregnancies for women well past menopause except to ascertain if a woman never had any pregnancies at all. Cancer is usually the primary possible diagnosis for a woman past menopause, so caregivers will want to focus assessment on this issue.
Are you sexually active?	Older women who have a new sexual partner may be vulnerable to STIs or may have questions or concerns about sexuality or sexual practices, issues they may have never dealt with in the past. As always, sensitive, individualized care that allows for enough time to address any issues is needed.

OBJECTIVE DATA

The examination of the gynecological system includes two examination techniques: inspection and palpation. The patient may be seated or in the supine position depending on patient's capability. The patient's position will determine the exact sequence of the examination, but one should develop a systematic approach that is used consistently for each examination.

Inspection

- External Genitalia configuration related to age, development
  - Labia majora/minora
  - Pubic hair distribution pattern
  - Presence of parasites/lesions
  - Bleeding, open areas, growths
  - Urethral meatus
  - Clitoris
- Vaginal bleeding
- Genital/pelvic injuries (trauma/assault)
- Prolapse
- Internal genitalia (vaginal walls, cervix [Pap test])

Palpation

- Inguinal lymph nodes
- Skene's glands/Bartholin's glands/urethra
- Muscle tone
- External structures (labia majora [assess bladder fullness if applicable])
- Bimanual palpation of external and internal pelvic organs

Percussion

- Only with distension to differentiate gas from bleeding

Auscultation

- With distension, assess bowel sounds

Level I to IV Examination

The Level I to Level IV examinations are performed on a continuum, which starts from a basic level to a more comprehensive level based on provider's abilities and knowledge as well as the patient's presentation and location. It may start at the outpatient setting progressing to the ED, hospital unit bed, critical care unit, or specialty unit. Frequently all the elements from basic to comprehensive exam are done in one setting like in a primary care setting or clinic.

The condition/illness of the patient is the primary consideration related to the type and amount of data needed to assess the patient's condition/illness/situation. The arrangement of skills into levels is for general purposes and is meant to be descriptive rather than prescriptive. The purpose of arranging into levels is to provide a framework to assist the learner in determining the appropriate data to collect.

Female Genitalia

	Level I	Level II	Level III	Level IV
Inspection	External genitalia configuration related to age, development Labia majora discharge Pubic hair distribution pattern Presence of parasites Presence of lesions	External genitalia bleeding, open areas, growths Labia minora Urethral meatus Clitoris	Vaginal bleeding Genital/pelvic injuries (trauma/assault) Prolapse Speculum exam to perform procedures or collect specimens from cervix and vagina if clinically applicable	Inspection of external genitalia, vaginal walls and cervix Speculum exam to perform procedures or collect specimens from cervix, vagina, or uterus if clinically applicable
Palpation		Skene's glands/ Bartholin's glands Muscle tone		Bimanual palpation of external and internal pelvic organs and palpation of inguinal lymph nodes
Percussion	Only with distension to differentiate gas from bleeding			
Auscultation	With distension, assess bowel sounds			

Inspection: Level I

The Level I exam begins with the overall inspection of the external genitalia in relation to the patient's age and development. It is necessary for the woman to separate her legs so that adequate visualization of the genitalia is possible, but she does not have to be on an examination table using stirrups. Any kind of bed can be used for a Level I exam. Nonsterile gloves are used for any gynecological exam.

Inspection Techniques and Expected Findings	Unexpected Findings
Initial inspection begins with observation of the overall appearance of the external genitalia (Figure 30-8). 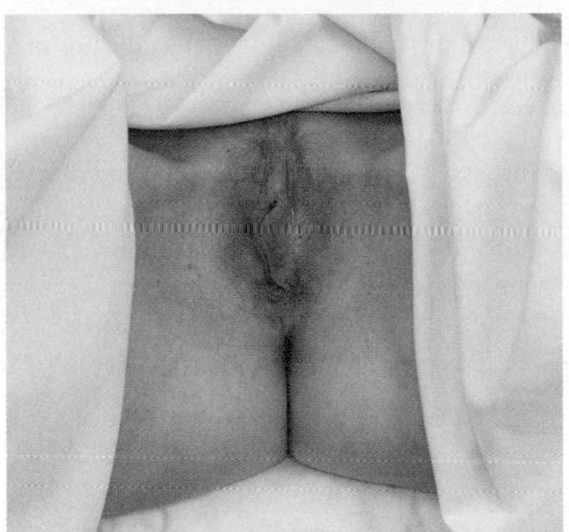 FIGURE 30-8 Inspection of external female genitalia	Note any unusual odors that may accompany various infections. Also observe of the presence of any unusual discharge. Three classic sources of abnormal vaginal discharge are Candida (yeast), bacterial vaginosis (BV) and/or trichomoniasis (a protozoa). Trichomoniasis is nearly always sexually transmitted (Figure 30-9); the other two may or may not be associated with sexual activity. Yeast discharge is usually thick, white and curdy like cottage cheese, and the vaginal area itches copiously. 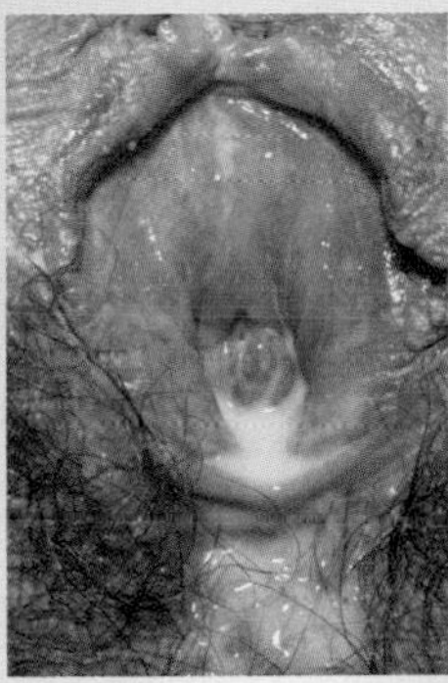 FIGURE 30-9 Trichomoniasis *Source:* Wellcome Image Library/ Custom Medical Stock BV discharge tends to be thin like water, gray, whitish, or yellowish, copious in amount, and with a characteristic unpleasant odor, often described as "fishy." Trichomonas is purulent and irritating, and often has a foamy, frothy appearance. Blood may be present secondary to accompanying cervicitis.
Make note of the pubic hair and its distribution. Pubic hair is coarser than scalp hair and ranges from relatively straight to curly. The pattern of hair growth is generally in the shape of an inverted triangle with the base of the triangle located horizontally across the lower pelvis from the points where the lower extremity meets the lower abdomen. There may also be a small train of hair that goes up towards the umbilicus. There are many variations in typical patterns related to race or ethnicity.	In the postoperative or postdelivery patient the hair may be absent due to shaving. It is not uncommon for women to shave or wax their pubic area (bikini wax), removing all of the hair or leaving a very small section.
Perform a closer inspection of the pubic hair. There should be no evidence of infestations.	The presence of parasites, (nits/lice) or burrowing tunnels (scabies) in an indicator of the presence of an infestation.
Inspect the labia majora for color, shape. and symmetry. It should be uniform in color and are often darker than the surrounding tissue. Each should appear to be smooth, well-formed, plump, closely approximated and symmetrical in appearance. They may also appear dry or moist (see Figure 30-8).	After a vaginal delivery, the labia majora may appear to be slightly shriveled with a slight gap between them. A darker red color may indicate an inflammation. Asymmetry may be indicative of swelling and edema resulting from infection.
Also inspect the labia majora for the presence of any lesions, rashes, or excoriations. You may observe sebaceous cysts, 1 cm nodules that are firm, nontender, and yellowish in color.	The presence of any of any lesions, rashes or excoriations is also indicative of inflammation or infection.
Inspect the perineal surface area, which should be smooth with even color distribution. There may be evidence of an episiotomy scar that may be midline or mediolateral.	Increased redness or presence of lesions is an unexpected finding.

Inspection: Level II

Inspection Techniques and Expected Findings	Unexpected Findings
This level of examination can be done with the woman lying on any kind of bed or table. An exam table with stirrups is not needed.	
Continue inspection by separating the labia majora with the thumb and index finger of one (gloved) hand. The labia minora are deep pink in color and should be moist and symmetrical in appearance and size (Figure 30-10).	A deeper pink/red color is an indicator of inflammation or infection.
With the labia minora separated, locate the urethral meatus, which may appear as an irregular opening or slit. It is midline and superior to the vaginal opening (see Figure 30-10).	Note the presence of any discharge or increased redness in the area, which may be due to repeated urinary tract infections. A caruncle may be present, which is a bright red polypoid nodule that protrudes from the urethral meatus. These are generally asymptomatic.

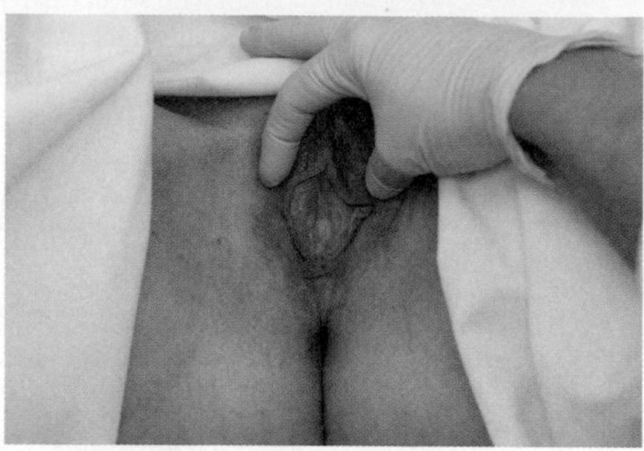

FIGURE 30-10 Separation of the labia

Inspection Techniques and Expected Findings	Unexpected Findings
Inspect the clitoris for size, which should be approximately 2 cm or less in length and 0.5 cm in diameter.	Enlargement may be an indication of a masculinizing condition.
The vaginal opening (introitus) appears as a narrow, vertical slit or as a larger opening. The tissues of the vaginal opening should be moist.	

Inspection: Level III

Inspection Techniques and Expected Findings	Unexpected Findings
This exam level primarily focuses on the presence of vaginal bleeding, pelvic pain, and visible trauma. The exam can be done with the woman lying on any kind of bed or table. Exam table with stirrups is not needed.	
Inspect the vulva, perineum, and anal area for evidence of nonvaginal bleeding.	Vulvar lesions or anal fissures may be present and the source of vaginal bleeding (Figure 30-11).

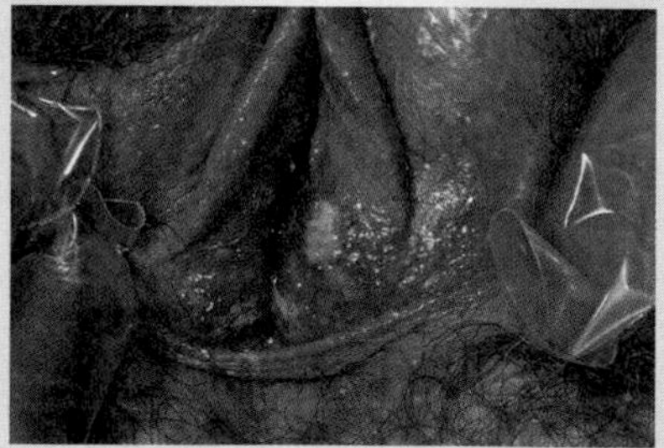

FIGURE 30-11 Vulvar lesions
Source: Dr. P. Marazzi/Science Source

Inspection Techniques and Expected Findings	Unexpected Findings
Inspect vagina with speculum for evidence of inflammatory or structural cervical or vaginal lesions. (See speculum insertion with Level IV examination.)	Cervical polyps, cervical ectropion, ulceration, or vaginal atrophy may be source of bleeding. If miscarriage is occurring, products of conception may be visible in upper vagina or through cervical opening.

Inspection Techniques and Expected Findings	Unexpected Findings
Observe for other systemic manifestations that may be present and a possible cause for the bleeding.	Pallor (conjunctiva, nail beds) present in anemia. Obesity, hair loss, brittle hair/nails, nonpitting edema present in hypothyroidism. Obesity, hirsutism, and acanthosis nigricans present in polycystic ovary syndrome (PCOS). Acne, male-patterned baldness, hirsutism, and clitoromegaly suggest excessive androgens. Acanthosis nigricans also associated with insulin resistance, which may also be associated with anovulation (Figure 30-12). Jaundice, hepatomegaly, ecchymosis and other manifestations of liver disease suggest hepatic dysfunction and associated coagulopathy as a possible cause for bleeding (Best Practice, 2012).

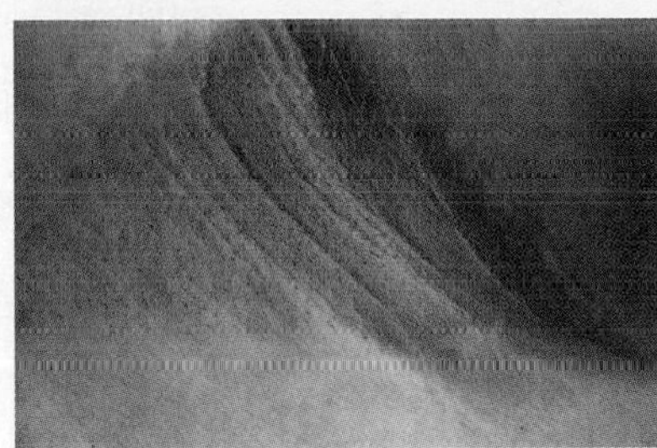

FIGURE 30-12 Acanthosis nigricans is an unexpected finding.
Source: Wellcome Image Library/Custom Medical Stock

PRACTICE POINT: Acanthosis Nigricans

The inner thighs and vulva are common places to first find acanthosis nigricans, which is a thickening and darkening of the skin. It often accompanies insulin resistance, and can be a marker of a patient with very high risk for type 2 diabetes. It is found in 40% of Native American teens, 13% of African American teens, 6% of Hispanic teens, and less than 1% of Caucasian teens. Obesity and insulin resistance in women often accompanies a syndrome called polycystic ovary syndrome, or PCOS. These women often ovulate irregularly and have issues with hirsutism and other androgenic features, like severe acne. Fertility can be an issue. If a provider sees acanthosis nigricans, he or she should use this finding as an entrée to have a health promotion discussion about prevention of type 2 diabetes. It would be appropriate to arrange for the woman to engage in diabetes prevention programs or activities (Habif, 2009).

Inspection Techniques and Expected Findings	Unexpected Findings
Inspect genital area for evidence of gynecologic trauma. Accidental genital trauma encompasses injury to the labia, vulva, vagina anogenital, and urogenital areas (Hall & Brown, 2009). Accidental trauma may result from blunt trauma (straddle injury, blows to the perineal area) penetrating injury, attempted self-abortion, and sexual assault.	Blunt trauma occurs primarily from motor vehicle accidents. A major concern with this type of trauma is a pelvic fracture, which may be life threatening due to massive hemorrhage. Crush injuries may also cause significant damage to the pelvis by sharp bone fragments penetrating the vagina and lower urinary tract. These injuries are commonly caused by horse riding accidents, with the horse falling and/or rolling onto the rider.
In the absence of external damage or injury, a speculum exam may be required to validate the presence of any lacerations. (See speculum insertion with Level IV examination.)	Straddle trauma occurs when the soft tissue of the vulva is compressed against a solid object such as a bicycle frame, fence, or monkey bars. This type of trauma generally results in abrasions, lacerations, and vulvar hematoma formation. Hematomas may be very painful and may result in urinary retention from pain and swelling of the tissues surrounding the urethra.

Inspection Techniques and Expected Findings	Unexpected Findings
Observe for the presence of vaginal injuries without any external evidence.	Penetrating injuries may also result from falling onto a pipe or fence, insufflation of the vagina with high pressure water, or from sexual intercourse. These types of injuries may present no external evidence of injury or damage. Over-distension of the vagina may result in deep vaginal lacerations which may cause considerable pain and hemorrhage. Injuries related to intercourse occur most commonly from the initial instance, a return to sexual activity after a period of abstinence, a congenital abnormality, deep penetration during an unusual position, drug or alcohol intoxication, brutality, and use of a foreign object. Penile piercings may also be the cause of such injuries. It is incumbent on the provider to determine whether these injuries occurred during consensual sex or if force or coercion were used by the partner.
Observe for other types of injuries.	Other causes of genital trauma include bites (human or animal), burns (scalds, flame, chemical), and genital piercings (clitoris, labia). Bites are associated with abrasions, lacerations, and contusions; burns are associated with partial- or full-thickness burns; and piercings are associated with pain, swelling, bleeding, as well as evidence of infection.
Observe for objective indicators of pain and investigate possible causes of severe abdominal pain.	Abdominal pain has a plethora of causes that is frequently related to GI organs; however, in gynecological causes, the patient frequently complains of pelvic pain that may or may not be accompanied by vaginal bleeding. Causes of pelvic pain may be related to abnormal pregnancies and infections.

PRACTICE POINT: Foreign Object Insertion

Insertion of a foreign object into the vagina is also a cause of genital trauma. The reason for the insertion may be difficult to ascertain, as the patient is often embarrassed about the situation. Inserting the foreign object may be due to "experimentation" of some sort, but it may also be due to self-harm. Injuries of this type may also be due to violence or abuse and it is necessary to determine if this was involved. If drugs or alcohol are involved, it is possible that the patient has no memory of what was inserted (Hall & Brown, 2009). Insertion of a foreign object into the vagina may also be related to an attempted self-abortion.

PRACTICE POINT: The Forensic Gynecological Exam

When a woman seeks care reporting that she has been raped, she will need a special kind of gynecological examination. She will need assessment for any injuries she reports, sensitive interpersonal care, preventative health care such as emergency contraception, referrals for gynecologic and psychologic follow-up care, and a special forensic examination designed to collect biologic specimens to be used as evidence. Once collected, this evidence must remain within a carefully documented chain of custody between the health care provider and law enforcement personnel.

The **forensic examination** is best done by someone who has received special training in how to collect and document all the evidence. An excellent program to accomplish this is to have nurses trained and on-call to do the exam when needed (SANE or Sexual Assault Nurse Examiners). The forensic exam needs to be done soon after the woman comes into care, but it can wait until the best trained provider is available. It is common to allow an on-call nurse provider an hour to arrive at the emergency setting. It is better to wait and have the best examination done, than to rush and end up with evidence that is of poor quality or is inadmissible in court because of documentation or chain of custody errors.

If there is no one at all with special training in the forensic exam available, the "rape kit" used to collect evidence is standardized and includes a paper with step-by-step directions. These directions must be followed to the letter. It is best to have an assistant of some kind reading the directions out loud and double checking that everything is collected and labeled properly. The rape kit can also be used to collect evidence from a male victim.

This exam usually takes over an hour to do well. It is best done in a private room with a door, away from the busyness and noise of an emergent setting. Once the exam has begun, the provider should NOT be interrupted to attend to other matters. So if the provider is also an "on-call" person at that time, someone else will need to become the "on-call" person until the exam is finished. The assistant can leave the room if truly necessary and should field any incoming telephone calls. Every emergency care setting should have a plan for how to maintain chain of custody for any kind of evidence. These procedures must be followed exactly as outlined.

Inspection: Level IV

The Level IV exam is essentially the pelvic exam that requires the use of a speculum and is performed to identify developmental or anatomic abnormalities, infections, neoplasms, ovarian cysts, uterine fibroids, and other conditions or disorders (Edelman, Anderson, Lai, Braner, & Tegtmeyer, 2007).

PRACTICE POINT: Use of the Examination Table with Leg Stirrups

A speculum exam is performed on an examination table with leg stirrups. The provider assists the woman to lie on the table with the head up to a level comfortable for her. A pillow may be used to increase comfort. The patient should be fully covered by a sheet or drape.

Place the feet into the stirrups one at a time. When the feet are positioned in the stirrups and the pull-out table is back in place, the back of the provider's hands are placed against the bottom of the table and the woman should scoot herself down the table to the edge until the provider's hands are felt. Adjust the length of the stirrups as needed to make the woman more comfortable.

Once the examination is finished, replace the drapes, pull out the small table at the bottom of the large table, and place the woman's legs, one at a time, onto the small table in the middle. Assist the woman to scoot herself backwards into a stable position. She may decide to sit up immediately in which case the pull-out table should be pushed back in. Or she may prefer to lie on the table and roll to the side to sit up; in that case the pull-out table is left out.

PRACTICE POINT: Leaving the Room

If the provider needs to leave the room for any reason once the exam has begun, first remove and discard the speculum (if it is in use at the time). Then assist the woman to change to a sitting position. NEVER leave the room with a woman still in the stirrups, and especially never leave with a speculum in place in her vagina.

Inspection Techniques and Expected Findings	Unexpected Findings
Select an appropriate-sized speculum based on the patient's parity, age, and the observed introitus, as well as the depth of the vagina as you assessed it (Figure 30-13).	

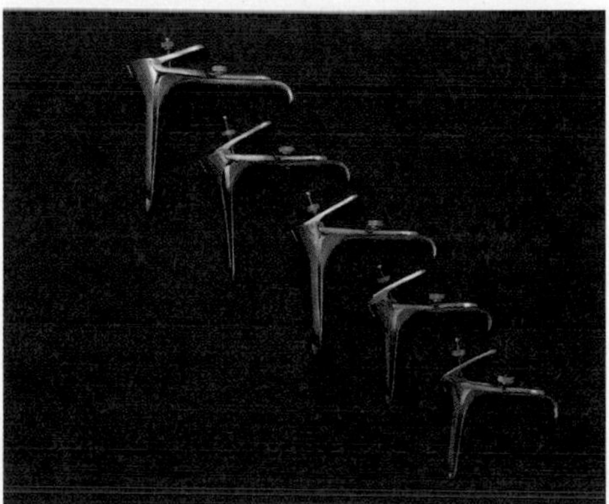

FIGURE 30-13 Vaginal specula

You may lubricate the speculum with warm water without disturbing tissues for samples that you will take. If you are NOT going to perform a Pap test or test for rupture of membranes, the speculum may be lubricated with water-based gel. A nonsterile speculum may be warmed with water, a heating pad or device, or the provider's hand. Holding a sterile speculum in the provider's hand for a short time helps to warm it up.

Inspection Techniques and Expected Findings	Unexpected Findings

PRACTICE POINT: Vaginal Specula

The speculum is a tool used to hold the vaginal walls open for visualization and examination of the cervix and vagina. Be familiar with the specula that are available at a clinical site. Practice putting the metal blades of the specula together, and how to adjust the blades with one hand. The goal is to avoid pinching or hurting the woman during the exam.

Vaginal specula can be made of stainless steel or plastic. Plastic specula are for one-time only use; however, metal specula can be cleaned, sterilized if needed, and reused many times. Even if a clinic predominately uses plastic specula, a few metal ones in the less frequently used sizes should be available. Plastic specula are clean enough for gynecologic exams, but cannot be sterilized.

Some plastic specula have a hollow handle designed to hold a specially designed very bright LED light. When using a metal or other brand of plastic specula, an external light source will be needed. These can be floor, table, or ceiling mounted lights of various designs. LED bulbs are much preferable to incandescent ones because the light is brighter and more easily focused upon the exact area needed. In an emergency or in low resource settings, an assistant can hold an ordinary flashlight.

Plastic specula generally come in sizes small-, medium-, and large-blade width. The blade length is standard for each width. Metal specula come in a much wider variety of blade lengths and widths. Pediatric specula are very small and made of metal.

In most cases, medium-sized will work for the majority of women; but some women, especially teens and older women require a small in order not to be in pain. There are also some women that require use of a large-sized to allow for adequate visualization. Some women will require a speculum that is longer but not wider. The provider should use palpation of the vagina before inserting the speculum in order to judge which size is needed.

It is not uncommon to try beginning the exam with the medium and then realize that a different size is needed. If that is the case, remove and discard the medium quickly and begin again with the better size.

Do your very best NOT to push, twist, and root around inside with a poorly sized speculum trying to find the cervix. Get help from a colleague if needed. Sometimes a given provider just cannot easily find the cervix for a particular woman, but a different person might be quickly successful.

Although it may sound counter intuitive, a metal speculum can be more flexible than a plastic one. The reason is that the metal speculum adjusts the opening size with a screw mechanism while the plastic ones use a series of preset notches. Some women may be very uncomfortable with the preset opening sizes. The metal ones can be adjusted very finely, just enough but not too much, which is often more comfortable.

The speculum portion is usually what worries a woman most as she thinks about a pelvic exam. And this portion usually what tends to cause the most discomfort because of the unnatural feeling of stretching in the vagina. It can be very helpful to let the woman handle the speculum in advance while she is sitting up and draped or clothed. Show her how the speculum opens and closes and is adjusted, and let her play with it herself. Explain to her why it is being used (simply to open the collapsed vaginal walls so that the cervix can be visualized and specimens can be taken), and assure her that you will be as fast as you possibly can be so the exam will only last a very short amount of time.

Check that all the needed instruments are placed in advance so they are readily accessible. The provider may prefer to do the whole exam alone or use an assistant according to patient/provider preference or clinic policy. Even if the assistant is not helping with the exam, if the assistant is female, her presence during the exam is appropriate and may be reassuring to the patient.

Just before starting the exam, remove the drape only as much as needed to do an effective exam. Adjust the light; if a floor or table light is being used direct it towards the woman's perineal area.

Begin the exam with inspection, using a gentle touch as needed to visualize external structures.

After inspection of the external genitalia, touch the woman's thigh, and inform her that the speculum will be inserted now.

Separate the labia and carefully insert the closed blades of the speculum at a slight angle, downward and in the direction of the cervix (Figure 30-14).

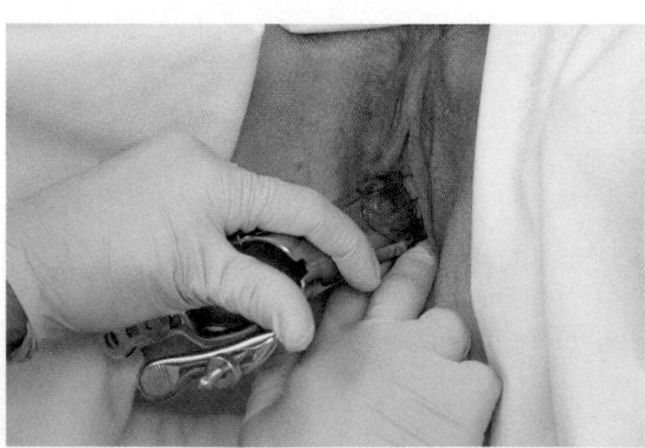

FIGURE 30-14 Insertion of speculum

Inspection Techniques and Expected Findings	Unexpected Findings

Carefully rotate the speculum so that the handle is pointing downwards (Figure 30-15a, b).

Gently open the blades by squeezing the handles of the blades together (Figure 30-15c). As the blades open you should observe the cervix, or the fornix.

Gently move or adjust the angle of the speculum so that the cervix is centered for optimal observation and sampling.

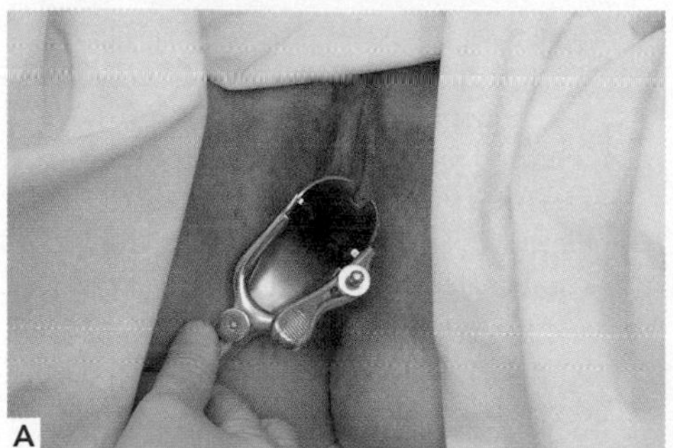

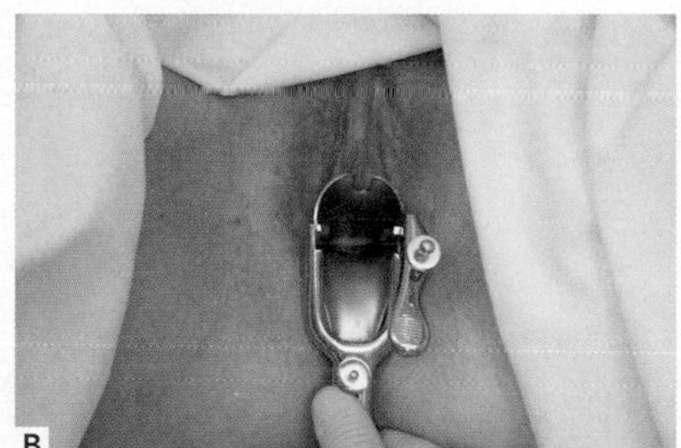

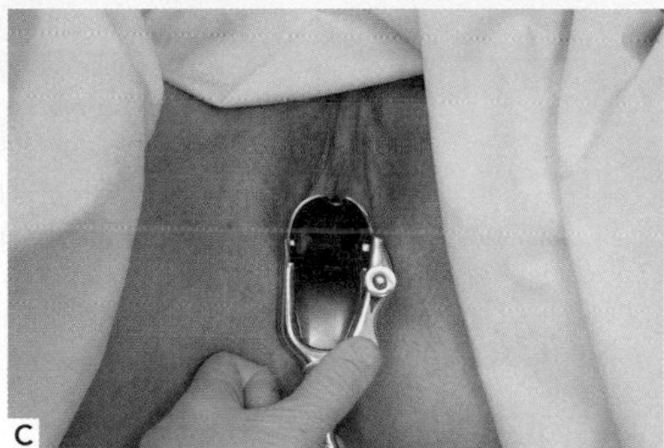

FIGURE 30-15A–C Rotation of speculum

The cervix is pink in color, which is evenly distributed, and positioned in the midline pointing in an anterior or posterior direction (Figure 30-16). The cervix may also project into the vagina 1–3 cm.

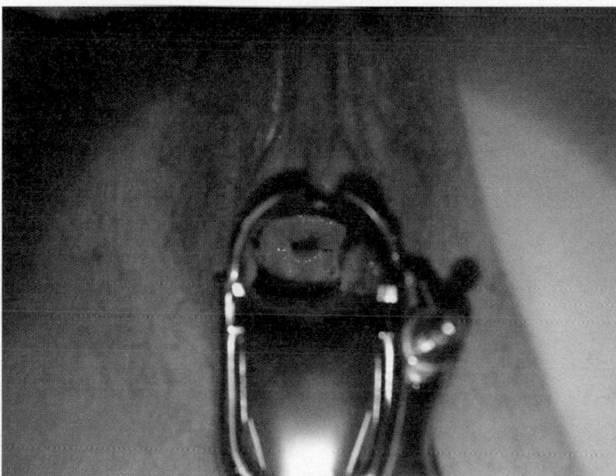

FIGURE 30-16 Healthy cervix

Inspection Techniques and Expected Findings	Unexpected Findings
The cervix may be bluish in color if the woman is pregnant.	Erythema that is symmetrical and circumscribed surrounding the os may be due to exposure of the columnar epithelium; however, it this is an initial finding it should be further explored, particularly if it is patchy or irregular. A pale cervix is an indicator of anemia. Severe cervicitis, usually secondary to an STI like chlamydia, is informally called sometimes a "hamburger cervix." This is easy to recognize. The surface of the cervix looks like raw, ground meat. It bleeds copiously and easily. Special swabs impregnated with silver nitrate can often stop the bleeding, but providers need to have those handy in the exam room. If the cervix bleeds heavily from the beginning of the exam, only test for STIs. Skip doing the Pap test at this time. Most likely the Pap results will return as either unreadable because of blood contamination and/or showing severe inflammation and therefore difficult to interpret regarding pre-cancerous changes.
To obtain cervical specimens for analysis, first remove any excess fluids or discharge from the cervical mucosa. Cover a sponge stick or large swab with a 2 × 2 and wipe any copious discharge off of the cervix (Figure 30-17). Obtain samples in this order: G/C, Pap, wet mount. Place swab for G/C in cervix for 30 seconds while rotating slowly; remove and place into the holding sleeve as directed on package.	Cotton swabs or sponge sticks leave fibers; gauze won't. Or follow specific package directions for the product being used.

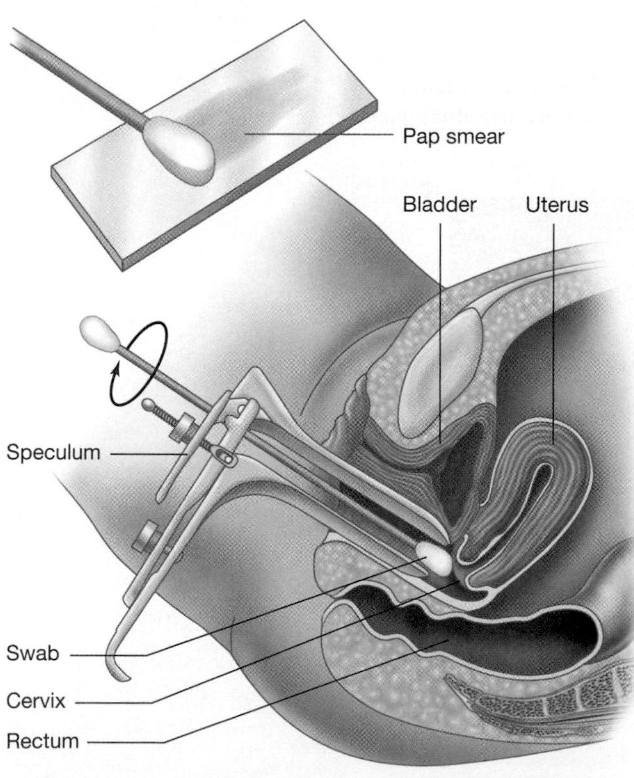

FIGURE 30-17 Obtaining a Pap smear

Inspection Techniques and Expected Findings	Unexpected Findings

PRACTICE POINT: Wet Prep

Examination of vaginal discharge: Examination of vaginal discharge under a microscope is commonly called a "wet prep." Vaginal discharge is collected into normal saline solution under some system specific to the setting (for example, by placing a swab into a small test tube containing the saline) and then transported to the laboratory. A wet slide with cover slip is then prepared. Potassium hydroxide (KOH) is applied to some of the specimen. If the problem is BV, a characteristic fishy odor may be immediately released. This will also kill bacteria and make any yeast spores more easily visible under the microscope.

In the wet specimen, trichomoniasis, if present, can be easily seen as a moving, crablike organism. In the KOH specimen, the dead body of the tiny animal may be visible. Yeast will be seen as fibrous or branching things and/or small, round characteristic spores. Bacterial vaginosis is diagnosed by observing characteristic "**clue cells**" which are large vaginal epithelial cells that have large amounts of small, round bacteria clinging to the outer membrane.

Other things may be observed under the microscope including sperm, white and red blood cells. Large amount of white blood cells may be suggestive of a more serious infection like chlamydia. Recently swab tests for office use (Affirm VPIII) have been developed to differentiate between BV and yeast.

Use the swab or "broom" to obtain cells by placing the slightly pointed center in the os and twisting it over the cervix to obtain tissue and then swish the swab or broom in the jar with commercial liquid medium until all tissue is removed, capping the specimen.

For the slide preparation, use the special wooden spatula by placing the more protruding portion in the cervix and rotating around and across the cervix, using the longer portion as the pivot. Remove and scrape the spatula across the bottom two-thirds of the slide to deposit tissue. Then place the small cylindrical brush in the cervix and rotate once, remove and rotate across the top one-third of the slide. Spray with fixative immediately.

Wet mount specimens may be obtained on a sterile cotton swab. The swab may then be placed in a laboratory tube holding about a ¼" of sterile saline (respiratory single use containers are easy) and either prepared by the provider or capped with the swab snapped below the edge of the tube and sent to the lab for wet mount evaluation.

Prepare a glass slide in the exam room. One slide (or one half of one slide) should have the specimen covered with a drop of saline and a cover slip. A second slide (or second half of one slide) should have KOH dropped onto the specimen.

Inspection Techniques and Expected Findings	Unexpected Findings
Smell the specimen as the KOH is being applied.	A "fishy" odor is a sign of bacterial vaginosis (BV).

Palpation: Level I

There are no structures that require palpation for a Level I exam.

Palpation: Level II

Palpation Techniques and Expected Findings	Unexpected Findings
Palpate the labia majora between the first finger and thumb for consistency and tenderness. The labia majora should feel homogenous in consistency and soft, without any tenderness or swelling.	Tenderness may be due to inflammation of the Bartholin's or Skene's glands.
Palpate Skene's glands, the urethra, and Bartholin's glands by first informing the patient of what you will be doing and that she will experience pressure exerted against her vaginal wall.	Pain or discharge generally indicates some type of infection, frequently gonococcal, but not always.

Palpation Techniques and Expected Findings	Unexpected Findings

To palpate the Skene's glands, insert the gloved index finger through the vaginal introitus into the vagina. It may be helpful to dip the gloved finger in warm water to provide some lubrication. Once inside the vagina, exert an upward pressure on the superior vaginal wall (urethra) and bring the finger forward while maintaining the pressure on the urethra. This procedure should not result in any pain or discharge (Figure 30-18).

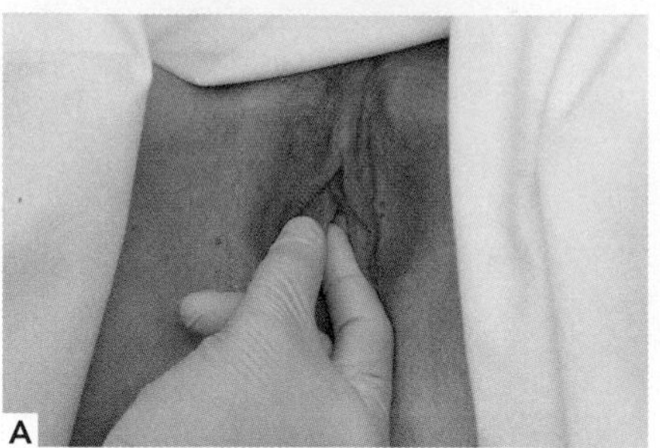
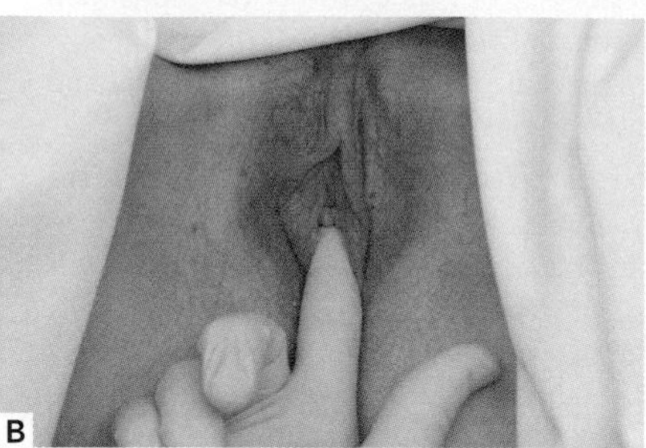

FIGURE 30-18A–B Palpation of **a)** Skene's glands and **b)** urethra

To palpate Bartholin's glands, palpate the lateral tissue surrounding the vaginal introitus. Inform the patient that she will feel pressure being exerted around the vaginal opening. Palpate the tissue between your index finger and thumb noting tissue consistency and pain. The tissue should be soft and smooth, without any discharge or pain. Palpate on both sides of the introitus (Figure 30-19).

Swelling, redness, pain, heat, and discharge are indicators of infection of the Bartholin's gland. The most common types of infection are staphylococcal or gonococcal. Any discharge should be cultured for identification and treatment.

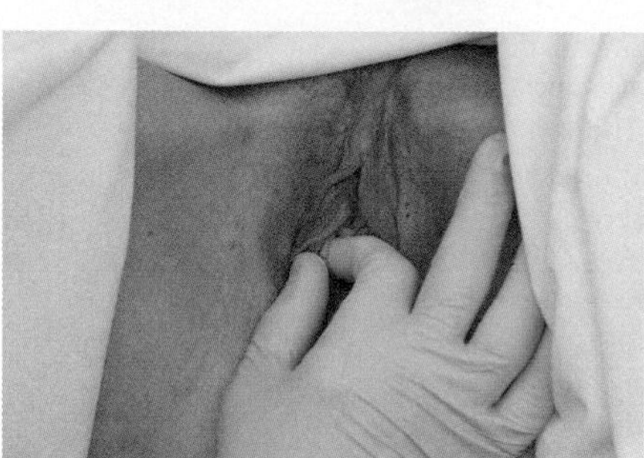

FIGURE 30-19 Palpation of Bartholin's glands

Assess muscle tone by asking the woman to contract her vaginal muscles around your fingers that have been placed inside the vagina. The muscles should contract tightly around the fingers. It may feel less tight in women who have given birth.

Separate the vaginal opening and ask the woman to bear down. There should not be any urine leaking from the urethra or any bulging noted.

Leaking of urine is associated with stress incontinence and bulging is the result of a cystocele, rectocele, or enterocele. It may also be caused by uterine prolapse.

Palpation: Level III

Palpation for the female reproductive organs would not be significantly different from abdominal palpation. No significant data obtained by abdominal palpation would help in differentiating reproductive organ alterations from other abdominal organ alterations.

Palpation: Level IV

Bimanual examination may be performed to determine if there are palpable internal lesions as the cause of bleeding.

The presence of genital tract pathology such as fibroids or adnexal masses, as well as pregnancy may be determined.

Sit or stand at the foot of the table positioned for better visualization. Lubricate the index and middle finger of the examining hand. For a smaller introitus, use only one finger. Touch the woman's leg and alert her to your entry. Insert the finger(s) by separating the labia, and press downwards to avoid the anterior structures (Figure 30-20).

Palpation Techniques and Expected Findings	Unexpected Findings

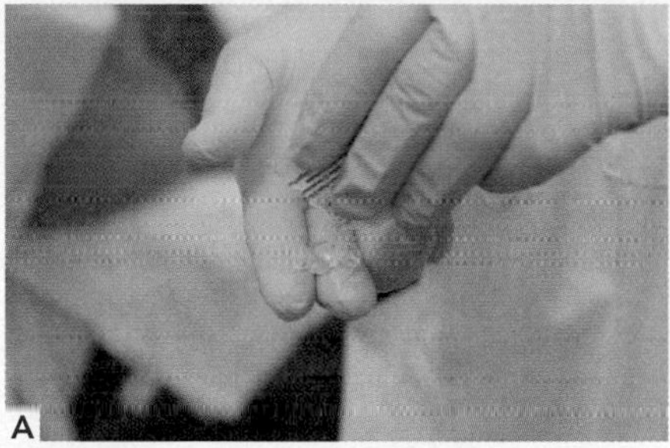

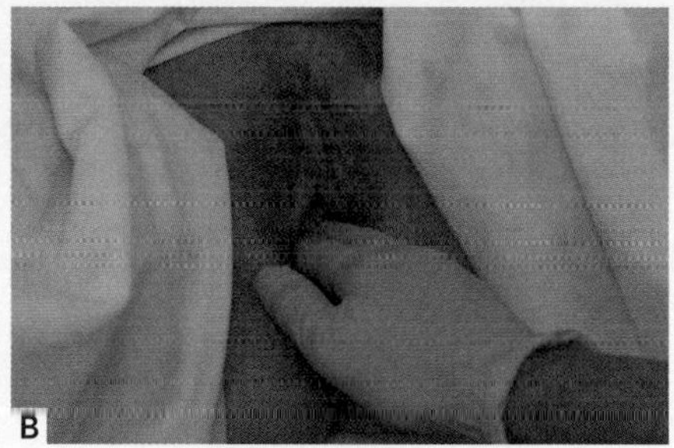

FIGURE 30-20A–B Lubricate gloves and insert fingers to begin the bimanual exam

Apply pressure to the posterior vaginal wall and have her bear down while you assess the anterior vaginal wall for any bulging or loss of urine from the urethra. See if the uterus descends.

While continuing to apply pressure, spread your fingers and have her bear down again as you look for bulges in the posterior wall.

Unexpected Findings: Bulging may indicate **cystocele** or **urethrocele**.

Put your fingers together and have her tighten around them (Kegels).

Unexpected Findings: This may indicate **rectocele.**

As you insert your fingers deeper, remember to think about whether you feel any cysts or growths.

As you reach the cervix, feel for size and shape. Grasp and move it. Severe pain is recorded as "cervical motion tenderness."

Unexpected Findings: Tenderness of the uterus may indicate the presence of fibroids, adenomyosis, endometriosis, or a pregnancy.

THINK LINK: Chandelier's Sign

The term "cervical motion tenderness" is a misnomer. It would more accurately be called "severe pain that is elicited when the cervix is touched." Informally practitioners call this the "chandelier sign" because the pain cause by the provider causes the woman to practically leap off the table towards the ceiling. If a pelvic exam causes a woman to show some discomfort, mild expressions of pain, or statements indicating that pressure is the issue, do not call this "cervical motion tenderness." Instead consider how one is performing the exam (one's technique.) Perhaps the provider is causing a bit more discomfort than is warranted by not doing the examination as gently as possible.

Palpate the uterus for size, shape, and contour (Figure 30-21).

- Place the other hand on the abdomen below the umbilicus, halfway between umbilicus and pubis.

Unexpected Findings: An enlarged uterus may indicate fibroids or pregnancy.

Push down and towards the pubis with the abdominal hand while your fingers in the vagina move from either side of the cervix towards the anterior surface of the cervix and push down on the cervix. This should raise the uterus towards the abdominal hand (**anteflexed** or **anteverted**).

Unexpected Findings: If you palpate an ovary in a postmenopausal woman, this is ALWAYS a concern and needs immediate follow up to check for cancer.

- If not, try sliding the cervical fingers under the cervix and pressing up on the cervix as the abdominal hand pushes down towards the pubis and the vaginal hand. (**retroverted/retroflexed**).

Unexpected Findings: If neither maneuver works, the uterus is retroverted and you need to use the fornices to feel as much of the uterus above the cervix as you can.

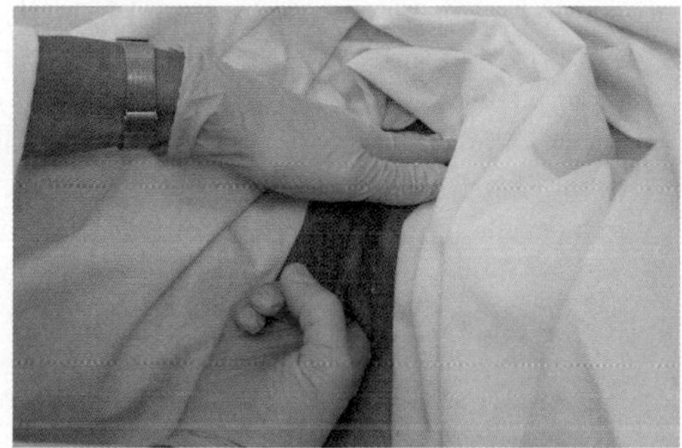

FIGURE 30-21 Palpation of uterus

Palpation Techniques and Expected Findings	Unexpected Findings
Palpate the adnexa for size, shape, tenderness or pain. Place both vaginal fingers in the fornix on the side you are assessing. Move the abdominal hand to a point about 3–4" off of the midline where you have been palpating from towards the side you wish to assess. Push upwards with the vaginal fingers as you push downwards and obliquely with the abdominal hand. The adnexa are almond-sized and will slip between the two examining hands. If you can't feel them, chart as "not felt."	An ovarian tumor (but not an ectopic pregnancy) may be palpated in the adnexa. This portion of the examination is most likely to cause the greatest discomfort because of the pressure that is needed for adequate palpation. Be sure to distinguish discomfort inherent in the procedure from true pain caused by some abnormality.
Remove the examining fingers at this time, smoothly.	

THINK LINK:* *Transgendered Persons

People who have decided to undergo gender change need especially sensitive care. An individual may seek care at any point during the change process. A woman who is transitioning into being a man (F to M) is most likely to seek gynecological care. Many of these men have had "top surgery" (breast removal) but decide against "bottom surgery" (removal of the female organs and construction of a kind of penis via plastic procedures) because this kind of surgical treatment is more extensive, expensive, painful, and complicated, and often not that effective at this point in time. Therefore, an F to M person who has transitioned as much as he intends may very well still have a uterus and vagina. He would still need to consider regular Pap test screening and might develop gynecological organ problems the same as any woman might. The use of high doses of male hormones will make his menstrual periods stop, prevent him from getting pregnant, and will probably prevent most common gynecologic problems, but such problems are not impossible as long as the actual organs are intact. He will continue to be vulnerable to STIs, and cancers of the female organs should remain a consideration.

A person who has transitioned from male to female (M to F) may have had plastic surgery to construct external female genitalia, but she will not have the internal organs. She will also remain vulnerable to STIs. She may feel more comfortable seeking general health care in a gynecological setting because of provider sensitivity, but will probably need minimal gynecological assessment and therapeutics.

Upon first meeting with a transgendered person, it is appropriate for a provider to ask in a very sensitive, nonjudgmental manner about how much of the total transition process the individual has already undergone and about plans for future additional transition procedures. Then the provider can update the information over time as appropriate.

Percussion: Levels I-IV
Auscultation: Levels I-IV

Percussion and auscultation are not included in a typical physical examination of the female reproductive organs, however as identified in the assessment level table on page 980, there may be instances where abdominal assessment techniques may be helpful.

DOCUMENTATION

Outpatient visit: Annual exam on an existing patient

Patient presenting for yearly physical stating "I think I want to try using the pill." No other complaints related to reproductive structures. She reports satisfaction with intercourse and has not experienced any pain or other difficulties concerning sexual activity. New male partner shortly after last visit 1 year ago, and has been using Today Sponge and condoms. Has never used hormonal contraceptives. Expresses concern that with more frequent intercourse, odds of pregnancy will increase; also some "irritation" today secondary to Today Sponge use, "and I might be smelly down there."

Menstrual triad: 13/31/4; denies pain, clotting, or heavy bleeding. Denies pain with urination; BM QOD without straining. Nulligravida. Monogamous relationship; no prior history per pt of STI or urinary problems in last year. Is able to identify major STIs and how to identify manifestations of them.

Pelvic Exam:

External: Mons with expected hair distribution (triangle) and no lesions noted. Labia hair removed via waxing per patient. External genitalia with typical female configuration. Labia majora equal, smooth without masses or lesions. Labia minora without lesions, smooth and moist. BUS (Bartholin's Urethra Skene's) no redness and swelling of area around glands, no pain with palpation and without any discharge. Internal: Vaginal rugae present, tissue deep pink and moist. Thin grey discharge seen on vaginal walls and pooled near posterior fornix. Cervix easily visualized; nulliparous in appearance without lesions or discharge. Pap smear for ThinPrep, GC/Chlamydia and swab for wet mount taken.

Bimanual: Uterus smooth, mobile. Anteverted. Adnexa palpable on left, not on right. Rectal exam deferred—no hemorrhoids noted visually.

Electronic Charting

Expectations of Electronic Charting

Electronic charting should accommodate the entire reproductive assessment, including related information such as sexual activity, birth control, and protection measures for STIs. Documentation should accommodate age-appropriate developmental assessments. Ideally, the system should accommodate modifiable graphics of the internal and external reproductive system.

Patients may be embarrassed about aspects of the reproductive assessment. Electronic charting should provide appropriate measures to protect patient privacy and confidentiality. Certain aspects such as sexually transmitted infections may have special data privacy protections, depending on your institution's policies.

Electronic charting systems are increasingly accommodating genomic information. Reproductive counseling may soon include counseling patients on the basis of genome-wide data stored in the EHR.

Comprehensive EHRs provide advanced features linking episodes of care such as routine examinations, prenatal visits, inpatient records, and neonatal records. Such EHRs may also provide decision support features that guide providers to use evidence-based standards or that provide alerts about specific risks (Jolles et al., 2012). Interoperability between outpatient and inpatient records has been shown to improve quality outcomes for women's reproductive health (Deily et al., 2013).

Limitations of Electronic Charting

While electronic charting is increasingly integrated into health care, the technology is not equally well developed in all areas. The particular charting system in use may or may not have structured documentation in place for all parts of the female reproductive assessment. Despite regulatory and funding initiatives, and evidence that electronic charting can support improved patient care in many aspects of health care, little research has been conducted about electronic health records in the areas of women's health and perinatal care (Jolles et al., 2012).

Documentation may need to be developed within your charting system, or you may need to document on unstructured forms such as free-text clinical notes. Unstructured documentation limits the ability to access data for longitudinal care, and to re-use data for research or quality improvement (Roth et al., 2009).

Summary

- Complete assessment of the female genital/reproductive system generally does not begin until puberty and the onset of menses. Postmenopause, reproductive function ceases; however, the need for assessment of the reproductive system does not change.
- The female genital/reproductive system consists of external structures and internal organs, which are primarily involved with reproductive functions. Anatomic and physiological alterations may be present that interfere or prevent the reproductive organs from functioning appropriately.
- Assessment of the female genital/reproductive structures and organs is carried out primarily through inspection and palpation. Examination of the internal structures requires the use of a vaginal speculum which provides for visualization of these structures.
- Expected findings of the female genital/reproductive structure and organs would be that they were correctly in place without any visual or felt evidence of pathological alterations.
- In addition to the standard elements of the history component, information related to the woman's sexuality is also obtained.
- Subjective and objective data obtained from the history and physical is documented in a way that correctly and appropriately describes the individual and unique characteristics of the female patient and are in agreement with each other.

Review Questions

1. The parent of a 12-year-old female tells the provider that she is concerned because her daughter is developing breasts. Which response would be most appropriate to give the mother?
   1. "Well, she is on the young side, isn't she? We will have her hormones checked."
   2. "Are you concerned that she will be having sex soon?"
   3. "The development of breasts in girls her age is typical."
   4. "This may be a sign that she is eating too many prepared foods."
2. A 42-year-old woman asks the provider if it is appropriate for her to stop using birth control because she hasn't had a period for about 8 months. How should the provider respond to this question?
   1. "No, menopause does not occur until age 50. You will need to continue to use birth control until then."
   2. "No, you would not be considered infertile until 12 months have passed since your last period."
   3. "Yes, if you feel that your periods have permanently stopped, then it is advisable to stop using birth control."
   4. "Yes, because it is unlikely that you would conceive if your periods have become irregular."
3. The provider is teaching a patient recently diagnosed with pelvic inflammatory disease (PID). The patient asks how she could have gotten this infection. What information should the provider give to the patient? (Select all that apply.)
   1. The infection may have been due to a droplet contact in a public restroom.
   2. The infection is most likely sexually transmitted caused by gonorrhea or Chlamydia.
   3. The female reproductive system is open, making the entry of the organism into the pelvis easy.
   4. Pelvic inflammatory disease has no definitive cause.
   5. The infection arises from normal flora of the reproductive tract entering the pelvis.

4. A student provider is asked to teach a high school health class about the birth process with a group of pregnant teens. Which structures would the student address as being part of the female internal reproductive tract through which the baby will pass during birth? (Select all that apply.)
   1. labia minora
   2. Bartholin's glands
   3. vaginal vestibule
   4. cervical os
   5. vagina
5. A woman tells the provider that she is concerned about her risk for ovarian cancer. How could the provider determine the woman's level of risk?
   1. Perform a speculum examination.
   2. Complete a comprehensive family history.
   3. Use the CAGE assessment to determine alcohol use.
   4. Palpate the patient's abdomen.
6. The provider is conducting a Level II physical assessment of the reproductive tract of an asymptomatic female. Which skills of examination would the provider utilize in conducting this examination? (Select all that apply.)
   1. inspection
   2. palpation
   3. direct percussion
   4. blunt percussion
   5. auscultation
7. When examining the reproductive tract of a female patient the provider suspects that the patient has an infection caused by Candida if the following is present on inspection?
   1. bloody drainage from the vagina
   2. watery discharge from the vagina, with an odor
   3. white, thick discharge from the vagina
   4. pelvic pain during the examination
8. The provider is conducting a speculum examination of a female patient's reproductive tract. The provider notes that the cervical os is irregular in shape and slitlike. The provider suspects that the patient
   1. has an infection.
   2. had a child.
   3. is pregnant.
   4. is a victim of sexual abuse.
9. The provider is about to conduct an interview with a young woman whose chief complaint is that she has not had a menstrual period in 6 months. Her pregnancy test is negative. Which question is important to ask this patient?
   1. "How old were you when your periods began?"
   2. "Do you smoke cigarettes?"
   3. "Can you tell me about your exercise habits?"
   4. "Do you have any allergies?"
10. The provider has completed an assessment of a female patient with a probable Bartholin's cyst. Which documentation by the provider is consistent with this diagnosis in this otherwise healthy patient?
    1. "Temperature 101 degrees F orally; patient complains of pain 8/10 on palpation of the lower abdomen."
    2. "Afebrile. Lesions noted around the cervical os on speculum examination. No complaints of pain."
    3. "Afebrile. Labia noted to be edematous on the right. Erythema noted in the area. Patient notes pain in the labial area."
    4. "Copious amounts of white, cheesy vaginal discharge. Patient in acute pain, 9/10 during palpation of the abdomen."

Conditions and Disorders

SEXUALLY TRANSMITTED INFECTIONS (STI)

Condyloma Acuminatum

Also called genital warts, these are wartlike lesions that result from HPV (types 6 and 11) infection. From a global perspective, HPV is the most common STI. There is equal distribution in genders with highest rates among 17–33 years of age.

Pathophysiology

- Basal layer of skin invaded by HPV virus; virus penetrates skin resulting in mucosal microabrasions.
- Virus enters a latent stage without any signs or symptoms and lasts from a month to years.
- When latent period ends, there is production of viral DNA, capsids, and particles that infect the host cells, which then develop into characteristic lesions.

Subjective Data

- Generally asymptomatic
- May be itching and bleeding at infection site

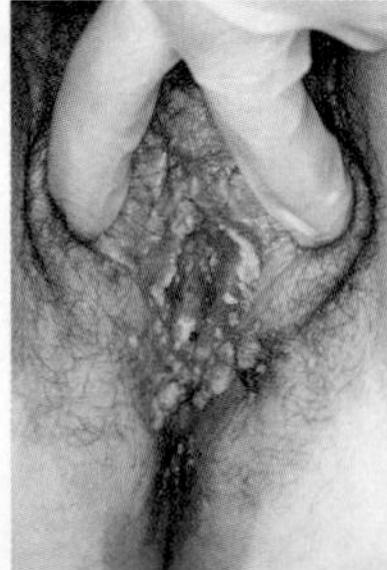

FIGURE 30-22 Genital warts
Source: Kallista Images/CMSP

Objective Data

- Flesh-colored, whitish pink to reddish brown discrete nodules/tumors
- Most common sites include vulva, cervix, perineum, and perianal regions.
- Nodules/tumors may occur singly or as clusters, which may enlarge to form cauliflower-like lesions.

Genital Herpes (Herpes Simplex)

This is a highly infectious viral invasion of the genital area. It is transmitted from individual to individual during sexual activity (genital or oral).

Pathophysiology

- Herpes simplex virus (HSV-1 or HSV-2) invades local cells and may or may not result in an immediate appearance of the infection.
- Once the virus invades a body, it remains there throughout one's lifetime. Most of the time it is inactive, but periodically becomes active and causes another outbreak. Each outbreak may be less severe and shorter in duration. The majority (85%) of infected individuals will experience recurring outbreaks.

Subjective Data

- Pain of variable intensity, decreasing with each incident

Other symptoms that may be present (commonly with initial instance) include the following:

- Fever, muscle aches, headaches, vaginal discharge, painful urination, swollen and tender lymph nodes

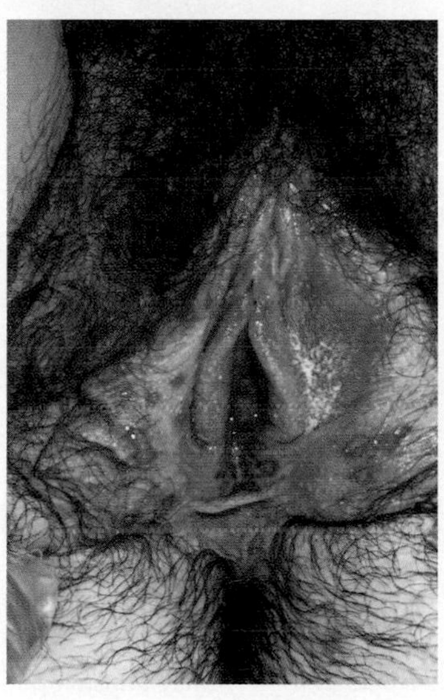

FIGURE 30-23 Genital herpes
Source: Wellcome Image Library/Custom Medical Stock

Objective Data

- Formation of blisters that open, forming tiny ulcers on the surface of the skin
- In females, lesions commonly in the vagina, but may appear around the os. (Internal lesions are not visible except with speculum.)

PRACTICE POINT: Condoms

The use of condoms during sexual activity does not completely prevent the spread of HSV as lesions may be located elsewhere in the genital area and not just on the penis. Even though an infected individual may not have manifestations of an outbreak, the virus can still be transmitted.

Syphilis

This is a sexually transmitted infection, caused by the bacteria *Treponema pallidum* that is usually passed from one to another during sexual activity, but can still be transmitted in the absence of symptoms. Untreated, syphilis generally progresses through three distinct stages.

Syphilis is still easily treated with penicillin, unlike other infectious diseases that are developing resistance to antibiotics.

Pathophysiology

- *T. pallidum* penetrates chafed skin or mucous membranes. Results in development of chancre at site of entry. Men are more likely to contract syphilis than women.

Subjective Data

- No significant symptoms during initial stage.

Objective Data

- Initial manifestation is the presence of a painless crater like chancre (lesion) at the site of infection, usually on the genitals. More obvious on penis and not obvious

- After disappearance of chancre, progresses into second stage; 4–10 weeks after initial lesion.
- The second stage is the latent stage and lasts about 1–2 years. There may be relapses associated with the symptoms of the second stage. After more than 2 years after the beginning of the latent phase, there may not be any symptoms and one is noninfectious; however it may be transmitted through blood transfusion.
- About one-third of individuals in the latent stage will progress into the third (tertiary) stage. This may not occur until years or decades later. In this stage, significant irreversible damage to the heart, skin, brain, and bones occurs.

- Multiple nonspecific symptoms: fever, joint pain, muscle aches, sore throat, flu like symptoms, headaches, loss of appetite, hair loss, swollen lymph nodes
- No specific symptoms except when relapse occurs.
- Symptoms dependent on organ(s) affected and severity of damage.

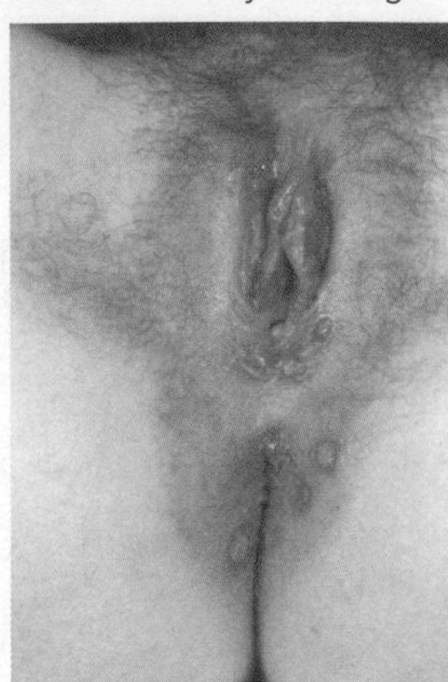

FIGURE 30-24 Syphilitic chancres
Source: CDC

on female is lesion in the vagina. Initial appearance about 2 weeks after infection, may last 3–6 weeks with spontaneous healing.

- Appearance of flat, round, or oval papules covered with gray exudate (condyloma latum), total body rash that includes palms/soles,
- Signs dependent on organ(s) affected and severity of damage.

Gonorrhea

This is one of the most common STI that is passed from person to person with sexual activity (genital, oral, anal). Rates of infection have decreased; however, it still remains the second-most common reportable disease in the United States. An infected woman may transmit gonorrhea to her newborn during vaginal delivery. *Nissereia gonorrhea* is developing resistance to conventional antibiotics and there is a major concern that eventually gonorrhea may become untreatable.

Pathophysiology

- Caused by infection with *Neisseria gonorrhea.*

Subjective Data

- Approximately 30%–40% of infected women have no symptoms.
- Sensation of needing to urinate often.
- Itching, burning of vagina with thick, yellow-green discharge
- Bleeding between periods

Objective Data

- Vaginal discharge
- Elevated white blood cell count

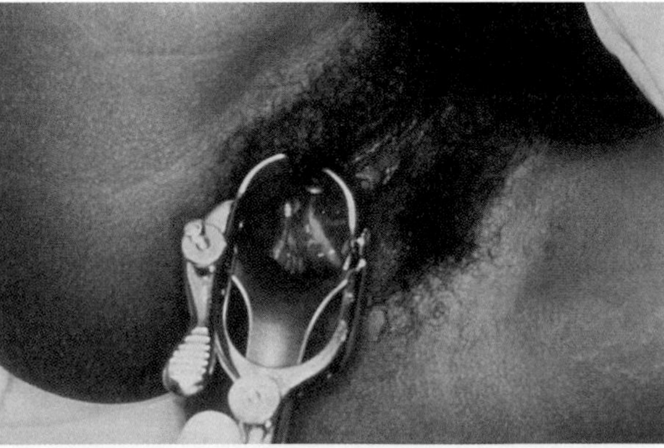

FIGURE 30-25 An infection of the cervix caused by gonorrhea
Source: CDC

Chlamydia (Mucopurulent Cervicitis)

This is the most common STI in the United States, with an estimated 2.8 million individuals affected. Young adults, 24 years and younger, are the most commonly affected group. Treatment with antibiotics results in 95% cure rate. In women, 10%–40% will progress to PID and 5% of women with PID will develop a type of liver disease (perihepatitis).

Pathophysiology

- *Chlamydia trachomatis* is the causative bacterium.
- In women, bacteria initially infect the cervix and urethra.

Subjective Data

Burning sensation during urination. If progresses to PID, symptoms associated with it including the following:

- Pelvic and/or abdominal pain
- Fever
- Unusual or heavy, foul smelling vaginal discharge
- Painful intercourse
- Painful urination
- Irregular menstrual cycles
- Abnormal uterine bleeding

Objective Data

- Purulent vaginal discharge with tenderness in genital area
- Skene's/Bartholin's glands may become inflamed/infected.

EXTERNAL CONDITIONS

Bartholin's Cyst

Also called **Bartholin's abscess**, this is a cyst that often forms as a result of inflammation or trauma. Approximately 2% of reproductive aged-women will experience swelling of one or both Bartholin's glands. There is no predominance in any particular ethnic group or race. *Neisseria gonorrhea* or *Chlamydia trachoma* frequently the cause of infection. *Escherichia coli* have also been implicated as a causative infectious agent.

Pathophysiology

- A Bartholin's cyst forms when the opening of the duct becomes obstructed, causing fluid to build up within the gland.
- Bartholin's abscess may be due to a primary infection of the gland or infection of the cyst.

Subjective Data

- Often asymptomatic unless it becomes quite large, then may cause pain and painful intercourse.
- Acute, rapid progression, vulvar pain when walking or standing, painful intercourse There may be a sudden relief of pain that is associated with a purulent discharge (spontaneous rupture).

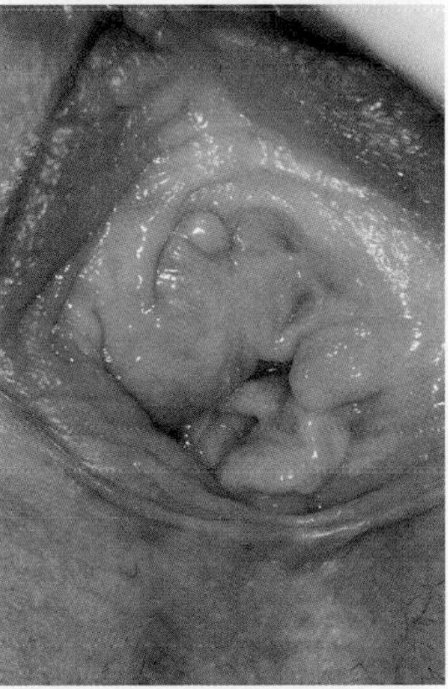

FIGURE 30-26 Bartholin's cyst
Source: Dr. P. Marazzi/Science Source

Objective Data

- Labial swelling on affected side
- Acute, painful, erythematous labial swelling Cellulitis may be present in some instances. May have fever, but not in healthy women.

INTERNAL CONDITIONS

Prolapsed Uterus

This is the collapse or herniation of uterus into or beyond the vagina.

Pathophysiology

- The muscles that support the uterus and maintain its position within the pelvic cavity often weaken due to childbirth or difficult deliveries. Additionally, the loss of estrogen with aging contributes to this weakening and as a result, the uterus may collapse (prolapse) into the vaginal canal.
- The degree of prolapse may be a slight sagging to falling completely through the vaginal canal, extending out of the vagina.

Subjective Data

- Sensation of fullness or pressure in pelvic area
- Low back pain
- Sensation of something coming out of vagina
- Painful intercourse
- Difficulty with urination or bowel movements
- Difficulty walking

Objective Data

Four stages of collapse:

- **First degree:** Cervix sags into the vagina.
- **Second degree:** Cervix adheres to the opening of the vagina.
- **Third degree:** Cervix protrudes through the vagina.
- **Fourth degree:** Entire uterus protrudes through the vagina and is completely visible.

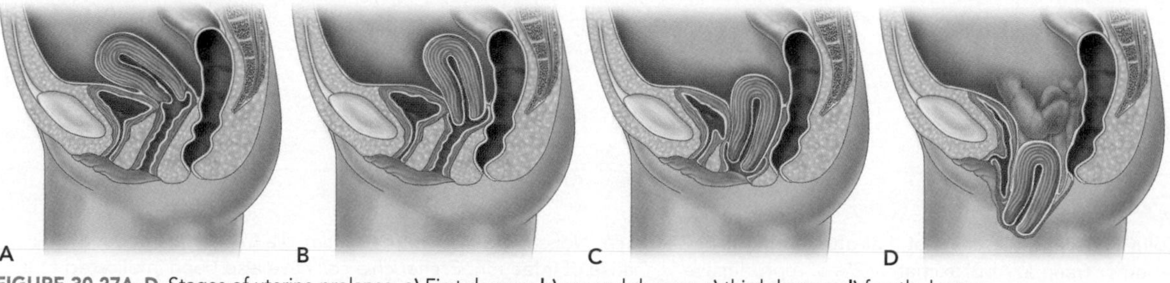

FIGURE 30-27A–D Stages of uterine prolapse. **a)** First degree; **b)** second degree; **c)** third degree; **d)** fourth degree

Endometriosis

This is the result of endometrial tissue that is distributed outside the uterus throughout the pelvic area, commonly the ovaries and bowel.

Pathophysiology

- The tissue responds to hormonal influence as if it were within the uterus causing it to enlarge, breakdown, and bleed.
- The bleeding tissue remains in the abdomen, causing inflammation, irritation, and eventually forms scar tissue.

Subjective Data

- Pain (menstrual, intercourse, bowel movements, urination)
- Bleeding (heavy periods, breakthrough)
- Infertility
- Fatigue, diarrhea, constipation, bloating, nausea (with menstrual cycle)

Objective Data

- No specific findings.
- With palpation, palpable cysts or nodules may have formed, which may be palpated if large enough.
- Diagnosis confirmed with laparoscopy.

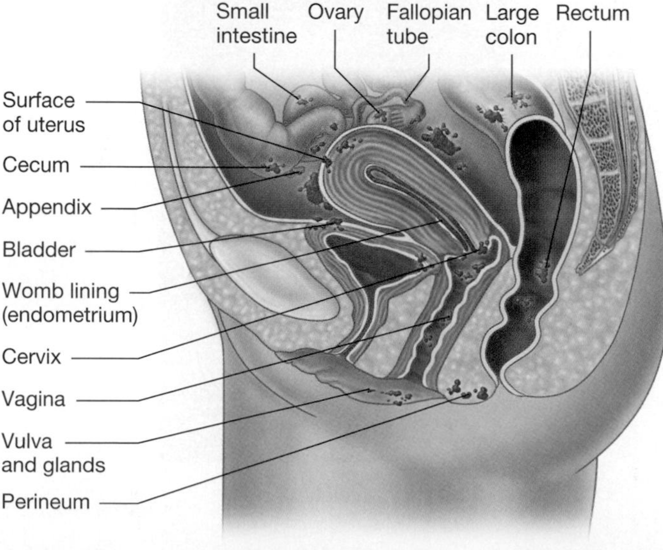

FIGURE 30-28 Sites of endometriosis

Rectocele

A rectocele is a collapse of the front wall of the rectum into the vaginal canal. The upright position of humans is one factor that allows for increased weight and pelvic pressure to lead to weakening of the pelvic muscles.

Pathophysiology

- A weakening of the thin wall of fibrous tissue (fascia) that separates the rectum from the vagina is the primary cause of a rectocele.
- The weakening is frequently related to childbirth or other processes that exert pressure on the fascia.

Subjective Data

- Difficulty with having a bowel movement with the need to push on the bulge in the vagina to help evacuate the rectum
- Sensation of fullness or pressure within the rectum along with the feeling that the rectum has not been completely evacuated after the bowel movement
- Sensation of loss of vaginal tone during intercourse

Objective Data

- Visualization of collapsed rectum into vagina during pelvic exam

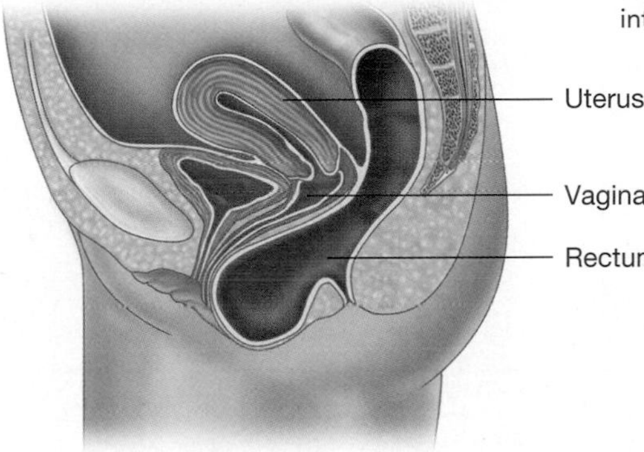

FIGURE 30-29 Rectocele

Cystocele

This is the collapse of the bladder into the vagina. Straining of the muscles during childbirth or with chronic constipation, violent coughing, and heavy lifting all contribute to weakening and stretching of the pelvic muscles.

Pathophysiology

- A weakness and stretching of the supportive tissue between the bladder and vagina allows for the collapse of the bladder into the vagina.

Subjective Data

- Sensation of fullness or pressure in pelvic area and vagina, particularly when standing for extended periods
- Increased discomfort when straining, coughing, bearing down, or lifting
- Sensation of not completely emptying bladder after urinating
- Frequent bladder infections
- Pain and/or urinary leakage during sexual intercourse

Objective Data

- Visualization of prolapsed bladder into vagina during pelvic exam

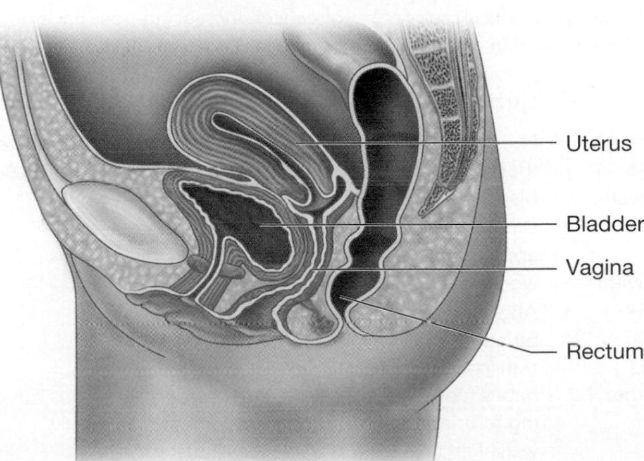

FIGURE 30-30 Cystocele

Pelvic Inflammatory Disease (PID)

This is an infection of a woman's pelvic organs including the uterus, Fallopian tubes, ovaries, and cervix. The two most common conditions associated with PID are sexually transmitted infections (STI)—gonorrhea and chlamydia. It may take as long as 2–3 months for manifestations of PID to occur. Over 1 million women are affected by PID annually with 25% of these requiring hospitalization. PID is a common cause of female infertility. The infection/inflammation of the Fallopian tubes creates the formation of scar tissue that can block the tubes and prevent an ovum from being fertilized by sperm as well as preventing it from being transported into the uterus. Sexually active greatest adolescent females and women younger than 25 are at the greatest risk for PID.

Pathophysiology

- Bacteria travel up from the vagina to the pelvic organs.
- Normal bacteria within vagina and on cervix may also be a cause of PID.

Subjective Data

- Symptoms are not always present and even when present, may be mild.
- Most common symptom is lower abdominal pain.

Other symptoms include the following:

- Fever (100.4 or >)
- Unusual or heavy, foul smelling vaginal discharge
- Painful intercourse
- Painful urination
- Irregular menstrual cycles
- Abnormal uterine bleeding
- Upper right abdomen pain

Objective Data

- Abnormal discharge from vagina
- Palpation of abscesses in the vicinity of ovaries and Fallopian tubes

Salpingitis

For all intents and purposes, salpingitis is synonymous with PID, although in some instances it may be a separate instance without infection/inflammation of other organs. It is described as either chronic or acute.

Pathophysiology

- Salpingitis is caused by the same organisms that cause PID.
- The process is the same as PID, beginning with a cervical or vaginal infection that ascends to the Fallopian tubes.
- Retrograde flow of blood from the uterus into Fallopian tubes during menstruation may carry organisms with it, initiating the infection/inflammation.

Subjective Data

- Constant lower quadrant pain, characteristically dull or cramping; may intensify with motion or intercourse
- Vaginal bleeding and/or discharge; nausea, vomiting, fever may also be present.

Objective Data

- Tenderness related to cervical motion/touch
- Tenderness in lower abdomen (adnexa) to palpation

Ovarian Cancer

This type of cancer is frequently undetected until it has spread within the pelvis and abdomen, which at this stage is difficult to treat. Women who are at high risk for developing ovarian cancer are those with inherited genetic mutation, family history, prior diagnosis of cancer, increasing age, have never been pregnant, and received hormone replacement therapy during menopause.

Pathophysiology

- Healthy cells mutate into cancer-producing cells that are nonfunctional, invasive, and grow rapidly. There are three types of ovarian cancers, depending on what type of cell cancer originated from.
- Epithelial—cancer cells from in the thin layer of tissue that covers the outside of the ovaries; most common type of ovarian cancer.
- Germ cell—cancer cells form in the egg producing cells; more common in younger women.
- Stromal—cancer cells form in ovarian tissue that secretes hormones (estrogen, progesterone, and testosterone).

Subjective Data

- Nonspecific symptoms that are commonly associated with digestive and bladder alterations
- When symptoms of ovarian cancer appear, they persist and gradually worsen.
- Abdominal pressure (fullness, swelling, bloating), pelvic pain, persistent indigestion (gas, nausea), changes in bowel habits (constipation), sensation of needing to urinate, loss of appetite, increasing waist line (tighter fitting clothes), lack of energy, low back pain

Objective Data

- Positive images of tumors on ultrasound
- Palpation of enlarged ovary in abdomen

Fibroids (Myomas)

Uterine fibroids are benign tumors that are composed of the same type of muscle as the uterine wall (myometrium). Despite this, they are much denser than the typical muscle. In most instances, if fibroids not causing any problems, there is no need to remove them. There is a rare cancerous form of fibroids (leiomysarcoma) that grows rapidly, and should be removed even if it's not causing problems. In some instances, the presence of fibroids may be a cause for recurrent miscarriages or making it difficult to achieve a pregnancy.

Pathophysiology

- The exact cause of fibroids is unknown. Suspected causes are genetic abnormalities, altered growth factor expression, vascular system abnormalities, and response of tissue to injury.
- Family history does seem to have a role in fibroid development.

Subjective Data

- Symptoms are related to number, size, and location of fibroids. Often there are no symptoms.
- If symptoms present, include heavy menstrual bleeding, prolonged menstrual bleeding, menstrual abdominal cramping, and pressure on bladder causing frequency, urgency, and incontinence with possible obstruction; rectal pressure/pain with bowel movements. Lower pelvic/abdominal pain.

Objective Data

- Presence of palpable firm, irregular tumors in abdomen during exam.

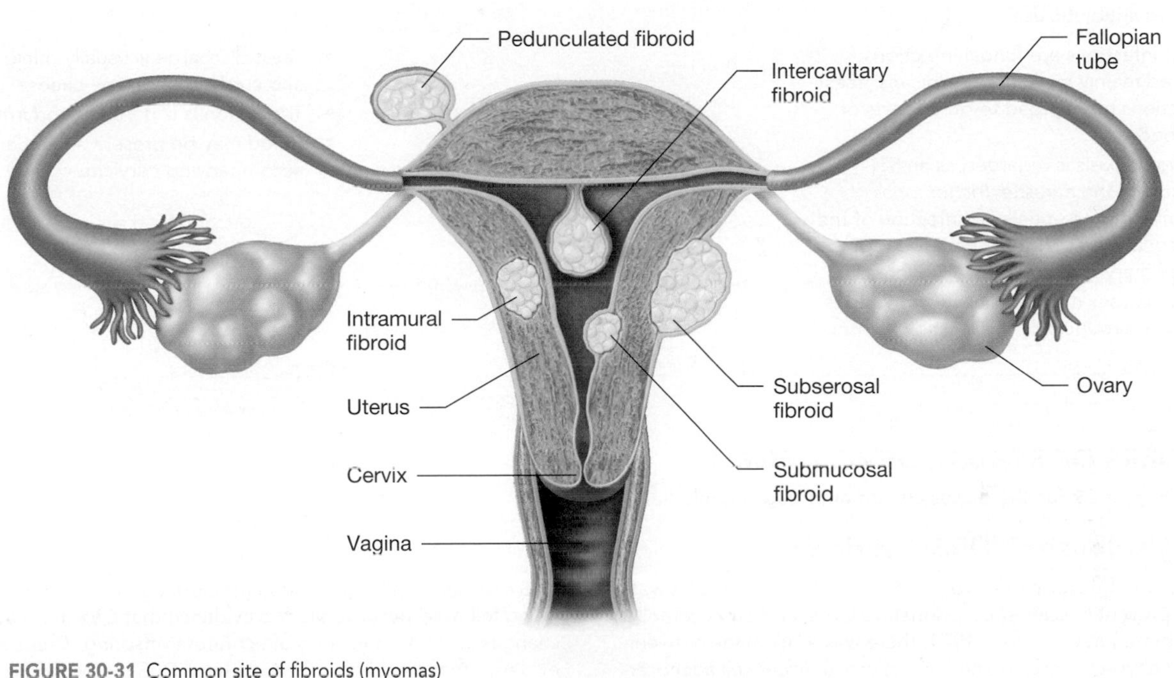

FIGURE 30-31 Common site of fibroids (myomas)

Atrophic Vaginitis

This is thinning and inflammation of the vaginal walls caused by a reduction of absence of estrogen during and after menopause.

Pathophysiology

- A physiologic reduction in estrogen production occurs prior to and throughout menopause. It also occurs with removal of or damage to the ovaries from radiation, chemotherapy, hormone therapy for breast cancer. It is also possible to occur during breastfeeding.

Subjective Data

- Vaginal dryness/itching, urinary urgency, burning, incontinence, infections; discomfort and/or bleeding with intercourse
- Possible vaginal discharge

Objective Data

- Vaginal mucosa becomes dry and pale, or could be reddened with the presence of petechiae and superficial erosions.
- There may also be vaginal discharge that may be white, gray, yellow/green, or blood tinged. It may also be watery, varying in amount, but not profuse.

Vaginitis (Vaginal Infections)

This is an inflammation of the vagina that is characterized by discharge, odor, irritation, or itching. There are many causes of vaginitis and frequently women use a variety of over the counter medications to self-treat. Vaginitis is frequently caused by infections, but may also be caused by hormonal changes and trauma.

Pathophysiology

- Most vaginitis is caused by three infections: bacterial vaginosis, yeast infection, and trichomoniasis.
- Yeast spores and the bacillus strains that cause BV (*Prevotella sp.* and *Mobiluncus sp., G. vaginalis,* and *Mycoplasma hominis*) can be found in minute amounts in normal vaginal flora if looked for. Infections occur when overgrowth happens secondary to vaginal pH changes that result in a more alkaline environment than normal and/or when normal flora are destroyed by factors such as antibiotic use.
- Yeast infections are fungal infections caused mainly by *Candida albicans*. Yeast infections may spread to other parts of the body.
- Trichomoniasis is regarded as an STI caused by the parasite *Trichomonas vaginlis*. It is essentially an infection of the urinary and genital tract, with the vagina the primary site of infection in women.
- Other causes may be allergies to various hygiene products or household cleansers.

Subjective Data

- Vaginal discharge
- Vaginal odor
- Vaginal irritation, or itching
- The sensation of burning with urination as well as itching around the outside of the vagina may also be present.

Objective Data

- Examination of the discharge under a microscope is necessary to diagnosis the problem accurately; however, many experienced providers, especially if laboratory support is not immediately available, will treat based only on symptoms and visual examination of the gross discharge.
- Abnormal vaginal discharge with an unpleasant (fishlike) odor. Discharge is usually white or gray and may be watery.
- Yeast discharge is usually think, white, and curdy like cottage cheese.
- Trichomonas is purulent and irritating.
- Blood may be present secondary to accompanying cervicitis.

DISORDERS OF SEXUAL DEVELOPMENT

Refer to Chapter 29 for the discussion on ambiguous genitalia.

Diethylstilbestrol (DES) Syndrome

DES is a synthetic form of estrogen. From 1940 to 1971, DES was used to prevent miscarriages, premature labor, and other complications in pregnant women. In 1971, there was a link made between DES and a type of cervical and vaginal cancer (clear cell adenocarcinoma) in a small group of women. However, DES was still used in European countries until the early 1980s, so immigrant women of childbearing age may have been exposed in utero after 1971 (Schrager & Potter, 2004). Female children of women who were given DES are also at risk for developing the same type of cancer as well as breast cancer. Fertility difficulties have also been linked to DES exposure. Third-generation (granddaughters) females are also being followed because there is evidence that DES may cause changes in DNA, which may affect future offspring. There is some evidence that men whose mothers used DES during pregnancy have an increased risk of testicular abnormalities, including undescended testicles or development of cysts in the epididymis (Palmer et al., 2009). It is still unclear whether these men have an increased risk for developing testicular or prostate cancer but there has not been any evidence that DES exposure causes infertility (Hatch, 2013).

Pathophysiology

- DES is an endocrine-disrupting chemical that is known to cause cancer, birth defects, and other abnormalities. These types of chemicals and their effects are most severe if exposure happens during fetal development.

Subjective Data

- Infertility
- Vaginal spotting
- Dysfunctional uterine bleeding
- Abnormal Pap smear
- Abnormal vaginal discharge
- Painful intercourse

Objective Data

- Cervical cell alterations
- Premature delivery
- Neonatal death
- Ectopic pregnancy
- Miscarriage (second trimester)
- Preeclampsia
- Structural alterations of uterus, vagina, and cervix

VULVAR DERMATOLOGIC CONDITIONS

Lichen Sclerosus, Lichen Planus, and Lichen Simplex Chronicus

- Lichen sclerosus is an inflammatory skin condition of unknown origin.
- Lichen planus is inflammation of mucous membranes in any part of the body including the vulvar and/or vaginal area.
- Lichen simplex chronicus is a skin condition that affects the vulva and many other areas of skin on the whole body.

Women with any of these conditions are often diagnosed after years of suffering because they think the conditions are one of the more common types of vaginitis and because many providers are not familiar with these problems. Treatment is lifelong. Flare-ups may happen. All are benign in the sense that none is cancerous or lead to cancer, but all can have significant, very negative impacts on the woman's life.

Pathophysiology	Subjective Data	Objective Data
• **Lichen sclerosus** seems to have a genetic component and is probably an autoimmune response to some irritant. It is most common in prepubertal girls or postmenopausal women so low estrogen is probably a mediating factor. Women with this condition often have other autoimmune disorders and/or thyroid conditions. It may be triggered by some prescription drugs including diuretics.	• Itching, burning, pain • The woman has often been treated (often numerous times) for other vulvar conditions like vaginal yeast without getting any relief. The condition may have gone on for years before the correct diagnosis is made.	• The vulvar skin tissue is characteristically white or silver, blanched, crinkly or shiny. The white area may be a small patch or may cover the whole area. A characteristic "figure-8" pattern may be seen. Skin changes secondary to itching including small fissures, swelling, excoriation, and purpura, may be seen. If the condition is long standing, there may be changes in the vulvar architecture including fusion of the labia minora and majora and burying the clitoral hood underneath scar tissue. The vagina is not affected. A biopsy is needed to confirm the diagnosis and to rule out vulvar cancer.
• Etiology of **lichen planus** is also unknown. It is an autoimmune disorder.	• Soreness, burning, itching, dyspareunia, dysuria, vaginal discharge. • The woman may also have these symptoms in other places with mucous membranes such as the mouth and gums.	• Bright red, eroded skin, which is very tender to touch. • There may be a lacy, white border around the area. Advanced cases may have the same architecture changes as Lichen sclerosus. A biopsy is needed for diagnosis.
• **Lichen simplex chronicus** is a chronic itch-scratch-itch-scratch cycle. The original trigger may or may not be present. The cycle may have begun years before the woman is seen.	• Intractable, uncontrollable itching, burning or pain	• Vulvar skin is thickened, edematous, hypertrophic, and leathery. Color varies, but the white patches of lichen scerlosus are not seen. Architecture remains normal. Biopsy not needed for diagnosis, but may be needed to rule out other conditions.

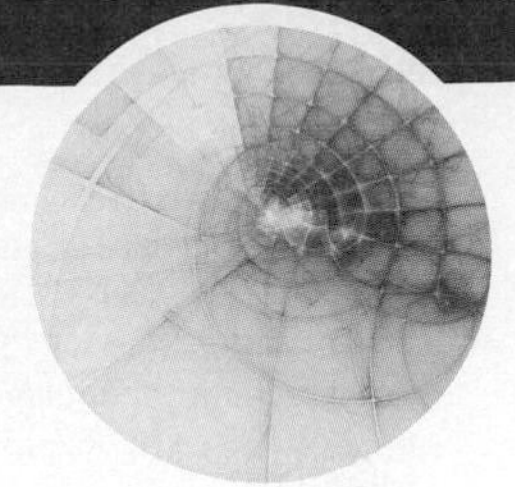

Appendix A

Chapter 1 References

* Indicates bibliographic reference

American Pain Foundation. (2010). Provisions from national pain care policy act included in health care reform bill to promote improved pain care. Retrieved June 17, 2010, from www.painfoundation.org

Cheatham, M. L. (2008). The death of George Washington: An end to the controversy. *The American Surgeon, 74*, 770–774.

Edwards, R. E., Daniel, M. A., Doleys, M., Fillingim, R. B., & Lowery, D. (2001). Ethnic difference in pain tolerance: Clinical implications for chronic pain; population. *Psychosomatic Medicine, 63*, 316–323.

Elliott, L. (2005). *Medieval Medicine and the plague* (pp. 316–323). New York, NY: Crabtree Publishing.

Giddens, J. F. (2007). A survey of physical assessment techniques performed by RNs: Lessons for nursing education. *Journal of Nursing Education, 46*(2).

Knox, R. (2010). The fading art of the physical exam. Retrieved September 12, 2012, from http://www.npr.org/templates/story/story.php?storyId=129931999&ps=cprs

Laine, C. (2002). The annual physical examination: Ritual or necessary routine? *Annals of Internal Medicine, 136*(9), 701–703.

Lambert, T. (2012). A brief history of medicine. Retrieved September 14, 2012, from http://www.localhistories.org/medicine.html

McCain, R. F. (1965). Nursing by assessment—not intuition. *American Journal of Nursing, 65*, 82–84.

Mehrotra, A., Zaslavsky, A. M., & Ayanian, J. Z. (2007). Preventive health examinations and preventive gynecological examinations in the United States. *Archives of Internal Medicine, 167*(17), 1876–1883.

Nelson-Hogan, D. (2008). Talking with Patricia Matthews-Juarez. *The Pain Practitioner, 18*(4), 8–11.

Payne, R. (2008). The role of culture, spirituality, and healing in the contexts of African-American culture and end-of-life care. *The Pain Practitioner, 18*(4), 14–16.

Prochazka, A. V., Lundahl, K., Pearson, W., Oboler, S. K., & Anderson, R. J. (2005). Support of evifence-based guidelines for the annual physical examination. *Archives of Internal Medicine, 165*(June 27), 1347–1352.

Robinson, L., Smith, M., & Segal, J. (2012). Healing emotional and psychological trauma: Symptoms, treatment, and recovery. Retrieved November,07, 2012, from http://www.helpguide.org/mental/emotional_psychological_trauma.htm

Secrest, J. A., Norwood, B. R., & DuMont, P. M. (2005). Physical assessment skills: A descriptive study of what is taught and what is practiced. *Journal of Professional Nursing, 21*(2), 114–118.

Sweet, V. (1999). Hildegard of bingen and the greening of medieval medicine. *Bulletin of the History of Medicin, 73*(3), 381–403.

Tiner, J. H. (1999). *Louis Pasteur–founder of modern Medicine* (2nd ed.) (p. 111). Milford: MI: Mott Media.

Vadakan, V.V. (2004). The asphyxiating and exsanguination death of George Washington. *The Permanente Journal, 8*(2), 76–79.

Verghese, A., Charlton, B. S., Cotter, B., & Kugler, J. (2011). A history of physical examination texts and the conception of bedside diagnosis. *Transactions of the American Clinical and Climatological Association, 122*, 290–307.

Chapter 2 References

Bekelman, D. B., Parry, C., Curlin, F. A., Yamashita, T.E., Fairclough, D. L., & Wamboldt, S. (2010). A comparison of two spirituality instruments and their relationship with depression and quality of life in chronic heart failure. *Journal of Pain and Symptom Management, 39*(3), 515–526.

Berlin, E.A., & Eisenberg, L. (1983). A teaching framework for cross-cultural health care. *The Western Journal of Medicine, 139*, 934–938.

California Health Advocates. (2012, 04/07). Are you practicing cultural humility? The key to success in cultural competence. *Medicare: Poilicy, Advocacy and Education*. Retrieved November 12, 2012, from http://www.cahealthadvocates.org/news/disparities/2007/are-you.html

Foster, J. (2009). Cultural humility and the importnce of long-term relationships in international partnerships. *Journal of Obstetrical Gynecologic and Neonatal Nursing, 38*(1), 100–107. doi: 10.1111/j.1552-6909.2008.00313.x

Fox, R.C. (2005). Cultural competence and the culture of medicine. *New England Journal of Medicine, 353*(13), 1316–1319.

Kleinman, A., Eisenberg, L., & Good, B. (1978). Culture, illness and care: Clinical lessons from anthropoloigic and cross-cultural research. *Annals of Internal Medicine, 88*, 251–258.

Office of Minority Health. (2010, 10/19/2005). What is cultural competency? Retrieved January 15, 2010, from http://minority health.hhs.gov/templates/browse aspx?iv=2%iv IID=11

Ondash, E., & Dibble, S. (2006). The importance of cultural awareness in patient care. *Nursezone.com*. Retrieved January 12, 2010, from http://www.nursezone.com/printArticle.expx?articleID=21922

Puchalski, C.M. (2001). The role of spirituality in health care. *BUMC Proceedings, 14*, 352–357.

Quappe, S., & Cantatore, S. (2005). What is cultural awareness, anyway? How do I build it? Retrieved January 12, 2010, from www.culturosity.com/articles/whatisculturalawareness

Spector, R.E. (2009). *Cultural diversity in health and illness* (7th ed.). Upper Saddle River: New Jersey: Prentice Hall.

Tanyi, R.A., McKenzie, M., & Chapek, C. (2009). How family practice physicians, nurse practitioners, and physician assistants incorporate spiritual care in practice. *Journal of the American Academy of Nurse Practitioners, 21*(2009), 690–697.

Tervalon, M., & Murray-Garcia, J. (1998). Cultural humility versus cultural competence: A critical distinction in defining physician training outcomes in multicultural education. *Journal of Health Care for the Poor and Underserved, 9*(2), 117–125.

U. S. Department of Health and Human Services. (2005). What is cultural competency?

*Weber, J., & Kelly, J. (2010). *Health assessment in nursing* (4th ed.). Philadelphia: Lippincott Williams & Wilkins.

Chapter 3 References

Abbasi, K. (2011). A riot of divergent thinking. *Journal of the Royal Society of Medicine, 104*, 391. doi: 10.1458/jrsm.2011.11k038

Ali, M. (n.d.). Intuition in servitude and analysis. Retrieved January 7, 2008, from www.majidalimd.com/intuitio.htm

Avis, M., & Freshwater, D. (2006). Evidence for practice, epistomology, and critical reflection. *Nursing Philosophy, 7*(4), 216–224.

Banning, M. (2007). A review of clinical decision making: Models and current research. *Journal of Clinical Nursing*. doi: 10.1111/j.1365-2702.2006.0179.x

Bednarz, T. F. (2012). Correctly framing problems pinpoints the right solution. *Leaders to Leaders* Retrieved November 26, 2012, from http://blog.majoriumbusinesspress.com/2012/04/12/correctly-framing-problems-pinpoints-the-right-solution/

Billay, D., Myrick, F., Luhanga, F., & Yonge, O. (2007). A pragmatic view of intuitive knowledge in nursing practice. *Nursing Forum, 42*(3), 147–155.

Bowen, J. L. (2006). Educational strategies to promote clinical diagnostic reasoning. *New England Journal of Medicine, 355*(21), 2217–2225.

Carnevali, D.L., & Thomas, M.D. (1993). *Diagnostic reasoning and treatment decision making in nursing*. Philadelphia: J.B. Lippincott.

Carpenito-Moyet, L.J. (2008). *Nursing diagnosis: Application to clinical practice*. Philadelphia: Lippincott Williams & Wilkins.

Crandall, B., & Wears, R.L. (2008). Expanding perspectives on misdiagnosis. *The American Journal of Medicine, 121*(5A [supplement]), S30–S33.

Crespo, K. E., Torres, J. E., & Recio, M. E. (2004). Reasoning process characteristics in the diagnostic skills of beginnner, competent, and expert dentists. *Journal of Dental Education, 68*(12).

Croskerry, P. (2003). The importance of cognitive errors in diagnosis and stragegies to minimize them. *Academic Medicine, 78*(8), 775–780.

Croskerry, P., & Norman, G. (2008). Overconfidence in clinical decision making. *The American Journal of Medicine, 121*(5A [supplement]), S24–S29.

Dillon, P.M. (2007). *Nursing health assessment: A critical thinking, case studies approach*. Philadelphia: F.A. Davis.

Elder, W., Rakel, D., Heitkemper, M., Hustedde, C., Harazduk, N., Gerik, S., & Haramati, A. (2007). Using complementary and alternative medicine curricular elements to foster medical student awareness. *Academic Medicine, 82*(10), 951–955.

Ely, J. W., Graber, M. L., & Croskerry, P. (2011). Checklists to reduce diagnostic errors. *Academic Medicine, 86*(3), 307–313.

Fletcher, L., & Carruthers, P. (2012). Metacognition and reasoning. *Philosophical Transactions of the Royal Society, 367*, 1366–1378. doi: 10.1098/rstb.2011.0413

Forneris, S. G., & Peden-McAlpine, C. (2007). Evaluation of a reflective learning intervention to improve critical thinking in novice nurses. *Journal of Advanced Nursing, 57*(4), 410–421.

Gigerenzer, G., & Gaissmaier, W. (2011). Heuristic decision making. *Annual Review of Psychology, 62*, 451–482. doi: 10.1146/annurev-psych-120709-145346

Graber, M. L., Franklin, N., & Gordon, R. (2005). Diagnostic error in internal medicine. *Journal of the American Medical Association, 165*(July 11), 1493–1499.

Green, C. (2000). *Critical thinking in nursing: Case studies across the curriculum*. Upper Saddle River:NJ: Prentice Hall Health.

Hare, W. (2004). Open-minded inquiry: A glossery of key concepts. *Inquiry: Critical Thinking Across Disciplines, 23*(3), 37–41.

Hoffman, K. A., Aitken, L. M., & Duffield, C. (2009). A comparison of novice and expert nurses' cue collection during clinical decision-making: Veral protocol analysis. *International Journal of Nursing Studies, 46*, 1335–1344.

Johnson, B. M., & Webber, P. B. (2005). *An introduction to theory and reasoning in nursing*. Philadelphia: Lippincott Williams & Wilkins.

Jolly, B., & Atkinson, K. (2009). To err is human. *Medical Education, 44*, 15–16.

Kuhn, G.J. (2002). Diagnostic errors. *Academic Emergency Medicine, 9*, 740–750.

Levett-Jones, T., Hoffman, K., Dempsey, J., Yeun-Sim Jeong, S., Noble, D., Norton, C. A., . . . Hickey, N. (2010). The "five rights" of clinical reasoning: An education model to enhance nursing student's ability to identify and manage clinically "at risk" patients. *Nurse Education Today, 30*, 515–520.

Mamede, S., & Schmidt, H.G. (2004). The structure of reflective practice in medicine. *Medical Education, 38*, 1302–130.

Mamede, S., Schmidt, H.G., & Rikers, R. (2007). Diagnostic errors and reflective practice in medicine. *Journal of Evaluation in Clinical Practice, 13*, 138–145.

Mann, K., Gordon, J., & MacLeod, A. (2009). Reflection and reflective practice in health professions education: A systematic review. *Advances in Health Science Education, 14*, 595–621.

Mast, M. S. (2007). On the importance of nonverbal communication in the physician–patient interaction. *Patient Education and Counseling, 67*, 315–318. doi: 10.1016.j.pec.2007.03.005

Moulton, C., Regher, G., Myopoulos, M., & MacRae, H.M. (2007). Slowing down when you should: A new model of expert judgment. *Academic Medicine, 82*(10 [supplement]), S109–S116.

Norman, G.R. (2010). Diagnostic error and clinical reasoning. *Medical Education, 44*, 94–100.

olde Hartman, T. C., & van Ravesteijn, H. J. (2008). 'Well doctor, it is all about how life is lived': Cues as a tool in the medical consultation. *Mental Health in Family Medicine, 5*, 183–187.

O'Reilly, P. (1993). Barriers to effective clinical decision making in nursing. Retrieved January 4, 2008, from www.cianhealth.nsw.gov.au/hospilic/stvincents/1993/a04.html

Paletz, S. B. F., & Peng, K. (2009). Problem finding and contradiction: Examining the relationship between naive dialectical thinking, ethnicity, and creativity. *Creativity Research Journal, 21*(2–3), 139–151. doi: 10.1080/10400410902858683

Paul, R., & Elder, L. (2001). *The minature guide to critial thinking*. Dillon Beach, CA: Foundation for Critical Thinking.

Paul, R., & Elder, L. (2012). *Critical thinking: Tools for taking charge of your learning and your life* (3rd ed.). Upper Saddle River: New Jersey: Prentice Hall.

Reason, J. (2000). Human error: Models and management. *British Medical Journal, 320*, 768–770.

Roter, D. L., Frankel, R. M., Hall, J. A., & Sluyter, D. (2006). The expression of emotion through nonverbal behavior in medical visits: Mechanisms and outcomes. *Journal of General Internal Medicine, 21*(Suppl), S28–S34. doi: 10.1111/j.1525-1497.2006.00306.x

Rudolph, J. W., & Morrison, J. B. (2008). Sidestepping superstitious learning, ambiguity, and other roadblocks: A feedback model of diagnostic problem solving. *The American Journal of Medicine, 121*(5A [supplement]), S34–S37.

Schiff, G. D. (2008). Minimizing diagnostic errors: The importance of follow-up and feedback. *The American Journal of Medicine, 121*(5A [supplement]), S38–S42.

Scott, I. (2009). Errors in clinical reasoning: Causes and remedial strategies. *British Medical Journal, 339*(4 July), 22–25.

Shin, R.S., Lee, J.H., Young, J., & Kim, K.H. (2006). Critical thinking dispositions in baccalaureate nursing students. *Journal of Advanced Nursing, 56*(2), 182–189.

Simmons, B. (2010). Clinical reasoning: Concept analysis. *Journal of Advanced Nursing, 66*(5), 1151–1158. doi: 10.1111/j.1365-2648.2010.05262.x

Simpson, E., & Courtney, M. (2007). A framework guiding critical thinking through reflective journal documentation: A middle eastern experience. *International Journal of Nursing Practice, 13*, 203–208.

Singh, H., Naik, A. D., Rao, R., & Petersen, L. A. (2007). Reducing diagnostic errors through effective communication: Harnessing the power of information technology. *Journal of General Internal Medicine, 23*(4), 489–494. doi: 10.1007/s11606-007-0393-z

Tanner, C. A. (2006). Thinking like a nurse: A research-based model of clinical judgment in nursing. *Journal of Nursing Education, 45*(6), 204–211.

Wilkinson, J.M. (2012). *Nursing process and critical thinking*. Upper Saddle River:NJ: Pearson.

Winters, B.D., Aswani, M.S., & Pronovost, P.J. (2011). Commentary: Reducing diagnostic errors: Another role for checklists? *Academic Medicine, 86*(3), 279–281.

Chapter 4 References

Beck, R. S., Daughtridge, R., & Sloane, P. D. (2002). Physician-patient communication in the primary care office: A systematic review. *Journal of the American Board of Family Practice, 15*(1), 25–38.

Bernstein, M. (2012). Teaching medical students about patient modesty. Retrieved from http://patientprivacyreview.blogspot.com/2012/01/teaching-medical-students-about-patient.html

*Brodaty, H., Kemp, N. M., & Low, L. (2004). Characteristics of the GPCOG, a screening tool for cognitive impairment. *International Journal of Geriatric Psychiatry, 19*, 870–874. doi: 10.1002/gps.1167

Coulenan, J. L., & Block, M. R. (2006). *The medical interview: Mastering skills for clinical practice* (5th ed.). Philadelphia: F.A. Davis.

Davis, M. A. (2009). A perspective on cultivating clinical empathy. *Complementary Therapies in Clinical Practice, 15*, 76–79. doi: 10.1016/j.ctcp.2009.01.001

Deering, C. G. (1999). To speak or not to speak: Self discolsure with patients. *American Journal of Nursing, 99*(1), 34–38.

Gany, F., Leng, J., Shapiro, E., Abramson, D., Motola, I., Shield, D. C., & Changrani, J. (2007). Patient satisfaction with different interpreting methods: A randomized controlled trial. *Journal of General Internal Medicine, 22*(suppl 2), 312–318. doi: 10.1007/s11606-007-0360-8

Goleman, D. (2001). Emotional intelligence: Issues in pardigm building. In C. Chernis & D. Goleman (Eds.). *The emotionally intelligent workplace* (pp. 13–26). San Francisco: Jossey-Bass.

Halpern, J. (2003). What is clinical empathy? *Journal of General Internal Medicine, 18*(8), 670–674. doi: 10.1046/j.1525-149732003.21017.x

Henderson, J. (2011). History of modesty, part 2. Retrieved November 11, 2012 from, http://patientprivacyreview.blogspot.com/2011/02/history-of-modesty-part-2.html

Hudelson, P. (2005). Improving patient-provider communication: Insights from interpreters. *Family Practice, 22*, 311–316.

Hull, S. K., & Broquet, K. (2007, June 2007). How to manage difficult patient encounters. *Family Practice Management Website.* Retrieved November 28, 2012, from www.aafp.org/fpm

Ioannidou, F., & Konstantikaki, V. (2008). Empathy and emotional intelligence? What is it really about? *International Journal of Caring Sciences, 1*(3), 118–123.

Karliner, L. S., Jacobs, E. A., Chen, A. H., & Mutha, S. (2007). Do professional interpreters improve cllinical care for patients with limited English profeciency? A systematic review of the literature. *Health Research and Educational Trust, 42*(2), 728–754.

*Levensky, E.R., Forcehimes, A., O"Donohue, W.T., & Beitz, K. (2007). Motivational interviewing. *American Journal of Nursing, 107*(10), 50–58.

Marck, P. (1990). Therapeutic reciprocity, a caring phenomenon. *Advances in Nursing Science, 13*(1), 49–59.

Olsen, P. (2007). Ethical cautions for nurses. *American Journal of Nursing, 107*(7), 75.

Pacala, J. T., & Yueh, B. (2012). Heaqring defecits in the older adult. *Journal of Amerrican Medical Association, 307*(11), 1185–1194.

*Rollnick, S., & Miller, W. R. (1995). What is motivational interviewing? *Behavioural and Cognitive Psychotherapy, 23*(4), 325–334.

Rosenberg, E., Leanza, Y., & Seller, R. (2007). Doctor-patient communication in primary care with an interpreter: Physician perceptions of professional and family interpreters. *Patient Education and Counseling, 67*, 286–292. doi: 10.1016/j.pec.2007.03.011

Ryde, K., Friedrichsen, M., & Strang, P. (2006). Crying: A for to balance emotions among cancer patients in a palliative home care. *Palliative and Supportive Care, 5*, 51–59. doi: 10.1017/S1478951507070071

Selph, R. B., Shiang, J., Engelberg, R., Curtis, J. R., & White, D. B. (2008). Empathy and life support decisions in the intensive care units. *Journal of General Internal Medicine, 23*(9), 1311–1317. doi: 10.1007/s11606-008-0643-8

Smith, R. C. (2002). *Patient-centered interviewing: An evidence-based method* (2nd ed.). Philadelphia: Lippincott Williams & Wilkins.

Stratton, T. D., Elam, C. L., Murphy-Spencer, C. L., & Quinlavin, S. L. (2005). Emotional intelligence and clinical skills: Preliminary results from a comprehensive clinical performance evaluation. *Academic Medicine, 80*(10 supplement), S34–S37.

Vivaldelli, J. (2007). Therapeutic reciprocity: A union through pain. *American Journal of Nursing, 107*, 74–76.

Chapter 5 References

Achkar, E. (2006). The death of the chief complaint or how gerd replaced heartburn. *American Journal of Gastroenterology, 101*, 1719–1720.

Anderson, R. S., Hansen, R. P., Sondergaard, J., & Bro, F. (2008). Learning based on ptient case reviews: An interview study. *BMC Medical Education, 8*(43). doi: 10.1186/1472-6920-8-43

Barrier, P. A., Li, J.C., & Jensen, N. M. (2003). Two words to improve physician–patient communication: What else? *Mayo Clinic Proceedings, 78*, 211–214.

Bell, R. A., Kravitz, R. L., Thom, D., Krupat, E., & Azari, R. (2002). Unmet expectations for care and the patient-physician relationship. *Journal of General Internal Medicine, 17*, 817–824.

Benbassat, J., & Baumal, R. (2004). What is empathy, and how can it be promoted during clinical clerkships? *Academic Medicine, 79*(9), 832–839.

Dwamena, F. C., Fortin VI, A. H., & Smith, R. C. (2005). Patient-centered interviewing. In L. M. Tierney & M. C. Henderson (Eds.). *The patient history: Evidence-based approach* (pp. 9–16). New York: McGraw Hill Medical.

Dyche, L., & Swiderski, D. (2005). The effect of physician solicitation on ability to identify patient concerns. *Journal of General Internal Medicine, 20*, 267–270. doi: 10.1111/j.1525-1497.2005.40266.x

Fitzgerald, F. T. (2005). History: Art and science. In L. M. Tierney Jr. & M. C. Henderson (Eds.), *The patient history: Evidence-based approach* (pp. 3–4). New York: Lange Medical Books/McGraw Hill.

Fortin VI, A. H., Dwamena, F. C., Frankel, R. M., & Smith, R. C. (2012). *Smith's patient centered interviewing: An evidence-based method* (3rd ed.). New York: McGraw Hill Medical.

Fortin VI, A. H., Dwamena, F. C., & Smith, R. C. (2012, 11/08/11). Patient-centered interviewing. *UpToDate*. Retrieved December 12, 2012, from http://www.uptodate.com/contents/patient-centered-interviewing

Franzini, L., Taylor, W., Elliott, M. N., Cuccaro, P., Tortolero, S. R., Gilliland, M. J., . . . Schuster, M. A. (2010). Neighborhood characteristics favorable to outdoor physical activity: Disparities by socioeconomic and ratial/ethnic composition. *Health and Place, 16*, 267–274. doi: 10.1016/j.healthplace.2009.10.009

Gordon, M. (2009). *Manual of nursing diagnosis* (12th ed.). Sudbury, MA: Jones and Bartlett.

Halpern, J. (2012). Gathering the patient's story and clinical empathy. *The Permanente Journal, 16*(1).

Haskard-Zolnierek, K. B., & DiMatteo, M. R. (2009). Physician communication and patient adherence to treatment: A meta-analaysis. *Medical Care, 47*(8), 826–834. doi: 10.1097/MLR.0b013e31819a5acc.

Hatem, D. S., Barrett, S. V., Hewson, M., Steele, D., Purwono, U., & Smith, R. (2007). Teaching the medical interview: Methods and key learning issues in a faculty development course. *Journal of General Internal Medicine, 22*(12), 18–24. doi: 10.1007/s11606-007-0408-9

Hupcey, J. E. (2000). Feeling safe: The psychosocial needs of ICU patients. *Journal of Nursing Scholarship, 32*(4), 361–367.

Kravitz, H. L., & Kravitz, R.L. (2005). Subtleties of medical history taking. In L. M. Tierney & M. C. Henderson (Eds.). *The patient history: Evidence-based approach* (pp. 5–7). New York. McGraw Hill Medical.

Lein, C., & Wills, C.E. (2007). Using patient-centered interviewing skills to manage complex patient encounters in primary care. *Journal of the American Academy of Nurse Practitioners, 19*, 215–220. doi: 10.1111/j.1745-7599.2007.00217.x

Lyles, J. S., Dwamena, F. C., Lein, C., & Smith, R. C. (2001). Evidence-based patient-centered interviewing. *Journal of Clinical Outcomes Medicine, 8*(7), 28–34.

Margalit, A. P., Glick, S. M., Bengassat, J., & Cohen, A. (2004). Effect of a biopsychosocial approach on patient satisfaction and patterns of care. *Journal of General Internal Medicine, 19*, 485–491.

Meriläinen, M., Kyngäs, H., & Ala-Kokko, T. (2010). 24-hour intensive care: An observational study of an environment and events. *Intensive and Critical Care Nursing, 26*, 246–253. doi: 10.1016/j.iccn.2010.06.003

Pollack, K. I., Alexander, m S. C., Tulkdy, J. A., Lyna, P., Coffman, C. J., Dolor, R. J., . . . Ostbye, T. (2011). Physician empathy and listening: Assciations with patient satisfaction and autonomy. *Journal of the American Board of Family Medicine, 24*(6), 665–672. doi: 10.3100/jabfm.2011.06.110025

Quine, S., & Morrell, S. (2008). Feeling sale in one's neighbourhood: Variation by location among older australians. *Australian Journal of Rural Health, 16*, 115–116. doi: 10.1111/j.1440-1584.2008.00960.x

Rouf, E., Chumley, H., & Dobbie, A. (2009). Patient-centered interviewing and student performance in a comprhensive clinical skills examination: Is there an association? *Patient Education and Counseling, 754*, 11–15. doi: 10.1016/j.pec.2008.09.016

Schapira, L., Tulsky, J., Buckman, R., & Pollack, K. I. (2008). Communication: What do patients want and need? *Journal of Oncology Practice, 4*(5). doi:10.1200/JOP.0856501

Smith, R.C. (2002). *Patient-centered interviewing: An evidence-based method* (2nd ed.). Philadelphia: Lippincott Williams & Wilkins.

Stewart, M., Brown, J. B., Donner, A., McWhinney, I. R., Oats, J., Weston, W. W., & Jordan, J. (2000). The impact of patient-centered care on outcomes. *The Journal of Family Practice, 49*(9), 796–804.

Strayer, D.L., Drews, F.A., & Crouch, D.J. (2006). A comparison of the cell phone driver and the drunk driver. *Human Factors, 48*(2), 381–391.

*Wilkinson, J.M. (2012). *Nursing process and critical thinking.* Upper Saddle River:NJ: Pearson.

Chapter 6 References

Anderson, R. C., Fagan, M. J., & Sebastian, J. (2001). Teaching the students the art and science of physical diagnosis. *The American Journal of Medicine, 110*(April 1), 419–423.

Duvivier, R. J., van Dalen, J., Muijtjens, A. M., Moulaert, V., van der Vleuten, C., & Scherpbier, A. (2011). The role of deliberate practice in the acquisition of clinical skills. *BMC Medical Education, 11:101*. doi: 10.1186/1472-6920-11-101

Feddock, C. A. (2007). The lost art of clinical skills. *The American Journal of Medicine, 120*(4), 374–378. doi: 10.1016/j.amjmed.2007.01.023

Garden, G. (2005). Physical examination in psychiatric practice. *Advances in Psychiatric Treatment, 11*, 142–149. doi: 10.1192/apt.11.2.142

Junger, J., Schafer, S., Roth, C., Shchellerberg, D., Ben-David, M. F., & Nikendi, C. (2005). Effects of basic clinical skills training on objective structured clinical examination performance. *Medical Education, 39*, 1015–1020. doi: 10.1111/j.1365-2929-2005.02266.x

Omori, D. M., Wong, R. Y., Antonelli, M. A. S., & Hemmer, P. A. (2005). Introduction to clinical medicine: A time for consensus and integration. *The American Journal of Medicine, 118*(2), 189–194. doi: 10.1016/j.amjmed.2004.11.017

Chapter 7 References

Al-Majid, S., & Waters, H. (2008). The biological mechanisms of cancer-related skeletal muscle wasting: The role of progressive resistance exercise. *Biological Research in Nursing, 10*(1), 7–20.

Alvarez, N. (2009, 6/16/2009). Tremors *e Medicine Health*. Retrieved December 21, 2009, from http://www.emedicinehealth.com/script/main.art.asp?articlekey=101182&pf=3&page=1

Brannon, G. E. (2009, Feb 4, 2008). History and mental status examination. *eMedicine from WebMD*. Retrieved December 30, 2009, from http://emedicine.medscape.com/article/293402-pring

Brodaty, H., Kemp, N. M., & Low, L. (2004). Characteristics of the gpcog, a screening tool for cognitive impairment. *International Journal of Geriatric Psychiatry, 19*, 870–874. doi: 10.1002/gps.1167

Colberg, S., Somma, C., & Sechrist, S. (2008). Physical activity participation may offset some of the negative impact of diabetes on cognitive function. *Journal of the American Medical Directors Association, 9*(6), 434–438.

Evans, B., Crogan, N., & Greenberg, E. (2008). Lessons learned in clinical research: Using the mmse with older mexican american nursing home residents. *Journal of the American Psychiatric Nurses Association 14*, 373–378.

Fearon, K, Strasser, F., Anker, S.D., Bosaeus, I., Bruera, E., Fainsinge, R.L., . . . Baracos, V.E. (2011). Definition and classification of cancer cachexia: An international consensus. *Lancet Oncology, 12*, 489–495. doi: 10.1016/S1470-2045(10)70218-7

Feldt, K., & Oh, H. (2000). Pain and hip fracture outcomes for older adults. *Orthopaedic Nursing, 19*(6), 35–44.

Folstein, M., Folstein, M., & McHugh, P. (1975). Mini-mental state: A practical method of grading the cognitive state of patients for the clinician. *Journal of Psychiatric Research, 12*, 189–198.

*Galvin, J. E., Roe, C. M., Powlishta, K. K., Coats, M. A., Muich, S. J., Grant, E., Morris, J. C. (2005). The ad8: A brief informant interview to detect dementia. *Neurology, 65*(August), 559–564. doi: 10.1212/01.wnl.0000172958.95282.2a

Galvin, J. E., & Sadowsky, C. H. (2012). Practical guidelines for the recognition and diagnosis of dementia. *Journal of the American Board of Family Medicine, 25*(3), 367–382. doi: 10.3122/jabfm.2012.03.100181

Hawlay, J.S. (2011, 06/06/2011). Pediatric tourette syndrome. *Medscape Reference Drugs, Diseases & Procedures*. Retrieved July 8, 2011, from http://emedicine.medscape.com/article/289457-overview

Kneisl, C. R., & Trigoboff, E. (2013). *Contemporary psychiatric-mental health nursing* (third ed.). Upper Saddle River, NJ: Pearson.

Lenk, K., Schuler, G., & Adams, V. (2010). Skeletal muscle wasting in cachexia and sarcopenia:

Molecular pathophysiology and impact of exercise training. *Journal of Cachexia, Sarcopenia and Muscle, 1*, 9–21. doi: 10.1007/s13539-010-0007-1

Maddigan, S., Farris, K., Keating, N., Wiens, C., & Johnson, J. (2003). Predictors of older adults' capacity for medication management in a self-medication program: A retrospective chart review. *Journal of Aging & Health, 15*(2), 332–352.

Mitchell, A. J. (2009). A meta-analysis of the accuracy of the mini-mental state examination in the detection of dementia and mild cognitive impairment. *Journal of Psychiatric Research, 43*, 411–431. doi: 10.1016/j.psychires.2008.04.014

Olai, L., Omne-Ponten, M., Borgquist, L., & Svardsudd, K. (2007). Prognosis assessment in stroke patients at discharge from hospital. *Age & Ageing, 36*(2), 184–189.

Parker, C., & Philip, I. .(2004). Screening for cognitive impairment among older people in black and minority ethnic groups. *Age & Ageing, 33*(5), 5447–5452.

Resnick, B. (2003). Health promotion practices of older adults: Model testing. *Public Health Nursing, 20*(1), 2–12.

Satre, D., Knight, B., Dickson-Fuhrmann, E., & Jarvik, L. (2004). Substance abuse treatment initiation among older adults in the get smart program: Effects of depression and cognitive status. *Aging & Mental Health, 8*(4), 346–354.

Scafuza, M., Almeida, O. P., Vallada, H. P., Tasse, W. A., & Menezes, P. R. (2009). Limitations of the mini-mental state examination for screening dementia in a community with low socioeconomic status. *European Archives of Psychiatry and Clinical Neuroscience, 259*, 8–15. doi: 10.1007/s00406-008-0827-6

Tariq, S. H., Tumosa, N., Chibnall, J. T., Perry III, H. M., & Morley, J. E. (2006). The Saint Louis University mental status (slums) examination for detecting mild cognitive impiarment and dementia is more sensitive than the mini-mental status examination (mmse): A pilot study. *American Journal of Geriatric Psychiatry, 14*, 900–910.

Townsend, M. C. (2009). Mental status assessment. In M. C. Townsend (Ed.), *Psychiatric mental health nursing: Concepts in evidence-based practice*. Philadelphia: F.A.Davis.

University of Portsmouth. (2008). Learning from the dead: What facial muscles can tell us about our emotion. *ScienceDaily.* Retrieved January 06, 2009, from http://www.sciencedaily.com/releases/2008/06/080616205044.htm

Waller, B.M., Cray, J.J., & Burrows, A.M. (2008). Selection for universal facial emotion. *Emotion, Jun 8*(3), 435–439.

Wood, R., Giuliano, K., Bignell, C., & Pritham, W. (2006). Assessing cognitive ability in research: Use of mmse with minority populations and elderly adults with low education levels. *Journal of Gerontological Nursing, 32*(4), 45–54.

Chapter 8 References

Akuma, A. O. (Jordan, S.). Pain management in neonates; a survey of nurses and doctors. *Journal of Advanced Nursing, 68*(6), 1288–1301. doi: 10.1111/j.1365-2648.2011.0587.x

Al-Atiyyat, N. M. H. (2009). Cultural diversity and cancer pain. *Journal of Hospice and Palliative Nursing, 11*(3), 154–164.

American Pain Foundation. (2010). Provisions from national pain care policy act included in health care reform bill to promote improved pain care. Retrieved June 17, 2010, from www.painfoundation.org

Anand, K. J. S. (2013). Assessment of neonatal pain. *UpToDate.* http://www.uptodate.com/contents/assessment-of-neonatal-pain?topic

Argoff, C. E., & Carberg, B. H. (2005). Chronic pain management in the elderly: Linking mechanisms and guidelines to the realities of clinical practice. *Geriatrics: Better Medicine for Midlife and Beyond.* Retrieved January 11, 2013, from http://geriatrics.modernmedicine.com/geriatrics/data/articlestandard/geriatrics/452005/193711/article.pdf

Arif-Rahu, M., Fisher, D., & Matsuda, Y. (2012). Biobehavioral measures for pain in the pediatric patient. *Pain Management Nursing, 13*(3), 157–168. doi: 10.1016/j.pmn.2010.10.036

Badr, L. K., Abdallah, B., Hawari, M., Sidani, S., Kassar, M., Nakad, P., & Breidi, J. (2010). Determinants of premature infant pain responses to heel sticks. *Pediatric Nursing, 36*(3), 129–136.

Baker, T. A., & Green, C. R. (2005). Intrarace differences among black and white americans presenting for chronic pain management: The influence of age, physical health, and psychosocial factors. *Pain Medicine, 6*(1), 29–38.

Beggs, S., Currie, G., Salter, M. W., Fitzgerald, M., & Walker, S. M. (2011). Priming of adult pain responses by neonatal pain experience: Maintenance by central neuroimmune activity. *Brain, 135*(2), 404–417. doi: 10.1093/brain/awr288

Breivik, H., Borchgrevink, P.C., Allen, S.M., Rosseland, L.A., Romundstad, L., Breivik, E.K., . . . Stubhaug, A. (2008). Assessment of pain. *British Journal of Anaesthesia, 101*(1), 17–24.

Callin, S., & Bennett, M.I. (2008). Assessment of neuropathic pain. *Continuing Education in Anaesthesia, Critical Care & Pain, 8*(6), 210–213. doi: 10.1093/bjaceaccp/mkn037

Cavalieri, T. A. (2007). Managing pain in geriatric paitnets. *Journal of the American Osteopathic Association, 107*(supp 4), ES10–ES16.

Chen, H., Lamer, T. J., Rho, R. H., Marshall, K. A., Sitzman, B. T., Ghazi, S. M., & Brewer, R. P. (2004). Contemporary management of neuropathic pain for the primary care physician. *Mayo Clinic Proceedings, 79*(12), 1533–1545.

Cherny, N. I. (2007). Cancer pain: Principles of assessment and syndromes. In A. M. Berger, J. J. L. Shuster & J. H. V. Roenn (Eds.). *Principles and practice of palliative care and supportive oncology* (3rd ed.) (pp. 3–26). Philadelphia: Lippincott Williams & Wilkins.

Cignacco, E., Hamers, J., vanLingen, R. A., Stoffel, L., Buchi, S., Muller, R., . . . Nelle, M. (2009). Neonatal procedural pain exposure and pain management in ventilated preterm infants during the first 14 days of life. *Swiss Medical Weekly, 139*(15–16), 226–232.

Davis, C. (2011, 04/19/2011). *Fever in adults.* Retrieved June 27, 2011, from http://www.emedicinehealth.com/fever_in_adults/article_em.htm

Diaz, M., & Becker, D. E. (2010). Thermoregulation: Physiological and clinical considerations during sedation and general anesthesia. *Anesthesia Progress, 57*(1), 25–33.

Dubin, A. E., & Patapoutian, A. (2010). Nociceptors: The sensors of the pain pathway. *The Journal of Clinical Investigation, 120*(11), 3760–3772. doi: 10.1172/JCI42843

Elliott, D. (2009). Pain management in the elderly. *Practical Pain Management, 9*. http://www.practicalpainmanagement.com

Giamberadino, M. A. (2005). Visceral pain. *Pain Clinical Updates (International Association for the Study of Pain), 13*(6), 1–6.

Gordon, D.B., Dahl, J.L., Miaskowski, C., McCarberg, B., Todd, K.H., Paice, J.A., . . . Carr, D.B. (2005). American pain society recommendation for improving the quality of acute and cancer pain management. *Archives of Internal Medicine, 165*, 1574–1580.

Gyland, E. A. (2012). Infant pain assessment: A quality improvement project in a level III neonatal intensive care unit in northeast Florida. *Newborn & Infant Nursing Reviews, 12*(1), 44–50. doi: 10.1053/j.nainr.2011.12.007

Haanpaa, M., & Treede, R. (2010). Diagnosis and classification of neuropathic pain. *Pain Clinical Updates (International Association for the Study of Pain), 18*(7), 1–6.

Hastie, B. A., Riley, J. L., & Fillingim, R. B. (2005). Ethnic diufferences and responses to pain in healthy young adults. *Pain Medicine, 6*(1), 61–71.

Helms, J. E., & Barone, C. L. (2008). Physiology and treatment of pain. *Critical Care Nurse, 28*(6), 38–50.

Hicks, R. (2013, 05/28/2012). Normal body temperature. *Boots WebMD.* Retrieved January 2, 2013, from http://www/webmd.boots.com/a-to-zguides/normal-body-temperature

Hildebrandt, B., Wust, P., Ahlers, O., Dieing, A., Sreenivasa, G., Kerner, T., . . . Riess, H. (2002). The cellular and molecular basis of hyperthermia. *Critical Reviews in Oncology/Hematology, 43*, 33–56.

Hintzsche, H., Riese, T., & Stopper, H. (2012). Hyperthermia-induced micronucleus formation in a human keratinocyte cell line. *Mutation Research, 738–739*, 71–74. doi: 10.1016/j.mrfmmmm.2012.08.004

Huether, S. E., & Defriez, C. B. (2006). Pain, temperature regulation, sleep, and sensory function. In K. L. McCance & S. E. Huether (Eds.), *Pathophysiology: The Biological Basis for Disease in Adults and Children* (pp. 447–489). St. Louis: Elsevier Mosby.

Jensen, M. P., Dworkin, R. H., Gammaitoni, A. R., Olaleye, D. O., Oleka, N., & Galer, B. S. (2005). Assessment of pain quality in chronic neuropathic and nociceptive pain clinical trials with the neuropathic pain scale. *The Journal of Pain, 6*(2), 98–106.

Jermyn, R. T., Janora, D. M., & Surve, S. A. (2010). Assessment and classification of pain in the elderly patient. *Clinical Geriatrics, 18*(8), 16–19.

Knochel, J.P. (2010, February, 2010). Heatstroke. *Heatillness: Merck Manual professional* Retrieved May 20, 2010, from http://www.merck.com/mmpe/sec21/ch318/ch318d.html

Lago, P., Garetti, E., Merazzi, D., Pieragostini, L., Ancora, G., Pirelli, A., & Bellieni, C. V. (2009). Guidelines for procedural pain in the newborn. *Acta Paediatrica, 98*, 932–939. doi: 10.1111/j.1651-2227.2009.0129.x

Lasch, K.E. (2002). Culture and pain. *Pain Clinical Updates (International Association for the Study of Pain), 10*(5). Retrieved from http://www.iasp-pain.org/AM/AMTemplate.cfm?Section=Home&CONTENTID=7578&TEMPLATE=/CM/ContentDisplay.cfm&SECTION=Home

*Lepock, J. P. (2003). Cellular effects of hyperthermia: Relevance to the minimum dose for thermal damage. *International Journal of Hyperthermia, 19*(3), 252–266.

Litman, R. S. (2013, 08/27/2012). Susceptibility to malignant hyperthermia. *Up To Date.* Retrieved January 06, 2013, from http://www.uptodate.com/contents/susceptibility-to-malignant-hyperthermia

Litman, R. S., Flood, C.D., Kaplan, R. F., Kim, Y. L., & Tobin, J. R. (2008). Postoperative malignant hyperthermia. *Anesthesiology, 109*(5), 825–829.

Lowery, C. L., Hardman, M. P., Manning, N., Clancy, B., Hall, R. W., & ANand, K. J. S. (2007). Neurodevelopmental changes of fetal pain. *Seminars in Perinatology, 31*, 275–282. doi: 10.1053/j.semperi.2007.07.004

*Mancuso, T., & Burns, J. (2009). Ethical concerns in the management of pain in the neonate. *Pediatric Anesthesia, 10*, 953–957. doi: 10.1111/j.1460-9592.2009.03144x

Mayo Clinic Staff. (2010, Nov 10, 2009). Phantom pain. *Mayo Clinic.com*. Retrieved June 14, 2010, from http://www.mayoclinic.com/health/phantom-pain/DS00444/METHOD=print

Melzack, R., & Wall, P. D. (1965). Pain mechanisms: A new theory. *Science, 150*(19), 971–979. doi: 10.1126/science.150.3699.971

Mularski, R. A., White-Chu, F., Overbay, D., Miller, L., Asch, S. M., & Ganzini, L. (2006). Measuring pain as the 5th vital sign does not improve quality of pain management. *Journal of General Internal Medicine, 21*, 607–612. doi: 10.1111/j.1525-1497.2006.00415.x

Nair, S. U., & Lundbye, J. B. (2011). The use of hypothremia therapy in cardiac arrest survivors. *Therapeutic Hypothermia and Temperature Management, 1*(1), 9–21. doi: 10.1089/ther.2010.0002

Nelson-Hogan, D. (2008). Talking with Patricia Matthews-Juarez. *The Pain Practitioner, 18*(4), 8–11.

Oliveria, C. R. D., dos Santos, C. S., Nogueira, C. S., & Mainardes, E. J. (2007). Spinal anesthesia in a patient with congenital insensitivity to pain with anhidrosis. *Anesthesia & Analgesia, 104*(6), 1561–1562.

Patel, N. B. (2010). Physiology of pain. In A. Kopf & N. B. Paterl (Eds.). *Guide to pain management in low-resource settings* (pp. 13–17). Seattle: International Asociation for the Study of Pain.

*Payne, R. (2008). The role of culture, spirituality, and healing in the contexts of african-american culture and end of life care. *The Pain Practitioner, 18*(4), 14–16.

Powell, R. A., Downing, J., Ddungu, H., & Mwangi-Powell, F. N. (2010). Pain history and pain assessment. In A. Kopf & N. B. Patel (Eds.), *Guide to pain management in low-resource management* (pp. 67–78). Seattle: International Association for the Study of Pain.

Ranger, M., Johnston, C. C., & Anand, K. J. S. (2007). Current controversies regarding pain assessment in neonates. *Seminars in Perinatology, 31*, 283–288.

Rosenberg, H., Davis, M. A., James, D., Pollock, N., & Stowell, K. (2007). Malighant hyperthermia. *Orphanant Journal of Rare Diseases, 2*(21). doi: 10.1186/1750-1172-2-21

Santacroce, L., Diomede, L., Gagliardi, S., & Balducci, L. (2010, Feb 21, 2010). Oaraneoplastic syndromes. *eMedicine*. Retrieved 18 June, 2010, from http://emedicine.medscape.com/article/280744-print

Simons, S. H. P., & Tibboel, D. (2006). Pain perception development and maturation. *Seminars in Fetal & Neonatal Medicine, 11*, 227–231. doi: 10.1016/j.siny.2006.02.010

Singh, M. K., Patel, J., Gallagher, R. M., Childers, M. K., Salcido, R., & Talavera, F. (2013, 06/27/2012). Chronic pain syndrome. *Medscape Reference Drugs, Diseases & Procedures*. Retrieved January 8, 2013, from http://www.emedicine.medscape.com/article/130834-overview

Slater, R., Canteralla, A., Franck, L., & Fitzgerald, M. (2008). Who well do clinical pain assessment tools reflect pain in infants? *PLoS Medicine, 5*(6), 0928–0933. doi: 10.1371/journal.pmed.0050129

Srouji, R., Ratnapalan, S., & Schneeweiss, S. (2010). Pain in children: Assessment and nonpharmacological management. *International Journal of Pediatrics, 2010*. doi: 10.1155/2010/474838

Stevens, B., Johnston, C., Taaddio, A., Gibbins, S., & Yamada, J. (2010). The premature infant pain profile: Evaluation 13 years after development. *Clinical Journal of Pain, 26*(9), 813–830.

Sund-Levander, M., & Grodzinsky, E. (2010). What is the evidence base for the assessment and evaluation of body temperature? *Nursing times.net, 106*. Retrieved January 1, 2009, from http://www.nursingtimes.net/what-is-the-evidence-base-for-the-assessment-and-evaluation-of-body-temperature/5010223.article

Warne, D. (2008). Pain management in American Indian communities. *The Pain Practitioner, 18*(4), 18–27.

Weiner, D. K. (2007). Office management of chronic pain in the elderly. *The American Journal of Medicine, 120*(4), 306–315. doi: 10.1016/j.amjmed.2006.05.048

Yamada, J., Stinson, J., Lambda, J., Dickson, A., McGrath, P. J., & Stevens, B. (2008). A review of systematic reviews on pain interventions in hospitalized infants. *Pain Research & Management, 13*(5), 413–420.

Zwakhalen, S. M. G., Hamers, J. P. H., Abu-Saad, H. H., & Berger, M. P. F. (2006). Pain in elderly people with severe dementia: A systematic review of behavioural pain assessment tools. *BMC Geriatrics, 6*(3). doi: 10.1186/1471-2318-6-3

Chapter 9 References

AHIMA e-HIM Work Group on Maintaining the Legal EHR (AHIMA workgroup). (2005). Update: Maintaining a legally sound health record—paper and electronic. *Journal of the American Health Information Management Association (AHIMA), 76*(10), 64A–L. Retrieved December 1, 2012, from http://library.ahima.org/xpedio/groups/public/documents/ahima/bok1_028509.hcsp?dDocName=bok1_028509

American Medical Informatics Association (AMIA). (2012a). What is informatics? Retrieved October 16, 2012, from www.amia.org

American Medical Informatics Association (AMIA). (2012b). The Clinical Informatics Subspecialty. Retrieved October 16, 2012, from www.amia.org/clinical-informatics-medical-subspecialty

American Nurses Association (ANA). (2008). Nursing informatics: Scope and standards of practice. Silver Spring, MD: American Nurses Association.

Austin, S. (2006). "Ladies and gentleman of the jury, I present the nursing documentation." *Nursing, 36*(1), 56–62.

Centers for Medicare & Medicaid Services (CMS). (2011). Quality Measures: Overview. Retrieved November 23, 2011, from www.cms.gov/qualitymeasures/

Cheng, F., Gilchrist, A., Robinson, K.M., & Paul, L. (2009).The risk and consequences of clinical miscoding due to inadequate medical documentation: a case study of the impact on health services funding. *The HIM Journal, 38*(1), 35–46.

Cipriano, P. (2011). Transforming care through health information technology: A conversation with Dr. Farzad Mostashari, National Coordinator for Health Information Technology. *American Nurse Today, 6*(11), 8–9.

Coulehan, J. L., & Block, M. R. (2006). The medical interview: Mastering skills for clinical practice (5th ed.). Philadelphia: F.A. Davis.

Currell, R., & Urquhart, C. (2006). Nursing record systems: Effects on nursing practice and health care outcomes. *Cochrane Database of Systematic Reviews*, Issue 3. Art. No.: CD002099 in The Cochrane Library 2006, issue 4. New York: John Wiley & Sons.

Cusack, C. M., Hripcsak, G., Bloomrosen, M., Rosenbloom, S. T., Weaver, C. A., Wright, A., . . . Mamykina, L. (2012). The future state of clinical data capture and documentation: a report from AMIA's 2011 Policy Meeting. *Journal of the American Medical Informatics Association*. doi: 10.1136/amiajnl-2012-001093

DeShazo, J.P., LaVallie, D.L., & Wolf, F.M. (2009). Publication trends in the medical informatics literature: 20 years of "medical informatics" in MeSH. *BMC Medical Informatics and Decision Making, 9*:7. PMCID: PMC2652453. Retrieved October 16, 2012, from www.biomedcentral.com/1472-6947/9/7/

Frank-Stromborg, M., & Olsen, S. J. (2004). Instruments for clinical healthcare research, third edition. Sudbury, MA: Jones and Bartlett.

Geibert, R. (2006). Using diffusion of innovation concepts to enhance implementation of an electronic health record to support evidence-based practice. *Nursing Administration Quarterly, 30*(3), 203–210,

Greenes, R. A. (2007). Clinical decision support: The road ahead. Boston: Elsevier.

Hall, K.L., Feng, A.X., Moser, R.P., Stokols, D., & Taylor, B.K. (2008). Moving the science of team science forward. *American Journal of Preventive Medicine, 35*(2S), S243–S249.

Hanson, J. L., Stephens, M. B., Pangaro, L. N., & Gimbel, R. W. (2012). Quality of outpatient clinical notes: A stakeholder definition derived through qualitative research. *BMC Health Services Research, 12*(1), 407. doi:10.1186/1472-6963-12-407. Epub ahead of print. Retrieved November 28, 2012, from www.biomedcentral.com/content/pdf/1472-6963-12-407.pdf

Harrington, L., Choromanski, L., Biddle, N., & Acosta, K. (2011). Documentation of others' work in the electronic health record. *Critical Care Nurse, 31*(3), 84–86.

Hersh, W. (2009). A stimulus to define informatics and health information technology. *BMC Medical Informatics and Decision Making, 9*:24. PMCID: PMC2695439. Retrieved October 16, 2012, from www.biomedcentral.com/1472-6947/9/24

HHS (U. S. Department of Health and Human Services). (n.d.) *Understanding Health Information Privacy*. Retrieved June 19, 2012, from www.hhs.gov/ocr/privacy/hipaa/understanding/index.html

Holroyd-Leduc, J.M., Lorenzetti, D., Straus, S.E., Sykes, L., & Quan, H. (2011). The impact of the electronic medical record on the structure, process, and outcomes within primary care: A systematic review. *Journal of the American Medical Informatics Association, 18*, 732–737.

Joint Commission. (2011). Facts about the official "do not use" list of abbreviations. Retrieved July 12, 2011, from www.jointcommission.org/facts_about_the_official_/

Karsh, B., Weinger, M. B., Abbott, P. A., & Wears, R. L. (2010). Health information technology: Fallacies and sober realities. *Journal of the American Medical Informatics Association, 17*, 617–623.

Kawamoto, K., Houlihan, C. A., Balas, E. A., & Lobach, D. F. (2005). Improving clinical practice using clinical decision support systems: A systematic review of trials to identify features critical to success. *BMJ, 330*, 765. Epub 2005 Mar 14. doi: http://dx.doi.org/10.1136/bmj.38398.500764.8F

Lewis, N. (2012). EHR implementation still costs too much. *Healthcare InformationWeek*, July 9 2012. Retrieved December 1, 2012, from www.informationweek.com/healthcare/electronic-medical-records/ehr-implementation-still-costs-too-much/240003310

Mitre Corporation (Mitre). (2006). *Electronic Health Records Overview*. Research report to the National Institutes of Health National Center for Research Resources. Retrieved June 19, 2012, from www.himss.org/content/files/Code 180 MITRE Key Components of an EHR.pdf

Monarch, K. (2007). Documentation, part 1: Principles for self-protection. *American Journal of Nursing, 107*(7), 58–60.

Monegain, B. (2009). HIPAA violators could face fines of up to $1.5 million. *Healthcare IT news, Nov 2, 2009*. Retrieved November 28, 2012, from www.healthcareitnews.com/news/hipaa-violators-could-face-fines-15m

Nurses Service Organization (NSO). (2012). Charting by exception: The legal risks. Retrieved November 30, 2012, from www.nso.com/nursing-resources/article/68.jsp

Osborn, K. S., Wraa, C. E., & Watson, A. B. (2010). Medical-surgical nursing: Preparation for practice. Upper Saddle River, NJ: Pearson.

Osheroff, J. A., Teich, J. M., Middleton, B., Steen, E.B., Wright, A., Detmer, D. E., (2007). A roadmap for national action on clinical decision support. *Journal of the American Medical Informatics Association 14*, 141–145.

Rebbeck, T.R., Paskett, E., & Sellers, T.A. (2010). Fostering transdisciplinary science. *Cancer epidemiology, biomarkers & prevention, 19*, 1149. doi: 10.1158/1055-9965. Retrieved October 16, 2012, from http://cebp.aacrjournals.org/content/19/5/1149.full

Rodriguez-Vera, F. J., Marin, Y., Sanshez, A., Borrachero, C., & Pujol, E. (2002). Illegible handwriting in medical records. *Journal of the Royal Society of Medicine, 95*(11), 545–546.

Siegler, E. L. (2010). The evolving medical record. *Annals of Internal Medicine, 153*(10), 671–677.

Shortliffe, E.H., & Cimino, J.J. (Eds). (2006). Biomedical informatics: Computer applications in health care and biomedicine (3rd ed). New York: Springer.

Titler, M.G. (2008). Chapter 7: The evidence for evidence-based practice implementation. In RG Hughes, Ed. *Patient safety and quality: An evidence based handbook for nurses*. Rockville, MD: Agency for Healthcare Research and Quality.

Wasserman, R. C. (2011). Electronic medical records (EMRs), epidemiology, and epistemology: Reflections on EMRs and future pediatric clinical research. *Academic Pediatrics, 11*(4), 280–287.

Chapter 10 References

Boos, S. C., & Endom, E. E. (2013, 05/28/2013). Differential diagnosis of suspected child abuse. *UpToDate*. Retrieved 10/15, 2013, from http://www.uptodate.com/contents/differential-diagnosis-of-suspected-child-abuse?topicKey=EM%2F6601&elapsedTimeMs=8&view=print&displayedView=full

Bower, R. (2010). Development and developmental assessment. *ACNR, 10*(1), 18–21.

Bronfenbrenner, U., & Morris, P. A. (2006). The bioecological model of human development. In W. Damon & R. M. Lerner (Eds.), *Handbook of child psychology, Vol. 1: Theoretical models of human development* (6th ed., pp. 793–828). New York: Wiley.

Cao, H., Li, X., & Liu, J. (2012). An updated review of the efficacy of cupping therapy. *PLoS ONE, 7*(2), 14. http://www.ncbi.nlm.nih.gov/pmc/articles/PMC3289625/ doi:10.1371/journal.pone.0031

Casey, J. (2012, 02/09/11). Evaluation of pediatric development [normal]. *Learn Pediatrics*. Retrieved October 25, 2012, from http://learnpediatrics.com/body-systems/nervous-syste/evaluation-of-pediatric-development-normal/

Chess, S., Thomas, A., & Birch, H. G. (1968). *Your Child Is A Person: A Psychological Approach To Childhood Without Guilt*. New York: The Viking Press.

Council on Children with Disabilities. (2006). Identifying infants and young children with develomental disorders in the medical home: An algorithm for developmental surveillance and screening. *Pediatrics, 118*(1), 405–420.

Drutz, J. E. (2013, 06/20/2012). The pediatric physical examination: General principles and standard measurements. *UpToDate*. Retrieved January 24, 2013, from http://www.uptodate.com/contents/the-pediatric-physical-examination-general-principles-and-standard-measurements?topicKey=PEDS%2F2865&elapsedTimeMs=4&view=print&displayedView=full

Duderstadt, K. G. (2006). *Pediatric physical examination: An illustrated handbooki*. St. Louis: Mosby/Elsevier.

Eisenberg, N., Spinrad, T. L., & Eggum, N.D. (2010). Emotion-related self-regulation and its relation to children's maladjustment. *Annual Review of Psychology, 6*(April 27), 495–525. doi: 10.1146/annurev.clinpsy.121208.131208

Ermertcan, A. T., & Ertan, P. (2010). Skin manifestations of child abuse. *Indian Journal of Dermatology, Venereology and Leprology, 76*(4), 317–326.

Grist, C. L., & McCord, D. M. (2010). Individual differences in preschool children: Temperament or personality? *Infant and Child Development* (p. 11). doi:10.1002/icd.663

Hockenberry, M. J., & Wilson, D. L. (2012). *Wong's essentials of pediatric nursing* (9th ed.). St. Louis: Elsevier.

Juckett, G. (2005). Cross-cultural medicine. *American Family Physician, 72*(11), 2267–2274.

Judy, K. (2011). Unintentional Injuries in Pediatrics. *Pediatrics in Review, 32*(10), 431–439. doi: 10.1542/pir.32-10-431

Keogh, B.K. (2013, ND). How temperament affects parents, children, and family life. *Great Schools*. Retrieved January 24, 2013, from http://www.greatschools.org/special-education/health/941-temperament-affects-parents-children-family.gs

Kotagal, S. (2012, 03/22/2012). Detailed neurologic assessment of infants and children. *UpToDate*. Retrieved October 25, 2012, from http://www.uptodate.com/contents/detailed-neurologic-assessment-of-infants-and-children

Kristal, J. (2005). *The temperament perspective: Working with children's behavioral styles*. New York: Paul H. Brookes.

Perry, S. E., Hockenberry, M. J., Lowdermilk, M. J., & Wilson, D. L. (2009). *Maternal child nursing care* (4th ed.). St. Louis: Elsevier.

Ringwalt, S. (2008). Developmental screening and assessment instruments with an emphasis on social and emotional development for young children ages birth through five. Retrieved October 25, 2012 from http://www.nectac.org/~pdfs/pubs/screening.pdf

Rothbart, M. K. (2007). Termperament, development, and personality. *Current Directions in Psychological Science, 16*(4), 207–212. doi: 10.1111/j.1467-8721.2007.00505.x

Rothbart, M. K., & Rueda, M. R. (2005). The developmental of effortful control. In U. Mayr, E. Awh & S. Keele (Eds.), *Developing individuality in the human brain: A tribute to Michael I. Posner* (pp. 167–188). Washington D. C.: American Psychological Association.

Schwebel, D. C., & Barton, B. K. (2005). Contribution of multiple risk factors to child injury. *Journal of Pediatric Psychology, 30*(7), 553–561. doi: 10.1093/jpepsy/jsio42

Schwebel, D. C., & Bounds, M. L. (2003). The role of parents and temperament on children's estimation of physical ability: Links to unintentional injury prevention. *Journal of Pediatric Psychology, 28*(7), 507–518. doi: 10.1093/jpepsy/jsg041

Schwebel, D. C., & Gaines, J. (2007). Pediatric unintentional injury: Behavioral risk factors and implications for prevention. *Journal of Developmental & Behavioral Pediatrics, 28*(3), 245–254.

Wahlstrom, D., Collins, P., White, T., & Luciana, M. (2010). Developmental changes in dopamine neurotransmission in adolescence: Behavioral implications and issues in assessment. *Brain and Cognition, 72*(1), 146–159. doi: http://dx.doi.org/10.1016/j.bandc.2009.10.013

Chapter 11 References

Benediktsson, I., McDonald, S. W., Vekved, M., McNeil, D. A., Dolan, S. M., & Tough, S. C. (2013). Comparing CenteringPregnancy® to standard prenatal care plus prenatal education. *BMC Pregnancy and Childbirth, 13*(Suppl 1), S5.

Berghella, V., Iams, J. D., Reedy, N. J., Oshiro, B. T., & Wachtel, J. S. (2011). Quality improvement opportunities in prenatal care. *Toward Improving the Outcomes of Pregnancy III*. Retrieved March 12, 2013, from http://www.marchofdimes.com/#

Clark, M. B., & Clark, D. A. (2012). Meconium aspiration syndrome. *Medscape Reference Drugs, Diseases & Procedures*. Retrieved September 25, 2012, from http://emedicine.medscape.com/article/974110-overview

Fanaroff, A. A. (2008). Meconium aspiration syndrome: Historical aspects. *Journal of Perinatology, 28*(Supplement), S3–S7. doi: 10.1038/jp.2008.162

Jansson, L. M., & Velez, M. (2012). Neonatal abstinance syndrome. *Current Opinion in Pediatrics, 24*(2), 252–258. doi: 10.1097/MOP.013e32834fdc3a

Lothian, J. L. (2008). The journey of becoming a mother. *Journal of Perinatology, 17*(4), 43–47. doi: 10.1624/105812408X364071

Low, L. K., Seng, J. S., & Miller, J. M. (2008). Use of the optimality index—United States in perinatal clinical research: A validation study. *Journal of Midwifery and Women's Health, 53*(4), 302–309. doi: 10.1016/j.jmwh.2008.01.009

Molloy, A. M., Kirke, P. N., Troendle, J. F., Burke, H., Sutton, M., Brody, L. C., . . . Mills, J. L. (2009). Maternal Vitamin B12 Status and Risk of Neural Tube Defects in a Population With High Neural Tube Defect Prevalence and No Folic Acid Fortification. *Pediatrics, 123*(3), 917–923. doi: 10.1542/peds.2008–1173

*Monchek, R. & Wiedaseck, S. (2012). Gestational trophoblastic disease. An overview. *Journal of Midwifery and Women's Health, 57*, 255–259.

Murphy, P. A., & Fulerton, J. T. (2006). Development of the optimality index as a new approach to evaluating outcomes of maternity care. *Journal of Obstetrical Gynecologic and Neonatal Nursing, 35*, 770–778. doi: 10.1111/J.1552-6909.2006.00105.x

Murphy, P. A., & Fullerton, J. (2001). Measuring outcomes of midwifery care: Development of an instrument to assess optimality. *Journal of Midwifery and Women's Health, 46*(5), 274–278.

Rising, S. S., Kennedy, H. P., & Klima, C. S. (2004). Redesigning prenatal care through centering pregnancy. *Journal of Midwifery and Women's Health, 49*(5), 398–404. doi: 10.1016/j.mwh.2004.04.018

Roberts, L., Gulliver, B., Fisher, J., & Cloves, K. G. (2010). The coping labor algorithim: An alternative pain assessment tool for the laboring woman. *Journal of Midwifery and Women's Health, 55*, 107–116.

The Joint Commission. (2013). Specifications Manual for Joint Commission National Quality Measures (v2013A1). Oak Brook, IL.

U. S. Department of Health and Human Services. (2009). *Healthy people 2020 summary of objectives*. Washington D.C.: U. S. Government Printing Services.

Welch, L. G., & Miller, L. A. (2012, 10/08). Emotional and educational components of pregnancy. *The Global Library of Women's Medicine*. Retrieved October 11, 2012, from www.glowm.com.

Chapter 12 References

Academy of Nutrition and Dietetics. (2013, 02/14/2013). Healthy aging. Retrieved from http://www.eatright.org/search.aspx?search=Healthy%20Aging

Adelman, R. D., Greene, M. G., & Charon, R. (1991). Issues in physician-elderly interaction. *Ageing and Society, 11*(Part 2), 127–148.

Agency for Healthcare Research and Quality. (2008). Healthcare cost and utilization project facts and figures 2008. Statistics on hospital-based care in the United States. Retrieved from http://www.hcup us.ahrq.gov/reports/factsandfigures/2008/section1_TOC.jsp

American Geriatrics Society. (2012). American geriatrics society update beers criteria for potentially inappropriate meddication use in older adults. Retrieved October 1, 2012, from http://www.americangeriatrics.org/files/documents/beers/2012BeersCriteris_JAGS.pdf

American Psychological Association. (2005). Growing mental and behavioral health concerns facing older Americans. Retrieved September 29, 2012, from http://www.apa.org/about/gr/issues/aging/growing-concerns.aspx

Arnold, E. (2004). Sorting out the 3s: Delerium, dementia, depression. *Nursing 04, 6*, 36–42.

Bastable, S.B. (2008). *Nurse as educator-principles of teaching and learning for nursing practice*. Sudbury, MA: Jones and Bartlett Publishers.

Beyth, R. J., & Short, R. I. (2007). *Drugs for the geriatric patient*. St. Louis: Elsevier Mosby.

Boltz, M., Capezuti, E., Fulmer, T., Zwicker, D., & O'Meara, M. A. (2012). *Evidence based geriatric nursing protocols for best practice* (4th ed.). New York, NY: Springer Publishing.

Bowling, A. (2007). Honor your father and mother? Ageism in medicine. *The British Journal of General Practice, 57*(538), 347–348.

Brown, A., & Draper, P. (2003). Elements of a language mode often experienced by older adults. *Journal of Advanced Nursing, 41*(1), 15–21.

Butler, R. (1989). Dispelling ageism. The cross-dutting intervention. *Annals of the American Political and Social Science, 503*, 138–147.

Centers for Disease Control and Prevention. (2012a, July 13, 2012). Immunization schedules: Immunization schedules for adults in easy-to-read formats. Retrieved from http://www.cdc.gov/vaccines/schedules/easy-to-read/adult.html#print

Centers for Disease Control and Prevention. (2012b, July 13, 2012). Seasonal influenza (flu). What you should know and do this flu season if you are 65 years and older. Retrieved from http://www.cdc.gov/flu/about/disease/65over.htm

Cutilli, C. C. (2007). Health literacy in geriatric patients: An integrative review of the literature. *Orthopaedic Nursing, 26*(1), 43–48.

Ellis, G. I., & Langhorne, P. (2005). Comprehensive geriatric assessment for older hospital patients. *British Medical Bulletin, 71*(1), 45–49.

Ellis, G., Whitehead, M. A., Robinson, D., O'Neill, D., & Langhorne, P. (2011). Comprehensive geriatric assessment for older adults admitted to hospital: Meta analysis of randomised controlled trials. *British Medical Journal, 343*, doi:org/10.1136/bmj.d6553..

Engelhardt, J., Toseland, R., Gao, J., & Banks, S. (2006). Long-term effects of geriatric outpatient evaluation and management on cost, health care utilization and survival. *Research on Social Work Practice, 16*(1), 20–21.

Erikson, E., & Erikson, J. M. (1997). *The ninth stage: The life cycle completed*. New York, NY: W. W. Norton & Company Ltd.

Federal Interagency Forum on Aging-Related Statistics. (2012). Older americans 2012: Key indicators of well-being. Washington DC: U. S. Government Printing Office. Retrieved from http://agingstats.gov/agingstatsdotnet/main_site/default.aspx.

First Consulting Group. (2007). *When I'm 64: How boomers will change health care*. Chicago: American Hospital Association.

Fulmer, T. (2007). How to try this: Fulmer spices. *Amercan Journal of Nursing, 107*(10), 40–48.

Gallop Poll. (2010). Religion. Retrieved October 9, 2012, from http://www.gallup.com/poll/1690/Religion.aspx

Gaskamp, C., Sutter, R., & Meraviglia, M. (2008). Evidence based guideline: Promoting spirituality to terminally ill older adults. *Journal of Gerontolological Nursing, 34 [Jul]*(7), 8–14.

Halter, J. B., Ouslander, J. G., Tinetti, M. E., Studenski, S., High, K. P., & Asthana, S. (2009). *Hazzard's geriatric Medicine and gerontology* (6th ed.). New York, NY: McGraw Hill.

Hartford Institute for Geriatric Nursing. Retrieved September 3, 2013, from http://www.hartfordign.org and http://www.hartfordign.org.

Herr, K. (2010). Pain in the older adult: An imperative across all health care settings. *Pain Management Nursing, 11* (2 Supplement), S1–S10.

Horgas, A.L., Elliott, A. F., & Mariske, M. (2009). Pain assessment in persons with dementia: Relationship between self-report and behavioral observation. *Journal of the American Geriatrics Society, 57*(1), 126–132.

Inouye, S. K., Studenski, S., Tinetti, M. E., & Kuchel, G. A. (2007). Geriatric syndromes: Clinical, research, and policy implications of a core geriatric concept. *Journal of the American Geriatric Society, 55*(5), 780–781.

Institute of Medicine. (2008). Retooling for an aging america: Building the health care workforce. Retrieved September 22, 2012, from http://www.iom.edu/Reports.aspx?Search=Retooling

*Jin, K. (2010). Modern biological theories of aging. *Aging and Disease, 1*(2), 72–72.

Kunter, M., Greenberg, E., Jin, Y., & Paulsen, C. (2006). *The health literacy of America's adults: Results from the 2003 national assessment of adult literacy* (Vol. NCES 2006-483). Washington D.C.: U. S. Department of Education National Center for Education Statistics.

Lange, J. W. (2012). *The nurse's role in promoting optimal health of older adults*. Philadelphia, PA: F. A. Davis.

Mauk, K. L. (2008). Myths of aging, gerontology update. Retrieved from http://www.rehabnurse.org/pdf/GeriatricMyths.pdf

McAuliffe, L., Nay, R., O'Donnell, M., & Fetherstonhaugh, D. (2009). Pain assessment in older people with dementia: Literature review. *Journal of Advanced Nursing, 65(Jan)*(1), 2–10.

Montgomery, J., Mitty, E., & Flores, S. (2008). Resident condition change: Should I call 911? *Geriatric Nursing, 29*(3), 1.

Murray, R.B., Zentner, J.P., & Yakimo, R. (2009) *Health promotion strategies through the life span*. Upper Saddle River, NJ: Pearson.

National Institutes of Health. (2011). *Dietary supplement fact sheet: Vitamin B_{12}*. Retrieved from http://ods.od.nih.gov/factsheets/VitaminB12-HealthProfessional/

Nelson, T. (2005). Ageism: Fear against our future self. *Journal of Social Issues, 61*(2), 207–221.

Nielsen-Bohlman, L., Panzer, A., & Kindig, D. (2004). *Health literacy: A prescription to end confusion*. Washington D.C.: National Academy Press.

Office of Disease Prevention and Health Promotion. (2012). Get active. *Quick guide to healthy living*. Retrieved from http://healthfinder.gov/prevention/ViewTopic.aspx?topicId=22

Olenek, K., Skowronski, T., & Schmaltz, D. (2003). Geriatric nursing assessment. *Journal of Gerontological Nursing, 8*, 5–9.

Onega, L. L. (2013, 2013). The Modified Caregiver Strain Index (MCSI). *Try This*. 2013, from http://consultgerirn.org/uploads/File/trythis/try_this_14.pdf

Pascala, JT., & Sullivan, GM. (2004). *Geriatrics review syllabus* (7th ed.) Syllabus/Book 1. New York, N.Y: American Geriatrics Society.

Pioneer Network. (2012). Elderspeak. Retrieved September 27, 2012, from http://www.pioneernetwork.net/CulturalChange/Elderspeak

Reardon, C. (2012). The changing face of older adult substance abuse. *Social Work Today, 12*(1), 8.

Robinson, L., deBenedictis, T., & Segal, J. (June 2012). Elder abuse and neglect: Warning signs, risk factors, prevention and help. Retrieved September 26, 2012, from http://www.helpguide.org/mental/elder_abuse_physical_emotional_sexual_neglect.htm

Rosenthal, R. A., & Kravic, S. M. (2004). Assessment and management of the geriatric patient. *Critical Care Medicine, 32*(4 Suppl), S92–S105.

Rubenstein, L. Z. (1995). An overview of comprehensive geriatric assessment: Rationale, history, program models, basic components. In R. Bernabei, L. Z. Rubenstein & D. Wieland (Eds.), *Geriatric assessment techonology: The state of the art*. New York, NY: Springer.

Ryan, E. B., Bourhis, R. Y., & Knops, U. (1991). Evaluative perceptions of patronizing speech addressed to elders. *Psychology and Aging, 6*(3), 442–450.

Salzman, B. (2006). Myths and realities of aging. *Care Management Journal, 7*(3), 141–150.

*Tabloski, P. A. (2010). *Gerontological nursing*. (2nd ed.). Upper Saddle River, NJ: Pearson.

U. S. Department of Health and Human Services. (2009). *Healthy people 2020 summary of objectives*. Washington D.C.: U. S. Government Printing Services.

United States Census Bureau. (2012). 2010 census shows America's diversity. Retrieved from http://www.census.gov/newsroom/releases/archives/2010_census/cb11-cn125.html

Chapter 13 References

*Administration on Aging. Older Americans Act. Retrieved July 20, 2010, from http://www.aoa.gov/AoARoot/AoA_Programs/OAA/index.aspx

*Andrews, Y. N.,& Castellanos, V. H. (2003). Development of a method for estimation of food and fluid intakes by nursing assistants in long-term care facilities: A pilot study. *Journal of the American Dietetic Association. 103,* 873–877.

Applegate, D. (2013, 02/17/2008). Anth 300 Forensic Anthropology Lab 12: Stature Estimation. Retrieved 10/18, 2013, from http://people.wku.edu/darlene.applegate/forensic/lab12/lab 12.html

Argiles, J. M. (2005). Cancer-associated malnutrition. *European Journal of Oncology Nursing. 9*(2), S39–S50.

*Brodie, D. A. (1988). Techniques of measurement of body composition. Part I. *Sports Medicine. 5*, 11–40.

Byrd, J., Langford, A., Paden, S. J., Plackemeier, W., Seidelman, C., Valla, M., & Wills, R. (2011). Scale consistency study: How accurate are in patient hospital scales? *Nursing. 41*(11), 21–24

*Castellanos, V. H., & Andrews, Y. N. (2002). Inherent flaws in a method of estimating meal intake commonly used in long-term-care facilities. *Journal of the American Dietetic Association..102*, 826–830.

*Centers for Disease Control. *Adult BMI Chart.* Retrieved July 20, 2010, from http://www.health.gov/dietaryguidelines/dga2005/document/html/chapter3.htm. May 30, 2000

*Charney, P., & Malone, A. M. (2009). *ADA Pocket Guide to Nutritional Assessment*. (2nd ed.). Chicago, IL: American Dietetic Association.

*Chumlea, W. C., & Roche, A. F. (1987). *Nutritional assessment of the elderly through anthropometry*. Columbus, OH: Ross Laboratories.

Chumlea, W. C., Guo, S. S., & Steinbaugh, M. L. (1994). Prediction of stature from knee height for black and white adults and children with application to mobility-impaired or handicapped persons. *Journal of the American Dietetic Association. 94*(12), 1385–1388.

Coats, K. G., Morgan, S. L., Bartolucci, A. A., & Weinsier, R. L. (1993). Hospital-associated malnutrition: a reevaluation 12 years later. *Journal of the American Dietetic Association. 93*(1), 27–33.

Committee on National Statistics, Division of Behavioral and Social Sciences and Education, National Research Council. Washington, DC: National Academies Press. 2006.

Committee on Nutritional Status During Pregnancy and Lactation, Institute of Medicine. Nutrition During Lactation. 1991. National Academies Press, National Academy of Sciences. Washington, DC

Drewnowski, A., & Specter, S. E. (2004). Poverty and obesity: The role of energy density and energy cost. *American Journal of Clinical Nutrition. 79*, 6–16.

*Felton, D. Food/Fluid Intake Form Policy and Observation Record Form. Retrieved July 20, 2010, from http://www.rd411.com/index.php?option=com_content&view=article&id=1164:foodfluid-intake-form-policy-and-observation-record-form&catid=117:clinical-policies&Itemid=382

Feinman, L., & Lieber, C. S. (1992). Nutrition: Medical problems of alcoholism. In Lieber, C.S., (Ed.), *Medical and Nutritional Complications of Alcoholism: Mechanisms in Management* (pp. 515–530). New York: Plenum Publishing Corp.

Fischer, J., & Johnson, M. A. (1990).. Low body weight and weight loss in the aged. *Journal of the American Dietetic Association. 90*, 1697–1706.

Flegal, K. M., Graubard, B. I., Williamson, D. F., & Gail, M. H. (2005). Excess deaths associated with underweight, overweight, and obesity. *Journal of the American Medical Association. 293*, 1861–1867.

French, S. A., Wall, M., & Nathan, R. (2010). Household income differences in food sources and food items purchased. *International Journal of Behavioral Nutrition and Physical Activity. 7*(1), 77–84.

Guzman, M. A. (2010). Diet and chronic diseases: INCAP studies of atherosclerosis and coronary heart disease. *Food and Nutrition Bulletin. 31*(1), 141–51.

*Hager, M. H. (2006). Hospital therapeutic diet orders and the Centers for Medicare & Medicaid Services: Steering through regulations to provide quality nutrition care and avoid survey citations. *Journal of the American Dietetic Association. 106*(2), 198–204.

*Hammond, K. A. (1999). The nutrition dimension of physical assessment. *Nutrition. 15*(5), 411–419.

Jackson, A. S., & Pollock, M. L. (1978). Generalized equations for predicting body density. *British Journal of Nutrition. 40*, 497.

Jackson, A. S., Pollock, M. L., & Ward, A. (1980). Generalized equations for predicting body density of women. *Medicine and Science in Sports and Exercise. 12*, 175–182.

Joint Commission on Accreditation of Healthcare Organizations. Standard FAQ details: Nutritional, functional, and pain assessments and screens. Retrieved December 19, 2011, from http://www.jointcommission.org/standards_information/jcfaqdetails.aspx?StandardsFaqId=208&ProgramId=1. Revised 11/24/2008

Jensen, M. B., & Hassov, I. (2000). Nutrition and rehabilitation after discharge from the hospital: Accelerating the rehabilitation with nutrition and physical training. *Nutrition. 16*(7–8), 619–621.

Joosten, K. F., & Hulst, J. M. (2008). Prevalence of malnutrition in pediatric hospital patients. *Current Opinion in Pediatrics. 20*(5), 590–596.

Ludwig, D. S. (2011). Technology, diet, and the burden of chronic disease. *Journal of the American Medical Association. 305*(13), 1352–1353.

Mangels, A. R., Messina, V., & Melina, V. (2003). Position of the American Dietetic Association and Dietitians of Canada: Vegetarian diets. *Journal of the American Dietetic Association. 103*(6), 748–765.

Marsano, L., & McClain, C. J. (1989). Effects of alcohol on electrolytes and minerals. *Alcohol Health & Research World. 13*(3), 255–260.

*Merck Manual Online Medical Library: Dehydration. Standard basal metabolic rates used for calculating maintenance fluid requirements. Retrieved July 20, 2010, from http://www.merck.com/mmpe/sec19/ch276/ch276b.html#CIHJBJCJ. Content last modified 03/13.

National Cholesterol Education Program (2001). Third report of the expert panel on decision, evaluation and treatment of high blood cholesterol in adults. Bethesda, MD: U. S. Department of Health and Human Services, Public Health Service; National Institutes of Health; National Heart, Lung and Blood Institute.

Nestle Health Science. (2013, 2006). MNA [Mini nutritional assessment]. Retrieved 10/18, 2013, from http://www.nestle-nutrition.com/Clinical_Resources/Mini_Nutritional_Assessment.aspx

*Nutrient Intake Analysis (Calorie Count). Retrieved July 20, 2010, from http://www.rd411.com/index.php?option=com_content&view=article&id=286:nutrient-intake-analysis-calorie-count&catid=117:clinical-policies&Itemid=382. Last Review Date 11/10.

* Panel on Macronutrients, Panel on the Definition of Dietary Fiber, Subcommittee on Upper Reference Level of Nutrients, Subcommittee on Interpretation and Uses of Dietary Reference Intakes, Standing Committee on Scientific Evaluation of Dietary Reference Intakes. (2002). Dietary reference intakes for energy, carbohydrate, fiber, fat, fatty acids, cholesterol, protein, amino acids. Washington DC: National Academy Press.

Pronsky, Z. M., Crowe, J., Elbe, D., Young, V., Roberts, W., Epstein, S. (2012). Food-medication interactions handbook (17th ed.). Birchrunville, PA: Food-Medication Interactions.

Ramsey, J. C., Smithard, D. G., & Kalra, L. (2003). Early assessments of dysphagia and aspiration risk in acute stroke patients. *Stroke. 34*, 1252–1257.

Sánchez-García, S., García-Peña, C., Duque-López, M. X., Juárez-Cedillo, T., Cortés-Núñez, A. R., & Reyes-Beaman, S. (2007). Anthropometric measures and nutritional status in a healthy elderly population. *Biomed Central Public Health. 7*, 2.

Siri, W. E. (1961). Body composition from fluid spaces and density: Analysis of methods. In Brozek, J., & Henzchel, A. *Techniques for measuring body composition* (pp. 224–244). Washington: National Academy of Sciences.

Sitoh, Y. Y., Lee, A., Phua, S. Y., Lieu, P. K., & Chan, S. P. (2000). Bedside assessment of swallowing: A useful screening tool for dysphagia in an acute geriatric ward. *Singapore Medical Journal. 41*(8), 376–381.

*Standing Committee on the Scientific Evaluation of Dietary Reference Intakes, Food and Nutrition Board, Institute of Medicine. (2000.) Dietary reference intakes for vitamin c, vitamin e, selenium and carotenoids. Washington, DC: National Academy Press.

Story, M., Kaphingst, K. M., Robinson-O'Brien, R., & Glanz, K. (2008). Creating healthy food and eating environments: Policy and environmental approaches. *The Annual Review of Public Health. 29*, 253–272.

Teixeira, J., Mota, T.,& Fernandes, J. C. (2011). Nutritional evaluation of alcoholic inpatients admitted for alcohol detoxification. *Alcohol and Alcoholism. 46*(5), 558–60.

The Joint Commission. (2008). Nutritional, functional, and pain assessments and screens *Standard FAQ details*. Oak Brook, IL.

Tortora, G. J., & Derrickson, B.H. (2011). *Principles of anatomy and physiology* (13th ed.). Hoboken, NJ: Wiley Publications.

*U. S. Department of Agriculture National Agricultural Library, Food and Nutrition Center. Dietary Guidance. Retrieved July 20, 2010, from http://fnic.nal.usda.gov/nal_display/index.php?info_center–4&tax_level=2&tax_subject=256&topic_id=1342

U.S. Department of Health and Human Services. (2009). *Healthy people 2020 summary of objectives.* Washington D.C.: U.S. Government Printing Services.

U.S. Department of Health and Human Services. (2009b). *Nutrition and weight status.* Washington D.C.: U.S. Government Printing Services Retrieved from http://www.healthypeople.gov/2020/topicsobjectives2020/overview.aspx?topicId=29

U. S. Department of Health and Human Services. 1988. The surgeon general's report on nutrition and health. Washington DC: U. S. Government Printing Office

*U. S. Department of Health and Human Services, Centers for Medicare and Medicaid Services. Minimum data set 3.0 for nursing homes and swing bed providers. Retrieved July 20, 2010, from https://www.cms.gov/NursingHomeQualityInits/25_NHQIMDS30.asp#TopOfPage

Ver Ploeg, M., Breneman, V., Farrigan, T., Hamrick, K., Hopkins, D., Kaufman, P., et al. (2009). Access to affordable and nutritious food—Measuring and understanding food deserts and their consequences: Report to Congress. Administrative Publication No. (AP-036).

Wagner, P. D. (2008). Possible mechanisms underlying the development of cachexia in COPD. *European Respiratory Journal. 31*(3), 492–501.

Chapter 14 References

Alcoholism: Clinical & Experimental Research. (2009). Low to mederate, not heavy, drinking releases "feel-good" endorphins in the brain. Retrieved February 1, 2013, from http://www.sciencedaily.com/releases/2009/03/090319161503.htm

Anda, R. F., Felitti, V. J., Bremmer, J. D., Walker, J. D, Whitfield, C., Perry, B. D., et. al. (2006). The enduring effects of abuse and related adverse experiences in childhood. *European Archives of Psychiatry and Clinical Neuroscience, 256*(3), 174–186. doi: 10.1007/s00406-005-0624-4

Babor, T. F., Higgins-Biddle, J. C., Saunders, J. B., & Monteiro, M. G. (2001). The alcohol use disorders identification test: Guidelines for use in primary care. Retrieved from http://whqlibdoc.who.int/hq/2001/who_msd_msb_01.6a.pdf

Barrocas, A. L., Hankin, B. L., Young, J. F., & Abela, J. R. Z. (2012). Rates of nonsuidical self-injury in youths: Age, sex, and behavioral methods in a community sample. *Pediatrics, 130*(1), 39–45. doi: 10.1542/peds.2011-2094

Benuto, L. (2010). What determines healthy sexuality: Variance is the spice of life. *Sexuality and Sexual Problems.* Retrieved from http://www.mentalhelp.net/poc/view_doc.php?type=doc&id=29690&cn=10

Black, M. C., Basile, K. C., Breiding, J., Smith, S. G., Walters, M. L., Merrick, M. T., et. al. (2011). The national intimate partner and sexual violence survey: 2010 summary report. Retrieved from www.cdc.gov/violenceprevention/nisvs/

Cabinum-Foeller, E. (2012, 01/2011). Abusive head trauma (shaken baby syndrome). *KidsHealth from Nemours.* Retrieved June 15, 2012, from http://kidshealth.org/PageManager.jsp?dn=KidsHealth&lic=1&p0s=107

Centers for Disease Control and Prevention. (2010a). Consequences. *Intimate Partner Violence.* Retrieved from http://www.cdc.gov/ViolencePrevention/intimatepartnerviolence/consequences

Centers for Disease Control and Prevention. (2010b). Definitions. *Intimate Partner Violence.* Retrieved from http://www.cdc.gov/ViolencePrevention/intimatepartnerviolence/definition

Centers for Disease Control and Prevention. (2010c). Risk and protective factors. *Intimate Partner Violence.* Retrieved from http://www.cdc.gov/ViolencePrevention/intimatepartnerviolence/riskprotectivefactors.html

Centers for Disease Control and Prevention. (2012). *Cost estimates of violent deaths: Figures and tables.* Atlanta, GA: Centers for Disease Control and Prevention.

Child Welfare Information Gateway. (2008a). Long-term consequences of child abuse and neglect. Retrieved June 13, 2012, from www.childwelfare.gov/pubs/factsheets/lont_term_consequences.cfm

Child Welfare Information Gateway. (2008b). What is chld abuse and neglect? Retrieved June 15, 2012, from www.childwelfare.gov/pubs/factsheets/whatiscan.cfm

Cichocki, M. (2013, 09/03/2010). Am I at risk for HIV infection? What infections am I at risk for? *Health AIDS/HIV.* Retrieved 09/03, 2013, from http://aids.about.com/od/hivaidsstats/f/infectionrisk.htm

Contet, C., Kieffer, B., & Before, K. (2004). Mu opioid receptor: A gateway to drug addiction. *Current Opinion in Neurobiology, 14,* 370–378. doi: 10.1016/j.conb.2004.05.005

Corso, P. S., Mercy, J. A., Simon, T. R., Finkelstein, E. A., & Miller, T.R. (2007). Medical costs and productivity losses due to interpersonal and self-directed violence in the United States. *American Journal of Preventive Medicine, 32*(6), 474–482. doi: 10.1016/j.amepre.2007.02.010

Counseling Resource Research Staff. (2013, 06/27/2012). Michigan Alcohol Screening Test [MAST], Revised. Retrieved 10/17, 2013, from http://counsellingresource.com/lib/quizzes/drug-testing/alcohol-mast/

Crosby, A. E., Buckner, A. V., & Taylor, B. D. (2011). Addressing self-directed violence prevention for preventive medicine practitioners. *American Journal of Lifestyle Medicine, 5*(Sept/Oct), 418–427. doi: 10.1177/1559827611410020

Crosby, A. E., Han, B., Ortega, L. A. G., Parks, S. E., & Gfroerer, J. (2011). Suicidal thoughts and behaviors among adults aged 18 years–United States, 2008–2009. *Morbidity and Mortality Weekly Report, 60*(13), 1–11.

De Leo, D., & Krysinska, K. E. (2008). Suicide and self directed violene. In K. Heggenhougen & S. Quah (Eds.), *International encyclopedia of public health* (1 ed., Vol. 6, pp. 267–275). San Diego: Elsevier, Inc.

Delima, J., & Vimpani, G. (2011). The neurobiological effects of childhood maltreatment. *Family Matters, 89,* 42–52.

DiazGranados, N., Ibrahim, L. A., Brutsche, N. E., Ameli, R., Henter, I. D., Luckenbaugh, D. A., et al. (2010). Rapid resolution of suicidal ideation after a single infusion of an *n*-methyl-d-aspartate antagonist in patients with treatment-resistant major depressive disorder. *Journal of Clinical Psychiatry, 71*(12), 1605–1611. doi: 10.4088/JCP.09m05327blu

Engs, R.C. (2003, n.d.). What are addictive behaviors? Retrieved June 25, 2010, from http://www.indiana..edu~engs/hints/addictive eb.html

Feltenstein, M. W., & See, R. E. (2008). The neurocircuitry of addiction: An overview. *British Journal of Pharmacology, 154,* 261–274. doi: 10.1038/bjp.2008.51

Fowler, J. C. (2012). Suicide risk assessment in clinical practice: Pragmatic guidelines for imperfect assessments. *Psychotherapy, 49*(1), 81–90. doi: 10.1037/a0026148

Garrett, F. P. (2009). The addictive process. *Psychiatry and Wellness.* Retrieved June 25, 2010, from http://www.bma-wellness.com/addictions/addictions.html

Glenn, C. R., & Klonsky, E. D. (2008). Social context during non-suicidal self injury indicates suicide risk. *Personalilty and Individual Differences, 46,* 25–29. doi: 10.1016/j.paid.2008.08.020

Gregoire, A. (1999). Abc of sexual health: Assessing and managing male sexual problems. *British Journal of Medicine. 318*(3), 315–317.

Gruber, J., Roth, B., & Daley, C. (2010, October 31, 2005). Alcoholism. *eMedicine Health.* Retrieved June 28, 2010, from http://www.emedicinehealth.com/script/main/art.asp?articlekey=58899pf=3&pages=1

Hepburn, L., Azrael, D., Molnar, B., & Miller, M. (2012). Bullying and suicidal behaviors among urban high school youth. *Journal of Adolescent Health, 51,* 93–95. doi: 10.1016/j.adohealth.2011.12.014

Holi, M. M., Pelkonen, M., Karlsson, L., Kiviruusu, O., Ruuttu, T., Heila, H., et al. (2005). Psychometric properties and clinical utility of the scale for suidical ideation (ssi) in adolescents. *BMC Psychiatry, 5*(8). doi: 10.1186/1471-244X-5-8

Horesh, N., Nachshoni, T., Wolmer, L., & Toren, P. (2009). A comparison of life events in suicidal and nonsuicidal adolescents and young adults with major depression and borderline personality disorder. *Comprehensive Psychiatry, 50,* 496–502. doi: 10.1016/j.comppsych.2009.01.006

Kianpoor, M., & Bakhshani, N. (2012). Trauma, dissociation, and high-risk behaviors. *International Journal of High Risk Behaviors and Addiction, 1*(1), 9–13. doi: 10.5814/ijhrba.4624

Kneisl, C. R., & Trigoboff, E. (2013). *Contemporary psychiatric-mental health nursing* (3d ed.). Upper Saddle River, NJ: Pearson.

Koob, G. F., & Simon, E. J. (2009). The neurobiology of addiction: Where we have been and where we are going. *Journal of Drug Issues, 39*(1), 115–132.

Krebs, L.U. (2007). Sexual assessment: Research and clinical. *Nursing Clinics of North America, 42,* 515–529.

Krebs, L. U. (2008). Sexual assessment in cancer care: Concepts, methods and strategies for success. *Seminars in Oncology Nursing, 24*(2 [May]), 80–90.

Krug, E. G., Dahlberg, L. L., Mercy, J. A., Zwi, A. B., & Lozano, R. (2002). World report on violence and health. Geneva: World Health Organization.

*Laux, J. M., Newman, I., & Brown, R. (2004). The Michigan alcoholism screening test (MAST): A statistical analysis. *Measurement and evaluation in counseling and development, 36*(January 1). Retrieved from http://www.accessmylibrary.com/article-1G1-115562442/michigan-alcoholism-screening-test.html

Lofthouse, N., & Yager-Schweller, J. (2009). Nonsuicidal self-injury and suicide risk among adolescents. *Current Opinion in Pediatrics, 21,* 641–645. doi: 10.1097/MOP.0b0113e2683306825

Marich-Merkin, J. (2011). Sexual addiction. *Course #9627.* Retrieved September 20, 2012, from http://www.netce.com/719/Course_9627.pdf

Martin, P. R., Singleton, C. K., & Stuemhofel, S.H. (2004). The role of thiamine deficiency in alcoholic brain disease. *National Institute of Alcohol Abuse and Alcoholism.* http://pubs.niaaa.nih.gov/publications/arh27-2/134-142.htm

Mayo Clinic Staff. (2010, December 11, 2008). Alcohol poisoning. Retrieved July 15, 2010, from http://www.mayoclinic.com/health/alcohol-poisoning/DS00861/METHOD=print

McKeown, N. J., & West, P. L. (2010, March 18, 2010). Withdrawal syndromes. *eMedicine Emergency Medicine.* Retrieved July 13, 2010, from http://emedicine/medscape.com/article/819502-print

MedicineNet. (2012, August 25, 2008). Shaken baby syndrome (sbs). Retrieved June 15, 2012, from http://www.medicinenet.com/script/main/art.asp?articlekey=92125

Muehlenkamp, J. J., Engel, S. G., Wadeson, A., Crosby, R. D., Wonderlich, S. A., Simonich, H., et al. (2008). Emotional states preceding and following acts of non-suicidal self-injury in bulemia nervosa patients. *Behaviour Research and Therapy, 47*, 83–87. doi: 10.1016/j.brat.2008.10.011

Nguyen-Khoa, D., Cope, D. W., Busschots, G., & Vallee, P. A. (2010). Beriberi (thiamine deficiency). *eMedicine from Web MD.* Retrieved July 1, 2010, from http://emedicine.medscape.com/article/116930-print

Nusbaum, M. R. H., & Hamilton, C. D. (2002). The proactive sexual health history. *American Family Physician, 66*(9), 1705–1713.

Pakpreo, P. (2005). Why do we take a sexual history? *Virtual Mentor, 7*(10). http://virtualmentor.ama-assn.org/2005/10/medul-0510.html

Pettit, J. W., Garza, M. J., Grover, K. E., Schatte, D. J., Morgan, S. T., Halper, A, et al. (2009). Factor structure and psychometric properties of the modified scale for suicidal ideation among suicidal youth. *Depression and Anxiety, 26*(8). doi: 10.1002/da.20575

Posner, K., Brown, G. K., Stanley, B., Brent, D. A., Yershova, K. V., Oquendo, M. A., et al. (2011). The Columbia-suicide severity rating scale: Initial validity and internal consistency findings from three multisite studies and adolescents and adults. *American Journal of Psychiatry, 168*(12), 1266–1277.

Posner, K., Oquendo, M. A., Gould, M., Stanley, B., & Davies, Mark. (2007). Columbia classification algorithm for suicide assessment (c-casa): Classification of suicidal events in the FDA's pediatric suicidal risk analysis of antidepressants. *American Journal of Psychiatry, 164*(7), 1035–1043.

Raue, P. J., Brown, E. L., Meyers, B. S., Schulberg, H. C., & Bruce, M. L. (2006). Does every allusion to possible suicide require the same response? *The Journal of Family Practice, 55*(7).

Rhodes, K .V., Frankel, R. M., Levinthall, N., Prenoveau, E., Bailey, J., & Levinson, W. (2007). "You're not a victim of domestic violence, are you?" Provider–patient communication about domestic violence. *Annals of Internal Medicine, 147*(9), 620–627.

Robinson, L., de Benedictis, T., & Segal, J. (2012, April 2012). Elder abuse and neglect: Warning signs, risk factors, prevention and help. Retrieved June 18, 2012, from http://www.helpguide.org/mental/elder_abuse_physical_emotional_sexual_neglect.htm

Sellas, M. I., & Krouse, L. H. (2012, June 08, 2011). Elder abuse. *Medscape Reference Drugs, Diseases & Procedures.* Retrieved June 18, 2012, from http://www.emedicine.medscape.com/article/805727

Shell, J.A. (2007). Including sexuality in your nursing practice. *Nursing Clinics of North America, 42*, 685–696.

Smith, M., & Segal, J. (2012, June 2012). Cutting and self-harm: Self-injury help, support and treatment. Retrieved September 21, 2012, from http://www.helpguide.org/mental/self_injury.htm

Springer, K. W., Sheridan, J., Kuo, D., & Carnes, M. (2007). Long-term physical and mental health consequences of childhood physical abuse: Results from a large population-based sample of men and women. *Child Abuse & Neglect, 31*, 517–530.

Subramanya, S. B., Subramanian, V. S., & Said, H. M. (2010). Chronic alcohol consumption and intestinal thiamin absorption: Effects on physiological and molecular parameters of the uptake process. *American Journal of Gastrointestinal and Liver Physiology, 299*, G23–G31.

Teicher, Martin H., Anderson, Carl M., & Polcari, Ann. (2012). Childhood maltreatment is associated with reduced volume in the hippocampal subfields ca3, dentate gyrus, and subiculum. *Proceedings of the National Academy of Sciences*. doi: 10.1073/pnas.1115396109

Thompson, W., Lande, R. G., & Kalapatapu, R. K. (2010, December 15, 2009). Alcoholism. *eMedicine Specialties.* Retrieved June 28, 2010, from http://emedicine.medscape.com/article/285913-print

U. S. Department of Health and Human Services. (2009). *Healthy people 2020 summary of objectives*. Washington DC: U. S. Government Printing Services.

Vonghia, L., Leggio, L., Ferrulli, A., Bertini, M., Gasbarrini, G., & Addolorato, G. (2008). Acute alcohol intoxication. *European Journal of Internal Medicine, 19*, 561–567.

Whitlock, J., Eckenrode, J., & Silverman, D. (2006). Self-injurious behaviors in a college population. *Pediatrics, 117*(6), 1939–1948. doi: 10.1542/peds.2005-2543

Wilmoth, M. C. (2007). Sexuality: A critical component of quality of life in chronic disease. *Nursing Clinics of North America, 42*, 507–514.

Woolf, L. M. (1998). *Elder abuse and neglect*. Gerontology. Webster University. Retrieved from http://www.webster.edu/~woolflm/abuse.html

World Health Organization. (2002). Gender and human rights. *Sexual and Reproductive Health.* http://www.who.int/reproductivehealth/topics/gender_rights/sexual_health/en/index.html

Young, K. A., Gobrogge, K. L., & Wang, Z. (2011). The role of mesocorticolimbic dopamine in regulating interactions between drugs of abuse and social behavior. *Neuroscience & Biobehavioral Reviews, 35*, 498–515. doi: 10.1016/j.neubiorev.2010.06.004

Chapter 16 References

Abdullah, L., & Abbas, O. (2011). Common nail changes and disorders in older people: Diagnosis and management. *Canadian Family Physician, 57*(February), 173–181.

American Cancer Society. (2011). Cancer facts & figures: 2011. Retrieved October 31, 2012, from http://www.cancer.org/acs/groups/content/@epidemiologysurveilance/documents/document/acspc-029771.pdf

American Cancer Society. (2012). Melanoma skin cancer overview. Retrieved October 31, 2012, from http://www.cancer.org/cancer/skincancer-melanoma/overviewguide/index

Antaya, J. (2012, 05/20/2013). Infantile hemangioma. *Medscape.* Retrieved from http://emedicine.medscape.com/article/1083849-overview

Baade, P. D., English, D. R., Youl, P. H., McPherson, M., Elwood, J. M., & Aitken, J. F. (2006). The relationship between melanoma thickness and time to diagnosis in a large population based study. *Archives of Dermatology*, 142, 1422–1427.

Bigal, M. E., Ashina, S., Burnstein, R., L., R. M., Buse, D., Serrano, D., & Lipton, R. B. (2008). Prevalance and characteristics of allodynia in headache sufferers: A population study. *Neurology, 70*(17 [April 22]), 1525-1533. doi: 10.1212/01.wnl.0000310645.31020.b1

Cancer Reference Information. (n.d.). What are the risk factors for squamous and basal cell skin cancer? Detailed Guide: Skin Cancer—Basal and Squamous Cell. Retrieved October 4, 2007, from http://www.cancer.org/docroot/CRI/content/CRI_2_4_2X_What_are _the_risk _fact

Czerkasij, V. (2007). What's getting under your skin? *Men in Nursing, 2*(3), 12–16.

Dawson, J. S. (2007). Relationship between smoking and wrinkles clarified. Retrieved October 9, 2007, from http://student,bmj.com/back_issues/0501/news/136b.html

DelRosso, J. Q., & Kim, G. K. (2009). Seborrheic dermatitis and *malassezia species*: How are they related? *The Journal of Clinical Aesthetic Dermatology, 2*(11), 14–18.

Edlich, R. F., Drake, D. B., & Long III, W. B. (2011, February 04, 2010). Thermal burns. *Medscape Reference Drugs, Diseases and Procedures.* Retrieved July 12, 2011, from http://emedicine.medscape.com/article12782

Fried, R. G., & Wechsler, A. (2006). Psychological problems in the acne patient. *Dermatologic Therapy, 19*, 237–240.

Garcia-Albea, V, & Limaye, K. (2012). The clinical conundrum of pruritus. *Journal of Dermatology Nurses' Association, 4*(2), 97–105. doi: 10.1097/JDN.0b013e31824abb10

*Habif, T. P. (1996). *Clinical dermatology*. St. Louis: Mosby.

Hettiaratchy, S., & Dziewulski, P. (2004). Abc of burns: Pathophysiology and types of burns. *British Medical Journal, 328*(12 June), 1427–1429.

Hilmer, A. M., Hanneken, S., Ritzman, S., Becker, T., Freudenberg, J., Brockschmidt, F.E., et al. (2005). Genetic variation in the human androgen receptor gene is the major determinant of common early-onset androgenetic alopecia. *American Journal of Human Genetics, 77*, 140–148.

Ikoma, A., Steinhoff, M., Stander, S., Yosipovitch, G., & Schmelz, M. (2006). The neurobiology of itch. *Neuroscience, 7*, 535–547. doi: 10.1038/nrn1950

Janda, M., Youl, P. H., Lowe, J. B., Baade, P. D., Elwood, M., Ring, I. T., et al. (2006). What motivates men age ≥ 50 years to participate in a screening program for melanoma? *Cancer 2006, 107*, 815–823.

Kaplan, P. D., Polefka, T., Grove, G., Daly, S., Jumbelic, L., Harper, D.,et al. (2011). Grey hair: Clinical investigation into changes in hair fibres with loss of pigmentation in a photoprotected population. *International Journal of Cosmetic Science, 33*, 171–182. doi: 10.1111/j.1468-2494.2010.00614.x

Kim, B. S. (2012, April 04, 2012). Atopic dermatitis clinical presentation. *Medscape Reference Drugs, Diseases & Procedures.* Retrieved November 1, 2012, from http://emedicine.medscape.com/article/1049085-overview#a0101

*Liu, W., Dowling, J. P., Murray, W. K., McArthur, G. A., Thompson, J. F., Wolfe, R., et al. (2006). Rate of growth in melanomas: Characteristics and associations of rapidly growing melanomas. *Archives of Dermatology, 142*, 1551–1558.

Martini, F. H., & Nath, J. L. (2009). *Fundamentals of anatomy and physiology*. San Francisco: Pearson Benjamin Cummings.

Mathew, N. T., Kailasam, J., & Seifert, T. (2004). Clinical recognition of allodynia in migraine. *Neurology, 63*, 848–852.

McLaughlin, M. R., O'Connor, N. R., & Ham, P. (2008). Nerwborn skin: Part ii. Birthmarks. *American Family Physician, 77*(1), 56–60.

*Moore, M. M., Geller, A. C., Zhang, Z., Hayes, B. B., Bergstrom, K., Graves, J. E., et al. (2006). Skin cancer examination teaching in US medical education. *Archives of Dermatolgy, 142*, 439–444.

Mounsey, A. L., & Reed, S.W. (2009). Diagnosing and treating hair loss. *American Family Physician, 80*(4), 356–362.

Murphy-Lavoie, H., & LeGros, T. L. (2010). Emergent diagnosis of the unknown rash: An algorithmic approach. *Emergency Medicine, March*, 6–17.

Pomeranz, M. K. (2013, December 11, 2012). The skin, hair, nails, and mucous membranes during pregnncy. *UpToDate.* Retrieved May 04, 2013, from http://www.uptodate.com/contents/the-skin-hair-nails-and-mucous-membranes-during-pregnancy?topicKey=OBGYN%2F456&elapsedTimeMs=5&vie

Rager, E. L., Bridgeford, E. P., & Ollia, D. W. (2005). Cutaneous melanoma: Update on prevention, screening, diagnosis, and treatment. *American Family Physician, 72*(2), 269–276.

Robinson, J. K., & Turrisi, R. (2006). Skills training to learn discrimination of ABCDE criteria by those at risk for developing melanoma. *Archives of Dermatology, 142*, 447–452.

Robinson, J. K., Fisher, S. G., & Turrisi, R. J. (2002). Predictors of skin self-examination performance. *Cancer 2002, 95*, 135–146.

Robinson, J. K., Turrisi, R., & Stapleton, J. (2007). Efficacy of a partner assistance intervention designed to increase skin self-examination performance. *Archives of Dermatology, 143*, 37–41.

Selden, S. T. (2012, March 23, 2012). Seborrheic dermatitis. *Medscape Reference Drugs, Diseases & Procedures.* Retrieved November 2, 2012, from http://emedicine.medscape.com/article/1108312-overview#a0104

Seidel, H. M., Ball, J. B., Dains, J. E., & Benedict, G.W. (2006). *Mosby's guide to physical examination.* St. Louis: Mosby Elsevier.

Taylor, S. T., & Zirwas, M. J. & Sood, A. (2012, August 1, 2011). Pruritus. *Disease Management Project.* Retrieved November 6, 2012, from http://www.clevelandclinicmeded.com/medicalpubs/diseasemanagement/dermatology/pruritus-itch/

Tunzi, M., & Gray, G. R. (2007). Common skin conditions during pregnancy. *American Family Physician, 75*(2), 211–218.

U. S. Department of Health and Human Services. (2009). *Healthy people 2020 summary of objectives.* Washington DC: U. S. Government Printing Services.

Wedro, B. C. (2011, October 28, 2008). First aid for burns. *MedicineNet.* Retrieved July 12, 2011, from http://www.medicinenet.com/script/main/art.asp?articlekey=306

Wilkin, J., Dahl, M., Detmar, M., Drake, L., Liang, M. H., Odom, R., & Powell, F. (2004). Standard grading system for rosacea: report of the National Rosacea Society Expert Committee on the classification and staging of rosacea. *Journal of the American Academy of Dermatology, 50*(6), 907–912. doi: http://dx.doi.org/10.1016/j.jaad.2004.01.048

Yosipovitch, G., & Bernhard, J. D. (2013). Chronic pruritus. *The New England Journal of Medicine, 368*(17), 1625–1634. doi: 10.1056/NEJMcp1208814

Chapter 17 References

Aegidius, K., Zwart, J., Hagen, K., & Stovner, L. (2009). The effect of pregnancy and parity on headache prevalence: The head-hunt study. *Headache, 49*, 851–859. doi: 10.1111/j.1526-4610.2009.01438.x

Agamanopolis, D. P. (2011, September 2010). Traumatic brain inury and increased intracranial pressure. *Neuropathology: An Illustrated Interactive Course for Medical Students and Residents.* Retrieved May 19, 2011, from http://www.neuropathologyweb.org/chapter4/chapter4bContusions_dai_sbs.html

Basaria, Shehzad, & Cooper, David S. (2005). Amiodarone and the thyroid. *The American Journal of Medicine, 118*(7), 706–714. doi: http://dx.doi.org/10.1016/j.amjmed.2004.11.028

Cabinum-Foeller, E. (2011, January 2011). Shaken baby/shaken impact syndrome. *KidsHealth from Nemours.* Retrieved May 23, 2011, from http://kidshealth.org/parent/medical/brain/shaken.html

Clinch, C. R. (2001). Evaluation of headaches in adults. *American Family Physician, 63*(4), 685–692.

Dawodu, S. T. (2011, March 30, 2009). Traumatic brain injury (TBI)—Definition, epidemiology, pathophysiology. *Medscape Reference.* Retrieved May 19, 2011, from http://emedicine.medscape.com/article/326510-overview#showall

Devereaux, M. (2009). Neck pain. *Medical Clinics of North America, 93*, 273–284. doi: 10.1016/j.mcna.2008.11.001

Ercan, I., Ozdemir, S. T., Etoz, A., Sigirli, D., Tubbds, R. S., Loukas, M., et al. (2008). Facial asymmetry in young healthy subjects evaluated by statistical shape analysis. *Journal of Anatomy, 213*, 663–669. doi: 10.1111/j.1469-7580.2008.01002.x

Faul, M., Likang, X., Wald, M. M., & Coronado, V. G. (2010). Traumatic brain injury in the United States: Emergency department visits, hospitalizations and deaths 2002–2006. Retrieved from ww.cdc.gov/TraumaticBrainInjury

Goldenberg, L.M.C. (2000). Thyroid disease in later life. *Thyrobulletin, 10*(4). Retrieved from thyroid.ca website: http://www.thyroid.ca/e4g.php

Kumar, A., & Karthikeyan, K. (2012). Madarosis: A marker of many maladies. *International Journal of Trichology, 4*(1), 3–18. doi: 10.4103/0974-7753.96079

Kwon, T. G., Park, H. S., Ryoo, H. M., & Lee, S. H. (2006). A comparison of carniofacial morphology in patients with and without facial symmetry—A three-dimensional analysis with computed tomography. *International Journal of Oral & Maxillofacial Surgery, 35*, 43–48. doi: 10.1016/ijom.2005.04.006

MacGregor, E. Anne. (2012). Headache in pregnancy. *Neurologic Clinics, 30*(3), 835–866. doi: http://dx.doi.org/10.1016/j.ncl.2012.04.001

Mohandas, R., & Gupta, V. K. (2003). Managing thyroid dysfunction in the elderly. *Posgraduate Medicine, 113*(5), 54–68,100.

Nayak, B., & Burman, K. (2006). Thyrotoxicosis and thyroid storm. *Endocrinology and Metabolism Clinics of North America, 35*, 663–686.

Uður, E, Meral., C., Karademir, F., Süleymanoðlu, S, Aydýnöz, S., & Göçmen, Ý. (2007). The effects of long-term carbamazepine, phenobarbital and valproic acid therapy on thyroid and parathyroid functions. *Gulhane Medical Journal, 49*(4), 222–225.

Pangilinan Jr, P. H., Kellyh, B. M., & Hurnyak, J. E. (2013, October 26, 2012). Classification and complications of traumatic brain injury. *Medscape Reference Drugs, Diseases & Procedures.* Retrieved May 13, 2013, from http://emedicine.medscape.com/article/326643-overview

Rehman, S. U., Cope, D. W., Senseney, A. D., & Brezesinski, W. (2005). Thyroid disorders in elderly patients. *Southern Medical Journal, 2005*(5), 543–549.

*Ronthal, M. (2013, 09/13/2012). Bell's palsy: Pathogenesis, clinical features, and diagnosis in adults. *UpToDate.* Retrieved October 4, 2013, from http://www.uptodate.com/contents/bells-palsy-pathogenesis-clinical-features-and-diagnosis-in-adults?topicKey=NEURO%2F5281&elapsedTimeMs=4&source=see_link&view=print&displayedView=full#

Ross, D. S. (2012, 05/14/2012). Beta blockers in the treatment of hyperthyroidism. *UpToDate.* Retrieved September 12, 2013, from http://www.uptodate.com/contents/beta-blockers-in-the-treatment-of-hyperthyroidism

Surks, M. I. (2013, 04/11/2012). Lithium and the thyroid. *UpToDate* Retrieved September 12, 2013, from http://www.uptodate.com/contents/lithium-and-the-thyroid

Tahboub, Rundsarah, & Arafah, Baha M. (2009). Sex steroids and the thyroid. *Best Practice & Research Clinical Endocrinology & Metabolism, 23*(6), 769–780. doi: http://dx.doi.org/10.1016/j.beem.2009.06.005

Taylor, D. C., Khoromi, S., & Zachariah, S.B. (2013, 11/30/2012). Bell's palsy. *Medscape Reference.* Retrieved October 09, 2013, from http://emedicine.medscape.com/article/1146903-overview#aw2aab6b2b5

U. S. Department of Health and Human Services. (2009). *Healthy people 2020 summary of objectives.* Washington DC: U. S. Government Printing Services.

Chapter 18 References

*Arroyo, J. G. (2013, 02/28/2013). Age-related macular degeneration: Clinical presentation, etiology, and diagnosis. *UpToDate.* Retrieved October 04, 2013, from http://www.uptodate.com/contents/age-related-macular-degeneration-clinical-presentation-etiology-and-diagnosis.

*Bok, D. (1993). The retinal pigment: A versatile partner in vision [supp]. *Journal of Cell Science, 17*, 189–195.

Brown, J. C., & Sunness, J. S. (2006). Pregnancy and the mother's eye. In W. Tasman & E. A. Jaeger (Eds.), *Duane's ophthalmology* (Vol. 5). Philadelphia: Lippincott Williams & Wilkins.

Bustos, D. E. (2011, April 27, 2010). Diabetic retinopathy. *Medline Plus.* Retrieved May 31, 2011, from http://www.nlm.nih.gov/medlineplus/ency/article/001212.htm

Chen, J., & Smith, L. E. H. (2006). Retinopathy of prematurity. *Angiogenesis, 10*, 133–140. doi: 10.1007/s10456-007-9066-0

College of Optomitrists. (2005). 10 reasons for having an eye examination. Retrieved November 11, 2007, from www.college-optomitrists.org/index.aspx/pcms/site

Dahl, A. A. (2013, 05/20/2011). Macular degeneration. *Medicine Net.com.* Retrieved October 09, 2013, from http://www.medicinenet.com/macular_degeneration/article.htm

Datta, S., Shankar, B., & Segal, S. (2010). *Obstetric anesthesia handbook* (5th ed.). New York: Springer.

Duderstadt, K. G. (2006). *Pediatric physical examination: An illustrated handbook.* St. Louis: Mosby/Elsevier.

Emanuele, N., Sacks, J., Klein, R., Reda, D., Anderson, R., Duckworth, W., & Abraira, C. (2005). Ethnicity, race, and baseline retinopathy correlates in the veterans affairs diabetes trial. *Diabetes Care, 28*(8), 1954–1958. doi: 10.2337/diacare.28.8.1954

Fraser, C. E., & D'Amico, D. J. (2013, 03/18/2013). Classification and clinical features of diabetic retinopathy. *UpToDat.e* Retrieved September 13, 2013, from http://www.uptodate.com/contents/classification-and-clinical-features-of-diabetic-retinopathy?topicKey=ENDO%2F1783&elapsedTimeMs=3&view=print&displayedView=full#

Friedman, D. S. (2004). Prevalence of open angle glaucoma among adults in the US Arch Ophthalmol. *122*, 532. Retrieved from http://www.uptodate.com.laneproxy.stanford.edu/contents/open-angle-glaucoma-epidemiology-clinical-presentation-and-diagnosis/abstract/5

*Heimmel. (2008). Ocular injuries in basketball and baseball: What are the risks and how can we prevent them? *Current Sports Medicine Reports, 7*(5), 284–288.

Hughes, B. M., & Moinfar, N. (2008, 1/04/2007). Hypertension. Retrieved 1/22, 2008, from http://www.emedicine.com/oph/topic4888.htm

Kawamura, S., & Tachibanaki, S. (2008). Rod and cone photoreceptors: Molecular basis of the difference in their physiology. *Comparative Biochemistry and Physiology Part A: Molecular & Integrative Physiology, 150*(4), 369–377. doi: http://dx.doi.org/10.1016/j.cbpa.2008.04.600

Klimanskaya, I., Hipp, J., Rezai, K. A., West, M., Atala, A., & Lanza, R. (2004). Deviation and comparative assessment of retinal pigment epithelium using transcriptonics. *Cloning and Stem Cells, 6*(3), 217–245.

Kruszelnicki, K. S. (2007). Pregnancy and eyesight. *Dr. Karl's Homework.* Retrieved December 20, 2007, from http://www.abc.net.au/science/k2/homework/s95613.htm

Lobach, D. F., Silvey, G. M., Macri, J. M., Hunt, M., Kacmaz, R. O., & Lee, P. P. (2005). Identifying and overcoming obstacles to point-of-care data collection for eye care professionals. Proceedings of the AMIA Annual Symposium, 465–469.

Lowther, G. E., & Lindsell, L. (n.d.). Eye examination. Retrieved November 11, 2007, from http://www/opt.indiana.edu.clinics/pt_educ/iexam/main.htm

Martini, F. H., & Nath, J. L. (2009). *Fundamentals of anatomy and physiology.* San Francisco: Pearson Benjamin Cummings.

Mayo Clinic Staff. (2006, February 11, 2010). Diabetic retinopathy. Retrieved November 30, 2007, from www.mayoclinic.com/health/diabetic-retinopathy/DS00447

Mayo Clinic Staff. (2007, August 26, 2010). Macular degeneration. Retrieved May 31, 2011, from http://www.mayoclinic.com/health/macular-degeneration/DS00284

*National Eye Institute. (2011, March 2010). Facts about retinopathy of prematurity. Retrieved June 01, 2011, from http://www.nei.nih.gov/health/rop/rop.asp

Paine, D. A., & Randleman, . J. B. (2007, March 18, 2008). Cataracts. *eMedicineHealth.* Retrieved May 31, 2011, from http://www.emedicinehealth.com/script/main/art.asp?articlekey=588

Pons, M. E., & Garcia-Valenzuela, E. (2007, 04/20/2007). Macular degeneration. *eMedicine Health.* Retrieved 11/11, 2007, from http://www.emedicinehealth.com/script/main/art.asp?articlekey=58819

Reing, C. S. & Wayne, N. J. (2006). Transitioning to EMR takes time but pays off: What you can learn from one practice's experience with transitioning to electronic medical records. Review of Ophthalmology, *13*(8). Retrieved from http://www.revophth.com/index.asp?page=1_996.htm

Rodriguez, J. O., Lavina, A. M., & Agarwal, A. (2003). Prevention and treatment of common eye injuries in sports. *American Family Physician, 67*(7), 1481–1488.

Seidel, H.M., Ball, J.W., Dains, J.E., & Benedict, G.W. (2006). Mosby's guide to physical examination. St. Louis: Mosby Elsevier.

Sheppared, J.D. (2011, September 29, 2008). Macular degeneration. Retrieved June 2, 2011, from http://www.emedicinehealth.com/macular_degeneration/article_em.htm

Shoji, T., Sakurai, Y., Sato, H., Chihara, E., & Takeuchi, M. (2011). Do type 2 diabetes patients without diabetic retinopathy or subjects with impaired fasting glucose have impaired colour vision? The okubo color study report. *Diabetic Medicine, 28*(7), 865–871. doi: 10.1111/j.1464-5491.2011.03290.x

Sowka, J. W., Gerwood, A. S., & Kabat, A. G. (2009). Hypertensive retinopathy. *Review of Optometry, April 15, 2009*(Supplement), 37A–39A.

Sparrow, J. R., Hicks, D., & Hamel, C. P. (2010). The retinal pigment epithelium in health and disease. *Current Molecular Medicine, 10*(9), 802–823. doi: 10.2174/156652410793937813

Spoerl, E., Zubaty, V., Raiskup-Wolf, F., & Pillunat, L. (2007). Oestrogen-induced changes in biomechanics in the cornea as a possible reason for keratcetasia. *British Journal of Ophthalmology, 91*(11), 1547–1550. doi: 10.1136/bjo.2007.124388

St. Luke's Eye. (2011). Cataracts. Retrieved May 31, 2011, from http://www.stlukeseye.com/conditions/cataracts.html

Strauss, O. (2005). The retinal pigment epithelium in visual function. *Physiological Review, 85*, 845–881. doi: 10.1152/physrev.00021.2004

U. S. Department of Health and Human Services. (2009). Healthy people 2020 *summary of objectives.* Washington DC: U. S. Government Printing Services.

Williams, M. E. (2006). Examining the eyes of an older adult. *Medscape Family Medicine.* Retrieved June 2, 2011, from http://ww.medscape.org/viewaartidcle/547645_print

Wilson, C., Horton, M., Cavallerano, J., & Aiello, L. M. (2005). Addition of primary care-based retinal imaging technology to an existing eye care professional referral program increased the rate of surveillance and treatment of diabetic retinopathy. *Diabetes Care, 28*(2), 318–322.

Wong, T.Y., & Mcintosh, R. (2005). Hypertensive retinopathy signs as risk indicators of cardiovascular morbidity and mortality. *British Medical Bulletin*, 73/74, 57–70

Wong, T., & Mitchell, P. (2007). The eye in hypertension. *Lancet, 369*(February 3), 425–435.

Chapter 19 References

Adcock, L. M., & Freysdottir, D. (2013, January 24, 2013). Screening the newborn for hearing loss. *UpToDate.* Retrieved May 21, 2013, from http://www.uptodate.com/contents/screening-the-newborn-for-hearing-loss?topicKey=PEDS%2F4985&elapsedTimeMs=4&view=print&displayedView=full#

Balentine, J. (2011, November 10, 2008). Meniere's disease (Meniere disease). *MedicineNet.com.* Retrieved June 14, 2011, from http://www.medicinenet.com/meniere_disease/article.htm

Berke, J. (2007, March 30, 2011). Top causes of deafness and hearing loss in children. Retrieved June 13, 2011, from http://deafness.about.com/od/medicalcauses/tp/topcauses.htm?p=1

Beyea, S. C. (2007). Noise: A distraction, interruption, and safety hazard. *AORN Journal, 86*(2), 281–285.

Bhattacharyya, N. (2011, January 21, 2009). Auditory brainstem auditory audiometry. *Medscape Reference: Drugs, Diseases & Procedures.* Retrieved June 9, 2011, from http://emedicine.medscape.com/article/836277

Bonilla, A. (2011, May 17, 2011). Pediatric microtia surgery. *Medscape Reference Drugs, Conditions & Procedures.* Retrieved June 08, 2011, from http://emedicine.medscape.com/article/995953

Bristol ENT Partnership. (2010, ND). Otoscopy. Retrieved October 09, 2013, from http://www.entbristol.co.uk/otoscopy.php

Broughton, Shelley S., Meyerhoff, William E., & Cohen, Stanley B. (2004). Immune-mediated inner ear disease: 10-year experience. *Seminars in Arthritis and Rheumatism, 34*(2), 544–548. doi: http://dx.doi.org/10.1016/j.semarthrit.2004.07.001

Buxton, O. M., Ellenbogen, J. M., Wang, W., Carbelleira, A., O'Connor, S., Cooper, D., et al. (2012). Sleep disruption due to hospital noises. *Annals of Internal Medicine, 157*(3), 170–179.

Centers for Disease Control and Prevention. (2013). *Hearing loss, facts.* Atlanta, GA: Retrieved from http://www.cdc.gov/NCBDDD/hearingloss/facts.html

Chanin, L. R. (2011, October 27, 10). Understanding ear infection—prevention. *WebMD.* Retrieved June 13, 2011, from http://www.webmd.com/cold-and-flu/ear-infection/understanding-otitis-media-prevention

Cunha, J. P. (2011, December 14, 2007). Cauliflower ear. *MedicineNet.com.* Retrieved June 14, 2011, from http://www.medicinenet.com/cauliflower_ear/article.htm

Cunha, J. P., & Decicco, M. (2011, February 22, 2008). Tinnitus. *eMedicinehealth.* Retrieved June 13, 2011, from http://www.emedicinehealth.com/tinnitus/article_em.htm

Davison, S. P., Bosley, N. B., & Sandel IV, H. D. (2011, September 19, 2008). Ear reconstruction and salvage procedures. *Medscape Reference Drugs, Diseases and Procedures.* Retrieved June 14, 2011, from http://emedicine.medscape.com/article/1288828-overview

Delaney, A. M., & Ruth, R. A. (2011a, June 15, 2010). Newborn hearing screening. *Medscape Reference: Drugs, Conditions & Procedures.* Retrieved June 06, 2011, from http://emedicine.medscape.com/article/836646-overview

Delaney, A. M., & Ruth, R. A. (2011b, June 15, 2010). Newborn hearing screening. *Medscape Reference: Drugs, Diseases & Procedures.* Retrieved June 09, 2011, from http://emedicine.medscape.com/article/836646-overview

Department of Otolaryngology Head and Neck Surgery. (2007). Hearing loss. Retrieved June 10, 2011, from http://www.entcolumbia.org/hearloss.html

Donaldson, J. D. (2011, February 02, 2010). Middle ear, acute otitis media, medical treatment. *Medscape Reference Drugs, Diseses & Procedures.* Retrieved June 09, 2011, from http://emedicine.medscapecom/article/859316

Eaton, D. A., & Murray, A. D. (2011, September 03, 2009). Complications of otitis media. *Medscape Reference: Drugs, Diseases & Peocedures.* Retrieved June 10, 2011, from http://emedicine/medscape.com/article/860323

Evrengül, H., Dursunoğlu, D., Kaftan, A., Zoghi, M., Tanrıverdi, H., Zungur, M., & Kılıç, M. (2004). Bilateral diagonal earlobe crease and coronary artery disease: A significant association. *Dermatology, 209*(4), 271–275.

Funk, E., & Gelbard, A. (2010). ENT complaints in pregnancy. Part 2: The ear and the throat. *Obstetric and Gynecologic Management, 22*(9), 28–40.

Gault, David. (2008). Post traumatic ear reconstruction. *Journal of Plastic, Reconstructive & Aesthetic Surgery, 61, Supplement 1*(0), S5–S12. doi: http://dx.doi.org/10.1016/j.bjps.2008.09.015

Ghosh, A., Harrison, M., & Body, R. (2006). Myringotomy in traumatic haemotympanum. *Emergency Medical Journal, 23*, 805–806

Ginzel, K. H., Maritz, G. S., Marks, D. F., Neuberger, M., Pauly, J. R., Polito, J. R., et al. (2007). Critical review: Nicotine for the fetus, the infant and the adolescent? *Journal of Health Psychology, 12*(2), 215–224. doi: 10.1177/1359105307074240

Gopen, Q., Keithley, E. M., & Harris, J. P. (2006). Mechanisms underlying autoimmune inner ear disease. *Drug Discovery Today: Disease Mechanisms, 3*(1), 137–142. doi: http://dx.doi.org/10.1016/j.ddmec.2006.02.006

Graven, S. N., & Browne, J. V. (2008). Auditory development in the fetus and infant. *Newborn & Infant Nursing Reviews 8*(4), 187–193. doi: 10.1053/j.nainr.2008.10.010

Gray, L. (2011). Chapter 12: Auditory system: Structure and function. *The vertebrate hair cell: Mechanoreceptor mechanism, tip links, K+ and Ca2+ channels.* Retrieved from http://neuroscience.uth.tmc.edu/s/2/chapter12.html

Harris, Tom. How Hearing Works. (30 March 2001). *HowStuffWorks.com.* Retrieved October 4, 2013, http://science.howstuffworks.com/life/human-biology/hearing.htm

Hartley, D., Rochtchina, E., Newall, P., Golding, M., & Mitchell, P. (2010). Use of hearing aids and assistive listening devices in an older australian population. *Journal of the American Academy of Audiology, 21*(10), 642–653. doi: 10.3766/jaaa.21.10.4.

Hepper, P. G., & Shahidullah, B. S. (1994). Development of fetal hearing. *Archives of Disease in Childhood, 71*, F81–F87.

HermanMiller Healthcare. (2006). Sound practices: Noise control. *Research Summary/2006*, 1–9. Retrieved from http://www.hermanmiller.com/MarketFacingTech/hmc/research_summaries/pdfs/wp_Sound_Practices.pdf

Juang, D. F., Lee, C. H., Yang, T., & Chang, M. C. (2010). Noise pollution and its effects on medical care workers and patients in hospitals. *International Journal of Environmental Science and Technology, 7*(4), 705–716.

Kelley, P. E., & Scholes, M. A. (2007). Microtia and congenital aural atresia. *Otolaryngological Clinics of North America, 40*, 61–80. doi: 10.1016/j.otc.2006.10.003

Kibby, J. E., & Mersch, J. (2011, July 23, 2008). Newborn infant hearing screening. *MedicineNet.com.* Retrieved June 09, 2011, from http://www.medicinenet.com/newborn_infant_hearing_screening/article.htm

Li, J. C. (2011, May 18, 2011). Inner ear, meniere disease, medical treatment. *Medscape Reference Drugs, Diseases & Procedures.* Retrieved June 14, 2011, from http://emedicine.medscape.com/article856547

Lin, S. J. (2011, December 21, 2009). Ear, prominent ear. *Medscape reference: Drugs, conditions & procedures.* Retrieved June 06, 2011, from http://emedicine.medscape.com/article/1290275-overview

Malloy, K. M., & Hollander, J. E. (2013, January 23, 2013). Assessment and management of auricle (ear) lacerations. *UpToDate.* Retrieved May 24, 2013, from http://uptodate.com/contents/assessment-and-management-of-auricle-lacerations

Martini, F. H., & Nath, J. L. (2009). *Fundamentals of anatomy and physiology.* San Francisco: Pearson Benjamin Cummings.

Mayo Clinic Staff. (2011, July 31, 2010). Tinnitus. *MayoClinichealth.* Retrieved June 13, 2011, from http://ww.mayoclinic.com/health/tinnitus/DS0365

Mazer, S. E. (2012). Creating a culture of safety: Reducing hospital noise. *Biomedical Instrumentation & Technology, September/October*(350–355).

Morlet, T. (2011, January 2011). Auditory processing disorder. *KidsHealth.* Retrieved June 13, 2011, from http://kidshealth.org/parent/medical/ears/central_auditory.html

Natal, B. L., & Chao, J. H. (2011, February 10, 2011). Otitis media in emergency medicine. *Medscape Reference: Drugs, Diseases & Procedures.* Retrieved June 09, 2011, from http://emedicine.medscape.com/article/764006

National Institute for Occupational Safety and Health. (2001). *Work related hearing loss.* (2001-103). Washington DC: US Government Printing Office. Retrieved from http://www.cdc.gov/niosh/docs/2001-103/.

Park, S. S. (2011, March 25, 2010). External ear, aural atresia. *Medscape Reference Drugs, Diseases & Procedures.* Retrieved June 08, 2011, from http://emedicine.medscape.com/article/845632-overview#showall

Perlstein, D. (2011). Otitis media (middle ear infection or inflammation). *MedicineNet.* Retrieved June 06, 2011, from http://www.medicinenet.com/otitis_media/article.htm

Pirozzo, S., Papinczak, T., & Glasziou, P. (2003). Whispered voiced test for screening for hearing impairment in adults and children: Systematic review. *British Medical Journal, 327*(October), 967–971.

Quail, G. (2005). Atypical facial pain: A diagnostic challenge. *Australian Family Physician, 34*(8), 641–645.

Ruben, R. J. (2011, April 2007). Hearing loss and deafness. *Merck Manual Home Edition.* Retrieved June 10, 2011, from http://www.merckmanuals.com/home/sec19/ch218/ch218a.html

Saunders, M. (2003). Otoscopy tutorial. *University of Bristol ENT.* Retrieved February 7, 2008, from www.bristol.ac.uk/Depts/ENT/otoscopu_tutorial.htm

Stachler, R. J., Chandrasekhar, S. S., Archer, S. M., Rosenfeld, R. M., Schwartz, S. R., Barrs, D. M., et. al. (2012). Clinical practice guidelines: Sudden hearing loss. *Otolaryngology—Head and Neck Surgery, 146*(S1), S1–S35. doi: 10.1177/0194599812436449

Stokowski, L. A. (2008). The inhospitable: No peace, no quiet. *MedscapeCME Nurses.* Retrieved June 09, 2011, from http://www.medscape.org/viewarticle/574813

The Joint Commission. (2013, April 08, 2013). Medical device alarm safety in hospitals. *The Joint Commission Sentinel Event Alert,* Issue 50. Retrieved May 22, 2013, from http://www.pwrnewmedia.com/2013/joint_commission/medical_alarm_safety/downloads/SEA_50_alarms.pdf

Thompson, B. L., Levitt, P., & Stanwood, G. D. (2009). Prenatal exposure to drugs: Effects on brain development and inplications for policy and education. *Nature Review Neuroscience, 10*(4), 303–312. doi: 10.1038/nrn2598

*Thrasher III, R. D. (2011, October 26, 2009). Middle ear, otitis media with effusion. *Medscape Reference Drugs, Diseases & Procedures.* Retrieved June 10, 2011, from http://emedicine.medscape.com/article/858990

Turner, K., Jones, A., & Handa, A. (2000). Emergency management of head injuries. *Student British Medical Journal, 8*, 140–142.

U. S. Department of Health and Human Services. (2009). Healthy people 2020 *summary of objectives.* Washington DC: U. S. Government Printing Services.

Waseem, M., & Aslam, M. (2011). Otitis media. *Medscape reference: Drugs, conditions & procedures.* Retrieved June 06, 2011, from http://emedicine.medscape.com/article/994656-overview

Wedro, B. C. (2011, January 29, 2011). Dizziness (dizzy). *MedicineNet.* Retrieved June 14, 2011, from http://www.medicinenet.com/dizziness_dizzy/article.htm

Yoon, T. (2008). Testing for hearing loss—The Weber and Rinne test. Retrieved January 15, 2008, from www.associatedcontent.com/pop_print.shtml?content_type=article&content_type_id=1.

Zamani, R., & Shaw, P. (2011, January 13, 2000). Ear infections (otitis media) and hearing loss in young children. *Health and Safety Notes California Childcare Health Program.* Retrieved June 10, 2011, from www.ucsfchildcarehealth.org

Yates, P. D., & Shahram, A., Chapter 49, otitis media. Lalwani AK: CURRENT Diagnosis & Treatment in Otolaryngology—Head & Neck Surgery, 2e. Retrieved from http://www.accessmedicine.com/content.aspx?aID=2830428.

Chapter 20 References

*Agency for Healthcare Research and Quality. (2001, February 2001). *Diagnosis and management of dental caries.* Retrieved May 23, 2008, from http://www.ahrq.gov/clinic.epcsums/dentsumm.htm

Aligne, C. A., Moss, M. E., Auinger, P., & Weitzman, M. (2003). Association of pediatric dental caries with passive smoking. *The Journal of the American Medical Association, 289*(10), 1258–1264.

American Cancer Society. (2007, September 28, 2007). *Treatment options by stage.* Retrieved May 23, 2008, from http://www.cancer.org/docroot/CRI/content/CRI_2_4_4X_Treatment_Options_by_Stage_60.a

*Ball, J. W., & Bindler, R. C. (2008). *Pediatric Nursing: Caring for Children* (4th ed.). Upper Saddle River; New Jersey: Pearson Prentice Hall.

Biavati, M. J., & Rocha-Worley, G. (2006, November 14, 2006). *Cleft palate.* Retrieved May 27, 2008, from http://ww.emedicine.com.ent/topic136.htm

Carstensen, T. K., & Fraser, W. R. (2006). *Periodontal (gum) disease.* Retrieved May 23, 2008, from http://www.emedicinehealth.com/script/main/art.asp?articlekey=58937&pf=3&page=1

Carver, A. P., & Morphis, L. (2006). Body piercing and its complications. *Nurse Practitioner Journal* (January).

Centers for Disease Control and Prevention. (2005). *Preventinag dental caries.* Retrieved May 23, 2008, from http://www.cdc.gov/print.co?url=http://ww/cdc/gov/nccdphp/publications/factsheets/prevention

Chao, M. T. (2013, 11/28/2012). Sports-related facial trauma. *Medscape Reference.* Retrieved September 16, 2013, from http://emedicine.medscape.com/article/1284288-overview

Douglas, D. (2008, May 7, 2008). *Gum disease, inflammation risky for pregnant women.* Retrieved May 23, 2008, from http://www.nlm.mih.gov/medlineplus/print/news/fullstory_64317.html

Duderstadt, K. G. (2006). *Pediatric Physical Examination: An Illustrated Handbook*. St. Louis: Mosby/Elsevier.

English, J. D., Buschang, P. H., & Throckmorton, G. S. (2002). Does malocclusion affect masticatory performance? *Angle Orthodontist, 72*(1), 21–27.

*Evans, J. A., & Rothenhaus, T. (2007, Nov 28, 2007). *Epistaxis*. Retrieved June 16, 2008, from http://www.emedicine.com?EMERG/topic806.htm

Grayson, C. E. (2005, February 17, 2005). *Gingivitis*. Retrieved May 23, 2008, from http://www.medicinenet.com/script/mainart.asp?ariclekey=376&pf=3&page=1

Hanioka, Takashi, Nakamura, Etsuko, Ojima, Miki, Tanaka, Keiko, & Aoyama, Hitoshi. (2008). Dental caries in 3-year-old children and smoking status of parents. *Paediatric and Perinatal Epidemiology, 22*(6), 546–550. doi: 10.1111/j.1365-3016.2008.00950.x

London, M. L., Laedwig, P. A. W., Ball, J. W., & Bindler, R. C. (2007). *Maternal & Child Nursing Care*. Upper Saddle River; New Jersey: Pearson Prentice Hall.

López, N. J., Da Silva, I. , Ipinza, J. , & Gutiérrez, J. (2005). Periodontal therapy reduces the rate of preterm low birth weight in women with pregnancy-associated gingivitis. *Journal of Periodontology, 76*(11 Suppl), 2144–2153.

Mangione, S. (2008). *Physical diagnosis secrets*. Philadelphia: Mosby.

March of Dimes. (2007). *Cleft lip and cleft palate: Quick references and fact sheet*. Retrieved May 27, 2008, from http://www.maarchofdimes.com/printableArticles/14332_1210.asp

Maupoime, G, Shulman, J. D., Medina-Solis, C. E., & Ladeinde, O. (2010). Is there a reationship between asthma and dental caries?: A critical review of the literature. *The Journal of the American Dental Association, 141*(9), 1061–1074.

Mayo Clinic Staff. (2006, July 14, 2006). *Oral and throat cancer*. Retrieved May 23, 2008, from http://www.mayoclinic.com/print/oral-and-throat-cancer/DS00349/DSECTION=all&METHOD=p

Mayo Clinic Staff. (2008). *Cleft lip and cleft palate*. Retrieved May 27, 2008, from http://www.mayoclinic.com/print/cleft-palate/DS00738/METHOD=print&DSECTION=all

Meltzer, D. I. (2005). Complications of body piercing. *American Family Physician, 72*(10), 2029–2034, 2035–2026.

Messahel, A., & Musgrove, B. (2009). Infective complications of tattooing and skin piercing. *Journal of Infection and Public Health, 2*, 7–13.

National Cancer Institute. (2004, September 8, 2004). *What you need to know about oral cancer*. Retrieved May 23, 2008, from http://www.cancer.gov/cancertopics/wyntk/oral/allpages/print

Nield-Gehrig, J. S., & Willman, D. E. (2007). Foundations of periodontics for the dental hygienist. Philadelphia: Lippncott Williams & Wilkins.

Parker, Samantha E., Mai, Cara T., Canfield, Mark A., Rickard, Russel, Wang, Ying, Meyer, Robert E., . . . for the National Birth Defects Prevention, Network. (2010). Updated national birth prevalence estimates for selected birth defects in the United States, 2004–2006. *Birth Defects Research Part A: Clinical and Molecular Teratology, 88*(12), 1008–1016. doi: 10.1002/bdra.20735

Peng, L. F., Kazzi, A. A., Peng, W., & Cheng, R. (2007, September 26, 2007). *Dental, Infections*. Retrieved June 16, 2008, from http://www.emedicine.com/emerg/topic128.htm

*Preidt, R. (2008). *HPV ties to better tongue, tonsil cancer outcomes*. Retrieved May 23, 2008, from http://www.nlm.nih.gov/medlineplus/news/fullstory_64616.html

Slayton, Rebecca L. (2012). Exposure to secondhand smoke may cause dental caries in children. *Journal of Evidence-Based Dental Practice, 12*(1), 8–9. doi: http://dx.doi.org/10.1016/j.jebdp.2011.12.004

Torpy, J. M. (2006). Periodontal disease. *Journal of the American Medical Association, 299*, 598.

Wolf, D., Foulds, M., & Daya, H. (2006). Antenatal carbimazole and choanal atresis. *Archives of Otolaryngology Head and Neck Surgery, 132*, 1009–1011.

Chapter 21 References

Aspinall, R., Del Guidice, G., Effros, R. B., Grubeck-Loebenstein, B., & Sambhara, S. (2007). Challenges for vaccination in the elderly. *Immunity & Ageing, 4*(9).

Ballow, M., Notarangelo, L., Grimbacher, B., Cunningham-Rundles, C., Stein, M., Helbert, M., . . . Franco, J. L. (2009). Immunodeficiencies. *Clinical & Experimental Immunology, 158*, 14–22. doi: 10.1111/j.1365-2249.2009.04023.x

Bonilla, F. A. (2013, 06/11/2013). Severe combined innumodeficiency [scid]: An overview. *UpToDate*. Retrieved September 17, 2013, from http://www.uptodate.com/contents/severe-combined-immunodeficiency-scid-an-overview?topicKey=ALLRG%2F3955&elapsedTimeMs=4&view=print&displayedView=full#

Gow, K. W. (2008). *Lymph node disorders*. Retrieved March 20, 2008, from http://www.emedicine.com/ped/TOPIC2975.HTM

Grethlein, S., & Perez, J. A. (2006, May 17, 2006). *Mucosal-associated lymphoid tissue*. Retrieved March 11, 2008, from http://www.emedicine,com/med/topic3204.htm

Kugler, M. (2007). *Severe combined innumodeficiency*. Retrieved March 25, 2008, from http://rarediseases.about.com/od/immunodedisorders/a/scid/htm?p=1

Lymph Notes. (2007). *Understanding the lymphatic system*. Retrieved February 19, 2008, from http://www.lymphnotes.com/article/php/id/151/

McCaughey, B. (2006, November 14, 2006). To catch a deadly germ. *The New York Times*.

Merck Manual of Geriatrics. (2008). *Infectious disease (Ageing and the immune system)*. Retrieved March 20, 2008, from http://www.merck.com/mkgr/mmg/sec16/ch131/ch131b.jsp

Modi, S. (2007). *How the lymphatic system works*. Retrieved March 10, 2008, from http://www.thenakedscientists.com/HTML/articles/article/thelymphaticsystem-1

Nield, L. S., & Kemat, D. K. (2004). Lymphadenopathy in children: When and how to evaluate. *Clinical Pediatrics, 43*, 25–33.

Revis, D. R. (2005, October 25, 2007). *Lymphedema*. Retrieved March 12, 2008, from http://www.emedicine.com/MED/topic2722.htm

Rossy, K. M., & Scheinfeld, N. S. (2013, 05/06/2013). Lymphedema. *Medscape* Retrieved October 5, 2013, from http://emedicine.medscape.com/article/1087313-overview

Secord, E. A. (2005). *Severe combined immunodeficiency*. Retrieved March 25, 2008, from http://www.emedicine.com/med/topic2214.htm

Stoppler, M. C. (2006, September 28, 2006). *8 causes of night sweats*. Retrieved March 20, 2008, from http://www.medicinenet.com/script/main/art.asp?articlekey=57394&pf=3&page=1

U. S. Department of Health and Human Services. (2000). *Healthy people 2010*. In Health and Human Services (Ed.) (2nd. ed.): U. S. Government Printing Services.

U. S. Department of Health and Human Services. (2009). Healthy people 2020 *summary of objectives*. Washington DC: U. S. Government Printing Services.

Viera, A. J., Bond, M. M., & Yates, S. W. (2003). Diagnosing night sweats. *American Family Physician, 67*(5), 1019–1024.

Williams, M. E. (2007, September 25, 2007). *Assessment of the neck and lymph nodes in the elderly patient*. Retrieved March 20, 2008, from http://www.medscape.com/viewprogram/7808_pnt

Chapter 22 References

*Armstrong, K., Moye, E., Williams, S., Berlin, J. A., & Reynolds, E. E. (2007). Screening mammography in women 40 to 49 years of age: A systematic review for the American college of physicians. *Annals of Internal Medicine, 146*(7), 516–526. doi: 10.7326/0003-4819-146-7-200704030-00008

*Brenner, R. James, & Parisky, Yuri. (2007). Alternative breast-imaging approaches. *Radiologic Clinics of North America, 45*(5), 907–923. doi: http://dx.doi.org/10.1016/j.rcl.2007.06.006

*Byrd, D. R., Dunnwald, L. K., Mankoff, D. A. , Anderson, B. O., Moe, R. E. , Yeung, R. S., Eary, J. F. (2001). Internal mammary lymph node drainage patterns in patients with breast cancer documented by breast lymphoscintigraphy. *Annals of Surgical Oncology, 8*(3), 234–240.

*Cho, E., Chen, W. Y., Hunter, D. J., & et al. (2006). Red meat intake and risk of breast cancer among premenopausal women. *Archives of Internal Medicine, 166*(20), 2253–2259. doi: 10.1001/archinte.166.20.2253

*Clemons, M., & Goss, P. (2001). Estrogen and the risk of breast cancer. *New England Journal of Medicine, 344*(23), 1804–1804. doi: doi:10.1056/NEJM200106073442318

*Colton, T., Greenberg, E., Noller, K., & et al. (1993). Breast cancer in mothers prescribed diethylstilbestrol in pregnancy: Further follow-up. *JAMA, 269*(16), 2096–2100. doi: 10.1001/jama.1993.03500160

*Eliassen, A., Colditz, G. A., Rosner, B., Willett, W. C., & Hankinson, S. E. (2006). Adult weight change and risk of postmenopausal breast cancer. *JAMA, 296*(2), 193–201. doi: 10.1001/jama.296.2.193

(FDA U. S. Food and Drug Administration). (2013). Medical devices (selenia dimensions 3d system-p08003). Silver Spring MD: U. S. Department of Health and Human Services. Retrieved from http://www.fda.gov/MedicalDevices/ProductsandMedicalProcedures/DeviceApprovalsandClearances/Recently-ApprovedDevices/ucm246400.htm

*Feigelson, Heather Spencer, Jonas, Carolyn R., Teras, Lauren R., Thun, Michael J., & Calle, Eugenia E. (2004). Weight gain, body mass index, hormone replacement therapy, and postmenopausal breast cancer in a large prospective study. *Cancer Epidemiology Biomarkers & Prevention, 13*(2), 220–224. doi: 10.1158/1055-9965.epi-03-0301

*Hamajima, N., Hirose, K., Tajima, K., Rohan, T., Calle, E. E., Heath Jr., C. W., . . . Meirik, O. (2002). Alcohol, tobacco and breast cancer - collaborative reanalysis of individual data from 53 epidemiological studies, including 58 515 women with breast cancer and 95 067 women without the disease. *Br J Cancer, 87*(11), 1234–1245. doi: org/10.1038/sj.bjc.6600596

*Hartmann, L. C., Sellers, T. A., Frost, M. H., Lingle, W. L., Degnim, A. C., Ghosh, K., . . . Visscher, Daniel W. (2005). Benign breast disease and the risk of breast cancer. *New England Journal of Medicine, 353*(3), 229–237. doi:10.1056/NEJMoa044383

*Henderson, T. O., Amsterdam, A., Hudson, M. M., Meadows, A. T., P., Neglia. J., Diller, L. R., Oeffinger, K. C. . (2010). Surveillance for breast cancer in women treated with chest radiation for a childhood, adolescent or young adult cancer: A report from the children's oncology group. *Annals of Internal Medicine, 152*(7), 444–W154. doi: 10.1059/0003-4819-152-7-201004060-00009

Hoover, R. N., Hyer, M., Pfeiffer, R. M., Adam, E., Bond, B., Cheville, A. L., . . . Troisi, R. (2011). Adverse health outcomes in women exposed in utero to diethylstilbestrol. *New England Journal of Medicine, 365*(14), 1304–1314. doi:10.1056/NEJMoa1013961

*Hulka, B. S., & Stark, A. T. (1995). Breast cancer: Cause and prevention. *The Lancet, 346*(8979), 883–887. doi: http://dx.doi.org/10.1016/S0140-6736(95)92713-1

*Jemal, A., Bray, F., Center, M. M., Ferlay, J., Ward, E., & Forman, D. (2011). Global cancer statistics. *CA: A Cancer Journal for Clinicians, 61*(2), 69–90. doi: 10.3322/caac.20107

*Jemal, A., Siegel, R., Xu, J., & Ward, E. (2010). Cancer statistics, 2010. *CA: A Cancer Journal for Clinicians, 60*(5), 277–300. doi: 10.3322/caac.20073

*McTiernan, A., Martin, C. F., Peck, J. D., Aragaki, A. K., Chlebowski, R. T., Pisano, E. D., . . . Investigators, for the Women's Health Initiative Mammogram Density Study. (2005). Estrogen-plus-progestin use and mammographic density in postmenopausal women: Women's health initiative randomized trial. *Journal of the National Cancer Institute, 97*(18), 1366–1376. doi: 10.1093/jnci/dji279

*Morimoto, L. M., White, E., Chen, Z., Chlebowski, R. T., Hays, J., Kuller, L., McTiernan, A. (2002). Obesity, body size, and risk of postmenopausal breast cancer: The women's health initiative (United States). *Cancer Causes & Control, 13*, 741–751.

*Moss, S. M., Cuckle, H., Evans, A., Johns, L., Waller, M., & Bobrow, L. (2006). Effect of mammographic screening from age 40 years on breast cancer mortality at 10 years' follow-up: A randomised controlled trial. *The Lancet, 368*(9552), 2053–2060. doi: http://dx.doi.org/10.1016/S0140-6736(06)69834-6

Nelson, H. D., Tyne, K., Naik, A., Bougatsos, C., Chan, B. K., & Humphrey, L. (2009). Screening for breast ccancer: An update for the U. S. Preventive services task force. *Annals of Internal Medicine, 151*(10), 727–737. doi: 10.7326/0003-4819-151-10-200911170-00009

*Parkin, D. M., Bray, F., Ferlay, J., & Pisani, P. (2005). Global cancer statistics, 2002. *CA: A Cancer Journal for Clinicians, 55*(2), 74–108.

*Rajukumar, S. V., & C., Hartmann L. (1999). Screening mammography in women aged 40–49 years. *Medicine, 78*(6), 410–416.

Ronquillo, J. G., Li, C., & Lester, W. T. (2012). Genetic testing behavior and reporting patterns in electronic medical records for physicians trained in a primary care specialty or subspecialty. *Journal of the American Medical Informatics Association.* doi: 10.1136/amiajnl-2011-000621

*Russo, J. (2013, 04/03/2013). Breast development and morphology. *UpToDate*, Retrieved from http://www.uptodate.com/contents/breast-development-and-morphology.

*Russo, I. H., & Russo, J. (1998). Role of hormones in mammary cancer initiation and progression. *Journal of Mammary Gland Biology and Neoplasia, 3*(1), 49–61

*Russo, J., Hu, Y. F., Silva, I. D. C. G., & Russo, I. H. (2001). Cancer risk related to mammary gland structure and development. *Microscopy Research and Technique, 52*(2), 204–223. doi: 10.1002/1097-0029(20010115)52:2<204::AID-JEMT1006>3.0.CO;2-F

*Russo, J., & Russo, I. H. (1987). In M. C. Neville & C. W. Daniel (Eds.), *The mammary gland: Development, regulation, and function* (pp. 648). New York NY: Springer.

*Sasco, Annie J., Lowenfels, Albert B., & Jong, Pieternel Pasker-De. (1993). Review article: Epidemiology of male breast cancer. A meta-analysis of published case-control studies and discussion of selected aetiological factors. *International Journal of Cancer, 53*(4), 538–549. doi:10.1002/ijc.2910530403

*Saslow, D., Boetes, C., Burke, W., Harms, S., Leach, M. O., Lehman, C. D., . . . Russell, C. A. . (2007). American cancer society guidelines for breast screening with MRI as an adjunct to mammography. *CA: A Cancer Journal for Clinicians, 57*(2), 75–89.

Smith, R. L., Pruthi, S., & Fitzpatrick, L. A. (2004). Evaluation and management of breast pain. *Mayo Clinic Proceedings, 79*(12), 1487–1598.

Tundia, N. L., Kelton, C. M. L., Cavanaugh, T. M., Guo, J. J., Hanseman, D. J., & Heaton, P.C. (2012). The effect of electronic medical record system sophistication on preventive healthcare for women. *Journal of the American Medical Informatics Association.* doi: 10.1136/amiajnl-2012-001099

Verloop, J., van Leeuwen, F. E., Helmerhorst, T. J. M., van Boven, H. H., & Rookus, M. A. (2010). Cancer risk in des daughters. *Cancer Causes & Control, 21*(7), 999–1007. doi: 0.1007/s10552-010-9526-5

U. S. Department of Health and Human Services. (2009). *Healthy people 2020 summary of objectives.* Washington DC: U. S. Government Printing Services.

Chapter 23 References

*Abbasi, K. (2011). A riot of divergent thinking. *Journal of the Royal Society of Medicine, 104*, 391. doi: 10.1458/jrsm.2011.11k038

*Bidwell, J. L., & Pachner, R. W. (2005). Hemoptysis: Diagnosis and management. *American Family Physician, 72*(7), 1253–1260.

*Cataletto, M.E. (2006). Obesity-hypoventilation syndrome and pulmonary consequences of obesity. *E-Medicine: Instant access to the minds of Medicine*. Retrieved from www.emedicine.com/ped/topic1627.htm

Cataletto, M.E., & Hertz, M. E. (2013, 09/23/2013). Pediatric obesity-hypoventilation syndrome. *Medscape*. Retrieved October 08, 2013, from http://emedicine.medscape.com/article/1002703-overview

Centers for Disease Control and Prevention (CDC). (2002). Annual smoking-attributable mortality, years of potential life lost, and economic costs—United States. *MMWR, 41*(300), 1–5. Retrieved from www.cdc.gov/mmwr/preview/mmwhrhtml/mm5425a1.htm

Centers for Disease Control and Prevention. (2013). *Economic facts about U. S. tobacco production and use.* Atlanta, GA: CDC. Retrieved from http://www.cdc.gov/tobacco/data_statistics/fact_sheets/economics/econ_facts/

*Centers for Disease Control and Prevention. (2011). *Quitting smoking among adults–United States, 2001–2010.* Atlanta GA: US Government. Retrieved from http://www.cdc.gov/mmwr/preview/mmwrhtml/mm6044a2.htm?s_cid=%20mm6044a2.htm_w

*Cincinnati Childrens Hospital Medical Center. (2004). Pectus excavatum. Retrieved from www.cincinnatichildrens.org/health/info/chest/diagnose/pectus-excavatum.htm

*Chang, R.C. (2005). Histoplasmosis. *E-Medicine: Instant access to the minds of Medicine.* Retrieved from www.emedicine.com/MED/topic1021.htm

*Christenbury, T.L. (2007). Patients "kick the habit" with nurses' help. *Men in Nursing, 2*(2), 15–21.

Farzan, S. (1997). Cough and sputum production. In S. Farzan & D. Farzan (Eds.), *A Concise Handbook of Respiratory Diseases* (4th ed., pp. 492). Saddleback, NJ: Prentice Hall.

Fiore, M. C., Jaén, C. R., Baker, T. B., Bailey, W. C., Benowitz, N. L., Curry, S. J., . . . Wewers, M. E. . (2008). *Treating tobacco use and dependence: 2008 update.Clinical practice guideline.* Rockville MD. Retrieved from http://www.ahrq.gov/professionals/clinicians-providers/guidelines-recommendations/tobacco/clinicians/update/treating_tobacco_use08.pdf.

Gardiner, R.M. (2004). Computerized clinical decision-support in respiratory care. *Respiratory Care, 49*, 378–386.

*Health Encyclopedia–Diseases and Conditions. (2001). Pigeon-breeders disease. *USA Today.* Retrieved from www.Healthscout.com.ency.68/300/main/html

Hebra, A. (2005). Pectus excavatum. *E-Medicine: Instant access to the minds of Medicine.* Retrieved from www.emedicine.com/ped/topic2558/htm

Hegewald, M. J., & Crapo, R. O. (2011). Respiratory Physiology in Pregnancy. *Clinics in Chest Medicine, 32*(1), 1–13. doi: http://dx.doi.org/10.1016/j.ccm.2010.11.001

Kamanger, N. (2013, 09/30/2013). Hypersensitivity pneumonitis. *Medscape Reference Drugs, Diseases and Procedures.* Retrieved 11/15, 2013, from http://emedicine.medscape.com/article/299174-overview

Karnani, N. G., Reisfield, G. M., & Wilson, G. R. (2005). Evaluation of chronic dyspnea. *American Family Physician, 71*(8), 1529–1538.

Kubin, L., Alheid, G. F., Zuperku, E. J., & McCrimmon, D. R. (2006). Central pathways of pulmonary and lower airway vagal afferants. *Journal of Applied Physiology, 101*(2), 618–627. doi: 10.1152/japplphysiol.00252.2006

Kuilboer, M. M., van Wijk, M. A., Mosseveld, M., van der Does, E., de Jongste, J. C., Overbeek, S. E., . . . van der Lei, J. . (2006). Computed critiquing integrated into daily clinical practice affects physicians' behavior—A randomized clinical trial with AsthmaCritic. *Methods of Information in Medicine, 45*, 447–454.

Madeppa, T., & Sharma, S. (2013, 03/30/2012). Atelectasis. *Medscape Reference Drugs, Diseases & Procedures.* Retrieved September 19, 2013, from http://emedicine.medscape.com/article/296468-overview

Mancini, M. C. (2013, 08/13/2012). Blunt chest trauma. *Medscape.* Retrieved 12/16, 2013, from http://emedicine.medscape.com/article/428723-overview#showall

Martini, F. H., & Nath, J. L. (2009). *Fundamentals of anatomy and physiology.* San Francisco: Pearson Benjamin Cummings.

Mayo Clinic Staff. (2006). Valley fever. Retrieved from www.mayoclinic.com/health/valleyfever/DS00695/DSection=3

Meisel, J. L., & Cottrell, D. (2013, 01/07/2013). Differential diagnosis of chest pain in adults. *UpToDate.* Retrieved September 19, 2013, from http://www.uptodate.com/contents/differential-diagnosis-of-chest-pain-in-adults

Muscari, M. E. (2005). *Pediatric nursing* (4th Edition ed.). Philadelphia: Lippincott Williams & Wilkins.

Polat, H., & Guler, I. (2004). A simple computer-based measurement and analysis system of pulmonary auscultation sounds. *Journal of Medical Systems, 28,* 665–672.

Ramanuja, S., & Kelkar, P. (2009). Habit cough. *Annals of Allergy, Asthma & Immunology, 102*(2), 91–95. doi: http://dx.doi.org/10.1016/S1081-1206(10)60235-9

*Rubenstein, L. Z. (1995). An overview of comprehensive geriatric assesment: Rationale, history, program models, basic components. In L. Z. Rubenstein, D. Wieland & R. Bernabei (Eds.), *Geriatric assessment technology: The state of the art.* New York, NY: Springer.

Schwartzstein, R. M. (2013, 09/05/2012). Approach to the patient with dyspnea. *UpToDate.* Retrieved September 20, 2013, from http://www.uptodate.com/contents/approach-to-the-patient-with-dyspnea?source=see_link

Seller, R. H. (2007). *Differential diangosis of common complaints* (5th ed.). Philadelphia: Saunders Elsevier.

Shiber, J. R., & Santana, J. (2006). Dyspnea. *The Medical clinics of North America, 90,* 453–479. doi: 10.1016/j.mcna.2005.11.006

Stochkendahl, M. J., & Christensen, H. W. (2010). Chest pain in focal musculoskeletal disorders. *Medical Clinics of North America, 94,* 259–273. doi: 10.1016/j.mcna.2010.01.007

Suratt, P. M. (2013, 05/15/2012). Pathogenesis of obesity hyperventilation syndrome. *UpToDate.* Retrieved 11/15, 2013, from http://www.uptodate.com/contents/pathogenesis-of-obesity-hypoventilation-syndrome?source=see_link

Thun, M. J., Carter, B. D., Feskanich, D., Freedman, N. D., Prentice, R., Lopez, A. D., . . . Gapstur, S. M. (2013). 50-Year Trends in Smoking-Related Mortality in the United States. *New England Journal of Medicine, 368*(4), 351–364. doi: doi:10.1056/NEJMsa1211127

U. S. Department of Health and Human Services. (2009). *Healthy people 2020 summary of objectives.* Washington DC: U. S. Government Printing Services.

U. S. Department of Health and Human Services. (2012). *Preventing tobacco use among youth and young adults: A report of the surgeon general.* Washington DC: U. S. Goverment Printing Office. Retrieved from http://www.ncbi.nlm.nih.gov/books/NBK99237/pdf/TOC.pdf.

Vinker, S., Kaiserman, I., Waitman, D. A., Blackman, S., & E., Kitai. (2006). Prescription of ocular beta-blockers in patients with obstructive pullomary disease: Does a central electronic medical record make a difference? *Clinical Drug Investigation, 26,* 495–450.

Weinberger, S. E. (2013, 06/06/2013). Etiology and evaluation of hemoptysis in adults. *UpToDate.* Retrieved September 20, 2013, from http://www.uptodate.com/contents/etiology-and-evaluation-of-hemoptysis-in-adults

Yasushi, O., Keiji, M., S., H., Yoshihiro, O., Yoshihiro, K., Kazue, K., & Mikio, O. (2011). Nutritional deficits in elderly smokers with respiratory symptoms that do not fulfill the criteria for COPD *International Journal of Chronic Obstructive Pulmonary Disease, 2011*(6), 679–683. doi: 10.2147/COPD.S25293

Chapter 24 References

American Heart Association. (2009, N.D.,). Congenital heart defects. Retrieved November 6, 2009, from http://www.americanheart.org/print_presenter.jhtml?identifier=4565

Beinart, S. C. (2012, 06/13/12). Junctional rhythm. *Medscape Reference Drugs, Diseases, & Procedures* Retrieved September 07, 2012, from http://emedicine.medscape.com/article/155146-overview

Budzikowski, A. S., Corsello, A.C., Daubert, J.P., & Shah, H. (2009, June 17, 2009). Third-degree atrioventricular block. *eMedicine* Retrieved November 24, 2009, from http://emedicine.medscape.com/article/1602007-print

Centers for Disease Control and Prevention. (2012, June 7, 2012). Childhood obesity facts Retrieved August 17, 2012, from http://www.cdc.gov/healthyyouth/obesity/facts/htm

Chin, T. K., Chin, E. M., Siddiqui, T., & Sundell, A. (2012, May 30, 2012). Rheumatic heart disease. *Medscape Reference Drugs, Diseases & Procedures* Retrieved July 09, 2012, from http://emedicine.medscape.com/article/891897-overview

Clarke, R., Bennett, D. A., Parish, S., Verhof, P., Dotsch-Klerk, M., Lathrop, M., . . . Peto, R. (2012). Homocysteine and coronary heart disease: Meta-analysis of mthfr case-control studies, avoiding publication bias. *PLoS Medicine, 9*(2), e1001177. doi: 10.1371/journal.pmed.1001177

Dowshen, S. (2009, July 2009). Type 2 diabetes: What is it. *KidsHealth* Retrieved October 30, 2009, from http://kidshealth/org/PageManager.jsp?dn=KidsHealth&llic=1&ps

Earnest, M. B., & Tadros, P. N. (2007). St-segment elevation myocardial infarction: What role for anticoagulants and antiplatelet agents? *Consultant, 47*(4), 1–7.

Fenton, D.E. (2009, October 9, 2009). Myocardial infarction. *eMedicine Emergency Medicine* Retrieved December 3, 2009, from http://emedicine.medscape.com/article759321-print

Giovino, G. A., Mirza, S. A., Samat, J. M., Gupta, P. C., Jarvis, M. J., Bhala, N., . . . Asma, S. (2012). Tobacco use in 3 billion individuals from 16 countries: An analysis of nationally representative cross-sectional household surveys. *Lancet, 380*(August 18), 668–679.

Kim, Y. J., & Park, H. A. (2005). Analysis of nursing records of cardiac-surgery patients. *International Journal of Medical Informatics, 74,* 952–959.

Ladewig, P. A. W., London, M. L., & Davidson, M. R. (2010). *Contemporary maternal-newborn nursing care* (7th ed.). Upper Saddle River, NJ: Pearson Education.

Levin, M. (2009, 4/28/2008). Infectious endocarditis. *Medline Plus.* Retrieved November 13, 2009, from http://www.nlm.nih.gov/medlineplus/print/ency/article/000681.htm

Lyon, R. A., Rees, P. S. C., Prasad, S., Poole-Wilson., P. A., & Harding, S.E. (2008). Stress (taksosubo) cardiomyopathy–A novel pathyphysiological hypothesis to explain catecholamine-induced myocardial stunjning. *Nature Clinical Practice Cardiovascular Medicine, 5*(1), 22–29. doi: 10.1038/npcardio 1066

Mangione, S. (2008). *Physical diagnosis secrets.* Philadelphia: Mosby.

Morbidity and Mortality Weekly Report. (2012, Oct 14, 2011). Prevalence of coronary heart disease–United States, 2006–2010 Retrieved August 16, 2012, from http://www.cdc.gov/mmwr/preview/mmwrhtml/mm6040a1.html

Mosca, L., Benjamin, E. J., Berra, K., Bezanson, J. L., Dolor, R. J., Lloyd-Jones, Donald M., . . . Wenger, N. K. (2011). Effectiveness-based guidelines for the prevention of cardiovascular disease in women–2011 update: A guideline from the American heart association. *Circulation, 123,* 1243–1262. doi: 10.1161/CIR.0

National Heart, Lung, and Blood Institute. (2012). Morbidity & mortality: 2012 chart book on cardiovascular, lung, and blood diseases. Retrieved August 16, 2012, from http://www.nhlbi.nih.gov/resources/docs/2012_ChartBook.pdf

Ogbru, Omudhome. (2009, September 9, 2008). Medications and drugs: Statins. *MedicineNet.com.* Retrieved October 23, 2009, from http://www.medicinenet.com/script/main/art.asp?articlekey+18510

Ogden, C .L., Carroll, M. D., Kit, B. K., & Flegal, K. M. (2012). Prevalence of obesity in the united states, 2009-2010. *NCHS Data Brief, 82*(Jan 2012), 1–8.

Petterson, G., & Thomas, J. (2010, 07/10.). Infective endocarditis *HealthHub from Cleveland Clinic.* Retrieved September 07, 2012, from http://my.clevelandclinic.org/heart/disorders/valve.sbe.aspx

U. S. Department of Health and Human Services. (2009). Healthy people 2020 *summary of objectives.* Washington DC: U. S. Government Printing Services.

Vaccarino, V. (2006). Angina and cardiac care: Are there gender differences and if so, why? *Circulation, 113,* 467–469. doi: 10.1161/CIRCULATIONAHA.105.602284

Vivian, E. M. (2006). Type 2 diabetes in children and adolescents–The next epidemic. *Current Medical Research and Opinion, 22,* 297–306. http://www.medscape.com/viewarticle

Wierzbicki, A. S. (2007). Homocysteine and cardiovascular disease: A review of the evidence. *Diabetes and Vascular Disease Research, 4,* 143–149. doi: 10.31321dvdr.2007.033

World Health Organization. (2012, September 2011). Cardiovascular diseases (cvds), Retrieved August 16, 2012, from http://www.who.int/mediacentre/factsheets/fs317/en/index.html

Chapter 25 References

Aboyans, V., Criqui, M. H., Denenberg, J. O., Knoke, J. D., Ridker, P. M., & Fronek, A. (2006). Risk factors for progression of peripheral arterial disease in large and small vessels. *Circulation, 113,* 2623–2629. doi: 10.1161/CIRCULATIONAHA.105.608679

Aquarius, A. E., DeVries, J., & Van Berge Henegouwen, D. P. (2006). Clinical indicators and psychosocial aspects of peripheral arterial disease. *Archives of Surgery, 141,* 161–166.

Assar, A. N., & Zarins, C. K. (2009). Ruptured abdominal aortic aneurysm: A surgical emergency with many clinical presentations. *Postgraduate Medicine, 85,* 268–273. doi: 140.1136/pgmj.2008.074666

Bartholomew, J. R., Schaffer, J. L., & McCormick, G. F. (2011). Air travel and venous thromboembolism: Minimizing the risk. *Cleveland Clinic Journal of Medicine, 78*(2), 111–120.

Bezanson, J. L., Strickland, O. L., Kinney, M. R., & Weintraub, W. S. (2002). Assessing data adequacy for clinical research: reliability and validity of a surgical database. *Journal of Nursing Measurement, 10*(2), 155–164.

Cevallos, M. (2012, June 07, 2011). DASH taks top honors in U. S. news diet ranking, *Los Angeles Times*. Retrieved from http://articles.latimes.com/print/2011/jun/07/news/la-heb-dash-diet

Cook, D. J., & Simel, D. L. (2009). Does this patient have abnormal central venous pressure? In D. L. Simel & D. Rennie (Eds.), *The rational clinical examination: Evidence-based clinical diagnosis* (pp. 744). New York: McGraw Medical.

Das, A. M., & Khayat, R. (2009). Hypertension in obstructive sleep apnea: risk and therapy. *Expert Review of Cardiovascular Therapy, 7*(6), 619–626. doi: 10.1586/erc.09.25

Gey, D. C., Lesho, E. P., & Manngold, J. (2004). Management of peripheral arterial disease. *American Family Physician, 69*(3), 525–532.

Khan, T. H., Farooqui, F. A., & Niazi, K. (2008). Critical review of the Ankle Brachial Index. *Current Cardiology Reviews, 4*(2), 101–106.

Lizka, H. A., Mainous, A. G., King, D. E., Everett, C. J., & Egan, B. M. (2005). Prehypertension and cardiovascular morbidity. *Annals of Family Medicine, 3*(4), 294–299. doi: 10.1370/afm.312

Mangione, S. (2008). *Physical diagnosis secrets.* Philadelphia: Mosby.

Maviglia, S. M., Teich, J. M., Fiskio, J., & Bates, D. W. (2001). Using an electronic medical record to identif oppoprtunities to imporve compliance with cholesterol guidelines. *Journal of General Internal Medicine, 16*, 531–537.

Mohler III, E. R., & Olin, J. W. (2013, 08/13/2013). Thromboangiitis obliterans (Buerger's disease). *UpToDate.* Retrieved September 22, 2013, from http://www.uptodate.com/contents/thromboangiitis-obliterans-buergers-disease

Moss, A. J., Liebling, W., Austin, W. O., & Adams, F. H. (1957). Determining blood pressure in infants: Use of the flush technique. *California Medicine, 87*(3), 166–167.

Muscari, M. E. (2005). *Pediatric nursing* (4th ed.). Philadelphia: Lippincott Williams & Wilkins.

National Institues of Health. (2001). *The DASH Diet.* Washington DC: U. S. Department of Health and Human Services.

O'Hare, J. L., & Earnshaw, J. J. (2008). Practical advice for the treatment of venous disease in the elderly. *Phlebology, 23*, 101–102. doi: 10.1258/phleb.2007.007080

Palm, M. D., Trizna, Z., & Goldman, M. P. (2011, Jan 15 2009). Thrombophlebitis. *Medscape Reference Drugs, Diseases & Procedures.* Retrieved November 22, 2011, from http://emedicine.medscape. com/article/1086399

Patel, J., Landers, K., Li, H., Mortimer, R. H., & Richard, K. (2011). Thyroid hormones and fetal neurological development. *Journal of Endocrinology, 209*, 1–8.

Pearce, W. H. (2011, Oct 28, 2009). Abdominal aortic aneurysm. *Medscape Reference.* Retrieved November 28, 2011, from http://emedicine.medscape.com/article/463354-overview

Raskob, G. E., Silverstein, R., Bratzler, D. W., Heit, J. A., & White, R. H. (2010). Surveillance for Deep Vein Thrombosis and Pulmonary Embolism: Recommendations from a National Workshop. *American Journal of Preventive Medicine, 38*(4, Supplement), S502–S509. doi: http://dx.doi.org/10.1016/j.amepre.2010.01.010

Rehring, T. F., Stolpart, R. S., Sandhoff, B. G., J. A., Merenichm, & Hollis Jr., H. W. (2006). Effect of a clinical pharmacy service on lipid control in patients with peripheral artery disease. *Journal of Vascular Surgery, 43*, 1205–1210.

Rinckenbach, S, Albertini, J. N., Thaveau, F., Steinmetz, E., Camin, A., Ohanessian, L., . . . Kretz, J. G. (2010). Prehospital treatment of infrarenal ruptured abdominal aortic aneurysms: A multicentric analysis. *Annals of Vascular Surgery, 24*(3), 308–314. doi: 10.1016/j.avsg.2009.08.011

Sakalihasan, N., Limet, R., & Defawe, O. D. (2005). Abdominal aortic aneurysm. *Lancet, 365*(April 30), 1577–1589.

Saultz, A., Mathews, E. L., Saultz, J. W., & Judkins, D. (2010). Does hypercoagulopathy testing benefit patients with DVT? *The Journal of Family Practice, 59*(5), 291–294.

Shammas, N., W. (2007). Epidemiology, classification, and modifiablel risk factors or peripheral vascular disease. *Vascular Health and Risk Management, 3*(2), 229–234.

Shamsham, F., & Mitchell, J. (2000). Essentials of the diagnosis of heart failure. *American Family Physician, 61*(5), 1319–1328.

Shapiro, A. D. (2001). An overview of thrombophilia. *Hemaware, 6*(5), 13–16.

Sontheimer, D. L. (2006). Peripheral vascular disease: Diagnosis and treatment. *American Family Physician, 73*, 1971–1976.

Tau, G. Z., & Peterson, B. S. (2012). Normal development of brain circuits. *Neuropsychopharmacology, 35*, 147–168. doi: 10.1038/npp.2009.115

U. S. Department of Health and Human Services. (2009). *Healthy people 2020 summary of objectives.* Washington DC: U. S. Government Printing Services.

*Wiese, J. (2000). The abdominojugular reflux sign. *The American Journal of Medicine, 109*, 59–61.

Chapter 26 References

Berne, R. M., & Levy, M. N. (2002). *Principles of Physiology*. St. Louis: Mosby.

Chiu, S.-L., & Cline, H. T. (2010). Insulin receptor signaling in the development of neuronal structure and function *Neural Development* (Vol. 5).

*Centers for Disease Control and Prevention. (2003). *Glascow coma scale.* Washington, DC: US Government Printing Office. Retrieved from http://emergency.cdc.gov/masscasualties/gscale.asp.

Cruz-Flores, S., Rabinstein, A., Biller, J., Elkind, S. V., Griffith, P., Gorelick, P. B., . . . Valderrama, A. L. (2011). Racial-ethnic disparities in stroke care: The American experience: A statement for healthcare professionals from the American heart associateion/American stroke association. *Stroke, 42*, 2091–2116. doi: 10.1161/STR.0b013e3182213e24

*Faul, M., Xu, L., Wald, M. M., & Coronado, V. G. (2010). *Traumatic brain injury in the United States: Emergency department visits, hospitalizations, and deaths 2002–2006.* Retrieved February 8, 2011, from http://www.cdc.gov/traumaticbraininjury/pdf/blue_book.pdf

Glynn, L. M., & Sandman, C. A. (2011). Prenatal origins of neurological development: A critical period for fetus and mother. *Current Directions in Psychological Science, 20*(6), 384–389. doi: 10.1177/0963721411422506

Kim, P., Leckman, J. F., Mayes, L. C., Feldman, R., Wang, X., & Swain, J. E. (2010). The plasticity of human maternal brain: Longitudinal changes in brain anatomy during the early postpartum period. *Behavioral Neuroscience, 124*(5), 695–700. doi: 10.1037/a0020884

Kinsley, C. H., & Meyer, E. A. (2010). The construction of the maternal brain: Theoretical comment on Kim et al. (2010). *Behavioral Neuroscience, 124*(5), 710–714. doi: 10.1037/a0021057

Members, Writing Group, Roger, Véronique L., Go, Alan S., Lloyd-Jones, Donald M., Benjamin, Emelia J., Berry, Jarett D., . . . Turner, Melanie B. (2012). Heart disease and stroke statistics—2012 update: A report from the American heart association. *Circulation, 125*(1), e2–e220. doi: 10.1161/CIR.0b013e31823ac046

Merck Manual, Professional Edition. (2005). Introduction: Stupor and coma. Retrieved May 16, 2007, from http://www. merck.com/mmpe/print/sec16/ch212/ch212a.html

Nor, A.M., McAllister, C., Louw, S.J., Dyker, A.G., Davis, M., Jenkinson, D., & Ford, G.A. (2004). Agreement between ambulance paramedic and physician recorded neurological signs with face arm speech test (fast) in acute stroke patients *Stroke, 35*, 1355–1368. http://stroke.ahsjournals.org/cgi/content/full/35/6/1355?maxtoshow=&HITS=10&hits=10 doi:01.STR.0000128529.63156.C5V1

Nor, S.M., McAllister, C., Louw, S.J., Dyker, A.G, Davis, M., & Jenkinson, D. (2004). Face, arm, speech tests allows for quick, accurate stroke diagnosis. American Stroke Association (Publication no. NR04-1246 [Stroke/Ford]). Retrieved Februray 26, 2007, from http://www.strokeassociation.org/presenter.jhtml?identifier=3021505

Oommen, K. (2013, 02/28/2013). Neurological history and physical examination. *Medscape Reference Drugs, Diseases & Procedures.* Retrieved September 22, 2013, from http://emedicine.medscape.com/article/1147993-overview#showall

Russell, S, & Triola, M. (2006). The precise neurological exam. Retrieved February 13, 2007, from http://endeavor.med.nyu.edu/neurosurgery/index.html

Sacco, R.L., Adams, R., Albers, G., Alberts, M.J., Benavente, O., Furie, K., . . . Tomsick, T. (2006). Guidelines for prevention of stroke in patients with ischemic stroke or transient ischemic attack. *Stroke, 37*, 577–617.

Sandman, C. A., Davis, E. P., Buss, C., & Glynn, L. M. (2011). Prenatal programming of human neurological function. *International Journal of Peptides, 2011*(Article ID 837596), 9. doi: 10.1155/2011/837596

Santacruz, K. S., & Swagerty, D. (2001). Early diagnosis of dementia. *American Family Physician, 63*(4), 703–713, 717–708.

Stephan, Alexander H., Barres, Ben A., & Stevens, Beth. (2012). The complement system: An unexpected role in synaptic pruning during development and disease. *Annual Review of Neuroscience, 35*(1), 369–389. doi: doi:10.1146/annurev-neuro-061010-113810

Stiles, J., & Jernigan, T. L. (2010). The basics of brain development. *Neuropsychological Review, 20*, 327–348. doi: 10.1007/s11065-010-9148-4

*Tamas Freund and Szabolcs Kali (2008) Interneurons. *Scholarpedia, 3*(9):4720.

*Teasdale, G.T. (1974). Assessment of coma and impaired consciousness: A practical scale. *Lancet, 2*, 81–84.

U. S. Department of Health and Human Services. (2009). Healthy people 2020 *summary of objectives.* Washington DC: U. S. Government Printing Services.

Yang, M. (2004). Newborn neurologic examination Retrieved February 19, 2007, from http://www.neurology.org/cgi/content/full/62/7/E15

Zieve, D., & Hoch, D. B. (2012, 6/16/2010). Spinal cord trauma. Retrieved March 3, 2012, from *http://www.ncbi.nlm.nih.gov/pubmedhealth/PMH0002061*

Chapter 27 References

*Abraham, I. (2000). Low back pain management. *The Clinical Advisor, September 2000*, 35–49.

American Association of Clinical Chemistry. (2006, August 17, 2006). *Lab tests online: Osteoporosis.* Retrieved August 1, 2008, from http://www.labtestsonline.org/understanding/conditions/osteoporosis

Arar, N. H., Wang, & Pugh, J. A. (2006). Self-care communication during medical encounters: Implications for future electronic medical records. *Perspectives in Health Information Mangement* (Vol. 3).

Bhangle, S., Sapru, S., & Panush, R. S. (2009). Back pain made simple: An approach based on principles and evidence. *Cleveland Clinic Journal of Medicine, 76*(7), 393–399. doi: 10.3949/ccjm.76a.08099

Bhatti, N. S., & Ertl, J. P. (2005, Dec 9, 2005). *Hip fracture.* Retrieved October 23, 2008, from http://www.emedicine.com/sports/topic48.htm

Brunner, L. C., & Kuo, T. Y. (2003). Hip fractures in adults. *American Family Physician, 67*, 537–542.

*Calis, M., Akgun, K., Birtane, M., Karacan, I., Calis, H., & Tuzun, F. (2000). Diagnostic values of clinical diagnostic tests in subacromial impingement syndrome. *Annals of Rheumatic Disorders, 59*, 44–47.

Cleveland Clinic. (2008, 3/27/2008). *Muscular dystrophies.* Retrieved October 7, 2008, from http://my.clevelandclinic.org/disorders/Muscular_Dystrophy/htm

*Clinical Practice Guidelines for Nurses in Primary Care. (2005, 03/17/2005). *Chapter 7–Musculoskeletal System.* Retrieved June 18, 2008, from http://www.hc-sc.gc.ca/fniah-spnia/pubs/services_nursing-infirm/2000_clin-guie/chap_07a-eng.php

Do, T. (2007, Mar 30, 2007). *Muscular dystrophy.* Retrieved October 7, 2008, from http://www.emedicine.com/orthoped/TOPIC418.HTM

*Drezner, J. A., & Herring, S. A. (2001). Managing low-back pain: Steps to optimize function and hasten return to activity. *The Physician and Sports Medicine, 29*(8), 37–43.

Duderstadt, K. G. (2006). *Pediatric Physical Examination: An Illustrated Handbook.* St. Louis: Mosby/Elsevier.

Galatz, L. M. (2010). Physical examination of the shoulder In J. F. Sarwark (Ed.). *Essentials of musculoskeletal care* (4th ed.). Rosemont, IL: American Academy of Orthopedic Surgeons.

Goldenberg, D. L. (2013, 08/07/2013). Clinical manifestations and diagnosis of fibromyalgia in adults. *UpToDate.* Retrieved September 25, 2013, from http://www.uptodate.com/contents/clinical-manifestations-and-diagnosis-of-fibromyalgia-in-adults

Hobar, C. (2005). *Osteoporosis.* Retrieved August 1, 2008, from http://www.emedicine.com/MED/topic1693.htm

Hugle, T., Geurts, J., Nuesch, C., Muller-Gerbe, M., & Valderrabano, V. (2012). Aging and Osteoarthritis: An Inevitable Encounter? *Journal of Aging Research, 2012*, 7. doi: 10.1155/2012/950192

Kinkade, S. (2007). Evaluation and treatment of acute back pain. *American Family Physician, 75*(8), 1181–1188.

*Liu, C.-C., Lin, Y.-C., Lo, C.-P., & Chang, T.-P. (2011). Cauda equina syndrome and dural ectasia: rare manifestations in chronic ankylosing spondylitis. *British Journal of Radiology, 84*(1002), e123–e125. doi: 10.1259/bjr/45816561

Lubar, D., White, P. H., Callahan, L. F., Chang, R. W., Helmick, C. G., Lappin, D. R., . . . Waterman, M. B. (2010). *A National Public Health Agenda for Osteoarthritis 2010.* Atlanta: Centers for Disease Control Retrieved from http://www.cdph.ca.gov/programs/capp/Documents/National%20Public%20Health%20Agenda%20for%20Osteoarthritis.pdf.

Mayo Clinic Staff. (2007, June 25, 2007). *Fibromyalgia.* Retrieved October 8, 2008, from http://www.mayoclinic.com/print/fibromyalgia/DS00079

Mosley-Williams, A., & Williams, C. (2005). Computer applications in clinical practice. *Current Opinion in Rheumatology, 17*(2), 124–127.

National Osteoporosis Foundation. (2008, n.d.). *Fast facts on osteoporosis.* Retrieved October 22, 2008, from http://www.nof.org/oseoporosis/diseasefacts.htm

Peh, W. C. G. (2005). *Ankylosing spondylitis.* Retrieved October 7, 2008, from http://emedicine.com/RADIO/topic41.htm

*Phillips, T. G., Reibach, A. M., & Sloiany, W. P. (2004). Diagnosis and management of scaphoid fractures. *American Family Physician, 70*, 879–884.

Plotkin, H., & Pattekar, M. A. (2008, May 8, 2008). *Osteogenesis imperfecta.* Retrieved October 8, 2008, from http://www/emedicine.com/ped/topic1674.htm

Preidt, R. (2008). Docs issue guideline on screening for osteoporosis in men. MedicineNet.com.

Rao, S. S., & Cherukuri, M. (2006). Management of hip fracture: The family physician's role. *American Family Physician, 73*, 2195–2200, 2201–2192.

*Rauch, D. (2007, May 2, 2007). *Simian crease—Overview.* Retrieved October 23, 2008, from http://www.umm.edu/ency/article/003290/htm

*Scanlon, V. C., & Sanders, T. (2007). *Essentials of Anatomy and Physiology* (2nd ed.). Philadelphia: F.A. Davis.

Sheil, W. C. (2008). *Ankylosing spondylitis.* Retrieved October 7, 2008, from http://www.medicinenet.com/script/main/art.asp?articlekey

Simons, S. M., Kruse, D., & Dixon, J. B. (2013, 10/23/2012). Shoulder impingement syndrome. *UpToDate.* Retrieved September 25, 2013, from http://www.uptodate.com/contents/shoulder-impingement-syndrome

Walker, D. J., & Kay, L. J. (2002). Musculoskeletal examination for medical students: The need to agree what we teach. *Rheumatology, 41*, 1221–1223.

*Wheeler, A. H. (2007, July 9, 2007). *Pathophysiology of chronic back pain.* Retrieved August 1, 2008, from http://www.emedicine.com/neuro/topic516.htm

Wheeler, S. G., Wopf, J. E., Staiger, T. O., & Deyo, R. A. (2013, 08/15/2013). Approach to the diagnosis and evaluation of low back pain in adults. *UpToDate.* Retrieved September 24, 2013, from http://www.uptodate.com/contents/approach-to-the-diagnosis-and-evaluation-of-low-back-pain-in-adults?topicKey=PC%2F7782&elapsedTimeMs=0&source=search_result&searchTerm=chronic+back+pain&selectedTitle=2~150&view=print&displayedView=full#

Winfield, J. (2007, August 15, 2007). *Fibromyalgia.* Retrieved October 8, 2008, from http://www.emedicine.com/med/TOPIC790.HTM

*Woodward, T. W., & Best, T. M. (2000). The painful shoulder: Part 1. Clinical evaluation. *American Family Physician, 61*, 3079–3088.

Chapter 28 References

Atreja, A., Achker, J. P., Jain, A.K., Harris, C. M., & Lasher, C. M. (2008). Using technology to promote gastrointestinal outcomes research: A case for electronic health records. *American Journal of Gastroenterology, 103*(9), 2171–2178.

Beveridge, L. A., Davey, P. G., Phillips, G., & McMurdo, M. E. T. (2011). Optimal management of urinary tract infections in older people. *Clinical Interventions in Aging, 6*, 173–180.

Brendolan, A., Rosado, M.M., Ccarsetti, R., Selleri, L., & Dear, T.N. (2007). Development and function of the mammalian spleen. *BioEssays, 29*, 166–177.

Buggs, A.M., & Lim, J.K. (2009, July 12, 2006). Hepatitis. Retrieved February 10, 2009, from http://emedicine.medscape.com/article/775507

Cacebe, E.C., Mehta, V.K., & Fisher, G. (2013, July 22, 2013). Gastric cancer. *Medscape Reference Drugs, Diseases & Procedures.* Retrieved August 13, 2013, from http://emedicine.medscape.com/article/278744-overview

Centers for Disease Control and Prevention. (2009, January 7, 2009). Obesity and overweight: Introduction. Retrieved January 16, 2009, from http://www.cdc.gov/ncdphp/dnpa/obesity/

Chang, Su-Hsin, Beason, Tracey S., Hunleth, Jean M., & Colditz, Graham A. (2012). A systematic review of body fat distribution and mortality in older people. *Maturitas, 72*(3), 175–191. doi: http://dx.doi.org/10.1016/j.maturitas.2012.04.004

Croke, B., & Sampson, D. (2012). Nonalcoholic fatty liver disease: Implications for clinical practice and health promotion. *Journal for Nurse Practitioners, 8*(1), 45–50.

Davenport, K. P., Blanco, F. C., & Sandler, A. D. (2012). Neuroblastoma, Wilm's tumor, hepatoblastoma, rhabdomyosarcoma, and saccroccygeal teratoma. *Surgical Clinics of North America, 92*, 745–767. doi: 10.1016/j.suc.2012.03.004

Dienstag, J. L. (2013). Acute viral hepatitis. In D. L. Longo & A. S. Fauci (Eds.), *Harrison's gastroenterology and hepatology* (2nd ed.). New York: McGraw-Hill.

Doerr, S.E. (2009, September 8, 2008). Pilonidal cyst. *eMedicine Health: Practical Guide to Health.* Retrieved March 10, 2009, from http://emedicinehealth.com/script/main/art.asp?article

*Dome, J. S., & Huff, V. (2013). Wilms tumor overview. In U. O. Washington (Ed.), *GeneReviews (Internet)* (Vol. Sept 19). Seattle WA: University of Washington.

Duderstadt, K. G. (2006). *Pediatric physical examination: An illustrated handbook.* St. Louis: Mosby/Elsevier.

Evers, D.B. (2006). Alterations of digestive function in children. In K. L. McCance & S. E. Huether (Eds.), *Pathophysiology: The biologic basis for disease in adults and children* (5th ed., pp. 1447–1470). St. Louis: Elsevier Mosby.

Fingerote, R.J. (2009, October 25, 2005). Colon cancer. *eMedicineHealth.* Retrieved January 26, 2009, from http://www.emedicinehealth.com/script/main/art.asp?

Gangloff, J.M. (2007). Liver cancer: More cases, more causes. *Cure, 6*(2), 34–40.

Gosnell, M. (2008). Killer fat: Not all fats are equal. *Discover, February 28.* Retrieved from http://discovermagazine.com/2007/feb/visceral-fat/article_view?b_start:int=2&-C=

Gund, S., & Zieve, D. (2009). Medical encyclopedia: Colon cancer. *Medline Plus.* Retrieved January 24, 2009, from http://www.nlm.nih.gov/medlineplus/ency/article/000262.htm

Hajar, N., Castell, D. O., Ghomrawi, H., Rackett, R., & Hila, H. (2012). Impedance ph confirms the relationship between GERD and BMI. *Digestie Diseases and Sciences, 57*(7). doi: 10.1007/s10620-012-2131-6

Heffernan, B. (2013). Irish team makes major breakthrough on children's cancer. Retrieved August 19, 2013, from http://www.independent.ie/

irish-news/irish-team-makes-major-break-through-on-childrens-cancer-29497104.html

Heidelbaugh, J. J., & Bruderly, M. (2006). Cirrhosis and chronic liver failure: Part I. Diagnosis and evaluation. *American Family Physician, 74*, 756–762,781.

Ko, Edmund Y., & Ritchey, Michael L. (2009). Current management of wilms' tumor in children. *Journal of Pediatric Urology, 5*(1), 56–65. doi: http://dx.doi.org/10.1016/j.jpurol.2008.08.007

Khoury, G., & Deeba, S.S. (2009, January 26, 2009). Pancreatitis. *eMedicine Emergency Medicine.* Retrieved February 12, 2099, from http://emedicine.medscape.com/article775867

Kuo, T., & Fisher, G. (Producer). (2009, February 12, 2009). Pancreatic cancer. *eMedicineHealth.* Retrieved from http://emediocinehealth.com

Lee, D. (2009, December 1, 2005). Cirrhosis (cirrhosis of the liver). *MedicineNet.com.* Retrieved February 10, 2009, from http://www.medicinenet.com

Marks, D. (2009, February 15, 2008). Gastroesophageal reflux disease (GERD, acid reflux, heartburn). *MedicineNet.com.* Retrieved 2 February, 2009, from http://www.medicinenet.com

Marks, J.W. (2009, February 19, 2008). Hiatal hernia. *MedicineNet.com.* Retrieved February 19, 2009, from http://www.medicinenet.com

Matrana, M. R., & Margolin, D. A. (2009). Epidemiology and pathophysiology of diverticular disease. *Clinics in Colon and Rectal Surgery, 22*(3), 141–146. doi: 10.1055/s-0029-1236157. ISSN 1531-0043

Mayo Clinic Staff. (2009, August 23, 2008). Pyloric stenosis. *MayoClinic.com: Tools for healthier lives.* Retrieved February 23, 2009, from http://www.mayoclinic.com/health/pyloric-stenosis/DS00815

Mayr, M., & Schmid, R. M. (2010). Pancreatic cancer and depression: Myth and truth. *BMC Cancer, 10.* doi: 10.1186/1471-2407-10-569

Moore, G.A., Hawley, D.A., & Bradley, P. (2009). Hepatitis c: Studying stigma. *Gastroenterology Nursing, 31*(5), 346–352.

National Cancer Institute. (2009, ND). Obesity and cancer: Questions and answers. Retrieved January 22, 2009, from http://www.cancer.gov/cancertopics/factsheet/Risk/Obesity

National Institute of Health. (2013). *Crohn's disease* (12-3410). Bethesda, MD: Retrieved from http://digestive.niddk.nih.gov/ddiseases/pubs/crohns/#causes.

Neu, J., & Walker, A. (2011). Necrotizing enterocolitis. *The New England Journal of Medicine, 364*(3), 255–264.

Orzano, A. J., Strickland, P. O., Tallia, A. F., Hudson, S., Balasubramanian, B., Nutting, P. A., & Crabtree, B. F. (2007). Improving outcomes for high risk diabetics using information systems. *Journal of the American Board of Family Medicine, 20*(3), 245–251.

Parikh, J. A., Yermilov, I., McGory, M. L., Ko, C. Y., & Maggard, M. A. (2007). How much do standardized forms improve the documentation of quality of care? *Journal of Surgical Research, 143*(1), 158–163.

Qureshi, W. A. (2009, February 28, 2006). Hiatal hernia. *eMedicine.* Retrieved February 19, 2009, from http://emedicine.medscape.com/article/178393

Ritz, P. (2000). Physiology of aging with respect to gastrointestinal, circulatory and immune system changes and their significance for energy and protein metabolism. *European Journal of Clinical Nutrition, 54*(Suppl 3), S21–S25.

Rosen, N.G., & Beals, D.A. (2009, April 19, 2007). Inperforate anus. *eMedicine from WebMD.* Retrieved March 10, 2009, from http://emedicine,medscape.com/article929904

Sarkar, Fazlul H., Banerjee, Sanjeev, & Li, Yiwei. (2007). Pancreatic cancer: Pathogenesis, prevention and treatment. *Toxicology and Applied Pharmacology, 224*(3), 326–336. doi: http://dx.doi.org/10.1016/j.taap.2006.11.007

Seller, R. H. (2007). *Differential diangosis of common complaints* (5th ed.). Philadelphia: Saunders Elsevier.

Stuart, K. E., & Stadler, Z. (2013, 11/26/2012). Primary hepatic carcinoma. *Medscape Reference Drugs, diseases & Procedures.* Retrieved August 14, 2013, from http://emedicine.medscape.com/article/282814-overview

Tarn, C., & Goodwin, A. K. (2005). Molecular rerserarch directions in the management of gastrointestinal stromal tumors. *Current Treatment Options in Oncology, 6*(6), 473–486.

Tendler, D. A. (2013, 09/26/2012). Pathogenesis of nonalcoholic fatty liver disease. *UpToDate.* Retrieved 09/25, 2013, from http://www.uptodate.com/contents/pathogenesis-of-nonalcoholic-fatty-liver-disease

U. S. Department of Health and Human Services. (2000). *Healthy people 2010.* U. S. Government Printing Services.

Udeani, J., & Reinberg, S.R. (2009, August 22, 2008). Abdominal trauma, blunt. *eMedicine.* Retrieved January 19, 2009, from www.emedicine.medscape.com

Vogelzangs, N., Kritchevsky, S.B., Beekman, T.F., Newman, A.B., Satterfield, S., Simonsick, E.M., . . . Penninx, B.W.J.H. (2008). Depressive symptoms and change in abdominal obesity in older adults. *Archives of General Psychiatry, 65*(12), 1386–1393.

Vorvick, L. (2009, June 03, 2008). Medical encyclopedia: Acute cholesystitis. Retrieved February 10, 2009, from http://www.nlm.gov/medlineplus/ency/article/000264.htm

Whang, Edward E, Ashley, Stanley W, & Zinner, Michael J. (2008). Small intestine. F. C. Brunicardi, D. K. Andersen, T. R. Billiar, D. L. Dunn, J. G. Hunter, J. B. Matthews, R. E. Pollock & S. I. Schwartz (Eds.), *Schwartz's Principles of Surgery, 8th Edition.* Retrieved from http://www.accessmedicine.com/content.aspx?aID=809514

White, M.J., & Counselman, F.L. (2009, ND). Troubleshooting acute abdominal pain. *Emergency Medicine.* Retrieved January 20, 2009, from http://www.emedmag.com.html/pre/cov/covers/011502.asp

Whittington, E. (2005). The science behind obesity: Is there a cancer link? *Cure, 4*(3), 52–59.

Chapter 29 References

Al-Qudah, H.S., Al-Omer, O., Parraga-Marquez, M., Santucci, R.A., & Wanlheim, P.S. (2009, Mar 3, 2008). Priaprism. *eMedicine from WebMD.* Retrieved May 26, 2009, from http://emedicine.medscape.com

*Allen, L. (2009). Disorders of sexual development. *Obstetric and Gynecological Clinics of North America, 36*, 25–45.

American Cancer Society. (2013, 01/07/2013). Penile cancer. Retrieved August 30, 2013, from http://www.cancer.org/acs/groups/cid/documents/webcontent/003132-pdf.pdf

Armstrong, M.L., Caliendo, C., & Roberts, A.E. (2006). Genital piercings: What is known and what people with genital piercings tell us. *Urologic Nursing, 26*(2), 176–179.

Brosman, S.A. (2013, 09/27/2012). Penile cancer. *eMedicine Specialties.* Retrieved August 30, 2013, from http://emedicine.medscape/com/article/446554-overview

Chen, H. (2009). Klinefelter's syndrome. *eMedicine Pediatrics: Genetic and Metabolic Disease.* Retrieved June 19, 2009, from http://emedicine.medscape.com/article/945649-print

Clayton, P.C., & Trueman, J.A. (2000). Leptin and puberty. *Archives of Disease in Childhood, 83*, 1–4.

Docimo, S.G., Silver, R.I., & Cromie, W. (2000). The undescended testicle: Diagnosis and management. *American Family Physician, 62*, 2037–2044, 2047–2038.

*Dougherty, C.M., Richard, A. J., & Carey, M.J. (2009). Priaprism. *eMedicine from WebMD.* Retrieved May 26, 2009, from http://emedicine.medscape.com

Gatti, .M., Kirsch, A.J., & Snyder, H.M. (2009, Nov 1 2007). Hypospadius. *eMedicine Pediatrics: Surgery.* Retrieved June 09, 2009, from http://www.emedicine.medscape.com

Griffin, R.M. (2003, ND). All about genital peircing. *WebMD: Better information, better health.* Retrieved July 29, 2009, from http://ww.webmd.com/skin-beauty/guide/all-about-genital-piercing

Gross, G., & Pfister, H. (2004). Role of human papillomavirus in penile cancer, penile intraepithelial squamous cell newplasias and in genital warts. *Medical Microbiology and Immunology, 193*(1), 35–44.

Hakenberg, O. W., & Protzel, C. (2012). Chemotherapy in penile cancer. *Therapeutic Advances in Urology, 4*(3), 133–138. doi: 10.1177/1756287212441235

Harris, J.W.R. (1998). Male genital pain syndrome. *Dematologic Clinics, 16*(4), 779–782.

Hitti, M. (2007). Obesity may up prostate cancer deaths. Retrieved March 20, 2009, from http://www.webmd.com/prostate-cancer/news/20070315/Obesity-may-up-prostate-cancer-deaths

Hutcheson, J., & Snyder III, H. M. (2012, 01/11/2012). Ambiguous genitalia and intersexuality. *Medscape Reference Drugs, Diseases & Procedures.* Retrieved September 10, 2012, from emedicine.medscape.com/article/1015520-overview

Keoghane, S. R., & Sullivan, M. E. (2010). Investigating and managing chronic scrotal pain. *British Medical Journal, 341*(11 Dec), 1263–1266. doi: 10.1136/bmj.c6716

*Kick, K. (1997). Disorders of the male reproductive system. In L. O. Burrell, M. J. M. Gerlach & P. B.S. (Eds.), *Adult nursing: Acute and community care* (2nd ed., pp. 1769–1795). Stamford, CT: Appleton & Lange.

Kim, H. (2007). Regulation of gonadatropin-releasing hormone gene expression. *Seminars in Reproductive Medicine, 25*(5), 313–325. doi: 10.1055/s-2007-984737

Lee, Vien H. Y., Lee, Leo T. O., & Chow, Billy K. C. (2008). Gonadotropin-releasing hormone: Regulation of the gnrh gene. *FEBS Journal, 275*(22), 5458–5478. doi: 10.1111/j.1742-4658.2008.06676.x

Leibovitch, Ilan, & Mor, Yoram. (2005). The vicious cycling: Bicycling related urogenital disorders. *European Urology, 47*(3), 277–287. doi: http://dx.doi.org/10.1016/j.eururo.2004.10.024

Lewis, R.A. (2007, May 1, 2007). Ambiguous genitalia—overview. Retrieved June 17, 2009, from www.umm.edu

Mann, D.R., & Plant, T.M. (2002). Leptin and pubertal development. *Seminars in Reproductive Medicine, 20*(2), 93–102.

Mayo Clinic Staff. (2009, March 20, 2009). Prostate cancer. Retrieved March 20, 2009, from http://www.mayoclinic.com/health/prostate-cancer/ds00043

Medical College of Georgia. (2005, May 23). Obesity is risk factor for aggressive prostate cancer. Retrieved March 20, 2009, from http://www.sciencedaily.com/releases/2005/05/050523091709.htm

Meltzer, D.I. (2005). Complications of body piercing. *American Family Physician, 72*(10), 2029–2034.

Meyer, D. (2000). Body piercing: Old traditions creating new challenges. *Journal of Emergency Nursing, 26*(6), 2029–2036.

National Cancer Institute. (2009, May 5 2008). Penile canter treatment (pdq): Health professional version. Retrieved June 10, 2009, from http://www.cancer.gov

Nishihara, R. (2000). When genital pain coours in adolescent boys, what conditions should we be thinking about? *Western Journal of Medicine, 172*(March).

Nolan, V.G., Wyszynski, D.F., Farrer, L.A., & Steinberg, M.H. (2005). Hemolysis-associated priaprism in sickle cell disease. *Blood, 106*(9), 3264–3267.

Oneill, P. (2009). Prostate cancer. Retrieved March 20, 2009, from http://ww.medicinenet.com

Pinon, R.. (2002). *Biology of human reproduction*. Portland, OR: University Science Books.

Pizzocaro, G., Algaba, F., Horenblas, S., Solsona, E., Tana, S., Van Der Poel, H., & Watkin, N. A. (2010). Eau penile cancer guidelines 2009. *European Urology, 57*, 1002–1012. doi: 10.1016/j.eururo.2010.01.039

Pourbagher, M.A., Turunc, T., Pourbagher, A., Guvel, S., & Koc, Z. (2005). Peyronie disease involving the entire tunica albuginea of the penis. *Journal of Ultrasound Medicine, 24*, 387–389.

Rosen, Alexandre, Jayram, Gautam, Drazer, Michael, & Eggener, Scott E. (2011). Global trends in testicular cancer incidence and mortality. *European Urology, 60*(2), 374–379. doi: http://dx.doi.org/10.1016/j.eururo.2011.05.004

Roth, C.P., Lim, Y., Pevnick, J.M., Asch, S.M., & McGlynn, E.A. (2009). The challenge of measuring quality of care from the electronic health record. *American Journal of Medical Quality OnlineFirst, May 29*(doi:10.1177). http://ajm.sagepub.com/cgi/rapidpdf/1062860609336627v1.pdf

Rupp, T.J., & Zwanger, M. (2009). Testicular torsion. *eMedicine Emergency Medicine*. Retrieved May 20, 2009, from www.emedicine.medscape.com

Rutters, F., Nieuwenhuizen, A. G., Verhoef, S. P. M., Lemmens, S. G. T., Vogels, N., & Westerterp-Plentenga, M. S. (2009). The relationship between leptin, gonadotropic hormones, and body composition during puberty in a dutch children cohort. *European Journal of Endocrinology, 160*, 973–978. doi: 10.1530/EJE-08-0762

Santucci, R.A., & Broghammer, J.A. (2009, August 14, 2006). Penile fracture and trauma. *eMedicine from WebMD*. Retrieved May 22, 2009, from emedicine.medscape.com

Soni, H.C., & Hardin, E. (2009, Oct 16, 2005). Prostate cancer. *eMedicineHealth: Practical Guide to Health*. Retrieved March 20, 2009, from http://www.emedicinehealth.com

Spanierman, C. (2009, May 15, 2007). Testicular torsion. *eMedicineHealth: Practical guide to health* Retrieved 12 April, 2009, from www.eMedicinehealth.com

*Speroff, L., & Fritz, M.A. (2005). *Clinical gynecologic endocrinology and infertility* (7th ed.). Philadelphia: Lippincott Williams & Wilkins.

Steele, G. S., Richie, J. P., Oh, W. K., & Michaelson, M. D. (2013, 06/12/2013). Clinical manifestations, diagnosis, and staging of testicular gem cerll tumors. *UpToDate*. Retrieved August 30, 2013, from http://www.uptodate.com/contents/clinical-manifestations-diagnosis-and-staging-of-testicular-germ-cell-tumors?topicKey=ONC%2F2980&elapsedTimeMs=4&source=see_link&view=print&displayedView=full#

Swerdlow, A. J., Scheomaker, M. J., Higgins, C. D., Wright, A. F., & Jacobs, P. A. (2005). Cancer incidence and mortality in men with klinfelter syndrome: A cohort study. *Journal of the National Cancer Institute, 97*(6). doi: 10.1093/jnci/dji240

Thomas, J.J., Santucci, R.A., & Morey, A.F. (2007). Genitourinary injury. In L. Flint, J. W. Merideth, C. W. Schwab, D. D. Trunkey, L. Rue & P. A. Taheri (Eds.), *Trauma: Contemporary principles and therapy*. Philadelphia Lippincott Williams & Wilkins.

*Trojian, T. H., Lishnak, T. S., & Heiman, D. (2009). Epididymitis and orchitis: An overview. *American Family Physician, 79*(7), 583–587.

U. S. Department of Health and Human Services. (2009). Healthy people 2020 *summary of objectives*. Washington DC: U. S. Government Printing Services.

Van Howe, R. S., & Hodgest, F. M. (2006). The carcinogenicity of smegma: Debunking a myth. *Journal of the European Academy of Dermatology and Venerology, 20*(9), 1046–1054. doi: 10.1111/j.1468-3083.2006.01653.x

Wise, Lauren A., Cramer, Daniel W., Hornstein, Mark D., Ashby, Rachel K., & Missmer, Stacey A. (2011). Physical activity and semen quality among men attending an infertility clinic. *Fertility and Sterility, 95*(3), 1025–1030. doi: http://dx.doi.org/10.1016/j.fertnstert.2010.11.006

Chapter 30 References

*American Cancer Society. (2013, 05/03/2013). American cancer society guidelines for the early detection of cancer Retrieved October 09, 2013, from http://www.cancer.org/healthy/findcancerearly/cancerscreeningguidelines/american-cancer-society-guidelines-for-the-early-detection-of-cancer

*American College of Obstetricians and Gynecologists. (2012, Nov.) Practice bulletin number 131: Screening for cervical cancer, 1–18.

Best Practice. (2012, Aug 23, 2011). Assessment of vaginal bleeding. *Best Practice*. Retrieved July 13, 20121, from http://bestpractice.bmj.com/best-practice/monograph/1166/diagnosis/guidelines/html

Burd, L., Cotsonas-Hassler, T. M., Martsolf, J. T., & Kerbashian, J. (2003). Recognition and famagement of fetal alcohol syndrome. *Neurotoxicology and Tetratology, 25*, 681–688. doi: 10.1016/j.ntt2003.07.020

Cannon, M. J., Dominique, Y., O'Leary, L. A., Sniezek, J. E., & Floyd, R. L. (2012). Characteristics and behaviors of mothers who have a child with fetal alcohol syndrome. *Neurotoxicology and Tetratology, 34*, 90–95. doi: 10.1013/j.ntt.2011.09.010

*Cox, K.J. & Neville, C.E. (2012). Assessment and management options for women with vulvodynia. *Journal of Midwifery & Women's Health, 57*, 231–240

Deily, M.E., Hu, T., Terrizzi, S., Chou, S.Y., Meyerhoefer, C.D. (2013). The impact of health information technology adoption by outpatient facilities on pregnancy outcomes. *Health Services Research, 48*(1), 70–94.

Edelman, A., Anderson, J., Lai, S., Braner, D., & Tegtmeyer. (2007). Pelvic examination. *The New England Journal of Medicine, 356*(26).

Hall, S., & Brown, D. J. G. (2009). Management of female genital trauma. *Trauma, 11*, 133–138. doi: 10.1177/1460408609104154

Habif, T. P. (2009) Clinical Dermatology: A Color Guide to Diagnosis and Therapy (5th Ed.). Philadelphia: Mosby.

Hatch, E. E. (2013, 06/04/2013). Outcome and follow-up of diethylstilbestrol (DESdes) exposed individuals. *UpToDate*. Retrieved September 26, 2013, from http://www.uptodate.com/contents/outcome-and-follow-up-of-diethylstilbestrol-des-exposed-individuals

Jolles, D. R., Brown, W. W., & King, K. B. (2012). Electronic health records and perinatal quality: A call to midwives. *Journal of Midwifery & Women's Health, 57*(4), 315–320.

*Koroma, L. & Stewart, L. (2012). Infertility: Evaluation and initial management. *Journal of Midwifery & Women's Health, 57*, 614–621.

Kesmodel, U. S., Bertrand, J. , Stovring, H., Skarpness, B., Denny, C. H., Mortensen, E. L., & Group, the Lifestyle During Pregnancy Study. (2012). The effect of different alcohol drinking patterns in early to mid pregnancy on the child's intelligence, attention, and executive function. *BJOG An International Journal of Obstetrics and Gynaecology, 1191*, 1180–1190. doi: 10.1111/j.1471-0528.2012.03393.x

*Mark, H., Jordan, E.T., Cruz, J., & Warren, N. (2012). What's new in sexually transmitted infection mangment: Changes in the 2010 guidelines from the Centers for Disease Control and Prevention. *Journal of Midwifery & Women's Health, 57*, 276–284.

*Mashburn, J. (2012) Vaginal infections update. *Journal of Midwifery & Women's Health, 57*, 629–634.

*Murphy, J. & Mark, H. (2012). Cervical cancer screening in the era of human papillomavirus testing and vaccination. *Journal of Midwifery & Women's Health, 57*, 569–576.

Palmer, J. R. , Herbst, A. L. , Noller, K. L. , Boggs, D. A., Troisi, R. , Titus-Ernstoff, L., . . . Hoover, R. N. (2009). Urogenital abnormalities in men exposed to diethylstilbestrol in utero: A cohort study. *Environmental Health, 8*(37). doi: 10.1186/1476-069X-8-37

*Rice, K.E. Secrist, J.R., Woodrow, E.L., Hallock, L.M. & Neal, J.L. (2012). Etilogy, diagnosis and management of uterine leimyomas. *Journal of Midwifery & Women's Health, 57*, 241–247.

Roth, C.P., Lim, Y., Pevnick, J.M., Asch, S.M., & McGlynn, E.A. (2009). The challenge of measuring quality of care from the electronic health record. *American Journal of Medical Quality OnlineFirst*, published on May 29, 2009 as doi:10.1177/1062. Retrieved June 29, 2009, from http://ajm.sagepub.com/cgi/rapidpdf/1062860609336627v1.pdf

Schrager, S., & Potter, B. E. (2004). Diethylstilbestrol exposure. *American Family Physician, 69*(10), 2395–2400.

*Thorstensen, K.A. & Birenbaum, D. L. (2012). Recognition and management of vulvar dermatologic conditions: Lichen sclerosus, lichen planus and lichen simplex chronicus. *Journal of Midwifery & Women's Health, 57*, 260–275.

U. S. Department of Health and Human Services. (2009). *Healthy people 2020* summary of objectives. Washington DC: U. S. Government Printing Services.

Index

B

C

D

E

F

G

H

J

K

L

M

P

Q

R

T

U

V